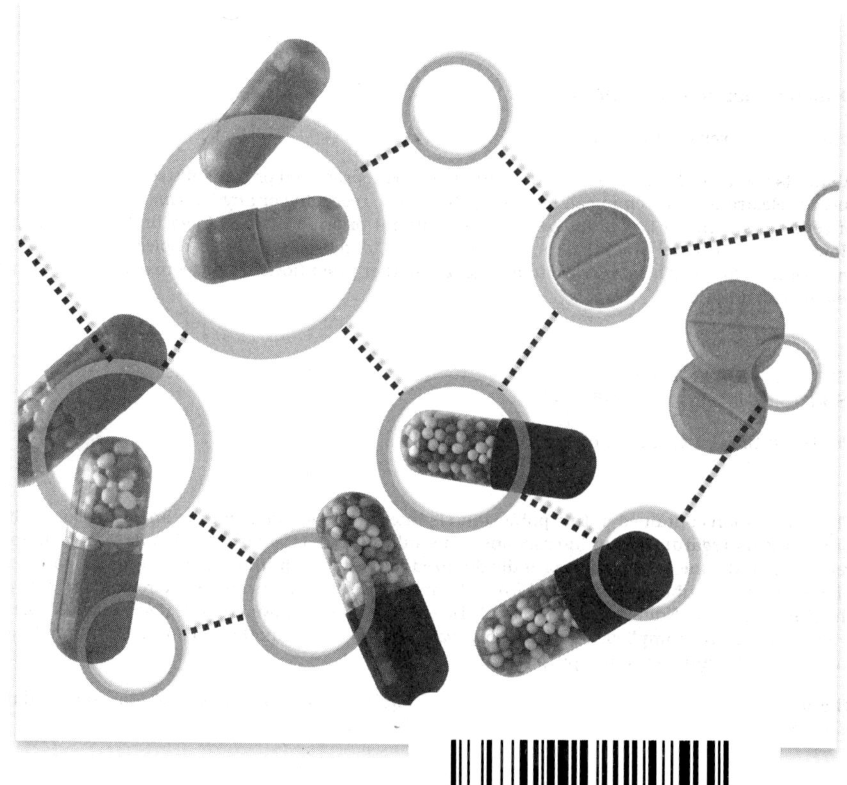

David S. Tatro, PharmD

Drug Interaction Facts™

THE AUTHORITY ON DRUG INTERACTIONS

2014

Facts & Comparisons®

Drug Interaction Facts™ 2014

ISBN-10: 1-57439-354-5
ISBN-13: 978-1-57439-354-5

Printed in the United States of America

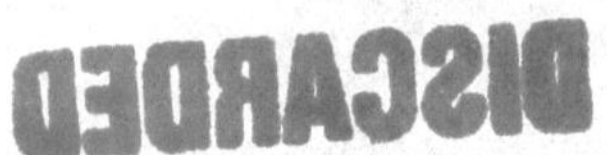

Wolters Kluwer Health
77 Westport Plaza, Suite 450
St. Louis, Missouri 63146-3125
Phone 314/392-0000 • 800/223-0554
Fax 314/392-0160
www.factsandcomparisons.com

Drug Interaction Facts™

Editor

David S. Tatro, PharmD
Drug Information Analyst
San Carlos, California

Facts & Comparisons® Publishing Group

Drug Interaction Facts™ Editorial Review Panel

Facts & Comparisons® Editorial Advisory Panel

Table of Contents

Preface

Wolters Kluwer Health is proud to publish *Drug Interaction Facts*™ as an authoritative resource providing current drug interaction information in a concise and practical manner. This reference continues the Facts & Comparisons® line of practical, up-to-date drug information with the superb database developed by the Editor and Editorial Review Panel.

The Data: *Drug Interaction Facts*™ is based on the most current published biomedical information and has been critically evaluated to ensure the accuracy and proper interpretation of the data. The Editorial Group places a strong emphasis on establishing the clinical *relevance* of the data to make its practical utility a priority. This information is intended to supplement the knowledge of health care professionals regarding drug interactions; it is advisory only and is not intended to replace sound clinical judgment or individualized patient care.

Practical Utility: In the ongoing development of this reference, we place an emphasis on the presentation of the data to enhance therapeutic decision making. For your convenience, the index includes the significance rating for each interaction next to each entry. In addition, each individual monograph is designed to represent a logical progression of information, allowing the practitioner easy review of the desired information.

1. A significance rating provides a relative ranking of the interaction.
2. The significance of the interaction is divided into three categories:

   Onset - Severity - Documentation
3. The interaction is then summarized into its practical components:

   Effects - what will happen
   Mechanism - why it will happen
   Management - how to prevent or manage the effects of the interaction
4. Detail is provided in the Discussion concerning the available data and how assessments were made.
5. References are provided for in-depth research, if desired.

Up-to-date: The medical literature is continually monitored to identify significant new drug interaction information. The loose-leaf format of *Drug Interaction Facts*™ with quarterly supplements assures the user that the information remains up-to-date. Also available, and updated quarterly, is the *Drug Interaction Facts*™ *on Disk* program. This electronic version contains every monograph found in the book, but allows you to enter up to 20 drugs at a time to check for multiple interactions more efficiently. Finally, *Drug Interaction Facts*™ is updated monthly as part of the *Facts & Comparisons eAnswers* family of on-line products.

Drug Interaction Facts™ has been designed to meet your needs. Your comments and suggestions, as always, are encouraged.

Renée M. Wickersham
Process Analysis Manager

How To Use *Drug Interaction Facts*™

Index

1. The index is the key to locating interaction monographs. Three types of entries will be found:

   Generic names – all interactions referenced (eg, Propranolol)
   Class names – all interactions referenced (eg, Beta-Adrenergic Blockers)
   Trade names – cross referenced to generic listings (eg, *Inderal*)

2. The index also identifies the significance rating of each interaction.

Features of Drug Interaction Monographs

1. **Drugs or drug classes** that may interact.

2. **Drugs** – Known and potentially interacting drugs are listed. Common trade names are given for ease of reference.

3. **Significance** –

   Significance rating – Summary of Severity and Documentation

   Onset

   - ☐ Rapid – within 24 hours
   - ☐ Delayed – days to weeks

   Severity

   - ☐ Major – life-threatening or permanent damage
   - ☐ Moderate – deterioration of patient's status
   - ☐ Minor – bothersome or little effect

   Documentation

   The confidence that an interaction *can* occur. This evaluation is based on supporting biomedical literature. The Discussion in each monograph provides specific comments on the data reviewed.

   - ☐ Established – proven to occur in well-controlled studies
   - ☐ Probable – very likely, but not proven clinically
   - ☐ Suspected – may occur; some good data, but needs more study
   - ☐ Possible – could occur, but data are very limited
   - ☐ Unlikely – doubtful; no good evidence of a clinical effect

4. **Effects** – Pharmacologic effects and clinical manifestations.

5. **Mechanism** – How the interaction occurs.

6. **Management** – Recommendations for appropriate action to prevent or respond to an interaction.

7. **Discussion** – Brief review of published data and selected primary references.

Introduction

As the development of new and more potent drugs continues, determining the interactive potential of an increasingly large number of possible drug combinations becomes more complex. Pharmacists and physicians cannot be expected to know the clinical consequences of all potential drug interactions. Therefore, this reference is designed to provide comprehensive information on drug-drug and drug-food interactions in a quick reference format to enhance therapeutic decision making.

Drug Interactions

A drug-drug interaction may be defined as the pharmacologic or clinical response to the administration of a drug combination different from that anticipated from the known effects of the 2 agents when given alone. The clinical result of a drug-drug interaction may manifest as *antagonism* (ie, $1 + 1 < 2$), *synergism* (ie, $1 + 1 > 2$), or *idiosyncratic* (ie, a response unexpected from the known effects of either agent).

Drug Interaction Facts attempts to present all drug-drug and drug-food interactions that have been reasonably well documented to occur in humans. Recently, we began including significant and well-documented interactions with herbal products as well. Simple additive or antagonistic effects anticipated to occur based on known pharmacologic activity are not necessarily included. For example, the additive blood pressure lowering effects of combining two antihypertensive agents or obvious antagonistic effects of beta-blockers and isoproterenol will not be considered drug interactions.

Incidence of Drug Interactions

The clinical effects of any interaction, no matter how well documented, do not occur in every patient or at the same degree of intensity. The incidence and degree of severity of an interaction depend on both patient-related factors and information about the effects of the interaction (eg, dose-dependency, route). Patient-related factors (eg, disease process, impairment of organ function) must be individually assessed. Incidence data are included in the Discussion section of each monograph when available.

Editorial Review

Information has been compiled from primary biomedical literature. With few exceptions, only data from human subjects are considered. The Editorial Review Panel and the Editor critically evaluate all studies as to the appropriateness of the methods, procedures, and statistical analyses used. These interdisciplinary groups, comprised of physicians, pharmacologists, and clinical pharmacists, provide an authoritative consensus about the clinical relevance of the published information.

Index

A comprehensive index references all drug interaction monographs by generic drug name and by drug class name. Selected product trade names are included with cross-references to the generic listing. All interactions are indexed, with their significance rating, under both interacting drug names.

The Drug Interaction Monograph

Drug interaction monographs are arranged alphabetically according to the principal drug affected. Each drug interaction is presented in a one-page monograph, with information in a uniform format for easy reference.

Each drug interaction monograph is divided into the following sections: Interacting drugs, including generic and trade names; clinical significance (significance rating, onset, severity, and documentation); effects, mechanism, and management; and a discussion with primary references.

Interacting Drugs

Monographs are titled by generic drug names (eg, cimetidine) or as a drug class monograph (eg, protease inhibitors) when pharmacologic or pharmacokinetic similarities suggest that a group of drugs interacts in a similar manner. By grouping drugs and screening by interaction class rather than individual drugs, the number of distinct interactions is reduced to several hundred instead of several thousand.

When an interaction monograph references an interaction class (eg, protease inhibitors), a list of interacting members of the drug class appears directly below the drug class name. The list includes drugs that have been reported to interact, as well as those likely to interact, based on pharmacologic or pharmacokinetic characteristics. Known interacting drugs are designated with an asterisk (*). For example, cimetidine is known to inhibit the hepatic metabolism of diazepam, chlordiazepoxide, and their demethylated metabolites. In the *Benzodiazepine-Cimetidine* monograph, both diazepam and chlordiazepoxide are designated with an asterisk in the list of interacting drugs. Other benzodiazepines (eg, clonazepam, quazepam) that undergo dealkylation and hydroxylation via the hepatic microsomal enzyme system are expected to interact and, therefore, are listed as interacting drugs.

Conversely, oxazepam, lorazepam, and temazepam, which are benzodiazepines that are primarily metabolized by glucuronidation, do not interact with cimetidine; therefore, they are not included in the list of interacting drugs. Noninteracting members of a drug class are listed in the discussion when information indicates that a drug does not, or is not likely to, interact.

Significance

When evaluating any potential drug interaction, a primary concern is the clinical relevance or significance of the interaction. Significance relates to the type and magnitude of the effect and, subsequently, to the necessity of monitoring the patient or altering therapy to avoid potentially adverse consequences.

The primary factors that define clinical significance include: SIGNIFICANCE RATING; the time of ONSET of the effects of the interaction; the potential SEVERITY of the interaction; and the DOCUMENTATION that an interaction occurs clinically. The following discussion defines the guidelines used to designate the Onset, Severity, and Documentation levels assigned to each drug interaction.

Significance Rating 1 2 3 4 5

A number 1 through 5 will be assigned to each interaction monograph, based on the Editorial Group's assessment of the interaction's Severity and Documentation (defined below).

1 is a severe and well-documented interaction.

5 is an interaction of no more than unlikely or possible documentation.

The formula for these number ratings is given in the following table:

Significance Rating	Severity	Documentation
1	Major	Suspected or >
2	Moderate	Suspected or >
3	Minor	Suspected or >
4	Major/Moderate	Possible
5	Minor	Possible
	Any	Unlikely

Onset

How rapidly the clinical effects of an interaction can occur determines the urgency with which preventive measures should be instituted to avoid the consequences of the interaction. Two levels of onset are used:

Rapid: The effect will be evident within 24 hours of administration of the interacting drug. *Immediate action is necessary to avoid the effects of the interaction.*

Delayed: The effect will not be evident until the interacting drug is administered for a period of days or weeks. *Immediate action is not required.*

Severity

The potential severity of the interaction is particularly important in assessing the risk vs benefit of therapeutic alternatives. With appropriate dosage adjustments or modification of the administration schedule, the negative effects of most interactions can be avoided. Three degrees of severity are defined:

Major: The effects are potentially life-threatening or capable of causing permanent damage.

Moderate: The effects may cause a deterioration in a patient's clinical status. Additional treatment, hospitalization, or an extended hospital stay may be necessary.

Minor: The effects are usually mild; consequences may be bothersome or unnoticeable but should not significantly affect the therapeutic outcome. Additional treatment is usually not required.

Documentation

Documentation determines the degree of confidence that an interaction can cause an altered clinical response. This scale represents the Editorial Group's evaluation of the quality and clinical relevance of the primary literature supporting the occurrence of an interaction. However, multiple factors can influence whether even a well-documented interaction occurs in a particular patient. The documentation does not address the incidence or frequency of the interaction; it is also independent of the potential severity of the effect of the interaction.

The following guidelines are used to establish the five Documentation levels:

Established: Proven to occur in well-controlled studies.

- An altered pharmacologic effect *has been demonstrated in well-controlled human studies* ... or ...
- A pharmacokinetic interaction *has been demonstrated in well-controlled human studies.* An altered pharmacologic response is expected based on the magnitude of the kinetic effect; clinical observations support the occurrence of the interaction.

Probable: Very likely but not proven clinically.

- A pharmacokinetic interaction has been demonstrated in well-controlled studies. Based on the magnitude of the kinetic changes and the known plasma level-response relationship of the affected drug, an altered pharmacologic response will *probably* occur ... or ...
- When controlled human experimentation is impractical, well-designed animal experiments confirm an interaction that is suggested by multiple case reports or uncontrolled studies.

Suspected: May occur; some good data; needs more study.

- A pharmacokinetic interaction has been demonstrated in well-controlled studies. Although an altered pharmacologic response *might be expected to occur* based on the magnitude of the kinetic changes, *no firm conclusion can be drawn* because a plasma level-response relationship has not been established for the affected drug ... or ...
- An altered pharmacologic response has been reported in multiple case reports or repeated uncontrolled clinical studies.

Possible: Could occur, but data are very limited.

- Although a pharmacokinetic interaction has been demonstrated, the kinetic changes are of such magnitude that it is *not possible to predict* if an altered response will occur ... or ...
- The evidence is divided as to whether an interaction exists ... or ...
- An altered pharmacologic response is suggested by limited data.

Unlikely: Doubtful; no good evidence of an altered clinical effect.

- A pharmacokinetic interaction has been demonstrated; however, based on the magnitude of kinetic change, a *pharmacologic alteration is unlikely* ... or ...
- *The bulk of documentation is of poor quality* or does not favor the existence of an interaction.
- In spite of reports of an interaction, well-controlled studies refute the existence of a clinically relevant interaction.

Drug interactions assigned Documentation levels of "Established," "Probable," or "Suspected" are considered to be reasonably well substantiated and have a significance rating of "1," "2," or "3." It is the opinion of the Editorial Group that these interactions have a reasonable probability of occurring.

Drug interactions assigned a Significance Rating of "4" or "5" have a Documentation level of "Possible" or "Unlikely" and are not substantiated. Because there is insufficient evidence supporting the existence of a clinically relevant interaction, prospective screening is probably not warranted. If an unanticipated effect occurs, the information in these monographs will be useful in reviewing what is known about these potential interactions.

Effects

Information concerning the pharmacologic effects of the interaction (eg, "the anticoagulant effects of oral anticoagulants are increased") and the clinical findings (eg, "possibly with bleeding") is included in this section. The interaction may lead to symptoms of drug toxicity or loss of therapeutic efficacy of one or both drugs. In some instances, the interacting combination will lead to effects that are unexpected based on the pharmacology of either drug.

The interactive potential of certain drug combinations may persist up to several days after one of the interacting drugs has been discontinued. Information concerning the duration of interactive potential is included in this section.

Mechanism

A brief description of the pharmacodynamic (eg, "decreased receptor sensitivity") or pharmacokinetic (eg, "decreased metabolism") mechanism by which an interacting drug affects the action of another drug is provided in this section.

Management

This section provides clinical management suggestions (eg, "may need a lower anticoagulant dose" or "give tetracycline at least 1 hour before antacids") so that the clinician can properly manage an interacting drug combination to prevent potential detrimental effects. Monitoring parameters are included when appropriate. Alternative therapy suggestions are provided when possible. Because of patient-, disease-, and drug-related variables, it is frequently impossible to provide specific management recommendations. Modification or alteration of the therapeutic regimen must be based on the practitioner's clinical assessment of each individual situation.

Discussion

A brief review and assessment of the studies used to document the interaction are provided to promote a better understanding of the incidence and magnitude of the interaction (eg, "in a controlled study of 6 patients, 5 developed severe hemorrhagic complications").

References

The principal references documenting the interaction are listed at the end of each monograph following the discussion. With few exceptions, only primary reference sources are used.

Principles of Drug Interactions

by Edward A. Hartshorn, PhD, and David S. Tatro, PharmD

A drug-drug interaction can be defined as the phenomenon that occurs when the effects or pharmacokinetics of a drug are altered by prior administration or coadministration of a second drug. The operational definition of drug interactions may also vary. Some restrict the term drug-drug interaction to adverse reactions and do not include beneficial interactions (eg, ampicillin and probenecid). Others view drug-drug interactions as only a part of the larger phenomenon of drug interactions, which includes interactions of drugs with foods (eg, fatty meals and griseofulvin), endogenous substances (eg, sulfonamides and bilirubin in neonates), herbals (eg, ginseng), environmental and industrial chemicals (eg, organophosphate insecticides and succinylcholine), and laboratory tests (eg, penicillins and *Clinitest*). *Drug Interaction Facts* is primarily comprised of adverse interactions that represent some clinical concern; it includes drug-drug interactions and drug-food interactions, while the herbal supplements and food edition includes herb-drug and food-drug interactions.

A drug interaction pair typically consists of the:

- object drug
- precipitant drug

The activity of the "object" drug is altered; the drug causing this change is the "precipitant" drug.[1] Other terms used have been "index drug" and "interacting drug," respectively.[2] *Drug Interaction Facts* is arranged alphabetically by object drug or object drug class. Occasionally, a drug may be an object drug in one interaction (eg, phenytoin-cimetidine) and a precipitant drug in another interaction (eg, doxycycline-phenytoin); rarely, both interacting drugs are affected by each other (eg, chloramphenicol-phenobarbital). With most pharmacologic interactions, there may be no object or precipitant drug, but simply a synergistic or antagonistic effect with both drugs (eg, concurrent use of several drugs with CNS depressant actions may result in excessive CNS depression).

Types of Drug Interactions

Drug interactions are frequently characterized as either pharmacokinetic or pharmacodynamic.

Pharmacokinetic

Pharmacokinetic interactions are those in which one drug alters the rate or extent of absorption, distribution, or elimination (metabolism or excretion) of another drug. This is most commonly measured by a change in one or more kinetic parameters, such as peak serum concentration, area under the concentration-time curve, half-life, total amount of drug excreted in urine, etc.

Pharmacodynamic

Pharmacodynamic interactions are those in which one drug induces a change in a patient's response to a drug without altering the object drug's pharmacokinetics. That is, one may see a change in drug action without altered plasma concentration. An example of this change is the increase in the toxicity of digoxin produced by potassium-wasting diuretics. Pharmacological interactions, that is, concurrent use of two or more drugs with similar or opposing pharmacological actions (eg, use of alcohol with an antianxiety drug and a hypnotic or antihistamine), are a form of pharmacodynamic interactions. Some clinicians suggest that such reactions are not drug interactions and, indeed, most are not unless an adverse reaction is reported.

Mechanisms of Drug Interactions

Pharmacokinetic

Altered Absorption: Most interactions involving altered drug absorption occur in the gut. There are many mechanisms by which drugs could theoretically alter the absorption of another drug, including altered splanchnic blood flow, gut motility, gut pH, drug solubility, gut metabolism, gut flora, or gut mucosa. However, most of the clinically important interactions involve formation of a nonabsorbable complex by either chelation (eg, tetracycline or ciprofloxacin and di- or trivalent cations), adsorption (eg, lincomycin and kaolin-pectin), or ion exchange (eg, cholestyramine-warfarin). Exceptions are the increase in digoxin absorption or decreased efficacy of estrogen-containing oral contraceptives following administration of antibiotics that alter the bacterial flora of the gut. In addition, drugs may be excreted back into the GI lumen by P-glycoprotein, a product of the multidrug resistant gene that lowers intracellular drug concentrations by acting as an energy (ie, ATP)-dependent drug efflux pump.[3-5] Numerous drugs are potential substrates for the P-glycoprotein transporter (see table 1). P-glycoprotein is found in high amounts in normal tissues, including the large and small intestine, kidneys, liver (ie, biliary hepatocytes), and endothelial cells at the blood-brain barrier.[5-9] Drugs or herbal products that inhibit or induce (eg, St. John's wort and Yohimbine) P-glycoprotein (see table 2) may increase or decrease plasma concentrations of P-glycoprotein substrate. Thus, P-glycoprotein may be involved in many drug interactions occurring in the GI tract, liver, and kidney. The oral administration of a drug that is a substrate for P-glycoprotein may be secreted back into the GI lumen by P-glycoprotein.[9] Along the GI tract, P-glycoprotein concentrations are lowest in the stomach and highest in the colon.[4] If a drug is a substrate of P-glycoprotein in the GI tract, uptake from the intestine will be incomplete (ie, decreasing drug levels).[6-8] Coadministration of digoxin (eg, *Lanoxin*) and rifampin (eg, *Rifadin*) may result in a decrease in digoxin plasma concentrations. The induction of intestinal P-glycoprotein by rifampin and the subsequent secretion of digoxin back into the GI tract by P-glycoprotein has been implicated as a major mechanism of this drug interaction.[10] In eight healthy volunteers, rifampin treatment increased intestinal P-glycoprotein content 3.5-fold, which correlated with the area under the plasma concentration-time curve after oral but not IV digoxin administration.[10]

Table 1. Substrates for P-Glycoprotein[3-6,9-19,67-69]

Aliskiren (*Tekturna*)	Estradiol (eg, *Estrace*)	Ondansetron (*Zofran*)
Ambrisentan (*Letairis*)	Etonogestrel (*Implanon*)	Paclitaxel (eg, *Taxol*)
Amiodarone (eg, *Cordarone*)	Etoposide (eg, *Vepesid*)	Progesterone (eg, *Prometrium*)
Boceprevir (*Victrelis*)	Felodipine (*Plendil*)	Promethazine (eg, *Phenergan*)
Chlorpromazine (eg, *Thorazine*)	Fexofenadine (*Allegra*)	Propranolol (eg, *Inderal*)
Clarithromycin (*Biaxin*)	Fluphenazine (eg, *Prolixin*)	Quinidine
Colchicine (eg, *Colcrys*)	Hydrocortisone (eg, *Cortef*)	Ranolazine (*Ranexa*)
Cyclosporine (eg, *Neoral*)	Indinavir (*Crixivan*)	Reserpine
Dactinomycin (*Cosmegen*)	Itraconazole (*Sporanox*)	Risperidone (eg, *Risperdal*)
Daunorubicin (eg, *Cerubidine*)	Ketoconazole (eg, *Nizoral*)	Ritonavir (eg, *Norvir*)
Dexamethasone (eg, *Decadron*)	Lidocaine (eg, *Xylocaine*)	Rivaroxaban (*Xarelto*)
Digoxin (eg, *Lanoxin*)	Linagliptin (*Tradjenta*)	Romidepsin (*Istodax*)
Diltiazem (eg, *Cardizem*)	Linezolid (*Zyvox*)	Saquinavir (eg, *Fortovase*)
Doxorubicin (eg, *Adriamycin*)	Loperamide (eg, *Imodium*)	Saxagliptin (*Onglyza*)
Erythromycin (eg, *E-Mycin*)	Lovastatin (eg, *Mevacor*)	Silodosin (*Rapaflo*)
	Mefloquine (*Lariam*)	Sirolimus (*Rapamune*)
	Mifepristone (*Mifeprex*, RU486)	Tacrolimus (*Prograf*)
	Mitoxantrone (*Novantrone*)	Tamoxifen (eg, *Nolvadex*)
	Nelfinavir (*Viracept*)	Telaprevir (*Incivek*)
	Nicardipine (eg, *Cardene*)	Teniposide (*Vumon*)
	Nifedipine (eg, *Procardia*)	Testosterone (*Delatestryl*)
	Nilotinib (*Tasigna*)	Tipranavir (*Aptivus*)
		Trifluoperazine
		Verapamil (eg, *Calan*)
		Vemurafenib (*Zelboraf*)
		Vinblastine (eg, *Velban*)
		Vincristine (eg, *Vincasar PFS*)

Table 2. Inducers and Inhibitors of P-Glycoprotein†[3,4,6,7,10,12-14,17,18,66,68,69]

Inducers	Inhibitors
Levothyroxine (eg,*Synthroid*)	Amiodarone (eg, *Cordarone*)
Rifampin (eg, *Rifadin*)	Atorvastatin (*Lipitor*)
Ritonavir (eg, *Norvir*)	Boceprevir (*Victrelis*)
St. John's wort	Chlorpromazine (eg, *Thorazine*)
Yohimbine	Clarithromycin (*Biaxin*)
	Crizotinib (*Xalkori*)
	Cyclosporine (eg, *Neoral*)
	Diltiazem (eg, *Cardizem*)
	Erythromycin (eg, *E-Mycin*)
	Felodipine (*Plendil*)
	Fluphenazine (eg, *Prolixin*)
	Hydrocortisone (eg, *Cortef*)
	Indinavir (*Crixivan*)
	Itraconazole (*Sporanox*)
	Ketoconazole (eg, *Nizoral*)
	Lidocaine (eg, *Xylocaine*)
	Mefloquine (*Lariam*)
	Mifepristone (*Mifeprex*)
	Nelfinavir (*Viracept*)
	Nicardipine (eg, *Cardene*)
	Nifedipine (eg, *Procardia*)
	Nilotinib (*Tasigna*)
	Progesterone (eg, *Prometrium*)

Table 2. Inducers and Inhibitors of P-Glycoprotein† [3,4,6,7,10,12-14,17,18,66,68,69]	
Inducers	Inhibitors
	Propranolol (eg, *Inderal*)
	Quinidine
	Ranolazine (*Ranexa*)
	Reserpine
	Ritonavir (eg, *Norvir*)
	Saquinavir (eg, *Fortovase*)
	Schisandra sphenanthera
	Sirolimus (*Rapamune*)
	Tacrolimus (*Prograf*)
	Tamoxifen (eg, *Nolvadex*)
	Telaprevir (*Incivek*)
	Testosterone (*Delatestryl*)
	Ticagrelor (*Brilinta*)
	Trifluoperazine
	Vemurafenib (*Zelboraf*)
	Verapamil (eg, *Calan*)

† If reference is not listed, then the package insert applies.

Altered Distribution:
Protein Binding – Once absorbed, a drug is carried via the blood to tissues and receptor sites. The amount of drug available to bind to the receptor is determined by the absorption, metabolism, excretion, and binding to inactive sites, as well as the affinity of the drug for the receptors and the drug's intrinsic activity. Of great concern are those drugs that are highly bound to plasma albumin and the potential for drug displacement from albumin binding sites upon coadministration of another highly bound drug. This is the mechanism used to explain many interactions, such as warfarin-phenylbutazone or phenytoin-valproic acid. Displacement of a drug from its inactive binding site (such as albumin) may increase the serum concentration of the free (and active) drug without any marked change in total serum concentration. However, displacement interactions may rarely be clinically important because of the rapid attainment of a new steady state. Some highly bound precipitant drugs also have enzyme inhibiting properties; therefore, the mechanism for the interaction is not clear (eg, warfarin and sulfamethoxazole-trimethoprim).

Receptor Binding – Binding sites other than albumin are occasionally important in drug interactions. For example, quinidine displaces digoxin from binding sites in skeletal muscle, increasing the serum concentration of digoxin (quinidine also alters the renal excretion of digoxin).

Displacement of drugs from their receptor sites is generally a pharmacologic effect rather than a drug interaction. Thus, a beta-blocker, such as propranolol, may displace a beta-agonist, such as terbutaline, from beta-$_2$ receptors and increase the likelihood of precipitating an asthmatic attack. Beta-blockers may produce an imbalance in response to sympathomimetics, such as epinephrine. Beta-receptor blockade may result in an excessive alpha (hypertensive) response.

Altered Metabolism: To produce a systemic effect, most drugs must reach receptor sites, which means they must be able to cross the lipid plasma membranes. Therefore, most drugs must be somewhat lipid-soluble. The role of metabolism is to change these active lipid-soluble compounds to inactive water-soluble substances that can be efficiently excreted. Enzymes, many of which are concentrated in the smooth surface of the endothelium of liver cells ("hepatic microsomal enzymes"), first oxidize, demethylate, hydrolyze, etc, the drug (phase I or "asynthetic" phase). Then, large water-soluble molecules (eg, glucuronic acid, sulfate) are attached to the drug (phase II or "synthetic" phase) to form the usually inactive water-soluble metabolite.

An important group of hepatic microsomal enzymes are the "mixed function oxidases," characterized by the cytochrome P450 isoenzymes. They are responsible for the oxidation of many drugs, such as warfarin, phenytoin, quinidine, tolbutamide, and cyclosporine. These mixed-function oxidases are the enzymes most commonly reported to be "induced" by other drugs.

Based on the current classification scheme, the entire group of cytochrome P450 enzymes represents a superfamily (CYP) consisting of families designated by an Arabic or Roman numeral (eg, CYP2 or CYPII) and subfamilies designated by a capital letter (eg, CYP2D or CYPIID), according to the similarity of amino acid sequences of the encoded P450 isozyme protein. The individual gene is designated by an Arabic numeral (eg, CYP2D6 or CYPIID6). Of the CYP genes that have been identified, families CYP1, CYP2, and CYP3 appear to be involved primarily with drug metabolism; however, the specific CYP isozyme responsible for the oxidation of most drugs is unknown. A number of drugs have been identified, in vivo and in vitro, as substrates, inhibitors, and inducers of metabolism by the CYP enzymes (see table 3).

Use of Table 3 – A drug that inhibits a CYP isozyme (see Enzyme Inhibition) may decrease the metabolism and increase serum concentrations of drugs that are substrates for that isozyme. Thus, propafenone inhibits CYP2D6 and has been reported to decrease the metabolism of metoprolol, a beta-blocker metabolized by the CYP2D6 isozyme. Conversely, a drug that induces a CYP isozyme (see Enzyme Induction) may increase the metabolism and decrease serum concentrations of drugs that are substrates for that isozyme. For example, carbamazepine induces CYP2C9 and has been reported to increase metabolism and decrease serum concentrations of phenytoin. When concurrent use of at least one drug is being considered, the table may be used to identify a potential risk for the occurrence of a drug interaction. This knowledge can be useful for health care providers selecting drug therapy and managing patients. By way of illustration, when there are no clinical data, if a drug interaction caused by enzyme inhibition is suspected based on drugs listed in the table, it may be prudent to start with a conservative dose of the object drug and carefully monitor the response of the patient as therapy is initiated and the drug dosage is titrated. However, there are limitations to extrapolating from the table. Even though in vitro interaction studies may indicate a possible interaction between two drugs, a drug interaction may not occur in vivo. For example, in vitro studies have shown that montelukast is a potent CYP2C8 inhibitor; however, in an in vivo clinical drug interaction study involving montelukast and rosiglitazone (a CYP2C8 substrate), montelukast did not inhibit CYP2C8.[65] Enzyme inhibitors or inducers vary quantitatively in their affinity for enzymes; for example, with inhibition of the CYP2D6 isozyme, fluoxetine > sertraline > fluvoxamine. However, when inhibition of CYP2C19 is considered, the affinity of fluvoxamine is greater than fluoxetine, and fluoxetine affinity is greater than sertraline.[18] Other factors that make predicting clinically important drug interactions more difficult are genetic polymorphism (ie, rapid vs poor metabolizers), interpatient variability, the amount of object drug undergoing metabolism, whether the metabolite is active or inactive, and the therapeutic index of the object drug. Therefore, clinical studies are needed to verify and determine the clinical importance of suspected drug interactions. In the absence of these data, the table may be useful as an additional tool in the management of patient care.

Table 3. Inhibitors, Inducers, and Substrates of Cytochrome P450 Enzymes†[1,2,20-64]

CYP Enzyme	Inhibitor	Inducer	Substrate	
1A2	Anastrozole Cimetidine (weak) Ciprofloxacin Citalopram (weak) Diethyldithiocarbamate Enoxacin Erythromycin Fluvoxamine Grapefruit Juice* Mexiletine Mibefradil Mirtazapine (weak) Norfloxacin Propranolol Ritonavir Sildenafil (weak) Tacrine Ticlopidine (moderate) Vemurafenib (moderate)	Charbroiled food Cigarette smoke Modafinil Omeprazole Phenobarbital Primidone Rifampin	Acetaminophen Aprepitant (minor) Asenapine Bortezomib Caffeine Cinacalcet Clozapine (major) Cyclobenzaprine Diazepam Doxepin (minor) Duloxetine Eltrombopag Erlotinib (minor) Estradiol Febuxostat Fluvoxamine Haloperidol Imatinib (minor) Isotretinoin Lidocaine Lomefloxacin Melatonin (major) Methadone Mexiletine (minor) Mirtazapine Naproxen Ofloxacin Olanzapine Ondansetron Phenacetin Propafenone	Propranolol Riluzole Ritonavir Ramelteon (major) Roflumilast Romidepsin (minor) Ropinirole Ropivacaine (major) Tacrine Tamoxifen Testosterone Theophylline (major) Tizanidine TCAs (demethylation) Amitriptyline Clomipramine Desipramine Imipramine Nortriptyline Verapamil R-Warfarin Zileuton Ziprasidone (minor) Zolmitriptan Zolpidem
2A6	Diethyldithiocarbamate Ketoconazole Methoxsalen Miconazole Pilocarpine Ritonavir		Dexmedetomidine Ritonavir Tamoxifen	
2B6	Diethyldithiocarbamate Orphenadrine Prasugrel (weak) Quazepam	Modafinil Phenobarbital Phenytoin Primidone	Bupropion Cyclophosphamide Efavirenz Ifosfamide	Efavirenz Methadone Prasugrel Quinine (minor) Romidepsin (minor) Sorafenib Tamoxifen

Table 3. Inhibitors, Inducers, and Substrates of Cytochrome P450 Enzymes†[1,2,20-64]

CYP Enzyme	Inhibitor	Inducer	Substrate	
2C8-10	Amiodarone (2C9) Anastrozole (2C8/2C9) Chloramphenicol (2C9) Cimetidine (2C9) Delavirdine (2C9) Diclofenac (2C9) Diethyldithiocarbamate (2C8) Disulfiram (2C9) Efavirenz (2C9) Fluconazole (2C9) Fluoxetine (2C9) Flurbiprofen (2C9) Fluvastatin (2C9) Fluvoxamine (2C9) Gemfibrozil (2C8) Ketoprofen (2C9) Lapatinib (2C8) Metronidazole (2C9) Miconazole (2C9) Modafinil (2C9) Montelukast (2C8) Nateglinide (2C9) Nilotinib (2C8, 2C9) Omeprazole (2C8) Phenylbutazone (2C9) Ritonavir (2C9) Sertraline (suspected) Sildenafil (2C9; weak) Sulfonamides (2C9) Sulfadiazine (2C9) Sulfamethizole (2C9) Sulfamethoxazole (2C9) Sulfinpyrazone (2C9) Ticlopidine (2C9; weak) Toremifene (2C9; weak) Trimethoprim (2C9) Troglitazone (2C9) Voriconazole (2C9) Zafirlukast (2C9)	Bosentan (2C9) Carbamazepine (2C9) Ethanol (2C9) Etravirine (2C9) Phenobarbital (2C8) Phenytoin (2C9) Primidone (2C8) Rifampin (2C9) Rifapentine (2C8/2C9)	Azilsartan (2C9) Barbiturates Hexobarbital (2C9) Mephobarbital (2C9) Benzphetamine (2C8) Bortezomib (2C9) Bosentan (2C9) Carvedilol (2C9) Celecoxib (2C9) Dapsone (2C9) Diazepam (2C8) Diclofenac (2C8/2C9) Dronabinol (2C9) Eltrombopag (2C8) Etravirine (2C9) Febuxostat (2C8/2C9) Fluoxetine (2C9) Flurbiprofen (2C9) Fluvastatin (2C9) Glimepiride (2C9) Glipizide (2C9) Glyburide (2C9) Ibuprofen (2C9) Imatinib (2C9; minor) Indomethacin (2C9) Irbesartan (2C9) Isotretinoin (2C8) Lapatinib (2C8; minor) Losartan (2C9) Mefenamic Acid (2C9) Melatonin (2C9; Meloxicam (2C9) minor) Mephenytoin (2C9) Mirtazapine (2C9) Montelukast (2C9) Naproxen (2C9) Nateglinide (2C9) Omeprazole (2C8) Paclitaxel (2C8; major) Phenytoin (2C9) Pioglitazone (2C8) Piroxicam (2C9) Pitavastatin (2C8 slight; 2C9 slight) Prasugrel (2C9) Quinine (2C8 minor; 2C9 minor) Ramelteon (2C9; minor) Retinoic acid (2C8) Repaglinide (2C8) Ritonavir (2C9) Rosiglitazone (2C8; 2C9; minor) Rosuvastatin (2C9) Sertraline (2C9)	Sildenafil (2C9) Sitagliptin (2C8; minor) Sorafenib (2C8) Suprofen (2C9) Terbinafine (2C9) Tetrahydrocannabinol (2C9) Tolbutamide (2C8/2C9) Torsemide (2C9) Treprostinil (2C8) TCAs Amitriptyline (2C9) Imipramine (2C9) Voriconazole (2C9) S-Warfarin (2C9) Zileuton (2C9)

Table 3. Inhibitors, Inducers, and Substrates of Cytochrome P450 Enzymes†[1,2,20-64]

CYP Enzyme	Inhibitor	Inducer	Substrate	
2C18-19	Cimetidine (2C19) Citalopram (2C19; weak) Delavirdine (2C19) Efavirenz (2C19) Felbamate (2C19) Fluoxetine (2C19) Fluvoxamine (2C19) Ketoconazole (2C19) Modafinil (2C19) Omeprazole (2C19) Ritonavir (2C19) Sildenafil (2C19; weak) Telmisartan (2C19) Ticlopidine (2C19) Tolbutamide (2C19) Tranylcypromine (2C19) Troglitazone (2C19) Voriconazole (2C19)	Bosentan (2C19*) Etravirine (2C19) Rifampin (2C19)	Ambrisentan (2C19) Arformoterol (2C19; minor) Atomoxetine (2C19; minor) Bortezomib (2C19) Carisoprodol (2C19) Chloramphenicol (2C19) Cilostazol (2C19) Citalopram (2C19) Clopidogrel (2C19) Cyclophosphamide (2C19) Desmethyldiazepam (2C19) Diazepam (2C19) Divalproex Sodium (2C19) Esomeprazole (2C19) Etravirine (2C19) Hexobarbital (2C19) Imatinib (2C19; minor) Indomethacin (2C19) Lansoprazole (2C19) Lapatinib (2C19; minor) Melatonin (2C19; minor) Mephenytoin (2C19) S-Mephenytoin (2C19) R-Mephobarbital (2C19) Naproxen (2C18) Nelfinavir (2C19) Nilutamide (2C19) Omeprazole (2C19) Pantoprazole (2C19) Phenobarbital (2C19) Phenytoin(2C19) Piroxicam (2C18)	Prasugrel (2C19) Primidone (2C19) Progesterone (2C19) Proguanil (2C19) Propranolol (2C19) Quinine (2C19) Rabeprazole (2C19) Retinoic Acid (2C18) Ritonavir (2C19) Romidepsin (2C19; minor) Rosuvastatin (2C19) Sertraline (2C19) S-Tetrahydrocannabinol (2C18) Tolbutamide (2C19) TCAs Amitriptyline (2C19) Clomipramine (2C19) Imipramine (2C19) Valproic Acid (2C19) Vilazodone (2C19; minor) S-Warfarin (2C18; minor) Ziprasidone

Table 3. Inhibitors, Inducers, and Substrates of Cytochrome P450 Enzymes†[1,2,20-64]

CYP Enzyme	Inhibitor	Inducer	Substrate	
2D6	Amiodarone Asenapine (weak) Black cohosh (weak) Chloroquine Cimetidine (weak) Citalopram (weak) Codeine Delavirdine Desvenlafaxine Dextropropoxyphene Doxepin Doxorubicin Escitalopram Febuxostat (weak) Fluoxetine Fluphenazine Fluvoxamine Gold seal Haloperidol Lomustine Methadone Methylnaltrexone (weak) Mibefradil Mirtazapine (weak) Nefazodone Nilotinib Norfluoxetine Norfluvoxamine Paroxetine Perphenazine Primaquine Propafenone Propranolol Quinidine Ranitidine Ritonavir Sertraline (suspected) Sildenafil (weak) Thioridazine Ticlopidine Venlafaxine Vinblastine Vinorelbine Yohimbine	Not affected by common inducers	Almotriptan Amphetamine Arformoterol Aripiprazole Asenapine Atomoxetine Bortezomib Carvedilol Chloroquine (possible) Chlorpheniramine Chlorpromazine Cinacalcet Citalopram Clozapine Codeine Cyclobenzaprine Darifenacin Debrisoquin Delavirdine Dexfenfluramine Dextromethorphan Dolasetron Donepezil Doxepin (major) Encainide Flecainide Fluoxetine Fluphenazine Halofantrine Haloperidol Hydrocodone Hydroxyamphetamine Iloperidone Imatinib (minor) Ivermectin (minor) Labetalol Maprotiline Methamphetamine Metoprolol Mexiletine (major) Mirtazapine Morphine Nortriptyline Olanzapine Ondansetron Oxaminiquine Oxycodone Paroxetine Penbutolol Pentazocine Propranolol Quinine (minor) Ranolazine (minor) Simvastatin	Perphenazine Phenformin Primaquine (possible) Propafenone Propoxyphene Propranolol (minor) Risperidone Ritonavir Ropivacaine Selegiline Sertraline Sparteine Tamoxifen Thioridazine Timolol Tolterodine (major) Tramadol Trazodone Tamsulosin Tetrabenazine (major) TCAs (hydroxylation) Amitriptyline Clomipramine Desipramine Doxepin Imipramine Nortriptyline Protriptyline Trimipramine Venlafaxine Vilazodone (2D6; minor) Ziprasidone Zolpidem
2E1	Diethyldithiocarbamate Disulfiram Garlic oil Kava Ritonavir Rufinamide (weak) Sildenafil (weak)	Ethanol Isoniazid St. John's wort	Acetaminophen Chlorzoxazone Dapsone Enflurane Eszopiclone Ethanol (minor) Halothane Ivermectin (minor) Isoflurane	Isoniazid Methoxyflurane Ondansetron Quinine (minor) Ritonavir Sevoflurane Tamoxifen Theophylline
3A3	Cimetidine Nefazodone (suspected) Ranitidine		Erythromycin Midazolam	

Table 3. Inhibitors, Inducers, and Substrates of Cytochrome P450 Enzymes†[1,2,20-64]

CYP Enzyme	Inhibitor	Inducer	Substrate	
3A4	Amprenavir	Aprepitant	Acetaminophen	Miconazole
	Anastrozole	Bosentan	Alfentanil	Midazolam
	Aprepitant	Carbamazepine	Alfuzosin	Mifepristone
	Atazanavir	Efavirenz	Aliskiren	Mirtazapine
	Boceprevir	Etravirine	Almotriptan	Modafinil
	Cimetidine	Glucocorticoids	Alprazolam	Mometasone
	Clarithromycin	Desvenlafaxine	Ambrisentan	Montelukast
	Clotrimazole	Dexamethasone	Amiodarone	Nateglinide
	Conivaptan	Prednisone	Amlodipine	Navelbine
	Crizotinib (moderate)	Macrolide Antibiotics	Aprepitant	Nefazodone
	Danazol	Modafinil	Aripiprazole	Nelfinavir
	Darunavir	Phenobarbital	Asenapine	Nevirapine
	Dasatinib	Phenylbutazone	Astemizole	Nicardipine
	Delavirdine	Phenytoin	Atazanavir	Nifedipine
	Diethyldithiocarbamate	Primidone	Atorvastatin	Nilotinib
	Diltiazem	Rifabutin	Benzphetamine	Nimodipine
	Efavirenz	Rifampin	Bromocriptine	Nisoldipine
	Erythromycin	Rifapentine	Busulfan	Nitrendipine
	Fluconazole	Rufinamide (weak)	Carbamazepine	Omeprazole
	Fluoxetine	St. John's wort	Cerivastatin	Ondansetron
	Fluvoxamine	Sulfinpyrazone	Chlorpromazine	Paclitaxel (minor)
	Golden seal	Vemurafenib	Cilostazol	Pimozide
	Grapefruit Juice		Cinacalcet	Pioglitazone
	Indinavir		Cisapride	Prasugrel
	Itraconazole		Citalopram	Progesterone
	Ketoconazole		Clarithromycin	Propafenone
	Lapatinib		Clindamycin	Quazepam
	Linagliptin (weak to moderate)		Clonazepam	Quetiapine
	Mibefradil		Clozapine	Quinidine
	Miconazole		Cocaine	Quinine
	Mifepristone		Codeine	Ramelteon (minor)
	Mirtazapine (weak)		Colchicine	Ranolazine (major)
	Nefazodone		Conivaptan	Rifabutin
	Nelfinavir		Crizotinib	Rilpivirine
	Nevirapine		Cyclobenzaprine	Ritonavir
	Nilotinib		Cyclophosphamide	Rivaroxaban
	Norfloxacin		Cyclosporine	Roflumilast
	Norfluoxetine		Dapsone	Romidepsin (major)
	Paroxetine		Darifenacin	Ropivacaine (minor)
	Posaconazole		Darunavir	Salmeterol
	Propranolol		Dasatinib	Saquinavir
	Quinine		Delavirdine	Saxagliptin
	Quinidine		Desvenlafaxine	Sertraline
	Ranitidine		Dexamethasone	Sibutramine
	Ritonavir		Dextromethorphan	Sildenafil
	Saquinavir		Diazepam	Silodosin
	Schisandra		Digoxin	Simvastatin
	Sertraline		Diltiazem	Sirolimus
	Sildenafil (weak)		Disopyramide	Sitagliptin
	Telaprevir		Docetaxel	Sufentanil
	Telithromycin		Dolasetron	Sunitinib
	Ticagrelor		Donepezil	Tacrolimus
	Troglitazone		Doxepin (minor)	Tamoxifen
	Troleandomycin		Doxorubicin	Tamsulosin
	Voriconazole		Dronabinol	Telaprevir (major)
	Zafirlukast		Dronedarone	Telithromycin (major)
			Dutasteride	Temsirolimus
			Efavirenz	Teniposide
			Eplerenone	Terfenadine
			Erlotinib (major)	Testosterone
			Erythromycin	Theophylline (minor)
			Esomeprazole	Tiagabine
			Eszopiclone	Ticagrelor (major)
			Ethinyl Estradiol	Tipranavir
			Ethosuximide	Tolterodine

Table 3. Inhibitors, Inducers, and Substrates of Cytochrome P450 Enzymes† [1,2,20-64]				
CYP Enzyme	Inhibitor	Inducer	Substrate	
3A4			Etoposide Etravirine Exemestane Felodipine Fentanyl Fexofenadine Glyburide Granisetron Halofantrine Hydrocortisone Ifosfamide Iloperidone Imatinib (major) Indinavir Irinotecan Isradipine Itraconazole* Ivermectin (major) Ixabepilone Ketoconazole Lansoprazole Lapatinib (major) Lercanidipine Lidocaine Loratadine Losartan Lovastatin Lurasidone Maraviroc Mefloquine Methadone Mibefradil Micafungin (minor)	Tolvaptan Toremifene Tretinoin Triazolam TCAs (demethylation) Amitriptyline Clomipramine Imipramine Troglitazone Troleandomycin Vandetanib Vemurafenib Venlafaxine Verapamil Vilazodone (major) Vinblastine Vincristine Voriconazole R-Warfarin Yohimbine Zileuton Ziprasidone (major) Zolpidem (major) Zonisamide
3A5-7	Boceprevir (3A5) Clotrimazole Crizotinib (3A5; moderate) Golden seal (eA5) Ketoconazole Metronidazole Miconazole Troleandomycin	Modafinil Phenobarbital Phenytoin Primidone Rifampin	Brentuximab Crizotinib Ethinyl Estradiol Lapatinib Lovastatin (3A5) Midazolam (3A5) Nifedipine (3A5) Quinidine Rivaroxaban Romidepsin	Terfenadine Testosterone Ticagrelor Triazolam Vinblastine Vincristine

† If reference is not listed, then the package insert applies.
* Effect uncertain or minimal.

Enzyme Induction – Enzyme induction is a stimulated increase in enzyme activity. The increase in enzyme activity is caused by an increase in the amount of enzyme present; therefore, because synthesis of enzymes requires time, enzyme induction is delayed. Approximately 400 drugs and chemicals (eg, insecticides, chemicals in cigarette smoke, certain vegetables) are enzyme inducers in animals. Clinically, phenobarbital, phenytoin, carbamazepine, and rifampin are the enzyme inducers of greatest interest. For drugs whose metabolism is stimulated by enzyme inducers, the dose may need to be increased upon initiation of inducer therapy and decreased when the inducer is discontinued. Drugs whose action has been clinically altered by enzyme inducers include warfarin, oral contraceptives, chloramphenicol, cyclosporine, disopyramide, doxycycline, griseofulvin, metronidazole, mexiletine, quinidine, theophylline, and verapamil (see table 3).

Enzyme Inhibition – Enzyme inhibition of drug-metabolizing enzymes generally decreases the rate of metabolism of the object drug. This is likely to result in increased serum concentrations of the object drug and, if the drug has a narrow therapeutic index, potential drug toxicity. Drug-metabolizing enzymes may become saturated when at least two drugs using the same metabolic pathway are administered, resulting in a decrease in the rate of metabolism of one or both drugs (eg, fluoxetine-imipramine). On the other hand, certain drugs may bind to an enzyme system and inhibit enzyme function (eg, cimetidine binds to certain isoenzymes of cytochrome P450). Cimetidine and erythromycin are the enzyme inhibitors most frequently reported in clinically important interactions. Other enzyme inhibitors include isoniazid, verapamil, chloramphenicol, ketoconazole, allopurinol, amiodarone, disulfiram, and the monoamine oxidase (MAO) inhibitors (see table 3).

Altered Excretion: Interactions involving altered excretion generally involve altered active transport in the tubules (eg, probenecid-penicillin; methotrexate-NSAIDs; quinidine-digoxin) or a pH effect on the passive transport of weak acids or weak bases. In the latter case, changes in urine pH appear to clinically affect the excretion of relatively few drugs; these include phenobarbital, salicylates, flecainide, quinidine, and amphetamine. A change in sodium presentation to the kidney (eg, use of diuretics, low-salt diet) alters the excretion (and serum level) of lithium. If a drug is a substrate of P-glycoprotein (see table 1) in the renal proximal tubules, active secretion into the urine results.[6-8] A drug that inhibits P-glycoprotein (see table 2) in the renal tubules could decrease the elimination of a P-glycoprotein substrate (increasing plasma concentrations of the substrate).[9] For example, quinidine blocks P-glycoprotein-mediated excretion in the proximal tubules of the kidney. The increase in digoxin plasma concentrations that occurs with coadministration of quinidine may be caused in part by inhibition of P-glycoprotein-mediated transport of digoxin into the renal proximal tubules, which may decrease digoxin excretion.[14] Quinidine-induced inhibition of P-glycoprotein in the GI tract and hepatic biliary system also may contribute to elevated digoxin plasma levels.[5] Inhibition of P-glycoprotein by quinidine as one of the mechanisms of this interaction is strongly supported by experimental data in mice.[14] A similar mechanism has been ascribed to increased plasma digoxin concentrations occurring with coadministration of verapamil (eg, *Calan*).[7]

Pharmacodynamic

Important pharmacologic/pharmacodynamic interactions include additive CNS depression, additive anticholinergic effect, potentiation of neuromuscular blockade, additive cardiac depression, changes in various components of the coagulation system, and changes in blood sugar.

Interpretation and Intervention

The incidence of adverse reactions caused by drug interactions is unknown. In many instances of administration of "interacting drugs," the patient only needs to be monitored with the knowledge of the potential changes caused by the interaction. In some cases, it may be prudent to alter the dose of the object drug when therapy by the precipitant drug is initiated or discontinued. Rarely, it may be necessary to change one of the drug pairs to a noninteracting agent, if available (eg, cimetidine to another H_2 antagonist). Inform the physician if potentially dangerous (clinically important) drug combinations are ordered (characterized in *Drug Interaction Facts* by significance ratings of "1," "2," or "3"). The patient may be alerted to watch for symptoms that denote an adverse effect.

Those drugs that are most likely to result in dangerous effects if their action is markedly altered are those with a narrow therapeutic index. Many of these are also used chronically and are metabolized by the hepatic mixed-function oxidase enzyme system; such agents include digoxin, phenytoin, carbamazepine, aminoglycosides, warfarin, theophylline, lithium, and cyclosporine.

Many patients may receive potentially interacting drugs without evidence of an adverse effect. It has not been possible to distinguish any clear-cut characteristics that determine who will or will not experience an adverse drug interaction. It appears that patients with multiple illnesses and those taking many drugs are the most susceptible. The elderly population often fits this description; therefore, many case reports involve elderly subjects receiving multiple drugs.

Circumventing an Interaction

Many drug interactions can be avoided if adequate precautions are taken. Monitoring therapy and making appropriate adjustments in the drug regimen may circumvent a potentially serious drug interaction. Hospitalized patients frequently receive warfarin with an interacting agent without clinical consequences. In this setting, the patient's prothrombin times are monitored frequently and appropriate adjustments are made in the warfarin dosage. However, to avoid possible bleeding or the risk of exacerbating the condition being treated, care must be taken if the interacting drug is discontinued after the patient leaves the hospital.

Beneficial Interactions

In some instances, drug interactions may be clinically useful. Coadministration of probenecid and penicillin enhances the effectiveness of the antibiotic. These drugs are frequently coadministered to the patient's therapeutic advantage.

Determining Clinical Importance

Animal Studies: These studies may not be extrapolative to humans. On a mg/kg basis, animals frequently receive much higher doses than humans.

Anecdotal Case Reports: As with clinical studies, the quality of observed events varies considerably. However, case reports usually require additional controlled studies to determine their clinical importance. One must be able to rule out other explanations for the observed event.

Healthy Volunteers: Studies of healthy volunteers or small numbers of patients may not allow adequate evaluation of a potential interaction. Some pharmacokinetic interactions may be determined in healthy volunteers but may not be clinically important in patients. Conversely, healthy volunteers may not exhibit an interaction that is observed in patients.

Magnitude of Effect: Based upon the magnitude of the effect of a drug interaction, studies may fail to identify or accurately describe a potential drug interaction. The clinical manifestations of a drug interaction are highly situational. Factors that may interfere with assessing the degree of effect include:

Order of Administration – The patient is stabilized on the precipitant drug when the object drug is started. In this instance, no interaction may be observed unless the precipitant drug is discontinued. Thus, if a patient has been receiving cimetidine before warfarin treatment is initiated, no interaction would be observed.

However, if cimetidine was discontinued after the warfarin dosage was stabilized, a higher anticoagulant dose might be required.

Treatment Duration – Some drug interactions occur almost immediately while others may not become evident for days or months. An interaction with a delayed onset may not be observed if the study time is too short. For example, neurotoxicity associated with coadministration of lithium and carbamazepine may not be observed for several days.

Adequate Dose – Many drug interactions are dose-related. Thus, high-dose salicylates (eg, aspirin more than 3 g/day) antagonize the uricosuric action of probenecid, but occasional low doses do not.

Dosage Form – The effects of food on drug absorption must be considered on an individual product basis. For example, although food can be ingested with many theophylline preparations, *Theo-24* taken less than 1 hour before a high-fat meal may result in increased theophylline absorption and peak serum concentrations.

Preexisting Patient Status – Preexisting patient status may determine the observability of a drug interaction. Two important factors that may play a role in whether a patient develops evidence of an adverse experience because of a drug interaction are the current serum level of the object drug and the individual's responsiveness to enzyme induction or inhibition (diagram 1).

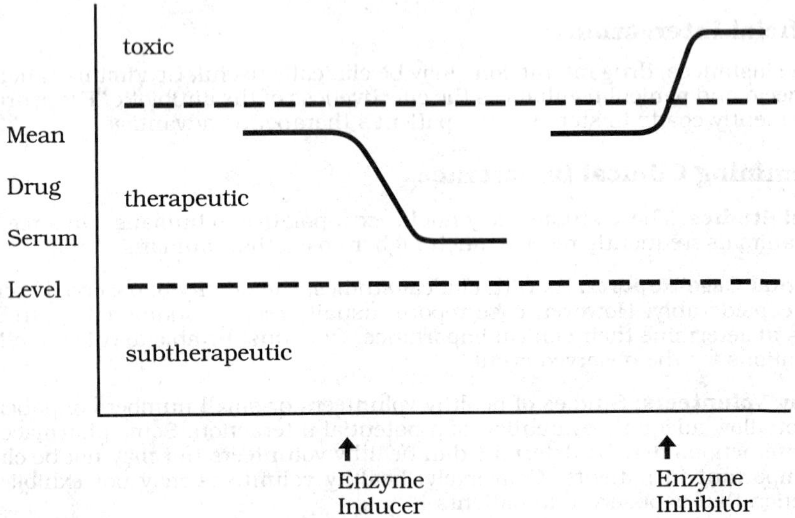

Diagram 1. Mean drug blood level response to an enzyme inducer or enzyme inhibitor

If the subject's drug blood level is in the upper therapeutic range, a moderate decrease in blood level in response to an enzyme inducer would probably result in a new level still within the therapeutic range. However, even a mild response to an enzyme inhibitor is likely to increase the drug level into the toxic range. This is complicated by the variation in individual responsiveness to an enzyme inducer or inhibitor. A study may report a 50% mean increase in object drug serum concentration in response to an enzyme inhibitor, but the individual responsiveness in the study may range from 0% to 300%. Patients whose drug serum concentration changed by 300% would be in jeopardy.

Multiple Drugs – In a preliminary study, the presence of propylene glycol in IV nitroglycerin preparations was reported to interfere with the anticoagulant effect of heparin. Subsequent reports demonstrated that the effect on heparin was caused by the nitroglycerin component. As the number of drugs present in a situation increases, it will become more difficult to identify the interacting sources, if any exist.

Extrapolation to Related Drugs: Not all members of a drug class may interact in the same manner. Cimetidine inhibits the microsomal enzymes involved in the metabolism of diazepam; however, famotidine does not appear to affect diazepam metabolism. In addition, cimetidine does not affect oxazepam metabolism.

Variability in Patient Response: In well-controlled drug interaction studies, it is not unusual to find wide variations in patient responses to the same drug regimen. The factors listed below account for some of the variability.

Age – The very young and the elderly may be at increased risk for interactions. Studies indicate that about 25% of all prescription drugs dispensed are prescribed to elderly patients; elderly patients also use OTC medications extensively. Furthermore, elderly patients may have other chronic diseases or decreased organ function (eg, renal, hepatic). However, regardless of age, monitor drug therapy more closely in any patient with decreased organ function.

Genetics – For example, the toxicity seen with the inhibitory effect of isoniazid on the metabolism of phenytoin appears to be most important in slow acetylators of isoniazid.

Disease States – Disease states (eg, impaired renal function, hepatic dysfunction, hypoalbuminemia) may influence the response to various drugs used concurrently.

There are 3 ways diseases can alter how a patient is affected by an interaction:

1. Primary disease effects - Altered physiology caused by the disease affects the outcome of the interaction (eg, the additive ototoxicity of aminoglycosides and ethacrynic acid is increased in the presence of renal failure).

2. Secondary disease effects - Some diseases dictate different drug usage by:
   - requiring different dosages
   - requiring various durations of therapy (eg, titration)
   - using different administration regimens
   - requiring additional drug therapy
   - treatment vs prophylaxis

3. Pharmacology - One pharmacological aspect of a drug interacts with another agent.

Alcohol Consumption – Acute alcohol intolerance (disulfiram reaction) has occurred in patients consuming alcohol while taking other drugs, including cefoperazone and cefotetan. Chronic alcoholism may cause changes that affect drug metabolism, primarily enzyme induction.

Smoking – Smoking increases the activity of drug-metabolizing enzymes in the liver. Smoking stimulates the metabolism of theophylline and mexiletine. Smokers may require larger doses of these drugs to maintain therapeutic serum levels.

Diet – Diet can affect drug absorption (eg, milk and tetracycline), action (eg, tyramine-containing foods and MAO inhibitors), and elimination (eg, protein diet and urinary pH).

Environmental Factors – Environmental factors (eg, some pesticides) may alter the effects of liver-metabolizing enzymes.

Particularly Susceptible Patients –

- elderly patients
- patients with acute illness
- patients with unstable diseases
- drug treatment-dependent patients
- patients with renal or hepatic disease
- patients with multiple prescribing physicians

Mean Values: For drug interactions that occur in a small number of patients, there may be no difference in average response between the control group and the study group. However, if one analyzes the results for individual patients, there may be a clinically important change in a few subjects. Some patients show a 5-fold increase in serum digoxin levels during coadministration of quinidine, while in others, the effect is minimal.

Therapeutic Index: Routinely monitor patients receiving drugs with a narrow therapeutic index (eg, cyclosporine, digoxin, phenytoin, theophylline, warfarin) for possible drug interactions. Drug interactions in this category may be life-threatening or have serious clinical consequences.

Conclusion

Health care professionals need to be aware of drug interaction resources that identify immediacy and severity of interactions, and be able to describe the result of the potential interaction and suggest appropriate interventions. It is also incumbent on the health care professional to be able to apply the available literature to a situation. The professional must be able to individualize recommendations based on patient-specific parameters. Although some authorities suggest adverse reactions resulting from drug interactions may be less frequent than originally believed, the health care professional should protect the patient against harmful effects of drugs, particularly when they can be anticipated and prevented.

References

1 Aronson JK, et al. Adverse drug interactions. *BMJ.* 1981;282:288.
2 McInnes GT, et al. Drug interactions that matter: A critical reappraisal. *Drugs.* 1988;36:83.
3 von Moltke LL, Greenblatt DJ. Drug transporters in psychopharmacology – are they important? *J Clin Psychopharmacol.* 2000;20:291-294.
4 Zhang Y, Benet LZ. The gut as a barrier to drug absorption: combined role of cytochrome P450 3A and P-glycoprotein. *Clin Pharmacokinetic.* 2001;40:159-168.
5 Fromm MF. P-glycoprotein: a defense mechanism limiting oral bioavailability and CNS accumulation of drugs. *Int J Clin Pharmacol Ther.* 2000;38:69-74.
6 Yu DK. The contribution of P-glycoprotein to pharmacokinetic drug-drug interactions. *J Clin Pharmacol.* 1999;39:1203-1211.
7 Verschraagen M, Koks CHW, Schellens JHM, et al. P-glycoprotein system as a determinant of drug interactions: the case of digoxin-verapamil. *Pharmacol Res.* 1999;40:301-306.

[8] Tanigawara Y. Role of P-glycoprotein in drug disposition. *Ther Drug Monit.* 2000;22:137-140.
[9] Matheny CJ, Lamb MW, Brouwer KLR, et al. Pharmacokinetic and pharmacodynamic implications of P-glycoprotein modulation. *Pharmacotherapy.* 2001;21:778-796.
[10] Greiner B, Eichelbaum M, Fritz P, et al. The role of intestinal P-glycoprotein in the interaction of digoxin and rifampin. *J Clin Invest.* 1999;104:147-153.
[11] Abernethy DR, Flockhart DA. Molecular basis of cardiovascular drug metabolism: implications for predicting clinically important drug interactions. *Circulation.* 2000;101:1749-1753.
[12] von Moltke LL, Greenblatt DJ. Drug transporters revisited. *J Clin Psychopharmacol.* 2001;21:1-3.
[13] Sadeque AJM, Wandel C, He H, et al. Increased drug delivery to the brain by P-glycoprotein inhibition. *Clin Pharmacol Ther.* 2000;68:231-237.
[14] Fromm MF, Kim RB, Stein CM, et al. Inhibition of P-glycoprotein-mediated drug transport: a unifying mechanism to explain the interaction between digoxin and quinidine. *Circulation.* 1999;99:552-557.
[15] Hamman MA, Bruce MA, Haehner-Daniels BD, et al. The effect of rifampin administration on the disposition of fexofenadine. *Clin Pharmacol Ther.* 2001;69:114-121.
[16] Masuda S, Uemoto S, Hasida T, et al. Effect of intestinal P-glycoprotein on daily tacrolimus trough level in a living-donor small bowel recipient. *Clin Pharmacol Ther.* 2000;68:98-103.
[17] Dürr D, Stieger B, Kullak-Ublick GA, et al. St. John's wort induces intestinal P-glycoprotein/ MDR1 and intestinal and hepatic CYP3A4. *Clin Pharmacol Ther.* 2000;68:598-604.
[18] Woodland C, Ito S, Koren G. A model for the prediction of digoxin-drug interactions at the renal tubular cell level. *Ther Drug Monit.* 1998;20:134-138.
[19] Levêque D, Jehl F. P-glycoprotein and pharmacokinetics. *Anticancer Res.* 1995;15:331-336.
[20] Halliday RC, et al. An investigation of the interaction between halofantrine, CYP2D6 and CYP3A4: studies with human liver microsomes and heterologous enzyme expression systems. *Br J Clin Pharmacol.* 1995;40:369-378.
[21] Ko JW, et al. In vitro inhibition of the cytochrome P450 (CYP450) system by the anti-platelet drug ticlopidine: potent effect on CYP2C19 and CYP2D6. *Br J Clin Pharmacol.* 2000;49:343-351.
[22] Cupp MJ, et al. Cytochrome P450: new nomenclature and clinical implications. *Am Fam Physician.* 1998;57:107-116.
[23] Caraco Y. Genetic determinants of drug responsiveness and drug interactions. *Ther Drug Monit.* 1998;20:517-524.
[24] Arlander E, et al. Metabolism of ropivacaine in humans is medicated by CYP1A2 and to a minor extent by CYP3A4: an interaction study with fluvoxamine and ketoconazole as in vivo inhibitors. *Clin Pharmacol Ther.* 1998;64:484-491.
[25] Abdel-Rahman SM, et al. Investigation of terbinafine as a CYP2D6 inhibitor in vivo. *Clin Pharmacol Ther.* 1999;65:465-472.
[26] Tanaka M, et al. Stereoselective pharmacokinetics of pantoprazole, a proton pump inhibitor, in extensive and poor metabolizers of S-mephenytoin. *Clin Pharmacol Ther.* 2001;69:108-113.
[27] Hylund R, Roe EG, Jones BC, Smith DA. Identification of the cytochrome P450 enzymes involved in the N-demethylation of sildenafil. *Br J Clin Pharmacol.* 2001;51:239-248.
[28] Greenblatt DJ, von Moltke LL, Harmatz JS, Shader RI. Human cytochromes and some newer antidepressants: kinetics, metabolism, and drug interactions. *J Clin Psychopharmacol.* 1999;19(suppl 1):23S-35S.
[29] Facciola G, Hidestrand M, von Bahr C, Tybring G. Cytochrome P450 isoforms involved in melatonin metabolism in human liver microsomes. *Eur J Clin Pharmacol.* 2001;46:881-888.
[30] Tatro DS. Understanding drug interactions. *Drug Newsletter.* 1988;7:57-59.
[31] Tatro DS. Cytochrome P450 enzyme drug interactions. *Drug Newsletter.* 1995;14:59-60.
[32] Mullen WJ, et al. Pharmaceuticals and the cytochrome P450 isoenzymes: A tool for decision making. *Pharm Practice News.* 1998;25:20-24.
[33] Miners JO, et al. Cytochrome P4502C9: An enzyme of major importance in human drug metabolism. *Br J Clin Pharmacol.* 1998;45:525-538.
[34] Gantmacher J, et al. Interaction between warfarin and oral terbinafine. *BMJ.* 1998;317:205.
[35] Michalets EL. Clinically significant cytochrome P-450 drug interactions – author's reply. *Pharmacotherapy.* 1998;18:892-893.
[36] Bailey DG, et al. Grapefruit juice-drug interactions. *Br J Clin Pharmacol.* 1998;46:101-110.
[37] Nakajima M, et al. Involvement of CYP 1A2 in mexiletine metabolism. *Br J Clin Pharmacol.* 1998;46:55-62.
[38] Jefferson JW. Drug interactions – friend or foe? *J Clin Psychiatry.* 1998;59(suppl 4):37-47.
[39] Michalets EL. Update: Clinically significant cytochrome P-450 drug interactions. *Pharmacotherapy.* 1998;18:84-112.
[40] Nemeroff CB, et al. Newer antidepressants and the cytochrome p450 system. *Am J Psychiatry.* 1996;153:311-320.

[41] Bertz RJ, et al. Use of in vitro and in vivo data to estimate the likelihood of metabolic pharmacokinetic interactions. *Clin Pharmacokinet.* 1997;32:210-258.
[42] Goldberg RJ. The P-450 system. *Arch Fam Med.* 1996;5:406-412.
[43] Teteishi T, et al. Omeprazole does not affect measured CYP3A4 activity using the erythromycin breath test. *Br J Clin Pharmacol.* 1995;40:411-412.
[44] Spatzenegger M, et al. Clinical importance of hepatic cytochrome P450 in drug metabolism. *Drug Metab Rev.* 1995;27:397-417.
[45] Flockhart DA. Drug Interactions: Cytochrome P450 Drug Interaction Table. Indiana University School of Medicine (2007). http://medicine.iupui.edu/clinpharm/ddis/table.asp. Accessed 9/28/2011.
[46] Gurley BJ, et al. Cytochrome P450 phenotype ratios for predicting herb-drug interactions in humans. *Clin Pharmacol Ther* 2002;72(3):276-287.
[47] Gurley BJ, et al. In vivo effects of goldenseal, kava kava, black cohosh, and valerian on human cytochrome P450 1A2, 2D6, 2E1, and 3A4/5 phenotypes. *Clin Pharmacol Ther.* 2005;77(5):415-426.
[48] Karonen T, et al. Gemfibrozil markedly increases the plasma concentrations of montelukast: A previously unrecognized role for CYP2C8 in the metabolism of montelukast. *Clin Pharmacol Ther.* 2010;88(2):323-230.
[49] Andrèn L, et al. Interaction between a commercially available St. John's wort product (*Movina*) and atorvastatin in patients with hypercholesterolemia. *Eur J Clin Pharmacol.* 2007;63(10):913-916.
[50] Johne A, et al. Pharmacokinetic interaction of digoxin with an herbal extract from St. John's wort (*Hypericum perforatum*). *Clin Pharmacol Ther.* 1999;66(4):338-345.
[51] Dresser GK, et al. St. John's wort induces intestinal and hepatic CYP3A4 and P-glycoprotein in healthy volunteers. *Clin Pharmacol Ther.* 2001;69(2):P23.
[52] Mathijssen RH, et al. Effects of St. John's wort on irinotecan metabolism. *J Natl Cancer Inst.* 2002;94(16):1247-1249.
[53] Mueller SC, et al. The extent of induction of CYP3A4 by St. John's wort varies among products and is linked to hyperforin dose. *Eur J Clin Pharmacol.* 2006,62(1):29-36.
[54] Hafner V, et al. Effect of simultaneous induction and inhibition of CYP3A by St. John's wort and ritonavir on CYP3A activity. *Clin Pharmacol Ther.* 2010:87(2):191-196.
[55] Lantz MS, et al. St. John's wort and antidepressant drug interactions in the elderly. *J Geriatr Psychiatry Neurol.* 1999;12(1):7-10.
[56] Piscitelli SC, et al. Indinavir concentrations and St. John's wort. *Lancet.* 2000;355(9203):547-548.
[57] de Maat MM, et al. Drug interaction between St. John's wort and nevirapine. *AIDS.* 2001;15(3):420-421.
[58] Smith M, et al. An open trial of nifedipine-herb interactions: nifedipine with St. John;s wort, ginseng or *Ginkgo biloba. Clin Pharmacol Ther.* 2001;69(2):P86.
[59] Wang LS, et al. St. John's wort induces both cytochrome P450 3A4-catalyzed sulfoxidation and 2C19-dependent hydroxylation of omeprazole. *Clin Pharmacol Ther.* 2004;75(3):191-197.
[60] Kawaguchi A, et al. Drug interaction between St. John's wort and quazepam. *Br J Clin Pharmacol.* 2004;58(4):403-410.
[61] Sugimoto KI, et al. Different effects of St. John's wort on the pharmacokinetics of simvastatin and pravastatin. *Clin Pharmacol Ther.* 2001;70:518-524.
[62] Tannergren C, et al. St. John's wort decreases the bioavailability of R- and S-verapamil through induction of first-pass metabolism. *Clin Pharmacol Ther.* 2004;75(4):298-309.
[63] Robertson P, et al. Effect of modafinil on the pharmacokinetics of ethinyl estradiol and triazolam in healthy volunteers. *Clin Pharmacol Ther.* 2002;71(1):46-56.
[64] Package insert for the product named.
[65] *Singulair* [package insert]. Whitehouse Station, NJ: Merck & Co Inc; December 2010.
[66] Siegmund W, Altmannsberger S, Paneitz A, et al. Effect of levothyroxine administration on intestinal P-glycoprotein expression: Consequences for drug disposition. *Clin Pharmacol Ther* 2002;72(3):256-264.
[67] Nakagami T, et al. Effect of verapamil on pharmacokinetics and pharmacodynamics of risperidone: In vivo evidence of involvement of P-glycoprotein in risperidone disposition. *Clin Pharmacol Ther.* 2005;78(1):43-51.
[68] Bolhuis MS, et al. Clarithromycin significantly increases linezolid serum concentrations. *Antimicrobial Agents Chemotherapy.* 2010;54(12):5418.
[69] Xing HW, et al. Effects of *Schisandra sphenanthera* extract on the pharmacokinetics of tacrolimus in healthy volunteers. *Br J Clin Pharmacol.* 2007;64(4):469-475.

Drug-induced Prolongation of the QT Interval and Torsades de Pointes

The QT interval is the period between the beginning of the QRS complex and the end of the T wave.[1] Thus, it is the estimate of the time interval between the earliest ventricular depolarization and the latest ventricular repolarization.[1] Because the QT interval is affected by changes in the heart rate, corrections are usually made to the QT interval for these changes (QTc).[1-3] There is no commonly accepted definition of a normal or prolonged QTc interval. The Committee for Proprietary Medicinal Products has suggested ranges for normal (ie, men less than 430 msec, women less than 450 msec), borderline (ie, men 430 to 450 msec, women 450 to 470 msec), and prolonged (ie, men greater than 450 msec, women greater than 470 msec) QTc intervals.[4] Moderate and clinically important increases in the QT interval over baseline have been considered to be 15% and 25% increases, respectively.[1]

Numerous drugs, representing a wide range of pharmacologic classes, have been implicated in prolonging the QT interval. Concern about serious and possibly fatal consequences of drug combinations that may cause prolongation of the QT interval has led to contraindicating the use of many drug pairs, even though coadministration may not have been studied. The potential of bepridil (*Vascor*), astemizole (*Hismanal*), grepafloxacin (*Raxar*), and terfenadine (*Seldane*) to prolong the QT interval played an important role in their removal from the market.

The precise mechanism by which QT interval prolongation (ie, long QT syndrome [LQTS]) occurs is unknown; however, it appears to be related to ion exchange (eg, outward repolarizing potassium current, inward depolarizing calcium or sodium current).[1,5-7] Class III antiarrhythmic agents prolong the QT interval by blocking potassium flow.[6] A prolonged QT interval may be congenital (eg, genetic) or acquired (eg, drug-induced).[2,4,5,7] In some instances, patients may have an underlying predisposition toward a prolonged QT interval (eg, longer than normal QT interval before drug administration).[5]

Drug-induced prolongation of the QT interval may be suspected if there are dose-related changes in the QT interval, the same drug causes QT prolongation in a number of patients, or prolonged QT interval recurs when a patient is rechallenged.[1] Drug-induced QT prolongation may be prevented by 1) not exceeding the recommended drug dose; 2) limiting use of the drug in patients with preexisting heart disease; 3) avoiding coadministration of agents that increase plasma levels of the drug in question; 4) avoiding concurrent use of other medications that prolong the QT interval; and 5) identification and correction of risk factors (eg, hypokalemia) before giving a drug known to prolong the QT interval.[8]

A great deal of attention has been focused on drug-induced prolongation of the QT interval and association of the prolongation with life-threatening ventricular arrhythmias, especially torsades de pointes. Torsades de pointes, meaning "twisting of points," refers to a ventricular arrhythmia in which the QRS complexes change amplitude and contour, appearing to twist around the isoelectric line on the electrocardiogram (ECG).[5,7] In patients who develop drug-induced torsades de pointes, the QT interval measured prior to drug exposure tends to be longer than in patients who receive the drug safely.[5,7] In patients with drug-induced torsades de pointes, ventricular repolarization is prolonged and characterized by marked prolongation of the QT interval (greater than 500 msec) and QTc interval (greater than 470 msec) of the ECG.[7] In individuals with a drug-induced increase in the QTc interval of more than 65 msec above normal (ie, greater than 500 msec), the risk of torsades de pointes may be greater than 3%.[3,4] This risk of torsades de pointes increases greatly when the QT interval exceeds 600 msec.[1] In the presence of a prolonged QT interval, women are at greater risk than men of developing torsades de pointes.[2,3,5,6]

Amiodarone (eg, *Cordarone*)[5,7] prolongs the QT interval but rarely causes torsades de pointes.[1] However, class I antiarrhythmic agents (eg, procainamide) are more likely to cause torsades de pointes but have a moderate effect on the QT interval.[1] Drug interactions may further prolong the QT interval and increase the risk of life-threatening cardiac arrhythmias, including torsades de pointes.[7] Thus, administration of cisapride (*Propulsid*), which prolongs the QT interval, with an inhibitor of cytochrome P450 (CYP) 3A4 (eg, grapefruit products, erythromycin) may increase cisapride plasma levels and the risk of life-threatening cardiac arrhythmias.[9]

Identification and correction of risk factors (eg, hypokalemia) before giving a drug known to prolong the QT interval or cause torsades de pointes are important in preventing drug-induced torsades de pointes.[7] Agents that prolong the QT interval are contraindicated in patients with a history of drug-induced torsades de pointes.[7]

Summary: Numerous drugs from a wide range of pharmacologic classes can prolong the QT interval and precipitate torsades de pointes. However, the consequences of QT interval prolongation and the occurrence of torsades de pointes can be minimized or prevented by identification and correction of risk factors. Use of drugs that prolong the QT interval is contraindicated in patients with a history of torsades de pointes.

Drugs reported to prolong the QT interval[1,2,4-8,10-14,16-53]

Analgesics
- Celecoxib (*Celebrex*)*
- Methadone (eg, *Dolophine*)*
- Oxycodone (eg, *OxyContin*)

Anesthetic agents
- Enflurane (eg, *Ethrane*)
- Isoflurane (eg, *Forane*)
- Halothane[c]

Antiarrhythmic agents
- Dronedarone (*Multaq*)[b]
- Class IA
  - Disopyramide (eg, *Norpace*)*
  - Procainamide*
  - Quinidine*
- Class IC
  - Flecainide (eg, *Tambocor*)*[a]
  - Propafenone (eg, *Rythmol*)*[b]
- Class III
  - Amiodarone (eg, *Cordarone*)*[b]
  - Bretylium*[c]
  - Dofetilide (*Tikosyn*)*[b]
  - Ibutilide (eg, *Corvert*)*[b]
  - Sotalol (eg, *Betapace*)*[b]

Anticholinergics
- Fesoterodine (*Toviaz*)[b]
- Solifenacin (*Vesicare*)*[b]
- Tolterodine (*Detrol*)[b]

Anticonvulsants
- Felbamate (eg, *Felbatol*)*
- Fosphenytoin (eg, *Cerebyx*)

Antiemetics
- Dolasetron (*Anzemet*)[b]
- Droperidol*[b]
- Granisetron (eg, *Granisol*)[b]
- Ondansetron (eg, *Zofran*)

Antihistamines
- Desloratadine (*Clarinex*)[b] (overdose)
- Diphenhydramine (eg, *Benadryl*)*
- Fexofenadine (eg, *Allegra*)
- Hydroxyzine (eg, *Vistaril*)

Anti-infectives
- Amantadine (eg, *Symmetrel*)*
- Antimalarials
  - Mefloquine[b]
  - Quinine (*Qualaquin*)*
- Antiretrovirals
  - Atazanavir(*Reyataz*)[b]
  - Efavirenz (*Sustiva*)*
  - Nelfinavir (*Viracept*)*[b]
  - Rilpivirine (*Edurant*)[b]
- Antivirals
  - Foscarnet[b]
- Azole antifungal agents
  - Fluconazole (eg, *Diflucan*)*[b]
  - Itraconazole (eg, *Sporanox*)
  - Ketoconazole (eg, *Nizoral*)
  - Voriconazole (eg, *Vfend*)*[b]
- Chloroquine (eg, *Aralen*)*
- Clindamycin (eg, *Cleocin*)
- Ketolides
  - Telithromycin (*Ketek*)[b]
- Macrolides and related antibiotics
  - Azithromycin (eg, *Zithromax*)[b]
  - Clarithromycin (eg, *Biaxin*)*[b]
  - Erythromycin (eg, *Ery-Tab*)*[b]
  - Troleandomycin
- Nalidixic acid[c]
- Pentamidine (eg, *Pentam*)*
- Quinolones
  - Ciprofloxacin (eg, *Cipro*)[b]
  - Gatifloxacin*[b]
  - Gemifloxacin (*Factive*)[b]
  - Levofloxacin (eg, *Levaquin*)*[a,b]
  - Moxifloxacin (*Avelox*)[b]
  - Ofloxacin*[b]
  - Sparfloxacin[b,c]
- Telavancin (*Vibativ*)[b]
- Trimethoprim/Sulfamethoxazole (eg, *Bactrim*)*

Antineoplastics
- Arsenic trioxide (*Trisenox*)*[b]
- Bendamustine (*Treanda*)[b] (overdose)
- Crizotinib (*Xalkori*)[b]

Dasatinib (*Sprycel*)[b]
Doxorubicin (eg, *Adriamycin*)
Lapatinib (*Tykerb*)[b]
Nilotinib (*Tasigna*)
Pazopanib (*Votrient*)[b]
Romidepsin (*Istodax*)[b]
Sunitinib (*Sutent*)[b]
Tamoxifen
Vandetanib (*Caprelsa*)[b]

Bronchodilators
Albuterol (eg, *Proventil*)[b]
Formoterol (*Foradil*)[b]
Isoproterenol
Levalbuterol (eg, *Xopenex*)[b]
Salmeterol (*Serevent*)[b]
Terbutaline[b]

Calcium channel blockers
Isradipine (eg, *DynaCirc*)
Nicardipine (eg, *Cardene*)

Contrast media
Ionic contrast media*
Non-ionic contrast media
Gadobenate (*MultiHance*)[b]
Iohexol (*Omnipaque*)
Perflutren (eg, *Definity*)[b]

Corticosteroids
Prednisolone (eg, *Prelone*)
Prednisone*

Diuretics
Furosemide (eg, *Lasix*)
Indapamide

GI agents
Cisapride (*Propulsid*)*[b]
Famotidine (eg, *Pepcid*)*

Immunosuppressants
Tacrolimus (eg, *Prograf*)*[b] (postmarketing)

Miscellaneous
Alfuzosin (eg, *Uroxatral*)[b]
Apomorphine (*Apokyn*)[b]
Fingolimod (*Gilenya*)[b]
Galantamine (eg, *Razadyne*)
Levomethadyl[c]
Moexipril/Hydrochlorothiazide (eg, *Uniretic*)
Octreotide (eg, *Sandostatin*)[b]
Oxytocin (eg, *Pitocin*; IV bolus)
Papaverine (eg, *Para-Time*)*
Probucol*[c]
Ranolazine (*Ranexa*)[b]
Sibutramine[c]
Tetrabenazine (*Xenazine*)[b]
Toremifene (*Fareston*)
Vardenafil (*Levitra*)[b]
Vasopressin (eg, *Pitressin*)*

Psychotropics
Asenapine (*Saphris*)[b]
Atomoxetine (*Strattera*)[b]
Benzisoxazoles
Iloperidone (*Fanapt*)[b]
Paliperidone (*Invega*)[b]
Risperidone (eg, *Risperdal*)[b] (overdose)
Ziprasidone (*Geodon*)[b]
Droperidol*
Haloperidol (eg, *Haldol*)*
Lithium (eg, *Lithobid*)*
Maprotiline*
Mirtazapine (eg, *Remeron*)[b]
Phenothiazines
Chlorpromazine*
Fluphenazine*
Perphenazine
Thioridazine*[b]
Trifluoperazine
Pimozide (*Orap*)*[b]
Quetiapine (*Seroquel*)[b]
SSRIs[d]
Citalopram (eg, *Celexa*)*[b]
Escitalopram (*Lexapro*)[b]
Fluoxetine (eg, *Prozac*)*[a]
Paroxetine (eg, *Paxil*)*
Sertraline (eg, *Zoloft*)*[a,b] (postmarketing)
SNRIs[d]
Venlafaxine (eg, *Effexor*)[b] (postmarketing)
Trazodone (eg, *Oleptro*)
Tricyclic antidepressants
Amitriptyline*
Clomipramine (eg, *Anafranil*)
Desipramine (eg, *Norpramin*)*
Doxepin (eg, *Silenor*)*
Imipramine (eg, *Tofranil*)*
Nortriptyline (eg, *Pamelor*)

Serotonin 5-HT$_1$ agonists
Naratriptan (eg, *Amerge*)
Sumatriptan (eg, *Imitrex*)[b]
Zolmitriptan (*Zomig*)[b]

Skeletal muscle relaxants
Tizanidine (eg, *Zanaflex*)[b] (animals)

* Drugs for which torsades de pointes has also been reported.[2,7,19,23,36,42,51]
a Association unclear.[23]
b QT, QTc, and/or torsades de pointes association listed in FDA approved product labeling.[36]
c Not available in the United States.
d SSRIs = selective serotonin reuptake inhibitors; SNRIs = serotonin-norepinephrine reuptake inhibitors.

Drug-induced Prolongation of the QT Interval and Torsades de Pointes

Factors that increase the risk of torsades de pointes[3,5-7,25,26,42,43]

- Administration of drugs that prolong the QT interval
- Altered nutritional states (eg, anorexia nervosa, liquid protein diet)
- Baseline QTc interval greater than 460 msec
- Coadministration of certain drugs that prolong QT interval with drugs metabolized by CYP3A4
- Congenital LQT syndrome
- Female gender
- Electrolyte imbalance (eg, hypokalemia, hypomagnesemia)
- Liver disease
- Hypothyroidism
- Nervous system injury (eg, stroke, subarachnoid hemorrhage)
- Preexisting cardiac disease (eg, congestive heart failure, heart failure, ventricular hypertrophy)
- Renal disease
- Slow heart rate (ie, bradyarrhythmia)

References

[1] Thomas M, et al. The dilemma on the prolonged QT interval in early drug studies. *Br J Clin Pharmacol.* 1996;41:77-81.
[2] Towbin JA, et al. Molecular biology and the prolonged QT syndromes. *Am J Med.* 2001;110:385-398.
[3] Malik M, et al. Evaluation of drug-induced QT interval prolongation: implications for drug approval and labelling. *Drug Saf.* 2001;24:323-351.
[4] Owens RC. Risk assessment for antimicrobial agent-induced QTc interval prolongation and torsades de pointes. *Pharmacotherapy.* 2001;21:301-319.
[5] Viskin S. Long QT syndromes and torsade de pointes. *Lancet.* 1999;354:1625-1633.
[6] De Ponti F, et al. QT-interval prolongation by non-cardiac drugs: lessons to be learned from recent experience. *Eur J Clin Pharmacol.* 2000;56:1-18.
[7] Tamargo J. Drug-induced torsade de pointes: from molecular biology to bedside. *Jpn J Pharmacol.* 2000;83:1-19.
[8] Yap YG, et al. Risk of torsades de pointes with non-cardiac drugs. *BMJ.* 2000;320:1158-1159.
[9] Tatro DS, ed. *Drug Interaction Facts.* St. Louis, MO: Wolters Kluwer Health, Inc. 2006.
[10] Thomas AR, et al. Prolongation of the QT interval related to cisapride-diltiazem interaction. *Pharmacotherapy.* 1998;18:381-385.
[11] Lannini PB, et al. Gatifloxacin-induced QTc prolongation and ventricular tachycardia. *Pharmacotherapy.* 2001;21:361-362.
[12] *Zagam* [package insert]. Collegeville, PA: Rhone-Poulenc Rorer Pharmaceuticals Inc.; January 1997.
[13] Pinto YM, et al. QT lengthening and life-threatening arrhythmias associated with fexofenadine. *Lancet.* 1999;353:980.
[14] Giraud T. QT lengthening and arrhythmias associated with fexofenadine. *Lancet.* 1999;353:2072.
[15] Pinto YM, et al. QT lengthening and arrhythmias associated with fexofenadine. *Lancet.* 1999;353:2072-2073.
[16] De Ponti F, et al. Non-antiarrhythmic drugs prolonging the QT interval: Considerable use in seven countries. *Br J Clin Pharmacol.* 2002;54:171-177.
[17] Crouch MA, et al. Clinical relevance and management of drug-related QT interval prolongation. *Pharmacotherapy.* 2003;23:881-908.
[18] Varriale P. Fluoxetine (*Prozac*) as a cause of QT prolongation. *Arch Intern Med* 2001;26:612.
[19] Lannini PB, et al. Risk of torsades de pointes with non-cardiac drugs. *BMJ.* 2001;322:46-47.
[20] Abernethy DR, et al. Loratadine and terfenadine interaction with nefazodone: both antihistamines are associated with QTc prolongation. *Clin Pharmacol Ther.* 2001;69:96-103.
[21] Hatta K, et al. The association between intravenous haloperidol and prolonged QT interval. *J Clin Psychopharmacology.* 2001;21:257-261.
[22] Hartigan-Go K, et al. Concentration-related pharmacodynamic effects of thioridazine and its metabolites in humans. *Clin Pharmacol Ther.* 1996;60:543-553.
[23] Woosley RL. Drugs that prolong the QT interval and/or induce torsades de pointes. http://www.qtdrugs.org. Accessed September 28, 2011; updated July 14, 2011.
[24] Goernig M, et al. Iohexol contrast medium induces QT prolongation in amiodarone patients. *Br J Clin Pharmacol.* 2004;58:96-98.
[25] Amankwa K, et al. Torsades de pointes associated with fluoroquinolones: importance of concomitant risk factors. *Clin Pharmacol Ther.* 2004;75:242-247.

[26] Owens RC. QT prolongation with antimicrobial agents. *Drugs.* 2004;64:1091-1124.
[27] Krantz MJ, et al. Dose-related effects of methadone on QT prolongation in a series of patients with torsade de pointes. *Pharmacotherapy.* 2003;23:802-805.
[28] Charbit B, et al. QT interval prolongation after oxytocin bolus during surgical induced abortion. *Clin Pharmacol Ther.* 2004;76:359-364.
[29] Lee KW, et al. Famotidine and long QT syndrome. *Am J Cardiol.* 2004;93:1325-1327.
[30] Khazan M, et al. Probable case of torsades de pointes induced by fluconazole. *Pharmacotherapy.* 2002;22:1632-1637.
[31] Pathak A, et al. Celecoxib-associated torsade de pointes. *Ann Pharmacother.* 2002;36:1290-1291.
[32] Castillo R, et al. Efavirenz-associated QT prolongation and torsade de pointes arrhythmia. *Ann Pharmacother.* 2002;36:1006-1008.
[33] Hoehns JD, et al. Torsades de pointes associated with chlorpromazine: case report and review of associated ventricular arrhythmias. *Pharmacotherapy.* 2001;21:871-883.
[34] Wysowski DK, et al. Cisapride and fatal arrhythmia. *N Engl J Med.* 1996;335:290-291.
[35] Reilly JG, et al. QTc-interval abnormalities and psychotropic drug therapy in psychiatric patients. *Lancet.* 2000;355:1048-1052.
[36] Package insert for the product listed.
[37] Williams NE, et al. Drug-induced QT prolongation and torsade de pointes. *Hospital Pharmacy.* May 2003. Wall chart.
[38] Piguet V, et al. QT interval prolongation in patients on methadone with concomitant drugs. *J Clin Psychopharmacol.* 2004;24:446-448.
[39] Gil M, et al. QT prolongation and torsades de pointes in patients infected with human immunodeficiency virus and treated with methadone. *Am J Cardiol.* 2003;92:995-997.
[40] Krantz MJ, et al. Effects of buprenorphine on cardiac repolarization in a patient with methadone-related torsades de pointes. *Pharmacotherapy.* 2005;25:611-614.
[41] Bertino JS, et al. Gatifloxacin-associated corrected QT interval prolongation, torsades de pointes, and ventricular fibrillation in patients with known risk factors. *Clin Infect Dis.* 2002;34:861-863.
[42] Glassman AH, et al. Antipsychotic drugs: Prolonged QTc interval, torsades de pointes, and sudden death. *Am J Psychiatry.* 2001;158:1774-1782.
[43] Roden DM. Drug-induced prolongation of the QT interval. *N Engl J Med.* 2004;350:1013-1022.
[44] Krantz MJ, Lowery CM, Martell BA, Gourevitch MN, Arnsten JH. Effects of methadone on QT-interval dispersion. *Pharmacotherapy.* 2005;25(11):1523-1529.
[45] Harrison-Woolrych M, Clark DW, Hill GR, Rees MI, Skinner JR. QT interval prolongation associated with sibutramine treatment. *Br J Clin Pharmacol.* 2006;61(4):464-469.
[46] Fanoe S, Jensen GB, Sjøgren P, Korsgaard MP, Grunnet M. Oxycodone is associated with dose-dependent QTc prolongation in patients and low-affinity inhibiting of hERG activity in vitro. *Br J Clin Pharmacol.* 2009;67(2):172-179.
[47] McMahon JH, Grayson ML. Torsades de pointes in a patient receiving fluconazole for cerebral cryptococcosis. *Am J Health Syst Pharm.* 2008;65(7):619-623.
[48] Knorr JP, Moshfeghi M, Sokoloski MC. Ciprofloxacin-induced QT-interval prolongation. *Am J Health Syst Pharm.* 2008;65(6):547-551.
[49] Fisher AA, Davis MW. Prolonged QT interval, syncope, and delirium with galantamine. *Ann Pharmacother.* 2008;42(2):278-283.
[50] Skjervold B, Bathen J, Spigset O. Methadone and the QT interval: relations to the serum concentrations of methadone and its enantiomers (R)-methadone and (S)-methadone. *J Clin Pscyhopharmacol.* 2006;26(6):687-689.
[51] Pham CP, de Feiter PW, van der Kuy PH, van Mook WN. Long QTc interval and torsades de pointes caused by fluconazole. *Ann Pharmacother.* 2006;40(7):1456-1461.
[52] Bloomfield DM, Kost JT, Ghosh K, et al. The effect of moxifloxacin on QTc and implications for the design of thorough QT studies. *Clin Pharmacol Ther.* 2008;84(4):475-480.
[53] Stringer J, Welsh C, Tommasello A. Methadone-associated Q-T interval prolongation and torsades de pointes. *Am J Health Syst Pharm.* 2009;66(9):825-833. Erratum in *Am J Health Syst Pharm.* 2010;67(2):94.

The Effects of Cigarette Smoking on Drug Therapy

The potential for the pharmacokinetics or pharmacodynamics of a drug to be altered by cigarette smoking is significant. Many people may be affected by this issue because cigarette smoking is so prevelant. Smoke contains over 3,000 identified chemicals. Some of the components of cigarettes are capable of enzyme induction (eg, nicotine, polyhalogenated insecticides, cadmium) while other components act as enzyme inhibitors (eg, carbon monoxide, hydrogen cyanide, nicotine).[1,2] Cigarette smoking induces CYP-450 1A1 and 1A2 while inhibiting CYP2A6.[2] Nicotine and other gaseous (eg, formaldehyde, nitric oxide, nitrogen dioxide) and particulate (eg, aldehydes, ketones, nicotine) constituents of cigarette smoke can affect the pharmacokinetics and pharmacodynamics of numerous drugs.[3,4]

Induction of liver enzymes by polynuclear aromatic hydrocarbons in cigarettes can increase drug metabolism. This is the most common mechanism by which smoking alters the pharmacokinetics of a drug.[1,3,4] Dosage requirements are increased in patients receiving drugs affected by this mechanism. The effects of smoking on drug metabolism are greater in younger smokers (ie, younger than 40 years of age) than in older individuals. The effects of smoking on drug metabolism may persist for months after smoking cessation.[1,5-7] Clinically important alterations in drug metabolism occur more frequently in subjects smoking more than 20 cigarettes daily, compared with those smoking fewer.[1,3,4]

In addition to the other components of cigarette smoke, the pharmacological effects of nicotine may increase or antagonize the effects of other drugs,[4] which may also be clinically relevant in individuals using transdermal nicotine patches. Assessing the clinical importance of the action of smoking on drug treatment is difficult because the number of patients evaluated is often small and, in some instances, the results of multiple studies are equivocal. Controlled trials are necessary to determine if smoking causes a clinically important effect on drug kinetics. These studies should focus on drugs with a narrow therapeutic index (eg, theophylline). If smoking is suspected of affecting the pharmacokinetics or pharmacodynamics of a drug, dosage adjustment may be necessary. One approach to management, but often the most difficult to achieve, is smoking cessation. However, if an individual stops smoking, it is necessary to consider the effects smoking cessation may have on the plasma concentrations of drugs they are currently taking. Elevated plasma concentrations of clozapine (3,004 ng/mL) occurred in a patient 6 days after a 16-day stay in a hospital in which smoking was prohibited.[8] Drugs that may be affected by smoking are listed in Table 1.

Summary: Cigarette smoking may interfere with the pharmacokinetics and pharmacodynamics of numerous drugs. Induction of liver enzymes, CYP1A1 and CYP1A2, is the most common mechanism by which smoking alters drug metabolism. Other components in cigarettes may act to inhibit CYP2A6 metabolism. The effects of smoking on drug metabolism may persist for months after smoking cessation. In addition, the pharmacologic effects of nicotine may increase or antagonize the effects of drugs. Close monitoring of the clinical response to drug therapy and dosage adjustments may be necessary in individuals who start or stop smoking.

Table 1: Drugs Affected by Cigarette Smoking

Drug	Summary	Ref
Acetaminophen (eg, *Tylenol*)	*Mechanism:* Increased hepatic metabolism. *Effect:* Results of studies have been variable, indicating that smoking has no effect or decreases acetaminophen serum concentrations. Clinical importance is unknown but is suspected to be minimal.	4
Adenosine (eg, *Adenocard*)	*Mechanism:* Unknown. *Effect:* Nicotine increases the cardiovascular effects of adenosine. Lower doses may be needed in patients receiving nicotine.	9,10
Amitriptyline	*Mechanism:* Increased hepatic metabolism. *Effect:* Amitriptyline concentrations may be reduced in smokers, resulting in possible decreased efficacy.	11

The Effects of Cigarette Smoking on Drug Therapy

Table 1: Drugs Affected by Cigarette Smoking		
Drug	Summary	Ref
Ascorbic acid (Vitamin C)	*Mechanism*: Unknown. *Effect*: Cigarette smokers have lower serum ascorbic acid concentrations than nonsmokers. Vitamin C requirements may be about 2 times greater in smokers than nonsmokers. In subjects smoking fewer than 20 cigarettes daily, ascorbic acid concentrations were 25% lower than in nonsmokers and 40% lower in those smoking 20 cigarettes or more daily. Similar findings occurred with cigar or pipe smokers.	12,13
Beclomethasone (*QVAR*)	*Mechanism*: Unknown. However, cysteinyl leukotriene production may play a role. *Effect*: The effect of smoking on response to inhaled beclomethasone in individuals with mild asthma was evaluated in nonsmokers and smokers (10 to 40 cigarettes/day). In smokers with mild asthma, the response to inhaled beclomethasone was diminished compared with nonsmokers.	14
Caffeine	*Mechanism*: Increased caffeine hepatic metabolism (CYP1A2). *Effect*: The $t_{1/2}$ of caffeine is shorter and the body clearance is increased in smokers. Nicotine also decreases the stimulant effects of caffeine. This may be a reason why higher consumption of coffee is reported among smokers.	2,15,16
Chlordiazepoxide (eg, *Librium*)	*Mechanism*: Increased hepatic metabolism and/or decreased end-organ response is suspected. *Effect*: Decreased drowsiness. Drowsiness with chlordiazepoxide was reported to be highest in nonsmokers, intermediate in patients smoking 20 or fewer cigarettes daily, and lowest in patients smoking more than 20 cigarettes daily. However, the effects observed in patients may be age-related.	3,4,17,18
Chlorpromazine	*Mechanism*: Increased hepatic metabolism and/or decreased end-organ response is suspected. *Effect*: Drowsiness with chlorpromazine was reported to be highest in nonsmokers, intermediate in patients smoking 20 or fewer cigarettes daily, and lowest in patients smoking more than 20 cigarettes daily. However, the effects observed in patients may be age-related. Drowsiness increased as the dose of the drug increased, irrespective of smoking. Peak plasma concentrations and AUC were decreased in smokers. Hypotension as an adverse reaction of chlorpromazine was reported to be directly related to the number of cigarettes smoked by patients, being observed less frequently the greater the number of cigarettes smoked. Increased chlorpromazine adverse reactions and serum levels were reported in a patient who abruptly stopped smoking.	3,4,19-23
Chlorzoxazone (eg, *Paraflex*)	*Mechanism*: Increased hepatic metabolism (CYP2E1). *Effect*: Cigarette smoking increased oral clearance of chlorzoxazone 24% (range, −10% to 71%).	2
Cilostazol (eg, *Pletal*)	*Mechanism*: Unknown. *Effect*: Population pharmacokinetic analysis indicates that smoking decreases cilostazol exposure approximately 20%.	24
Cimetidine (eg, *Tagamet*)	*Mechanism*: Unknown. *Effect*: Decreased rate of ulcer healing. Sucralfate (eg, *Carafate*) is not affected by smoking and may be a suitable alternative.	4

Table 1: Drugs Affected by Cigarette Smoking		
Drug	Summary	Ref
Clozapine (eg, *Clozaril*)	*Mechanism*: Increased hepatic metabolism (CYP1A2). *Effect*: Elevated clozapine plasma concentrations were reported in 2 patients as a consequence of smoking cessation. In 1 patient, clozapine plasma concentrations of 3,004 ng/mL were measured 6 days after a 16-day hospital stay in which smoking was prohibited. In another patient, smoking cessation resulted in extreme sedation and fatigue within 2 weeks; there was a 3-fold increase in clozapine levels. A 35-year-old man successfully treated with clozapine 700 to 725 mg daily for 7 years developed tonic-clonic seizures followed by stupor and coma after abruptly stopping smoking. Clozapine 425 mg daily was successfully reinstituted. In a study of 11 hospitalized patients receiving stable clozapine doses, there was a 72% mean increase in clozapine levels after a hospital-wide nonsmoking policy was implemented. Smoking 7 to 12 cigarettes daily may be sufficient for maximum induction of clozapine metabolism. Nonsmokers may require a 50% lower starting dose of clozapine than smokers.	8,25-27
Contraceptives, hormonal	*Mechanism*: Increased hepatic metabolism. *Effect*: Although a decrease in hormonal contraceptive effectiveness is possible, an increase in failure rates has not been reported. Smoking has an antiestrogenic effect, which may contribute to the decreased incidence of endometrial cancer, increased incidence of osteoporosis, and early menopause. Also, smoking increases the risk of cardiovascular adverse reactions (eg, stroke) associated with hormonal contraceptive use. Patients taking hormonal contraceptives should avoid smoking.	4,28-31
Dexamethasone (eg, *Decadron*)	*Mechanism*: Unknown. *Effect*: Although smoking does not affect the pharmacokinetics of dexamethasone, it does appear to antagonize the suppressive effects of dexamethasone on adrenocortical secretion.	32,33
Diazepam (eg, *Valium*)	*Mechanism*: Increased hepatic metabolism and/or decreased end-organ response is suspected. *Effect*: Findings have indicated that smoking has no effect or reduces diazepam serum concentrations, decreasing drowsiness. Drowsiness was highest in nonsmokers, intermediate for patients smoking 20 or fewer cigarettes daily, and lowest for patients smoking more than 20 cigarettes daily. However, the effects observed in patients may be age-related.	3,4,18,34
Duloxetine (*Cymbalta*)	*Mechanism*: Unknown. *Effect*: Duloxetine bioavailability may be reduced by about 33%. However, dosage alterations are not recommended.	35
Flecainide (*Tambocor*)	*Mechanism*: Increased hepatic metabolism is suspected. *Effect*: Serum flecainide levels may be decreased, increasing flecainide dosage requirements. Smokers (10 or more cigarettes daily) with premature ventricular contractions required higher doses of flecainide than nonsmokers. Because the optimal dose is determined by titration, flecainide therapy in smokers should be adjusted accordingly.	36
Fluvoxamine (eg, *Luvox CR*)	*Mechanism*: Increased hepatic metabolism is suspected. *Effect*: In a single-dose study, fluvoxamine serum levels were 32% lower in smokers compared with nonsmokers.	37

The Effects of Cigarette Smoking on Drug Therapy

Table 1: Drugs Affected by Cigarette Smoking		
Drug	Summary	Ref
Furosemide (eg, *Lasix*)	*Mechanism*: Nicotine increases the secretion of antidiuretic hormone, which inhibits diuresis. *Effect*: Decreased furosemide effectiveness. However, because tolerance to the effect of smoking develops, an interaction is not expected in chronic smokers.	4,38
Glutethimide†	*Mechanism*: Unknown. *Effect*: In a study of 7 patients who smoked, elevated serum glutethimide concentrations were reported.	4,39
Haloperidol (eg, *Haldol*)	*Mechanism*: Induction of glucuronyl transferase, the major metabolic pathway of haloperidol, in smokers is suspected. *Effect*: In studies of schizophrenic patients, haloperidol plasma concentrations were lower in smokers than nonsmokers. In addition, patients who smoked were treated with higher doses of haloperidol than nonsmokers.	40-43
Heparin	*Mechanism*: Unknown. *Effect*: In 5 smokers, the elimination of heparin was faster, the $t_{1/2}$ was shorter, and the dosage requirement was increased, compared with 15 nonsmokers.	44
Imipramine (eg, *Tofranil*)	*Mechanism*: Increased hepatic metabolism. *Effect*: Compared with nonsmokers, a smoker's imipramine serum level may be reduced 45%, which may result in a decrease in efficacy.	45
Insulin (eg, *Novolin*)	*Mechanism*: Decreased subcutaneous insulin absorption resulting from peripheral vasoconstriction, as well as increased catecholamine and cortisol release in smokers. *Effect*: Insulin requirements may be increased by 30% in heavy smokers. Monitor blood glucose levels closely and make adjustments in insulin dosage as necessary in diabetic patients who start or stop smoking.	4,46,47
Irinotecan (*Camptosar*)	*Mechanism*: Increased metabolism is suspected. *Effect*: Cigarette smoking lowers both the exposure to irinotecan and treatment-induced neutropenia (particularly grade 3 to 4 neutropenia), indicating possible treatment failure.	48
Lidocaine (eg, *Xylocaine*)	*Mechanism*: Increased hepatic metabolism is suspected. *Effect*: Results of studies vary. The clinical importance has not been determined.	4,49
Lorazepam (eg, *Ativan*)	*Mechanism*: Unknown. *Effect*: Limited data indicate that lorazepam clearance is increased in smokers. The clinical importance of this finding has not been assessed.	50
Meperidine (eg, *Demerol*)	*Mechanism*: Increased hepatic metabolism. *Effect*: Decreased analgesia has been observed; however, the effect may not occur for several weeks.	4
Meprobamate (eg, *Miltown*)	*Mechanism*: Increased hepatic metabolism. *Effect*: In vitro studies have reported a decrease in efficacy. Human studies are needed to determine the clinical importance of these findings.	4
Morphine (eg, *MS Contin*)	*Mechanism*: Increased hepatic metabolism. *Effect*: Decreased analgesia has been observed, but the effect may not occur for several weeks.	4
Nortriptyline (eg, *Aventyl*)	*Mechanism*: Limited data do not support an interaction. *Effect*: Findings indicate smoking either reduces nortriptyline serum levels or has no effect.	4,11,51

Table 1: Drugs Affected by Cigarette Smoking		
Drug	Summary	Ref
Olanzapine (*Zyprexa*)	*Mechanism*: Increased metabolism (CYP1A2) is suspected. *Effect*: Olanzapine plasma concentrations and antipsychotic effects were decreased in smokers, compared with nonsmokers. The olanzapine plasma concentration-to-dose ratio was 5-fold lower in smokers than nonsmokers. A 30-year-old man was successfully treated with olanzapine during hospitalization. After discharge, his smoking increased from 12 to 80 cigarettes daily. After 10 days, his olanzapine plasma levels were decreased and his delusions of persecution, hostility level, and aggressive behavior worsened. Smoking 7 to 12 cigarettes daily may be sufficient for maximum induction of olanzapine metabolism. Nonsmokers may require a 50% lower starting dose of olanzapine than smokers.	27,52-54
Pentazocine (*Talwin*)	*Mechanism*: Increased hepatic metabolism (40% greater in smokers than nonsmokers). *Effect*: Possible decrease in analgesia; smokers may require higher doses of pentazocine than nonsmokers.	4,55
Propofol (eg, *Diprivan*)	*Mechanism*: Unknown. *Effect*: Compared with nonsmokers, cigarette smokers required higher concentrations of propofol to produce sedation and loss of consciousness. This may affect management of smokers undergoing propofol sedation.	56
Propoxyphene (eg, *Darvon*)	*Mechanism*: Increased hepatic metabolism is suspected. *Effect*: Analgesia and adverse reactions may be decreased. In nonsmokers, propoxyphene was ineffective in 10% of patients, compared with 15% of patients smoking 20 or fewer cigarettes daily and 20% of patients smoking more than 20 cigarettes daily. Smokers may need a higher dose of propoxyphene.	3,57
Propranolol (eg, *Inderal*)	*Mechanism*: Increased metabolism and catecholamine release in smokers. *Effect*: Smoking may decrease the $t_{1/2}$ and increase the body clearance of propranolol. Serum propranolol concentrations may decrease, increasing the dosage requirement. Also, smoking may interfere with the efficacy of propranolol in the treatment of angina pectoris.	58,59
Quinine	*Mechanism*: Increased hepatic metabolism is suspected. *Effect*: Compared with nonsmokers, quinine clearance was nearly 80% greater in smokers, possibly producing subtherapeutic quinine serum levels. The clinical importance of the effect of smoking on quinine remains to be determined.	60
Ranitidine (eg, *Zantac*)	*Mechanism*: Unknown. *Effect*: Decreased rate of ulcer healing. Sucralfate (eg, *Carafate*) is not affected by smoking and may be a suitable alternative.	4
Tacrine (*Cognex*)	*Mechanism*: Increased metabolism (CYP1A2) is suspected. *Effect*: The manufacturer reports that tacrine plasma levels are 33% lower in smokers compared with nonsmokers. The elimination $t_{1/2}$ is 2.1 hours in smokers compared with 3.2 hours in nonsmokers.	61,62

The Effects of Cigarette Smoking on Drug Therapy

Table 1: Drugs Affected by Cigarette Smoking		
Drug	Summary	Ref
Theophylline (eg, *Theochron*)	*Mechanism*: Increased hepatic metabolism. *Effect*: Decreased effectiveness of theophylline, increasing the dosage requirement. Smoking decreases the $t_{½}$ and serum concentration of theophylline while increasing clearance. The effects of smoking on theophylline metabolism seem to be greater in younger subjects than in those older than 40 years of age. Because theophylline has a narrow therapeutic index, patient monitoring and dosage adjustment are advised if smoking habits are altered. In a study of theophylline toxicity, the incidence of adverse reactions was 13% in nonsmokers, 11% in patients smoking 20 or fewer cigarettes daily, and 7% in those who smoked more heavily. The effects of smoking on theophylline appear to be due to the polyaromatic hydrocarbons and not nicotine and may persist for months after smoking cessation.	1,4,7,63-68
Thioridazine	*Mechanism*: Increased thioridazine metabolism (possibly CYP1A2). *Effect*: In 76 patients receiving thioridazine, the dose-corrected, steady-state plasma level of thioridazine was decreased 46% in 58 smokers compared with 18 nonsmokers.	69
Tizanidine (eg, *Zanaflex*)	*Mechanism*: Increased tizanidine metabolism (possibly CYP1A2). *Effect*: In a study of healthy smokers and nonsmokers, tizanidine plasma levels and pharmacologic effects were decreased in smokers compared with nonsmokers.	70
Tolbutamide (eg, *Orinase*)	*Mechanism*: Unknown. *Effect*: Cardiac arrhythmia was reported in a smoker taking tolbutamide. On rechallenge, smoking appeared to potentiate premature ventricular contractions associated with high serum concentrations of tolbutamide.	71
Verapamil (eg, *Calan*)	*Mechanism*: Possible inhibition of metabolism (CYP1A2). *Effect*: In 12 healthy smokers, verapamil and norverapamil AUC and C_{max} were decreased 0.61- and 0.85-fold, respectively, compared with 12 nonsmokers.	72
Warfarin (eg, *Coumadin*)	*Mechanism*: It is suspected that the vitamin K in tobacco may inhibit the effect of warfarin on vitamin K–dependent clotting factors. *Effect*: A 34-year-old man was unsuccessfully treated with warfarin (up to 30 mg/day), and the INR never stabilized over a 4.5-year period while he was using smokeless tobacco. When he stopped using tobacco, his INR increased from 1.1 to 2.3 within 1 week. If a patient receiving warfarin stops or starts smoking, monitor coagulation parameters.	73,74

† Not available in the United States.

References

1. Jusko WJ. Influence of cigarette smoking on drug metabolism in man. *Drug Metab Rev.* 1979;9(2):221-236.
2. Benowitz NL, et al. Effects of cigarette smoking and carbon monoxide on chlorzoxazone and caffeine metabolism. *Clin Pharmacol Ther.* 2003;74 (5):468-474.
3. Miller RR. Effects of smoking on drug action. *Clin Pharmacol Ther.* 1977;22(5 pt 2):749-756.
4. Miller LG. Recent developments in the study of the effects of cigarette smoking on clinical pharmacokinetics and clinical pharmacodynamics. *Clin Pharmacokinet.* 1989;17(2):90-108.
5. Greenblatt DJ, et al. Diazepam disposition determinants. *Clin Pharmacol Ther.* 1980;27(3):301-312.
6. Vestal RE, et al. Effects of age and cigarette smoking on propranolol disposition. *Clin Pharmacol Ther.* 1979;26(1):8-15.

[7] Hunt SN, et al. Effect of smoking on theophylline disposition. *Clin Pharmacol Ther.* 1976;19(5 pt 1):546-551.
[8] Bondolfi G, et al. Increased clozapine plasma concentrations and side effects induced by smoking cessation in 2 CYP1A2 genotyped patients. *Ther Drug Monit.* 2005;27(4):539-543.
[9] Smits P, et al. Nicotine enhances the circulatory effects of adenosine in human beings. *Clin Pharmacol Ther.* 1989;46(3):272-278.
[10] Sylvén C, et al. Nicotine enhances angina pectoris-like chest pain and atrioventricular blockade provoked by intravenous bolus of adenosine in healthy volunteers. *J Cardiovasc Pharmacol.* 1990;16(6):962-965.
[11] Linnoila M, et al. Effect of alcohol consumption and cigarette smoking on antidepressant levels of depressed patients. *Am J Psychiatry.* 1981;138(6):841-842.
[12] Pelletier O. Vitamin C and cigarette smokers. *Ann NY Acad Sci.* 1975;58:156-166.
[13] Murata A. Smoking and vitamin C. *World Rev Nutr and Diet.* 1991;64:31-57.
[14] Lazarus SC, et al. Smoking affects response to inhaled corticosteroids or leukotriene receptor antagonists in asthma. *Am J Respir Crit Care Med.* 2007;175(8):783-790.
[15] Parsons WD, et al. Effect of smoking on caffeine clearance. *Clin Pharmacol Ther.* 1978;24(1):40-45.
[16] Rose JE, et al. Psychophysiological interactions between caffeine and nicotine. *Pharmacol Biochem Behav.* 1991;38(2):333-337.
[17] Desmond PV, et al. No effect of smoking on metabolism of chlordiazepoxide. *N Engl J Med.* 1979;300(4):199-200.
[18] Boston Collaborative Drug Surveillance Program. Clinical depression of the central nervous system due to diazepam and chlordiazepoxide in relation to cigarette smoking and age. *N Engl J Med.* 1973;288(6):277-280.
[19] Pantuck EJ, et al. Cigarette smoking and chlorpromazine disposition and actions. *Clin Pharmacol Ther.* 1982;31(4):533-538.
[20] Stimmel GL, et al. Chlorpromazine plasma levels, adverse effects, and tobacco smoking: Case Report. *J Clin Psychiatry.* 1983;44(11):420-422.
[21] Swett C Jr. Drowsiness due to chlorpromazine in relation to cigarette smoking. *Arch Gen Psychiatry.* 1974;31(8):211-213.
[22] Swett C Jr, et al. Hypotension due to chlorpromazine. *Arch Gen Psychiatry.* 1977;34(6):661-663.
[23] Swett C Jr. Side effects of chlorpromazine in relation to cigarette smoking. *Psychopharmacol Bull.* 1977;13:57-58.
[24] *Pletal* [package insert]. Rockville, MD: Otsuka America Pharmaceutical, Inc.; 2005.
[25] Meyer JM. Individual changes in clozapine levels after smoking cessation: Results and a predictive model. *J Clin Psychopharmacol.* 2001;21(6):569-574.
[26] Skogh E, et al. Could discontinuing smoking be hazardous for patients administered clozapine medication? A case report. *Ther Drug Monit.* 1999;21(5):580-582.
[27] Haslemo T, et al. The effect of variable cigarette consumption on the interaction with clozapine and olanzapine. *Eur J Clin Pharmacol.* 2006;62(11):1049-1053.
[28] Goldbaum GM, et al. The relative impact of smoking and oral contraceptive use on women in the United States. *JAMA.* 1987;258(10):1339-1342.
[29] Collaborative Group for the Study of Stroke in Young Women. Oral contraceptives and stroke in young women. *JAMA.* 1975;231(7):718-722.
[30] Kanarkowski R, et al. Pharmacokinetics of single and multiple doses of ethinyl estradiol and levonorgestrel in relation to smoking. *Clin Pharmacol Ther.* 1988;43(1):23-31.
[31] Crawford FE, et al. Oral contraceptive steroid plasma concentrations in smokers and nonsmokers. *Br Med J.* 1981;282:1829-1830.
[32] Kershbaum A, et al. Smoking effect on dexamethasone suppression test. *Clin Res.* 1969;17:287.
[33] Rose JQ, et al. Effect of smoking on prednisone, prednisolone, and dexamethasone pharmacokinetics. *J Pharmacokinet Biopharm.* 1981;9(1):1-14.
[34] Ochs HR, et al. Kinetics of diazepam, midazolam, and lorazepam in cigarette smokers. *Chest.* 1985;87(2):223-226.
[35] *Cymbalta* [package insert]. Indianapolis, IN: Eli Lilly and Company; 2007.
[36] Holtzman JL, et al. Identification of drug interactions by meta-analysis of premarketing trials: The effect of smoking on the pharmacokinetics and dosage requirements for flecainide acetate. *Clin Pharmacol Ther.* 1989;46(1):1-8.
[37] Spigset O, et al. Effect of cigarette smoking on fluvoxamine pharmacokinetics in humans. *Clin Pharmacol Ther.* 1995;58(4):399-403.
[38] Vapaatalo HI, et al. Effect of cigarette smoking on diuresis induced by furosemide. *Ann Clin Res.* 1971;3:159-162.
[39] Crow JW, et al. Glutethimide and 4-OH glutethimide: Pharmacokinetics and effect on performance in man. *Clin Pharmacol Ther.* 1977;22(4):458-464.

[40] Pan L, et al. Effects of smoking, CYP2D6 genotype, and concomitant drug intake on the steady state plasma concentrations of haloperidol and reduced haloperidol in schizophrenic inpatients. *Ther Drug Monit.* 1999;21(5):489-497.
[41] Shimoda, K, et al. Lower plasma levels of haloperidol in smoking than in nonsmoking schizophrenic patients. *Ther Drug Monit.* 1999;21(3):293-296.
[42] Perry PJ, et al. Haloperidol dosing requirements: the contribution of smoking and nonlinear pharmacokinetics. *J Clin Psychopharmacol.* 1993;13(1):46-51.
[43] Jann MW, et al. Effects of smoking on haloperidol and reduced haloperidol plasma concentrations and haloperidol clearance. *Psychopharmacology.* 1986;90(4):468-470.
[44] Cipolle RJ, et al. Heparin kinetics: Variables related to disposition of dosage. *Clin Pharmacol Ther.* 1981;29(3):387-393.
[45] Perel JM, et al. Pharmacodynamics of imipramine in depressed patients. *Psychopharmacol Bull.* 1975;11:16-18.
[46] Klemp P, et al. Smoking reduces insulin absorption from subcutaneous tissue. *Br Med J.* 1982;284:237.
[47] Madsbad S, et al. Influence of smoking on insulin requirement and metabolic status in diabetes mellitus. *Diabetes Care.* 1980;3(1):41-343.
[48] van der Bol JM, et al. Cigarette smoking and irinotecan treatment: pharmacokinetic interaction and effects on neutropenia. *J Clin Oncol.* 2007;25(19):2719-2726.
[49] Huet PM, et al. Effects of smoking and chronic hepatitis B on lidocaine and indocyanine green kinetics. *Clin Pharmacol Ther.* 1980;28(2):208-215.
[50] Greenblatt DJ, et al. Lorazepam kinetics in the elderly. *Clin Pharmacol Ther.* 1979;26(1):103-113.
[51] Norman TR, et al. Cigarette smoking and plasma nortriptyline levels. *Clin Pharmacol Ther.* 1977;21(4):453-456.
[52] Carrillo JA, et al. Role of the smoking-induced cytochrome P450 (CYP)1A2 and polymorphic CYP2D6 in steady-state concentrations of olanzapine. *J Clin Psychopharmacol.* 2003;23(2):119-127.
[53] Gex-Fabry M, et al. Therapeutic drug monitoring of olanzapine: The combined effect of age, gender, smoking, and comedication. *Ther Drug Monit.* 2003;25(1):46-53.
[54] Chiu CC, et al. Heavy smoking, reduced olanzapine levels, and treatment effects: A case report. *Ther Drug Monit.* 2004;26(5):579-581.
[55] Vaughan DP, et al. The influence of smoking on the inter-subject variation in pentazocine elimination. *Br J Clin Pharmacol.* 1976;3:279-283.
[56] Lysakowski C, et al. The effect of cigarette smoking on the hypnotic efficacy of propofol. *Anaesthesia.* 2006;61(9):826-831.
[57] Boston Collaborative Drug Surveillance Program. Decreased clinical efficacy of propoxyphene in cigarette smokers. *Clin Pharmacol Ther.* 1973;14(2):259-263.
[58] Gardner SK, et al. Effect of smoking on the elimination of propranolol hydrochloride. *Int J Clin Pharmacol Ther Toxicol.* 1980;18(10):421-424.
[59] Fox K, et al. Interaction between cigarettes and propranolol in treatment of angina pectoris. *Br Med J.* 1980;281:191-193.
[60] Wanwimolruk S, et al. Cigarette smoking enhances the elimination of quinine. *Br J Clin Pharmacol.* 1993;36:610-614.
[61] Welty D, et al. The effect of smoking on the pharmacokinetics and metabolism of Cognex in healthy volunteers. *Pharm Res.* 1993;10:S-334.
[62] *Cognex* [package insert]. Morris Plains, NJ: Parke-Davis; October 17, 2000.
[63] Jusko WJ, et al. Enhanced biotransformation of theophylline in marihuana and tobacco smokers. *Clin Pharmacol Ther.* 1978;24(4):406-410.
[64] Powell JR, et al. The influence of cigarette smoking and sex on theophylline disposition. *Am Rev Resp Dis.* 1977;116:17-23.
[65] Ogilvie RI. Smoking and theophylline dose schedules. *Ann Intern Med.* 1978;88(2):263-264.
[66] Pfeifer HJ, et al. Clinical toxicity of theophylline in relation to cigarette smoking. *Chest.* 1978;73(4):455-559.
[67] Jenne J, et al. Decreased theophylline half-life in cigarette smokers. *Life Sci.* 1975;17(2):195-198.
[68] Talseth T, et al. Aging, cigarette smoking and oral theophylline requirement. *Eur J Clin Pharmacol.* 1981;21:33-37.
[69] Berecz R, et al. Thioridazine steady-state plasma concentrations are influenced by tobacco smoking and CYP2D6, but not by the CYP2C9 genotype. *Eur J Clin Pharmacol.* 2003;59(1):45-50.
[70] Backman JT, et al. Effects of gender and moderate smoking on the pharmacokinetics and effects of the CYP1A2 substrate tizanidine. *Eur J Clin Pharmacol.* 2008;64(1):17-24.
[71] Poffenbarger PL, et al. Tolbutamide, smoking, and cardiac arrhythmia. *JAMA.* 1980;244(8):811-812.

[72] Fuhr U, et al. Effects of grapefruit juice and smoking on verapamil concentrations in steady state. *Eur J Clin Pharmacol.* 2002;58(1):45-53.
[73] Kuykendall JR, et al. Possible warfarin failure due to interaction with smokeless tobacco. *Ann Pharmacother.* 2004;38(4):595-597.
[74] Evans M, et al. Increase in international normalized ratio after smoking cessation in a patient receiving warfarin. *Pharmacotherapy.* 2005;25(11):1656-1659.

Standard Abbreviations

Abbreviation	*Meaning*
ACE	angiotensin-converting enzyme
AIDS	acquired immunodeficiency syndrome
ALT	alanine aminotransferase
AST	aspartate aminotransferase
AUC	area under the curve
BP	blood pressure
bpm	beats per minute
CBC	complete blood cell count
cc	cubic centimeter
Ccr	creatinine clearance
CDC	Centers for Disease Control and Prevention
CHF	congestive heart failure
cm^2	square centimeter(s)
cm^3	cubic centimeter(s)
C_{max}	maximum effective plasma concentration
C_{min}	minimum effective plasma concentration
CNS	central nervous system
CrCl	creatinine clearance
CT	computed tomography
CV	cardiovascular
CYP	cytochrome P-450
dL	deciliter (100 mL)
DMSO	dimethyl sulfoxide
ECG	electrocardiogram
eg	for example
ELISA	enzyme-linked immunosorbent assay
ER	extended-release
et al	for 2 or more coauthors or coworkers
Fab	fragment of immunoglobulin G involved in antigen binding
FDA	Food and Drug Administration
g	gram
GI	gastrointestinal
h	hour
HDL	high-density lipoprotein
Hgb	hemoglobin
HIV	human immunodeficiency virus
HMG-CoA	3-hydroxy-3-methylglutaryl coenzyme A
hr	hour
ie	that is

Abbreviation	*Meaning*
IM	intramuscular
INR	international normalized ratio
IV	intravenous
kg	kilogram
L	liter
LDL	low-density lipoprotein
m	meter
m^2	square meter
MAOI	monoamine oxidase inhibitor
mcg	microgram
mg	milligram
MI	myocardial infarction
min	minute
mL	milliliter
mm	millimeter
mm Hg	millimeters of mercury
mo	month
msec	millisecond
ng	nanogram
NNRT	nonnucleoside reverse transcriptase
NSAID	nonsteroidal anti-inflammatory drugs
OC	oral contraceptive
OM3	omega-3-acid ethyl esters
OTC	over-the-counter (nonprescription)
oz	ounce
PABA	paraaminobenzoic acid
PDE5	phosphodiesterase type 5
pg	picogram
P-gp	P-glycoprotein
pH	negative logarithm of the hydrogen ion concentration
ppm	parts per million
PT	prothrombin time
RBC	red blood cell
RDA	recommended dietary allowance
Scr	serum creatinine
sec	second
SRI	serotonin reuptake inhibitor
SSRI	selective serotonin reuptake inhibitor
$t_{1/2}$	half-life
T_4	thyroxine
TCA	tricyclic antidepressant

Standard Abbreviations

Abbreviation	Meaning
T_{max}	time to reach maximum concentration
TSH	thyroid-stimulating hormone
US	United States
WBC	white blood cell
WHO	World Health Organization
wk	week
yr	year

DRUG MONOGRAPHS

Abacavir — *Ethanol*

Abacavir* (*Ziagen*)	Ethanol* (Alcohol, Ethyl Alcohol)

Significance	Onset	Severity	Documentation
5	☐ Rapid	☐ Major	☐ Established
	■ **Delayed**	☐ Moderate	☐ Probable
		■ **Minor**	☐ Suspected
			☐ Possible
			■ **Unlikely**

Effects ABACAVIR plasma concentrations may be increased.

Mechanism ETHANOL may interfere with ABACAVIR metabolism by alcohol dehydrogenase.

Management Based on available data, no alteration in ABACAVIR dose is needed.

Discussion

A pharmacokinetic interaction between abacavir and ethanol was evaluated in 25 HIV-infected men.[1] In an open-label, randomized, 3-way crossover study, each patient received 600 mg of abacavir alone, 0.7 g/kg of ethanol alone, and abacavir 600 mg with ethanol 0.7 g/kg. Abacavir did not affect the pharmacokinetics of ethanol. However, ethanol increased the area under the plasma concentration-time curve of abacavir 41%, increased peak plasma concentration 15% (from 3.6 to 4.13 mcg/mL), and prolonged the half-life 26% (from 1.42 to 1.79 hours). The magnitude of the increase in abacavir plasma concentrations was not considered clinically important.

[1] McDowell JA, et al. *Antimicrob Agents Chemother.* 2000;44:1686.

* Asterisk indicates drugs cited in interaction reports.

ACE Inhibitors — Antacids

ACE Inhibitors	Antacids
Captopril* (eg, *Capoten*)	Aluminum Hydroxide/Magnesium Hydroxide (eg, *Maalox*)

Significance	Onset	Severity	Documentation
5	■ **Rapid**	□ Major	□ Established
	□ Delayed	□ Moderate	□ Probable
		■ **Minor**	□ Suspected
			■ **Possible**
			□ Unlikely

Effects Antihypertensive effectiveness of CAPTOPRIL may be reduced.

Mechanism GI absorption of CAPTOPRIL may be decreased.

Management If an interaction is suspected, consider separating CAPTOPRIL dose from food or ANTACID administration by 1 to 2 hours.

Discussion

In a study of 10 patients, administration of a single dose of captopril 50 mg after 50 mL of antacid and breakfast reduced the bioavailability of captopril by 42% and 56%, respectively.[1] Although food and antacids similarly decrease bioavailability, there are no data to indicate that the efficacy of captopril is compromised by this interaction. See also ACE Inhibitors-Food.

[1] Mantyla R, et al. *Int J Clin Pharmacol Ther Toxic* 1984;22:626.

* Asterisk indicates drugs cited in interaction reports.

ACE Inhibitors — Capsaicin

ACE Inhibitors		Capsaicin
Benazepril (*Lotensin*)	Lisinopril (eg, *Prinivil*)	Capsaicin* (*Zostrix*)
Captopril* (eg, *Capoten*)	Quinapril (*Accupril*)	
Enalapril (*Vasotec*)	Ramipril (*Altace*)	
Fosinopril (*Monopril*)		

Significance	Onset	Severity	Documentation
5	■ **Rapid**	□ Major	□ Established
	□ Delayed	□ Moderate	□ Probable
		■ **Minor**	□ Suspected
			■ **Possible**
			□ Unlikely

Effects CAPSAICIN may cause or exacerbate coughing associated with ACE INHIBITOR treatment and vice versa.

Mechanism Unknown.

Management Advise patients receiving an ACE INHIBITOR of the possibility of a cough being induced if topical CAPSAICIN is prescribed or vice versa.

Discussion

In a double-blind, randomized investigation in 16 healthy volunteers, pretreatment with captopril 25 mg intensified the cough induced by capsaicin inhalation when compared to pretreatment with a placebo.[1] Although capsaicin is not used by inhalation as a medication, a 53-year-old female patient maintained on an ACE inhibitor for several years complained of cough following the topical application of capsaicin 0.075% cream to her lower extremities.[2] The patient had not experienced a cough while receiving the ACE inhibitor alone. However, it was not determined if the patient could have experienced the cough with application of capsaicin alone.

Additional studies are needed to determine if capsaicin may produce or exacerbate coughing in patients receiving an ACE inhibitor.

[1] Morice AH, et al. *Lancet*. 1987;2:1116.

[2] Hakas JF Jr. *Ann Allergy*. 1990;65:322.

* Asterisk indicates drugs cited in interaction reports. Based on pharmacologic and pharmacokinetic considerations, similar interactions may occur with other drugs that are listed.

ACE Inhibitors — Everolimus

ACE Inhibitors		Everolimus
Benazepril (eg, *Lotensin*)	Perindopril (eg, *Aceon*)	Everolimus* (eg, *Afinitor*)
Captopril	Quinapril (eg, *Accupril*)	
Enalapril* (eg, *Vasotec*)	Ramipril* (eg, *Altace*)	
Fosinopril	Trandolapril (eg, *Mavik*)	
Lisinopril (eg, *Prinivil*)		
Moexipril (eg, *Univasc*)		

Significance	Onset	Severity	Documentation
2	□ Rapid	□ Major	□ Established
	■ **Delayed**	■ **Moderate**	□ Probable
		□ Minor	■ **Suspected**
			□ Possible
			□ Unlikely

Effects The risk of angioedema, including life-threatening edema of the tongue, may be increased.

Mechanism Unknown.

Management Coadminister with caution. If angioedema occurs, treat appropriately; consider discontinuing one or both drugs if angioedema persists or recurs.

Discussion

Lingual angioedema was reported in 6 of 114 patients after being switched from cyclosporine and tacrolimus to everolimus.[1] When angioedema occurred, the patients had been receiving concomitant treatment with enalapril or ramipril as part of their treatment regimens. Although angioedema has been reported with ACE inhibitor therapy, the occurrence of the angioedema was clearly associated with the start of everolimus therapy. Angioedema occurred within 2 to 41 days after the initiation of everolimus therapy. In 5 of 6 patients, lingual angioedema resolved with antiallergic treatment. In 1 patient, 2 severe episodes of lingual angioedema occurred, and everolimus therapy had to be discontinued. Angioedema was reported in 13 of 71 patients receiving an ACE inhibitor and everolimus concurrently in another study.[2] The median onset of angioedema was 2 months, but in 1 patient it occurred in 6 months. All patients recovered with steroid therapy. No further episodes of angioedema occurred after discontinuation of the ACE inhibitor. In a retrospective study of 309 renal transplant patients receiving everolimus or sirolimus, 137 patients were also receiving an ACE inhibitor.[3] Nine patients (6.6%) developed angioedema after a mean period of 123 days of concurrent therapy. The incidence of angioedema was lower in patients receiving an ACE inhibitor alone (2.1%) or either everolimus or sirolimus alone (1.2%). See ACE Inhibitors-Sirolimus.

[1] Fuchs U, et al. *Transplantation.* 2005;79(8):981.
[2] Fiocchi R, et al. *J Heart Lung Transplant.* 2009;28(2)(suppl):S308.
[3] Duerr M, et al. *Clin J Am Soc Nephrol.* 2010;5(4):703.

* Asterisk indicates drugs cited in interaction reports. Based on pharmacologic and pharmacokinetic considerations, similar interactions may occur with other drugs that are listed.

ACE Inhibitors — *Food*

Captopril* (eg, *Capoten*)	Food*

Significance	Onset	Severity	Documentation
2	■ **Rapid**	□ Major	□ Established
	□ Delayed	■ **Moderate**	□ Probable
		□ Minor	■ **Suspected**
			□ Possible
			□ Unlikely

Effects Antihypertensive effectiveness of CAPTOPRIL may be decreased by FOOD.

Mechanism GI absorption of CAPTOPRIL may be decreased by FOOD.

Management Administer CAPTOPRIL 1 hour before meals.

Discussion

In a randomized, crossover study in 12 healthy subjects, administration of captopril 100 mg immediately after a standard meal resulted in a 35% to 40% reduction in the bioavailability of the drug when compared with administration under fasting conditions.[1] In another randomized, crossover study, 10 healthy subjects were given a single 50 mg oral dose of captopril after fasting and following a meal.[2] Food decreased captopril bioavailability by more than 50% and the hypotensive activity of the drug was delayed. More recent randomized crossover studies in hypertensive patients suggest that food does not influence the hemodynamic effects of captopril and does not diminish the blood pressure reduction attained with the drug.[4,5]

Although the recent investigations suggest that food is unlikely to alter the effects of captopril, additional studies of this potential interaction are needed. Until this question is resolved, it is advisable to administer captopril 1 hour before meals.

Food does not reduce the GI absorption of enalapril[3] (*Vasotec*) or lisinopril (eg, *Zestril*).

[1] Singhvi SM, et al. *J Clin Pharmacol.* 1982;22:135.
[2] Mantyla R, et al. *Int J Clin Pharmacol Ther Toxicol.* 1984;22:626.
[3] Swanson BN, et al. *J Pharm Sci.* 1984;73:1655.
[4] Ohman KP, et al. *J Cardiovasc Pharmacol.* 1985;7:S20.
[5] Salvetti A, et al. *J Cardiovasc Pharmacol.* 1985;7:S25.

* Asterisk indicates drugs cited in interaction reports.

ACE Inhibitors — *Indomethacin*

Benazepril (*Lotensin*)	Moexipril (*Univasc*)	Indomethacin* (eg, *Indocin*)
Captopril* (eg, *Capoten*)	Perindopril (*Aceon*)	
Enalapril* (*Vasotec*)	Quinapril (*Accupril*)	
Fosinopril (*Monopril*)	Ramipril (*Altace*)	
Lisinopril (eg, *Prinivil*)	Trandolapril (*Mavik*)	

Significance	Onset	Severity	Documentation
2	■ **Rapid** □ Delayed	□ Major ■ **Moderate** □ Minor	□ Established ■ **Probable** □ Suspected □ Possible □ Unlikely

Effects The hypotensive effect of ACE INHIBITORS may be reduced.

Mechanism Inhibition of prostaglandin synthesis.

Management Monitor BP. Discontinue INDOMETHACIN or use an alternative antihypertensive agent if an interaction is suspected.

Discussion

Both healthy and hypertensive patients show a reduction in BP and an increase in urinary prostaglandin excretion and plasma renin activity when given captopril. These changes are blunted or completely abolished after the inhibition of endogenous prostaglandin synthesis by indomethacin in low-renin or volume-dependent hypertensive patients.[1-7] In a randomized, double-blind, multicenter study, 105 hypertensive patients on captopril (50 mg twice daily) received indomethacin (75 mg) for 1 week.[9] Compared with the control period, 67% of patients receiving captopril experienced an increase in diastolic BP. There was a slight rise in the 24-hour systolic (4.6 mmHg) and diastolic (2.7 mmHg) BPs. Loss of antihypertensive effect also has been reported in a 48-year-old man receiving enalapril 10 mg/day following 4 days of indomethacin 100 mg/day.[8] Severe hypertension persisted until indomethacin was discontinued. In a double-blind, crossover study, 18 elderly hypertensive patients taking enalapril received indomethacin (50 mg) or placebo daily for 3 weeks.[10] Compared with placebo, indomethacin resulted in a rise in systolic (10 mmHg) and diastolic (4.9 mmHg) BPs.

1 Abe K, et al. *Clin Sci.* 1980;59:141s.
2 Abe K, et al. *Tohoku J Exp Med.* 1980;132:117.
3 Ogihara T, et al. *Clin Pharmacol Ther.* 1981;30:328.
4 Moore TJ, et al. *Hypertension.* 1981;3:168.
5 Fujita T, et al. *Clin Exp Hypertens.* 1981;3:939.
6 Salvetti A, et al. *Clin Sci.* 1982;63:261s.
7 Silberbauer K, et al. *Br J Clin Pharmacol.* 1982;14:87S.
8 Ahmad S. *South Med J.* 1991;84:411.
9 Conlin PR, et al. *Hypertension.* 2000;36:461.
10 Morgan TO, et al. *Am J Hypertens.* 2000;13:1161.

* Asterisk indicates drugs cited in interaction reports. Based on pharmacologic and pharmacokinetic considerations, similar interactions may occur with other drugs that are listed.

ACE Inhibitors — *NSAIDs, COX-2 Selective Inhibitors*

ACE Inhibitors	NSAIDs, COX-2 Selective Inhibitors
Lisinopril* (eg, *Prinivil*)	Rofecoxib*†

Significance	Onset	Severity	Documentation
4	□ Rapid	□ Major	□ Established
	■ **Delayed**	■ **Moderate**	□ Probable
		□ Minor	□ Suspected
			■ **Possible**
			□ Unlikely

Effects The hypotensive effect of LISINOPRIL may be reduced.

Mechanism Unknown.

Management Closely monitor BP when starting or stopping ROFECOXIB.

Discussion

Increased BP was reported in a 59-year-old man during concurrent treatment with lisinopril and the nonsteroidal anti-inflammatory cyclooxygenase-2 (COX-2) selective inhibitor rofecoxib.[1] The patient's mildly elevated BP had been successfully managed (baseline 130 to 135/80 to 85 mm Hg) for 5 years with lisinopril 10 mg/day. Rofecoxib 25 mg/day was started for joint pain. After 5 weeks of treatment, the patient's BP was found to be 168/98 mm Hg at a routine office visit; rofecoxib was discontinued. Four days later, his BP was 128/83 mm Hg and averaged 127/78 mm Hg over the next 18 days. The patient experienced increased joint pain and rofecoxib was resumed. Within 2 days, his BP measurements increased and averaged 143/89 mm Hg over the next 2 weeks. BP measurements were brought into baseline range when the dose of lisinopril was increased to 20 mg/day. In a randomized, double-blind, placebo-controlled study, celecoxib 200 mg twice daily or placebo were given to 178 hypertensive patients whose BP was controlled by lisinopril.[2] There was no difference in 24-hour ambulatory BP measurements between the groups.

[1] Brown CH. *Ann Pharmacother.* 2000;34(12):1486.

[2] White WB, et al. *Hypertension.* 2002;39(4):929.

* Asterisk indicates drugs cited in interaction reports.
† Not available in the United States.

ACE Inhibitors × Phenothiazines

ACE Inhibitors		Phenothiazines	
Benazepril (eg, *Lotensin*)	Lisinopril (eg, *Prinivil*)	Chlorpromazine*	Promethazine (eg, *Phenergan*)
Captopril*	Quinapril (eg, *Accupril*)	Fluphenazine	Thioridazine
Enalapril (eg, *Vasotec*)	Ramipril (eg, *Altace*)	Perphenazine	Trifluoperazine
Fosinopril		Prochlorperazine (eg, *Compro*)	

Significance	Onset	Severity	Documentation
4	■ **Rapid**	□ Major	□ Established
	□ Delayed	■ **Moderate**	□ Probable
		□ Minor	□ Suspected
			■ **Possible**
			□ Unlikely

Effects The pharmacologic effects of ACE INHIBITORS may be increased.

Mechanism Additive or synergistic pharmacologic activity.

Management Use this combination with caution. If hypotension occurs, supportive treatment may be necessary.

Discussion

During concurrent treatment with captopril and chlorpromazine (administered for an acute psychotic episode), a 49-year-old man developed marked hypotension with postural intolerance.[1] Subsequently, the patient's supine and standing blood pressures were evaluated while he received captopril 6.25 mg twice daily with chlorpromazine 200 mg 3 times daily, chlorpromazine alone 200 mg 3 times daily, or no drug therapy. Administration of chlorpromazine alone produced an asymptomatic decrease in supine blood pressure from 220/120 to 190/110 mm Hg. Coadministration of both drugs caused a further reduction in supine blood pressure of 84/32 mm Hg (ie, from 190/110 to 106/78 mm Hg) and an additional decrease upon standing from 106/78 to 66/48 mm Hg. In the absence of therapy, no postural hypotension was observed. Long-term studies are needed to determine if this interaction would persist with long-term therapy.

[1] White WB. *Arch Intern Med.* 1986;146(9):1833.

* Asterisk indicates drugs cited in interaction reports. Based on pharmacologic and pharmacokinetic considerations, similar interactions may occur with other drugs that are listed.

ACE Inhibitors — *Probenecid*

Benazepril (eg, *Lotensin*)	Lisinopril (eg, *Prinivil*)	Probenecid*
Captopril*	Quinapril (eg, *Accupril*)	
Enalapril (eg, *Vasotec*)	Ramipril (eg, *Altace*)	
Fosinopril		

Significance	Onset	Severity	Documentation
5	☐ Rapid	☐ Major	☐ Established
	■ **Delayed**	☐ Moderate	☐ Probable
		■ **Minor**	☐ Suspected
			☐ Possible
			■ **Unlikely**

Effects Increased duration of action of ACE INHIBITORS.

Mechanism Reduced renal elimination of ACE INHIBITORS by PROBENECID.

Management If an interaction is suspected, monitor blood pressure and reduce the ACE INHIBITOR dose accordingly.

Discussion

In 4 healthy adults, pretreatment with oral probenecid resulted in increased captopril blood levels and decreased total clearance.[1] Despite these changes, there were no adverse effects or important changes noted in the physical, electrocardiographic, or clinical laboratory findings in any of these subjects. Because the correlation of blood levels to hemodynamic effects with captopril is poor and there are no data available in hypertensive patients, the clinical importance of this interaction is unknown. There are no data available with other ACE inhibitors.

[1] Singhvi SM, et al. *Clin Pharmacol Ther.* 1982;32(2):182.

* Asterisk indicates drugs cited in interaction reports. Based on pharmacologic and pharmacokinetic considerations, similar interactions may occur with other drugs that are listed.

ACE Inhibitors — Rifampin

Enalapril* (eg, *Vasotec*)	Rifampin* (eg, *Rifadin*)

Significance	Onset	Severity	Documentation
4	■ **Rapid**	□ Major	□ Established
	□ Delayed	■ **Moderate**	□ Probable
		□ Minor	□ Suspected
			■ **Possible**
			□ Unlikely

Effects The pharmacologic effects of ENALAPRIL may be decreased, resulting in a decrease in antihypertensive control.

Mechanism Unknown.

Management Consider monitoring BP in patients receiving this combination. If hypertension occurs, alternative antihypertensive treatment may be necessary.

Discussion

An increase in BP occurred in a 35-year-old man with essential hypertension during treatment with enalapril and rifampin.[1] The patient was treated with streptomycin, oxytetracycline, and rifampin 300 mg twice daily for a *Brucella abortus* infection. During administration of these antibiotics, therapy was continued with enalapril 15 mg twice daily, warfarin, bendroflumethiazide, acebutolol, dipyridamole, metoclopramide, and an antacid-containing aluminum hydroxide with magnesium carbonate and sodium alginate. On day 4, following the start of antibiotic therapy, the patient's BP elevated; by days 5 and 6, his BP was significantly greater ($P < 0.05$) than it had been prior to antibiotic treatment. Because an interaction between enalapril and rifampin was suspected, rifampin was discontinued for 4 days, then restarted. The AUC of enalapril was reduced by 4% during coadministration of rifampin. Zero to 7 hours after enalapril administration, the AUC of enalaprilat (the active metabolite of enalapril) was reduced by 31% by rifampin.

Additional studies are needed to determine the clinical importance of this possible interaction.

[1] Kandiah D, et al. *Eur J Clin Pharmacol.* 1988;35(4):431.

* Asterisk indicates drugs cited in interaction reports.

ACE Inhibitors — Salicylates

ACE Inhibitors		Salicylates	
Benazepril (eg, *Lotensin*)	Perindopril (*Aceon*)	Aspirin* (eg, *Bayer*)	Magnesium Salicylate (eg, *Doan's*)
Captopril*	Quinapril (eg, *Accupril*)	Bismuth Subsalicylate (eg, *Pepto-Bismol*)	Salsalate
Enalapril* (eg, *Vasotec*)	Ramipril* (eg, *Altace*)		
Fosinopril	Trandolapril (eg, *Mavik*)		
Lisinopril* (eg, *Prinivil*)			
Moexipril (eg, *Univasc*)			

Significance	Onset	Severity	Documentation
2	■ **Rapid**	□ Major	□ Established
	□ Delayed	■ **Moderate**	□ Probable
		□ Minor	■ **Suspected**
			□ Possible
			□ Unlikely

Effects The hypotensive and vasodilator effects of the ACE INHIBITOR may be reduced.

Mechanism Inhibition of prostaglandin synthesis.

Management If both agents are necessary, monitor BP and hemodynamic parameters. If an adverse effect on hemodynamic parameters is noted, consider one of the following options: reduce ASPIRIN dosage to less than 100 mg/day, convert to nonaspirin antiplatelet agent, or continue ASPIRIN and convert patient from ACE INHIBITOR to angiotensin-receptor blocker.

Discussion

In 18 patients with severe heart failure, a single dose of aspirin 350 mg appeared to attenuate the vasodilator and other prostaglandin-dependent effects of enalapril for more than 24 hours.[1] No clinical deterioration was noted in this 3-day study. Although reports regarding this interaction are contradictory, some extrapolations can be made: low-dose aspirin (less than 100 mg/day) may cause fewer interactions; the interaction may occur in patients with hypertension, coronary artery disease, or heart failure; and interindividual susceptibilities are probable.[2-6] No adverse effect was seen with coadministration of ACE inhibitors and aspirin in heart failure[7-11]; however, in 1 study, mortality was higher in patients receiving ACE inhibitors and aspirin in doses of 325 mg or more daily.[9] Studies are needed to assess the effects of long-term aspirin administration and lower doses of aspirin (eg, 81 mg/day) on ACE inhibitor therapy.[2,3,12,13]

1 Hall D, et al. *J Am Coll Cardiol.* 1992;20(7):1549.
2 Stys T, et al. *Arch Intern Med.* 2000;160(10):1409.
3 Nawarskas JJ, et al. *Pharmacotherapy.* 2000;20(6):698.
4 Peterson JG, et al. *Cleve Clin J Med.* 2001;68(6):569.
5 Cleland JG, et al. *Curr Opin Nephrol Hypertens.* 2001;10(5):625.
6 MacIntrye IM, et al. *Cardiovasc Drugs Ther.* 2005;19(4):261.
7 Teo KK, et al. *Lancet.* 2002;360(9339):1037.
8 Harjai KJ, et al. *Int J Cardiol.* 2003;88(2-3):207.
9 Guazzi M, et al. *Arch Intern Med.* 2003;163(13):1574.
10 Pedone C, et al. *Drugs Aging.* 2005;22(7):605.
11 Levy PD, et al. *Am Heart J.* 2010;159(2):222.
12 Nawarskas JJ, et al. *Pharmacotherapy.* 1998;18(5):1041.
13 Song KH, et al. *Ann Pharmacother.* 1999;33(3):375.

* Asterisk indicates drugs cited in interaction reports. Based on pharmacologic and pharmacokinetic considerations, similar interactions may occur with other drugs that are listed.

ACE Inhibitors — Sirolimus

ACE Inhibitors		Sirolimus
Benazepril (eg, *Lotensin*)	Perindopril (eg, *Aceon*)	Sirolimus* (*Rapamune*)
Captopril	Quinapril (eg, *Accupril*)	
Enalapril (eg, *Vasotec*)	Ramipril* (eg, *Altace*)	
Fosinopril	Trandolapril (eg, *Mavik*)	
Lisinopril (eg, *Prinivil*)		
Moexipril (eg, *Univasc*)		

Significance	Onset	Severity	Documentation
2	☐ Rapid	☐ Major	☐ Established
	■ **Delayed**	■ **Moderate**	☐ Probable
		☐ Minor	■ **Suspected**
			☐ Possible
			☐ Unlikely

Effects The risk of angioedema, including life-threatening tongue edema, may be increased.

Mechanism Unknown.

Management Coadminister with caution. If angioedema occurs, treat appropriately and consider discontinuing one or both drugs if angioedema persists or recurs.

Discussion

Edema of the tongue was reported in 5 renal transplant patients during concomitant administration of high doses of ramipril (5 mg daily) and sirolimus (5 mg daily).[1] Two weeks after discontinuing ramipril, edema resolved. Three months later, ramipril 2.5 mg daily was reintroduced without recurrence of tongue edema. See ACE Inhibitors-Everolimus interaction.

In a retrospective study of 309 renal transplant patients receiving sirolimus or everolimus, 137 patients were also receiving an ACE inhibitor.[2] Nine patients (6.6%) developed angioedema after a mean period of 123 days of concurrent therapy. The incidence of angioedema was lower in patients receiving an ACE inhibitor alone (2.1%) or either sirolimus or everolimus alone (1.2%).

1 Stallone G, et al. *Nephrol Dial Transplant.* 2004;19(11):2906.

2 Duerr M, et al. *Clin J Am Soc Nephrol.* 2010;5(4):703.

* Asterisk indicates drugs cited in interaction reports. Based on pharmacologic and pharmacokinetic considerations, similar interactions may occur with other drugs that are listed.

ACE Inhibitors — *Tizanidine*

ACE Inhibitors		Tizanidine
Benazepril (eg, *Lotensin*)	Perindopril (eg, *Aceon*)	Tizanidine* (eg, *Zanaflex*)
Captopril	Quinapril (eg, *Accupril*)	
Enalapril (eg, *Vasotec*)	Ramipril (eg, *Altace*)	
Fosinopril (eg, *Monopril*)	Trandolapril (eg, *Mavik*)	
Lisinopril* (eg, *Prinivil*)		
Moexipril (eg, *Univasc*)		

Significance	Onset	Severity	Documentation
4	■ **Rapid**	□ Major	□ Established
	□ Delayed	■ **Moderate**	□ Probable
		□ Minor	□ Suspected
			■ **Possible**
			□ Unlikely

Effects The pharmacologic effects of the ACE INHIBITOR may be increased, possibly resulting in severe hypotension.

Mechanism Unknown.

Management Use this combination with caution and closely monitor patients. If hypotension occurs, supportive treatment may be necessary.

Discussion

Severe hypotension was reported in a 48-year-old woman receiving lisinopril after tizanidine was added to her treatment regimen.[1] The patient was admitted to the hospital after a sudden change in consciousness caused by a midbrain and pons hemorrhage. Also, on admission, she had decerebrate posturing. Her BP was approximately 160/100 mm Hg. To reduce the risk of stroke and to control her BP, amlodipine (eg, *Norvasc*), nimodipine (eg, *Nimotop*), labetalol (eg, *Trandate*), and lisinopril 10 mg/day were added successively. Her BP decreased to 135/85 mm Hg. After 3 weeks of hospitalization, tizanidine 2 mg was started to treat increased muscle tone associated with the decerebrate rigidity. Within 2 hours of administering tizanidine, her BP decreased from 130/85 to 66/42 mm Hg. Dopamine was administered, and tizanidine and the antihypertensive medications were stopped. Within 5 hours, her BP was 120/50 mm Hg. Dopamine was discontinued 20 hours later. When the patient's BP was approximately 152/85 mm Hg (42 hours later), tizanidine and the antihypertensive agents, excluding lisinopril, were resumed without incidence. Hypotension developed in a 10-year-old boy who had been receiving lisinopril for the previous 10 months to control hypertension.[2] The hypotension occurred after tizanidine was started for the treatment of spasticity. An 85-year-old man developed severe hypotension (60/32 mm Hg) and bradycardia (37 bpm) 2 days after starting tizanidine. He was on multiple drugs, including lisinopril.[3]

[1] Kao CD, et al. *Ann Pharmacother.* 2004;38(11):1840.
[2] Johnson TR, et al. *J Child Neurol.* 2000;15(12):818.
[3] Publow SW, et al. *Am J Health Syst Pharm.* 2010;67(19):1606.

* Asterisk indicates drugs cited in interaction reports. Based on pharmacologic and pharmacokinetic considerations, similar interactions may occur with other drugs that are listed.

ACE Inhibitors — Trimethoprim

ACE Inhibitors		Trimethoprim	
Benazepril* (eg, *Lotensin*)	Perindopril* (eg, *Aceon*)	Trimethoprim* (eg, *Primsol*)	Trimethoprim/ Sulfamethoxazole* (eg, *Bactrim*)
Captopril*	Quinapril* (eg, *Accupril*)		
Enalapril* (eg, *Vasotec*)	Ramipril* (eg, *Altace*)		
Fosinopril* (eg, *Monopril*)	Trandolapril* (eg, *Mavik*)		
Lisinopril* (eg, *Prinivil*)			
Moexipril* (eg, *Univasc*)			

Significance	Onset	Severity	Documentation
2	☐ Rapid	☐ Major	☐ Established
	■ **Delayed**	■ **Moderate**	☐ Probable
		☐ Minor	■ **Suspected**
			☐ Possible
			☐ Unlikely

Effects The risk of hyperkalemia may be increased, especially in elderly patients.

Mechanism ACE INHIBITORS and TRIMETHOPRIM may act additively or synergistically to inhibit renal excretion of potassium.

Management If coadministration cannot be avoided, closely monitor potassium plasma concentrations and clinical response. Adjust the ACE INHIBITOR dose as needed.

Discussion

In a case control study spanning 14 years, the risk of hyperkalemia-associated hospitalization in patients 66 years and older who were being treated with trimethoprim/ sulfamethoxazole and an ACE inhibitor or angiotensin II receptor antagonists was assessed.[1] During the study period, 4,248 admissions involving hyperkalemia occurring within 14 days of antibiotic exposure were identified.[1] Coadministration of an ACE inhibitor or angiotensin II receptor antagonist and trimethoprim/ sulfamethoxazole was associated with a nearly 7-fold increased risk of hyperkalemia-associated hospitalization compared with amoxicillin (eg, *Amoxil*). Other comparator antibiotics were not associated with this risk.

[1] Antoniou T, et al. *Arch Intern Med.* 2010;170(12):1045.

* Asterisk indicates drugs cited in interaction reports.

Acetaminophen — *Anticholinergics*

Acetaminophen	Anticholinergics	
Acetaminophen* (eg, *Tylenol*)	Atropine*	Methscopolamine (*Pamine*)
	Belladonna	Orphenadrine (eg, *Norflex*)
	Benztropine (eg, *Cogentin*)	Oxybutynin (eg, *Ditropan*)
	Clidinium (*Quarzan*)	Procyclidine (*Kemadrin*)
	Dicyclomine (eg, *Bentyl*)	Propantheline* (eg, *Pro-Banthine*)
	Glycopyrrolate* (eg, *Robinul*)	Scopolamine (eg, *Scopace*)
	Hyoscyamine (eg, *Anaspaz*)	Trihexyphenidyl (eg, *Artane*)
	Mepenzolate (*Cantil*)	

Significance	Onset	Severity	Documentation
5	■ **Rapid**	□ Major	□ Established
	□ Delayed	□ Moderate	□ Probable
		■ **Minor**	□ Suspected
			■ **Possible**
			□ Unlikely

Effects The onset of ACETAMINOPHEN effect may be delayed or decreased slightly, but the ultimate pharmacological effect is not affected by ANTICHOLINERGICS.

Mechanism A slight delay in the absorption of ACETAMINOPHEN from the GI tract is apparently caused by decreased GI motility induced by ANTICHOLINERGICS.

Management ACETAMINOPHEN and ANTICHOLINERGICS may be coadministered with little or no clinical risk.

Discussion

In a study involving 6 subjects, the time to peak acetaminophen concentration in plasma was more than doubled to 160 minutes and the maximum plasma concentration was reduced by one-third when IV propantheline 30 mg was administered 15 minutes before a 1.5 g oral dose of acetaminophen.[1] The 24-hour urinary excretion of acetaminophen was not affected. Rate, but not ultimate extent, of absorption was influenced by IV propantheline. Another study involving oral and IV butropium bromide (anticholinergic) suggested a variable effect on gastric emptying time and the potential rate of acetaminophen absorption in patients with gastric ulcer.[2] A study involving 60 women, 30 pregnant in their first trimester, suggested that 0.3 mg or less IV glycopyrrolate decreased gastric emptying and delayed the absorption of acetaminophen. Atropine IV (maximum dose, 0.6 mg) did not produce a similar effect.[3]

[1] Nimmo J, et al. *BMJ*. 1973;1:587.
[2] Harasawa S, et al. *Tokai J Exp Clin Med*. 1982;7:551.
[3] Clark JM, et al. *Br J Anaesth*. 1983;55:1195.

* Asterisk indicates drugs cited in interaction reports. Based on pharmacologic and pharmacokinetic considerations, similar interactions may occur with other drugs that are listed.

Acetaminophen — *Barbiturates*

Acetaminophen		Barbiturates	
Acetaminophen* (eg, *Tylenol*)		Amobarbital (*Amytal*)	Pentobarbital (eg, *Nembutal*)
		Aprobarbital (*Alurate*)	Phenobarbital*
		Butabarbital (eg, *Butisol*)	Primidone* (eg, *Mysoline*)
		Butalbital	Secobarbital (eg, *Seconal*)
		Mephobarbital (*Mebaral*)	

Significance	Onset	Severity	Documentation
4	☐ Rapid	☐ Major	☐ Established
	■ **Delayed**	■ **Moderate**	☐ Probable
		☐ Minor	☐ Suspected
			■ **Possible**
			☐ Unlikely

Effects The potential hepatotoxicity of ACETAMINOPHEN may be increased when large or chronic doses of BARBITURATES are coadministered. The therapeutic effects of ACETAMINOPHEN may be reduced with BARBITURATE therapy.

Mechanism BARBITURATES may induce hepatic microsomal enzymes that accelerate the metabolism of ACETAMINOPHEN, which could lead to abnormally high levels of hepatotoxins.

Management Risk is greatest when ACETAMINOPHEN overdosage accompanies regular BARBITURATE use. At usual oral therapeutic doses no special adjustment or monitoring is required.

Discussion

In 16 subjects overdosed on acetaminophen, 8 had consumed alcohol or barbiturates for at least 3 weeks prior to acetaminophen poisoning.[1] The group taking hepatic enzyme inducers had a significantly higher level of hepatic injury; 2 died in hepatic coma and 1 developed acute tubular necrosis. A 13-year-old girl receiving chronic phenobarbital therapy overdosed on acetaminophen 6 to 9 g and phenobarbital 500 to 1000 mg.[2] Extensive hepatic necrosis, degeneration of renal tubules, and cerebral cortex damage occurred; she died 8 days after ingestion. In 6 subjects on chronic seizure medication and 6 normal subjects, the elimination rate and total body clearance of acetaminophen were higher in the epileptics, but not significantly.[3] Acetaminophen 20 mg/kg was administered orally to 15 patients taking chronic antiseizure medication or rifampin; minor changes in the pharmacokinetics of acetaminophen were noted, but no significant increase in hepatotoxic metabolites occurred.[4] Other studies suggest a potentiation of acetaminophen hepatotoxicity by phenobarbital.[5,6] Hepatotoxic risk appears to be very low when oral acetaminophen is coadministered with barbiturates. Chronic acetaminophen use with hepatic microsomal enzyme inducers remains to be studied.

[1] Wright N, et al. *Scot Med J.* 1973;18:56.
[2] Wilson JT, et al. *Am J Dis Child.* 1978;132:466.
[3] Perucca E, et al. *Br J Clin Pharmacol.* 1979;7:201.
[4] Prescott LF, et al. *Br J Clin Pharmacol.* 1981;12:149.
[5] Pirotte JH. *Ann Intern Med.* 1984;101:403.
[6] Douidar SM, et al. *J Pharmacol Exp Ther.* 1987;240:578.

* Asterisk indicates drugs cited in interaction reports. Based on pharmacologic and pharmacokinetic considerations, similar interactions may occur with other drugs that are listed.

Acetaminophen — *Beta-Blockers*

Acetaminophen* (eg, *Tylenol*)	Propranolol* (eg, *Inderal*)

Significance	Onset	Severity	Documentation
5	☐ Rapid ■ **Delayed**	☐ Major ☐ Moderate ■ **Minor**	☐ Established ☐ Probable ☐ Suspected ■ **Possible** ☐ Unlikely

Effects The pharmacologic effects of ACETAMINOPHEN may be increased.

Mechanism PROPRANOLOL appears to inhibit the enzyme systems responsible for the glucuronidation and oxidation of ACETAMINOPHEN.

Management Based on currently available documentation, no special precautions are necessary.

Discussion

In a double-blind, crossover study involving 10 healthy volunteers, propranolol reduced the clearance of acetaminophen 14%.[1] Each subject was given placebo or propranolol 160 mg/day for 5 days. Venous blood samples were drawn at varying intervals for 24 hours after a single oral dose of acetaminophen 500 mg, and plasma levels of acetaminophen and its metabolites were measured. Propranolol caused a significant ($P < 0.05$) increase in the half-life (from 2.7 to 3.4 hours) and a significant ($P < 0.05$) decrease in acetaminophen clearance (from 364 to 313 mL/min). In addition, the fractional clearance of the glucuronide, cysteine, and mercapturate metabolites of acetaminophen, but not the sulfate conjugate, was ($P < 0.05$) reduced.

Additional studies are needed to determine the clinical significance of this possible interaction.

[1] Baraka OZ, et al. *Br J Clin Pharmacol.* 1989;28:230P.

* Asterisk indicates drugs cited in interaction reports.

Acetaminophen — *Carbamazepine*

Acetaminophen* (eg, *Tylenol*)	Carbamazepine* (eg, *Tegretol*)

Significance	Onset	Severity	Documentation
4	□ Rapid	□ Major	□ Established
	■ **Delayed**	■ **Moderate**	□ Probable
		□ Minor	□ Suspected
			■ **Possible**
			□ Unlikely

Effects The potential hepatotoxicity of ACETAMINOPHEN may be increased when large or chronic doses of CARBAMAZEPINE are administered concurrently. The therapeutic effects of ACETAMINOPHEN may be reduced with simultaneous CARBAMAZEPINE therapy.

Mechanism CARBAMAZEPINE may induce hepatic microsomal enzymes that accelerate the metabolism of ACETAMINOPHEN. An unusually high rate of ACETAMINOPHEN metabolism could lead to abnormally high levels of metabolites toxic to the liver.

Management Risk appears greatest when ACETAMINOPHEN overdosage accompanies regular CARBAMAZEPINE use. At usual oral therapeutic doses of ACETAMINOPHEN and CARBAMAZEPINE, no dosage adjustment is generally required.

Discussion

A 17-year-old girl developed hepatic failure requiring liver transplantation following ingestion of 7 to 8 g acetaminophen in a suicide attempt.[5] The patient had been taking 300 mg daily of carbamazepine for mood stabilization and was malnourished because of binge/purging-type anorexia nervosa. Carbamazepine alters acetaminophen metabolism.[1-4] Carbamazepine induces hepatic microsomal enzymes, thus accelerating acetaminophen metabolism. The liver toxicity of acetaminophen seems to be related to an increased formation of toxic metabolites and depletion of hepatic glutathione. The importance of this interaction at usual doses administered intermittently, rather than chronically, is not well defined.

1 Perucca E, et al. *Br J Clin Pharmacol* 1979;7:201.
2 Prescott LF, et al. *Br J Clin Pharmacol* 1981;12:149.
3 Miners JO, et al. *Clin Pharmacol Ther* 1984;35:480.
4 Smith JAE, et al. *Human Toxicol* 1986;5:383.
5 Young CR, et al. *J Clin Psychiatry* 1998;59:622.

* Asterisk indicates drugs cited in interaction reports.

Acetaminophen — *Contraceptives, Hormonal*

Acetaminophen* (eg, *Tylenol*)	Contraceptives, Oral* (eg, *Ortho-Novum*)

Significance	Onset	Severity	Documentation
5	□ Rapid ■ **Delayed**	□ Major □ Moderate ■ **Minor**	□ Established □ Probable □ Suspected ■ **Possible** □ Unlikely

Effects The onset of ACETAMINOPHEN's effect may be delayed or decreased slightly, but the ultimate pharmacological effect does not appear to be affected by combination ORAL CONTRACEPTIVES.

Mechanism Increase in glucuronidation, resulting in increased plasma clearance and a decreased half-life of ACETAMINOPHEN.

Management Oral ACETAMINOPHEN and combination ORAL CONTRACEPTIVES may be coadministered with little or no significant clinical risk at therapeutic dosage levels.

Discussion

Numerous studies report an increased rate of acetaminophen metabolism when a combination oral contraceptive (OC) is taken concurrently.[1-6] Elimination half-life of acetaminophen decreases 21% to 30% in users of combination OCs. Use of such OCs has been associated with metabolic clearance rates of acetaminophen that are 15% to 64% above baseline rates, depending on the dose of acetaminophen.[1,2,4] OCs appear to increase acetaminophen metabolism primarily by increasing glucuronidation, although other metabolic processes may be affected to lesser degrees.

The clinical significance of this interaction is not great at usual dosage levels. Risk is theoretically increased when high doses of acetaminophen are ingested concurrently with estrogen/progestin OC therapy. This could result in an increased formation of toxic metabolites and depletion of hepatic glutathione.

1 Abernethy DR, et al. *Obstet Gynecol.* 1982;60:338.
2 Mitchell MC, et al. *Clin Pharmacol Ther.* 1983;34:48.
3 Miners JO, et al. *Br J Clin Pharmacol.* 1983;16:503.
4 Ochs HR, et al. *Pharmacology.* 1984;28:188.
5 Baciewicz AM. *Ther Drug Monit.* 1985;7:26.
6 Farrell GC. *Med J Aust.* 1986;145:600.

* Asterisk indicates drugs cited in interaction reports.

Acetaminophen — *Ethanol*

Acetaminophen* (eg, *Tylenol*)	Ethanol*

Significance	Onset	Severity	Documentation
2	□ Rapid ■ **Delayed**	□ Major ■ **Moderate** □ Minor	□ Established □ Probable ■ **Suspected** □ Possible □ Unlikely

Effects Chronic consumption of ETHANOL may increase the risk of ACETAMINOPHEN-induced liver damage.

Mechanism Induction of hepatic microsomal enzymes by chronic ETHANOL consumption may be associated with ACETAMINOPHEN-induced hepatotoxicity when ACETAMINOPHEN is ingested during an ETHANOL-free period, but this mechanism has not been substantiated.

Management Caution patients who consume ETHANOL chronically and in excess about this potential interaction; advise them to avoid regular and excessive ACETAMINOPHEN use or avoid chronic use of ETHANOL.

Discussion

Because either chronic acetaminophen or alcohol ingestion may cause hepatotoxicity, a cause-and-effect relationship is difficult to establish for this interaction. Nevertheless, hepatotoxicity has occurred in chronic alcoholics following moderate to excessive dose levels of acetaminophen.[1-10] An open-label, randomized, crossover study in 10 healthy subjects investigated the formation of the hepatotoxic metabolite of acetaminophen (ie, N-acetyl-p-benzoquine imine) following ingestion of acetaminophen 500 mg 8 hours after a 6-hour infusion of ethanol or dextrose 5% in water.[11] Hepatic microsomal enzyme induction by chronic alcohol ingestion may increase liver toxicity induced by acetaminophen and its toxic metabolites when acetaminophen is ingested during an ethanol-free period.

Controlled studies are needed to substantiate the mechanism and clinical importance of this interaction.

[1] Wrights N, et al. *Scott Med J.* 1973;18(2):56.
[2] Emby DJ, et al. *S Afr Med J.* 1977;51(7):208.
[3] McClain CJ, et al. *JAMA.* 1980;244(3):251.
[4] Licht H, et al. *Ann Intern Med.* 1980;92(4):511.
[5] Lieber CS. *Pharmacol Biochem Behav.* 1983;18(suppl 1):181.
[6] Dietz AJ Jr, et al. *J Clin Pharmacol.* 1984;24(4):205.
[7] Leist MH, et al. *J Clin Gastroenterol.* 1985;7(1):55.
[8] Seeff LB, et al. *Ann Intern Med.* 1986;104(3):399.
[9] Lesser PB, et al. *Dig Dis Sci.* 1986;31(1):103.
[10] Kartsonis A, et al. *Ann Intern Med.* 1986;105(1):138.
[11] Thummel KE, et al. *Clin Pharmacol Ther.* 2000;67(6):591.

* Asterisk indicates drugs cited in interaction reports.

Acetaminophen — *Exenatide*

Acetaminophen* (eg, *Tylenol*)	Exenatide* (*Byetta*)

Significance	Onset	Severity	Documentation
5	☐ Rapid ■ **Delayed**	☐ Major ☐ Moderate ■ **Minor**	☐ Established ☐ Probable ☐ Suspected ■ **Possible** ☐ Unlikely

Effects The onset of ACETAMINOPHEN effect may be delayed, but the extent of absorption is not altered.

Mechanism EXENATIDE slows gastric emptying, delaying ACETAMINOPHEN GI absorption.

Management Administer ACETAMINOPHEN at least 1 hour prior to or 4 hours after EXENATIDE to minimize a delay in the onset of the ACETAMINOPHEN effect.

Discussion

The effects of exenatide administration on the pharmacokinetics of acetaminophen were evaluated in 39 healthy subjects.[1] Using a randomized, single-blind, placebo-controlled design, each subject received oral acetaminophen 1,000 mg elixir with subcutaneous placebo from 1 hour before to 4 hours after receiving subcutaneous exenatide 10 mcg. Compared with placebo, administration of exenatide reduced the acetaminophen C_{max} by 37% to 56%, reduced the AUC by 11% to 24%, and delayed the time to reach C_{max} from 0.6 to 4.2 hours.

[1] Blasé E, et al. *J Clin Pharmacol.* 2005;45(5):570.

* Asterisk indicates drugs cited in interaction reports.

Acetaminophen — *Hydantoins*

Acetaminophen	Hydantoins	
Acetaminophen* (eg, *Tylenol*)	Ethotoin (*Peganone*)	Mephenytoin†
	Fosphenytoin (*Cerebyx*)	Phenytoin* (eg, *Dilantin*)

Significance	Onset	Severity	Documentation
2	☐ Rapid	☐ Major	☐ Established
	■ **Delayed**	■ **Moderate**	☐ Probable
		☐ Minor	■ **Suspected**
			☐ Possible
			☐ Unlikely

Effects The potential hepatotoxicity of ACETAMINOPHEN may be increased when chronic doses of HYDANTOINS are coadministered. The therapeutic effects of ACETAMINOPHEN may be reduced with simultaneous HYDANTOIN therapy.

Mechanism HYDANTOINS may induce hepatic microsomal enzymes that increase the metabolism of ACETAMINOPHEN to hepatotoxic metabolites.

Management The risk of hepatotoxicity is greatest when chronic dosing or overdosage with ACETAMINOPHEN accompanies regular HYDANTOIN use. Generally, no special dosage adjustment or monitoring is required at the usual therapeutic doses of ACETAMINOPHEN and HYDANTOINS.

Discussion

Hydantoins alter acetaminophen metabolism.[1-5] Hydantoins apparently induce hepatic microsomal enzymes, thus accelerating acetaminophen metabolism. One study revealed that, in 6 patients on chronic anticonvulsant therapy, acetaminophen clearance was 46% faster and half-life was 28% shorter in the group receiving anticonvulsants compared with 12 controls[5]; other studies have confirmed this observation.[5,6]

Toxicity of acetaminophen depends largely upon the rate of formation of hepatotoxic metabolites and the rate of depletion of hepatic glutathione.[4] Hepatic microsomal enzyme inducers (eg, hydantoins) may place patients who overdose on acetaminophen or chronically consume therapeutic doses of acetaminophen at increased risk of hepatotoxicity.

Additional controlled studies are needed to assess the clinical importance of this potential interaction.

[1] Perucca E, et al. *Br J Clin Pharmacol.* 1979;7(2):201.
[2] Cunningham JL, et al. *Br J Clin Pharmacol.* 1981;11(6):591.
[3] Prescott LF, et al. *Br J Clin Pharmacol.* 1981;12(2):149.
[4] Prescott LF, et al. *Am J Med.* 1983;75(5A):113.
[5] Miners JO, et al. *Clin Pharmacol Ther.* 1984;35(4):480.
[6] Minton NA, et al. *Hum Toxicol.* 1988;7(1):33.

* Asterisk indicates drugs cited in interaction reports. Based on pharmacologic and pharmacokinetic considerations, similar interactions may occur with other drugs that are listed.
† Not available in the United States.

Acetaminophen — *Isoniazid*

Acetaminophen* (eg, *Tylenol*)	Isoniazid* (eg, *Nydrazid*)

Significance	Onset	Severity	Documentation
5	☐ Rapid	■ **Major**	☐ Established
	■ **Delayed**	☐ Moderate	☐ Probable
		☐ Minor	☐ Suspected
			☐ Possible
			■ **Unlikely**

Effects Hepatotoxicity has been reported.

Mechanism Unknown.

Management If coadministration cannot be avoided, monitor patients for evidence of liver damage.

Discussion

The effects of isoniazid on the metabolism of acetaminophen were studied in 10 healthy volunteers who received isoniazid 300 mg/day for 7 days and acetaminophen 500 mg the day before starting isoniazid (day 0), on the seventh day of isoniazid administration, and 2 days after the last dose of isoniazid (day 9).[1] Compared with days 0 and 9, all of the oxidative metabolites of acetaminophen were decreased on day 7. However, the clearance of acetaminophen through nonoxidative pathways was not affected. Isoniazid inhibited the clearance of the glutathione and catechol metabolites of acetaminophen 69.7% and 62.2%, respectively, and decreased total clearance 15%. Within 2 days of discontinuation of isoniazid, acetaminophen metabolism returned to baseline. There were an equal number of rapid and slow acetylators of isoniazid in the study population. The effect of isoniazid on acetaminophen metabolism is small and would not be expected to be of clinical importance. Because isoniazid interferes with the formation of the toxic metabolite of acetaminophen, patients ingesting an acute or chronic overdose of the drug could experience a beneficial effect, helping to prevent hepatotoxicity. These findings are contradictory to 6 case reports of hepotoxicity in patients receiving acetaminophen plus isoniazid[2,3] or acetaminophen plus isoniazid, rifampin, and pyrazinamide.[4] Two cases involved intentional large doses of acetaminophen (ie, 6 and 11.5 g), while 3 cases involved short-term use of normal doses of acetaminophen.[2-4]

Because both drugs are potentially hepatotoxic, additional studies are needed to determine if the observed reaction is due to an interaction. An unknown amount of acetaminophen was ingested by 1 patient.[3]

[1] Epstein MM, et al. *Br J Clin Pharmacol.* 1991;31(2):139.

[2] Murphy R, et al. *Ann Intern Med.* 1990;113(10):799.

[3] Moulding TS, et al. *Ann Intern Med.* 1991;114(5):431.

[4] Nolan CM, et al. *Chest.* 1994;105(2):408.

* Asterisk indicates drugs cited in interaction reports.

Acetaminophen — *Probenecid*

Acetaminophen* (eg, *Tylenol*)	Probenecid*

Significance	Onset	Severity	Documentation
5	☐ Rapid	☐ Major	☐ Established
	■ **Delayed**	☐ Moderate	☐ Probable
		■ **Minor**	☐ Suspected
			■ **Possible**
			☐ Unlikely

Effects PROBENECID may increase the therapeutic effectiveness of ACETAMINOPHEN slightly.

Mechanism PROBENECID may reduce the degradation and urinary excretion of the glucuronide metabolite of ACETAMINOPHEN.

Management No clinical interventions appear necessary at usual dosage levels of ACETAMINOPHEN and PROBENECID.

Discussion

Probenecid 500 mg every 6 hours caused a decrease in IV acetaminophen 650 mg clearance from approximately 329 to approximately 178 mL/min and increased elimination half-life from approximately 2.51 to approximately 4.3 hours (71%).[2] The renal elimination of the glucuronide metabolite of acetaminophen during 24 hours was decreased (from 260 to 84 mg/day). In addition, probenecid has been shown to inhibit acetaminophen secretion into saliva.[3] This interaction may not occur with other uricosurics. For example, sulfinpyrazone has increased acetaminophen metabolism.[1] See Acetaminophen-Sulfinpyrazone. The clinical relevance of this potential interaction at usual oral dosage levels is poorly defined. More data are required to define and clarify significance.

[1] Miners JO, et al. *Clin Pharmacol Ther.* 1984;35:480.

[2] Abernethy DR, et al. *J Pharmacol Exp Ther.* 1985;234:345.

[3] Kamali F, et al. *J Pharm Pharmacol.* 1987;39:150.

* Asterisk indicates drugs cited in interaction reports.

Acetaminophen — *Rifamycins*

Acetaminophen	Rifamycins	
Acetaminophen* (eg, *Tylenol*)	Rifampin* (eg, *Rifadin*)	Rifapentine (*Priftin*)
	Rifabutin (*Mycobutin*)	

Significance	Onset	Severity	Documentation
4	☐ Rapid	☐ Major	☐ Established
	■ **Delayed**	■ **Moderate**	☐ Probable
		☐ Minor	☐ Suspected
			■ **Possible**
			☐ Unlikely

Effects The therapeutic effectiveness of ACETAMINOPHEN as an analgesic/antipyretic may be decreased slightly by RIFAMYCINS. RIFAMYCINS may enhance ACETAMINOPHEN toxicity.

Mechanism RIFAMYCINS may induce hepatic microsomal enzymes that accelerate the breakdown of ACETAMINOPHEN to potentially hepatoxic metabolites.

Management Risk is greatest when ACETAMINOPHEN overdosage accompanies regular RIFAMYCIN use. Risk at usual therapeutic doses of ACETAMINOPHEN and RIFAMYCINS has not been determined. Consider closer monitoring for hepatotoxicity in patients receiving this combination.

Discussion

A limited number of studies suggest that rifampin increases acetaminophen glucuronidation and decreases its half-life.[1,2] The relevance of this information to the clinician has yet to be determined.

Accelerated metabolism of acetaminophen to hepatotoxic metabolites and subsequent depletion of hepatic glutathione by rifampin may pose a clinical risk in some patients. A case of severe hepatotoxicity occurred 2 days after starting rifampin 600 mg twice daily in a 32-year-old woman who had been taking, and continued to take, 2 to 4 g/day of acetaminophen for several weeks.[3] Controlled studies are needed to further define the clinical risk of this potential interaction in acute and chronic dosing situations.

[1] Prescott LF, et al. *Br J Clin Pharmacol.* 1981;12:149.
[2] Bock KW, et al. *Eur J Clin Pharmacol.* 1987;31:677.
[3] Stephenson I, et al. *Am J Gastroenterol.* 2001;96:1310.

* Asterisk indicates drugs cited in interaction reports. Based on pharmacologic and pharmacokinetic considerations, similar interactions may occur with other drugs that are listed.

Acetaminophen — *Sulfinpyrazone*

Acetaminophen* (eg, *Tylenol*)	Sulfinpyrazone* (eg, *Anturane*)

Significance	Onset	Severity	Documentation
2	☐ Rapid	☐ Major	☐ Established
	■ **Delayed**	■ **Moderate**	☐ Probable
		☐ Minor	■ **Suspected**
			☐ Possible
			☐ Unlikely

Effects SULFINPYRAZONE may increase the risk of hepatotoxicity from ACETAMINOPHEN and reduce its therapeutic effects.

Mechanism SULFINPYRAZONE may induce hepatic microsomal enzymes that accelerate the metabolism of ACETAMINOPHEN. An unusually high rate of ACETAMINOPHEN metabolism could lead to abnormally high levels of metabolites toxic to the liver.

Management The risk of hepatotoxicity is greatest when ACETAMINOPHEN overdosage accompanies regular SULFINPYRAZONE use. At usual oral therapeutic doses of ACETAMINOPHEN and SULFINPYRAZONE, no special dosage adjustment or monitoring is generally required.

Discussion

Sulfinpyrazone pretreatment of 800 mg/day for 1 week, followed by an oral dose of acetaminophen 1 g, increased acetaminophen clearance 22.8% and decreased elimination $t_{1/2}$ 18.8%.[1] The clinical importance of accelerated acetaminophen metabolism is poorly defined.

Toxicity of acetaminophen apparently depends upon the rate of formation of hepatotoxic metabolites and the rate of depletion of hepatic glutathione. Patients who receive hepatic microsomal enzyme inducers (eg, sulfinpyrazone) and who overdose on acetaminophen or consume therapeutic doses of acetaminophen chronically may be at increased risk of hepatotoxicity.

The clinical importance of this potential interaction at usual dosage levels is poorly defined. This interaction may not occur with other uricosurics. For example, probenecid has been shown to decrease acetaminophen metabolism.[2] Controlled studies are needed to assess the clinical importance of this potential interaction relative to liver toxicity and possible reduction in the therapeutic response to acetaminophen.

[1] Miners JO, et al. *Clin Pharmacol Ther.* 1984;35:480.

[2] Abernethy DR, et al. *J Pharmacol Exp Ther.* 1985;234:345.

* Asterisk indicates drugs cited in interaction reports.

Acitretin — *Ethanol*

Acitretin*
(*Soriatane*)

Ethanol*
(Alcohol, Ethyl Alcohol)

Significance	Onset	Severity	Documentation
1	☐ Rapid	■ **Major**	☐ Established
	■ **Delayed**	☐ Moderate	☐ Probable
		☐ Minor	■ **Suspected**
			☐ Possible
			☐ Unlikely

Effects Increased duration of teratogenic potential in women.

Mechanism ETHANOL increases the transesterification of ACITRETIN to etretinate.

Management ETHANOL is contraindicated in women of reproductive potential taking ACITRETIN and for 2 months after stopping therapy.

Discussion

Acitretin is a metabolite of etretinate.† Major human fetal abnormalities have been reported with administration of acitretin and etretinate. The manufacturer of acitretin states that there is clinical evidence that concomitant ingestion of acitretin and ethanol is associated with etretinate formation, which has a longer elimination $t_{½}$ than acitretin.[1] The longer $t_{½}$ of etretinate increases the duration of teratogenic potential in women. To eliminate acitretin from the body, thereby removing the substrate for transesterification to etretinate, women must not ingest ethanol during treatment with acitretin or for 2 months after stopping therapy. In cases in which etretinate is formed, as occurs with concurrent use of acitretin and ethanol, it may take 2 to 3 years to eliminate 98% of the etretinate. In 1 patient who was reported to have sporadically consumed alcoholic beverages, etretinate was found in the plasma and subcutaneous fat 52 months after she completed acitretin therapy (cumulative dose, 9,900 mg).[2]

The basis for this monograph is information on file with the manufacturer. Because of the seriousness of the problems, clinical evaluation of this interaction in humans is not likely to be forthcoming.

1 *Soriatane* [package insert]. Nutley, NJ: Roche Pharmaceuticals; August 1997.

2 Maier H, et al. *Lancet.* 1996;348:1107.

* Asterisk indicates drugs cited in interaction reports.
† Not available in the United States.

Acyclovir — *Mycophenolate*

Acyclovir		Mycophenolate	
Acyclovir* (eg, *Zovirax*)	Valacyclovir* (*Valtrex*)	Mycophenolate Mofetil* (*CellCept*) Mycophenolate Mofetil Hydrochloride (*CellCept*)	Mycophenolate Sodium (*Myfortic*)

Significance	Onset	Severity	Documentation
5	□ Rapid ■ **Delayed**	□ Major □ Moderate ■ **Minor**	□ Established □ Probable □ Suspected ■ **Possible** □ Unlikely

Effects ACYCLOVIR plasma concentrations may be elevated, increasing the pharmacologic effects.

Mechanism Unknown. However, decreased renal clearance of ACYCLOVIR may be partly involved.

Management Based on available clinical data, no special precautions are needed in patients with healthy kidney function.

Discussion

The effects of mycophenolate mofetil on the pharmacokinetics of acyclovir and valacyclovir, a prodrug of acyclovir, were studied in 15 healthy men.[1] In a prospective, open-label, single-dose, crossover study, each subject received acyclovir 800 mg, valacyclovir 2 g, or mycophenolate mofetil 1 g alone. In addition, each subject received acyclovir or valacyclovir with mycophenolate mofetil. Each treatment was administered in a randomized sequence separated by a 7-day washout period. Coadministration of mycophenolate mofetil and acyclovir increased the acyclovir C_{max} 40%, the time to reach the C_{max} 0.38 hours, and the AUC 31%. In addition, the acyclovir $t_{1/2}$ was decreased 11% and the renal clearance was reduced 19%. Coadministration of mycophenolate mofetil and valacyclovir decreased the time to reach the acyclovir C_{max} by 0.5 hours. Acyclovir did not affect the pharmacokinetics of mycophenolic acid or its inactive glucuronide conjugate (MPAG); however, valacyclovir decreased the AUC of MPAG 12%.

Additional studies in patients with impaired renal function are warranted.

[1] Gimenez F, et al. *Clin Pharmacokinet.* 2004;43(10):685.

* Asterisk indicates drugs cited in interaction reports. Based on pharmacologic and pharmacokinetic considerations, similar interactions may occur with other drugs that are listed.

Acyclovir — *Probenecid*

Acyclovir* (eg, *Zovirax*)	Valacyclovir* (*Valtrex*)	Probenecid*

Significance	Onset	Severity	Documentation
3	■ **Rapid** □ Delayed	□ Major □ Moderate ■ **Minor**	□ Established □ Probable ■ **Suspected** □ Possible □ Unlikely

Effects PROBENECID may increase ACYCLOVIR serum concentrations, increasing the therapeutic effects and adverse reactions.

Mechanism PROBENECID apparently inhibits renal tubular secretion of ACYCLOVIR.

Management The dosage of ACYCLOVIR and VALACYCLOVIR may need to be reduced if ACYCLOVIR toxicity develops.

Discussion

A 1-hour IV infusion of acyclovir 5 mg/kg was administered to 3 volunteers with normal renal function before and after oral administration of probenecid 1 g.[1] After probenecid administration, there was a 32% decline in renal clearance, a 40% increase in AUC, and an 18% increase in the terminal plasma $t_{1/2}$ of acyclovir.

Valacyclovir is a prodrug of acyclovir. The manufacturer reports that probenecid enhances the bioconversion of valacyclovir to acyclovir.[2] Consequently, peak plasma acyclovir concentrations are increased 23%, while the ensuing renal clearance of acyclovir is decreased 33%. In an open-label, randomized, crossover study, 12 men were given oral valacyclovir 1 g alone or 2 hours after probenecid 1 g.[3] Compared with controls, valacyclovir mean C_{max} and AUC increased 23% and 22%, respectively, while acyclovir mean C_{max} and AUC increased 22% and 48%, respectively.

The clinical importance of this possible interaction requires further clarification. However, because acyclovir has a wide therapeutic range, no acute toxicity is expected.

[1] Laskin OL, et al. *Antimicrob Agents Chemother.* 1982;21(5):804.
[2] *Valtrex* [package insert]. Philadelphia, PA: GlaxoSmithKline; June 1995.
[3] De Bony F, et al. *Antimicrob Agents Chemother.* 2002;46(2):458.

* Asterisk indicates drugs cited in interaction reports.

Acyclovir — *Zidovudine*

Acyclovir* (eg, *Zovirax*)	Zidovudine* (*Retrovir*)

Significance	Onset	Severity	Documentation
5	■ **Rapid**	□ Major	□ Established
	□ Delayed	□ Moderate	□ Probable
		■ **Minor**	□ Suspected
			□ Possible
			■ **Unlikely**

Effects When ACYCLOVIR is added to ZIDOVUDINE therapy, severe drowsiness and lethargy may occur.

Mechanism Unknown.

Management Chronic mucocutaneous herpes simplex infections are common in AIDS patients; therefore, this drug combination is likely. If severe lethargy occurs, consider reducing ACYCLOVIR dosage. Withdrawal may be necessary.

Discussion

A 30-year-old man with acquired immunodeficiency syndrome (AIDS) developed persistent fever after being treated with trimethoprim-sulfamethoxazole (TMP-SMZ; eg, *Septra*) for *Pneumocystis carinii* pneumonia.[1] He developed severe herpes simplex infection of the lips and was treated with parenteral acyclovir 250 mg every 8 hours. Zidovudine (AZT) was begun, 200 mg every 4 hours, 3 days after acyclovir because of persistent fever; within 1 hour the patient noted severe lethargy and fatigue which continued for 3 days despite switching to oral acyclovir 200 mg every 4 hours. Discontinuation of acyclovir resulted in patient alertness returning to baseline. The patient agreed to be rechallenged. Within 30 minutes of the initiation of infusion, he felt a sense of overwhelming fatigue and had to be roused from sleep 1 and 3 hours later. Sedation and lethargy were not reported as side effects in 515 patients receiving both acyclovir and zidovudine as part of a multicenter AIDS cohort study.[2] However, a prolonged survival rate was reported with early administration of acyclovir in patients receiving zidovudine.

This is not an unusual drug combination in patients with AIDS.

[1] Bach MC. *N Engl J Med* 1987;316:547.

[2] Stein DS, et al. *Ann Intern Med* 1994;121:100.

* Asterisk indicates drugs cited in interaction reports.

Adenosine — *Dipyridamole*

Adenosine* (*Adenocard*)	Dipyridamole* (eg, *Persantine*)

Significance	Onset	Severity	Documentation
2	■ **Rapid**	□ Major	□ Established
	□ Delayed	■ **Moderate**	□ Probable
		□ Minor	■ **Suspected**
			□ Possible
			□ Unlikely

Effects The pharmacologic effects of ADENOSINE may be potentiated by DIPYRIDAMOLE. Profound bradycardia may follow rapid bolus ADENOSINE administration.

Mechanism Possible inhibition of ADENOSINE metabolism or transport.

Management Due to the short half-life of ADENOSINE, no special precautions appear necessary when using ADENOSINE to terminate supraventricular tachycardia. If ADENOSINE infusions are given to simulate exercise during cardiac imaging, a reduction in the initial infusion rate is indicated. Titrate the doses according to response.

Discussion

Two studies involving healthy volunteers describe a potentiation of the pharmacologic effects of adenosine by dipyridamole.[1,3] In both studies, infusions of adenosine increased heart rate, systolic blood pressure, respiratory rate and skin temperature. The doses needed to achieve these effects were lower with dipyridamole pretreatment. More side effects were noted during concurrent administration of both drugs. Oral dipyridamole 400 mg/day has increased intrinsic adenosine levels, indicating that dipyridamole may alter intrinsic adenosine metabolism.[4] In contrast to continuous infusions, rapid bolus injections of adenosine decrease heart rate.[2] In two patients who developed spontaneous supraventricular tachycardia while taking dipyridamole, administration of adenosine 40 mcg/kg produced marked bradycardia in one of the patients. Empirically reducing the dose of adenosine to 10 mcg/kg in the second patient was effective in restoring sinus rhythm. The mean effective dose in both patients was 1 mg compared with 8.8 mg in five patients not receiving dipyridamole.

These findings suggest that empiric reduction in adenosine dose may be needed. However, additional clinical experience is needed before definite recommendations can be made.

[1] Biaggioni I, et al. *Life Sci* 1986;39:2229.
[2] Watt AH, et al. *Br J Clin Pharmacol* 1986;21:227.
[3] Conradson TBG, et al. *Acta Physiol Scand* 1987;129:387.
[4] German DC, et al. *Clin Pharmacol Ther* 1989;45:80.

* Asterisk indicates drugs cited in interaction reports.

Adenosine — *Nicotine*

Adenosine* (eg, *Adenocard*)	Nicotine Polacrilex* (eg, *Nicorette*)

Significance	Onset	Severity	Documentation
5	■ **Rapid** □ Delayed	□ Major □ Moderate ■ **Minor**	□ Established □ Probable □ Suspected ■ **Possible** □ Unlikely

Effects NICOTINE may enhance the cardiovascular effects of ADENOSINE. Angina-like pain induced by rapid ADENOSINE injections may be increased by NICOTINE.

Mechanism Unknown.

Management No special precautions appear necessary when ADENOSINE is given to terminate supraventricular tachycardia. In other situations, such as electrophysiologic studies and stress testing, advise patients to refrain from chewing NICOTINE gum. Lower ADENOSINE doses may be needed.

Discussion

Two pharmacologic studies substantiate an enhancement of the cardiovascular effects of adenosine by administration of nicotine gum to healthy volunteers.[1,2] In 1 trial, the increase in heart rate occurring with slow infusion of adenosine was potentiated by nicotine gum.[1] The typical increase in diastolic BP that occurs during nicotine exposure was blunted by adenosine. The second study involved 7 healthy volunteers who were given increasing bolus injections of adenosine until they developed angina-like chest pain.[2] In comparison to a baseline evaluation, subjects reported increased pain during concurrent nicotine gum chewing. In addition, more subjects developed AV block that was of longer duration during nicotine administration. These data suggest that patients using nicotine gum may respond to a lower dose of adenosine. Additional clinical experience is needed.

[1] Smits P, et al. *Clin Pharmacol Ther.* 1989;46:272. [2] Sylven C, et al. *J Cardiovasc Pharmacol.* 1990;16:962.

* Asterisk indicates drugs cited in interaction reports.

Adenosine		*Theophyllines*
Adenosine* (eg, *Adenocard*)	Aminophylline* Oxtriphylline (eg, *Choledyl SA*)	Theophylline* (eg, *Theo-Dur*)

Significance	Onset	Severity	Documentation
2	■ **Rapid** □ Delayed	□ Major ■ **Moderate** □ Minor	□ Established □ Probable ■ **Suspected** □ Possible □ Unlikely

Effects THEOPHYLLINES may antagonize the cardiovascular effects of ADENOSINE.

Mechanism Unknown. However, THEOPHYLLINES may antagonize ADENOSINE receptors.

Management The efficacy of standard doses of ADENOSINE to terminate supraventricular tachycardia may be reduced. Assess response and repeat with larger doses as needed.

Discussion

A pharmacologic interaction between methylxanthines (eg, theophylline, caffeine) and adenosine has been demonstrated in healthy volunteers.[1,2] Theophylline blunted or obliterated the elevation in heart rate, minute ventilation, skin temperature, and systolic BP that usually occurs with systemic infusion of adenosine.[1,2] Local infusion of adenosine usually causes pain and vasodilation. In experiments using direct instillation of adenosine into the brachial artery of volunteers, theophylline reduced the vasodilatory effect of adenosine, providing evidence that theophylline antagonizes the action of adenosine and that the effect may be due to antagonism of local adenosine receptors.[3,4]

While adenosine infusions increase heart rate, rapid IV administration causes bradycardia, possibly by a direct action on cardiac adenosine receptors. Therapeutically, this action is used to terminate paroxysmal supraventricular tachycardia. Although there are no studies of a possible antagonism of adenosine by methylxanthines in this clinical setting, the results from the studies cited indicate that higher adenosine doses may be required. In addition, adenosine is used as a pharmacologic stress test with thallium myocardial scanning. Patients who have taken theophylline or consumed caffeine-containing beverages cannot be studied and must be rescheduled.

1 Maxwell DL, et al. *Acta Physiol Scand.* 1987;131:459.
2 Biaggioni I, et al. *J Pharmacol Exp Ther.* 1991;258:588.
3 Taddei S, et al. *Clin Pharmacol Ther.* 1990;48:144.
4 Smits P, et al. *Clin Pharmacol Ther.* 1990;48:410.

* Asterisk indicates drugs cited in interaction reports. Based on pharmacologic and pharmacokinetic considerations, similar interactions may occur with other drugs that are listed.

Albendazole — *Food*

Albendazole* (*Albenza*)	Grapefruit Juice*

Significance	Onset	Severity	Documentation
5	■ **Rapid**	□ Major	□ Established
	□ Delayed	□ Moderate	□ Probable
		■ **Minor**	□ Suspected
			■ **Possible**
			□ Unlikely

Effects ALBENDAZOLE plasma concentrations may be elevated, increasing the risk of adverse effects.

Mechanism Inhibition of ALBENDAZOLE metabolism (CYP3A4) in the small intestine by GRAPEFRUIT JUICE is suspected.

Management Patients may require a lower dose of ALBENDAZOLE when taken with GRAPEFRUIT JUICE. Advise patients taking ALBENDAZOLE to avoid GRAPEFRUIT PRODUCTS and to take ALBENDAZOLE with a liquid other than GRAPEFRUIT JUICE.

Discussion

The effect of grapefruit juice on the metabolism of albendazole was studied in 6 healthy men.[1] Each subject received a single oral dose of albendazole 10 mg/kg with water or double-strength grapefruit juice 250 mL. Compared with water, grapefruit juice increased the AUC and peak plasma concentrations of albendazole 3.1- and 3.2-fold, respectively. Unexpectedly, grapefruit juice shortened the $t_{½}$ of albendazole 46%.

[1] Nagy J, et al. *Am J Trop Med Hyg.* 2002;66(3):260.

* Asterisk indicates drugs cited in interaction reports.

Albendazole — *Praziquantel*

Albendazole* (*Albenza*)	Praziquantel* (*Biltricide*)

Significance	Onset	Severity	Documentation
4	☐ Rapid	☐ Major	☐ Established
	■ **Delayed**	■ **Moderate**	☐ Probable
		☐ Minor	☐ Suspected
			■ **Possible**
			☐ Unlikely

Effects Plasma concentrations of both ALBENDAZOLE and PRAZIQUANTEL may be elevated, increasing their pharmacologic effects and risk of adverse reactions.

Mechanism Unknown.

Management Monitor the clinical response and adjust treatment as needed.

Discussion

The potential for a 2-way pharmacokinetic interaction between albendazole and praziquantel was studied in 9 healthy volunteers.[1] Using a 3-phase, randomized, crossover design, each subject received a single dose of albendazole 400 mg, a single dose of praziquantel 1,500 mg, and coadministration of albendazole 400 mg and praziquantel 1,500 mg. Coadministration of albendazole and praziquantel increased the C_{max} and AUC of the albendazole active metabolite, (+)-albendazole sulfoxide, approximately 139% and 162%, respectively, compared with albendazole alone. Coadministration increased the C_{max} and AUC of (−)-(R)-praziquantel approximately 56% and 65%, respectively, compared with praziquantel alone.

[1] Lima RM, et al. *Br J Clin Pharmacol.* 2011;71(4):528.

* Asterisk indicates drugs cited in interaction reports.

Alfentanil — *Erythromycin*

Alfentanil* (eg, *Alfenta*)	Erythromycin* (eg, *Ery-Tab*)

Significance	Onset	Severity	Documentation
4	■ **Rapid**	□ Major	□ Established
	□ Delayed	■ **Moderate**	□ Probable
		□ Minor	□ Suspected
			■ **Possible**
			□ Unlikely

Effects The pharmacologic effects of ALFENTANIL may be increased.

Mechanism ERYTHROMYCIN is suspected to inhibit the metabolism of ALFENTANIL.

Management Consider administering a lower dose of ALFENTANIL or an alternative narcotic. Monitor patients for prolonged or recurrent respiratory depression and sedation.

Discussion

Among 30 patients studied, an isolated case of unexpected prolonged sedation occurred with alfentanil administration.[1] No causative factor was identified; however, the patient had received erythromycin concurrently. In another study involving 6 healthy volunteers, a 7-day course of erythromycin decreased the clearance and increased the elimination $t_{½}$ of a single dose of alfentanil.[2] Each individual received alfentanil 50 mcg/kg infused over a 5-minute period 3 times: 1 dose with no other medication (control dose); 1 dose 90 minutes after a single oral dose of erythromycin 500 mg; and 1 dose after a course of erythromycin 500 mg twice daily for 7 days. Naloxone (eg, *Narcan*) 0.4 mg was administered, and an additional 0.4 mg was mixed with alfentanil to block its sedative and respiratory depressant effects. Blood samples were drawn before and up to 8 hours after the start of the infusion. Following the 7-day course of antibiotic, the alfentanil clearance was decreased and the elimination $t_{½}$ was prolonged significantly ($P < 0.05$ and $P < 0.01$, respectively). While 2 subjects were affected minimally, the clearance was reduced 50% and the elimination $t_{½}$ nearly doubled in 2 other subjects during this phase of the investigation. No consistent changes were noted in heart rates, blood pressures, or respiratory rates during the study; however, nausea and a pale, distressed appearance were observed in 3 patients after the alfentanil dose that followed the 7-day course of erythromycin. A subsequent case report of unexpected, prolonged respiratory depression in a patient who received alfentanil for anesthetic induction and erythromycin preoperatively lends clinical support to the severity of this potential interaction.[3]

[1] Yate PM, et al. *Br J Anaesth.* 1986;58:1091.
[2] Bartkowski RR, et al. *Clin Pharmacol Ther.* 1989;46:99.
[3] Bartkowski RR, et al. *Anesthesiology.* 1990;73:566.

* Asterisk indicates drugs cited in interaction reports.

Alfentanil — *Ethanol*

Alfentanil* (eg, *Alfenta*)	Ethanol* (Alcohol, Ethyl Alcohol)

Significance	Onset	Severity	Documentation
2	■ **Rapid** □ Delayed	□ Major ■ **Moderate** □ Minor	□ Established □ Probable ■ **Suspected** □ Possible □ Unlikely

Effects Chronic ETHANOL consumption may produce a pharmacodynamic tolerance to ALFENTANIL.

Mechanism Unknown.

Management Patients who regularly consume ETHANOL may need higher doses of ALFENTANIL.

Discussion

The effects of ethanol ingestion on the pharmacodynamics of alfentanil were studied in 2 groups of women undergoing surgery for primary breast cancer.[1] Six patients in group 1 had an average daily consumption of ethanol 20 to 40 g (approximately two to four 3 oz glasses of wine). The patients in group 2 consumed more than 60 g of ethanol annually. Premedication consisted of oral temazepam (eg, *Restoril*) and atropine. Pancuronium was administered to prevent muscle rigidity. Nitrous oxide and an alfentanil infusion were initiated simultaneously. The average total alfentanil requirement to produce adequate anesthesia (somatic and autonomic control) was significantly higher ($P < 0.005$) in group 1 than in group 2 (3.7 vs 1.9 mcg/kg/min). The plasma alfentanil concentration, for which there is a 50% probability that a therapeutic response will occur during surgery, was significantly higher ($P < 0.001$) in group 1 than in group 2 (522 vs 208 ng/mL). The average plasma concentration at extubation in patients who did not need naloxone was significantly higher ($P < 0.005$) in group 1 than in group 2 (372 vs 176 ng/mL).

[1] Lemmens HJ, et al. *Anesthesiology*. 1989;71:669.

* Asterisk indicates drugs cited in interaction reports.

Aliskiren — *Atorvastatin*

Aliskiren* (*Tekturna*)	Atorvastatin* (eg, *Lipitor*)

Significance	Onset	Severity	Documentation
4	□ Rapid	□ Major	□ Established
	■ **Delayed**	■ **Moderate**	□ Probable
		□ Minor	□ Suspected
			■ **Possible**
			□ Unlikely

Effects ALISKIREN plasma concentrations may be elevated, increasing the pharmacologic effects and risk of adverse reactions.

Mechanism Increased absorption of ALISKIREN resulting from inhibition of P-gp expression by ATORVASTATIN.

Management Based on available data, no special precautions are needed.

Discussion

The potential interaction between atorvastatin and aliskiren was evaluated in 20 healthy subjects.[1] In an open-label, multiple-dose study, atorvastatin (80 mg daily) increased the aliskiren (300 mg daily) AUC and C_{max} 47% and 50%, respectively, compared with aliskiren alone. Aliskiren decreased the atorvastatin C_{max} 23%. The AUC of the active atorvastatin metabolite, o-hydroxy-atorvastatin, was reduced 11%. Adjustments to the starting dose of aliskiren are not likely to be needed.

[1] Vaidyanathan S, et al. *J Clin Pharmacol.* 2008;48(11):1323.

* Asterisk indicates drugs cited in interaction reports.

Aliskiren — *Azole Antifungal Agents*

Aliskiren* (*Tekturna*)	Itraconazole* (eg, *Sporanox*)	Ketoconazole* (eg, *Nizoral*)

Significance	Onset	Severity	Documentation
2	☐ Rapid ■ **Delayed**	☐ Major ■ **Moderate** ☐ Minor	☐ Established ☐ Probable ■ **Suspected** ☐ Possible ☐ Unlikely

Effects ALISKIREN plasma concentrations may be elevated, increasing the pharmacologic effects and risk of adverse reactions.

Mechanism Increased absorption of ALISKIREN resulting from inhibition of P-gp expression by certain AZOLE ANTIFUNGAL AGENTS. In addition, AZOLE ANTIFUNGAL AGENTS may inhibit ALISKIREN metabolism (CYP3A4).

Management Avoid coadministration of ALISKIREN and ITRACONAZOLE.[1,2] No ALISKIREN dose adjustment is needed in patients receiving ALISKIREN and KETOCONAZOLE concurrently.[1,3] However, close clinical monitoring is warranted.

Discussion

The potential interaction between ketoconazole and aliskiren was evaluated in 20 healthy subjects.[3] In an open-label, multiple-dose study, ketoconazole (200 mg twice daily) increased the aliskiren (300 mg daily) AUC and C_{max} 76% and 81%, respectively, compared with aliskiren alone. Coadministration of ketoconazole decreased aliskiren apparent total clearance from the plasma 43%. Adverse reactions were similar in patients receiving aliskiren alone compared with coadministration of aliskiren and ketoconazole. The effects of itraconazole on the pharmacokinetics of aliskiren were studied in a randomized, crossover study of 11 healthy subjects.[2] Each subject received itraconazole 200 mg as an initial dose followed by 100 mg twice daily for 5 days. On day 3, a single dose of aliskiren 150 mg was administered. Compared with giving aliskiren alone, coadministration of itraconazole increased the aliskiren C_{max} and AUC 5.8- and 6.5-fold, respectively. The aliskiren elimination $t_{½}$ was not affected. Plasma renin activity 24 hours after aliskiren administration was 68% lower during coadministration of itraconazole and aliskiren compared with aliskiren alone.

[1] *Tekturna* [package insert]. East Hanover, NJ: Novartis Pharmaceuticals Corporation; February 2011.
[2] Tapaninen T, et al. *J Clin Pharmacol.* 2011;51(3):359.
[3] Vaidyanathan S, et al. *J Clin Pharmacol.* 2008;48(11):1323.

* Asterisk indicates drugs cited in interaction reports.

Aliskiren — *Cyclosporine*

Aliskiren*	Cyclosporine*
(*Tekturna*)	(eg, *Neoral*)

Significance	Onset	Severity	Documentation
2	☐ Rapid	☐ Major	☐ Established
	■ **Delayed**	■ **Moderate**	☐ Probable
		☐ Minor	■ **Suspected**
			☐ Possible
			☐ Unlikely

Effects ALISKIREN plasma concentrations may be elevated, increasing the pharmacologic effects and risk of adverse reactions.

Mechanism Inhibition of P-gp–mediated efflux transport in the intestine by CYCLOSPORINE is suspected.

Management Avoid coadministration.[1]

Discussion

The effect of cyclosporine on the pharmacokinetics of aliskiren was evaluated in 8 healthy patients.[2] In an open-label, single-dose study, each subject received a single dose of aliskiren 75 mg alone, coadministration of aliskiren 75 mg with cyclosporine 200 mg, and aliskiren 75 mg with cyclosporine 600 mg. Coadministration of aliskiren and cyclosporine increased the aliskiren AUC and C_{max} approximately 4- to 5-fold and 2.5-fold, respectively. The mean $t_{½}$ of aliskiren increased from 25 to 45 hours. Coadministration of aliskiren and cyclosporine increased the number of adverse reactions, primarily hot flashes and GI symptoms. Aliskiren did not affect the pharmacokinetics of cyclosporine.

[1] *Tekturna* [package insert]. East Hanover, NJ: Novartis Pharmaceuticals Corporation; October 2011.

[2] Rebello S, et al. *J Clin Pharmacol.* 2011;51(11):1549.

* Asterisk indicates drugs cited in interaction reports.

Aliskiren — *Food*

Aliskiren* (*Tekturna*)	Apple Juice* Grapefruit Juice*	Orange Juice*

Significance	Onset	Severity	Documentation
2	☐ Rapid ■ **Delayed**	☐ Major ■ **Moderate** ☐ Minor	☐ Established ☐ Probable ■ **Suspected** ☐ Possible ☐ Unlikely

Effects

ALISKIREN plasma concentrations and pharmacologic effects may be decreased.

Mechanism

Inhibition of organic anion–transporting polypeptide 2B1 (OATP2B1)–mediated absorption of ALISKIREN from the GI lumen by APPLE JUICE, GRAPEFRUIT JUICE, and ORANGE JUICE is suspected.

Management

Advise patients taking ALISKIREN to avoid APPLE JUICE, GRAPEFRUIT products (including GRAPEFRUIT JUICE), and ORANGE JUICE, and to take ALISKIREN with a liquid other than these juices. Caution patients taking ALISKIREN not to use nonprescription or herbal products without consulting their health care provider.

Discussion

Apple juice – In a randomized, crossover study, the effects of apple juice on the pharmacokinetics of aliskiren were evaluated in 12 healthy volunteers.[1] Each subject ingested 200 mL of apple juice or water 3 times daily for 5 days. On day 3, a single oral dose of aliskiren 150 mg was administered. Compared with water, apple juice decreased aliskiren C_{max} and AUC by 84% and 63%, respectively. The renal clearance and $t_{½}$ of aliskiren were not altered. Plasma renin activity was 67% higher at 24 h after apple juice ingestion compared with water.

Grapefruit juice – In a randomized, crossover study, the effects of grapefruit juice on the pharmacokinetics of aliskiren were evaluated in 11 healthy volunteers.[2] Each subject ingested 200 mL of grapefruit juice or water 3 times per day for 5 days. On day 3, subjects took a single dose of aliskiren 150 mg. Compared with water, taking aliskiren with grapefruit juice decreased the aliskiren C_{max} and AUC by 81% and 61%, respectively, and reduced the elimination $t_{½}$ from 26.1 to 23.6 h. In a crossover study, 28 healthy subjects received a single oral dose of aliskiren 300 mg with 300 mL of water or grapefruit juice.[3] Compared with water, grapefruit juice decreased the mean AUC and C_{max} of aliskiren 38% and 61%, respectively.

Orange juice – In a randomized, crossover study, the effects of orange juice on the pharmacokinetics of aliskiren were evaluated in 12 healthy volunteers.[1] Each subject ingested 200 mL of orange juice or water 3 times daily for 5 days. On day 3, a single oral dose of aliskiren 150 mg was administered. Compared with water, orange juice decreased aliskiren C_{max} and AUC by 80% and 62%, respectively. The renal clearance and $t_{½}$ of aliskiren were not altered. Plasma renin activity was 87% higher at 24 h after orange juice ingestion compared with water.

[1] Tapaninen T, et al. *Br J Clin Pharmacol.* 2011;71(5):718.
[2] Tapaninen T, et al. *Clin Pharmacol Ther.* 2010;88(3):339.
[3] Rebello S, et al. *Eur J Clin Pharmacol.* 2012;68(5):697.

* Asterisk indicates drugs cited in interaction reports.

Aliskiren — Rifamycins

Aliskiren* (*Tekturna*)	Rifabutin (*Mycobutin*)	Rifapentine (*Priftin*)
	Rifampin* (eg, *Rifadin*)	

Significance	Onset	Severity	Documentation
4	☐ Rapid	☐ Major	☐ Established
	■ **Delayed**	■ **Moderate**	☐ Probable
		☐ Minor	☐ Suspected
			■ **Possible**
			☐ Unlikely

Effects ALISKIREN plasma concentrations may be reduced, decreasing the pharmacologic effects.

Mechanism Increased metabolism (CYP3A4) and induction of P-gp in the intestine by RIFAMPIN are suspected, resulting in increased metabolism and decreased GI absorption of ALISKIREN.

Management Monitor blood pressure response to ALISKIREN when RIFAMYCINS are started or stopped. Adjust the ALISKIREN dose as needed.

Discussion

The effects of rifampin on the pharmacokinetics and pharmacodynamics of aliskiren were studied in 12 healthy volunteers.[1] Using a randomized, crossover design, each subject received rifampin 600 mg or placebo once daily for 5 days. On day 6, a single dose of aliskiren 150 mg was administered. Pretreatment with rifampin reduced the aliskiren C_{max} and AUC 39% and 56%, respectively, compared with placebo. Rifampin did not affect aliskiren elimination t½ or renal clearance. Plasma renin activity 24 hours after taking aliskiren was 61% higher after pretreatment with rifampin compared with placebo.

[1] Tapaninen T, et al. *Eur J Clin Pharmacol.* 2010;66(5):497.

* Asterisk indicates drugs cited in interaction reports. Based on pharmacologic and pharmacokinetic considerations, similar interactions may occur with other drugs that are listed.

Aliskiren — *Verapamil*

Aliskiren* (*Tekturna*)	Verapamil* (eg, *Isoptin*)

Significance	Onset	Severity	Documentation
4	☐ Rapid ■ **Delayed**	☐ Major ■ **Moderate** ☐ Minor	☐ Established ☐ Probable ☐ Suspected ■ **Possible** ☐ Unlikely

Effects ALISKIREN plasma concentrations may be elevated, increasing the pharmacologic effects and risk of adverse reactions.

Mechanism Inhibition of ALISKIREN metabolism (CYP3A4) and/or P-gp transport is suspected.

Management No dosage adjustments appear to be necessary. Consider monitoring blood pressure more frequently during coadministration of ALISKIREN with VERAPAMIL and when coadministration is started or stopped.

Discussion

The effect of verapamil on the pharmacokinetics of aliskiren was studied in 18 healthy subjects.[1] Each subject received a single dose of aliskiren 300 mg alone and after 8 days of treatment with verapamil 240 mg daily. Compared with giving aliskiren alone, pretreatment with verapamil increased aliskiren C_{max} and AUC approximately 2-fold. Single-dose administration of aliskiren did not alter the verapamil plasma concentration to a clinically important degree.

[1] Rebello S, et al. *J Clin Pharmacol.* 2011;51(2):218.

* Asterisk indicates drugs cited in interaction reports.

Allopurinol — *ACE Inhibitors*

Allopurinol* (eg, *Zyloprim*)	Captopril* Enalapril* (eg, *Vasotec*)

Significance	Onset	Severity	Documentation
4	☐ Rapid ■ **Delayed**	■ **Major** ☐ Moderate ☐ Minor	☐ Established ☐ Probable ☐ Suspected ■ **Possible** ☐ Unlikely

Effects The risk of hypersensitivity reactions may be higher when ALLOPURINOL and CAPTOPRIL or ENALAPRIL are given together than when each drug is administered alone.

Mechanism Unknown.

Management Hypersensitivity reactions are unpredictable if there has been no previous reaction to either drug. If manifestations of hypersensitivity develop, discontinue both drugs. Manage symptoms of the hypersensitivity reaction.

Discussion

Two cases have been reported involving a suspected hypersensitivity reaction in patients receiving allopurinol and the ACE inhibitor captopril.[1,2] Severe hypersensitivity reactions have been reported with captopril and allopurinol when given alone.[3-6] A 50-year-old man taking enalapril and furosemide (eg, *Lasix*) experienced symptoms of anaphylaxis and severe coronary spasm within 20 minutes of taking allopurinol.[7] The potential allopurinol-captopril interaction requires verification.

[1] Pennell DJ, et al. *Lancet.* 1984;1(8374):463.
[2] Samanta A, et al. *Lancet.* 1984;1(8378):679.
[3] Lang PG Jr. *South Med J.* 1979;72(11):1361.
[4] Lupton GP, et al. *J Am Acad Dermatol.* 1979;1(4):365.
[5] Burkle WS, et al. *Drug Intell Clin Pharm.* 1979;13(4):218.
[6] Hande KR, et al. *Am J Med.* 1984;76(1):47.
[7] Ahmad S. *Chest.* 1995;108(2):586.

* Asterisk indicates drugs cited in interaction reports.

Allopurinol ✕ *Aluminum Salts*

Allopurinol	Aluminum Salts	
Allopurinol* (eg, *Zyloprim*)	Aluminum Hydroxide* (eg, *Amphojel*)	Kaolin-Pectin (eg, *Kaodene*)
	Attapulgite (eg, *K-pek*)	Magaldrate (eg, *Riopan*)

Significance	Onset	Severity	Documentation
4	■ **Rapid**	□ Major	□ Established
	□ Delayed	■ **Moderate**	□ Probable
		□ Minor	□ Suspected
			■ **Possible**
			□ Unlikely

Effects The pharmacologic effects of ALLOPURINOL may be decreased.

Mechanism Unknown. However, GI absorption of ALLOPURINOL may be decreased by ALUMINUM SALTS.

Management If an interaction is suspected, administer ALLOPURINOL at least 3 hours before the ALUMINUM SALT.

Discussion

Coadministration of aluminum hydroxide and allopurinol decreased the activity of allopurinol in 3 patients on chronic hemodialysis.[1] The patients were receiving aluminum hydroxide 5.7 g/day and allopurinol 300 mg/day. All patients had elevated uric acid concentrations (12.3 to 25.7 mg/dL). When serum uric acid levels did not decrease with allopurinol administration, allopurinol was given 3 hours prior to antacid ingestion. After 1 to 2 months of treatment with this modified dosing regimen, uric acid levels decreased in all patients. The amount of the decrease ranged from about 40% to 65%. A rechallenge in 1 patient involving coadministration of both drugs produced a rise in serum uric acid concentration to 13.4 mg/dL.

Because of the small number of patients involved, consider these data preliminary. Additional studies are needed.

[1] Weissman I, et al. *Ann Intern Med.* 1987;107(5):787.

* Asterisk indicates drugs cited in interaction reports. Based on pharmacologic and pharmacokinetic considerations, similar interactions may occur with other drugs that are listed.

Allopurinol — *Probenecid*

Allopurinol* (eg, *Zyloprim*)	Probenecid*

Significance	Onset	Severity	Documentation
5	☐ Rapid	☐ Major	☐ Established
	■ **Delayed**	☐ Moderate	☐ Probable
		■ **Minor**	☐ Suspected
			■ **Possible**
			☐ Unlikely

Effects ALLOPURINOL combined with PROBENECID produces a beneficial drug-drug interaction. The combination may increase the uric acid–lowering effect of ALLOPURINOL.

Mechanism The metabolism of PROBENECID may be impaired by ALLOPURINOL, thereby prolonging the t½ of the uricosuric. Also, PROBENECID may enhance the renal clearance of oxipurinol, the primary metabolite of ALLOPURINOL.

Management No particular dosing or monitoring precautions other than those associated with the use of each drug alone are required.

Discussion

The coadministration of allopurinol and probenecid does not need to be avoided; it generally appears to be a beneficial combination.[1-3] The deleterious effects of this drug combination are not apparent through the published literature.[4-6]

[1] Yue TF, et al. *Am J Med.* 1964;37:885.
[2] Rundles RW, et al. *Ann Intern Med.* 1966;64(2):229.
[3] Stocker SL, et al. *Clin Pharmacokinet.* 2008;47(2):111.
[4] Elion GB, et al. *Am J Med.* 1968;45(1):69.
[5] Tjandramaga TB, et al. *Pharmacology.* 1972;8(4):259.
[6] Horwitz D, et al. *Eur J Clin Pharmacol.* 1977;12(2):133.

* Asterisk indicates drugs cited in interaction reports.

Allopurinol — *Thiazide Diuretics*

Allopurinol	Thiazide Diuretics	
Allopurinol* (eg, *Zyloprim*)	Bendroflumethiazide	Hydroflumethiazide (eg, *Saluron*)
	Chlorothiazide* (eg, *Diuril*)	Indapamide
	Chlorthalidone (eg, *Thalitone*)	Methyclothiazide (eg, *Enduron*)
	Hydrochlorothiazide* (eg, *HydroDIURIL*)	Metolazone (eg, *Zaroxolyn*)

Significance	Onset	Severity	Documentation
5	☐ Rapid	■ **Major**	☐ Established
	■ **Delayed**	☐ Moderate	☐ Probable
		☐ Minor	☐ Suspected
			☐ Possible
			■ **Unlikely**

Effects THIAZIDE DIURETICS coadministered with ALLOPURINOL therapy have been associated with an increase in the incidence of hypersensitivity reactions to ALLOPURINOL.

Mechanism Unknown.

Management If a hypersensitivity reaction to ALLOPURINOL develops, assess the clinical status of the patient to determine the causative agent. Alter therapy as needed.

Discussion

A rare but potentially severe hypersensitivity reaction from allopurinol is well documented.[1-6] When these symptoms of hypersensitivity (eg, fever, chills, eosinophilia, pruritus, maculopapular rash, hepatic and renal toxicity) occur, it is usually within 4 weeks of initiating allopurinol therapy and may last for several weeks. Allopurinol toxicity and hypersensitivity have been associated with use in patients with renal insufficiency. Allopurinol toxicity/hypersensitivity also has been associated with the combined use of allopurinol and thiazide diuretics.[1] The cause-effect relationship is poorly defined. In 8 volunteers, hydrochlorothiazide 50 mg/day was evaluated to determine the extent to which it might affect the renal clearance and $t_{1/2}$ of oxipurinol, the major metabolite of allopurinol.[7] No change in oxipurinol renal clearance or $t_{1/2}$ was noted. Allopurinol hypersensitivity is apparently related more to individual susceptibility and renal insufficiency than concurrent use of thiazide diuretics. Evidence that thiazides predispose to allopurinol hypersensitivity reactions is lacking. Observations suggesting a causal relationship appear to be coincidental and remain unsubstantiated.

1 Mills RM Jr. *JAMA.* 1971;216(5):799.
2 Young JL Jr, et al. *Arch Intern Med.* 1974;134(3):553.
3 Lang PG Jr. *South Med J.* 1979;72(11):1361.
4 Burkle WS. *Drug Intell Clin Pharm.* 1979;13:218.
5 Lupton GP, et al. *J Am Acad Dermatol.* 1979;1(4):365.
6 Hande KR, et al. *Am J Med.* 1984;76(1):47.
7 Hande KR, et al. *Am J Med Sci.* 1986;292(4):213.

* Asterisk indicates drugs cited in interaction reports. Based on pharmacologic and pharmacokinetic considerations, similar interactions may occur with other drugs that are listed.

Alosetron — *Fluvoxamine*

Alosetron* (*Lotronex*)	Fluvoxamine* (eg, *Luvox*)

Significance	Onset	Severity	Documentation
2	☐ Rapid ■ **Delayed**	☐ Major ■ **Moderate** ☐ Minor	☐ Established ☐ Probable ■ **Suspected** ☐ Possible ☐ Unlikely

Effects ALOSETRON plasma concentrations may be elevated, increasing the risk of adverse reactions.

Mechanism Inhibition of ALOSETRON metabolism (CYP1A2) by FLUVOXAMINE.

Management Coadministration of ALOSETRON and FLUVOXAMINE is contraindicated.

Discussion

The effects of fluvoxamine on the pharmacokinetics of alosetron were studied in 40 healthy women.[1] All subjects received fluvoxamine in escalating dosages from 50 to 200 mg/day for 16 days. Alosetron 1 mg was administered on the last day. Pretreatment with fluvoxamine increased mean alosetron plasma concentrations approximately 6-fold and prolonged the $t_{1/2}$ approximately 3-fold.

The basis for this monograph is information on file with the manufacturer. Clinical data are needed to further assess this interaction.

[1] *Lotronex* [package insert]. San Diego, CA: Prometheus Laboratories, Inc; February 2008.

* Asterisk indicates drugs cited in interaction reports.

Alpha-1 Adrenergic Blockers ⨯ Azole Antifungal Agents

Alpha-1 Adrenergic Blockers		Azole Antifungal Agents	
Alfuzosin* (eg, *Uroxatral*)	Tamsulosin* (eg, *Flomax*)	Itraconazole* (eg, *Sporanox*)	Ketoconazole* (eg, *Nizoral*)
Silodosin* (*Rapaflo*)			

Significance	Onset	Severity	Documentation
2	☐ Rapid ■ **Delayed**	☐ Major ■ **Moderate** ☐ Minor	☐ Established ☐ Probable ■ **Suspected** ☐ Possible ☐ Unlikely

Effects ALFUZOSIN and SILODOSIN blood concentrations may be elevated, increasing pharmacologic effects and adverse reactions.

Mechanism AZOLE ANTIFUNGAL AGENTS may inhibit the hepatic metabolism (CYP3A4) of ALFUZOSIN or SILODOSIN.

Management Coadministration of ALFUZOSIN or SILODOSIN and ITRACONAZOLE or KETOCONAZOLE is contraindicated.

Discussion

Repeat administration of ketoconazole 400 mg once daily increased tamsulosin C_{max} and AUC 2.2- and 2.8-fold, respectively, after a single dose of tamsulosin 0.4 mg compared with giving tamsulosin alone.[1] The terminal $t_{½}$ of tamsulosin increased from 10.5 to 11.8 hours. There were no clinically important changes in hemodynamic responses during orthostatic stress testing. Repeat administration of ketoconazole 400 mg increased alfuzosin C_{max} and AUC 2.3- and 3.2-fold, respectively, after a single dose of alfuzosin 10 mg.[2] Because of the increased exposure to alfuzosin and silodosin, potent inhibitors of CYP3A4 (eg, itraconazole, ketoconazole) should not be coadministered with alfuzosin or silodosin. Coadministration of a single dose of silodosin 8 mg with ketoconazole 400 mg increased the silodosin C_{max} and AUC 3.8- and 3.2-fold, respectively.[3] Similarly, coadministration of silodosin with ketoconazole 200 mg increased the silodosin C_{max} and AUC 3.7- and 2.9-fold, respectively.[3]

1 Troost J, et al. *Br J Clin Pharmacol.* 2011;72(2):247.
2 *Uroxatral* [package insert]. New York, NY: Sanofi-Synthelabo Inc; June 2003.
3 *Rapaflo* [package insert]. Corona, CA: Watson Pharmaceuticals Inc; September 2008.

* Asterisk indicates drugs cited in interaction reports.

Alpha-1 Adrenergic Blockers — *Ethanol*

Doxazosin (eg, *Cardura*)	Tamsulosin (eg, *Flomax*)	Ethanol* (Alcohol, Ethyl Alcohol)
Prazosin* (eg, *Minipress*)	Terazosin	

Significance	Onset	Severity	Documentation
2	■ **Rapid**	□ Major	□ Established
	□ Delayed	■ **Moderate**	□ Probable
		□ Minor	■ **Suspected**
			□ Possible
			□ Unlikely

Effects Increased risk of hypotension, particularly in patients who are deficient in aldehyde dehydrogenase (often noted in patients who flush after ALCOHOL ingestion).

Mechanism It is suspected that inhibition of the sympathetic nervous system by ALPHA-1 ADRENERGIC BLOCKERS may accentuate ALCOHOL-induced hypotension.

Management Advise patients taking ALPHA-1 ADRENERGIC BLOCKERS, particularly those patients who flush after ALCOHOL ingestion, to avoid ALCOHOL.

Discussion

The effects of prazosin on alcohol-induced BP changes were studied in 10 Japanese men with mild hypertension.[1] Each patient received alcohol 1 mL/kg or an isocaloric drink before and after 5 to 7 days of treatment with prazosin 1 mg 3 times daily. Before prazosin administration, alcohol ingestion reduced BP. Alcohol-induced hypotension was augmented by prazosin administration.

[1] Kawano Y, et al. *Am J Hypertens.* 2000;13(3):307.

* Asterisk indicates drugs cited in interaction reports. Based on pharmacologic and pharmacokinetic considerations, similar interactions may occur with other drugs that are listed.

Alpha-1 Adrenergic Blockers — *HCV Protease Inhibitors*

Alfuzosin* (eg, *Uroxatral*)	Silodosin (*Rapaflo*)	Boceprevir* (*Victrelis*)	Telaprevir* (*Incivek*)

Significance	Onset	Severity	Documentation
2	☐ Rapid ■ **Delayed**	☐ Major ■ **Moderate** ☐ Minor	☐ Established ☐ Probable ■ **Suspected** ☐ Possible ☐ Unlikely

Effects ALPHA-1 ADRENERGIC BLOCKER plasma concentrations may be elevated, increasing the pharmacologic effects and risk of adverse reactions (eg, hypotension, cardiac arrhythmias).

Mechanism ALPHA-1 ADRENERGIC BLOCKER metabolism (CYP3A) may be inhibited by HEPATITIS C VIRUS (HCV) PROTEASE INHIBITORS.

Management Coadministration of ALFUZOSIN and HCV PROTEASE INHIBITORS is contraindicated.[1,2]

Discussion

Concurrent use of strong CYP3A4 inhibitors, such as boceprevir, may elevate alfuzosin or silodosin plasma concentrations, increasing the risk of serious adverse effects (eg, hypotension).[1,2] Concomitant use of alfuzosin and boceprevir or telaprevir is contraindicated.

The basis for this monograph is information on file with the manufacturer. Published clinical data are needed to further assess this interaction. Because of the seriousness of the cardiac problem, clinical evaluation of the interaction in humans is not likely to be forthcoming.

[1] *Victrelis* [package insert]. Whitehouse Station, NJ: Schering Corporation; May 2011.

[2] *Incivek* [package insert]. Cambridge, MA: Vertex Pharmaceuticals Incorporated; May 2011.

* Asterisk indicates drugs cited in interaction reports. Based on pharmacologic and pharmacokinetic considerations, similar interactions may occur with other drugs that are listed.

Alpha-1 Adrenergic Blockers	*Macrolide Antibiotics*
Silodosin* (*Rapaflo*)	Clarithromycin* (eg, *Biaxin*)

Significance	Onset	Severity	Documentation
2	☐ Rapid ■ **Delayed**	☐ Major ■ **Moderate** ☐ Minor	☐ Established ☐ Probable ■ **Suspected** ☐ Possible ☐ Unlikely

Effects SILODOSIN plasma concentrations may be elevated, increasing the pharmacologic effects and adverse reactions.

Mechanism CLARITHROMYCIN may inhibit the hepatic metabolism (CYP3A4) of SILODOSIN.

Management Coadministration of SILODOSIN and CLARITHROMYCIN is contraindicated.

Discussion

Administration of strong CYP3A4 inhibitors (eg, clarithromycin) may increase silodosin C_{max} and AUC.[1] Because of the increased risk of exposure to silodosin, strong inhibitors of CYP3A4 (eg, clarithromycin) are contraindicated.

[1] *Rapaflo* [package insert]. Corona, CA: Watson Pharmaceuticals Inc; September 2008.

* Asterisk indicates drugs cited in interaction reports.

Alpha-1 Adrenergic Blockers — Protease Inhibitors

Alfuzosin* (eg, *Uroxatral*)	Silodosin* (*Rapaflo*)	Ritonavir* (*Norvir*)

Significance	Onset	Severity	Documentation
2	☐ Rapid ■ **Delayed**	☐ Major ■ **Moderate** ☐ Minor	☐ Established ☐ Probable ■ **Suspected** ☐ Possible ☐ Unlikely

Effects ALFUZOSIN and SILODOSIN blood concentrations may be elevated, increasing the pharmacologic and adverse reactions.

Mechanism PROTEASE INHIBITORS may inhibit the hepatic metabolism (CYP3A4) of ALFUZOSIN or SILODOSIN.

Management Coadministration of ALFUZOSIN or SILODOSIN and RITONAVIR is contraindicated.

Discussion

Administration of potent CYP3A4 inhibitors (eg, ritonavir) may increase alfuzosin C_{max} and AUC.[1,2] Because of the increased risk of exposure to alfuzosin or silodosin, do not coadminister potent inhibitors of CYP3A4 (eg, ritonavir) with alfuzosin or silodosin.

1 *Uroxatral* [package insert]. New York, NY: Sanofi-Synthelabo Inc; June 2003.

2 *Rapaflo* [package insert]. Corona, CA: Watson Pharmaceuticals Inc; September 2008.

* Asterisk indicates drugs cited in interaction reports.

Alpha-1 Adrenergic Blockers — Serotonin Reuptake Inhibitors

Alpha-1 Adrenergic Blockers	Serotonin Reuptake Inhibitors	
Tamsulosin* (eg, *Flomax*)	Duloxetine (*Cymbalta*)	Paroxetine* (eg, *Paxil*)
	Fluoxetine (eg, *Prozac*)	

Significance	Onset	Severity	Documentation
4	□ Rapid	□ Major	□ Established
	■ **Delayed**	■ **Moderate**	□ Probable
		□ Minor	□ Suspected
			■ **Possible**
			□ Unlikely

Effects TAMSULOSIN plasma concentrations may be elevated, increasing the pharmacologic effects and risk of adverse reactions.

Mechanism Certain SEROTONIN REUPTAKE INHIBITORS may inhibit the metabolism (CYP2D6) of TAMSULOSIN.

Management Monitor the clinical response to TAMSULOSIN. If an interaction is suspected, adjust the TAMSULOSIN dose as needed.

Discussion

The effects of paroxetine on the pharmacokinetics and pharmacodynamics of tamsulosin were studied in 24 healthy men.[1] Using an open-label, randomized, crossover design, each subject received a single oral dose of tamsulosin 0.4 mg alone or during administration of paroxetine 10 mg once daily for 3 days, then paroxetine 20 mg once daily for 9 days, and finally, paroxetine 10 mg once daily for 3 days to taper out the regimen. On day 11 of paroxetine administration, a single oral dose of tamsulosin 0.4 mg was administered. Compared with giving tamsulosin alone, pretreatment with paroxetine increased the mean C_{max} and AUC of tamsulosin 1.34- and 1.64-fold, respectively. The terminal $t_{½}$ of tamsulosin increased from 11.4 to 15.3 hours. There were no clinically important changes in hemodynamic responses during orthostatic stress testing.

[1] Troost J, et al. *Br J Clin Pharmacol.* 2011;72(2):247.

* Asterisk indicates drugs cited in interaction reports. Based on pharmacologic and pharmacokinetic considerations, similar interactions may occur with other drugs that are listed.

Alpha-1 Adrenergic Blockers — *Tadalafil*

Alfuzosin* (eg, *Uroxatral*)	Silodosin* (*Rapaflo*)	Tadalafil* (eg, *Cialis*)
Doxazosin* (eg, *Cardura*)	Tamsulosin* (eg, *Flomax*)	
Prazosin* (eg, *Minipress*)	Terazosin*	

Significance	Onset	Severity	Documentation
2	■ **Rapid**	□ Major	□ Established
	□ Delayed	■ **Moderate**	□ Probable
		□ Minor	■ **Suspected**
			□ Possible
			□ Unlikely

Effects The BP-lowering effect of ALPHA-1 ADRENERGIC BLOCKERS may be increased.

Mechanism Additive pharmacologic effects.

Management Ensure that patients are stable on ALPHA-1 ADRENERGIC BLOCKER therapy prior to starting TADALAFIL therapy, and start TADALAFIL at the lowest recommended dose.[1]

Discussion

In separate double-blind, randomized studies, the effect of placebo or tadalafil 20 mg on the hypotensive effect of doxazosin and the effect of placebo or tadalafil 10 to 20 mg on the hypotensive effect of tamsulosin were evaluated in healthy men.[2] A single dose of placebo or tadalafil was administered after each subject was pretreated for 7 days with doxazosin 8 mg/day or tamsulosin 0.4 mg/day. Tadalafil 20 mg augmented the hypotensive effect of doxazosin. The mean maximal decrease in standing systolic BP was 9.8 mm Hg greater with coadministration of tadalafil and doxazosin compared with placebo and doxazosin. Doses of tadalafil 10 and 20 mg did not affect the hypotensive effect of tamsulosin. In a study in healthy men, coadministration of tamsulosin 0.4 mg/day and tadalafil 5 mg/day was well tolerated.[3] However, coadministration of tadalafil 5 mg/day with increasing dosages of doxazosin of up to 4 mg/day resulted in a low incidence of hypotension compared with coadministration of placebo and doxazosin.

1 *Cialis* [package insert]. Indianapolis, IN: Eli Lilly & Co; January 2008.
2 Guillaume M, et al. *J Clin Pharmacol.* 2007;47(10):1303.
3 Kloner RA, et al. *J Urol.* 2004;172(5 Pt 1):1935.

* Asterisk indicates drugs cited in interaction reports.

Alteplase — *Anticoagulants*

Alteplase* (*Activase*)	Warfarin* (eg, *Coumadin*)

Significance	Onset	Severity	Documentation
1	■ **Rapid**	■ **Major**	☐ Established
	☐ Delayed	☐ Moderate	☐ Probable
		☐ Minor	■ **Suspected**
			☐ Possible
			☐ Unlikely

Effects Risk of serious bleeding may be increased.

Mechanism Additive or synergistic effects.

Management Combined use is contraindicated.

Discussion

Alteplase therapy is contraindicated in patients with acute ischemic stroke in situations when there is a known bleeding diathesis, including concomitant use of oral anticoagulants (eg, warfarin), because of an increased risk of bleeding that could result in disability or death.[1] In a retrospective study, alteplase administration for ischemic stroke to patients taking warfarin with INRs below 1.7 resulted in hemorrhagic stroke in 30.8% of cases, compared with 3.2% in patients not taking warfarin.[2]

[1] *Activase* [package insert]. South San Francisco, CA: Genentech Inc; May 3, 2002.

[2] Prabhakaran S, et al. *Arch Neurol.* 2010;67(5):559.

* Asterisk indicates drugs cited in interaction reports.

Alteplase — *Heparin*

Alteplase* (*Activase*)	Heparin*

Significance	Onset	Severity	Documentation
1	■ **Rapid**	■ **Major**	□ Established
	□ Delayed	□ Moderate	□ Probable
		□ Minor	■ **Suspected**
			□ Possible
			□ Unlikely

Effects Risk of serious bleeding may be increased.

Mechanism Additive or synergistic effects.

Management Combined use is contraindicated.

Discussion

Alteplase therapy in patients with acute ischemic stroke is contraindicated in situations in which there is a known bleeding diathesis, including administration of heparin within 48 hours preceding the onset of stroke and when activated partial thromboplastin time (APTT) is elevated at presentation, because of an increased risk of bleeding that could result in disability or death.[1]

The basis for this monograph is information on file with the manufacturer. Because of the seriousness of the possible reaction, clinical evaluation of this interaction in humans is not likely to be forthcoming.

[1] *Activase* [package insert]. South San Francisco, CA: Genentech Inc; May 3, 2002.

* Asterisk indicates drugs cited in interaction reports.

Alteplase — *Nitroglycerin*

Alteplase* (tPA; *Activase*)	Nitroglycerin* (eg, *Nitrostat*)

Significance	Onset	Severity	Documentation
1	■ **Rapid**	■ **Major**	□ Established
	□ Delayed	□ Moderate	■ **Probable**
		□ Minor	□ Suspected
			□ Possible
			□ Unlikely

Effects Plasma tissue-type plasminogen activator (tPA) antigen concentrations are decreased, indicating impairment of the thrombolytic effect of ALTEPLASE (tPA).

Mechanism NITROGLYCERIN may enhance hepatic blood flow, facilitating hepatic metabolism of tPA.

Management Avoid use of NITROGLYCERIN with tPA. If NITROGLYCERIN is considered critical, use the lowest effective dose, realizing that less than optimal thrombolytic effect may be achieved with tPA. Be prepared to pursue alternative therapies to achieve reperfusion.

Discussion

In a nonrandomized study, 11 patients were treated with tPA plus saline solution (group I), and 36 patients received tPA plus IV nitroglycerin (group II).[1] All patients received aspirin 165 mg on admission and tPA 100 mg infused over 3 hours followed by a 5000 U heparin bolus and 1000 U/hr infusion. Reperfusion occurred in 91% of group I and 44% of group II patients. Mean tPA plasma antigen concentrations were lower and plasminogen activator inhibitor-1 concentrations were higher in group II than in group I patients. These differences persisted for more than 6 hours after tPA infusion. In a controlled study, 60 patients were randomized to receive tPA alone (group A, 33 patients) or tPA plus nitroglycerin infused at 100 mcg/min (group B, 27 patients).[2] All patients were given a 5000 U heparin bolus and aspirin 300 mg followed by tPA 100 mg infused over 3 hours. A heparin infusion followed the tPA infusion in all patients. Group A patients reperfused faster (20 vs 38 minutes), more often (76% vs 56%), and had fewer reocclusions (24% vs 53%) than group B patients. Group A patients also had higher peak plasma levels of tPA and fewer in-hospital adverse events.

[1] Nicolini FA, et al. *Am J Cardiol.* 1994;74:662.

[2] Romeo F, et al. *Am Heart J.* 1995;130:692.

* Asterisk indicates drugs cited in interaction reports.

Amantadine — *Bupropion*

Amantadine* (*Symmetrel*)	Bupropion* (eg, *Wellbutrin*)

Significance	Onset	Severity	Documentation
4	☐ Rapid ■ **Delayed**	☐ Major ■ **Moderate** ☐ Minor	☐ Established ☐ Probable ☐ Suspected ■ **Possible** ☐ Unlikely

Effects Increased risk of neurotoxicity.

Mechanism Possibly synergistic or additive central dopamine effects.

Management Observe the patient for symptoms of neurotoxicity. If neurotoxicity occurs, it may be necessary to discontinue both drugs.

Discussion

The nursing home records of 8 depressed patients receiving bupropion (75 to 200 mg/day) were reviewed.[1] Three of 6 patients who had received bupropion and amantadine concurrently developed symptoms of neurotoxicity (eg, restlessness, agitation, gross motor tremors, ataxia, gait disturbances, dizziness, vertigo). Symptoms were sufficiently severe in 2 patients that hospitalization was required. In all 3 patients, symptoms resolved within 72 hours of discontinuing amantadine and bupropion.

Additional documentation is needed to determine if the reaction was the result of amantadine therapy alone or a drug interaction.

[1] Trappler B, et al. *J Clin Psychiatry*. 2000;61:61.

* Asterisk indicates drugs cited in interaction reports.

Amantadine — *Quinine Derivatives*

Amantadine* (eg, *Symmetrel*)	Quinidine*	Quinine*

Significance	Onset	Severity	Documentation
4	■ **Rapid**	□ Major	□ Established
	□ Delayed	■ **Moderate**	□ Probable
		□ Minor	□ Suspected
			■ **Possible**
			□ Unlikely

Effects Serum AMANTADINE concentrations may be elevated in men but not women. The risk of AMANTADINE toxicity (eg, ataxia, mental confusion) may be increased.

Mechanism QUININE DERIVATIVES may inhibit renal clearance of AMANTADINE in men.

Management Consider monitoring patients for CNS side effects if these agents are coadministered.

Discussion

The effects of oral quinidine or quinine on the renal clearance of amantadine in 18 healthy volunteers were investigated in a randomized, crossover study.[1] Subjects consisted of 5 men and 4 women from 27 to 39 years of age and 4 men and 5 women from 60 to 72 years of age. Subjects received 3 mg/kg amantadine the evening before receiving quinidine 200 mg, quinine 200 mg, or no additional drug. Renal clearance of amantadine was inhibited by quinidine or quinine only in men and was not affected by age. In the absence of drug administration, renal clearance of amantadine was not affected by gender or age.

Additional studies are needed to confirm the gender difference reported for this drug interaction and to determine the effects of multiple dosing.

[1] Gaudry SE, et al. *Clin Pharmacol Ther.* 1993;54:23.

* Asterisk indicates drugs cited in interaction reports.

Amantadine — *Thiazide Diuretics*

Amantadine	Thiazide Diuretics	
Amantadine* (eg, *Symmetrel*)	Bendroflumethiazide (*Naturetin*)	Indapamide (eg, *Lozol*)
	Benzthiazide (eg, *Exna*)	Methyclothiazide (eg, *Enduron*)
	Chlorothiazide (eg, *Diuril*)	Metolazone (eg, *Zaroxolyn*)
	Chlorthalidone (eg, *Hygroton*)	Polythiazide (*Renese*)
	Hydrochlorothiazide* (eg, *HydroDiuril*)	Quinethazone (*Hydromox*)
	Hydroflumethiazide (eg, *Saluron*)	Trichlormethiazide (eg, *Naqua*)

Significance	Onset	Severity	Documentation
4	☐ Rapid ■ **Delayed**	☐ Major ■ **Moderate** ☐ Minor	☐ Established ☐ Probable ☐ Suspected ■ **Possible** ☐ Unlikely

Effects THIAZIDE diuretics may increase the risk for developing adverse effects from AMANTADINE if given concurrently.

Mechanism Unknown.

Management Approaches to management are discontinuation of the THIAZIDE diuretic, lowering the dose of AMANTADINE, or discontinuing AMANTADINE and substituting another drug.

Discussion

One case of a suspected interaction between amantadine and *Dyazide* (hydrochlorothiazide plus triamterene) has been reported.[1] In this case, a 61-year-old male receiving amantadine 300 mg/day for Parkinson's disease began receiving *Dyazide* (one tablet twice daily) for edema 1 week before hospital admission with agitation, ataxia, visual hallucinations, myoclonus and mental confusion. Symptoms cleared within 48 hours of discontinuing amantadine and *Dyazide*. A 14–day rechallenge study was conducted to determine the likelihood that a drug-drug interaction led to the symptoms requiring hospitalization. On days 1 through 14, amantadine 100 mg/day was administered. *Dyazide* was added to the regimen on day 7 (two times daily) and continued through day 14. Amantadine plasma levels increased from 156 mg/mL before *Dyazide* to 243 mg/mL on days 13 and 14. Urinary excretion of amantadine also declined with *Dyazide* therapy.

One or both ingredients (triamterene/hydrochlorothiazide) of *Dyazide* may predispose to amantadine toxicity by reducing clearance and increasing plasma concentrations of amantadine.

Further studies are needed to objectively confirm this suspected interaction and identify whether triamterene or hydrochlorothiazide is the etiological factor.

[1] Wilson TW, et al. *Can Med Assoc J* 1983;129:974.

* Asterisk indicates drugs cited in interaction reports. Based on pharmacologic and pharmacokinetic considerations, similar interactions may occur with other drugs that are listed.

Amantadine / *Triamterene*

Amantadine* (eg, *Symmetrel*)	Triamterene* (*Dyrenium*)

Significance	Onset	Severity	Documentation
4	☐ Rapid ■ **Delayed**	☐ Major ■ **Moderate** ☐ Minor	☐ Established ☐ Probable ☐ Suspected ■ **Possible** ☐ Unlikely

Effects TRIAMTERENE, a potassium-sparing diuretic, may increase the risk for developing adverse effects from AMANTADINE if given concurrently.

Mechanism Unknown.

Management Approaches to management are discontinuation of the TRIAMTERENE-containing diuretic, lowering the dose of AMANTADINE or discontinuing AMANTADINE and substituting another drug.

Discussion

One case of a suspected interaction between amantadine and *Dyazide* (triamterene plus hydrochlorothiazide) has been reported.[1] In this case, a 61-year-old male receiving amantadine 300 mg/day for Parkinson's disease began receiving *Dyazide* (one tablet twice daily) for edema 1 week before hospitalization with agitation, ataxia, visual hallucinations, myoclonus and mental confusion. Symptoms cleared within 48 hours of discontinuing amantadine and *Dyazide*. A 14-day rechallenge study was conducted to determine the likelihood that a drug-drug interaction led to the symptoms requiring hospitalization. On days 1 through 14, amantadine 100 mg/day was administered. *Dyazide* was added to the regimen on day 7 (two times daily) and continued through day 14. Amantadine plasma levels increased from 156 ng/mL before *Dyazide* to 243 ng/mL on days 13 and 14. Urinary excretion of amantadine also declined with *Dyazide* therapy.

One or both ingredients (triamterene/hydrochlorothiazide) of *Dyazide* may predispose patients to amantadine toxicity by reducing clearance and increasing plasma concentrations of amantadine. Further studies are needed to objectively confirm this suspected interaction and identify whether triamterene, hydrochlorothiazide or related diuretics is the etiological factor.

[1] Wilson TW, et al. *Can Med Assoc J* 1983;129:974.

* Asterisk indicates drugs cited in interaction reports.

Amantadine — *Trimethoprim*

Amantadine	Trimethoprim
Amantadine*	Trimethoprim (eg, *Primsol*)
	Trimethoprim/ Sulfamethoxazole* (eg, *Bactrim*)

Significance	Onset	Severity	Documentation
4	☐ Rapid	☐ Major	☐ Established
	■ **Delayed**	■ **Moderate**	☐ Probable
		☐ Minor	☐ Suspected
			■ **Possible**
			☐ Unlikely

Effects Coadministration of these drugs may cause acute mental confusion.

Mechanism AMANTADINE and TRIMETHOPRIM may inhibit renal clearance of each other, producing increased serum levels.

Management Consider monitoring patients for CNS adverse effects if these agents are coadministered.

Discussion

Short-term mental confusion occurred in an 84-year-old man receiving amantadine and trimethoprim-sulfamethoxazole concurrently.[1] The patient had a history of chronic obstructive pulmonary disease, Parkinson disease, and chronic atrial fibrillation. He had been receiving amantadine 100 mg twice daily and digoxin (eg, *Lanoxin*) 0.125 mg/day for at least 2 years. The patient developed symptoms of bronchitis and was given trimethoprim-sulfamethoxazole double strength twice daily. Within 72 hours, he returned with symptoms of mental confusion. Neurological examination revealed some cogwheel rigidity and a resting tremor. Amantadine and trimethoprim-sulfamethoxazole were discontinued and, within 24 hours, the mental status of the patient returned to baseline.

Additional studies are needed to determine the clinical significance of this possible drug interaction.

[1] Speeg KV, et al. *Am J Med Sci.* 1989;298(6):410.

* Asterisk indicates drugs cited in interaction reports. Based on pharmacologic and pharmacokinetic considerations, similar interactions may occur with other drugs that are listed.

Ambrisentan — Azole Antifungal Agents

Ambrisentan	Azole Antifungal Agents	
Ambrisentan* (*Letairis*)	Fluconazole (eg, *Diflucan*)	Posaconazole (*Noxafil*)
	Itraconazole (eg, *Sporanox*)	Voriconazole (eg, *Vfend*)
	Ketoconazole* (eg, *Nizoral*)	

Significance	Onset	Severity	Documentation
5	□ Rapid	□ Major	□ Established
	■ **Delayed**	□ Moderate	□ Probable
		■ **Minor**	□ Suspected
			□ Possible
			■ **Unlikely**

Effects AMBRISENTAN plasma concentrations may be elevated; however, clinically important effects on the efficacy and safety of AMBRISENTAN are unlikely.

Mechanism Inhibition of AMBRISENTAN metabolism (CYP3A4) by AZOLE ANTIFUNGAL AGENTS.

Management Based on available data, no special precautions are needed.

Discussion

The effects of ketoconazole on the pharmacokinetics of ambrisentan and its oxidative metabolite, 4-hydroxymethyl ambrisentan, were studied in 16 healthy men.[1] In an open-label, nonrandomized, 2-period study, each subject received a single dose of ambrisentan 10 mg alone and after 4 days of receiving ketoconazole 400 mg once daily. Compared with giving ambrisentan alone, coadministration of ketoconazole increased the ambrisentan AUC and C_{max} approximately 35% and 20%, respectively. The AUC and C_{max} of the 4-hydroxymethyl ambrisentan metabolite were decreased 4% and 16.5%, respectively. Coadministration of ambrisentan and ketoconazole was well tolerated. See also Bosentan-Azole Antifungal Agents.

[1] Richards DB, et al. *J Clin Pharmacol.* 2009;49(6):719.

* Asterisk indicates drugs cited in interaction reports. Based on pharmacologic and pharmacokinetic considerations, similar interactions may occur with other drugs that are listed.

Ambrisentan — *Cyclosporine*

Ambrisentan* (*Letairis*)	Cyclosporine* (eg, *Neoral*)

Significance	Onset	Severity	Documentation
4	☐ Rapid ■ **Delayed**	☐ Major ■ **Moderate** ☐ Minor	☐ Established ☐ Probable ☐ Suspected ■ **Possible** ☐ Unlikely

Effects AMBRISENTAN plasma concentrations may be elevated, increasing the pharmacologic effects and risk of adverse reactions.

Mechanism Unknown.

Management Limit the daily oral dose of AMBRISENTAN to 5 mg in patients receiving CYCLOSPORINE.

Discussion

Using an open-label, parallel-treatment design, the effects of cyclosporine (100 to 150 mg twice daily) on the pharmacokinetics of ambrisentan 5 mg daily and the effects of ambrisentan on the pharmacokinetics of cyclosporine were evaluated in 50 healthy volunteers.[1] Cyclosporine increased the ambrisentan AUC and C_{max} 2- and 1.5-fold, respectively, compared with placebo. Ambrisentan administration resulted in marginal increases in cyclosporine AUC and C_{max} compared with placebo. Twice as many subjects experienced adverse reactions when both drugs were coadministered compared with giving either drug alone. All adverse reactions were considered mild (eg, flushing, headache, nausea).

[1] Spence R, et al. *Clin Pharmacol Ther.* 2010;88(4):513.

* Asterisk indicates drugs cited in interaction reports.

Aminoglycosides — *Cephalosporins*

Aminoglycosides		Cephalosporins	
Amikacin	Neomycin	Cefazolin	Ceftazidime* (eg, *Fortaz*)
Gentamicin* (eg, *Garamycin*)	Tobramycin* (eg, *Tobi*)	Cefotaxime (eg, *Claforan*)	Ceftizoxime (*Cefizox*)
Kanamycin		Cefotetan	Ceftriaxone (eg, *Rocephin*)
		Cefoxitin	Cefuroxime (eg, *Zinacef*)

Significance	Onset	Severity	Documentation
2	☐ Rapid	☐ Major	☐ Established
	■ **Delayed**	■ **Moderate**	☐ Probable
		☐ Minor	■ **Suspected**
			☐ Possible
			☐ Unlikely

Effects Nephrotoxicity may be increased. Bactericidal activity against certain pathogens may be enhanced.

Mechanism Unknown.

Management Monitor AMINOGLYCOSIDE levels and kidney function closely. If renal dysfunction develops, reduce the dosage or discontinue 1 or both drugs and use alternative agents.

Discussion

Cephalothin appears to interact most adversely with parenteral aminoglycosides. Drug-induced nephrotoxicity seems more frequent with gentamicin and cephalothin than with other combinations.[1-11] Objective evidence that other parenteral cephalosporins interact with aminoglycosides to produce clinically significant nephrotoxicity is lacking.[1-3,5,7-15] Synergistic bactericidal antimicrobial activity with parenteral aminoglycosides and cephalosporins against selected organisms is well documented.[16-22] Although ceftazidime and tobramycin appear to compete for renal elimination in normal renal function, kinetic parameter changes are of little clinical significance.[22]

1 Fillastre R, et al. *Br Med J.* 1973;2(5863):396.
2 Klastersky J, et al. *JAMA.* 1974;227(1):45.
3 Bloomfield CD, et al. *Cancer.* 1974;34(2):431.
4 Harrison WO, et al. *Antimicrob Agents Chemother.* 1975;8(2):209.
5 Cabanillas F, et al. *Arch Intern Med.* 1975;135(6):850.
6 Klastersky J, et al. *Antimicrob Agents Chemother.* 1975;7(5):640.
7 Fanning WL, et al. *Antimicrob Agents Chemother.* 1976;10(1):80.
8 Plager JE. *Cancer.* 1976;37(4):1937.
9 Hansen MM, et al. *Acta Med Scand.* 1977;201(5):463.
10 Wade JC, et al. *Lancet.* 1978;2(8090):604.
11 Schimpff SC, et al; EORTC Int Antimicrob Ther Project Group. *J Infect Dis.* 1978;137(1):14.
12 Brown AE, et al. *Antimicrob Agents Chemother.* 1982;21(4):592.
13 Kuhlmann J, et al. *Infection.* 1982;10(4):233.
14 Mondorf AW, et al. *Infection.* 1983;11(suppl 1):S57.
15 Aronoff GR, et al. *Antimicrob Agents Chemother.* 1990;34(6):1139.
16 Van der Auwera P, et al. *Antimicrob Agents Chemother.* 1986;30(1):122.
17 Braveny I, et al. *Eur J Clin Microbiol.* 1986;5(1):119.
18 Wagenvoort JH, et al. *Arzneimittelforschung.* 1986;36(9):1301.
19 Giamarellou H. *Am J Med.* 1986;80(6B):126.
20 Bergeron MG, et al. *Antimicrob Agents Chemother.* 1986;29(2):379.
21 Pascual-Lopez A, et al. *Int J Clin Pharmacol Res.* 1987;7(1):45.
22 Bingen E, et al. *Infection.* 1988;16(2):121.

* Asterisk indicates drugs cited in interaction reports. Based on pharmacologic and pharmacokinetic considerations, similar interactions may occur with other drugs that are listed.

Aminoglycosides — *Enflurane*

Aminoglycosides		Enflurane
Amikacin (eg, *Amikin*)	Neomycin (eg, *Mycifradin*)	Enflurane* (eg, *Ethrane*)
Gentamicin* (eg, *Garamycin*)	Netilmicin (*Netromycin*)	
Kanamycin (eg, *Kantrex*)	Tobramycin* (eg, *Nebcin*)	

Significance	Onset	Severity	Documentation
4	■ **Rapid**	□ Major	□ Established
	□ Delayed	■ **Moderate**	□ Probable
		□ Minor	□ Suspected
			■ **Possible**
			□ Unlikely

Effects The nephrotoxicity of AMINOGLYCOSIDES may be increased.

Mechanism Unknown.

Management Other than the usual monitoring of renal function, no special precautions are necessary.

Discussion

The urinary excretion of alanine aminopeptidase (AAP), an indicator of proximal renal tubular damage, was measured in 18 patients before and after enflurane anesthesia with and without coadministration of gentamicin or tobramycin to determine whether enflurane increased the potential for aminoglycoside nephrotoxicity.[1] Ten patients received 0.5% to 1% enflurane alone for an average of 106 minutes; 8 patients received 0.75% to 1.25% enflurane for an average of 154 minutes, plus an aminoglycoside; and 4 patients, receiving neither enflurane nor an aminoglycoside, served as the control group. Two days postoperatively, urinary AAP excretion was significantly higher ($P < 0.025$) than preoperative levels in both groups of patients receiving enflurane. In addition, patients treated concurrently with an aminoglycoside had significantly greater AAP excretion ($P < 0.005$) than did patients receiving enflurane alone. However, no clinical evidence of renal impairment was demonstrated in patients receiving enflurane alone or in combination with an aminoglycoside. No postoperative changes in AAP excretion were observed in the control group. Since a group receiving aminoglycosides alone was not included, additional studies are needed to determine whether the increase in the urinary AAP excretion is a predictor of clinically significant renal damage.

[1] Motuz DJ, et al. *Anesth Analg.* 1988;67:770.

* Asterisk indicates drugs cited in interaction reports. Based on pharmacologic and pharmacokinetic considerations, similar interactions may occur with other drugs that are listed.

Aminoglycosides — *Loop Diuretics*

Aminoglycosides		Loop Diuretics	
Amikacin (eg, *Amikin*)	Netilmicin (*Netromycin*)	Bumetanide (eg, *Bumex*)	Furosemide* (eg, *Lasix*)
Gentamicin* (eg, *Garamycin*)	Streptomycin*	Ethacrynic Acid* (*Edecrin*)	Torsemide (*Demadex*)
Kanamycin* (eg, *Kantrex*)	Tobramycin* (eg, *Nebcin*)		

Significance	Onset	Severity	Documentation
1	■ **Rapid**	■ **Major**	□ Established
	□ Delayed	□ Moderate	□ Probable
		□ Minor	■ **Suspected**
			□ Possible
			□ Unlikely

Effects Auditory toxicity may be increased. Hearing loss of varying degrees may occur. Irreversible hearing loss has occurred.

Mechanism Not known. Possibly synergistic auditory toxicity.

Management Perform baseline hearing testing and periodic monitoring. Avoid excessive doses. Reduced doses of 1 or both drugs may be necessary in patients with renal insufficiency.

Discussion

Both aminoglycosides and loop diuretics may produce ototoxicity when given alone.[13] Experimental data suggest that a synergistic effect results when a parenteral aminoglycoside is combined with a loop diuretic.[1-9,11] Furthermore, the ototoxicity appears to be related to dose and serum concentrations of the respective drugs.[10,11] Risk of ototoxicity is increased further in renal insufficiency.[7] Irreversible hearing loss appears to be more likely with the aminoglycoside/loop diuretic combination than with either drug administered alone.[3,12]

[1] Mathog RH, et al. *N Engl J Med.* 1969;280:1223.
[2] Meriwether WD, et al. *JAMA.* 1971;216:795.
[3] West BA, et al. *Arch Otolaryngol.* 1973;98:32.
[4] Prazma J, et al. *Ann Otol Rhinol Laryngol.* 1974;83:111.
[5] Brummett RE, et al. *Acta Otolaryngol.* 1975;80:86.
[6] Quick CA, et al. *Ann Otol Rhinol Laryngol.* 1975;84:94.
[7] Quick CA. *Ann Otol Rhinol Laryngol.* 1976;85:776.
[8] Ohtani I, et al. *ORL.* 1978;40:216.
[9] Brummett RE, et al. *J Clin Pharmacol.* 1981;21:628.
[10] Lawson DH, et al. *J Clin Pharmacol.* 1982;22:254.
[11] Kaka JS, et al. *Drug Intell Clin Pharm.* 1984;18:235.
[12] Rybak LP. *Laryngoscope.* 1985;95(suppl 38):1.
[13] Bates DE, et al. *Ann Pharmacother.* 2002;36:446.

* Asterisk indicates drugs cited in interaction reports. Based on pharmacologic and pharmacokinetic considerations, similar interactions may occur with other drugs that are listed.

Aminoglycosides — *NSAIDs*

Aminoglycosides		NSAIDs	
Amikacin* (*Amikin*)	Netilmicin (*Netromycin*)	Diclofenac (eg, *Cataflam*)	Meclofenamate (eg, *Meclomen*)
Gentamicin* (eg, *Garamycin*)	Streptomycin	Etodolac (*Lodine*)	Mefenamic Acid (*Ponstel*)
Kanamycin (*Kantrex*)	Tobramycin* (eg, *Nebcin*)	Fenoprofen (eg, *Nalfon*)	Nabumetone (*Relafen*)
		Flurbiprofen (*Ansaid*)	Naproxen (eg, *Naprosyn*)
		Ibuprofen* (eg, *Motrin*)	Oxaprozin (*Daypro*)
		Indomethacin* (eg, *Indocin*)	Piroxicam (*Feldene*)
		Ketoprofen (eg, *Orudis*)	Sulindac (*Clinoril*)
		Ketorolac (*Toradol*)	Tolmetin (eg, *Tolectin*)

Significance	Onset	Severity	Documentation
2	☐ Rapid ■ **Delayed**	☐ Major ■ **Moderate** ☐ Minor	☐ Established ☐ Probable ■ **Suspected** ☐ Possible ☐ Unlikely

Effects Plasma AMINOGLYCOSIDE concentrations may be elevated.

Mechanism NSAIDs may cause an accumulation of AMINOGLYCOSIDES by reducing the glomerular filtration rate.

Management Avoid this combination if possible. If concomitant use cannot be avoided, reduce the AMINOGLYCOSIDE dose prior to starting an NSAID. Monitor renal function and AMINOGLYCOSIDE serum levels. Adjust AMINOGLYCOSIDE dose based on monitored parameters.

Discussion

The effects of indomethacin administration on amikacin and gentamicin serum concentrations were prospectively evaluated in 20 preterm infants with patent ductus arteriosus.[1] IV indomethacin therapy was started at 4 to 16 days postnatal age, after at least 3 days of aminoglycoside therapy. Both trough and peak aminoglycoside concentrations were elevated in association with indomethacin therapy. Trough amikacin concentrations increased 29% while gentamicin levels increased 48%. Peak amikacin levels increased 17% compared with 33% for gentamicin. Serum creatinine increased 17% (from 0.94 to 1.1 mg/dL) after indomethacin was administered. Six infants developed hyponatremia. Four children with cystic fibrosis, who were receiving ibuprofen, developed transient renal failure after aminoglycoside therapy was started for exacerbation of lung disease.[2] Two patients had elevated aminoglycoside levels. Levels were not reported in the remaining 2 patients.

[1] Zarfin Y, et al. *J Pediatr.* 1985;106:511.

[2] Kovesi TA, et al. *N Engl J Med.* 1998;338:65.

* Asterisk indicates drugs cited in interaction reports. Based on pharmacologic and pharmacokinetic considerations, similar interactions may occur with other drugs that are listed.

Aminoglycosides — *Penicillins*

Amikacin* (*Amikin*)	Netilmicin* (*Netromycin*)	Ampicillin* (eg, *Principen*)	Penicillin G* (eg, *Pfizerpen*)
Gentamicin* (eg, *Garamycin*)	Streptomycin	Mezlocillin* (*Mezlin*)	Piperacillin* (*Pipracil*)
Kanamycin (eg, *Kantrex*)	Tobramycin* (eg, *Nebcin*)	Nafcillin	Ticarcillin* (*Ticar*)
		Oxacillin	

Significance	Onset	Severity	Documentation
2	□ Rapid ■ **Delayed**	□ Major ■ **Moderate** □ Minor	□ Established ■ **Probable** □ Suspected □ Possible □ Unlikely

Effects Certain parenteral PENICILLINS may inactivate certain AMINOGLYCOSIDES.

Mechanism Unknown.

Management Do not mix parenteral AMINOGLYCOSIDES and PENICILLINS in the same solution. Monitor AMINOGLYCOSIDE concentrations and renal function. Adjust the dosage as needed.

Discussion

The synergism of these antibiotics is well documented.[1-11,14-18] However, some aminoglycosides are more subject to inactivation by certain penicillins. The problem may be greatest when they are combined in vitro. With parenteral administration, dilution appears to attenuate a physichemical incompatibility. Tobramycin and gentamicin are affected more by penicillins than netilmicin or amikacin.[8,9,12,17] Gentamicin inactivation may be greater with ticarcillin therapy than with mezlocillin or piperacillin.[13] In vivo inactivation of aminoglycosides by penicillins appears to be related to decreased renal function. In one patient, tobramycin clearance was greatly increased by administration of piperacillin.[18] Use of this combination in individuals with moderate to severe renal insufficiency warrants close monitoring and possible dosage adjustments.[1-4,10,11] Concurrent use of tobramycin and ticarcillin in patients with normal renal function may result in clinically unimportant reductions in tobramycin serum concentrations.[19]

1 Riff L, et al. *Arch Intern Med.* 1972;130:887.
2 Davies M, et al. *Antimicrob Agents Chemother.* 1975;7:431.
3 Ervin FR, et al. *Antimicrob Agents Chemother.* 1976;9:1004.
4 Weibert R, et al. *Trans Am Soc Artif Intern Organs.* 1976;22:439.
5 Murillo J, et al. *JAMA.* 1979;241:2401.
6 Krajdan A, et al. *Arch Intern Med.* 1980;140:1668.
7 Russo ME. *Am J Hosp Pharm.* 1980;37:702.
8 Henderson JL, et al. *Am J Hosp Pharm.* 1981;38:1167.
9 Pickering LK, et al. *J Pharmacol Exp Ther.* 1981;217:345.
10 Russo ME, et al. *Clin Nephrol.* 1981;15:175.
11 Thompson MI, et al. *Antimicrob Agents Chemother.* 1982;21:268.
12 Matzke GR, et al. *Clin Pharmacol Ther.* 1985;37:210.
13 Viollier AF, et al. *J Antimicrob Chemother.* 1985;15:597.
14 Fuursted K. *Acta Pathol Microbiol Immunol Scand.* 1987;95:351.
15 Lorian V, et al. *Diagn Microbiol Infect Dis.* 1988;11:163.
16 Bingen E, et al. *Infection.* 1988;16:121.
17 Halstenson CE, et al. *Antimicrob Agents Chemother.* 1990;34:128.
18 Uber WE, et al. *DICP.* 1991;25:357.
19 Roberts GW, et al. *Br J Clin Pharmacol.* 1993;36:372.

* Asterisk indicates drugs cited in interaction reports. Based on pharmacologic and pharmacokinetic considerations, similar interactions may occur with other drugs that are listed.

Aminoglycosides — *Vancomycin*

Aminoglycosides		Vancomycin
Amikacin* (eg, *Amikin*)	Netilmicin (*Netromycin*)	Vancomycin* (eg, *Vancocin*)
Gentamicin* (eg, *Garamycin*)	Streptomycin	
Kanamycin (eg, *Kantrex*)	Tobramycin* (eg, *Nebcin*)	

Significance	Onset	Severity	Documentation
4	☐ Rapid	☐ Major	☐ Established
	■ **Delayed**	■ **Moderate**	☐ Probable
		☐ Minor	☐ Suspected
			■ **Possible**
			☐ Unlikely

Effects Each drug is associated with a risk of nephrotoxicity when used alone. The risk may be increased when the two agents are given concurrently.

Mechanism Unknown.

Management Monitor renal function and serum drug concentrations. Adjust dosage of AMINOGLYCOSIDE or VANCOMYCIN if necessary.

Discussion

Some studies suggest that the incidence of nephrotoxicity associated with the combination of aminoglycoside plus vancomycin is greater than that resulting from either drug administered alone.[1-3] Other studies do not support this observation.[4-6,8] Renal toxicity allegedly associated with an aminoglycoside-vancomycin combination may also be related to undefined patient factors or the individual drugs. In addition, in patients receiving aminoglycosides and vancomycin, increased risk of nephrotoxicity was observed in patients with one or more of the following risk factors: Neutropenia, peritonitis, liver disease, concomitant amphotericin B (eg, *Fungizone*) treatment, increased age and male sex.[7] The risk of nephrotoxicity from this drug combination needs to be further defined.

[1] Farber BF, et al. *Antimicrob Agents Chemother* 1983;23:138.
[2] Odio C, et al. *J Pediatr* 1984;105:491.
[3] Dean RP, et al. *J Pediatr* 1985;106:861.
[4] Nahata MC. *Chemotherapy* 1987;33:302.
[5] Swinney VR, et al. *J Pediatr* 1987;110:497.
[6] Goren MP, et al. *Pediatr Infect Dis J* 1989;8:278-82.
[7] Pauly DJ, et al. *Pharmacotherapy* 1990;10:378.
[8] Munar MY, et al. *J Clin Pharmacol* 1991;31:618.

* Asterisk indicates drugs cited in interaction reports. Based on pharmacologic and pharmacokinetic considerations, similar interactions may occur with other drugs that are listed.

Aminoquinolines — *Aluminum Salts*

Aminoquinolines	Aluminum Salts	
Chloroquine* (eg, *Aralen*)	Aluminum Carbonate (*Basaljel*)	Attapulgite (eg, *Donnagel*)
	Aluminum Hydroxide (eg, *Amphojel*)	Kaolin-Pectin* (eg, *Kaodene*)
	Aluminum Phosphate (*Phosphaljel*)	Magaldrate (eg, *Riopan*)

Significance	Onset	Severity	Documentation
5	□ Rapid	□ Major	□ Established
	■ **Delayed**	□ Moderate	□ Probable
		■ **Minor**	□ Suspected
			■ **Possible**
			□ Unlikely

Effects ALUMINUM SALTS may decrease the absorption and the therapeutic effect of CHLOROQUINE.

Mechanism Oral ALUMINUM SALTS may adsorb CHLOROQUINE.

Management Separating doses of CHLOROQUINE and ALUMINUM SALTS by 2 to 4 hours may prevent adsorption of CHLOROQUINE.

Discussion

A single in vitro study and one randomized, crossover study in six healthy volunteers suggest that kaolin (eg, Fuller's earth, aluminum silicate, terra alba) administered with chloroquine diphosphate may decrease chloroquine absorption and plasma levels.[1,2] Findings are inconclusive relative to clinical significance. Controlled studies are needed to determine the significance of this potential interaction.

[1] McElnay JC, et al. *J Trop Med Hyg* 1982;85:153. [2] McElnay JC, et al. *J Trop Med Hyg* 1982;85:159.

* Asterisk indicates drugs cited in interaction reports. Based on pharmacologic and pharmacokinetic considerations, similar interactions may occur with other drugs that are listed.

Aminoquinolines — *Cimetidine*

Chloroquine* (eg, *Aralen*)	Cimetidine* (eg, *Tagamet*)

Significance	Onset	Severity	Documentation
3	☐ Rapid ■ **Delayed**	☐ Major ☐ Moderate ■ **Minor**	☐ Established ☐ Probable ■ **Suspected** ☐ Possible ☐ Unlikely

Effects The pharmacologic effects of CHLOROQUINE may be increased.

Mechanism The metabolism of CHLOROQUINE may be decreased due to inhibition of hepatic mixed function oxidases by CIMETIDINE.

Management May need a lower CHLOROQUINE dose during CIMETIDINE coadministration.

Discussion

In a randomized, controlled study involving ten healthy male volunteers, cimetidine reduced the oral clearance rate of chloroquine.[1] Subjects were randomly assigned to two sets of five patients (control and test groups). Each control subject received two chloroquine tablets (total of 300 mg base) 8 hours after an overnight fast. The test group received oral cimetidine 400 mg at bedtime for 4 days; on the test day, they received chloroquine base 300 mg. In the test patients, compared with the control subjects, cimetidine administration was associated with a 53% decrease in the oral clearance of chloroquine, a 49% increase in the elimination half-life, and a 57% increase in the apparent volume of distribution. In addition, there was a 47% reduction in chloroquine metabolism. The reduction in clearance was associated with altered kinetics of the major metabolite of chloroquine.

Until the relative contributions of chloroquine and its major metabolite to efficacy and toxicity are known, the clinical significance of this possible interaction cannot be assessed.

[1] Ette EI, et al. *J Clin Pharmacol* 1987;27:813.

* Asterisk indicates drugs cited in interaction reports.

Aminoquinolines		**Magnesium Salts**
Chloroquine* (eg, *Aralen*)	Magaldrate (eg, *Riopan*) Magnesium Carbonate (eg, *Marblen*) Magnesium Citrate Magnesium Gluconate Magnesium Hydroxide (eg, *Milk of Magnesia*)	Magnesium Oxide (eg, *Mag-Ox*) Magnesium Sulfate (eg, *Epsom Salts*) Magnesium Trisilicate*

Significance	Onset	Severity	Documentation
3	□ Rapid ■ **Delayed**	□ Major □ Moderate ■ **Minor**	□ Established □ Probable ■ **Suspected** □ Possible □ Unlikely

Effects Oral MAGNESIUM SALTS may decrease the absorption and therapeutic effect of CHLOROQUINE or other oral AMINOQUINOLINES. The antacid activity of MAGNESIUM SALTS may also be reduced.

Mechanism Oral MAGNESIUM SALTS administered with CHLOROQUINE (and possibly other AMINOQUINOLINES) may adsorb CHLOROQUINE. The same mechanism may impair the antacid potency of MAGNESIUM SALTS.

Management Separating doses of CHLOROQUINE and MAGNESIUM SALTS by 2 to 4 hours may prevent the adsorption of CHLOROQUINE. It may be necessary to increase the dose of CHLOROQUINE.

Discussion

Two in vitro studies and one randomized, crossover study in six healthy volunteers suggest that magnesium trisilicate (available only in combination antacid products) administered with chloroquine diphosphate may decrease chloroquine absorption and plasma levels.[1-3] Decreased antacid efficacy of magnesium trisilicate is also a possibility. Findings are inconclusive relative to clinical significance. Controlled studies are needed to objectively and conclusively determine the significance of potential interactions between chloroquine (and other aminoquinolines) and magnesium trisilicate (and other magnesium salts).

[1] Khalil SAH. *J Pharm Sci* 1977;66:289.
[2] McElnay JC, et al. *J Trop Med Hyg* 1982;85:153.
[3] McElnay JC, et al. *J Trop Med Hyg* 1982;85:159.

* Asterisk indicates drugs cited in interaction reports. Based on pharmacologic and pharmacokinetic considerations, similar interactions may occur with other drugs that are listed.

Aminoquinolines | *Methylene Blue*

Chloroquine*
(eg, *Aralen*)

Methylene Blue*
(eg, *Urolene Blue*)

Significance	Onset	Severity	Documentation
5	☐ Rapid ■ **Delayed**	☐ Major ☐ Moderate ■ **Minor**	☐ Established ☐ Probable ☐ Suspected ■ **Possible** ☐ Unlikely

Effects CHLOROQUINE whole blood concentrations may be slightly decreased.

Mechanism Unknown.

Management Based on available data, no special precautions are needed.

Discussion

In a randomized, placebo-controlled investigation, 24 healthy individuals received a 3-day course of chloroquine with twice daily placebo or methylene blue 130 mg.[1] The men received chloroquine phosphate 1,000 mg on the first 2 days and 500 mg on day 3, while women received chloroquine 750 mg on the first 2 days and 375 mg on day 3. Compared with taking chloroquine with placebo, coadministration of methylene blue decreased the chloroquine AUC (normalized to body weight) 21% and the AUC of the desethylchloroquine metabolite of chloroquine (normalized to body weight) 35%. The metabolic ratio between chloroquine and the metabolite was not changed. The magnitude of the reduction in chloroquine exposure was not expected to be clinically important.

[1] Rengelshausen J, et al. *Eur J Clin Pharmacol.* 2004;60:709.

* Asterisk indicates drugs cited in interaction reports.

Amiodarone — *Cimetidine*

Amiodarone* (*Cordarone*)	Cimetidine* (eg, *Tagamet*)

Significance	Onset	Severity	Documentation
4	☐ Rapid	☐ Major	☐ Established
	■ **Delayed**	■ **Moderate**	☐ Probable
		☐ Minor	☐ Suspected
			■ **Possible**
			☐ Unlikely

Effects Levels of AMIODARONE and its active metabolite may be elevated, increasing the pharmacologic and toxic effects.

Mechanism Unknown. However, CIMETIDINE may inhibit the hepatic metabolism of AMIODARONE by the cytochrome P450 oxidase system.

Management Consider monitoring serum AMIODARONE levels when initiating CIMETIDINE therapy. Adjust the dose of AMIODARONE accordingly.

Discussion

Cimetidine increased serum amiodarone levels in 8 of 12 patients receiving both drugs concomitantly.[1] The potential interaction was studied in 12 patients receiving amiodarone 200 mg twice daily for at least 6 months. Each patient was given cimetidine 300 mg 4 times daily for 1 week. After 1 week of concurrent treatment with amiodarone and cimetidine, amiodarone levels increased from 1.4 to 1.93 mcg/mL, while levels of the desethylamiodarone metabolite increased from 1.41 to 2.17 mcg/mL.

Documentation for this possible interaction consists of an abstract. More substantive data are needed to evaluate the clinical importance of this reported interaction.

[1] Hogan C, et al. *J Clin Pharmacol.* 1988;28:909.

* Asterisk indicates drugs cited in interaction reports.

Amiodarone — *Diltiazem*

Amiodarone* (eg, *Cordarone*)	Diltiazem* (eg, *Cardizem*)

Significance	Onset	Severity	Documentation
4	☐ Rapid ■ **Delayed**	■ **Major** ☐ Moderate ☐ Minor	☐ Established ☐ Probable ☐ Suspected ■ **Possible** ☐ Unlikely

Effects Sinus arrest and life-threatening low cardiac output may occur.

Mechanism Unknown. However, because both agents affect myocardial contractility and sinus and atrioventricular nodal function, additive pharmacologic effects may occur. Also, AMIODARONE is known to inhibit the metabolism of a number of other drugs; therefore a pharmacokinetic interaction and additive pharmacodynamic effects may occur.

Management Monitor patients for cardiotoxicity when AMIODARONE and DILTIAZEM are coadministered, particularly during the loading phase of AMIODARONE therapy.

Discussion

A 61-year-old woman with cardiomyopathy, compensated congestive heart failure (CHF), paroxysmal atrial fibrillation, and ventricular arrhythmias developed sinus arrest and life-threatening low cardiac output with oliguria when amiodarone was added to her treatment regimen of diltiazem and furosemide (eg, *Lasix*).[1] The patient had been hospitalized because of intractable atrial and ventricular arrhythmias. All previous drugs, other than furosemide and oral potassium, had been discontinued. Trials with mexiletine (eg, *Mexitil*), procainamide (eg, *Procanbid*), quinidine, and verapamil (eg, *Calan*) were discontinued because of intolerable side effects or failure to control the arrhythmias. Oral diltiazem 90 mg every 6 hours was started to reduce systemic ventricular resistance and to control the ventricular response in atrial fibrillation. After 4 days, malignant ventricular arrhythmias persisted, and oral amiodarone treatment was initiated with a loading dose of 600 mg every 12 hours. On the fourth day of combined therapy, the patient suddenly developed sinus arrest and a severe low cardiac output with oliguria. Both drugs were discontinued, and hemodynamic stability was achieved with ventricular pacing at a rate of 80 and high-dose dopamine (eg, *Intropin*). Four days later, amiodarone was reinstated at 200 mg/day. The patient was later discharged on amiodarone 400 mg/day and furosemide 160 mg/day. At her 1-month follow-up, she was in normal sinus rhythm with no evidence of CHF.

[1] Lee TH, et al. *Am Heart J.* 1985;109:163.

* Asterisk indicates drugs cited in interaction reports.

Amiodarone | **Fentanyl**

Amiodarone*
(eg, *Cordarone*)

Fentanyl*
(eg, *Sublimaze*)

Significance	Onset	Severity	Documentation
1	■ **Rapid**	■ **Major**	□ Established
	□ Delayed	□ Moderate	□ Probable
		□ Minor	■ **Suspected**
			□ Possible
			□ Unlikely

Effects Profound bradycardia, sinus arrest, and hypotension have occurred.

Mechanism Unknown.

Management Monitor hemodynamic function and administer inotropic, chronotropic, and pressor support as indicated. The bradycardia is usually unresponsive to atropine. Large doses of vasopressors (eg, epinephrine, phenylephrine) have been used.

Discussion

Administration of fentanyl as an anesthetic caused serious complications in patients receiving amiodarone.[1-5] A 54-year-old man receiving amiodarone developed bradycardia, hypotension, and marked reduction in cardiac output during coronary artery surgery for which fentanyl anesthesia was given.[1] The patient was treated with multiple pressor agents, including simultaneous infusions of epinephrine, norepinephrine, and metaraminol. In addition, the patient required prolonged hemodynamic support. A 71-year-old woman receiving amiodarone experienced sinus arrest and repeated episodes of bradycardia following administration of fentanyl.[4] The patient recovered following treatment with ephedrine IV, isoproterenol boluses, and infusion. A 33-year-old pregnant patient receiving amiodarone for intractable ventricular arrhythmias was given epidural fentanyl and chloroprocaine for regional anesthesia prior to a Cesarean section.[5] She developed hypotension that was successfully managed with phenylephrine. In a retrospective investigation, patients who had received amiodarone and fentanyl concurrently were compared with patients who had not received amiodarone[3]; the amiodarone group had more episodes of low systemic vascular resistance. In addition, more patients receiving amiodarone required hemodynamic support with intra-arterial balloon placement. Of the patients receiving amiodarone plus fentanyl, 66% developed bradycardia, complete heart block, or became pacemaker dependent compared with 17% of the patients receiving fentanyl alone.

Whether the observed effects are specific to fentanyl anesthesia or the result of anesthesia in general remains to be determined; however, caution is warranted.

[1] Gallagher JD, et al. *Anesthesiology*. 1981;55(2):186.
[2] MacKinnon G, et al. *Can J Surg*. 1983;26(4):355.
[3] Liberman BA, et al. *Can Anaesth Soc J*. 1985;32(6):629.
[4] Navalgund AA, et al. *Anesth Analg*. 1986;65(4):414.
[5] Koblin DD, et al. *Anesthesiology*. 1987;66(4):551.

* Asterisk indicates drugs cited in interaction reports.

Amiodarone — *Food*

Amiodarone* (eg, *Cordarone*)	Grapefruit Juice*

Significance	Onset	Severity	Documentation
4	■ **Rapid**	□ Major	□ Established
	□ Delayed	■ **Moderate**	□ Probable
		□ Minor	□ Suspected
			■ **Possible**
			□ Unlikely

Effects AMIODARONE plasma concentrations may be increased.

Mechanism Inhibition of AMIODARONE metabolism (CYP3A4) by GRAPEFRUIT JUICE is suspected.

Management Avoid administration of AMIODARONE with GRAPEFRUIT JUICE. Caution patients to take AMIODARONE with liquids other than GRAPEFRUIT JUICE.

Discussion

The effects of grapefruit juice ingestion on the pharmacokinetics of amiodarone were studied in 11 healthy, nonsmoking, male adults.[1] Each subject received amiodarone (approximately 17 mg/kg) with water and simultaneously with 300 mL of grapefruit juice followed by 300 mL of grapefruit juice 3 and 9 hours after amiodarone administration. Compared with water, administration of amiodarone with grapefruit juice increased the amiodarone AUC by 50% and the C_{max} by 84%. The T_{max} and $t_{½}$ of amiodarone were not altered. Grapefruit juice completely inhibited the production of N-desethylamiodarone, a major, active metabolite of amiodarone. No differences were observed for ECG measurements and arterial pressure data between the baseline period and ingestion of amiodarone with grapefruit juice. An 83-year-old woman with a history of MI and atrial fibrillation was seen in the emergency department with postprandial syncope and palpitations.[2] After cardioversion with IV amiodarone, the ECG showed marked QT prolongation associated with ventricular arrhythmias, including torsades de pointes, which required immediate electrical cardioversion and IV lidocaine. After 24 hours, there was no recurrence of the ventricular arrhythmias. The patient's history revealed that she had been drinking grapefruit juice in large quantities (1 to 1.5 L/day).

[1] Libersa CC, et al. *Br J Clin Pharmacol.* 2000;49(4):373.

[2] Agosti S, et al. *Am J Emerg Med.* 2012;30(1):248.e5.

* Asterisk indicates drugs cited in interaction reports.

Amiodarone — *Iohexol*

Amiodarone* (eg, *Cordarone*)	Iohexol* (eg, *Omnipaque 140*)

Significance	Onset	Severity	Documentation
4	■ **Rapid**	■ **Major**	□ Established
	□ Delayed	□ Moderate	□ Probable
		□ Minor	□ Suspected
			■ **Possible**
			□ Unlikely

Effects The risk of life-threatening cardiac arrhythmias may be increased.

Mechanism Unknown.

Management Until more data are available, avoid concurrent use of AMIODARONE and IOHEXOL. If coadministered, carefully monitor patients and be prepared to treat any new arrhythmias.

Discussion

The ECG findings of patients taking amiodarone who underwent cardiac catheterization and received iohexol contrast media were analyzed in a retrospective investigation.[1] Routine ECG recordings were available on the day of cardiac catheterization and the following day for 21 patients taking amiodarone and receiving iohexol. The ECG recordings were compared with 21 age-matched patients who underwent cardiac catheterization and received iohexol but not amiodarone. The QT intervals corrected for heart rate (QTc) were increased (from an average of 433 to 480 msec) after catheterization in patients receiving amiodarone. A QTc prolongation of more than 500 msec was not observed in any patient receiving amiodarone before catheterization. However, 6 of the 21 patients had a severely lengthened QTc interval (more than 500 msec) after catheterization. No change in the QTc interval occurred in the control group. See Drug-induced Prolongation of the QT Interval and Torsades de Pointes.

[1] Goernig M, et al. *Br J Clin Pharmacol.* 2004;58:96.

* Asterisk indicates drugs cited in interaction reports.

Amiodarone — *Metronidazole*

Amiodarone* (eg, *Cordarone*)	Metronidazole* (eg, *Flagyl*)

Significance	Onset	Severity	Documentation
4	☐ Rapid ■ **Delayed**	■ **Major** ☐ Moderate ☐ Minor	☐ Established ☐ Probable ☐ Suspected ■ **Possible** ☐ Unlikely

Effects AMIODARONE plasma concentrations may be elevated, increasing the risk of toxicity, including QT interval prolongation and torsades de pointes.

Mechanism METRONIDAZOLE inhibition of AMIODARONE metabolism (CYP3A4) is suspected.

Management Until more data are available, avoid coadministration of AMIODARONE and METRONIDAZOLE.

Discussion

A 71-year-old woman with a history of coronary artery bypass grafting and paroxysmal atrial fibrillation was started on metronidazole 500 mg 3 times daily for antibiotic-associated pseudomembranous colitis.[1] On hospital admission, her ECG demonstrated a QTc interval of 440 msec. After experiencing atrial fibrillation, she was given amiodarone IV (450 mg bolus followed by 900 mg/day). Two days later, conversion to sinus rhythm occurred, and the ECG showed a prolonged QTc interval (625 msec). Subsequently, she experienced sustained polymorphic torsades de pointes ventricular tachycardia, which required defibrillation to restore sinus rhythm. Amiodarone and metronidazole were discontinued immediately. During the next 6 days, the QTc interval decreased gradually to the initial value without clinically important arrhythmias. See also, Drug-Induced Prolongation of the QT Interval and Torsades de Pointes.

[1] Kounas SP, et al. *Pacing Clin Electrophysiol.* 2005;28:472.

* Asterisk indicates drugs cited in interaction reports.

Amiodarone — *Orlistat*

Amiodarone* (eg, *Cordarone*)	Orlistat* (*Xenical*)

Significance	Onset	Severity	Documentation
4	☐ Rapid ■ **Delayed**	☐ Major ■ **Moderate** ☐ Minor	☐ Established ☐ Probable ☐ Suspected ■ **Possible** ☐ Unlikely

Effects AMIODARONE plasma concentrations may be reduced slightly.

Mechanism AMIODARONE absorption may be decreased.

Management Monitor patients for a decrease in AMIODARONE response.

Discussion

The effects of orlistat on the pharmacokinetics of amiodarone were studied in 2 parallel treatment groups.[1] One group of 16 healthy volunteers received amiodarone 1,200 mg after being pretreated with orlistat 120 mg 3 times daily. A second group received amiodarone after pretreatment with a matching placebo 3 times daily. Compared with placebo administration, orlistat reduced the AUC and C_{max} of amiodarone 27% and 23%, respectively.

[1] Zhi J, et al. *J Clin Pharmacol.* 2003;43:428.

* Asterisk indicates drugs cited in interaction reports.

Amiodarone — *Protease Inhibitors*

Amiodarone	Protease Inhibitors	
Amiodarone* (eg, *Cordarone*)	Amprenavir (*Agenerase*)	Nelfinavir* (*Viracept*)
	Atazanavir* (*Reyataz*)	Ritonavir* (*Norvir*)
	Indinavir* (*Crixivan*)	Saquinavir (eg, *Fortovase*)
	Lopinavir/Ritonavir (*Kaletra*)	

Significance	Onset	Severity	Documentation
1	□ Rapid	■ **Major**	□ Established
	■ **Delayed**	□ Moderate	□ Probable
		□ Minor	■ **Suspected**
			□ Possible
			□ Unlikely

Effects Increases in plasma AMIODARONE concentrations may occur, increasing the risk of AMIODARONE toxicity.

Mechanism PROTEASE INHIBITORS may inhibit the metabolism (cytochrome P450 3A4 [CYP3A4]) of AMIODARONE.

Management RITONAVIR and NELFINAVIR are contraindicated in patients receiving AMIODARONE. Because other PROTEASE INHIBITORS may interact similarly, carefully monitor AMIODARONE plasma levels and the patient for AMIODARONE toxicity. Be prepared to adjust the dose of AMIODARONE.

Discussion

Ritonavir[1] and nelfinavir[2] are expected to produce large increases in amiodarone plasma levels, increasing the risk of toxicity. Elevated plasma levels of amiodarone may cause QT prolongation and serious cardiac arrhythmias.[3] Amiodarone is metabolized by the CYP3A4 isozyme; drugs that inhibit amiodarone metabolism may produce an increase in amiodarone plasma levels. Studies using human liver microsomes have shown that CYP3A is a major isoform in ritonavir metabolism.[1] Therefore, coadministration of ritonavir and amiodarone is contraindicated. After starting antiretroviral prophylaxis, which included indinavir 800 mg 3 times/day, in a 38-year-old man stabilized on amiodarone 200 mg/day, amiodarone levels increased 44% (from 0.9 to 1.3 mg/L).[4] Amiodarone levels gradually decreased following discontinuation of antiretroviral therapy.

The basis for this monograph is information on file with the manufacturer.[1,2,5] Published clinical data are needed to further assess this interaction. However, because of the seriousness of the cardiac problems associated with this drug combination, clinical evaluation of this interaction in humans is not likely to be forthcoming.

1 *Norvir* [package insert]. Abbott Park, IL: Abbott Laboratories; 2001.
2 *Viracept* [package insert]. La Jolla, CA: Agouron Pharmaceuticals, Inc.; 2002.
3 Thomas M, et al. *Br J Clin Pharmacol.* 1996;41:77.
4 Lohman JJ, et al. *Ann Pharmacother.* 1999;33:645.
5 *Reyataz* [package insert]. Princeton, NJ: Bristol-Myers Squibb Co.; 2003.

* Asterisk indicates drugs cited in interaction reports. Based on pharmacologic and pharmacokinetic considerations, similar interactions may occur with other drugs that are listed.

Amiodarone		***Rifamycins***
Amiodarone* (eg, *Cordarone*)	Rifabutin (*Mycobutin*) Rifampin* (eg, *Rifadin*)	Rifapentine (*Priftin*)

Significance	Onset	Severity	Documentation
4	□ Rapid ■ **Delayed**	■ **Major** □ Moderate □ Minor	□ Established □ Probable □ Suspected ■ **Possible** □ Unlikely

Effects Serum concentrations of AMIODARONE and its active metabolite may be decreased, reducing its pharmacologic effect.

Mechanism Possible increased AMIODARONE metabolism (CYP3A4) induced by RIFAMYCINS.

Management Closely monitor AMIODARONE serum concentrations when starting or stopping a RIFAMYCIN.

Discussion

A possible drug interaction between amiodarone and rifampin was reported in a 33-year-old woman with a history of congenital heart disease, atrial arrhythmia, and ventricular arrhythmia.[1] She was treated with amiodarone 400 mg/day, an epicardial pacing system, and an implantable cardioverter defibrillator. Other medications the patient was receiving included bumetanide, digoxin (eg, *Lanoxin*), famotidine (eg, *Pepcid*), hydralazine, isosorbide dinitrate (eg, *Isordil Titradose*), losartan (*Cozaar*), magnesium oxide (eg, *Mag-G*), metoprolol (eg, *Lopressor*), and potassium chloride (eg, *K-Dur*). She was started on doxycycline (eg, *Doryx*) 200 mg/day and rifampin 600 mg/day to suppress a methicillin-resistant staphylococcal infection. One month prior to starting rifampin, serum concentrations of amiodarone and its active metabolite desethylamiodarone (DEA) were 0.5 and 0.7 mg/L, respectively. The patient was admitted to the hospital with palpitations and implantable cardioverter-defibrillator shock approximately 5 weeks after starting rifampin. The serum amiodarone concentration was 0.3 mg/L, and DEA levels were undetectable. Her amiodarone dosage was increased to 400 mg twice daily. Two months later, she returned to the hospital with complaints of palpitations. Amiodarone and DEA serum concentrations were 0.4 and 0.6 mg/L, respectively. Rifampin was discontinued, and 2 weeks later, amiodarone and DEA concentrations were 1.2 and 1 mg/L, respectively. Subsequently, the dosage of amiodarone was decreased to 600 mg/day. One month later, amiodarone and DEA concentrations were 1.6 and 1.3 mg/L, respectively. Resolution of amiodarone-induced cornea verticillata (corneal deposits) occurred in an 83-year-old man while taking rifampin concurrently.[2] This was associated with subtherapeutic amiodarone concentrations. Cornea verticillata returned 4 months after rifampin was discontinued.

[1] Zarembski DG, et al. *Pharmacotherapy.* 1999;19(2):249.

[2] Mehta S, et al. *Cornea.* 2012;31(1):81.

* Asterisk indicates drugs cited in interaction reports. Based on pharmacologic and pharmacokinetic considerations, similar interactions may occur with other drugs that are listed.

Amiodarone — *Zolpidem*

Amiodarone* (eg, *Cordarone*)	Zolpidem* (*Ambien*)

Significance	Onset	Severity	Documentation
4	☐ Rapid ■ **Delayed**	■ **Major** ☐ Moderate ☐ Minor	☐ Established ☐ Probable ☐ Suspected ■ **Possible** ☐ Unlikely

Effects The risk of life-threatening cardiac arrhythmias, including torsades de pointes, may be increased.

Mechanism Unknown. However, interference with AMIODARONE metabolism because of competitive inhibition for the same isozyme (CYP3A4) by ZOLPIDEM is suspected.

Management Until more information is available, coadminister these agents with caution and closely monitor cardiac function.

Discussion

A 67-year-old woman with a history of prosthetic mitral valve and CHF was admitted to the emergency department with complaints of palpitations.[1] Three weeks earlier she was started on zolpidem for insomnia. On admission, her baseline ECG showed sinus rhythm with left bundle branch block, premature ventricular complexes, and a QTc interval of 440 msec. Amiodarone was started as a 450 mg bolus followed by 900 mg daily. Four days later, the patient developed torsades de pointes ventricular tachycardia that degenerated to ventricular fibrillation and required defibrillation to restore sinus rhythm. Marked QTc interval prolongation of 565 msec was recorded prior to the episode, and amiodarone and zolpidem were withdrawn. Subsequently, over the following days, the QTc interval gradually decreased to initial values.

[1] Letsas KP, et al. *Cardiology*. 2006;105(3):146.

* Asterisk indicates drugs cited in interaction reports.

Amlodipine — *Diltiazem*

Amlodipine* (eg, *Norvasc*)	Diltiazem* (eg, *Cardizem*)

Significance	Onset	Severity	Documentation
4	☐ Rapid ■ **Delayed**	☐ Major ■ **Moderate** ☐ Minor	☐ Established ☐ Probable ☐ Suspected ■ **Possible** ☐ Unlikely

Effects AMLODIPINE plasma concentrations may be elevated, increasing the pharmacologic effects and adverse reactions.

Mechanism Unknown.

Management In patients receiving AMLODIPINE, carefully monitor BP when DILTIAZEM is started or stopped. Be prepared to adjust the AMLODIPINE dose as needed.

Discussion

The effects of diltiazem on the pharmacokinetics and pharmacodynamics of amlodipine were studied in 8 elderly patients with essential hypertension.[1] In an open-label investigation, each patient received amlodipine 5 mg on day 1 and day 14 with or without pretreatment with diltiazem 180 mg/day for 3 days. Pretreatment with diltiazem increased the peak concentration of amlodipine 57% (from 3 to 4.7 ng/mL) and the AUC 57%. Compared with administration of amlodipine alone, pretreatment with diltiazem further decreased the systolic, diastolic, and standing BPs.

[1] Sasaki M, et al. *Eur J Clin Pharmacol.* 2001;57(1):85.

* Asterisk indicates drugs cited in interaction reports.

Amlodipine — *Food*

Amlodipine* (eg, *Norvasc*)	Grapefruit Juice*

Significance	Onset	Severity	Documentation
5	■ **Rapid**	□ Major	□ Established
	□ Delayed	□ Moderate	□ Probable
		■ **Minor**	□ Suspected
			■ **Possible**
			□ Unlikely

Effects AMLODIPINE serum concentrations may be elevated, increasing pharmacologic effects and adverse reactions.

Mechanism Possibly caused by inhibition of AMLODIPINE metabolism.

Management Avoid coadministration.

Discussion

Data are conflicting. The effects of grapefruit juice on the pharmacokinetics and pharmacodynamics of amlodipine were studied in 12 healthy men.[1] Utilizing a randomized, open, crossover study design, the effect of taking a single dose of amlodipine 5 mg with 250 mL of grapefruit juice was compared with taking the drug with a glass of water. Giving the calcium channel blocker with grapefruit juice increased the C_{max} of amlodipine from 2.7 to 3.1 ng/L and the AUC 14%; however, the variation in C_{max} and AUC between subjects was approximately 2-fold. There were no differences in BP or heart rate between the 2 treatments. In a randomized, 4-way, crossover study, 20 healthy men received amlodipine 10 mg orally or IV with 240 mL of water or grapefruit juice.[2] No differences in amlodipine pharmacokinetics or pharmacodynamics were found between concurrent ingestion with water or grapefruit juice. See also Felodipine-Food, Nifedipine-Food, and Nisoldipine-Food.

[1] Josefsson M, et al. *Eur J Clin Pharmacol.* 1996;51(2):189.

[2] Vincent J, et al. *Br J Clin Pharmacol.* 2000;50(5):455.

* Asterisk indicates drugs cited in interaction reports.

Amlodipine — *Protease Inhibitors*

Amlodipine* (eg, *Norvasc*)	Atazanavir (*Reyataz*)
	Fosamprenavir (*Lexiva*)
	Indinavir* (*Crixivan*)
	Lopinavir/Ritonavir (*Kaletra*)
	Nelfinavir (*Viracept*)
	Ritonavir* (*Norvir*)
	Saquinavir (*Invirase*)
	Tipranavir (*Aptivus*)

Significance	Onset	Severity	Documentation
4	☐ Rapid	☐ Major	☐ Established
	■ **Delayed**	■ **Moderate**	☐ Probable
		☐ Minor	☐ Suspected
			■ **Possible**
			☐ Unlikely

Effects AMLODIPINE plasma concentrations may be elevated, increasing the pharmacologic and pharmacodynamic effects and adverse reactions.

Mechanism Inhibition of AMLODIPINE metabolism (CYP3A) by the PROTEASE INHIBITOR.

Management Monitor AMLODIPINE clinical response and adverse reactions when PROTEASE INHIBITORS are started or stopped. Adjust the dose as needed.

Discussion

The potential for a 2-way pharmacokinetic drug interaction between indinavir plus ritonavir and amlodipine was evaluated in 18 healthy HIV-seronegative subjects.[1] Each subject received amlodipine 5 mg daily for days 1 through 7 and 20 through 26. In addition, each subject received indinavir 800 mg and ritonavir 100 mg every 12 hours on days 8 through 26. Indinavir plus ritonavir increased the median amlodipine AUC 90%. The steady-state AUCs of indinavir and ritonavir were not affected by amlodipine.

[1] Glesby MJ, et al. *Clin Pharmacol Ther.* 2005;78(2):143.

* Asterisk indicates drugs cited in interaction reports. Based on pharmacologic and pharmacokinetic considerations, similar interactions may occur with other drugs that are listed.

Amphotericin B — *Foscarnet*

Amphotericin B* (eg, *Amphotec*)	Foscarnet* (*Foscavir*)

Significance	Onset	Severity	Documentation
4	☐ Rapid	☐ Major	☐ Established
	■ **Delayed**	■ **Moderate**	☐ Probable
		☐ Minor	☐ Suspected
			■ **Possible**
			☐ Unlikely

Effects The risk of renal toxicity may be increased.

Mechanism These agents may have additive or synergistic nephrotoxic effects.

Management If coadministration cannot be avoided, aggressive hydration with close monitoring of renal function is warranted.

Discussion

Three men with advanced AIDS developed renal insufficiency within 4 to 5 days of starting combined therapy with amphotericin B and foscarnet.[1] Amphotericin B was discontinued within 5 to 11 days in all patients. In addition, foscarnet was discontinued in 1 patient, while being continued for 4 to 7 months in the other patients. Renal function improved in 1 patient and returned to baseline values in the remaining patients.

Because nephrotoxicity can occur with either agent, additional documentation is needed.

[1] Zaman MM, et al. *Clin Infect Dis.* 1996;22(2):378.

* Asterisk indicates drugs cited in interaction reports.

Amygdalin — *Ascorbic Acid*

Amygdalin*	Ascorbic Acid*

Significance	Onset	Severity	Documentation
1	■ **Rapid**	■ **Major**	□ Established
	□ Delayed	□ Moderate	□ Probable
		□ Minor	■ **Suspected**
			□ Possible
			□ Unlikely

Effects Risk of life-threatening cyanide toxicity may be increased.

Mechanism Unknown; however, in vitro, ASCORBIC ACID increases conversion of AMYGDALIN to cyanide and reduces body stores of cysteine, which detoxifies cyanide.

Management Avoid concurrent use of AMYGDALIN and ASCORBIC ACID.

Discussion

A 68-year-old woman with cancer was seen in the emergency department with seizures and severe lactic acidosis shortly after ingesting amygdalin 3 g.[1] In addition to her conventional treatment, the patient had been taking ascorbic acid 4,800 mg daily and complementary/alternative medicines, including amygdalin. The patient was treated for cyanide toxicity with hydroxocobalamin IV and responded rapidly. Although the FDA has banned the use of the synthetic form of amygdalin, laetrile, for cancer treatment in the United States, amygdalin has been used as complementary/alternative medicine by patients with cancer.

[1] Bromley J, et al. *Ann Pharmacother.* 2005;39(9):1566.

* Asterisk indicates drugs cited in interaction reports.

Angiotensin II Receptor Antagonists — *Trimethoprim*

Angiotensin II Receptor Antagonists		Trimethoprim	
Candesartan* (*Atacand*)	Olmesartan* (*Benicar*)	Trimethoprim* (eg, *Primsol*)	Trimethoprim/ Sulfamethoxazole* (eg, *Bactrim*)
Eprosartan* (*Teveten*)	Telmisartan* (*Micardis*)		
Irbesartan* (*Avapro*)	Valsartan* (*Diovan*)		
Losartan* (eg, *Cozaar*)			

Significance	Onset	Severity	Documentation
2	☐ Rapid ■ **Delayed**	☐ Major ■ **Moderate** ☐ Minor	☐ Established ☐ Probable ■ **Suspected** ☐ Possible ☐ Unlikely

Effects The risk of hyperkalemia may be increased, especially in elderly patients.

Mechanism ANGIOTENSIN II RECEPTOR ANTAGONISTS and TRIMETHOPRIM may act additively or synergistically to inhibit renal excretion of potassium.

Management If coadministration cannot be avoided, closely monitor potassium plasma concentrations and clinical response. Adjust the ANGIOTENSIN II RECEPTOR ANTAGONIST dose as needed.

Discussion

In a case control study spanning 14 years, the risk of hyperkalemia-associated hospitalization in patients 66 years and older who were being treated with trimethoprim/ sulfamethoxazole and an ACE inhibitor or angiotensin II receptor antagonist was assessed.[1] During the study period, 4,248 admissions involving hyperkalemia occurring within 14 days of antibiotic exposure were identified.[1] Coadministration of an ACE inhibitor or angiotensin II receptor antagonist and trimethoprim-sulfamethoxazole was associated with a nearly 7-fold increased risk of hyperkalemia-associated hospitalization compared with amoxicillin (eg, *Amoxil*). Other comparator antibiotics were not associated with this risk.

[1] Antoniou T, et al. *Arch Intern Med.* 2010;170(12):1045.

* Asterisk indicates drugs cited in interaction reports.

Angiotensin II Receptor Antagonists — *Valproic Acid*

Angiotensin II Receptor Antagonists	Valproic Acid	
Losartan* (eg, *Cozaar*)	Divalproex Sodium (eg, *Depakote*) Valproate Sodium (eg, *Depacon*)	Valproic Acid* (eg, *Depakene*)

Significance	Onset	Severity	Documentation
4	□ Rapid ■ **Delayed**	□ Major ■ **Moderate** □ Minor	□ Established □ Probable □ Suspected ■ **Possible** □ Unlikely

Effects The antihypertensive effect of LOSARTAN may be decreased because of reduced exposure to the active carboxylic acid metabolite (E3174).

Mechanism Inhibition of LOSARTAN metabolism (CYP2C9) to its metabolite E3174 by VALPROIC ACID.

Management Closely monitor BP response and renal function (including potassium concentrations) in patients receiving LOSARTAN when the dose of VALPROIC ACID is started, stopped, or changed. Because olmesartan (*Benicar*) is not metabolized after absorption from the GI tract, it may not interact with VALPROIC ACID.

Discussion

The effect of valproic acid on losartan metabolism was evaluated in 9 patients with a history of generalized or partial seizures.[1] Patients received valproic acid based on their clinical need (mean dose of 200 mg/day for the first week and 400 mg/day for the following 4 weeks). Each patient received a single oral dose of losartan 25 mg 2 days prior to valproic acid treatment and after dose 1, week 1, and week 4 of valproic acid treatment. The ratio of losartan to the carboxylic acid metabolite (E3174) was not different on day 1 or week 1 of valproic acid treatment compared with administration of losartan alone. However, the ratio increased from 0.6 to 1.09 after 4 weeks of valproic acid treatment, indicating an inhibitory effect of valproic acid on losartan metabolism (CYP2C9 enzyme). The degree of metabolic inhibition correlated with steady-state valproic acid plasma concentrations.

[1] Gunes A, et al. *Basic Clin Pharmacol Toxicol.* 2007;100(6):383.

* Asterisk indicates drugs cited in interaction reports. Based on pharmacologic and pharmacokinetic considerations, similar interactions may occur with other drugs that are listed.

Antacids | ***Enteral Nutrition***

Antacids	Enteral Nutrition
Aluminum Hydroxide (eg, *Amphojel*)	Enteral Nutrition, High Molecular Protein*
Aluminum/Magnesium Hydroxide* (eg, *Maalox*)	

Significance	Onset	Severity	Documentation
2	☐ Rapid	☐ Major	☐ Established
	■ **Delayed**	■ **Moderate**	☐ Probable
		☐ Minor	■ **Suspected**
			☐ Possible
			☐ Unlikely

Effects Risk of esophageal obstruction may be increased.

Mechanism Formation of a protein-aluminum complex that is not degraded by pepsin or low pH.

Management ENTERAL NUTRITION with high molecular protein solutions should not be mixed with or followed by aluminum-containing ANTACIDS. If an ANTACID is needed, separate the administration time from the ENTERAL NUTRITION by as much time as possible, and flush the feeding tube beforehand.

Discussion

Esophageal obstruction was reported in 3 patients receiving enteral feeding with a high-protein liquid nutrient and an aluminum-containing antacid to prevent stress ulcer.[1] The antacid was administered intermittently through the feeding tube. On removal of the feeding tube, esophageal plugs were found in the patients. Analysis of the plugs by atomic mass absorption determined the presence of aluminum.

[1] Valli C, et al. *Lancet.* 1986;1(8483):747.

* Asterisk indicates drugs cited in interaction reports. Based on pharmacologic and pharmacokinetic considerations, similar interactions may occur with other drugs that are listed.

Antiarrhythmic Agents | Macrolide & Related Antibiotics

Antiarrhythmic Agents		Macrolide & Related Antibiotics	
Amiodarone* (eg, *Cordarone*)	Procainamide* (eg, *Procanbid*)	Azithromycin* (eg, *Zithromax*)	Erythromycin* (eg, *Ery-Tab*)
Bretylium*	Quinidine*	Clarithromycin* (eg, *Biaxin*)	Telithromycin* (*Ketek*)
Disopyramide* (eg, *Norpace*)	Sotalol* (eg, *Betapace*)		
Dofetilide* (*Tikosyn*)			

Significance	Onset	Severity	Documentation
1	☐ Rapid ■ **Delayed**	■ **Major** ☐ Moderate ☐ Minor	☐ Established ☐ Probable ■ **Suspected** ☐ Possible ☐ Unlikely

Effects The risk of life-threatening cardiac arrhythmias, including torsades de pointes, may be increased.[1-3]

Mechanism An additive or synergistic increase in the QT interval may result.

Management Use certain MACROLIDE ANTIBIOTICS with caution[2] and avoid TELITHROMYCIN[3] in patients receiving class IA and class III ANTIARRHYTHMIC AGENTS.

Discussion

Dose-related prolongation of the QT interval and torsades de pointes occur with sotalol therapy.[2] Therefore, administer sotalol with caution in conjunction with drugs known to prolong the QT interval, such as certain macrolide antibiotics (eg, clarithromycin, erythromycin).[1,2] In addition, because telithromycin has the potential to prolong the QT interval, which may increase the risk of ventricular arrhythmias including torsades de pointes, avoid telithromycin in patients receiving class IA (eg, procainamide, quinidine) or class III (eg, dofetilide, sotalol) antiarrhythmic agents.[1,3] However, in a study of 24 women receiving sotalol and telithromycin, no increase in QTc occurred.[4] In fact, there was a greater increase in the QTc with administration of sotalol plus placebo. QT prolongation was reported in a 68-year-old woman during amiodarone and azithromycin coadministration.[5] She had been receiving amiodarone 200 mg/day for paroxysmal atrial fibrillation for more than 1 year. On day 3 of azithromycin therapy, she experienced intermittent dizziness, and her ECG showed sinus bradycardia with marked prolongation of the QT interval and increased QT dispersion. Four days after discontinuing azithromycin, the QT interval and QT dispersion were at baseline. See Drug-induced Prolongation of the QT Interval and Torsades de Pointes.

[1] Thomas M, et al. *Br J Clin Pharmacol.* 1996;41(2):77.
[2] *Betapace* [package insert]. Wayne, NJ: Berlex Laboratories; 2000.
[3] *Ketek* [package insert]. Kansas City, MO: Aventis Pharmaceuticals, Inc; June 2004.
[4] Démolis JL, et al. *Br J Clin Pharmacol.* 2005;60(2):120.
[5] Samarendra P, et al. *Pacing Clin Electrophysiol.* 2001;24(10):1572.

* Asterisk indicates drugs cited in interaction reports.

Antiarrhythmic Agents | **Quinolones**

Antiarrhythmic Agents		Quinolones	
Amiodarone* (eg, *Cordarone*)	Ibutilide* (*Corvert*)	Gatifloxacin* (*Zymar*)	Moxifloxacin* (*Avelox*)
Bretylium*	Procainamide* (eg, *Procanbid*)	Levofloxacin* (*Levaquin*)	Ofloxacin* (eg, *Floxin*)
Disopyramide* (eg, *Norpace*)	Quinidine*		
Dofetilide* (*Tikosyn*)	Sotalol* (eg, *Betapace*)		

Significance	Onset	Severity	Documentation
1	☐ Rapid ■ **Delayed**	■ **Major** ☐ Moderate ☐ Minor	☐ Established ☐ Probable ■ **Suspected** ☐ Possible ☐ Unlikely

Effects The risk of life-threatening cardiac arrhythmias, including torsades de pointes, may be increased.[1]

Mechanism Unknown.

Management Avoid GATIFLOXACIN, LEVOFLOXACIN, MOXIFLOXACIN, and OFLOXACIN in patients receiving class IA and class III ANTIARRHYTHMIC AGENTS.

Discussion

Moxifloxacin,[2] gatifloxacin,[3] and ofloxacin[4] may prolong the QTc interval; avoid administering these drugs to patients receiving class IA or class III antiarrhythmic agents. The effects of a single dose of ciprofloxacin 1,500 mg, levofloxacin 1,000 mg, and moxifloxacin 800 mg on the QT and QTc intervals were compared with placebo in 48 healthy subjects.[5] Compared with placebo, each of the fluoroquinolones produced statistically significant increases in the QT and QTc intervals. The changes in the QT and QTc intervals were greatest with moxifloxacin. Levofloxacin has been associated with torsades de pointes[6]; however, the association is unclear. In a study of 9 healthy volunteers, ofloxacin increased the procainamide AUC 27%, increased the C_{max} from 4.8 to 5.8 mcg/mL, and decreased the plasma clearance 21%.[7] In addition, procainamide renal clearance was reduced 30%, resulting in a 12% decrease in the 24-hour recovery of unchanged procainamide. Renal clearance of the active metabolite of procainamide, N-acetyl procainamide (NAPA), increased 18%, resulting in a 23% increase in the 24-hour recovery of NAPA. See also Procainamide-Ciprofloxacin and Drug-Induced Prolongation of the QT Interval and Torsades de Pointes.

1 Thomas M, et al. *Br J Clin Pharmacol.* 1996;41(2):77.
2 *Avelox* [package insert]. West Haven, CT: Bayer Corporation; November 2000.
3 *Tequin* [package insert]. Princeton, NJ: Bristol-Myers Squibb Company; March 2001.
4 *Floxin* [package insert]. Raritan, NJ: Ortho-McNeil Pharmaceuticals, Inc; March 2003.
5 Noel GJ, et al. *Clin Pharmacol Ther.* 2003;73(4):292.
6 Arizona Center for Education and Research on Therapeutics. University of Arizona Health Sciences Center Web site. http://www.torsades.org. Accessed January 3, 2008.
7 Martin DE, et al. *J Clin Pharmacol.* 1996;36(1):85.

* Asterisk indicates drugs cited in interaction reports.

Anticholinergics — *Amantadine*

Anticholinergics		Amantadine
Atropine (eg, *Sal-Tropine*)	Methscopolamine (eg, *Pamine*)	Amantadine* (eg, *Symmetrel*)
Belladonna	Orphenadrine* (eg *Norflex*)	
Benztropine* (eg, *Cogentin*)	Oxybutynin (eg, *Ditropan*)	
Biperiden* (*Akineton*)	Procyclidine (*Kemadrin*)	
Clidinium	Propantheline (eg, *Pro-Banthine*)	
Dicyclomine (eg, *Bentyl*)	Scopolamine (eg, *Scopace*)	
Glycopyrrolate (eg, *Robinul*)	Trihexyphenidyl* (eg, *Trihexy-2*)	
Hyoscyamine (eg, *Anaspaz*)		
Mepenzolate (*Cantil*)		

Significance	Onset	Severity	Documentation
4	□ Rapid	□ Major	□ Established
	■ **Delayed**	■ **Moderate**	□ Probable
		□ Minor	□ Suspected
			■ **Possible**
			□ Unlikely

Effects The ANTICHOLINERGIC adverse reactions may be increased.

Mechanism Probably additive or synergistic toxicity.

Management If an interaction is suspected, consider decreasing the dose of the ANTICHOLINERGIC agent during coadministration of AMANTADINE. Monitor the patient's response and adjust the dosage accordingly.

Discussion

In patients receiving amantadine and anticholinergic agents, possible potentiation of anticholinergic adverse reactions, including nocturnal confusion and hallucinations, has been reported.[1-3] These reactions disappear when the dose of the anticholinergic agent is reduced.[1]

Because these reactions can occur with administration of anticholinergic agents alone, controlled studies are needed to verify a definite interaction between these drugs.

[1] Schwab RS, et al. *JAMA.* 1969;208(7):1168.
[2] Parkes JD, et al. *Lancet.* 1971;1(7709):1083.
[3] Postma JU, et al. *J Am Geriatr Soc.* 1975;23(5):212.

* Asterisk indicates drugs cited in interaction reports. Based on pharmacologic and pharmacokinetic considerations, similar interactions may occur with other drugs that are listed.

Anticholinergics — *Betel Nut*

Anticholinergics		Betel Nut
Benztropine (eg, *Cogentin*)	Procyclidine* (*Kemadrin*)	Betel Nut*
Biperiden (*Akineton*)	Trihexyphenidyl (eg, *Trihexy-2*)	

Significance	Onset	Severity	Documentation
4	☐ Rapid	☐ Major	☐ Established
	■ **Delayed**	■ **Moderate**	☐ Probable
		☐ Minor	☐ Suspected
			■ **Possible**
			☐ Unlikely

Effects Extrapyramidal symptoms may occur.

Mechanism Antagonism of the anticholinergic action of ANTICHOLINERGICS by the active ingredient in BETEL NUT (ie, arecoline, which mimics acetylcholine at muscarinic and nicotinic receptors) is suspected.

Management Patients using ANTICHOLINERGICS should avoid concomitant use of BETEL NUT.

Discussion

Two patients developed severe extrapyramidal symptoms during concurrent use of procyclidine and heavy consumption of betel nut.[1] One patient, a 51-year-old man with chronic schizophrenia, had remained stable for 2 years on fluphenazine decanoate and procyclidine 5 mg twice daily, which he was taking to control occasional extrapyramidal symptoms. After the patient experienced marked rigidity, bradykinesia, and jaw tremor, he admitted to chewing betel nut. He stopped chewing betel nut and 7 days later his stiffness and abnormal movements subsided. The second patient had a 12-year history of a schizoaffective disorder and had been receiving flupenthixol† for the previous year. Upon returning from India, the patient complained of marked stiffness, tremor, and akathisia. The symptoms had not been relieved by procyclidine 20 mg/day, which he took during the previous month. The patient admitted to heavy consumption of betel nut during his trip to India. He stopped chewing betel nut and his symptoms resolved over the next 4 days. Both patients displayed the characteristic red stains on their teeth that are associated with chewing betel nut.

[1] Deahl M. *Mov Disord.* 1989;4(4):330.

* Asterisk indicates drugs cited in interaction reports. Based on pharmacologic and pharmacokinetic considerations, similar interactions may occur with other drugs that are listed.
† Not available in the United States.

Anticholinesterases — *Corticosteroids*

Anticholinesterases		Corticosteroids	
Ambenonium Chloride (*Mytelase*)	Neostigmine* (eg, *Prostigmin*)	Betamethasone (eg, *Celestone*)	Hydrocortisone* (eg, *Cortef*)
Edrophonium (*Enlon*)	Pyridostigmine* (eg, *Mestinon*)	Corticotropin* (*Acthar HP*)	Methylprednisolone* (eg, *Medrol*)
		Cortisone*	Prednisolone* (eg, *Prelone*)
		Cosyntropin (eg, *Cortrosyn*)	Prednisone (eg, *Sterapred*)
		Dexamethasone (eg, *Baycadron*)	Triamcinolone (eg, *Kenalog*)
		Fludrocortisone	

Significance	Onset	Severity	Documentation
1	□ Rapid ■ **Delayed**	■ **Major** □ Moderate □ Minor	□ Established ■ **Probable** □ Suspected □ Possible □ Unlikely

Effects CORTICOSTEROIDS antagonize the effects of ANTICHOLINESTERASES in myasthenia gravis. Profound muscular depression relatively refractory to ANTICHOLINESTERASES has occurred.

Mechanism Unknown.

Management Occasional long-term benefits from CORTICOSTEROID therapy in myasthenia gravis occur. Consequently, combined use may be attempted under supervised conditions and with ready availability of life-support systems.

Discussion

Several investigators have reported severe deterioration in muscle strength in patients with myasthenia gravis given corticosteroids.[1-4] Typically, the deterioration began 2 days after therapy and became maximal at approximately 7 days. Patients were relatively refractory to acetylcholinesterase inhibitors, and in some cases required mechanical ventilation. Despite this adverse reaction, long-term improvement above baseline muscle strength has also been described.[4] Alternate-day prednisone therapy has been advocated as safer.[5]

The mechanism remains unclear. Using in vitro muscle preparations or evoked potentials in patients, hydrocortisone or corticotropin had no immediate effect on neuromuscular transmission. No changes occurred in the function of nerve or muscle fibers.[3] However, hydrocortisone antagonized neostigmine and pyridostigmine in rat muscle preparation.[6]

1 Millikan CH, et al. *Neurology*. 1951;1(2):145.
2 Grob D, et al. *Bull Johns Hopkins Hosp*. 1952;91(2):124.
3 Namba T. *Arch Neurol*. 1972;26(2):144.
4 Brunner NG, et al. *Neurology*. 1972;22(6):603.
5 Warmolts JR, et al. *Lancet*. 1970;2(7684):1198.
6 Patten BM, et al. *Neurology*. 1974;24(5):442.

* Asterisk indicates drugs cited in interaction reports. Based on pharmacologic and pharmacokinetic considerations, similar interactions may occur with other drugs that are listed.

Anticoagulants		*Acai Berry Juice*
Warfarin* (eg, *Coumadin*)		Acai Berry Juice*

Significance	Onset	Severity	Documentation
4	□ Rapid ■ **Delayed**	□ Major ■ **Moderate** □ Minor	□ Established □ Probable □ Suspected ■ **Possible** □ Unlikely

Effects The risk of fluctuations in the INR of patients receiving WARFARIN may be increased.

Mechanism Vitamin K present in the formulation may inhibit the effect of WARFARIN on vitamin K–dependent clotting factors. Glucosamine present in the formulation may have additive pharmacologic effects when administered with WARFARIN.

Management Because WARFARIN has a narrow therapeutic index, advise patients taking WARFARIN to avoid the blended ACAI BERRY JUICE, *MonaVie Active*. Caution patients receiving WARFARIN against using herbal products without consulting their health care provider and to report any unusual bruising.

Discussion

The amount of the blended acai berry juice (*MonaVie Active*) recommended for daily consumption, 30 mL twice daily, contains vitamin K 16 to 25 mcg.[1] This is less than the amount expected to affect warfarin. The *MonaVie Active* recommended for daily consumption also contains glucosamine 600 mg. It is not known if this amount of glucosamine is sufficient to affect warfarin therapy. Although the interaction of warfarin with the blended acai berry juice (*MonaVie Active*) has not been studied, it is suspected that potential fluctuations in the INR in patients receiving warfarin may occur.

[1] Katcher S, et al. *Am J Health Syst Pharm.* 2010;67(2):107.

* Asterisk indicates drugs cited in interaction reports.

Anticoagulants — *Acarbose*

Warfarin* (eg, *Coumadin*)	Acarbose* (eg, *Precose*)

Significance	Onset	Severity	Documentation
4	□ Rapid ■ **Delayed**	□ Major ■ **Moderate** □ Minor	□ Established □ Probable □ Suspected ■ **Possible** □ Unlikely

Effects The anticoagulant effect of WARFARIN may be increased.

Mechanism Unknown.

Management Monitor anticoagulant function when ACARBOSE is started or stopped. Adjust the dose of WARFARIN as needed.

Discussion

A possible drug interaction between warfarin and acarbose was reported in a 66-year-old man.[1] The patient had a history of a cerebrovascular accident, for which he was receiving warfarin 42.5 mg/week. In addition, he had hypertension, coronary artery disease, diabetes mellitus, and peripheral vascular disease. The patient was receiving fosinopril (eg, *Monopril*), hydrochlorothiazide (eg, *Microzide*), glipizide (eg, *Glucotrol*), regular insulin (eg, *Humulin R*), and diphenhydramine (eg, *Benadryl*). Acarbose was started at 25 mg daily for week 1, 25 mg twice daily in week 2, and 25 mg 3 times daily in week 3. The patient's INR had been 2.53 to 3.13 for the previous 10 months. Four days before initiating acarbose therapy, the INR was 3.09, and after 2 weeks of acarbose therapy the INR increased to 4.85. Warfarin therapy was withheld for 1 day and then resumed at 40 mg/week. Subsequently, acarbose was discontinued, and after 7 and 14 days, the INR was 3.28 and 2.84, respectively.

[1] Morreale AP, et al. *Am J Health Syst Pharm.* 1997;54(13):1551.

* Asterisk indicates drugs cited in interaction reports.

Anticoagulants		**Acetaminophen**
Warfarin* (eg, *Coumadin*)		Acetaminophen* (eg, *Tylenol*)

Significance	Onset	Severity	Documentation
2	□ Rapid ■ **Delayed**	□ Major ■ **Moderate** □ Minor	□ Established ■ **Probable** □ Suspected □ Possible □ Unlikely

Effects

ACETAMINOPHEN (APAP) appears to increase the antithrombotic effect of oral ANTICOAGULANTS in a dose-dependent manner. The interaction may not be clinically important with low-dose, infrequent use (no more than six 325 mg tablets/wk) of APAP.

Mechanism

Possible augmentation of vitamin K antagonism by APAP or a metabolite.[1]

Management

Limit APAP use and monitor coagulation parameters 1 to 2 times/wk when APAP is started or stopped, particularly if more than 2,275 mg/wk is consumed. Be prepared to adjust the ANTICOAGULANT dose as necessary.

Discussion

Controlled studies and case reports[1-8] are conflicting. Most reports found little or no increase in coagulation parameters. One case reported an increase in PT from 13 to 23 seconds in conjunction with hematuria and gingival bleeding following addition of APAP (48 tablets over 10 days).[9] A second case reported 2 episodes of elevated INR (8.5 and 12) and bleeding in 1 patient following the addition of APAP-containing analgesics (14 g over 7 days, 14 g over 8 days) to a stable warfarin dose.[10] A 72-year-old man on a stable dose of acenocoumerol[†] experienced a drop in INR when APAP 1 to 2 g/day was stopped.[11] His INR returned to baseline when APAP was restarted. In a case-controlled study investigating factors associated with INR elevations higher than 6, APAP ingestion was an independent risk factor.[12] The effect appears to be dose-related. Daily ingestion of APAP 325 to 650 mg raised the risk of elevating the INR 3.5-fold, while daily ingestion of at least 1,250 mg increased the risk 10-fold. In a study of 11 patients on a stable warfarin regimen, APAP 4 g/day raised the INR after 4 days, increasing the risk of bleeding.[13] In a study of 20 healthy volunteers, APAP 4 g/day for 2 wk did not affect anticoagulation of a single dose of warfarin 20 mg.[7] However, in a study of patients taking warfarin who had stable INRs, administration of APAP 2 or 4 g daily produced higher mean INRs than placebo.[14] A study using a large postmortem toxicology database suggests the risk of fatal bleeding in patients taking warfarin and acetaminophen is 4.6 times higher compared with taking acetaminophen alone and 2.7 times higher compared with taking warfarin alone.[15] In a study with 45 patients taking warfarin, administration of acetaminophen 2 or 3 g daily increased the mean INR 0.7 and 0.67, respectively, by the third day of combined therapy.[16] Other risk factors[12] (eg, diarrhea) or concurrent diseases that alter APAP metabolism[8] may play a role in this interaction.

1 Gebauer MG, et al. *Pharmacotherapy.* 2003;23(1):109.
2 Antlitz AM, et al. *Curr Ther Res Clin Exp.* 1968;10(10):501.
3 Antlitz AM, et al. *Curr Ther Res Clin Exp.* 1969;11(6):360.
4 Udall JA. *GP.* 1969;40(1):117.
5 Udall JA. *J R Coll Physicians Lond.* 1970;77:20.
6 Boeijinga JJ, et al. *Lancet.* 1982;1(8270):506.
7 Kwan D, et al. *J Clin Pharmacol.* 1999;39(1):68.
8 Lehmann DE. *Pharmacotherapy.* 2000;20(12):1464.
9 Bartle WR, et al. *JAMA.* 1991;265(10):1260.
10 Fitzmaurice DA, et al. *Postgrad Med J.* 1997;73(861):439.
11 Bagheri H, et al. *Ann Pharmacother.* 1999;33(4):506.
12 Hylek EM, et al. *JAMA.* 1998;279(9):657.
13 Mahé I, et al. *Br J Clin Pharmacol.* 2005;59(3):371.
14 Parra D, et al. *Pharmacotherapy.* 2007;27(5):675.
15 Launiainen T, et al. *Eur J Clin Pharmacol.* 2010;66(1):97.
16 Zhang Q, et al. *Eur J Clin Pharmacol.* 2011;67(3):309.

* Asterisk indicates drugs cited in interaction reports.
† Not available in the United States.

Anticoagulants — *Allopurinol*

Warfarin* (eg, *Coumadin*)	Allopurinol* (eg, *Zyloprim*)

Significance	Onset	Severity	Documentation
4	☐ Rapid ■ **Delayed**	☐ Major ■ **Moderate** ☐ Minor	☐ Established ☐ Probable ☐ Suspected ■ **Possible** ☐ Unlikely

Effects ALLOPURINOL may enhance the ANTICOAGULANT action of some oral ANTICOAGULANTS, but probably not that of WARFARIN.

Mechanism Inhibition of hepatic metabolism by ALLOPURINOL is suspected.

Management The interaction is unpredictable. However, consider monitoring anticoagulation parameters and adjusting the oral ANTICOAGULANT dose as needed.

Discussion

Data are conflicting. A pharmacokinetic study of 6 healthy volunteers showed a prolongation in the dicumarol† t½ from 51 to 152 hours.[1] However, another study found only a modest increase in 1 of 3 patients.[2] When comparing these 2 studies, the baseline dicumarol t½ was different, suggesting a methodological error. Warfarin has been studied in combination with allopurinol in healthy volunteers.[2,3] No alteration in warfarin pharmacokinetics was detected. A single case report of PT prolongation after the administration of allopurinol to a patient receiving warfarin was inconclusive.[4] In a drug surveillance program, 1,835 patients receiving allopurinol were monitored. Three patients developed an increased anticoagulant effect while taking concurrent warfarin.[5] Because of limited data, a drug interaction could not be proven. Another coumarin derivative, phenprocoumon,† is also suspected of interacting with allopurinol. Two cases were reported in which the serum levels of phenprocoumon increased. Bleeding occurred in 1 of the cases.[6]

The effect of allopurinol on oral anticoagulants appears to be drug-specific. Further controlled studies are needed to verify this interaction with warfarin. Caution is required with other coumarins.

1 Vesell ES, et al. *N Engl J Med.* 1970;283(27):1484.
2 Pond SM, et al. *Aust N Z J Med.* 1975;5(4):324.
3 Rawlins MD, et al. *Br J Pharmacol.* 1973;48(4):693.
4 Self TH, et al. *Lancet.* 1975;2(7934):557.
5 McInnes GT, et al. *Ann Rheum Dis.* 1981;40(3):245.
6 Jähnchen E, et al. *Klin Wochenschr.* 1977;55(15):759.

* Asterisk indicates drugs cited in interaction reports.
† Not available in the United States.

Anticoagulants — *Aminoglutethimide*

Anisindione (*Miradon*)	Warfarin* (eg, *Coumadin*)	Aminoglutethimide* (*Cytadren*)
Dicumarol†		

Significance	Onset	Severity	Documentation
2	□ Rapid	□ Major	□ Established
	■ **Delayed**	■ **Moderate**	□ Probable
		□ Minor	■ **Suspected**
			□ Possible
			□ Unlikely

Effects — WARFARIN's action to decrease prothrombin levels may be reduced.

Mechanism — Increased WARFARIN metabolic clearance, probably because of liver microsomal enzyme induction.

Management — Monitor prothrombin time when adding or stopping AMINOGLUTETHIMIDE. Tailor WARFARIN doses as needed.

Discussion

A higher than normal warfarin requirement was noted in patients receiving aminoglutethimide for breast cancer.[1,2] In a pharmacokinetic investigation of two such cases, the clearance of warfarin rose from 0.0011 L/kg or 0.0013 L/kg to 0.0037 L/kg or 0.0067 L/kg, respectively. Consequently, higher warfarin doses were needed to maintain therapeutic anticoagulation.[3] In another study, the effects of low (125 mg BID) versus high (250 mg QID) aminoglutethimide doses on warfarin pharmacokinetics were investigated in nine women. Using R- or S-warfarin isomers, results indicated an equal increase in the metabolic rate of either warfarin isomer. Considerable interpatient variability existed. Furthermore, in two patients who received low-dose aminoglutethimide for 4 weeks followed by the high dose, there was a further increase in warfarin clearance.[4]

While these studies are strongly suggestive of an interaction, they involved few patients. The mechanism has been postulated as hepatic microsomal enzyme induction based on the chemical similarity of aminoglutethimide to glutethimide. The latter is a known hepatic enzyme inducer. Further characterization of this interaction awaits larger controlled studies.

[1] Murray RML, et al. *Med J Aust* 1981;1:179.
[2] Bruning PF, et al. *Lancet* 1983;2:582.
[3] Lonning PE, et al. *Cancer Chemother Pharmacol* 1984;12:10.
[4] Lonning PE, et al. *Cancer Chemother Pharmacol* 1986;17:177.

* Asterisk indicates drugs cited in interaction reports. Based on pharmacologic and pharmacokinetic considerations, similar interactions may occur with other drugs that are listed.
† Not available in the United States.

Anticoagulants — Aminoglycosides

Anticoagulants		Aminoglycosides	
Anisindione (*Miradon*) Dicumarol†	Warfarin* (eg, *Coumadin*)	Kanamycin (*Kantrex*) Neomycin* (eg, *Mycifradin*)	Paromomycin* (*Humatin*)

Significance	Onset	Severity	Documentation
5	□ Rapid ■ **Delayed**	□ Major □ Moderate ■ **Minor**	□ Established □ Probable □ Suspected ■ **Possible** □ Unlikely

Effects A small rise in WARFARIN-induced hypoprothrombinemia may occur.

Mechanism Unknown. Interference in the absorption of dietary vitamin K is suspected.

Management No special precautions are generally needed. However, malnourished patients could theoretically be more susceptible to this interaction and should be monitored more carefully.

Discussion

The possibility of an interaction between neomycin and warfarin has been postulated on the basis of altered vitamin K gut flora production or malabsorption caused by oral neomycin.[1,2,5] However, clinical evidence to substantiate the interaction and its significance is very limited. No reports of bleeding exist.

In one case reported with paromomycin, no change in warfarin requirements was noted.[3] Likewise, in a study of the cholesterol-lowering effect of neomycin, no change in dose requirements for oral anticoagulants was reported, albeit no details were provided.[7] Conversely, in a study of the effect of several drugs on warfarin therapy, an average 5.6 second prolongation in the PT time was noted in six of ten patients.[6]

Udall performed several experiments in 10 healthy anticoagulated volunteers. Vitamin K did not reverse anticoagulation if instilled directly into the colon, whereas it readily did so if given orally. There was a minimal effect of oral neomycin (4 g/day x 3 weeks) on PT time. Similarly, there was a minimal effect of vitamin K-free diet in non-coagulated individuals. However, in one anticoagulated patient, this diet caused the PT time to rise over 40 seconds. The effect of neomycin on warfarin anticoagulation is minimal and probably unrelated to colonic gut flora vitamin K production. Yet when dietary vitamin K was curtailed, the effect of neomycin in a single patient was greater.[4] The latter situation deserves further study.

[1] Haden HT. *Arch Int Med* 1957;100:986.
[2] Jacobson ED, et al. *JAMA* 1961;175:187.
[3] Messinger WJ, et al. *Angiology* 1965;16:29.
[4] Udall JA. *JAMA* 1965;194:127.
[5] Faloon WW, et al. *Ann NY Acad Sci* 1966;132:879.
[6] Udall JA. *Clin Med* 1970 Aug;77:20.
[7] Schade RWB, et al. *Acta Med Scand* 1976;199:175.

* Asterisk indicates drugs cited in interaction reports. Based on pharmacologic and pharmacokinetic considerations, similar interactions may occur with other drugs that are listed.

† Not available in the United States.

Anticoagulants — **Amiodarone**

Warfarin*
(eg, *Coumadin*)

Amiodarone*
(eg, *Cordarone*)

Significance	Onset	Severity	Documentation
1	☐ Rapid ■ **Delayed**	■ **Major** ☐ Moderate ☐ Minor	■ **Established** ☐ Probable ☐ Suspected ☐ Possible ☐ Unlikely

Effects Hypoprothrombinemic effect of oral ANTICOAGULANTS is augmented by concomitant AMIODARONE therapy.

Mechanism AMIODARONE inhibits the metabolism (CYP1A2, CYP2C9) of the R- and S-enantiomers of WARFARIN.[1,2]

Management Monitor INR closely during first 6 to 8 weeks of AMIODARONE therapy. In patients receiving AMIODARONE maintenance doses of 100, 200, 300, or 400 mg/day, reduce the WARFARIN dose by approximately 25%, 30%, 35%, or 40%, respectively,[2] but a 30% to 50% reduction in WARFARIN dose is typically required.[3] The effect may persist for 1.5 to 4 months after discontinuing AMIODARONE, necessitating continual WARFARIN adjustment.[4]

Discussion

In case reports, amiodarone has potentiated the effects of warfarin.[4-8] Bleeding was noted in some patients. In 9 patients, the addition of amiodarone doubled the PT; 5 patients had bleeding after 3 to 4 weeks.[4] Consequently, the warfarin dose was reduced 33%. One trial documented a nonlinear correlation between amiodarone doses and the warfarin dose needed to maintain a therapeutic PT.[9] Despite the difference in weekly warfarin dose (23 vs 38 mg control), warfarin plasma levels were the same in 19 patients, suggesting metabolic inhibition.[9] In a pharmacokinetic investigation, 8 patients had their warfarin clearance decrease from 4.71 to 2.65 L/day.[10] Another study of 8 patients showed a 44% increase in PT at 2 weeks, requiring subsequent decrease in warfarin dose from 5.99 to 4.12 mg/day at 4 weeks.[11] In a retrospective study, more patients receiving warfarin plus amiodarone had an INR greater than 5, compared with patients receiving warfarin alone.[12] The INR values greater than 5 were most common during the first 12 weeks of concurrent treatment with warfarin and amiodarone, necessitating a warfarin dosage reduction.

[1] O'Reilly RA, et al. *Clin Pharmacol Ther.* 1987;42(3):290.
[2] Sanoski CA, et al. *Chest.* 2002;121(1):19.
[3] Rotmensch HH, et al. *Med Clin North Am.* 1988;72(2):321.
[4] Martinowitz U, et al. *N Engl J Med.* 1981;304(11):671.
[5] Rees A, et al. *Br Med J.* 1981;282(6278):1756.
[6] Serlin MJ, et al. *Br Med J.* 1981;283(6283):58.
[7] Hamer A, et al. *Circulation.* 1982;65(5):1025.
[8] Woeber KA, et al. *West J Med.* 1999;170(1):49.
[9] Almog S, et al. *Eur J Clin Pharmacol.* 1985;28(3):257.
[10] Watt AH, et al. *Br J Clin Pharmacol.* 1985;20(6):707.
[11] Kerin NZ, et al. *Arch Intern Med.* 1988;148(8):1779.
[12] Lu Y, et al. *Am J Health Syst Pharm.* 2008;65(10):947.

* Asterisk indicates drugs cited in interaction reports.

Anticoagulants | *Androgens (17-alkyl)*

Anticoagulants	Androgens (17-alkyl)	
Warfarin* (eg, *Coumadin*)	Danazol* Fluoxymesterone (eg, *Androxy*) Methyltestosterone* (eg, *Android*)	Oxandrolone (eg, *Oxandrin*) Oxymetholone* (*Anadrol-50*)

Significance	Onset	Severity	Documentation
1	☐ Rapid ■ **Delayed**	■ **Major** ☐ Moderate ☐ Minor	☐ Established ■ **Probable** ☐ Suspected ☐ Possible ☐ Unlikely

Effects The hypoprothrombinemic effect of oral ANTICOAGULANTS is potentiated by 17-ALKYL ANDROGENS.

Mechanism Unknown.

Management Avoid the combination if possible. When adding ANDROGENIC OR ANABOLIC STEROIDS, oral ANTICOAGULANT dose requirements will be reduced. Monitor anticoagulation parameters (eg, PT) and tailor doses as needed.

Discussion

Multiple cases exist of 17-alkylated testosterone derivatives causing warfarin requirements to decrease. The interaction has been reported with methandrostenolone†,[1-4] norethandrolone,[5] 17-alpha methyltestosterone,[5] ethylestrenol,[5] oxymetholone,[4,6-9] and methenolone†,[3] including some cases of bleeding. Additionally, 2 related steroid molecules, danazol and stanozolol, have increased the sensitivity to warfarin.[10-13] Danazol[10,11] prolonged the PT up to 168 seconds and caused serious bleeding. Giving dicumarol and norethandrolone† concurrently did not modify anticoagulant levels or vitamin K–dependent clotting factors.[14] Bleeding has been reported with acenocoumarol† and oxymetholone,[15] phenprocoumon† and methyltestosterone,[16] and phenindione† with ethylestrenol†,[17] or oxymetholone.[9]

Despite the fact that non-17-alkylated androgens appear to be safer, at least 1 case report has described a similar interaction.[18]

1 Pyorala K, et al. *Scand J Clin Lab Invest.* 1963;15:367.
2 Murakami M, et al. *Jpn Circ J.* 1965;29:243.
3 Pyorala K, et al. *Ann Med Exp Fenn.* 1965;43(2):95.
4 Dresdale FC, et al. *J Med Soc NJ.* 1967;64(11):609.
5 Pyorala K, et al. *Lancet.* 1963;2:360.
6 Edwards MS, et al. *Lancet.* 1971;2(7717):221.
7 Robinson BH, et al. *Lancet.* 1971;1(7713):1356.
8 Ekert H, et al. *Lancet.* 1971;2(7724):609.
9 Longridge RG, et al. *Lancet.* 1971;2(7715):90.
10 Goulbourne IA, et al. *Br J Obstet Gynecol.* 1981;88(9):950.
11 Small M, et al. *Scott Med J.* 1982;27(4):331.
12 Acomb C, et al. *Pharm J.* 1985;234:73.
13 Meeks ML, et al. *Ann Pharmacother.* 1992;26(5):641.
14 Schrogie JJ, et al. *Clin Pharmacol Ther.* 1967;8(1):70.
15 De Oya JC, et al. *Lancet.* 1971;2(7718):259.
16 Husted S, et al. *Eur J Clin Pharmacol.* 1976;10:209.
17 Vere DW, et al. *Lancet.* 1968;2(7562):281.
18 Lorentz SM, et al. *Clin Pharm.* 1985;4(3):332.

* Asterisk indicates drugs cited in interaction reports. Based on pharmacologic and pharmacokinetic considerations, similar interactions may occur with other drugs that are listed.

† Not available in the United States.

Anticoagulants × *Androgens (Non-17-alkyl Derivatives)*

Anticoagulants	Androgens (Non-17-alkyl Derivatives)
Warfarin* (eg, *Coumadin*)	Testosterone* (eg, *Delatestryl*)

Significance	Onset	Severity	Documentation
4	☐ Rapid ■ **Delayed**	☐ Major ■ **Moderate** ☐ Minor	☐ Established ☐ Probable ☐ Suspected ■ **Possible** ☐ Unlikely

Effects TESTOSTERONE may enhance the hypoprothrombinemic effect of oral ANTICOAGULANTS.

Mechanism Unknown.

Management Monitor coagulation parameters and tailor the dose of oral ANTICOAGULANTS as needed.

Discussion

There is limited information regarding this interaction. One report found that testosterone did not affect warfarin anticoagulation in 4 patients. However, no details were provided.[1] A single case report described a 69-year-old woman who received a topical testosterone propionate 2% ointment applied to the vulvar area.[2] Her PT rose from 16.8 to 29.4 seconds after 2 weeks. Along with warfarin dose reduction, the patient decreased use of the ointment. Subsequently, her prothrombin ratio became subtherapeutic. Her warfarin dose was then increased, but she also resumed use of the ointment. Her prothrombin ratio again rose to 2.8. The testosterone serum level was measured at 5,667 pg/mL or approximately 10 times the level obtained 3 months after she stopped using the ointment, proving that the testosterone was absorbed systemically. While the rechallenge features of this case are suggestive of an interaction, well-designed trials are necessary to determine clinical importance.

[1] Edwards MS, et al. *Lancet.* 1971;2(7717):221.

[2] Lorentz SM, et al. *Clin Pharm.* 1985;4(3):332.

* Asterisk indicates drugs cited in interaction reports.

Anticoagulants	**Antineoplastic Agents**	
Warfarin* (eg, *Coumadin*)	Capecitabine* (*Xeloda*)	Etoposide* (eg, *VePesid*)
	Carboplatin* (eg, *Paraplatin*)	Fluorouracil* (eg, *Adrucil*)
	Cisplatin* (eg, *Platinol-AQ*)	Gemcitabine* (eg, *Gemzar*)
	Cyclophosphamide* (eg, *Cytoxan*)	Paclitaxel* (eg, *Taxol*)

Significance	Onset	Severity	Documentation
1	☐ Rapid ■ **Delayed**	■ **Major** ☐ Moderate ☐ Minor	☐ Established ☐ Probable ■ **Suspected** ☐ Possible ☐ Unlikely

Effects The anticoagulant effect of WARFARIN may be increased.

Mechanism Possible protein displacement, inhibition of WARFARIN metabolism, or inhibition of clotting-factor synthesis.

Management Carefully monitor coagulation parameters during and after chemotherapy. Adjust WARFARIN dosage as needed.

Discussion

In patients receiving warfarin, increased PT was reported after discontinuing[1] or adding cyclophosphamide.[2,3] Fluorouracil increased the effect of warfarin.[4-10] Fluctuating INR was reported in a patient receiving fluorouracil after starting warfarin.[11] A possible delayed interaction may occur with each repeated 5-fluorouracil chemotherapy cycle.[10] Fifteen days after the first course of a carboplatin/etoposide regimen, elevated INR and GI bleeding occurred in a patient stabilized on warfarin.[12] Etoposide plus vindesine† prolonged PT.[4] A patient receiving warfarin experienced a posttreatment rise in INR after each cycle of paclitaxel/carboplatin.[13] Another patient required a 16% dose reduction in warfarin while receiving 2 cycles of gemcitabine.[14] Coadministration of warfarin and capecitabine has been associated with altered coagulation parameters and bleeding (including death).[15-18] In some patients, increases in PT and INR occurred several days or several months after starting and within 1 month after stopping capecitabine. In 4 patients receiving capecitabine and given a single dose of warfarin 20 mg, the AUC of S-warfarin increased 57%; R-warfarin was not affected.[16] Coadministration of warfarin and cisplatin resulted in an elevated INR in 2 patients.[19]

1 Tashima CK. *South Med J.* 1979;72(5):633.
2 Booth BW, et al. *N Engl J Med.* 1981;305(3):170.
3 Ward K, et al. *Cancer Treat Rep.* 1984;68(5):817.
4 Seifter EJ, et al. *Cancer Treat Rep.* 1985;69(2):244.
5 Wajima T, et al. *Am J Hematol.* 1992;40(3):238.
6 Brown MC. *Pharmacotherapy.* 1997;17(3):631.
7 Kolesar JM, et al. *Pharmacotherapy.* 1999;19(12):1445.
8 Brown MC. *Chemotherapy.* 1999;45(5):392.
9 Aki Z, et al. *Am J Gastroenterol.* 2000;95(4):1093.
10 Davis DA, et al. *Pharmacotherapy.* 2005;25(3):442.
11 Carabino J, et al. *Am J Health Syst Pharm.* 2002;59(9):875.
12 Le AT, et al. *Ann Pharmacother.* 1997;31(9):1006.
13 Thompson ME, et al. *Ann Oncol.* 2003;14(3):500.
14 Kinikar SA, et al. *Pharmacotherapy.* 1999;19(11):1331.
15 *Xeloda* [package insert]. Nutley, NJ: Roche Laboratories; September 2001.
16 Camidge R, et al. *J Clin Oncol.* 2005;23(21):4719.
17 Janney LM, et al. *Ann Pharmacother.* 2005;39(9):1546.
18 Yildirim Y, et al. *Int J Clin Pharmacol Ther.* 2006;44(2):80.
19 Yano R, et al. *Ann Pharmacother.* 2011;45(10):e55.

* Asterisk indicates drugs cited in interaction reports.
† Not available in the United States.

Anticoagulants | **Aprepitant**

Warfarin*
(eg, *Coumadin*)

Aprepitant*
(*Emend*)

Significance	Onset	Severity	Documentation
4	☐ Rapid ■ **Delayed**	☐ Major ■ **Moderate** ☐ Minor	☐ Established ☐ Probable ☐ Suspected ■ **Possible** ☐ Unlikely

Effects The anticoagulant effect of WARFARIN may be decreased.

Mechanism Induction of S(-)WARFARIN metabolism (CYP2C9) by APREPITANT is suspected.

Management In patients receiving WARFARIN, closely monitor coagulation parameters for 14 days following the initiation of each 3-day APREPITANT cycle.

Discussion

The effect of aprepitant on the pharmacokinetics and pharmacodynamics of warfarin was evaluated in 22 healthy volunteers.[1] Using a double-blind, placebo-controlled, randomized, 2-period, parallel-group design, each subject was individually titrated to an INR ranging from 1.3 to 1.8. Subsequently, warfarin was administered for an additional 8 days. On days 1 to 3, warfarin was coadministered with placebo or aprepitant 125 mg on day 1, and 80 mg on days 2 and 3. Compared with placebo, trough concentrations of the pharmacologically active S(-) warfarin enantiomer decreased on days 5 to 8, with a maximum decrease of 34% on day 8, during coadministration of aprepitant. In addition, there was an 11% mean maximum decrease in the INR on day 8 after aprepitant administration compared with placebo.

[1] Depré M, et al. *Eur J Clin Pharmacol.* 2005;61(5-6):341.

* Asterisk indicates drugs cited in interaction reports.

Anticoagulants | **Argatroban**

Warfarin* (eg, *Coumadin*)	Argatroban*

Significance	Onset	Severity	Documentation
2	☐ Rapid ■ **Delayed**	☐ Major ■ **Moderate** ☐ Minor	☐ Established ☐ Probable ■ **Suspected** ☐ Possible ☐ Unlikely

Effects Abnormal prolongation of the PT and INR, increasing the risk of bleeding.

Mechanism Unknown; however, both WARFARIN and ARGATROBAN increase the INR.

Management Closely monitor coagulation parameters when starting or stopping ARGATROBAN. Adjust the WARFARIN or ARGATROBAN dose as needed. Do not use a loading dose of WARFARIN in patients receiving ARGATROBAN.[1] Measure the INR daily during coadministration of these agents.[1]

Discussion

Coadministration of argatroban, which can independently increase the INR, and warfarin resulted in prolongation of the PT and INR.[1] It is recommended that the INR should be measured daily during coadministration of warfarin and argatroban.[1] The potential for a pharmacokinetic interaction between argatroban and warfarin was studied in a randomized, crossover investigation in 12 healthy volunteers.[2] Each subject received both drugs, a single dose of warfarin 7.5 mg orally, or argatroban 1.25 mcg/kg/min IV for 100 hours. PT was prolonged similarly when argatroban was given alone and with warfarin. No pharmacokinetic interaction was detected between argatroban and warfarin. Prolonged anticoagulation, as measured by the INR, was reported in a 32-year-old morbidly obese woman 19 days after she received her last dose of warfarin and 20 days after argatroban discontinuation.[3]

[1] *Argatroban* [package insert]. North Chicago, IL: Abbott Laboratories; April 3, 2002.
[2] Brown PM, et al. *Am J Health Syst Pharm.* 2002;59(21):2078.
[3] Shapiro NL, et al. *Pharmacotherapy.* 2006;26(12):1806.

* Asterisk indicates drugs cited in interaction reports.

Anticoagulants — *Ascorbic Acid*

Warfarin*
(eg, *Coumadin*)

Ascorbic Acid*
(eg, *Ascocid*)

Significance	Onset	Severity	Documentation
5	□ Rapid	□ Major	□ Established
	■ **Delayed**	■ **Moderate**	□ Probable
		□ Minor	□ Suspected
			□ Possible
			■ **Unlikely**

Effects The anticoagulation actions of WARFARIN may be reduced.

Mechanism Unknown.

Management No clinical interventions appear to be necessary unless the patient is taking large (more than 5 to 10 g/day) ASCORBIC ACID doses.

Discussion

The possibility of an interaction between warfarin and ascorbic acid is suggested by 2 case reports. In 1 case, no details on the ascorbic acid dose were available. The patient presented with decreasing PT despite increased warfarin dosage.[1] In the second case, a woman previously stabilized on warfarin 5 mg/day presented with a baseline PT of 12 seconds and thrombophlebitis. This patient required warfarin 25 mg/day to regain anticoagulation. She admitted to consumption of approximately 16 g/day of ascorbic acid.[2]

In other controlled investigations, this effect of ascorbic acid on anticoagulation could not be reproduced either in rabbits,[3] dogs,[4] or man.[3,5] In 1 study, 19 patients received ascorbic acid 3, 5, or 10 g/day for a week after a control warfarin stabilization period.[5] No clinically important variations in PT were noted with any ascorbic acid dose. However, plasma warfarin levels did decrease in most patients. This effect was attributed to possible warfarin malabsorption because of ascorbic acid-induced diarrhea.

Current data on this interaction are very limited.

1 Rosenthal G. *JAMA*. 1971;215(10):1671.
2 Smith EC, et al. *JAMA*. 1972;221(10):1166.
3 Hume R, et al. *JAMA*. 1972;219(11):1479.
4 Weintraub M, et al. *Toxicol Appl Pharmacol*. 1974;28(1):53.
5 Feetam CL, et al. *Toxicol Appl Pharmacol*. 1975;31(3):544.

* Asterisk indicates drugs cited in interaction reports.

Anticoagulants — *Atovaquone*

Warfarin* (eg, *Coumadin*)	Atovaquone* (*Mepron*)

Significance	Onset	Severity	Documentation
4	☐ Rapid ■ **Delayed**	☐ Major ■ **Moderate** ☐ Minor	☐ Established ☐ Probable ☐ Suspected ■ **Possible** ☐ Unlikely

Effects Anticoagulant effect of WARFARIN may be transiently increased.

Mechanism ATOVAQUONE may displace WARFARIN from protein-binding sites.

Management Monitor anticoagulant activity for 10 days after starting or discontinuing ATOVAQUONE and adjust the WARFARIN dose as needed.

Discussion

A 53-year-old HIV-infected man was prescribed warfarin 5 mg (target INR, 2.5) daily for 12 months after being diagnosed with idiopathic deep vein thrombosis and bilateral pulmonary emboli.[1] Seven days after starting atovaquone for *Pneumocystis jiroveci* pneumonia prophylaxis, the INR increased from 2.3 to 3.5. The INR remained supratherapeutic (4.2) despite a 5% decrease in the warfarin dose. One dose of warfarin was withheld, and the total weekly warfarin dose was decreased another 10%. Atovaquone was discontinued 8 days later. The following day, the INR decreased to 1.7. The total weekly warfarin dose was increased 5% 8 days later. No further INR values were obtained because the patient completed the 12-month course of warfarin therapy. No signs or symptoms of hemorrhage were reported while the INR was supratherapeutic.[1]

[1] Hidalgo K, et al. *Ann Pharmacother.* 2011;45(1):e3.

* Asterisk indicates drugs cited in interaction reports.

Anticoagulants × *Azole Antifungal Agents*

Anticoagulants	Azole Antifungal Agents	
Warfarin* (eg, *Coumadin*)	Econazole* (eg, *Spectazole*)	Ketoconazole* (eg, *Nizoral*)
	Fluconazole* (eg, *Diflucan*)	Miconazole* (eg, *Micatin*)
	Itraconazole* (eg, *Sporanox*)	Voriconazole* (*Vfend*)

Significance	Onset	Severity	Documentation
1	☐ Rapid	■ **Major**	■ **Established**
	■ **Delayed**	☐ Moderate	☐ Probable
		☐ Minor	☐ Suspected
			☐ Possible
			☐ Unlikely

Effects The anticoagulant effect of WARFARIN may be increased.

Mechanism Inhibition of WARFARIN metabolism.

Management Monitor PT and INR values frequently (eg, every 2 days) when adding or discontinuing an AZOLE ANTIFUNGAL AGENT. Adjust the WARFARIN dose as needed.

Discussion

Studies and case reports document that azole antifungal agents increase the anticoagulant effect of warfarin.[1-8] Patients well controlled on warfarin developed bleeding complications,[4,5] bruising,[4,9-11] increased PT,[3,10] or increased INR[4,12] after treatment with fluconazole,[3] itraconazole,[4] ketoconazole,[10] econazole,[13,14] or miconazole topical cream,[15] gel,[5,12] and vaginal suppositories.[16] Miconazole inhibits warfarin hydroxylation, decreasing warfarin enantiomers and increasing PT response 4- to 5-fold.[6] In 15 volunteers, fluconazole 200 mg for 7 days prolonged the PT versus time curve.[7] In another report, 7 patients experienced a 16% to 64% increase in PT after the addition of fluconazole 200 mg/day.[7] In a patient with chronic renal insufficiency, fluconazole increased the INR from 2.7 to 5.2 despite a reduction and subsequent discontinuation of warfarin.[8] A case-control epidemologic study reported a 2-fold increase in risk of GI bleeding in patients exposed to fluconazole while receiving warfarin.[17] In 14 volunteers, voriconazole 300 mg twice daily increased the anticoagulant effect of a single dose of warfarin 30 mg.[18] Thus, it appears that all azole antifungal agents interact with warfarin; however, some may have a greater potential to interact than others.

1 Brass C, et al. *Antimicrob Agents Chemother.* 1982;21(1):151.
2 Lazar JD, et al. *Rev Infect Dis.* 1990;12(suppl 3):S327.
3 Seaton TL, et al. *DICP.* 1990;24(12):1177.
4 Yeh J, et al. *BMJ.* 1990;301(6753):669.
5 Shenfield GM, et al. *Aust N Z J Med.* 1991;21(6):928.
6 O'Reilly RA, et al. *Clin Pharmacol Ther.* 1992;51(6):656.
7 Crussell-Porter LL, et al. *Arch Intern Med.* 1993;153(1):102.
8 Gericke KR. *Pharmacotherapy.* 1993;13(5):508.
9 Ortin M, et al. *Ann Pharmacother.* 1999;33(2):175.
10 Smith AG. *Br Med J.* 1984;288(6412):188.
11 Lansdorp D, et al. *Br J Clin Pharmacol.* 1999;47(2):225.
12 Silingardi M, et al. *Thromb Haemost.* 2000;83(5):794.
13 Lang PG Jr, et al. *J Am Acad Dermatol.* 2006;55(5)(suppl):S117.
14 Alexandra JF, et al. *Ann Intern Med.* 2008; 148(8):633.
15 Devaraj A, et al. *BMJ.* 2002;325(7355):77.
16 Thirion DJ, et al. *Pharmacotherapy.* 2000;20(1):98.
17 Schelleman H, et al. *Clin Pharmacol Ther.* 2008; 84(5):581.
18 Purkins L, et al. *Br J Clin Pharmacol.* 2003;56(suppl 1):24.

* Asterisk indicates drugs cited in interaction reports.

Anticoagulants — *Barbiturates*

Anticoagulants	Barbiturates	
Dicumarol*†	Amobarbital* (*Amytal*)	Pentobarbital
Warfarin* (eg, *Coumadin*)	Butabarbital (eg, *Butisol*)	Phenobarbital* (eg, *Solfoton*)
	Butalbital	Primidone (eg, *Mysoline*)
	Mephobarbital (*Mebaral*)	Secobarbital* (*Seconal*)

Significance	Onset	Severity	Documentation
1	□ Rapid	■ **Major**	■ **Established**
	■ **Delayed**	□ Moderate	□ Probable
		□ Minor	□ Suspected
			□ Possible
			□ Unlikely

Effects BARBITURATES reduce the effects of ANTICOAGULANTS.

Mechanism Increased metabolic clearance of ANTICOAGULANTS, probably caused by induction of hepatic microsomal enzymes.

Management Patients receiving BARBITURATES will need modification of their ANTICOAGULANT dose. Monitor ANTICOAGULANT action and adjust doses as needed. Termination of BARBITURATE therapy will result in decreased ANTICOAGULANT requirements. Monitor patients for several weeks. Consider using a benzodiazepine.[1]

Discussion

The use of phenobarbital increased dicumarol dose requirements 33% in 8 patients[2]; a similar effect occurred with hexobarbital,[†3] apparently because of enzyme induction.[4] Phenobarbital reduced the plasma dicumarol levels in 5 of 7 patients. Similar changes occurred with warfarin.[5-8] Bleeding has been attributed to discontinuation of phenobarbital therapy in at least 3 patients. In 2 other patients who died from bleeding due to excessive anticoagulation, the discontinuation of other unspecified barbiturates was a possible cause.[6] Other barbiturates also have been reported to interact with warfarin. Amobarbital[9] and secobarbital[8-10] reduced warfarin t½ and mean PT. Instability in the dose of oral anticoagulants was noted in patients taking hypnotic barbiturates.[11] It appears that barbiturates alter the pharmacokinetics of warfarin but not the pharmacodynamics.[12]

[1] Orme M, et al. *Br Med J.* 1972;3(5827):611.
[2] Goss JE, et al. *N Engl J Med.* 1965;273(20):1094.
[3] Aggeler PM, et al. *J Lab Clin Med.* 1969;74(2):229.
[4] Cucinell SA, et al. *Clin Pharmacol Ther.* 1965;6:420.
[5] Robinson DS, et al. *J Pharmacol Exp Ther.* 1966;153:250.
[6] MacDonald MG, et al. *JAMA.* 1968;204(2):97.
[7] MacDonald MG, et al. *Clin Pharmacol Ther.* 1969;10(1):80.
[8] Udall JA. *Am J Cardiol.* 1975;35(1):67.
[9] Robinson DS, et al. *Ann Intern Med.* 1970;72(6):853.
[10] O'Reilly RA, et al. *Clin Pharmacol Ther.* 1980;28(2):187.
[11] Williams JR, et al. *Q J Med.* 1976;45(177):63.
[12] Chan E, et al. *Clin Pharmacol Ther.* 1994;56(3):286.

* Asterisk indicates drugs cited in interaction reports. Based on pharmacologic and pharmacokinetic considerations, similar interactions may occur with other drugs that are listed.
† Not available in the United States.

Anticoagulants — *Bee Pollen*

Warfarin* (eg, *Coumadin*)	Bee Pollen*

Significance	Onset	Severity	Documentation
4	☐ Rapid ■ **Delayed**	■ **Major** ☐ Moderate ☐ Minor	☐ Established ☐ Probable ☐ Suspected ■ **Possible** ☐ Unlikely

Effects The anticoagulant effect of WARFARIN may be increased.

Mechanism Unknown. However, flavonoids found in BEE POLLEN may be involved.

Management Because WARFARIN has a narrow therapeutic index, advise patients taking WARFARIN to avoid concurrent ingestion of BEE POLLEN. Caution patients against using herbal products or dietary supplements without consulting their health care provider and to report any signs of unexplained bleeding.

Discussion

Bee pollen consists of plant pollen combined with plant nectar and bee saliva that are packed by the bee into small pellets for use as a food source.[1] A 71-year-old man taking warfarin 47.5 mg/week was seen at an anticoagulant clinic for routine warfarin monitoring.[2] His INR value was 7.1 (therapeutic range, 2 to 3). During the previous 9 months, all his medications and herbal supplement dosages had been stable and his INR ranged from 1.9 to 3.3. The patient had begun taking 1 teaspoon of bee pollen granules twice daily 1 month prior to the clinic visit in which his INR was greatly elevated. Warfarin was withheld, and 3 days later his INR was 3.7. Warfarin was withheld a fourth day and then restarted. Because the patient wanted to continue ingesting bee pollen, the weekly dose of warfarin was decreased by 5 mg/week (11%) from his previous maintenance dose. The patient continued taking warfarin and bee pollen and was seen in the clinic 7 days later with an INR of 2.6. During the next 7 months, all INR values were within or near the therapeutic range.

[1] DerMarderosian A, Beutler JA, eds. Bee Pollen. *The Review of Natural Products*. St. Louis, MO: Wolters Kluwer Health Inc; 2010.

[2] Hurren KM, et al. *Am J Health Syst Pharm.* 2010;67(23):2034.

* Asterisk indicates drugs cited in interaction reports.

Anticoagulants — *Beta-Blockers*

Warfarin*
(eg, *Coumadin*)

Propranolol*
(eg, *Inderal*)

Significance	Onset	Severity	Documentation
4	☐ Rapid	☐ Major	☐ Established
	■ **Delayed**	■ **Moderate**	☐ Probable
		☐ Minor	☐ Suspected
			■ **Possible**
			☐ Unlikely

Effects PROPRANOLOL may increase the anticoagulant effect of WARFARIN.

Mechanism Unknown.

Management No clinical interventions are required at this time. If an interaction is suspected, monitor PT.

Discussion

The possibility of an interaction between warfarin and propranolol was suggested by the ability of propranolol to inhibit the metabolism of certain drugs (eg, antipyrine) and by a single case report.[1] The case involved a thyrotoxic patient on warfarin who received propranolol 80 mg twice daily. His PT increased as measured by the British corrected ratio but remained within the therapeutic range. Subsequent investigations have been limited by study design. The pharmacokinetic and pharmacodynamic alterations to a single dose of warfarin 15 mg by propranolol, atenolol (eg, *Tenormin*), or metoprolol (eg, *Lopressor*) were evaluated in 6 volunteers.[2] While propranolol increased the warfarin AUC 16% and warfarin C_{max} 23%, there was no effect on PT or plasma clotting factor VII. Neither atenolol nor metoprolol produced any changes. In another study involving 6 volunteers, propranolol 80 mg twice daily caused a small but statistically significant increase in the trough warfarin levels.[3] There was no effect on warfarin protein binding, and there was no alteration in the PT.[3] Despite these findings, at therapeutic warfarin doses, even small variations in warfarin levels could result in more important changes in the PT because of the shape of the dose-response curve for warfarin. Neither atenolol nor metoprolol have affected the pharmacodynamic effects of acenocoumarin†[4] or phenprocoumon.†[5] Beta-adrenergic blockers that are not highly lipophilic appear to have less potential to interact with oral anticoagulants. Controlled studies in patients therapeutically anticoagulated are needed to support this interaction.

[1] Bax ND, et al. *Drugs.* 1983;25(suppl 2):121.
[2] Bax ND, et al. *Br J Clin Pharmacol.* 1984;17(5):553.
[3] Scott AK, et al. *Br J Clin Pharmacol.* 1984;17(5):559.
[4] Mantero F, et al. *Br J Clin Pharmacol.* 1984;17(suppl 1):94S.
[5] Spahn H, et al. *Br J Clin Pharmacol.* 1984;17(suppl 1):97S.

* Asterisk indicates drugs cited in interaction reports.
† Not available in the United States.

Anticoagulants			**Bosentan**
Warfarin* (eg, *Coumadin*)		Bosentan* (*Tracleer*)	
Significance	Onset	Severity	Documentation
2	☐ Rapid ■ **Delayed**	☐ Major ■ **Moderate** ☐ Minor	☐ Established ■ **Probable** ☐ Suspected ☐ Possible ☐ Unlikely

Effects The effects of WARFARIN may be decreased.

Mechanism Induction of WARFARIN metabolism (CYP2C9 and CYP3A4) by BOSENTAN is suspected.

Management In patients receiving WARFARIN, carefully monitor coagulation parameters when the dose of BOSENTAN is started, stopped, or changed. Adjust the WARFARIN dose as needed.

Discussion

A decrease in the INR was reported in a 35-year-old woman stabilized on warfarin after the addition of bosentan to her treatment regimen.[1] The patient had been stabilized on warfarin (27.5 mg weekly) for 3 months with an INR within the therapeutic range (2 to 3). Her INR decreased to 1.7 ten days after starting bosentan (62.5 mg twice daily). The INR remained decreased over the next 5 weeks, despite weekly increases in the warfarin dose to 57.5 mg/week. At this point, the INR increased above the therapeutic range (above 3) for 3 weeks, and it was necessary to decrease the warfarin dose. Subsequently, during coadministration with bosentan, the INR was maintained in the therapeutic range with a dose of warfarin 45 mg/week. After starting bosentan in a 52-year-old woman stabilized on warfarin, it was necessary to increase the warfarin dose 43% to maintain a therapeutic INR.[2] The effects of bosentan on the pharmacokinetics and pharmacodynamics of warfarin were studied in 12 healthy men.[3] Using a double-blind, placebo-controlled, randomized, 2-way crossover design, each subject received a single oral dose of warfarin 26 mg in the morning of day 6 of bosentan (500 mg twice daily for 10 days) treatment and on day 6 of placebo administration. Compared with placebo, bosentan decreased the maximal PT and the AUC of PT and factor VII activity on average 23% and 38%, respectively.

[1] Murphey LM, et al. *Ann Pharmacother.* 2003;37(7-8):1028.

[2] Spangler ML, et al. *Clin Ther.* 2010;32(1):53.

[3] Weber C, et al. *J Clin Pharmacol.* 1999;39(8):847.

* Asterisk indicates drugs cited in interaction reports.

Anticoagulants — *Carbamazepine*

Warfarin* (eg, *Coumadin*)	Carbamazepine* (eg, *Tegretol*)

Significance	Onset	Severity	Documentation
2	□ Rapid ■ **Delayed**	□ Major ■ **Moderate** □ Minor	□ Established ■ **Probable** □ Suspected □ Possible □ Unlikely

Effects The anticoagulant effect of WARFARIN may be diminished during CARBAMAZEPINE coadministration.

Mechanism Induction of hepatic metabolism of ANTICOAGULANTS by CARBAMAZEPINE is suspected.

Management Monitor coagulation parameters when starting or stopping CARBAMAZEPINE therapy in patients receiving WARFARIN. Adjust the WARFARIN dose as needed.

Discussion

Limited evidence suggests an interaction between warfarin and carbamazepine. Two patients taking warfarin were studied after therapy with carbamazepine.[1] One of these patients had a reversal of anticoagulation, as measured by the prothrombin-proconvertin percentage, from 20% to 90% after 2 weeks. With discontinuation of carbamazepine, the prothrombin-proconvertin percentage decreased to 50%. Also, there was a decrease in warfarin plasma levels from 2.8 to 1.5 mg/L. Similar findings were observed in the second patient. An additional single-dose warfarin pharmacokinetic study demonstrated a reduction in warfarin $t_{1/2}$ in 2 of 3 patients. The pharmacokinetics of warfarin in 5 patients also receiving carbamazepine were compared with those of warfarin in 54 patients not receiving an interacting drug.[2] Warfarin clearance was higher in patients taking carbamazepine. In addition, in patients cotreated with carbamazepine, the average warfarin dosage was 9 mg/day compared with 3.86 mg/day in patients not receiving an interacting drug. In another report, a patient who stopped carbamazepine demonstrated a PT equal to 5 times the control value.[3] In 1 patient, prolongation of PT to nearly 6 times the control value was associated with ecchymosis.[4] In another patient, complete reversal of anticoagulation occurred with carbamazepine 200 mg twice daily.[5] Other case reports illustrate similar changes.[6,7]

Further controlled investigations are necessary to fully evaluate this interaction.

1 Hansen JM, et al. *Clin Pharmacol Ther.* 1971;12(3):539.
2 Herman D, et al. *Eur J Clin Pharmacol.* 2006;62(4):291.
3 Ross JR, et al. *Br Med J.* 1980;280(6229):1415.
4 Denbow CE, et al. *South Med J.* 1990;83(8):981.
5 Kendall AG, et al. *Ann Intern Med.* 1981;94(2):280.
6 Massey EW. *Ann Neurol.* 1983;13(6):691.
7 Parrish RH, et al. *Pharmacotherapy.* 2006;26(11):1650.

* Asterisk indicates drugs cited in interaction reports.

Anticoagulants — *Cephalosporins*

Anticoagulants	Cephalosporins	
Warfarin* (eg, *Coumadin*)	Cefamandole*†	Cefoxitin*
	Cefazolin*	Ceftriaxone* (eg, *Rocephin*)
	Cefoperazone*†	
	Cefotetan*	

Significance	Onset	Severity	Documentation
2	☐ Rapid	☐ Major	☐ Established
	■ **Delayed**	■ **Moderate**	☐ Probable
		☐ Minor	■ **Suspected**
			☐ Possible
			☐ Unlikely

Effects The anticoagulant effect of WARFARIN is increased.

Mechanism Unknown.

Management WARFARIN doses may need to be reduced during administration of parenteral CEPHALOSPORINS. Monitor PTs and tailor dose accordingly.

Discussion

Increased sensitivity to warfarin in patients receiving parenteral cefazolin,[1,2] cefoxitin,[3] and ceftriaxone[4] is postulated on the basis of alterations in coagulation observed in patients receiving the cephalosporins alone. Bleeding was associated with marked prolongation in PT, suggesting an effect on vitamin K–dependent coagulation factors. All patients had severe renal dysfunction. In some patients, drug accumulation occurred, but in others, doses were adjusted to account for renal dysfunction. In 1 case,[2] bleeding time was also prolonged, suggesting an effect on platelet function. Coagulopathy was reported with cefamandole,[5] moxalactam,[†6] cefoperazone,[7] and cefotetan.[8] A retrospective analysis of nonuremic neutropenic patients receiving various combinations of antibiotics showed PT prolongation in patients receiving azlocillin[†] in combination with cefoxitin.[9] However, no episodes of bleeding were detected and there was no change in the activated partial thromboplastin time. One study has evaluated the effect of nonmethylthiotetrazole chain cephalosporins on warfarin anticoagulation.[10] Patients (n = 60) were randomized to receive cefamandole, cefazolin, or vancomycin (eg, *Vancocin*) as prophylaxis. Warfarin levels were equal in the 3 groups. The PT percent activity was lower for the 2 cephalosporins compared with vancomycin, but the percent change from the baseline was only different for cefamandole, indicating that cefazolin had an intermediate effect on warfarin anticoagulation. Elevated INR was reported in a 67-year-old woman receiving long-term warfarin therapy on 2 occasions following administration of ceftriaxone.[11]

[1] Lerner PI, et al. *N Engl J Med.* 1974;290(23):1324.
[2] Khaleeli M, et al. *Blood.* 1976;48(5):791.
[3] Reddy J, et al. *N Z Med J.* 1980;92(672):378.
[4] Haubenstock A, et al. *Lancet.* 1983;1(8335):1215.
[5] Rymer W, et al. *DICP.* 1980;14:780.
[6] Brown RB, et al. *Arch Intern Med.* 1986;146(11):2159.
[7] Freedy HR Jr, et al. *DICP.* 1986;20(4):281.
[8] Conjura A, et al. *Ann Intern Med.* 1988;108(4):643.
[9] Fainstein V, et al. *J Infect Dis.* 1983;148(4):745.
[10] Angaran DM, et al. *Ann Surg.* 1987;206(2):155.
[11] Clark TR, et al. *Am J Health Syst Pharm.* 2011;68(17):1603.

* Asterisk indicates drugs cited in interaction reports.
† Not available in the United States.

Anticoagulants		***Chamomile***
Warfarin* (eg, *Coumadin*)		Chamomile*

Significance	Onset	Severity	Documentation
4	☐ Rapid ■ **Delayed**	■ **Major** ☐ Moderate ☐ Minor	☐ Established ☐ Probable ☐ Suspected ■ **Possible** ☐ Unlikely

Effects The risk of bleeding may be increased.

Mechanism Unknown.

Management Because WARFARIN has a narrow therapeutic index, patients receiving WARFARIN should avoid CHAMOMILE except in modest doses. Caution patients to consult their health care provider before using nonprescription medicines or herbal products.

Discussion

A 70-year-old woman receiving warfarin for a mechanical mitral valve experienced multiple internal hemorrhages after using chamomile.[1] She was seen in the emergency department with a cough, expectoration of yellow sputum, and difficulty sleeping. She was diagnosed with an upper respiratory tract infection and discharged without antibiotics. Her INR at that visit was 3.6. She returned with similar symptoms 5 days later. In addition, she had dyspnea on exertion, bilateral pedal edema, and ecchymosis in her perineal area, across her lower abdomen, and over her left hip (INR was 7.9). She was admitted to the hospital and given 3 units of packed RBCs and 2 units of fresh frozen plasma. Her hemorrhages ultimately resolved, and the warfarin dose was adjusted to achieve a stable INR. Questioning revealed that, after her initial discharge from the emergency department, she applied a chamomile-based lotion (1 teaspoon to each leg 4 to 5 times/day) for her pedal edema. In addition, to soothe her sore throat, she drank 4 to 5 cups/day of chamomile tea prepared from dried chamomile leaves. Although she had been taking other medications, including amiodarone (eg, *Cordarone*), her drug regimen had been stable for 3 years without previous hemorrhage.

[1] Segal R, et al. *CMAJ*. 2006;174(9):1281.

* Asterisk indicates drugs cited in interaction reports.

Anticoagulants — *Chitosan*

Warfarin* (eg, *Coumadin*)	Chitosan*

Significance	Onset	Severity	Documentation
4	☐ Rapid	☐ Major	☐ Established
	■ **Delayed**	■ **Moderate**	☐ Probable
		☐ Minor	☐ Suspected
			■ **Possible**
			☐ Unlikely

Effects The anticoagulant effect of WARFARIN may be increased.

Mechanism CHITOSAN contains positively charged amino groups that may bind to negatively charged lipid and bile components, reducing GI absorption.[1] Interference with vitamin K absorption from the GI tract is suspected.[2]

Management Because WARFARIN has a narrow therapeutic index, patients receiving WARFARIN should avoid using CHITOSAN. Caution patients receiving WARFARIN to consult their health care provider before using nonprescription or herbal products.

Discussion

Chitin is a cellulose-like biopolymer found mainly in exoskeletons of marine invertebrates and arthropods, such as shrimp, crabs, or lobsters.[1] Chitosan is deacetylated chitin. Potentiation of the anticoagulant effect of warfarin was reported in an 83-year-old man during coadministration of chitosan.[2] The patient had hypertensive cardiovascular disease, type 2 diabetes, and chronic atrial fibrillation complicated by left atrial thrombus formation, and he had been taking warfarin 2.5 mg/day for over 1 year. His INR was maintained in the target range of 2 to 3. When the INR increased to above the target range despite a decrease in the warfarin dosage to 1.25 mg/day, the patient was hospitalized for evaluation. It was determined that he had begun self-medicating with chitosan 1,200 mg twice daily. Vitamin K was administered parenterally and chitosan was discontinued. The INR decreased to 1.63. Against medical advice, the patient restarted chitosan and the INR increased to 4.47 to 5.6 over a 3-month period. Chitosan was discontinued and the INR remained in the target range thereafter.

[1] DerMarderosian A, Beutler JA, eds. *The Review of Natural Products*. St. Louis, MO: Wolters Kluwer Health; 2004.

[2] Huang SS, et al. *Ann Pharmacother*. 2007;41(11):1912.

* Asterisk indicates drugs cited in interaction reports.

Anticoagulants — Chloral Hydrate

Dicumarol*†	Chloral Hydrate*
Warfarin* (eg, *Coumadin*)	(eg, *Somnote*)

Significance	Onset	Severity	Documentation
3	☐ Rapid	☐ Major	☐ Established
	■ **Delayed**	☐ Moderate	■ **Probable**
		■ **Minor**	☐ Suspected
			☐ Possible
			☐ Unlikely

Effects CHLORAL HYDRATE may enhance the hypoprothrombinemic response to oral ANTICOAGULANTS. However, this effect is usually small and transient.

Mechanism Trichloroacetic acid, a metabolite of CHLORAL HYDRATE, displaces WARFARIN from its binding sites.

Management Monitor anticoagulant activity during the first several days of concurrent therapy and adjust the WARFARIN dose as needed. Benzodiazepines do not appear to affect anticoagulant control and are safe alternatives.[1]

Discussion

In 10 healthy volunteers receiving chloral betaine (metabolized to chloral hydrate), the response to a single warfarin dose indicated no effect on PT despite a reduced warfarin $t_{1/2}$.[2] However, another small study reported an increased PT even with warfarin dose reduction after chloral hydrate.[3] The effect was attributed to concentration-dependent displacement of warfarin from its protein binding sites by trichloroacetic acid.[4] A fall in total plasma warfarin levels without a change in anticoagulation has been seen after chloral hydrate therapy in patients maintained on oral anticoagulants.[5] In experiments lasting 3 to 8 weeks, chloral betaine insignificantly altered warfarin anticoagulation.[6] One study found increased warfarin sensitivity in 5 of 8 subjects during the start of warfarin therapy. Conversely, during the long-term experiment, PT did not differ.[7] These results agree with the Boston Collaborative Drug Surveillance Program, wherein 32 patients who received daily chloral hydrate therapy used lower warfarin doses during the first 4 days of therapy. However, maintenance dosages were similar (6.3 vs 6.8 mg/day in no chloral hydrate vs chloral hydrate groups, respectively).[8] Because PT variations appear small and transient, chloral hydrate appears safe to use with warfarin.[9] This interaction has also been reported with chloral hydrate and dicumarol coadministration.[10]

1 Orme M, et al. *Br Med J.* 1972;3(5827):611.
2 MacDonald MG, et al. *Clin Pharmacol Ther.* 1969;10(1):80.
3 Sellers EM, et al. *N Engl J Med.* 1970;283(16):827.
4 Sellers EM, et al. *Ann NY Acad Sci.* 1971;179:213.
5 Breckenridge A, et al. *Clin Sci.* 1971;40(4):351.
6 Griner PF, et al. *Ann Intern Med.* 1971;74(4):540.
7 Udall JA. *Ann Intern Med.* 1974;81(3):341.
8 Boston Collaborative Drug Surveillance Program. *N Engl J Med.* 1972;286(2):53.
9 Udall JA. *Am J Cardiol.* 1975;35(1):67.
10 Cucinell SA, et al. *JAMA.* 1966;197(5):366.

* Asterisk indicates drugs cited in interaction reports.
† Not available in the United States.

Anticoagulants ✕ Chloramphenicol

Anisindione (*Miradon*)	Warfarin* (eg, *Coumadin*)	Chloramphenicol* (eg, *Chloromycetin*)
Dicumarol*†		

Significance	Onset	Severity	Documentation
2	☐ Rapid	☐ Major	☐ Established
	■ **Delayed**	■ **Moderate**	☐ Probable
		☐ Minor	■ **Suspected**
			☐ Possible
			☐ Unlikely

Effects Anticoagulation action of oral ANTICOAGULANTS may be enhanced by CHLORAMPHENICOL.

Mechanism Possible inhibition of hepatic metabolism of oral ANTICOAGULANTS.

Management Monitor anticoagulation parameters and adjust WARFARIN doses as needed.

Discussion

Chloramphenicol and other antimicrobials may impair coagulation. There are several case reports of bleeding in patients who received either parenteral or oral chloramphenicol alone or with other antimicrobials. Most of these patients were very ill and deprived of dietary sources of vitamin K; administration of vitamin K restored coagulation.[1,4,6] Similar potentiation of anticoagulation has been reported in patients receiving oral anticoagulants,[2] including a case evaluation of the international normalized ratio to 8.92 following 11 days of therapy with chloramphenicol eye drops.[8] Suppression of colonic bacteria by the antibiotics may be the cause of this reaction because colonic bacteria synthesize vitamin K. It is presumed that in the absence of dietary vitamin K, normal synthesis of clotting factors relies upon intestinal bacterial vitamin K sources. However, administration of vitamin K directly into the cecum of anticoagulated patients did not reverse anticoagulation.[3] Conversely, parenteral vitamin K readily reversed anticoagulation. Additionally, chloramphenicol inhibits hepatic enzymes that are responsible for the metabolism of several drugs. In 4 patients receiving chloramphenicol and dicumarol, chloramphenicol prolonged the half-life of dicumarol by 2 to 4 times.[5] In a well-designed rat model study, chloramphenicol reduced warfarin clearance approximately 70% irrespective of the warfarin enantiomer. There was no effect on plasma warfarin binding.[7] Caution is warranted when using chloramphenicol and oral anticoagulants because of the potential inhibition of warfarin metabolism and possible general antimicrobial effects on vitamin K bioavailability.

1 Haden HT. *Arch Intern Med* 1957;100:986.
2 Magid E. *Scand J Clin Lab Invest* 1962;14:565.
3 Udall JA. *JAMA* 1965;194:127.
4 Klippel AP, et al. *Arch Surg* 1968;96:266.
5 Christensen LK, et al. *Lancet* 1969;2:1397.
6 Matsaniotis N, et al. *Arch Dis Child* 1970;45:586.
7 Yacobi A, et al. *J Pharmacol Exp Ther* 1984;231:80.
8 Leone R, et al. *Ann Pharmacother* 1999;33:114.

* Asterisk indicates drugs cited in interaction reports. Based on pharmacologic and pharmacokinetic considerations, similar interactions may occur with other drugs that are listed.
† Not available in the United States.

Anticoagulants ✕ Cholestyramine

Dicumarol†	Cholestyramine*
Warfarin* (eg, *Coumadin*)	(eg, *Questran*)

Significance	Onset	Severity	Documentation
2	□ Rapid	□ Major	□ Established
	■ **Delayed**	■ **Moderate**	■ **Probable**
		□ Minor	□ Suspected
			□ Possible
			□ Unlikely

Effects The anticoagulant effect of oral ANTICOAGULANTS may be decreased by CHOLESTYRAMINE.

Mechanism Reduced oral ANTICOAGULANT absorption and possibly increased elimination. Refer to discussion.

Management Separate administration of these agents by at least 3 hours. Monitor ANTICOAGULANT activity and tailor oral ANTICOAGULANT doses as needed.

Discussion

Cholestyramine binds bile acids and many other substances and could reduce the bioavailability of oral anticoagulants. A pharmacokinetic and pharmacodynamic interaction was demonstrated in animal experiments[1] and in humans.[2,3,8,9] In vitro, cholestyramine tightly binds 95% of a warfarin dose.[1] Mean plasma warfarin concentrations and hypoprothrombinemic effects were reduced whether cholestyramine was administered with or 3 hours prior to a single warfarin dose.[3] The effect was smaller with separation of the administration times.[3] Similarly, cholestyramine 8 g 3 times daily administered 30 minutes after warfarin decreased plasma warfarin levels (2.7 vs 5.6 mcg/mL). However, administration 6 hours after warfarin did not reduce plasma warfarin levels (4.7 vs 5.6 mcg/mL) nor did it affect the prothrombin time.[2] Decreased oral absorption in the presence of cholestyramine has also been demonstrated for phenprocoumon.[†4,6,7] Another investigator has found that the half-life of parenterally administered warfarin is reduced by oral cholestyramine as a result of increased total warfarin clearance.[9] This suggests that cholestyramine may also interrupt enterohepatic recirculation of warfarin.

In a single-dose, placebo-controlled study, colestipol had no effect on plasma phenprocoumon levels in the 4 volunteers studied.[5] Likewise, colestipol had less binding of phenprocoumon in vitro compared with cholestyramine; nonetheless, it does bind phenprocoumon.[5] In another small, single-dose study, colestipol reduced the relative absorption of warfarin to 95% vs 68% for cholestyramine.[8] It seems prudent to observe the same precautions for colestipol as for cholestyramine.

1 Gallo DG, et al. *Proc Soc Exp Biol Med* 1965;120:60.
2 Kuentzel WP, et al. *Clin Res* 1970;18:594.
3 Robinson DS, et al. *Clin Pharmacol Ther* 1971;12:491.
4 Hahn K-J, et al. *Eur J Clin Pharmacol* 1972;4:142.
5 Harvengt C, et al. *Eur J Clin Pharmacol* 1973;6:19.
6 Meinertz T, et al. *Clin Pharmacol Ther* 1977;21:731.
7 Meinertz T, et al. *BMJ* 1977;2:439.
8 Hunninghake DB, et al. *Fed Proc* 1977;36:996.
9 Jahnchen E, et al. *Br J Clin Pharmacol* 1978;5:437.

* Asterisk indicates drugs cited in interaction reports. Based on pharmacologic and pharmacokinetic considerations, similar interactions may occur with other drugs that are listed.
† Not available in the United States.

Anticoagulants — *Cisapride*

Warfarin* (eg, *Coumadin*)	Cisapride*† (*Propulsid*)

Significance	Onset	Severity	Documentation
4	☐ Rapid ■ **Delayed**	☐ Major ■ **Moderate** ☐ Minor	☐ Established ☐ Probable ☐ Suspected ■ **Possible** ☐ Unlikely

Effects Hypoprothrombinemic effect of WARFARIN may be enhanced, increasing the risk of bleeding.

Mechanism Unknown.

Management Monitor anticoagulant function when CISAPRIDE dosage is started, stopped, or changed. Adjust the dose of WARFARIN as needed.

Discussion

Hypoprothrombinemia was reported in a 75-year-old man during coadministration of warfarin and cisapride.[1] The patient had a history of gastroesophageal reflux disease, hyperlipidemia, and tissue heart-valve replacement. He had been receiving warfarin for 3 years. While taking warfarin 4 mg/day for several months, the INR was 2.2 to 2.5. Therapy with cisapride 10 mg 4 times daily was started, and 3 weeks later the INR was measured at 10.7. Warfarin therapy was withheld for 2 days. The INR decreased to 2.3 and warfarin was restarted at 3 mg/day. There had been no alterations in the patient's diet, alcohol or nonprescription drug use, or adherence to his medication. The only change that occurred was that metoclopramide (eg, *Reglan*) was discontinued when therapy with cisapride was initiated.

[1] Raburn M. *Am J Health Syst Pharm.* 1997;54(3):320.

* Asterisk indicates drugs cited in interaction reports.
† Available from the manufacturer on a limited-access protocol.

Anticoagulants — **Clopidogrel**

Warfarin* (eg, *Coumadin*)	Clopidogrel* (*Plavix*)

Significance	Onset	Severity	Documentation
2	☐ Rapid ■ **Delayed**	■ **Major** ☐ Moderate ☐ Minor	☐ Established ☐ Probable ■ **Suspected** ☐ Possible ☐ Unlikely

Effects The risk of nonfatal and fatal bleeding may be increased with combined therapy.

Mechanism Unknown.

Management When indicated, coadminister with caution. Closely monitor coagulation parameters and the patient for bleeding events.

Discussion

In a large, observational cohort study, the risk of nonfatal and fatal bleeding was estimated in more than 118,000 patients with atrial fibrillation and during their posthospital therapy with warfarin, aspirin, clopidogrel, and combinations of these drugs.[1] The incidence of bleeding with coadministration of clopidogrel and warfarin was 13.9% per patient-year and 15.7% per patient-year with coadministration of clopidogrel, warfarin, and aspirin, compared with 3.9% per patient-year with warfarin monotherapy. Most bleeding events were GI. It was found that combining aspirin or clopidogrel with warfarin monotherapy greatly increased the risk of fatal and nonfatal bleeding without demonstrating a benefit in prevention of ischemic stroke. See also Clopidogrel/Salicylates.

[1] Hansen ML, et al. *Arch Intern Med.* 2010;170(16):1433.

* Asterisk indicates drugs cited in interaction reports.

Anticoagulants — *Colesevelam*

Warfarin* (eg, *Coumadin*)	Colesevelam* (*Welchol*)

Significance	Onset	Severity	Documentation
4	☐ Rapid ■ **Delayed**	☐ Major ■ **Moderate** ☐ Minor	☐ Established ☐ Probable ☐ Suspected ■ **Possible** ☐ Unlikely

Effects WARFARIN plasma concentrations may be reduced, decreasing the anticoagulant effect.

Mechanism COLESEVELAM may bind with WARFARIN in the GI tract, decreasing WARFARIN absorption.

Management In patients receiving WARFARIN, frequently monitor the INR when COLESEVELAM is started and periodically thereafter.[1]

Discussion

In an open-label, single-dose, crossover study, 24 subjects received warfarin 10 mg with and without colesevelam 4.5 g.[2] Simultaneous administration of warfarin with colesevelam did not alter the pharmacokinetics of warfarin compared with giving warfarin alone. However, reports during postmarketing surveillance indicate a reduced INR may occur in patients receiving warfarin and colesevelam. In patients receiving warfarin and colesevelam, frequently monitor the INR when colesevelam is started and periodically thereafter. Because postmarketing reports are voluntary and from a population of uncertain size, it is not possible to reliably estimate the frequency or establish a causal relationship to drug exposure.[1]

[1] *Welchol* [package insert]. Parsippany, NJ: Daiichi Sakyo Inc; February 2010.

[2] Donovan JM, et al. *Cardiovasc Drugs Ther.* 2000; 14(6):681.

* Asterisk indicates drugs cited in interaction reports.

Anticoagulants	***Contraceptives, Hormonal***
Warfarin (eg, *Coumadin*)	Contraceptives, Oral* (eg, *Ortho-Novum*)

Significance	Onset	Severity	Documentation
5	□ Rapid	□ Major	□ Established
	■ **Delayed**	■ **Moderate**	□ Probable
		□ Minor	□ Suspected
			□ Possible
			■ **Unlikely**

Effects ORAL CONTRACEPTIVES (OCs) may be thrombogenic in rare instances.

Mechanism Unknown.

Management No clinical interventions appear necessary. However, women requiring ANTICOAGULANTS may have a relative contraindication for OCs.

Discussion

The data for this interaction are contradictory. Following a 20-day course of a norethindrone/mestranol contraceptive, the anticoagulant response to a single dose of dicumarol† was decreased in 3 of 4 healthy women.[1] A single dose of phenprocoumon† was administered to 7 healthy women on long-term OCs and to 7 healthy women as controls.[2] Although phenprocoumon clearance was greater in the OC group, there was no difference in the hypoprothrombinemic effect. Conversely, in another study using nicoumalone,† the PT was higher, and the daily dose of anticoagulant was lower during coadministration with OCs, indicating a potentiation of the anticoagulant effect.[3]

The majority of cautions regarding a possible drug interaction are extrapolated from the observed effects of OCs alone on coagulation parameters and the risk of thromboembolic disease. Controversy exists as to the mechanism by which OCs may predispose patients to the formation of thrombi. Changes occur in many tests that measure platelet function, coagulation, and fibrinolysis. The clinical importance of these changes is unknown. OCs also appear to increase the level of clotting factors, but these factors circulate in inactive states and do not necessarily represent a hypercoagulable state.[4] Other factors, such as smoking or exercise, may alter the risk for thromboembolism. Reviewers have concluded that risk of thrombosis with OCs is small because of the low estrogen content in currently available agents and the avoidance of their use by women at risk of thromboembolic disease.[5] Whether OCs modify the pharmacological actions of oral anticoagulants remains unknown.

1 Schrogie JJ, et al. *Clin Pharmacol Ther.* 1967;8(5):670.
2 Mönig H, et al. *Br J Clin Pharmacol.* 1990;30(1):115.
3 de Teresa E, et al. *Br Med J.* 1979;2(6200):1260.
4 Mammen EF. *Am J Obstet Gynecol.* 1982;142(6, pt 2):781.
5 Notelovitz M. *Clin Obstet Gynecol.* 1985;28(1):73.

* Asterisk indicates drugs cited in interaction reports. Based on pharmacologic and pharmacokinetic considerations, similar interactions may occur with other drugs that are listed.
† Not available in the United States.

Anticoagulants — *Corticosteroids*

Anticoagulants	Corticosteroids	
Warfarin* (eg, *Coumadin*)	Betamethasone (eg, *Celestone*)	Fludrocortisone
	Budesonide (eg, *Pulmicort*)	Hydrocortisone (eg, *Cortef*)
	Corticotropin* (*Acthar HP*)	Methylprednisolone* (eg, *Medrol*)
	Cortisone*	Prednisolone (eg, *Prelone*)
	Cosyntropin (eg, *Cortrosyn*)	Prednisone* (eg, *Sterapred*)
	Dexamethasone* (eg, *Baycadron*)	Triamcinolone (eg, *Kenalog*)

Significance	Onset	Severity	Documentation
2	□ Rapid	□ Major	□ Established
	■ **Delayed**	■ **Moderate**	□ Probable
		□ Minor	■ **Suspected**
			□ Possible
			□ Unlikely

Effects CORTICOSTEROIDS may reduce ANTICOAGULANT dose requirements and occasionally induce hypercoagulation that could oppose ANTICOAGULANT action.

Mechanism Unknown.

Management Monitor ANTICOAGULANT activity and adjust the dose as needed when a CORTICOSTEROID is started or stopped.

Discussion

Data conflict. Early reports indicate reduced anticoagulant dose requirements during corticosteroid administration.[1-3] Bleeding was reported in 1 patient receiving ethyl biscoumacetate† after corticotropin 20 mg/day was started. In 10 patients on stable dosages of fluindione† or acenocoumarol,† a single injection of methylprednisolone 500 to 1,000 mg over 1 hr increased the mean INR from 2.75 to 8.04, compared with 5 patients taking the corticosteroid alone.[4] The maximum increase occurred after a mean of 92 hr. Similarly, dexamethasone 40 mg/day increased the INR from an average of 2.75 to 5.22 in 9 patients taking fluindione or warfarin.[5] There were 2 cases of reduced clotting time and increased ethyl biscoumacetate requirements after either cortisone or corticotropin,[6] indicating an antagonism of the anticoagulant effect.[7] In 32 patients stabilized on warfarin, an increase in INR from a mean of 2.33 to 3.57 occurred following glucocorticoid therapy.[8] The change was measured on average 6.7 days after starting corticosteroid therapy. The increase was above the therapeutic INR goal in 62.5% of the patients and resulted in warfarin dosage adjustments in 16 patients. One case of nosebleed was reported. These reports indicate that corticosteroids have a variable effect on oral anticoagulant therapy, depending on genetic factors[9]; disease process; and the steroid, dose, and route of administration.

1 Gerisch RA, et al. *Harper Hosp Bull.* 1961;19:197.
2 Sievers J, et al. *Cardiologia.* 1964;45:65.
3 Brozovi c M, et al. *Br J Haematol.* 1973;24(5):579.
4 Costedoat-Chalumeau N, et al. *Ann Intern Med.* 2000;132(8):631.
5 Sellam J, et al. *Joint Bone Spine.* 2007;74(5):446.
6 Chatterjea JB, et al. *Br Med J.* 1954;2(4891):790.
7 Menczel J, et al. *J Lab Clin Med.* 1960;56:14.
8 Hazlewood KA, et al. *Ann Pharmacother.* 2006;40(12):2101.
9 Ruud E, et al. *Pediatr Blood Cancer.* 2008;50(3):710.

* Asterisk indicates drugs cited in interaction reports. Based on pharmacologic and pharmacokinetic considerations, similar interactions may occur with other drugs that are listed.
† Not available in the United States.

Anticoagulants — *Cranberry Juice*

Warfarin* (eg, *Coumadin*)	Cranberry Juice*

Significance	Onset	Severity	Documentation
1	□ Rapid	■ **Major**	□ Established
	■ **Delayed**	□ Moderate	□ Probable
		□ Minor	■ **Suspected**
			□ Possible
			□ Unlikely

Effects Increased risk of severe bleeding, including hemorrhage.

Mechanism Unknown.

Management Because WARFARIN has a narrow therapeutic index, advise patients to avoid concurrent ingestion of large amounts of CRANBERRY JUICE.

Discussion

Data are conflicting. Bleeding and an increased INR have been reported in at least 10 patients taking warfarin and drinking cranberry juice.[1-4] In an open-label, randomized, crossover study, 12 healthy men received a single dose of warfarin 25 mg alone and after 2 weeks of pretreatment with cranberry equivalent to 57 g of fruit/day.[5] Compared with giving warfarin alone, pretreatment with cranberry increased the INR AUC 30%. The Committee on Safety of Medicines (United Kingdom) has received reports of at least 7 cases of possible increases in warfarin activity in patients ingesting cranberry juice concurrently.[1] One patient whose INR increased dramatically (more than 50) died of hemorrhage 6 weeks after he started drinking cranberry juice.[1] An elevated INR (11) accompanied by postoperative bleeding problems (eg, several episodes of frank hematuria via the catheter, bright red postrectal bleeding from the anastomosis site) occurred in a patient receiving warfarin.[2] During ward rounds, the patient was noted to be drinking almost 2 L/day of cranberry juice, which was recommended by the patient's general practitioner 2 weeks earlier to alleviate recurrent urinary tract infections. The patient was advised to stop drinking the juice, and after 3 days, the INR stabilized to 3. Major bleeding and an elevated INR (more than 18) were reported in a 71-year-old man taking a stable warfarin dose (18 mg/wk) 2 weeks after he started drinking 24 oz of cranberry juice daily.[3] The INR increased on 2 occasions in a 46-year-old woman after consumption of 1,420 to 1,893 mL of cranberry juice cocktail daily.[6] At least 2 cases of increased INR have been reported in patients taking warfarin and ingesting cranberry sauce.[7,8] Nine additional case reports from the British Committee on Safety of Medicines are summarized in a review article that questions the validity of this interaction.[9] In a double-blind, randomized, crossover study, 7 men on stable doses of warfarin for 3 months ingested 250 mL of cranberry juice or cranberry juice placebo daily for 7 days.[10] Compared with the placebo, cranberry juice did not affect the INR of patients receiving warfarin. Lack of an interaction was reported in a similar study in 10 healthy volunteers.[11] In another report, consumption of 240 mL of cranberry juice daily by patients on stable warfarin dosages did not interfere with warfarin therapy.[12] Fatal internal hemorrhage was reported in an elderly man who consumed only pure cranberry juice (300 to 400 mL daily) for 2 weeks while maintaining his usual warfarin dose.[13] In 9 men on stable warfarin doses, 240 mL of cranberry juice twice daily for 7 days did not alter the pharmacokinetics of warfarin.[14]

1 Suvarna R, et al. *BMJ.* 2003;327(7429):1454.
2 Grant P. *J Heart Valve Dis.* 2004;13(1):25.
3 Rindone JP, et al. *Am J Ther.* 2006;13(3):283.
4 Paeng CH, et al. *Clin Ther.* 2007;29(8):1730.
5 Mohammed Abdul MI, et al. *Br J Pharmacol.* 2008;154(8):1691.
6 Hamann GL, et al. *Ann Pharmacother.* 2011;45(3):e17.
7 Mergenhagen KA, et al. *Am J Health Syst Pharm.* 2008;65(22):2113.
8 Haber SL, et al. *Consult Pharm.* 2012;27(1):58.
9 Zikria J, et al. *Am J Med.* 2010;123(5):384.
10 Li Z, et al. *J Am Diet Assoc.* 2006;106(12):2057.
11 Lilja JJ, et al. *Clin Pharmacol Ther.* 2007;81(6):833.
12 Ansell J, et al. *J Clin Pharmacol.* 2009;49(7):824.
13 Griffiths AP, et al. *J R Soc Promot Health.* 2008;128(6):324.
14 Mellen CK, et al. *Br J Clin Pharmacol.* 2010;70(1):139.

* Asterisk indicates drugs cited in interaction reports.

Anticoagulants — *Cyclosporine*

Warfarin* (eg, *Coumadin*)	Cyclosporine* (eg, *Sandimmune*)

Significance	Onset	Severity	Documentation
4	☐ Rapid ■ **Delayed**	■ **Major** ☐ Moderate ☐ Minor	☐ Established ☐ Probable ☐ Suspected ■ **Possible** ☐ Unlikely

Effects The effects of WARFARIN and CYCLOSPORINE may be decreased.

Mechanism Unknown.

Management Monitor ANTICOAGULANT parameters and CYCLOSPORINE blood concentrations. In addition, observe the clinical response of patients. Adjust the dose of either drug as needed.

Discussion

A possible drug interaction was reported in a 39-year-old man during coadministration of warfarin and cyclosporine.[1] One week after starting warfarin in a patient receiving cyclosporine, phenobarbital (eg, *Luminal*), magnesium supplements, and folic acid, the patient's reticulocyte count fell; subsequently, his hemoglobin and cyclosporine blood levels decreased. Upon increasing the cyclosporine dosage from 3 to 7 mg/kg/day, the patient's reticulocyte count, hemoglobin level, and cyclosporine blood concentration increased. With the increase in the cyclosporine dose, the prothrombin activity increased from 17% to 64%, and it was necessary to increase the warfarin dose to maintain therapeutic range of anticoagulation. It was not determined whether phenobarbital contributed to the drug interaction. In contrast, in a report of a patient receiving cyclosporine and the anticoagulant acenocoumarol,[†] the effects of the anticoagulant and cyclosporine were increased.[2] See also Cyclosporine-Barbiturates and Anticoagulants-Barbiturates.

Controlled studies are needed to evaluate this possible drug interaction and to determine the clinical importance.

[1] Snyder DS. *Ann Intern Med.* 1988;108(2):311.

[2] Campistol JM, et al. *Nephron.* 1989;53(3):291.

* Asterisk indicates drugs cited in interaction reports.
† Not available in the United States.

Anticoagulants		***Danshen***
Warfarin* (eg, *Coumadin*)		Danshen*

Significance	Onset	Severity	Documentation
2	☐ Rapid	☐ Major	☐ Established
	■ **Delayed**	■ **Moderate**	☐ Probable
		☐ Minor	■ **Suspected**
			☐ Possible
			☐ Unlikely

Effects Increased ANTICOAGULANT effects of WARFARIN.

Mechanism Unknown.

Management Caution patients to consult their health care provider regarding the use of nonprescription or herbal products and to report any signs of bleeding. Monitor clotting parameters more frequently when patients on oral ANTICOAGULANTS ingest substances with undocumented effects.

Discussion

The anticoagulant effect of warfarin was reported to be increased in 2 patients as a result of ingestion of danshen, a Chinese herbal medicine used for a variety of complaints, particularly cardiovascular complaints.[1,2] The first patient was a 43-year-old female who underwent percutaneous transvenous mitral valvuloplasty.[1] The patient was taking warfarin, furosemide (eg, *Lasix*), and digoxin (eg, *Lanoxin*). Her warfarin dose was 2.5 to 3.5 mg/day to maintain an international normalized ratio (INR) of 1.5 to 3. When her INR was 1.35, the warfarin dose was increased to 4 mg/day. Seven weeks later, she was seen in the emergency department. Her INR was more than 5.62. During this interval, she had received mefenamic acid (*Ponstel*) and theophylline (eg, *Theo-Dur*) for 2 days and herbal medicines every other day for nearly a month. The herbal medication (a main component was identified as danshen) and warfarin were discontinued. Subsequent to stopping the herbal product, her INR stabilized on warfarin 3 mg/day. The second patient, a 62-year-old man, was started on warfarin following mitral valve replacement.[2] Four weeks after surgery he was stable on warfarin 5 mg/day. Two weeks later he was found to have a pleural effusion from which 4.5 L of nonclotted blood was drained (INR more than 8.4). He had started taking danshen daily 2 weeks before this hospitalization. Subsequent to discontinuing danshen, his INR again stabilized on warfarin 5 mg/day.

The ingredients of many herbal products are not standardized. It is unclear if herbal products contain ingredients other than those listed on the label or purported to be present that could affect coagulation or interact with warfarin. See also Anticoagulants-Ginseng.

[1] Yu CM, et al. *J Intern Med* 1997;241:337.

[2] Izzat MB, et al. *Ann Thorac Surg* 1998;66:941.

* Asterisk indicates drugs cited in interaction reports.

Anticoagulants — *Dextrothyroxine*

Anticoagulants		Dextrothyroxine
Anisindione (*Miradon*)	Warfarin* (eg, *Coumadin*)	Dextrothyroxine*† (*Choloxin*)
Dicumarol*†		

Significance	Onset	Severity	Documentation
1	☐ Rapid ■ **Delayed**	■ **Major** ☐ Moderate ☐ Minor	☐ Established ■ **Probable** ☐ Suspected ☐ Possible ☐ Unlikely

Effects DEXTROTHYROXINE increases the hypoprothrombinemic effect of oral ANTICOAGULANTS.

Mechanism Unknown.

Management Reduced oral ANTICOAGULANT doses are needed when coadministered with DEXTROTHYROXINE. Monitor ANTICOAGULANT activity, and tailor doses as needed.

Discussion

Ten of 11 patients receiving dicumarol required dose reduction because of prolonged prothrombin time (PT) during concurrent administration of dextrothyroxine.[1] These observations were confirmed in a study of 8 healthy volunteers who received dextrothyroxine 8 mg/day. The anticoagulant response to a single dicumarol dose was increased.[3] An investigation of 11 patients who received dextrothyroxine reported a reduction in weekly warfarin dose between 2.5 and 30 mg because of PT prolongation. PT achieved values as high as 59 seconds during the first week of dextrothyroxine therapy. One patient suffered a leg hematoma and required hospitalization.[2] In 3 other patients receiving dextrothyroxine without anticoagulants, a 2-second prolongation in the PT was reported.[2]

Dextrothyroxine did not affect the metabolic rate of dicumarol in humans.[3] Using a single-patient study, an increase in warfarin affinity for its receptor was postulated.[4] Alternately, it has been shown in dogs that the rate of prothrombin degradation is increased by dextrothyroxine.[5]

[1] Jones RJ, et al. *Circulation* 1961;24:164.
[2] Owens JC, et al. *N Engl J Med* 1962;266:76.
[3] Schrogie JJ, et al. *Clin Pharmacol Ther* 1967;8:70.
[4] Solomon HM, et al. *Clin Pharmacol Ther* 1967;8:797.
[5] Weintraub M, et al. *J Lab Clin Med* 1973;81:273.

* Asterisk indicates drugs cited in interaction reports. Based on pharmacologic and pharmacokinetic considerations, similar interactions may occur with other drugs that are listed.
† Not available in the United States.

Anticoagulants — *Diflunisal*

Anisindione (*Miradon*)	Warfarin* (eg, *Coumadin*)	Diflunisal* (*Dolobid*)
Dicumarol†		

Significance	Onset	Severity	Documentation
5	☐ Rapid	☐ Major	☐ Established
	■ **Delayed**	☐ Moderate	☐ Probable
		■ **Minor**	☐ Suspected
			■ **Possible**
			☐ Unlikely

Effects Discontinuation of DIFLUNISAL therapy may result in loss of anticoagulation. Additionally, DIFLUNISAL has some antiplatelet and gastric irritant effects which may predispose to bleeding in patients receiving oral ANTICOAGULANTS.

Mechanism Unknown.

Management No special precautions appear necessary.

Discussion

Diflunisal is a nonsteroidal anti-inflammatory agent that strongly binds to albumin. The potential displacement of oral anticoagulants was investigated in vitro using phenprocoumon.† Diflunisal increased phenprocoumon's free fraction in a dose-dependent manner but increased it to a lesser extent than phenylbutazone.[2] In studies using human subjects, three patients on acenocoumarol (not available in the US) had increased prothrombin times. However, there was no effect on two patients taking phenprocoumon.[1] The potential interaction with warfarin was studied using five healthy volunteers. Diflunisal 500 mg twice a day for 2 weeks did not change anticoagulation. There was a decrease in total warfarin levels and an increase in the free warfarin fraction as expected from protein displacement. The active free warfarin concentration probably did not change. Upon discontinuation of diflunisal, patients gradually lost their anticoagulation, which was unexpected. It was noticed that the unbound fraction returned to normal more quickly than the total warfarin concentration.[3] It must be noted that the warfarin doses in the study were small and the patients were healthy. It is unknown if higher warfarin doses in actual patients may interact differently with diflunisal.

In addition, diflunisal decreases platelet function and increases fecal blood loss when used at higher doses (1,000 mg twice a day). The effect at 500 mg twice a day is variable while there is no effect with 250 mg twice a day.[4] This could predispose anticoagulated patients to bleeding.

[1] Tempero KF, et al. *Br J Clin Pharmacol* 1977;4(Suppl 1):31S.
[2] Verbeeck RK, et al. *Biochem Pharmacol* 1980;29:571.
[3] Serlin MJ, et al. *Clin Pharmacol Ther* 1980;28:493.
[4] Green D, et al. *Clin Pharmacol Ther* 1981;30:378.

* Asterisk indicates drugs cited in interaction reports. Based on pharmacologic and pharmacokinetic considerations, similar interactions may occur with other drugs that are listed.
† Not available in the United States.

Anticoagulants — *Disopyramide*

Anticoagulants	Disopyramide
Dicumarol*†	Disopyramide*
Warfarin*	(eg, *Norpace*)
(eg, *Coumadin*)	

Significance	Onset	Severity	Documentation
5	□ Rapid	□ Major	□ Established
	■ **Delayed**	□ Moderate	□ Probable
		■ **Minor**	□ Suspected
			□ Possible
			■ **Unlikely**

Effects Decreased prothrombin time after discontinuation of DISOPYRAMIDE therapy.

Mechanism Unknown.

Management No clinical interventions appear required.

Discussion

In a single case report, a 58-year-old man with congestive heart failure discontinued disopyramide 100 mg every 6 hours because of hypotension.[1] The patient had been receiving warfarin 3 mg/day for at least 4 weeks. A previously stable prothrombin time decreased from 24 to 15 seconds. However, this potential drug interaction has also been explained due to an improved cardiac function and improved hepatic perfusion which improves the synthesis or release of clotting factors.[2] Because disopyramide has negative inotropic effects, and because the patient was on a low warfarin dose, this is a plausible explanation. In a small study, Sylven demonstrated that patients who converted from atrial fibrillation to normal sinus rhythm had approximately 10% higher dicumarol requirements regardless of disopyramide or quinidine use.[3] Again this information supports a hemodynamic effect for changes in anticoagulation and argues against a drug-drug interaction.

[1] Haworth E, et al. *BMJ* 1977;2:866.
[2] Ryll C, et al. *DICP* 1979;13:260.
[3] Sylven C, et al. *BMJ* 1983;286:1181.

* Asterisk indicates drugs cited in interaction reports.
† Not available in the United States.

Anticoagulants — *Disulfiram*

Warfarin* (eg, *Coumadin*)	Disulfiram* (*Antabuse*)

Significance	Onset	Severity	Documentation
2	☐ Rapid	☐ Major	☐ Established
	■ **Delayed**	■ **Moderate**	■ **Probable**
		☐ Minor	☐ Suspected
			☐ Possible
			☐ Unlikely

Effects DISULFIRAM may increase the anticoagulant effects of WARFARIN.

Mechanism Unknown.

Management Monitor anticoagulation parameters, and tailor the dosage of WARFARIN as needed.

Discussion

An interaction between warfarin and disulfiram was initially reported in a 45-year-old man. Prolongation in his PT to 47 seconds and bleeding were noted on 3 separate occasions after he began disulfiram therapy.[1] In another report, a patient's warfarin dose was reduced in preparation for disulfiram 500 mg/day. The patient was adequately anticoagulated, but when his disulfiram dose was reduced to 250 mg/day, an increase in warfarin also was needed.[2] This suggests a dose-dependent effect of disulfiram upon warfarin anticoagulation. When a single dose of warfarin was administered after disulfiram 250 to 500 mg/day to healthy volunteers, the anticoagulant's effect was potentiated, and the mean warfarin AUC increased 27%.[3,4] Coadministration of these drugs for 21 days increased anticoagulation as measured by reduction in percent prothrombin activity. The plasma warfarin level rose from 2.5 to 3.1 mcg/mL.[4,5] In a study of effects on the individual warfarin enantiomers, S-warfarin increased PT, whereas the R-enantiomer did not have an effect. Disulfiram did not affect the warfarin AUC of either enantiomer.[6] It was concluded that the increase in PT observed during disulfiram therapy is not caused by a pharmacokinetic interaction but involves an effect on warfarin's pharmacodynamics. Further study is needed.

[1] Rothstein E. *JAMA*. 1968;206:1574.
[2] Rothstein E. *JAMA*. 1972;221:1052.
[3] O'Reilly RA. *Clin Res*. 1971;19:180.
[4] O'Reilly RA. *Ann Intern Med*. 1973;78:73.
[5] O'Reilly RA. *Clin Res*. 1972;20:185.
[6] O'Reilly RA. *Clin Pharmacol Ther*. 1981;29:332.

* Asterisk indicates drugs cited in interaction reports.

Anticoagulants — *Dong Quai*

Warfarin* (eg, *Coumadin*)	Dong Quai*

Significance	Onset	Severity	Documentation
4	☐ Rapid	☐ Major	☐ Established
	■ **Delayed**	■ **Moderate**	☐ Probable
		☐ Minor	☐ Suspected
			■ **Possible**
			☐ Unlikely

Effects The anticoagulant effects of WARFARIN may be increased.

Mechanism Unknown.

Management Caution patients to consult their health care provider regarding the use of nonprescription or herbal products and to report any signs of bleeding. Monitor clotting parameters more frequently when patients on oral ANTICOAGULANTS ingest substances with undocumented effects.

Discussion

An increase in anticoagulant parameters was reported in a patient taking warfarin and dong quai.[1] A 46-year-old woman with a history of rheumatic heart disease, stroke, and atrial fibrillation was maintained on warfarin 5 mg/day with an INR of 2 to 3. After she ingested 2 to 3 servings of collard greens, her INR decreased to 1.89. No adjustments were made in her warfarin dosage. One month later, her INR was 4.04 without evidence of bleeding. The warfarin dosage was withheld for 1 day, then resumed at 5 mg/day. The patient missed her appointment the next week and did not return for 1 month. When she returned, her INR was 4.9. The patient stated that she had been taking dong quai 565 mg 1 to 2 times daily for 1 month. The patient was instructed to skip 1 day of warfarin therapy, then resume taking warfarin 5 mg/day and to discontinue dong quai. Two weeks later, the patient's INR was 3.41. Four weeks after stopping dong quai, her INR was 2.48.

The ingredients of many herbal products are not standardized. It is unclear if herbal products contain ingredients other than those listed on the label or purported to be present that could affect coagulation or interact with warfarin. See also Anticoagulants-Danshen, Anticoagulants-Ginkgo Biloba, Anticoagulants-Ginseng.

[1] Page RL 2nd, et al. *Pharmacotherapy*. 1999;19:870.

* Asterisk indicates drugs cited in interaction reports.

Anticoagulants — *Echinacea*

Warfarin*
(eg, *Coumadin*)

Echinacea*

Significance	Onset	Severity	Documentation
5	☐ Rapid ■ **Delayed**	☐ Major ☐ Moderate ■ **Minor**	☐ Established ☐ Probable ☐ Suspected ■ **Possible** ☐ Unlikely

Effects WARFARIN concentrations may be reduced, decreasing the anticoagulant effect.

Mechanism Unknown.

Management Based on available data, no special precautions are needed. However, monitor INR more closely whenever a dietary supplement is started or stopped.

Discussion

The effects of echinacea on the pharmacokinetics and pharmacodynamics of warfarin were studied in 11 healthy men.[1] Using an open-label, randomized, crossover design, each subject received a single oral dose of warfarin 25 mg before and after 2 weeks of receiving echinacea (containing *Echinacea angustifolia* root 600 mg and *Echinacea purpurea* root 675 mg; standardized to contain total alkamides 5.75 mg). Compared with taking warfarin alone, pretreatment with echinacea slightly increased the apparent clearance of the more active (S)-warfarin enantiomer and did not affect the pharmacokinetics of (R)-warfarin. The increase in (S)-warfarin clearance was not associated with a clinically important effect on warfarin pharmacodynamics, and there was no clinically relevant change in INR. In addition, platelet aggregation was not altered.

[1] Abdul MI, et al. *Br J Clin Pharmacol.* 2010;69(5):508.

* Asterisk indicates drugs cited in interaction reports.

Anticoagulants — *Enteral Nutrition*

Warfarin* (eg, *Coumadin*)	Enteral Nutrition* (eg, *Ensure*)

Significance	Onset	Severity	Documentation
4	☐ Rapid ■ **Delayed**	☐ Major ■ **Moderate** ☐ Minor	☐ Established ☐ Probable ☐ Suspected ■ **Possible** ☐ Unlikely

Effects The ANTICOAGULANT effect of WARFARIN may be decreased during administration of ENTERAL NUTRITION.

Mechanism Binding of WARFARIN to proteins in the ENTERAL NUTRITION products is suspected.

Management Monitor coagulation parameters closely, especially when ENTERAL NUTRITION products are started or discontinued. Be prepared to adjust the WARFARIN dose or withhold ENTERAL NUTRITION for 1 hour before and after WARFARIN administration.

Discussion

Warfarin resistance has been reported in patients receiving enteral nutrition products. The temporal association between the decrease in the warfarin anticoagulant effect and enteral feeding supports the interaction.[1,2] A need to increase the warfarin dosage to maintain adequate anticoagulation during enteral feeding, followed by an increase in PT after the feeding was discontinued, has been reported.[1] In some cases, after enteral nutrition was started, the PT decreased in patients who had been receiving stable warfarin doses for years. In vitro investigation has demonstrated that enteral feeding products can bind warfarin, possibly leading to a reduction in bioavailability.[2] In a small observational study, withholding enteral feeding for 1 hour before and after warfarin administration appeared to prevent the interaction.[3] In patients receiving warfarin, vitamin K is usually not included in the enteral nutrition formulation.

[1] Howard PA, et al. *J Am Diet Assoc.* 1985;85(6):713.
[2] Penrod LE, et al. *Arch Phys Med Rehabil.* 2001;82(9):1270.
[3] Dickerson RN, et al. *Pharmacotherapy.* 2008;28(3):308.

* Asterisk indicates drugs cited in interaction reports.

Anticoagulants — *Erlotinib*

Anticoagulants	Erlotinib
Warfarin* (eg, *Coumadin*)	Erlotinib* (*Tarceva*)

Significance	Onset	Severity	Documentation
4	□ Rapid ■ **Delayed**	■ **Major** □ Moderate □ Minor	□ Established □ Probable □ Suspected ■ **Possible** □ Unlikely

Effects The anticoagulant effect of WARFARIN may be enhanced, increasing the risk of bleeding.

Mechanism Unknown.

Management In patients receiving WARFARIN, closely monitor anticoagulant function when starting or stopping ERLOTINIB. Adjust the WARFARIN dose as needed.

Discussion

An elevated INR was reported in a 47-year-old man receiving warfarin after erlotinib was added to his treatment regimen.[1] The patient was stabilized on warfarin 2.5 mg daily for the treatment of a venous thromboembolism. His INR was stable between 2.1 and 3.2 for at least 8 weeks before erlotinib was added to his non–small cell lung cancer treatment regimen. The patient's INR value increased to 5.3 seven days after starting erlotinib. The INR continued to increase to 9.1 despite withholding warfarin for 2 days, and the patient developed an elbow hematoma. His anticoagulation reversed after administration of subcutaneous phytonadione (vitamin K_1). Erlotinib was discontinued and the next day his INR was 2.4.

[1] Thomas KS, et al. *Am J Health Syst Pharm.* 2010;67(17):1426.

* Asterisk indicates drugs cited in interaction reports.

Anticoagulants — Estrogens

Anticoagulants		Estrogens	
Anisindione (*Miradon*)	Warfarin (eg, *Coumadin*)	Conjugated Estrogens* (eg, *Premarin*) Esterified Estrogens (eg, *Estratab*) Estradiol* (eg, *Estrace*) Estrogenic Substance (eg, *Gynogen*)	Estrone (eg, *Aquest*) Estropipate (eg, *Ogen*) Ethinyl Estradiol* (*Estinyl*) Quinestrol (*Estrovis*)

Significance	Onset	Severity	Documentation
4	☐ Rapid ■ **Delayed**	☐ Major ■ **Moderate** ☐ Minor	☐ Established ☐ Probable ☐ Suspected ■ **Possible** ☐ Unlikely

Effects ESTROGENS affect several coagulation and fibrinolysis tests and, at high doses, could increase the risk of thromboembolism. Consequently, the benefit from oral ANTICOAGULANTS could be diminished by ESTROGEN.

Mechanism Unknown.

Management Because of a lack of clinical correlation between coagulation tests and the actual risk of thromboembolism, no clinical interventions should be necessary.

Discussion

Evidence for a direct interaction between estrogens used in replacement therapy and oral anticoagulants is very limited.[1-8] Higher estrogen doses seem to have a more concrete effect (see Anticoagulants-Contraceptives, Oral). However, no direct interaction studies have been performed with estrogens when used for the control of menopausal symptoms. In postmenopausal women receiving mestranol, fibrinogen and plasminogen were increased, but fibrin split products were the same,[2] indicating no alteration in the coagulability of blood. However, several other studies have reported a hypercoagulable state.[3-7]

The clinical importance of these test alterations has been questioned.[9] However, the use of small doses, as in oral (or transdermal)[10] estrogen replacement therapy, is likely to cause small and clinically unimportant effects.[11]

1 Schrogie JJ, et al. *Clin Pharmacol Ther.* 1967;8:670.
2 Beller FK, et al. *Obstet Gynecol.* 1972;39:775.
3 von Kaulla E, et al. *Am J Obstet Gynecol.* 1975;122:688.
4 Coope J, et al. *Br Med J.* 1975;4:139.
5 Davies T, et al. *Thromb Haemost.* 1976;35:403.
6 Stangel JJ, et al. *Obstet Gynecol.* 1977;49:314.
7 Poller L, et al. *Br Med J.* 1977;1:935.
8 de Teresa E, et al. *Br Med J.* 1979;2:1260.
9 Mammen EF. *Am J Obstet Gynecol.* 1982;142(6 pt 2):781.
10 De Lignieres B, et al. *J Clin Endocrinol Metab.* 1986;62:536.
11 Notelovitz M. *Clin Obstet Gynecol.* 1985;28:73.

* Asterisk indicates drugs cited in interaction reports. Based on pharmacologic and pharmacokinetic considerations, similar interactions may occur with other drugs that are listed.

Anticoagulants — *Ethanol*

Warfarin* (eg, *Coumadin*)	Ethanol* (Alcohol, Ethyl Alcohol)

Significance	Onset	Severity	Documentation
4	□ Rapid ■ **Delayed**	□ Major ■ **Moderate** □ Minor	□ Established □ Probable □ Suspected ■ **Possible** □ Unlikely

Effects The chronic consumption of ETHANOL in high amounts may increase the clearance of WARFARIN. However, moderate or small amounts of ETHANOL may either increase or not alter the anticoagulant effect of WARFARIN.

Mechanism Unknown.

Management No clinical interventions appear necessary. The alcohol content in medicinal products is not likely to alter anticoagulation in patients receiving oral ANTICOAGULANTS. However, ETHANOL consumption could affect oral ANTICOAGULANT therapy in other ways.

Discussion

A patient drinking 50 mL of whiskey/day experienced changes in anticoagulation and warfarin levels when stopping or restarting alcohol consumption.[1] Discontinuation of alcohol use resulted in decreased warfarin levels and loss of anticoagulation. This patient had preexisting liver disease, which could explain his sensitivity to the small amount of alcohol. Another patient consuming an estimated 5.35 g of alcohol every other day had an increase in INR from an average of 2.18 to 8.[2] Alcoholic patients using 250 g of alcohol/day or more have markedly increased warfarin clearance compared with healthy nonalcoholic patients. The $t_{1/2}$ of warfarin was 26.5 hours in alcoholics vs 41.1 hours in normal subjects.[3] Despite these changes, anticoagulation was not affected.[3,4] Presumably, alcoholics have some liver damage that makes them sensitive to lower warfarin levels.

In other controlled investigations using patients or healthy subjects anticoagulated with warfarin, neither PT nor warfarin levels were affected by daily consumption of small to moderate amounts of alcohol.[5-7] Given the levels of ethanol consumed in these studies, it appears unlikely that the amount of alcohol typically present in medicinal products would affect anticoagulant therapy. Likewise, an occasional small amount of alcohol with a meal probably poses no risk. However, if alcohol is consumed to a state of inebriation, it could result in bleeding secondary to accidental injuries. Furthermore, in alcoholics, sensitivity to warfarin and other anticoagulants may be increased because of possible liver damage.

[1] Breckenridge A, et al. *Ann NY Acad Sci*. 1971;179:421.
[2] Havrda DE, et al. *Pharmacotherapy*. 2005;25:303.
[3] Kater RM, et al. *Am J Med Sci*. 1969;258:35.
[4] Waris E. *Ann Med Exp Biol Fenn*. 1963;41:45.
[5] Udall JA. *Clin Med*. 1970;77:20.
[6] O'Reilly RA. *Am J Med Sci*. 1979;277:189.
[7] O'Reilly RA. *Arch Intern Med*. 1981;141:458.

* Asterisk indicates drugs cited in interaction reports.

Anticoagulants | *Ethchlorvynol*

Warfarin* (eg, *Coumadin*)	Ethchlorvynol* (*Placidyl*)

Significance	Onset	Severity	Documentation
2	☐ Rapid	☐ Major	☐ Established
	■ **Delayed**	■ **Moderate**	☐ Probable
		☐ Minor	■ **Suspected**
			☐ Possible
			☐ Unlikely

Effects ETHCHLORVYNOL may reduce the hypoprothrombinemic effect of oral ANTICOAGULANTS.

Mechanism Unknown.

Management Monitor anticoagulation parameters and tailor dosages as needed. Alternatively, consider the use of a benzodiazepine hypnotic in place of ETHCHLORVYNOL.

Discussion

Six postmyocardial infarct patients treated with dicumarol (not available in the US) for 2 weeks were given ethchlorvynol 1 g/day. Anticoagulation, as measured by the Quick index, was reduced. Furthermore, the same study reported a 62-year-old man receiving dicumarol who suffered hematuria following temporary discontinuation of ethchlorvynol.[1] In 1 patient receiving griseofulvin (eg, *Fulvicin*) and warfarin, the administration of ethchlorvynol produced additional loss of anticoagulation, but no details were provided.[2] This information, although scant, indicates that ethchlorvynol may antagonize the effects of oral anticoagulants. The interaction between ethchlorvynol and oral anticoagulants needs further study.

Benzodiazepines are considered safe for use in anticoagulated patients.[3] A benzodiazepine hypnotic should be used in place of ethchlorvynol in patients receiving oral anticoagulants.

[1] Johansson SA. *Acta Med Scand.* 1968;184:297.
[2] Cullen SI, et al. *JAMA.* 1967;199:582.
[3] Orme M, et al. *Br Med J.* 1972;3:611.

* Asterisk indicates drugs cited in interaction reports.

Anticoagulants — *Felbamate*

Warfarin* (eg, *Coumadin*)	Felbamate* (*Felbatol*)

Significance	Onset	Severity	Documentation
4	☐ Rapid	☐ Major	☐ Established
	■ **Delayed**	■ **Moderate**	☐ Probable
		☐ Minor	☐ Suspected
			■ **Possible**
			☐ Unlikely

Effects The anticoagulant effects of WARFARIN may be increased.

Mechanism Unknown.

Management Monitor coagulation parameters more frequently when FELBAMATE is started or stopped. Be prepared to adjust the WARFARIN dose as needed.

Discussion

An increase in the INR was associated with the addition of felbamate to the drug regimen of a 62-year-old man receiving warfarin 35 mg/week.[1] The patient also had been receiving carbamazepine (eg, *Tegretol*) and phenobarbital (eg, *Solfoton*) for generalized tonic-clonic seizures. The patient's INR increased from a range of 2.5 to 3.5 to 7.8 two weeks after the initiation of felbamate therapy (2,400 mg/day increased to 3200 mg/day after 2 weeks). When felbamate was started, carbamazepine and phenobarbital therapy were discontinued. It was necessary to decrease the dose of warfarin to 2.5 mg/day to maintain the INR within the target range. The increase in the anticoagulant effects of warfarin may have resulted from discontinuing carbamazepine and phenobarbital, rather than from the addition of felbamate to the patient's treatment regimen.

Controlled studies are needed to determine whether this interaction is caused by coadministration of warfarin and felbamate. See also Anticoagulants-Carbamazepine and Anticoagulants-Barbiturates.

[1] Tisdel KA, et al. *Ann Pharmacother.* 1994;28:805.

* Asterisk indicates drugs cited in interaction reports.

Anticoagulants		***Fibric Acids***
Warfarin* (eg, *Coumadin*)	Clofibrate*† Fenofibrate* (eg, *Tricor*)	Gemfibrozil* (eg, *Lopid*)

Significance	Onset	Severity	Documentation
1	□ Rapid ■ **Delayed**	■ **Major** □ Moderate □ Minor	■ **Established** □ Probable □ Suspected □ Possible □ Unlikely

Effects FIBRIC ACIDS may increase the hypoprothrombinemic effects of oral ANTICOAGULANTS. Bleeding and death have occurred. Warfarin plasma levels are not affected.[1-5]

Mechanism Coagulation factor synthesis may be affected.

Management If combined use cannot be avoided, monitor INR frequently when a FIBRIC ACID is started or stopped. Be prepared to adjust the ANTICOAGULANT dose. Advise patients to immediately report unusual bleeding or bruising.

Discussion

Case reports and controlled studies document an interaction between clofibrate and phenindione[†,6] dicumarol[†,7], and warfarin.[1-5] Episodes of bleeding and death caused by hemorrhage,[6,8] elevations in PT,[9] and the need for reduction in anticoagulant dose[7,10] have been reported. Clofibrate displaced warfarin from protein binding sites,[3,11] but the effect was small. An effect on the S-enantiomer, but not in the R-enantiomer, of warfarin was noted in 1 study.[4] In 8 volunteers, therapy with warfarin and clofibrate reduced levels of factors II and X.[12] Case reports describe an increased anticoagulant effect with or without bleeding when gemfibrozil is started in patients receiving warfarin.[13,14] Two weeks after starting gemfibrozil 1.2 g daily, a 38-year-old woman experienced an increased PT and excessive menstrual bleeding, which resolved upon decreasing the warfarin dose from 5 to 2.5 mg daily.[15] Two patients receiving warfarin experienced elevations in their INR after starting fenofibrate.[16] One patient who also experienced hematuria was rechallenged twice with fenofibrate, resulting in elevations of INR in both instances. A patient stabilized on warfarin 6 mg daily experienced grossly elevated INR and rectal bleeding 1 month after converting from gemfibrozil therapy to fenofibrate.[17] In contrast, gemfibrozil 600 mg twice daily appears to have limited effects on single-dose warfarin 10 mg in healthy subjects.[18]

1 Pyörälä K, et al. *Ann Med Intern Fenn.* 1968;57(4):157.
2 O'Reilly RA, et al. *Thromb Diath Haemorrh.* 1972;27(2):309.
3 Pond SM, et al. *Aust N Z J Med.* 1975;5(4):324.
4 Bjornsson TD, et al. *J Pharmacokinet Biopharm.* 1977;5(5):495.
5 Bjornsson TD, et al. *J Pharmacol Exp Ther.* 1979;210(3):316.
6 Williams GE, et al. *J Atheroscler Res.* 1963:3:658.
7 Schrogie JJ, et al. *Clin Pharmacol Ther.* 1967;8(1):70.
8 Solomon RB, et al. *N Y State J Med.* 1973;73(15):2002.
9 Udall JA. *Clin Med.* 1970;77:20.
10 Eastham RD. *Br Med J.* 1973;2(5865):554.
11 Veronich K, et al. *J Pharm Sci.* 1979;68(12):1515.
12 Bjornsson TD, et al. *J Pharmacol Exp Ther.* 1979;210(3):322.
13 Dixon DL, et al. *Pharmacotherapy.* 2009;29(6):744.
14 Rindone JP, et al. *Chest.* 1998;114(2):641.
15 Ahmad S. *Chest.* 1990;98(4):1041.
16 Ascah KJ, et al. *Ann Pharmacother.* 1998;32(7-8):765.
17 Aldridge MA, et al. *Pharmacotherapy.* 2001;21(7):886.
18 Lilja JJ, et al. *Br J Clin Pharmacol.* 2005;59(4):433.

* Asterisk indicates drugs cited in interaction reports.
† Not available in the United States.

Anticoagulants | **Fish Oil**

Warfarin* (eg, *Coumadin*)	Fish Oil*

Significance	Onset	Severity	Documentation
4	☐ Rapid	☐ Major	☐ Established
	■ **Delayed**	■ **Moderate**	☐ Probable
		☐ Minor	☐ Suspected
			■ **Possible**
			☐ Unlikely

Effects The anticoagulant effect of WARFARIN may be increased by FISH OIL ingestion.

Mechanism Unknown; however, FISH OIL may interfere with vitamin K–dependent clotting factors or affect platelet aggregation.

Management Evaluate patients for potential risk and monitor INR more closely when FISH OIL supplementation is started, stopped, increased, or decreased. Caution patients against using herbal products without consulting a health care provider and to report any signs of bleeding.

Discussion

An elevated INR was reported in a 67-year-old woman taking a fish oil product and warfarin.[1] The patient's INR was in the therapeutic range (2 to 3) for 5 months while she was receiving warfarin 1.5 mg daily. During this time, she started taking fish oil 1 g daily without any change in INR. However, 1 week after increasing her fish oil dose to 2 g daily, her INR increased from 2.8 to 4.3. Her weekly warfarin dose was reduced and she decreased the fish oil dose to 1 g daily. Eight days after these changes were implemented, a subtherapeutic INR (1.6) measurement was obtained. The warfarin dosage was changed to the original regimen (1.5 mg daily) and the INR remained in the therapeutic range.

[1] Buckley MS, et al. *Ann Pharmacother.* 2004;38(1):50.

* Asterisk indicates drugs cited in interaction reports.

Anticoagulants — *Food*

Warfarin*
(eg, *Coumadin*)

Food*

Significance	Onset	Severity	Documentation
4	☐ Rapid ■ **Delayed**	☐ Major ■ **Moderate** ☐ Minor	☐ Established ☐ Probable ☐ Suspected ■ **Possible** ☐ Unlikely

Effects The anticoagulant effects of WARFARIN may be decreased by certain FOODS.

Mechanism Vitamin K–rich vegetables may antagonize WARFARIN activity. Some FOODS may interfere with WARFARIN absorption.

Management Minimize or avoid consumption of vitamin K–containing FOODS or nutritional supplements.

Discussion

Resistance to the hypoprothrombinemic effect of warfarin caused by the ingestion of vitamin K–rich vegetables has been reported.[1,2] However, warfarin's anticoagulant effects also have been reduced by ingestion of foods low in vitamin K content.[3] Two patients previously stabilized on warfarin experienced dramatic reduction in INR following ingestion of avocado.[3] Eliminating avocado from their diet resulted in a return of adequate anticoagulation. One patient demonstrated the same loss of anticoagulant control following avocado ingestion a second time. Avocado contains low amounts of vitamin K. See also Anticoagulants-Vitamin K.

[1] Kempin SJ. *N Engl J Med.* 1983;308(20):1229.
[2] Karlson B, et al. *Acta Med Scand.* 1986;220(4):347.
[3] Blickstein D, et al. *Lancet.* 1991;337(8746):914.

* Asterisk indicates drugs cited in interaction reports.

Anticoagulants — *Gefitinib*

Warfarin* (eg, *Coumadin*)	Gefitinib* (*Iressa*)

Significance	Onset	Severity	Documentation
2	□ Rapid	□ Major	□ Established
	■ **Delayed**	■ **Moderate**	□ Probable
		□ Minor	■ **Suspected**
			□ Possible
			□ Unlikely

Effects The anticoagulant effect of WARFARIN may be potentiated, increasing the risk of bleeding.

Mechanism Unknown.

Management In patients receiving WARFARIN, closely monitor coagulation parameters when GEFITINIB is started or stopped. Adjust the WARFARIN dose as needed.

Discussion

The anticoagulant effects of warfarin were increased in a patient during coadministration of gefitinib.[1] The patient, a 74-year-old woman, was receiving warfarin to prevent thromboembolic events. Upon diagnosis with carcinoma of the lung, she was started on gefitinib 250 mg/m^2 daily. At that time, the patient was receiving warfarin 4 mg daily (INR approximately 2). After starting gefitinib therapy, the warfarin dose was decreased to 3 mg daily; however, the INR increased to 2.4. The daily warfarin dose was decreased to 2.5 mg and the INR returned to the target value of 2. In a second patient who received warfarin and gefitinib, no interaction occurred. In a retrospective chart review, 6 of 12 patients receiving gefitinib and warfarin concurrently had an elevated PT/INR.[2] Liver dysfunction was associated with the PT/INR elevation.

[1] Onoda S, et al. *Jpn J Clin Oncol.* 2005;35(8):478.

[2] Arai S, et al. *Int J Clin Oncol.* 2009;14(4):332.

* Asterisk indicates drugs cited in interaction reports.

Anticoagulants — *Ginkgo biloba*

Anticoagulants	Ginkgo biloba
Warfarin* (eg, *Coumadin*)	Ginkgo biloba*

Significance	Onset	Severity	Documentation
4	☐ Rapid ■ **Delayed**	■ **Major** ☐ Moderate ☐ Minor	☐ Established ☐ Probable ☐ Suspected ■ **Possible** ☐ Unlikely

Effects The risk of bleeding may be increased.

Mechanism Possible additive or synergistic ANTICOAGULANT effects may occur.

Management Caution patients to avoid concurrent use of WARFARIN and GINKGO BILOBA because of potentially life-threatening bleeding complications.

Discussion

Intracerebral hemorrhage was reported in a 78-year-old woman taking warfarin and *Ginkgo biloba*.[1] The patient, who had been taking warfarin for 5 years following coronary artery bypass surgery, developed severe apraxia, a marked change in her mild to moderate cognitive deficits, and an inability to feed herself. A CT scan showed a left parietal hemorrhage, and her PT was 16.9. The patient was hospitalized and anticoagulation was allowed to reverse. She was eventually transferred to a rehabilitation hospital, at which time her daughter admitted that she had been giving her mother *Ginkgo biloba* for 2 months prior to the event. In a double-blind, crossover study, 21 patients on stable warfarin regimens received *Ginkgo biloba* 100 mg or placebo for 4 weeks.[2] There were no changes in INR or weekly warfarin dose and no bleeding episodes during *Ginkgo biloba* ingestion. Bleeding disorders also have been reported in patients receiving *Ginkgo biloba* in the absence of warfarin.[3,4] In an open-label study in 12 healthy men, pretreatment for 7 days with recommended doses of *Ginkgo biloba* from herbal medicine products did not affect clotting status or the pharmacokinetics or pharmacodynamics of a single dose of warfarin 25 mg.[5] See also Anticoagulants-Danshen, Anticoagulants-Dong Quai, and Anticoagulants-Ginseng.

[1] Matthews MK Jr. *Neurology*. 1998;50(6):1933.
[2] Engelsen J, et al. *Thromb Haemost*. 2002;87(6):1075.
[3] Rowin J, et al. *Neurology*. 1996;46(6):1775.
[4] Gilbert GJ. *Neurology*. 1997;48(4):1137.
[5] Jiang X, et al. *Br J Clin Pharmacol*. 2005;59(4):425.

* Asterisk indicates drugs cited in interaction reports.

Anticoagulants — *Ginseng*

Warfarin* (eg, *Coumadin*)	Ginseng*

Significance	Onset	Severity	Documentation
4	☐ Rapid ■ **Delayed**	■ **Major** ☐ Moderate ☐ Minor	☐ Established ☐ Probable ☐ Suspected ■ **Possible** ☐ Unlikely

Effects Anticoagulant effects of WARFARIN may be decreased. Thrombotic events could occur.

Mechanism Unknown.

Management Avoid this combination if possible. If combined use cannot be avoided, closely monitor anticoagulation parameters when starting or stopping GINSENG in patients receiving WARFARIN. Adjust the WARFARIN dose as needed.

Discussion

Reports are conflicting. A possible interaction between warfarin and ginseng has been reported in 2 patients.[1,2] A 47-year-old man with a mechanical heart valve had been receiving warfarin for the previous 5 years.[1] His warfarin dose had remained stable at 5 mg/day, with 7.5 mg administered every Tuesday. The patient's INR was 3.1 four weeks before he started taking ginseng capsules 3 times/day to boost his energy level. Two weeks later, his INR had decreased to 1.5, and the ginseng was discontinued. The INR returned to 3.3 in 2 weeks. No thrombotic episode occurred. The ginseng was the only change in the patient's regimen. A 58-year-old man on a stable warfarin regimen experienced a drop in INR to 1.4 and a thrombosis on his mechanical bileaflet aortic valve following self-medication with a ginseng-containing product.[2] In a randomized, double-blind, placebo-controlled study in 20 healthy volunteers receiving warfarin 5 mg/day for 3 days, 14 days of pretreatment with ginseng 1 g twice daily decreased the peak INR, INR AUC, warfarin AUC, and warfarin C_{max}.[3] In a randomized, open-label, crossover study in 12 healthy men, 7 days of pretreatment with ginseng extract (*Panax ginseng* root 0.5 g plus ginsenosides 8.93 mg) did not affect the pharmacokinetics or pharmacodynamics of warfarin.[4] In an open-label study, 25 patients with newly diagnosed ischemic stroke were randomized into 2 groups.[5] One group (13 patients) received only warfarin 2 mg/day for 7 days followed by 5 mg/day for 7 days. The second group (12 patients) received the same warfarin regimen plus *Panax ginseng* 0.5 g aqueous extract 3 times daily. There was no difference in peak values and INR and PT AUC in patients taking warfarin and *Panax ginseng* concurrently compared with taking warfarin alone. No changes in INR were found when warfarin was administered with Korean red ginseng compared with placebo.[6] See also Anticoagulants-Danshen, Anticoagulants-Dong Quai, and Anticoagulants-*Ginkgo biloba*.

[1] Janetzky K, et al. *Am J Health Syst Pharm.* 1997;54(6):692.
[2] Rosado MF. *Cardiology.* 2003;99(2):111.
[3] Yuan CS, et al. *Ann Intern Med.* 2004;141(1):23.
[4] Jiang X, et al. *Br J Clin Pharmacol.* 2004;57(5);592.
[5] Lee SH, et al. *J Altern Complement Med.* 2008;14(6):715.
[6] Lee YH, et al. *Int J Cardiol.* 2010;145(2):275.

* Asterisk indicates drugs cited in interaction reports.

Anticoagulants — *Glucagon*

Warfarin* (eg, *Coumadin*)	Glucagon* (eg, *Glucagen*)

Significance	Onset	Severity	Documentation
2	□ Rapid	□ Major	□ Established
	■ **Delayed**	■ **Moderate**	■ **Probable**
		□ Minor	□ Suspected
			□ Possible
			□ Unlikely

Effects The anticoagulant effect of WARFARIN may be enhanced in patients receiving sustained doses of GLUCAGON (bleeding may occur).

Mechanism Unknown.

Management Monitor patients receiving WARFARIN and GLUCAGON concurrently daily for prothrombin activity and signs of bleeding. Adjust doses as needed.

Discussion

Twenty-four patients with myocardial contractile failure receiving warfarin and glucagon were evaluated retrospectively. Of 13 patients who received glucagon in doses of 50 mg or more for 2 days, 8 demonstrated excessive inhibition of prothrombin activity, and 3 had evidence of bleeding. Most of these patients were receiving multiple drugs. The severity of heart failure was not described in the affected patients.[1] It is unknown if a similar effect can be expected in patients without heart failure. Closely monitor patients receiving warfarin and prolonged doses of glucagon for excessive inhibition of prothrombin activity and signs of bleeding.

[1] Koch-Weser J. *Ann Intern Med.* 1970;72(3):331.

* Asterisk indicates drugs cited in interaction reports.

Anticoagulants — *Glucosamine*

Anticoagulants	Glucosamine
Warfarin* (eg, *Coumadin*)	Glucosamine*

Significance	Onset	Severity	Documentation
4	☐ Rapid	☐ Major	☐ Established
	■ **Delayed**	■ **Moderate**	☐ Probable
		☐ Minor	☐ Suspected
			■ **Possible**
			☐ Unlikely

Effects The anticoagulant effect of WARFARIN may be increased, increasing the risk of bleeding.

Mechanism Possible additive pharmacologic effect with WARFARIN and high-dose GLUCOSAMINE-CHONDROITIN.[1]

Management If coadministration of GLUCOSAMINE and WARFARIN cannot be avoided, closely monitor the INR and be prepared to adjust the WARFARIN dose when starting or stopping GLUCOSAMINE. Caution patients receiving WARFARIN against using herbal products without consulting their health care provider and to report any signs of bleeding or unusual bruising.

Discussion

A possible drug interaction between warfarin and glucosamine-chondroitin was reported in a 69-year-old man stabilized on warfarin 47.5 mg/week.[2] The patient's INR had been maintained in the target range of 2 to 3 for 4 months. He started self-treatment with 6 capsules daily of a product containing glucosamine hydrochloride 500 mg, sodium chondroitin sulfate 400 mg, and manganese ascorbate. His INR increased from 2.58 before starting glucosamine-chondroitin to 4.52 four weeks after it was started. The weekly warfarin dose was reduced to 40 mg and the INR decreased to 2.15. With continued use of glucosamine-chondroitin, his INR was maintained in the target range for 3 months with no further changes in the warfarin dose. Additional cases of increased INR in patients receiving concurrent warfarin and glucosamine have been reported in the literature and are listed in the WHO adverse drug reaction database.[3] The INR frequently decreases or returns to the therapeutic range when glucosamine is discontinued or the dose is reduced.

[1] Scott GN. *Am J Health Syst Pharm.* 2004;61(11):1186.
[2] Rozenfeld V, et al. *J Health Syst Pharm.* 2004;61(3):306.
[3] Knudsen JF, et al. *Pharmacotherapy.* 2008;28(4):540.

* Asterisk indicates drugs cited in interaction reports.

Anticoagulants		*Glutethimide*
Warfarin* (eg, *Coumadin*)	Glutethimide*	

Significance	Onset	Severity	Documentation
2	☐ Rapid	☐ Major	☐ Established
	■ **Delayed**	■ **Moderate**	■ **Probable**
		☐ Minor	☐ Suspected
			☐ Possible
			☐ Unlikely

Effects Inhibition of prothrombin activity may be impaired. Inadequate therapeutic response to coumarin ANTICOAGULANTS may occur.

Mechanism GLUTETHIMIDE appears to increase the clearance of coumain ANTICOAGULANTS by stimulation of hepatic microsomal enzymes.

Management Monitor PT carefully if GLUTETHIMIDE is added to coumarin ANTICOAGULANT therapy or if GLUTETHIMIDE is withdrawn from concomitant therapy; anticoagulant therapy will likely need adjustment. Alternative sedative therapy (eg, benzodiazepines) may be appropriate.

Discussion

Controlled studies of patients and volunteers have documented an inhibition of the anticoagulant response to warfarin in the majority of cases when glutethimide is administered.[1,2] Decreases in warfarin plasma concentrations and $t_{1/2}$ have also been described in patients and volunteers after glutethimide administration, which probably accounts for the decreased pharmacologic response.[3,4] The pattern of kinetic changes suggests an increase in metabolic clearance due to increased hepatic microsomal enzyme activity similar to phenobarbital.[2]

Alternative therapy may include benzodiazepines, which do not appear to interfere with the anticoagulant response to or the metabolism of warfarin.[3]

[1] Orme M, et al. *Br Med J.* 1972;3(5827):611.
[2] Udall JA. *Am J Cardiol.* 1975;35(1):67.
[3] Corn M. *Thromb Diath Haemorrh.* 1966;16(3):606.
[4] MacDonald MG, et al. *Clin Pharmacol Ther.* 1969;10(1):80.

* Asterisk indicates drugs cited in interaction reports.

Anticoagulants — *Griseofulvin*

Warfarin* (eg, *Coumadin*)	Griseofulvin* (eg, *Grisactin 500*)

Significance	Onset	Severity	Documentation
2	□ Rapid	□ Major	□ Established
	■ **Delayed**	■ **Moderate**	□ Probable
		□ Minor	■ **Suspected**
			□ Possible
			□ Unlikely

Effects The anticoagulant activity of WARFARIN may be decreased.

Mechanism Unknown.

Management In patients stabilized on WARFARIN therapy, monitor anticoagulant parameters more frequently when GRISEOFULVIN dosage is altered. Adjust the WARFARIN dosage accordingly.

Discussion

A small number of case reports of patients stabilized on warfarin have documented decreased prothrombin times when griseofulvin was administered.[1,3] In 1 controlled study, 4 of 10 patients with vascular disease receiving warfarin demonstrated a decreased prothrombin time.[2] Additional studies are needed to identify mechanisms and risk factors for this interaction.

[1] Cullen SI, et al. *JAMA*. 1967;199:582.
[2] Udall JA. *Clin Med*. 1970;77:20.
[3] Okino K, et al. *Drug Intell Clin Pharm*. 1986;20:291.

* Asterisk indicates drugs cited in interaction reports.

Anticoagulants — *Histamine H_2 Antagonists*

Warfarin* (eg, *Coumadin*)	Cimetidine* (eg, *Tagamet*)

Significance	Onset	Severity	Documentation
1	□ Rapid ■ **Delayed**	■ **Major** □ Moderate □ Minor	■ **Established** □ Probable □ Suspected □ Possible □ Unlikely

Effects Increase in WARFARIN effects; possible hemorrhage.

Mechanism Stereoselective inhibition of the hepatic metabolism of the less potent (R)-warfarin enantiomer.[11,12,20,23,24]

Management Avoid this combination if possible; alternative H_2-ANTAGONISTS, such as nizatidine, appear unlikely to interact. If this combination is used, monitor anticoagulation parameters and tailor WARFARIN doses as needed.

Discussion

Multiple case reports describe prolongation of the prothrombin time (PT) with moderate to severe bleeding following the introduction of cimetidine to warfarin-treated patients.[2,4-8] Cimetidine produces a 20% increase in PT and clotting time.[1] Seven volunteers showed PT prolongation as a result of a decrease in warfarin clearance.[3] Only 7 of 14 patients had significant PT prolongation associated with increases in the warfarin levels, while the remainder had either minimal or no change.[15] There also may be a dose-dependent effect.[17,20] The effect of cimetidine on acenocoumarol has been variable with one report of inhibition of the (R)-isomer[14] and another of no effect.[13] In one study, both cimetidine and ranitidine reduced warfarin clearance but cimetidine had a greater effect.[9] Excessive hypoprothrombinemia occurred in a patient on warfarin when the dose of ranitidine was increased from 300 to 600 mg/day.[22] By contrast, others have found no pharmacokinetic or pharmacodynamic changes with ranitidine.[7,10,16] Based on currently available data, it is unlikely that there is a clinically important interaction between ranitidine and warfarin. In volunteers, nizatidine had no effect on PT or warfarin levels.[19,21] Similarly, famotidine is not expected to interact because it does not bind with the cytochrome P450 enzyme system.[18,21]

[1] Flind AC. *Br Med J.* 1978;2:1367.
[2] Silver BA, et al. *Ann Intern Med.* 1979;90:348.
[3] Serlin MJ, et al. *Lancet.* 1979;2:317.
[4] Hetzel D, et al. *Lancet.* 1979;2:639.
[5] Wallin BA, et al. *Ann Intern Med.* 1979;90:993.
[6] Devanesen S. *Med J Aust.* 1981;1:537.
[7] Serlin MJ, et al. *Br J Clin Pharmacol.* 1981;12:791.
[8] Kerley B, et al. *Can Med Assoc J.* 1982;126:116.
[9] Desmond PV, et al. *Clin Pharmacol Ther.* 1984;35:338.
[10] O'Reilly RA. *Arch Intern Med.* 1984;144:989.
[11] Choonara IA, et al. *Br J Clin Pharmacol.* 1986;21:271.
[12] Toon S, et al. *Br J Clin Pharmacol.* 1986;21:245.
[13] Thijssen HH, et al. *Eur J Clin Pharmacol.* 1986;30:619.
[14] Gill TS, et al. *Br J Clin Pharmacol.* 1986;21:564P.
[15] Bell WR, et al. *Arch Intern Med.* 1986;146:2325.
[16] Toon S, et al. *Eur J Clin Pharmacol.* 1987;32:165.
[17] Sax MJ, et al. *Clin Pharm.* 1987;6:492.
[18] Sax MJ. *Pharmacotherapy.* 1987;7:110S.
[19] Cournot A, et al. *J Clin Pharmacol.* 1988;28:1120.
[20] Hunt BA, et al. *Pharmacotherapy.* 1989;9:184.
[21] Hussey EK, et al. *Drug Intell Clin Pharm.* 1989;23:675.
[22] Baciewicz AM, et al. *Ann Intern Med.* 1990;112:76.
[23] Niopas I, et al. *Br J Clin Pharmacol.* 1991;32:508.
[24] Niopas I, et al. *Eur J Clin Pharmacol.* 1999;55:399.

* Asterisk indicates drugs cited in interaction reports.
† Not available in the United States.

Anticoagulants — *HMG-CoA Reductase Inhibitors*

Warfarin* (eg, *Coumadin*)	Fluvastatin* (*Lescol*)	Rosuvastatin* (*Crestor*)
	Lovastatin* (eg, *Mevacor*)	Simvastatin* (eg, *Zocor*)

Significance	Onset	Severity	Documentation
1	□ Rapid	■ **Major**	□ Established
	■ **Delayed**	□ Moderate	■ **Probable**
		□ Minor	□ Suspected
			□ Possible
			□ Unlikely

Effects The anticoagulant effect of WARFARIN may increase.

Mechanism Decreased S- and R-WARFARIN clearance by inhibition of CYP2C9 and CYP3A4 metabolism, respectively.[1]

Management Monitor ANTICOAGULANT parameters when starting or discontinuing coadministration of an HMG-CoA REDUCTASE INHIBITOR. Atorvastatin (*Lipitor*)[2] and pravastatin (eg, *Pravachol*)[3] do not appear to interact with WARFARIN.

Discussion

Several reports of bleeding and PT elevations in patients taking warfarin and lovastatin have been published; however, it was not established if these events were caused by a drug interaction.[4] Elevation of PT and bleeding were reported in 2 patients on stable warfarin regimens, to which lovastatin 20 mg/day was added.[5] One patient developed rectal bleeding 3 wk after starting lovastatin; the other patient developed epistaxis and hematuria 10 days after starting lovastatin. In both patients, the PT was elevated. The warfarin dose was reduced in both cases with resolution of bleeding and return of the PT to the therapeutic range. Seven cases of an apparent interaction between warfarin and fluvastatin have been reported.[6-8] Decreasing the dose of warfarin was necessary to maintain the INR or PT within the desired range after starting or increasing the dose of fluvastatin. Warfarin requirements returned to pre-fluvastatin levels in 3 patients when fluvastatin was discontinued.[7,8] Simvastatin 20 mg/day did not potentiate warfarin-induced anticoagulation in 1 patient.[9] Forty-six patients on stable warfarin regimens and pravastatin were converted to simvastatin.[10] Average INR increased from 2.4 to 2.7, while the warfarin dose did not change. In a study of 29 patients on stable warfarin regimens, the addition of simvastatin increased the INR 27% and decreased the mean daily warfarin dose 9%.[11] A patient on long-term warfarin therapy developed bruising, hematuria, and light-headedness, and in 4 wk, her INR increased from 2 to 8 after starting rosuvastatin.[12] Compared with placebo, pretreatment with rosuvastatin 40 mg/day increased the average INR 19% after a single dose of warfarin 25 mg.[13] In patients on chronic warfarin therapy, both rosuvastatin 10 and 80 mg increased the INR to more than 4.[13] However, in another study, rosuvastatin 40 mg daily did not affect the anticoagulant effect of warfarin.[14] Long-term use of HMG-CoA reductase inhibitors may decrease bleeding events in patients treated with warfarin.[15] In an 82-yr-old woman stabilized on warfarin and receiving atorvastatin, the INR increased from 2.6 to more than 8 after atorvastatin was changed to simvastatin.[16] Despite vitamin K treatment, she developed a cerebral hemorrhage and died.

1 Sconce EA, et al. *J Thromb Haemost.* 2006;4(6):1422.
2 Stern R, et al. *J Clin Pharmacol.* 1997;37(11):1062.
3 Pan HY. *Eur J Clin Pharmacol.* 1991;40(suppl 1):S15.
4 Tobert JA. *Am J Cardiol.* 1988;62(15):28J.
5 Ahmad S. *Arch Intern Med.* 1990;150(11):2407.
6 Trilli LE, et al. *Ann Pharmacother.* 1996;30(12):1399.
7 Kline SS, et al. *Ann Pharmacother.* 1997;31(6):790.
8 Andrus MR. *Pharmacotherapy.* 2004;24(2):285.
9 Gaw A, et al. *Lancet.* 1992;340(8825):979.
10 Lin JC, et al. *J Clin Pharmacol.* 1999;39(1):86.
11 Hickmott H, et al. *Thromb Haemost.* 2003;89(5):949.
12 Barry M. *Lancet.* 2004;363(9405):328.
13 Simonson SG, et al. *J Clin Pharmacol.* 2005;45(8):927.
14 Jindal D, et al. *Eur J Clin Pharmacol.* 2005;61(9):621.
15 Douketis JD, et al. *Am J Med.* 2007;120(4):369.e9.
16 Westergren T, et al. *Ann Pharmacother.* 2007;41(7):1292.

* Asterisk indicates drugs cited in interaction reports.

Anticoagulants		***Ifosfamide***
Warfarin* (eg, *Coumadin*)	Ifosfamide* (eg, *Ifex*)	

Significance	Onset	Severity	Documentation
4	☐ Rapid ■ **Delayed**	☐ Major ■ **Moderate** ☐ Minor	☐ Established ☐ Probable ☐ Suspected ■ **Possible** ☐ Unlikely

Effects The anticoagulant effect of WARFARIN may increase.

Mechanism Unknown. However, inhibition of WARFARIN metabolism and displacement of WARFARIN from its protein-binding site by IFOSFAMIDE are suspected to be involved.

Management Monitor PTs when starting or discontinuing concurrent IFOSFAMIDE administration.

Discussion

Disturbances in the INR (therapeutic range, 2.5 to 3.5) were observed in 3 patients receiving warfarin concurrently with the combination of ifosfamide and mesna (eg, *Mesnex*).[1] A 16-year-old girl was given warfarin 4 mg/day for 2 months for a left femoral vein thrombosis. Her INR was stable. Forty-eight hours after the start of IV chemotherapy with etoposide (eg, *VePesid*), cisplatin, and ifosfamide/mesna (both in a dose of 3 g/m^2), the INR increased to 8.4. The second patient, a 61-year-old woman with advanced breast cancer, received warfarin 4 mg/day for an axillary vein thrombosis. Her INR was stable at 2.3. IV chemotherapy consisted of doxorubicin (eg, *Adriamycin*) and ifosfamide 5 g/m^2 as a 24-hour infusion preceded by an IV bolus of mesna 1 g/m^2. In addition, over a 32-hour period beginning with the ifosfamide infusion, the patient received mesna 4 g/m^2. Forty-eight hours after the start of chemotherapy, the INR increased to 7.5. The INR decreased to 1.3 on discontinuation of warfarin. Five days after the completion of chemotherapy, the INR remained below 2, even though the patient was receiving warfarin 10 mg/day. Subsequently, the INR remained stable and within the therapeutic range with warfarin 4 mg/day. The third patient, a 25-year-old man, received warfarin 4 mg/day following partial resection of a retroperitoneal malignancy. The INR was stable at 2.1. Chemotherapy consisted of IV bolus injections of doxorubicin and vincristine (eg, *Vincasar*) followed by ifosfamide 9 g/m^2 plus mesna 10.5 g/m^2 infused simultaneously over 72 hours. Forty-eight hours after starting chemotherapy, the INR was 5.5. Warfarin was discontinued and restarted 2 days later at a dose of 4 mg/day. The INR remained stable. Three weeks later, he received a second course of chemotherapy; within 3 days of initiation of treatment, the INR increased from 2.8 to 4.8. See also Anticoagulants-Antineoplastic Agents.

[1] Hall G, et al. *Postgrad Med J.* 1990;66(780):860.

* Asterisk indicates drugs cited in interaction reports.

Anticoagulants — *Influenza Virus Vaccine*

Warfarin* (eg, *Coumadin*) | Influenza Virus Vaccine* (eg, *Fluzone*)

Significance	Onset	Severity	Documentation
4	☐ Rapid	■ **Major**	☐ Established
	■ **Delayed**	☐ Moderate	☐ Probable
		☐ Minor	☐ Suspected
			■ **Possible**
			☐ Unlikely

Effects The anticoagulant activity of WARFARIN may be enhanced in some patients receiving the INFLUENZA VACCINE.

Mechanism Unknown.

Management In patients receiving WARFARIN, begin monitoring the INR within 7 days after administering the VACCINE.

Discussion

The observation that viral infections[1] and the influenza vaccine[2] can decrease CYP-450 enzyme activity led to further investigations evaluating plasma levels and prothrombin activity in patients and volunteers. In 1 case, an 81-year-old man taking warfarin for 12 years developed hematemesis and melena associated with a PT of 36 seconds 10 days after receiving the influenza vaccine. As a follow-up, the investigators conducted a study that demonstrated an increase in PTs over a previous 12-month control period in 4 of 8 patients.[3] A 64-year-old man taking warfarin who had a relatively stable INR (1.4 to 4.7) for 6 months suffered a fatal cranial bleed; his INR was higher than 15 approximately 4.5 weeks after vaccination with an influenza virus vaccine.[4] A case-control study of 90 patients reported an increase in INR from an average of 2.79 to 3.35 occurring 7 to 10 days after receiving the vaccine.[5] By contrast, the control group of 45 patients who were not vaccinated did not have a change in INR. Subsequent studies in a total of 134 subjects have failed to document any change in PTs.[6-10] Adverse reactions to warfarin were not increased in a total of 45 institutionalized patients given the influenza vaccine.[9,11] Additionally, kinetic evaluations including warfarin $t_{1/2}$[3] and steady-state plasma levels[8] have not demonstrated changes.[3,8,12,13]

The consistency of numerous negative studies suggests that this interaction is unlikely.

[1] Chang KC, et al. *Lancet.* 1978;1(8074):1132.
[2] Kramer P, et al. *N Engl J Med.* 1981;305(21):1262.
[3] Kramer P, et al. *Clin Pharmacol Ther.* 1984;35(3):416.
[4] Carroll DN, et al. *Ann Pharmacother.* 2009;43(4):754.
[5] Paliani U, et al. *Haematologica.* 2003;88(5):599.
[6] Lipsky BA, et al. *Ann Intern Med.* 1984;100(6):835.
[7] Farrow PR, et al. *J Infect.* 1984;9(2):157.
[8] Scott AK, et al. *Br J Clin Pharmacol.* 1985;19:144P.
[9] Gomolin IH, et al. *J Am Geriatr Soc.* 1985;33(4):269.
[10] Bussey HI, et al. *Drug Intell Clin Pharm.* 1988;22(3):198.
[11] Patriarca PA, et al. *N Engl J Med.* 1983;308(26):1601.
[12] Bussey HI, et al. *Drug Intell Clin Pharm.* 1986;20(6):460.
[13] Gomolin IH. *CMAJ.* 1986;135(1):39.

* Asterisk indicates drugs cited in interaction reports.

Anticoagulants — *Isoniazid*

Warfarin* (eg, *Coumadin*)	Isoniazid* (eg, *Nydrazid*)

Significance	Onset	Severity	Documentation
4	☐ Rapid ■ **Delayed**	☐ Major ■ **Moderate** ☐ Minor	☐ Established ☐ Probable ☐ Suspected ■ **Possible** ☐ Unlikely

Effects The anticoagulant activity of WARFARIN may be enhanced when ISONIAZID is administered.

Mechanism Unknown.

Management Consider the possibility of an increased response to WARFARIN when ISONIAZID is administered. Monitor PTs and adjust the dose as needed.

Discussion

Case reports and animal studies have conflicting data. One study reported that a 35-year-old man, who was well controlled on warfarin and isoniazid 300 mg, developed clinical bleeding and excessive hypoprothrombinemia after an increase to isoniazid 600 mg/day.[1] Another study reported a case of increased warfarin dose requirements in a patient receiving rifampin and isoniazid 300 mg/day.[2] No cases of drug interaction have been reported at the usual dose of isoniazid 300 mg.

[1] Rosenthal AR, et al. *JAMA*. 1977;238(20):2177.

[2] Almog S, et al. *South Med J*. 1988;81(10):1304.

* Asterisk indicates drugs cited in interaction reports.

Anticoagulants — **Leflunomide**

Warfarin*
(eg, *Coumadin*)

Leflunomide*
(eg, *Arava*)

Significance	Onset	Severity	Documentation
4	☐ Rapid ■ **Delayed**	☐ Major ■ **Moderate** ☐ Minor	☐ Established ☐ Probable ☐ Suspected ■ **Possible** ☐ Unlikely

Effects The ANTICOAGULANT effect of WARFARIN may be increased, resulting in an increased risk of bleeding.

Mechanism Inhibition of WARFARIN metabolism (CYP2C9) by the active metabolite of LEFLUNOMIDE is suspected.

Management In patients receiving WARFARIN, closely monitor coagulation parameters when starting, stopping, or changing the dose of LEFLUNOMIDE. Adjust the WARFARIN dose as needed.

Discussion

A possible drug interaction between warfarin and leflunomide was reported in a 49-year-old man with resistant rheumatoid arthritis.[1] The patient was started on leflunomide at the recommended loading dose of 100 mg/day for 3 days. His INR was stable for the previous year while he was receiving warfarin. Two days prior to starting leflunomide, his INR was 3.4. After the second dose of leflunomide, the patient developed gross hematuria and was hospitalized; his INR was 11. Warfarin was discontinued, and the hematuria resolved several hours after admission. The INR remained elevated for the next 2 days. On day 3, the dose of leflunomide was changed to the maintenance dose (20 mg/day). In addition, the patient was given vitamin K 1 mg IV and, 12 hours later, the INR decreased to 1.9. Warfarin therapy was resumed at a lower dose (1 mg/day), which maintained the INR within the recommended range. At least 300 reports of an elevated INR during coadministration of warfarin and leflunomide have been noted.[1] An elevated INR (7.3) was reported in a 61-year-old woman receiving long-term warfarin therapy after leflunomide was started.[2] It was necessary to decrease the warfarin dosage 22% (from 36 to 28 mg/wk) to maintain a therapeutic INR of 2 to 3.

[1] Lim V, et al. *BMJ.* 2002;325(7376):1333.

[2] Chonlahan J, et al. *Pharmacotherapy.* 2006;26(6):868.

* Asterisk indicates drugs cited in interaction reports.

Anticoagulants		***Loop Diuretics***
Warfarin* (eg, *Coumadin*)	Ethacrynic Acid* (*Edecrin*) Furosemide* (eg, *Lasix*)	Torsemide* (eg, *Demadex*)

Significance	Onset	Severity	Documentation
4	☐ Rapid ■ **Delayed**	☐ Major ■ **Moderate** ☐ Minor	☐ Established ☐ Probable ☐ Suspected ■ **Possible** ☐ Unlikely

Effects The anticoagulant activity of WARFARIN may be enhanced by coadministration of certain LOOP DIURETICS.

Mechanism LOOP DIURETICS may increase free WARFARIN plasma concentrations because of displacement from albumin-binding sites. TORSEMIDE may inhibit S-WARFARIN metabolism (CYP2C9).

Management Monitor prothrombin activity more frequently when LOOP DIURETICS are administered with WARFARIN. Lower WARFARIN doses may be required.

Discussion

Displacement of warfarin from albumin-binding sites by ethacrynic acid has occurred in vitro.[1] Following 4 to 15 days of ethacrynic acid treatment, a single case of increased hypoprothrombinemia was reported in a patient previously stabilized on warfarin.[2] A 43-year-old woman stabilized on warfarin (INR 2.5 to 3.5) developed an elevated INR (6.2) 1 week after starting torsemide.[3]

Studies of healthy volunteers have not demonstrated any evidence of increased warfarin plasma levels or anticoagulant response when usual doses of bumetanide (*Bumex*) or furosemide were coadministered.[4,5]

A single-dose study in rats utilizing large doses of furosemide 5 to 10 mg/kg demonstrated increased free concentrations of warfarin, more rapid plasma clearance, and enhanced anticoagulant effects.[6] Additional multiple-dose studies with furosemide are needed.

1 Sellers EM, et al. *Clin Pharmacol Ther.* 1970;11(4):524.
2 Petrick RJ, et al. *JAMA.* 1975;231(8):843.
3 Bird J, et al. *Ann Pharmacother.* 2008;42(12):1893.
4 Nilsson CM, et al. *J Clin Pharmacol.* 1978;18(2-3):91.
5 Nipper H, et al. *J Clin Pharmacol.* 1981;21(11-12, pt 2):654.
6 Ogiso T, et al. *J Pharmacobiodyn.* 1982;5(10):829.

* Asterisk indicates drugs cited in interaction reports.

Anticoagulants		Macrolide & Related Antibiotics	
Warfarin* (eg, *Coumadin*)		Azithromycin* (eg, *Zithromax*)	Erythromycin* (eg, *Ery-Tab*)
		Clarithromycin* (eg, *Biaxin*)	Telithromycin* (*Ketek*)

Significance	Onset	Severity	Documentation
1	☐ Rapid	■ **Major**	☐ Established
	■ **Delayed**	☐ Moderate	■ **Probable**
		☐ Minor	☐ Suspected
			☐ Possible
			☐ Unlikely

Effects The anticoagulant effect of oral ANTICOAGULANTS may be increased. Hemorrhage has occurred.

Mechanism The total body clearance of WARFARIN is reduced.

Management Monitor anticoagulant parameters and adjust the dose frequently when MACROLIDE and RELATED ANTIBIOTICS are started or stopped. It may be necessary to monitor and adjust the ANTICOAGULANT dosage for several days after stopping MACROLIDE and RELATED ANTIBIOTICS.

Discussion

Case reports document an interaction between warfarin and erythromycin,[1-6] clarithromycin,[7-9] and azithromycin.[10-13] Often, bleeding complications were associated with elevations in clotting parameters. PT prolongation may occur with small doses of erythromycin,[14] within days of starting therapy and increase despite stopping warfarin.[5] In all case reports, treatment included vitamin K, which corrected the excessive anticoagulation. Controlled studies[15-18] with erythromycin found a 14% reduction in warfarin clearance and a 9.4% increase in blood levels. While these changes are small, caution is warranted because of the magnitude of the problems encountered. Other studies found no interaction between warfarin and azithromycin.[19,20] Elevated INR, hemoptysis, and blood-stained mucus were reported in a 73-year-old man receiving long-term treatment with warfarin (stable INR values, 2.8 to 3.5) 4 days after starting telithromycin 800 mg/day.[21] The next day, the INR was 11. Telithromycin was discontinued, and the previous warfarin dose was restarted. His INR was stable between 2.8 and 3.3.

1 Bartle WR. *Arch Intern Med.* 1980;140(7):985.
2 O'Donnell D. *Med J Aust.* 1989;150(3):163.
3 Schwartz J, et al. *South Med J.* 1983;76(1):91.
4 Husserl FE. *Arch Intern Med.* 1983;143(9):1831.
5 Sato RI, et al. *Arch Intern Med.* 1984;144(12):2413.
6 Parker DL, et al. *Am J Health Syst Pharm.* 2010;67(1):38.
7 Oberg KC. *Pharmacotherapy.* 1998;18(2):386.
8 Gooderham MJ, et al. *Ann Pharmacother.* 1999;33(7-8):796.
9 Dandekar SS, et al. *J R Soc Med.* 2001;94(11):583.
10 Woldtvedt BR, et al. *Ann Pharmacother.* 1998;32(2):269.
11 Foster DR, et al. *Pharmacotherapy.* 1999;19(7):902.
12 Williams D, et al. *Am J Health Syst Pharm.* 2003;60(3):274.
13 Shrader SP, et al. *Pharmacotherapy.* 2004;24(7):945.
14 Hassell D, et al. *South Med J.* 1985;78(8):1015.
15 Schwartz J, et al. *Drug Intell Clin Pharm.* 1983;17:438.
16 Bachmann K, et al. *Pharmacology.* 1984;28(3):171.
17 Weibert RT, et al. *Clin Pharmacol Ther.* 1987;41(2):224.
18 Weibert RT, et al. *Clin Pharm.* 1989;8(3):210.
19 Beckey NP, et al. *Pharmacotherapy.* 2000;20(9):1055.
20 McCall KL, et al. *Pharmacotherapy.* 2004;24(2):188.
21 Kolilekas L, et al. *Ann Pharmacother.* 2004;38(9):1424.

* Asterisk indicates drugs cited in interaction reports.

Anticoagulants — *Magnesium Salts*

Anticoagulants	Magnesium Salts	
Dicumarol*†	Magaldrate (eg, *Riopan*)	Magnesium Oxide (eg, *Mag-Ox 400*)
	Magnesium Carbonate	Magnesium Sulfate
	Magnesium Citrate	Magnesium Trisilicate*
	Magnesium Gluconate	
	Magnesium Hydroxide* (eg, *Milk of Magnesia*)	

Significance	Onset	Severity	Documentation
4	☐ Rapid	☐ Major	☐ Established
	■ **Delayed**	■ **Moderate**	☐ Probable
		☐ Minor	☐ Suspected
			■ **Possible**
			☐ Unlikely

Effects MAGNESIUM SALTS may increase the anticoagulant activity of DICUMAROL, but this has not been demonstrated in human studies.

Mechanism Possible increase in absorption of MAGNESIUM-DICUMAROL chelate.[1]

Management If an interaction is suspected, monitor PTs and adjust the dose as needed.

Discussion

Increased plasma concentrations of dicumarol have occurred in humans when the drug is administered with magnesium hydroxide[1] and in animals when coadministered with magnesium hydroxide or magnesium oxide.[1,2] Increased anticoagulant effects were noted in a study with dogs[2] but not with human volunteers.[1] Aluminum hydroxide did not increase the absorption of dicumarol, while magnesium hydroxide did.[1,2]

Warfarin (eg, *Coumadin*) plasma levels and hypoprothrombinemic action were not altered by aluminum hydroxide, magnesium hydroxide,[1] or their combination[3] in studies of human volunteers. Magnesium trisilicate increased warfarin absorption 19% in an in vitro study,[4] but the results have not been confirmed in humans or animals.

There are no case reports of bleeding or inadequate response to oral anticoagulants associated with magnesium salts.[5]

1 Ambre JJ, et al. *Clin Pharmacol Ther.* 1973;14(2):231.
2 Akers MA, et al. *J Pharm Sci.* 1973;62(3):391.
3 Robinson DS, et al. *Clin Pharmacol Ther.* 1971;12(3):491.
4 McElnay JC, et al. *Br Med J.* 1978;2(6145):1166.
5 D'Arcy PF, et al. *Drug Intell Clin Pharm.* 1987;21(7-8):607.

* Asterisk indicates drugs cited in interaction reports. Based on pharmacologic and pharmacokinetic considerations, similar interactions may occur with other drugs that are listed.
† Not available in the United States.

Anticoagulants — *Mefloquine*

Anticoagulants	Mefloquine
Warfarin* (eg, *Coumadin*)	Mefloquine*

Significance	Onset	Severity	Documentation
4	☐ Rapid ■ **Delayed**	■ **Major** ☐ Moderate ☐ Minor	☐ Established ☐ Probable ☐ Suspected ■ **Possible** ☐ Unlikely

Effects The anticoagulant effect of WARFARIN may be increased.

Mechanism Possible displacement of drug from plasma proteins.

Management In patients receiving WARFARIN, monitor anticoagulant parameters more closely during coadministration of MEFLOQUINE. Adjust the WARFARIN dosage as needed.

Discussion

In 2 patients stabilized on warfarin therapy, prolonged PT and bleeding occurred after mefloquine 250 mg/wk was added to their treatment regimen.[1]

[1] Loefler I. *J Travel Med.* 2003;10(3):194.

* Asterisk indicates drugs cited in interaction reports.

Anticoagulants		**Menthol**
Warfarin* (eg, *Coumadin*)		Menthol*

Significance	Onset	Severity	Documentation
4	☐ Rapid ■ **Delayed**	☐ Major ■ **Moderate** ☐ Minor	☐ Established ☐ Probable ☐ Suspected ■ **Possible** ☐ Unlikely

Effects Anticoagulant effects of WARFARIN may be decreased.

Mechanism Unknown.

Management Caution patients taking warfarin to avoid use of MENTHOL. If MENTHOL is ingested, closely monitor anticoagulant parameters when MENTHOL usage is started or stopped. Adjust the WARFARIN dose as needed.

Discussion

Menthol is a volatile oil found in peppermint. A possible interaction of WARFARIN with menthol cough drops (eg, *Halls*) was reported in a 57-year-old man.[1] Prior to cardioversion for atrial fibrillation, the patient was receiving warfarin 7 mg/day. At this dosage, his INR values were stable in the range of 2.28 to 2.68 for 3 weeks. Approximately 1 week later, the INR decreased to 1.45. Although the patient was receiving numerous other medications, there were no medication changes for the 3 months prior to warfarin therapy, and the patient denied changes to his medication regimen or diet. The patient stated that he had developed a flu-like illness and had been taking about 6 menthol cough drops daily for 4 days. The warfarin dosage was increased to 7 mg 3 days/wk and then 8 mg 4 days/wk (53 mg/wk). He discontinued the menthol cough drops, and the INR increased to 2.22. The warfarin dosage was reduced to 52 mg/wk. The INR was 3.06 two weeks later, and the warfarin dosage was decreased to 7 mg/day. The next week, the INR was 2.92. A 46-year-old man taking warfarin 50 mg/wk experienced a decrease in the INR from 2.6 to 1.6 while taking 8 to 10 menthol cough drops daily.[2] The INR remained at 1.6 for 3 weeks, despite incremental increases in the warfarin dose. Five days after stopping the cough drops, the INR increased from 1.6 to 2.9 and remained stable on a weekly dose of warfarin 40 mg.

[1] Kassebaum PJ, et al. *Ann Pharmacother.* 2005;39(2):365.

[2] Coderre K, et al. *Pharmacotherapy.* 2010;30(1):110.

* Asterisk indicates drugs cited in interaction reports.

Anticoagulants		*Mesalamine*
Warfarin* (eg, *Coumadin*)		Mesalamine* (eg, *Pentasa*)

Significance	Onset	Severity	Documentation
4	□ Rapid ■ **Delayed**	□ Major ■ **Moderate** □ Minor	□ Established □ Probable □ Suspected ■ **Possible** □ Unlikely

Effects The anticoagulant effect of WARFARIN may be decreased.

Mechanism Unknown.

Management Monitor anticoagulant parameters when starting, stopping, or changing the dose of MESALAMINE. If an interaction is suspected, it may be necessary to discontinue MESALAMINE.

Discussion

Failure to attain a hypoprothrombinemic effect to warfarin was reported in a 51-year-old woman after she started mesalamine 800 mg 3 times daily for a cecal ulcer.[1] The patient had been receiving warfarin 5 mg/day for deep venous thrombosis (DVT). At this dose of warfarin, her INR was 2 to 3. Other medications she was receiving included famotidine (eg, *Pepcid*), isradipine (eg, *DynaCirc*), lisinopril (eg, *Prinivil*), and lorazepam (eg, *Ativan*). Four weeks after starting mesalamine, the patient was admitted to the hospital with DVT. Her INR was 0.9. Six days later, her INR reached a peak of 1.7. Plasma warfarin concentration was undetectable. Mesalamine was discontinued, and the next day, the patient's INR was 1.8, increasing to 2.1 after 2 days.

Additional studies are needed to confirm this possible drug interaction.

[1] Marinella MA. *Ann Pharmacother.* 1998;32:841.

* Asterisk indicates drugs cited in interaction reports.

Anticoagulants	*Methylphenidate*
Dicumarol†	Methylphenidate* (eg, *Ritalin*)

Significance	Onset	Severity	Documentation
5	□ Rapid ■ **Delayed**	□ Major □ Moderate ■ **Minor**	□ Established □ Probable □ Suspected □ Possible ■ **Unlikely**

Effects The anticoagulant action of ETHYL BISCOUMACETATE may possibly be enhanced.

Mechanism Unknown.

Management No management interventions appear required at this time.

Discussion

Results from two controlled studies are conflicting. One study[1] reported an increased half-life of ethyl biscoumacetate† in four volunteers when preceded by methylphenidate 20 mg/day for 3 to 5 days. A second study[2] was unable to duplicate the results and found no change in ethyl biscoumacetate half-life or effect on prothrombin time in 12 volunteers.

Interactions with other coumarin oral anticoagulants have not been reported.

[1] Garrettson LK, et al. *JAMA* 1969;207:2053.

[2] Hague DE, et al. *Clin Pharmacol Ther* 1971;12:259.

* Asterisk indicates drugs cited in interaction reports. Based on pharmacologic and pharmacokinetic considerations, similar interactions may occur with other drugs that are listed.

† Not available in the United States.

Anticoagulants — *Metronidazole*

Warfarin* (eg, *Coumadin*)	Metronidazole* (eg, *Flagyl*)

Significance	Onset	Severity	Documentation
1	☐ Rapid ■ **Delayed**	■ **Major** ☐ Moderate ☐ Minor	■ **Established** ☐ Probable ☐ Suspected ☐ Possible ☐ Unlikely

Effects The anticoagulant effect of WARFARIN may be enhanced; hemorrhage could occur.

Mechanism Liver metabolism of the S(−) enantiomorph of racemic WARFARIN may be decreased by METRONIDAZOLE.

Management Monitor patients more frequently and educate regarding signs and symptoms of bleeding whenever METRONIDAZOLE and WARFARIN are coadministered. A lower dose of WARFARIN may be required.

Discussion

One study investigated the effects of 7 days of treatment with metronidazole 750 mg/day on the plasma concentration and hypoprothrombinemia of 1.5 mg/kg single doses of racemic warfarin, S(-) warfarin 0.75 mg/kg and R(+) warfarin 1.5 mg/kg. The mean plasma level and hypoprothrombinemic response were increased by both racemic and S(-) warfarin, but not by the R(+) enantiomorph.[1] Animal studies (rats) have confirmed the inhibitory effect of metronidazole on S(-) warfarin metabolism and also identified additional enhancement of free warfarin concentration and pharmacodynamic effects upon coagulation.[4] Two case reports, both with significant bleeding and elevations of prothrombin time, have established the serious potential of this interaction in patients.[2,3]

This interaction appears likely to occur in most patients receiving this drug combination. Advise short course or alternative therapy when metronidazole is considered.

[1] O'Reilly RA. *N Engl J Med* 1976;295:354.
[2] Kazmier FJ. *Mayo Clin Proc* 1976;51:782.
[3] Dean RP, et al. *DICP* 1980;14:864.
[4] Yacobi A, et al. *J Pharmacol Exp Ther* 1984;231:72.

* Asterisk indicates drugs cited in interaction reports.

Anticoagulants — *Mineral Oil*

Anisindione (*Miradon*)	Warfarin (eg, *Coumadin*)	Mineral Oil*

Significance	Onset	Severity	Documentation
5	☐ Rapid	☐ Major	☐ Established
	■ **Delayed**	■ **Moderate**	☐ Probable
		☐ Minor	☐ Suspected
			☐ Possible
			■ **Unlikely**

Effects The action of ANTICOAGULANTS may be enhanced.

Mechanism Unknown; however, MINERAL OIL may cause a vitamin K deficiency because of malabsorption or decreased bacterial synthesis.

Management If necessary, recommend other laxatives to patients taking ANTICOAGULANTS.

Discussion

Decreased prothrombin concentration occurred in 7 of 10 patients receiving daily doses of mineral oil for several weeks.[2] Other case reports demonstrated a return to normal prothrombin concentration when mineral oil was stopped and oral or parenteral vitamin K was administered.[1] No interactions with oral anticoagulants have been reported. Further studies are necessary before a significant interaction can be claimed.

[1] Javert CT, et al. *Am J Obstet Gynecol* 1941;42:409.

[2] Becker GL. *Am J Dig Dis* 1952;19:344.

* Asterisk indicates drugs cited in interaction reports. Based on pharmacologic and pharmacokinetic considerations, similar interactions may occur with other drugs that are listed.

Anticoagulants — *Mitotane*

Anisindione (*Miradon*)	Mitotane* (*Lysodren*)
Dicumarol†	
Warfarin* (eg, *Coumadin*)	

Significance	Onset	Severity	Documentation
4	☐ Rapid	☐ Major	☐ Established
	■ **Delayed**	■ **Moderate**	☐ Probable
		☐ Minor	☐ Suspected
			■ **Possible**
			☐ Unlikely

Effects ANTICOAGULANT requirement may be increased.

Mechanism MITOTANE may increase the hepatic metabolism of oral ANTICOAGULANTS.

Management Monitor the response to the oral ANTICOAGULANT. It may be necessary to adjust the dose of ANTICOAGULANT when starting, stopping or changing the dose of MITOTANE.

Discussion

The warfarin dosage requirements in a 58-year-old woman increased during concurrent administration of mitotane therapy for stage IV adrenal carcinoma.[1] The patient was initially stabilized on an alternate day regimen of warfarin 5 and 2.5 mg. Over a 2.5-month period, while receiving mitotane 4 g/day, her warfarin dosage requirement gradually increased to 12.5 mg/day.

Controlled studies are needed to assess the clinical importance of this possible interaction.

[1] Cuddy PG, et al. *South Med J* 1986;79:387.

* Asterisk indicates drugs cited in interaction reports. Based on pharmacologic and pharmacokinetic considerations, similar interactions may occur with other drugs that are listed.

† Not available in the United States.

Anticoagulants — *Moricizine*

Warfarin* (eg, *Coumadin*)	Moricizine* (*Ethmozine*)

Significance	Onset	Severity	Documentation
4	☐ Rapid	■ **Major**	☐ Established
	■ **Delayed**	☐ Moderate	☐ Probable
		☐ Minor	☐ Suspected
			■ **Possible**
			☐ Unlikely

Effects The hypoprothrombinemic effect of WARFARIN may be increased.

Mechanism Unknown.

Management Monitor International Normalization Ratio or prothrombin time, and observe the patient for signs of bleeding when adding or changing the dose of MORICIZINE.

Discussion

Documentation for this possible interaction consists of a single case report.[1] Concurrent administration of moricizine and warfarin reportedly produced hematuria and a prolonged prothrombin time (PT) in a 69-year-old woman. The patient presented to the emergency department with right upper quadrant pain of 2 days duration. Six hours prior to admission, the pain had become more severe, and the patient had frank hematuria as well as two episodes of bloody emesis. At the time of admission, the patient was receiving digoxin (eg, *Lanoxin*) 0.25 mg/day, captopril (*Capoten*) 12.5 mg twice daily, prednisone (eg, *Deltasone*) 5 mg every other day, warfarin 7.5 mg/day and moricizine 300 mg three times daily (started 4 days prior to admission). The patient had been maintained on warfarin with PTs between 15 to 20 seconds over approximately 4 months. On hospital admission, gross hematuria was present and the PT was 41 seconds (PT ratio, 3.4). Moricizine and warfarin were discontinued and the patient was treated with a total dose of oral phytonadione (*Mephyton*) 35 mg. Within 48 hours, PT measured 14 seconds (PT ratio, 1.2). In a second report, a clinically significant interaction could not be demonstrated in 12 healthy volunteers given a single 25 mg dose of warfarin 14 days before and after starting moricizine, 250 mg every 8 hours.[2] Additional studies are needed to confirm this potential interaction.

[1] Serpa MD, et al. *Ann Pharmacother* 1992;26:127.

[2] Benedek IH, et al. *J Clin Pharmacol* 1992;32:558.

* Asterisk indicates drugs cited in interaction reports.

Anticoagulants — *Myrrh*

Anticoagulants	Myrrh
Warfarin* (eg, *Coumadin*)	Myrrh*

Significance	Onset	Severity	Documentation
4	□ Rapid	□ Major	□ Established
	■ **Delayed**	■ **Moderate**	□ Probable
		□ Minor	□ Suspected
			■ **Possible**
			□ Unlikely

Effects The anticoagulant effect of WARFARIN may be decreased.

Mechanism Unknown.

Management Because WARFARIN has a narrow therapeutic index, avoid concurrent use of MYRRH. Caution patients against using herbal products without consulting a health care provider.

Discussion

Commiphora molmol, a thorny shrub, serves as a source of myrrh. A 57-year-old man with an INR of 2.4 and taking a stable dosage of warfarin 3 mg/day experienced a decrease in his INR to 0.9 within 1 week of self-medicating with an aqueous extract of myrrh.[1] The patient was admitted to the hospital and treated with heparin, while continuing with warfarin 3 mg/day. After his INR returned to acceptable limits, the patient was discharged and instructed to avoid herbal medications.

[1] Al Faraj S. *Ann Trop Med Parasitol.* 2005;99(2):219.

* Asterisk indicates drugs cited in interaction reports.

Anticoagulants | ***Nalidixic Acid***

Warfarin*
(eg, *Coumadin*)

Nalidixic Acid*†

Significance	Onset	Severity	Documentation
2	☐ Rapid ■ **Delayed**	☐ Major ■ **Moderate** ☐ Minor	☐ Established ☐ Probable ■ **Suspected** ☐ Possible ☐ Unlikely

Effects The anticoagulant effects of WARFARIN may be enhanced by NALIDIXIC ACID; hemorrhage could occur.

Mechanism Displacement of WARFARIN from binding sites on plasma proteins. The sustained nature of this interaction indicates another mechanism is also involved.

Management Monitor patients more closely during coadministration of WARFARIN and NALIDIXIC ACID. A decreased dose of WARFARIN may be required.

Discussion

Three case reports, one with soft tissue bleeding, have described increased prothrombin times up to 45 seconds in previously well-controlled warfarin-treated patients.[1-3] An in vitro study demonstrated increased free concentrations of warfarin with the addition of nalidixic acid to a buffered solution of human albumin.[4]

[1] Hoffbrand BI. *Br Med J.* 1974;2(5920):666.
[2] Potasman I, et al. *Ann Intern Med.* 1980;92(4):571.
[3] Leor J, et al. *Ann Intern Med.* 1987;107(4):601.
[4] Sellers EM, et al. *Clin Pharmacol Ther.* 1970;11(4):524.

* Asterisk indicates drugs cited in interaction reports.
† Not available in the United States.

Anticoagulants — *Nevirapine*

Warfarin* (eg, *Coumadin*)	Nevirapine* (eg, *Viramune*)

Significance	Onset	Severity	Documentation
2	☐ Rapid	☐ Major	☐ Established
	■ **Delayed**	■ **Moderate**	☐ Probable
		☐ Minor	■ **Suspected**
			☐ Possible
			☐ Unlikely

Effects The anticoagulant effect of WARFARIN may be decreased.

Mechanism Induction of WARFARIN metabolism (CYP2C9) by NEVIRAPINE is suspected.

Management Monitor coagulation parameters when starting or stopping NEVIRAPINE. Adjust the WARFARIN dose as needed.

Discussion

Increased warfarin dosage requirements were reported in 3 HIV-infected men during coadministration of nevirapine.[1] The first patient, a 38-year-old man with severe primary pulmonary hypertension, had been treated with warfarin 2.5 mg/day for 2 years. His INR was 2.1 to 2.4. After starting treatment with nevirapine, his INR dropped to 1.3. An increase in the warfarin dosage to 5 mg/day resulted in an increase in the INR to 2. A few days later, when the patient was not receiving nevirapine, his warfarin dosage was reduced to 2.5 mg/day. A 28-year-old patient who was receiving nevirapine was started on warfarin for deep vein thrombosis. In spite of administration of warfarin up to 17 mg/day, the PT did not drop less than 65%. After stopping nevirapine, a dosage of warfarin 5 mg daily was sufficient to stabilize the PT and INR in the therapeutic range. When nevirapine was restarted, warfarin 12 mg/day was needed to maintain anticoagulation within the therapeutic range. A 39-year-old man with deep vein thrombosis had an INR of 1.18 during coadministration of warfarin 12.5 mg/day and nevirapine. After discontinuing nevirapine, warfarin 7.5 mg/day was sufficient to maintain the INR in the therapeutic range (INR, 3.47). A 39-year-old man with an 11-year history of HIV infection receiving a drug regimen that included nevirapine required warfarin 20 mg/day for treatment of a newly developed pulmonary embolus and deep venous thrombosis.[2] When the antiretroviral regimen was changed and nevirapine was excluded, the daily dosage of warfarin was reduced to 12.5 mg. See also Anticoagulants-NNRT Inhibitors.

[1] Dionisio D, et al. *AIDS*. 2001;15(2):277.

[2] Fulco PP, et al. *Pharmacotherapy*. 2008;28(7):945.

* Asterisk indicates drugs cited in interaction reports.

Anticoagulants		*Niacin*
Warfarin* (eg, *Coumadin*)		Niacin* (eg, *Niaspan*)

Significance	Onset	Severity	Documentation
4	☐ Rapid ■ **Delayed**	☐ Major ■ **Moderate** ☐ Minor	☐ Established ☐ Probable ☐ Suspected ■ **Possible** ☐ Unlikely

Effects The anticoagulant effect of WARFARIN may be increased, resulting in an increased risk of bleeding.

Mechanism Unknown.

Management Closely monitor anticoagulant activity when starting, stopping, or changing the dose of NIACIN. Adjust the WARFARIN dose as needed.

Discussion

A 69-year-old woman receiving a stable dose of warfarin 2.5 mg daily was seen in the anticoagulant clinic with an INR of 12.3.[1] The previous week, her extended-release niacin dose was increased from 500 to 1,000 mg daily. The patient had been receiving extended-release niacin 500 mg for 3 months without it affecting the INR. The previous INR was 2.4. Warfarin was withheld and niacin was discontinued. Two days later, the INR was 4.8. The warfarin dose was titrated to a maintenance dose of 2.5 mg daily and the INR was 2.3.

[1] Christopher A, et al. *Ann Pharmacother.* 2011;45(11):e58.

* Asterisk indicates drugs cited in interaction reports.

Anticoagulants | **NNRT Inhibitors**

Warfarin* (eg, *Coumadin*)	Delavirdine (*Rescriptor*)	Efavirenz* (*Sustiva*)

Significance	Onset	Severity	Documentation
4	☐ Rapid ■ **Delayed**	☐ Major ■ **Moderate** ☐ Minor	☐ Established ☐ Probable ☐ Suspected ■ **Possible** ☐ Unlikely

Effects Increased risk of bleeding.

Mechanism Inhibition of WARFARIN metabolism (CYP2C9) by EFAVIRENZ is suspected.

Management Carefully monitor ANTICOAGULANT parameters and adjust the WARFARIN dose as needed.

Discussion

A possible interaction between warfarin and efavirenz was reported in a 34-year-old woman with HIV.[1] The patient was on a stable antiretroviral regimen that included efavirenz. After developing extensive deep vein thrombosis, she underwent placement of a vena cava filter and was started on a mean daily dose of warfarin 5 mg. Her INR was in the therapeutic range (2 to 3). Twenty-two days after discharge, the patient was readmitted with macrohematuria, an INR of 7, and thrombocytopenia. Warfarin treatment was withheld, and vitamin K was administered. The bleeding stopped, and the INR normalized. The patient was discharged with a mean daily dose of warfarin 1.25 mg and normalized platelet count. See also Anticoagulants-Nevirapine.

[1] Bonora S, et al. *Clin Infect Dis*. 2008;46(1):146.

* Asterisk indicates drugs cited in interaction reports. Based on pharmacologic and pharmacokinetic considerations, similar interactions may occur with other drugs that are listed.

Anticoagulants — *NSAIDs*

Anticoagulants	NSAIDs	
Warfarin* (eg, *Coumadin*)	Diclofenac (eg, *Cataflam*)	Meclofenamate*
	Etodolac	Mefenamic Acid (*Ponstel*)
	Fenoprofen* (eg, *Nalfon*)	Nabumetone*
	Flurbiprofen (eg, *Ansaid*)	Naproxen* (eg, *Naprosyn*)
	Ibuprofen* (eg, *Motrin*)	Oxaprozin (eg, *Daypro*)
	Indomethacin* (eg, *Indocin*)	Piroxicam* (eg, *Feldene*)
	Ketoprofen*	Sulindac* (eg, *Clinoril*)
	Ketorolac	Tolmetin*

Significance	Onset	Severity	Documentation
1	☐ Rapid	■ **Major**	☐ Established
	■ **Delayed**	☐ Moderate	■ **Probable**
		☐ Minor	☐ Suspected
			☐ Possible
			☐ Unlikely

Effects Increased ANTICOAGULANT activity and risk of bleeding.[1-9]

Mechanism Gastric irritation and decreased platelet function contribute.

Management Monitor patients closely and instruct them to report signs and symptoms of bleeding to their health care provider.

Discussion

A large retrospective study of patients 65 yr of age and older receiving oral anticoagulants and non-aspirin NSAIDs reported a 13-fold increase in their risk of hemorrhagic peptic ulcers compared with patients not using NSAIDs.[10] The risk of hemorrhagic peptic ulcer increased 4-fold during use of oral anticoagulants and NSAIDs compared with use of either agent alone. In a study of small or large bowel bleeding with NSAID use, NSAIDs increased the risk of bleeding about 2.5 times.[7] A retrospective cohort study of 35,548 patients found that coadministration of NSAIDs and warfarin increased the risk of GI bleeding compared with taking warfarin alone (hazard ratio, 3.58).[11] In a 1-yr observational study, concurrent use of NSAIDs and coumarin anticoagulants greatly increased the risk of bleeding compared with coumarin alone.[12] PTs have been altered during use of warfarin and indomethacin,[13-15] ketoprofen,[16] meclofenamate,[17] nabumetone,[18] fenoprofen[18] (increased INR),[19] naproxen,[20,21] piroxicam,[22] or sulindac.[23-25] Others found that etodolac,[26] tolmetin,[27] ketoprofen,[28] or indomethacin[29,30] did not affect anticoagulant activity or decrease prothrombin activity (eg, naproxen).[31] See Anticoagulants-NSAIDs (COX-2 Selective).

1 Mielke CH, et al. *Int Congr Ser.* 1975;372:200.
2 McIntyre BA, et al. *Clin Pharmacol Ther.* 1978;24(5):616.
3 Fisherman EW, et al. *Ann Allergy.* 1978;41(2):75.
4 Pemberton RE, et al. *Dig Dis Sci.* 1979;24(1):53.
5 Brogden RN, et al. *Drugs.* 1981;22(3):165.
6 Dahl SL, et al. *Pharmacotherapy.* 1982;2(2):80.
7 Langman MJ, et al. *Br Med J (Clin Res Ed).* 1985;290(6465):347.
8 Schulman S, et al. *Br J Rheumatol.* 1989;28(1):46.
9 Gabb GM. *Med J Aust.* 1996;164(11):700.
10 Shorr RI, et al. *Arch Intern Med.* 1993;153(14):1665.
11 Cheetham TC, et al. *Ann Pharmacother.* 2009; 43(11):1765.
12 Knijff-Dutmer EA, et al. *Ann Pharmacother.* 2003;37(1):12.
13 Self TH, et al. *Lancet.* 1975;2(7934):557.
14 Self TH, et al. *Drug Intell Clin Pharm.* 1978;12:580.
15 Chan TY. *Br J Clin Pract.* 1997;51(3):177.
16 Flessner MF, et al. *JAMA.* 1988;259(3):353.
17 Baragar FD, et al. *Curr Ther Res Clin Exp.* 1978;23(suppl 4):S51.
18 Kim KY, et al. *Ann Pharmacother.* 2003;37(2):212.
19 Dennis VC, et al. *Pharmacotherapy.* 2000;20(2):234.
20 Slattery JT, et al. *Clin Pharmacol Ther.* 1979;25(1):51.
21 Jain A, et al. *Clin Pharmacol Ther.* 1979;25(1):61.
22 Rhodes RS, et al. *Drug Intell Clin Pharm.* 1985;19(7-8):556.
23 Carter SA. *Lancet.* 1979;2(8144):698.
24 Ross JR, et al. *Lancet.* 1979;2(8151):1075.
25 Loftin JP, et al. *J Clin Pharmacol.* 1979;19(11-12):733.
26 Ermer JC, et al. *Clin Pharmacol Ther.* 1994;55(3):305.
27 Whitsett TL, et al. *Int Congr Ser.* 1975;372:160.
28 Mieszczak C, et al. *Eur J Clin Pharmacol.* 1993;44(2):205.
29 Vesell ES, et al. *J Clin Pharmacol.* 1975;15(7):486.
30 Pullar T, et al. *Scott Med J.* 1983;28(1):42.
31 Petersen PB, et al. *Scand J Rheumatol.* 1979;8(1):54.

* Asterisk indicates drugs cited in interaction reports. Based on pharmacologic and pharmacokinetic considerations, similar interactions may occur with other drugs that are listed.

Anticoagulants		*NSAIDs (COX-2 Selective)*	
Warfarin* (eg, *Coumadin*)		Celecoxib* (*Celebrex*)	Rofecoxib*†

Significance	Onset	Severity	Documentation
1	☐ Rapid ■ **Delayed**	■ **Major** ☐ Moderate ☐ Minor	☐ Established ■ **Probable** ☐ Suspected ☐ Possible ☐ Unlikely

Effects Increased ANTICOAGULANT effects of WARFARIN.

Mechanism Unknown.

Management If coadministration cannot be avoided, carefully monitor ANTICOAGULANT parameters when the dose of the NSAID is started, stopped, or changed.

Discussion

Several case reports document an increase in INR (some with bleeding) in warfarin-treated patients given celecoxib or rofecoxib.[1-7] A 73-yr-old woman was receiving celecoxib 200 mg/day, warfarin 5 mg/day, captopril (eg, *Capoten*), digoxin (eg, *Lanoxin*), diltiazem, furosemide (eg, *Lasix*), levothyroxine (eg, *Levothroid*), oxycodone/acetaminophen (eg, *Percocet*), and trazodone (eg, *Oleptro*).[1] The only medication or dosage change during the previous 3 years was celecoxib, which was started 5 wk prior to hospital admission. The patient denied using alcohol, OTC medications, or herbal products. Prior to admission, the patient's INR was 4.4; upon admission, her INR was 5.68. Warfarin and celecoxib were withheld during her hospital stay. Fresh frozen plasma and vitamin K were administered to normalize the INR. Rechallenge with warfarin and celecoxib was not performed. An increase in INR (3.1 to 5.8) was also reported in an 88-yr-old woman (stabilized on warfarin 40 mg/wk) 1 wk after adding celecoxib 200 mg/day to her treatment regimen and in a 71-yr-old man (INR, 2.1 to 4) 7 days after starting celecoxib.[2,3] GI bleeding occurred in the latter case. During celecoxib administration, it was necessary to reduce the warfarin dosage 25% to achieve an INR of 3. In contrast, other studies found celecoxib had no effect on the INR,[8] PT,[9] or steady-state pharmacokinetics[9] of warfarin. In a study of 39 volunteers, rofecoxib increased R-warfarin AUC 27% to 40% and likely was responsible for small increases in the INR (5% to 11%).[10] In a case-control study of patients admitted to the hospital with GI hemorrhage, there appeared to be a similar risk for hemorrhage with celecoxib or rofecoxib as compared with nonselective NSAIDs.[11] This is in contrast with a retrospective cohort study of 35,548 patients that found a lower risk of GI bleeding with COX-2 selective NSAIDs (hazard ratio 1.75 vs warfarin alone) compared with nonselective NSAIDs (hazard ratio 3.58 vs warfarin alone).[12] See also Anticoagulants-NSAIDs.

[1] Mersfelder TL, et al. *Ann Pharmacother.* 2000;34(3):325.
[2] Haase KK, et al. *Ann Pharmacother.* 2000;34(5):666.
[3] Linder JD, et al. *South Med J.* 2000;93(9):930.
[4] Stading JA, et al. *Am J Health Syst Pharm.* 2001;58(21):2076.
[5] Schaefer MG, et al. *Am J Health Syst Pharm.* 2003;60(13):1319.
[6] Stoner SC, et al. *J Am Geriatr Soc.* 2003;51(5):728.
[7] Malhi H, et al. *Postgrad Med J.* 2004;80(940):107.
[8] Dentali F, et al. *Ann Pharmacother.* 2006;40(7-8):1241.
[9] Karim A, et al. *J Clin Pharmacol.* 2000;40(6):655.
[10] Schwartz JI, et al. *Clin Pharmacol Ther.* 2000;68(6):626.
[11] Battistella M, et al. *Arch Intern Med.* 2005;165(2):189.
[12] Cheetham TC, et al. *Ann Pharmacother.* 2009;43(11):1765.

* Asterisk indicates drugs cited in interaction reports.
† Not available in the United States.

Anticoagulants — *Omega-3-Acid Ethyl Esters*

Warfarin* (eg, *Coumadin*)	Omega-3-Acid Ethyl Esters* (eg, *Lovaza*)

Significance	Onset	Severity	Documentation
4	☐ Rapid ■ **Delayed**	■ **Major** ☐ Moderate ☐ Minor	☐ Established ☐ Probable ☐ Suspected ■ **Possible** ☐ Unlikely

Effects OMEGA-3-ACID ETHYL ESTERS combined with WARFARIN may increase the risk of serious bleeding.

Mechanism Unknown; however, additive ANTICOAGULANT effects may be involved.

Management If coadministration of these agents cannot be avoided, use with caution and closely monitor patients. Advise patients of the possible risk of increased bleeding.

Discussion

A 75-year-old man experienced a minor fall when a stool he was sitting on tipped.[1] He was brought to the emergency department (ED) after developing a headache and experiencing decreased coordination, trouble walking, and slurred speech. His current regimen included warfarin (7.5 mg 4 days/wk and 5 mg 3 days/wk), aspirin 81 mg/day, and OTC omega-3-acid ethyl esters 6 g/day. The patient's most recent INR was 2.8 (target range, 2 to 3), measured 1 month before the fall. At the time he was seen in the ED, his INR was 3.2. Results of a CT scan disclosed an acute large right subdural hematoma that measured 3 cm. The patient's coagulopathy was treated with fresh frozen plasma and vitamin K. He underwent a craniotomy for drainage and evacuation of the hematoma. He was discharged to a rehabilitation facility, and warfarin was restarted at 7.5 mg/day until the INR was higher than 2.5. Subsequently, he was placed on a maintenance dosage of warfarin 7.5 mg 3 days/week plus 5 mg 4 days/week. The patient was instructed not to resume taking omega-3-acid ethyl esters or aspirin. A 65-year-old man with pulmonary thromboembolism was stabilized on warfarin.[2] His INR ranged between 2 and 3. Subsequently, he was prescribed trazodone and fish oil (omega-3 fatty acids), and he was later admitted to the ED with an INR and PT of 6.08 and 36 seconds, respectively. All medications were stopped and his INR returned to normal within 2 days. Warfarin was restarted at the previous dose while the other drugs were not resumed. His INR was within the desired range 2 weeks later. See Anticoagulants-Trazodone.

[1] McClaskey EM, et al. *Pharmacotherapy.* 2007;27(1):152.

[2] Jalili M, et al. *Arch Med Res.* 2007;38(8):901.

* Asterisk indicates drugs cited in interaction reports.

Anticoagulants — *Omeprazole*

Warfarin* (eg, *Coumadin*)	Omeprazole* (eg, *Prilosec*)

Significance	Onset	Severity	Documentation
4	☐ Rapid ■ **Delayed**	☐ Major ■ **Moderate** ☐ Minor	☐ Established ☐ Probable ☐ Suspected ■ **Possible** ☐ Unlikely

Effects The hypoprothrombinemic effects of WARFARIN may be increased.

Mechanism Stereoselective inhibition of the hepatic metabolism of the less potent R-WARFARIN enantiomer.

Management Monitor ANTICOAGULANT parameters when starting or stopping OMEPRAZOLE. Adjust the WARFARIN dose accordingly.

Discussion

In a double-blind, randomized, crossover trial, the effects of coadministration of omeprazole 20 mg/day on the plasma concentration and anticoagulation action of warfarin were studied in 21 healthy men.[1] Warfarin is a racemic mixture of 2 enantiomers, S- and R-warfarin, that differ in anticoagulant potency. The anticoagulant effect of S-warfarin is 3 to 6 times greater than that of R-warfarin. The anticoagulant effect and the plasma concentrations of the enantiomers were measured. To determine the dosage requirement for the vitamin K-dependent coagulation factors to decrease to within 10% to 20% of the normal range, warfarin alone was administered for 3 weeks prior to the crossover study. The final dose determined (2.5 to 8.125 mg/day) was maintained throughout the crossover phase. The addition of omeprazole to the dosage regimen had no effect on the mean concentration of the more active S-warfarin but did result in a small (12%) but statistically significant increase in the mean R-warfarin concentration (from 490 to 548 ng/mL). It was not necessary to adjust the warfarin dosage in any subject. The small effect of omeprazole on the anticoagulation activity of warfarin would not be expected to be clinically significant. In another double-blind, randomized, crossover study, 28 patients stabilized on warfarin were given omeprazole 20 mg or placebo for 3 weeks.[2] Concentrations of R-warfarin increased 9.5% while S-warfarin concentrations were not affected. Coagulation times were not changed. A single case report indicates that certain individuals may exhibit clinically important increases in hypoprothrombinemic effects of warfarin after prolonged omeprazole therapy (20 mg/day for 2 weeks).[3]

Additional studies are needed to determine whether a larger, yet still therapeutic, dose of omeprazole would have a more pronounced effect on warfarin activity.

[1] Sutfin T, et al. *Ther Drug Monit.* 1989;11:176.
[2] Unge P, et al. *Br J Clin Pharmacol.* 1992;34:509.
[3] Ahmad S. *South Med J.* 1991;84:674.

* Asterisk indicates drugs cited in interaction reports.

Anticoagulants ✕ *Orlistat*

Warfarin* (eg, *Coumadin*)	Orlistat* (*Xenical*)

Significance	Onset	Severity	Documentation
4	☐ Rapid	☐ Major	☐ Established
	■ **Delayed**	■ **Moderate**	☐ Probable
		☐ Minor	☐ Suspected
			■ **Possible**
			☐ Unlikely

Effects The anticoagulant effects of WARFARIN may be increased.

Mechanism Unknown.

Management Monitor coagulation parameters more frequently, especially during the first month, when ORLISTAT is started or stopped. Be prepared to adjust the WARFARIN dose as needed.

Discussion

An increase in the INR was reported in a 66-year-old man receiving warfarin after orlistat was added to the treatment regimen.[1] The patient had been receiving warfarin for 2.5 years, and his INR had been stable for over 1 year on a dose of warfarin 5 and 6 mg on alternate days. He had a history of hypertension that was being treated with amlodipine (eg, *Norvasc*) and perindopril (*Aceon*). He also had type 2 diabetes mellitus that was being controlled by diet. The patient was started on orlistat 120 mg 3 times/day for weight reduction. An increase in the INR to 4.7 was noted 18 days after starting orlistat. During this time, the patient reduced the quantity of food he consumed, particularly fatty foods because they upset his stomach. Warfarin was withheld for 2 days and restarted at 5 mg/day; however, his INR remained elevated. Subsequently, the INR was maintained satisfactorily on a warfarin dose of 3 mg/day. In 12 healthy volunteers, administration of a single 30 mg warfarin dose on day 11 of orlistat administration (120 mg 3 times/day) did not alter the pharmacokinetics or pharmacodynamics of warfarin.[2]

[1] MacWalter RS, et al. *Ann Pharmacother.* 2003;37:510. [2] Zhi J, et al. *J Clin Pharmacol.* 1996;36:659.

* Asterisk indicates drugs cited in interaction reports.

Anticoagulants × Penicillins

Warfarin* (eg, *Coumadin*)		Ampicillin (eg, *Principen*) Dicloxacillin* Nafcillin* Oxacillin	Penicillin G (eg, *Pfizerpen*) Piperacillin Ticarcillin* (*Ticar*)

Significance	Onset	Severity	Documentation
2	□ Rapid ■ **Delayed**	□ Major ■ **Moderate** □ Minor	□ Established □ Probable ■ **Suspected** □ Possible □ Unlikely

Effects Large IV doses of PENICILLINS can increase the bleeding risks of ANTICOAGULANTS by prolonging bleeding time. Conversely, NAFCILLIN and DICLOXACILLIN have been associated with WARFARIN resistance, which may persist for 3 weeks or more following discontinuation of the antibiotic.

Mechanism WARFARIN-induced hypoprothrombinemia in conjunction with PENICILLIN-induced inhibition of adenosine diphosphonate–mediated platelet aggregation. Possible hepatic enzyme induction for NAFCILLIN- and DICLOXACILLIN-induced WARFARIN resistance.

Management Monitor for bleeding when giving high-dose IV PENICILLINS and oral ANTICOAGULANTS concurrently. In patients receiving NAFCILLIN or DICLOXACILLIN, monitor coagulation parameters on initiation and for at least 3 weeks following discontinuation of the antibiotic.

Discussion

High doses of penicillins, especially ticarcillin, can prolong bleeding time and decrease platelet function. Bleeding episodes have occurred in numerous patients and in volunteers during controlled studies.[1-9] Renal dysfunction may increase bleeding risks caused by decreased penicillin elimination and the hemostatic defects associated with uremia.[4,5] Prothrombin activity does not appear to be altered.[1,2] Bleeding risk is associated with increased template bleeding time, rather than with hypoprothrombinemia. Nafcillin and dicloxacillin may inhibit warfarin activity.[10-16] Controlled studies are needed.

1 Brown CH 3rd, et al. *N Engl J Med.* 1974;291(6):265.
2 Brown CH 3rd, et al. *Antimicrob Agents Chemother.* 1975;7(5):652.
3 Brown CH 3rd, et al. *Blood.* 1976;47(6):949.
4 Andrassy K, et al. *Lancet.* 1976;2(7994):1039.
5 Andrassy K, et al. *Thromb Haemost.* 1976;36(1):115.
6 Dijkmans BA, et al. *J Antimicrob Chemother.* 1980;6(4):554.
7 Gentry LO, et al. *Antimicrob Agents Chemother.* 1981;19(4):532.
8 Alexander DP, et al. *Antimicrob Agents Chemother.* 1983;23(1):59.
9 Davis RL, et al. *J Pediatr.* 1991;118(2):300.
10 Qureshi GD, et al. *Ann Intern Med.* 1984;100(4):527.
11 Krstenansky PM, et al. *Clin Pharm.* 1987;6(10):804.
12 Shovick VA, et al. *DICP.* 1991;25(6):598.
13 Taylor AT, et al. *J Fam Pract.* 1994;39(2):182.
14 Mailloux AT, et al. *Ann Pharmacother.* 1996;30(12):1402.
15 Lacey CS. *Ann Pharmacother.* 2004;38(5):898.
16 Kim KY, et al. *Pharmacotherapy.* 2007;27(10):1467.

* Asterisk indicates drugs cited in interaction reports. Based on pharmacologic and pharmacokinetic considerations, similar interactions may occur with other drugs that are listed.

Anticoagulants ✕ **Pomegranate Juice**

Warfarin* (eg, *Coumadin*)	Pomegranate Juice*

Significance	Onset	Severity	Documentation
4	☐ Rapid	☐ Major	☐ Established
	■ **Delayed**	■ **Moderate**	☐ Probable
		☐ Minor	☐ Suspected
			■ **Possible**
			☐ Unlikely

Effects Increased risk of bleeding.

Mechanism Unknown; however, inhibition of WARFARIN metabolism (CYP2C9) by POMEGRANATE JUICE is suspected.

Management Because WARFARIN has a narrow therapeutic index, patients should limit or avoid concurrent ingestion of POMEGRANATE JUICE. If POMEGRANATE JUICE cannot be avoided, the patient should drink a consistent amount and notify their health care provider if the amount consumed changes. Monitor INR more frequently if POMEGRANATE JUICE is started or discontinued.

Discussion

A possible interaction between warfarin and pomegranate juice was reported in a 64-year-old woman being treated for deep vein thrombosis.[1] The patient had been receiving warfarin 4 mg/day for several months. Her INRs were stable in the therapeutic range at 2 to 3. During this time the patient was drinking 1 glass of pomegranate juice 2 to 3 times a week. Subsequently, she stopped ingesting pomegranate juice and her INR became subtherapeutic at 1.7. In order to maintain therapeutic anticoagulation, it was necessary to increase her weekly warfarin dosage from 4 mg daily to 6 mg on 1 day of the week and 4 mg on the other days of the week. Her next 2 INR measurements were therapeutic at 2.1.

[1] Komperda KE. *Pharmacotherapy*. 2009;29(8):1002.

* Asterisk indicates drugs cited in interaction reports.

Anticoagulants		**Progestins**	
Warfarin* (eg, *Coumadin*)		Levonorgestrel* (eg, *Plan B*)	
Significance	Onset	Severity	Documentation
4	☐ Rapid ■ **Delayed**	☐ Major ■ **Moderate** ☐ Minor	☐ Established ☐ Probable ☐ Suspected ■ **Possible** ☐ Unlikely

Effects The anticoagulant activity of WARFARIN may be enhanced by LEVONORGESTREL.

Mechanism Unknown.

Management In patients receiving WARFARIN, monitor INR frequently while LEVONORGESTREL is being administered for emergency contraception. Be prepared to adjust the WARFARIN dose.

Discussion

A 35-year-old woman on a stable dosage of warfarin 7 mg/day experienced an increase in INR (from a range of 2 to 3 to 8.1) 3 days after receiving 2 doses of levonorgestrel 0.75 mg for emergency contraception.[1] Warfarin therapy was withheld for 2 days and her INR decreased to 2.1. She resumed warfarin at 5 mg/day and no bleeding problems were noted.

[1] Ellison J, et al. *BMJ.* 2000;321(7273):1382.

* Asterisk indicates drugs cited in interaction reports.

Anticoagulants — *Propafenone*

Warfarin* (eg, *Coumadin*)	Propafenone* (eg, *Rythmol*)

Significance	Onset	Severity	Documentation
4	☐ Rapid ■ **Delayed**	☐ Major ■ **Moderate** ☐ Minor	☐ Established ☐ Probable ☐ Suspected ■ **Possible** ☐ Unlikely

Effects The effects of WARFARIN may be increased.

Mechanism Unknown. However, PROPAFENONE is suspected to inhibit the hepatic metabolism of WARFARIN.

Management During coadministration of these drugs, monitor the PT and adjust the WARFARIN dose accordingly.

Discussion

The effect of propafenone 225 mg 3 times/day on the pharmacokinetic and pharmacologic effects of warfarin 5 mg/day was studied in 8 healthy volunteers.[1] Each drug was administered alone for 1 week, followed by coadministration for 1 week, and the effect of each treatment on the PT was evaluated. During coadministration of propafenone, the mean steady-state warfarin plasma concentration increased almost 39%. A similar increase in peak warfarin plasma concentration was measured. When propafenone and warfarin were coadministered, the PT increased significantly ($P < 0.01$). In 3 of the 8 patients, there was little change in PT, whereas it doubled in 2 patients and increased by an intermediate degree in the remaining patients.

The clinical relevance of these findings remains to be determined.

[1] Kates RE, et al. *Clin Pharmacol Ther.* 1987;42(3):305.

* Asterisk indicates drugs cited in interaction reports.

Anticoagulants — *Propoxyphene*

Warfarin* (eg, *Coumadin*)	Propoxyphene* (eg, *Darvon*)

Significance	Onset	Severity	Documentation
4	☐ Rapid	☐ Major	☐ Established
	■ **Delayed**	■ **Moderate**	☐ Probable
		☐ Minor	☐ Suspected
			■ **Possible**
			☐ Unlikely

Effects The anticoagulation induced by WARFARIN may be potentiated by PROPOXYPHENE. Hemorrhage could occur.

Mechanism Unknown.

Management Monitor PT more frequently. Decreases in WARFARIN dosage may be required.

Discussion

Bleeding and excessive hypoprothrombinemia has occurred in several patients receiving warfarin and propoxyphene with acetaminophen (eg, *Darvocet-N*).[1-3] Acetaminophen (eg, *Tylenol*) alone increased PT in 1 study of 50 patients receiving maintenance doses of warfarin in an anticoagulation clinic.[4] Controlled evaluations of propoxyphene alone and warfarin are lacking. Thus, the precipitant drug in these case reports is unclear.

Until further evaluations clarify the causative agent, closely monitor patients receiving warfarin concurrently with propoxyphene or its combination products.

[1] Orme M, et al. *Br Med J.* 1976;1(6003):200.
[2] Jones RV. *Br Med J.* 1976;1(6007):460.
[3] Smith R, et al. *Drug Intell Clin Pharm.* 1984;18(10):822.
[4] Antlitz AM, et al. *Curr Ther Res Clin Exp.* 1968;10(10):501.

* Asterisk indicates drugs cited in interaction reports.

Anticoagulants | **Protease Inhibitors**

Anticoagulants	Protease Inhibitors	
Warfarin* (eg, *Coumadin*)	Atazanavir (*Reyataz*)	Nelfinavir (*Viracept*)
	Fosamprenavir (*Lexiva*)	Ritonavir* (*Norvir*)
	Indinavir* (*Crixivan*)	Saquinavir (*Invirase*)
	Lopinavir/Ritonavir* (*Kaletra*)	

Significance	Onset	Severity	Documentation
4	☐ Rapid	☐ Major	☐ Established
	■ **Delayed**	■ **Moderate**	☐ Probable
		☐ Minor	☐ Suspected
			■ **Possible**
			☐ Unlikely

Effects The anticoagulant effect of WARFARIN may be decreased.

Mechanism Unknown.

Management Observe the patient's clinical response and carefully monitor anticoagulant function when a PROTEASE INHIBITOR is started or stopped. Adjust the WARFARIN dose as needed.

Discussion

A decrease in the anticoagulant effect of warfarin was reported in a 27-year-old woman after the addition of ritonavir to her drug regimen.[1] She was receiving warfarin 12.5 mg/day and had an INR between 2 and 3. Eight weeks after warfarin therapy was started, treatment with ritonavir 400 mg twice daily was initiated. Over the next few weeks, the INR decreased, and it was necessary to almost double the warfarin dose to maintain the INR within the therapeutic range. Ritonavir was discontinued approximately 3 months later because of adverse reactions. Within 1 week of stopping ritonavir, the INR increased more than 3-fold, and a downward adjustment in warfarin dosage was necessary. In another case report, a 50-year-old asymptomatic HIV-positive man experienced a decrease in the anticoagulant effect of warfarin while receiving either indinavir or ritonavir.[2] A 46-year-old HIV-infected man receiving acencoumarol† experienced a profound decrease in INR 8 days after stavudine (eg, *Zevit*), lamivudine (*Epivir*), and ritonavir (600 mg twice daily) were added to the regimen.[3] Ritonavir was discontinued when the target INR could not be achieved, even after the acencoumarol dose was increased 300%. With respect to the time course of this interaction, the optimal time to start monitoring clotting factors cannot be determined from the data presented. Warfarin resistance occurred in a 42-year-old man with HIV after starting lopinavir/ritonavir.[4] To maintain a therapeutic INR, the warfarin dose was increased from 5.5 mg/day at baseline to 13 mg/day. Similar warfarin resistance was observed in a 66-year-old man after lopinavir/ritonavir was added to his treatment regimen.[5] Use of fosamprenavir in 3 warfarin-treated patients did not affect the INR.[6]

[1] Knoell KR, et al. *Ann Pharmacother.* 1998;32(12):1299.
[2] Gatti G, et al. *AIDS.* 1998;12(7):825.
[3] Llibre JM, et al. *Ann Pharmacother.* 2002;36(4):621.
[4] Hughes CA, et al. *CMAJ.* 2007;177(4):357.
[5] Bonora S, et al. *Clin Infect Dis.* 2008;46(1):146.
[6] Honda H, et al. *Int J STD AIDS.* 2009;20(6):441.

* Asterisk indicates drugs cited in interaction reports. Based on pharmacologic and pharmacokinetic considerations, similar interactions may occur with other drugs that are listed.
† Not available in the United States.

Anticoagulants — *Quilinggao*

Warfarin* (eg, *Coumadin*)	Quilinggao*

Significance	Onset	Severity	Documentation
4	□ Rapid	□ Major	□ Established
	■ **Delayed**	■ **Moderate**	□ Probable
		□ Minor	□ Suspected
			■ **Possible**
			□ Unlikely

Effects Increased risk of bleeding.

Mechanism Additive or synergistic anticoagulant effects.

Management In patients receiving ANTICOAGULANT therapy, closely monitor anticoagulant function when starting or stopping an herbal product, especially if the ingredients are not known (eg, QUILINGGAO). Caution patients taking ANTICOAGULANTS against use of herbal products or dietary supplements without consulting their health care provider and to report unusual bruising or any signs of bleeding.

Discussion

Loss of anticoagulant control with bleeding occurred in a 61-year-old man taking warfarin and ingesting quilinggao ("essence of tortoise shell"), a product containing various herbal ingredients.[1] The patient had been well controlled on 3 and 3.5 mg of warfarin on alternate days (INR ranging from 1.6 to 2.8). Five days after changing brands of quilinggao, the patient noticed bleeding. He continued to ingest quilinggao until he was seen in the clinic 4 days later. At that time, his INR was greater than 6, and he complained of gum bleeding and epistaxis over the preceding 3 days. Warfarin therapy was withheld and 3 days later the INR decreased to 2.9. The INR was 1.9 on day 5 when warfarin was restarted. After discharge, the patient began ingesting a third brand of quilinggao daily. After 4 days, his INR increased to 5.2, and warfarin therapy was withheld again. The INR decreased to 1.9 over the next 5 days and warfarin was restarted.

There are many brands of quilinggao. Not all brands contain components that interact with warfarin. Some brands may contain ingredients such as *beimu* (which inhibits platelet aggregation), *chishao* (a glycopeptide structurally similar to heparin that displays anticoagulant activity), *jinyinhua* (which inhibits platelet function), and *jishi* (a coumarin compound with antiplatelet activity).[1] The ingredients of many herbal products are not standardized. It is unclear if herbal products contain ingredients other than those listed on the label or purported to be present that could affect coagulation or interact with warfarin.

[1] Wong AL, et al. *Ann Pharmacother.* 2003;37:836.

* Asterisk indicates drugs cited in interaction reports.

Anticoagulants	*Quinine Derivatives*
Warfarin* (eg, *Coumadin*)	Quinidine* Quinine* (*Qualaquin*)

Significance	Onset	Severity	Documentation
1	☐ Rapid ■ **Delayed**	■ **Major** ☐ Moderate ☐ Minor	☐ Established ☐ Probable ■ **Suspected** ☐ Possible ☐ Unlikely

Effects Anticoagulation may be potentiated by QUININE DERIVATIVES. Hemorrhage may occur.

Mechanism QUININE DERIVATIVES may inhibit the hepatically synthesized clotting factors.

Management Monitor INR and adjust the WARFARIN dose as indicated. A lower dose of WARFARIN may be required when QUININE DERIVATIVES are coadministered.

Discussion

Hypoprothrombinemia can be induced by quinine and prevented by coadministration of vitamin K.[1] Numerous case reports have documented excessive hypoprothrombinemia and bleeding in patients previously controlled on warfarin when quinine or quinidine therapy was instituted.[2-4] Retrospective evaluation[5] and controlled studies[6,7] in patients receiving warfarin have not confirmed changes in warfarin dose requirements or PTs.

1 Pirk LA, et al. *J Am Med Assoc.* 1945;128(15):1093.
2 Jarnum S. *Scand J Clin Lab Invest.* 1954;6(2):91
3 Koch-Weser J. *Ann Intern Med.* 1968;68(3):511.
4 Gazzaniga AB, et al. *N Engl J Med.* 1969;280(13):711.
5 Jones FL Jr. *Ann Intern Med.* 1968;69(5):1074.
6 Udall JA. *J R Coll Physicians Lond.* 1970;77:20.
7 Sylvén C, et al. *Br Med J (Clin Res Ed).* 1983;286(6372):1181.

* Asterisk indicates drugs cited in interaction reports.

Anticoagulants		**Quinolones**	
Warfarin* (eg, *Coumadin*)		Ciprofloxacin* (eg, *Cipro*) Gatifloxacin* (*Zymar*) Levofloxacin* (*Levaquin*)	Moxifloxacin* (*Avelox*) Norfloxacin* (*Noroxin*) Ofloxacin* (eg, *Floxin*)

Significance	Onset	Severity	Documentation
1	□ Rapid ■ **Delayed**	■ **Major** □ Moderate □ Minor	□ Established ■ **Probable** □ Suspected □ Possible □ Unlikely

Effects Increased ANTICOAGULANT effect of WARFARIN.

Mechanism Unknown.

Management If possible, choose a non-QUINOLONE antibiotic. Monitor ANTICOAGULANT activity more frequently when QUINOLONES are started or stopped and adjust the WARFARIN dose accordingly.

Discussion

PT prolongation was reported when warfarin and norfloxacin were coadministered.[1,2] Increased PT and a lethal pontine hemorrhage occurred in 1 patient.[1] No interaction was detected when 10 volunteers taking norfloxacin 400 mg twice daily for 9 days were given a midtrial dose of warfarin 30 mg.[3] Case reports describe an interaction between ciprofloxacin and warfarin.[2,4-10] The PT typically was prolonged after a few days of therapy in patients stabilized on warfarin. In 2 cases, marked PT and INR elevation with bleeding occurred.[4,10] Another patient had a bleeding complication with a small prolongation.[6] In 16 patients receiving ciprofloxacin and low-dose warfarin, a 22% PT prolongation occurred in 1 patient.[11,12] In a double-blind study of 34 patients, ciprofloxacin 750 mg twice daily for 12 days increased levels of R-warfarin, while decreasing factors II and VII.[13] Two cases of excessive anticoagulation were described when ofloxacin was administered with warfarin.[9,14] In 1 case, the PT was 78 seconds with gross hematuria.[9] Levofloxacin did not increase the PT in healthy subjects receiving warfarin.[15] INR values were increased in a retrospective review of 21 patients receiving warfarin after treatment with levofloxacin.[16] After adding levofloxacin to stable warfarin regimens, 11 cases of elevated INR occurred, including some with serious bleeding complications and death.[17-20] At least 9 cases of elevated INR, including 1 with bleeding, were reported in patients on chronic warfarin therapy given moxifloxacin.[21-23] In elderly patients receiving levofloxacin and warfarin, the rate of bleeding did not differ from that of control patients.[24] A markedly elevated PT was reported in an 88-year-old man taking warfarin 4 days after starting gatifloxacin.[25] Prolonged-release ciprofloxacin did not alter warfarin pharmacokinetics or pharmacodynamics.[26]

1 Linville T, et al. *Ann Intern Med.* 1989;110(9):751.
2 Jolson HM, et al. *Arch Intern Med.* 1991;151(5):1003.
3 Rocci ML Jr, et al. *J Clin Pharmacol.* 1990;30(8):728.
4 Mott FE, et al. *Ann Intern Med.* 1989;111(6):542.
5 Kamada AK. *DICP.* 1990;24(1):27.
6 Linville D II, et al. *Am J Med.* 1991;90(6):765.
7 Dugoni-Kramer BM. *DICP.* 1991;25(12):1397.
8 Renzi R, et al. *Am J Emerg Med.* 1991;9(6):551.
9 Baciewicz AM, et al. *Ann Intern Med.* 1993;119(12):1223.
10 Byrd DC, et al. *J Am Board Fam Pract.* 1999;12(6):486.
11 Rindone JP, et al. *Clin Pharm.* 1991;10(2):136.
12 Bianco TM, et al. *Pharmacotherapy.* 1992;12(6):435.
13 Israel DS, et al. *Clin Infect Dis.* 1996;22(2):251.
14 Leor J, et al. *Ann Intern Med.* 1988;109(9):761.
15 Liao S, et al. *J Clin Pharmacol.* 1996;36(11):1072.
16 Mercadal Orfila G, et al. *Pharm World Sci.* 2009;31(2):224.
17 Ravnan SL, et al. *Pharmacotherapy.* 2001;21(7):884.
18 Gheno G, et al. *Eur J Clin Pharmacol.* 2001;57(5):427.
19 Jones CB, et al. *Ann Pharmacother.* 2002;36(10):1554.
20 Vadlamudi RS, et al. *South Med J.* 2007;100(7):720.
21 Elbe DH, et al. *Ann Pharmacother.* 2005;39(2):361.
22 Arnold LM, et al. *Pharmacotherapy.* 2005;25(6):904.
23 Yildiz F, et al. *Heart Vessels.* 2008;23(4):286.
24 Stroud LF, et al. *Am J Med.* 2005;118(12):1417.
25 Chock AW, et al. *Am J Health Syst Pharm.* 2006;63(16):1539.
26 Washington C, et al. *J Clin Pharmacol.* 2007;47(10):1320.

* Asterisk indicates drugs cited in interaction reports.

Anticoagulants — *Retinoids*

Warfarin* (eg, *Coumadin*)	Isotretinoin* (eg, *Accutane*)

Significance	Onset	Severity	Documentation
4	☐ Rapid ■ **Delayed**	☐ Major ■ **Moderate** ☐ Minor	☐ Established ☐ Probable ☐ Suspected ■ **Possible** ☐ Unlikely

Effects Anticoagulant effect of WARFARIN may be decreased.

Mechanism Unknown.

Management Carefully monitor coagulation parameters when ISOTRETINOIN is started or stopped. Adjust the WARFARIN dose as needed.

Discussion

A possible drug interaction between warfarin and isotretinoin was reported in a 61-year-old man.[1] The patient had been maintained on warfarin 2.5 mg daily for 2 to 3 years and reported an INR in the therapeutic range during that time. Upon being evaluated for a sudden facial eruption, consisting of multiple, small follicular pustules, from which *Klebsiella* spp. were isolated, he was started on oral cefpodoxime proxetil (*Vantin*) 200 mg twice daily and isotretinoin 30 mg daily. After starting this regimen, the patient's INR decreased, and it was necessary to increase the warfarin dose to 3.75 mg daily in order to maintain the INR within the therapeutic range. Cefpodoxime was discontinued after 10 days. Isotretinoin therapy was continued and the INR remained stable. Upon discontinuation of isotretinoin, after 40 days of treatment, the INR increased and warfarin was reduced to the 2.5 mg daily pretreatment dosage. Etretinate, a retinoic acid analogue therapy for psoriasis (not available in the United States), has been reported to decrease the anticoagulant effect of warfarin.[2]

Additional studies are needed to determine if acitretin (*Soriatane*) interacts similarly with warfarin.

[1] Fiallo P. *Br J Dermatol.* 2004;150:164.

[2] Ostlere LS, et al. *Br J Dermatol.* 1991;124:505.

* Asterisk indicates drugs cited in interaction reports.

Anticoagulants			***Ribavirin***
Warfarin* (eg, *Coumadin*)		Ribavirin* (eg, *Rebetol*)	
Significance	Onset	Severity	Documentation
4	□ Rapid ■ **Delayed**	□ Major ■ **Moderate** □ Minor	□ Established □ Probable □ Suspected ■ **Possible** □ Unlikely

Effects The anticoagulant action of WARFARIN may be decreased.

Mechanism Unknown.

Management In patients receiving WARFARIN therapy, closely monitor the anticoagulant activity, especially during the first 4 weeks, after starting or stopping RIBAVIRIN. Adjust the WARFARIN dose as needed.

Discussion

Decreased anticoagulant activity was reported in a 61-year-old man during coadministration of warfarin and ribavirin.[1] Following a heart valve replacement, the patient was receiving warfarin 45 mg/week, which maintained the INR between 1.8 and 2.3. After hepatitis C was diagnosed, a 1-year course of therapy with interferon alfa-2b (*Intron A* [3 MIU 3 times weekly]) and ribavirin (600 mg twice daily) was started. During the first month of coadministration of warfarin and the antiviral therapy, it was necessary to progressively increase the warfarin dose from 45 to 62.5 mg/week in order to maintain the INR in the target range. Over the next 11 months, the dose of warfarin stabilized at 57 mg/week. Three weeks after discontinuing interferon and ribavirin, the INR increased from 2.2 to 3.4. To maintain the INR in the target range, it was necessary to decrease the dose of warfarin to 47.5 mg/week. To determine if the interaction was casued by ribavirin, and not interferon, a rechallenge with ribavirin 1,000 mg/day for 4 weeks was conducted while the warfarin dose was kept constant at 52.5 mg/week. During this period, the INR decreased slowly from 2.6 to 1.8. When ribavirin was discontinued, the INR increased despite a reduced warfarin dose.

[1] Schulman S. *Ann Pharmacother*. 2002;36:72.

* Asterisk indicates drugs cited in interaction reports.

Anticoagulants — *Rifamycins*

Anticoagulants	Rifamycins	
Dicumarol†	Rifabutin (*Mycobutin*)	Rifapentine* (*Priftin*)
Warfarin* (eg, *Coumadin*)	Rifampin* (eg, *Rifadin*)	

Significance	Onset	Severity	Documentation
2	□ Rapid	□ Major	■ **Established**
	■ **Delayed**	■ **Moderate**	□ Probable
		□ Minor	□ Suspected
			□ Possible
			□ Unlikely

Effects RIFAMPIN decreases the anticoagulation action of WARFARIN.

Mechanism Increased hepatic microsomal enzyme metabolism of WARFARIN by RIFAMYCINS appears responsible.

Management Increased dosage of ANTICOAGULANTS may be needed when RIFAMYCINS are coadministered. Monitor anticoagulant parameters frequently when starting or stopping RIFAMYCINS. Be prepared to adjust the ANTICOAGULANT dose. Monitoring and adjusting the ANTICOAGULANT dose may be necessary for several weeks after discontinuing the RIFAMYCIN.

Discussion

Several controlled studies have demonstrated that rifampin increases warfarin elimination and decreases hypoprothrombinemia.[1-4] Increased activity of the hepatic microsomal cytochrome P450 enzyme system responsible for warfarin metabolism appears to be the mechanism involved.[3] Case reports have documented 50%[5,6] to 200%[7] increases in warfarin dosage requirements with coadministration of rifampin. Hematuria was reported when rifampin was discontinued and phenprocoumon† was administered at the same dose.[8]

1 O'Reilly RA. *Ann Intern Med.* 1974;81(3):337.
2 O'Reilly RA. *Ann Intern Med.* 1975;83(4):506.
3 Heimark LD, et al. *Clin Pharmacol Ther.* 1987;42(4):388.
4 Almog S, et al. *South Med J.* 1988;81(10):1304.
5 Romankiewicz JA, et al. *Ann Intern Med.* 1975;82(2):224.
6 Self TH, et al. *Chest.* 1975;67(4):490.
7 Lee CR, et al. *Pharmacotherapy.* 2001;21(10):1240.
8 Boekhout-Mussert RJ, et al. *JAMA.* 1974;229(14):1903.

* Asterisk indicates drugs cited in interaction reports. Based on pharmacologic and pharmacokinetic considerations, similar interactions may occur with other drugs that are listed.
† Not available in the United States.

Anticoagulants	*Rifaximin*
Warfarin* (eg, *Coumadin*)	Rifaximin* (*Xifaxan*)

Significance	Onset	Severity	Documentation
4	☐ Rapid	☐ Major	☐ Established
	■ **Delayed**	■ **Moderate**	☐ Probable
		☐ Minor	☐ Suspected
			■ **Possible**
			☐ Unlikely

Effects The anticoagulant effect of WARFARIN may be decreased.

Mechanism Unknown.

Management Monitor anticoagulant activity when RIFAXIMIN is started or stopped and adjust the WARFARIN dose as needed.

Discussion

A 49-year-old woman experienced a decrease in the anticoagulant effect of warfarin after starting concurrent treatment with rifaximin.[1] The patient had been taking warfarin 7.5 mg daily for approximately 5 months with a target INR of 2 to 3.5. Five days after starting rifaximin 400 mg 3 times daily for small intestine bacterial overgrowth, her INR decreased to 1.2 and remained suppressed throughout the course of rifaximin therapy despite incremental increases in her warfarin dosage (up to 15 mg/day). She completed the course of rifaximin treatment and 12 days later the INR was supratherapeutic at 4.2. The warfarin dose was titrated to the baseline dose and an INR in the therapeutic range was achieved. Similar results were obtained with a subsequent rifaximin rechallenge.

[1] Hoffman JT, et al. *Ann Pharmacother*. 2011;45(5):e25.

* Asterisk indicates drugs cited in interaction reports.

Anticoagulants — *Ropinirole*

Anticoagulants	Ropinirole
Warfarin* (eg, *Coumadin*)	Ropinirole* (eg, *Requip*)

Significance	Onset	Severity	Documentation
4	☐ Rapid ■ **Delayed**	☐ Major ■ **Moderate** ☐ Minor	☐ Established ☐ Probable ☐ Suspected ■ **Possible** ☐ Unlikely

Effects The anticoagulant effect of WARFARIN may be increased.

Mechanism Unknown.

Management In patients receiving WARFARIN, closely monitor anticoagulant parameters when starting, stopping, or changing the dose of ROPINIROLE. Adjust the WARFARIN dose as needed.

Discussion

In a patient stabilized on warfarin 4 mg/day, an increase in the INR occurred 9 days after starting ropinirole 0.25 mg 3 times/day.[1] He was being maintained on warfarin, levodopa/carbidopa (eg, *Sinemet*), and doxazosin (eg, *Cardura*). His INR had been stable (range, 1.8 to 2.6) for approximately 15 months. Nine days after starting ropinirole, his INR had increased to 4.6. There were no signs of bleeding. Warfarin therapy was withheld for 4 days, then restarted at 2 mg/day (INR, 1.2). The warfarin dosage was increased to 3 mg/day (INR 1.7). Ropinirole was discontinued because of GI adverse reactions, and the INR decreased to 1.4, necessitating an increase in the warfarin dosage to 4 mg/day.

[1] Bair JD, et al. *Ann Pharmacother.* 2001;35(10):1202.

* Asterisk indicates drugs cited in interaction reports.

Anticoagulants — *Royal Jelly*

Anticoagulants	Royal Jelly
Warfarin* (eg, *Coumadin*)	Royal Jelly*

Significance	Onset	Severity	Documentation
4	☐ Rapid ■ **Delayed**	■ **Major** ☐ Moderate ☐ Minor	☐ Established ☐ Probable ☐ Suspected ■ **Possible** ☐ Unlikely

Effects The risk of bleeding may be increased.

Mechanism Unknown.

Management Because WARFARIN has a narrow therapeutic index, patients should avoid concurrent ingestion of ROYAL JELLY. Caution patients to consult their health care provider regarding the use of nonprescription medicines or herbal products and to report unusual bruising or bleeding. Monitor clotting parameters more frequently when patients on oral ANTICOAGULANTS ingest substances with undocumented effects.

Discussion

A possible interaction between warfarin and royal jelly was reported in an 87-year-old man.[1] The patient had stage IV-A follicular non-Hodgkin lymphoma, atrial fibrillation, and hypertension. He was receiving long-term therapy with several drugs, including warfarin 2.5 mg 6 days per week and warfarin 5 mg 1 day per week. His drug therapy had been stable during the preceding 3 months and his INR ranged from 1.9 to 2.4 (therapeutic range, 2 to 3). Four weeks after being seen for a routine anticoagulant management visit, the patient went to the emergency department with hematuria. On hospital admission, his INR was 6.88, which increased to 7.29 during his hospital stay. The patient admitted that 1 week earlier he had started taking royal jelly (a milky white secretion produced by the hypopharyngeal and mandibular glands of worker honeybees). After treatment with vitamin K and maintenance fluids, his INR was 3.2. The patient was discharged on his previous dosage of warfarin and his INR remained stable.

[1] Lee NJ, et al. *Pharmacotherapy*. 2006;26(4):583.

* Asterisk indicates drugs cited in interaction reports.

Anticoagulants — *Salicylates*

Warfarin* (eg, *Coumadin*)	Aspirin* (eg, *Bayer*)	Methyl Salicylate*†

Significance	Onset	Severity	Documentation
1	☐ Rapid ■ **Delayed**	■ **Major** ☐ Moderate ☐ Minor	■ **Established** ☐ Probable ☐ Suspected ☐ Possible ☐ Unlikely

Effects ANTICOAGULANT activity may be enhanced. The adverse reactions of ASPIRIN on gastric mucosa and platelet function also may increase the possibility of hemorrhage.

Mechanism See Discussion.

Management If concurrent use cannot be avoided, frequently monitor INR and adjust the ANTICOAGULANT dose accordingly when SALICYLATE therapy is started or stopped. Instruct patients to report unusual bleeding or bruising if ASPIRIN or topical SALICYLATES and ANTICOAGULANTS are coadministered.

Discussion

Controlled studies in patients receiving oral anticoagulants consistently demonstrated enhanced anticoagulant activity when aspirin dosages exceeded 3 g/day.[1-4] Platelet aggregation is inhibited in large and small aspirin doses.[5,6] Severe hypoprothrombinemia and bleeding episodes have been caused by large doses of aspirin.[7,8] Studies associated increased bleeding risk, especially GI, with 500 mg/day[9,10] but only minor risk with 100 mg/day, which was accompanied by a reduction in mortality.[11] Low-dose aspirin 75 mg/day plus low-intensity warfarin (INR, 1.5) is associated with slightly greater minor and intermediate bleeding than low-dose aspirin or low-intensity warfarin alone.[12] In patients with ischemic strokes, no differences in bleeding rates were found when short-term use of aspirin plus warfarin or heparin was compared with anticoagulant use alone.[13] However, in patients receiving warfarin, aspirin, and clopidogrel (*Plavix*), 9.2% developed clinically important bleeding.[14] A meta-analysis of 10 studies comparing coadministration of aspirin and oral anticoagulant therapy with oral anticoagulant therapy alone found an increased risk of major bleeding with no clinical benefit (except in patients with mechanical heart valves) with coadministration of aspirin and oral anticoagulant therapy.[15] A study of patients with GI bleeding reported an association between the bleeding and use of warfarin plus aspirin compared with either drug alone.[16] Nonacetylated salicylates had a lack of antiplatelet effects and were associated with a low incidence of bleeding.[5] Salicylic acid is detected in blood following topical use of salicylates.[17,18] Potentiation of warfarin anticoagulation following topical use of ointment,[13] gel,[19] medicated oil,[20] and analgesic balm[21] containing methyl salicylate (oil of wintergreen) has been reported. See also Heparin-Salicylates.

1 Quick AJ, et al. *J Pharmacol Exp Ther.* 1960;128:95.
2 Watson RM, et al. *Circulation.* 1961;24:613.
3 Udall JA. *J R Coll Physicians Lond.* 1970;77:20.
4 O'Reilly RA, et al. *Ann N Y Acad Sci.* 1971;179:173.
5 Weiss HJ, et al. *J Clin Invest.* 1968;47(9):2169.
6 Zucker MB, et al. *J Lab Clin Med.* 1970;76(1):66.
7 Barrow MV, et al. *Arch Intern Med.* 1967;120(5):620.
8 Fausa O. *Acta Med Scand.* 1970;188(5):403.
9 Dale J, et al. *Am Heart J.* 1980;99(6):746.
10 Chesebro JH, et al. *Am J Cardiol.* 1983;51(9):1537.
11 Turpie AG, et al. *N Engl J Med.* 1993;329(8):524.
12 Meade TW, et al. *Thromb Haemost.* 1992;68(1):1.
13 Fagan SC, et al. *Ann Pharmacother.* 1994;28(4):441.
14 Orford JL, et al. *Am Heart J.* 2004;147(3):463.
15 Dentali F, et al. *Arch Intern Med.* 2007;167(2):117.
16 Delaney JA, et al. *CMAJ.* 2007;177(4):347.
17 Chow WH, et al. *J R Soc Med.* 1989;82(8):501.
18 Morra P, et al. *Ann Pharmacother.* 1996;30(9):935.
19 Joss JD, et al. *Ann Pharmacother.* 2000;34(6):729.
20 Tam LS, et al. *Aust N Z J Med.* 1995;25(3):258.
21 Chan TY. *Pharmacoepidemiol Drug Saf.* 2009;18(5):420.

* Asterisk indicates drugs cited in interaction reports.
† Not available in the United States.

Anticoagulants — *Selegiline*

Warfarin* (eg, *Coumadin*)	Selegiline* (eg, *Eldepryl*)

Significance	Onset	Severity	Documentation
4	□ Rapid ■ **Delayed**	□ Major ■ **Moderate** □ Minor	□ Established □ Probable □ Suspected ■ **Possible** □ Unlikely

Effects WARFARIN's anticoagulant effect and risk of bleeding may be increased.

Mechanism Inhibition of WARFARIN's metabolism by SELEGILINE is suspected.

Management Monitor coagulation parameters when SELEGILINE is started or stopped and adjust the WARFARIN dose as needed.

Discussion

An increase in INR was reported in a 49-year-old woman receiving warfarin after selegiline was added to her treatment regimen.[1] The patient had been receiving escalating doses of warfarin for 2 months for the prevention of a venous thromboembolism after orthopedic surgery. Despite the escalating doses of warfarin, her INR was subtherapeutic (less than 2). The patient's INR increased to 9 five days after starting transdermal selegiline. The warfarin dose was withheld for 2 days, selegiline was withheld, and the patient received oral phytonadione 2.5 mg. Subsequently, her INR was 1.4.

[1] Ensor CR, et al. *Hosp Pharm.* 2010;45(6):478.

* Asterisk indicates drugs cited in interaction reports.

Anticoagulants — *Serotonin Reuptake Inhibitors*

Anticoagulants	Serotonin Reuptake Inhibitors	
Warfarin* (eg, *Coumadin*)	Citalopram* (eg, *Celexa*)	Fluvoxamine* (eg, *Luvox*)
	Duloxetine* (*Cymbalta*)	Paroxetine* (eg, *Paxil*)
	Escitalopram (eg, *Lexapro*)	Sertraline (eg, *Zoloft*)
	Fluoxetine* (eg, *Prozac*)	

Significance	Onset	Severity	Documentation
2	☐ Rapid	☐ Major	☐ Established
	■ **Delayed**	■ **Moderate**	☐ Probable
		☐ Minor	■ **Suspected**
			☐ Possible
			☐ Unlikely

Effects Increased ANTICOAGULANT effects of WARFARIN.

Mechanism Unknown.

Management Monitor ANTICOAGULANT parameters for at least 10 days when starting or stopping an SRI in patients receiving WARFARIN. Adjust the dose of WARFARIN as needed. The effect of the interaction may persist for several weeks after discontinuing DULOXETINE.[1]

Discussion

Available data conflict. Loss of anticoagulant control with warfarin (ie, increase in INR) occurred in 2 patients following administration of fluoxetine 20 mg/day.[2] The INR returned to baseline after stopping fluoxetine. An 83-year-old man stabilized on warfarin (INR, 2 to 3) developed an elevated INR of 4.8 eight days after starting fluoxetine 10 mg/day.[3] He died 9 days later of a cerebral hemorrhage, despite an INR of 3. These case reports are in contrast to a controlled study of 6 patients on stable warfarin regimens in whom addition of fluoxetine 20 mg/day for 21 days did not cause a change in clotting parameters.[4] Bleeding episodes have been reported in patients receiving fluoxetine alone.[5,6] An unspecific bleeding tendency occurred in 5 of 27 patients several days after initiating treatment with warfarin and paroxetine.[7] In a study in 12 healthy men, citalopram did not alter warfarin pharmacokinetics.[8] In contrast, gingivorrhea and an INR greater than 15 were noted 10 days after citalopram 20 mg/day was added to a stable acenocoumarol† regimen.[9] A 79-year-old woman stabilized on warfarin and citalopram had an elevated INR of 3.7 five days after fluvoxamine 50 mg/day was substituted for citalopram.[10] In a 44-year-old woman, duloxetine increased the warfarin effect, which persisted for 36 days after discontinuing warfarin.[1] In a retrospective study of 100 patients receiving warfarin, concurrent use with an SSRI was associated with an increased risk of any bleeding event (odds ratio, 2.6) and major bleeding (odds ratio, 4.4) compared with patients taking warfarin without an antidepressant.[11]

1 Glueck CJ, et al. *JAMA*. 2006;295(13):1517.
2 Woolfrey S, et al. *BMJ*. 1993;307(6898):241.
3 Dent LA, et al. *Pharmacotherapy*. 1997;17(1):170.
4 Ford MA, et al. *J Clin Psychopharmacol*. 1997;17(2):110.
5 Yaryura-Tobias JA, et al. *Am J Psychiatry*. 1991;148(7):949.
6 Aranth J, et al. *Am J Psychiatry*. 1992;149(3):412.
7 Bannister SJ, et al. *Acta Psychiatr Scand Suppl*. 1989;350:102.
8 Priskorn M, et al. *Br J Clin Pharmacol*. 1997;44(2):199.
9 Borrás-Blasco J, et al. *Ann Pharmacother*. 2002;36(2):345.
10 Limke KK, et al. *Ann Pharmacother*. 2002;36(12):1890.
11 Cochran KA, et al. *Ther Drug Monit*. 2011;33(4):433.

* Asterisk indicates drugs cited in interaction reports. Based on pharmacologic and pharmacokinetic considerations, similar interactions may occur with other drugs that are listed.
† Not available in United States.

Anticoagulants | **Shengmai-Yin**

Warfarin* (eg, *Coumadin*)	Shengmai-Yin*

Significance	Onset	Severity	Documentation
4	☐ Rapid ■ **Delayed**	■ **Major** ☐ Moderate ☐ Minor	☐ Established ☐ Probable ☐ Suspected ■ **Possible** ☐ Unlikely

Effects The anticoagulant effect of WARFARIN may be increased.

Mechanism Unknown.

Management Instruct patients receiving WARFARIN to avoid SHENGMAI-YIN. Because WARFARIN has a narrow therapeutic index, advise patients to consult their health care provider before using nonprescription or herbal products.

Discussion

Shengmai-yin is a Chinese combination herbal product containing hongsheng (red ginger), maidong (liriope), and wuweizi (*Schisandra chinensis*).[1] It has been used for coronary heart disease, cardiogenic shock, and septic shock. A 71-year-old man was on a stable warfarin regimen (2.25 mg daily) with an INR ranging between 1.8 and 2.2 after heart valve replacement surgery. Seven days after starting ingestion of shengmai-yin 10 mL daily, he was admitted to the intensive care unit because of consciousness disturbance. His INR was 5.08. A CT revealed an intracerebral hematoma. Both warfarin and shengmai-yin were withheld and vitamin K was administered. Two days after admission, a craniotomy was performed to remove the hematoma. He was confused and restless for 2 days before showing progressive recovery in his consciousness level as well as motor and verbal functions. The patient was subsequently discharged with an INR of 2 and a warfarin 2.25 mg daily regimen and advised not to take shengmai-yin or other herbal products.

[1] Su Q, et al. *Yonsei Med J.* 2010;51(5):793.

* Asterisk indicates drugs cited in interaction reports.

Anticoagulants — *Sorafenib*

Warfarin* (eg, *Coumadin*)	Sorafenib* (*Nexavar*)

Significance	Onset	Severity	Documentation
4	☐ Rapid ■ **Delayed**	■ **Major** ☐ Moderate ☐ Minor	☐ Established ☐ Probable ☐ Suspected ■ **Possible** ☐ Unlikely

Effects The pharmacologic effects of WARFARIN may be increased, increasing the risk of bleeding.

Mechanism Unknown.

Management Monitor coagulation parameters and adjust the WARFARIN dose as needed when starting or stopping SORAFENIB.

Discussion

A 70-year-old man stabilized on warfarin 36 mg/week experienced an elevated INR and hemorrhage after sorafenib 200 mg/day was added to his treatment regimen.[1] One month after starting sorafenib, the patient's PT was 84.8 and the INR was 39.5. Twelve days earlier, the INR was 2.9. The patient was admitted to the hospital with lower-extremity hemorrhage diagnosed as warfarin toxicity. Sorafenib was discontinued and warfarin was held. Subsequently, the patient was stabilized on warfarin 36 mg/week with therapeutic INR values. He was restarted on sorafenib 200 mg daily because of progression of his metastatic disease. Approximately 2 weeks later, his INR increased to 4.7 and sorafenib was discontinued permanently.

[1] Moretti LV, et al. *Am J Health Syst Pharm.* 2009;66(23):2123.

* Asterisk indicates drugs cited in interaction reports.

Anticoagulants — *Spironolactone*

Warfarin* (eg, *Coumadin*)	Spironolactone* (eg, *Aldactone*)

Significance	Onset	Severity	Documentation
5	□ Rapid ■ **Delayed**	□ Major □ Moderate ■ **Minor**	□ Established □ Probable □ Suspected ■ **Possible** □ Unlikely

Effects The hypoprothrombinemic effect of WARFARIN may be decreased.

Mechanism Diuretic-induced hemoconcentration of clotting factors may be responsible.

Management Monitor anticoagulation parameters and tailor the dose as needed. Increased WARFARIN dosage may be required.

Discussion

A study of 9 men demonstrated a decreased hypoprothrombinemic response and an increased hematocrit following 8 days of spironolactone 200 mg/day and a single dose of warfarin 1.5 mg/kg. No change in warfarin plasma levels was observed.[1] The decrease in warfarin action was associated with the hemoconcentration of clotting factors.

[1] O'Reilly RA. *Clin Pharmacol Ther.* 1980;27(2):198.

* Asterisk indicates drugs cited in interaction reports.

Anticoagulants		**St. John's Wort**
Anisindione†	Warfarin*	St. John's Wort*
Dicumarol†	(eg, *Coumadin*)	

Significance	Onset	Severity	Documentation
2	□ Rapid	□ Major	□ Established
	■ **Delayed**	■ **Moderate**	□ Probable
		□ Minor	■ **Suspected**
			□ Possible
			□ Unlikely

Effects The ANTICOAGULANT effect may be decreased.

Mechanism Increased metabolism (CYP2C9) or inhibition of absorption of the ANTICOAGULANT is suspected.

Management Caution patients to consult their health care provider before using nonprescription or herbal products. If use of ST. JOHN'S WORT cannot be avoided, closely monitor coagulation parameters when ST. JOHN'S WORT is started or stopped. Adjust the ANTICOAGULANT dose as needed.

Discussion

At least 7 cases of decreased anticoagulant effect of warfarin, as measured by the INR, have been reported to the Medical Products Agency in Uppsala, Sweden.[1] Most patients received stable doses of warfarin prior to taking St. John's wort. The INR returned to target values after increasing the dose of warfarin or discontinuing St. John's wort. The effect of St. John's wort on the AUC of the anticoagulant phenprocoumon† was studied in 10 healthy men.[2] In a randomized, single-blind, placebo-controlled, crossover study, each subject received St. John's wort extract 900 mg/day or placebo for 11 days. On day 11, a single dose of phenprocoumon 12 mg was administered. Compared with placebo, administering phenprocoumon with St. John's wort resulted in a 17% decrease in the mean AUC (from 218.9 to 180.8 mcg•hr/L) of the anticoagulant. Using a randomized, open-label, crossover design, the effects of St. John's wort extract (*Hypericum perforatum* 1 g) on the pharmacokinetics and pharmacodynamics of warfarin were studied in 12 healthy subjects.[3] Each subject received a single dose of warfarin 25 mg alone and after 14 days of pretreatment with St. John's wort. Compared with giving warfarin alone, pretreatment with St. John's wort decreased the warfarin AUC and $t_{½}$ and increased the apparent total clearance, leading to a reduction in the pharmacologic effect of warfarin.

The ingredients of many herbal products are not standardized. It is unclear if herbal products contain ingredients other than those listed on the label or purported to be present that could interact with anticoagulants.

[1] Yue QY, et al. *Lancet.* 2000;355:576.
[2] Maurer A, et al. *Eur J Clin Pharmacol.* 1999;55:A22.
[3] Jiang X, et al. *Br J Clin Pharmacol.* 2004;57:592.

* Asterisk indicates drugs cited in interaction reports. Based on pharmacologic and pharmacokinetic considerations, similar interactions may occur with other drugs that are listed.
† Not available in the United States.

Anticoagulants — *Sucralfate*

Warfarin* (eg, *Coumadin*)	Sucralfate* (eg, *Carafate*)

Significance	Onset	Severity	Documentation
5	☐ Rapid ■ **Delayed**	☐ Major ☐ Moderate ■ **Minor**	☐ Established ☐ Probable ☐ Suspected ■ **Possible** ☐ Unlikely

Effects The hypoprothrombinemic effect of WARFARIN may be decreased.

Mechanism SUCRALFATE may reduce WARFARIN absorption.

Management Monitor anticoagulation parameters and adjust the WARFARIN dose as needed. If unable to use alternative peptic ulcer therapy, consider separating the doses of SUCRALFATE and WARFARIN by at least 2 hours.

Discussion

Three case reports associated a failure to achieve therapeutic anticoagulation with sucralfate administration.[1-3] Warfarin plasma concentrations were decreased in the first 2 patients.[1] In both cases, therapy was being initiated or restarted.[1,2] In the third case, the patient's anticoagulation was adequately controlled while on concurrent treatment with sucralfate and warfarin (doses separated by 2 hr).[3] A reduction in PTs, necessitating an increase in warfarin dose, occurred when sucralfate and warfarin were administered at the same time. Warfarin sensitivity was re-established when the doses were separated again. Warfarin plasma levels were not measured. Two controlled evaluations in patients stabilized on warfarin reported no effect of 14 days of sucralfate administration on prothrombin activity or plasma warfarin concentrations.[4,5]

1 Mungall D, et al. *Ann Intern Med.* 1983;98:557.
2 Braverman SE, et al. *Drug Intell Clin Pharm.* 1988;22:913.
3 Parrish RH, et al. *Ann Pharmacother.* 1992;26:1015.
4 Neuvonen PJ, et al. *Br J Clin Pharmacol.* 1985;20:178.
5 Talbert RL, et al. *Drug Intell Clin Pharm.* 1985;19:456.

* Asterisk indicates drugs cited in interaction reports.

Anticoagulants — *Sulfinpyrazone*

Warfarin* (eg, *Coumadin*)	Sulfinpyrazone*†

Significance	Onset	Severity	Documentation
1	☐ Rapid	■ **Major**	■ **Established**
	■ **Delayed**	☐ Moderate	☐ Probable
		☐ Minor	☐ Suspected
			☐ Possible
			☐ Unlikely

Effects The anticoagulant activity of WARFARIN will likely be enhanced; hemorrhage could occur.

Mechanism Liver degradations of the S-WARFARIN enantiomorph are impaired by the SULFINPYRAZONE sulfide metabolite.[1]

Management Monitor coagulation parameters closely. Expect to decrease the WARFARIN dose when SULFINPYRAZONE treatment is initiated, and increase the dosage when SULFINPYRAZONE is discontinued.

Discussion

Multiple case reports involving 9 separate patients have documented enhanced hypoprothrombinemia and bleeding episodes when sulfinpyrazone was administered to patients stabilized on warfarin.[2-8] A controlled study with racemic warfarin reported enhanced hypoprothrombinemia in 5 subjects, which was not associated with changes in warfarin protein binding or plasma levels.[9] When the separate R- and S-warfarin enantiomorphs were studied, a selective inhibition of the CYP-450–mediated oxidation of S-warfarin was demonstrated.[10,11] This selective inhibition of CYP-450 may be mediated by the sulfide metabolite of sulfinpyrazone rather than sulfinpyrazone itself.[1]

Although only 1 case of a biphasic enhancement followed by antagonism of warfarin's anticoagulant effects has been reported,[12] expect this interaction to occur in the majority of patients. Warfarin dose reductions of 50% may be required to avoid excessive bleeding risks.

Phenprocoumon† therapy does not appear to be altered by sulfinpyrazone.[13]

1 He M, et al. *Drug Metab Dispos.* 1995;23(6):659.
2 Mattingly D, et al. *Br Med J.* 1978;2(6154):1786.
3 Davis JW, et al. *N Engl J Med.* 1978;299(17):955.
4 Weiss M. *Lancet.* 1979;1(8116):609.
5 Bailey RR, et al. *Lancet.* 1980;1(8162):254.
6 Gallus A, et al. *Lancet.* 1980;1(8167):535.
7 Jamil A, et al. *Chest.* 1981;79(3):375.
8 Thompson PL, et al. *Med J Aust.* 1981;1(1):41.
9 Miners JO, et al. *Eur J Clin Pharmacol.* 1982;22(4):327.
10 O'Reilly RA. *Circulation.* 1982;65(1):202.
11 Toon S, et al. *Clin Pharmacol Ther.* 1986;39(1):15.
12 Nenci GG, et al. *Br Med J (Clin Res Ed).* 1981;282(6273):1361.
13 O'Reilly RA. *Arch Intern Med.* 1982;142(9):1634.

* Asterisk indicates drugs cited in interaction reports.
† Not available in the United States.

Anticoagulants		**Sulfonamides**	
Warfarin* (eg, *Coumadin*)		Sulfamethizole*† Sulfamethoxazole*† Sulfasalazine* (eg, *Azulfidine*)	Sulfisoxazole*† Trimethoprim/ Sulfamethoxazole* (eg, *Septra*)
Significance	Onset	Severity	Documentation
1	☐ Rapid ■ **Delayed**	■ **Major** ☐ Moderate ☐ Minor	■ **Established** ☐ Probable ☐ Suspected ☐ Possible ☐ Unlikely

Effects The anticoagulant effect of WARFARIN may be enhanced, resulting in hemorrhage.

Mechanism Unclear. However, TRIMETHOPRIM/SULFAMETHOXAZOLE appears to inhibit hepatic metabolism of S-WARFARIN.

Management Monitor the anticoagulant action of WARFARIN and adjust the dose as necessary.

Discussion

Case histories[1-6] and controlled studies[7-9] have demonstrated a potentially serious drug interaction between warfarin and trimethoprim/sulfamethoxazole. Controlled studies in volunteers receiving 7 days of trimethoprim 320 mg/sulfamethoxazole 1,600 mg prior to single doses of warfarin 1.5 mg/kg demonstrated increased hypoprothrombinemia.[7,8] Warfarin plasma levels were increased, although only when the more potent S-warfarin enantiomorph was administered.[3] Whether trimethoprim or sulfamethoxazole was responsible for the elevation of S-warfarin is unclear. In an epidemiologic study of patients taking warfarin, administration of trimethoprim/sulfamethoxazole increased the risk of GI bleeding by an odds ratio of 1.68.[10] In 2 case reports, coadministration of sulfisoxazole and warfarin was associated with hypoprothrombinemia and bleeding complications, including hemoptysis, hematuria, and gingival bleeding.[11,12] In another study, sulfamethizole was associated with increased warfarin $t_{1/2}$ and decreased clearance rates in 2 patients.[13] A 37-year-old woman required an increase in her warfarin dose (from 30 to 75 mg/wk) to maintain a therapeutic INR following addition of sulfasalazine 4 g/day to her stable warfarin regimen.[14] Warfarin requirements returned to baseline following discontinuation of sulfasalazine. In contrast, in a 60-year-old man, sulfasalazine potentiated the anticoagulant effect of warfarin.[15]

1 Barnett DB, et al. *Br Med J.* 1975;1(5958):608.
2 Hassall C, et al. *Lancet.* 1975;2(7945):1155.
3 Tilstone WJ, et al. *Postgrad Med J.* 1977;53(621):388.
4 Errick JK, et al. *Am J Hosp Pharm.* 1978;35(11):1399.
5 Greenlaw CW. *Am J Hosp Pharm.* 1979;36(9):1155.
6 Kaufman JM, et al. *Urology.* 1980;16(6):601.
7 O'Reilly RA, et al. *Ann Intern Med.* 1979;91(1):34.
8 O'Reilly RA. *N Engl J Med.* 1980;302(1):33.
9 Fischer HD, et al. *Arch Intern Med.* 2010;170(7):617.
10 Schelleman H, et al. *Clin Pharmacol Ther.* 2008;84(5):581.
11 Self TH, et al. *Circulation.* 1975;52(3):528.
12 Sioris LJ, et al. *Arch Intern Med.* 1980;140(4):546.
13 Lumholtz B, et al. *Clin Pharmacol Ther.* 1975;17(6):731.
14 Teefy AM, et al. *Ann Pharmacother.* 2000;34(11):1265.
15 Hall S, et al. *J Clin Pharm Ther.* 2011;36(2):246.

* Asterisk indicates drugs cited in interaction reports.
† Not available in the United States.

Anticoagulants — *Tamoxifen*

Warfarin* (eg, *Coumadin*)	Tamoxifen*

Significance	Onset	Severity	Documentation
1	☐ Rapid ■ **Delayed**	■ **Major** ☐ Moderate ☐ Minor	☐ Established ☐ Probable ■ **Suspected** ☐ Possible ☐ Unlikely

Effects The hypoprothrombinemic effect of oral ANTICOAGULANTS may be increased, possibly with bleeding.

Mechanism Unknown.

Management If an interaction is suspected, consider decreasing the dose of oral ANTICOAGULANTS during coadministration of TAMOXIFEN. Monitor PT and adjust the dose accordingly.

Discussion

A life-threatening reaction attributed to the coadministration of tamoxifen and warfarin has been reported in a 65-year-old woman.[1] The patient had been treated with warfarin for 11 years following an aortic valve replacement. The total weekly dose ranged from 27 to 28.5 mg, producing a PT of 23 to 34 seconds (control, 12 seconds). After a mastectomy for breast cancer, the patient was started on tamoxifen 10 mg twice daily. Three days later, the patient's PT was 39 seconds (control, 14 seconds). Three weeks later, her PT was 75.6 seconds (control, 14 seconds), believed to be caused by a 5-day course of trimethoprim/sulfamethoxazole (eg, *Septra*). The warfarin dose was left unchanged. After 3 more weeks, the patient was admitted to the hospital with hematemesis, abdominal pain, and hematuria. Her PT was 206 seconds (control, 14 seconds). Fresh frozen plasma was administered, and warfarin treatment was discontinued until her PT returned to the therapeutic range. Within 12 hours following admission, the patient's hematuria and hematemesis stopped. Five days after admission, warfarin therapy was restarted. Upon discharge, the patient's weekly warfarin dosage was 17.5 mg, PT was stable at 34 to 37 seconds (control, 14 seconds), and tamoxifen treatment was continued. Thus, to achieve the same hypoprothrombinemic effect as prior to tamoxifen treatment, the warfarin dose in this patient was decreased approximately 40%. A 43-year-old woman stabilized on warfarin 5 mg/day was given tamoxifen 40 mg/day.[2] The next day her PT increased from 19 to 38 seconds, resulting in titration of the warfarin dosage to 1 mg/day. A review of medical records identified 5 additional patients who received warfarin and tamoxifen. Complications developed in 2 patients. One developed a subdural hematoma and the other patient developed severe hematuria. In another report, a medical review of patients receiving warfarin and tamoxifen identified 5 of 22 patients with increased anticoagulation.[3]

[1] Lodwick R, et al. *Br Med J (Clin Res Ed)*. 1987;295(6606):1141.
[2] Tenni P, et al. *BMJ*. 1989;298(6666):93.
[3] Ritchie LD, et al. *BMJ*. 1989;298(6682):1253.

* Asterisk indicates drugs cited in interaction reports.

Anticoagulants — *Terbinafine*

Warfarin* (eg, *Coumadin*)	Terbinafine* (eg, *Lamisil*)

Significance	Onset	Severity	Documentation
4	☐ Rapid ■ **Delayed**	■ **Major** ☐ Moderate ☐ Minor	☐ Established ☐ Probable ☐ Suspected ■ **Possible** ☐ Unlikely

Effects The effects of the oral ANTICOAGULANT may be decreased.

Mechanism Possibly caused by induction of hepatic metabolism.

Management Carefully monitor coagulation parameters when TERBINAFINE is started or stopped. Adjust the ANTICOAGULANT dose as needed.

Discussion

A possible drug interaction has been reported in a patient receiving warfarin and oral terbinafine.[1] A 68-year-old woman was being maintained on warfarin 5.5 mg/day for mitral valve disease. Her INR was stable between 2 and 3. Other medications the patient was receiving included glyburide (eg, *DiaBeta*), metformin (eg, *Glucophage*), furosemide (eg, *Lasix*), and spironolactone (eg, *Aldactone*), the doses of which had not been changed during the previous 2 years. The patient was started on a 3-month course of terbinafine 250 mg/day for the treatment of tinea unguium. While still receiving warfarin 5.5 mg/day, her INR decreased from 2.1 to 1.1 over a 28-day period. Over the next 3 weeks, her warfarin dose was increased to 7.5 mg/day (INR 2 to 3). After 12 weeks of therapy, terbinafine was discontinued, and over the next 4 weeks, the dose of warfarin was gradually decreased to 5.5 mg/day. Others have questioned the reasons for the change in this patient's INR.[2,3] A 71-year-old patient stabilized on warfarin 5 mg/day experienced GI bleeding 32 days after starting terbinafine.[4] At the time of admission for the GI bleed, coagulation indices were above the therapeutic range. The warfarin dose was decreased to 2.5 mg/day alternating with 5 mg/day while the 12-week course of terbinafine was completed. In a study involving 16 healthy subjects, terbinafine 250 mg was administered for 14 days, and on day 8, a single dose of warfarin 30 mg was administered.[5] No interaction was observed. In postmarketing surveillance, no interaction occurred in 26 patients receiving warfarin and terbinafine concurrently.[6]

1 Warwick JA, et al. *BMJ.* 1998;316(7129):440.
2 Gantmacher J, et al. *BMJ.* 1998;317(7152):205.
3 Clarke MF, et al. *BMJ.* 1998;317(7152):205.
4 Gupta AK, et al. *Dermatology.* 1998;196(2):266.
5 Guerret M, et al. *Pharmacotherapy.* 1997;17(4):767.
6 O'Sullivan DP, et al. *Br J Clin Pharmacol.* 1996;42(5):559.

* Asterisk indicates drugs cited in interaction reports.

Anticoagulants — *Tetracyclines*

Anticoagulants	Tetracyclines	
Warfarin* (eg, *Coumadin*)	Demeclocycline (eg, *Declomycin*)	Oxytetracycline (eg, *Terramycin*)
	Doxycycline* (eg, *Vibramycin*)	Tetracycline (eg, *Sumycin*)
	Minocycline (eg, *Minocin*)	

Significance	Onset	Severity	Documentation
1	☐ Rapid	■ **Major**	☐ Established
	■ **Delayed**	☐ Moderate	☐ Probable
		☐ Minor	■ **Suspected**
			☐ Possible
			☐ Unlikely

Effects The action of WARFARIN may be increased.

Mechanism TETRACYCLINES may directly affect hemostasis.[1-3]

Management Monitor ANTICOAGULANT parameters frequently and adjust the WARFARIN dose accordingly if these agents must be coadministered. Instruct patients regarding the early signs and symptoms of bleeding.

Discussion

Several cases of increased INR and bleeding have been reported in patients receiving warfarin and doxycycline concurrently.[4-8] A serious hemorrhage was attributed to a 10-day course of doxycycline in a patient who had been maintained on warfarin without incident during the preceding 15 months.[4] The hemorrhage was successfully treated by warfarin discontinuation, vitamin K administration, and blood transfusions. After discharge, warfarin requirements returned to prehemorrhage doses. Two additional patients stabilized on oral anticoagulants experienced bleeding and elevated PTs after receiving doxycycline.[6] The anticoagulant dosage requirements returned to prehemorrhage doses following discontinuation of doxycycline. A 69-year-old woman stabilized on warfarin for 7 months experienced a serious retroperitoneal bleeding episode and elevated INR (7.22) 6 days after starting doxycycline 100 mg twice daily.[7] Therapy included vitamin K administration as well as transfusion with fresh frozen plasma and packed red blood cells. Warfarin was not restarted. Increased hypoprothrombinemia has also been attributed to combination therapy with warfarin and a tetracycline-plus-nystatin product.[5]

Antibiotics (including tetracyclines) may have independent effects on hemostasis,[1-3] making the interpretation of an interaction with oral anticoagulants difficult. Eradication of vitamin K–producing gut bacteria by antibiotics may contribute to the increased anticoagulant effect of warfarin; however, dietary sources of vitamin K may be more important.[9]

[1] Bell WN, et al. *J Clin Pathol.* 1955;8(2):173.
[2] Haden HT. *AMA Arch Intern Med.* 1957;100(6):986.
[3] Magid E. *Scand J Clin Lab Invest.* 1962;14:565.
[4] Westfall LK, et al. *Am J Hosp Pharm.* 1980;37(12):1620.
[5] O'Donnell D. *Med J Aust.* 1989;150(3):163.
[6] Caraco Y, et al. *Ann Pharmacother.* 1992;26(9):1084.
[7] Baciewicz AM, et al. *Arch Intern Med.* 2001;161(9):1231.
[8] Hasan SA. *Cornea.* 2007;26(6):742.
[9] Udall JA. *JAMA.* 1965;194(2):127.

* Asterisk indicates drugs cited in interaction reports. Based on pharmacologic and pharmacokinetic considerations, similar interactions may occur with other drugs that are listed.

Anticoagulants	*Thiazide Diuretics*	
Warfarin* (eg, *Coumadin*)	Bendroflumethiazide Chlorothiazide (eg, *Diuril*) Chlorthalidone* (eg, *Thalitone*) Hydrochlorothiazide (eg, *HydroDIURIL*) Hydroflumethiazide (eg, *Saluron*)	Indapamide (eg, *Lozol*) Methyclothiazide (eg, *Enduron*) Metolazone (eg, *Zaroxolyn*) Polythiazide

Significance	Onset	Severity	Documentation
4	☐ Rapid ■ **Delayed**	☐ Major ■ **Moderate** ☐ Minor	☐ Established ☐ Probable ☐ Suspected ■ **Possible** ☐ Unlikely

Effects The action of oral ANTICOAGULANTS may be decreased.

Mechanism Higher plasma concentrations of clotting factors as a result of diuretic-induced volume contraction has been proposed.

Management Consider monitoring coagulation indices during combined use of oral ANTICOAGULANTS and THIAZIDE DIURETICS. ANTICOAGULANT doses may need to be increased.

Discussion

The hypoprothrombinemic response observed after a single dose of warfarin alone was decreased after chlorthalidone was administered with the warfarin dose and for 1 week thereafter.[1] Because there were no changes in plasma warfarin concentrations, this effect was attributed to the volume contraction and increased plasma clotting protein concentrations resulting from chlorthalidone administration. In contrast, 3 weeks of chlorothiazide administration had no effect on the hypoprothrombinemic response to single doses of warfarin.[2] Clinical oral anticoagulant failures attributed to coadministration of thiazide diuretics have not been documented.

[1] O'Reilly RA, et al. *Ann NY Acad Sci.* 1971;179:173.
[2] Robinson DS, et al. *Ann Intern Med.* 1970;72(6):853.

* Asterisk indicates drugs cited in interaction reports. Based on pharmacologic and pharmacokinetic considerations, similar interactions may occur with other drugs that are listed.

Anticoagulants — *Thioamines*

Warfarin* (eg, *Coumadin*)	Methimazole* (eg, *Tapazole*) Propylthiouracil*

Significance	Onset	Severity	Documentation
1	☐ Rapid ■ **Delayed**	■ **Major** ☐ Moderate ☐ Minor	☐ Established ☐ Probable ■ **Suspected** ☐ Possible ☐ Unlikely

Effects The action of oral ANTICOAGULANTS may be changed during coadministration of THIOAMINES.

Mechanism Unknown.

Management Monitor coagulation indices and observe for clinical signs of excessive or subtherapeutic responses to oral ANTICOAGULANTS during coadministration of THIOAMINES. Adjust the oral ANTICOAGULANT dosage as necessary.

Discussion

Disappearance of vitamin K–dependent clotting factors is increased in hyperthyroidism and, as a result, the hypoprothrombinemic response to oral anticoagulants occurs earlier and to a greater extent than in euthyroidism.[1] This response may decrease as hyperthyroidism is corrected with thioamines. Higher doses of oral anticoagulants may be necessary.[2-4]

In isolated cases, the use of thioamines has been associated with hypoprothrombinemia and clinical bleeding.[5-8] The mechanism is unknown. Although this appears to occur rarely, thioamines could add to the hypoprothrombinemic response to oral anticoagulants. This was considered a possible explanation in 1 case in which an unexpectedly excessive response to warfarin occurred in a patient receiving propylthiouracil.[9]

[1] Loeliger EA, et al. *Thromb Diath Haemorrh.* 1964;10:267.
[2] Vagenakis AG, et al. *Johns Hopkins Med J.* 1972;131(1):69.
[3] Busenbark LA, et al. *Ann Pharmacother.* 2006;40(6):1200.
[4] Akin F, et al. *Blood Coagul Fibrinolysis.* 2008;19(1):89.
[5] Greenstein RH. *JAMA.* 1960;173:1014.
[6] Naeye RL, et al. *Am J Clin Pathol.* 1960;34(3):254.
[7] Gilbert DK. *JAMA.* 1964;189:855.
[8] Gotta AW, et al. *Anesthesiology.* 1972;37(5):562.
[9] Self T, et al. *JAMA.* 1975;231(11):1165.

* Asterisk indicates drugs cited in interaction reports.

Anticoagulants		*Thiopurines*	
Warfarin* (eg, *Coumadin*)		Azathioprine* (eg, *Imuran*)	Mercaptopurine* (eg, *Purinethol*)

Significance	Onset	Severity	Documentation
2	□ Rapid ■ **Delayed**	□ Major ■ **Moderate** □ Minor	□ Established □ Probable ■ **Suspected** □ Possible □ Unlikely

Effects The action of WARFARIN may be decreased.

Mechanism Unknown; however, THIOPURINES have been reported to increase the synthesis or activation of prothrombin,[1] as well as reduce plasma WARFARIN concentrations.[2]

Management Monitor ANTICOAGULANT parameters frequently when the dose of THIOPURINES is started, stopped, or changed. Adjust the WARFARIN dose accordingly.

Discussion

Reduction of hypoprothrombinemic effect has been reported during maintenance warfarin therapy and has been associated with concomitant use of 6-mercaptopurine[3] or azathioprine.[4-6] During 2 successive courses of 6-mercaptopurine administration, a patient required increases in warfarin doses to compensate for a diminishing hypoprothrombinemic response.[7] After completion of each 6-mercaptopurine cycle, the hypoprothrombinemic response was regained, and the warfarin dose could be reduced to previous amounts. A 52-year-old woman receiving azathioprine and warfarin required warfarin 14 to 17 mg daily to maintain a PT of 16 to 18 seconds and was controlled for 6 years.[4] Following discontinuation of azathioprine, bleeding and an elevated PT (32 seconds) occurred. After recovery, control was maintained on warfarin 5 mg/day. A 30-year-old woman was stabilized on warfarin 20 mg/day and azathioprine 150 mg/day.[5] On 2 occasions, the warfarin dose needed to be decreased following reduction in the azathioprine dose. When the azathioprine dosage was increased back to 150 mg/day, it was necessary to increase the warfarin dosage to 17 mg/day. A 50-year-old woman receiving warfarin 40 mg/week required warfarin dosages of up to 150 mg/week after starting azathioprine 100 mg/day.[3] When azathioprine was withdrawn, her INR was maintained with warfarin 30 mg/week. A 41-year-old woman receiving warfarin 5 mg/day required a dosage of 12 mg/day to reach the target INR after starting azathioprine 150 mg/day.[2] A 25% increase in warfarin dosage was required to achieve a therapeutic INR in a patient receiving a 12-week cycle of mercaptopurine.[8] A reduction in warfarin dosage was needed when the mercaptopurine cycle was completed.

[1] Martini A, et al. *J Pharmacol Exp Ther.* 1977;201(3):547.
[2] Walker J, et al. *J Rheumatol.* 2002;29(2):398.
[3] Rotenberg M, et al. *Ann Pharmacother.* 2000;34(1):120.
[4] Singleton JD, et al. *Am J Med.* 1992;92(2):217.
[5] Rivier G, et al. *Am J Med.* 1993;95(3):342.
[6] Vazquez SR, et al. *Ann Pharmacother.* 2008;42(7):1118.
[7] Spiers AS, et al. *Lancet.* 1974;2(7874):221.
[8] Martin LA, et al. *Pharmacotherapy.* 2003;23(2):260.

* Asterisk indicates drugs cited in interaction reports.

Anticoagulants	***Thyroid Hormones***	
Dicumarol† Warfarin* (eg, *Coumadin*)	Levothyroxine* (eg, *Synthroid*) Liothyronine* (eg, *Cytomel*)	Liotrix (*Thyrolar*) Thyroid (eg, *Armour Thyroid*)

Significance	Onset	Severity	Documentation
1	□ Rapid ■ **Delayed**	■ **Major** □ Moderate □ Minor	□ Established ■ **Probable** □ Suspected □ Possible □ Unlikely

Effects The anticoagulant action of oral ANTICOAGULANTS is amplified during coadministration of THYROID HORMONES.

Mechanism A more rapid disappearance of vitamin K–dependent clotting factors as a result of THYROID HORMONE administration has been proposed, but not clearly established.

Management Closely observe for clinical signs of bleeding and monitor coagulation indices. Oral ANTICOAGULANT doses may need to be decreased during administration of THYROID HORMONES. Conversely, oral ANTICOAGULANT doses may need to be increased if concurrent THYROID HORMONE administration is discontinued.

Discussion

In isolated case reports,[1,2] reductions of maintenance oral anticoagulant doses of 50% to 400% were necessary after initiation of replacement thyroid hormone therapy for severe hypothyroidism. In a case involving a 13-year-old girl,[2] the need for oral anticoagulant dosage adjustment became apparent after she presented with a subdural hematoma and subarachnoid hemorrhage. Consistent with these findings have been cases of excessive hypoprothrombinemic responses to oral anticoagulants in thyrotoxic patients.[3,4] In a study involving 7 subjects with myxedema,[5] the anticoagulant response to a single 40 mg/m^2 dose was markedly enhanced after 3 to 6 months of thyroid replacement therapy. No changes in warfarin pharmacokinetic indices were recorded, suggesting that the mechanism of this interaction is more likely caused by metabolic changes as a result of thyroid hormone administration. Disappearance of vitamin K–dependent clotting factors is increased in hyperthyroidism, and, as a result, the hypoprothrombinemic response to oral anticoagulants occurs earlier and to a greater extent than in euthyroidism.[6]

1 Walters MB. *Am J Cardiol.* 1963;11:112.
2 Costigan DC, et al. *Clin Pediatr.* 1984;23(3):172.
3 Vagenakis AG, et al. *Johns Hopkins Med J.* 1972;131(1):69.
4 Self T, et al. *JAMA.* 1975;231(11):1165.
5 Rice AJ, et al. *Am J Med Sci.* 1971;262(4):211.
6 Loeliger EA, et al. *Thromb Diath Haemorrh* 1963;10:267.

* Asterisk indicates drugs cited in interaction reports. Based on pharmacologic and pharmacokinetic considerations, similar interactions may occur with other drugs that are listed.
† Not available in the United States.

Anticoagulants — *Tigecycline*

Warfarin* (eg, *Coumadin*)	Tigecycline* (*Tygacil*)

Significance	Onset	Severity	Documentation
5	☐ Rapid ■ **Delayed**	☐ Major ☐ Moderate ■ **Minor**	☐ Established ☐ Probable ☐ Suspected ■ **Possible** ☐ Unlikely

Effects The anticoagulant effect of WARFARIN may be decreased.

Mechanism A decrease in the fraction of unbound warfarin (ie, an increase in protein binding) is suspected.

Management Based on available information, no special precautions are needed. Routine monitoring of WARFARIN anticoagulant activity is recommended.

Discussion

The potential for an interaction between tigecycline and warfarin was evaluated in 8 healthy men.[1] In an open-label, nonrandomized study, each subject received a single oral dose of warfarin 25 mg alone and after 5 days of treatment with IV tigecycline (100 mg loading dose followed by 50 mg every 12 hours). Warfarin is a racemic mixture of S- and R-warfarin. The S-warfarin enantiomer has greater anticoagulant activity. Warfarin did not affect the pharmacokinetics of tigecycline. However, pretreatment with tigecycline increased the AUC of R- and S-warfarin 68% and 29%, respectively, and decreased the clearance 40% and 23%, respectively, compared with giving warfarin alone. The t½ of R-warfarin was increased 61%. Tigecycline did not alter the anticoagulant effect of warfarin.

[1] Zimmerman JJ, et al. *Pharmacotherapy*. 2008;28(7):895.

* Asterisk indicates drugs cited in interaction reports.

Anticoagulants — *Tolterodine*

Warfarin* (eg, *Coumadin*)	Tolterodine* (*Detrol*)

Significance	Onset	Severity	Documentation
4	☐ Rapid	☐ Major	☐ Established
	■ **Delayed**	■ **Moderate**	☐ Probable
		☐ Minor	☐ Suspected
			■ **Possible**
			☐ Unlikely

Effects The anticoagulant effect of WARFARIN may be increased.

Mechanism Unknown.

Management Closely monitor anticoagulant parameters when starting or stopping TOLTERODINE therapy in patients receiving WARFARIN. Adjust the WARFARIN dose as needed. Counsel the patient to look for signs and symptoms of bleeding during concurrent use of these agents.

Discussion

Prolonged INRs were reported in 2 patients following the addition of tolterodine to their warfarin regimen.[1] Both patients were receiving stable dosages of warfarin 5 mg/day for stroke prophylaxis in association with atrial fibrillation. Tolterodine 2 mg/day was started in both patients for urinary disorders. One patient received a 56-day course of levofloxacin (*Levaquin*) therapy for prostatitis, which was completed 1 week prior to the start of tolterodine. Minor fluctuations in the INR were noted during this course of therapy. It was only necessary to withhold 1 dose of warfarin near the completion of levofloxacin therapy. Other medications the patients were receiving remained unchanged. In 1 patient, the INR increased from 3.1 to 6.1 during 14 days of tolterodine therapy. The patient discontinued tolterodine the day before a routine clinic visit because of a lack of benefit. Warfarin therapy was withheld for 3 consecutive doses, resulting in an INR of 1.2. In the second patient, the INR increased from a range of 1.5 to 2 to 7.4 after 8 days of tolterodine therapy. That patient stopped taking tolterodine 2 days prior to his clinic visit because the drug was not controlling his urinary symptoms. Three dosages of warfarin 5 mg/day were withheld, and the INR returned to 1.8. In both patients, warfarin was restarted and produced INR values similar to those determined prior to tolterodine administration.

[1] Colucci VJ, et al. *Ann Pharmacother.* 1999;33(11):1173.

* Asterisk indicates drugs cited in interaction reports.

Anticoagulants — *Tramadol*

Anticoagulants	Tramadol
Warfarin* (eg, *Coumadin*)	Tramadol* (eg, *Ultram*)

Significance	Onset	Severity	Documentation
2	☐ Rapid ■ **Delayed**	☐ Major ■ **Moderate** ☐ Minor	☐ Established ☐ Probable ■ **Suspected** ☐ Possible ☐ Unlikely

Effects The effect of the oral ANTICOAGULANT may be increased.

Mechanism Unknown.

Management Carefully monitor coagulation values when TRAMADOL is started or stopped. Adjust the ANTICOAGULANT dose as needed.

Discussion

Increased anticoagulant effects of warfarin[1-3] and bleeding have been reported.[1] A 61-year-old woman receiving warfarin after mitral valve replacement experienced extensive bruising following the addition of tramadol to her treatment regimen.[1] The patient complained of a 1-day history of a large ecchymosis covering approximately 35% of the surface of her upper arm. Her current therapy consisted of warfarin 5 mg 3 times a week and 7.5 mg 4 times a week, which had not been changed during the preceding 3 months. Approximately 2 weeks prior to the bruising episode, the patient was started on tramadol 50 mg every 6 hours for musculoskeletal pain. She continued this dosage until 2 to 3 days prior to the occurrence of the ecchymosis. The PT was 39.6 seconds, and the INR was 10.6. Because therapy with tramadol had been completed, warfarin therapy was stopped until the INR returned to the therapeutic range. Within 3 days, warfarin was resumed at 5 mg/day and, while monitoring the INR, the dose of warfarin was gradually increased from 2.5 to 5 mg weekly to the dose she had been receiving before tramadol therapy was initiated. A 76-year-old man receiving warfarin 5 mg/day was prescribed tramadol 50 mg 3 times daily.[2] After 1 month, his INR had increased from 3.5 to 7.31. The INR returned to the initial range after temporarily stopping warfarin and discontinuing tramadol. A 65-year-old man stabilized on warfarin 60 mg/week was started on tramadol 50 mg twice daily.[3] The INR increased from 2.5 to 6.14 with no signs of bleeding. Therapy with warfarin plus tramadol was successfully continued after a 30% reduction in the warfarin dose.

[1] Sabbe JR, et al. *Pharmacotherapy.* 1998;18:871.
[2] Scher ML, et al. *Ann Pharmacother.* 1997;31:646
[3] Dumo PA, et al. *Pharmacotherapy.* 2006;26:1654.

* Asterisk indicates drugs cited in interaction reports.

Anticoagulants — *Trastuzumab*

Warfarin* (eg, *Coumadin*)	Trastuzumab* (*Herceptin*)

Significance	Onset	Severity	Documentation
4	☐ Rapid	☐ Major	☐ Established
	■ **Delayed**	■ **Moderate**	☐ Probable
		☐ Minor	☐ Suspected
			■ **Possible**
			☐ Unlikely

Effects The risk of bleeding may be increased.

Mechanism Unknown.

Management Monitor anticoagulant parameters when starting or stopping TRASTUZUMAB and adjust the ANTICOAGULANT dose.

Discussion

Hypoprothrombinemia was reported in 2 patients with locally advanced breast cancer when trastuzumab was added to their warfarin regimen.[1] One patient had been receiving warfarin 5 and 7.5 mg on alternate days for approximately 9 years (INR range, 2.1 to 2.8). The patient was started on IV trastuzumab (loading dose 4 mg/kg, then 2 mg/kg weekly) when an enlarged axillary soft tissue mass was found to overexpress HER2/neu. The patient experienced severe epistaxis after 10 doses of trastuzumab (PT, 27 seconds; INR, 6). The second patient had been treated with induction chemotherapy after mastectomy, radiation, and 8 additional chemotherapy cycles. Six months later, the patient was treated with additional chemotherapy and autologous stem-cell transplantation for pulmonary metastases. During the transplant, superior vena cava syndrome and a right axillary vein thrombosis required administration of heparin and warfarin. Subsequently, the patient was discharged from the hospital on warfarin 7 mg/day (INR range, 2.2 to 2.6). Her original tumor was found to strongly overexpress HER2/neu, and the patient was treated with trastuzumab. The patient reported bruising, epistaxis, and bleeding for several minutes after clipping her nails following 8 doses of trastuzumab (PT, 24 seconds; INR, 5.8). Both patients were treated with fresh frozen plasma and vitamin K, and warfarin was discontinued. In the first patient, warfarin was restarted at a reduced dose.

The manufacturer of trastuzumab conducted a search on a large patient database in which 469 women with HER2-overexpressing metastatic breast cancer treated for the first time for metastatic disease were randomized to receive chemotherapy with and without trastuzumab.[2] More patients were treated with trastuzumab plus chemotherapy than chemotherapy alone and for a longer period, allowing more opportunities for bleeding events to be reported. Mild to moderate severe bleeding occurred, and nosebleeds were the most common complication. The rates of bleeding events were similar for patients receiving chemotherapy with and without trastuzumab and with or without anticoagulants.

[1] Nissenblatt MJ, et al. *JAMA*. 1999;282:2299.

[2] Stewart SJ. *JAMA*. 1999;282:2300.

* Asterisk indicates drugs cited in interaction reports.

Anticoagulants × *Trazodone*

Anticoagulants	Trazodone
Warfarin* (eg, *Coumadin*)	Trazodone*

Significance	Onset	Severity	Documentation
2	☐ Rapid	☐ Major	☐ Established
	■ **Delayed**	■ **Moderate**	☐ Probable
		☐ Minor	■ **Suspected**
			☐ Possible
			☐ Unlikely

Effects The hypoprothrombinemic effect of WARFARIN may be decreased. Suboptimal anticoagulation with possible exacerbation of the disease being treated may occur.

Mechanism Unknown.

Management Monitor ANTICOAGULANT parameters frequently when starting or stopping TRAZODONE and be prepared to adjust ANTICOAGULANT dose. Avoid as-needed use of TRAZODONE in patients receiving ANTICOAGULANTS.

Discussion

A case report suggests that trazodone may reduce the anticoagulant effect of warfarin.[1,2] A 40-year-old woman receiving warfarin 6.4 mg/day following a mitral valve replacement was treated with trazodone for severe depression.[1] Coinciding with an increase in trazodone dosage, the PT and partial thromboplastin time decreased 30% and 18%, respectively. These parameters returned to their initial values when the daily dose of the anticoagulant was increased to 7.5 mg. When trazodone was discontinued, the warfarin dose was decreased to 6.4 mg/day. Retrospective chart review of 75 patients receiving warfarin and trazodone concurrently identified 3 patients with a probable interaction.[2] In 2 cases, addition of trazodone 50 or 100 mg at bedtime resulted in a reduction of INR and PT while on a stable warfarin regimen. Trazodone was continued in both patients and the warfarin dose was increased (ie, from 40 to 50 mg/wk in the patient receiving trazodone 100 mg; 45 to 65 mg/wk in the patient receiving trazodone 50 mg) to regain anticoagulant control. The third patient had stopped taking trazodone and the INR and PT increased, necessitating a reduction in the warfarin dose. The INR and PT decreased when trazodone was resumed. A 65-year-old man with pulmonary thromboembolism was stabilized on warfarin.[3] His INR ranged between 2 and 3. Subsequently, he was prescribed trazodone and fish oil (omega-3 fatty acids), and he later presented to the emergency department with an INR and PT of 6.08 and 36 seconds, respectively. All medications were stopped and his INR returned to normal within 2 days. Warfarin was restarted at the previous dose while the other drugs were not resumed. His INR was within the desired range 2 weeks later. See Anticoagulants-Omega-3-Acid Ethyl Esters.

[1] Hardy JL, et al. *CMAJ* 1986;135(12):1372.
[2] Small NL, et al. *Ann Pharmacother* 2000;34(6):734.
[3] Jalili M, et al. *Arch Med Res.* 2007;38(8):901.

* Asterisk indicates drugs cited in interaction reports.

Anticoagulants ✕ *Tricyclic Antidepressants*

Anticoagulants	Tricyclic Antidepressants	
Dicumarol*†	Amitriptyline*	Imipramine (eg, *Tofranil*)
	Amoxapine	Nortriptyline* (eg, *Pamelor*)
	Clomipramine (eg, *Anafranil*)	Protriptyline (eg, *Vivactil*)
	Desipramine (eg, *Norpramin*)	Trimipramine (*Surmontil*)
	Doxepin (eg, *Sinequan*)	

Significance	Onset	Severity	Documentation
2	☐ Rapid	☐ Major	☐ Established
	■ **Delayed**	■ **Moderate**	☐ Probable
		☐ Minor	■ **Suspected**
			☐ Possible
			☐ Unlikely

Effects TRICYCLIC ANTIDEPRESSANTS (TCAs) may increase the t½ or bioavailability of DICUMAROL, possibly resulting in increased anticoagulation actions.

Mechanism Impairment of DICUMAROL's liver degradation by the TCA is possible. Increased DICUMAROL absorption may also be involved.

Management Monitor PTs and observe patients for signs of bleeding. The dose of DICUMAROL may need to be decreased.

Discussion

In 1 study, 6 volunteers received a single dose of dicumarol 4 mg/kg after 8 days of nortriptyline 0.2 mg/kg 3 times daily.[1] Nortriptyline prolonged the t½ of dicumarol from 35.3 to 105.7 hours. In another study, a single dose of dicumarol 200 mg was taken after 9 days of amitriptyline or nortriptyline in 4 subjects.[2] The bioavailability of dicumarol was increased, which was associated with a prolongation of its t½. The t½ of warfarin was not affected by amitriptyline or nortriptyline in 1 study involving 12 subjects.[2] It is not known if anisindione[†] would interact with TCAs.

[1] Vesell ES, et al. *N Engl J Med.* 1970;283(27):1484.

[2] Pond SM, et al. *Clin Pharmacol Ther.* 1975;18(2):191.

* Asterisk indicates drugs cited in interaction reports. Based on pharmacologic and pharmacokinetic considerations, similar interactions may occur with other drugs that are listed.

† Not available in the United States.

Anticoagulants		*Thiazolinediones*
Warfarin* (eg, *Coumadin*)	Pioglitazone* (eg, *Actos*) Rosiglitazone* (*Avandia*)	Troglitazone*†

Significance	Onset	Severity	Documentation
4	☐ Rapid ■ **Delayed**	■ **Major** ☐ Moderate ☐ Minor	☐ Established ☐ Probable ☐ Suspected ■ **Possible** ☐ Unlikely

Effects The effect of the oral ANTICOAGULANT may be increased or decreased.

Mechanism Unknown.

Management Carefully monitor coagulation parameters when THIAZOLIDINEDIONE therapy is started or stopped. Adjust the ANTICOAGULANT dose as needed.

Discussion

Data are conflicting.[1,2] A possible drug interaction was reported in a 51-year-old man during coadministration of warfarin and troglitazone.[1] The patient was admitted to the hospital for a repeat femoral-popliteal arterial bypass graft. He had received a mechanical aortic valve 18 years previously, and at the time of admission he was receiving warfarin 45 mg weekly to prevent thromboembolism. Troglitazone 200 mg daily for 2 weeks followed by 400 mg daily was started to improve control of the patient's diabetes. Five days before initiating troglitazone therapy, the patient's INR was 3.3, and 22 days later the INR had increased to 5.5. When the dose of warfarin was reduced to 32.5 mg weekly, the INR decreased to 2.8. The patient was maintained at this dose of warfarin while receiving troglitazone 400 mg daily. During the suspected interaction, he did not experience bleeding or increased bruising. Decreased INR was reported in 2 patients well controlled on long-term warfarin therapy.[2] One patient, an 84-year-old woman, was receiving a maintenance dose of warfarin (goal INR, 2 to 3) for approximately 1 year when pioglitazone 15 mg daily was started. Approximately 12 weeks after starting pioglitazone, the INR was 1.2. Subsequently, it was necessary to increase the warfarin dose from 8.5 to 16 mg/wk to maintain the INR from 1.9 to 3.2. The second patient, a 76-year-old man, was receiving a maintenance dose of warfarin (goal INR, 1.5 to 2) for approximately 18 months when rosiglitazone 4 mg daily was started. By week 4, the INR was 1.1. A therapeutic INR was achieved after the warfarin dose was increased from 24 to 42 mg/wk. At this warfarin dose the INR was maintained at 1.7 to 2.6.

[1] Plowman BK, et al. *Am J Health Syst Pharm.* 1998;55(10):1071.

[2] Hoffmann TK, et al. *Ann Pharmacother.* 2006;40(5):994.

* Asterisk indicates drugs cited in interaction reports.
† Not available in the United States.

Anticoagulants — *Ubiquinone*

Anticoagulants	Ubiquinone
Warfarin* (eg, *Coumadin*)	Ubiquinone* (Coenzyme Q_{10})

Significance	Onset	Severity	Documentation
4	☐ Rapid ■ **Delayed**	☐ Major ■ **Moderate** ☐ Minor	☐ Established ☐ Probable ☐ Suspected ■ **Possible** ☐ Unlikely

Effects The anticoagulant effects of WARFARIN may be reduced.

Mechanism Unknown; however, UBIQUINONE is closely related to vitamin K,[1] which reduces the action of WARFARIN.

Management Because WARFARIN has a narrow therapeutic index, avoid concomitant use of UBIQUINONE. If combined use cannot be avoided, monitor INR more frequently and be prepared to adjust the WARFARIN dose when UBIQUINONE is started or stopped.

Discussion

There have been reports of 3 patients who experienced a decrease in their INR after ubiquinone was added to their warfarin regimen.[2] Two patients had been receiving warfarin therapy for several years before starting ubiquinone. All patients experienced a drop in INR after starting ubiquinone, which reversed when ubiquinone was stopped. However, in a double-blind, placebo-controlled, crossover study, no changes in INR or weekly warfarin dose were reported in 21 patients receiving stable warfarin doses and given coenzyme Q_{10} (100 mg daily) or placebo for 4 weeks.

The ingredients of many herbal products are not standardized. It is unclear if herbal products contain ingredients other than those listed on the label or purported to be present that could interact with anticoagulants.

[1] Engelsen J, et al. *Thromb Haemost.* 2002;87(6):1075. [2] Spigset O. *Lancet.* 1994;344(8933):1372.

* Asterisk indicates drugs cited in interaction reports.

Anticoagulants — *Valproic Acid*

Anticoagulants	Valproic Acid	
Warfarin* (eg, *Coumadin*)	Divalproex Sodium* (eg, *Depakote*)	Valproic Acid* (eg, *Depakene*)
	Valproate Sodium* (eg, *Depacon*)	

Significance	Onset	Severity	Documentation
4	☐ Rapid	☐ Major	☐ Established
	■ **Delayed**	■ **Moderate**	☐ Probable
		☐ Minor	☐ Suspected
			■ **Possible**
			☐ Unlikely

Effects The hypoprothrombinemic effect of WARFARIN may be transiently increased.

Mechanism Possible displacement of WARFARIN from its protein-binding sites by VALPROIC ACID.

Management Consider monitoring the patient for increased anticoagulant response to WARFARIN during the first week of concurrent therapy.

Discussion

A case of a transient increase in the response to warfarin has been reported in a 68-year-old female patient.[1] While receiving ibuprofen (eg, *Motrin*) 400 to 800 mg/day and warfarin 2.5 and 5 mg on alternate days, the patient's PT ratio stabilized between 1.5 and 2, and her INR stabilized between 2.5 and 3.5. Fluphenazine 5 mg once daily and valproic acid 250 mg twice daily were added to the patient's regimen. The PT ratio increased to 2, and INR increased to 3.9 on the morning after her first dose of valproic acid. The patient's warfarin dosage underwent numerous adjustments to maintain the PT ratio and INR within the desired range. When the patient was discharged from the hospital, her PT ratio and INR were stable on a drug regimen that consisted of valproic acid 500 mg twice daily, fluphenazine 5 mg/day, and warfarin 2.5 and 5 mg on alternate days. A 71-year-old woman receiving long-term warfarin therapy experienced a rapid increase in INR (from 3.4 to 7.6) following an IV loading dose of valproic acid.[2] No new major bleeding occurred; however, vitamin K was used to reverse anticoagulation. A 42-year-old woman receiving divalproex 1,000 mg daily underwent a mechanical heart valve replacement and was started on warfarin 2.5 mg daily.[3] By day 4, the INR was 5.4 and she was treated with frozen plasma.

[1] Guthrie SK, et al. *J Clin Psychopharmacol.* 1995;15(2):138.
[2] Yoon HW, et al. *Neurocrit Care.* 2011;15(1):182.
[3] Nadkarni A, et al. *J Card Surg.* 2011;26(5):492.

* Asterisk indicates drugs cited in interaction reports.

Anticoagulants — *Vitamin E*

Anisindione (*Miradon*)	Warfarin* (eg, *Coumadin*)	Vitamin E*

Significance	Onset	Severity	Documentation
1	☐ Rapid	■ **Major**	☐ Established
	■ **Delayed**	☐ Moderate	☐ Probable
		☐ Minor	■ **Suspected**
			☐ Possible
			☐ Unlikely

Effects The action of oral ANTICOAGULANTS may be increased by coadministration of VITAMIN E.

Mechanism VITAMIN E may interfere with vitamin K–dependent clotting factors, thereby adding to the effects of oral ANTICOAGULANTS.

Management Closely observe for signs of an excessive hypoprothrombinemic response to oral ANTICOAGULANTS and monitor coagulation indices during coadministration of VITAMIN E. Lower ANTICOAGULANT doses may be required.

Discussion

A patient who had been stabilized on a maintenance dose of warfarin presented with a markedly prolonged PT and bleeding 2 months after self-initiating vitamin E supplementation (1,200 units/day or less).[1,2] After stabilization, the patient was rechallenged with vitamin E 800 units/day. Within 6 weeks, the PT became progressively prolonged, vitamin K–dependent clotting factors decreased, and bleeding recurred. It has been suggested that doses of vitamin E more than 400 units/day are necessary for this additive hypoprothrombinemic effect to occur.[3,4]

1 Corrigan JJ Jr., et al. *JAMA*. 1974;230(9):1300.
2 *Nutr Rev*. 1982;40(6):180.
3 Schrogie JJ. *JAMA*. 1975;232(1):19.
4 Corrigan JJ, et al. *Am J Clin Nutr*. 1981;34(9):1701.

* Asterisk indicates drugs cited in interaction reports. Based on pharmacologic and pharmacokinetic considerations, similar interactions may occur with other drugs that are listed.

Anticoagulants — Vitamin K

Anticoagulants	Vitamin K
Warfarin* (eg, *Coumadin*)	Vitamin K*

Significance	Onset	Severity	Documentation
2	☐ Rapid	☐ Major	■ **Established**
	■ **Delayed**	■ **Moderate**	☐ Probable
		☐ Minor	☐ Suspected
			☐ Possible
			☐ Unlikely

Effects Oral ANTICOAGULANT action is attenuated or reversed, leading to possible thrombus formation. Decreased VITAMIN K intake may increase the effect of ANTICOAGULANTS.

Mechanism VITAMIN K may inhibit the effect of WARFARIN on VITAMIN K–dependent clotting factors.

Management Avoid or minimize variable consumption of foods or nutritional supplements containing VITAMIN K. Monitor coagulation indices and observe for signs of thrombus formation or bleeding during variable VITAMIN K ingestion. Oral ANTICOAGULANT doses may need to be altered.

Discussion

Vitamin K interferes with the hypoprothrombinemic effect of oral anticoagulants.[1] Resistance to oral anticoagulants linked to the vitamin K content in foods, green tea,[2] black tea,[3] and nutritional supplements has been reported.[4-21] Response to oral anticoagulants is usually regained after discontinuation of vitamin K–containing products. However, administration of vitamin K for anticoagulation reversal may cause transient warfarin resistance for up to 3.5 weeks.[22] Diets high or low in vitamin K alter INR in anticoagulated patients.[23] Serious clinical consequences have been reported rarely. In 1 case, coronary artery thromboemboli and acute MI were attributed to the loss of the hypoprothrombinemic response to warfarin during enteral feeding with a vitamin K–containing product.[14] In another case, thrombosis of an aortic valve prosthesis occurred.[18] Snacks containing *Olestra* have vitamin K 80 mg/oz of snack food.[24] Reduction of vitamin K dietary intake in a patient previously stabilized with warfarin resulted in bleeding complications associated with marked INR elevation. A daily warfarin dose reduction was necessary to maintain a therapeutic INR.

1 Andersen P, et al. *Acta Med Scand.* 1975;198(4):269.
2 Taylor JR, et al. *Ann Pharmacother.* 1999;33(4):426.
3 Parker DL, et al. *Ann Pharmacother.* 2009;43(1):150.
4 O'Reilly RA, et al. *N Engl J Med.* 1980;303(3):160.
5 Lader E, et al. *Ann Intern Med.* 1980;93(2):373.
6 Michaelson R, et al. *Clin Bull.* 1980;10(4):171.
7 Westfall LK. *Drug Intell Clin Pharm.* 1981;15(2):131.
8 Lee M, et al. *Ann Intern Med.* 1981;94(1):140.
9 Zallman JA, et al. *Am J Hosp Pharm.* 1981;38(8):1174.
10 Parr MD, et al. *Clin Pharm.* 1982;1(3):274.
11 Griffith LD, et al. *Crit Care Med.* 1982;10(11):799.
12 Kempin SJ. *N Engl J Med.* 1983;308(20):1229.
13 Watson AJ, et al. *Br Med J (Clin Res Ed).* 1984;288(6416):557.
14 Walker FB IV. *Arch Intern Med.* 1984;144(10):2089.
15 Howard PA, et al. *J Am Diet Assoc.* 1985;85(6):713.
16 Karlson B, et al. *Acta Med Scand.* 1986;220(4):347.
17 Martin JE, et al. *JPEN J Parenter Enteral Nutr.* 1989;13(2):206.
18 Chow WH, et al. *Postgrad Med J.* 1990;66(780):855.
19 Pedersen FM, et al. *J Intern Med.* 1991;229(6):517.
20 Kurnik D, et al. *Thromb Haemost.* 2004;92(5):1018.
21 Ducharlet KN, et al. *Australas J Aging.* 2011;30(1):41.
22 Fugate SE, et al. *Pharmacotherapy.* 2004;24(9):1213.
23 Franco V, et al. *Am J Med.* 2004;116(10):651.
24 Harrell CC, et al. *JAMA.* 1999;282(12):1133.

* Asterisk indicates drugs cited in interaction reports.

Antineoplastic Agents — *Thiazide Diuretics*

Antineoplastic Agents		Thiazide Diuretics	
Cyclophosphamide*	Methotrexate* (eg, *Rheumatrex*)	Bendroflumethiazide	Indapamide
Fluorouracil* (eg, *Adrucil*)		Chlorothiazide* (eg, *Diuril*)	Methyclothiazide
		Chlorthalidone* (eg, *Thalitone*)	Metolazone (eg, *Zaroxolyn*)
		Hydrochlorothiazide* (eg, *Microzide*)	Polythiazide
		Hydroflumethiazide	Trichlormethiazide*

Significance	Onset	Severity	Documentation
4	☐ Rapid	☐ Major	☐ Established
	■ **Delayed**	■ **Moderate**	☐ Probable
		☐ Minor	☐ Suspected
			■ **Possible**
			☐ Unlikely

Effects THIAZIDES may prolong antineoplastic-induced leukopenia.

Mechanism Unknown.

Management Consider alternative antihypertensive therapy in patients receiving this combination of chemotherapy.

Discussion

In 14 women with breast cancer and leukopenia, granulocyte counts rose more slowly when thiazides were taken concurrently with antineoplastic therapy.[1] All patients received a combination of cyclophosphamide 600 mg/m^2, methotrexate 50 mg/m^2, and 5-fluorouracil 500 mg/m^2 administered IV every 21 days. Thiazides were administered daily to each of these patients for 3 cycles of chemotherapy, discontinued for 3 cycles, and then reinstituted. The granulocyte count was lower during thiazide therapy than without thiazides.

[1] Orr, LE. *Drug Intell Clin Pharm.* 1981;15(12):967.

* Asterisk indicates drugs cited in interaction reports. Based on pharmacologic and pharmacokinetic considerations, similar interactions may occur with other drugs that are listed.

Apomorphine / Selective 5-HT3 Receptor Antagonists

Apomorphine	Selective 5-HT3 Receptor Antagonists	
Apomorphine* (*Apokyn*)	Alosetron* (*Lotronex*)	Ondansetron* (eg, *Zofran*)
	Dolasetron* (*Anzemet*)	Palonosetron* (*Aloxi*)
	Granisetron* (eg, *Kytril*)	

Significance	Onset	Severity	Documentation
2	■ **Rapid**	□ Major	□ Established
	□ Delayed	■ **Moderate**	□ Probable
		□ Minor	■ **Suspected**
			□ Possible
			□ Unlikely

Effects The risk of profound hypotension and loss of consciousness may be increased.

Mechanism Unknown.

Management Coadministration of APOMORPHINE and SELECTIVE 5-HT$_3$ RECEPTOR (5-HT$_3$) ANTAGONISTS is contraindicated.

Discussion

Profound hypotension and loss of consciousness have been reported with concomitant use of apomorphine and ondansetron. Therefore, the concurrent use of apomorphine with 5-HT$_3$ antagonists is contraindicated.[1]

The basis for this monograph is information on file with the manufacturer. Published clinical data are needed to further assess this interaction.

[1] *Apokyn* [package insert]. Brisbane, CA: Ipsen Group; July 2010.

* Asterisk indicates drugs cited in interaction reports.

Aripiprazole — *Azole Antifungal Agents*

Aripiprazole	Azole Antifungal Agents	
Aripiprazole* (*Abilify*)	Fluconazole (eg, *Diflucan*)	Posaconazole (*Noxafil*)
	Itraconazole* (eg, *Sporanox*)	Voriconazole (eg, *Vfend*)
	Ketoconazole* (eg, *Nizoral*)	

Significance	Onset	Severity	Documentation
2	☐ Rapid	☐ Major	☐ Established
	■ **Delayed**	■ **Moderate**	☐ Probable
		☐ Minor	■ **Suspected**
			☐ Possible
			☐ Unlikely

Effects ARIPIPRAZOLE plasma concentrations may be elevated, increasing the pharmacologic effects and adverse reactions.

Mechanism Certain AZOLE ANTIFUNGAL AGENTS may inhibit the hepatic metabolism (CYP3A4) of ARIPIPRAZOLE.

Management When KETOCONAZOLE or ITRACONAZOLE are coadministered with ARIPIPRAZOLE, reduce the ARIPIPRAZOLE dose to 50% of the normal dose. When the AZOLE ANTIFUNGAL AGENT is discontinued, increase the dose of ARIPIPRAZOLE.[1]

Discussion

Aripiprazole has been evaluated in premarketing clinical trials using double-blind, comparative and noncomparative, open-label studies.[2] Coadministration of ketoconazole 200 mg daily for 14 days with a single dose of aripiprazole 15 mg increased the AUC of aripiprazole and its active metabolite 63% and 77%, respectively.[1] Itraconazole can be expected to have a similar effect on aripiprazole.[1] In a pharmacokinetic study, 27 healthy men were given itraconazole 100 mg daily for 21 days and aripiprazole 3 mg on days 8 to 21.[3] Itraconazole increased aripiprazole plasma concentrations and prolonged the $t_{1/2}$ from 65 to 78 hours.

1 *Abilify* [package insert]. Princeton, NJ: Bristol-Myers Squibb Company; May 2004.

2 Cha YJ, et al. Written communication. Bristol-Myers Squibb Company; September 30, 2004.

3 Koue T, et al. *Biol Pharm Bull.* 2007;30(11):2154.

* Asterisk indicates drugs cited in interaction reports. Based on pharmacologic and pharmacokinetic considerations, similar interactions may occur with other drugs that are listed.

Aripiprazole — *Carbamazepine*

Aripiprazole* (*Abilify*)

Carbamazepine* (eg, *Tegretol*)

Significance	Onset	Severity	Documentation
2	☐ Rapid ■ **Delayed**	☐ Major ■ **Moderate** ☐ Minor	☐ Established ☐ Probable ■ **Suspected** ☐ Possible ☐ Unlikely

Effects ARIPIPRAZOLE plasma concentrations may be reduced, decreasing the pharmacologic effects.

Mechanism CARBAMAZEPINE may induce the hepatic metabolism (CYP3A4) of ARIPIPRAZOLE.

Management When CARBAMAZEPINE is added to ARIPIPRAZOLE therapy, double the ARIPIPRAZOLE dosage.[1,2] Make additional dosage adjustments based on clinical evaluation. When CARBAMAZEPINE is discontinued, decrease the dosage of ARIPIPRAZOLE.[1]

Discussion

According to the manufacturer of aripiprazole, the drug was evaluated in premarketing clinical trials using double-blind, comparative and noncomparative, open-label studies.[2] Coadministration of carbamazepine 200 mg twice daily with a single dose of aripiprazole 30 mg decreased the C_{max} and AUC of aripiprazole and its active metabolite, dehydro-aripiprazole, approximately 70%.[1] In an open-label pharmacokinetic study, the effects of carbamazepine on aripiprazole were evaluated in 6 men with schizophrenia or schizoaffective disorder.[3] Subjects received aripiprazole 30 mg daily for 14 days, and then carbamazepine (titrated to 8 to 12 mg/L) was started. The addition of carbamazepine decreased aripiprazole AUC and C_{max} 71% and 66%, respectively, compared with aripiprazole monotherapy. Similarly, in 18 patients with schizophrenia, coadministration of carbamazepine for 1 week decreased mean aripiprazole levels 64%.[4] There was no worsening of schizophrenia symptoms.

1 *Abilify* [package insert]. Princeton, NJ: Bristol-Myers Squibb Company; May 2004.

2 Cha YJ, et al. Written communication. Bristol-Myers Squibb Company; September 2004.

3 Citrome L, et al. *J Clin Psychopharmacol.* 2007;27(3):279.

4 Nakamura A, et al. *Ther Drug Monit.* 2009;31(5):575.

* Asterisk indicates drugs cited in interaction reports.

Aripiprazole — *Haloperidol*

Aripiprazole* (*Abilify*)	Haloperidol* (eg, *Haldol*)

Significance	Onset	Severity	Documentation
4	☐ Rapid	☐ Major	☐ Established
	■ **Delayed**	■ **Moderate**	☐ Probable
		☐ Minor	☐ Suspected
			■ **Possible**
			☐ Unlikely

Effects Both worsening and improvement in psychotic symptoms have been reported.

Mechanism The dopamine D_2 agonist properties of ARIPIPRAZOLE may interfere with dopamine D_2 antagonist properties of HALOPERIDOL.

Management Closely monitor the clinical response of patients during coadministration of ARIPIPRAZOLE and HALOPERIDOL. Be prepared to adjust therapy as needed.

Discussion

Both worsening[1] and improvement[2] of schizophrenic symptoms have been reported with coadministration of aripiprazole and haloperidol. A 30-year-old man with schizophrenia was hospitalized with poorly controlled psychotic symptoms (eg, paranoia associated with aggressive outbursts).[1] At admission, the patient had been taking aripiprazole 10 mg/day and haloperidol 5 mg twice daily for about 3 weeks. The aripiprazole dosage was increased to 30 mg/day; however, the patient became more paranoid and aggressive. The dosage of haloperidol was increased to 10 mg twice daily for 4 days. There was marginal improvement in his psychotic symptoms and an absence of extrapyramidal symptoms. A pharmacodynamic interaction was suspected and aripiprazole was discontinued. Over the next 4 days, the patient's psychotic symptoms and agitation improved, and he was discharged. In another report, when a 41-year-old man with schizophrenia and poorly controlled psychotic symptoms (eg, auditory hallucinations, delusions of persecution) did not achieve full recovery from his psychosis after aripiprazole 15 mg/day administration, haloperidol 2.5 mg/day was added to his treatment regimen.[2] Complete remission was not achieved, and the dosage of haloperidol was increased to 5 mg/day and then to 7.5 mg/day over the next 3 months. At this time, the auditory hallucinations were gone. The patient was still in remission after 1 year.

[1] Burke MJ, et al. *Ann Clin Psychiatry*. 2006;18(2):129.
[2] Kuo J, et al. *Clin Neuropharmacol*. 2008;31(3):173.

* Asterisk indicates drugs cited in interaction reports.

Aripiprazole — *Lithium*

Aripiprazole* (*Abilify*)	Lithium* (eg, *Lithobid*)

Significance	Onset	Severity	Documentation
4	☐ Rapid ■ **Delayed**	■ **Major** ☐ Moderate ☐ Minor	☐ Established ☐ Probable ☐ Suspected ■ **Possible** ☐ Unlikely

Effects The risk of neuroleptic malignant syndrome (NMS) may be increased.

Mechanism Unknown.

Management Closely monitor patients for adverse reactions. NMS requires immediate medical attention, including withdrawal of therapy, supportive care, and, if needed, treatment with dantrolene (eg, *Dantrium*).

Discussion

Moderate to severe NMS was reported in a patient with bipolar disorder during coadministration of aripiprazole and lithium.[1] The patient was started on valproic acid (eg, *Depakene*) and aripiprazole during his fifth hospitalization in 4 years. Subsequently, the patient was switched from valproic acid to lithium, which was titrated to a dosage of 600 mg twice daily. Aripiprazole 5 mg daily was titrated slowly to 15 mg twice daily. Approximately 3 weeks after admission, the patient complained of weakness, stiff muscles, stiffness in his back, and neck rigidity. He exhibited bilateral tremor in his upper extremities. He was febrile, had labile BP, and displayed a creatine phosphokinase elevation to 7,928 units/L (from 228 units/L). His plasma myoglobin (4.12 ng/mL) was well above the normal range. The patient was diagnosed with NMS. Aripiprazole was discontinued, and lithium was withheld. Over the next 4 days, his physical symptoms improved, and the laboratory values decreased. Lithium was restarted, and the patient was discharged 3 days later.

[1] Ali S, et al. *J Clin Psychopharmacol.* 2006;26(4):434.

* Asterisk indicates drugs cited in interaction reports.

Aripiprazole — *Protease Inhibitors*

Aripiprazole	Protease Inhibitors	
Aripiprazole* (*Abilify*)	Atazanavir (*Reyataz*)	Nelfinavir (*Viracept*)
	Darunavir* (*Prezista*)	Ritonavir* (*Norvir*)
	Fosamprenavir (*Lexiva*)	Saquinavir (*Invirase*)
	Indinavir (*Crixivan*)	Tipranavir (*Aptivus*)
	Lopinavir/Ritonavir (*Kaletra*)	

Significance	Onset	Severity	Documentation
2	☐ Rapid	☐ Major	☐ Established
	■ **Delayed**	■ **Moderate**	☐ Probable
		☐ Minor	■ **Suspected**
			☐ Possible
			☐ Unlikely

Effects ARIPIPRAZOLE plasma concentrations may be elevated, increasing the pharmacologic effects and risk of adverse reactions.

Mechanism Inhibition of ARIPIPRAZOLE metabolism (CYP3A4) by PROTEASE INHIBITORS.

Management Closely monitor the patient and ARIPIPRAZOLE plasma concentrations when a PROTEASE INHIBITOR is coadministered. Be prepared to adjust the ARIPIPRAZOLE dose as needed when a PROTEASE INHIBITOR is started or stopped. When ARIPIPRAZOLE and a strong CYP3A4 inhibitor, such as ritonavir, are given concurrently, consider a 50% reduction in the ARIPIPRAZOLE dose.[1]

Discussion

Strong CYP3A4 inhibitors can decrease aripiprazole metabolism, resulting in increased plasma concentrations.[1] Because ritonavir is a strong CYP3A4 inhibitor, it is anticipated that coadministration of aripiprazole with ritonavir may elevate aripiprazole plasma concentrations and increase the risk of adverse reactions. Increased aripiprazole plasma concentrations were reported in a 43-year-old HIV-positive man who had been receiving darunavir and ritonavir concomitantly.[2] A month after the aripiprazole dose was increased to 50 mg daily, the patient developed confusion and loss of coordination. One week later, he was seen in the emergency department with back pain, blurred vision, cough, fever, headache, and neck stiffness. His symptoms improved with pain control and IV fluids. He was discharged a couple of days after admission. Subsequently, treatment with aripiprazole 50 mg daily, darunavir 800 mg daily, and ritonavir 100 mg daily was reinstated. A random steady-state aripiprazole concentration obtained 49 days after discharge was 1,100 ng/mL (therapeutic concentration 100 to 200 ng/mL).

[1] *Abilify* [package insert]. Princeton, NJ: Bristol-Myers Squibb Company; 2010.

[2] Aung GL, et al. *Ann Pharmacother.* 2010;44(11):1850.

* Asterisk indicates drugs cited in interaction reports. Based on pharmacologic and pharmacokinetic considerations, similar interactions may occur with other drugs that are listed.

Aripiprazole — *Quinidine*

Aripiprazole* (*Abilify*)	Quinidine*

Significance	Onset	Severity	Documentation
2	☐ Rapid ■ **Delayed**	☐ Major ■ **Moderate** ☐ Minor	☐ Established ☐ Probable ■ **Suspected** ☐ Possible ☐ Unlikely

Effects ARIPIPRAZOLE plasma concentrations may be elevated, increasing the pharmacologic effects and adverse reactions.

Mechanism QUINIDINE may inhibit the hepatic metabolism (CYP2D6) of ARIPIPRAZOLE.

Management When QUINIDINE is coadministered with ARIPIPRAZOLE, reduce the ARIPIPRAZOLE dose to 50% of the normal dose. When QUINIDINE is discontinued, increase the dose of ARIPIPRAZOLE.[1]

Discussion

According to the manufacturer of aripiprazole, the drug has been evaluated in premarketing clinical trials using double-blind, comparative and noncomparative, open-label studies.[2] Coadministration of quinidine 166 mg daily for 13 days with a single dose of aripiprazole 10 mg increased the AUC of aripiprazole 112% but decreased the AUC of its active metabolite, dehydro-aripiprazole, 35%.[1]

The basis for this monograph is information on file with the manufacturer. Published clinical data are needed to further assess this interaction.

[1] *Abilify* [package insert]. Princeton, NJ: Bristol-Myers Squibb Company; May 2004.

[2] Cha YJ, et al. Written communication. Bristol-Myers Squibb Company; September 30, 2004.

* Asterisk indicates drugs cited in interaction reports.

Aripiprazole — *Serotonin Reuptake Inhibitors*

Aripiprazole* (*Abilify*)	Escitalopram (eg, *Lexapro*)	Nefazodone
	Fluoxetine (eg, *Prozac*)	Paroxetine* (eg, *Paxil*)
	Fluvoxamine* (eg, *Luvox*)	Sertraline* (eg, *Zoloft*)

Significance	Onset	Severity	Documentation
2	☐ Rapid	☐ Major	☐ Established
	■ **Delayed**	■ **Moderate**	☐ Probable
		☐ Minor	■ **Suspected**
			☐ Possible
			☐ Unlikely

Effects ARIPIPRAZOLE plasma concentrations may be elevated, increasing the pharmacologic effects and adverse reactions.

Mechanism SRIs may inhibit the metabolism (CYP2D6 and/or CYP3A4) of ARIPIPRAZOLE.

Management Monitor the clinical response to ARIPIPRAZOLE when starting or stopping SRIs and adjust the ARIPIPRAZOLE dose as needed.

Discussion

In an open-label study, the effect of fluvoxamine or paroxetine on the pharmacokinetics of aripiprazole was evaluated in 27 healthy men (13 CYP2D6 extensive metabolizers and 14 CYP2D6 intermediate metabolizers).[1] Each subject received aripiprazole 3 mg before and after steady-state plasma concentrations of paroxetine (20 mg daily) or fluvoxamine (100 mg daily) were achieved. Coadministration of paroxetine increased aripiprazole C_{max} and AUC approximately 40% and 136%, respectively, in extensive metabolizers, and approximately 25% and 29%, respectively, in intermediate metabolizers. Fluvoxamine increased the aripiprazole C_{max} and AUC approximately 39% and 63%, respectively, in extensive metabolizers, and approximately 26% and 64%, respectively, in intermediate metabolizers.

[1] Azuma J, et al. *Eur J Clin Pharmacol.* 2012;68(1):29.

* Asterisk indicates drugs cited in interaction reports. Based on pharmacologic and pharmacokinetic considerations, similar interactions may occur with other drugs that are listed.

Aromatase Inhibitors — *Tamoxifen*

Letrozole* (*Femara*)	Tamoxifen* (eg, *Soltamox*)

Significance	Onset	Severity	Documentation
4	☐ Rapid ■ **Delayed**	☐ Major ■ **Moderate** ☐ Minor	☐ Established ☐ Probable ☐ Suspected ■ **Possible** ☐ Unlikely

Effects LETROZOLE plasma concentrations may be reduced, decreasing the antitumor efficacy of LETROZOLE.

Mechanism Induction of LETROZOLE metabolism (CYP3A4) by TAMOXIFEN is suspected.

Management Monitor patient response during coadministration of these agents. Sequential therapy may be preferable to coadministration.

Discussion

The effects of tamoxifen on the pharmacokinetics and pharmacodynamics of letrozole were evaluated in 12 patients with locally advanced or locoregional recurrent or metastatic breast cancer.[1] Patients received letrozole 2.5 mg daily alone for 6 weeks and in combination with tamoxifen 20 mg/day for the subsequent 6 weeks. Compared with administration of letrozole alone, the AUC was decreased almost 38% during coadministration of tamoxifen. The AUC after 6 weeks and after 4 to 8 months of concurrent therapy was the same. However, suppression of estradiol, estrone, and estrone sulfate was not affected by concomitant treatment with letrozole and tamoxifen. Letrozole does not appear to affect the pharmacokinetics of tamoxifen.[2]

[1] Dowsett M, et al. *Clin Cancer Res.* 1999;5(9):2338. [2] Ingle JN, et al. *Clin Cancer Res.* 1999;5(7):1642.

* Asterisk indicates drugs cited in interaction reports.

Artemether — *Food*

Artemether*	Grapefruit Juice*

Significance	Onset	Severity	Documentation
3	☐ Rapid	☐ Major	☐ Established
	■ **Delayed**	☐ Moderate	☐ Probable
		■ **Minor**	■ **Suspected**
			☐ Possible
			☐ Unlikely

Effects GRAPEFRUIT JUICE may increase the bioavailability of ARTEMETHER.

Mechanism Unknown.

Management Based on available data, no special precautions are necessary. Ingestion of ARTEMETHER with GRAPEFRUIT JUICE may increase the activity of ARTEMETHER.

Discussion

A study of the effect of grapefruit juice on the bioavailability of artemether illustrates the occurrence of a possible interaction.[1] The study was a randomized, 2-phase, crossover investigation involving 8 healthy men who took artemether 100 mg with water or double-strength grapefruit juice once daily for 5 days. The mean AUC of artemether and the mean peak plasma concentration after the last dose on day 5 were approximately 33% of that on day 1 (without a change in the elimination $t_{½}$) after ingestion with water and grapefruit juice. Grapefruit juice increased the peak concentration and AUC of artemether 2-fold on day 1 and 5. Four hours after artemether ingestion with water, 3 subjects on day 1 and 6 subjects on day 5 had undetectable artemether blood levels, while with grapefruit juice, none of the subjects on day 1 and 3 subjects on day 5 had undetectable levels. There was a 2-fold increase in the peak concentration and AUC of the artemether active metabolite dihydroartemisinin with grapefruit juice. However, there was no change in the expected time-dependent reduction in bioavailability.

[1] van Agtmael MA, et al. *Clin Pharmacol Ther.* 1999;66(4):408.

* Asterisk indicates drugs cited in interaction reports.

Artemether/Lumefantrine — *Protease Inhibitors*

Artemether/Lumefantrine* (*Coartem*)	Lopinavir/Ritonavir* (*Kaletra*)	Ritonavir (*Norvir*)

Significance	Onset	Severity	Documentation
4	☐ Rapid	☐ Major	☐ Established
	■ **Delayed**	■ **Moderate**	☐ Probable
		☐ Minor	☐ Suspected
			■ **Possible**
			☐ Unlikely

Effects ARTEMETHER/LUMEFANTRINE pharmacologic effects and adverse reactions may be increased.

Mechanism Inhibition of LUMEFANTRINE metabolism by certain PROTEASE INHIBITORS is suspected.

Management Based on available data, no special precautions are needed.

Discussion

In an open-label study, the effects of lopinavir/ritonavir on the pharmacokinetics of artemether/lumefantrine were evaluated in 10 healthy volunteers.[1] Each subject received artemether 80 mg/lumefantrine 480 mg twice daily on days 1 to 4 and 28 to 31. On days 14 to 41, lopinavir 400 mg/ritonavir 100 mg twice daily was administered. Lumefantrine AUC was increased 2- to 3-fold by lopinavir/ritonavir administration. There was a trend toward decreases in artemether C_{max} and AUC that did not reach statistical significance.

Additional studies are needed to determine the clinical importance of this interaction.

[1] German P, et al. *J Acquir Immune Defic Syndr.* 2009;51(4):424.

* Asterisk indicates drugs cited in interaction reports. Based on pharmacologic and pharmacokinetic considerations, similar interactions may occur with other drugs that are listed.

Atazanavir — *Histamine H_2 Antagonists*

Atazanavir* (*Reyataz*)	Cimetidine (eg, *Tagamet*)	Nizatidine (eg, *Axid*)
	Famotidine* (eg, *Pepcid*)	Ranitidine* (eg, *Zantac*)

Significance	Onset	Severity	Documentation
4	□ Rapid	□ Major	□ Established
	■ **Delayed**	■ **Moderate**	□ Probable
		□ Minor	□ Suspected
			■ **Possible**
			□ Unlikely

Effects ATAZANAVIR plasma concentrations may be reduced, which may decrease the efficacy and result in development of resistance.

Mechanism Decreased solubility and GI absorption of ATAZANAVIR due to the increased gastric pH from administration of the HISTAMINE H_2 ANTAGONIST.

Management Administer ATAZANAVIR plus ritonavir (*Norvir*) once daily with food and simultaneously with, and/or at least 10 hours after, the dose of the HISTAMINE H_2 ANTAGONIST.[1]

Discussion

The effects of ranitidine on ritonavir-boosted atazanavir were studied in HIV-negative healthy adults. Subjects received atazanavir 300 mg and ritonavir 100 mg daily for 15 days.[2] On day 11, a single dose of ranitidine 150 mg was administered 1 hour before breakfast, while ritonavir-boosted atazanavir was administered 30 minutes after the start of a moderate-fat meal. Compared with taking ritonavir-boosted atazanavir alone, ranitidine administration reduced the atazanavir AUC 48%. In the same study, a different group of subjects received lopinavir/ritonavir (*Kaletra*) with ranitidine. Neither lopinavir nor ritonavir pharmacokinetics were affected. When atazanavir 400 mg daily was administered simultaneously with famotidine 40 mg twice daily, atazanavir plasma concentrations were substantially decreased.[1] In a survey of electronic medical records at 10 HIV clinics, mean atazanavir trough concentrations were inadequate in 4 of 19 patients receiving histamine H_2 antagonists, even though 2 of the 4 patients were receiving ritonavir-boosted atazanavir.[3]

1 *Reyataz* [package insert]. Princeton, NJ: Bristol-Myers Squibb Company; September 2008.
2 Klein CE, et al. *J Clin Pharmcol.* 2008;48(5):553.
3 Khanlou H, et al. *J Acquir Immune Defic Syndr.* 2005;39(4):503.

* Asterisk indicates drugs cited in interaction reports. Based on pharmacologic and pharmacokinetic considerations, similar interactions may occur with other drugs that are listed.

Atazanavir — *Indinavir*

Atazanavir* (*Reyataz*)	Indinavir* (*Crixivan*)

Significance	Onset	Severity	Documentation
2	☐ Rapid ■ **Delayed**	☐ Major ■ **Moderate** ☐ Minor	☐ Established ☐ Probable ■ **Suspected** ☐ Possible ☐ Unlikely

Effects The risk of hyperbilirubinemia may be increased.

Mechanism Additive or potentiated adverse reactions, leading to hyperbilirubinemia.

Management Coadministration of ATAZANAVIR and INDINAVIR is contraindicated.[1]

Discussion

Atazanavir and indinavir are associated with indirect (unconjugated) hyperbilirubinemia. Because of this potentially serious adverse reaction, the manufacturer of atazanavir states that coadministration of atazanavir and indinavir is contraindicated.[1]

The basis for this monograph is information on file with the manufacturer. Published clinical data are needed to further assess this interaction.

[1] *Reyataz* [package insert]. Princeton, NY: Bristol-Myers Squibb Company; 2008.

* Asterisk indicates drugs cited in interaction reports.

Atazanavir — *Rifamycins*

Atazanavir* (*Reyataz*)	Rifabutin (*Mycobutin*)	Rifapentine* (*Priftin*)
	Rifampin* (eg, *Rifadin*)	

Significance	Onset	Severity	Documentation
2	☐ Rapid	☐ Major	☐ Established
	■ **Delayed**	■ **Moderate**	■ **Probable**
		☐ Minor	☐ Suspected
			☐ Possible
			☐ Unlikely

Effects RIFAMYCINS may reduce ATAZANAVIR plasma concentrations, decreasing the efficacy.

Mechanism RIFAMYCINS may induce the metabolism (CYP3A4) of ATAZANAVIR.

Management Avoid concurrent use of ATAZANAVIR in patients receiving a RIFAMYCIN. If coadministration cannot be avoided, use with extreme caution.

Discussion

The effects of rifampin on the pharmacokinetics of atazanavir were evaluated in an open-label, single-arm study in 10 healthy HIV-negative men.[1] Each subject received atazanavir 300 mg every 12 hours without rifampin, atazanavir 300 mg every 12 hours with rifampin 600 mg every 24 hours, and atazanavir 400 mg every 12 hours with rifampin 600 mg every 24 hours. Compared with administering atazanavir alone, coadministration of rifampin reduced plasma concentrations of atazanavir 300 mg every 12 hours and 400 mg every 12 hours more than 18- and 7-fold, respectively. In both instances, adequate atazanavir plasma exposure was not maintained. In a study in 3 HIV-infected patients with tuberculosis treated with a rifampin-containing regimen and antiretroviral therapy, which included nucleoside reverse transcriptase inhibitors plus atazanavir 300 mg once daily and ritonavir (*Norvir*) 100 mg daily, atazanavir concentrations were subtherapeutic more than 50% of the time.[2] It has been recommended that rifapentine be used with extreme caution, if at all, in patients receiving protease inhibitors.[3] See also Indinavir-Rifamycins, Ritonavir-Rifamycins, and Saquinavir-Rifamycins.

[1] Acosta EP, et al. *Antimicrob Agents Chemother.* 2007;51(9):3104.
[2] Mallolas J, et al. *HIV Med.* 2007;8(2):131.
[3] *Priftin* [package insert]. Bridgewater, NJ: Sanofi-Aventis US LLC; December 2006.

* Asterisk indicates drugs cited in interaction reports. Based on pharmacologic and pharmacokinetic considerations, similar interactions may occur with other drugs that are listed.

Atazanavir — *Tetracyclines*

Atazanavir* (*Reyataz*)	Minocycline* (eg, *Minocin*)

Significance	Onset	Severity	Documentation
4	☐ Rapid	☐ Major	☐ Established
	■ **Delayed**	■ **Moderate**	☐ Probable
		☐ Minor	☐ Suspected
			■ **Possible**
			☐ Unlikely

Effects ATAZANAVIR plasma concentrations may be reduced by MINOCYCLINE, decreasing the pharmacologic effects.

Mechanism Unknown.

Management Until additional information is available, it would be prudent to avoid using MINOCYCLINE in patients receiving ATAZANAVIR.

Discussion

The effect of minocycline on the pharmacokinetics of atazanavir was studied in 12 HIV-infected subjects.[1] Each subject received atazanavir 300 mg/ritonavir 100 mg daily alone and with minocycline 100 mg twice daily. Compared with receiving atazanavir/ritonavir alone, coadministration of minocycline reduced the atazanavir AUC, C_{min}, and C_{max} by 37%, 50%, and 25%, respectively. Minocycline did not alter ritonavir concentrations.

Additional studies are needed to determine if minocycline would alter plasma concentrations of other protease inhibitors and to determine the clinical importance of this interaction.

[1] DiCenzo R, et al. *Antimicrob Agents Chemother.* 2008;52(9):3035.

* Asterisk indicates drugs cited in interaction reports.

Atomoxetine — *MAOIs*

Atomoxetine	MAOIs	
Atomoxetine* (*Strattera*)	Isocarboxazid* (*Marplan*)	Rasagiline* (*Azilect*)
	Linezolid* (*Zyvox*)	Selegiline* (eg, *Eldepryl*)
	Phenelzine* (eg, *Nardil*)	Tranylcypromine* (eg, *Parnate*)

Significance	Onset	Severity	Documentation
1	■ **Rapid** □ Delayed	■ **Major** □ Moderate □ Minor	□ Established □ Probable ■ **Suspected** □ Possible □ Unlikely

Effects Increased risk of serious or fatal reactions, including hyperthermia, autonomic instability with possible rapid fluctuations of vital signs, and mental status changes.

Mechanism Possibly altered brain monoamine concentrations.

Management Coadministration is contraindicated. After discontinuing an MAOI, allow at least 2 weeks before administering ATOMOXETINE. Allow at least 2 weeks after discontinuing ATOMOXETINE before giving an MAOI.

Discussion

There have been reports of serious, sometimes fatal, reactions including hyperthermia, rigidity, myoclonus, autonomic instability with possible rapid fluctuations of vital signs, and mental status changes (ie, extreme agitation progressing to delirium and coma) with coadministration of drugs that alter brain monoamine concentrations and MAOIs.[1] Some cases presented with signs and symptoms resembling neuroleptic malignant syndrome. These reactions may occur when these agents (ie, atomoxetine plus an MAOI) are given concomitantly or in close proximity.

The basis for this monograph is information on file with the manufacturer. Because of the seriousness of possible adverse reactions, clinical evaluation of this interaction in humans is not likely to be forthcoming.

[1] *Strattera* [package insert]. Indianapolis, IN: Eli Lilly and Co; September 3, 2003.

* Asterisk indicates drugs cited in interaction reports.

Atomoxetine / Serotonin Reuptake Inhibitors

Atomoxetine* (*Strattera*)	Fluoxetine (eg, *Prozac*)	Paroxetine* (eg, *Paxil*)

Significance	Onset	Severity	Documentation
2	☐ Rapid ■ **Delayed**	☐ Major ■ **Moderate** ☐ Minor	☐ Established ☐ Probable ■ **Suspected** ☐ Possible ☐ Unlikely

Effects ATOMOXETINE plasma concentrations may be elevated, increasing the pharmacologic effects and adverse reactions.

Mechanism Certain SEROTONIN REUPTAKE INHIBITORS may inhibit the metabolism (CYP2D6) of ATOMOXETINE.

Management In patients receiving ATOMOXETINE, closely monitor the patient when the dose of certain SEROTONIN REUPTAKE INHIBITORS is started, stopped, or changed. Adjust the dose of ATOMOXETINE as needed.

Discussion

The effect of paroxetine on atomoxetine metabolism was studied, and the effect of atomoxetine on the pharmacokinetics of paroxetine was investigated.[1] In a single-blind, 2-period, sequential study, 14 healthy subjects who were extensive CYP-450 metabolizers received oral atomoxetine (20 mg) every 12 hr for 9 doses in period 1. In period 2, paroxetine 20 mg was given once daily with placebo every 12 hr on days 1 through 11. Starting on the morning of day 12 and continuing through the morning of day 17, paroxetine (once daily) was given with atomoxetine 20 mg every 12 hr. Paroxetine administration increased the atomoxetine C_{max} approximately 3.5-fold, AUC 6.5-fold, and $t_{½}$ 2.5-fold. After coadministration of atomoxetine and paroxetine, there was an increase in the N-desmethylatomoxetine and decrease in the 4-hydroxyatomoxetine metabolites of atomoxetine. Atomoxetine did not alter the pharmacokinetics of paroxetine. The results supported the conclusion that inhibition of CYP2D6 by paroxetine markedly affected atomoxetine disposition, resulting in atomoxetine pharmacokinetics similar to poor metabolizers of CYP2D6 substrates.

[1] Belle DJ, et al. *J Clin Pharmacol.* 2002;42(11):1219.

* Asterisk indicates drugs cited in interaction reports. Based on pharmacologic and pharmacokinetic considerations, similar interactions may occur with other drugs that are listed.

Atorvastatin — *Protease Inhibitors*

Atorvastatin	Protease Inhibitors	
Atorvastatin* (*Lipitor*)	Amprenavir (*Agenerase*)	Nelfinavir (*Viracept*)
	Indinavir (*Crixivan*)	Ritonavir* (*Norvir*)
	Lopinavir/Ritonavir (*Kaletra*)	Saquinavir* (*Invirase*)

Significance	Onset	Severity	Documentation
2	☐ Rapid	☐ Major	☐ Established
	■ **Delayed**	■ **Moderate**	☐ Probable
		☐ Minor	■ **Suspected**
			☐ Possible
			☐ Unlikely

Effects ATORVASTATIN plasma levels may be elevated, increasing the risk of adverse reactions (eg, rhabdomyolysis).

Mechanism Inhibition of ATORVASTATIN first-pass metabolism (CYP3A4) in the GI tract is suspected.

Management Carefully monitor patients receiving ATORVASTATIN for adverse reactions when PROTEASE INHIBITOR therapy, especially ritonavir plus saquinavir, is started.

Discussion

The effects of ritonavir coadministered with saquinavir on the pharmacokinetics of atorvastatin were evaluated in 14 HIV-seronegative volunteers.[1] Using a randomized, open-label design, patients were administered atorvastatin 40 mg/day from days 1 through 4 and 15 through 18. Subjects received ritonavir (300 mg twice daily from days 4 to 8 and 400 mg twice daily from days 8 through 18) plus saquinavir (400 mg twice daily from days 4 through 18). Administration of ritonavir plus saquinavir increased the AUC of total active atorvastatin 73%. See Pravastatin-Protease Inhibitors and Simvastatin-Protease Inhibitors.

[1] Fichtenbaum CJ, et al. *AIDS.* 2002;16(4):569.

* Asterisk indicates drugs cited in interaction reports. Based on pharmacologic and pharmacokinetic considerations, similar interactions may occur with other drugs that are listed.

Azathioprine — *Mercaptopurine*

Azathioprine* (eg, *Imuran*)	Mercaptopurine* (eg, *Purinethol*)

Significance	Onset	Severity	Documentation
1	□ Rapid ■ **Delayed**	■ **Major** □ Moderate □ Minor	□ Established □ Probable ■ **Suspected** □ Possible □ Unlikely

Effects Risk of developing life-threatening myelosuppression, including pancytopenia, may be increased. Leukocyte, erythrocyte, and platelet depletion may occur.

Mechanism Additive bone marrow suppression.

Management Avoid coadministration of these agents.

Discussion

A patient being treated for Crohn disease died after developing profound myelosuppression and sepsis while receiving azathioprine 150 mg daily and 6-mercaptopurine 100 mg daily.[1] Unaware that another health care provider had prescribed azathioprine, 6-mercaptopurine was prescribed. The patient took both medications as directed. Because 6-mercaptopurine is an active metabolite of azathioprine, they share pharmacologic and toxic effects. Thus, myelosuppression may occur with either drug alone or in combination.

[1] ISMP. *ISMP Medication Safety Alert.* Huntingdon Valley, PA: ISMP; June 29, 2006.

* Asterisk indicates drugs cited in interaction reports.

Azole Antifungal Agents — *Ascorbic Acid*

Itraconazole* (eg, *Sporanox*)	Ascorbic Acid* (eg, *Vita-C*)

Significance	Onset	Severity	Documentation
4	■ **Rapid**	□ Major	□ Established
	□ Delayed	■ **Moderate**	□ Probable
		□ Minor	□ Suspected
			■ **Possible**
			□ Unlikely

Effects ASCORBIC ACID-CONTAINING BEVERAGES may elevate itraconazole plasma concentrations, increasing therapeutic effects and risk of adverse reactions.

Mechanism ASCORBIC ACID-CONTAINING BEVERAGES may facilitate itraconazole solubility, increasing GI absorption.

Management Unless itraconazole is being administered with an ASCORBIC ACID-CONTAINING BEVERAGE to increase the bioavailability of the antifungal agent, instruct patients to take ITRACONAZOLE with water.

Discussion

In 12 healthy subjects, administration of itraconazole 200 mg with an acidic (2.7 pH) beverage containing 500 mg of vitamin C increased the itraconazole AUC and C_{max} approximately 49% and 56%, respectively, compared with giving itraconazole alone. In addition, administration with the vitamin C-containing beverage increased the AUC and C_{max} of the active metabolite of itraconazole, 7-hydroxyitraconazole, approximately 40% and 44%, respectively.[1] See Azole Antifungal Agents-Food.

[1] Bae SK, et al. *J Clin Pharmacol.* 2011;51(3):444.

* Asterisk indicates drugs cited in interaction reports.

Azole Antifungal Agents — Didanosine

Itraconazole* (eg, *Sporanox*)	Ketoconazole* (eg, *Nizoral*)	Didanosine* (eg, *Videx*)	
Significance	Onset	Severity	Documentation
2	■ **Rapid** □ Delayed	□ Major ■ **Moderate** □ Minor	□ Established □ Probable ■ **Suspected** □ Possible □ Unlikely

Effects The therapeutic effects of AZOLE ANTIFUNGAL AGENTS may be decreased.

Mechanism The buffers in DIDANOSINE chewable tablets appear to decrease the absorption of AZOLE ANTIFUNGAL AGENTS.

Management Administer the AZOLE ANTIFUNGAL AGENT at least 2 hours before DIDANOSINE chewable tablets.

Discussion

Relapse of cryptococcal meningitis occurred in a 35-year-old man during coadministration of itraconazole and didanosine tablets.[1] To determine if didanosine had interfered with itraconazole absorption, the patient received 6 itraconazole 100 mg capsules and 2 chewable didanosine 100 mg tablets concomitantly. The next day, he was given 6 itraconazole 100 mg capsules without concurrent didanosine. Evaluation of the itraconazole plasma concentration indicated that didanosine delayed (and probably decreased) the absorption of the antifungal agent. When administered with didanosine, itraconazole was not detected in the plasma sample 2 hours after the dose was given, and a peak concentration of 1.4 mcg/mL was measured after 8 hours. In contrast, when given alone, the peak serum itraconazole concentration was 1.6 mcg/mL within 2 hours of administration. The patient's relapse was attributed to inadequate absorption of itraconazole, possibly because of changes in gastric pH caused by the buffers in the didanosine tablet formulation. In 6 healthy subjects, simultaneous administration of itraconazole 200 mg and didanosine 300 mg resulted in undetectable itraconazole levels.[2] Twelve men seropositive for HIV received didanosine 375 mg twice daily alone, ketoconazole 200 mg/day alone, or 1 dose of ketoconazole 2 hours before receiving didanosine for 4 days.[3] Ketoconazole administration decreased the AUC of didanosine 8%. When ketoconazole was given 2 hours prior to didanosine, no changes in the pharmacokinetics of ketoconazole were observed.

[1] Moreno F, et al. *JAMA*. 1993;269(12):1508.
[2] May DB, et al. *Pharmacotherapy*. 1994;14(5):509.
[3] Knupp CA, et al. *J Clin Pharmacol*. 1993;33(10):912.

* Asterisk indicates drugs cited in interaction reports.

Azole Antifungal Agents — **Food**

Itraconazole* (eg, *Sporanox*)	Cola Beverages* Grapefruit Juice*	Orange Juice*

Significance	Onset	Severity	Documentation
2	■ **Rapid**	□ Major	□ Established
	□ Delayed	■ **Moderate**	□ Probable
		□ Minor	■ **Suspected**
			□ Possible
			□ Unlikely

Effects

COLA – May increase ITRACONAZOLE serum levels.

GRAPEFRUIT/ORANGE JUICE – May reduce plasma levels and therapeutic effects of ITRACONAZOLE.

Mechanism

COLA – Increased ITRACONAZOLE solubility and absorption.

GRAPEFRUIT JUICE – Decreased ITRACONAZOLE absorption (capsule) or inhibited gut wall metabolism (CYP3A4 [solution]).

ORANGE JUICE – Unknown.

Management

COLA – In hypochlorhydric patients taking gastric acid suppressants, COLA may increase ITRACONAZOLE bioavailability.

GRAPEFRUIT/ORANGE JUICE – Should not be ingested with ITRACONAZOLE.

Discussion

Cola beverages – Taking itraconazole with cola beverages increased itraconazole bioavailability in fasting subjects,[1] AIDS patients,[2] and healthy volunteers taking ranitidine (eg, *Zantac*).[3] In 12 healthy subjects, administration of itraconazole 200 mg with 240 mL of cola increased the itraconazole AUC and C_{max} approximately 76% and 92%, respectively, compared with giving itraconazole alone.[4] In addition, cola increased the AUC and C_{max} of the active metabolite of itraconazole, 7-hydroxyitraconazole, approximately 57% and 41%, respectively.

Grapefruit/Orange juice – Compared with water, taking itraconazole immediately after breakfast with double-strength grapefruit juice reduced the mean itraconazole AUC 43% and increased T_{max} from 4 to 5.5 h.[5] Grapefruit juice reduced the mean AUC of the active hydroxymetabolite of itraconazole 47% and increased the mean T_{max} from 5 to 7 h. In contrast, drinking regular-strength grapefruit juice (240 mL for 2 days) increased itraconazole AUC 17% and reduced the oral clearance 14% when itraconazole was taken as an oral solution (200 mg per 20 mL).[6] In 22 healthy men taking itraconazole, the pharmacokinetics were not altered by grapefruit juice.[7] In contrast, another study found small pharmacokinetic changes only in women.[8] Orange juice reduced itraconazole AUC 58%, $t_{½}$ 44%, and C_{max} 79%.

1 Jaruratanasirikul S, et al. *Eur J Clin Pharmacol.* 1997;52(3):235.
2 Lange D, et al. *Curr Ther Res.* 1997;58(3):202.
3 Lange D, et al. *J Clin Pharmacol.* 1997;37(6):535.
4 Bae SK, et al. *J Clin Pharmacol.* 2011;51(3):444.
5 Penzak SR, et al. *Ther Drug Monit.* 1999;21(3):304.
6 Gubbins PO, et al. *Pharmacotherapy.* 2004;24(4):460.
7 Kawakami M, et al. *Int J Clin Pharmacol Ther.* 1998;36(6):306.
8 Gubbins PO, et al. *Eur J Clin Pharmacol.* 2008;64(3):293.

* Asterisk indicates drugs cited in interaction reports.

Azole Antifungal Agents — *Histamine H_2 Antagonists*

Itraconazole* (eg, *Sporanox*)	Posaconazole (*Noxafil*)	Cimetidine* (eg, *Tagamet*)	Nizatidine (eg, *Axid*)
Ketoconazole* (eg, *Nizoral*)		Famotidine (eg, *Pepcid*)	Ranitidine* (eg, *Zantac*)

Significance	Onset	Severity	Documentation
2	□ Rapid	□ Major	□ Established
	■ **Delayed**	■ **Moderate**	□ Probable
		□ Minor	■ **Suspected**
			□ Possible
			□ Unlikely

Effects The effects of ITRACONAZOLE and KETOCONAZOLE may be attenuated. CIMETIDINE levels may increase slightly.

Mechanism Decreased AZOLE ANTIFUNGAL AGENT bioavailability caused by reduced tablet dissolution in the presence of higher gastric pH. ITRACONAZOLE may inhibit active tubular secretion of CIMETIDINE by inhibiting active transport (eg, P-glycoprotein).

Management Consider discontinuing one of the agents. If KETOCONAZOLE must be used, give glutamic acid hydrochloride 680 mg 15 min prior to KETOCONAZOLE administration.[1]

Discussion

Ketoconazole 200 mg/day was ineffective in treating cryptococcal suppurative arthritis in a case report.[2] Therapy included sodium bicarbonate, aluminum oxide, and cimetidine. The patient responded to cimetidine discontinuation and sodium bicarbonate and aluminum oxide administration 2 hr after the ketoconazole dose. One study found that cimetidine decreased ketoconazole plasma levels when given 2 hr before ketoconazole,[2] while an in vitro study showed that ketoconazole dissolution was directly related to pH.[3] At pH 2 or 3, dissolution was more than 85% after 5 min, compared with 10% after 60 min at pH 6. In 12 healthy volunteers, cimetidine 300 mg and sodium bicarbonate 2 g given prior to ketoconazole 200 mg orally reduced ketoconazole C_{max} from 4.37 to 0.32 mcg/mL in control patients.[1] The 24-hr AUC was reduced 92%. In 6 healthy men, ranitidine 150 mg orally every 12 hr for 2 days then 2 hr prior to administration of ketoconazole 400 mg resulted in a 95% reduction in ketoconazole bioavailability when compared with a control period.[4] Because alteration of gastric acidity appears to decrease GI dissolution of ketoconazole, this interaction may occur with omeprazole (eg, *Prilosec*) and antacids. Eight healthy subjects received cimetidine 36 mg/hr by IV infusion for 4 hr alone and after pretreatment with itraconazole 400 mg/day for 4 days.[5] Compared with infusion of cimetidine alone, itraconazole pretreatment increased the cimetidine AUC 25%. See Ketoconazole-Antacids.

[1] Lelawongs P, et al. *Clin Pharm.* 1988;7(3):228.
[2] Van Der Meer JW, et al. *J Antimicrob Chemother.* 1980;6(4):552.
[3] Carlson JA, et al. *Am J Hosp Pharm.* 1983;40(8):1334.
[4] Piscitelli SC, et al. *Antimicrob Agents Chemother.* 1991;35(9):1765.
[5] Karyekar CS, et al. *J Clin Pharmacol.* 2004;44(8):919.

* Asterisk indicates drugs cited in interaction reports. Based on pharmacologic and pharmacokinetic considerations, similar interactions may occur with other drugs that are listed.

Azole Antifungal Agents — *NNRT Inhibitors*

Azole Antifungal Agents		NNRT Inhibitors	
Fluconazole* (eg, *Diflucan*) Itraconazole* (eg, *Sporanox*)	Ketoconazole (eg, *Nizoral*)	Delavirdine (*Rescriptor*) Efavirenz* (*Sustiva*)	Nevirapine* (*Viramune*)

Significance	Onset	Severity	Documentation
2	☐ Rapid ■ **Delayed**	☐ Major ■ **Moderate** ☐ Minor	☐ Established ☐ Probable ■ **Suspected** ☐ Possible ☐ Unlikely

Effects AZOLE ANTIFUNGAL AGENT plasma concentrations may be reduced, decreasing the efficacy, while NNRT INHIBITOR concentration may be elevated, increasing the risk of toxicity.

Mechanism Increased hepatic metabolism (CYP3A4) of the AZOLE ANTIFUNGAL AGENT and/or induction of P-glycoprotein activity are suspected. NNRT INHIBITOR metabolism may be inhibited.

Management Carefully monitor AZOLE ANTIFUNGAL AGENT plasma levels and the clinical status of the patient for any signs of a decrease or failure in response to the AZOLE ANTIFUNGAL AGENT or NNRT toxicity. If an interaction is suspected, consider a change in dose or alternative therapy.

Discussion

The effects of itraconazole and nevirapine on the pharmacokinetics of each other were studied in a 2-way crossover investigation in 12 healthy volunteers.[1] Itraconazole did not affect the pharmacokinetics of nevirapine. However, coadministration of itraconazole 200 mg and nevirapine 200 mg once daily for 7 days decreased the C_{max} and AUC of itraconazole 38% and 61%, respectively, and shortened the $t_{½}$ from 27.1 to 18.6 hours, compared with giving itraconazole alone. A decrease in response to itraconazole and undetectable plasma levels occurred in a 42-year-old man during coadministration of efavirenz.[2] The patient's response to itraconazole and itraconazole plasma levels increased after efavirenz was discontinued and atazanavir (*Reyataz*) was started. In a retrospective review, 4 patients with histoplasmosis who were receiving itraconazole 200 to 400 mg/day plus efavirenz or nevirapine had subtherapeutic itraconazole levels (less than 0.05 mcg/mL).[3] After changing to a protease inhibitors–based regimen, 3 of the patients achieved therapeutic itraconazole levels. In a pharmacological study, patients receiving nevirapine were given fluconazole 200 mg 3 times a week for cryptococcal prophylaxis.[4] In 27 patients receiving fluconazole, the nevirapine AUC increased 29% compared with 22 patients receiving placebo. The increase in nevirapine concentrations were not associated with increased hepatotoxicity. See also Voriconazole-Efavirenz.

[1] Jaruratanasirikul S, et al. *Eur J Clin Pharmacol.* 2007;63(5):451.
[2] Koo HL, et al. *Clin Infect Dis.* 2007;45(6):e77.
[3] Andrade RA, et al. *Ann Pharmacother.* 2009;43(5):908.
[4] Wakeham K, et al. *J Antimicrob Chemother.* 2010;65(2):316.

* Asterisk indicates drugs cited in interaction reports. Based on pharmacologic and pharmacokinetic considerations, similar interactions may occur with other drugs that are listed.

Azole Antifungal Agents — Proton Pump Inhibitors

Azole Antifungal Agents		Proton Pump Inhibitors	
Itraconazole* (eg, *Sporanox*)	Posaconazole* (*Noxafil*)	Esomeprazole (*Nexium*)	Pantoprazole (eg, *Protonix*)
Ketoconazole* (eg, *Nizoral*)		Lansoprazole (eg, *Prevacid*)	Rabeprazole (*AcipHex*)
		Omeprazole* (eg, *Prilosec*)	

Significance	Onset	Severity	Documentation
2	■ **Rapid**	□ Major	□ Established
	□ Delayed	■ **Moderate**	■ **Probable**
		□ Minor	□ Suspected
			□ Possible
			□ Unlikely

Effects Plasma levels of certain AZOLE ANTIFUNGAL AGENTS may be reduced, decreasing the pharmacologic effect.

Mechanism The bioavailability of certain AZOLE ANTIFUNGAL AGENTS may be decreased because of a possible reduction in tablet dissolution in the presence of a high gastric pH.

Management If possible, avoid this combination. If combined use cannot be avoided, the AZOLE ANTIFUNGAL AGENT can be taken with hydrochloric acid 0.1 to 0.2 N or an acidic beverage (eg, *Coca-Cola*, *Pepsi*) to increase AZOLE ANTIFUNGAL AGENT absorption. Increasing the dose of the AZOLE ANTIFUNGAL AGENT has been recommended but not studied.[1]

Discussion

The effectiveness of a commercial acidic beverage (eg, *Coca-Cola*; pH 2.5) in improving ketoconazole absorption in omeprazole-induced achlorhydria was studied in 9 healthy volunteers.[2] Each subject received a) ketoconazole 200 mg taken with water (control), b) omeprazole 60 mg followed 6 to 8 h later by ketoconazole 200 mg taken with water, and c) omeprazole 60 mg followed 6 to 8 h later by ketoconazole 200 mg taken with 240 mL of *Coca-Cola*. Ketoconazole levels were highest in the control period (4.1 mcg/mL) and lowest in omeprazole-induced achlorhydria (treatment B; 0.8 mcg/mL); ketoconazole bioavailability was decreased more than 80%. Absorption of ketoconazole during treatment C was increased approximately 65% compared with treatment B. Serum ketoconazole levels were higher when taken with *Coca-Cola* in the presence of omeprazole-induced achlorhydria (2.4 mcg/mL) but were lower than during the control period. The AUC was 10-fold greater during treatment C than B ($P < 0.05$). However, some subjects experienced no increase or only slight increases in the bioavailability of ketoconazole when taken during treatment C. In 11 healthy volunteers, itraconazole 200 mg on days 1 and 15 and omeprazole 40 mg on days 2 to 15 reduced itraconazole AUC and C_{max} 64% and 66%, respectively.[1] In a 58-year-old man, posaconazole plasma concentrations decreased from about 1.3 to 0.8 mg/L after 3 days of omeprazole 40 mg/day administration.[3] In a retrospective analysis of posaconazole levels in 17 cardiothoracic transplant patients, use of proton pump inhibitors was correlated with lower posaconazole levels and a higher risk of fungal prophylaxis failure.[4]

1 Jaruratanasirikul S, et al. *Eur J Clin Pharmacol.* 1998;54(2):159.
2 Chin TW, et al. *Antimicrob Agents Chemother.* 1995;39(8):1671.
3 Alffenaar JW, et al. *Clin Infect Dis.* 2009;48(6):839.
4 Shields RK, et al. *Antimicrob Agents Chemother.* 2011;55(3):1308.

* Asterisk indicates drugs cited in interaction reports. Based on pharmacologic and pharmacokinetic considerations, similar interactions may occur with other drugs that are listed.

Azole Antifungal Agents — *Quinolones*

Fluconazole* (eg, *Diflucan*) Itraconazole (eg, *Sporanox*)	Ketoconazole (eg, *Nizoral*)	Levofloxacin* (eg, *Levaquin*)	Moxifloxacin (*Avelox*)

Significance	Onset	Severity	Documentation
4	☐ Rapid ■ **Delayed**	■ **Major** ☐ Moderate ☐ Minor	☐ Established ☐ Probable ☐ Suspected ■ **Possible** ☐ Unlikely

Effects The risk of QTc interval prolongation and development of torsades de pointes may be increased.

Mechanism Potassium channel blockade by these agents is suspected.

Management If possible, consider alternative therapy. If this combination cannot be avoided, closely monitor the patient for QTc interval prolongation.

Discussion

A 53-year-old man who was dependent on hemodialysis developed QTc interval prolongation and torsades de pointes during coadministration of fluconazole and levofloxacin.[1] Levofloxacin was considered to be the causative agent, and it was discontinued after the patient had received a total of 8 doses over 14 days. The QTc interval remained prolonged the next day; fluconazole was discontinued after a total of 2 doses. The QTc interval remained prolonged for 12 days following the episode of torsades de pointes before returning to the normal range. The patient had a normal electrolyte panel prior to and immediately after the development of torsades de pointes.

[1] Gandhi PJ, et al. *Am J Health Syst Pharm.* 2003;60(23):2479.

* Asterisk indicates drugs cited in interaction reports. Based on pharmacologic and pharmacokinetic considerations, similar interactions may occur with other drugs that are listed.

Azole Antifungal Agents — *Rifamycins*

Azole Antifungal Agents		Rifamycins	
Fluconazole* (eg, *Diflucan*)	Ketoconazole* (eg, *Nizoral*)	Rifabutin* (*Mycobutin*)	Rifapentine (*Priftin*)
Itraconazole* (eg, *Sporanox*)	Posaconazole* (*Noxafil*)	Rifampin* (eg, *Rifadin*)	

Significance	Onset	Severity	Documentation
1	☐ Rapid	■ **Major**	☐ Established
	■ **Delayed**	☐ Moderate	■ **Probable**
		☐ Minor	☐ Suspected
			☐ Possible
			☐ Unlikely

Effects Plasma levels of AZOLE ANTIFUNGAL AGENTS may be decreased. Ketoconazole may decrease RIFAMYCIN levels; itraconazole may increase rifabutin levels.

Mechanism RIFAMYCINS may induce metabolism of AZOLE ANTIFUNGAL AGENTS. Ketoconazole may interfere with RIFAMYCIN absorption; itraconazole may inhibit rifabutin metabolism.

Management If concurrent use cannot be avoided, monitor antimicrobial activity, and adjust the dosages as needed.

Discussion

The AUC and C_{max} of ketoconazole were decreased up to 82% by long-term rifampin therapy.[1-7] Rifampin reduced the $t_{½}$ and AUC of fluconazole 20% and 23%, respectively.[8] Similar results occurred in 40 patients with AIDS.[9] In 3 patients receiving fluconazole, rifampin was associated with a relapse of cryptococcal meningitis, which also can occur with fluconazole alone.[10] A patient experienced a 47% decrease in fluconazole levels after receiving rifampin.[10] Marked reductions in fluconazole levels were seen in 2 patients given rifampin.[11] Eight patients experienced lower or undetectable itraconazole levels during rifampin and isoniazid treatment, compared with itraconazole alone.[7,12] Treatment failure occurred in 4 patients. When rifampin was discontinued, 2 patients improved and itraconazole levels remained the same or increased. In 6 healthy volunteers and 3 patients with AIDS, rifampin treatment resulted in lower or undetectable serum itraconazole levels.[13] In a 20-year-old man, rifampin administration decreased posaconazole levels up to 80%.[14] Ketoconazole decreased rifampin levels and AUC approximately 50% in 1 patient.[3] There was no effect when administration times were separated by 12 hours. Other studies found ketoconazole[6] and fluconazole[15] do not affect rifampin. Increased rifabutin levels and uveitis occurred in a patient after adding itraconazole to 1 stable rifabutin regimen.[16]

1 Brass C, et al. *Antimicrob Agents Chemother.* 1982;21(1):151.
2 Drouhet E, et al. *Am J Med.* 1983;74(1B):30.
3 Engelhard D, et al. *N Engl J Med.* 1984;311(26):1681.
4 Meunier F. *Eur J Clin Microbiol.* 1986;5(1):103.
5 Abadie-Kemmerly S, et al. *Ann Intern Med.* 1988;109(10):844.
6 Doble N, et al. *J Antimicrob Chemother.* 1988;21(5):633.
7 Tucker RM, et al. *Clin Infect Dis.* 1992;14(1):165.
8 Apseloff G, et al. *J Clin Pharmacol.* 1991;31(4):358.
9 Panomvana Na Ayudhya D, et al. *Clin Pharmacokinet.* 2004;43(11):725.
10 Coker RJ, et al. *BMJ.* 1990;301(6755):818.
11 Nicolau DP, et al. *Ann Pharmacother.* 1995;29(10):994.
12 Blomley M, et al. *Lancet.* 1990;336(8725):1255.
13 Jaruratanasirikul S, et al. *J Antimicrob Chemother.* 1996;38(5):877.
14 Hohmann C, et al. *Clin Infect Dis.* 2010;50(6):939.
15 Jaruratanasirikul S, et al. *Eur J Clin Pharmacol.* 1998;54(2):155.
16 Lefort A, et al. *Ann Intern Med.* 1996;125(11):939.

* Asterisk indicates drugs cited in interaction reports. Based on pharmacologic and pharmacokinetic considerations, similar interactions may occur with other drugs that are listed.

Barbiturate Anesthetics — **Ketamine**

Thiopental* (*Pentothal*)	Ketamine* (eg, *Ketalar*)

Significance	Onset	Severity	Documentation
5	■ **Rapid**	□ Major	□ Established
	□ Delayed	□ Moderate	□ Probable
		■ **Minor**	□ Suspected
			■ **Possible**
			□ Unlikely

Effects The hypnotic effect of THIOPENTAL may be antagonized.

Mechanism Unknown.

Management Monitor patients. Adjust the dose of THIOPENTAL as needed.

Discussion

The effects of an analgesic dose of ketamine 4 mg/kg IV on the subhypnotic dose of IV thiopental were studied in women.[1] In the initial phase of the investigation, the dose-response curves of ketamine and thiopental were determined separately. In the second phase, the dose-response curve of thiopental in patients pretreated with a previously determined subhypnotic dose of ketamine was established. The study population consisted of 392 women undergoing minor gynecological surgery (eg, dilation and curettage) or minor orthopedic surgery. Patients in each group were comparable in age, body weight, and obesity index. The dose at which 50% of the patients receiving ketamine lost consciousness (ulcerogenic dose in 50% [UD_{50}]) was calculated to be 0.697 mg/kg. The UD_{50} for thiopental was 2.365 mg/kg. The UD_{50} for thiopental when administered with ketamine was 1.473 mg/kg. Based on isobologram analysis, the UD_{50} would have been anticipated to be near 1 mg/kg. Thus, the findings indicated an antagonism between the analgesic dose (subhypnotic dose) of ketamine and the hypnotic effects of thiopental.

[1] Manani G, et al. *Eur J Anaesthesiol.* 1992;9(1):43.

* Asterisk indicates drugs cited in interaction reports.

Barbiturate Anesthetics — *Narcotic Analgesics*

Barbiturate Anesthetics		Narcotic Analgesics	
Methohexital (*Brevital*)	Thiopental* (eg, *Pentothal*)	Alfentanil* (*Alfenta*)	Morphine* (eg, *Duramorph*)
Thiamylal (*Surital*)		Buprenorphine (*Buprenex*)	Nalbuphine (eg, *Nubain*)
		Butorphanol (*Stadol*)	Opium (eg, *Paregoric*)
		Codeine	Oxycodone (*Roxicodone*)
		Fentanyl* (eg, *Sublimaze*)	Oxymorphone (*Numorphan*)
		Hydrocodone (eg, *Vicodin*)	Pentazocine (eg, *Talwin*)
		Hydromorphone (eg, *Dilaudid*)	Propoxyphene (eg, *Darvon*)
		Levorphanol (*Levo-Dromoran*)	Sufentanil (eg, *Sufenta*)
		Meperidine* (eg, *Demerol*)	
		Methadone (eg, *Dolophine*)	

Significance	Onset	Severity	Documentation
2	■ **Rapid**	□ Major	□ Established
	□ Delayed	■ **Moderate**	□ Probable
		□ Minor	■ **Suspected**
			□ Possible
			□ Unlikely

Effects The dose of THIOPENTAL required to induce anesthesia may be reduced in the presence of NARCOTIC ANALGESICS. Apnea may be more common with this combination.

Mechanism Drug actions may be additive.

Management No additional precautions other than those routinely used in anesthesia appear necessary.

Discussion

Thirty patients undergoing outpatient oral surgery procedures were premedicated with atropine 0.4 mg and 40 to 60 mg alphaprodine (*Nisentil*, not available in the US), a narcotic analgesic chemically related to meperidine; 30 control patients received only atropine premedication. Approximately 45 minutes later, anesthesia was induced with thiopental sodium. Patients premedicated with the narcotic required 40% less thiopental to achieve induction. In the treatment group, 13 patients were apneic at the time of induction, versus one in the control group. Respiratory rate was lower in the treatment group, both prior to and at the induction point.[2] This study agreed with earlier observations of five patients which showed increased respiratory depression from a combination of thiopental and morphine or meperidine compared with any of the drugs used alone.[1] Fentanyl and alfentanil pretreatment have also reduced the dose of thiopental required for induction.[4] Antagonism of the analgesic effect of meperidine by thiopental and phenobarbital has been reported.[3] The clinical significance is difficult to determine because the doses were subtherapeutic. The additive pharmacologic effects of these drugs are frequently used therapeutically.

[1] Eckenhoff JE, et al. *Anesthesiology*. 1958;19:240.
[2] DeLapa RJ. *J Oral Surg*. 1960;18:163.
[3] Dundee JW. *Br J Anaesth*. 1960;32:407.
[4] Dundee JW, et al. *Anaesthesia*. 1986;41:159.

* Asterisk indicates drugs cited in interaction reports. Based on pharmacologic and pharmacokinetic considerations, similar interactions may occur with other drugs that are listed.

Barbiturate Anesthetics — *Phenothiazines*

Barbiturate Anesthetics		Phenothiazines	
Methohexital* (*Brevital*)	Thiopental*	Chlorpromazine* (eg, *Thorazine*)	Promethazine* (eg, *Phenergan*)
		Perphenazine*	Trifluoperazine*
		Prochlorperazine* (eg, *Compazine*)	Triflupromazine* (*Vesprin*)

Significance

3

Onset	Severity	Documentation
■ **Rapid**	□ Major	□ Established
□ Delayed	□ Moderate	□ Probable
	■ **Minor**	■ **Suspected**
		□ Possible
		□ Unlikely

Effects Preanesthesia administration of PHENOTHIAZINES may increase the frequency and severity of neuromuscular excitation and hypotension in patients who receive BARBITURATE ANESTHESIA. The significance of this interaction is variable depending on the specific PHENOTHIAZINE and BARBITURATE ANESTHETIC combination.

Mechanism Unknown.

Management Avoid preanesthetic administration of PROMETHAZINE in patients who receive METHOHEXITAL or THIOPENTAL anesthesia. Use other PHENOTHIAZINES with caution in combination with these BARBITURATE ANESTHETICS.

Discussion

An increase in the incidence and severity of excitatory phenomena and hypotension has been reported in patients receiving phenothiazines prior to methohexital anesthesia.[1,2] One study reported a definite correlation between the incidence of excitatory phenomena and the antianalgesic effect of the phenothiazine combined with methohexital. Excitatory phenomena were reported in 25% of patients who received phenothiazines with some analgesic action (eg, promazine [not available in the US]), 36% of patients who received mildly antianalgesic phenothiazines (eg, prochlorperazine), and 69% of patients who received strongly antianalgesic phenothiazines (eg, promethazine).[1] Only strongly antianalgesic phenothiazines have been reported to increase the incidence of excitatory phenomena when combined with thiopental.[3] Phenothiazines have not been reported to affect the incidence of respiratory complications when combined with barbiturate anesthetics.[2]

[1] Moore J, et al. *Anaesthesia.* 1961;16:50.
[2] Dundee JW, et al. *Br J Anaesth.* 1961;33:382.
[3] Dundee JW, et al. *Br J Anaesth.* 1964;36:106.

* Asterisk indicates drugs cited in interaction reports.

Barbiturate Anesthetics — Probenecid

Thiopental*	Probenecid*

Significance	Onset	Severity	Documentation
3	■ **Rapid**	□ Major	□ Established
	□ Delayed	□ Moderate	■ **Probable**
		■ **Minor**	□ Suspected
			□ Possible
			□ Unlikely

Effects The anesthesia produced by THIOPENTAL may be extended or achieved at lower doses.

Mechanism Unknown.

Management The dose of THIOPENTAL used for induction may be reduced. However, because of the short duration (ie, minutes) of this drug, no other precautions other than those routinely used during anesthesia appear necessary.

Discussion

Pretreatment with probenecid has been reported to prolong thiopentone-induced anesthesia (as measured by loss of eyelid reflex) 26% to 109%.[1] In a double-blind study, 86 patients undergoing minor gynecologic surgery (laparotomy or suction curettage) received probenecid 3 hours prior to the procedure. Patients were premedicated with atropine and then assigned to 1 of 3 groups: Group I (n = 20) received thiopental IV 4 mg/kg after probenecid 0.5 g; Group II (n = 20) received thiopental 7 mg/kg after probenecid 0.5 g; Group III (n = 46) received thiopental 7 mg/kg plus meperidine and either 0.5 or 1 g probenecid. Pretreatment with probenecid prolonged the mean duration of anesthesia 109% in Group I (2.1 to 4.4 minutes), 26% in Group II (3 to 3.8 minutes), 65% in the Group III patients treated with probenecid 0.5 g, and 46% in the Group III patients who received probenecid 1 g. Pretreatment with probenecid did not influence the depth of anesthesia, the incidence of apnea, or heart rate and blood pressure changes. In a study of patients undergoing minor gynecological surgery, pretreatment with probenecid 1 g reduced the dose of thiopental required to induce sleep from 5.3 mg/kg in the control group (n = 52) to 4.2 mg/kg (n = 54).[2] Additional studies in other patient groups are necessary to clarify the clinical importance of this interaction.

[1] Kaukinen S, et al. *Br J Anaesth* 1980;52:603.

[2] McMurray TJ, et al. *Proceedings of the BPS, 7-9 Sept, 1983*;224P.

* Asterisk indicates drugs cited in interaction reports.

Barbiturate Anesthetics — *Sulfonamides*

Barbiturate Anesthetics	Sulfonamides
Thiopental* (*Pentothal*)	Sulfisoxazole* (*Gantrisin*)

Significance	Onset	Severity	Documentation
5	■ **Rapid**	□ Major	□ Established
	□ Delayed	□ Moderate	□ Probable
		■ **Minor**	□ Suspected
			■ **Possible**
			□ Unlikely

Effects SULFISOXAZOLE may enhance the anesthetic effects of THIOPENTAL.

Mechanism Unknown.

Management Consider a reduced dose of THIOPENTAL in patients who are receiving SULFISOXAZOLE.

Discussion

Thiopental 0.1 mg/kg was administered to 48 patients undergoing neurosurgery. Each patient also received placebo or a 40% sulfisoxazole solution prior to thiopental, and a blinded observer assessed the response to anesthesia.[1] The mean dose required to achieve hypnosis and anesthesia, the total dose of thiopental received, the duration of thiopental administration, and the time until waking were all significantly shorter in the sulfisoxazole group.

[1] Csogor SI, et al. *Br J Anaesth.* 1970;42:988.

* Asterisk indicates drugs cited in interaction reports.

Barbiturates — *Felbamate*

Phenobarbital* (*Solfoton*)	Primidone (eg, *Mysoline*)	Felbamate* (*Felbatol*)

Significance	Onset	Severity	Documentation
4	□ Rapid ■ **Delayed**	□ Major ■ **Moderate** □ Minor	□ Established □ Probable □ Suspected ■ **Possible** □ Unlikely

Effects Serum PHENOBARBITAL concentrations may be increased, possibly producing toxicity.

Mechanism Inhibition of PHENOBARBITAL metabolism.

Management Consider monitoring serum PHENOBARBITAL concentrations and observing the patients for changes in clinical response when starting, stopping, or altering the dose of FELBAMATE. Adjust the anticonvulsant dose as indicated.

Discussion

A 23-year-old man with a history of seizures had been taking phenobarbital 230 mg/day, thioridazine, and valproic acid for 3 months prior to starting felbamate 3600 mg/day.[1] At the time felbamate treatment was initiated, the dose of phenobarbital was decreased to 200 mg/day, while the dose of valproic acid was reduced to 500 mg/day. Five weeks following the addition of felbamate therapy, the patient was admitted to the hospital with a 1-week history of increasing anorexia, ataxia, and lethargy. His serum phenobarbital concentration was 68 mcg/mL. Prior to felbamate treatment, his phenobarbital concentrations had been 45 and 48 mcg/mL. Phenobarbital was stopped for 3 days and then restarted at 150 mg/day while felbamate and valproic acid were continued. The patient was discharged with a phenobarbital concentration of 58 mcg/mL and diminished symptoms of neurotoxicity. In a double-blind, placebo-controlled study of 24 healthy volunteers, the addition of felbamate 240 mg/day to a daily phenobarbital dose of 100 mg resulted in a 22% increase in the phenobarbital AUC and a 24% increase in peak plasma concentration compared with placebo administration.[2] Phenobarbital total body clearance was decreased 28% while renal clearance was unchanged. Felbamate plasma concentrations were also noted to be lower (38 mcg/mL) in these subjects than in patients in another study (60 mcg/mL) who were taking felbamate 2400 mg/day without phenobarbital.

[1] Gidal BE, et al. *Ann Pharmacother.* 1994;28:455.

[2] Reidenberg P, et al. *Clin Pharmacol Ther.* 1995;58:279.

* Asterisk indicates drugs cited in interaction reports. Based on pharmacologic and pharmacokinetic considerations, similar interactions may occur with other drugs that are listed.

Barbiturates — MAOIs

Barbiturates	MAOIs	
Amobarbital* (*Amytal*)	Isocarboxazid (*Marplan*)	Tranylcypromine* (*Parnate*)
	Phenelzine* (*Nardil*)	

Significance	Onset	Severity	Documentation
5	■ **Rapid**	☐ Major	☐ Established
	☐ Delayed	■ **Moderate**	☐ Probable
		☐ Minor	☐ Suspected
			☐ Possible
			■ **Unlikely**

Effects MAOIs may enhance the sedative effects of BARBITURATES.

Mechanism Unknown.

Management Closely monitor patients receiving MAOIs for oversedation when BARBITURATES are administered.

Discussion

A 20-year-old woman was receiving the MAOI tranylcypromine 10 mg 3 times daily for a few weeks following a suicide attempt, when she received an IM injection of amobarbital sodium 250 mg.[1] She became ataxic 1 hour later and fell to the floor, hitting her head. Over the next several hours she felt nauseous and dizzy, began vomiting, and became semicomatose. She remained semicomatose for 36 hours but gradually improved over the subsequent weeks. Both a brain concussion and drug interaction were suspected. Subsequent animal studies produced inconsistent results but raised the possibility that monoamine oxidase inhibitors might enhance barbiturate-induced sedation.[1,2]

[1] Domino EF, et al. *Am J Psychiatry*. 1962;118:941.

[2] Findlay JW, et al. *J Pharm Pharmacol*. 1981;33:45.

* Asterisk indicates drugs cited in interaction reports. Based on pharmacologic and pharmacokinetic considerations, similar interactions may occur with other drugs that are listed.

Barbiturates — *Phenacemide*

Barbiturates	Phenacemide
Phenobarbital*	Phenacemide*†
Primidone* (eg, *Mysoline*)	

Significance	Onset	Severity	Documentation
5	□ Rapid	□ Major	□ Established
	■ **Delayed**	□ Moderate	□ Probable
		■ **Minor**	□ Suspected
			■ **Possible**
			□ Unlikely

Effects PHENACEMIDE may increase BARBITURATE serum concentrations.

Mechanism Unknown.

Management None required. If BARBITURATE serum concentrations seem unusually high in a patient who also is receiving PHENACEMIDE, this interaction may be suspected.

Discussion

A collection of case reports of seven patients who were receiving either primidone or phenobarbital suggests that phenobarbital serum concentrations may increase when ethylphenacemide is added to the therapy.[1]

[1] Huisman JW, et al. *Epilepsia*. 1970;11:207.

* Asterisk indicates drugs cited in interaction reports.
† Not available in the United States.

Barbiturates — *Propoxyphene*

Barbiturates		Propoxyphene
Pentobarbital* (eg, *Nembutal*)	Primidone (eg, *Mysoline*)	Propoxyphene* (eg, *Darvon*)
Phenobarbital*		

Significance	Onset	Severity	Documentation
5	☐ Rapid	☐ Major	☐ Established
	■ **Delayed**	☐ Moderate	☐ Probable
		■ **Minor**	☐ Suspected
			■ **Possible**
			☐ Unlikely

Effects Serum levels of BARBITURATES may increase, resulting in enhanced actions.

Mechanism Unknown. Hepatic metabolism of BARBITURATES may be reduced.

Management No clinical interventions other than routine clinical monitoring appear required with short-term or occasional use of this combination. However, chronic administration of the combination may require dosage adjustment.

Discussion

Chronic phenobarbital monotherapy given to four patients for epilepsy had an average 20% (range, 8% to 29%) increase in serum trough phenobarbital levels after the addition of propoxyphene, 65 mg three times daily for 6 days.[2] Because sampling was discontinued at the same time as propoxyphene therapy was discontinued, further increases in serum levels of this long half-life drug may not have been detected. The acute administration of propoxyphene to pentobarbital-treated rats significantly prolonged pentobarbital-induced sleep times. This was presumed to be due to inhibition of metabolism, because no change in absorption could be detected.[1] However, chronic administration of propoxyphene in this rat model showed it to be a potent inducer of its own metabolism.

Additional studies are necessary to determine the clinical significance, if any, of this interaction.

[1] Peterson GR, et al. *Life Sci* 1978;22:2087.

[2] Hansen BS, et al. *Acta Neurol Scand* 1980;61:357.

* Asterisk indicates drugs cited in interaction reports. Based on pharmacologic and pharmacokinetic considerations, similar interactions may occur with other drugs that are listed.

Barbiturates — *Pyridoxine*

Barbiturates	Pyridoxine
Phenobarbital* Primidone (eg, *Mysoline*)	Pyridoxine* (eg, *Nestrex*)

Significance	Onset	Severity	Documentation
5	□ Rapid ■ **Delayed**	□ Major □ Moderate ■ **Minor**	□ Established □ Probable □ Suspected ■ **Possible** □ Unlikely

Effects PYRIDOXINE may decrease the serum concentration of concurrent PHENOBARBITAL, possibly resulting in a decreased therapeutic effect of PHENOBARBITAL.

Mechanism Unknown, but may be related to an increase in the activity of pyridoxal-phosphate-dependent enzymes that are involved in the biotransformation of PHENOBARBITAL.

Management If decreased plasma levels of PHENOBARBITAL or a decreased response occurs during concurrent PYRIDOXINE, the dose of PHENOBARBITAL may need to be increased.

Discussion

In one study, five patients receiving long-term phenobarbital were given pyridoxine 200 mg/day for 4 weeks.[1] Phenobarbital levels decreased in each patient by 35% to 53%. The clinical significance of this interaction was not determined.

[1] Hansson O, et al. *Lancet* 1976;1:256.

* Asterisk indicates drugs cited in interaction reports. Based on pharmacologic and pharmacokinetic considerations, similar interactions may occur with other drugs that are listed.

Barbiturates — *Quinine*

Phenobarbital*

Significance	Onset	Severity	Documentation
4	☐ Rapid	☐ Major	☐ Established
	■ **Delayed**	■ **Moderate**	☐ Probable
		☐ Minor	☐ Suspected
			■ **Possible**
			☐ Unlikely

Effects Serum PHENOBARBITAL concentrations may be elevated, increasing the pharmacologic and adverse effects.

Mechanism Possible inhibition of PHENOBARBITAL metabolism.

Management In patients receiving PHENOBARBITAL, observe the clinical response of the patient when starting or stopping QUININE therapy. Adjust the PHENOBARBITAL dose as needed.

Discussion

The effects of oral quinine 600 mg on the pharmacokinetics of phenobarbital 120 mg were studied in six healthy volunteers.[1] Quinine administration increased peak serum phenobarbital concentrations by 34.8% and the area under the plasma concentration-time curve by 44.7%. Controlled studies are needed to determine the clinical importance of this drug interaction.

[1] Amabeoku GJ, et al. *East Afr Med J.* 1993;70:90.

* Asterisk indicates drugs cited in interaction reports.

Barbiturates — *Rifamycins*

Barbiturates		Rifamycins	
Amobarbital (*Amytal*)	Phenobarbital* (eg, *Luminal*)	Rifabutin (*Mycobutin*)	Rifampin* (eg, *Rifadin*)
Butabarbital (eg, *Butisol*)	Primidone (eg, *Mysoline*)		
Butalbital	Secobarbital (*Seconal*)		
Pentobarbital (*Nembutal*)			

Significance	Onset	Severity	Documentation
5	□ Rapid	□ Major	□ Established
	■ **Delayed**	□ Moderate	□ Probable
		■ **Minor**	□ Suspected
			■ **Possible**
			□ Unlikely

Effects Coadministration of RIFAMPIN and BARBITURATES may result in an increased rate of BARBITURATE metabolism and resultant reduced actions.

Mechanism RIFAMPIN may stimulate liver microsomal enzymes, resulting in more rapid degradation of BARBITURATES.

Management When RIFAMPIN is added to the regimen of a patient receiving a BARBITURATE, monitor the patient for changes in clinical status and plasma BARBITURATE levels. The BARBITURATE dosage may need to be raised.

Discussion

Several studies have documented that coadministration of rifampin and hexobarbital significantly shortened the elimination $t_{½}$ and increased the oral clearance of hexobarbital.†[1-5] This is confirmed in young adult and elderly volunteers.[5] The effects of rifampin on the metabolism of other barbiturates have not been determined.[6] Further studies are necessary to clarify this interaction.

1 Zilly W, et al. *Eur J Clin Pharmacol.* 1975;9(2-3):219.
2 Zilly W, et al. *Eur J Clin Pharmacol.* 1977;11(4):287.
3 Breimer DD, et al. *Clin Pharmacol Ther.* 1977;21(4):470.
4 Richter E, et al. *Eur J Clin Pharmacol.* 1980;17(3):197.
5 Smith DA, et al. *Pharmacotherapy.* 1989;9:183.
6 Baciewicz AM, et al. *Arch Intern Med.* 1984;144(8):1667.

* Asterisk indicates drugs cited in interaction reports. Based on pharmacologic and pharmacokinetic considerations, similar interactions may occur with other drugs that are listed.

† Not available in the United States.

Barbiturates — *Valproic Acid*

Phenobarbital* (eg, *Luminal*)	Primidone (eg, *Mysoline*)	Divalproex Sodium (eg, *Depakote*)	Valproic Acid* (eg, *Depakene*)

Significance	Onset	Severity	Documentation
2	□ Rapid ■ **Delayed**	□ Major ■ **Moderate** □ Minor	■ **Established** □ Probable □ Suspected □ Possible □ Unlikely

Effects Plasma BARBITURATE concentrations may be elevated, increasing the pharmacologic and adverse effects.

Mechanism VALPROIC ACID may decrease the hepatic metabolism of BARBITURATES.

Management When VALPROIC ACID is added to the therapeutic regimen of a patient receiving a BARBITURATE, monitor the patient and the serum BARBITURATE concentration. BARBITURATE dosage may need to be decreased in some patients.

Discussion

Phenobarbital metabolism is reduced by valproic acid.[1-11] In one study, a 30% reduction in phenobarbital dose was necessary when valproic acid was administered concurrently.[4] A study of valproic acid–induced changes in phenobarbital elimination parameters reported an increase in phenobarbital $t_{½}$ from 96 to 142 hours, a decrease in plasma clearance rate from 4.2 to 3 mL/h/kg, no change in renal clearance, a decrease in metabolic clearance from 3.3 to 2 mg/h/kg, fraction of dose excreted unchanged increased from 0.22 to 0.33, and the fraction of dose metabolized decreased from 0.78 to 0.67.[7] One study reported that the serum level/dose ratio of phenobarbital increased 50.9% in adults and 112.5% in children when sodium valproate was added to the treatment regimen, suggesting that age may affect the magnitude of this interaction.[10]

1 Völzke E, et al. *Epilepsia.* 1973;14(2):185.
2 Schobben F, et al. *Eur J Clin Pharmacol.* 1975;8(2):97.
3 Windorfer A, et al. *Acta Paediatr Scand.* 1975;64(5):771.
4 Gram L, et al. *Epilepsia.* 1977;18(2):141.
5 Wilder BJ, et al. *Neurology.* 1978;28(9 Pt 1):892.
6 Patel IH, et al. *Clin Pharmacol Ther.* 1980;27(4):515.
7 Bruni J, et al. *Neurology.* 1980;30(1).94.
8 Kapetanović IM, et al. *Clin Pharmacol Ther.* 1981;29(4):480.
9 Suganuma T, et al. *J Pediatr.* 1981;99(2):314.
10 Fernandez de Gatta MR, et al. *Ther Drug Monit.* 1986;8(4):416.
11 Bourgeois BF. *Am J Med.* 1988;84(1A):29.

* Asterisk indicates drugs cited in interaction reports. Based on pharmacologic and pharmacokinetic considerations, similar interactions may occur with other drugs that are listed.

Benzodiazepines — *Antacids*

Benzodiazepines		Antacids	
Chlordiazepoxide*	Temazepam* (eg, *Restoril*)	Aluminum Hydroxide (eg, *Alternagel*)	Magnesium Hydroxide (eg, *Milk of Magnesia*)
Clorazepate* (eg, *Tranxene*)	Triazolam* (eg, *Halcion*)	Aluminum Hydroxide/ Magnesium Hydroxide* (eg, *Maalox*)	
Diazepam* (eg, *Valium*)			

Significance	Onset	Severity	Documentation
5	■ **Rapid**	□ Major	□ Established
	□ Delayed	□ Moderate	□ Probable
		■ **Minor**	□ Suspected
			■ **Possible**
			□ Unlikely

Effects A decrease or delay in the sedative effect of single doses of some BENZODIAZEPINES may occur.

Mechanism Unknown.

Management No special precautions are needed.

Discussion

Several studies report this interaction.[1-11] Administration of an aluminum hydroxide–containing antacid enhanced the sedative properties of diazepam in one trial,[2] while a subsequent study of both aluminum hydroxide/magnesium hydroxide and *Maalox* revealed lower diazepam C_{max}.[6] When slow-release diazepam was administered with *Maalox*, no effects on absorption were observed.[9]

Clorazepate demonstrated a slower absorption and lower C_{max} when administered with *Maalox*.[4] In a single-dose trial, *Maalox* administration delayed or decreased the patients' subjective ratings of the effects of clorazepate.[7] No differences in steady-state concentrations of clorazepate were found when administered long-term with *Maalox*.[8]

For chlordiazepoxide, administration with *Maalox* resulted in delays in the rate of absorption and decreases in the patients' subjective ratings of drug effect.[3]

In 2 trials of patients with end-stage renal disease (ESRD), aluminum hydroxide gel resulted in no effects on the absorption of temazepam[11] but increased the C_{max} and AUC of triazolam.[10] This is not likely to warrant an empiric dosage decrease because triazolam concentrations are typically lower in patients with ESRD.

1 Greenblatt DJ, et al. *Clin Pharmacol Ther.* 1976;19(2):234.
2 Nair SG, et al. *Br J Anaesth.* 1976;48(12):1175.
3 Greenblatt DJ, et al. *Am J Psychiatry.* 1977;134(5):559.
4 Chun AHC, et al. *Clin Pharmacol Ther.* 1977;22(3):329.
5 Abruzzo CW, et al. *J Pharmacokinet Biopharm.* 1977;5(4):377.
6 Greenblatt DJ, et al. *Clin Pharmacol Ther.* 1978;24(5):600.
7 Shader RI, et al. *Clin Pharmacol Ther.* 1978;24(3):308.
8 Shader RI, et al. *Clin Pharmacol Ther.* 1982;31(2):180.
9 Locniskar A, et al. *J Clin Pharmacol.* 1984;24(5-6):255.
10 Kroboth PD, et al. *Br J Clin Pharmacol.* 1985;19(6):839.
11 Kroboth PD, et al. *Clin Pharmacol Ther.* 1985;37(4):453.

* Asterisk indicates drugs cited in interaction reports. Based on pharmacologic and pharmacokinetic considerations, similar interactions may occur with other drugs that are listed.

Benzodiazepines — *Aprepitant*

Benzodiazepines		Aprepitant
Alprazolam (eg, *Xanax*)	Estazolam	Aprepitant* (*Emend*)
Chlordiazepoxide	Flurazepam	
Clonazepam (eg, *Klonopin*)	Midazolam*	
Clorazepate (eg, *Tranxene*)	Quazepam (*Doral*)	
Diazepam (eg, *Valium*)	Triazolam (eg, *Halcion*)	

Significance	Onset	Severity	Documentation
4	☐ Rapid	☐ Major	☐ Established
	■ **Delayed**	■ **Moderate**	☐ Probable
		☐ Minor	☐ Suspected
			■ **Possible**
			☐ Unlikely

Effects Plasma concentrations of certain BENZODIAZEPINES may be elevated, increasing the pharmacologic effects and adverse reactions.

Mechanism Inhibition of BENZODIAZEPINE metabolism (CYP3A4) by APREPITANT is suspected.

Management Closely monitor patients taking certain BENZODIAZEPINES for increased reactions (eg, CNS depression) when APREPITANT is coadministered.

Discussion

The effects of aprepitant on the pharmacokinctics of midazolam were studied in 16 healthy men.[1] In an open-label, randomized, single-period study, 8 subjects received either aprepitant 125 mg on day 1 and 80 mg/day on days 2 to 5, or aprepitant 40 mg on day 1 and 25 mg/day on days 2 to 5. All subjects received an oral dose of midazolam 2 mg 3 to 7 days before aprepitant administration and 1 hour after aprepitant on days 1 and 5. Compared with administration of midazolam alone, the aprepitant 125 and 80 mg regimen increased the AUC 2.3-fold on day 1 and 3.3-fold on day 5, while increasing the $t_{½}$ of midazolam from 1.7 to 3.3 hours on both days 1 and 5. The midazolam C_{max} was increased 1.5- and 1.9-fold on days 1 and 5, respectively. The aprepitant 40 and 25 mg regimen did not affect the pharmacokinetics of midazolam. The effects of a single dose of aprepitant 125 mg on the pharmacokinetics of midazolam 2 mg IV were evaluated in 12 healthy subjects.[2] The geometric mean AUC of midazolam increased nearly 46% and the $t_{½}$ increased from 3.7 to 5.2 hours. The effect was considered to be of modest clinical importance.

[1] Majumdar AK, et al. *Clin Pharmacol Ther.* 2003;74(2):150.

[2] Majumdar AK, et al. *J Clin Pharmacol.* 2007;47(6):744.

* Asterisk indicates drugs cited in interaction reports. Based on pharmacologic and pharmacokinetic considerations, similar interactions may occur with other drugs that are listed.

Benzodiazepines (Ox.) | **Azole Antifungal Agents**

Alprazolam* (eg, *Xanax*)	Estazolam	Fluconazole* (eg, *Diflucan*)	Posaconazole* (*Noxafil*)
Chlordiazepoxide*	Flurazepam	Itraconazole* (eg, *Sporanox*)	Voriconazole* (eg, *Vfend*)
Clonazepam (eg, *Klonopin*)	Midazolam*	Ketoconazole*	
Clorazepate (eg, *Tranxene-T*)	Quazepam* (*Doral*)		
Diazepam* (eg, *Valium*)	Triazolam* (eg, *Halcion*)		

Significance	Onset	Severity	Documentation
	☐ Rapid	■ **Major**	■ **Established**
	■ **Delayed**	☐ Moderate	☐ Probable
		☐ Minor	☐ Suspected
			☐ Possible
			☐ Unlikely

Effects Increased and prolonged CNS depression and psychomotor impairment, possibly continuing for several days after the AZOLE ANTIFUNGAL AGENT is stopped.[1,2]

Mechanism Decreased oxidative metabolism (CYP3A4) of certain BENZODIAZEPINES and the first-pass effect of TRIAZOLAM.

Management Use of oral MIDAZOLAM with ITRACONAZOLE is contraindicated. Use of oral ALPRAZOLAM[3] or TRIAZOLAM with ITRACONAZOLE or KETOCONAZOLE is contraindicated. When using FLUCONAZOLE, consider giving a lower BENZODIAZEPINE dose or a BENZODIAZEPINE metabolized by glucuronidation (eg, lorazepam [eg, *Ativan*], temazepam[4] [eg, *Restoril*]). Warn patients about increased and prolonged sedative effects.

Discussion

Itraconazole 200 mg/day for 4 days increased the AUC of midazolam 10-fold and triazolam 27-fold, the $t_{1/2}$ of midazolam from 2.9 to 7.9 h and triazolam from 3.3 to 22.3 h, and the serum level of each benzodiazepine 3-fold.[5,6] Similar results occurred with ketoconazole,[5-8] but not quazepam.[9] Giving ketoconazole before a single dose of triazolam increased the $t_{1/2}$ of triazolam from 4 to 17.7 h and decreased clearance 9-fold.[10] Itraconazole[11] and ketoconazole[12] increased the AUC of alprazolam 13- and 14-fold, respectively. A single dose of ketoconazole and chlordiazepoxide IV decreased chlordiazepoxide clearance 20% and the volume of distribution 26%, while giving ketoconazole for 5 days decreased chlordiazepoxide clearance 38%.[13] Oral ketoconazole increased IV and oral midazolam AUC 5- and 16-fold, respectively.[14] Midazolam clearance decreased 84%, and total bioavailability increased 25% to 80%. Fluconazole increased the AUC of midazolam oral (but not IV)[15-17] and triazolam.[18] While both fluconazole oral and IV increase midazolam levels, the effect is greatest with fluconazole oral.[19] Fluconazole IV increased midazolam plasma levels 0- to 4-fold in 10 patients receiving stable infusions of midazolam.[20] Voriconazole decreased midazolam clearance 72%, resulting in an increase in $t_{1/2}$ from 2.8 to 8.3 h.[21] Fluconazole oral and voriconazole oral increased diazepam AUC 157% and 110%, respectively.[22] Posaconazole oral increased the AUC of midazolam IV or oral between 4.6- to 6.5-fold.[23]

1 Neuvonen PJ, et al. *Clin Pharmacol Ther.* 1996;60(3):326.
2 Backman JT, et al. *Eur J Clin Pharmacol.* 1998;54(1):53.
3 *Niravam* [package insert]. Philadelphia, PA: Azur Pharma Inc; June 2012.
4 Ahonen J, et al. *Ther Drug Monit.* 1996;18(2):124.

[5] Olkkola KT, et al. *Clin Pharmacol Ther.* 1994;55(5):481.
[6] Varhe A, et al. *Clin Pharmacol Ther.* 1994;56(6, pt 1):601.
[7] Tham LS, et al. *Ther Drug Monit.* 2006;28(2):255.
[8] Stoch SA, et al. *J Clin Pharmacol.* 2009;49(4):398.
[9] Kato K, et al. *Ther Drug Monit.* 2003;25(4):473.
[10] Greenblatt DJ, et al. *Lancet.* 1995;345(8943):191.
[11] Yasui N, et al. *Psychopharmacology (Berl.).* 1998;139(3):269.
[12] Greenblatt DJ, et al. *Clin Pharmacol Ther.* 1998;64(3):237.
[13] Brown MW, et al. *Clin Pharmacol Ther.* 1985;37(3):290.
[14] Tsunoda SM, et al. *Clin Pharmacol Ther.* 1999;66(5):461.
[15] Olkkola KT, et al. *Anesth Analg.* 1996;82(3):511.
[16] Varhe A, et al. *Br J Clin Pharmacol.* 1996;42(4):465.
[17] von Moltke LL, et al. *J Clin Pharmacol.* 1996;36(9):783.
[18] Varhe A, et al. *Br J Clin Pharmacol.* 1996;41(4):319.
[19] Ahonen J, et al. *Eur J Clin Pharmacol.* 1997;51(5):415.
[20] Ahonen J, et al. *Acta Anaesthesiol Scand.* 1999;43(5):509.
[21] Saari TI, et al. *Clin Pharmacol Ther.* 2006;79(4):362.
[22] Saari TI, et al. *Eur J Clin Pharmacol.* 2007;63(10):941.
[23] Krishna G, et al. *Clin Ther.* 2009;31(2):286.

* Asterisk indicates drugs cited in interaction reports. Based on pharmacologic and pharmacokinetic considerations, similar interactions may occur with other drugs that are listed.

Benzodiazepines (Ox.) — *Berberine*

Alprazolam (eg, *Xanax*)	Estazolam	Berberine*
Chlordiazepoxide	Flurazepam	
Clonazepam (eg, *Klonopin*)	Midazolam*	
Clorazepate (eg, *Tranxene-T*)	Quazepam (*Doral*)	
Diazepam (eg, *Valium*)	Triazolam (eg, *Halcion*)	

Significance	Onset	Severity	Documentation
4	☐ Rapid	☐ Major	☐ Established
	■ **Delayed**	■ **Moderate**	☐ Probable
		☐ Minor	☐ Suspected
			■ **Possible**
			☐ Unlikely

Effects BENZODIAZEPINE plasma concentrations may be elevated, increasing the pharmacologic effects and risk of adverse reactions.

Mechanism Inhibition of hepatic metabolism (CYP3A4) of BENZODIAZEPINES that undergo oxidative metabolism is suspected.

Management Advise patients taking certain BENZODIAZEPINES to avoid BERBERINE.

Discussion

The effects of berberine (a plant alkaloid found in herbs such as goldenseal) on the pharmacokinetics of midazolam were evaluated in 17 healthy men.[1] Using a randomized, crossover design, each subject received either placebo or berberine 300 mg 3 times daily for 14 days. Midazolam 2 mg was administered before and at the end of the 14 days. Compared with placebo, berberine ingestion increased the C_{max} and AUC of midazolam 38% and 37%, respectively. The T_{max} and $t_{1/2}$ of midazolam were prolonged from 3.03 to 3.66 hours and 0.66 to 0.99 hours, respectively, after berberine ingestion. The oral clearance of midazolam was decreased 27% by berberine.

[1] Guo Y, et al. *Eur J Clin Pharmacol.* 2012;68(2):213.

* Asterisk indicates drugs cited in interaction reports. Based on pharmacologic and pharmacokinetic considerations, similar interactions may occur with other drugs that are listed.

Benzodiazepines — *Beta-Blockers*

Benzodiazepines		Beta-Blockers	
Chlordiazepoxide Clonazepam (eg, *Klonopin*) Clorazepate* (eg, *Tranxene*)	Diazepam* (eg, *Valium*) Flurazepam Triazolam (eg, *Halcion*)	Metoprolol* (eg, *Lopressor*)	Propranolol* (eg, *Inderal*)

Significance	Onset	Severity	Documentation
5	☐ Rapid ■ **Delayed**	☐ Major ☐ Moderate ■ **Minor**	☐ Established ☐ Probable ☐ Suspected ■ **Possible** ☐ Unlikely

Effects Effects of certain BENZODIAZEPINES may be increased by lipophilic BETA-BLOCKERS.

Mechanism Inhibition of BENZODIAZEPINE hepatic metabolism by BETA-BLOCKERS has been proposed.

Management Consider using a BETA-BLOCKER that does not interfere with BENZODIAZEPINE hepatic metabolism (eg, atenolol).

Discussion

The combination of propranolol and diazepam has been beneficial in treating anxiety in some patients.[1] In volunteers, adding either lipophilic beta-blocker (propranolol or metoprolol) to diazepam further affected certain indices of alertness and reaction in some subjects, although the magnitude of effect was usually slight.[2,3] Also, adverse reactions were reported slightly more often with the combination of metoprolol or propranolol with diazepam than with diazepam alone. The number of adverse reactions observed with the combination of atenolol and diazepam was not different than those observed with diazepam alone.[2]

In 3 small pharmacokinetic studies,[3-5] the clearance of diazepam and its metabolite desmethyldiazepam was decreased 12% to 18% when combined with propranolol or metoprolol. The diazepam AUC increased by similar magnitudes during coadministration of metoprolol or propranolol in another study.[2] These effects on diazepam and desmethyldiazepam clearance have not been observed with atenolol,[2] nor have propranolol or metoprolol affected the clearance of lorazepam (eg, *Ativan*), alprazolam (eg, *Xanax*),[4] or bromazepam.[†6] Oxazepam clearance was unaffected by propranolol or labetalol (eg, *Trandate*).[7]

[1] Hallstrom C, et al. *Br J Psychiatry.* 1981;139:417.
[2] Hawksworth G, et al. *Br J Clin Pharmacol.* 1984;17(suppl 1):69S.
[3] Klotz U, et al. *Eur J Clin Pharmacol.* 1984;26(2):223.
[4] Ochs HR, et al. *Clin Pharmacol Ther.* 1984;36(4):451.
[5] Ochs HR, et al. *J Clin Pharmacol.* 1986;26:556.
[6] Scott AK, et al. *Eur J Clin Pharmacol.* 1991;40(4):405.
[7] Sonne J, et al. *Br J Clin Pharmacol.* 1990;29(1):33.

* Asterisk indicates drugs cited in interaction reports. Based on pharmacologic and pharmacokinetic considerations, similar interactions may occur with other drugs that are listed.

† Not available in the United States.

Benzodiazepines — *Carbamazepine*

Alprazolam* (eg, *Xanax*)	Midazolam*	Carbamazepine* (eg, *Tegretol*)
Clonazepam* (eg, *Klonopin*)		

Significance	Onset	Severity	Documentation
2	□ Rapid	□ Major	□ Established
	■ **Delayed**	■ **Moderate**	□ Probable
		□ Minor	■ **Suspected**
			□ Possible
			□ Unlikely

Effects The pharmacologic effects of certain BENZODIAZEPINES may be decreased.

Mechanism Induction of BENZODIAZEPINE metabolism (CYP3A4).

Management Monitor for a decrease in BENZODIAZEPINE clinical response during coadministration of CARBAMAZEPINE. If an interaction is suspected, consider using a higher dose of the BENZODIAZEPINE.

Discussion

A 32-year-old man with atypical bipolar disorder and disabling panic attacks exhibited a 55% reduction in plasma alprazolam concentrations and a deterioration in his clinical condition after starting carbamazepine.[1] In a study of 6 epileptic patients and 7 control subjects receiving carbamazepine or phenytoin and oral midazolam, the $t_{½}$, AUC, and C_{max} of midazolam were decreased 94%, 92%, and 42%, respectively, compared with control subjects.[2] The sedative effects were greatly reduced in the epileptic patients receiving carbamazepine or phenytoin. Pharmacokinetic modeling was conducted with 7 healthy men given oral midazolam before and with carbamazepine for 16 days.[3] Based on this modeling, carbamazepine increased gut-wall extraction of midazolam from 43% to 66% and increased clearance 42%, compared with giving midazolam alone. Mean steady-state clonazepam plasma levels and elimination $t_{½}$ decreased nearly 30% over a 3-week period after initiation of carbamazepine in 7 volunteers.[4] In a retrospective analysis, coadministration of clonazepam and carbamazepine resulted in a 22% increase in clonazepam clearance and a 20.5% decrease in carbamazepine clearance.[5] Another study found that carbamazepine plasma levels were not affected by 6 weeks of clonazepam coadministration.[6]

[1] Arana GW, et al. *J Clin Psychiatry.* 1988;49(11):448.
[2] Backman JT, et al. *Epilepsia.* 1996;37(3):253.
[3] Magnusson MO, et al. *Clin Pharmacol Ther.* 2008;84(1):52.
[4] Lai AA, et al. *Clin Pharmacol Ther.* 1978;24(3):316.
[5] Yukawa E, et al. *J Clin Psychopharmacol.* 2001;21(6):588.
[6] Johannessen SI, et al. *Acta Neurol Scand.* 1977;55(6):506.

* Asterisk indicates drugs cited in interaction reports.

Benzodiazepines — *Cholestyramine*

Lorazepam* (eg, *Ativan*)	Cholestyramine* (eg, *Questran*)

Significance	Onset	Severity	Documentation
5	■ **Rapid**	□ Major	□ Established
	□ Delayed	□ Moderate	□ Probable
		■ **Minor**	□ Suspected
			□ Possible
			■ **Unlikely**

Effects CHOLESTYRAMINE, administered with neomycin, increases the clearance of oral and IV LORAZEPAM.

Mechanism Unknown. However, interference with enterohepatic recycling of LORAZEPAM glucuronide is possible.

Management No special precautions are needed.

Discussion

In a study of 7 healthy volunteers, radiolabeled lorazepam was given IV at the same time as an oral dose of non-labeled lorazepam. Pharmacokinetic parameters were determined before and after treatment with neomycin 1 g every 6 hours (started the day before lorazepam) given with cholestyramine 4 g every 4 hours (started 4 hours after lorazepam). Cholestyramine and neomycin were given empirically to interfere with enterohepatic recirculation of lorazepam glucuronide, the major metabolite of lorazepam. The clearance of both IV and oral lorazepam was more rapid following cholestyramine and neomycin administration. The $t_{1/2}$ of IV lorazepam decreased from 19.7 to 16 hours, while that of oral lorazepam declined from 15.8 to 11.7 hours, indicating that the metabolite normally undergoes enterohepatic recirculation.[1] Although both neomycin and cholestyramine were used in this study, an in vitro experiment demonstrated that cholestyramine binds 74% of lorazepam glucuronide as measured through equilibrium dialysis using physiologic fluid simulation and expected in vivo drug concentrations.[2] These data suggest that the primary effect was due to cholestyramine, although neomycin appears to contribute.

No information exists on impairment of the clinical effects of lorazepam as a result of this drug interaction. Based on the magnitude of the change and the apparent need to have both neomycin and cholestyramine given together, it is unlikely that the interaction would result in significant morbidity.

[1] Herman RJ, et al. *Clin Pharmacol Ther.* 1989;46(1):18. [2] Herman RJ, et al. *Pharm Res.* 1991;8(4):538.

* Asterisk indicates drugs cited in interaction reports.

Benzodiazepines (Ox.) — *Cimetidine*

Alprazolam* (eg, *Xanax*)	Estazolam	Cimetidine* (eg, *Tagamet*)
Chlordiazepoxide*	Flurazepam* (eg, *Dalmane*)	
Clonazepam (*Klonopin*)	Midazolam*	
Clorazepate* (eg, *Tranxene*)	Quazepam (*Doral*)	
Diazepam* (eg, *Valium*)	Triazolam* (eg, *Halcion*)	

Significance	Onset	Severity	Documentation
3	■ **Rapid**	□ Major	□ Established
	□ Delayed	□ Moderate	■ **Probable**
		■ **Minor**	□ Suspected
			□ Possible
			□ Unlikely

Effects Serum levels of some BENZODIAZEPINES may be increased. Certain actions, especially sedation, may be enhanced.

Mechanism Inhibition of hepatic oxidative metabolism due to enzyme inhibition; other mechanisms may be involved.[1-4]

Management Monitor for increased/prolonged sedation. Warn patients of possible impairment of judgment and reflexes. Reduce the BENZODIAZEPINE dose as needed. Use of BENZODIAZEPINES not metabolized by oxidation may avoid the interaction.

Discussion

Benzodiazepines that undergo oxidative metabolism have reduced clearance (30% to 63%), longer half-lives, and higher serum levels with this combination.[2,3,5-16] Onset is rapid and sustained, but returns to baseline if cimetidine is stopped for 48 h.[8] Effects may be more pronounced in elderly patients with baseline impairment in clearance.[11] Reports of increased bioavailability of some agents reflect decreased first-pass metabolism rather than enhanced GI absorption.[4,7,11,12] While increased duration of sedation has occurred,[6,7,10,17,18] benzodiazepines undergoing hepatic glucuronidation (lorazepam [eg, *Ativan*], oxazepam, and temazepam [eg, *Restoril*]) do not interact.[1,7,13,19] Studies with midazolam show no effect[20] or effects comparable with diazepam.[20-22] Nizatidine (eg, *Axid*) or famotidine (eg, *Pepcid*) do not appear to interact.[14,23]

1 Patwardhan RV, et al. *Gastroenterology.* 1980;79(5 pt 1):912.
2 Greenblatt DJ, et al. *N Engl J Med.* 1984;310(25):1639.
3 Pourbaix S, et al. *Int J Clin Pharmacol Ther Toxicol.* 1985;23(8):447.
4 Fee JP, et al. *Clin Pharmacol Ther.* 1987;41(1):80.
5 Desmond PV, et al. *Ann Intern Med.* 1980;93(2):266.
6 Klotz U, et al. *N Engl J Med.* 1980;302(18):1012.
7 Klotz U, et al. *Eur J Clin Pharmacol.* 1980;18(6):517.
8 Patwardhan RV, et al. *Gastroenterology.* 1981;81(3):547.
9 Klotz U, et al. *Clin Pharmacol Ther.* 1981;30(4):513.
10 Gough PA, et al. *Br J Clin Pharmacol.* 1982;14(5):739.
11 Divoll M, et al. *J Am Geriat Soc.* 1982;30(11):684.
12 Abernethy DR, et al. *Psychopharmacol.* 1983;80(3):275.
13 Greenblatt DJ, et al. *J Clin Pharmacol.* 1984;24(4):187.
14 Locniskar A, et al. *J Clin Pharmacol.* 1986;26(4):299.
15 Friedman H, et al. *J Clin Pharmacol.* 1988;28(3):228.
16 Andersson T, et al. *Eur J Clin Pharmacol.* 1990;39(1):51.
17 Parker WA, et al. *DICP.* 1984;18(12):980.
18 Britton ML, et al. *Drug Intell Clin Pharm.* 1985;19(9):666.
19 Greenblatt DJ, et al. *J Pharm Sci.* 1984;73(3):399.
20 Greenblatt DJ, et al. *Anesth Analg.* 1986;65(2):176.
21 Salonen M, et al. *Acta Pharmacol Toxicol.* 1986;58(2):91.
22 Sanders LD, et al. *Anaesthesia.* 1993;48(4):286.
23 Klotz U. *Scand J Gastroenterol.* 1987;136(suppl):18.

* Asterisk indicates drugs cited in interaction reports. Based on pharmacologic and pharmacokinetic considerations, similar interactions may occur with other drugs that are listed.

Benzodiazepines — *Cisapride*

Benzodiazepines	Cisapride
Diazepam* (eg, *Valium*)	Cisapride*† (*Propulsid*)

Significance	Onset	Severity	Documentation
5	■ **Rapid**	□ Major	□ Established
	□ Delayed	□ Moderate	□ Probable
		■ **Minor**	□ Suspected
			■ **Possible**
			□ Unlikely

Effects The rate of absorption of DIAZEPAM may be increased, causing a faster onset of action. The effect usually does not persist with multiple dosing.

Mechanism Accelerated absorption of DIAZEPAM because of increased GI motility produced by CISAPRIDE.

Management Caution patients about the faster initial onset of DIAZEPAM action, but that a clinically important effect is not expected with multiple dosing.

Discussion

In a randomized, double-blind, placebo-controlled trial, the effects of cisapride administration on the pharmacokinetics of diazepam were studied in 8 healthy volunteers.[1] Following the IV administration of cisapride 8 mg or placebo, subjects received an orange drink containing diazepam 10 mg in solution. Cisapride administration increased stomach emptying time. The peak serum concentration of diazepam increased from 368.6 to 433.5 mcg/L, and the AUC increased from 253 to 328 mcg•h/L during the first hour after drinking the diazepam solution with cisapride coadministration compared with placebo. However, the AUC of diazepam at 48 hours was not significantly altered. The changes in the pharmacokinetics of diazepam were associated with accentuation of the slowing in patients' reaction time response to visual stimuli during the first 45 minutes after drinking the diazepam solution; however, there was no significant difference in reaction time after 1 hour. The onset of response to diazepam may be increased by administration of cisapride, but because the overall bioavailability of diazepam is not affected, a clinically important effect is not expected to occur with multiple dosing of diazepam.

[1] Bateman DN. *Eur J Clin Pharmacol.* 1986;30(2):205.

* Asterisk indicates drugs cited in interaction reports.
† Available from the manufacturer on a limited-access protocol.

Benzodiazepines (Ox.) — *Clotrimazole*

Alprazolam (eg, *Xanax*)	Estazolam	Clotrimazole*
Chlordiazepoxide	Flurazepam	
Clonazepam (eg, *Klonopin*)	Midazolam*	
Clorazepate (eg, *Tranxene*)	Quazepam (*Doral*)	
Diazepam (eg, *Valium*)	Triazolam (eg, *Halcion*)	

Significance	Onset	Severity	Documentation
4	□ Rapid	□ Major	□ Established
	■ **Delayed**	■ **Moderate**	□ Probable
		□ Minor	□ Suspected
			■ **Possible**
			□ Unlikely

Effects Plasma concentrations of certain oral BENZODIAZEPINES may be elevated, increasing the pharmacologic effects and risk of adverse reactions (eg, increased sedation).

Mechanism Inhibition of presystemic metabolism (CYP3A4) of certain BENZODIAZEPINES by oral CLOTRIMAZOLE.

Management Monitor the clinical response of the patient when CLOTRIMAZOLE is started or stopped. Adjust the BENZODIAZEPINE dose as needed.

Discussion

The effects of clotrimazole troches on the pharmacokinetics of midazolam oral and IV were studied in 10 healthy subjects.[1] In a randomized, crossover study, each subject received oral midazolam 2 mg or IV midazolam 0.025 mg/kg alone or 1 hour after the last dose of clotrimazole troches 10 mg 3 times daily for 5 days. Compared with receiving oral midazolam alone, pretreatment with clotrimazole decreased the oral clearance of midazolam 37% and increased the AUC 61%. Clotrimazole did not alter the pharmacokinetics of IV midazolam.

[1] Shord SS, et al. *Br J Clin Pharmacol.* 2010;69(2):160.

* Asterisk indicates drugs cited in interaction reports. Based on pharmacologic and pharmacokinetic considerations, similar interactions may occur with other drugs that are listed.

Benzodiazepines — *Clozapine*

Benzodiazepines		Clozapine
Clonazepam (eg, *Klonopin*)	Flurazepam*	Clozapine* (eg, *Clozaril*)
Diazepam* (eg, *Valium*)	Lorazepam* (eg, *Ativan*)	

Significance	Onset	Severity	Documentation
1	■ **Rapid**	■ **Major**	□ Established
	□ Delayed	□ Moderate	□ Probable
		□ Minor	■ **Suspected**
			□ Possible
			□ Unlikely

Effects The pharmacologic or toxic effects of certain BENZODIAZEPINES may be increased.

Mechanism Unknown.

Management Consider monitoring vital signs and observing patients for excessive adverse reactions when CLOZAPINE and BENZODIAZEPINES are coadministered.

Discussion

Marked sedation and excessive salivation have occurred in patients during coadministration of clozapine and benzodiazepines.[1,2] Two patients became acutely agitated while taking clozapine 100 mg/day.[2] To treat the agitation, 1 patient received lorazepam 2 mg IM. Within 95 minutes, the patient experienced marked sedation, salivation, and ataxia. The second patient was given 3 doses of lorazepam 1 mg orally over 24 hours. The next day, the patient was lethargic, pale, drooling, and ataxic. Both patients required assistance in order to walk. Two hours after discontinuation of lorazepam each patient was alert. In 1 patient, rechallenge with lorazepam while receiving clozapine 350 mg/day resulted in calming without sedation. In a second report, 4 patients collapsed and lost consciousness while taking diazepam, flurazepam, or lorazepam during coadministration with clozapine.[1] In addition, patients experienced severe sedation, excessive salivation, hypotension, toxic delirium, or respiratory arrest. Death of a 43-year-old man was attributed to respiratory arrest possibly due to coadministration of clozapine and a benzodiazepine regimen (ie, lorazepam plus flunitrazepam†).[3]

[1] Grohmann R, et al. *Psychopharmacology (Berl)*. 1989;99(suppl):S109.
[2] Cobb CD, et al. *Am J Psychiatry*. 1991;148(11):1606.
[3] Klimke A, et al. *Am J Psychiatry*. 1994;151(5):780.

* Asterisk indicates drugs cited in interaction reports. Based on pharmacologic and pharmacokinetic considerations, similar interactions may occur with other drugs that are listed.
† Not available in the United States.

Benzodiazepines (Gluc.) | **Contraceptives, Hormonal**

Lorazepam* (eg, *Ativan*)	Temazepam* (eg, *Restoril*)	Contraceptives, Oral* (eg, *Ortho-Novum*)
Oxazepam*		

Significance	Onset	Severity	Documentation
5	□ Rapid ■ **Delayed**	□ Major □ Moderate ■ **Minor**	□ Established □ Probable □ Suspected ■ **Possible** □ Unlikely

Effects The coadministration of combination ORAL CONTRACEPTIVES and certain BENZODIAZEPINES may result in an increased BENZODIAZEPINE clearance rate.

Mechanism Combination ORAL CONTRACEPTIVES may stimulate the rate of BENZODIAZEPINE glucuronidation. The exact mechanism is unknown.

Management Monitor patients receiving combination ORAL CONTRACEPTIVES concurrently with these BENZODIAZEPINES for clinical signs and symptoms suggesting an alteration in the BENZODIAZEPINE dose.

Discussion

One study of 7 women taking combination OCs for at least 6 months compared with 8 matched controls reported that after a single dose of lorazepam or oxazepam the group receiving OCs showed a reduced $t_{1/2}$ for lorazepam (57%) and oxazepam (36%) as well as an increase in both plasma clearance and volume of distribution.[1] A second study based on single doses of lorazepam and temazepam reported a decrease in $t_{1/2}$ compared with controls of 12.8 versus 16.5 h and 8 versus 13.3 h, respectively.[2] However, a third study reported no difference in the $t_{1/2}$ of single doses of lorazepam and oxazepam when administered to women taking OCs for at least 3 months compared with controls.[3]

Additional data suggest that women taking combination OCs are more sensitive to psychomotor impairment resulting from benzodiazepine administration and that these changes are not explained by pharmacokinetic alterations.[4] However, this study does not address at what point during the menstrual cycle the evaluations were performed. This may be pertinent because a study of diazepam (eg, *Valium*) suggests that both motor and cognitive impairment may fluctuate based on the day of the menstrual cycle on which the woman is evaluated.[5]

[1] Patwardhan RV, et al. *Hepatology*. 1983;3(2):248.
[2] Stoehr GP, et al. *Clin Pharmacol Ther*. 1984;36(5):683.
[3] Abernethy DR, et al. *Clin Pharmacol Ther*. 1983;33(5):628.
[4] Kroboth PD, et al. *Clin Pharmacol Ther*. 1985;38(5):525.
[5] Ellinwood EH, et al. *Clin Pharmacol Ther*. 1984;35(3):360.

* Asterisk indicates drugs cited in interaction reports.

Benzodiazepines (Ox.) — *Contraceptives, Hormonal*

Benzodiazepines (Ox.)		Contraceptives, Hormonal
Alprazolam* (eg, *Xanax*)	Halazepam	Contraceptives, Oral* (eg, *Ortho-Novum*)
Chlordiazepoxide*	Midazolam*	
Clonazepam (eg, *Klonopin*)	Prazepam	
Clorazepate (eg, *Tranxene*)	Quazepam (*Doral*)	
Diazepam* (eg, *Valium*)	Triazolam* (eg, *Halcion*)	
Flurazepam		

Significance	Onset	Severity	Documentation
3	☐ Rapid	☐ Major	☐ Established
	■ **Delayed**	☐ Moderate	☐ Probable
		■ **Minor**	■ **Suspected**
			☐ Possible
			☐ Unlikely

Effects Coadministration of combination HORMONAL CONTRACEPTIVES and certain BENZODIAZEPINES that undergo oxidation may result in a prolongation of BENZODIAZEPINE $t_{1/2}$.

Mechanism Combination HORMONAL CONTRACEPTIVES may inhibit hepatic mixed-function oxidases, leading to a decrease in BENZODIAZEPINE oxidation rate.

Management Observe patients receiving this combination for any clinical signs and symptoms that suggest a reduction in the BENZODIAZEPINE dose is indicated.

Discussion

Studies examining the potential drug interaction between combination OCs and diazepam[1,2] or chlordiazepoxide[3,4] reported a prolongation of diazepam and chlordiazepoxide $t_{1/2}$ compared with controls.[1,2] None of these studies reported statistically significant changes in volume of distribution or plasma protein binding.[1-4] Conflicting data have been reported regarding alprazolam. One study reported inhibition of alprazolam metabolism by OCs, while another study reported no interaction.[5,6] In 9 healthy women who took a combination contraceptive or placebo for 10 days before a single midazolam 7.5 mg oral dose, midazolam AUC was increased an average of 21% compared with placebo.[7] Similar results were reported in a study that enrolled 34 obese women.[8] Additional data suggest that women taking OCs are more sensitive to psychomotor impairment resulting from benzodiazepine administration and that these changes are not explained by pharmacokinetic alterations.[9] However, this study does not address at what point during the menstrual cycle the evaluations were performed. This may be pertinent because the study of diazepam suggests that both motor and cognitive impairment may fluctuate based on the day of the menstrual cycle on which the woman is evaluated.[10]

1 Giles HG, et al. *Eur J Clin Pharmacol.* 1981;20(3):207.
2 Abernethy DR, et al. *N Engl J Med.* 1982;306(13):791.
3 Roberts RK, et al. *Clin Pharmacol Ther.* 1979;25(6):826.
4 Patwardhan RV, et al. *Hepatology.* 1983;3(2):248.
5 Stoehr GP, et al. *Clin Pharmacol Ther.* 1984;36(5):683.
6 Scavone JM, et al. *J Clin Pharmacol.* 1988;28(5):454.
7 Palovaara S, et al. *Br J Clin Pharmacol.* 2000;50(4):333.
8 Edelman A, et al. *Br J Clin Pharmacol.* 2012;74(3):510.
9 Kroboth PD, et al. *Clin Pharmacol Ther.* 1985;38(5):525.
10 Ellinwood EH, et al. *Clin Pharmacol Ther.* 1984;35(3):360.

* Asterisk indicates drugs cited in interaction reports. Based on pharmacologic and pharmacokinetic considerations, similar interactions may occur with other drugs that are listed.

Benzodiazepines — *Danshen*

Diazepam (eg, *Valium*)	Triazolam (eg, *Halcion*)	Danshen*
Midazolam*		
Quazepam (*Doral*)		

Significance	Onset	Severity	Documentation
4	☐ Rapid	☐ Major	☐ Established
	■ **Delayed**	■ **Moderate**	☐ Probable
		☐ Minor	☐ Suspected
			■ **Possible**
			☐ Unlikely

Effects MIDAZOLAM plasma concentrations may be reduced, decreasing the pharmacologic effect.

Mechanism Increased GI metabolism (CYP3A4) of oral MIDAZOLAM by DANSHEN.

Management If DANSHEN cannot be avoided, coadminister with caution. Monitor the clinical response of patients and adjust the MIDAZOLAM dose as needed.

Discussion

The effect of danshen on the pharmacokinetics of oral midazolam was studied in 12 healthy men.[1] Using a sequential, open-label, 2-period design, each subject received a single dose of midazolam 15 mg before and after 14 days of receiving danshen extract 4 g 3 times daily. Compared with giving midazolam alone, pretreatment with danshen increased midazolam oral clearance 35.4% and reduced the C_{max} and AUC 31.1% and 27%, respectively. The midazolam t½ was not changed.

[1] Qiu F, et al. *Br J Clin Pharmacol.* 2010;69(6):656.

* Asterisk indicates drugs cited in interaction reports. Based on pharmacologic and pharmacokinetic considerations, similar interactions may occur with other drugs that are listed.

Benzodiazepines — *Deferasirox*

Midazolam*	Deferasirox* (*Exjade*)

Significance	Onset	Severity	Documentation
4	☐ Rapid ■ **Delayed**	☐ Major ■ **Moderate** ☐ Minor	☐ Established ☐ Probable ☐ Suspected ■ **Possible** ☐ Unlikely

Effects MIDAZOLAM plasma concentrations may be reduced, decreasing the pharmacologic effect.

Mechanism DEFERASIROX may increase the metabolism (CYP3A4) of MIDAZOLAM.

Management Monitor the clinical response of patients. If an interaction is suspected, adjust the MIDAZOLAM dose as needed.

Discussion

The effects of deferasirox on the pharmacokinetics of midazolam were studied in 22 healthy subjects.[1] A single dose of midazolam 5 mg oral solution was administered alone and after 5 days of deferasirox 30 mg/kg daily. Compared with giving midazolam alone, pretreatment with deferasirox decreased midazolam exposure (AUC) and C_{max} 9.8% and 22%, respectively. Other midazolam pharmacokinetic parameters were not altered by deferasirox administration. Although the effects of deferasirox on the midazolam AUC and C_{max} were modest, more pronounced effects may occur in the clinical setting.[1]

[1] Skerjanec A, et al. *J Clin Pharmacol.* 2010;50(2):205.

* Asterisk indicates drugs cited in interaction reports.

Benzodiazepines (Gluc.) — *Diflunisal*

Benzodiazepines (Gluc.)		Diflunisal
Lorazepam (eg, *Ativan*)	Temazepam (eg, *Restoril*)	Diflunisal* (eg, *Dolobid*)
Oxazepam* (eg, *Serax*)		

Significance	Onset	Severity	Documentation
5	■ **Rapid**	□ Major	□ Established
	□ Delayed	□ Moderate	□ Probable
		■ **Minor**	□ Suspected
			■ **Possible**
			□ Unlikely

Effects DIFLUNISAL may decrease the bioavailability of OXAZEPAM; however, a clinically important interaction appears unlikely.

Mechanism DIFLUNISAL may displace OXAZEPAM from plasma protein binding sites, thereby increasing presystemic hepatic extraction and decreasing systemic availability. Also, the glucuronides of DIFLUNISAL and OXAZEPAM may compete for tubular secretion.

Management Because a clinically important interaction is unlikely, dosage adjustment of either agent is probably not necessary.

Discussion

In 6 healthy men, a single dose of oxazepam 30 mg was administered following diflunisal 500 mg twice daily for 9 days.[1] The peak plasma concentration and AUC of diflunisal decreased 38% and 16%, respectively. The AUC and elimination $t_{½}$ of oxazepam glucuronide increased 38%. The clinical importance of this interaction was not established.

It is not known if benzodiazepines metabolized by oxidation would interact similarly with diflunisal. The other benzodiazepines that are metabolized by glucuronidation (lorazepam and temazepam) may interact in a similar manner to oxazepam.

[1] van Hecken AM, et al. *Br J Clin Pharmacol.* 1985;20:225.

* Asterisk indicates drugs cited in interaction reports. Based on pharmacologic and pharmacokinetic considerations, similar interactions may occur with other drugs that are listed.

Benzodiazepines — *Diltiazem*

Benzodiazepines		Diltiazem
Diazepam* (eg, *Valium*)	Triazolam* (eg, *Halcion*)	Diltiazem* (eg, *Cardizem*)
Midazolam* (eg, *Versed*)		

Significance	Onset	Severity	Documentation
2	■ **Rapid**	□ Major	□ Established
	□ Delayed	■ **Moderate**	■ **Probable**
		□ Minor	□ Suspected
			□ Possible
			□ Unlikely

Effects Effects of certain BENZODIAZEPINES may be increased, producing increased CNS depression and prolonged effects.

Mechanism DILTIAZEM may decrease metabolism of certain BENZODIAZEPINES and decrease first-pass effect of TRIAZOLAM.

Management Give a lower dose of the BENZODIAZEPINE. Caution the patient about increased and prolonged sedative effects.

Discussion

The effects of oral diltiazem 60 mg 3 times/day for 2 days on the pharmacokinetics and pharmacodynamics of a single 15 mg oral dose of midazolam were studied in a double-blind, placebo-controlled, randomized, crossover investigation in 9 healthy volunteers.[1] The AUC for midazolam increased 275%, while the peak midazolam concentration doubled, and the elimination $t_{1/2}$ was prolonged 49%. The changes in midazolam pharmacokinetics were accompanied by prolonged and deep sedative effects. In 30 patients undergoing coronary artery bypass grafting, diltiazem increased the midazolam mean concentration-time curve and $t_{1/2}$ 24% and 43%, respectively, compared with placebo.[2] In a study involving 10 healthy volunteers, diltiazem 60 mg increased mean AUC, elimination $t_{1/2}$, and peak plasma concentration of triazolam 0.25 mg when compared with placebo.[3] Similar changes in triazolam pharmacokinetics were noted in another study of 7 healthy volunteers who received triazolam after 3 days of diltiazem or placebo.[4] Increased and prolonged pharmacodynamic effects were noted in both studies. In a randomized, double-blind, crossover study, 13 healthy volunteers were given placebo or 200 mg diltiazem orally for 3 days before and 7 days after a single 2 mg oral dose of diazepam.[5] Diltiazem increased diazepam AUC 24% and $t_{1/2}$ by 42% compared with placebo. No pharmacodynamic changes were noted with this small dose of diazepam. With this drug interaction, midazolam and triazolam should not be treated as short-acting agents.[3]

[1] Backman JT, et al. *Br J Clin Pharmacol.* 1994;37:221.
[2] Ahonen J, et al. *Anesthesiology.* 1996;85:1246.
[3] Varhe A, et al. *Clin Pharmacol Ther.* 1996;59:369.
[4] Kosuge K, et al. *Br J Clin Pharmacol.* 1997;43:367.
[5] Kosuge K, et al. *Drug Metab Dispos.* 2001;29:1284.

* Asterisk indicates drugs cited in interaction reports.

Benzodiazepines (Ox.) — *Disulfiram*

Benzodiazepines (Ox.)		Disulfiram
Alprazolam* (eg, *Xanax*)	Diazepam* (eg, *Valium*)	Disulfiram* (eg, *Antabuse*)
Chlordiazepoxide* (eg, *Librium*)	Flurazepam	
Clonazepam (eg, *Klonopin*)	Quazepam (*Doral*)	
Clorazepate (eg, *Tranxene*)	Triazolam (eg, *Halcion*)	

Significance	Onset	Severity	Documentation
3	☐ Rapid	☐ Major	☐ Established
	■ **Delayed**	☐ Moderate	☐ Probable
		■ **Minor**	■ **Suspected**
			☐ Possible
			☐ Unlikely

Effects Possible increase in CNS-depressant actions.

Mechanism DISULFIRAM may inhibit the hepatic metabolism of BENZODIAZEPINES that undergo oxidation.

Management If increased CNS-depressant effects occur during coadministration of these agents, the dose of BENZODIAZEPINE may need to be decreased.

Discussion

In 1 study, 6 healthy subjects received a single IV dose of chlordiazepoxide 50 mg, oral diazepam 0.143 mg/kg, and oral oxazepam 0.429 mg/kg after 12 to 14 days of disulfiram 500 mg/day therapy.[1] The plasma clearance of chlordiazepoxide and diazepam decreased 54% and 41%, respectively, and the plasma clearance of the active N-desmethyl metabolites also decreased. Oxazepam and lorazepam (eg, *Ativan*), benzodiazepines metabolized by glucuronidation, were not affected by disulfiram coadministration.[2] Temazepam (eg, *Restoril*) is also not likely to interact with disulfiram. One study in alcoholic patients failed to demonstrate a change in single-dose pharmacokinetics after 2 weeks of disulfiram treatment.[3]

[1] MacLeod SM, et al. *Clin Pharmacol Ther.* 1978;24(5):583.
[2] Sellers EM, et al. *Arzneimittelforschung.* 1980;30(5a):882.
[3] Diquet B, et al. *Eur J Clin Pharmacol.* 1990;38(2):157.

* Asterisk indicates drugs cited in interaction reports. Based on pharmacologic and pharmacokinetic considerations, similar interactions may occur with other drugs that are listed.

Benzodiazepines — *Echinacea*

Midazolam*	Echinacea*

Significance	Onset	Severity	Documentation
4	☐ Rapid ■ **Delayed**	☐ Major ■ **Moderate** ☐ Minor	☐ Established ☐ Probable ☐ Suspected ■ **Possible** ☐ Unlikely

Effects MIDAZOLAM plasma concentrations may be reduced, decreasing the effect.

Mechanism ECHINACEA may increase MIDAZOLAM's hepatic metabolism (CYP3A) while inhibiting intestinal metabolism (CYP3A).

Management Avoid ECHINACEA use in patients receiving MIDAZOLAM.

Discussion

Results are conflicting. The effects of echinacea (*Echinacea purpurea* root) on CYP-450 activity were assessed by administering the probe drug midazolam (CYP3A).[1] Twelve subjects received midazolam (5 mg oral and 0.05 mg/kg IV) alone and after 8 days of pretreatment with echinacea 400 mg 4 times daily. Echinacea increased the systemic clearance of IV midazolam 34% and decreased the AUC 23%. The oral clearance of midazolam was not affected by echinacea; however, the oral availability of midazolam was increased 50%. Hepatic and intestinal availability of midazolam were altered in opposite directions; the hepatic availability decreased 18%, while intestinal availability increased 85%. Others found a minimal effect of echinacea on midazolam levels.[2] The discrepancy may be caused by the differences in study design. In 1 study, the echinacea product was an extract from echinacea root,[2] whereas in the second study the echinacea product was a whole plant extract.[1] In another study, 13 healthy subjects received a single oral dose of midazolam 8 mg syrup before and after 28 days of *E. purpurea* 250 mg (fresh extract).[3] Pretreatment with echinacea decreased the AUC and increased the oral clearance of midazolam compared with taking midazolam alone.

The ingredients of many herbal products are not standardized. It is unclear if herbal products contain ingredients other than those listed on the label or purported to be present that could interact with midazolam.

[1] Gorski JC, et al. *Clin Pharmacol Ther.* 2004;75(1):89.
[2] Gurley BJ, et al. *Clin Pharmacol Ther.* 2004;76(5)428.
[3] Penzak SR, et al. *Pharmacotherapy.* 2010;30(8):797.

* Asterisk indicates drugs cited in interaction reports.

Benzodiazepines | **Fluoxetine**

Alprazolam* (eg, *Xanax*)
Diazepam* (eg, *Valium*)
Midazolam*

Fluoxetine* (eg, *Prozac*)

Significance	Onset	Severity	Documentation
5	☐ Rapid	☐ Major	☐ Established
	■ **Delayed**	☐ Moderate	☐ Probable
		■ **Minor**	☐ Suspected
			■ **Possible**
			☐ Unlikely

Effects Increased pharmacologic effects of BENZODIAZEPINES.

Mechanism Hepatic metabolism of BENZODIAZEPINES may be decreased because of microsomal enzyme inhibition.

Management Based on present evidence, no specific recommendations can be made. If the effects of the BENZODIAZEPINE are increased, decrease the dose as needed.

Discussion

In 6 healthy men, coadministration of diazepam and fluoxetine decreased the clearance and increased the t½ of diazepam.[1] Patients received diazepam 10 mg or fluoxetine 60 mg in combination or with placebo. Psychomotor performance tests were conducted on each subject before and at varying intervals for 12 hr after they received diazepam, fluoxetine, or placebo. The plasma levels of diazepam and its active metabolite, N-desmethyldiazepam, were higher following fluoxetine administration compared with placebo. After fluoxetine pretreatment, the AUC for diazepam was larger, the t½ was longer, and the plasma clearance was decreased, resulting in higher plasma concentrations of diazepam. Although there was an apparent pharmacokinetic interaction, no clinical effects were demonstrated by the psychomotor tests used. Because diazepam and its N-desmethyl metabolite are pharmacologically active, the total active benzodiazepines (eg, diazepam plus N-desmethyldiazepam) would be quantitated as similar in the presence or absence of fluoxetine administration. Thus, no clinically important interaction was observed. There was considerable variation in individual response, and no statistical analysis was applied to the data. In a study of 24 healthy subjects, multiple doses of fluoxetine 60 mg/day for 8 days did not alter the pharmacokinetics of triazolam (eg, *Halcion*) 0.25 mg.[2] Fluoxetine prolonged the t½ of alprazolam (from 17 to 20 hr) and reduced the clearance 21%.[3] In the same study, fluoxetine increased absorption of clonazepam (eg, *Klonopin*) but did not affect clearance. The clinical consequences of these pharmacokinetic changes were not assessed. In vitro inhibition of midazolam metabolism also has been demonstrated.[4] A study comparing the effects of fluoxetine on alprazolam found a small increase in alprazolam t½ but no change in pharmacodynamics.[5]

[1] Lemberger L, et al. *Clin Pharmacol Ther.* 1988;43:412.
[2] Wright CE, et al. *Pharmacotherapy.* 1992;12:103.
[3] Greenblatt DJ, et al. *Clin Pharmacol Ther.* 1992;52:479.
[4] von Moltke LL, et al. *J Clin Pharmacol.* 1996;36:783.
[5] Hall J, et al. *J Clin Psychopharmacol.* 2003;23:349.

* Asterisk indicates drugs cited in interaction reports.

Benzodiazepines — *Fluvoxamine*

Alprazolam* (eg, *Xanax*)	Estazolam	Fluvoxamine*
Chlordiazepoxide (eg, *Librium*)	Flurazepam	
Clonazepam (eg, *Klonopin*)	Midazolam	
Clorazepate (eg, *Tranxene*)	Quazepam* (*Doral*)	
Diazepam* (eg, *Valium*)	Triazolam (eg, *Halcion*)	

Significance	Onset	Severity	Documentation
3	☐ Rapid ■ **Delayed**	☐ Major ☐ Moderate ■ **Minor**	☐ Established ☐ Probable ■ **Suspected** ☐ Possible ☐ Unlikely

Effects Reduced clearance, prolonged $t_{½}$, and increased serum concentrations of certain BENZODIAZEPINES may occur. Sedation or ataxia may be increased.

Mechanism FLUVOXAMINE appears to inhibit the oxidative hepatic metabolism of BENZODIAZEPINES.

Management Observe patients for increased or prolonged sedation or other evidence of CNS impairment. A reduced BENZODIAZEPINE dosage or longer dosing interval may be needed. Use of a BENZODIAZEPINE not metabolized by oxidation, such as lorazepam (eg, *Ativan*), may avoid this interaction.

Discussion

The effects of fluvoxamine 100 to 150 mg/day on the pharmacokinetics of oral diazepam 10 mg/day were studied in 8 healthy volunteers.[1] Compared with the control period, fluvoxamine decreased the oral clearance of diazepam 65%, while increasing the mean C_{max} 32% (from 108 to 143 ng/mL), increasing the AUC 180%, and prolonging the $t_{½}$ 131% (from 51 to 118 hr).[1] Fluvoxamine may inhibit the N-desmethylation of diazepam to its active metabolite. In another study, fluvoxamine increased alprazolam plasma levels 100%, and the $t_{½}$ was prolonged from 20 to 34 hr, resulting in reductions in psychomotor performance within 10 days.[2] The dosage of a benzodiazepine that undergoes oxidative metabolism (eg, alprazolam) may need to be reduced during coadministration of fluvoxamine.[1,2] In 12 volunteers, fluvoxamine did not change plasma levels of quazepam but decreased levels of its active metabolite.[3] The pharmacokinetics of lorazepam, which is metabolized by conjugation, were not affected by coadministration of fluvoxamine.[1] The pharmacokinetics of fluvoxamine do not appear to be altered.

[1] Perucca E, et al. *Clin Pharmacol Ther.* 1994;56(5):471.
[2] Fleishaker JC, et al. *Eur J Clin Pharmacol.* 1994;46(1):35.
[3] Kanda H, et al. *J Clin Pharmacol.* 2003;43(12):1392.

* Asterisk indicates drugs cited in interaction reports. Based on pharmacologic and pharmacokinetic considerations, similar interactions may occur with other drugs that are listed.

Benzodiazepines — *Food*

Diazepam* (eg, *Valium*)	Triazolam* (eg, *Halcion*)	Grapefruit Juice*
Midazolam*		
Quazepam* (*Doral*)		

Significance	Onset	Severity	Documentation
2	■ **Rapid**	□ Major	□ Established
	□ Delayed	■ **Moderate**	■ **Probable**
		□ Minor	□ Suspected
			□ Possible
			□ Unlikely

Effects The pharmacologic effects of certain BENZODIAZEPINES may be increased and the onset delayed.

Mechanism Inhibition of first-pass enteric metabolism (CYP3A4) of certain BENZODIAZEPINES. Patients with liver cirrhosis may be more dependent on CYP3A4 intestinal metabolism of MIDAZOLAM than patients with normal liver function.[1]

Management Avoid coadministration. Caution patients to take BENZODIAZEPINES that undergo first-pass metabolism with a liquid other than GRAPEFRUIT JUICE (GFJ) and that effects can last up to 72 hr after a single glass of GFJ.[2] Alprazolam (eg, *Xanax*) does not appear to be affected by GFJ.[3]

Discussion

Diazepam – GFJ increased diazepam AUC 3.2-fold, C_{max} 1.5-fold, and delayed the time to reach the peak level (T_{max}) from 1.5 to 2.06 hr.[4]

Midazolam – GFJ increased midazolam AUC 106% and decreased the AUC of the hydroxylmidazolam metabolite 25%.[1] Giving GFJ 15 or 60 min before midazolam increased C_{max} 56%, T_{max} 79%, AUC 52%, and bioavailability 11%.[5] Performance on the digit symbol substitution test (DSST) was increased. GFJ did not affect IV midazolam pharmacokinetics. Flavonoids in GFJ may inhibit midazolam metabolism.[6] GFJ increased midazolam C_{max} and AUC 1.3- and 1.5-fold, respectively, and reduced oral clearance 28%.[7]

Quazepam – GFJ increased the C_{max} and AUC of quazepam and the active metabolite 2-oxoquazepam.[8] Sedative effects were not enhanced.[8]

Triazolam – GFJ increased the triazolam C_{max} 1.3-fold, AUC 1.5-fold, and delayed the T_{max} from 1.6 to 2.5 hr.[9] GFJ ingestion for 7 days before a dose of triazolam increased the AUC 143% compared with 49% when triazolam was taken with GFJ.[10] Performance on the DSST was decreased.[8] Sedative effects were not enhanced. Others studies have shown minor increases in the effects of midazolam[11] or slight drowsiness.[7]

1 Andersen V, et al. *Br J Clin Pharmacol.* 2002;54(2):120.
2 Greenblatt DJ, et al. *Clin Pharmacol Ther.* 2003;74(2):121.
3 Yasui N, et al. *Psychopharmacology.* 2000;150(2):185.
4 Ozdemir M, et al. *Eur J Drug Metab Pharmacokinet.* 1998;23(1):55.
5 Kupferschmidt HH, et al. *Clin Pharmacol Ther.* 1995;58(1):20.
6 Ha HR, et al. *Eur J Clin Pharmacol.* 1995;48(5):367.
7 Farkas D, et al. *J Clin Pharmacol.* 2007;47(3):286.
8 Sugimoto K, et al. *Eur J Clin Pharmacol.* 2006;62(3):209.
9 Hukkinen SK, et al. *Clin Pharmacol Ther.* 1995;58(2):127.
10 Lilja JJ, et al. *Eur J Clin Pharmacol.* 2000:56(5):411.
11 Vanakoski J, et al. *Eur J Clin Pharmacol.* 1996;50(6):501.

* Asterisk indicates drugs cited in interaction reports.

Benzodiazepines — *Ginkgo biloba*

Alprazolam* (eg, *Xanax*)	Midazolam*	Ginkgo biloba*

Significance	Onset	Severity	Documentation
5	□ Rapid ■ **Delayed**	□ Major □ Moderate ■ **Minor**	□ Established □ Probable □ Suspected ■ **Possible** □ Unlikely

Effects ALPRAZOLAM and MIDAZOLAM AUC may be altered by GINKGO BILOBA.

Mechanism Unknown.

Management Be prepared for evidence of a change in ALPRAZOLAM or MIDAZOLAM efficacy. Adjust the ALPRAZOLAM or MIDAZOLAM dose as needed.

Discussion

Data are conflicting. The effects of *Ginkgo biloba* extract on the pharmacokinetics of alprazolam were studied in 12 healthy volunteers.[1] Each subject received alprazolam 2 mg before and after 14 days of taking *Ginkgo biloba* extract 120 mg twice daily. Compared with administration of alprazolam alone, pretreatment with *Ginkgo biloba* decreased the alprazolam AUC 17%. However, the elimination $t_{½}$ of alprazolam was not affected, indicating a lack of effect of *Ginkgo biloba* on alprazolam metabolism (via the CYP3A4 pathway). In an open-label, randomized, crossover study in healthy volunteers receiving *Ginkgo biloba* and midazolam, *Ginkgo biloba* did not inhibit or induce CYP3A activity.[2] In a study in 13 healthy volunteers, a single oral dose of midazolam 8 mg was given before and after administering *Ginkgo biloba* 120 mg standardized extract twice daily for 28 days.[3] Pretreatment with *Ginkgo biloba* decreased the midazolam AUC 34% compared with giving midazolam alone. In another study, the effects of *Ginkgo biloba* extract (eg, *Ginkgold*) on the pharmacokinetics of midazolam were studied in 10 healthy men.[4] Each subject received oral midazolam 8 mg alone and after taking *Ginkgo biloba* extract 120 mg 3 times daily for 28 days. Compared with taking midazolam alone, pretreatment with *Ginkgo biloba* increased the midazolam AUC 25% and decreased the oral clearance 26%.

[1] Markowitz JS, et al. *J Clin Psychopharmacol.* 2003;23(6):576.
[2] Zadoyan G, et al. *Eur J Clin Pharmacol.* 2012;68(5):553.
[3] Penzak SR, et al. *J Clin Pharmacol.* 2008;48(6):671.
[4] Uchida S, et al. *J Clin Pharmacol.* 2006;46(11):1290.

* Asterisk indicates drugs cited in interaction reports.

Benzodiazepines — *Goldenseal*

Midazolam*	Goldenseal*

Significance	Onset	Severity	Documentation
4	☐ Rapid ■ **Delayed**	☐ Major ■ **Moderate** ☐ Minor	☐ Established ☐ Probable ☐ Suspected ■ **Possible** ☐ Unlikely

Effects MIDAZOLAM plasma concentrations may be elevated, possibly resulting in excessive CNS depressant effect.

Mechanism Inhibition of MIDAZOLAM metabolism (CYP3A4) by GOLDENSEAL.

Management Advise patients taking MIDAZOLAM to avoid concurrent use of GOLDENSEAL and to consult their health care provider before using herbal products.

Discussion

The effects of goldenseal on the pharmacokinetics of midazolam were studied in 16 healthy subjects.[1] Each individual received goldenseal (standardized to contain isoquinoline alkaloids 24.1 mg per capsule) 3 times daily for 14 days. Midazolam 8 mg was administered prior to the start of goldenseal administration and 2 hours after the last dose of goldenseal. Compared with taking midazolam alone, pretreatment with goldenseal; prolonged the $t_{½}$ from 2.01 to 3.15 hours, decreased the oral clearance 35.7%, and increased the midazolam AUC and C_{max} approximately 62.5% and 40.7%, respectively.

[1] Gurley BJ, et al. *Clin Pharmacol Ther.* 2008;83(1):61.

* Asterisk indicates drugs cited in interaction reports.

Benzodiazepines — *HCV Protease Inhibitors*

Alprazolam* (eg, *Xanax*) Midazolam*	Triazolam* (eg, *Halcion*)	Boceprevir* (*Victrelis*)	Telaprevir* (*Incivek*)

Significance	Onset	Severity	Documentation
1	☐ Rapid ■ **Delayed**	■ **Major** ☐ Moderate ☐ Minor	☐ Established ☐ Probable ■ **Suspected** ☐ Possible ☐ Unlikely

Effects MIDAZOLAM and TRIAZOLAM plasma concentrations may be elevated, increasing the pharmacologic effects and risk of severe sedation and prolonged respiratory depression.

Mechanism BENZODIAZEPINE metabolism (CYP3A) may be inhibited by HEPATITIS C VIRUS (HCV) PROTEASE INHIBITORS.

Management Coadministration of TRIAZOLAM or oral MIDAZOLAM and HCV PROTEASE INHIBITORS is contraindicated. Close clinical monitoring for respiratory depression and prolonged sedation is recommended when ALPRAZOLAM or IV MIDAZOLAM are coadministered with HCV PROTEASE INHIBITORS.[1,2] Consider a lower BENZODIAZEPINE dose.

Discussion

Pretreatment with boceprevir or telaprevir increased the AUC of oral midazolam approximately 5.3- and 9-fold, respectively.[1,2] Coadministration of triazolam or oral midazolam and boceprevir or telaprevir is contraindicated. Close clinical monitoring is warranted when parenteral midazolam and boceprevir or telaprevir are coadministered. Consider reducing the dose of midazolam. In an open-label study of 24 healthy volunteers, oral pretreatment with telaprevir 750 mg every 8 hours increased the AUC of a single IV dose of midazolam 0.5 mg and a single oral dose of midazolam 2 mg approximately 5- and 13-fold, respectively.[3]

[1] *Victrelis* [package insert]. Whitehouse Station, NJ: Schering Corporation; May 2011.

[2] *Incivek* [package insert]. Cambridge, MA: Vertex Pharmaceuticals Incorporated; May 2011.

[3] Garg V, et al. *J Clin Pharmacol.* 2012;52(10):1566.

* Asterisk indicates drugs cited in interaction reports.

Benzodiazepines — HMG-CoA Reductase Inhibitors

Benzodiazepines		HMG-CoA Reductase Inhibitors
Alprazolam (eg, *Xanax*)	Flurazepam	Atorvastatin* (eg, *Lipitor*)
Chlordiazepoxide	Midazolam*	
Clonazepam (eg, *Klonopin*)	Quazepam (*Doral*)	
Diazepam (eg, *Valium*)	Triazolam (eg, *Halcion*)	
Estazolam		

Significance	Onset	Severity	Documentation
4	☐ Rapid	☐ Major	☐ Established
	■ **Delayed**	■ **Moderate**	☐ Probable
		☐ Minor	☐ Suspected
			■ **Possible**
			☐ Unlikely

Effects The effects of certain BENZODIAZEPINES may be increased and prolonged.

Mechanism Decreased oxidative metabolism (CYP3A4) of certain BENZODIAZEPINES by ATORVASTATIN is suspected.

Management In patients receiving long-term treatment with ATORVASTATIN, consider the possibility of increased respiratory depression and prolonged sedation if BENZODIAZEPINES are administered.

Discussion

The effects of atorvastatin on the pharmacokinetics of midazolam were studied in 14 patients undergoing general anesthesia for elective surgery.[1] Seven patients had not received atorvastatin. Five patients were receiving atorvastatin 10 mg daily, 1 was receiving 20 mg daily, and 1 was receiving 40 mg daily. Each patient received midazolam 0.15 mg/kg IV administered over 1 minute. In patients taking long-term atorvastatin, the clearance of midazolam was decreased approximately 33% and the AUC was increased approximately 41% compared with patients who had not received atorvastatin. However, in another study using 11 healthy volunteers, neither atorvastatin, pitavastatin (*Livalo*), nor simvastatin (eg, *Zocor*) affected the pharmacokinetics of midazolam or its metabolite, 1′-hydroxymidazolam.[2]

[1] McDonnell CG, et al. *Anaesthesia.* 2003;58(9):899.

[2] Kokudai M, et al. *J Clin Pharmacol.* 2009;49(5):568.

* Asterisk indicates drugs cited in interaction reports. Based on pharmacologic and pharmacokinetic considerations, similar interactions may occur with other drugs that are listed.

Benzodiazepines (Ox.) — *Isoniazid*

Benzodiazepines (Ox.)		Isoniazid
Alprazolam (eg, *Xanax*)	Flurazepam (eg, *Dalmane*)	Isoniazid* (eg, *Nydrazid*)
Chlordiazepoxide (eg, *Librium*)	Halazepam (*Paxipam*)	
Clonazepam (eg, *Klonopin*)	Prazepam	
Clorazepate (eg, *Tranxene*)	Quazepam (*Doral*)	
Diazepam* (eg, *Valium*)	Triazolam* (eg, *Halcion*)	
Estazolam (eg, *ProSom*)		

Significance	Onset	Severity	Documentation
5	☐ Rapid	☐ Major	☐ Established
	■ **Delayed**	☐ Moderate	☐ Probable
		■ **Minor**	☐ Suspected
			■ **Possible**
			☐ Unlikely

Effects By decreasing clearance, ISONIAZID may enhance the actions of certain BENZODIAZEPINES.

Mechanism ISONIAZID may inhibit the oxidative hepatic metabolism of BENZODIAZEPINES.

Management If excessive BENZODIAZEPINE effects appear, consider reducing the dose.

Discussion

Nine healthy subjects were administered a single IV dose of diazepam 5 or 7.5 mg with and without isoniazid 180 mg/day pretreatment in a randomized, controlled fashion.[1] Isoniazid induced no change in diazepam volume of distribution; however, diazepam half-life was increased 25% (34.1 to 45.4 hr), and clearance was reduced 26%. In another study of 6 healthy volunteers on the same regimen of isoniazid,[2] the elimination half-life of triazolam was prolonged by a similar magnitude, and the oral clearance of triazolam was observed to increase about 40%. In this study, isoniazid did not affect the metabolic clearance of oxazepam.

These studies suggest that isoniazid inhibits the metabolic clearance of benzodiazepines that undergo oxidative metabolism and not those that undergo glucuronidation (eg, oxazepam [eg, *Serax*], lorazepam [eg, *Ativan*], temazepam [eg, *Restoril*]). The clinical importance of this interaction has yet to be established.

[1] Ochs HR, et al. *Clin Pharmacol Ther.* 1981;29:671.

[2] Ochs HR, et al. *Br J Clin Pharmacol.* 1983;16:743.

* Asterisk indicates drugs cited in interaction reports. Based on pharmacologic and pharmacokinetic considerations, similar interactions may occur with other drugs that are listed.

Benzodiazepines — Kava

Benzodiazepines		Kava
Alprazolam* (eg, *Xanax*)	Halazepam (*Paxipam*)	Kava*
Chlordiazepoxide (eg, *Librium*)	Lorazepam (eg, *Ativan*)	
Clonazepam (eg, *Klonopin*)	Midazolam (*Versed*)	
Clorazepate (eg, *Tranxene*)	Oxazepam (eg, *Serax*)	
Diazepam (eg, *Valium*)	Quazepam (*Doral*)	
Estazolam (eg, *ProSom*)	Temazepam (eg, *Restoril*)	
Flurazepam (eg, *Dalmane*)	Triazolam (eg, *Halcion*)	

Significance	Onset	Severity	Documentation
4	☐ Rapid	☐ Major	☐ Established
	■ **Delayed**	■ **Moderate**	☐ Probable
		☐ Minor	☐ Suspected
			■ **Possible**
			☐ Unlikely

Effects CNS side effects may be increased.

Mechanism Additive or synergistic effects caused by action on the same CNS receptor is suspected.

Management It would be prudent to caution patients to avoid concomitant use of BENZODIAZEPINES and KAVA.

Discussion

A semicomatose state was reported in a 54-year-old man during concurrent use of alprazolam and kava.[1] Upon admission to the hospital, the patient was lethargic and disoriented. His medications at that time included alprazolam, cimetidine (eg, *Tagamet*), and terazosin (*Hytrin*). Several hours after admission, the patient became more alert and stated that he had been taking a "natural tranquilizer" containing kava for the previous 3 days.

The ingredients of many herbal products are not standardized. It is unclear if herbal products contain ingredients other than those listed on the label or purported to be present that could interact with benzodiazepines.

[1] Almeida JC, et al. *Ann Intern Med.* 1996;125:940.

* Asterisk indicates drugs cited in interaction reports. Based on pharmacologic and pharmacokinetic considerations, similar interactions may occur with other drugs that are listed.

Benzodiazepines ✕ *Loxapine*

Benzodiazepines	Loxapine
Lorazepam* (eg, *Ativan*)	Loxapine* (eg, *Loxitane*)

Significance	Onset	Severity	Documentation
4	■ **Rapid**	□ Major	□ Established
	□ Delayed	■ **Moderate**	□ Probable
		□ Minor	□ Suspected
			■ **Possible**
			□ Unlikely

Effects The pharmacologic or toxic effects of LORAZEPAM may be increased.

Mechanism Unknown.

Management Consider monitoring vital signs during coadministration of these agents.

Discussion

A 35-year-old woman developed respiratory depression 2 hours after treatment with loxapine 25 mg orally and lorazepam 2 mg orally.[1] The patient was lethargic, with respirations as slow as 4 breaths/min and irregular with occasional episodes of apnea. Oxygen was administered, and the patient was observed for 12 hours in the intensive care unit. Her recovery was uneventful. Two additional patients are described in whom the coadministration of loxapine and lorazepam was followed by excessive stupor and a reduction in respiratory rate.[2] One of the patients, a 41-year-old woman, also experienced hypotension and was brought to the emergency room in an agitated state with hyperactive psychomotor behavior, labile affect, pressured speech, loose associations, and paranoid ideation. She was treated orally with loxapine 50 mg. However, after 50 minutes, there was no change in her mental status, and she was administered lorazepam 2 mg IM. The patient was asleep within 15 minutes. Two hours later, she responded to painful stimuli but did not react to vigorous shaking. Her supine BP was 80/palpable, heart rate was 60 and regular, and respirations were sonorous and irregular at a rate of 8 breaths/min. Over the next several hours, the patient's respiratory rate and BP slowly returned to normal. The second patient, a 23-year-old man, was seen in the emergency room exhibiting hyperactive and agitated motor behavior, pressured speech, labile affect, and aggressive thought content. The patient was given loxapine 50 mg but remained uncooperative and agitated and, after 30 minutes, was administered lorazepam 1 mg IM. The patient was asleep within 10 minutes, and attempts to awaken him after 1 hour revealed eye opening with localized withdrawal to pain and incomprehensible speech. This stuporous state persisted for about 3 hours. All 3 patients were previously treated with similar or higher doses of loxapine alone without incident.

[1] Cohen S, et al. *J Clin Psychopharmacol.* 1987;7(3):199.

[2] Battaglia J, et al. *J Clin Psychopharmacol.* 1989;9(3):227.

* Asterisk indicates drugs cited in interaction reports.

Benzodiazepines (Ox.) | **Macrolide & Related Antibiotics**

Alprazolam* (eg, *Xanax*)	Midazolam*	Clarithromycin* (eg, *Biaxin*)	Telithromycin* (*Ketek*)
Diazepam* (eg, *Valium*)	Triazolam* (eg, *Halcion*)	Erythromycin* (eg, *Ery-Tab*)	Troleandomycin*†

Significance	Onset	Severity	Documentation
2	■ **Rapid**	□ Major	□ Established
	□ Delayed	■ **Moderate**	□ Probable
		□ Minor	■ **Suspected**
			□ Possible
			□ Unlikely

Effects Increased CNS depression and prolonged sedation.

Mechanism Decreased metabolism of certain BENZODIAZEPINES,[1,2] including inhibition of intestinal CYP3A4 activity.[3]

Management Caution patients about increased or prolonged sedation. Reduce the BENZODIAZEPINE dose as needed. BENZODIAZEPINES undergoing conjugative metabolism, including lorazepam (eg, *Ativan*), oxazepam (eg, *Serax*), and temazepam (eg, *Restoril*), are unlikely to interact.[4] Azithromycin (eg, *Zithromax*) does not alter MIDAZOLAM metabolism[5,6] but may delay its absorption.[7]

Discussion

Erythromycin has been reported to decrease triazolam oral clearance and volume of distribution, prolong the elimination $t_{1/2}$, and increase the C_{max}.[8] Erythromycin pretreatment reduced the clearance and $t_{1/2}$ of oral and IV midazolam.[9] Psychomotor testing changes correlated with changes in midazolam kinetics. Erythromycin IV produced elevated midazolam levels and marked sedation in a child receiving oral midazolam.[10] Similarly, prolonged sedation has been reported in a child receiving oral midazolam and oral erythromycin.[11] Benzodiazepine metabolism may be decreased after the first dose of erythromycin.[12] Erythromycin pretreatment produced similar pharmacokinetic effects with single doses of alprazolam[2] and diazepam.[13] In 16 healthy subjects, clarithromycin increased the AUC of oral midazolam 7-fold and IV midazolam 3-fold while doubling the sleep time.[14] The increase was greatest in women. In a study of elderly volunteers, clarithromycin increased the $t_{1/2}$ of IV midazolam from 3.2 to 13 h and increased the AUC of both oral and IV midazolam.[15] Telithromycin increased the AUC of IV and oral midazolam 2- and 6-fold, respectively.[16]

1 Wood M. *Br J Anaesth.* 1991;67(1):131.
2 Yasui N, et al. *Clin Pharmacol Ther.* 1996;59(5):514.
3 Pinto AG, et al. *Clin Pharmacol Ther.* 2005;77(3):178.
4 Luurila H, et al. *Ther Drug Monit.* 1994;16(6):548.
5 Mattila MJ, et al. *Eur J Clin Pharmacol.* 1994;47(1):49.
6 Yeates RA, et al. *Int J Clin Pharmacol Ther.* 1996;34(9):400.
7 Backman JT, et al. *Int J Clin Pharmacol Ther.* 1995;33(6):356.
8 Phillips JP, et al. *J Clin Psychopharmacol.* 1986;6(5):297.
9 Olkkola KT, et al. *Clin Pharmacol Ther.* 1993;53(3):298.
10 Hiller A, et al. *Br J Anaesth.* 1990;65(6):826.
11 Senthilkumaran S, et al. *Indian Pediatr.* 2011;48(11):909.
12 Mattila MJ, et al. *Pharmacol Toxicol.* 1993;73(3):180.
13 Luurila H, et al. *Pharmacol Toxicol.* 1996;78(2):117.
14 Gorski JC, et al. *Clin Pharmacol Ther.* 1998;64(2):133.
15 Quinney SK, et al. *Br J Clin Pharmacol.* 2008;65(1):98.
16 *Ketek* [package insert]. Kansas City, MO: Aventis Pharmaceuticals Inc; 2004.

* Asterisk indicates drugs cited in interaction reports.
† Not available in the United States.

Benzodiazepines — *Modafinil*

Benzodiazepines	Modafinil	
Midazolam*	Armodafinil* (*Nuvigil*)	Modafinil* (*Provigil*)
Triazolam* (eg, *Halcion*)		

Significance	Onset	Severity	Documentation
2	☐ Rapid	☐ Major	☐ Established
	■ **Delayed**	■ **Moderate**	☐ Probable
		☐ Minor	■ **Suspected**
			☐ Possible
			☐ Unlikely

Effects TRIAZOLAM and MIDAZOLAM plasma levels may be reduced, decreasing the pharmacologic effects.

Mechanism Induction of GI (major) and hepatic (minor) metabolism (CYP3A4/5) of TRIAZOLAM and MIDAZOLAM by MODAFINIL is suspected.

Management Closely observe the patient's clinical response to TRIAZOLAM or MIDAZOLAM when MODAFINIL is started or stopped. Adjust the BENZODIAZEPINE dose as needed.

Discussion

The effects of daily administration of modafinil on the pharmacokinetics of a single-dose of triazolam were studied in 41 healthy women.[1] In a randomized, placebo-controlled, single-blind, single-period study, each subject was randomized to 1 of 2 treatment groups. Each subject received a single dose of triazolam 0.125 mg. The next day, subjects received modafinil 200 mg/day for 7 days, followed by 400 mg/day for 21 days. A second dose of triazolam 0.125 mg was given on the last day of modafinil administration. The protocol for the second group was the same as for the first, except subjects received matching placebo in place of modafinil for 28 days. Thirty-nine subjects completed the study. Modafinil decreased triazolam AUC 59% compared with an 8% increase with placebo, and decreased the mean peak plasma level 42% compared with a 7% increase with placebo. In addition, modafinil increased the triazolam elimination rate constant 51% and decreased the triazolam $t_{1/2}$ 35% compared with a 4% decrease in the elimination rate constant and a 4% increase in $t_{1/2}$ with placebo. Oral and IV midazolam were administered to 17 healthy volunteers before and after treatment with armodafinil (the R-enantiomer of modafinil) for 4 weeks.[2] Armodafinil reduced the AUC of IV and oral midazolam 17% and 32%, respectively.

[1] Robertson P Jr, et al. *Clin Pharmacol Ther.* 2002;71(1):46.

[2] Darwish M, et al. *Clin Pharmacokinet.* 2008;47(1):61.

* Asterisk indicates drugs cited in interaction reports.

Benzodiazepines (Ox.) — *Nefazodone*

Benzodiazepines (Ox.)		Nefazodone
Alprazolam* (eg, *Xanax*)	Flurazepam (eg, *Dalmane*)	Nefazodone* (*Serzone*)
Chlordiazepoxide (eg, *Librium*)	Halazepam (*Paxipam*)	
Clonazepam (eg, *Klonopin*)	Prazepam	
Clorazepate (eg, *Tranxene*)	Quazepam (*Doral*)	
Diazepam (eg, *Valium*)	Triazolam* (eg, *Halcion*)	
Estazolam (eg, *ProSom*)		

Significance	Onset	Severity	Documentation
3	☐ Rapid	☐ Major	■ **Established**
	■ **Delayed**	☐ Moderate	☐ Probable
		■ **Minor**	☐ Suspected
			☐ Possible
			☐ Unlikely

Effects Possible increase in CNS-depressant effects.

Mechanism Inhibition of hepatic metabolism (cytochrome P450 3A4) of BENZODIAZEPINES undergoing oxidative metabolism.

Management Monitor for increased or decreased CNS effects of BENZODIAZEPINES when NEFAZODONE therapy is started or stopped, respectively. An agent that is not eliminated by oxidative metabolism (eg, lorazepam [eg, *Ativan*]) may be a suitable alternative.

Discussion

In healthy subjects, nefazodone was more likely to interact with benzodiazepines undergoing oxidative metabolism than those eliminated by conjugative metabolism.[1-4] Compared with giving alprazolam 1 mg twice daily alone, 7 days of administration with nefazodone 200 mg twice daily increased the steady-state alprazolam peak plasma concentration 60%, the half-life of alprazolam 105%, and the area under the plasma concentration-time curve (AUC) of alprazolam 98%.[3] Peak levels and AUC of the 4-hydroxy-metabolite of alprazolam were decreased 36% and 28%, respectively. In addition, nefazodone potentiated the effects of alprazolam on psychomotor performance and sedation.[1] Compared with giving triazolam 0.25 mg/day alone, nefazodone 200 mg twice daily increased the peak plasma level of triazolam 66.5%, the mean AUC 290%, and the half-life 359%.[2] In addition, nefazodone increased and sustained triazolam effects on psychomotor performance and sedation.[1] Neither triazolam nor alprazolam affected the pharmacokinetics of nefazodone.[1,2] Nefazodone does not appear to interact with lorazepam.[1,4]

[1] Kroboth PD, et al. *J Clin Psychopharmacol.* 1995;15:306.

[2] Barbhaiya RH, et al. *J Clin Psychopharmacol.* 1995;15:320.

[3] Greene DS, et al. *J Clin Psychopharmacol.* 1995;15:399.

[4] Greene DS, et al. *J Clin Psychopharmacol.* 1995;15:409.

* Asterisk indicates drugs cited in interaction reports. Based on pharmacologic and pharmacokinetic considerations, similar interactions may occur with other drugs that are listed.

Benzodiazepines — *NNRT Inhibitors*

Benzodiazepines		NNRT Inhibitors	
Alprazolam* (eg, *Xanax*)	Triazolam* (eg, *Halcion*)	Delavirdine* (*Rescriptor*)	Efavirenz* (*Sustiva*)
Midazolam* (*Versed*)			

Significance	Onset	Severity	Documentation
2	☐ Rapid	☐ Major	☐ Established
	■ **Delayed**	■ **Moderate**	☐ Probable
		☐ Minor	■ **Suspected**
			☐ Possible
			☐ Unlikely

Effects The pharmacologic effects of certain BENZODIAZEPINES may be increased and the duration prolonged, leading to protracted sedation and respiratory depression.

Mechanism NON-NUCLEOSIDE REVERSE TRANSCRIPTASE (NNRT) INHIBITORS may inhibit the hepatic metabolism (CYP3A4) of the BENZODIAZEPINE.

Management Do not administer certain BENZODIAZEPINES concomitantly with NNRT INHIBITORS.

Discussion

Because of possible competition for metabolism, do not use the benzodiazepines listed above in patients receiving the NNRT inhibitors delavirdine and efavirenz.[1,2] Concomitant administration of delavirdine or efavirenz with alprazolam, midazolam, or triazolam may lead to increased plasma concentrations of the benzodiazepine and create the potential for serious adverse reactions (eg, prolonged sedation and respiratory depression).

The basis for this monograph is information on file with the manufacturers. Published clinical data are needed to further assess this interaction. However, because of the seriousness of this interaction, clinical evaluation in humans is not likely to be forthcoming.

[1] Product Information. Delavirdine (*Rescriptor*). Upjohn Company. April 1997.

[2] Product Information. Efavirenz (*Sustiva*). DuPont Pharmaceuticals. September 1998.

* Asterisk indicates drugs cited in interaction reports.

Benzodiazepines (Ox.) — *Omeprazole*

Benzodiazepines (Ox.)		Omeprazole
Alprazolam (eg, *Xanax*)	Flurazepam* (eg, *Dalmane*)	Omeprazole* (eg, *Prilosec*)
Chlordiazepoxide (eg, *Librium*)	Halazepam (*Paxipam*)	
Clonazepam (eg, *Klonopin*)	Midazolam (*Versed*)	
Clorazepate (eg, *Tranxene*)	Prazepam	
Diazepam* (eg, *Valium*)	Quazepam (*Doral*)	
Estazolam (eg, *ProSom*)	Triazolam* (eg, *Halcion*)	

Significance	Onset	Severity	Documentation
3	☐ Rapid	☐ Major	☐ Established
	■ **Delayed**	☐ Moderate	☐ Probable
		■ **Minor**	■ **Suspected**
			☐ Possible
			☐ Unlikely

Effects Reduced clearance, prolonged t½, and increased serum levels of certain BENZODIAZEPINES may occur. Certain actions, especially sedation or ataxia, may be enhanced.

Mechanism Decreased oxidative metabolism of BENZODIAZEPINES.

Management Monitor for prolonged sedation or evidence of CNS impairment. Reduce BENZODIAZEPINE dosage or increase dosing intervals as needed. BENZODIAZEPINES not metabolized by oxidation may not interact.

Discussion

Healthy subjects received omeprazole 40 mg/day orally for 9 days.[1] On day 7, diazepam 0.1 mg/kg was infused over 5 min. Diazepam levels following omeprazole were higher in each subject compared with giving diazepam alone. Serum levels of desmethyldiazepam, the major metabolite of diazepam, increased more slowly, and peak levels after 3 days were lower following omeprazole treatment. Omeprazole decreased the total systemic plasma clearance of diazepam 55% and increased the elimination t½ an average of 130% in each subject. In 12 healthy subjects, omeprazole 20 mg/day for 7 days decreased diazepam clearance 27%, increased plasma t½ 36%, and delayed the appearance of desmethyldiazepam when compared with placebo.[2] The degree of enzyme inhibition by omeprazole appears to be dose-related. A decrease in diazepam clearance and prolongation of diazepam and desmethyldiazepam t½s were greater in 8 white subjects given omeprazole 40 mg/day concurrently, compared with 7 Chinese subjects.[3] Additional studies are needed to determine the mechanism for these interethnic differences. Two cases of acute ataxia were attributed to a triazolam-omeprazole interaction.[4]

[1] Gugler R, et al. *Gastroenterology.* 1985;89:1235.
[2] Andersson T, et al. *Eur J Clin Pharmacol.* 1990;39:51.
[3] Caraco Y, et al. *Clin Pharmacol Ther.* 1995;58:62.
[4] Martí-Massó JF, et al. *Ann Pharmacother.* 1992;26:429.

* Asterisk indicates drugs cited in interaction reports. Based on pharmacologic and pharmacokinetic considerations, similar interactions may occur with other drugs that are listed.

Benzodiazepines — *Paroxetine*

Benzodiazepines	Paroxetine
Oxazepam* (eg, *Serax*)	Paroxetine* (eg, *Paxil*)

Significance	Onset	Severity	Documentation
5	☐ Rapid	☐ Major	☐ Established
	■ **Delayed**	☐ Moderate	☐ Probable
		■ **Minor**	☐ Suspected
			■ **Possible**
			☐ Unlikely

Effects The CNS effects of OXAZEPAM may be increased.

Mechanism Unknown.

Management If an interaction is suspected, decreasing the dose of OXAZEPAM during coadministration of PAROXETINE may be necessary.

Discussion

The objective and subjective psychomotor effects of a single, oral dose of oxazepam 30 mg were compared in 11 healthy volunteers before and after 9 to 12 days of oral administration of paroxetine 30 mg/day.[1] The dose of oxazepam impaired psychomotor function and caused subjective feelings of sedation (eg, subjects felt less alert, less attentive, less energetic, less strong, less clear-headed). The only sedative effect of oxazepam that was potentiated to a statistically significant amount by paroxetine was the subjective assessment of strength. In contrast, paroxetine produced some improvement in performance. Other studies have found no interaction between paroxetine and diazepam[2,3] or paroxetine and alprazolam.[4]

Controlled trials are needed to determine whether the combined effects of administering paroxetine and benzodiazepines are greater than giving either agent alone.

[1] McClelland GR, et al. *Br J Clin Pharmacol.* 1987;23:117P.
[2] Bannister SJ, et al. *Acta Psychiatr Scand Suppl.* 1989;350:102.
[3] Cooper SM, et al. *Acta Psychiatr Scand Suppl.* 1989;350:53.
[4] Calvo G, et al. *J Clin Psychopharmacol.* 2004;24:268.

* Asterisk indicates drugs cited in interaction reports.

Benzodiazepines — *Probenecid*

Benzodiazepines		Probenecid
Chlordiazepoxide (eg, *Librium*)	Midazolam* (*Versed*)	Probenecid* (eg, *Benemid*)
Clorazepate (eg, *Tranxene*)	Oxazepam (eg, *Serax*)	
Diazepam (eg, *Valium*)	Prazepam	
Estazolam (eg, *ProSom*)	Quazepam (*Doral*)	
Flurazepam (eg, *Dalmane*)	Temazepam (eg, *Restoril*)	
Lorazepam* (eg, *Ativan*)	Triazolam (eg, *Halcion*)	

Significance	Onset	Severity	Documentation
4	■ **Rapid**	□ Major	□ Established
	□ Delayed	■ **Moderate**	□ Probable
		□ Minor	□ Suspected
			■ **Possible**
			□ Unlikely

Effects A more rapid onset or more prolonged BENZODIAZEPINE effect may occur with PROBENECID administration.

Mechanism PROBENECID interference with BENZODIAZEPINE conjugation in the liver is suspected.

Management Be prepared for a more rapid onset of BENZODIAZEPINE effect. Also observe for clinical signs of BENZODIAZEPINE accumulation (eg, increasing sedation, lethargy) during concurrent administration of PROBENECID. The BENZODIAZEPINE dose may need to be reduced.

Discussion

One group of investigators recorded induction times of 85 seconds after 0.3 mg/kg of midazolam in presurgical patients pretreated with probenecid, compared with 109 seconds in presurgical patients who did not receive probenecid.[2,3] In addition, the proportion of patients asleep within 3 minutes of midazolam administration was 80% of those pretreated with probenecid compared with 66% of those who did not receive probenecid. In a group of nine volunteer subjects, the clearance of lorazepam decreased by nearly 50% and the elimination half-life increased accordingly when probenecid preceded lorazepam administration.[1]

[1] Abernethy DR, et al. *J Pharmacol Exp Ther* 1985;234:345.

[2] Halliday NJ, et al. *Anaesthesia* 1985;40:763.

[3] Dundee JW, et al. *Eur J Anaesth* 1986; 3:247.

* Asterisk indicates drugs cited in interaction reports. Based on pharmacologic and pharmacokinetic considerations, similar interactions may occur with other drugs that are listed.

Benzodiazepines — *Propoxyphene*

Alprazolam* (eg, *Xanax*)	Diazepam* (eg, *Valium*)	Propoxyphene* (eg, *Darvon*)

Significance	Onset	Severity	Documentation
5	☐ Rapid	☐ Major	☐ Established
	■ **Delayed**	☐ Moderate	☐ Probable
		■ **Minor**	☐ Suspected
			■ **Possible**
			☐ Unlikely

Effects Additive CNS-depressant effects may occur.

Mechanism PROPOXYPHENE may inhibit the hepatic metabolism of certain BENZODIAZEPINES.

Management If additive CNS-depressant effects occur, the BENZODIAZEPINE dose may need to be decreased.

Discussion

Eight healthy subjects received a single 1 mg dose of alprazolam following propoxyphene 65 mg every 6 hours.[1] Propoxyphene significantly prolonged the half-life of alprazolam by 58% (11.6 to 18.3 hours) and reduced its total clearance by 38%. In six subjects propoxyphene prolonged the half-life of a single IV dose of diazepam by 12% and reduced its clearance by 15%; however, this was statistically insignificant. Lorazepam (eg, *Ativan*) was not affected by propoxyphene.

Although both alprazolam and diazepam are metabolized by oxidation, propoxyphene significantly decreases the hydroxylation of alprazolam but has less of an effect on the N-demethylation of diazepam. Lorazepam, metabolized by glucuronidation, is not affected by propoxyphene.

[1] Abernethy DR, et al. *Br J Clin Pharmacol.* 1985;19:51.

* Asterisk indicates drugs cited in interaction reports.

Benzodiazepines (Ox.) — *Protease Inhibitors*

Benzodiazepines (Ox.)		Protease Inhibitors	
Alprazolam* (eg, *Xanax*)	Estazolam*	Atazanavir* (*Reyataz*)	Nelfinavir* (*Viracept*)
Chlordiazepoxide	Flurazepam*	Darunavir* (*Prezista*)	Ritonavir* (*Norvir*)
Clonazepam (eg, *Klonopin*)	Midazolam*	Indinavir* (*Crixivan*)	Saquinavir* (*Invirase*)
Clorazepate* (eg, *Tranxene*)	Quazepam (*Doral*)	Lopinavir/Ritonavir* (*Kaletra*)	
Diazepam* (eg, *Valium*)	Triazolam* (eg, *Halcion*)		

Significance	Onset	Severity	Documentation
1	☐ Rapid	■ **Major**	☐ Established
	■ **Delayed**	☐ Moderate	☐ Probable
		☐ Minor	■ **Suspected**
			☐ Possible
			☐ Unlikely

Effects Possibly severe sedation and respiratory depression.

Mechanism Inhibition of the hepatic metabolism (CYP3A4) of BENZODIAZEPINES that undergo oxidative metabolism.

Management Certain BENZODIAZEPINES are contraindicated in patients taking PROTEASE INHIBITORS. MIDAZOLAM and TRIAZOLAM are contraindicated in patients taking ATAZANAVIR[1] or DARUNAVIR.[2]

Discussion

Large increases in serum concentrations of benzodiazepines that undergo oxidative metabolism (those metabolized by the CYP3A4 isozyme) may lead to severe sedation and respiratory depression. Studies using human liver microsomes have demonstrated that CYP3A is a major isoform in darunavir,[2] indinavir,[3] nelfinavir,[4] ritonavir,[5] and saquinavir[6] metabolism. Therefore, coadministration of these protease inhibitors with benzodiazepines metabolized by this enzyme is contraindicated. Prolonged sedation was reported in a 32-year-old patient who received IV midazolam for bronchoscopy after receiving saquinavir, but not after receiving midazolam alone.[7] Saquinavir decreased midazolam clearance 56%.[8] In the same study, oral midazolam bioavailability increased from 41% to 90%. Studies suggest extensive impairment of triazolam and alprazolam clearance by ritonavir.[9,10] In a prospective study of 28 patients infected with HIV, lopinavir-ritonavir decreased the hepatic clearance of midazolam 76.1%.[11] In 1 study, ritonavir caused more than a 20-fold increase in the triazolam AUC.[12] In a study of 16 healthy volunteers, ritonavir-boosted saquinavir markedly increased midazolam exposure.[13] In a pharmacokinetic study, both ritonavir and nelfinavir markedly inhibited IV midazolam clearance.[14] Prolonged sedation was reported in 9.8% of patients receiving IV midazolam concurrently with protease inhibitors, primarily ritonavir-boosted atazanavir or lopinavir, compared with 1.58% of patients not receiving the protease inhibitors.[15] Simultaneous administration of midazolam with the CYP3A inducer St. John's wort and inhibitor ritonavir increased the AUC of IV midazolam 180%, whereas the AUC of oral midazolam increased 412%.[16]

1 *Reyataz* [package insert]. Princeton, NJ: Bristol-Myers Squibb Co; 2003.
2 *Prezista* [package insert]. Raritan, NJ: Tibotec Therapeutics; June 2006.
3 *Crixivan* [package insert]. White House Station, NJ: Merck & Co Inc; 1996.
4 *Viracept* [package insert]. La Jolla, CA: Agouron Pharmaceuticals; 2002.
5 *Norvir* [package insert]. Abbott Park, IL: Abbott Laboratories; 2001.
6 *Fortovase* [package insert]. Nutley, NJ: Roche Laboratories Inc; 1997.
7 Merry C, et al. *AIDS*. 1997;11(2):268.
8 Palkama VJ, et al. *Clin Pharmacol Ther.* 1999;66(1):33.
9 Greenblatt DJ, et al. *J Clin Psychopharmacol.* 1999;19(4):293.
10 Greenblatt DJ, et al. *Clin Pharmacol Ther.* 2000;67(4):335.
11 Wyen C, et al. *Clin Pharmacol Ther.* 2008;84(1):75.
12 Culm-Merdek KE, et al. *Clin Pharmacol Ther.* 2006;79(3):243.
13 Schmitt C, et al. *Pharmacotherapy.* 2009;29(10):1175.
14 Kirby BJ, et al. *Drug Metab Dispos.* 2011;39(6):1070.
15 Hsu AJ, et al. *Pharmacotherapy.* 2012;32(6):538.
16 Hafner V, et al. *Clin Pharmacol Ther.* 2010;87(2):191.

* Asterisk indicates drugs cited in interaction reports. Based on pharmacologic and pharmacokinetic considerations, similar interactions may occur with other drugs that are listed.

Benzodiazepines — *Quinolones*

Benzodiazepines	Quinolones
Diazepam* (eg, *Valium*)	Ciprofloxacin* (eg, *Cipro*)

Significance	Onset	Severity	Documentation
5	☐ Rapid	☐ Major	☐ Established
	■ **Delayed**	☐ Moderate	☐ Probable
		■ **Minor**	☐ Suspected
			■ **Possible**
			☐ Unlikely

Effects The pharmacologic effects of DIAZEPAM may be increased.

Mechanism CIPROFLOXACIN may inhibit the metabolism of DIAZEPAM. In addition, CIPROFLOXACIN may alter the activity of DIAZEPAM by competitively binding to gamma-aminobutyric acid (GABA) receptor sites. BENZODIAZEPINES exert their pharmacologic activity by binding to the GABA receptor complex.

Management If increased CNS-depressant effects occur, it may be necessary to decrease the dose of DIAZEPAM.

Discussion

In a double-blind, placebo-controlled, crossover study, the effects of pretreatment with a 7-day course of oral ciprofloxacin 500 mg twice daily on the pharmacokinetics and pharmacodynamics of a single IV dose of diazepam 5 mg were investigated in 12 healthy volunteers.[1] Pretreatment with ciprofloxacin decreased the clearance of diazepam 37% and prolonged the $t_{1/2}$ 94%.

Additional studies are needed to determine the clinical importance of this interaction.

[1] Kamali F, et al. *Eur J Clin Pharmacol.* 1993;44(4):365.

* Asterisk indicates drugs cited in interaction reports.

Benzodiazepines — *Ranitidine*

Diazepam* (eg, *Valium*)	Triazolam* (eg, *Halcion*)	Ranitidine* (eg, *Zantac*)

Significance	Onset	Severity	Documentation
5	■ **Rapid** ☐ Delayed	☐ Major ☐ Moderate ■ **Minor**	☐ Established ☐ Probable ☐ Suspected ☐ Possible ■ **Unlikely**

Effects Effects of certain BENZODIAZEPINES may be impaired or enhanced. It is unlikely that the degree of change in BENZODIAZEPINE level would be clinically important.

Mechanism The bioavailability of certain BENZODIAZEPINES may be altered.

Management Monitor the clinical response of the patient. Staggering administration times may avoid an interaction.

Discussion

In 6 healthy volunteers, steady-state diazepam plasma levels were approximately 25% less after 10 days of diazepam 5 mg and ranitidine 300 mg/day, compared with levels after 10 days of diazepam 5 mg/day alone.[1] In 3 randomized, crossover studies involving a total of 19 healthy subjects,[2-4] peak midazolam plasma levels and bioavailability were higher after single doses of oral midazolam 15 mg preceded by ranitidine 150 mg every 12 hours (2 to 3 doses) than after oral midazolam 15 mg alone. In a randomized, placebo-controlled study that assessed the clinical effects of this interaction, the average time-to-peak hypnotic effect was faster and the percentage of drowsy patients was higher for the 32 patients who had received 2 doses of ranitidine 150 mg prior to a preoperative dose of oral midazolam 10 mg, compared with the 32 patients who had received only midazolam.[5] In a group of 12 volunteers, pretreatment with ranitidine 150 mg twice daily for 2 days produced a 27% increase in the bioavailability of triazolam 0.25 mg. This was not seen when triazolam was given IV.[6] Another study confirmed these results in young and older adults.[7] Similar pharmacokinetic and clinical effects were not observed with temazepam (eg, *Restoril*).[2,5] In a controlled trial involving 50 duodenal ulcer patients,[8] 96% of the patients receiving ranitidine 150 mg orally twice daily with prazepam† healed after 4 weeks of therapy compared with 75% of patients receiving ranitidine 150 mg twice daily and placebo 3 times daily. See also Benzodiazepines-Cimetidine.

1 Klotz U, et al. *Eur J Clin Pharmacol.* 1983;24(3):357.
2 Elliott P, et al. *Eur J Anaesthesiol.* 1984;1(3):245.
3 Greenblatt DJ, et al. *Anesth Analg.* 1986;65(2):176.
4 Fee JP, et al. *Clin Pharmacol Ther.* 1987;41(1):80.
5 Wilson CM, et al. *Br J Anaesth.* 1986;58(5):483.
6 Vanderveen RP, et al. *Clin Pharm.* 1991;10(7):539.
7 O'Connor-Semmes RL, et al. *Clin Pharmacol Ther.* 2001;70(2):126.
8 Hüscher C, et al. *Eur J Clin Pharmacol.* 1985;28(2):177.

* Asterisk indicates drugs cited in interaction reports.
† Not available in the United States.

Benzodiazepines (Ox.) — *Rifamycins*

Benzodiazepines (Ox.)		Rifamycins	
Alprazolam (eg, *Xanax*)	Estazolam	Rifabutin (*Mycobutin*)	Rifapentine (*Priftin*)
Chlordiazepoxide (eg, *Librium*)	Flurazepam	Rifampin* (eg, *Rifadin*)	
Clonazepam (eg, *Klonopin*)	Midazolam*		
Clorazepate (eg, *Tranxene*)	Quazepam (*Doral*)		
Diazepam* (eg, *Valium*)	Triazolam* (eg, *Halcion*)		

Significance	Onset	Severity	Documentation
2	□ Rapid	□ Major	□ Established
	■ **Delayed**	■ **Moderate**	□ Probable
		□ Minor	■ **Suspected**
			□ Possible
			□ Unlikely

Effects The pharmacologic effects of certain BENZODIAZEPINES may be decreased.

Mechanism The oxidative metabolism (CYP-450) of BENZODIAZEPINES may be increased.

Management Monitor the clinical response to the BENZODIAZEPINE when starting or stopping a RIFAMYCIN. Adjust the dose as needed.

Discussion

In an open study of 21 healthy men, the pharmacokinetics of diazepam and its metabolites were investigated before and after administration of rifampin 600 or 1,200 mg/day for 7 days.[1] Rifampin increased urinary excretion of diazepam about 300%, while the elimination $t_{1/2}$ decreased approximately 250%; these changes were independent of the rifampin dose. In 7 patients with active pulmonary or renal tuberculosis receiving isoniazid (eg, *Nydrazid*), rifampin 450 to 600 mg/day, ethambutol (eg, *Myambutol*) orally or IV, and a single IV dose of diazepam 5 to 7.5 mg, diazepam renal clearance increased more than 300%, while $t_{1/2}$ was reduced to less than 33% in triple-therapy patients.[2] Conversely, rifampin had no effect on temazepam pharmacokinetics.[3] In 10 healthy volunteers, pretreatment with rifampin decreased oral midazolam AUC 96%, peak serum levels 94%, and elimination $t_{1/2}$ from 3.1 to 1.3 hours.[4] The pharmacodynamic effects of midazolam were markedly decreased from those observed with placebo. Another study found similar effects.[5] In 10 healthy volunteers, rifampin markedly decreased triazolam plasma levels (88%) and $t_{1/2}$ (46%).[6] In addition, the triazolam psychomotor tests were reduced. In a study of 24 healthy volunteers, rifampin administration resulted in an increase in lorazepam systemic clearance in each type of patient.[7] However, the UGT2B15*2 genotype polymorphism was a major determinant of interindividual variability. Oral rifamixin (*Xifaxan*) did not affect the pharmacokinetics of oral or IV midazolam or its major metabolite.[8]

1 Ohnhaus EE, et al. *Clin Pharmacol Ther.* 1987;42(2):148.
2 Ochs HR, et al. *Clin Pharmacol Ther.* 1981;29(5):671.
3 Brockmeyer NH, et al. *Int J Clin Pharmacol Ther Toxicol.* 1990;28(9):387.
4 Backman JT, et al. *Clin Pharmacol Ther.* 1996;59(1):7.
5 Backman JT, et al. *Eur J Clin Pharmacol.* 1998;54(1):53.
6 Villikka K, et al. *Clin Pharmacol Ther.* 1997;61(1):8.
7 Chung JY, et al. *Clin Pharmacol Ther.* 2005;77(6):486.
8 Pentikis HS, et al. *Pharmacotherapy.* 2007;27(10):1361.

* Asterisk indicates drugs cited in interaction reports. Based on pharmacologic and pharmacokinetic considerations, similar interactions may occur with other drugs that are listed.

Benzodiazepines		***St. John's Wort***
Alprazolam* (eg, *Xanax*)	Midazolam*	St. John's Wort*
Clonazepam (eg, *Klonopin*)	Quazepam* (*Doral*)	
Diazepam (eg, *Valium*)	Triazolam (eg, *Halcion*)	

Significance	Onset	Severity	Documentation
2	☐ Rapid	☐ Major	☐ Established
	■ **Delayed**	■ **Moderate**	☐ Probable
		☐ Minor	■ **Suspected**
			☐ Possible
			☐ Unlikely

Effects Plasma levels of certain BENZODIAZEPINES may be reduced, decreasing the pharmacologic effect.

Mechanism ST. JOHN'S WORT may induce the enzymes responsible for the hepatic and intestinal metabolism (CYP3A4) of certain BENZODIAZEPINES.[1-3] The extent of CYP3A4 induction depends on the hyperforin dose.[4]

Management Caution patients to inform their health care provider before using nonprescription or herbal products. If ST. JOHN'S WORT cannot be avoided, assess the response to the BENZODIAZEPINE when ST. JOHN'S WORT is started or stopped. Adjust the dose of the BENZODIAZEPINE as needed.

Discussion

Multiple, but not single, doses of St. John's wort appear to induce hepatic and intestinal CYP3A4 activity.[1-3] The effect of a single oral dose of St. John's wort (*Hypericum perforatum*) 900 mg or St. John's wort 300 mg 3 times/day for 14 days on the oral clearance of midazolam and systemic clearance of IV midazolam was assessed in 12 subjects.[1] A single dose of St. John's wort 900 mg had no effect on the pharmacokinetics of a single IV (0.05 mg/kg) or oral (5 mg) dose of midazolam, compared with water. In contrast, administration of St. John's wort 300 mg 3 times/day for 2 weeks decreased the oral availability of midazolam 39%, increased the oral clearance 109%, and decreased the AUC more than 50%. The AUC of IV midazolam was decreased 20%. In healthy volunteers, administration of St. John's wort 900 mg daily for 12 days decreased the AUC of oral and IV administration of midazolam 56% and 24%, respectively.[2] In 12 healthy volunteers, administration of St. John's wort 300 mg 3 times/day for 2 weeks decreased the AUC of an alprazolam 2 mg dose 54%.[3] Similarly, in 13 healthy subjects, administration of St. John's wort 300 mg 3 times/day for 14 days decreased the AUC and C_{max} of a quazepam 15 mg dose 25%.[5] St. John's wort did not affect the pharmacokinetics of quazepam. Simultaneous administration of midazolam with the CYP3A inducer St. John's wort and inhibitor ritonavir increased the AUC of IV midazolam 180%, whereas the AUC of oral midazolam increased 412%.[6]

[1] Wang Z, et al. *Clin Pharmacol Ther.* 2001;70(4):317.
[2] Dresser GK, et al. *Clin Pharmacol Ther.* 2001;69(2):P23.
[3] Markowitz JS, et al. *JAMA.* 2003;290(11):1500.
[4] Mueller SC, et al. *Eur J Clin Pharmacol.* 2006;62(1):29.
[5] Kawaguchi A, et al. *Br J Clin Pharmacol.* 2004;58(4):403.
[6] Hafner V, et al. *Clin Pharmacol Ther.* 2010;87(2):191.

* Asterisk indicates drugs cited in interaction reports. Based on pharmacologic and pharmacokinetic considerations, similar interactions may occur with other drugs that are listed.

Benzodiazepines / *Theophyllines*

Benzodiazepines		Theophyllines	
Alprazolam* (eg, *Xanax*)	Lorazepam (eg, *Ativan*)	Aminophylline*	Theophylline* (eg, *Theochron*)
Chlordiazepoxide (eg, *Librium*)	Midazolam*	Dyphylline (*Lufyllin*)	
Clonazepam (eg, *Klonopin*)	Oxazepam		
Clorazepate (eg, *Tranxene*)	Quazepam (*Doral*)		
Diazepam* (eg, *Valium*)	Temazepam (eg, *Restoril*)		
Estazolam	Triazolam (eg, *Halcion*)		
Flurazepam (Dalmane)			

Significance	Onset	Severity	Documentation
3	■ **Rapid**	□ Major	□ Established
	□ Delayed	□ Moderate	□ Probable
		■ **Minor**	■ **Suspected**
			□ Possible
			□ Unlikely

Effects The sedative effects of BENZODIAZEPINES may be antagonized by THEOPHYLLINES.

Mechanism Possibly an antagonistic action by competitive binding to intracerebral adenosine receptors.[1]

Management No special precautions appear necessary. Assess the clinical status of patients and tailor the dosage of the BENZODIAZEPINE as needed.

Discussion

Aminophylline has antagonized diazepam-induced sedation, somnolence, impairment in thinking, and psychomotor performance in various case reports and controlled studies including postoperative patients and healthy subjects.[2-6] The reversal of diazepam effects by aminophylline (1 to 12.7 mg/kg IV) occurred rapidly (usually within a few minutes) after rectal or IV aminophylline administration.[1-8] Diazepam pharmacokinetics did not appear to be altered. However, aminophylline prolonged the $t_{1/2}$ of midazolam in a small study.[9] In 1 report, coadministration of alprazolam and theophylline resulted in lower theophylline levels and AUC than those found in patients receiving theophylline alone.[10] Clinical correlation with these results was not reported.

Additional studies are needed to confirm this interaction and to determine whether theophylline interferes with other pharmacologic actions of diazepam.

1 Bonfiglio MF, et al. *Pharmacotherapy.* 1991;11(1):85.
2 Stirt JA. *Anesth Analg.* 1981;60(10):767.
3 Arvidsson SB, et al. *Lancet.* 1982;2(8313):1467.
4 Arvidsson S, et al. *Anesthesia.* 1984;39(8):806.
5 Meyer BH, et al. *Anesth Analg.* 1984;63(10):900.
6 Gallen JS. *Anesth Analg.* 1989;69(2):268.
7 Henauer SA, et al. *Eur J Clin Pharmacol.* 1983;25(6):743.
8 Mattila MJ, et al. *Med Biol.* 1983;61(6):337.
9 Bonfiglio MF, et al. *Pharmacotherapy.* 1996;16(6):1166.
10 Tuncok Y, et al. *Int J Clin Pharmacol Ther.* 1994;32(12):642.

* Asterisk indicates drugs cited in interaction reports. Based on pharmacologic and pharmacokinetic considerations, similar interactions may occur with other drugs that are listed.

Benzodiazepines — *Valproic Acid*

Benzodiazepines		Valproic Acid	
Alprazolam (eg, *Xanax*)	Lorazepam* (eg, *Ativan*)	Divalproex Sodium* (*Depakote*)	Valproic Acid* (eg, *Depakene*)
Chlordiazepoxide (eg, *Librium*)	Midazolam		
Clorazepate (eg, *Tranxene*)	Quazepam (*Doral*)		
Diazepam* (eg, *Valium*)	Triazolam (eg, *Halcion*)		
Flurazepam (eg, *Dalmane*)			

Significance	Onset	Severity	Documentation
4	☐ Rapid	☐ Major	☐ Established
	■ **Delayed**	■ **Moderate**	☐ Probable
		☐ Minor	☐ Suspected
			■ **Possible**
			☐ Unlikely

Effects Increased blood levels of certain BENZODIAZEPINES, resulting in increased CNS depression.

Mechanism VALPROIC ACID may decrease the oxidative liver glucuronidation metabolism of some BENZODIAZEPINES. Displacement of DIAZEPAM metabolites from plasma protein binding sites may also be responsible.

Management No interventions appear necessary. If an interaction is suspected, reduce the dose of the BENZODIAZEPINE.

Discussion

Diazepam 10 mg was administered IV to 6 healthy men to study the pharmacokinetic effects of oral sodium valproate 1,500 mg/day.[1] The level of unbound plasma diazepam increased approximately 2-fold, while the serum metabolite levels were lower during sodium valproate administration. In a controlled crossover study, the interaction between valproate and lorazepam was evaluated in 9 healthy volunteers.[2] Subjects received divalproex sodium 500 mg twice daily or placebo for 12 days and lorazepam 1 mg every 12 hours on days 6 through 9 and on the morning of day 10. Compared with placebo, divalproex sodium increased lorazepam C_{max} 8%, AUC 20%, and trough concentration 31%. There was no difference in sedation. The pharmacokinetics of valproate were not changed. Likewise, a study of 24 healthy volunteers demonstrated a decrease in systemic clearance of lorazepam.[3] However, the clearance and metabolite AUC ratios differed markedly among the various UGT2B15 genotypes. In 14 healthy volunteers, valproic acid reduced the clearance of lorazepam.[4] The UGT2B7 genotype appears to affect the interaction, especially in subjects who have UGT2B7 and UGT2B15 genotypes.

[1] Dhillon S, et al. *Br J Clin Pharmacol.* 1982;13(4):553.
[2] Samara EE, et al. *J Clin Pharmacol.* 1997;37(5):442.
[3] Chung JY, et al. *Clin Pharmacol Ther.* 2005;77(6):486.
[4] Chung JY, et al. *Clin Pharmacol Ther.* 2008;83(4):595.

* Asterisk indicates drugs cited in interaction reports. Based on pharmacologic and pharmacokinetic considerations, similar interactions may occur with other drugs that are listed.

Benzodiazepines — *Venlafaxine*

Diazepam* (eg, *Valium*)	Venlafaxine* (*Effexor*)

Significance	Onset	Severity	Documentation
5	☐ Rapid	☐ Major	☐ Established
	■ **Delayed**	☐ Moderate	☐ Probable
		■ **Minor**	☐ Suspected
			☐ Possible
			■ **Unlikely**

Effects DIAZEPAM AUC may be decreased.

Mechanism Unknown.

Management Based on available data, while a statistically significant interaction occurs, the magnitude of the effect is not sufficient to be clinically important.

Discussion

The possibility of a pharmacokinetic or pharmacodynamic interaction between diazepam and venlafaxine was evaluated in 18 healthy men.[1] Using a randomized, double-blind, crossover design, each subject received venlafaxine 50 mg every 8 hours or placebo for 10 days. On day 4, a single dose of placebo was administered; on day 5, a single dose of diazepam 10 mg was given. The single dose of diazepam did not have any significant effect on the pharmacokinetics of venlafaxine or the active metabolite of venlafaxine (O-desmethylvenlafaxine). Venlafaxine did not affect the maximum plasma concentration of diazepam or the time to reach the maximum concentration. However, there were statistically significant increases in the clearance of diazepam (from 24 to 26 mL/hr; $P = 0.007$) and volume of distribution (from 0.85 to 0.99 L/kg, $P = 0.02$), while the AUC for diazepam decreased (from 5,973 to 5,008 ng•hr/mL; $P = 0.02$). Because the diazepam AUC met bioequivalence criteria, the effects of venlafaxine on the pharmacokinetics of diazepam, while statistically significant, were not considered to be clinically important. Based on psychometric test results, no clinically important pharmacodynamic interaction was detected between diazepam and venlafaxine. In addition, venlafaxine had no effect on the pharmacokinetics of the active metabolite of diazepam, desmethyldiazepam.

Additional studies are needed to determine whether a clinically important interaction would occur with multiple dosing of diazepam (ie, at steady-state conditions) or whether benzodiazepines alter the pharmacokinetics of venlafaxine.

[1] Troy SM, et al. *J Clin Pharmacol.* 1995;35(4):410.

* Asterisk indicates drugs cited in interaction reports.

Benzodiazepines		***Verapamil***
Midazolam* (*Versed*)	Triazolam (*Halcion*)	Verapamil* (eg, *Calan*)

Significance	Onset	Severity	Documentation
4	■ **Rapid** □ Delayed	□ Major ■ **Moderate** □ Minor	□ Established □ Probable □ Suspected ■ **Possible** □ Unlikely

Effects Effects of certain BENZODIAZEPINES may be increased, producing increased CNS depression and prolonged effects.

Mechanism VERAPAMIL may decrease the metabolism of certain BENZODIAZEPINES and decrease the first-pass effect of TRIAZOLAM. See Discussion.

Management Consider giving a lower dose of the BENZODIAZEPINE. Caution the patient about an increased and prolonged sedative effect.

Discussion

The effects of oral verapamil 80 mg on the pharmacokinetics and pharmacodynamics of oral midazolam 15 mg were studied in a double-blind, placebo controlled, randomized, crossover investigation in nine healthy volunteers.[1] Each subject received verapamil or placebo three times daily for 2 days, and on the second day, they were given midazolam. The midazolam area under the concentration-time curve increased from 12 to 35 mcg•min/mL ($P < 0.001$), while the peak midazolam concentration doubled ($P < 0.01$), and the elimination half-life was prolonged by 41% ($P < 0.05$). The changes in midazolam pharmacokinetics were accompanied by prolonged and deep sedative effects.

Midazolam, triazolam and verapamil appear to be metabolized by the same cytochrome P450 3A isozyme. Therefore, to the extent that the mechanism involves inhibition of benzodiazepine metabolism, the interaction would occur whether the benzodiazepine was given orally or parenterally. If increased bioavailability is involved, the interaction would occur only with oral administration of the drug. When both mechanisms are involved, the magnitude of the interaction would be expected to be greater with the oral benzodiazepine than with the IV route. In the latter situation, bioavailability is complete, and the presystemic metabolism is avoided. With this drug interaction, midazolam should not be treated as a short-acting agent. Patients should be carefully monitored for deep and prolonged sedation.

[1] Backman JT, et al. *Br J Clin Pharmacol.* 1994;37:221.

* Asterisk indicates drugs cited in interaction reports. Based on pharmacologic and pharmacokinetic considerations, similar interactions may occur with other drugs that are listed.

Beta-Blockers — *Aluminum Salts*

Beta-Blockers		Aluminum Salts	
Atenolol* (eg, *Tenormin*)	Propranolol* (eg, *Inderal*)	Aluminum Carbonate (*Basaljel*)	Attapulgite (eg, *Donnagel*)
Metoprolol* (eg, *Lopressor*)	Sotalol* (*Betapace*)	Aluminum Hydroxide* (eg, *Amphojel*)	Kaolin (eg, *Kaodene*)
		Aluminum Phosphate (*Phosphaljel*)	Magaldrate (eg, *Riopan*)

Significance	Onset	Severity	Documentation
3	■ **Rapid**	□ Major	□ Established
	□ Delayed	□ Moderate	□ Probable
		■ **Minor**	■ **Suspected**
			□ Possible
			□ Unlikely

Effects Pharmacokinetic and pharmacologic effects of BETA-BLOCKERS may be altered by certain ALUMINUM SALTS.[3]

Mechanism The rate of gastric emptying may be decreased, leading to reduced bioavailability of BETA-BLOCKERS.

Management Separate the oral doses of BETA-BLOCKERS and ALUMINUM SALTS by at least 2 hours.

Discussion

In a randomized, crossover study, a single oral dose of propranolol 40 mg was administered to six healthy subjects alone and at 2-week intervals with aluminum hydroxide gel 30 mL. The mean plasma concentrations and the mean changes in exercise heart rate with or without coadministration of aluminum hydroxide gel were clinically insignificant.[5] Another study showed no absorption interaction between propranolol and aluminum hydroxide gel.[4] These studies were in contrast to investigations by others who reported a decrease in bioavailability of propranolol.[3] In another study,[2] an increase of 11% in the area under the plasma concentration-time curve (AUC) occurred when aluminum hydroxide antacid 30 mL was administered concomitantly with metoprolol in six healthy subjects, but a mean reduction of 57% in peak plasma concentration of atenolol was also reported.[1] Antacids affecting the rate of gastric emptying may have been the underlying mechanism. In a randomized, crossover study in six healthy subjects, peak sotalol concentration, AUC and cumulative urinary excretion were reduced when sotalol 160 mg was taken with magnesium-aluminum hydroxide 20 mL, but not when administered 2 hours before the antacid.[7] Higher heart rates were associated with the lower sotalol levels.

Additional studies are needed to determine the clinical importance of this interaction.[6]

1 Dobbs JH, et al. *Curr Ther Res.* 1977;21:887.
2 Regardh CG, et al. *Biopharm Drug Dispos.* 1981;2:79.
3 Kirch W, et al. *Clin Pharmacol Ther.* 1981;30:429.
4 McElnay JC, et al. *Br J Clin Pharmacol.* 1982;13:399.
5 Hong CY, et al. *Int J Clin Pharmacol Ther Toxicol.* 1985;23:244.
6 D'Arcy PF, et al. *DICP.* 1987;21:607. Review.
7 Läer S, et al. *Br J Clin Pharmacol.* 1997;43:269.

* Asterisk indicates drugs cited in interaction reports. Based on pharmacologic and pharmacokinetic considerations, similar interactions may occur with other drugs that are listed.

Beta-Blockers — Aminoglycosides

Nadolol* (eg, *Corgard*)	Neomycin* (eg, *Mycifradin*)

Significance	Onset	Severity	Documentation
5	■ **Rapid**	□ Major	□ Established
	□ Delayed	□ Moderate	□ Probable
		■ **Minor**	□ Suspected
			■ **Possible**
			□ Unlikely

Effects The rate of oral absorption and extrarenal elimination of NADOLOL may be increased by coadministration of oral ERYTHROMYCIN base and NEOMYCIN.

Mechanism Unknown. Probable interference with intraluminal fat digestion and increased biliary excretion of NADOLOL.

Management No precautions appear necessary.

Discussion

A crossover investigation was conducted to assess whether nadolol undergoes enterohepatic circulation.[1] Eight healthy subjects received oral nadolol 80 mg on two occasions at least 2 weeks apart. The first phase was a control. In another phase, the subjects received erythromycin base (eg, *E-Mycin*) 0.5 g and oral neomycin 0.5 g four times daily for 2 days before nadolol. After the antibiotics, nadolol area under the plasma concentration-time curve (AUC) was constant, percentage of nadolol recovered in urine fell to 12.7 ± 1.7%, nadolol half-life fell to 11.6 ± 1.3 hours from 17.3 ± 1.7 hours (33%), and mean peak nadolol concentration rose from 146 ± 15 to 397 ± 52 ng/mL (172% higher) on the average of 1 hour sooner. These results suggest that there is an enterohepatic circulation for nadolol and that antibiotics may increase the nadolol effect. The combination induced only small changes in resting arterial blood pressure and in resting pulse.

The assessment of the clinical significance requires more controlled data.

[1] du Souich P, et al. *Clin Pharmacol Ther*. 1983;33:585.

* Asterisk indicates drugs cited in interaction reports.

Beta-Blockers — *Amiodarone*

Carvedilol* (eg, *Coreg*)	Propranolol (eg, *Inderal*)	Amiodarone* (eg, *Cordarone*)
Metoprolol* (eg, *Lopressor*)		

Significance	Onset	Severity	Documentation
4	■ **Rapid**	□ Major	□ Established
	□ Delayed	■ **Moderate**	□ Probable
		□ Minor	□ Suspected
			■ **Possible**
			□ Unlikely

Effects The pharmacologic effects of METOPROLOL and possibly other BETA-BLOCKERS eliminated by hepatic metabolism (eg, PROPRANOLOL) may be increased.

Mechanism Decreased hepatic metabolism and diminished first-pass effect with increased bioavailability is suspected. CARVEDILOL metabolism is stereospecific. AMIODARONE inhibits S-CARVEDILOL metabolism.

Management No special precautions, other than the usual monitoring of cardiovascular status, appear to be necessary.

Discussion

Sinus bradycardia and hypotension developed in a 64-year-old woman shortly after the coadministration of metoprolol and amiodarone.[1] The patient had been hospitalized because of bursts of ventricular tachycardia. She had been receiving atenolol (eg, *Tenormin*) 100 mg/day. On hospital admission, her BP was 150/90 mm Hg, and her pulse rate was 75 bpm and regular. Amiodarone therapy was started at 1,200 mg/day, and the atenolol dosage was reduced to 50 mg/day. Five days later, the heart rate was 55 bpm, and atenolol was replaced with metoprolol 100 mg once daily. Three hours after the first dose of metoprolol, the patient experienced dizziness, weakness, and blurred vision. She was pale, sweating, and had an irregular pulse of 20 bpm. Her systolic BP was 60 mm Hg. The patient's sinus bradycardia did not respond to 2 IV doses of atropine 1 mg; however, following isoproterenol infusion, her BP increased to 100/70 mm Hg and her pulse accelerated to 90 bpm. Metoprolol was discontinued, and the patient recovered within 24 hours. Two large, randomized, double-blind, placebo-controlled studies (2,687 patients) of amiodarone in patients recovering from an MI failed to find any risk with concurrent beta-blocker therapy.[2] Rather, these studies determined that combined amiodarone/beta-blocker therapy resulted in fewer deaths than the use of either drug alone. Coadministration of amiodarone lowered the serum concentration to dose (C/D) ratio of S-carvedilol and increased mean S-carvedilol concentrations, compared with giving carvedilol alone.[3] The C/D ratio of R-carvedilol was not affected by amiodarone.

[1] Leor J, et al. *Am Heart J.* 1988;116(1, pt 1):206.
[2] Boutitie F, et al. *Circulation.* 1999;99(17):2268.
[3] Fukumoto K, et al. *Drug Metab Pharmacokinet.* 2005;20(6):423.

* Asterisk indicates drugs cited in interaction reports. Based on pharmacologic and pharmacokinetic considerations, similar interactions may occur with other drugs that are listed.

Beta-Blockers — *Anticholinergics*

Beta-Blockers	Anticholinergics	
Atenolol* (eg, *Tenormin*)	Atropine (eg, *Sal-tropine*)	Methscopolamine (eg, *Pamine*)
	Belladonna	Orphenadrine (eg, *Norflex*)
	Benztropine (eg, *Cogentin*)	Oxybutynin (eg, *Ditropan*)
	Clidinium	Propantheline* (eg, *Pro-Banthine*)
	Dicyclomine (eg, *Bentyl*)	Scopolamine (eg, *Scopace*)
	Glycopyrrolate (eg, *Robinul*)	Trihexyphenidyl (eg, *Trinexy-5*)
	Hyoscyamine (eg, *Anaspaz*)	
	Mepenzolate (*Cantil*)	

Significance	Onset	Severity	Documentation
4	■ **Rapid**	□ Major	□ Established
	□ Delayed	■ **Moderate**	□ Probable
		□ Minor	□ Suspected
			■ **Possible**
			□ Unlikely

Effects The bioavailability of ATENOLOL may be increased by the administration of ANTICHOLINERGICS.

Mechanism ANTICHOLINERGICS increase retention time of BETA-BLOCKERS in the stomach that may in turn enhance the dissolution and bioavailability of the drug.

Management If an increase in beta-blockade is suspected, tailoring the BETA-BLOCKER dose downward may be necessary.

Discussion

Oral propantheline 30 mg given 1.5 hours earlier prolonged the absorption of atenolol 100 mg and increased the AUC 36% in 6 healthy subjects studied in single-dose, randomized, crossover fashion.[1] Metoclopramide (eg, *Reglan*) 25 mg given 1 hour earlier did not affect the time course of plasma atenolol or its bioavailability. In another study of 4 healthy subjects given oral propranolol 80 mg with simultaneous IV injection of metoclopramide 10 mg and propantheline 30 mg, the peak plasma concentration of propranolol was lower with propantheline and higher with metoclopramide.[2] In contrast, propantheline and metoclopramide showed no significant effect on the bioavailability of metoprolol.[3] Similarly, the bioavailability of long-acting propranolol was not significantly affected by metoclopramide.[4] More studies are needed to determine the effect of anticholinergics on beta-blockers.

[1] Regårdh CG, et al. *Biopharm Drug Dispos.* 1981;2(1):79.
[2] Castleden CM, et al. *Br J Clin Pharmacol.* 1978;5(2):121.
[3] Briant RH, et al. *Eur J Clin Pharmacol.* 1983;25(3):353.
[4] Charles BG, et al. *Br J Clin Pharmacol.* 1981;11(5):517.

* Asterisk indicates drugs cited in interaction reports. Based on pharmacologic and pharmacokinetic considerations, similar interactions may occur with other drugs that are listed.

Beta-Blockers — *Anticholinesterases*

Beta-Blockers		Anticholinesterases	
Acebutolol (eg, *Sectral*)	Nadolol* (eg, *Corgard*)	Ambenonium (*Mytelase*)	Neostigmine* (eg, *Prostigmin*)
Betaxolol (eg, *Kerlone*)	Penbutolol (*Levatol*)	Edrophonium (*Enlon*)	Pyridostigmine (eg, *Mestinon*)
Carteolol	Pindolol		
Metoprolol (eg, *Lopressor*)	Propranolol* (eg, *Inderal*)		

Significance	Onset	Severity	Documentation
4	■ **Rapid**	□ Major	□ Established
	□ Delayed	■ **Moderate**	□ Probable
		□ Minor	□ Suspected
			■ **Possible**
			□ Unlikely

Effects The risk of severe and prolonged bradycardia may be increased when BETA-BLOCKERS and ANTICHOLINESTERASES are coadministered.

Mechanism Additive or synergistic pharmacologic effects.

Management Use with caution and carefully monitor the patient.

Discussion

A profound decrease in heart rate was reported in a 52-year-old man undergoing meniscectomy.[1] The patient was receiving propranolol for supraventricular tachycardia. Bradycardia occurred after a dose of neostigmine and atropine was administered and resolved with additional atropine administration. A 51-year-old woman taking nadolol for hypertension and angina pectoris developed prolonged and refractory bradycardia and hypotension after reversal of neuromuscular blockade with neostigmine and atropine.[2] Both patients were receiving other medications that may have contributed to their bradycardia.

[1] Sprague DH. *Anesthesiology.* 1975;42(2):208.

[2] Seidl DC, et al. *Anesth Analg.* 1984;63(3):365.

* Asterisk indicates drugs cited in interaction reports. Based on pharmacologic and pharmacokinetic considerations, similar interactions may occur with other drugs that are listed.

Beta-Blockers — Ascorbic Acid

Beta-Blockers	Ascorbic Acid
Propranolol* (eg, *Inderal*)	Ascorbic Acid*

Significance	Onset	Severity	Documentation
5	■ **Rapid** □ Delayed	□ Major □ Moderate ■ **Minor**	□ Established □ Probable □ Suspected □ Possible ■ **Unlikely**

Effects The pharmacologic effects of PROPRANOLOL may be decreased.

Mechanism Possible decreased GI absorption of PROPRANOLOL.

Management Consider monitoring the clinical response of patients, and adjust the PROPRANOLOL dose as needed.

Discussion

In a crossover study, the effect of ascorbic acid on the availability of propranolol was studied in 5 healthy men and women.[1] In the control period after an overnight fast, each subject received oral propranolol 80 mg. At least 1 month later, the same subjects were given a dose of ascorbic acid 2 g 30 minutes before receiving propranolol 80 mg. Compared with the control phase, ascorbic acid administration decreased the peak serum concentration of propranolol 28% (from 463 to 334 nmol/L) and the AUC of propranolol 37%, while increasing the time to reach the peak concentration (from 1.9 to 2.7 hours). In addition, ascorbic acid decreased the amounts of propranolol metabolites recovered in the urine. The heart rate decreased less when propranolol was given with ascorbic acid compared with taking the beta-blocker with water.

Additional studies are needed to determine the clinical importance of these changes.

[1] Gonzalez JP, et al. *Eur J Clin Pharmacol.* 1995;48(3-4):295.

* Asterisk indicates drugs cited in interaction reports.

Beta-Blockers — *Barbiturates*

Beta-Blockers		Barbiturates	
Alprenolol*†	Propranolol* (eg, *Inderal*)	Amobarbital (*Amytal*)	Phenobarbital* (eg, *Luminal*)
Metoprolol* (eg, *Lopressor*)		Butabarbital (*Butisol*)	Primidone (eg, *Mysoline*)
		Mephobarbital (eg, *Mebaral*)	Secobarbital (*Seconal*)
		Pentobarbital*	

Significance	Onset	Severity	Documentation
2	■ **Rapid**	□ Major	□ Established
	□ Delayed	■ **Moderate**	■ **Probable**
		□ Minor	□ Suspected
			□ Possible
			□ Unlikely

Effects Pharmacokinetic effects of certain BETA-BLOCKERS may be reduced by concomitant treatment with BARBITURATES.

Mechanism BARBITURATES enhance enzyme induction and hepatic first-pass extraction that may reduce oral bioavailability of certain BETA-BLOCKERS.

Management If an interaction is suspected, consider a higher BETA-BLOCKER dose during coadministration of BARBITURATES.

Discussion

Several studies have demonstrated that pretreatment with barbiturates markedly decreases the steady-state plasma concentrations of beta-adrenergic blockers, including propranolol, metoprolol, and alprenolol†.[1-7] In 1 study, 6 healthy subjects were given a single oral dose of alprenolol 200 mg or placebo before and after pentobarbital 100 mg for 10 days.[5] Plasma levels of alprenolol and its metabolite were decreased 40%, and exercise tachycardia inhibition by alprenolol was reduced from 14% to 10% after pentobarbital. In another study of 8 healthy subjects, oral pentobarbital 100 mg decreased the AUC of oral metoprolol 100 mg an average of 32%.[4] In contrast, the pharmacokinetic parameters of oral timolol (eg, *Blocadren*) with a small first-pass effect (15% to 20%) were not affected by phenobarbital.[8]

It appears that the pharmacokinetic changes reported may be responsible for a slight reduction in beta-adrenergic blockade.

[1] Alván G, et al. *J Pharmacokinet Biopharm.* 1977;5(3):193.
[2] Alván G, et al. *Clin Pharmacol Ther.* 1977;22(3):316.
[3] Sotaniemi EA, et al. *Clin Pharmacol Ther.* 1979;26(2):153.
[4] Haglund K, et al. *Clin Pharmacol Ther.* 1979;26(3):326.
[5] Collste P, et al. *Clin Pharmacol Ther.* 1979;25(4):423.
[6] Branch RA, et al. *Br J Clin Pharmacol.* 1984;17(suppl 1):77S.
[7] Seideman P, et al. *Br J Clin Pharmacol.* 1987;23(3):267.
[8] Mäntylä R, et al. *Eur J Clin Pharmacol.* 1983;24(2):227.

* Asterisk indicates drugs cited in interaction reports. Based on pharmacologic and pharmacokinetic considerations, similar interactions may occur with other drugs that are listed.
† Not available in the United States.

Beta-Blockers		***Bupropion***
Carvedilol (*Coreg*)	Propranolol (eg, *Inderal*)	Bupropion* (eg, *Wellbutrin*)
Labetalol (eg, *Trandate*)	Timolol (eg, *Blocadren*)	
Metoprolol* (eg, *Lopressor*)		

Significance	Onset	Severity	Documentation
4	□ Rapid ■ **Delayed**	□ Major ■ **Moderate** □ Minor	□ Established □ Probable □ Suspected ■ **Possible** □ Unlikely

Effects Plasma concentrations and cardiovascular effects (eg, bradycardia) of certain BETA-BLOCKERS may be increased.

Mechanism Inhibition of CYP2D6-mediated BETA-BLOCKER metabolism is suspected.

Management With certain BETA-BLOCKERS, carefully monitor patients when starting, stopping, or changing the dose of BUPROPION. Consider use of a BETA-BLOCKER not metabolized by CYP2D6 (eg, atenolol [eg, *Tenormin*]).

Discussion

A 56-year-old man with hypertension was on stable doses of metoprolol 75 mg and diltiazem (eg, *Cardizem*) twice daily for more than 1 year.[1] He was started on bupropion 150 mg twice daily for smoking cessation. Twelve days later, he presented with 24 hours of fatigue and dyspnea. A physical examination revealed a heart rate of 43 bpm, BP of 102/65, a mildly labored respiratory rate of 24, and pitting edema just above the ankles. The 3 medications were withheld, and by the next morning all symptoms resolved and normal sinus rhythm was restored. Metoprolol was restarted and, through 1 month of follow-up, the patient remained asymptomatic without bradycardia, dyspnea, or lower extremity edema.

[1] McCollum DL, et al. *Cardiovasc Drugs Ther.* 2004;18(4):329.

* Asterisk indicates drugs cited in interaction reports. Based on pharmacologic and pharmacokinetic considerations, similar interactions may occur with other drugs that are listed.

Beta-Blockers		Calcium Salts	
Atenolol* (eg, *Tenormin*)		Calcium Carbonate (eg, *Os-Cal 500*) Calcium Citrate (*Citracal*) Calcium Glubionate (*Neo-Calglucon*)	Calcium Gluconate Calcium Lactate Tricalcium Phosphate (*Posture*)

Significance	Onset	Severity	Documentation
4	■ **Rapid** □ Delayed	□ Major ■ **Moderate** □ Minor	□ Established □ Probable □ Suspected ■ **Possible** □ Unlikely

Effects CALCIUM SALTS may alter the pharmacokinetic parameters and decrease the pharmacologic effects of ATENOLOL.

Mechanism Impaired absorption of ATENOLOL in the GI tract, and possibly an increase in the area of volume of distribution.

Management When appropriate via monitoring, consider tailoring the dose of ATENOLOL upward.

Discussion

In an open, crossover study, six healthy subjects were administered one oral dose of atenolol 100 mg with and without calcium 500 mg (as the lactate, gluconate and carbonate salts).[1] The mean peak plasma levels of atenolol decreased by 51% and a reduction of 32.2% in the area under the plasma concentration-time curve were observed after calcium administration. The elimination half-life also increased by 43.6% as compared with atenolol administered alone.

Pharmacologically, a reduction in beta-adrenergic blockade, as measured by an inhibition of exercise-induced tachycardia, was demonstrated 12 hours after atenolol was administered with calcium salts.

The prolonged elimination half-life of atenolol appeared to compensate for the decrease in serum concentration observed earlier. During the 1-month treatment period, blood pressure values of those on atenolol alone were not significantly different from those on combination therapies.

More studies are needed to determine the clinical significance of this interaction in chronically treated patients.

[1] Kirch W, et al. *Clin Pharmacol Ther.* 1981;30:429.

* Asterisk indicates drugs cited in interaction reports. Based on pharmacologic and pharmacokinetic considerations, similar interactions may occur with other drugs that are listed.

Beta-Blockers — *Cholestyramine*

Propranolol* (eg, *Inderal*)	Cholestyramine* (eg, *Questran*)

Significance	Onset	Severity	Documentation
4	■ **Rapid**	□ Major	□ Established
	□ Delayed	■ **Moderate**	□ Probable
		□ Minor	□ Suspected
			■ **Possible**
			□ Unlikely

Effects The plasma concentration of PROPRANOLOL and metabolite were reduced, which may cause a diminished pharmacologic effect.

Mechanism PROPRANOLOL appears to bind with anionic exchange resins forming a complex that may decrease absorption in the GI tract.

Management Consider tailoring the dose of PROPRANOLOL upward when appropriate. Staggering administration time may prevent this interaction.

Discussion

Results from an early study using oral propranolol and a single dose of cholestyramine administered concomitantly in five type II hyperlipoproteinemia patients demonstrated no interference in terms of absorption or bioavailability of propranolol.[1] However, this was contradicted in a randomized and controlled study, in which 12 healthy male subjects were administered oral propranolol 120 mg and cholestyramine 8 g or equivalent doses of colestipol 10 g.[2] Six of the subjects received one dose of the anionic exchange resin; the remaining six received an additional dose of the resin. When two doses of either cholestyramine or colestipol were administered prior to propranolol, the peak plasma concentration and area under the concentration-time curve (AUC) for both propranolol and metabolite (4′-hydroxy propranolol) were reduced significantly. There was no significant difference between the pharmacologic effects of these two treatment groups. The peak plasma concentration of propranolol was also lowered by a single dose of cholestyramine, but a single dose of colestipol demonstrated a significant increase in AUC and peak plasma concentration of propranolol.

More multiple dose studies are needed to determine the clinical significance of this interaction.

[1] Schwartz DE, et al. *Clin Pharmacol Ther.* 1982;31:268.

[2] Hibbard DM, et al. *Br J Clin Pharmacol.* 1984;18:337.

* Asterisk indicates drugs cited in interaction reports.

Beta-Blockers — *Cimetidine*

Carvedilol (eg, *Coreg*)	Nebivolol* (*Bystolic*)	Cimetidine* (eg, *Tagamet*)
Labetalol (eg, *Trandate*)	Propranolol* (eg, *Inderal*)	
Metoprolol* (eg, *Lopressor*)	Timolol* (eg, *Blocadren*)	

Significance	Onset	Severity	Documentation
2	■ **Rapid**	□ Major	□ Established
	□ Delayed	■ **Moderate**	■ **Probable**
		□ Minor	□ Suspected
			□ Possible
			□ Unlikely

Effects Pharmacologic effects of BETA-BLOCKERS metabolized by CYP-450 pathway may be increased.

Mechanism CIMETIDINE may reduce hepatic first-pass extraction, decrease liver blood flow, and inhibit hepatic metabolism (CYP2D6) of certain BETA-BLOCKERS.

Management Monitor for beta-blockade when starting or stopping CIMETIDINE. Adjust BETA-BLOCKER dose as needed. Consider changing from CIMETIDINE to another histamine H_2-receptor antagonist (eg, famotidine [eg, *Pepcid*]).

Discussion

Cimetidine interferes with the oral and systemic clearance of propranolol.[1-7] A 33% reduction of liver blood flow occurred in subjects on chronic cimetidine therapy[3]; increases in propranolol plasma level of 1.5- to 3-fold have been reported.[1-5,8,9] Effects produced by single or divided daily doses of cimetidine appear to be the same.[10,11] A substantial reduction of resting pulse rate was reported in 1 study[3] and profound hypotension and sinus bradycardia were reported in another.[8] Other beta-blockers such as atenolol (eg, *Tenormin*), pindolol (eg, *Visken*), and nadolol (eg, *Corgard*) are not affected by cimetidine, apparently because of their diverse pharmacokinetic properties.[4,6,12-14] Conversely, cimetidine caused a slight prolongation of the elimination $t_{½}$ of atenolol[12] and a marked increase of metoprolol plasma level.[5,6] Other studies demonstrated no bioavailability changes in metoprolol in patients treated with cimetidine.[12,14] The conflict may be caused by the stereoselectivity of cimetidine on the less pharmacologically active (R)-metoprolol enantiomer.[15] In 12 healthy volunteers, coadministration of cimetidine with topical ocular timolol resulted in greater reductions in resting heart rate, intraocular pressure, and exercise tolerance than timolol alone.[16] In a study of 12 healthy men, although cimetidine inhibited nebivolol metabolism, it did not have an effect on resting BP or heart rate.[17]

[1] Reimann IW, et al. *Br J Clin Pharmacol.* 1981;12(6):785.
[2] Heagerty AM, et al. *Br Med J.* 1981;282(6280):1917.
[3] Feely J, et al. *N Engl J Med.* 1981;304(12):692.
[4] Reimann IW, et al. *Clin Pharmacol Ther.* 1982;32(6):749.
[5] Kirch W, et al. *Drugs.* 1983;25(suppl 2):127.
[6] Mutschler E, et al. *Br J Clin Pharmacol.* 1984;17(suppl 1):51S.
[7] Asgharnejad M, et al. *Clin Pharmacol Ther.* 1987;41:203.
[8] Donovan MA, et al. *Lancet.* 1981;1(8212):164.
[9] Duchin KL, et al. *Am Heart J.* 1984;108(4)(pt 2):1084.
[10] Donn KH, et al. *J Clin Pharmacol.* 1984;24(11-12):500.
[11] Asgharnejad M, et al. *J Clin Pharmacol.* 1988;28(4):339.
[12] Houtzagers JJ, et al. *Br J Clin Pharmacol.* 1982;14(1):67.
[13] Duchin KL, et al. *Br J Clin Pharmacol.* 1984;17(4):486.
[14] Ellis ME, et al. *Br J Clin Pharmacol.* 1984;17(suppl 1):59S.
[15] Toon S, et al. *Clin Pharmacol Ther.* 1988;43(3):283.
[16] Ishii Y, et al. *J Clin Pharmacol.* 2000;40(2):193.
[17] Kamali F, et al. *Br J Clin Pharmacol.* 1997;43(2):201.

* Asterisk indicates drugs cited in interaction reports. Based on pharmacologic and pharmacokinetic considerations, similar interactions may occur with other drugs that are listed.

Beta-Blockers | **Colestipol**

Propranolol* (eg, *Inderal*)	Colestipol* (eg, *Colestid*)

Significance	Onset	Severity	Documentation
4	■ **Rapid** □ Delayed	□ Major ■ **Moderate** □ Minor	□ Established □ Probable □ Suspected ■ **Possible** □ Unlikely

Effects The therapeutic and pharmacologic actions of PROPRANOLOL may be decreased.

Mechanism Possibly decreased GI absorption because of binding of PROPRANOLOL to nonabsorbable anionic exchange resins.

Management If BP control deteriorates, consider tailoring the PROPRANOLOL dose as needed.

Discussion

Six healthy volunteers received colestipol 10 g or cholestyramine 8 g two minutes prior to oral propranolol 120 mg. A second group of 6 subjects received an additional dose of these resins 12 hours prior to propranolol.[1] The 2-dose treatment with either colestipol or cholestyramine lowered the total AUC and the peak plasma level of propranolol. However, administration of colestipol alone was reported with an increase in total and peak concentration of propranolol. No difference was reported in the effects of these 2 regimens.

The clinical relevance of these findings remains to be determined.

[1] Hibbard DM, et al. *Br J Clin Pharmacol.* 1984;18(3):337.

* Asterisk indicates drugs cited in interaction reports.

Beta-Blockers ✕ *Contraceptives, Hormonal*

Acebutolol* (eg, *Sectral*)	Propranolol* (eg, *Inderal*)	Contraceptives, Oral* (eg, *Ortho-Novum*)
Metoprolol* (eg, *Lopressor*)		

Significance	Onset	Severity	Documentation
4	□ Rapid	□ Major	□ Established
	■ **Delayed**	■ **Moderate**	□ Probable
		□ Minor	□ Suspected
			■ **Possible**
			□ Unlikely

Effects The pharmacologic effects of certain BETA-BLOCKERS may be increased.

Mechanism ORAL CONTRACEPTIVES may decrease the first-pass metabolism of certain BETA-BLOCKERS by inhibition of hepatic microsomal enzymes.

Management Consider monitoring the patient and tailoring the dose of the BETA-BLOCKER as necessary.

Discussion

The pharmacokinetics of metoprolol were investigated in female volunteers with or without oral contraceptives (OCs) in 2 studies involving 23 and 27 healthy subjects, respectively.[1,2] The area under the plasma concentration-time curve (AUC) and peak plasma concentration (C_{max}) were higher in those taking OCs. In another study, 69 healthy women (with and without administration of low-dose estrogen OCs) were given a single oral dose of acebutolol 400 mg, metoprolol 100 mg, oxprenolol (not available in the US) 80 mg, or propranolol 80 mg.[3] Greater AUCs and higher peak plasma concentrations were demonstrated in patients administered metoprolol, oxprenolol, and propranolol in the OC group, but statistical significance was established only with metoprolol. A smaller AUC and lower C_{max} resulted with acebutolol but this finding was not statistically significant.

Further studies are needed.

[1] Kendall MJ, et al. *Br J Clin Pharmacol.* 1982;14:120.
[2] Jack DB, et al. *Eur J Clin Pharmacol.* 1982;23:37.
[3] Kendall MJ, et al. *Br J Clin Pharmacol.* 1984;17:87S.

* Asterisk indicates drugs cited in interaction reports.

Beta-Blockers — *Diltiazem*

Beta-Blockers		Diltiazem
Atenolol* (eg, *Tenormin*)	Pindolol* (eg, *Visken*)	Diltiazem* (eg, *Cardizem*)
Metoprolol* (eg, *Lopressor*)	Propranolol* (eg, *Inderal*)	

Significance	Onset	Severity	Documentation
2	■ **Rapid**	☐ Major	☐ Established
	☐ Delayed	■ **Moderate**	☐ Probable
		☐ Minor	■ **Suspected**
			☐ Possible
			☐ Unlikely

Effects The pharmacologic effects of certain BETA-BLOCKERS may be increased. Symptomatic bradycardia may occur.

Mechanism Possibly inhibition of oxidative metabolism of BETA-BLOCKERS and additive pharmacologic effects.

Management If an interaction is suspected, consider decreasing the dose of the BETA-BLOCKER. If bradycardia occurs, alternative therapy may be necessary.

Discussion

In a 2-way, crossover trial, the effect of diltiazem on a single oral dose of atenolol, metoprolol, or propranolol, administered 30 minutes after the tenth dose of diltiazem 30 mg 3 times daily, was studied in 13 healthy male volunteers.[1] Compared with placebo, mean plasma concentrations, elimination half-lives, area under the concentration-time curves, and peak plasma levels of propranolol and metoprolol increased after diltiazem administration. The time to reach the maximum concentration (t_{max}) was shorter for propranolol following diltiazem administration, but the t_{max} for metoprolol was not affected. Diltiazem did not alter the mean plasma level or pharmacokinetics of atenolol. After diltiazem administration, compared with the pretreatment groups, all 3 beta-blockers decreased pulse rate; however, only atenolol and metoprolol decreased systolic blood pressure. In 12 healthy volunteers, 6 days of coadministration of diltiazem and propranolol was associated with a 27% and 24% decrease in the clearance of d- and l-propranolol, respectively.[2] In an uncontrolled observation, symptomatic bradycardia occurred in patients treated with diltiazem and beta-blockers.[3] Four cases of symptomatic bradycardia requiring pacemaker insertion were reported in elderly patients taking diltiazem and a beta-blocker (eg, atenolol, metoprolol, propranolol) concurrently.[4] In a prospective review of 2574 admissions to a medical unit, 21 admissions resulted from an adverse cardiovascular event associated with coadministration of diltiazem and propranolol (13 cases), atenolol (5 cases), metoprolol (2 cases), or oxprenonol (not available in the US [1 case]).[5] Bradycardia appears to be most likely to occur in elderly subjects and in those with poor left ventricular function.

[1] Tateishi T, et al. *Eur J Clin Pharmacol.* 1989;36:67.
[2] Hunt BA, et al. *Clin Pharmacol Ther.* 1990;47:584.
[3] Sagie A, et al. *Clin Cardiol.* 1991;14:314.
[4] Yust I, et al. *Isr J Med Sci.* 1992;28:292.
[5] Edoute Y, et al. *J Cardiovasc Pharmacol.* 2000;35;556.

* Asterisk indicates drugs cited in interaction reports.

Beta-Blockers ✕ *Diphenhydramine*

Carvedilol (eg, *Coreg*)	Propranolol (eg, *Inderal*)	Diphenhydramine* (eg, *Benadryl*)
Labetalol (eg, *Trandate*)	Timolol	
Metoprolol* (eg, *Lopressor*)		

Significance	Onset	Severity	Documentation
2	☐ Rapid	☐ Major	☐ Established
	■ **Delayed**	■ **Moderate**	☐ Probable
		☐ Minor	■ **Suspected**
			☐ Possible
			☐ Unlikely

Effects Increased plasma concentrations and cardiovascular effects of certain BETA-BLOCKERS.

Mechanism Inhibition of CYP2D6-mediated BETA-BLOCKER metabolism.

Management With certain BETA-BLOCKERS, carefully monitor patients when DIPHENHYDRAMINE is started or stopped. Because DIPHENHYDRAMINE is available OTC, apprise patients of this potential interaction.

Discussion

The effects of diphenhydramine on the in vitro metabolism, pharmacokinetics, and pharmacodynamics of metoprolol were evaluated in extensive metabolizers (EMs) and poor metabolizers (PMs [ie, CYP2D6]) of metoprolol.[1] The study was a randomized, double-blind, crossover, placebo-controlled investigation involving 16 healthy, nonsmoking men. Ten subjects had high (EMs) and 6 had low (PMs) CYP2D6 activity. Each subject received a single oral dose of metoprolol 100 mg on day 3 of a 5-day course of either diphenhydramine 50 mg or placebo 3 times daily. The in vitro phase of the study demonstrated diphenhydramine to be a potent inhibitor of CYP2D6 metabolism of metoprolol to alpha-hydroxymetoprolol. In the in vivo phase, diphenhydramine did not affect the pharmacokinetics or pharmacodynamics of metoprolol in PMs. However, in EMs, diphenhydramine decreased the oral and nonrenal clearance of metoprolol 2-fold and the partial metabolic clearance of metoprolol to the hydroxy metabolite 2.5-fold. In addition, in EMs, diphenhydramine produced more pronounced and protracted metoprolol-related effects on heart rate, systolic BP, and Doppler-derived aortic blood flow peak velocity compared with EMs receiving placebo. A similar study of 20 women found diphenhydramine to have a greater effect on metoprolol pharmacokinetics in EMs compared with PMs.[2] Comparison of data from these 2 studies shows that EM CYP2D6 women have a greater increase in S-metoprolol AUC from diphenhydramine coadministration compared with men.[3]

[1] Hamelin BA, et al. *Clin Pharmacol Ther.* 2000;67(5):466.
[2] Sharma A, et al. *J Pharmacol Exp Ther.* 2005;313(3):1172.
[3] Sharma A, et al. *J Clin Pharmacol.* 2010;50(2):214.

* Asterisk indicates drugs cited in interaction reports. Based on pharmacologic and pharmacokinetic considerations, similar interactions may occur with other drugs that are listed.

Beta-Blockers	**Erythromycin**
Nadolol* (eg, *Corgard*)	Erythromycin* (eg, *Ery-Tab*)

Significance	Onset	Severity	Documentation
5	■ **Rapid** ☐ Delayed	☐ Major ☐ Moderate ■ **Minor**	☐ Established ☐ Probable ☐ Suspected ☐ Possible ■ **Unlikely**

Effects Pharmacokinetic profile may be altered, but therapeutic and pharmacologic effects are unpredictable based on present evidence.

Mechanism Unconfirmed, but possibly because of eradication of intestinal flora-induced hydrolysis and increased biliary elimination of NADOLOL by MACROLIDE ANTIBIOTICS.

Management No specific precautions appear necessary.

Discussion

In a sequential study, eight healthy subjects received oral nadolol 80 mg alone as a control.[1] The subjects then received erythromycin base 0.5 g and neomycin (eg, *Mycifradin*) 0.5 g four times daily orally for 2 days before nadolol. When poorly absorbable antibiotics were given, the mean peak plasma level was 170% higher and achieved 1 hour earlier, but the area under the nadolol plasma concentration-time curve and the renal clearance of nadolol were similar to that of the control. Conversely, a decrease in systolic blood pressure and a reduction of elimination half-life by 30% were achieved by nadolol compared with the control period. Similar results were obtained with neomycin alone before nadolol and direct evidence implicating erythromycin specifically in this interaction is lacking.

More data will be required before a clinical assessment can be made on this interaction or on other members of these groups.

[1] du Souich P, et al. *Clin Pharmacol Ther.* 1983;33:585.

* Asterisk indicates drugs cited in interaction reports.

Beta-Blockers — *Ethanol*

Propranolol* (eg, *Inderal*)	Ethanol*

Significance	Onset	Severity	Documentation
5	■ **Rapid**	□ Major	□ Established
	□ Delayed	□ Moderate	□ Probable
		■ **Minor**	□ Suspected
			■ **Possible**
			□ Unlikely

Effects The pharmacologic and therapeutic effects of this combination are difficult to anticipate (see discussion).

Mechanism Unknown. Acute ALCOHOL ingestion may reduce gastric motility, delay gastric emptying time and prolong the time interval for PROPRANOLOL to reach its absorption site in the small intestine.

Management It may be advisable to avoid this combination; however, precautions appear unnecessary.

Discussion

The additive effects of CNS inhibition by ethanol in combination with propranolol have been described.[1,2,9] In these studies, propranolol impaired the performance of psychomotor testing when used with ethanol. However, no significant changes in the absorption rate, absorption fraction and elimination of ethanol were observed.[3] In a controlled study of five normal subjects, administration of oral propranolol 80 mg with 60 mL of 50% ethanol resulted in a significant increase in maximum plasma concentration and elimination rate of propranolol.[4] Researchers investigated eight healthy subjects in another controlled study; plasma clearance of oral propranolol 80 mg increased by 26% when given with 32 to 72 mL absolute alcohol.[5] In contrast, a significant decrease in free propranolol clearance was also reported.[6] Despite the kinetic changes of propranolol in combination with alcohol, the inhibiting effect on heart rate of propranolol may be offset by the cardio-acceleratory effect of ethanol.[8] Another study investigated the interaction involving eight healthy subjects ingesting atenolol (eg, *Tenormin*) 100 mg and metoprolol (eg, *Lopressor*) 100 mg, all pretreated with 200 mL absolute alcohol. No significant kinetic changes were reported in either drug.[7] Similarly, the elimination of sotalol (not available in the US) was not affected by ethanol, but the hypotensive effect was increased.[5]

More studies are needed to define the effect of acute and chronic ethanol ingestion on the kinetics of other beta-adrenergic blockers.

[1] Noble EP, et al. *Fed Proc.* 1973;32;724.
[2] Khan MA, et al. *J Pharmacol Clin.* 1975;2:168.
[3] Svendsen TL, et al. *Eur J Clin Pharmacol.* 1978;13:91.
[4] Grabowski BS, et al. *Int J Clin Pharmacol Ther Toxicol.* 1980;18:317.
[5] Sotaniemi EA, et al. *Clin Pharmacol Ther.* 1981;29:705.
[6] Dorian P, et al. *Clin Pharmacol Ther.* 1982;31:219.
[7] Kirch W, et al. *Drugs.* 1983;25(Suppl 2):152.
[8] Dorian P, et al. *Eur J Clin Pharmacol.* 1984;27:209.
[9] Aucamp AK, et al. *S Afr Med J.* 1984;66:445.

* Asterisk indicates drugs cited in interaction reports.

Beta-Blockers | **Felodipine**

Metoprolol* (eg, *Lopressor*)	Felodipine* (*Plendil*)

Significance	Onset	Severity	Documentation
5	☐ Rapid	☐ Major	☐ Established
	■ **Delayed**	☐ Moderate	☐ Probable
		■ **Minor**	☐ Suspected
			■ **Possible**
			☐ Unlikely

Effects Serum METOPROLOL levels may be increased. The elevations appear to be slight and would not be expected to be clinically significant.

Mechanism Unknown.

Management No special precautions, other than the usual monitoring of cardiovascular status, appear to be necessary.

Discussion

In a double-blind crossover study, the possibility of a pharmacokinetic interaction between felodipine and metoprolol was investigated in eight healthy subjects.[1] In random order, patients received felodipine 10 mg twice daily plus metoprolol 100 mg twice daily, felodipine 10 mg twice daily plus placebo, or metoprolol 100 mg twice daily plus placebo for 5 days. The pharmacokinetics of felodipine were unchanged by the concurrent administration of metoprolol. However, the maximum plasma metoprolol concentration (C_{max}) and the area under the metoprolol concentration-time curve (AUC) over the first 12 hours after dosing were significantly ($P < 0.01$) increased by concomitant felodipine administration. The C_{max} for metoprolol increased from 807 to 1112 nmol/L, while the AUC increased from 5047 to 6600 nmol•hr/L. The minimum plasma metoprolol concentration, the time to reach maximum concentration, and the half-life for metoprolol were unchanged by concurrent felodipine administration. The mechanism for this interaction is unknown. Although felodipine administration may result in an increase in metoprolol plasma levels, these changes appear to be slight and, based on currently available information, the alterations would not be expected to have clinical consequences.

[1] Smith SR, et al. *Eur J Clin Pharmacol.* 1987;31:575.

* Asterisk indicates drugs cited in interaction reports.

Beta-Blockers — *Flecainide*

Acebutolol (*Sectral*)	Metoprolol (eg, *Lopressor*)	Flecainide* (*Tambocor*)
Betaxolol (*Kerlone*)	Penbutolol (*Levatol*)	
Carteolol (*Cartrol*)	Pindolol (eg, *Visken*)	
Labetalol (eg, *Trandate*)	Propranolol* (eg, *Inderal*)	

Significance	Onset	Severity	Documentation
4	□ Rapid	□ Major	□ Established
	■ **Delayed**	■ **Moderate**	□ Probable
		□ Minor	□ Suspected
			■ **Possible**
			□ Unlikely

Effects The pharmacologic effects of PROPRANOLOL (and possibly other beta-adrenergic blockers) and FLECAINIDE may be increased.

Mechanism Unknown; possibly inhibition of metabolism of both drugs as well as additive pharmacologic effects.

Management No special precautions, other than the usual monitoring of cardiovascular status, appear to be necessary.

Discussion

The effects of concurrent oral administration of flecainide and propranolol on cardiac function and the pharmacokinetics of each of these agents were studied in healthy volunteers.[1] Each subject was administered flecainide 200 mg twice daily on days 8 through 11 and 19 through 23 and propranolol 80 mg three times daily on days 1 through 11 and 23. The effects of both drugs on cardiac function were, at most, additive. However, propranolol increased the area under the concentration-time curve (AUC) of flecainide 1.2 times ($P < 0.01$) while flecainide increased the AUC of propranolol 1.31 times ($P < 0.05$). Neither drug affected the terminal plasma half-life of the other.

[1] Holtzman JL, et al. *Eur J Clin Pharmacol.* 1987;33:97.

* Asterisk indicates drugs cited in interaction reports. Based on pharmacologic and pharmacokinetic considerations, similar interactions may occur with other drugs that are listed.

Beta-Blockers — *Fluvoxamine*

Metoprolol* (eg, *Lopressor*)	Propranolol* (eg, *Inderal*)	Fluvoxamine*

Significance	Onset	Severity	Documentation
4	☐ Rapid ■ **Delayed**	☐ Major ■ **Moderate** ☐ Minor	☐ Established ☐ Probable ☐ Suspected ■ **Possible** ☐ Unlikely

Effects The pharmacologic effects of certain BETA-BLOCKERS may be increased.

Mechanism FLUVOXAMINE may inhibit the oxidative metabolism of BETA-BLOCKERS.

Management If an interaction is suspected, it may be necessary to adjust the dose of the BETA-BLOCKERS when starting, stopping, or changing the dose of FLUVOXAMINE. When starting therapy with a BETA-BLOCKER in patients receiving FLUVOXAMINE, consider giving a conservative dose of the BETA-BLOCKER, carefully titrating the dose.

Discussion

Administration of fluvoxamine 100 mg/day and propranolol 160 mg/day to healthy volunteers has caused a 2- to 17-fold (mean, 5-fold) increase in minimum plasma propranolol concentrations.[1] However, there was only a slight potentiation of the propranolol-induced reduction in heart rate (approximately 3 beats/minute) and a reduction in the exercise diastolic pressure.[1] The hypotensive effects of propranolol were not affected by fluvoxamine.[2] Bradycardia, hypotension, and orthostatic hypotension have been reported during coadministration of metoprolol and fluvoxamine. In contrast, the serum concentrations of atenolol (eg, *Tenormin*), a beta-blocker that does not undergo hepatic metabolism, were not affected by fluvoxamine administration. Nevertheless, there was a slight potentiation in the heart rate reduction action of atenolol and a slight antagonism in the BP-lowering effects of atenolol during exercise.[2,3]

This monograph is based on secondary references and information on file with the manufacturer. Published clinical data are needed to further assess this interaction.

[1] Van Harten J. *Clin Pharmacokinet.* 1993;24:203.
[2] Benfield P, et al. *Drugs.* 1986;32:313.
[3] Perucca E, et al. *Clin Pharmacokinet.* 1994;27:175.

* Asterisk indicates drugs cited in interaction reports.

Beta-Blockers — *Food*

Acebutolol* (eg, *Sectral*)	Atenolol* (eg, *Tenormin*)	Orange Juice*

Significance	Onset	Severity	Documentation
2	□ Rapid ■ **Delayed**	□ Major ■ **Moderate** □ Minor	□ Established □ Probable ■ **Suspected** □ Possible □ Unlikely

Effects ATENOLOL plasma concentrations and AUC may be reduced, decreasing the pharmacologic and pharmacodynamic effects.

Mechanism Unknown.

Management If ORANGE JUICE cannot be avoided in patients taking ATENOLOL, it may be necessary to adjust the ATENOLOL dosage or separate ATENOLOL administration and ORANGE JUICE ingestion by as much time as possible. The effect of GRAPEFRUIT JUICE on ACEBUTOLOL does not appear to be clinically important.

Discussion

The effect of orange juice ingestion on the pharmacokinetics of atenolol was studied in 10 healthy men.[1] Using a randomized, crossover design, each subject ingested 200 mL of orange juice or water 3 times daily for 3 days and twice on day 4. On the morning of day 3, each subject took atenolol 50 mg with an additional 200 mL of orange juice or water. Compared with water, taking atenolol with orange juice decreased the C_{max} and AUC of atenolol 49% and 40%, respectively. The time to reach the C_{max} and elimination $t_{1/2}$ of atenolol were not altered. The amount of atenolol excreted in the urine decreased 38%, but the renal clearance was not affected. The average heart rate was slightly higher when atenolol was taken with orange juice compared with water. In a similar investigation, the effects of grapefruit juice on the pharmacokinetics of acebutolol were studied.[2] Grapefruit juice decreased the acebutolol C_{max} 19% and AUC 7% compared with water. The $t_{1/2}$ of acebutolol was prolonged from 4 to 5.1 hours. Grapefruit juice decreased the AUC, C_{max}, and amount of diacetolol (the active metabolite of acebutolol) excreted in the urine 18%, 24%, and 20%, respectively, compared with water.

[1] Lilja JJ, et al. *Eur J Clin Pharmacol.* 2005;61:337.

[2] Lilja JJ, et al. *Br J Clin Pharmacol.* 2005;60:659.

* Asterisk indicates drugs cited in interaction reports.

Beta-Blockers — *Gefitinib*

Carvedilol (*Coreg*)	Propranolol (eg, *Inderal*)	Gefitinib* (*Iressa*)
Labetalol (eg, *Trandate*)	Timolol (eg, *Blocadren*)	
Metoprolol* (eg, *Lopressor*)		

Significance	Onset	Severity	Documentation
4	☐ Rapid	☐ Major	☐ Established
	■ **Delayed**	■ **Moderate**	☐ Probable
		☐ Minor	☐ Suspected
			■ **Possible**
			☐ Unlikely

Effects Plasma concentrations and cardiovascular effects of certain BETA-BLOCKERS may be increased.

Mechanism Inhibition of CYP2D6-mediated BETA-BLOCKER metabolism.

Management Based on available data, the magnitude of the interaction is not likely to be clinically important. If an interaction is suspected, be prepared to adjust treatment as needed.

Discussion

The effects of gefitinib on the pharmacokinetics of metoprolol were investigated in 18 patients with solid tumors.[1] In an open-label, nonrandomized study, each subject received metoprolol 50 mg alone and after receiving gefitinib 500 mg/day for 15 days (gefitinib 500 mg every 12 hours was given on day 1). Data from 3 patients were excluded from the pharmacokinetic analysis. Compared with administration of metoprolol alone, pretreatment with gefitinib increased the metoprolol C_{max} 10% and AUC 35%.

[1] Swaisland HC, et al. *Clin Pharmacokinet.* 2005;44:1067.

* Asterisk indicates drugs cited in interaction reports. Based on pharmacologic and pharmacokinetic considerations, similar interactions may occur with other drugs that are listed.

Beta-Blockers — *Haloperidol*

Propranolol* (eg, *Inderal*)	Haloperidol* (eg, *Haldol*)

Significance	Onset	Severity	Documentation
4	■ **Rapid**	■ **Major**	□ Established
	□ Delayed	□ Moderate	□ Probable
		□ Minor	□ Suspected
			■ **Possible**
			□ Unlikely

Effects Pharmacologic effects of both drugs may be increased.

Mechanism Probable synergistic pharmacologic activity.

Management Avoid this combination if possible. May need a lower dose of 1 or both drugs if coadministration is necessary.

Discussion

Haloperidol and propranolol have been documented to produce hypotensive effects individually. In a case report, a 48-year-old woman developed a severe hypotensive reaction on 3 separate occasions after coadministration of haloperidol 10 to 20 mg and propranolol 40 to 80 mg therapy. Cardiopulmonary resuscitation was instituted on 2 of the occasions but with no residual effects.[1] The hypotensive episodes were attributed to intrinsic, relaxant effects on peripheral blood vessels by haloperidol and a similar effect on peripheral blood vessels by propranolol.

No hypotensive episodes have been reported with the combination of haloperidol and other beta-adrenergic blockers.

[1] Alexander HE, et al. *JAMA*. 1984;252:87.

* Asterisk indicates drugs cited in interaction reports.

Beta-Blockers			*Hydralazine*
Metoprolol* (eg, *Lopressor*)	Propranolol* (eg, *Inderal*)	Hydralazine*	
Significance	Onset	Severity	Documentation
2	■ **Rapid** □ Delayed	□ Major ■ **Moderate** □ Minor	□ Established ■ **Probable** □ Suspected □ Possible □ Unlikely

Effects Serum levels and hence, pharmacologic effects of both drugs may be enhanced.

Mechanism HYDRALAZINE increases systemic availability of some BETA-BLOCKERS, probably by transient increase in splanchnic blood flow and decreasing first-pass hepatic metabolism.

Management Carefully monitor the patient when HYDRALAZINE is prescribed with any oral BETA-BLOCKER. Tailoring the dosage of either drug may be warranted.

Discussion

The beneficial therapeutic effects of combined hydralazine and beta-adrenergic blockers for treatment of hypertension are well documented.[1,2,12] Four studies using fasting subjects showed that a 50% to 110% increase in oral bioavailability[3,4,10,11] and peak plasma concentration (C_{max}) of propranolol may be increased up to 500%[7] in the presence of hydralazine. However, hydralazine has no effect on the bioavailability of slow-release propranolol[11] and on nonfasting subjects.[5] Other studies show that hydralazine increases the area under the plasma concentration-time curve (AUC) and C_{max} of metoprolol 38% and 88%, respectively.[13] This effect appears attributable to the transient change in hepatic blood flow and lipophilicity of propranol,[1] metoprolol, and oxprenolol (not available in the US).[3,6,9] Predictably, beta-blockers with low hepatic clearance or no first-pass metabolism such as acebutolol (eg, *Sectral*), atenolol (eg, *Tenormin*), and nadolol (eg, *Corgard*) do not exhibit interaction with hydralazine.[6-8] Propranolol may enhance AUC of hydralazine 59%,[5] but oxprenolol did not change "apparent hydralazine" kinetics.[8]

The exact mechanism of this interaction has not been elucidated. The correlation of plasma concentration of beta-blockers and pharmacologic effects have not been firmly established. Additional studies are needed to determine clinical relevance.

[1] Zacest R, et al. *N Engl J Med.* 1972;286:617.
[2] Guevara J, et al. *Curr Ther Res Clin Exp.* 1977;21:277.
[3] McLean AJ, et al. *Clin Pharmacol Ther.* 1980;27:726.
[4] Jackman GP, et al. *Clin Pharmacol Ther.* 1981;30:291.
[5] Schafer-Korting M, et al. *Eur J Clin Pharmacol.* 1982;21:315.
[6] Jack DB, et al. *Biopharm Drug Dispos.* 1982;3:47.
[7] McLean AJ, et al. *Drugs.* 1983;25 (Suppl 2):131.
[8] Hawksworth GM, et al. *Drugs.* 1983;25 (Suppl 2):136.
[9] Mantyla R, et al. *Eur J Clin Pharmacol.* 1983;24:227.
[10] Schneck DW, et al. *Clin Pharmacol Ther.* 1984;35:447.
[11] Byrne AJ, et al. *Br J Clin Pharmacol.* 1984;17:45S.
[12] Lewis RV, et al. *Med Toxicol.* 1986;1:343. Review.
[13] Lindeberg S, et al. *Eur J Clin Pharmacol.* 1988;35:131.

* Asterisk indicates drugs cited in interaction reports.

Beta-Blockers | **Hydroxychloroquine**

Beta-Blockers		Hydroxychloroquine
Carvedilol (*Coreg*)	Propranolol (eg, *Inderal*)	Hydroxychloroquine* (eg, *Plaquenil*)
Labetalol (eg, *Trandate*)	Timolol (eg, *Blocadren*)	
Metoprolol* (eg, *Lopressor*)		

Significance	Onset	Severity	Documentation
4	☐ Rapid	☐ Major	☐ Established
	■ **Delayed**	■ **Moderate**	☐ Probable
		☐ Minor	☐ Suspected
			■ **Possible**
			☐ Unlikely

Effects Plasma concentrations and cardiovascular effects of certain BETA-BLOCKERS may be increased.

Mechanism Inhibition of CYP2D6-mediated BETA-BLOCKER metabolism.

Management With certain BETA-BLOCKERS, carefully monitor patients when HYDROXYCHLOROQUINE is started or stopped. Consider use of an alternative BETA-BLOCKER (eg, atenolol [eg, *Tenormin*]).

Discussion

The effects of hydroxychloroquine on the activity of cytochrome P450 2D6 (CYP2D6) and on the metabolism of metoprolol were studied in 7 healthy male volunteers.[1] In a placebo-controlled, randomized, double-blind, 2-phase crossover design, each subject received 400 mg hydroxychloroquine or placebo twice daily for 8 days. Prior to the first study phase and on day 8, each subject received 20 mg of dextromethorphan (eg, *Benylin*) as a probe to test the CYP2D6 substrate. All subjects were classified as extensive metabolizers. However, 1 subject was a heterozygous extensive metabolizer while the remaining 6 subjects were homozygous. After administration of hydroxychloroquine, the phenotype of the heterozygous extensive metabolizer was changed to poor metabolizer. Each subject received 100 mg metoprolol on day 9. The area under the plasma concentration-time curve of metoprolol in the 6 homozygous extensive metabolizers increased 65% and the peak plasma concentration was 72% higher after hydroxychloroquine compared with placebo.

[1] Somer M, et al. *Br J Clin Pharmacol.* 2000;49:549.

* Asterisk indicates drugs cited in interaction reports. Based on pharmacologic and pharmacokinetic considerations, similar interactions may occur with other drugs that are listed.

Beta-Blockers | **Loop Diuretics**

Beta-Blockers	Loop Diuretics
Propranolol* (eg, *Inderal*)	Furosemide* (eg, *Lasix*)

Significance	Onset	Severity	Documentation
5	■ **Rapid**	□ Major	□ Established
	□ Delayed	□ Moderate	□ Probable
		■ **Minor**	□ Suspected
			□ Possible
			■ **Unlikely**

Effects The cardiovascular actions of PROPRANOLOL may be enhanced.

Mechanism Probably by reduction of extracellular fluid and alteration of PROPRANOLOL pharmacokinetic parameters.

Management No clinical intervention appears necessary. Monitor the cardiovascular status of the patient; tailor the dose of BETA-ADRENERGIC BLOCKERS as needed.

Discussion

Ten healthy volunteers were administered oral propranolol 40 mg and oral furosemide 25 mg as a single dose; this resulted in a 33% increase in propranolol plasma levels.[2] When 6 additional subjects were investigated, a 6-fold increase in isoproterenol dose was needed to increase heart rate 25% when given in the presence of a propranolol and furosemide combination. A higher incidence of propranolol side effects including bradycardia and hypotension are reported with this combination therapy.[1]

In contrast, furosemide did not significantly alter the pharmacokinetic parameters and antihypertensive effects of atenolol (eg, *Tenormin*).[3] More studies are needed to determine the clinical importance of a similar interaction between beta-blockers and other loop diuretics.

[1] Bravo EL, et al. *N Engl J Med.* 1975;292:66.
[2] Chiariello M, et al. *Clin Pharmacol Ther.* 1979;26:433.
[3] Kirch W, et al. *Clin Pharmacol Ther.* 1981;30:429.

* Asterisk indicates drugs cited in interaction reports.

Beta-Blockers — *MAOIs*

Beta-Blockers		MAOIs	
Metoprolol* (eg, *Lopressor*)	Pindolol* (eg, *Visken*)	Isocarboxazid (*Marplan*)	Tranylcypromine* (*Parnate*)
Nadolol* (eg, *Corgard*)		Phenelzine* (*Nardil*)	

Significance	Onset	Severity	Documentation
5	□ Rapid	□ Major	□ Established
	■ **Delayed**	□ Moderate	□ Probable
		■ **Minor**	□ Suspected
			■ **Possible**
			□ Unlikely

Effects Bradycardia or orthostatic hypotension may develop during coadministration of certain BETA-BLOCKERS and MAOIs.

Mechanism Unknown.

Management Consider monitoring pulse rate and BP during coadministration of these agents. Reducing the dose or discontinuing the BETA-BLOCKER may be necessary if symptomatic bradycardia occurs. Reducing the BETA-BLOCKER dose, followed by slowly increasing the dose, may reduce symptomatic hypotension.

Discussion

While receiving nadolol or metoprolol, 2 elderly patients with previously normal pulse rates developed bradycardia during coadministration of the MAOI phenelzine.[1] In both patients, the pulse rate decreased to 46 to 53 bpm while receiving phenelzine 60 mg daily and the beta-blocker. The bradycardia occurred 8 days after starting phenelzine in the patient receiving nadolol 40 mg/day and in 11 days in the patient receiving metoprolol 150 mg/day. When the dose of nadolol was decreased to 20 mg/day and the metoprolol was discontinued, the pulse rates in these patients increased to 70 to 80 bpm. A 29-year-old woman experienced pronounced orthostatic hypotension when pindolol 2.5 mg 3 times/day was added to augment the antidepressant effects of tranylcypromine 60 mg/day.[2] The pindolol dose was decreased to 2.5 mg twice daily until her BP stabilized and then was slowly increased to 5 mg 3 times/day.

[1] Reggev A, et al. *Psychosomatics*. 1989;30:106.

[2] Kraus RP. *J Clin Psychopharmacol*. 1997;17:225.

* Asterisk indicates drugs cited in interaction reports. Based on pharmacologic and pharmacokinetic considerations, similar interactions may occur with other drugs that are listed.

Beta-Blockers — Nefazodone

Beta-Blockers	Nefazodone
Propranolol* (eg, *Inderal*)	Nefazodone* (eg, *Serzone*)

Significance	Onset	Severity	Documentation
5	□ Rapid	□ Major	□ Established
	■ **Delayed**	□ Moderate	□ Probable
		■ **Minor**	□ Suspected
			□ Possible
			■ **Unlikely**

Effects The pharmacologic effects of PROPRANOLOL may be decreased by NEFAZODONE.

Mechanism Unknown.

Management Based on available data, the changes in PROPRANOLOL pharmacokinetics are not expected to be clinically important. Monitor the clinical response of the patient. If an interaction is suspected, adjust therapy as indicated.

Discussion

The effects of nefazodone on the pharmacokinetics and pharmacodynamics of propranolol were evaluated in 18 healthy men.[1] In an open-label, crossover design, subjects were randomly assigned 3 treatment periods: (1) nefazodone 200 mg, (2) propranolol 40 mg, and (3) nefazodone 200 mg plus propranolol 40 mg. The drugs were administered every 12 hr for 7 days. Nefazodone decreased the peak concentration of propranolol 29% and the AUC 14%, prolonged the $t_{1/2}$ of propranolol 1 hr and resulted in 1 extra day to achieve steady-state propranolol concentrations. The peak concentration and AUC of the hydroxymetabolite of propranolol were decreased 15% and 21%, respectively. Despite the decrease in serum propranolol concentrations, the exercise heart rate and exercise double product (heart rate in bpm × mm Hg) were reduced to a slightly greater extent during coadministration of nefazodone and propranolol, than with propranolol alone.

Based upon the pharmacodynamic findings of this study, the changes in propranolol pharmacokinetics may not be clinically important. Additional studies are needed.

[1] Salazar DE, et al. *J Clin Pharmacol.* 1995;35:1109.

* Asterisk indicates drugs cited in interaction reports.

Beta-Blockers		**Nicardipine**
Metoprolol* (eg, *Lopressor*)	Propranolol* (eg, *Inderal*)	Nicardipine* (eg, *Cardene*)

Significance	Onset	Severity	Documentation
4	■ **Rapid** □ Delayed	□ Major ■ **Moderate** □ Minor	□ Established □ Probable □ Suspected ■ **Possible** □ Unlikely

Effects The pharmacologic effects of PROPRANOLOL or METOPROLOL may be increased.

Mechanism Unknown. However, increased bioavailability due to decreased hepatic first-pass clearance is believed to be involved.

Management If an interaction is suspected, consider decreasing the dose of PROPRANOLOL or METOPROLOL.

Discussion

The effects of nicardipine on the pharmacokinetics and hemodynamics of propranolol were investigated in a randomized, single-dose study in 12 healthy volunteers.[1] Subjects were administered either oral propranolol 80 mg alone or with oral nicardipine 30 mg. Coadministration of nicardipine increased the peak serum concentration of propranolol by 80% and increased the area under the concentration-time curve (AUC) by 47% during the first 9 hours after administration. Heart rate decreased significantly more in subjects treated with propranolol alone ($P < 0.05$) but blood pressures were not different within the two groups. The increased AUC was attributed to a decrease in hepatic first-pass clearance of propranolol by nicardipine. These results were confirmed in a subsequent study.[3] In addition, the effects of nicardipine on sustained release propranolol were small in marked contrast to the effects of immediate release propranolol. In another study, nicardipine produced a slight but significant increase in metoprolol plasma concentrations (from 36 to 46 ng/mL) in extensive metabolizers but not in poor metabolizers of metoprolol.[2] The beta-blocking effects of metoprolol were not altered.

Additional studies are needed to determine the clinical importance of this possible interaction.

1 Schoors DF, et al. *Br J Clin Pharmacol.* 1990;29:497.
2 Laurent-Kenesi MA, et al. *Br J Clin Pharmacol.* 1993;36:531.
3 Vercruysse I, et al. *Eur J Clin Pharmacol.* 1995;49:121.

* Asterisk indicates drugs cited in interaction reports.

Beta-Blockers — Nifedipine

Beta-Blockers		Nifedipine
Acebutolol (eg, *Sectral*)	Nadolol (eg, *Corgard*)	Nifedipine* (eg, *Procardia*)
Atenolol* (eg, *Tenormin*)	Penbutolol (*Levatol*)	
Betaxolol (*Kerlone*)	Pindolol (eg, *Visken*)	
Bisoprolol (*Zebeta*)	Propranolol* (eg, *Inderal*)	
Carteolol (*Cartrol*)	Sotalol (eg, *Betapace*)	
Esmolol (*Brevibloc*)	Timolol (eg, *Blocadren*)	
Metoprolol* (eg, *Lopressor*)		

Significance	Onset	Severity	Documentation
4	■ **Rapid**	□ Major	□ Established
	□ Delayed	■ **Moderate**	□ Probable
		□ Minor	□ Suspected
			■ **Possible**
			□ Unlikely

Effects Pharmacologic effects of both drugs may be potentiated.

Mechanism Possible synergistic or additive effects.

Management Carefully monitor cardiac function of patients at greatest risk of cardiovascular side effects.

Discussion

Nifedipine exerts a negative inotropic effect but with little or no effect on atrioventricular (AV) conduction.[11] Beta-blockers also depress myocardial contractility and decrease AV conduction. Nifedipine stimulates an increase in sympathetic reflex as a result of direct peripheral vasodilation.[10] With beta-blockade, this elevated sympathetic tone may be overwhelmed by the negative inotropic effects and precipitate heart failure.[12] This combination may benefit patients with stable effort angina and essential hypertension.[7,12,14-16,18] However, additive adverse effects have been reported.[1-6,10,17,21] Based on animal data, cardiovascular side effects may be more prominent in subjects with preexisting left ventricular dysfunction, underlying myocardial conduction defects, and elevated drug levels.[13]

A pharmacokinetic interaction was not demonstrated in 2 studies between nifedipine and propranolol, metoprolol, or atenolol;[8,9] although, other studies have shown a slight increase in propranolol levels during absorption[20] and an increase in nifedipine bioavailability during coadministration.[19] In 1 of 338 patients, the addition of metoprolol to nifedipine had a short-term beneficial effect. See also Beta-Blockers/Verapamil.

[1] Opie LH, et al. *BMJ.* 1980;281:1462.
[2] Anastassiades CJ. *BMJ.* 1980;281:1251.
[3] Staffurth JS, et al. *BMJ.* 1981;282:225.
[4] Joshi PI, et al. *Br Heart J.* 1981;45:457.
[5] Robson RH, et al. *BMJ.* 1982;284:104.
[6] Anastassiades CJ. *BMJ.* 1982;284:506.
[7] Vanhaleweyk GL, et al. *Eur Heart J.* 1983;4(Suppl D):117. Review.
[8] Gangji D, et al. *Br J Clin Pharmacol.* 1984;17(Suppl 1):29S.
[9] Kendall MJ, et al. *Br J Clin Pharmacol.* 1984;18:331.
[10] Leon MB, et al. *Am J Cardiol.* 1985;55:69B. Review.
[11] Vetrovec GW, et al. *Am J Cardiol.* 1985;55:21E.
[12] Lam YWF, et al. *DICP.* 1986;20:187. Review.
[13] Hamann SR, et al. *J Cardiovasc Pharmacol.* 1987;10:182.
[14] Lubsen J, et al. *Am J Cardiol.* 1987;60:18A.
[15] Swales JD, et al. *Drugs.* 1988;35(Suppl 4):1.
[16] *BMJ.* 1988;296:468.
[17] MacLean D, et al. *Br J Clin Pharmacol.* 1988;25:425.
[18] Stanley NN, et al. *Eur J Clin Pharmacol.* 1988;34:543.
[19] Zylber-Katz E, et al. *Fundam Clin Pharmacol.* 1988;2:29.
[20] Bauer LA, et al. *Eur J Clin Pharmacol.* 1989;37:257.
[21] Edoute Y, et al. *J Cardiovasc Pharmacol.* 2000;35:556.

* Asterisk indicates drugs cited in interaction reports. Based on pharmacologic and pharmacokinetic considerations, similar interactions may occur with other drugs that are listed.

Beta-Blockers — *NSAIDs*

Beta-Blockers		NSAIDs	
Acebutolol (eg, *Sectral*)	Nadolol (eg, *Corgard*)	Ibuprofen* (eg, *Motrin*)	Naproxen* (eg, *Naprosyn*)
Atenolol* (eg, *Tenormin*)	Penbutolol (*Levatol*)	Indomethacin* (eg, *Indocin*)	Piroxicam* (eg, *Feldene*)
Betaxolol (*Kerlone*)	Pindolol* (eg, *Visken*)		
Bisoprolol (*Zebeta*)	Propranolol* (eg, *Inderal*)		
Carteolol (*Cartrol*)	Sotalol (eg, *Betapace*)		
Esmolol (*Brevibloc*)	Timolol (eg, *Blocadren*)		
Metoprolol (eg, *Lopressor*)			

Significance	Onset	Severity	Documentation
2	☐ Rapid	☐ Major	☐ Established
	■ **Delayed**	■ **Moderate**	■ **Probable**
		☐ Minor	☐ Suspected
			☐ Possible
			☐ Unlikely

Effects Impaired antihypertensive effect of BETA-BLOCKERS.

Mechanism NSAIDs may inhibit renal prostaglandin synthesis, allowing unopposed pressor systems to produce hypertension.[10]

Management Avoid this combination if possible. Monitor blood pressure and adjust the BETA-BLOCKER dose as needed. Consider using a noninteracting NSAID (eg, sulindac [eg, *Clinoril*]).[16]

Discussion

In a single-blind study, 7 hypertensive patients received propranolol or pindolol, placebo, beta-blocker plus indomethacin, then beta-blocker alone.[2] Indomethacin inhibited the antihypertensive effect. In a crossover study, indomethacin impaired the blood pressure response to oxprenolol (not available in US).[5] Similar results were reported with indomethacin and other beta-blockers.[1,3,4,6,7] Two women with preeclampsia receiving propranolol or pindolol became severely hypertensive after 3 and 5 days of therapy, respectively, for premature labor with indomethacin.[13] Piroxicam, sulindac,[11] and ibuprofen[12] may attenuate the antihypertensive effect of propranolol. However, in a crossover study, the hypotensive effect of atenolol was impaired by indomethacin but not by sulindac.[7] Neither sulindac nor naproxen affected blood pressure in atenolol-treated patients.[14] Indomethacin did not inhibit the ocular hypotensive effect of timolol (eg, *Timoptic*).[8,9] In a crossover study of 26 hypertensive patients controlled with labetolol (eg, *Normodyne*), indomethacin caused a slight increase in systolic and diastolic blood pressure, and sulindac caused a small increase in systolic blood pressure.[15]

1 Patak RV, et al. *Prostaglandins*. 1975;10:649.
2 Durao V, et al. *Lancet*. 1977;2:1005.
3 Lopez-Ovejero JA, et al. *Clin Sci Mol Med*. 1978;55:203S.
4 Watkins J, et al. *BMJ*. 1980;281:702.
5 Salvetti A, et al. *Eur J Clin Pharmacol*. 1982;22:197.
6 Mills EH, et al. *Aust N Z J Med*. 1982;12:478.
7 Salvetti A, et al. *Br J Clin Pharmacol*. 1984;17:108S.
8 Lichter M, et al. *Am J Ophthalmol*. 1984;98:79.
9 Mekki QA, et al. *Br J Clin Pharmacol*. 1985;19:523.
10 Webster J. *Drugs*. 1985;30:32. Review.
11 Alvarez CR, et al. *J Clin Pharmacol*. 1986;26:544.
12 Radack KL, et al. *Ann Intern Med*. 1987;107:628.
13 Schoenfeld A, et al. *Am J Obstet Gynecol*. 1989;161:1204.
14 Abate MA, et al. *DICP*. 1990;24:810.
15 Abate MA, et al. *Br J Clin Pharmacol*. 1991;31:363.
16 Pope JE, et al. *Arch Intern Med*. 1993;153:477. Review.

* Asterisk indicates drugs cited in interaction reports. Based on pharmacologic and pharmacokinetic considerations, similar interactions may occur with other drugs that are listed.

Beta-Blockers — *Penicillins*

Atenolol* (eg, *Tenormin*)	Ampicillin* (eg, *Principen*)

Significance	Onset	Severity	Documentation
2	■ **Rapid** □ Delayed	□ Major ■ **Moderate** □ Minor	□ Established □ Probable ■ **Suspected** □ Possible □ Unlikely

Effects Antihypertensive and antianginal effects of ATENOLOL may be impaired.

Mechanism The bioavailability of ATENOLOL may be decreased by impaired GI absorption induced by AMPICILLIN.

Management If an interaction is suspected, consider increasing the dose of ATENOLOL and monitor blood pressure closely. Administering AMPICILLIN in smaller, more divided doses and staggering administration times may avoid this interaction.

Discussion

Atenolol kinetics were investigated in 6 healthy subjects. After a single oral dose of atenolol 100 mg combined with ampicillin 1 g, the bioavailability of atenolol was reduced to 36% ± 5% compared with 60% ± 8% after monotherapy.[1] During long-term cotreatment, the bioavailability of atenolol fell to 24%. Mean peak plasma levels were lowered from 511 ± 59 ng/mL on monotherapy to 344 ± 33 ng/mL after ampicillin. The area under the plasma concentration-time curve, mean steady-state concentration, and urinary recovery were reduced; 12 hours after atenolol 100 mg and ampicillin 1 g, exercise tachycardia was significantly higher than after atenolol alone. During the 4-week treatment in 6 hypertensive patients, blood pressure levels of those on atenolol 100 mg/day alone were not different from those on the cotherapy with ampicillin 1 g/day. In another study, atenolol 50 mg plus ampicillin 250 mg followed by 4 additional ampicillin 250 mg doses over 24 hours post-atenolol resulted in a fall in atenolol bioavailability by 18.2%.[2]

Additional case reports indicate that beta-adrenergic blockers may potentiate anaphylactic reactions of penicillin by decreasing intracellular levels of cyclic-AMP, thereby enhancing the release of anaphylactic substances from mast cells.[3]

[1] Schafer-Korting M, et al. *Clin Pharmacol Ther.* 1983;33:283.

[2] McLean AJ, et al. *Br J Clin Pharmacol.* 1984;18:969.

[3] Berkelman RL, et al. *Ann Intern Med.* 1986;104:134.

* Asterisk indicates drugs cited in interaction reports.

Beta-Blockers			**Phenothiazines**
Pindolol* (eg, *Visken*)	Propranolol* (eg, *Inderal*)	Chlorpromazine* (eg, *Thorazine*)	Thioridazine*

Significance	Onset	Severity	Documentation
1	☐ Rapid ■ **Delayed**	■ **Major** ☐ Moderate ☐ Minor	☐ Established ■ **Probable** ☐ Suspected ☐ Possible ☐ Unlikely

Effects Patients may experience increased effects from either or both drugs, including increased risk of life-threatening cardiac arrhythmias with THIORIDAZINE.

Mechanism CHLORPROMAZINE may inhibit the first-pass hepatic metabolism of PROPRANOLOL and increase its pharmacologic effects. Certain BETA-BLOCKERS may inhibit the metabolism of THIORIDAZINE.

Management It may be necessary to decrease the dosage during coadministration; however, THIORIDAZINE is contraindicated in patients receiving PINDOLOL or PROPRANOLOL.[5]

Discussion

The kinetic interactions of oral propranolol and chlorpromazine were investigated in 5 volunteers.[1] Propranolol bioavailability was increased from 25% to 32%. Propranolol plasma levels were increased in three subjects and resulted in increased isoproterenol antagonism and lower renin activity. Ten hospitalized chronic schizophrenic patients were given chlorpromazine (mean dose, 6.7 mg/kg/day) alone and chlorpromazine plus propranolol (mean dose, 8.1 mg/kg/day) in two 7-week segments according to a randomized, crossover design.[2] Chlorpromazine plasma levels were 5-fold higher with propranolol coadministration. The serum levels of neuroleptics expressed as "chlorpromazine equivalents" and serum prolactin levels were elevated. Two other cases have been reported that implicate propranolol in causing an increased effect of chlorpromazine[3] and thioridazine.[4] It is not known whether other beta-blockers and phenothiazines interact in a similar manner.

[1] Vestal RE, et al. *Clin Pharmacol Ther.* 1979;25:19.
[2] Peet M, et al. *Br J Psychiatry.* 1981;139:112.
[3] Miller FA, et al. *Am J Psychiatry.* 1982;139:1198.
[4] Silver JM, et al. *Am J Psychiatry.* 1986;143:1290.
[5] Product information. Thioridazine (*Mellaril*). Novartis Pharmaceutical Corporation, June 2000.

* Asterisk indicates drugs cited in interaction reports.

Beta-Blockers — *Propafenone*

Metoprolol* (eg, *Lopressor*)	Propranolol* (eg, *Inderal*)	Propafenone* (eg, *Rythmol*)

Significance	Onset	Severity	Documentation
2	■ **Rapid** □ Delayed	□ Major ■ **Moderate** □ Minor	□ Established ■ **Probable** □ Suspected □ Possible □ Unlikely

Effects The pharmacologic effects of BETA-BLOCKERS metabolized by the liver may be increased.

Mechanism PROPAFENONE increases plasma BETA-BLOCKER level by decreasing first-pass metabolism and reducing systemic clearance. Both drugs are oxidized by the hepatic CYP-450 system, and PROPAFENONE appears to inhibit the metabolism of the BETA-BLOCKER.

Management Monitor cardiac function, and adjust the dose of the BETA-BLOCKER as needed.

Discussion

In 4 patients receiving metoprolol 150 to 200 mg/day for cardiovascular disease, there was a 2- to 5-fold increase in steady-state metoprolol levels following the addition of propafenone 450 mg/day to their treatment regimens. During coadministration of the drugs, 2 patients developed severe adverse reactions (nightmares and cardiac failure) that disappeared on dose reduction or discontinuation of metoprolol. In an open, randomized, crossover design, 6 healthy volunteers received metoprolol 50 mg, propafenone 150 mg, and a combination of metoprolol 50 mg and propafenone 150 mg.[1] All but one subject developed higher concentrations of metoprolol during administration of propafenone. In the presence of propafenone, the mean AUC for metoprolol increased, and the oral clearance decreased. In an investigation involving 12 healthy subjects, the effects of propafenone 675 mg/day on the pharmacokinetics and pharmacodynamics of propranolol 150 mg/day were studied.[2] Coadministration of propafenone and propranolol significantly increased the peak plasma propranolol concentration (from 102 to 187 ng/mL), the time to peak plasma concentration (from 2 to 3.1 hr), the half-life (from 3.7 to 4.8 hr), and the mean steady-state plasma concentration (from 63 to 134 ng/mL) of propranolol. In addition, combined administration of propafenone and propranolol significantly decreased supine systolic and diastolic BP 2.5% to 15.4%, respectively. Beta-blockers did not affect serum propafenone levels.

[1] Wagner F, et al. *Br J Clin Pharmacol.* 1987;24(2):213. [2] Kowey PR, et al. *J Clin Pharmacol.* 1989;29(6):512.

* Asterisk indicates drugs cited in interaction reports.

Beta-Blockers — *Quinidine*

Beta-Blockers		Quinidine
Atenolol* (eg, *Tenormin*)	Nebivolol (*Bystolic*)	Quinidine*
Carvedilol (eg, *Coreg*)	Propranolol* (eg, *Inderal*)	
Metoprolol* (eg, *Lopressor*)	Timolol* (eg, *Blocadren*)	

Significance	Onset	Severity	Documentation
2	■ **Rapid**	□ Major	□ Established
	□ Delayed	■ **Moderate**	□ Probable
		□ Minor	■ **Suspected**
			□ Possible
			□ Unlikely

Effects The effects of certain BETA-BLOCKERS may be increased in extensive metabolizers (EMs).

Mechanism Oxidative metabolism (CYP2D6) of certain BETA-BLOCKERS may be inhibited by QUINIDINE.

Management The oral BETA-BLOCKER dose may need to be tailored if excessive beta-blockade is noted. Advise patients receiving topical BETA-BLOCKER therapy to monitor their pulse more frequently and to notify their health care provider if slowing is noted.

Discussion

Five EMs and 5 poor metabolizers (PMs) of debrisoquine were administered oral metoprolol 100 mg alone and, 1 week later, they were given the same dose 2 hours after a single dose of quinidine 50 mg.[1] Quinidine caused a 3-fold increase of the total and active metoprolol (−) isomer concentration in EMs. Although 1 study demonstrated a reduction in propranolol clearance from 3,087 to 1,378 mL/min and an enhancement of beta-blockade,[2] other studies failed to show any kinetic interactions between quinidine and propranolol,[3-5] a beta-blocker that does not undergo polymorphic oxidative metabolism. Two cases of orthostatic hypotension have been reported in patients treated with quinidine and propranolol[6] or atenolol.[7] A 70-year-old man stabilized on quinidine 500 mg 3 times daily developed symptomatic bradycardia 12 weeks after starting timolol eye drops for glaucoma.[8] Bradycardia and other symptoms resolved when both drugs were discontinued but recurred when rechallenged. In a single-blind, crossover study, 13 healthy men received 2 drops of timolol in each nostril to simulate absorption of ocular application.[9] When timolol was administered after oral quinidine 50 mg, plasma timolol concentrations were higher, and heart rate was lower compared with baseline. Although changes were greatest in EMs, changes were also noted in PMs.

1 Leemann T, et al. *Eur J Clin Pharmacol.* 1986;29(6):739.
2 Zhou HH, et al. *Clin Pharmacol Ther.* 1990;47(6):686.
3 Kessler KM, et al. *Am Heart J.* 1978;96(5):627.
4 Kates RE, et al. *J Clin Pharmacol.* 1979;19(7):378.
5 Fenster P, et al. *Clin Pharmacol Ther.* 1980;27(4):450.
6 Loon NR, et al. *Am J Med.* 1986;81(6):1101.
7 Manolis AS, et al. *Am J Med.* 1987;82(5):1083.
8 Dinai Y, et al. *Ann Intern Med.* 1985;103(6)(pt 1):890.
9 Edeki TI, et al. *JAMA.* 1995;274(20):1611.

* Asterisk indicates drugs cited in interaction reports. Based on pharmacologic and pharmacokinetic considerations, similar interactions may occur with other drugs that are listed.

Beta-Blockers | *Quinolones*

Betaxolol (*Kerlone*)	Propranolol (eg, *Inderal*)	Ciprofloxacin* (*Cipro*)
Metoprolol* (eg, *Lopressor*)		

Significance	Onset	Severity	Documentation
4	□ Rapid	□ Major	□ Established
	■ **Delayed**	■ **Moderate**	□ Probable
		□ Minor	□ Suspected
			■ **Possible**
			□ Unlikely

Effects The pharmacologic effects of METOPROLOL and perhaps other BETA-BLOCKERS metabolized by cytochrome P450IID (eg, BETAXOLOL, PROPRANOLOL) may be increased.

Mechanism Unknown. However, CIPROFLOXACIN may decrease the oral clearance of METOPROLOL by inhibition of hepatic metabolism.

Management Consider monitoring cardiac function when CIPROFLOXACIN therapy is initiated or discontinued in patients receiving METOPROLOL.

Discussion

The effects of pretreatment with ciprofloxacin 500 mg every 12 hours for five doses on the pharmacokinetics of a single 100 mg oral dose of metoprolol was studied in seven healthy male subjects.[1] Administration of ciprofloxacin increased the area under the concentration-time curve (AUC) for (+) metoprolol from 136 to 210 ng•hr/mL (54%; $P < 0.05$) while the AUC of (−) metoprolol also significantly ($P < 0.05$) increased from 377 to 486 ng•hr/mL (29%). The oral clearance of (+) metoprolol was decreased from 698 to 429 L/hr (38.5%) while the clearance of (−) metoprolol was decreased from 176 to 154 L/hr (12.5%). Ciprofloxacin significantly ($P < 0.05$) increased the half-life of both isomers. Documentation for this possible interaction consists of an abstract. More substantive data are needed to evaluate the clinical significance of this reported interaction.

[1] Waite NM, et al. *Pharmacother.* 1990;10:236. Abstract.

* Asterisk indicates drugs cited in interaction reports. Based on pharmacologic and pharmacokinetic considerations, similar interactions may occur with other drugs that are listed.

Beta-Blockers | **Ranitidine**

Beta-Blockers	Ranitidine
Metoprolol* (eg, *Lopressor*)	Ranitidine* (eg, *Zantac*)

Significance	Onset	Severity	Documentation
5	☐ Rapid	☐ Major	☐ Established
	■ **Delayed**	☐ Moderate	☐ Probable
		■ **Minor**	☐ Suspected
			☐ Possible
			■ **Unlikely**

Effects Certain BETA-BLOCKERS' pharmacologic effects may be enhanced.

Mechanism Unknown.

Management No clinical interventions appear necessary.

Discussion

The pharmacokinetic parameters of metoprolol and atenolol (eg, *Tenormin*) were studied in six normal subjects after 7 days of oral administration of each drug alone (metoprolol 100 mg twice daily, atenolol 10 mg/day).[5] Intrasubject kinetic profiles of the drugs were compared after a further 7 days of coadministration with ranitidine 150 mg twice daily. The area under the metoprolol plasma concentration curve (AUC) was increased by 55% and its elimination half-life was 50% longer. The kinetics of atenolol were not significantly altered by ranitidine.[7] Data reported in this study have been questioned.[6,8] Beta-blockade activity of metoprolol measured by exercise-induced tachycardia did not show greater inhibition by ranitidine.[9] Similarly, other reports have indicated that ranitidine failed to alter the pharmacokinetics of propranolol[3,4] and model drug antipyrine.[1,2] Other studies also showed conflicting data on the disposition of metoprolol by ranitidine.[10,11]

The mechanism of kinetic interference of ranitidine on metoprolol are controversial and inconclusive; clinical significance is difficult to assess.

[1] Henry DA, et al. *BMJ.* 1980;281:775.
[2] Breen KJ, et al. *Clin Pharmacol Ther.* 1982;31:297.
[3] Reimann IW, et al. *Clin Pharmacol Ther.* 1982;32:749.
[4] Heagerty AM, et al. *BMJ.* 1982;284:1304.
[5] Spahn H, et al. *BMJ.* 1983;286:1546.
[6] Jack D, et al. *BMJ.* 1983;286:2064.
[7] Spahn H, et al. *BMJ.* 1983;287:838.
[8] Jack D, et al. *BMJ.* 1983;287:1218.
[9] Kirch W, et al. *Arch Toxicol.* 1984;7(Suppl):256.
[10] Kelly JG, et al. *Br J Clin Pharmacol.* 1985;19:219.
[11] Toon S, et al. *Clin Pharmacol Ther.* 1988;43:283.

* Asterisk indicates drugs cited in interaction reports.

Beta-Blockers — *Rifamycins*

Beta-Blockers		Rifamycins	
Atenolol* (eg, *Tenormin*)	Metoprolol* (eg, *Lopressor*)	Rifabutin (*Mycobutin*)	Rifapentine (*Priftin*)
Bisoprolol* (*Zebeta*)	Propranolol* (eg, *Inderal*)	Rifampin* (eg, *Rifadin*)	

Significance	Onset	Severity	Documentation
2	☐ Rapid ■ **Delayed**	☐ Major ■ **Moderate** ☐ Minor	☐ Established ☐ Probable ■ **Suspected** ☐ Possible ☐ Unlikely

Effects The pharmacologic effects of certain BETA-BLOCKERS may be reduced by RIFAMYCINS. May need a 3- to 4-week washout period for the enzyme induction effect to disappear.

Mechanism Induction of hepatic metabolism by RIFAMYCINS is suspected.

Management Close monitoring of therapeutic response (eg, BP) is essential. If the clinical condition deteriorates, a higher dose of BETA-BLOCKERS may be necessary.

Discussion

The effect of rifampin on the pharmacokinetic parameters of bisoprolol, metoprolol, and propranolol has been described.[1-4] Rifampin 600 mg/day for 3 weeks was given to 6 healthy men pretreated with oral propranolol 120 mg every 8 hours for 2 weeks.[2] Rifampin caused a 3-fold increase in oral clearance of propranolol, but elimination $t_{½}$ and extent of plasma binding were not affected. Increasing the daily dose of rifampin to 1,200 mg/day did not cause any additional change in the oral clearance of propranolol.[2] In a similar study, rifampin 600 mg/day was administered to 12 men (who were pretreated with metoprolol 100 mg/day) for 15 days.[1] The AUC of metoprolol was reduced, but the elimination rate constant was not affected. In a study of 6 healthy volunteers, rifampin decreased the C_{max} and increased the elimination of bisoprolol.[3] In a study of 9 healthy volunteers, rifampin slightly affected the pharmacokinetics of atenolol, decreasing serum levels and AUC 19%.[5]

Although a correlation between the plasma concentration and clinical effect of beta-adrenergic blockers has not been established, a marked reduction of steady-state concentration of beta-blockers resulting from long-term administration with rifampin may result in a decrease in pharmacologic effect of the beta-blockers. The clinical importance of the interaction between rifampin and bisoprolol remains to be determined.

[1] Bennett PN, et al. *Br J Clin Pharmacol.* 1982;13(3):387.
[2] Herman RJ, et al. *Br J Clin Pharmacol.* 1983;16(5):565.
[3] Kirch W, et al. *Eur J Clin Pharmacol.* 1986;31(1):59.
[4] Shaheen O, et al. *Clin Pharmacol Ther.* 1987;41:158.
[5] Lilja JJ, et al. *Basic Clin Pharmacol Toxicol.* 2006;98(6):555.

* Asterisk indicates drugs cited in interaction reports. Based on pharmacologic and pharmacokinetic considerations, similar interactions may occur with other drugs that are listed.

Beta-Blockers ✕ *Salicylates*

Beta-Blockers		Salicylates	
Acebutolol (eg, *Sectral*)	Metoprolol (eg, *Lopressor*)	Aspirin* (eg, *Bayer*)	Salsalate (eg, *Amigesic*)
Atenolol (eg, *Tenormin*)	Nadolol (eg, *Corgard*)	Bismuth Subsalicylate (eg, *Pepto-Bismol*)	Sodium Thiosalicylate
Betaxolol (*Kerlone*)	Penbutolol (*Levatol*)	Magnesium Salicylate (eg, *Doan's*)	
Bisoprolol (*Zebeta*)	Pindolol* (eg, *Visken*)		
Carteolol (*Cartrol*)	Propranolol* (eg, *Inderal*)		
Carvedilol* (*Coreg*)	Timolol (eg, *Blocadren*)		

Significance	Onset	Severity	Documentation
2	■ **Rapid**	□ Major	□ Established
	□ Delayed	■ **Moderate**	□ Probable
		□ Minor	■ **Suspected**
			□ Possible
			□ Unlikely

Effects The BP-lowering effects of BETA-BLOCKERS may be attenuated by SALICYLATES. In addition, the beneficial effects of BETA-BLOCKERS on left ventricular ejection fraction (LVEF) in patients with chronic heart failure may be attenuated.

Mechanism Hypertension: SALICYLATES may inhibit biosynthesis of prostaglandins involved in the antihypertensive activity of BETA-BLOCKERS. Heart failure: Unknown.

Management Hypertension: Monitor BP. If an interaction is suspected, consider lowering the dose of the SALICYLATE, changing to a nonsalicylate antiplatelet agent, or using alternative antihypertensive therapy. Heart failure: Monitor LVEF and the patient's clinical status. If an interaction is suspected, consider lowering the dose of SALICYLATE or changing to a nonsalicylate antiplatelet agent.

Discussion

Ten hypertensive male inpatients received pindolol 1 mg IV after a placebo and aspirin pretreatment (5 g in 24 hours).[1] Aspirin prevented the antihypertensive effect of pindolol. In 6 hospitalized men (2 slightly hypertensive, 4 normotensive), a single oral dose of aspirin 1 or 1.5 g attenuated the hypotensive action of propranolol 5 mg IV; diastolic BP actually increased. Aspirin did not affect the decrease in heart rate or cardiac contractility by either beta-blocker. In a retrospective evaluation of the Multicenter Oral Carvedilol Heart Failure Assessment trial, LVEF improved less (not statistically significant) in patients receiving concurrent aspirin.[2] There were no changes noted in heart rate or systolic BP responses. See also Beta-Blockers-NSAIDs.

[1] Sziegoleit W, et al. *Int J Clin Pharmacol Ther Toxicol.* 1982;20(9):423.

[2] Lindenfeld J, et al. *J Am Coll Cardiol.* 2001;38(7):1950.

* Asterisk indicates drugs cited in interaction reports. Based on pharmacologic and pharmacokinetic considerations, similar interactions may occur with other drugs that are listed.

Beta-Blockers — *Serotonin Reuptake Inhibitors*

Carvedilol* (eg, *Coreg*)	Nebivolol* (*Bystolic*)	Citalopram* (eg, *Celexa*)	Fluoxetine* (eg, *Prozac*)
Metoprolol* (eg, *Lopressor*)	Propranolol* (eg, *Inderal*)	Duloxetine* (*Cymbalta*)	Paroxetine* (eg, *Paxil*)
		Escitalopram* (*Lexapro*)	Sertraline* (eg, *Zoloft*)

Significance	Onset	Severity	Documentation
2	☐ Rapid	☐ Major	☐ Established
	■ **Delayed**	■ **Moderate**	☐ Probable
		☐ Minor	■ **Suspected**
			☐ Possible
			☐ Unlikely

Effects Excessive beta-blockade (bradycardia) may occur.

Mechanism Certain SRIs (FLUOXETINE, PAROXETINE) may inhibit the metabolism (CYP2D6) of certain BETA-BLOCKERS.[1]

Management Monitor for signs and symptoms of excessive beta-blockade. This interaction may be less likely to occur with BETA-BLOCKERS not metabolized by CYP2D6 (eg, atenolol [eg, *Tenormin*], sotalol [eg, *Betapace*]).

Discussion

Within 2 days of starting fluoxetine 20 mg/day, a 54-year-old man taking metoprolol 100 mg/day complained of lethargy and had a bradycardia of 36 bpm.[2] Fluoxetine was stopped, and over the next 5 days the heart rate returned to 64 bpm. Sotalol was substituted for metoprolol. One week later, fluoxetine was restarted without recurrence of the bradycardia. A 53-year-old man stabilized on propranolol 40 mg/day developed complete heart block 2 weeks after starting fluoxetine 20 mg/day.[3] A preexisting conduction system abnormality exacerbated by fluoxetine was not ruled out. Compared with placebo, pretreatment with paroxetine increased the metoprolol C_{max} 2-fold, prolonged the terminal $t_{½}$, and produced more sustained beta-blockade.[4] Similar findings were noted with metoprolol immediate- or extended-release doseforms when coadministered with paroxetine.[5,6] In a randomized, double-blind, crossover study in 10 patients with stable heart failure, the addition of fluoxetine (20 mg/day for 28 days) to a stable carvedilol regimen resulted in stereospecific inhibition of carvedilol metabolism.[7] Although the AUC of the R(+)-enantiomer increased 77%, no difference in heart rate, BP, or adverse reactions were noted between treatment groups compared with placebo. Sertraline did not alter the beta-blocking activity of atenolol in 10 healthy subjects.[8] Similar results were found in a study of 12 healthy volunteers during coadministration of carvedilol with paroxetine.[9] In a randomized, double-blind, placebo-controlled trial assessing 111 patients, addition of pindolol 7.5 mg/day to fluoxetine 20 mg/day increased the antidepressant effectiveness of fluoxetine.[10] In a study in healthy volunteers, duloxetine, escitalopram, and sertraline increased the metoprolol AUC.[11] The effect was greatest with duloxetine. Coadministration of paroxetine and nebivolol increased nebivolol C_{max} and AUC 2.3- and 6-fold, respectively.[12]

[1] Belpaire FM, et al. *Eur J Clin Pharmacol.* 1998;54(3):261.
[2] Walley T, et al. *Lancet.* 1993;341(8850):967.
[3] Drake WM, et al. *Lancet.* 1994;343(8894):425.
[4] Hemeryck A, et al. *Clin Pharmacol Ther.* 2000;67(3):283.
[5] Stout SM, et al. *J Clin Pharmacol.* 2011;51(3):389.
[6] Parker RB, et al. *Pharmacotherapy.* 2011;31(7):630.
[7] Graff DW, et al. *J Clin Pharmacol.* 2001;41(1):97.
[8] Ziegler MG, et al. *J Clin Psychiatry.* 1996;57(suppl 1):12.
[9] Stout SM, et al. *J Cardiovasc Pharmacol Ther.* 2010;15(4):373.
[10] Pérez V, et al. *Lancet.* 1997;349(9065):1594.
[11] Preskorn SH, et al. *J Clin Psychopharmacol.* 2007;27(1):28.
[12] Lindamood C, et al. *J Clin Pharmacol.* 2011;51(4):575.

* Asterisk indicates drugs cited in interaction reports.

Beta-Blockers — *Sulfinpyrazone*

Beta-Blockers		Sulfinpyrazone
Acebutolol (*Sectral*)	Nadolol (*Corgard*)	Sulfinpyrazone* (eg, *Anturane*)
Atenolol (*Tenormin*)	Oxprenolol*†	
Betaxolol (*Kerlone*)	Penbutolol (*Levatol*)	
Bisoprolol (*Zebeta*)	Pindolol (eg, *Visken*)	
Carteolol (*Cartrol*)	Propranolol (eg, *Inderal*)	
Metoprolol (eg, *Lopressor*)	Timolol (*Blocadren*)	

Significance	Onset	Severity	Documentation
4	☐ Rapid	☐ Major	☐ Established
	■ **Delayed**	■ **Moderate**	☐ Probable
		☐ Minor	☐ Suspected
			■ **Possible**
			☐ Unlikely

Effects The antihypertensive effects of BETA-BLOCKERS could be attenuated.

Mechanism SULFINPYRAZONE inhibition of prostaglandin synthesis responsible for antihypertensive action and accelerated BETA-BLOCKER metabolism are possible mechanisms.

Management Close monitoring of blood pressure may be necessary, and if an interaction is suspected, consider lowering or discontinuing SULFINPYRAZONE.

Discussion

In a double-blind crossover controlled study, the interference of antihypertensive effects of oxprenolol (not available commercially) by sulfinpyrazone was investigated.[1] Ten hypertensive patients were administered sulfinpyrazone 400 mg twice a day with oxprenolol 800 mg twice a day for 15 days. Oxprenolol significantly reduced blood pressure and heart rate when given alone, but blood pressure returned to pretreatment levels when combined with sulfinpyrazone. The ability of oxprenolol to reduce heart rate was not significantly influenced by the combination therapy.

Additional studies are needed to establish the clinical significance of the interference of sulfinpyrazone on other beta-adrenergic blockers.

[1] Ferrara LA, et al. *Eur J Clin Pharmacol.* 1986;29:717.

* Asterisk indicates drugs cited in interaction reports. Based on pharmacologic and pharmacokinetic considerations, similar interactions may occur with other drugs that are listed.
† Not available in the United States.

Beta-Blockers			**Thioamines**
Metoprolol* (eg, *Lopressor*)	Propranolol* (eg, *Inderal*)	Methimazole (*Tapazole*)	Propylthiouracil (PTU)

Significance	Onset	Severity	Documentation
2	☐ Rapid ■ **Delayed**	☐ Major ■ **Moderate** ☐ Minor	☐ Established ■ **Probable** ☐ Suspected ☐ Possible ☐ Unlikely

Effects The pharmacokinetic profiles of certain BETA-BLOCKERS may be altered and pharmacologic effects may be increased.

Mechanism Hyperthyroidism appears to cause increased clearance of BETA-BLOCKERS with a high extraction ratio. This may be the result of increased liver blood flow, first-pass metabolism and volume of distribution.

Management A dose reduction of BETA-ADRENERGIC BLOCKERS may be needed when a hyperthyroid patient becomes euthyroid.

Discussion

The kinetic profiles of the beta-blockers atenolol, propranolol, metoprolol, sotalol and practolol (not available in the US) have been studied in patients converted from hyperthyroid to euthyroid states.[1-10] The oral clearance of metoprolol, practolol and propranolol was increased 35% to 45% in patients with hyperactive thyroid conditions compared with patients with normal thyroid balance.[1,3-5,7-10] Conversely, the bioavailability of beta-blockers with substantial renal clearance like sotalol and atenolol was not significantly affected in hyperthyroid states.[8,9] A wide intersubject variation in plasma propranolol concentrations has been found after the same dose both in euthyroid and in hyperthyroid patients. In a study of 30 patients, the plasma propranolol concentration vs time curve (AUC) increased 92% after treatment of hyperthyroidism by surgery, antithyroid drugs or radioiodine.[5] A high variability of 2- to 3-fold increases in plasma propranolol concentrations has also been reported after therapeutically induced euthyroidism.[4] Additional factors such as age or smoking habits may account partially for the interindividual variation in plasma concentration.[4]

Despite the undefined correlation between plasma concentration and effect in beta-blockers, it is expected that the magnitude of plasma level increase in beta-blockers with a high liver extraction ratio may enhance the beta-blockade effect when patients are being rendered euthyroid from a hyperthyroid condition.

[1] Bell JM, et al. *Br J Clin Pharmacol.* 1977;4:79.
[2] Riddell JG, et al. *Clin Pharmacol Ther.* 1980;28:565.
[3] Feely J, et al. *Ann Intern Med.* 1981;94:472.
[4] Feely J, et al. *Br J Clin Pharmacol.* 1981;12:73.
[5] Feely J, et al. *Eur J Clin Pharmacol.* 1981;19:329.
[6] Tawara K, et al. *Eur J Clin Pharmacol.* 1981;19:197.
[7] Wells PG, et al. *Clin Res.* 1981;29:279A.
[8] Hallengren B, et al. *Eur J Clin Pharmacol.* 1982;21:379.
[9] Aro A, et al. *Eur J Clin Pharmacol.* 1982;21:373.
[10] Wells PG, et al. *Clin Pharmacol Ther.* 1983;33:603.

* Asterisk indicates drugs cited in interaction reports. Based on pharmacologic and pharmacokinetic considerations, similar interactions may occur with other drugs that are listed.

Beta-Blockers		***Thyroid Hormones***	
Metoprolol (eg, *Lopressor*)	Propranolol* (eg, *Inderal*)	Levothyroxine* (eg, *Synthroid*)	Liotrix (*Thyrolar*)
		Liothyronine (eg, *Cytomel*)	Thyroid (eg, *Armour Thyroid*)

Significance	Onset	Severity	Documentation
4	☐ Rapid	☐ Major	☐ Established
	■ **Delayed**	■ **Moderate**	☐ Probable
		☐ Minor	☐ Suspected
			■ **Possible**
			☐ Unlikely

Effects The actions of certain BETA-BLOCKERS may be impaired when a hypothyroid patient is converted to the euthyroid state.

Mechanism Possibly caused by a reduction in hepatic blood flow and hepatic microsomal enzyme activity in hypothyroidism.

Management No clinical interventions appear necessary.

Discussion

The increase in oral and systemic clearances of beta-blockers with a high extraction ratio such as propranolol and metoprolol in hyperthyroid states as compared with euthyroid states has been reported.[1-6] The underlying mechanism of this kinetic profile alteration was postulated to be an increase in hepatic blood flow and hepatic microsomal enzyme activity. However, the converse was not evident in hypothyroidism. A randomized study of 6 patients with a change in thyroid states from hypothyroid to euthyroid produced no change in the kinetic parameters of oral propranolol except that the elimination $t_{1/2}$ was 85% longer than in euthyroid states.[7] In a study involving 8 hyperthyroid and 4 hypothyroid patients who were administered oral propranolol 100 mg, no change in elimination $t_{1/2}$ and total plasma concentrations was found between the 2 groups.[8] However, other investigators reported a mean reduction of 40.9% in steady-state plasma propranolol concentration (propranolol 160 mg/day) in 6 hypothyroid patients rendered euthyroid by up to 0.15 mg/day of levothyroxine.[3] In another study, no alterations in free drug concentration and plasma protein binding of propranolol in hypothyroid and hyperthyroid states were reported.[9]

More studies are needed to determine the clinical importance of thyroid hormones on the effects of beta-adrenergic blockers.

1 Feely J, et al. *Ann Intern Med.* 1981;94(4) (pt 1):472.
2 Feely J, et al. *Br J Clin Pharmacol.* 1981;12(1):73.
3 Feely J, et al. *Eur J Clin Pharmacol.* 1981;19(5):329.
4 Hallengren B, et al. *Eur J Clin Pharmacol.* 1982;21(5):379.
5 Aro A, et al. *Eur J Clin Pharmacol.* 1982;21(5):373.
6 Wells PG, et al. *Clin Pharmacol Ther.* 1983;33(5):603.
7 Riddell JG, et al. *Clin Pharmacol Ther.* 1980;28(5):565.
8 Bell JM, et al. *Br J Clin Pharmacol.* 1977;4(1):79.
9 Kelly JG, et al. *Br J Clin Pharmacol.* 1978;6(2):123.

* Asterisk indicates drugs cited in interaction reports. Based on pharmacologic and pharmacokinetic considerations, similar interactions may occur with other drugs that are listed.

Beta-Blockers — *Verapamil*

Beta-Blockers		Verapamil
Acebutolol (eg, *Sectral*)	Nadolol (eg, *Corgard*)	Verapamil* (eg, *Calan*)
Atenolol* (eg, *Tenormin*)	Nebivolol (*Bystolic*)	
Betaxolol (*Kerlone*)	Penbutolol (*Levatol*)	
Carteolol (*Cartrol*)	Pindolol* (eg, *Visken*)	
Esmolol (eg, *Brevibloc*)	Propranolol* (eg, *Inderal*)	
Metoprolol* (eg, *Lopressor*)	Timolol* (eg, *Blocadren*)	

Significance	Onset	Severity	Documentation
1	■ **Rapid**	■ **Major**	□ Established
	□ Delayed	□ Moderate	■ **Probable**
		□ Minor	□ Suspected
			□ Possible
			□ Unlikely

Effects Effects of both drugs may be increased.

Mechanism Possible synergistic or additive effects. VERAPAMIL may inhibit oxidative metabolism of certain BETA-BLOCKERS.

Management Monitor cardiac function; reduce the doses as needed.

Discussion

In hypertension and unstable angina, combination therapy with beta-blockers and verapamil is generally effective and acceptable,[1-16] but profound untoward cardiovascular effects may manifest.[2,9,10,15-18] Risk factors include left ventricular dysfunction, AV conduction defects, and IV administration.[1,11] Both drugs possess direct negative inotropic and chronotropic effects.[17] Also, beta-blockade may predominate over the compensatory reflex mechanism from the direct peripheral vasodilation of verapamil. Verapamil has markedly increased metoprolol levels[11,14,16] but not atenolol,[11] while minimally affecting propranolol levels.[19,20] However, chronic verapamil use may increase atenolol levels and decrease d- and l-propranolol clearance.[21,22] In 12 healthy subjects, atenolol, metoprolol, and propranolol did not affect verapamil kinetics; however, heart rate was reduced. Beta-1 selective agents may be preferable.[23] Sinus nodal dysfunction caused by absorption of timolol ophthalmic drops (eg, *Timoptic*) has also been noted.[4,15,24] See also Beta-Blockers/Nifedipine.

1 Winniford MD, et al. *Am J Cardiol.* 1982;50(4):704.
2 Packer M, et al. *Circulation.* 1982;65(4):660.
3 Wayne VS, et al. *Aust N Z J Med.* 1982;12(4):285.
4 Sinclair NI, et al. *Med J Aust.* 1983;1(12):548.
5 Vanhaleweyk GL, et al. *Eur Heart J.* 1983;4(suppl D):117.
6 Eisenberg JN, et al. *Postgrad Med J.* 1984;60(708):705.
7 Findlay IN, et al. *Br Med J.* 1984;289(6451):1074.
8 Warrington SJ, et al. *Br J Clin Pharmacol.* 1984;17(suppl 1):37S.
9 Zatuchni J. *Heart Lung.* 1985;14(1):94.
10 Winniford MD, et al. *Am Heart J.* 1985;110(2):498.
11 McLean AJ, et al. *Am J Cardiol.* 1985;55(13)(pt 1):1628.
12 Leon MB, et al. *Am J Cardiol.* 1985;55(3):69B.
13 Dargie H, et al. *Am J Cardiol.* 1986;57(7):80D.
14 Keech AC, et al. *Am J Cardiol.* 1986;58(6):551.
15 Pringle SD, et al. *Br Med J.* 1987;294(6565):155.
16 McCourty JC, et al. *Br J Clin Pharmacol.* 1988;25(3):349.
17 Bailey DG, et al. *Clin Pharmacol Ther.* 1991;49(4):370.
18 Edoute Y, et al. *J Cardiovasc Pharmacol.* 2000;35(4):556.
19 Murdoch D, et al. *Br J Clin Pharmacol.* 1989;28:233P.
20 Murdoch DL, et al. *Br J Clin Pharmacol.* 1991;31(3):323.
21 Keech AC, et al. *Eur J Clin Pharmacol.* 1988;35(4):363.
22 Hunt BA, et al. *Clin Pharmacol Ther.* 1990;47(5):584.
23 Carruthers SG, et al. *Clin Pharmacol Ther.* 1989;46(4):469.
24 Minish T, et al. *J Emerg Med.* 2002;22(3):247.

* Asterisk indicates drugs cited in interaction reports. Based on pharmacologic and pharmacokinetic considerations, similar interactions may occur with other drugs that are listed.

Beta-Carotene — *Orlistat*

Beta-Carotene*	Orlistat* (eg, *Xenical*)

Significance	Onset	Severity	Documentation
3	☐ Rapid	☐ Major	☐ Established
	■ **Delayed**	☐ Moderate	☐ Probable
		■ **Minor**	■ **Suspected**
			☐ Possible
			☐ Unlikely

Effects Plasma levels of BETA-CAROTENE may be decreased.

Mechanism ORLISTAT may decrease the GI absorption of BETA-CAROTENE.

Management Based on available information, no special precautions are needed.

Discussion

The effect of orlistat on beta-carotene absorption was studied in an open-label, parallel, placebo-controlled, randomized, 2-way crossover investigation involving 48 healthy volunteers.[1] Each subject received a single oral dose of beta-carotene 0, 30, 60, or 120 mg on day 4 of treatment with orlistat 120 mg or placebo 3 times daily for 6 days. Compared with placebo, orlistat administration decreased the absorption of beta-carotene approximately 33% at all doses of beta-carotene.

[1] Zhi J, et al. *J Clin Pharmacol.* 1996;36(2):152.

* Asterisk indicates drugs cited in interaction reports.

Bisphosphonates — *Antacids*

Bisphosphonates		Antacids	
Alendronate* (eg, *Fosamax*)	Pamidronate* (eg, *Aredia*)	Aluminum Hydroxide* (eg, *Amphojel*)	Magnesium Hydroxide* (eg, *Milk of Magnesia*)
Etidronate* (eg, *Didronel*)	Risedronate* (*Actonel*)	Aluminum/Magnesium Hydroxide* (eg, *Riopan*)	
Ibandronate* (*Boniva*)	Tiludronate* (*Skelid*)		

Significance	Onset	Severity	Documentation
2	□ Rapid ■ **Delayed**	□ Major ■ **Moderate** □ Minor	□ Established □ Probable ■ **Suspected** □ Possible □ Unlikely

Effects BISPHOSPHONATE absorption may be decreased, reducing the pharmacologic effect.

Mechanism Decreased BISPHOSPHONATE GI absorption.

Management ALENDRONATE or RISEDRONATE should be taken at least 30 minutes before an aluminum and/or magnesium ANTACID is taken.[1,2] IBANDRONATE should be taken at least 60 minutes before an aluminum and/or magnesium ANTACID is taken.[3] Do not administer ETIDRONATE or TILUDRONATE within 2 hours before or after an aluminum and/or magnesium ANTACID is taken.[4,5]

Discussion

Because an antacid containing aluminum and/or magnesium is likely to decrease the absorption of bisphosphonates, these medicines should not be taken simultaneously.[1-6] To maximize absorption, the administration times should be separated (see Management section for recommended spacing of administration times). Administration of tiludronate 1 hour after an antacid containing aluminum-magnesium hydroxide decreased the tiludronate AUC and C_{max} approximately 49% and 53%, respectively.[6] In contrast, administration of tiludronate 2 hours before the antacid did not affect the AUC or C_{max} of tiludronate.

The basis for this monograph is information on file with the manufacturers.

1 *Fosamax* [package insert]. Whitehouse Station, NJ: Merck & Co, Inc; February 2006.
2 *Actonel* [package insert]. Cincinnati, OH: Procter & Gamble Pharmaceuticals, Inc; May 2007.
3 *Boniva* [package insert]. Nutley, NJ: Roche Laboratories, Inc; August 2006.
4 *Didronel* [package insert]. North Norwich, NY: OSG Norwich Pharmaceuticals, Inc; May 2005.
5 *Skelid* [package insert]. Melbourne, Australia: Mayne Pharma Pty Ltd; May 31, 2004.
6 Sansom LN, et al. *Bone*. 1995;17(5 suppl):479S.

* Asterisk indicates drugs cited in interaction reports.

Bisphosphonates — *Calcium Salts*

Bisphosphonates		Calcium Salts	
Alendronate* (eg, *Fosamax*)	Pamidronate* (eg, *Aredia*)	Calcium Acetate* (eg, *PhosLo*)	Calcium Gluconate* (eg, *Cal-Glu*)
Etidronate* (eg, *Didronel*)	Risedronate* (eg, *Actonel*)	Calcium Carbonate* (eg, *Os-Cal*)	Calcium Lactate* (eg, *Cal-Lac*)
Ibandronate* (eg, *Boniva*)	Tiludronate* (*Skelid*)	Calcium Citrate* (eg, *Calcitrate*)	Tricalcium Phosphate* (*Posture*)
		Calcium Glubionate* (*Calcionate*)	

Significance	Onset	Severity	Documentation
2	☐ Rapid	☐ Major	☐ Established
	■ **Delayed**	■ **Moderate**	☐ Probable
		☐ Minor	■ **Suspected**
			☐ Possible
			☐ Unlikely

Effects BISPHOSPHONATE absorption may be decreased, reducing the pharmacologic effect.

Mechanism Decreased BISPHOSPHONATE GI absorption.

Management Take ALENDRONATE or RISEDRONATE at least 30 minutes before taking a CALCIUM SALT.[1,2] Take IBANDRONATE at least 60 minutes before taking a CALCIUM SALT.[3] Do not take ETIDRONATE or TILUDRONATE within 2 hours before or after taking a CALCIUM SALT.[4,5]

Discussion

Because calcium is likely to decrease the absorption of bisphosphonates, do not administer simultaneously.[1-5] To maximize absorption, separate the administration times (see Management for recommended spacing of administration times).

The basis for this monograph is information on file with the manufacturers.

1 *Fosamax* [package insert]. Whitehouse Station, NJ: Merck & Co Inc; February 2006.
2 *Actonel* [package insert]. Cincinnati, OH: Procter & Gamble Pharmaceuticals Inc; May 2007.
3 *Boniva* [package insert]. Nutley, NJ: Roche Laboratories Inc; August 2006.
4 *Didronel* [package insert]. North Norwich, NY: OSG Norwich Pharmaceuticals Inc; May 2005.
5 *Skelid* [package insert]. Melbourne, Australia: Mayne Pharma Pty Ltd; May 31, 2004.

* Asterisk indicates drugs cited in interaction reports.

Bleomycin	**Brentuximab**
Bleomycin*	Brentuximab* (*Adcetris*)

Significance	Onset	Severity	Documentation
1	☐ Rapid ■ **Delayed**	■ **Major** ☐ Moderate ☐ Minor	☐ Established ☐ Probable ■ **Suspected** ☐ Possible ☐ Unlikely

Effects The risk of pulmonary toxicity may be increased.

Mechanism Unknown.

Management Coadministration is contraindicated.

Discussion

Concurrent use of brentuximab with bleomycin is contraindicated because of pulmonary toxicity.[1] In a clinical trial in which brentuximab and bleomycin were administered as part of a combination regimen, the rate of noninfectious pulmonary toxicity was higher than the historical incidence reported with bleomycin, dacarbazine, doxorubicin (eg, *Adriamycin*), and vinblastine. Patients reported cough and dyspnea. Interstitial infiltration and/or inflammation were seen on radiographs and CT imaging of the chest.

[1] *Adcetris* [package insert]. Bothell, WA: Seattle Genetics Inc; January 2012.

* Asterisk indicates drugs cited in interaction reports.

Bortezomib			***Azole Antifungal Agents***
Bortezomib* (*Velcade*)		Itraconazole* (eg, *Sporanox*)	Ketoconazole* (eg, *Nizoral*)

Significance	Onset	Severity	Documentation
4	□ Rapid ■ **Delayed**	□ Major ■ **Moderate** □ Minor	□ Established □ Probable □ Suspected ■ **Possible** □ Unlikely

Effects

BORTEZOMIB plasma concentrations may be elevated, increasing the pharmacologic effects and adverse reactions.

Mechanism

Inhibition of BORTEZOMIB metabolism (CYP3A4) by AZOLE ANTIFUNGAL AGENTS.

Management

Monitor the clinical response to BORTEZOMIB when AZOLE ANTIFUNGAL AGENTS are started or stopped. Monitor for BORTEZOMIB adverse reactions when BORTEZOMIB and AZOLE ANTIFUNGAL AGENTS are used concurrently. Adjust the BORTEZOMIB dose as needed.

Discussion

The effects of ketoconazole on the pharmacokinetics of bortezomib were evaluated in 12 patients with advanced solid tumors.[1] Using a prospective, open-label, randomized, crossover design, all patients received bortezomib 1 mg/m^2 IV on days 1, 4, 8, and 11 of two 21-day cycles. Patients were randomized to receive ketoconazole 400 mg at bedtime on days 6 through 9 of cycle 1 or 2. Compared with receiving bortezomib alone, coadministration of ketoconazole increased bortezomib exposure (AUC) 35%. The incidence of adverse reactions was similar for administration of bortezomib alone and with ketoconazole. Itraconazole may exacerbate bortezomib-induced peripheral neuropathy and thrombocytopenia.[2]

[1] Venkatakrishnan K, et al. *Clin Ther*. 2009;31(pt 2):2444.

[2] Iwamoto T, et al. *Pharmacotherapy*. 2010;30(7):661.

* Asterisk indicates drugs cited in interaction reports.

Bosentan — Azole Antifungal Agents

Bosentan* (*Tracleer*)	Fluconazole (eg, *Diflucan*)	Ketoconazole* (eg, *Nizoral*)
	Itraconazole (eg, *Sporanox*)	Voriconazole (eg, *Vfend*)

Significance	Onset	Severity	Documentation
2	□ Rapid	□ Major	□ Established
	■ **Delayed**	■ **Moderate**	□ Probable
		□ Minor	■ **Suspected**
			□ Possible
			□ Unlikely

Effects BOSENTAN plasma concentrations may be elevated, increasing the pharmacologic and adverse reactions (eg, headache).

Mechanism Inhibition of BOSENTAN metabolism (CYP3A4) by AZOLE ANTIFUNGAL AGENTS is suspected.

Management In patients receiving BOSENTAN, closely monitor the clinical response when AZOLE ANTIFUNGAL AGENT therapy is started or stopped. Observe patients for an increase in adverse reactions during coadministration of these agents.

Discussion

The effects of ketoconazole on the pharmacokinetics of bosentan were studied in 10 healthy men.[1] In a randomized, crossover study, each subject received bosentan 62.5 mg on day 1 followed by 62.5 mg twice daily for 5.5 days alone and with ketoconazole 200 mg once daily. Compared with administration of bosentan alone, coadministration of ketoconazole increased the bosentan AUC and C_{max} 2.3- and 2.1-fold, respectively. Headache occurred more frequently in patients receiving concomitant bosentan and ketoconazole.

[1] van Giersbergen PL, et al. *Br J Clin Pharmacol.* 2002;53(6):589.

* Asterisk indicates drugs cited in interaction reports. Based on pharmacologic and pharmacokinetic considerations, similar interactions may occur with other drugs that are listed.

Bosentan — *Cyclosporine*

Bosentan* (*Tracleer*)	Cyclosporine* (eg, *Neoral*)

Significance	Onset	Severity	Documentation
1	☐ Rapid	■ **Major**	☐ Established
	■ **Delayed**	☐ Moderate	☐ Probable
		☐ Minor	■ **Suspected**
			☐ Possible
			☐ Unlikely

Effects Trough concentrations of BOSENTAN may be elevated, increasing the risk of adverse reactions, while CYCLOSPORINE plasma levels may be decreased.

Mechanism BOSENTAN may increase the metabolism (CYP3A4) of CYCLOSPORINE, while CYCLOSPORINE may inhibit the metabolism (CYP3A4) of BOSENTAN.

Management Coadministration of CYCLOSPORINE and BOSENTAN is contraindicated.

Discussion

During the first day of cyclosporine and bosentan coadministration, trough concentrations of bosentan were increased approximately 30-fold.[1] Compared with bosentan alone, steady-state bosentan plasma levels were 3- to 4-fold higher when given with cyclosporine. Coadministration of cyclosporine and bosentan resulted in an approximate 50% decrease in cyclosporine plasma levels.

The basis for this monograph is information on file with the manufacturer. Published clinical data are needed to assess this interaction further. However, because of the increased risk of bosentan adverse reactions, clinical evaluation of this interaction in humans is not likely to be forthcoming.

[1] *Tracleer* [package insert]. South San Francisco, CA: Actelion Pharmaceuticals; 2001.

* Asterisk indicates drugs cited in interaction reports.

Bosentan — Glyburide

Bosentan* (*Tracleer*)	Glyburide* (eg, *DiaBeta*)

Significance	Onset	Severity	Documentation
1	☐ Rapid ■ **Delayed**	■ **Major** ☐ Moderate ☐ Minor	☐ Established ☐ Probable ■ **Suspected** ☐ Possible ☐ Unlikely

Effects Increased risk of elevated liver enzymes (eg, ALT, AST) resulting in serious liver injury. Plasma levels of BOSENTAN and GLYBURIDE may be decreased.

Mechanism BOSENTAN may increase the metabolism (CYP2C9 and CYP3A4) of GLYBURIDE. Other mechanisms may also be involved.[1]

Management Coadministration of BOSENTAN and GLYBURIDE is contraindicated. An alternative hypoglycemic agent is recommended.[2]

Discussion

Increased liver aminotransferases were observed in patients receiving concomitant bosentan and glyburide.[2] A possible pharmacokinetic interaction between bosentan and glyburide was studied in a randomized, 2-way, crossover investigation involving 12 healthy subjects.[3] Coadministration of bosentan and glyburide resulted in a decrease in the AUC of both drugs (40% for glyburide, 20% to 30% for bosentan and its metabolite). One case of elevated ALT (to 4-fold the upper limit of normal [ULN]) and 1 case of elevated AST (to 9-fold the ULN) and ALT (to 2-fold the ULN) occurred.

Additional studies are needed to resolve the decreased plasma levels of both drugs and the elevated liver enzymes.

[1] Personal communication. Actelion Pharmaceuticals; September 30, 2002.

[2] *Tracleer* [package insert]. South San Francisco, CA: Actelion Pharmaceuticals; 2001.

[3] van Giersbergen PL, et al. *Clin Pharmacol Ther.* 2002;71(4):253.

* Asterisk indicates drugs cited in interaction reports.

Bosentan — *Rifamycins*

Bosentan	Rifamycins	
Bosentan* (*Tracleer*)	Rifabutin (*Mycobutin*)	Rifapentine (*Priftin*)
	Rifampin* (eg, *Rifadin*)	

Significance	Onset	Severity	Documentation
4	□ Rapid	□ Major	□ Established
	■ **Delayed**	■ **Moderate**	□ Probable
		□ Minor	□ Suspected
			■ **Possible**
			□ Unlikely

Effects A transient increase in BOSENTAN trough concentration followed by a decrease in the concentration at steady state.

Mechanism Initially, RIFAMPIN may inhibit the hepatic uptake of BOSENTAN via organic anion-transporting polypeptide, then induce the hepatic metabolism (CYP2C9 and CYP3A4) of BOSENTAN.

Management Closely monitor patients receiving BOSENTAN when starting or stopping a RIFAMYCIN. Be prepared to adjust the BOSENTAN dose as needed.

Discussion

The effects of rifampin on the pharmacokinetics of bosentan were evaluated in 9 healthy men.[1] Using an open-label, randomized, crossover design, each individual received bosentan 125 mg twice daily for 6.5 days alone and with rifampin 600 mg daily. Compared with giving bosentan alone, coadministration of rifampin initially increased bosentan trough concentrations 5-fold. However, at steady state, coadministration of rifampin decreased the bosentan AUC 58%.

[1] van Giersbergen PL, et al. *Clin Pharmacol Ther.* 2007;81(3):414.

* Asterisk indicates drugs cited in interaction reports. Based on pharmacologic and pharmacokinetic considerations, similar interactions may occur with other drugs that are listed.

Bromocriptine — *Erythromycin*

Bromocriptine* (*Parlodel*)	Erythromycin Estolate* (eg, *Ilosone*)

Significance	Onset	Severity	Documentation
2	☐ Rapid	☐ Major	☐ Established
	■ **Delayed**	■ **Moderate**	☐ Probable
		☐ Minor	■ **Suspected**
			☐ Possible
			☐ Unlikely

Effects Serum BROMOCRIPTINE levels may be increased, resulting in an increase in the pharmacologic and toxic effects of BROMOCRIPTINE.

Mechanism Because ERYTHROMYCIN is known to inhibit hepatic metabolism of other drugs, increased bioavailability because of decreased hepatic first-pass metabolism may be involved.

Management Monitor the patient. If an interaction is suspected, adjust the dose of BROMOCRIPTINE accordingly.

Discussion

The effects of erythromycin on the pharmacokinetics of bromocriptine were studied in five healthy, nonsmoking male volunteers.[1] A dose of bromocriptine 5 mg was administered alone and after 4 days of treatment with erythromycin estolate 250 mg four times daily. Coadministration of erythromycin and bromocriptine significantly increased the area under the concentration-time curve of bromocriptine by 286% ($P = 0.025$) and increased the maximum serum concentration of bromocriptine by 4.6 times (from 465 to 2135 pg/mL). The time to reach the maximum serum concentration was not significantly altered. In addition, subjective side effects increased during coadministration of bromocriptine and erythromycin. With bromocriptine alone, three subjects experienced nausea and vomiting while all five subjects vomited following coadministration of erythromycin.

[1] Nelson MV, et al. *Clin Pharmacol Ther*. 1990;47:694.

* Asterisk indicates drugs cited in interaction reports.

Bromocriptine — *Phenothiazines*

Bromocriptine	Phenothiazines	
Bromocriptine* (*Parlodel*)	Chlorpromazine (eg, *Thorazine*)	Promethazine (eg, *Phenergan*)
	Fluphenazine (eg, *Prolixin*)	Propiomazine (*Largon*)
	Methotrimeprazine (*Levoprome*)	Thiethylperazine (*Torecan*)
	Perphenazine	Thioridazine*
	Prochlorperazine (eg, *Compazine*)	Trifluoperazine
	Promazine (eg, *Sparine*)	Triflupromazine (*Vesprin*)

Significance	Onset	Severity	Documentation
4	☐ Rapid	☐ Major	☐ Established
	■ **Delayed**	■ **Moderate**	☐ Probable
		☐ Minor	☐ Suspected
			■ **Possible**
			☐ Unlikely

Effects PHENOTHIAZINES may inhibit the effectiveness of BROMOCRIPTINE when employed for prolactin-secreting tumors.

Mechanism PHENOTHIAZINES may exert a dopamine receptor blockade that antagonizes the dopamine receptor-stimulating effect of BROMOCRIPTINE.

Management If possible, avoid PHENOTHIAZINE and BROMOCRIPTINE coadministration.

Discussion

In a clinical case report, a 40-year-old man underwent bromocriptine treatment for a prolactin-secreting chromophobe adenoma involving the basal hypothalamus and the right temporal lobe.[1] His serum prolactin levels increased by 2.5- to 5-fold and visual field deterioration was noted in two separate events 4 months apart when he received thioridazine 50 to 200 mg/day for paranoid schizophrenia. In a 42-year-old man with the same adenoma, the serum prolactin level increased 5- to 10-fold after thioridazine 200 mg/day was administered for 4 months.[2]

This anecdotal evidence implies that the phenothiazines, as dopamine antagonists, may impair the effectiveness of bromocriptine for treatment of certain prolactin-secreting tumors.

[1] Robbins RJ, et al. *Am J Med.* 1984;76:921.

[2] Weingarten JC, et al. *Gen Hosp Psychiatry.* 1985;7:364.

* Asterisk indicates drugs cited in interaction reports. Based on pharmacologic and pharmacokinetic considerations, similar interactions may occur with other drugs that are listed.

Bromocriptine — *Sympathomimetics*

Bromocriptine* (*Parlodel*)	Isometheptene* (eg, *Midrin*)

Significance	Onset	Severity	Documentation
4	■ **Rapid**	■ **Major**	□ Established
	□ Delayed	□ Moderate	□ Probable
		□ Minor	□ Suspected
			■ **Possible**
			□ Unlikely

Effects Exacerbation of BROMOCRIPTINE side effects, headaches, hypertension, and ventricular tachycardia have been reported during coadministration of SYMPATHOMIMETICS.

Mechanism Unknown.

Management Closely monitor patients.

Discussion

Severe worsening of bromocriptine-related adverse reactions have been reported in 3 patients following administration of a sympathomimetic.[1,2] Two patients were taking bromocriptine 2.5 mg twice daily.[1] The first woman had a history of vascular headaches. She presented 4 days postpartum with a severe progressive headache and nonpleuritic chest pain. A diagnosis of vascular headache was made, and the patient was given 2 capsules of a combination product containing isometheptene 65 mg, dichloralphenazone 100 mg, and acetaminophen 325 mg, followed by 1 capsule every hr until the headache resolved. Within 1 hr of taking the third capsule, the intensity of her headache increased. Upon arrival in the emergency department, her BP was 164/100 mm Hg with a pulse of 108 bpm. She was experiencing frequent premature ventricular complexes and short runs of ventricular tachycardia. The second woman had no history of hypertension or headache. She complained of a headache a few hr after delivery that was attributed to the epidural anesthesia. She was later started on a product containing phenylpropanolamine 75 mg and guaifenesin 400 mg twice daily for nasal drainage. After 2 doses, she experienced sudden vision loss and had 2 grand mal seizures. Her BP was 164/110 mm Hg, and her pulse was 130 bpm after the first seizure. She recovered slowly with supportive therapy. The third patient, a woman with no history of headache or hypertension, was prescribed bromocriptine 5 mg 3 times daily.[2] Two hr after taking her third dose of bromocriptine and 2 tablets of a combination rhinitis product that contained phenylpropanolamine 25 mg, she awoke with an intense headache and elevated BP (240/140 mm Hg). The bromocriptine and rhinitis medication were discontinued. She restarted bromocriptine 48 hr later and again experienced a severe headache and elevated BP (160/120 mm Hg).

[1] Kulig K, et al. *Obstet Gynecol.* 1991;78:941.
[2] Chan JC, et al. *Drug Invest.* 1994;8:254.

* Asterisk indicates drugs cited in interaction reports.

Bupivacaine — *Azole Antifungal Agents*

Bupivacaine* (eg, *Sensorcaine*)	Fluconazole (*Diflucan*)	Ketoconazole (eg, *Nizoral*)
	Itraconazole* (*Sporanox*)	

Significance	Onset	Severity	Documentation
5	☐ Rapid	☐ Major	☐ Established
	■ **Delayed**	☐ Moderate	☐ Probable
		■ **Minor**	☐ Suspected
			■ **Possible**
			☐ Unlikely

Effects BUPIVACAINE plasma levels may be elevated, possibly increasing the pharmacologic and adverse effects (eg, cardiotoxicity).

Mechanism Inhibition of BUPIVACAINE metabolism (CYP3A4) by the AZOLE ANTIFUNGAL AGENT is suspected. FLUCONAZOLE, especially 200 mg/day or greater, may inhibit CYP3A4.

Management Consider the possibility of increased local anesthetic effect of BUPIVACAINE in patients receiving an AZOLE ANTIFUNGAL AGENT.

Discussion

The effect of itraconazole on the pharmacokinetics of bupivacaine was studied in 7 healthy volunteers.[1] Each subject received 200 mg of itraconazole or a placebo orally for 4 days. On the fourth day, 0.3 mg/kg of racemic bupivacaine was given IV over 60 minutes. Compared with placebo, administration of itraconazole reduced the clearance of R-bupivacaine 21% and S-bupivacaine 25%. No other pharmacokinetic parameters were affected. No symptoms of toxicity or ECG changes were observed.

Additional studies are needed to assess the clinical importance of this interaction.

[1] Palkama VJ, et al. *Br J Anaesth.* 1999;83:659.

* Asterisk indicates drugs cited in interaction reports. Based on pharmacologic and pharmacokinetic considerations, similar interactions may occur with other drugs that are listed.

Buprenorphine — *Delavirdine*

Buprenorphine* (eg, *Buprenex*)	Delavirdine* (*Rescriptor*)

Significance	Onset	Severity	Documentation
5	☐ Rapid ■ **Delayed**	☐ Major ☐ Moderate ■ **Minor**	☐ Established ☐ Probable ☐ Suspected ■ **Possible** ☐ Unlikely

Effects BUPRENORPHINE plasma concentrations may be increased.

Mechanism Inhibition of BUPRENORPHINE hepatic metabolism (CYP3A4).

Management Based on available data, no special precautions are needed. However, be prepared to adjust the BUPRENORPHINE dose if an interaction is suspected.

Discussion

The effects of delavirdine on the pharmacokinetics of buprenorphine were studied in 10 opioid-dependent individuals and 15 matched controls.[1] The opioid-dependent individuals received buprenorphine/naloxone to determine buprenorphine pharmacokinetics followed by coadministration of delavirdine 600 mg twice daily for 7 days. Delavirdine increased the buprenorphine AUC approximately 325% and the C_{max} 241% while decreasing the AUC and C_{max} of the norbuprenorphine metabolite approximately 61% and 64%, respectively. However, despite these changes in buprenorphine and norbuprenorphine pharmacokinetics, no individual experienced symptoms of opiate adverse reactions. See Buprenorphine-NNRT Inhibitors and Methadone-NNRT Inhibitors.

[1] McCance-Katz EF, et al. *Clin Infect Dis.* 2006;43(suppl 4):S224.

* Asterisk indicates drugs cited in interaction reports.

Buprenorphine — *NNRT Inhibitors*

Buprenorphine* (eg, *Buprenex*)	Efavirenz* (*Sustiva*)	Nevirapine (*Viramune*)

Significance	Onset	Severity	Documentation
5	☐ Rapid ■ **Delayed**	☐ Major ☐ Moderate ■ **Minor**	☐ Established ☐ Probable ☐ Suspected ■ **Possible** ☐ Unlikely

Effects BUPRENORPHINE plasma concentrations may be reduced.

Mechanism Increased BUPRENORPHINE hepatic metabolism (CYP3A4).

Management Based on available data, no special precautions are needed. However, be prepared to adjust the BUPRENORPHINE dose if an interaction is suspected.

Discussion

The effects of efavirenz on the pharmacokinetics of buprenorphine were studied in 10 opioid-dependent individuals.[1] The opioid-dependent individuals received buprenorphine/naloxone to determine buprenorphine pharmacokinetics, followed by coadministration of efavirenz 600 mg daily for 15 days. Efavirenz decreased the buprenorphine AUC approximately 50% and the AUC of the norbuprenorphine metabolite 71%. However, despite the decrease in buprenorphine and norbuprenorphine exposure, no individual experienced symptoms of opiate withdrawal. See also Buprenorphine-Delavirdine and Methadone-NNRT Inhibitors.

[1] McCance-Katz EF, et al. *Clin Infect Dis.* 2006;43(suppl 4):S224.

* Asterisk indicates drugs cited in interaction reports. Based on pharmacologic and pharmacokinetic considerations, similar interactions may occur with other drugs that are listed.

Bupropion — *Baicalin*

Bupropion* (eg, *Wellbutrin*)	Baicalin*

Significance	Onset	Severity	Documentation
4	☐ Rapid	☐ Major	☐ Established
	■ **Delayed**	■ **Moderate**	☐ Probable
		☐ Minor	☐ Suspected
			■ **Possible**
			☐ Unlikely

Effects Plasma concentrations of the active metabolite of BUPROPION, hydroxybupropion, may be increased.

Mechanism BAICALIN may increase the metabolism of BUPROPION to hydroxybupropion by inducing the CYP2B6 isozyme.

Management Patients receiving BUPROPION should avoid taking BAICALIN. Caution patients taking BUPROPION not to use nonprescription or herbal products without consulting their health care provider.

Discussion

The effects of baicalin, a flavone glucuronide from the plant *Radix scutellariae*, on the pharmacokinetics of bupropion were studied in 17 healthy men.[1] Each subject received an oral dose of bupropion 150 mg alone and after receiving baicalin 500 mg 3 times daily for 14 days. Compared with taking bupropion alone, pretreatment with baicalin increased the hydroxybupropion C_{max} and AUC 73% and 87%, respectively. There was no change in the hydroxybupropion elimination $t_{½}$. In addition, baicalin increased the ratio of hydroxybupropion to bupropion AUC 63%. Baicalin administration did not affect bupropion pharmacokinetics. No adverse reactions were observed.

[1] Fan L, et al. *Eur J Clin Pharmacol.* 2009;65(4):403.

* Asterisk indicates drugs cited in interaction reports.

Bupropion — Carbamazepine

Bupropion*
(eg, *Wellbutrin*)

Carbamazepine*
(eg, *Tegretol*)

Significance	Onset	Severity	Documentation
2	☐ Rapid ■ **Delayed**	☐ Major ■ **Moderate** ☐ Minor	☐ Established ☐ Probable ■ **Suspected** ☐ Possible ☐ Unlikely

Effects Serum concentrations of BUPROPION may be decreased, reducing the pharmacologic effects.

Mechanism CARBAMAZEPINE increases the hepatic metabolism (CYP450 3A4) of BUPROPION.

Management Observe the clinical response of the patient. If an interaction is suspected, adjust therapy as indicated.

Discussion

In a placebo-controlled investigation involving patients with mood disorders, the effects of carbamazepine or valproic acid (eg, *Depakene*) on the pharmacokinetics of bupropion were studied.[1] Seven patients received placebo or carbamazepine, and 4 patients received placebo or valproic acid. When carbamazepine or valproic acid was administered, patients received either drug for at least 3 weeks to allow dosage titration and steady-state serum concentrations of carbamazepine or valproic acid to be reached. During each pharmacokinetic phase, a single oral dose of bupropion 150 mg was administered in a blind fashion. Carbamazepine therapy significantly decreased peak bupropion concentrations 87% (from 127 to 17 ng/mL; $P < 0.0001$) and AUC 90% (from 520 to 52 ng•hr/mL; $P < 0.0001$). In 5 of 12 patients receiving coadministration of carbamazepine and bupropion, bupropion concentrations were undetectable. Valproic acid did not affect the peak serum concentrations or AUC of bupropion; however, there was a trend toward earlier time to reach peak bupropion concentrations during valproic acid administration ($P < 0.01$). Overall, carbamazepine increased the metabolism of bupropion via hydroxylation. Valproic acid did not alter bupropion concentrations but increased concentrations of the hydroxymetabolite of bupropion.

Additional studies are needed to determine the safety and efficacy of concurrent bupropion and carbamazepine therapy.

[1] Ketter TA, et al. *J Clin Psychopharmacol.* 1995;15:327.

* Asterisk indicates drugs cited in interaction reports.

Bupropion | **Clopidogrel**

Bupropion*
(eg, *Wellbutrin*)

Clopidogrel*
(*Plavix*)

Significance	Onset	Severity	Documentation
4	☐ Rapid ■ **Delayed**	☐ Major ■ **Moderate** ☐ Minor	☐ Established ☐ Probable ☐ Suspected ■ **Possible** ☐ Unlikely

Effects BUPROPION plasma concentrations may be elevated, increasing the pharmacologic and adverse effects.

Mechanism Inhibition of BUPROPION first-pass metabolism (CYP2B6) by CLOPIDOGREL may occur.

Management Carefully monitor patients when BUPROPION and CLOPIDOGREL are coadministered. Be prepared to adjust the BUPROPION dosage when CLOPIDOGREL therapy is started or stopped.

Discussion

The effect of clopidogrel on the hydroxylation of bupropion was studied in 12 healthy men.[1] Using an open crossover design, each subject received a single oral dose of bupropion 150 mg alone or after pretreatment with clopidogrel 75 mg daily for 4 days. On the fourth day, bupropion was administered 1 hour after the last dose of clopidogrel. Compared with taking bupropion alone, clopidogrel increased the bupropion AUC 60%, and decreased the AUC of the hydroxybupropion metabolite 52% and the AUC ratio of hydroxybupropion to bupropion 68%. In addition, clopidogrel administration increased the C_{max} of bupropion 40% and decreased the oral clearance 26%. Clopidogrel did not alter the time to reach the C_{max} or the $t_{½}$ of bupropion.

[1] Turpeinen M, et al. *Clin Pharmacol Ther*. 2005;77:553.

* Asterisk indicates drugs cited in interaction reports.

Bupropion — *Efavirenz*

Bupropion* (eg, *Wellbutrin*)	Efavirenz* (*Sustiva*)

Significance	Onset	Severity	Documentation
4	☐ Rapid	☐ Major	☐ Established
	■ **Delayed**	■ **Moderate**	☐ Probable
		☐ Minor	☐ Suspected
			■ **Possible**
			☐ Unlikely

Effects BUPROPION plasma concentrations may be decreased, reducing the pharmacologic effects.

Mechanism Increased metabolism (CYP2B6) of BUPROPION by EFAVIRENZ is suspected.

Management Coadminister with caution. Monitor the clinical response of the patient when EFAVIRENZ is started or stopped. Adjust the BUPROPION dose as needed.

Discussion

The effect of efavirenz on the metabolism of bupropion was studied in 13 healthy subjects.[1] Using an open-label, 2-phase, sequential design, each subject received a single dose of sustained-release bupropion 150 mg before and after 14 days of pretreatment with efavirenz 600 mg daily at bedtime. Compared with giving bupropion alone, pretreatment with efavirenz decreased the bupropion AUC and C_{max} by 55% and 34%, respectively, and decreased the $t_{1/2}$ from approximately 8.6 to 4.7 hours.

[1] Robertson SM, et al. *J Acquir Immune Defic Syndr*. 2008;49(5):513.

* Asterisk indicates drugs cited in interaction reports.

Bupropion — *Guanfacine*

Bupropion* (eg, *Wellbutrin*)	Guanfacine* (*Tenex*)

Significance	Onset	Severity	Documentation
4	☐ Rapid ■ **Delayed**	☐ Major ■ **Moderate** ☐ Minor	☐ Established ☐ Probable ☐ Suspected ■ **Possible** ☐ Unlikely

Effects The risk of BUPROPION toxicity may be increased.

Mechanism Unknown.

Management Closely monitor patients. If an interaction is suspected, adjust therapy as needed.

Discussion

A generalized tonic-clonic seizure was reported in a 10-year-old girl during coadministration of bupropion and guanfacine.[1] The patient had no history of seizures and was receiving bupropion for attention deficit hyperactivity disorder and dysthymic disorder. She frequently exhibited angry and aggressive behavior. Bupropion therapy was started at 75 mg/day and increased in increments to 100 mg 3 times daily. Three weeks later, guanfacine 0.5 mg twice daily was added to her regimen because she was still aggressive, irritable, and inattentive. After 10 days, the dosage of guanfacine was increased to 0.5 mg 3 times daily. Ten days later, the patient experienced a generalized tonic-clonic seizure, and all medication was discontinued. She had no other seizures.

Additional documentation is needed to confirm this possible drug interaction.[2]

[1] Tilton P. *J Am Acad Child Adolesc Psychiatry.* 1998;37:682.

[2] Watson A. *J Am Acad Child Adolesc Psychiatry.* 1998;37:683.

* Asterisk indicates drugs cited in interaction reports.

Bupropion — *Linezolid*

Bupropion* (eg, *Wellbutrin*)	Linezolid* (*Zyvox*)

Significance	Onset	Severity	Documentation
4	■ **Rapid** ☐ Delayed	■ **Major** ☐ Moderate ☐ Minor	☐ Established ☐ Probable ☐ Suspected ■ **Possible** ☐ Unlikely

Effects Risk of hypertensive crisis may be increased.

Mechanism Unknown. However, it may be related to the MAOI effect of LINEZOLID.

Management Because coadministration of BUPROPION and traditional MAOIs is contraindicated, avoid concurrent use of BUPROPION and LINEZOLID until more clinical information is available.

Discussion

Intraoperative hemodynamic lability and severe intermittent hypertension were reported in a 57-year-old man receiving bupropion after linezolid was started.[1] The patient was on a stable regimen of bupropion for depression. He was admitted to the hospital for antibiotic therapy after being seen in the emergency department with evidence of a vascular graft infection. After trials with several antibiotics, the patient was started on linezolid for treatment of resistant, gram-positive organisms. Bupropion was continued during his hospital stay. After receiving linezolid for 24 hours, he was taken to the operating room (OR) for graft removal. In the OR he received propofol (eg, *Diprivan*), succinylcholine (eg, *Anectine*), isoflurane (eg, *Forane*), and fentanyl (eg, *Sublimaze*). During this intraoperative course, he experienced several episodes of severe hypertension (as high as 260/145 mm Hg), which resulted in admission to the intensive care unit (ICU). In the ICU, the patient had an unremarkable postoperative recovery. See also Bupropion-MAOIs.

[1] Marcucci C, et al. *Anesthesiology*. 2004;101:1487.

* Asterisk indicates drugs cited in interaction reports.

Bupropion — *MAOIs*

Bupropion	MAOIs	
Bupropion* (eg, *Wellbutrin*)	Isocarboxazid* (*Marplan*)	Rasagiline* (*Azilect*)
	Linezolid* (*Zyvox*)	Selegiline* (eg, *Eldepryl*)
	Phenelzine* (*Nardil*)	Tranylcypromine* (eg, *Parnate*)

Significance	Onset	Severity	Documentation
1	□ Rapid	■ **Major**	□ Established
	■ **Delayed**	□ Moderate	□ Probable
		□ Minor	■ **Suspected**
			□ Possible
			□ Unlikely

Effects Risk of acute BUPROPION toxicity may be increased.

Mechanism Unknown.

Management Coadministration of BUPROPION and MAOIs is contraindicated. Allow at least 14 days to elapse between discontinuing an MAOI and starting BUPROPION.

Discussion

Animal studies demonstrate that the acute toxicity of bupropion may be increased by the administration of the MAOI phenelzine.[1]

The basis for this monograph is information on file with the manufacturer. Because of the seriousness of the reaction, clinical evaluation of this interaction in humans is not likely to be forthcoming.

[1] *Wellbutrin* [package insert]. Research Triangle Park, NC: GlaxoSmithKline; September 2006.

* Asterisk indicates drugs cited in interaction reports.

Bupropion — *Rifamycins*

Bupropion*
(eg, *Wellbutrin*)

Rifampin*
(eg, *Rifadin*)

Significance	Onset	Severity	Documentation
2	☐ Rapid ■ **Delayed**	☐ Major ■ **Moderate** ☐ Minor	☐ Established ☐ Probable ■ **Suspected** ☐ Possible ☐ Unlikely

Effects BUPROPION plasma concentrations may be reduced, decreasing the therapeutic effect.

Mechanism Increased metabolism of BUPROPION (CYP2B6) is suspected.

Management In patients receiving BUPROPION, monitor for a decrease in clinical effect if RIFAMPIN is coadministered. Be prepared to adjust the BUPROPION dose as needed.

Discussion

The effects of rifampin on the pharmacokinetics of bupropion were evaluated in 16 healthy subjects.[1] Each subject received a single dose of sustained-release bupropion 150 mg alone and on day 8 of daily administration with rifampin 600 mg. Compared with taking bupropion alone, pretreatment with rifampin increased the clearance of bupropion more than 3-fold and decreased the $t_{½}$ from 15.9 to 8.2 hours. In addition, rifampin increased the C_{max} of the hydroxybupropion metabolite 28%, decreased the AUC 43%, and reduced the elimination $t_{½}$ from 21.9 to 10.7 hours.

[1] Loboz KK, et al. *Clin Pharmacol Ther.* 2006;80(1):75.

* Asterisk indicates drugs cited in interaction reports.

Bupropion — *Ritonavir*

Bupropion* (eg, *Wellbutrin*)	Lopinavir/Ritonavir* (*Kaletra*)	Ritonavir* (*Norvir*)

Significance	Onset	Severity	Documentation
4	☐ Rapid	☐ Major	☐ Established
	■ **Delayed**	■ **Moderate**	☐ Probable
		☐ Minor	☐ Suspected
			■ **Possible**
			☐ Unlikely

Effects BUPROPION levels may be reduced, decreasing the therapeutic effects.

Mechanism Unknown.

Management In patients coadministered BUPROPION and RITONAVIR, monitor the clinical response and be prepared to adjust the dosages of these agents.

Discussion

Ritonavir is expected to increase bupropion plasma levels.[1] However, a study in 7 healthy volunteers receiving ritonavir for 2 days found a non–statistically significant (20%) increase in bupropion AUC.[2] Administration of lopinavir/ritonavir to 12 volunteers for 2 weeks resulted in a 57% decrease in C_{max} and AUC of a single dose of sustained-release bupropion.[3] The effect of ritonavir high dose (600 mg twice daily) and low dose (100 mg twice daily) for 16 days on the pharmacokinetics of a single 150 mg dose of sustained-release bupropion was studied in 2 groups of healthy volunteers.[4] High-dose ritonavir reduced the bupropion AUC and C_{max} 62% and 67%, respectively, while low dose reduced the AUC and C_{max} 21% and 22%, respectively.

[1] *Norvir* [package insert]. Abbott Park, IL: Abbott Laboratories Pharmaceutical Division; January 2006.
[2] Hesse LM, et al. J *Clin Pharmacol.* 2006;46(5):567.
[3] Hogeland GW, et al. *Clin Pharmacol Ther.* 2007;81(1):69.
[4] Park J, et al. *J Clin Pharmacol.* 2010; 50(10):1180.

* Asterisk indicates drugs cited in interaction reports.

Bupropion | **Serotonin Reuptake Inhibitors**

Bupropion*
(eg, *Wellbutrin*)

Fluoxetine*
(eg, *Prozac*)

Significance	Onset	Severity	Documentation
4	☐ Rapid	☐ Major	☐ Established
	■ **Delayed**	■ **Moderate**	☐ Probable
		☐ Minor	☐ Suspected
			■ **Possible**
			☐ Unlikely

Effects The risk of delirium may be increased.

Mechanism Inhibition of metabolism (CYP2D6) of the active metabolite of BUPROPION, hydroxybupropion, by FLUOXETINE is suspected.

Management Coadminister BUPROPION and FLUOXETINE with caution; monitor patients closely for increased CNS adverse reactions, especially delirium.

Discussion

Delirium was reported in a 51-year-old man during coadministration of bupropion and fluoxetine.[1] Fluoxetine 20 mg/day titrated to 40 mg/day in 3 weeks was administered for major depressive disorder. Four weeks later, sustained-release bupropion 150 mg/day was added because of complaints of easy fatigue and loss of energy. Subsequently, the patient was admitted to the hospital with complaints of disorientation to time and place as well as impairment of attention and memory. All medications were discontinued and the patient was treated with IM haloperidol (eg, *Haldol*) and lorazepam (eg, *Ativan*). He gradually became oriented over a 2-day period.

[1] Chan CH, et al. *J Clin Psychopharmacol.* 2006;26(6):677.

* Asterisk indicates drugs cited in interaction reports.

Bupropion — *Ticlopidine*

Bupropion* (eg, *Wellbutrin*)	Ticlopidine*

Significance	Onset	Severity	Documentation
4	☐ Rapid	☐ Major	☐ Established
	■ **Delayed**	■ **Moderate**	☐ Probable
		☐ Minor	☐ Suspected
			■ **Possible**
			☐ Unlikely

Effects BUPROPION plasma concentrations may be elevated, increasing the pharmacologic effects and adverse reactions.

Mechanism Inhibition of BUPROPION first-pass metabolism (CYP2B6) by TICLOPIDINE may occur.

Management Carefully monitor patients when BUPROPION and TICLOPIDINE are coadministered. Be prepared to adjust the BUPROPION dosage when TICLOPIDINE therapy is started or stopped.

Discussion

The effect of ticlopidine on the hydroxylation of bupropion was studied in 12 healthy men.[1] Using an open, crossover design, each subject received a single oral dose of bupropion 150 mg alone or with ticlopidine 250 mg twice daily for 4 days. On the fourth day, bupropion was administered 1 hour after the last dose of ticlopidine. Compared with taking bupropion alone, ticlopidine increased the bupropion AUC 85%, and decreased the AUC of hydroxybupropion 84% and the AUC ratio of hydroxybupropion to bupropion 90%. Ticlopidine administration increased the C_{max} of bupropion 38% and decreased the oral clearance 36%. Ticlopidine did not alter the time to reach the C_{max} or the $t_{½}$ of bupropion.

[1] Turpeinen M, et al. *Clin Pharmacol Ther*. 2005;77(6):553.

* Asterisk indicates drugs cited in interaction reports.

Buspirone — *Azole Antifungal Agents*

Buspirone	Azole Antifungal Agents	
Buspirone* (eg, *BuSpar*)	Fluconazole (eg, *Diflucan*)	Ketoconazole (eg, *Nizoral*)
	Itraconazole* (eg, *Sporanox*)	Posaconazole (*Noxafil*)

Significance	Onset	Severity	Documentation
2	□ Rapid	□ Major	□ Established
	■ **Delayed**	■ **Moderate**	□ Probable
		□ Minor	■ **Suspected**
			□ Possible
			□ Unlikely

Effects Plasma BUSPIRONE concentrations may be elevated, increasing the pharmacologic effects and adverse reactions.

Mechanism Possibly because of inhibition, by the AZOLE ANTIFUNGAL AGENT, of the CYP3A4 isozyme responsible for first-pass metabolism of BUSPIRONE.

Management In patients receiving BUSPIRONE, closely observe the clinical response when an AZOLE ANTIFUNGAL AGENT dose is started, stopped, or changed. In patients receiving an AZOLE ANTIFUNGAL AGENT when BUSPIRONE is started, start with a conservative dose of BUSPIRONE and adjust as needed.

Discussion

Using a randomized, double-blind, placebo-controlled, crossover design, the possible pharmacodynamic and pharmacokinetic drug interactions of buspirone with itraconazole were evaluated in 8 healthy volunteers.[1] Each subject received doses of itraconazole 100 mg twice a day or placebo 3 times a day for 4 days. On day 4, buspirone 10 mg was administered. Pretreatment with itraconazole increased the AUC of buspirone approximately 19-fold, compared with placebo. The mean peak plasma concentrations of buspirone were increased approximately 13-fold (from 1 to 13.4 ng/mL) by itraconazole. Although there was wide interindividual variability, the interactions occurred in all subjects. The increase in plasma buspirone levels was accompanied by an increase in adverse reactions and impaired psychomotor performance. Another study in 6 healthy volunteers reported similar itraconazole-induced changes in buspirone pharmacokinetics compared with placebo.[2]

[1] Kivistö KT, et al. *Clin Pharmacol Ther.* 1997;62(3):348. [2] Kivistö KT, et al. *Pharmacol Toxicol.* 1999;84(2):94.

* Asterisk indicates drugs cited in interaction reports. Based on pharmacologic and pharmacokinetic considerations, similar interactions may occur with other drugs that are listed.

Buspirone — *Diltiazem*

Buspirone* (eg, *BuSpar*)	Diltiazem* (eg, *Cardizem*)

Significance	Onset	Severity	Documentation
2	☐ Rapid ■ **Delayed**	☐ Major ■ **Moderate** ☐ Minor	☐ Established ☐ Probable ■ **Suspected** ☐ Possible ☐ Unlikely

Effects The pharmacologic and adverse effects of BUSPIRONE may be increased.

Mechanism The bioavailability of BUSPIRONE may be enhanced as a result of reduced first-pass metabolism (CYP3A4) in the small intestine and liver.

Management Closely observe the clinical response of the patient to BUSPIRONE when DILTIAZEM is started or stopped. Adjust the BUSPIRONE dosage as needed. An antianxiety agent that is not metabolized by CYP3A4 (eg, lorazepam [eg, *Ativan*]) would not be expected to interact with DILTIAZEM. A dihydropyridine calcium channel blocker that does not inhibit CYP3A4 would not be expected to interact with BUSPIRONE.

Discussion

In a randomized, placebo-controlled, crossover trial, the effects of diltiazem on the pharmacokinetics and pharmacodynamics of buspirone were studied in 9 healthy volunteers.[1] Each subject received diltiazem 60 mg or placebo 3 times/day. After the fifth dose, buspirone 10 mg was administered. Diltiazem administration increased the AUC 5.5-fold and the C_{max} 4-fold (from 2.6 to 10.3 ng/mL). Diltiazem did not change the elimination $t_{½}$ of buspirone. The only pharmacodynamic effect of buspirone that changed was the subjective overall drug effect as measured with a visual analog scale. Nine subjects reported adverse effects during diltiazem administration compared with 2 during placebo administration.

[1] Lamberg TS, et al. *Clin Pharmacol Ther.* 1998;63:640.

* Asterisk indicates drugs cited in interaction reports.

Buspirone	***Fluoxetine***
Buspirone* (eg, *BuSpar*)	Fluoxetine* (eg, *Prozac*)

Significance	Onset	Severity	Documentation
4	☐ Rapid ■ **Delayed**	☐ Major ■ **Moderate** ☐ Minor	☐ Established ☐ Probable ☐ Suspected ■ **Possible** ☐ Unlikely

Effects BUSPIRONE's effects may be decreased. Paradoxical worsening of obsessive-compulsive disorder (OCD) or serotonin syndrome have been reported.

Mechanism FLUOXETINE is a selective inhibitor of serotonin neuronal reuptake and may block BUSPIRONE's serotonergic activity.

Management Consider avoiding concomitant use of these drugs. Observe patient for worsening status or serotonin syndrome.

Discussion

Apparent loss of anxiolytic action of buspirone (60 mg/day) was observed in a 35-year-old man following addition of fluoxetine 20 mg/day to his treatment regimen.[1] Although the patient also received trazodone (eg, *Desyrel*), a weak serotonin reuptake inhibitor, loss of the therapeutic effects of buspirone did not occur prior to the addition of fluoxetine treatment. A grand mal seizure occurred in a patient who had buspirone added to his fluoxetine therapy.[2] Euphoria and pressured speech occurred in 3 patients during coadministration of buspirone and fluoxetine.[3] It was not determined whether the patient's reactions were side effects of buspirone or caused by a drug interaction.

The addition of buspirone to the treatment regimen of patients receiving fluoxetine 80 mg/day for 7 to 48 weeks for OCD resulted in improvement and no reported side effects.[4,5] Buspirone also has been reported to enhance the antidepressant effectiveness of fluoxetine[6,7] and to enhance its effectiveness in treating symptoms of depersonalization.[8] However, a 31-year-old woman reported worsened OCD symptoms 3 days after initiation of buspirone 10 mg/day.[9] She had been treated with fluoxetine 20 mg/day with a mild response. Her reaction may have been idiosyncratic or caused by the low dose of fluoxetine. Symptoms suggestive of serotonin syndrome were reported in a 37-year-old man taking fluoxetine 20 mg/day and buspirone 60 mg/day.[10]

1 Bodkin JA, et al. *J Clin Psychopharmacol.* 1989;9:150.
2 Grady TA, et al. *J Clin Psychopharmacol.* 1992;12:70.
3 Lebert F, et al. *Am J Psychiatry.* 1993;150:167.
4 Markovitz PJ, et al. *Am J Psychiatry.* 1990;147:798.
5 Jenike MA, et al. *J Clin Psychiatry.* 1991;52:13.
6 Bakish D. *Can J Psychiatry.* 1991;36:749.
7 Dimitriou EC, et al. *J Clin Psychopharmacol.* 1998;18:465.
8 Abbas S, et al. *J Clin Psychiatry.* 1995;56:484.
9 Tanquary J, et al. *J Clin Psychopharmacol.* 1990; 10:377.
10 Manos GH. *Ann Pharmacother.* 2000;34:871.

* Asterisk indicates drugs cited in interaction reports.

Buspirone — *Fluvoxamine*

Buspirone* (*BuSpar*)	Fluvoxamine* (*Luvox*)

Significance	Onset	Severity	Documentation
3	☐ Rapid ■ **Delayed**	☐ Major ☐ Moderate ■ **Minor**	☐ Established ☐ Probable ■ **Suspected** ☐ Possible ☐ Unlikely

Effects BUSPIRONE plasma concentrations may be increased; however, these changes are probably of limited clinical importance.

Mechanism FLUVOXAMINE may inhibit BUSPIRONE metabolism (CYP3A4).

Management Monitor the patient's clinical response to BUSPIRONE during administration of FLUVOXAMINE and adjust the BUSPIRONE dose as needed.

Discussion

The effects of fluvoxamine on the hormonal and psychological responses to buspirone were studied in 11 healthy male volunteers.[1] Fluvoxamine administration was started at 50 mg/day and increased to a maximum dose of 150 mg/day. In a balanced-order, double-blind design, each subject received placebo and buspirone 30 mg on different days. Fluvoxamine administration resulted in a nearly 3-fold increase in plasma buspirone concentrations. Buspirone treatment caused an increase in plasma prolactin (PRL) and plasma growth hormone (GH) concentrations. The increase in PRL was enhanced by concomitant fluvoxamine administration, and the increase in GH was blunted by fluvoxamine treatment. The psychological responses to buspirone were also blunted by coadministration of fluvoxamine. In a controlled, 2-phase crossover study, the effects of fluvoxamine on buspirone were evaluated in 10 healthy volunteers.[2] After 5 days of fluvoxamine 100 mg/day or placebo, each subject received buspirone 10 mg. Compared with placebo, fluvoxamine increased the area under the plasma concentration-time curve of buspirone 2.4-fold and the peak plasma concentration 2-fold. No changes in psychomotor tests were detected. See also Buspirone-Fluoxetine.

[1] Anderson IM, et al. *Psychopharmacology.* 1996;128:74.

[2] Lamberg TS, et al. *Eur J Clin Pharmacol.* 1998;54:761.

* Asterisk indicates drugs cited in interaction reports.

Buspirone — *Food*

Buspirone* (*BuSpar*)	Grapefruit Juice*

Significance	Onset	Severity	Documentation
2	☐ Rapid ■ **Delayed**	☐ Major ■ **Moderate** ☐ Minor	☐ Established ■ **Probable** ☐ Suspected ☐ Possible ☐ Unlikely

Effects Plasma concentrations of BUSPIRONE may be elevated, increasing its pharmacologic and adverse effects.

Mechanism Possible inhibition of BUSPIRONE metabolism (CYP3A4) in the wall of the small intestine.

Management Avoid coadministration of BUSPIRONE with GRAPEFRUIT products. Caution patients to take BUSPIRONE with a liquid other than GRAPEFRUIT JUICE.

Discussion

The effect of grapefruit juice on the pharmacokinetics and pharmacodynamics of buspirone was studied in 10 healthy volunteers.[1] Using a randomized crossover design, each subject ingested either 200 mL of double-strength grapefruit juice or water 3 times daily for 2 days. On day 3, each subject received 10 mg buspirone with 200 mL double-strength grapefruit juice or water. In addition, grapefruit juice or water was taken ½ hour and 1½ hours after buspirone. Compared with water, grapefruit juice increased the mean peak concentration of buspirone approximately 4-fold, increased the mean area under the plasma concentration-time curve approximately 9-fold, prolonged the time to reach peak concentration from 0.75 to 3 hours, and increased the average half-life from 1.8 to 2.7 hours. Although there was considerable interindividual variability, the effects of grapefruit juice on buspirone pharmacokinetics were demonstrated in each subject. When evaluated with a visual analog scale to measure subjective drowsiness and overall subjective drug effect, the pharmacodynamic effect of buspirone was greater during the grapefruit phase than the water phase.

[1] Lilja JJ, et al. *Clin Pharmacol Ther.* 1998;64:655.

* Asterisk indicates drugs cited in interaction reports.

Buspirone — *Linezolid*

Buspirone* (eg, *BuSpar*)	Linezolid* (*Zyvox*)

Significance	Onset	Severity	Documentation
1	■ **Rapid** □ Delayed	■ **Major** □ Moderate □ Minor	□ Established □ Probable ■ **Suspected** □ Possible □ Unlikely

Effects Serotonin syndrome (eg, agitation, altered consciousness, ataxia, myoclonus, overactive, reflexes, shivering) may occur in some patients.

Mechanism Accumulation of serotonin in the CNS.

Management Unless patients are carefully observed for signs and symptoms of serotonin syndrome, LINEZOLID should not be coadministered with BUSPIRONE.[1]

Discussion

Unless patients are carefully observed for signs and symptoms of serotonin syndrome, do not coadminister linezolid with buspirone.[1]

The basis for this monograph is information on file with the manufacturer. Published clinical data are needed to further assess this interaction. However, due to the seriousness of this interaction, clinical evaluation in humans is not likely to be forthcoming.

[1] *Zyvox* [package insert]. New York, NY: Pharmacia & Upjohn Company; December 2009.

* Asterisk indicates drugs cited in interaction reports.

Buspirone — *Macrolide & Related Antibiotics*

Buspirone	Macrolide & Related Antibiotics	
Buspirone* (eg, *BuSpar*)	Clarithromycin (eg, *Biaxin*)	Telithromycin (*Ketek*)
	Erythromycin* (eg, *Ery-Tab*)	

Significance	Onset	Severity	Documentation
2	☐ Rapid	☐ Major	☐ Established
	■ **Delayed**	■ **Moderate**	☐ Probable
		☐ Minor	■ **Suspected**
			☐ Possible
			☐ Unlikely

Effects Plasma BUSPIRONE concentrations may be elevated, increasing the pharmacologic effects and adverse reactions.

Mechanism Inhibition of the CYP3A4 isozyme responsible for first-pass metabolism of BUSPIRONE is suspected.

Management In patients receiving BUSPIRONE, closely observe the response of the patient when a dose of MACROLIDE or RELATED ANTIBIOTIC is started, stopped, or changed. In patients receiving a MACROLIDE or RELATED ANTIBIOTIC when starting BUSPIRONE, start with a conservative BUSPIRONE dose. Adjust the BUSPIRONE dose as needed. Azithromycin (eg, *Zithromax*) is not metabolized by the CYP3A4 isozyme and is not expected to interact with buspirone.[1]

Discussion

Using a randomized, double-blind, placebo-controlled, crossover design, the possible pharmacodynamic and pharmacokinetic drug interactions of buspirone with erythromycin were evaluated in 8 healthy volunteers.[2] Each subject received oral doses of erythromycin base 500 mg or placebo 3 times a day for 4 days. On day 4, buspirone 10 mg was administered. Pretreatment with erythromycin increased the AUC of buspirone approximately 6-fold (from 3.3 to 19.5 ng•hr/mL) compared with placebo. The mean peak plasma concentrations of buspirone were increased approximately 5-fold (from 1 to 5 ng/mL) by erythromycin. Although there was wide interindividual variability, the interactions occurred in all subjects. The increase in plasma buspirone concentrations was accompanied by an increase in adverse reactions and impaired psychomotor performance.

[1] von Rosensteil NA, et al. *Drug Saf.* 1995;13(2):105.

[2] Kivistö KT, et al. *Clin Pharmacol Ther.* 1997;62(3):348.

* Asterisk indicates drugs cited in interaction reports. Based on pharmacologic and pharmacokinetic considerations, similar interactions may occur with other drugs that are listed.

Buspirone	***Protease Inhibitors***	
Buspirone* (eg, *BuSpar*)	Atazanavir (*Reyataz*)	Nelfinavir (*Viracept*)
	Fosamprenavir (*Lexiva*)	Ritonavir* (*Norvir*)
	Indinavir* (*Crixivan*)	Saquinavir (*Invirase*)
	Lopinavir/Ritonavir (*Kaletra*)	Tipranavir (*Aptivus*)

Significance	Onset	Severity	Documentation
4	□ Rapid	□ Major	□ Established
	■ **Delayed**	■ **Moderate**	□ Probable
		□ Minor	□ Suspected
			■ **Possible**
			□ Unlikely

Effects BUSPIRONE plasma concentrations may be elevated, increasing the pharmacologic effects and adverse reactions.

Mechanism Inhibition of BUSPIRONE metabolism (CYP3A4) by the PROTEASE INHIBITOR.

Management In patients receiving BUSPIRONE, closely observe the clinical response of the patient when the dose of the PROTEASE INHIBITOR is started, stopped, or changed.

Discussion

Parkinson-like symptoms occurred in a 54-year-old HIV-positive man after ritonavir 400 mg twice daily and indinavir 400 mg twice daily were added to his treatment regimen.[1] The patient had been receiving buspirone 75 mg daily for 2 years for depression when ritonavir and indinavir were started. Six to 8 weeks after starting ritonavir and indinavir, the patient experienced fatigue and worsening depression. In addition, he developed symptoms of Parkinson disease (eg, ataxia, dizziness, rigidity, shuffling gait, tremor). Ritonavir and indinavir were discontinued, and the buspirone dosage was decreased to 15 mg 3 times daily. Amprenavir 1,200 mg twice daily was started. Eight days after the change in his drug regimen, the dizziness and Parkinson symptoms subsided. Within 15 days of the changes, the patient felt less fatigue and reported improvement in his depression.

[1] Clay PG, et al. *Ann Pharmacother.* 2003;37(2):202.

* Asterisk indicates drugs cited in interaction reports. Based on pharmacologic and pharmacokinetic considerations, similar interactions may occur with other drugs that are listed.

Buspirone — *Rifamycins*

Buspirone	Rifamycins	
Buspirone* (eg, *Buspar*)	Rifabutin (*Mycobutin*)	Rifapentine (*Priftin*)
	Rifampin* (eg, *Rifadin*)	

Significance	Onset	Severity	Documentation
2	☐ Rapid	☐ Major	☐ Established
	■ **Delayed**	■ **Moderate**	■ **Probable**
		☐ Minor	☐ Suspected
			☐ Possible
			☐ Unlikely

Effects BUSPIRONE plasma concentrations and pharmacologic effects may be decreased.

Mechanism Induction of first-pass metabolism (CYP3A4) of BUSPIRONE by RIFAMYCINS.

Management In patients receiving BUSPIRONE, closely observe the clinical response when the dose of a RIFAMYCIN is started, stopped, or changed. Adjust the BUSPIRONE dose as needed.

Discussion

Using a randomized, placebo-controlled, crossover design, the effects of rifampin on the pharmacokinetics and pharmacodynamics of buspirone were investigated.[1] Ten healthy volunteers received rifampin 600 mg once daily or a matching placebo for 5 days. On the sixth day, buspirone 30 mg was administered. Compared with placebo, rifampin reduced the buspirone AUC 90%, peak plasma concentrations 87% (from 6.6 to 0.84 ng/mL), and the $t_{½}$ 54% (from 2.8 to 1.3 hours). Rifampin administration reduced the effects of buspirone on 3 of 6 psychomotor tests (postural sway test with eyes closed, subjective drowsiness, and overall drug effect). Following pretreatment with rifampin, none of the subjects had measurable plasma buspirone levels 6 hours after taking the drug, while levels could be measured up to 10 hours after ingestion in the placebo phase. Buspirone adverse reactions were more common in the placebo phase than in the rifampin phase. Another study with 6 healthy volunteers reported similar rifampin-induced changes in buspirone pharmacokinetics compared with placebo.[2]

[1] Lamberg TS, et al. *Br J Clin Pharmacol.* 1998;45(4):381.

[2] Kivistö KT, et al. *Pharmacol Toxicol.* 1999;84(2):94.

* Asterisk indicates drugs cited in interaction reports. Based on pharmacologic and pharmacokinetic considerations, similar interactions may occur with other drugs that are listed.

Buspirone — *Verapamil*

Buspirone* (*BuSpar*)	Verapamil* (eg, *Calan*)

Significance	Onset	Severity	Documentation
2	□ Rapid ■ **Delayed**	□ Major ■ **Moderate** □ Minor	□ Established □ Probable ■ **Suspected** □ Possible □ Unlikely

Effects The pharmacologic and adverse effects of BUSPIRONE may be increased.

Mechanism The bioavailability of BUSPIRONE may be enhanced as a result of reduced first-pass metabolism (CYP3A4) in the small intestine and liver.

Management Closely observe the clinical response of the patient to BUSPIRONE when VERAPAMIL is started or stopped. Adjust the dosage of BUSPIRONE as needed. An antianxiety agent that is not metabolized by CYP3A4 (eg, lorazepam [eg, *Ativan*]) would not be expected to interact with VERAPAMIL. A dihydropyridine calcium channel blocker that does not inhibit CYP3A4 would not be expected to interact with BUSPIRONE.

Discussion

In a randomized, placebo-controlled, crossover trial, the effects of verapamil on the pharmacokinetics and pharmacodynamics of buspirone were studied in 9 healthy volunteers.[1] Each subject received verapamil 80 mg or placebo 3 times daily. After the fifth dose, buspirone 10 mg was administered. Verapamil administration increased the AUC of buspirone 3.4-fold and the peak plasma concentration 3.4-fold (from 2.6 to 8.8 ng/mL). Verapamil did not change the elimination $t_{1/2}$ of buspirone. The only pharmacodynamic effect of buspirone that changed was the subjective overall drug effect.

[1] Lamberg TS, et al. *Clin Pharmacol Ther.* 1998 Jun;63(6):640.

* Asterisk indicates drugs cited in interaction reports.

Busulfan — *Azole Antifungal Agents*

Busulfan* (eg, *Myleran*)	Itraconazole* (*Sporanox*)

Significance	Onset	Severity	Documentation
2	☐ Rapid	☐ Major	☐ Established
	■ **Delayed**	■ **Moderate**	☐ Probable
		☐ Minor	■ **Suspected**
			☐ Possible
			☐ Unlikely

Effects ITRACONAZOLE may elevate BUSULFAN plasma levels, increasing the risk of toxicity (eg, pancytopenia).

Mechanism Unknown.

Management Monitor patients receiving BUSULFAN for increased toxicity. Be prepared to adjust the BUSULFAN dose as needed. When indicated, fluconazole (*Diflucan*) may be a safe alternative to ITRACONAZOLE.

Discussion

The pharmacokinetics and pharmacodynamics of busulfan in 13 bone marrow transplant patients were compared with 26 matched controls who received busulfan alone and 13 matched patients who received busulfan and fluconazole.[1] Fluconazole (6 mg/kg/day) did not affect the pharmacokinetics of busulfan. Compared with patients receiving busulfan (1 mg/kg every 6 hr) alone, coadministration of busulfan (1 mg/kg every 6 hr) and itraconazole (6 mg/kg/day) increased the mean busulfan AUC 25%, the steady-state peak concentration 33%, the steady-state concentration 25%, the $t_{½}$ 17%, and decreased the clearance 18%. Grade II-III regimen-related toxicity was experienced in 69% of the patients receiving busulfan and itraconazole concomitantly, compared with 38% of the patients receiving busulfan alone and 23% of the patients receiving busulfan and fluconazole concurrently.

Additional studies are needed to determine the clinical importance of this interaction and to assess if other azole antifungal agents interact similarly.

[1] Buggia I, et al. *Anticancer Res.* 1996;16:2083.

* Asterisk indicates drugs cited in interaction reports.

Busulfan — *Metronidazole*

Busulfan* (eg, *Myleran*)	Metronidazole* (eg, *Flagyl*)

Significance	Onset	Severity	Documentation
1	☐ Rapid ■ **Delayed**	■ **Major** ☐ Moderate ☐ Minor	☐ Established ☐ Probable ■ **Suspected** ☐ Possible ☐ Unlikely

Effects BUSULFAN trough concentrations may be elevated, increasing the risk of serious toxicity (eg, veno-occlusive disease [VOD], hemorrhagic cystitis).

Mechanism Unknown.

Management In patients receiving BUSULFAN, avoid coadministration of METRONIDAZOLE.

Discussion

The effect of metronidazole administration on busulfan trough concentrations was investigated in patients undergoing hematopoietic stem cell transplantation.[1] All patients received oral busulfan 1 mg/kg on days 9 through 5 prior to transplantation. Then, 24 hours after the last busulfan dose, patients were treated with cyclophosphamide (eg, *Cytoxan*) 60 mg/kg on days 4 and 3 prior to transplantation. In addition, 5 patients received oral metronidazole 400 mg 3 times/day during busulfan therapy to prevent *Clostridium difficile* infection before transplant and as prophylaxis after transplant against graft-versus-host disease. Nine patients received busulfan alone for the first 2 days of treatment, then metronidazole was started. A control group (10 patients) received busulfan alone. Coadministration of busulfan and metronidazole for 4 days increased busulfan trough concentrations 87% compared with the control group. In patients receiving metronidazole for days 3 and 4, busulfan concentrations increased 79%, compared with days 1 and 2 (busulfan alone). In patients receiving busulfan and metronidazole concomitantly for 4 days, all patients experienced elevated liver transaminases and bilirubin, 3 experienced VOD, 1 developed hemorrhagic cystitis, and 1 patient with VOD died with multiorgan failure. In patients receiving busulfan and metronidazole concurrently on days 3 and 4, 6 patients had elevated liver function tests, but no patient experienced VOD. A 7-year-old boy was being treated with several drugs, including busulfan for myeloid leukemia.[2] Initiation of therapy with metronidazole for presumed *C. difficile* infection resulted in a 46% decrease in busulfan clearance. The predicted busulfan AUC was exceeded by 86%. The last busulfan dose was not administered and metronidazole was discontinued once the drug interaction was recognized.

[1] Nilsson C, et al. *Bone Marrow Transplant.* 2003;31(6):429.

[2] Gulbis AM, et al. *Ann Pharmacother.* 2011;45(7-8):e39.

* Asterisk indicates drugs cited in interaction reports.

Cabergoline — *Macrolide & Related Antibiotics*

Cabergoline	Macrolide & Related Antibiotics	
Cabergoline*	Clarithromycin* (eg, *Biaxin*)	Telithromycin (*Ketek*)
	Erythromycin (eg, *Ery-Tab*)	

Significance	Onset	Severity	Documentation
2	□ Rapid	□ Major	□ Established
	■ **Delayed**	■ **Moderate**	□ Probable
		□ Minor	■ **Suspected**
			□ Possible
			□ Unlikely

Effects CABERGOLINE plasma concentrations may be elevated, increasing the risk of toxicity.

Mechanism Inhibition of P-gp and CABERGOLINE metabolism (CYP3A4) is suspected.

Management If coadministration cannot be avoided, carefully monitor the clinical response of patients, especially those with Parkinson disease who have shown levodopa induced psychosis or dyskinesia.

Discussion

In a randomized, crossover investigation, the effects of clarithromycin on cabergoline plasma concentrations were studied in 10 healthy men and 7 patients with Parkinson disease.[1] Healthy subjects received cabergoline 1 mg/day alone and with clarithromycin 400 mg/day for 6 days. Patients with Parkinson disease were on stable dosages of cabergoline, and plasma levels were evaluated before and after coadministration of clarithromycin 400 mg twice daily for 6 days and again 1 month later. In healthy subjects, clarithromycin increased the cabergoline C_{max} and AUC approximately 2.8- and 2.6-fold, respectively, compared with taking cabergoline alone. In patients with Parkinson disease, clarithromycin increased cabergoline plasma concentrations 1.7-fold. No dose-related serious adverse reactions were reported.

[1] Nakatsuka A, et al. *J Pharmacol Sci.* 2006;100(1):59.

* Asterisk indicates drugs cited in interaction reports. Based on pharmacologic and pharmacokinetic considerations, similar interactions may occur with other drugs that are listed.

Caffeine — *Cimetidine*

Caffeine*

Cimetidine*
(eg, *Tagamet*)

Significance	Onset	Severity	Documentation
5	□ Rapid ■ **Delayed**	□ Major □ Moderate ■ **Minor**	□ Established □ Probable □ Suspected ■ **Possible** □ Unlikely

Effects The effects of CAFFEINE may be enhanced when coadministered with CIMETIDINE.

Mechanism CIMETIDINE may impair the hepatic microsomal metabolism of CAFFEINE.

Management Clinical intervention does not appear necessary. With multiple dosing, CV or CNS toxicity could be expected.[1] If toxicity occurs, avoid or reduce CAFFEINE consumption.

Discussion

In a randomized, placebo-controlled study in 5 healthy subjects, pretreatment with cimetidine 1 g/day for 6 days reduced the systemic clearance of a single oral dose of anhydrous caffeine 300 mg.[2] The steady-state plasma caffeine level increased approximately 70%, and the mean AUC, $t_{1/2}$, and first-order elimination rate constant were all markedly altered. No change in apparent volume of distribution was noted. In a similar study, a 31% to 42% decrease in total body clearance and a 45% to 96% increase in elimination $t_{1/2}$ resulted from a single 2 mg/kg dose of oral caffeine in 6 smokers and 6 nonsmokers given cimetidine 1.2 g/day for 4 days.[1]

Both studies failed to determine the correlation between elevated plasma levels of caffeine and excessive CNS stimulation. More controlled studies are required to adequately clarify the clinical relevance of this interaction.

[1] May DC, et al. *Clin Pharmacol Ther.* 1982;31:656.

[2] Broughton LJ, et al. *Br J Clin Pharmacol.* 1981;12:155.

* Asterisk indicates drugs cited in interaction reports.

Caffeine ✕ *Contraceptives, Hormonal*

Caffeine* (eg, *NoDoz*)	Contraceptives, Oral* (eg, *Ortho-Novum*)

Significance	Onset	Severity	Documentation
3	☐ Rapid	☐ Major	☐ Established
	■ **Delayed**	☐ Moderate	☐ Probable
		■ **Minor**	■ **Suspected**
			☐ Possible
			☐ Unlikely

Effects The actions of CAFFEINE may be enhanced.

Mechanism ORAL CONTRACEPTIVES may impair the hepatic metabolism of CAFFEINE.

Management If CAFFEINE-related adverse CNS and cardiovascular effects are apparent, consider lowering or abstaining from CAFFEINE intake.

Discussion

A single oral dose of caffeine 250 mg was administered to 9 healthy women receiving oral contraceptive steroids (OCs) and 9 other women taking no OCs.[1] The elimination $t_{½}$ was 94% longer and total plasma clearance was 40% less in women on OCs. Volume of distribution and plasma binding were similar in both groups. In a similar study involving 9 healthy young women, OCs increased the AUC 100% and mean residue time by a factor of 2 at the end of a 6-week cycle.[2] Researchers studied the effects of chronic (longer than 3 months) administration of low dose (less than 50 mcg) estrogen OCs on 9 healthy women receiving a single oral dose of caffeine base 162 mg.[3] Elimination $t_{½}$ of caffeine was prolonged 46%, and a mean reduction of 66.6% in plasma clearance of caffeine compared with nonusers of OCs was noted.

A direct correlation of pharmacokinetic changes and pharmacologic effects was not investigated in these studies, but excess CNS and cardiovascular effects are likely to occur in OC users who indulge in excessive quantities of caffeine-containing substances. More data are needed to clarify the interaction of caffeine with estrogen-progestin or progestin-only OCs.

1 Patwardhan RV, et al. *J Lab Clin Med.* 1980;95:603.
2 Rietveld EC, et al. *Eur J Clin Pharmacol.* 1984;26:371.
3 Abernethy DR, et al. *Eur J Clin Pharmacol.* 1985;28:425.

* Asterisk indicates drugs cited in interaction reports.

Caffeine — *Disulfiram*

Caffeine* (eg, *NoDoz*)	Disulfiram* (*Antabuse*)

Significance	Onset	Severity	Documentation
4	☐ Rapid	☐ Major	☐ Established
	■ **Delayed**	■ **Moderate**	☐ Probable
		☐ Minor	☐ Suspected
			■ **Possible**
			☐ Unlikely

Effects Cardiovascular and CNS stimulation effects of CAFFEINE may be increased by DISULFIRAM.

Mechanism Possibly because of inhibition of CAFFEINE metabolism in liver microsomes.

Management No clinical interventions appear necessary. Consider CAFFEINE abstinence if signs of CAFFEINE toxicity occur (eg, CNS excitation, cardiovascular abnormalities).

Discussion

Ten healthy, nonsmoking men and 11 recovering alcoholics (9 men, 2 women) were studied to examine the kinetics of caffeine elimination.[1] In the healthy subjects, the total body clearance of caffeine decreased 30% and 29% after disulfiram 250 and 500 mg. In recovering alcoholics, the total body clearance of caffeine decreased 24%. The mean caffeine $t_{½}$ increased 39% and 34% in healthy subjects after disulfiram 250 and 500 mg and 29% in recovering alcoholics, respectively.

Although the kinetic changes of caffeine leading to higher concentrations of caffeine in tissue may predispose the patient to excessive cerebral and cardiac excitation, thus complicating alcohol withdrawal, more studies are needed to clarify the clinical significance of this interaction.

[1] Beach CA, et al. *Clin Pharmacol Ther.* 1986;39:265.

* Asterisk indicates drugs cited in interaction reports.

Caffeine — *Echinacea*

Caffeine* | Echinacea*

Significance	Onset	Severity	Documentation
5	☐ Rapid	☐ Major	☐ Established
	■ **Delayed**	☐ Moderate	☐ Probable
		■ **Minor**	☐ Suspected
			■ **Possible**
			☐ Unlikely

Effects CAFFEINE plasma concentrations may be increased, enhancing the effect.

Mechanism ECHINACEA may inhibit the metabolism (CYP1A2) of CAFFEINE.

Management If CAFFEINE-related adverse effects occur, consider decreasing CAFFEINE intake or discontinuing ECHINACEA.

Discussion

Results are conflicting. The effects of echinacea (*Echinacea purpurea* root) on cytochrome P-450 (CYP) activity were assessed by administering the probe drug caffeine (CYP1A2).[1] Twelve subjects received caffeine 20 mg alone and after 8 days of pretreatment with echinacea 400 mg 4 times/day. Compared with administering caffeine alone, echinacea reduced the oral clearance of caffeine 27% (more than 50% in 2 patients) and increased the peak plasma concentration 30%. Others found a minimal effect of echinacea on caffeine levels.[2] The discrepancy may be caused by differences in the study designs. In 1 study, the echinacea product was an extract from echinacea root,[2] while in the second study, the echinacea product was a whole plant extract.[2]

The ingredients of many herbal products are not standardized. It is unclear if herbal products contain ingredients, other than those listed on the label or purported to be present, that could interact with caffeine.

[1] Gorski JC, et al. *Clin Pharmacol Ther.* 2004;75:89.

[2] Gurley BJ, et al. *Clin Pharmacol Ther.* 2004;76:428.

* Asterisk indicates drugs cited in interaction reports.

Caffeine — *Menthol*

Caffeine* | Menthol*

Significance	Onset	Severity	Documentation
5	■ **Rapid** □ Delayed	□ Major □ Moderate ■ **Minor**	□ Established □ Probable □ Suspected ■ **Possible** □ Unlikely

Effects CAFFEINE absorption may be delayed by MENTHOL ingestion, blunting the heart-rate-slowing effect of CAFFEINE.

Mechanism Unknown.

Management Based on available data, no special precautions are needed.

Discussion

The effects of menthol on caffeine metabolism and pharmacological response to caffeine were measured in 11 healthy women.[1] Using a randomized, double-blind, crossover design, each subject received a single oral dose of caffeine 200 mg taken with a single oral dose of menthol 100 mg or placebo. Compared with placebo, menthol ingestion resulted in a 75% increase in the time to reach peak plasma concentrations of caffeine. The C_{max}, AUC, and terminal $t_{1/2}$ of caffeine were not affected by menthol. Cardiovascular data were analyzed in 9 subjects. Heart rate decreased in both phases of the study; however, the maximum decrease in heart rate was less during the menthol phase compared with placebo.

[1] Gelal A, et al. *Eur J Clin Pharmacol.* 2003;59:417.

* Asterisk indicates drugs cited in interaction reports.

Caffeine — *Propafenone*

Caffeine*	Propafenone (eg, *Rythmol*)

Significance	Onset	Severity	Documentation
5	■ **Rapid**	□ Major	□ Established
	□ Delayed	□ Moderate	□ Probable
		■ **Minor**	□ Suspected
			■ **Possible**
			□ Unlikely

Effects CAFFEINE plasma concentrations may be elevated, increasing the risk for proarrhythmic effects.

Mechanism PROPAFENONE may inhibit the metabolism (CYP1A2) of CAFFEINE.

Management Because CAFFEINE has intrinsic proarrhythmic activity, it should be used with caution in patients taking PROPAFENONE who have atrial fibrillation or flutter and especially in poor metabolizers of CYP2D6.

Discussion

The effects of propafenone on the pharmacokinetics of caffeine were studied in 8 healthy men.[1] Each subject received caffeine 300 mg alone and 2 hours after administration of propafenone 300 mg. Compared with taking caffeine alone, propafenone decreased caffeine clearance 35% and increased the elimination $t_{1/2}$ and C_{max} 54% and 6%, respectively. Caffeine plasma concentrations and clearance were greatest in one subject who was a poor metabolizer of CYP2D6. In individuals who are poor metabolizers of CYP2D6, propafenone levels may be increased 4- to 8-fold and the elimination $t_{1/2}$ prolonged 3-fold. In these individuals, inhibition of CYP1A2 metabolism may be of greater clinical importance than in subjects without the poor metabolizer phenotype. On average, 240 mL of brewed coffee contains 150 mg of caffeine.[2]

[1] Michaud V, et al. *Ther Drug Monit.* 2006;28(6):779.

[2] Wickersham RM, Novak KK, eds. *Drug Facts and Comparisons.* 60th ed. St. Louis, MO: Wolters Kluwer Health; 2006:942.

* Asterisk indicates drugs cited in interaction reports.

Caffeine — *Quinolones*

Caffeine	Quinolones	
Caffeine*	Ciprofloxacin* (eg, *Cipro*)	Ofloxacin* (*Floxin*)
	Enoxacin*	
	Norfloxacin* (*Noroxin*)	

Significance	Onset	Severity	Documentation
3	☐ Rapid	☐ Major	☐ Established
	■ **Delayed**	☐ Moderate	☐ Probable
		■ **Minor**	■ **Suspected**
			☐ Possible
			☐ Unlikely

Effects The pharmacologic effects of CAFFEINE may be increased.

Mechanism The hepatic metabolism of CAFFEINE is decreased by certain QUINOLONES.

Management Patients treated with certain QUINOLONES should limit use of CAFFEINE-containing medications and beverages. Restrict CAFFEINE intake if excessive CNS or cardiovascular effects occur.

Discussion

The effects of 3 quinolone antibacterial agents on the pharmacokinetics of caffeine were studied in 12 healthy men.[1,2] The pharmacokinetics of 2 single doses of oral caffeine citrate 220 to 230 mg were measured before and after several doses of ciprofloxacin 250 mg twice daily, enoxacin 400 mg twice daily, or ofloxacin 200 mg twice daily in a crossover design. Ofloxacin did not alter any of the parameters of caffeine. In contrast, ciprofloxacin decreased the total body clearance of caffeine, as reflected by increases in plasma elimination $t_{1/2}$ and AUC. However, ciprofloxacin did not affect the peak plasma caffeine level or the time to reach this peak. Similar changes occurred in 12 healthy subjects.[3] Enoxacin exerted the greatest effects on the pharmacokinetics of caffeine, decreasing total body clearance and increasing the elimination $t_{1/2}$ and AUC approximately 4- to 5-fold. In addition, enoxacin increased the peak plasma caffeine level. Except for a slight increase in $t_{1/2}$, norfloxacin 400 mg twice daily had no effect on caffeine pharmacokinetics.[4] However, in another study, norfloxacin 800 mg twice daily increased the AUC and decreased the plasma clearance of caffeine, although the elimination $t_{1/2}$ was not altered.[5] Temafloxacin†,[3] and ofloxacin[1,2,6] do not appear to affect caffeine pharmacokinetics. In 24 healthy volunteers, ciprofloxacin altered caffeine kinetics while flevoxacin† did not.[7] In 12 healthy volunteers, caffeine clearance was reduced 83% and 47% during administration of enoxacin and pefloxacin†, respectively.[8]

1 Staib AH, et al. *Drugs.* 1987;34(suppl 1):170.
2 Stille W, et al. *J Antimicrob Chemother.* 1987;20(5):729.
3 Mahr G, et al. *Clin Pharmacokinet.* 1992;22(suppl 1):90.
4 Harder S, et al. *Eur J Clin Pharmacol.* 1988;35(6):651.
5 Carbó M, et al. *Clin Pharmacol Ther.* 1989;45(3):234.
6 Barnett G, et al. *Eur J Clin Pharmacol.* 1990;39(1):63.
7 Nicolau DP, et al. *Drugs.* 1995;49(suppl 2):357.
8 Kinzig-Schippers M, et al. *Clin Pharmacol Ther.* 1999;65(3):262.

* Asterisk indicates drugs cited in interaction reports.
† Not available in the US.

Caffeine — *Sympathomimetics*

Caffeine*	Ephedrine*

Significance	Onset	Severity	Documentation
5	■ **Rapid**	□ Major	□ Established
	□ Delayed	□ Moderate	□ Probable
		■ **Minor**	□ Suspected
			■ **Possible**
			□ Unlikely

Effects Cardiovascular, metabolic, and hormonal responses may be increased slightly.

Mechanism Additive or synergistic effects are suspected.

Management Based on available data, no special precautions are needed.

Discussion

In 15 healthy subjects, the pharmacokinetics and pharmacodynamics of caffeine and ephedrine taken in combination were compared with those of each drug taken alone.[1] In a randomized, double-blind, crossover study, each subject received caffeine 200 mg, ephedrine 25 mg, both drugs, or placebo. Compared with placebo, caffeine alone increased mean systolic BP 9.1 mm Hg. Ephedrine alone did not increase systolic BP. In addition, the effects on heart rate, fasting glucose, insulin, lactate, free fatty acids, and subjective stimulant responses were intensified by coadministration of caffeine and ephedrine. However, the increased effects were slight. The pharmacokinetics of caffeine and ephedrine taken in combination were not different compared with those of each drug taken alone. One hour after concurrent ingestion of caffeine and ephedrine, there was a mean increase in systolic BP of 11.7 mm Hg, compared with placebo.

[1] Haller CA, et al. *Clin Pharmacol Ther.* 2004;75(4):259.

* Asterisk indicates drugs cited in interaction reports.

Calcium Salts		***Proton Pump Inhibitors***	
Calcium Carbonate* (eg, *Os-Cal 500*)		Esomeprazole (*Nexium*)	Pantoprazole (*Protonix*)
		Lansoprazole (*Prevacid*)	Rabeprazole (*Aciphex*)
		Omeprazole* (eg, *Prilosec*)	

Significance	Onset	Severity	Documentation
4	☐ Rapid	☐ Major	☐ Established
	■ **Delayed**	■ **Moderate**	☐ Probable
		☐ Minor	☐ Suspected
			■ **Possible**
			☐ Unlikely

Effects CALCIUM absorption may be reduced, decreasing the therapeutic effect.

Mechanism Decrease in pH-dependent CALCIUM absorption may be induced by coadministration of a PROTON PUMP INHIBITOR.

Management Consider increasing the CALCIUM dosage, especially in elderly patients, if an interaction is suspected with long-term PROTON PUMP INHIBITOR therapy.

Discussion

The effect of acid suppression by the proton pump inhibitor omeprazole on calcium absorption was evaluated in 18 women 65 years of age and older.[1] Using a randomized, double-blind, placebo-controlled, crossover design, each subject took omeprazole 20 mg or placebo every morning for 7 days and also received a multivitamin containing vitamin D 400 units daily. One week before each study day, calcium supplements were stopped. In women taking bisphosphonates or diuretics, these agents were withheld until the afternoon of each study day. Food was not eaten for 5 hours after the study drug. Following an overnight fast, each subject ingested omeprazole or placebo, the multivitamin, and elemental calcium 500 mg. Compared with placebo, omeprazole decreased fractional calcium absorption from 9.1% to 3.5%. The difference represented an average decrease of 41%. One patient experienced an increase in calcium absorption while taking omeprazole. If the results of this outlier were removed from analysis, the average decrease in calcium absorption was 61%.

[1] O'Connell MB, et al. *Am J Med.* 2005;118(7):778.

* Asterisk indicates drugs cited in interaction reports. Based on pharmacologic and pharmacokinetic considerations, similar interactions may occur with other drugs that are listed.

Calcium Salts — *Thiazide Diuretics*

Calcium Salts		Thiazide Diuretics	
Calcium Acetate (eg, *PhosLo*)	Calcium Gluconate (eg, *Cal-Glu*)	Chlorothiazide* (eg, *Diuril*)	Indapamide
Calcium Carbonate* (eg, *Os-Cal*)	Calcium Lactate (eg, *Cal-Lac*)	Chlorthalidone (eg, *Thalitone*)	Methyclothiazide
Calcium Chloride	Tricalcium Phosphate (*Posture*)	Hydrochlorothiazide* (eg, *Microzide*)	Metolazone (eg, *Zaroxolyn*)
Calcium Citrate (eg, *Citracal*)			
Calcium Glubionate (*Calcionate*)			

Significance	Onset	Severity	Documentation
4	☐ Rapid	☐ Major	☐ Established
	■ **Delayed**	■ **Moderate**	☐ Probable
		☐ Minor	☐ Suspected
			■ **Possible**
			☐ Unlikely

Effects Hypercalcemia and possible CALCIUM toxicity.

Mechanism Hypercalcemia, resulting from renal tubular reabsorption of CALCIUM, bone release of CALCIUM, or both, associated with THIAZIDE DIURETICS may be amplified by exogenous CALCIUM.

Management Monitor serum CALCIUM and observe for signs of hypercalcemia during concurrent use of CALCIUM SALTS and THIAZIDE DIURETICS, particularly in hyperparathyroid patients or in patients taking vitamin D.

Discussion

Thiazide-type diuretics may cause hypercalcemia by decreasing renal tubular calcium excretion by a direct action that increases distal tubular calcium reabsorption. In addition, thiazides may enhance the effect of parathyroid hormone and vitamin D on calcium mobilization from bone. Moderate increases in serum calcium concentrations have been observed during thiazide-type diuretic use in patients with normal parathyroid, hypoparathyroid, and hyperparathyroid function. However, this effect is inconsistent and is more likely to occur in hyperparathyroid patients or patients on vitamin D supplementation.[1-8] Milk-alkali syndrome developed in a patient during ingestion of chlorothiazide 500 mg/day and calcium carbonate 7.5 to 10 g/day.[9]

1 Brickman AS, et al. *J Clin Invest.* 1972;51(4):945.
2 Parfitt AM. *J Clin Invest.* 1972;51(7):1879.
3 Parfitt AM. *Ann Intern Med.* 1972;77(4):557.
4 Middler S, et al. *Metabolism.* 1973;22(2):139.
5 Popovtzer MM, et al. *J Clin Invest.* 1975;55(6):1295.
6 Ljunghall S, et al. *Scand J Urol Nephrol.* 1981;15(3):257.
7 Crowe M, et al. *Practitioner.* 1984;228(1389):312.
8 Santos F, et al. *Am J Dis Child.* 1986;140(2):139.
9 Gora ML, et al. *Clin Pharm.* 1989;8(3):227.

* Asterisk indicates drugs cited in interaction reports. Based on pharmacologic and pharmacokinetic considerations, similar interactions may occur with other drugs that are listed.

Carbamazepine | Azole Antifungal Agents

Carbamazepine* (eg, *Tegretol*)	Fluconazole* (eg, *Diflucan*)	Ketoconazole* (eg, *Nizoral*)
	Itraconazole (eg, *Sporanox*)	

Significance	Onset	Severity	Documentation
2	☐ Rapid	☐ Major	☐ Established
	■ **Delayed**	■ **Moderate**	☐ Probable
		☐ Minor	■ **Suspected**
			☐ Possible
			☐ Unlikely

Effects Plasma concentrations of CARBAMAZEPINE may be elevated, increasing clinical effects and adverse reactions.

Mechanism Possible inhibition of CARBAMAZEPINE metabolism (CYP3A4) by the AZOLE ANTIFUNGAL AGENT. FLUCONAZOLE, especially 200 mg/day or more, may inhibit CYP3A4.

Management Closely monitor CARBAMAZEPINE concentrations and observe the clinical response when an AZOLE ANTIFUNGAL AGENT is started or stopped.

Discussion

The effect of ketoconazole on plasma levels of carbamazepine and its active metabolite, carbamazepine-10,11-epoxide (CBZ-E), was studied in 8 epileptic patients.[1] All patients were stabilized on carbamazepine (range, 400 to 800 mg/day). Each patient received ketoconazole 200 mg/day for 6 days. Mean plasma concentrations of carbamazepine increased from 5.6 mcg/mL to 7 and 7.2 mcg/mL on days 7 and 10 of ketoconazole therapy, respectively. When ketoconazole treatment was stopped, the mean carbamazepine plasma level returned to pretreatment values (5.9 mcg/mL). No changes in plasma CBZ-E concentrations occurred. There were no signs or symptoms of carbamazepine toxicity or changes in seizure frequency during coadministration of carbamazepine and ketoconazole. A 33-year-old man on a stable dosage of carbamazepine 1,200 mg/day for seizure control developed stupor and his carbamazepine plasma level increased from 11.1 to 24.5 mcg/mL 3 days after starting fluconazole.[2] Fluconazole was discontinued and carbamazepine was held for 24 hours. The next day his symptoms had resolved. Carbamazepine was restarted without incident. A 38-year-old man on a stable dosage of carbamazepine 1,000 mg/day received IV fluconazole.[3] The carbamazepine level increased from 6 to 18 mcg/mL after 10 days of fluconazole. No signs or symptoms of toxicity were noted. A 40-year-old woman receiving carbamazepine 600 mg daily was prescribed fluconazole 150 mg daily.[4] Two days later she experienced symptoms of carbamazepine toxicity and carbamazepine levels increased from a baseline of 7.3 to 18 mcg/mL. One day after fluconazole was withdrawn, her symptoms disappeared and carbamazepine plasma levels decreased to 9 mcg/mL.

[1] Spina E, et al. *Ther Drug Monit.* 1997;19(5):535.
[2] Nair DR, et al. *Ann Pharmacother.* 1999;33(7-8):790.
[3] Finch CK, et al. *South Med J.* 2002;95(9):1099.
[4] Tsouli S, et al. *Psychiatry Clin Neurosci.* 2011;65(1):112.

* Asterisk indicates drugs cited in interaction reports. Based on pharmacologic and pharmacokinetic considerations, similar interactions may occur with other drugs that are listed.

Carbamazepine — *Barbiturates*

Carbamazepine	Barbiturates	
Carbamazepine* (eg, *Tegretol*)	Amobarbital (*Amytal*)	Pentobarbital (eg, *Nembutal*)
	Aprobarbital (*Alurate*)	Phenobarbital*
	Butabarbital (eg, *Butisol*)	Primidone* (eg, *Mysoline*)
	Butalbital	Secobarbital (eg, *Seconal*)
	Mephobarbital (*Mebaral*)	

Significance	Onset	Severity	Documentation
3	☐ Rapid	☐ Major	☐ Established
	■ **Delayed**	☐ Moderate	☐ Probable
		■ **Minor**	■ **Suspected**
			☐ Possible
			☐ Unlikely

Effects Decreased serum CARBAMAZEPINE concentrations, possibly resulting in loss of effectiveness.

Mechanism Increased rate of CARBAMAZEPINE clearance resulting from BARBITURATE induction of CARBAMAZEPINE hepatic metabolism (epoxidation).

Management Monitor serum CARBAMAZEPINE concentrations, and observe the patient for loss of CARBAMAZEPINE efficacy. Consider discontinuing the BARBITURATE or adjusting the dose of CARBAMAZEPINE as needed.

Discussion

Lower serum carbamazepine concentrations have been observed in patients treated for seizure disorders with carbamazepine and phenobarbital than when treated with carbamazepine alone. Pharmacokinetic investigations suggest that these observations result from phenobarbital induction of carbamazepine metabolism.[1-8,10] In addition, the rate of elimination of the epoxide metabolite, which may have antiseizure activity, is increased.[11] However, none of these studies reported a loss of carbamazepine efficacy.

In a case report, initial drug therapy with carbamazepine and primidone failed to achieve seizure control.[9] Increasing carbamazepine doses only slightly affected serum concentrations. Seizures were controlled after discontinuing primidone, resulting in an increase in serum carbamazepine concentrations. See also Primidone-Carbamazepine.

[1] Christiansen J, et al. *Acta Neurol Scand.* 1973;49:543.
[2] Cereghino JJ, et al. *Clin Pharmacol Ther.* 1975;18:733.
[3] Rane A, et al. *Clin Pharmacol Ther.* 1976;19:276.
[4] Eichelbaum M, et al. *Clin Pharmacol Ther.* 1979;26:366.
[5] McKauge L, et al. *Ther Drug Monit.* 1981;3:63.
[6] Eichelbaum M, et al. *Clin Pharmacokinet.* 1985;10:80.
[7] Riva R, et al. *Clin Pharmacokinet.* 1985;10:524.
[8] Tomson T, et al. *Ther Drug Monit.* 1987;9:117.
[9] Benetello P, et al. *Int J Clin Pharm Res.* 1987;7:165.
[10] Ramsey RE, et al. *Ther Drug Monit.* 1990; 12:235.
[11] Spina E, et al. *Ther Drug Monit.* 1991;13:109.

* Asterisk indicates drugs cited in interaction reports. Based on pharmacologic and pharmacokinetic considerations, similar interactions may occur with other drugs that are listed.

Carbamazepine — *Cimetidine*

Carbamazepine* (eg, *Tegretol*)	Cimetidine* (eg, *Tagamet*)

Significance	Onset	Severity	Documentation
2	□ Rapid	□ Major	□ Established
	■ **Delayed**	■ **Moderate**	□ Probable
		□ Minor	■ **Suspected**
			□ Possible
			□ Unlikely

Effects CARBAMAZEPINE plasma levels may increase; toxicity may result.

Mechanism CIMETIDINE inhibition of CARBAMAZEPINE hepatic metabolism.

Management Monitor serum CARBAMAZEPINE concentrations, and observe the patient for signs of toxicity after initiation of CIMETIDINE therapy. Adjust the dose accordingly.

Discussion

Since the first case linking carbamazepine toxicity to an interaction with cimetidine was reported,[1] the findings from clinical investigations of this interaction have been equivocal. A reduction in carbamazepine clearance was demonstrated in the reports in which steady-state serum carbamazepine concentrations had not been reached (ie, single-dose or short-term studies).[3-5] No effect or only transient decreases in carbamazepine clearance were observed in the trials in which cimetidine was withheld until steady-state serum carbamazepine concentrations were attained.[2,6,8]

This interaction appears to be of greater clinical importance when cimetidine is added to carbamazepine during the first 4 weeks of therapy. After steady-state serum carbamazepine concentrations are achieved, it appears that the effect of cimetidine on carbamazepine clearance decreases and is transient in nature. However, carbamazepine toxicity may still occur.[8] Ranitidine did not alter single-dose carbamazepine pharmacokinetics in 8 healthy subjects.[7]

[1] Telerman-Toppet N, et al. *Ann Intern Med.* 1981;94:544.
[2] Sonne J, et al. *Acta Neurol Scand.* 1983;68:253.
[3] MacPhee GJA, et al. *Br J Clin Pharmacol.* 1984;18:411.
[4] Webster LK, et al. *Eur J Clin Pharmacol.* 1984;27:341.
[5] Dalton MJ, et al. *Epilepsia.* 1985;26:127.
[6] Levine M, et al. *Neurology.* 1985;35:562.
[7] Dalton MJ, et al. *DICP.* 1985;19:941.
[8] Dalton MJ, et al. *Epilepsia.* 1986;27:553.

* Asterisk indicates drugs cited in interaction reports.

Carbamazepine — *Danazol*

Carbamazepine* (eg, *Tegretol*)	Danazol*

Significance	Onset	Severity	Documentation
2	☐ Rapid	☐ Major	☐ Established
	■ **Delayed**	■ **Moderate**	☐ Probable
		☐ Minor	■ **Suspected**
			☐ Possible
			☐ Unlikely

Effects Serum CARBAMAZEPINE concentrations may be increased, resulting in an increase in pharmacologic and toxic effects.

Mechanism DANAZOL inhibition of CARBAMAZEPINE metabolism.

Management Avoid this combination if possible. If both drugs are given, monitor CARBAMAZEPINE serum levels and observe patients for signs of toxicity after initiating DANAZOL therapy. In patients stabilized on CARBAMAZEPINE, it may be necessary to alter the dose when starting or stopping DANAZOL.

Discussion

Carbamazepine clearance was markedly reduced and elimination half-life was correspondingly prolonged after danazol was added to the drug regimen of a 34-year-old woman treated for partial seizures and endometriosis. Using radiolabeled carbamazepine, it was demonstrated that carbamazepine metabolism decreased during concurrent danazol therapy.[1] After the addition of danazol for fibrocystic breast disease in 6 women stabilized on antiepileptic drug regimens that included carbamazepine, 5 complained of neurotoxicity (eg, lethargy, ataxia); 2 patients required hospitalization. Serum carbamazepine concentrations increased by 38% to 123% within 30 days, while serum concentrations of the other antiepileptic drugs remained approximately the same. Symptoms improved and serum carbamazepine concentrations decreased when danazol was discontinued or carbamazepine doses were reduced.[2] In a 48-year-old woman stabilized on a regimen of carbamazepine/sodium valproate (eg, *Depakene*), carbamazepine serum concentrations doubled and clinical toxicity occurred 4 days after adding danazol.[3]

[1] Krämer G, et al. *Ther Drug Monit.* 1986;8(4):387.
[2] Zielinski JJ, et al. *Ther Drug Monit.* 1987;9(1):24.
[3] Hayden M, et al. *Med J Aust.* 1991;155(11-12):851.

* Asterisk indicates drugs cited in interaction reports.

Carbamazepine — *Diltiazem*

Carbamazepine* (eg, *Tegretol*)	Diltiazem* (eg, *Cardizem*)

Significance	Onset	Severity	Documentation
2	☐ Rapid	☐ Major	☐ Established
	■ **Delayed**	■ **Moderate**	☐ Probable
		☐ Minor	■ **Suspected**
			☐ Possible
			☐ Unlikely

Effects Serum CARBAMAZEPINE concentrations may be increased; CARBAMAZEPINE toxicity may result.

Mechanism DILTIAZEM inhibition of the metabolic degradation of CARBAMAZEPINE is suspected.

Management Monitor serum CARBAMAZEPINE levels, and observe patients for signs of CARBAMAZEPINE toxicity or a loss of therapeutic effect if DILTIAZEM is added to or discontinued from the treatment regimen. Be prepared to increase the CARBAMAZEPINE dose if DILTIAZEM is discontinued.

Discussion

Five case reports demonstrated a temporal relationship among the initiation of diltiazem, increases in serum carbamazepine concentrations, and the onset of symptoms consistent with carbamazepine toxicity.[1-3] Hospitalization was required for a 78-year-old woman. A 43-year-old man was subsequently treated with nifedipine (eg, *Procardia*), and serum carbamazepine levels were not affected. However, in a 60-year-old woman, discontinuation of diltiazem resulted in a drop in the carbamazepine serum concentration, which was associated with recurrence of seizure activity.[3] A 69-year-old woman stabilized on carbamazepine 300 mg/day for trigeminal neuralgia developed carbamazepine toxicity and elevated serum levels (14.4 mcg/mL) 2 weeks after starting diltiazem 120 mg/day. Carbamazepine levels returned to the therapeutic range, and toxicity resolved after stopping diltiazem.[4] A 64-year-old man stabilized on a regimen of carbamazepine 800 mg/day, perphenazine 40 mg/day, and diltiazem 180 mg/day experienced depression and a 54% (from 10.1 mcg/mL to 4 to 6 mcg/mL) decrease in carbamazepine serum concentration after diltiazem was discontinued.[5] Nifedipine does not appear to affect carbamazepine concentrations.[1,6] See Carbamazepine-Verapamil.

1 Brodie MJ, et al. *Br Med J (Clin Res Ed).* 1986;292(6529):1170.
2 Eimer M, et al. *Drug Intell Clin Pharm.* 1987;21(4)1:340.
3 Maoz E, et al. *Arch Intern Med.* 1992;152(12):2503.
4 Ahmad S. *Am Heart J.* 1990;120(6, pt 1):1485.
5 Gadde K, et al. *J Clin Psychopharmacol.* 1990;10(5):378.
6 Bahls FH, et al. *Neurology.* 1991;41(5):740.

* Asterisk indicates drugs cited in interaction reports.

Carbamazepine — *Efavirenz*

Carbamazepine* (eg, *Tegretol*)	Efavirenz* (*Sustiva*)

Significance	Onset	Severity	Documentation
4	☐ Rapid ■ **Delayed**	☐ Major ■ **Moderate** ☐ Minor	☐ Established ☐ Probable ☐ Suspected ■ **Possible** ☐ Unlikely

Effects Plasma concentrations of CARBAMAZEPINE and EFAVIRENZ may be reduced, decreasing the efficacy.

Mechanism CARBAMAZEPINE and EFAVIRENZ are suspected to induce the metabolism of each other.

Management When these agents are coadministered, closely monitor the clinical response of patients and adjust treatment as needed. Consider titration of CARBAMAZEPINE to a higher dose or selection of an alternative anticonvulsant. Also, a higher dose of EFAVIRENZ may be needed.

Discussion

Using a randomized, open-label, crossover design, the potential for an interaction between carbamazepine and efavirenz was evaluated in 26 healthy subjects.[1] One group of subjects received efavirenz 600 mg/day for 35 days. On days 15 through 35, carbamazepine titrated to 400 mg/day was coadministered with efavirenz. A second group of subjects received carbamazepine titrated to 400 mg/day for 35 days. On days 22 through 35, efavirenz 600 mg/day was coadministered with carbamazepine. Compared with giving efavirenz alone, coadministration of carbamazepine reduced the efavirenz AUC, C_{max}, and C_{min} approximately 36%, 21%, and 47%, respectively. Compared with giving carbamazepine alone, coadministration of efavirenz reduced the carbamazepine AUC, C_{max}, and C_{min} approximately 27%, 20%, and 35%, respectively. However, the effect of efavirenz on the pharmacokinetics of the active metabolite of carbamazepine, carbamazepine-10-11-epoxide, were minimal.

[1] Ji P, et al. *J Clin Pharmacol.* 2008;48(8):948.

* Asterisk indicates drugs cited in interaction reports.

Carbamazepine — *Felbamate*

Carbamazepine* (eg, *Tegretol*)	Felbamate* (*Felbatol*)

Significance	Onset	Severity	Documentation
2	☐ Rapid	☐ Major	☐ Established
	■ **Delayed**	■ **Moderate**	☐ Probable
		☐ Minor	■ **Suspected**
			☐ Possible
			☐ Unlikely

Effects Decreased CARBAMAZEPINE or FELBAMATE serum concentrations, possibly resulting in a loss of effectiveness.

Mechanism Unknown. Possibly increased metabolism of CARBAMAZEPINE or decreased conversion of the active epoxide metabolite of CARBAMAZEPINE to the diol metabolite. CARBAMAZEPINE may also increase the metabolism of FELBAMATE.

Management During any change in drug therapy, observe patients for changes in seizure control. The epoxide metabolite is active and may pharmacodynamically balance the decrease in CARBAMAZEPINE concentration. Also, in patients receiving FELBAMATE, carefully monitor concentrations if therapy with CARBAMAZEPINE is altered.

Discussion

Administration of felbamate to patients stabilized on monotherapy with carbamazepine decreased carbamazepine serum concentrations.[1] The effect was apparent after 1 week of concurrent felbamate and carbamazepine therapy and persisted during the entire treatment period. A plateau was reached during the 2 to 4 weeks of treatment and serum carbamazepine concentrations returned to initial values 2 to 3 weeks after felbamate was discontinued. The average decrease in carbamazepine concentration was 25% (range, 10% to 42%). The decrease in carbamazepine concentration was accompanied by marked increases in the active epoxide metabolite of carbamazepine (46% increase) and ratio of the epoxide metabolite to carbamazepine (100% increase). The effects of felbamate on carbamazepine and its metabolites have been studied in epileptic patients receiving concomitant phenytoin (eg, *Dilantin*) and carbamazepine.[2-4] Addition of felbamate produced a decrease in the serum carbamazepine concentration,[2-4] an increase in the carbamazepine epoxide metabolite concentration,[2,4] an increase in the epoxide/carbamazepine ratio,[4] and an increase in the epoxide/diol metabolites ratio.[4]

Carbamazepine also increases felbamate clearance, decreasing serum felbamate concentrations.[5] See also Hydantoins-Felbamate.

[1] Albani F, et al. *Epilepsia.* 1991;32(1):130.
[2] Fuerst RH, et al. *Epilepsia.* 1988;29(4):488.
[3] Graves NM, et al. *Epilepsia.* 1989;30(2):225.
[4] Wagner ML, et al. *Clin Pharmacol Ther.* 1993;53(5):536.
[5] Wagner ML, et al. *Epilepsia.* 1991;32(3):398.

* Asterisk indicates drugs cited in interaction reports.

Carbamazepine — *Fluoxetine*

Carbamazepine* (eg, *Tegretol*)	Fluoxetine* (eg, *Prozac*)

Significance	Onset	Severity	Documentation
2	☐ Rapid	☐ Major	☐ Established
	■ **Delayed**	■ **Moderate**	☐ Probable
		☐ Minor	■ **Suspected**
			☐ Possible
			☐ Unlikely

Effects Serum CARBAMAZEPINE levels may be increased, producing possible toxicity.

Mechanism Unknown. However, FLUOXETINE is known to inhibit the metabolism of other drugs, suggesting that this may be the mechanism.

Management Monitor serum CARBAMAZEPINE levels during coadministration of FLUOXETINE. Adjust the dose of CARBAMAZEPINE accordingly. Sertraline (eg, *Zoloft*) does not appear to interact with CARBAMAZEPINE and may be an alternative.[1]

Discussion

Two patients stabilized on carbamazepine therapy experienced increased serum carbamazepine levels and symptoms of carbamazepine toxicity when fluoxetine was added to their treatment regimens.[2] A 55-year-old woman had been receiving carbamazepine 1 g/day for 3 years. Plasma levels were 36 mcmol/L. One week after starting fluoxetine 20 mg/day, the patient experienced diplopia, blurred vision, tremor, and vertigo, which worsened over the following 2 weeks. The carbamazepine level was 48 mcmol/L. The dosage of carbamazepine was reduced to 800 mg/day and, except for the tremors, the patient's symptoms resolved over the next 2 weeks. A 45-year-old woman had been receiving carbamazepine 600 mg/day for 5 months and had a plasma level of 27 mcmol/L. Ten days after starting fluoxetine 20 mg/day, the patient had an exacerbation of previously experienced symptoms, including slurred speech, ataxia, and myoclonic leg movements. In addition, new symptoms of nausea, vomiting, vertigo, and tinnitus occurred. All symptoms increased in severity over the next 3 weeks. Fluoxetine was discontinued and, within 2 weeks, the symptoms of vertigo, tinnitus, and vomiting abated, and the remaining symptoms returned to their previous level of intensity. In 6 healthy men receiving carbamazepine 400 mg/day for 21 days and then carbamazepine plus fluoxetine 20 mg/day for 7 days, addition of fluoxetine produced a 27% increase in the carbamazepine AUC, a 31% increase in the carbamazepine 10,11-epoxide metabolite, and a 46% reduction in carbamazepine intrinsic clearance.[3] An in vitro study in human liver microsomes showed no inhibition of this carbamazepine metabolite with either fluoxetine or norfluoxetine.[4] Additional studies are needed to document the clinical importance of this possible interaction.

[1] Rapeport WG, et al. *J Clin Psychiatry.* 1996;57(suppl 1):20.
[2] Pearson HJ. *J Clin Psychiatry.* 1990;51(3):126.
[3] Grimsley SR, et al. *Clin Pharmacol Ther.* 1991;50(1):10.
[4] Gidal BE, et al. *Ther Drug Monit.* 1993;15(5):405.

* Asterisk indicates drugs cited in interaction reports.

Carbamazepine — *Fluvoxamine*

Carbamazepine* (eg, *Tegretol*)	Fluvoxamine* (eg, *Luvox*)

Significance	Onset	Severity	Documentation
4	☐ Rapid	☐ Major	☐ Established
	■ **Delayed**	■ **Moderate**	☐ Probable
		☐ Minor	☐ Suspected
			■ **Possible**
			☐ Unlikely

Effects Serum CARBAMAZEPINE concentrations may be increased, resulting in an increase in the pharmacologic and toxic effects.

Mechanism Unknown.

Management When starting therapy with CARBAMAZEPINE in patients receiving FLUVOXAMINE, consider giving a conservative dose of CARBAMAZEPINE and carefully titrating therapy. In patients stabilized on CARBAMAZEPINE, altering the dose when starting or stopping FLUVOXAMINE may be necessary. Monitor serum CARBAMAZEPINE concentrations, and observe patients for signs of toxicity. Sertraline does not appear to interact with CARBAMAZEPINE and may be an alternative.[1]

Discussion

Coadministration of fluvoxamine and carbamazepine may result in increased plasma carbamazepine concentrations and toxicity.[2,3] In 1 patient with bipolar depressive disorder receiving chronic treatment with carbamazepine 600 mg/day, trough plasma carbamazepine concentrations increased from 8 to 19 mcg/mL 1 week after starting fluvoxamine 100 mg/day.[3] In addition, the patient displayed signs of carbamazepine toxicity. Fluvoxamine was discontinued, and plasma carbamazepine concentrations returned to previous values in 10 days or less. A similar interaction has been reported in 3 other patients taking carbamazepine and fluvoxamine.[2] However, in a prospective study designed to investigate the interaction between carbamazepine and fluvoxamine, administration of fluvoxamine 100 mg/day to 7 epileptic patients receiving long-term treatment with carbamazepine 800 to 1,600 mg/day did not produce any changes in steady-state serum concentrations of carbamazepine or its active epoxide metabolite.[4]

1 Rapeport WG, et al. *J Clin Psychiatry.* 1996;57(suppl 1):20.
2 Fritze J, et al. *Acta Psychiatr Scand.* 1991;84(6):583.
3 Martinelli V, et al. *Br J Clin Pharmacol.* 1993;36(6):615.
4 Spina E, et al. *Ther Drug Monit.* 1993;15(3):247.

* Asterisk indicates drugs cited in interaction reports.

Carbamazepine — *Food*

Carbamazepine* (eg, *Tegretol*)	Grapefruit Juice*

Significance	Onset	Severity	Documentation
2	☐ Rapid	☐ Major	☐ Established
	■ **Delayed**	■ **Moderate**	☐ Probable
		☐ Minor	■ **Suspected**
			☐ Possible
			☐ Unlikely

Effects Serum CARBAMAZEPINE concentrations may be elevated, producing an increase in the pharmacologic effects and adverse reactions.

Mechanism Possibly due to inhibition of gut wall and hepatic metabolism (CYP3A4) of CARBAMAZEPINE.

Management Avoid coadministration of CARBAMAZEPINE with grapefruit products. Caution patients to take CARBAMAZEPINE with liquids other than GRAPEFRUIT JUICE.

Discussion

The effect of grapefruit juice on the bioavailability of carbamazepine was evaluated in 10 patients with epilepsy.[1] The study was a randomized, crossover design in which each patient received carbamazepine 200 mg 3 times daily for 3 to 4 weeks. On study days, the patients were given carbamazepine 200 mg with either 300 mL of grapefruit juice or water. Each treatment was separated by 2 days, and carbamazepine therapy was not interrupted. Compared with giving carbamazepine with water, administration with grapefruit juice increased the peak concentration of carbamazepine from 6.55 to 9.2 mcg/mL (40.4%), the trough concentration from 4.51 to 6.28 mcg/mL (39.2%), and the AUC by 40.8%. The time to reach the peak plasma carbamazepine concentration was not affected.

[1] Garg SK, et al. *Clin Pharmacol Ther.* 1998;64(3):286.

* Asterisk indicates drugs cited in interaction reports.

Carbamazepine — *Isoniazid*

Carbamazepine* (eg, *Tegretol*)	Isoniazid* (eg, *Nydrazid*)

Significance	Onset	Severity	Documentation
2	□ Rapid	□ Major	□ Established
	■ **Delayed**	■ **Moderate**	□ Probable
		□ Minor	■ **Suspected**
			□ Possible
			□ Unlikely

Effects CARBAMAZEPINE toxicity, ISONIAZID hepatotoxicity, or both may result.

Mechanism ISONIAZID is suspected to inhibit CARBAMAZEPINE metabolism, and CARBAMAZEPINE may increase ISONIAZID degradation to hepatotoxic metabolites.

Management Monitor serum CARBAMAZEPINE concentrations, and observe patients for toxicity. Adjust the dose of CARBAMAZEPINE as needed. Monitor liver function and consider discontinuing ISONIAZID if hepatotoxicity occurs.

Discussion

Reports are almost exclusively related to carbamazepine toxicity.[1-3] In 2 patients maintained on carbamazepine and other anticonvulsants, addition of isoniazid precipitated reactions consistent with carbamazepine toxicity in conjunction with toxic serum concentrations.[2,3] In both patients, symptoms resolved and serum carbamazepine levels returned to the therapeutic range after stopping isoniazid. A third patient had toxic reactions during administration of carbamazepine and isoniazid plus rifampin.[4] Addition of isoniazid for tuberculosis prophylaxis in 10 of 13 epileptic patients resulted in symptoms of carbamazepine toxicity.[1] Serum carbamazepine concentrations could be obtained from 3 patients; all were in the toxic range. Symptoms resolved and serum carbamazepine levels returned to baseline after reducing the carbamazepine dose 50%. Coadministration of isoniazid and other agents known to impair carbamazepine metabolism (eg, cimetidine [eg, *Tagamet*]) may potentiate isoniazid-induced carbamazepine toxicity.[5]

In one patient, serum liver enzyme concentrations increased within days of carbamazepine and isoniazid coadministration. Although serum liver enzymes continued to increase for 3 days after discontinuation of isoniazid, they ultimately returned to baseline.[3] Similar findings have been reported in another study.[6]

[1] Valsalan VC, et al. *Br Med J.* 1982;285(6337):261.
[2] Block SH. *Pediatrics.* 1982;69(4):494.
[3] Wright JM, et al. *N Engl J Med.* 1982;307(21):1325.
[4] Fleenor ME, et al. *Chest.* 1991;99(6):1554.
[5] García B, et al. *Ann Pharmacother.* 1992;26(6):841.
[6] Barbare JC, et al. *Gastroenterol Clin Biol.* 1986;10(6–7):523.

* Asterisk indicates drugs cited in interaction reports.

Carbamazepine — *Isotretinoin*

Carbamazepine* (eg, *Tegretol*)	Isotretinoin* (eg, *Accutane*)

Significance	Onset	Severity	Documentation
4	■ **Rapid**	□ Major	□ Established
	□ Delayed	■ **Moderate**	□ Probable
		□ Minor	□ Suspected
			■ **Possible**
			□ Unlikely

Effects The pharmacologic effects of CARBAMAZEPINE may be decreased.

Mechanism Unknown. Possible alteration of bioavailability and clearance of CARBAMAZEPINE or its metabolite by ISOTRETINOIN.

Management During concurrent treatment with these drugs, monitor CARBAMAZEPINE levels. Adjust the dose accordingly.

Discussion

A 23-year-old man with tonic–clonic epilepsy had been treated with carbamazepine 600 mg once daily for 4 years with good control of seizures and without adverse reactions.[1] During concurrent therapy with isotretinoin for severe acne, both the plasma and salivary carbamazepine AUCs decreased. The oral clearance of the antiepileptic agent increased during treatment with isotretinoin 1 mg/kg/day but not with 0.5 mg/kg/day. The ratio of plasma carbamazepine AUC to carbamazepine 10,11-epoxide AUC, an active metabolite, was 6.3 prior to isotretinoin treatment and 7 and 8.5 with isotretinoin 0.5 and 1 mg/kg/day, respectively. Saliva ratios were 3, 4, and 5.6, respectively.

[1] Marsden JR. *Br J Dermatol.* 1988;119(3):403.

* Asterisk indicates drugs cited in interaction reports.

Carbamazepine — *Levetiracetam*

Carbamazepine* (eg, *Tegretol*)	Levetiracetam* (*Keppra*)

Significance	Onset	Severity	Documentation
4	☐ Rapid	☐ Major	☐ Established
	■ **Delayed**	■ **Moderate**	☐ Probable
		☐ Minor	☐ Suspected
			■ **Possible**
			☐ Unlikely

Effects CARBAMAZEPINE toxicity, unrelated to elevated plasma concentrations, may occur.

Mechanism Unknown; however, a pharmacodynamic interaction is suspected.

Management Closely monitor patients receiving CARBAMAZEPINE for symptoms of toxicity when starting or increasing the dose of LEVETIRACETAM; possible CARBAMAZEPINE dose reduction or LEVETIRACETAM withdrawal may be needed.

Discussion

Carbamazepine toxicity was reported in 4 patients with severe refractory epilepsy after levetiracetam was added to their treatment regimen.[1] When levetiracetam was started, 3 patients receiving carbamazepine were taking at least 1 other medication, while the remaining patient was receiving carbamazepine monotherapy. In all patients, levetiracetam was started at 500 mg/day. Upon increasing the dosage of levetiracetam to 500 mg twice daily in 2 patients, 1,000 mg twice daily in 1 patient, and 1,500 mg/day in the remaining patient, disabling symptoms of carbamazepine toxicity (eg, ataxia, nystagmus, unsteady gait) occurred. The symptoms resolved in 3 patients when the carbamazepine dose was reduced. The fourth patient discontinued levetiracetam on her own accord. Neither carbamazepine nor carbamazepine-epoxide plasma concentrations were elevated. No changes in carbamazepine levels were seen in a study of 35 children who took carbamazepine plus levetiracetam for 14 weeks.[2] Toxicity was not reported.

[1] Sisodiya SM, et al. *Epilepsy Res.* 2002;48(3):217.

[2] Otoul C, et al. *Epilepsia.* 2007;48(11):2111.

* Asterisk indicates drugs cited in interaction reports.

Carbamazepine — *Loxapine*

Carbamazepine* (eg, *Tegretol*)	Loxapine* (eg, *Loxitane*)

Significance	Onset	Severity	Documentation
4	☐ Rapid ■ **Delayed**	☐ Major ■ **Moderate** ☐ Minor	☐ Established ☐ Probable ☐ Suspected ■ **Possible** ☐ Unlikely

Effects Serum concentrations of the epoxide metabolite of CARBAMAZEPINE may be increased, resulting in possible neurotoxicity.

Mechanism Increased metabolism of CARBAMAZEPINE or decreased elimination of CARBAMAZEPINE epoxide is suspected.

Management Observe patients for signs of neurotoxicity. If an interaction is suspected, the dose of CARBAMAZEPINE may need to be reduced. Because serum CARBAMAZEPINE levels may be normal or low, measurements of serum CARBAMAZEPINE and the epoxide metabolite concentrations would be helpful in monitoring patients.

Discussion

A possible drug interaction between carbamazepine and loxapine was reported in a 55-year-old man.[1] The patient had a history of chronic schizophrenia, hypertension, and myoclonic seizures. At the time carbamazepine (CBZ) was started, the patient was receiving loxapine 350 mg/day, imipramine (eg, *Tofranil*) 250 mg/day, enalapril (eg, *Vasotec*) 2.5 mg/day, and chlorthalidone (eg, *Hygroton*) 25 mg 3 times a week. In addition, the patient was receiving valproic acid (eg, *Depakene*) 750 mg/day; however, valproic acid therapy was stopped when carbamazepine 200 mg 3 times daily was initiated. Ten days after starting carbamazepine, the patient experienced neurotoxicity and the dosage was decreased to 100 mg twice daily. Ten days after the dosage adjustment, plasma concentrations of carbamazepine and the carbamazepine epoxide (CBZE) metabolite were 2.6 and 2 mcg/mL, respectively (CBZE/CBZ ratio, 0.76). Approximately 3 years later, the CBZE/CBZ ratio was virtually unchanged (0.71) and the patient had not experienced seizures or toxicity. Seven months later, loxapine therapy was discontinued and clozapine was started. Carbamazepine and CBZE concentrations obtained 1 month later were 3.3 and 0.6 mcg/mL, respectively (CBZE/CBZ, 0.18). Subsequently, in a retrospective review of 4 additional patients receiving carbamazepine and loxapine, the ratio of serum CBZE/CBZ concentrations was higher than expected.

[1] Collins DM, et al. *Ann Pharmacother.* 1993;27(10):1180.

* Asterisk indicates drugs cited in interaction reports.

Carbamazepine — *Macrolide Antibiotics*

Carbamazepine* (eg, *Tegretol*)	Clarithromycin* (*Biaxin*) Erythromycin* (eg, *Ery-Tab*)	Troleandomycin*† (*Tao*)

Significance	Onset	Severity	Documentation
1	■ **Rapid** □ Delayed	■ **Major** □ Moderate □ Minor	■ **Established** □ Probable □ Suspected □ Possible □ Unlikely

Effects CARBAMAZEPINE concentration/toxicity may be increased.

Mechanism Inhibition of CARBAMAZEPINE (CBZ) hepatic metabolism (CYP3A4), leading to decreased CBZ clearance.[4,15,17]

Management Avoid this combination if possible; otherwise, monitor CBZ levels, and closely observe the patient for toxicity. Consider stopping either drug, decreasing the CBZ dose or using an alternative macrolide (eg, azithromycin [*Zithromax*])[18] or anti-infective agent that is unlikely to interact.

Discussion

Elevated CBZ levels with toxicity (within 24 hours to a few days) have been reported in children and adults after initiation of erythromycin therapy. Hospitalization was often required and, in some cases, included immediate resuscitative measures. Symptoms and serum CBZ levels decreased upon discontinuation of erythromycin.[2,3,5-14,16,21] Clinical signs of CBZ toxicity were reported within 24 hours of troleandomycin (TOA) administration to 8 epileptic patients.[1] In 17 epileptic patients on CBZ 8 to 36 mg/kg/day, adding TOA 8 to 33 mg/kg/day caused acute toxicity within 24 to 48 hours.[2] When TOA was discontinued, symptoms subsided in 2 to 3 days. In a patient stabilized on CBZ, addition of clarithromycin 250 mg twice daily for 10 days increased CBZ levels 60% despite a 22% reduction in CBZ dose.[19] In 2 other cases, CBZ toxicity occurred with CBZ levels of 15 and 19 mcg/mL after starting clarithromycin.[20] Symptoms resolved after stopping clarithromycin. Introduction of clarithromycin as part of a *Helicobacter pylori* regimen resulted in elevations of serum CBZ levels in 2 previously well-controlled patients.[22] Neither patient developed symptoms, and in both, the CBZ levels returned to baseline after stopping clarithromycin.

1 Dravet C, et al. *Lancet.* 1977;1:810.
2 Mesdjian E, et al. *Epilepsia.* 1980;21:489.
3 Straughan J. *S Afr Med J.* 1982;61:420.
4 Wong YY, et al. *Clin Pharmacol Ther.* 1983;33:460.
5 Hedrick R, et al. *Ther Drug Monit.* 1983;5:405.
6 Vajda FJ, et al. *Med J Aust.* 1984;140:81.
7 Carranco E, et al. *Arch Neurol.* 1985;42:187.
8 Kessler JM. *S Afr Med J.* 1985;67:1038.
9 Wroblewski BA, et al. *JAMA.* 1986;255:1165.
10 Berrettini WH, et al. *J Clin Psychiatry.* 1986;47:147.
11 Jaster PJ, et al. *Neurology.* 1986;36:594.
12 Goulden KJ, et al. *J Pediatr.* 1986;109:135.
13 Zitelli BJ, et al. *Clin Pediatr.* 1987;26:117.
14 Woody RC. *Pediatr Infect Dis J.* 1987;6:578.
15 Barzaghi N, et al. *Br J Clin Pharmacol.* 1987;24:836.
16 Macnab AJ, et al. *Pediatrics.* 1987;80:952.
17 Miles MV, et al. *Ther Drug Monit.* 1989;11:47.
18 Hopkins S. *Am J Med.* 1991;91(Suppl 3A):3A.
19 Albani F, et al. *Epilepsia.* 1993;34:161.
20 Tatum WO, et al. *Hosp Pharm.* 1994;29:45.
21 Stafstrom CE, et al. *Arch Pediatr Adolesc Med.* 1995;149:99
22 Metz DC, et al. *Dig Dis Sci.* 1995;40:912.

* Asterisk indicates drugs cited in interaction reports.
† Not available in the United States.

Carbamazepine — *MAOIs*

Carbamazepine* (eg, *Tegretol*)	Isocarboxazid* (*Marplan*)	Phenelzine* (*Nardil*)
	Tranylcypromine* (*Parnate*)	

Significance	Onset	Severity	Documentation
1	☐ Rapid ■ **Delayed**	■ **Major** ☐ Moderate ☐ Minor	☐ Established ☐ Probable ■ **Suspected** ☐ Possible ☐ Unlikely

Effects Theoretical risk of severe side effects (eg, hyperpyrexia, hyperexcitability, muscle rigidity, seizures).

Mechanism Unknown.

Management On theoretical grounds, coadministration of CARBAMAZEPINE and an MONOAMINE OXIDASE INHIBITOR (MAOI) is contraindicated.[6] Discontinue the MAOI at least 14 days prior to administration of CARBAMAZEPINE.

Discussion

Although the product information for carbamazepine notes a theoretical risk of side effects when carbamazepine is coadministered with MAOIs, several case reports document some clinical success and no evidence of toxicity during concurrent use. Carbamazepine is structurally related to tricyclic antidepressants. Since hypertensive crisis, convulsions, and death have occurred with coadministration of tricyclic antidepressants and MAOIs, carbamazepine administration is contraindicated with MAOIs. Tranylcypromine was added to the treatment regimen of a 24-year-old man who was receiving carbamazepine and lithium (eg, *Eskalith*).[1] Tranylcypromine administration did not increase carbamazepine plasma levels or cause side effects. Subsequently, 2 other patients were reported who did not experience an increase in carbamazepine plasma levels or apparent toxicity when tranylcypromine was coadministered.[2] In another report, a 70-year-old woman did not experience a marked rise in carbamazepine plasma levels or toxicity during concurrent treatment with phenelzine and carbamazepine.[3] Ten patients receiving carbamazepine or carbamazepine plus lithium, tolerated the addition of an MAOI (ie, tranylcypromine or phenelzine) treatment without experiencing changes in carbamazepine levels or the occurrence of toxicity.[5] Others have reported that MAOIs differ in their effect on carbamazepine plasma levels to explain why 5 patients receiving tranylcypromine required a carbamazepine dose that was 2.3 times higher than the dose needed by 4 patients taking phenelzine and carbamazepine.[4] See also Tricyclic Antidepressants-MAOIs.

[1] Joffe RT, et al. *Arch Gen Psychiatry*. 1985;42:738.
[2] Lydiard RB, et al. *J Clin Psychopharmacol*. 1987;7:360.
[3] Yatham LN, et al. *Am J Psychiatry*. 1990;147:367.
[4] Barklage NE, et al. *J Clin Psychiatry*. 1992;53:258.
[5] Ketter TA, et al. *J Clin Psychiatry*. 1995;56:471.
[6] Product information. Carbamazepine (*Tegretol*). Novartis Pharmaceuticals Corporation, 1998.

* Asterisk indicates drugs cited in interaction reports.

Carbamazepine — *Metronidazole*

Carbamazepine* (eg, *Tegretol*)	Metronidazole* (eg, *Flagyl*)

Significance	Onset	Severity	Documentation
4	☐ Rapid	☐ Major	☐ Established
	■ **Delayed**	■ **Moderate**	☐ Probable
		☐ Minor	☐ Suspected
			■ **Possible**
			☐ Unlikely

Effects Serum CARBAMAZEPINE concentrations may be elevated, increasing the pharmacologic and toxic effects of CARBAMAZEPINE.

Mechanism Possible inhibition of CARBAMAZEPINE metabolism.

Management Observe the clinical response of the patient when starting or stopping METRONIDAZOLE. Monitoring serum CARBAMAZEPINE concentrations may be useful in patient management. Adjust the dose of CARBAMAZEPINE as indicated.

Discussion

Increased carbamazepine serum concentrations with signs of toxicity were observed in a 49-year-old woman with bipolar disorder during coadministration of metronidazole.[1] In addition to carbamazepine, the patient was receiving conjugated estrogen and alprazolam (eg, *Xanax*). Plasma carbamazepine concentrations had been stable for 1.5 years. The dose of carbamazepine was increased from 800 to 1000 mg/day, which subsequently produced a serum concentration of 9 mcg/mL. The patient was started on oral metronidazole 250 mg 3 times daily and trimethoprim/sulfamethoxazole (TMP-SMZ [eg, *Bactrim*]) for diverticulitis. When symptoms worsened, the dose of metronidazole was increased to 500 mg IV 3 times/day, and cefazolin (eg, *Kefzol*) 500 mg IV every 8 hours was started. TMP-SMZ was discontinued. Two days later the patient experienced dizziness, diplopia, and nausea (carbamazepine concentration, 14.3 mcg/mL). The patient was discharged on oral metronidazole, and she reduced her own dose of carbamazepine to 800 mg/day because of adverse effects. A month later, after increasing the dose of carbamazepine to 1000 mg/day, the serum concentration was 7.1 mcg/mL.

[1] Patterson BD. *Ann Pharmacother.* 1994;28:1303.

* Asterisk indicates drugs cited in interaction reports.

Carbamazepine — *Nefazodone*

Carbamazepine* (eg, *Tegretol*)	Nefazodone* (*Serzone*)

Significance	Onset	Severity	Documentation
1	☐ Rapid ■ **Delayed**	■ **Major** ☐ Moderate ☐ Minor	☐ Established ☐ Probable ■ **Suspected** ☐ Possible ☐ Unlikely

Effects Elevated serum CARBAMAZEPINE levels with possible increase in side effects and lower NEFAZODONE levels with possible decrease in efficacy.

Mechanism NEFAZODONE may inhibit the hepatic metabolism (cytochrome P450 3A4) of CARBAMAZEPINE, while CARBAMAZEPINE may induce the metabolism of NEFAZODONE.

Management Coadministration of CARBAMAZEPINE and NEFAZODONE is contraindicated.[3]

Discussion

Carbamazepine toxicity in 2 patients with DSM-IV bipolar disorder was reported following the addition of nefazodone to their treatment regimens.[1] In the first patient, nefazodone 100 mg twice daily for 1 week was started, then increased to 150 mg twice daily. After 15 days, the patient reported lightheadedness and ataxia. The carbamazepine serum level was 10.8 mcg/mL. The carbamazepine dose was decreased to 800 mg/day. However, the carbamazepine serum level remained elevated (10.2 mcg/mL). When the daily dose of carbamazepine was reduced to 600 mg, the serum level decreased to 7.4 mcg/mL and carbamazepine side effects disappeared. The second patient was receiving 1000 mg/day of carbamazepine when nefazodone 100 mg twice daily was started. The dose of nefazodone was increased to 150 mg twice daily and approximately 2 weeks later, the patient reported diminished depth perception, sedation, slurred speech, loss of appetite, and hypersomnia of 12 to 13 hours/night. The serum carbamazepine level was 15.1 mcg/mL. The carbamazepine dose was reduced to 200 mg 3 times daily and nefazodone was discontinued. Within 5 days, the serum carbamazepine level decreased to 5.8 mcg/mL. In a controlled study of 12 healthy volunteers, the area under the concentration-time curve (AUC) of carbamazepine increased 23% during coadminstration of nefazodone and after a 30-day period to allow for self-induction of carbamazepine metabolism.[2] In the same study, concurrent use of both drugs decreased nefazodone AUC 93%.

[1] Ashton AK, et al. *Am J Psychiatry*. 1996;153:733.
[2] Laroudie C, et al. *J Clin Psychopharmacol*. 2000;20:46.
[3] Product information. Nefazodone (*Serzone*). Bristol-Myers Squibb. 2001.

* Asterisk indicates drugs cited in interaction reports.

Carbamazepine — *Nicotinamide*

Carbamazepine* (eg, *Tegretol*)	Nicotinamide*

Significance	Onset	Severity	Documentation
4	☐ Rapid	☐ Major	☐ Established
	■ **Delayed**	■ **Moderate**	☐ Probable
		☐ Minor	☐ Suspected
			■ **Possible**
			☐ Unlikely

Effects Increased CARBAMAZEPINE serum concentrations with resulting toxicity may occur.

Mechanism Decreased CARBAMAZEPINE clearance as a result of NICOTINAMIDE inhibition of hepatic degradation has been proposed.

Management Monitor serum CARBAMAZEPINE concentrations and observe for signs of toxicity. Adjust the dose accordingly.

Discussion

Carbamazepine clearance decreased and serum concentrations increased after the addition of nicotinamide (niacinamide) to the treatment regimen of 2 epileptic children.[1] Both children were taking several antiseizure medications concurrently, making it difficult to discern an interaction between carbamazepine and nicotinamide.

[1] Bourgeois BF, et al. *Neurology.* 1982;32:1122.

* Asterisk indicates drugs cited in interaction reports.

Carbamazepine — *Piperine*

Carbamazepine* (eg, *Tegretol*)	Piperine*

Significance **5**

Onset	Severity	Documentation
☐ Rapid	☐ Major	☐ Established
■ **Delayed**	☐ Moderate	☐ Probable
	■ **Minor**	☐ Suspected
		■ **Possible**
		☐ Unlikely

Effects CARBAMAZEPINE concentrations may be elevated, increasing the pharmacologic effects and risk of adverse reactions.

Mechanism Unknown.

Management Caution patients receiving CARBAMAZEPINE to consult their health care provider before using herbal products or receiving other complementary/alternative therapies (eg, Ayurvedic medicine).

Discussion

Piperine is a major alkaloidal component of black pepper and long pepper. The effects of a single dose of piperine on the steady-state pharmacokinetics of carbamazepine were studied in 2 groups of 10 adult epileptic patients.[1] One group of patients was receiving carbamazepine 300 mg twice daily and the second group was receiving carbamazepine 500 mg twice daily for at least 2 months when a single dose of piperine 20 mg was administered. Patients received the piperine dose with their morning dose of carbamazepine. In patients who had been receiving carbamazepine 300 mg twice daily, piperine slightly increased the carbamazepine C_{max} and AUC (approximately 8% and 10%, respectively) compared with administering carbamazepine alone. When piperine was given to patients receiving carbamazepine 500 mg twice daily, the C_{max} and AUC increased 10% and 13%, respectively, while the T_{max} was decreased approximately 14% and the $t_{½}$ was prolonged 40%. The magnitude of these changes is not likely to be clinically important.

[1] Pattanaik S, et al. *Phytother Res.* 2009;23(9):1281.

* Asterisk indicates drugs cited in interaction reports.

Carbamazepine — *Probenecid*

Carbamazepine* (eg, *Tegretol*)	Probenecid*

Significance	Onset	Severity	Documentation
5	☐ Rapid	☐ Major	☐ Established
	■ **Delayed**	☐ Moderate	☐ Probable
		■ **Minor**	☐ Suspected
			■ **Possible**
			☐ Unlikely

Effects CARBAMAZEPINE plasma concentrations may be decreased slightly.

Mechanism Induction of CARBAMAZEPINE metabolism (CYP2C8 and CYP3A4) is suspected.

Management Based on available data, no special precautions are needed.

Discussion

The effects of probenecid on the pharmacokinetics of carbamazepine were studied in 10 healthy men.[1] Using a randomized, open-label, 2-way crossover design, each subject received probenecid 500 mg or a matching placebo twice daily for 10 days. On day 6, a single dose of carbamazepine 200 mg was administered. Compared with placebo, probenecid decreased the AUC of carbamazepine 19% while increasing the AUC of the carbamazepine 10,11-epoxide metabolite 33%. Probenecid increased the oral clearance of carbamazepine 26% and increased the AUC ratio of the epoxide metabolite to carbamazepine 45% (from 0.11 to 0.16). Probenecid had minimal effects on the recovery of the free and conjugated forms of carbamazepine and its metabolite in the urine.

[1] Kim KA, et al. *Eur J Clin Pharmacol.* 2005;61(4):275.

* Asterisk indicates drugs cited in interaction reports.

Carbamazepine — *Propoxyphene*

Carbamazepine* (eg, *Tegretol*)	Propoxyphene* (eg, *Darvon*)

Significance	Onset	Severity	Documentation
2	■ **Rapid** □ Delayed	□ Major ■ **Moderate** □ Minor	□ Established □ Probable ■ **Suspected** □ Possible □ Unlikely

Effects Increased CARBAMAZEPINE serum concentrations with resulting toxicity may occur.

Mechanism Inhibition of hepatic metabolism by PROPOXYPHENE may decrease CARBAMAZEPINE clearance.

Management Because of the potential for toxicity and the availability of alternative analgesics, avoid PROPOXYPHENE. If this combination is used, monitor serum CARBAMAZEPINE concentrations and observe patients for clinical signs of toxicity. Be prepared to adjust the CARBAMAZEPINE dose as needed.

Discussion

Five of 7 patients maintained on carbamazepine for neurological disorders reported symptoms of carbamazepine toxicity after taking propoxyphene 65 mg 3 times/day. In the 5 patients from whom serum carbamazepine levels could be obtained, increases ranged from 45% to 77%.[1] In another study, propoxyphene 65 mg 3 times/day was given to 8 patients who were maintained on carbamazepine. Subsequent serum carbamazepine levels in 6 patients revealed a mean increase of 66% over baseline; however, only 1 patient experienced carbamazepine toxicity.[2] Eight additional cases of carbamazepine toxicity following propoxyphene administration have been described.[3] Toxicity was associated with variable increases in levels up to 6-fold. Two patients were hospitalized, including 1 patient who became comatose within 24 hours after receiving 2 doses of propoxyphene. Elderly patients may be particularly sensitive and demonstrate signs of toxicity even with therapeutic carbamazepine serum levels.[4] Severe carbamazepine toxicity was reported in a patient maintained on carbamazepine within 2 days of starting propoxyphene napsylate 100 to 200 mg every 6 hours as needed.[5] The serum carbamazepine level increased to 25 mcg/mL from a baseline of 3.3 mcg/mL. After the clinical signs of toxicity resolved and steady-state serum carbamazepine levels were re-established, rechallenge with propoxyphene precipitated symptoms of carbamazepine toxicity, which again resolved after discontinuation of propoxyphene. Three other cases have been reported, but temporal relationships were not established.[6]

[1] Dam M, et al. *Acta Neurol Scand.* 1977;56:603.
[2] Hansen BS, et al. *Acta Neurol Scand.* 1980;61:357.
[3] Oles KS, et al. *Surg Neurol.* 1989;32:144.
[4] Bergendal L, et al. *Eur J Clin Pharmacol.* 1997;53:203.
[5] Kubacka RT, et al. *Clin Pharm.* 1983;2:104.
[6] Yu YL, et al. *Postgrad Med J.* 1986;62:231.

* Asterisk indicates drugs cited in interaction reports.

Carbamazepine — *Protease Inhibitors*

Carbamazepine	Protease Inhibitors	
Carbamazepine* (eg, *Tegretol*)	Amprenavir (*Agenerase*)	Nelfinavir* (*Viracept*)
	Atazanavir (*Reyataz*)	Ritonavir* (*Norvir*)
	Darunavir (*Prezista*)	Saquinavir* (eg, *Fortovase*)
	Fosamprenavir (*Lexiva*)	Tipranavir (*Aptivus*)
	Indinavir* (*Crixivan*)	
	Lopinavir/Ritonavir* (*Kaletra*)	

Significance	Onset	Severity	Documentation
2	■ **Rapid**	□ Major	□ Established
	□ Delayed	■ **Moderate**	□ Probable
		□ Minor	■ **Suspected**
			□ Possible
			□ Unlikely

Effects CARBAMAZEPINE levels may be elevated, increasing the risk of toxicity, while PROTEASE INHIBITOR levels may decrease, resulting in antiretroviral treatment failure.

Mechanism Inhibition of hepatic metabolism (CYP3A4) of CARBAMAZEPINE is suspected, while CARBAMAZEPINE may induce PROTEASE INHIBITOR metabolism (CYP3A4).

Management Closely monitor CARBAMAZEPINE serum levels when starting, stopping, or changing the dose of the PROTEASE INHIBITOR and observe the clinical response to PROTEASE INHIBITOR therapy. Adjust the dose as needed.

Discussion

In patients on stable carbamazepine doses, increased carbamazepine levels and signs of toxicity have been reported following the addition of lopinavir/ritonavir,[1] nelfinavir,[1] ritonavir,[2-4] or saquinavir[3,4] to the treatment regimen. On 2 occasions, a 20-year-old man with HIV and epilepsy, who was receiving carbamazepine 350 mg twice daily and zonisamide (eg, *Zonegran*), experienced nausea, vomiting, and elevated carbamazepine serum levels (17.8 mcg/mL on the first occasion and 16.3 mcg/mL on the second) after ritonavir was added to his anticonvulsant regimen.[2] After a 33% reduction in the doses of carbamazepine and zonisamide, the carbamazepine level decreased to 6.2 mcg/mL. After starting carbamazepine, antiretroviral therapy failure occurred in a 48-year-old HIV-positive man receiving indinavir, lamivudine (*Epivir*), and zidovudine (eg, *Retrovir*).[5] Before starting carbamazepine, indinavir levels were slightly below the lower limit of the mean population curve. During carbamazepine therapy, indinavir levels decreased. Indinavir levels were above mean population values approximately 2 weeks after discontinuing carbamazepine.

[1] Bates DE, et al. *Ann Pharmacother.* 2006;40:1190.
[2] Kato Y, et al. *Pharmacotherapy.* 2000;20:851.
[3] Berbel Garcia A, et al. *Clin Neuropharmacol.* 2000;23:216.
[4] Mateu-de Antonio J, et al. *Ann Pharmacother.* 2001;35:125.
[5] Hugen PW, et al. *Ann Pharmacother.* 2000;34:465.

* Asterisk indicates drugs cited in interaction reports. Based on pharmacologic and pharmacokinetic considerations, similar interactions may occur with other drugs that are listed.

Carbamazepine — *Quetiapine*

Carbamazepine* (eg, *Tegretol*)	Quetiapine* (*Seroquel*)

Significance	Onset	Severity	Documentation
2	☐ Rapid ■ **Delayed**	☐ Major ■ **Moderate** ☐ Minor	☐ Established ☐ Probable ■ **Suspected** ☐ Possible ☐ Unlikely

Effects Plasma concentrations of the active metabolite of CARBAMAZEPINE, carbamazepine-10,11-epoxide (CBZ-E), may be elevated, resulting in neurotoxicity. CARBAMAZEPINE may decrease QUETIAPINE serum levels.

Mechanism Unknown. However, CARBAMAZEPINE may increase QUETIAPINE metabolism (CYP3A4).

Management Observe patients for possible neurotoxicity or increased seizure activity if CARBAMAZEPINE and QUETIAPINE are coadministered. Consider monitoring CBZ-E levels. Also, monitor for a decrease in QUETIAPINE response. If an interaction is suspected, it may be necessary to discontinue CARBAMAZEPINE or QUETIAPINE. Because oxcarbazepine (eg, *Trileptal*) is not metabolized to CBZ-E, it may be a safe alternative.

Discussion

Two patients receiving carbamazepine experienced markedly elevated plasma levels of CBZ-E after starting quetiapine therapy (started at 100 mg/day and gradually increased to 700 mg/day).[1] In both patients, the CBZ-E:carbamazepine ratio increased. In 1 patient, CBZ-E levels returned to baseline after substituting oxcarbazepine for carbamazepine. In the second patient, levels returned to baseline after discontinuing quetiapine. During concurrent treatment with carbamazepine and quetiapine, the first patient experienced symptoms of agitation and ataxia that resolved when oxcarbazepine was started. The second patient was asymptomatic. In a retrospective study with 62 psychiatric patients receiving quetiapine, coadministration of carbamazepine lowered the concentration-to-dose ratio.[2] Similar findings were reported in a study of 39 patients.[3] In an open-label study, 18 psychiatric patients were titrated to quetiapine 300 mg twice daily, then titrated to carbamazepine 600 mg daily for 2 weeks.[4] Carbamazepine decreased the quetiapine C_{max} 80% (from 1,042 to 205 ng/mL) and increased the clearance 7.5-fold (from 65 to 483 L/hr). In a report of 3 cases, quetiapine plasma concentrations were not detectable during concomitant carbamazepine therapy.[5]

[1] Fitzgerald BJ, et al. *Pharmacotherapy.* 2002;22(11):1500.
[2] Hasselstrøm J, et al. *Ther Drug Monit.* 2004;26(5):486.
[3] Castberg I, et al. *J Clin Psychiatry.* 2007;68(10):1540.
[4] Grimm SW, et al. *Br J Clin Pharmacol.* 2006;61(1):58.
[5] Nickl-Jockschat T, et al. *Clin Neuropharmacol.* 2009;32(1):55.

* Asterisk indicates drugs cited in interaction reports.

Carbamazepine — *Quinine*

Carbamazepine* (eg, *Tegretol*)	Quinine*

Significance	Onset	Severity	Documentation
4	☐ Rapid	☐ Major	☐ Established
	■ **Delayed**	■ **Moderate**	☐ Probable
		☐ Minor	☐ Suspected
			■ **Possible**
			☐ Unlikely

Effects Serum CARBAMAZEPINE concentrations may be elevated, increasing the pharmacologic and adverse effects.

Mechanism Possible inhibition of CARBAMAZEPINE metabolism (CYP3A4).

Management In patients receiving CARBAMAZEPINE, monitor serum CARBAMAZEPINE concentrations and observe the clinical response of the patient when starting or stopping QUININE therapy. Adjust the CARBAMAZEPINE dose as needed.

Discussion

The effects of oral quinine 600 mg on the pharmacokinetics of carbamazepine 200 mg were studied in 6 healthy volunteers.[1] Quinine administration increased peak serum carbamazepine concentrations by 36.5% and the area under the plasma concentration-time curve by 51%.

Controlled studies are needed to determine the clinical importance of this drug interaction.

[1] Amabeoku GJ, et al. *East Afr Med J.* 1993;70:90.

* Asterisk indicates drugs cited in interaction reports.

Carbamazepine — *Ticlopidine*

Carbamazepine* (eg, *Tegretol*)	Ticlopidine* (*Ticlid*)

Significance	Onset	Severity	Documentation
4	☐ Rapid ■ **Delayed**	☐ Major ■ **Moderate** ☐ Minor	☐ Established ☐ Probable ☐ Suspected ■ **Possible** ☐ Unlikely

Effects Elevated CARBAMAZEPINE plasma levels with symptoms of toxicity may occur.

Mechanism Possible inhibition of CARBAMAZEPINE metabolism (CYP3A4).

Management Closely monitor patients receiving CARBAMAZEPINE when TICLOPIDINE is started or stopped. Plasma CARBAMAZEPINE concentrations may be useful in adjusting dosage.

Discussion

A possible drug interaction between carbamazepine and ticlopidine was reported in a 67-year-old male patient undergoing percutaneous transluminal coronary angioplasty (ie, coronary stenting).[1] The patient had a history of partial and generalized seizures and was receiving 600 mg of carbamazepine controlled release formulation twice daily. He had previously been treated with carbamazepine 700 mg twice daily; however, the dose was reduced following a possible diltiazem (eg, *Cardizem*) drug interaction, which included symptoms of dizziness and a decreased level of consciousness (ie, carbamazepine toxicity). Other medications the patient was receiving included aspirin and nitroglycerin (via a patch). One week prior to his revascularization procedure, ticlopidine 250 mg twice daily was started. Shortly thereafter, the patient again developed symptoms of carbamazepine toxicity. Within 1 hour of his morning ticlopidine dose, the patient experienced drowsiness and dizziness. Over the next 2 hours, he became ataxic and was unable to walk. The symptoms resolved over the next 6 hours. One week later, successful coronary stenting was performed. At this time, his carbamazepine plasma concentration (75 mol/L; therapeutic 25 to 50 mol/L) was nearly 75% higher than it had been 5 weeks previously. The next day the patient was discharged, receiving ticlopidine 250 mg twice daily and a reduced dose of carbamazepine (500 mg twice daily). His symptoms resolved. One week later, the carbamazepine concentration was 53 mol/L. Four weeks later, per post-stent procedure, ticlopidine was discontinued. Two weeks later, the carbamazepine concentration was 42 mol/L.

[1] Brown RIG, et al. *Can J Cardiol.* 1997;13:853.

* Asterisk indicates drugs cited in interaction reports.

Carbamazepine — Tricyclic Antidepressants

Carbamazepine	Tricyclic Antidepressants	
Carbamazepine* (eg, *Tegretol*)	Amitriptyline* Desipramine* (eg, *Norpramin*) Doxepin* (eg, *Silenor*)	Imipramine* (eg, *Tofranil*) Nortriptyline* (eg, *Pamelor*)

Significance	Onset	Severity	Documentation
2	☐ Rapid ■ **Delayed**	☐ Major ■ **Moderate** ☐ Minor	☐ Established ■ **Probable** ☐ Suspected ☐ Possible ☐ Unlikely

Effects Serum CARBAMAZEPINE (CBZ) levels may be elevated, increasing pharmacologic and toxic effects, while TRICYCLIC ANTIDEPRESSANT (TCA) levels may be decreased.

Mechanism TCAs may compete with CBZ for hepatic microsomal enzyme metabolism. CBZ may induce hepatic metabolism of TCAs.

Management Consider monitoring CBZ and TCA levels. Observe the patient for signs of toxicity or loss of therapeutic effect when either drug is added to or discontinued from the treatment regimen. Adjust the doses as needed.

Discussion

A 40-year-old woman stabilized on CBZ 800 mg daily (level, 7.7 mcg/mL) developed symptoms of CBZ toxicity (eg, acute nausea, vomiting, ataxia) and an elevated CBZ level (15 mcg/mL) following addition of desipramine (150 mg/day).[1] In a retrospective study of 36 children receiving imipramine, those who also received CBZ required a 38% larger mean dose of imipramine but had lower imipramine and desipramine levels.[2] In a comparison of 22 patients taking CBZ and doxepin or amitriptyline vs 25 patients given only an antidepressant, lower serum doxepin and amitriptyline levels (46% and 42%, respectively) were measured in those receiving CBZ concurrently.[3] Addition of CBZ 600 mg/day to a stable nortriptyline regimen (75 mg/day) resulted in a 60% reduction in serum nortriptyline concentration.[4] It was necessary to double the nortriptyline dose to reestablish therapeutic plasma levels. In a retrospective review of data collected over 10 years, CBZ decreased the concentration/dose ratio of both amitriptyline and nortriptyline approximately 50%.[5] In a study of 6 healthy volunteers, desipramine clearance was increased 31% during coadministration of CBZ 400 mg/day.[6] In 13 depressed patients receiving imipramine (2 mg/kg/day), addition of CBZ (400 mg/day) resulted in a 42% and 25% decrease in total imipramine and desipramine serum levels, respectively.[7] However, free imipramine and desipramine serum levels did not change.

[1] Lesser I. *J Clin Psychiatry*. 1984;45(8):360.
[2] Brown CS, et al. *J Clin Psychopharmacol*. 1990;10(5):359.
[3] Leinonen E, et al. *J Clin Psychopharmacol*. 1991;11(5):313.
[4] Brøsen K, et al. *Ther Drug Monit*. 1993;15(3):258.
[5] Jerling M, et al. *Ther Drug Monit*. 1994;16(1):1.
[6] Spina E, et al. *Psychopharmacology (Berl)*. 1995;117(4):413.
[7] Szymura-Oleksiak J, et al. *Psychopharmacology (Berl)*. 2001;154(1):38.

* Asterisk indicates drugs cited in interaction reports.

Carbamazepine — *Verapamil*

Carbamazepine* (eg, *Tegretol*)	Verapamil* (eg, *Calan*)

Significance	Onset	Severity	Documentation
2	☐ Rapid ■ **Delayed**	☐ Major ■ **Moderate** ☐ Minor	☐ Established ☐ Probable ■ **Suspected** ☐ Possible ☐ Unlikely

Effects Serum CARBAMAZEPINE levels may be increased, resulting in an increase in pharmacologic and toxic effects.

Mechanism VERAPAMIL appears to impair the hepatic metabolism of CARBAMAZEPINE.

Management Monitor serum CARBAMAZEPINE levels, and observe the patient for signs of CARBAMAZEPINE toxicity or loss of therapeutic effect if VERAPAMIL is added to or discontinued from the treatment regimen. CARBAMAZEPINE dose may need to be decreased 40% to 50% when administered with VERAPAMIL.

Discussion

Six patients, stabilized on carbamazepine 1,200 to 2,000 mg/day for refractory complex partial epilepsy and secondary generalized seizures, but otherwise healthy, were given verapamil 360 mg/day.[1] All patients reported symptoms of carbamazepine toxicity within 36 to 96 hours, which recurred with rechallenge. Resolution of symptoms occurred within a few days. Based on 5 patients, there was a mean 46% and 33% increase in total and free plasma carbamazepine concentrations, respectively, and a 36% decrease in the ratio of the principal 10,11-epoxide metabolite to carbamazepine. The carbamazepine AUC was increased 42% in 1 patient. Two other observations of this interaction also have been published.[1,2] Several other cases of neurotoxicity resulting from this combination have occurred.[3,4] Diltiazem also has increased carbamazepine serum concentrations, with accompanying neurotoxicity.[2,5] However, nifedipine (eg, *Procardia*) does not appear to affect carbamazepine levels.[2] See Carbamazepine-Diltiazem.

[1] Macphee GJ, et al. *Lancet.* 1986;1(8483):700.
[2] Brodie MJ, et al. *Br Med J (Clin Res Ed).* 1986;292(6529):1170.
[3] Price WA, et al. *J Clin Psychiatry.* 1988;49(2):80.
[4] Beattie B, et al. *Eur Neurol.* 1988;28(2):104.
[5] Eimer M, et al. *Drug Intell Clin Pharm.* 1987;21(4):340.

* Asterisk indicates drugs cited in interaction reports.

Carmustine — *Cimetidine*

Carmustine* (eg, *BiCNU*)	Cimetidine* (eg, *Tagamet*)

Significance	Onset	Severity	Documentation
1	☐ Rapid	■ **Major**	☐ Established
	■ **Delayed**	☐ Moderate	☐ Probable
		☐ Minor	■ **Suspected**
			☐ Possible
			☐ Unlikely

Effects CIMETIDINE may enhance the myelosuppressive effects of CARMUSTINE, possibly leading to toxicity.

Mechanism Undetermined, but additive bone marrow suppression or inhibition of metabolism of CARMUSTINE by CIMETIDINE are proposed.

Management Avoid coadministration unless no other options are available.

Discussion

Leukopenia and thrombocytopenia developed in 6 of 8 patients receiving carmustine, corticosteroids, and cimetidine, with nadirs well below those expected.[1] This was in contrast to a group of 40 patients who did not receive cimetidine and in whom only 6 patients had a similar hematologic response. The records of 40 patients receiving carmustine 80 mg/m^2/day for 3 days, cranial irradiation (6,000 radiation—absorbed dose over 6 weeks) and methylprednisolone 64 to 400 mg/day were analyzed.[2] In addition, 9 of these patients also received cimetidine 1,200 mg/day; however, a life-threatening neutropenia was recognized and cimetidine therapy stopped. The neutrophil nadir averaged 2,160/mm^3 for the patients not treated with cimetidine and 650/mm^3 for those who had received cimetidine. Bone marrow recovery also appeared delayed in these patients.

It has been proposed that cimetidine has additive effects on bone marrow suppression.[1,2] However, the mechanism could be an interference of carmustine metabolism by cimetidine.[3,4] Additional data are needed to define the mechanisms.

[1] Selker RG, et al. *N Engl J Med.* 1978;299(15):834.
[2] Volkin RL, et al. *Arch Intern Med.* 1982;142(2):243.
[3] Feagin OT. *Arch Intern Med.* 1982;142(10):1971.
[4] Dorr RT. *Arch Intern Med.* 1982;142(10):1971.

* Asterisk indicates drugs cited in interaction reports.

Caspofungin — *Cyclosporine*

Caspofungin* (*Cancidas*)	Cyclosporine* (eg, *Neoral*)

Significance	Onset	Severity	Documentation
4	☐ Rapid	☐ Major	☐ Established
	■ **Delayed**	■ **Moderate**	☐ Probable
		☐ Minor	☐ Suspected
			■ **Possible**
			☐ Unlikely

Effects The risk of hepatic function impairment may be increased.

Mechanism Unknown.

Management If these agents are coadministered, closely monitor liver function.

Discussion

In a retrospective study, the charts of 40 patients who received caspofungin and cyclosporine concurrently, for a median of 17 days, were reviewed.[1] Elevations in ALT or AST occurred in 35% of the patients. The AST elevations in 5 of these patients were considered to be at least possibly related to coadministration of caspofungin and cyclosporine, but no elevation was greater than 3.5 times the upper limit of normal. No ALT elevations were considered to be related to coadministration of caspofungin and cyclosporine. Two patients discontinued therapy due to hepatotoxicity possibly related to coadministration of caspofungin and cyclosporine. Three other retrospective studies indicate that clinically important hepatotoxicity with concomitant use of caspofungin and cyclosporine is rare[2,3] or does not occur.[4]

[1] Marr KA, et al. *Transpl Infect Dis*. 2004;6(3):110.
[2] Morrissey CO, et al. *Mycoses*. 2007;50(suppl 1):24.
[3] Christopeit M, et al. *Mycoses*. 2008;51(suppl 1):19.
[4] Saner F, et al. *Infection*. 2006;34(6):328.

* Asterisk indicates drugs cited in interaction reports.

Caspofungin — *Rifamycins*

Caspofungin* (*Cancidas*)	Rifampin* (eg, *Rifadin*)

Significance	Onset	Severity	Documentation
4	□ Rapid ■ **Delayed**	□ Major ■ **Moderate** □ Minor	□ Established □ Probable □ Suspected ■ **Possible** □ Unlikely

Effects CASPOFUNGIN plasma concentrations may be reduced, decreasing the therapeutic effect.

Mechanism Unknown.

Management Monitor patients for a decrease in CASPOFUNGIN activity when RIFAMPIN is coadministered. Be prepared to increase the CASPOFUNGIN dose as needed.

Discussion

The effects of rifampin on the pharmacokinetics of caspofungin were studied in an open-label, randomized, parallel investigation of healthy men.[1] Subjects received caspofungin 50 mg IV once daily for 14 days, coadministration of caspofungin and rifampin 600 mg orally once daily for 14 days, or rifampin for 28 days with caspofungin coadministered with rifampin on the last 14 days. When caspofungin and rifampin were started on the same day, rifampin increased the caspofungin AUC 61% on the first day. In contrast, after pretreatment with rifampin for 14 days or after 14 days of coadministration of caspofungin and rifampin, there was no change in the caspofungin AUC. However, compared with administration of caspofungin alone, coadministration of rifampin and caspofungin reduced the caspofungin trough concentrations approximately 30% on days 1 and 14. Rifampin plasma levels were not affected by caspofungin.

[1] Stone JA, et al. *Antimicrob Agents Chemother.* 2004;48(11):4306.

* Asterisk indicates drugs cited in interaction reports.

Cefprozil | *Anticholinergics*

Cefprozil	Anticholinergics	
Cefprozil* (eg, *Cefzil*)	Atropine (eg, *Sal-Tropine*)	Methscopolamine (*Pamine*)
	Belladonna	Orphenadrine (eg, *Norflex*)
	Benztropine (eg, *Cogentin*)	Oxybutynin (eg, *Ditropan*)
	Biperiden (*Akineton*)	Procyclidine (*Kemadrin*)
	Dicyclomine (eg, *Bentyl*)	Propantheline* (eg, *Pro-Banthine*)
	Glycopyrrolate (eg, *Robinul*)	Scopolamine (eg, *Scopace*)
	Hyoscyamine (eg, *Anaspaz*)	Trihexyphenidyl (eg, *Trihexy-5*)
	Mepenzolate (*Cantil*)	

Significance	Onset	Severity	Documentation
5	□ Rapid	□ Major	□ Established
	■ **Delayed**	□ Moderate	□ Probable
		■ **Minor**	□ Suspected
			■ **Possible**
			□ Unlikely

Effects CEFPROZIL plasma levels may be reduced slightly and the time to reach the peak level may be delayed.

Mechanism ANTICHOLINERGICS may slow gastric emptying, delaying absorption.

Management Based on available data, no special precautions are needed.

Discussion

The effects of propantheline on cis and trans isomers of cefprozil were studied in 15 healthy men.[1] Subjects received cefprozil 1 g under fasting conditions and 30 minutes after receiving propantheline 30 mg. Compared with fasting conditions, propantheline increased the mean residence time of both cefprozil isomers, reduced the C_{max} 20%, and delayed the time to reach the C_{max}. Other pharmacokinetic parameters were not altered.

[1] Shukla UA, et al. *J Clin Pharmacol.* 1992;32:725.

* Asterisk indicates drugs cited in interaction reports. Based on pharmacologic and pharmacokinetic considerations, similar interactions may occur with other drugs that are listed.

Cefprozil — *Metoclopramide*

Cefprozil* (eg, *Cefzil*)	Metoclopramide* (eg, *Reglan*)

Significance	Onset	Severity	Documentation
5	☐ Rapid ■ **Delayed**	☐ Major ☐ Moderate ■ **Minor**	☐ Established ☐ Probable ☐ Suspected ■ **Possible** ☐ Unlikely

Effects The time to reach CEFPROZIL peak plasma levels may be delayed slightly.

Mechanism METOCLOPRAMIDE increases GI motility, increasing the gastric emptying rate of CEFPROZIL.

Management Based on available data, no special precautions are needed.

Discussion

The effects of metoclopramide on cis and trans isomers of cefprozil were studied in 15 healthy men.[1] Subjects received cefprozil 1 g under fasting conditions and 30 minutes after receiving metoclopramide 30 mg. Compared with fasting conditions, metoclopramide decreased the mean residence time of both cefprozil isomers and reduced the time to reach the C_{max}. Other pharmacokinetic parameters were not altered.

[1] Shukla UA, et al. *J Clin Pharmacol.* 1992;32:725.

* Asterisk indicates drugs cited in interaction reports.

Cephalosporins — *Histamine H_2 Antagonists*

Cefpodoxime* (*Vantin*)	Cephalexin* (eg, *Keflex*)	Cimetidine (eg, *Tagamet*)	Nizatidine (eg, *Axid*)
Cefuroxime* (eg, *Ceftin*)		Famotidine (eg, *Pepcid*)	Ranitidine* (eg, *Zantac*)

Significance	Onset	Severity	Documentation
4	■ **Rapid**	□ Major	□ Established
	□ Delayed	■ **Moderate**	□ Probable
		□ Minor	□ Suspected
			■ **Possible**
			□ Unlikely

Effects HISTAMINE H_2 ANTAGONISTS may decrease the bioavailability of certain CEPHALOSPORINS.

Mechanism Unknown. Changes in gastric pH may affect drug absorption.

Management Although it is not likely that HISTAMINE H_2 ANTAGONISTS will affect the pharmacokinetics of CEFUROXIME and CEFPODOXIME to a clinically important extent, patients may be advised to take these CEPHALOSPORINS with meals to optimize absorption.

Discussion

A pharmacokinetic investigation was conducted using 6 healthy volunteers.[1] Serum cefuroxime levels were measured after a 1 g dose under 4 conditions: cefuroxime axetil alone, pretreatment with ranitidine 300 mg plus sodium bicarbonate, postprandial administration, and postprandial with ranitidine and sodium bicarbonate combined. Administration with sodium bicarbonate and ranitidine was intended to raise gastric pH. Cefuroxime C_{max} decreased from 7.3 to 4.3 mcg/mL and AUC decreased 43%. Food had the opposite effect and increased bioavailability above that seen when ingesting cefuroxime in the fasted state. Food also diminished the ranitidine/sodium bicarbonate effect, such that bioavailability was intermediate of that seen postprandially and in the fasted state. A similar effect was observed during coadministration of cefpodoxime proxetil and ranitidine.[2] With the exception of a delay in time to peak levels, ranitidine had minimal effects on the pharmacokinetics of cephalexin.[3]

These data are limited but suggest that a potentially clinically important decrease in cefuroxime and cefpodoxime levels could occur. Similar effects can be expected with other drugs that increase gastric pH, including omeprazole (eg, *Prilosec*) and antacids. Additional studies are needed.

[1] Sommers DK, et al. *Br J Clin Pharmacol.* 1984;18:535.
[2] Hughes GS, et al. *Clin Pharmacol Ther.* 1989;46:674.
[3] Madaras-Kelly K, et al. *J Clin Pharmacol.* 2004;44:1391.

* Asterisk indicates drugs cited in interaction reports. Based on pharmacologic and pharmacokinetic considerations, similar interactions may occur with other drugs that are listed.

Cetirizine | *Protease Inhibitors*

Cetirizine* (*Zyrtec*)	Ritonavir* (*Norvir*)

Significance	Onset	Severity	Documentation
5	☐ Rapid ■ **Delayed**	☐ Major ☐ Moderate ■ **Minor**	☐ Established ☐ Probable ☐ Suspected ■ **Possible** ☐ Unlikely

Effects CETIRIZINE exposure may be elevated, increasing the risk of side effects.

Mechanism Unknown.

Management Based on available data, no special precautions are needed.

Discussion

The potential for a pharmacokinetic interaction between cetirizine and ritonavir was evaluated in 16 healthy men.[1] In an open-label, crossover investigation, each subject received cetirizine (10 mg daily for 4 days) alone, ritonavir (dosage titration from 300 mg twice daily to 600 mg twice daily) alone, and cetirizine (10 mg daily) plus ritonavir (600 mg twice daily) for 4 days. Cetirizine did not affect the pharmacokinetics of ritonavir. However, compared with giving cetirizine alone, ritonavir administration increased the cetirizine AUC 42%, the elimination $t_{½}$ 53%, and the apparent volume of distribution 15%, while decreasing the apparent total body clearance 29%. No adverse reaction to the drugs was noted.

[1] Peytavin G, et al. *Eur J Clin Pharmacol.* 2005;61:267.

* Asterisk indicates drugs cited in interaction reports.

Charcoal Interactants — Charcoal

Charcoal Interactants		Charcoal	
Acetaminophen* (eg, *Tylenol*)	Phenothiazines*	Activated Charcoal*	Charcoal*
Barbiturates*	Propoxyphene* (eg, *Darvon*)		
Carbamazepine* (eg, *Tegretol*)	Salicylates*		
Citalopram* (*Celexa*)	Sulfones*		
Diazepam* (eg, *Valium*)	Sulfonylureas*		
Digitoxin*	Temazepam* (eg, *Restoril*)		
Digoxin* (eg, *Lanoxin*)	Tetracyclines*		
Fluoxetine* (eg, *Prozac*)	Theophyllines*		
Furosemide* (eg, *Lasix*)	Tricyclic Antidepressants*		
Glutethimide*	Valproic Acid* (eg, *Depakene*)		
Hydantoins*	Verapamil (eg, *Calan*)		
Ibuprofen (eg, *Motrin*)			
Methotrexate* (eg, *Rheumatrex*)			
Nizatidine* (eg, *Axid*)			

Significance	Onset	Severity	Documentation
2	☐ Rapid ■ **Delayed**	☐ Major ■ **Moderate** ☐ Minor	☐ Established ☐ Probable ■ **Suspected** ☐ Possible ☐ Unlikely

Effects CHARCOAL can reduce absorption of many drugs and actually remove drugs from the systemic circulation which will reduce the effectiveness or toxicity of a given agent.[1-12]

Mechanism CHARCOAL reduces the GI absorption of ingested drugs and adsorbs enterohepatically circulated drugs.

Management As an antidote, give ACTIVATED CHARCOAL 30 to 100 g as soon as possible. Multiple doses may enhance efficacy. Avoid as an antiflatulent/antidiarrheal.

Discussion

Activated charcoal 30 to 100 g, an antidote for drug overdoses, adsorbs drugs, impairing the GI absorption. If possible, administer activated charcoal within 1 to 2 hr of overdose; however, administration even hours after drug ingestion may interrupt enterohepatic circulation by "GI dialysis," for drugs so affected. When used therapeutically as multiple doses over 2 days or more, lowered drug plasma levels may result. Always consider an adsorptive interaction with charcoal products.

1 Neuvonen PJ. *Clin Pharmacokinet.* 1982;7:465.
2 Gadgil SD, et al. *Cancer Treat Rep.* 1982;66:1169.
3 Park GD, et al. *Arch Intern Med.* 1986;146:969.
4 Watson WA. *DICP.* 1987;21:160.
5 Knadler MP, et al. *Clin Pharmacol Ther.* 1987;42:514.
6 Kivisto KT, et al. *Br J Clin Pharmacol.* 1990;30:733.
7 Dolgin JG, et al. *DICP.* 1991;25:646.
8 Howard CE, et al. *Ann Pharmacother.* 1994;28:201.
9 Laine K, et al. *Pharmacol Toxicol.* 1996;79:270.
10 Lapatto-Reiniluoto D, et al. *Br J Clin Pharmacol.* 1999;48:148.
11 Yeates PJA, et al. *Br J Clin Pharmacol.* 2000;49:11.
12 Lapatto-Reiniluoto D, et al. *Eur J Clin Pharmacol.* 2000;56:285.

* Asterisk indicates drugs cited in interaction reports.

Chloral Hydrate — Loop Diuretics

Chloral Hydrate	Loop Diuretics	
Chloral Hydrate* (eg, *Aquachloral*)	Bumetanide (eg, *Bumex*)	Furosemide* (eg, *Lasix*)
	Ethacrynic Acid (eg, *Edecrin*)	Torsemide (*Demadex*)

Significance	Onset	Severity	Documentation
5	■ **Rapid**	□ Major	□ Established
	□ Delayed	□ Moderate	□ Probable
		■ **Minor**	□ Suspected
			□ Possible
			■ **Unlikely**

Effects Transient diaphoresis, hot flashes, hypertension, tachycardia, weakness and nausea may occur. This reaction has been observed rarely.

Mechanism Unknown.

Management Monitor for adverse effects after administration of LOOP DIURETICS in patients who have received CHLORAL HYDRATE within the previous 24 hours.

Discussion

Diaphoresis, hot flashes, labile blood pressure and a feeling of uneasiness shortly after administration of furosemide were described in six patients who had received chloral hydrate during the preceding 24 hours. The reaction occurred in one patient upon rechallenge.[1] A similar reaction was observed in an 8-year-old boy.[3]

In a large retrospective analysis of over 15,000 medical records in one hospital covering a period of 6 years, 1 definite reaction and 2 possible reactions after furosemide administration were recorded in 43 patients who had received chloral hydrate within the preceding 24 hours. No reactions occurred after furosemide administration in randomly selected patients who had received furosemide alone, chloral hydrate alone, or furosemide within 24 hours of flurazepam (eg, *Dalmane*) administration.[2]

[1] Malach M, et al. *JAMA*. 1975;232:638.
[2] Pevonka MP, et al. *DICP*. 1977;11:332.
[3] Dean RP, et al. *Clin Pharm*. 1991;10:385.

* Asterisk indicates drugs cited in interaction reports. Based on pharmacologic and pharmacokinetic considerations, similar interactions may occur with other drugs that are listed.

Chloramphenicol — *Acetaminophen*

Chloramphenicol*	Acetaminophen* (eg, *Tylenol*)

Significance	Onset	Severity	Documentation
5	☐ Rapid	☐ Major	☐ Established
	■ **Delayed**	☐ Moderate	☐ Probable
		■ **Minor**	☐ Suspected
			☐ Possible
			■ **Unlikely**

Effects No physiological effects have been reported.

Mechanism Unknown.

Management No clinical intervention appears warranted.

Discussion

Investigations of an interaction involving chloramphenicol and acetaminophen have produced equivocal results.[1-3,6] In one study of six patients, the plasma elimination half-life of chloramphenicol during a 6-hour study phase increased after injection of acetaminophen at hour 2.[1] In contrast, the steady-state plasma elimination half-life of chloramphenicol decreased in five children after the administration of acetaminophen.[3] In a third investigation,[2] no significant differences in chloramphenicol pharmacokinetic parameters were observed between 18 children receiving chloramphenicol with acetaminophen and those children receiving chloramphenicol without acetaminophen. None of the investigations accounted for other variables that could affect chloramphenicol pharmacokinetics or reported any manifestations of drug toxicity.[1-5]

A prospective pharmacokinetic study failed to demonstrate a significant interaction between oral acetaminophen 1 g every 6 hours and oral chloramphenicol 500 mg every 6 hours.[6]

Acetaminophen does not appear to interact with chloramphenicol.

1 Buchanan N, et al. *BMJ.* 1979;2:307.
2 Kearns GL, et al. *J Pediatr.* 1985;107:134.
3 Spika JS. *Arch Dis Childhood.* 1986;61:1121.
4 Choonara IA. *Arch Dis Childhood.* 1987;62:319.
5 Spika JS, et al. *Arch Dis Childhood.* 1987;62:1087.
6 Stein CM, et al. *Br J Clin Pharmacol.* 1989;27:262.

* Asterisk indicates drugs cited in interaction reports.

Chloramphenicol — *Barbiturates*

Chloramphenicol	Barbiturates	
Chloramphenicol*	Amobarbital (*Amytal*)	Pentobarbital (eg, *Nembutal*)
	Aprobarbital (*Alurate*)	Phenobarbital*
	Butabarbital (eg, *Butisol*)	Primidone (eg, *Mysoline*)
	Butalbital	Secobarbital (eg, *Seconal*)
	Mephobarbital (*Mebaral*)	

Significance	Onset	Severity	Documentation
4	☐ Rapid	☐ Major	☐ Established
	■ **Delayed**	■ **Moderate**	☐ Probable
		☐ Minor	☐ Suspected
			■ **Possible**
			☐ Unlikely

Effects CHLORAMPHENICOL efficacy may be reduced (decreased serum levels) while BARBITURATE effects may be enhanced. Effects may persist for days after BARBITURATES are withdrawn.

Mechanism The metabolism of CHLORAMPHENICOL may be increased and BARBITURATE metabolism decreased.

Management More CHLORAMPHENICOL may be required. Monitor antibiotic plasma levels and tailor dosage. If BARBITURATE intoxication manifests, perhaps lower barbiturate dose.

Discussion

With minor discrepancies, most patient and animal data indicate that coadministration of phenobarbital and chloramphenicol decreases antibiotic plasma levels.[1,2,4-8] Chloramphenicol plasma concentrations were decreased in two patients (ages 3 months and 7 months) being treated for meningitis when the combination was administered.[4] In 34 pediatric patients on chloramphenicol, six received phenobarbital which appeared to decrease peak and trough chloramphenicol serum levels by 35% and 44%, respectively.[6] Conversely, a 23-year-old epileptic stabilized on phenytoin (eg, *Dilantin*) and phenobarbital experienced CNS depression when chloramphenicol 48 mg/kg/day was administered.[3] Antiepileptic doses were reduced. Toxicity was attributed to increased phenobarbital levels caused by a 30% decrease in phenobarbital clearance.

Significant reductions in serum chloramphenicol levels occurred in neonates, but not in infants, who received concomitant phenobarbital therapy.[2] Other researchers observed similar results. However, when matched for postnatal and gestational age, concomitant phenobarbital had no effect on serum chloramphenicol levels or clearance.[7]

1 Palmer DL, et al. *Antimicrob Agents Chemother.* 1972;1:112.
2 Windorfer A Jr, et al. *Eur J Pediatr.* 1977;124:129.
3 Koup JR, et al. *Clin Pharmacol Ther.* 1978;24:571.
4 Bloxham RA, et al. *Arch Dis Child.* 1979;54:76.
5 Powell DA, et al. *J Pediatr.* 1981;98:1001.
6 Krasinski K, et al. *Pediatr Infect Dis.* 1982;1:232.
7 Mulhall A, et al. *J Antimicrob Chemother.* 1983;12:629.
8 Kearns GL, et al. *J Pediatr.* 1985;107:134.

* Asterisk indicates drugs cited in interaction reports. Based on pharmacologic and pharmacokinetic considerations, similar interactions may occur with other drugs that are listed.

Chloramphenicol — *Rifampin*

Chloramphenicol*	Rifampin* (eg, *Rifadin*)

Significance	Onset	Severity	Documentation
4	☐ Rapid	☐ Major	☐ Established
	■ **Delayed**	■ **Moderate**	☐ Probable
		☐ Minor	☐ Suspected
			■ **Possible**
			☐ Unlikely

Effects CHLORAMPHENICOL serum levels progressively decrease, possibly leading to decreased anti-infective action. These effects could continue for days after RIFAMPIN is withdrawn.

Mechanism CHLORAMPHENICOL metabolism may be increased due to induction of hepatic microsomal enzymes by RIFAMPIN.

Management The CHLORAMPHENICOL dose may need to be increased during RIFAMPIN coadministration if the expected therapeutic response is not forthcoming.

Discussion

Two pediatric patients, 2 and 5 years old, were given chloramphenicol succinate 100 mg/kg/day for 7 days to treat *Haemophilus influenzae* meningitis. During the last 4 days of this treatment, rifampin 20 mg/kg/day was added. This drug combination apparently caused a decrease in peak chloramphenicol serum levels in both patients (86% and 64%, respectively). A dose of 125 mg/kg/day chloramphenicol was required to reattain therapeutic serum levels. In two additional patients, chloramphenicol serum concentrations decreased by 75% and 94% after starting rifampin, despite an increase in chloramphenicol dosage.[2] Animal studies confirmed an increase in chloramphenicol total body clearance although there was a wide range in response.[1]

[1] Prober CG. *N Engl J Med.* 1985;312:788.
[2] Kelly HW, et al. *J Pediatr.* 1988;112:817.

* Asterisk indicates drugs cited in interaction reports.

Chlorzoxazone — *Disulfiram*

Chlorzoxazone* (eg, *Paraflex*)	Disulfiram* (eg, *Antabuse*)

Significance	Onset	Severity	Documentation
2	□ Rapid ■ **Delayed**	□ Major ■ **Moderate** □ Minor	□ Established ■ **Probable** □ Suspected □ Possible □ Unlikely

Effects Possible increase in CNS-depressant side effects.

Mechanism DISULFIRAM inhibits the hepatic metabolism of CHLORZOXAZONE.

Management If increased CNS-depressant side effects occur during concurrent administration of these agents, the dose of CHLORZOXAZONE may need to be decreased.

Discussion

The efficacy of a single oral dose of disulfiram as an inhibitor of cytochrome P450 2E1 (CYP 2E1) was investigated in 6 male volunteers.[1] This inhibitory action of disulfiram was assessed by the 6-hydroxylation of chlorzoxazone, a metabolic pathway catalyzed by CYP 2E1. In a crossover design, each subject received a single dose of chlorzoxazone 750 mg 10 hours after receiving either disulfiram 500 mg or no pretreatment drug. Pretreatment with disulfiram decreased chlorzoxazone elimination clearance from 3.28 to 0.49 mL/kg/min (85%; $P < 0.005$), prolonged the eliminatio n half-life from 0.92 to 5.1 hours (454%; $P < 0.001$), increased the peak plasma chlorzoxazone concentration from 10.3 to 20.6 mcg/mL (100%; $P < 0.001$), and decreased the formation clearance of 6-hydroxychlorzoxazone from 2.3 to 0.17 mL/kg/min (93%; $P < 0.005$). No important side effects were reported from chlorzoxazone alone or after disulfiram pretreatment.

Controlled, multiple-dose studies are needed to determine the clinical importance of this drug interaction.

[1] Kharasch ED, et al. *Clin Pharmacol Ther.* 1993;53:643.

* Asterisk indicates drugs cited in interaction reports.

Chlorzoxazone — *Food*

Chlorzoxazone* (eg, *Paraflex*)	Watercress*

Significance	Onset	Severity	Documentation
2	■ **Rapid**	□ Major	□ Established
	□ Delayed	■ **Moderate**	□ Probable
		□ Minor	■ **Suspected**
			□ Possible
			□ Unlikely

Effects Plasma concentrations of CHLORZOXAZONE may be elevated, increasing the therapeutic and adverse effects.

Mechanism Possibly due to inhibition of the hepatic metabolism (CYP2E1) of CHLORZOXAZONE by WATERCRESS.

Management Patients known to ingest WATERCRESS should be warned that the side effects (eg, CNS depression) of CHLORZOXAZONE may be increased.

Discussion

The effect of watercress, a vegetable rich in gluconasturtiin, on the metabolism of chlorzoxazone was studied in 10 healthy volunteers.[1] The effects of administration of isoniazid (eg, *Nydrazid*) on the pharmacokinetics of chlorzoxazone were evaluated as a control. In the first phase of the investigation, the metabolism of chlorzoxazone was studied after each subject ingested 1 dose of chlorzoxazone 500 mg. Six days later (phase 2), each subject ingested 50 g of watercress homogenate at 10 pm, and 1 dose of chlorzoxazone 500 mg at 9 am the next morning. In the third phase (starting 7 days after phase 2), each subject took isoniazid 300 mg/day for 7 days before taking a single dose of chlorzoxazone 500 mg. Ingestion of watercress increased the peak concentration of chlorzoxazone from 14.1 to 18.1 mcg/mL (28%), increased the area under the plasma concentration-time curve by 52%, and prolonged the mean plasma elimination half-life from 1.01 to 1.41 hours (40%).

[1] Leclercq I, et al. *Clin Pharmacol Ther.* 1998;64:144.

* Asterisk indicates drugs cited in interaction reports.

Chlorzoxazone — *Isoniazid*

Chlorzoxazone* (eg, *Paraflex*)	Isoniazid* (eg, *Nydrazid*)

Significance	Onset	Severity	Documentation
2	☐ Rapid ■ **Delayed**	☐ Major ■ **Moderate** ☐ Minor	☐ Established ☐ Probable ■ **Suspected** ☐ Possible ☐ Unlikely

Effects Plasma concentrations of CHLORZOXAZONE may be elevated, increasing the therapeutic and adverse reactions.

Mechanism Possible inhibition of the hepatic metabolism (CYP2E1) of CHLORZOXAZONE by ISONIAZID.

Management Caution patients taking ISONIAZID that the CNS-depressant effects of CHLORZOXAZONE may be increased. If the interaction is suspected, the dose of CHLORZOXAZONE may need to be decreased.

Discussion

The effect of watercress, a vegetable rich in gluconasturtiin, on the metabolism of chlorzoxazone was studied in 10 healthy volunteers.[1] The effects of isoniazid administration on the pharmacokinetics of chlorzoxazone were evaluated as a control. In phase 1 of the investigation, the metabolism of chlorzoxazone was studied after each subject ingested 1 dose of chlorzoxazone 500 mg. Six days later (phase 2), each subject ingested watercress homogenate 50 g at 10 PM and 1 dose of chlorzoxazone 500 mg at 9 AM the next day. In phase 3 (starting 7 days after phase 2), each subject took isoniazid 300 mg/day for 7 days before taking a single dose of chlorzoxazone 500 mg. Isoniazid administration increased the peak concentration of chlorzoxazone from 14.1 to 20.3 mcg/mL (44%), increased the AUC 125%, and prolonged the mean plasma elimination $t_{½}$ from 1.01 to 2.01 hours (99%).

[1] Leclercq I, et al. *Clin Pharmacol Ther.* 1998;64(2):144.

* Asterisk indicates drugs cited in interaction reports.

Cilostazol — *Food*

Cilostazol*
(eg, *Pletal*)

Grapefruit Juice*

Significance	Onset	Severity	Documentation
4	■ **Rapid**	□ Major	□ Established
	□ Delayed	■ **Moderate**	□ Probable
		□ Minor	□ Suspected
			■ **Possible**
			□ Unlikely

Effects CILOSTAZOL plasma concentrations may be elevated, increasing the pharmacologic effects and adverse reactions.

Mechanism GRAPEFRUIT may inhibit first-pass metabolism (CYP3A4) of CILOSTAZOL in the small intestine.

Management Avoid administration of CILOSTAZOL with GRAPEFRUIT products. Caution patients to take CILOSTAZOL with a liquid other than GRAPEFRUIT JUICE.

Discussion

Purpura was reported in a 79-year-old man taking cilostazol and aspirin after he began drinking grapefruit juice 200 mL every other day.[1] His purpura disappeared after he stopped drinking grapefruit juice even though cilostazol and aspirin were continued. The manufacturer of cilostazol warns that grapefruit juice ingestion can increase the C_{max} of cilostazol approximately 50%.[2] The AUC does not appear to be affected.

[1] Taniguchi K, et al. *J Clin Pharmacol Ther.* 2007;32(5):457.

[2] *Pletal* [package insert]. Rockville, MD: Otsuka America Pharmaceutical; 2006.

* Asterisk indicates drugs cited in interaction reports.

Cilostazol — *Ginkgo biloba*

Cilostazol* (eg, *Pletal*)	Ginkgo biloba*

Significance	Onset	Severity	Documentation
4	□ Rapid ■ **Delayed**	□ Major ■ **Moderate** □ Minor	□ Established □ Probable □ Suspected ■ **Possible** □ Unlikely

Effects GINKGO BILOBA does not appear to affect the antiplatelet activity of CILOSTAZOL; however, bleeding time may be prolonged.

Mechanism Additive or synergistic prolongation of bleeding time.

Management Until more data are available, caution patients taking CILOSTAZOL to avoid GINKGO BILOBA.

Discussion

In an open-label, randomized, crossover study, the effects of *Ginkgo biloba* on the pharmacodynamics of cilostazol were evaluated in 10 healthy men.[1] Each subject received single doses of cilostazol 100 mg, cilostazol 200 mg, *Ginkgo biloba* 120 mg, and *Ginkgo biloba* 240 mg alone plus coadministration of a single dose of cilostazol 100 mg and *Ginkgo biloba* 120 mg. Compared with administration of cilostazol alone, coadministration of *Ginkgo biloba* did not alter platelet aggregation, clotting time, or platelet count. However, with coadministration of cilostazol and *Ginkgo biloba*, bleeding time was prolonged.

[1] Aruna D, et al. *Br J Clin Pharmacol.* 2006;63(3):333.

* Asterisk indicates drugs cited in interaction reports.

Cilostazol — *Macrolide Antibiotics*

Cilostazol* (eg, *Pletal*)	Clarithromycin (eg, *Biaxin*)	Erythromycin* (eg, *Ery-Tab*)

Significance	Onset	Severity	Documentation
2	☐ Rapid ■ **Delayed**	☐ Major ■ **Moderate** ☐ Minor	☐ Established ☐ Probable ■ **Suspected** ☐ Possible ☐ Unlikely

Effects CILOSTAZOL plasma concentrations may be elevated, increasing the therapeutic and adverse effects.

Mechanism Certain MACROLIDE ANTIBIOTICS may inhibit the metabolism (CYP3A4) of CILOSTAZOL.

Management It may be necessary to decrease the dose of CILOSTAZOL during coadministration of certain MACROLIDE ANTIBIOTICS. Consider a dosage of CILOSTAZOL 50 mg twice daily in patients receiving one of these MACROLIDE ANTIBIOTICS.

Discussion

Using an open-label, nonrandomized, crossover design, the effect of erythromycin on the pharmacokinetics of cilostazol was studied in 16 healthy volunteers.[1] A single dose of cilostazol 100 mg was administered on days 1 and 15, while erythromycin 150 mg 3 times daily was administered on days 8 to 20. Coadministration of erythromycin increased the cilostazol peak plasma level 47% and AUC 73%. Of the 2 major circulating active metabolites of cilostazol, the peak plasma concentration and AUC of one metabolite increased 29% and 141%, respectively, while the peak plasma concentration of the second metabolite decreased 24%. There were no serious adverse reactions with administration of cilostazol alone or concurrently with erythromycin.

[1] Suri A, et al. *Clin Pharmacokinet.* 1999;37(suppl 2):61.

* Asterisk indicates drugs cited in interaction reports.

Cilostazol — *Omeprazole*

Cilostazol* (eg, *Pletal*)	Omeprazole* (eg, *Prilosec*)

Significance	Onset	Severity	Documentation
2	☐ Rapid ■ **Delayed**	☐ Major ■ **Moderate** ☐ Minor	☐ Established ☐ Probable ■ **Suspected** ☐ Possible ☐ Unlikely

Effects CILOSTAZOL plasma concentrations may be elevated, increasing the therapeutic and adverse effects.

Mechanism OMEPRAZOLE may inhibit the metabolism (CYP2C19) of CILOSTAZOL.

Management It may be necessary to decrease the dose of CILOSTAZOL during coadministration of OMEPRAZOLE. Consider a dosage of CILOSTAZOL 50 mg twice daily in patients receiving OMEPRAZOLE.

Discussion

Using an open-label, nonrandomized, crossover design, the effect of omeprazole on the pharmacokinetics of cilostazol was studied in 20 healthy volunteers.[1] A single dose of cilostazol 100 mg was administered on days 0 and 14, while omeprazole 40 mg/day was administered on days 7 to 18. Coadministration of omeprazole increased cilostazol peak plasma level 18% and AUC 26%. Of the 2 measurable active metabolites of cilostazol, the peak plasma concentration and AUC of one metabolite increased 29% and 69%, respectively, while the peak plasma concentration and AUC of the second metabolite decreased 22% and 31%, respectively. There were no serious adverse reactions with administration of cilostazol alone or concurrently with omeprazole.

[1] Suri A, et al. *Clin Pharmacokinet.* 1999;37(suppl 2):53.

* Asterisk indicates drugs cited in interaction reports.

Cimetidine — *Anticholinergics*

Cimetidine	Anticholinergics	
Cimetidine* (eg, *Tagamet*)	Anisotropine	Methantheline (*Banthine*)
	Atropine	Methscopolamine (*Pamine*)
	Belladonna	Orphenadrine (eg, *Norflex*)
	Benztropine (eg, *Cogentin*)	Oxybutynin
	Biperiden (*Akineton*)	Procyclidine (*Kemadrin*)
	Clidinium (*Quarzan*)	Propantheline* (eg, *Pro-Banthine*)
	Dicyclomine (eg, *Bentyl*)	Scopolamine
	Glycopyrrolate (eg, *Robinul*)	Tridihexethyl (*Pathilon*)
	Hyoscyamine (eg, *Anaspaz*)	Trihexyphenidyl (eg, *Artane*)
	Mepenzolate (*Cantil*)	

Significance	Onset	Severity	Documentation
5	□ Rapid ■ **Delayed**	□ Major □ Moderate ■ **Minor**	□ Established □ Probable □ Suspected □ Possible ■ **Unlikely**

Effects CIMETIDINE bioavailability may be reduced by concomitant use of ANTICHOLINERGICS.

Mechanism Unknown.

Management No actions appear warranted.

Discussion

In eight healthy volunteers, oral cimetidine bioavailability was reduced ≈ 20% when ingested 1 hour after propantheline 30 mg.[1] In contrast, a similar study showed that coadministration of propantheline and ranitidine (eg, *Zantac*) results in an increase in ranitidine bioavailability.[2]

The magnitude of effect for either cimetidine or ranitidine, independent of direction, is not likely to be clinically significant. Clinical cimetidine failure as a result of concomitant anticholinergic use has not been reported.

[1] Kanto J, et al. *Br J Clin Pharmacol.* 1981;11:629.
[2] Donn KH, et al. *Pharmacotherapy.* 1984;4:89.

* Asterisk indicates drugs cited in interaction reports. Based on pharmacologic and pharmacokinetic considerations, similar interactions may occur with other drugs that are listed.

Cimetidine — *Barbiturates*

Cimetidine	Barbiturates	
Cimetidine* (eg, *Tagamet*)	Amobarbital (*Amytal*)	Phenobarbital* (eg, *Solfoton*)
	Butabarbital (eg, *Butisol*)	Primidone (eg, *Mysoline*)
	Butalbital	Secobarbital (*Seconal*)
	Mephobarbital (*Mebaral*)	Thiopental* (eg, *Pentothal*)
	Pentobarbital	

Significance	Onset	Severity	Documentation
5	☐ Rapid	☐ Major	☐ Established
	■ **Delayed**	☐ Moderate	☐ Probable
		■ **Minor**	☐ Suspected
			☐ Possible
			■ **Unlikely**

Effects PHENOBARBITAL may reduce bioavailability of CIMETIDINE. CIMETIDINE use with THIOPENTAL infusions may result in higher than expected plasma PENTOBARBITAL concentrations.

Mechanism PHENOBARBITAL may affect absorption of CIMETIDINE or induce first-pass hepatic extraction. CIMETIDINE may either shunt THIOPENTAL metabolism to PENTOBARBITAL or inhibit metabolism of PENTOBARBITAL, resulting in accumulation.

Management No actions are necessary.

Discussion

The AUC of cimetidine decreased an average of 15% in 8 healthy subjects after they received phenobarbital for 3 weeks.[1] Nonrenal cimetidine elimination increased, but no other pharmacokinetic parameters changed. Phenobarbital may reduce oral cimetidine bioavailability by inhibiting absorption or inducing a first-pass hepatic extraction. Clinical cimetidine failures have not been reported.

Blood phenobarbital concentrations were higher than expected in a patient being treated with a continuous infusion of thiopental for seizure control.[2] Shunting of thiopental metabolism preferentially to pentobarbital or inhibition of pentobarbital metabolism as a result of concurrent cimetidine usage are possible explanations.

[1] Somogyi A, et al. *Eur J Clin Pharmacol.* 1981;19:343.

[2] Watson WA, et al. *Drug Intell Clin Pharm.* 1986;20:283.

* Asterisk indicates drugs cited in interaction reports. Based on pharmacologic and pharmacokinetic considerations, similar interactions may occur with other drugs that are listed.

Cimetidine — *Metoclopramide*

Cimetidine* (eg, *Tagamet*)	Metoclopramide* (eg, *Reglan*)

Significance	Onset	Severity	Documentation
5	☐ Rapid	☐ Major	☐ Established
	■ **Delayed**	☐ Moderate	☐ Probable
		■ **Minor**	☐ Suspected
			■ **Possible**
			☐ Unlikely

Effects Bioavailability of CIMETIDINE may be reduced.

Mechanism Reduced CIMETIDINE absorption as a result of faster gastric transit time during concurrent METOCLOPRAMIDE use has been postulated but not established.

Management If possible, administer CIMETIDINE at least 2 hours before METOCLOPRAMIDE. Observe for signs of CIMETIDINE treatment failure. If treatment failure occurs, consider discontinuing METOCLOPRAMIDE if other possible reasons for CIMETIDINE treatment failure have been excluded (eg, compliance, dose).

Discussion

Cimetidine and metoclopramide have been used in combination preoperatively to decrease the risk of aspiration pneumonitis (increased gastric pH greater than 2.5 and reduced gastric fluid volume less than 20 to 25 mL).[1-4] Metoclopramide has not reliably added to the effects of cimetidine. However, the addition of metoclopramide to cimetidine has been effective in the treatment of severe reflux esophagitis.[5]

In 2 studies involving a total of 16 healthy volunteers, the bioavailability of cimetidine decreased 22% to 30% when metoclopramide was ingested concurrently.[6,7] However, peak plasma cimetidine concentrations were not affected. Administering cimetidine 2 hours before metoclopramide 20 mg does not reduce the bioavailability of cimetidine.[8]

Clinically, cimetidine failure as a result of concurrent metoclopramide use has not been reported.

[1] Manchikanti L, et al. *Anesthesiology.* 1984;61:48.
[2] Rao TL, et al. *Anesth Analg.* 1984;63:1014.
[3] Pandit SK, et al. *Anaesthesia.* 1986;41:486.
[4] Lam AM, et al. *Can Anaesth Soc J.* 1986;33:773.
[5] Lieberman DA, et al. *Ann Intern Med.* 1986;104:21.
[6] Gugler R, et al. *Eur J Clin Pharmacol.* 1981;20:225.
[7] Kanto J, et al. *Br J Clin Pharmacol.* 1981;11:629.
[8] Barzaghi N, et al. *Eur J Clin Pharmacol.* 1989;37:409.

* Asterisk indicates drugs cited in interaction reports.

Cimetidine — *Probenecid*

Cimetidine* (eg, *Tagamet*)	Probenecid*

Significance	Onset	Severity	Documentation
5	■ **Rapid**	□ Major	□ Established
	□ Delayed	□ Moderate	□ Probable
		■ **Minor**	□ Suspected
			□ Possible
			■ **Unlikely**

Effects The therapeutic actions of CIMETIDINE may be increased; however, the effects appear to be transient and slight, indicating that the interaction is probably not clinically important.

Mechanism PROBENECID reduces the renal clearance of CIMETIDINE by decreasing the glomerular filtration rate (GFR) and the net secretory clearance.

Management Based on currently available documentation, no special precautions are necessary.

Discussion

In a 2-treatment, randomized, crossover design with 7 days separating each study period, the effects of the organic anion probenecid on renal excretion of the organic cation cimetidine were evaluated in 6 healthy men.[1] In the first phase of the study, subjects received cimetidine 300 mg IV. In the second treatment period, probenecid 500 mg every 6 hours for 13 doses preceded the IV administration of cimetidine 300 mg. In comparing the 2 treatment phases, there was no statistically significant difference in overall elimination, volume of distribution, AUC, $t_{½}$, or nonrenal clearance of cimetidine. In addition, the amount of cimetidine excreted unchanged in the urine was not significantly different in the 2 study groups. However, prior administration of probenecid significantly decreased the GFR (29%; $P < 0.01$) and the net secretory rate ($P < 0.05$) of cimetidine, resulting in a significant ($P < 0.01$) decrease in the renal clearance of cimetidine. The reduction in cimetidine renal clearance was most pronounced in the first hour following administration of cimetidine. These effects were transient and slight, indicating that the interaction is probably not clinically important.

[1] Gisclon LG, et al. *Clin Pharmacol Ther.* 1989;45(4):444.

* Asterisk indicates drugs cited in interaction reports.

Cinacalcet — *Azole Antifungal Agents*

Cinacalcet* (*Sensipar*)	Itraconazole (eg, *Sporanox*)	Posaconazole (*Noxafil*)
	Ketoconazole* (eg, *Nizoral*)	Voriconazole (*Vfend*)

Significance	Onset	Severity	Documentation
2	☐ Rapid	☐ Major	☐ Established
	■ **Delayed**	■ **Moderate**	☐ Probable
		☐ Minor	■ **Suspected**
			☐ Possible
			☐ Unlikely

Effects CINACALCET plasma concentrations may be elevated, increasing the pharmacologic effects and adverse reactions.

Mechanism Inhibition of CINACALCET metabolism (CYP3A4) by AZOLE ANTIFUNGAL AGENTS.

Management In patients receiving CINACALCET, monitor parathyroid hormone and calcium concentrations when starting or stopping an AZOLE ANTIFUNGAL AGENT, and observe patients for treatment-related adverse reactions. Adjust the dose of CINACALCET as needed.

Discussion

In an open-label, crossover investigation, the effects of ketoconazole on the pharmacokinetics of cinacalcet were evaluated in 20 healthy subjects.[1] Each subject received cinacalcet 90 mg alone and on day 5 of 7 days of ketoconazole 200 mg twice-daily administration. Compared with administration of cinacalcet alone, pretreatment with ketoconazole increased the cinacalcet AUC and mean C_{max} 2.3- and 2.2-fold, respectively. The time to reach the C_{max} was not affected. Treatment-related adverse reactions (eg, dizziness, headache, nausea, stomach pain, vomiting) were reported more frequently by patients receiving concurrent cinacalcet and ketoconazole compared with cinacalcet alone.

[1] Harris RZ, et al. *Clin Pharmacokinet.* 2007;46(6):495.

* Asterisk indicates drugs cited in interaction reports. Based on pharmacologic and pharmacokinetic considerations, similar interactions may occur with other drugs that are listed.

Cinoxacin — *Probenecid*

Cinoxacin*	Probenecid*

Significance	Onset	Severity	Documentation
5	☐ Rapid	☐ Major	☐ Established
	■ **Delayed**	☐ Moderate	☐ Probable
		■ **Minor**	☐ Suspected
			■ **Possible**
			☐ Unlikely

Effects Pharmacologic effects of CINOXACIN may be enhanced.

Mechanism Unknown.

Management Based on available data, no special precautions are needed.

Discussion

The effect of probenecid on the urinary excretion of cinoxacin was studied in 6 healthy men.[1] Cinoxacin 250 mg per 70 kg of body weight was infused IV for 1 hour, then 125 mg per 70 kg of body weight was infused for an additional 2 hours. Cinoxacin was administered alone and following pretreatment with oral probenecid. Compared with giving cinoxacin alone, probenecid administration increased cinoxacin serum levels 2-fold and prolonged the serum $t_{1/2}$ from 1.3 to 3.5 hours. Renal clearance of cinoxacin was reduced. Distribution of cinoxacin in the body was not altered.

[1] Rodriguez N, et al. *Antimicrob Agents Chemother.* 1979;15(3):465.

* Asterisk indicates drugs cited in interaction reports.

Cisapride — *Antiarrhythmic Agents*

Cisapride	Antiarrhythmic Agents	
Cisapride*†	Amiodarone* (eg, *Cordarone*)	Procainamide* (eg, *Pronestyl*)
	Bretylium*	Propafenone (eg, *Rythmol*)
	Disopyramide* (eg, *Norpace*)	Quinidine*
	Flecainide (eg, *Tambocor*)	Sotalol* (eg, *Betapace*)
	Ibutilide (*Corvert*)	

Significance	Onset	Severity	Documentation
1	☐ Rapid	■ **Major**	☐ Established
	■ **Delayed**	☐ Moderate	☐ Probable
		☐ Minor	■ **Suspected**
			☐ Possible
			☐ Unlikely

Effects The risk of life-threatening cardiac arrhythmias, including torsades de pointes, may be increased.

Mechanism Possible additive prolongation of the QT interval.

Management CISAPRIDE is contraindicated in patients receiving class Ia and class III ANTIARRHYTHMIC AGENTS.

Discussion

QT interval prolongation, torsades de pointes, cardiac arrest, and sudden death have occurred in patients receiving cisapride.[1] Frequently, patients had risk factors that may have predisposed them to arrhythmias (ie, concomitant medications known to prolong the QT interval). Thus, cisapride is contraindicated in patients taking concurrent medications known to prolong the QT interval and increase the risk of arrhythmia, such as class Ia (eg, quinidine) and class III (eg, sotalol) antiarrhythmic agents.[1,2] Certain antiarrhythmic agents cause a dose-related increase in the QT interval (eg, flecainide, ibutilide, propafenone); until more data are available, avoid use of these agents in patients receiving cisapride.

In 9 hospitalized patients with arrhythmias, coadministration of cisapride 2.5 mg and disopyramide 100 mg 3 times daily resulted in increased gastric emptying time, higher peak plasma disopyramide concentrations, a 2-fold higher disopyramide apparent rate constant, and a 2-fold shorter lag time of disopyramide, compared with giving disopyramide alone.[3]

The basis for this monograph is information on file with the manufacturer. Because of the seriousness of the cardiac problems, clinical evaluation of this interaction in humans is not likely to be forthcoming.

[1] *Propulsid* [package insert]. Titusville, NJ: Janssen Pharmaceutica; September 1998.
[2] Thomas M, et al. *Br J Clin Pharmacol.* 1996;41(2):77.
[3] Kuroda T, et al. *J Pharmacobiodyn.* 1992;15(8):395.

* Asterisk indicates drugs cited in interaction reports. Based on pharmacologic and pharmacokinetic considerations, similar interactions may occur with other drugs that are listed.
† Available from the manufacturer on a limited-access protocol.

Cisapride — *Aprepitant*

Cisapride*† | Aprepitant* (*Emend*) | Fosaprepitant* (*Emend*)

Significance	Onset	Severity	Documentation
1	☐ Rapid	■ **Major**	☐ Established
	■ **Delayed**	☐ Moderate	☐ Probable
		☐ Minor	■ **Suspected**
			☐ Possible
			☐ Unlikely

Effects The risk of life-threatening cardiac arrhythmias may be increased.

Mechanism APREPITANT may inhibit the metabolism (CYP3A4) of CISAPRIDE.

Management Coadministration of APREPITANT or FOSAPREPITANT and CISAPRIDE is contraindicated.

Discussion

Although not studied, coadministration of aprepitant with cisapride may increase cisapride plasma concentrations, resulting in QT prolongation and increasing the risk of cardiac arrhythmias. Coadministration of cisapride and aprepitant or fosaprepitant is contraindicated by the manufacturer.[1,2]

The basis for this monograph is information on file with the manufacturer. Published clinical data are needed to further assess this interaction. Because of the seriousness of the cardiac problem, clinical evaluation of this interaction in humans is not likely to be forthcoming.

[1] *Emend* PO [package insert]. Whitehouse Station, NJ: Merck & Co, Inc; May 2003.

[2] *Emend* IV [package insert]. Whitehouse Station, NJ: Merck & Co, Inc; January 2008.

* Asterisk indicates drugs cited in interaction reports.
† Available from the manufacturer on a limited-access protocol.

Cisapride — *Azole Antifungal Agents*

Cisapride	Azole Antifungal Agents	
Cisapride*†	Fluconazole* (eg, *Diflucan*)	Miconazole* (eg, *Monistat*)
	Itraconazole* (eg, *Sporanox*)	Posaconazole* (*Noxafil*)
	Ketoconazole* (eg, *Nizoral*)	Voriconazole* (*Vfend*)

Significance	Onset	Severity	Documentation
1	□ Rapid	■ **Major**	□ Established
	■ **Delayed**	□ Moderate	□ Probable
		□ Minor	■ **Suspected**
			□ Possible
			□ Unlikely

Effects Increased CISAPRIDE plasma concentrations with cardiotoxicity may occur.

Mechanism AZOLE ANTIFUNGAL AGENTS may inhibit the hepatic metabolism (CYP3A4) of CISAPRIDE. FLUCONAZOLE, especially 200 mg/day or greater, may inhibit CYP3A4.

Management AZOLE ANTIFUNGAL AGENTS are contraindicated in patients receiving CISAPRIDE.

Discussion

Cisapride is metabolized primarily by the CYP-450 3A4 isozyme (CYP3A4).[1,2] Drugs that inhibit this isozyme may lead to increased plasma cisapride concentrations. Life-threatening cardiac arrhythmias, including torsades de pointes, QT prolongation, ventricular tachycardia, and ventricular fibrillation, have been reported in patients taking cisapride with drugs that inhibit CYP3A4, including azole antifungals.[3,4] Coadministration of cisapride with fluconazole, itraconazole, ketoconazole, miconazole, posaconazole,[5] or voriconazole[6] is contraindicated.[2]

The basis for this monograph is information on file with the manufacturer. Published clinical data are needed to further assess this interaction. Because of the seriousness of the cardiac problems, clinical evaluation of this interaction in humans is not likely to be forthcoming. Animal studies are needed and are more likely to be performed.

[1] Communication from Janssen Pharmaceutica. October 14, 1995.
[2] *Propulsid* [package insert]. Titusville, NJ: Janssen Pharmaceutica; 1995.
[3] Wysowski DK, et al. *N Engl J Med.* 1996;335(4):290.
[4] Pettignano R, et al. *Crit Care Med.* 1996;24(7):1268.
[5] *Noxafil* [package insert]. Kenilworth, NJ: Schering Corporation; October 2006.
[6] *Vfend* [package insert]. New York, NY: Pfizer Inc; November 2006.

* Asterisk indicates drugs cited in interaction reports.
† Available from the manufacturer on a limited-access protocol.

Cisapride		*Carbonic Anhydrase Inhibitors*	
Cisapride*† (*Propulsid*)		Acetazolamide* (eg, *Diamox*) Dichlorphenamide*	Methazolamide*

Significance	Onset	Severity	Documentation
1	☐ Rapid ■ **Delayed**	■ **Major** ☐ Moderate ☐ Minor	☐ Established ☐ Probable ■ **Suspected** ☐ Possible ☐ Unlikely

Effects The risk of life-threatening cardiac arrhythmias, including torsades de pointes, may be increased.

Mechanism Possibly additive prolongation of the QT interval because of electrolyte loss.

Management CISAPRIDE is contraindicated in patients who may experience a rapid reduction in plasma potassium, such as those receiving CARBONIC ANHYDRASE INHIBITORS.

Discussion

Prolongation of the QT interval, torsades de pointes, cardiac arrest, and sudden death have occurred in patients receiving cisapride.[1] Frequently, patients had risk factors that may have predisposed them to arrhythmias, for example, uncorrected electrolyte disorders (eg, hypokalemia, hypomagnesemia). Thus, cisapride administration is contraindicated in those patients who might experience a rapid reduction of plasma potassium, such as those patients receiving a potassium-wasting diuretic in acute settings.[1] Hypokalemia with carbonic anhydrase inhibitors (eg, acetazolamide) may develop in patients with severe cirrhosis or with interference of adequate oral electrolyte intake.

The basis for this monograph is information on file with the manufacturer. Because of the seriousness of the cardiac problems, clinical evaluation of this interaction in humans is not likely to be forthcoming.

[1] *Propulsid* [package insert]. Titusville, NJ: Janssen Pharmaceutica; September 1998.

* Asterisk indicates drugs cited in interaction reports.
† Available from the manufacturer on a limited-access protocol.

Cisapride — *Diltiazem*

Cisapride*† (*Propulsid*)	Diltiazem* (eg, *Cardizem*)

Significance	Onset	Severity	Documentation
4	☐ Rapid ■ **Delayed**	■ **Major** ☐ Moderate ☐ Minor	☐ Established ☐ Probable ☐ Suspected ■ **Possible** ☐ Unlikely

Effects Increased CISAPRIDE plasma concentrations with possible cardiotoxicity.

Mechanism Inhibition of hepatic metabolism (CYP3A4) of CISAPRIDE by DILTIAZEM is suspected.

Management Until additional information is available, avoid coadministration of these agents. If therapy is necessary, carefully monitor the ECG. Metoclopramide (eg, *Reglan*) may be a safer alternative to CISAPRIDE.

Discussion

A possible drug interaction has been reported in a 45-year-old woman during coadministration of cisapride and diltiazem.[1] The patient was referred to the emergency department with acute onset of shortness of breath and dyspnea. She had a medical history that included steroid-dependent asthma, hypertension, CHF, diabetes mellitus, and gastroesophageal reflux disease. The patient had experienced 2 near-episodes of syncope 3 weeks prior to admission. She was receiving albuterol inhaler (eg, *Ventolin*), cisapride 20 mg/day, doxepin (eg, *Sinequan*), fluoxetine (eg, *Prozac*), furosemide (eg, *Lasix*), glyburide (eg, *DiaBeta*), ipratropium inhaler (eg, *Atrovent*), isosorbide mononitrate (eg, *Imdur*), omeprazole (eg, *Prilosec*), potassium chloride (eg, *K-Dur*), and prednisone (eg, *Deltasone*). Her ECG revealed a prolonged QT interval. It was suspected that the prolonged QT interval was caused by multiple drug interactions, particularly between cisapride and diltiazem. Cisapride was discontinued and replaced with metoclopramide. Subsequent cardiac monitoring did not show an abnormal cardiac rhythm. Her QT interval 2 months later was normal.

[1] Thomas AR, et al. *Pharmacotherapy*. 1998;18(2):381.

* Asterisk indicates drugs cited in interaction reports.
† Available from the manufacturer on a limited-access protocol.

Cisapride — *Fluoxetine*

Cisapride*† (*Propulsid*)	Fluoxetine* (eg, *Prozac*)

Significance	Onset	Severity	Documentation
5	☐ Rapid	☐ Major	☐ Established
	■ **Delayed**	☐ Moderate	☐ Probable
		■ **Minor**	☐ Suspected
			☐ Possible
			■ **Unlikely**

Effects CISAPRIDE plasma concentrations may be reduced.

Mechanism Unknown.

Management Based on available data, no special precautions are necessary.

Discussion

The effects of fluoxetine on the pharmacokinetics and pharmacodynamics of cisapride were studied in 12 healthy men.[1] Each subject received cisapride 10 mg 4 times daily for 6 days, fluoxetine 20 mg daily for 6 days, and cisapride 10 mg 4 times daily plus fluoxetine 20 mg daily for 6 days. Compared with taking cisapride alone, coadministration of fluoxetine decreased cisapride plasma concentrations approximately 35% and 23% after coadministration for 3 days and 6 days, respectively. There was no clinically important change in the QTc interval during administration of cisapride alone or in combination with fluoxetine.

[1] Zhao Q, et al. *Pharmacotherapy*. 2001;21(2):149.

* Asterisk indicates drugs cited in interaction reports.
† Available from the manufacturer on a limited-access protocol.

Cisapride — *Food*

Cisapride*†
(*Propulsid*)

Grapefruit Juice*

Significance	Onset	Severity	Documentation
1	■ **Rapid**	■ **Major**	□ Established
	□ Delayed	□ Moderate	□ Probable
		□ Minor	■ **Suspected**
			□ Possible
			□ Unlikely

Effects Elevated CISAPRIDE plasma concentrations with increased risk of adverse reactions, including life-threatening cardiac arrhythmias (eg, torsades de pointes).

Mechanism GRAPEFRUIT JUICE may inhibit intestinal first-pass metabolism (CYP3A4) of CISAPRIDE.

Management CISAPRIDE is contraindicated in patients receiving GRAPEFRUIT JUICE. Advise patients not to take CISAPRIDE with any GRAPEFRUIT product.

Discussion

The effect of grapefruit juice ingestion on the pharmacokinetics of oral cisapride was investigated in 14 healthy volunteers.[1] On 2 separate occasions, each subject received, in random order, cisapride 10 mg with either 250 mL of water or grapefruit juice. Coadministration of cisapride with grapefruit juice increased the mean peak plasma concentration of cisapride 34% and prolonged the mean time to reach the peak concentration 37% in all but 2 subjects. In addition, the mean AUC of cisapride was increased 39% in all but 1 subject. There was considerable interindividual variation in the effect of grapefruit juice on the AUC and peak concentration of cisapride. The $t_{1/2}$ of cisapride was not affected. Urinary recovery of norcisapride, the major metabolite of cisapride, was unchanged by grapefruit juice ingestion. No subject experienced a change in heart rate, BP, or QTc interval after administration of cisapride with water or grapefruit juice. In 10 healthy volunteers, taking cisapride 10 mg with 200 mL of double-strength grapefruit juice increased the AUC and peak concentration of cisapride 81% and 144%, respectively, and prolonged the time to reach the peak concentration from 1.5 to 2.5 hours and the elimination $t_{1/2}$ from 6.8 to 8.4 hours, compared with taking cisapride with water.[2]

[1] Gross AS, et al. *Clin Pharmacol Ther.* 1999;65(4):395. [2] Kivistö KT, et al. *Clin Pharmacol Ther.* 1999;66(5):448.

* Asterisk indicates drugs cited in interaction reports.
† Available from the manufacturer on a limited-access protocol.

Cisapride — *HCV Protease Inhibitors*

Cisapride		HCV Protease Inhibitors	
Cisapride*† (*Propulsid*)		Boceprevir* (*Victrelis*)	Telaprevir* (*Incivek*)

Significance	Onset	Severity	Documentation
1	□ Rapid ■ **Delayed**	■ **Major** □ Moderate □ Minor	□ Established □ Probable ■ **Suspected** □ Possible □ Unlikely

Effects CISAPRIDE plasma concentrations may be elevated, increasing the pharmacologic effects and risk of life-threatening cardiac arrhythmias, including torsades de pointes.

Mechanism CISAPRIDE metabolism (CYP3A) may be inhibited by HEPATITIS C VIRUS (HCV) PROTEASE INHIBITORS.

Management Coadministration of CISAPRIDE and HCV PROTEASE INHIBITORS is contraindicated.[1,2]

Discussion

Concurrent use of strong CYP3A4 inhibitors, such as boceprevir, may elevate cisapride plasma concentrations, increasing the risk of serious adverse effects (eg, life-threatening cardiac arrhythmias).[1,2] Concomitant use of cisapride and boceprevir or telaprevir is contraindicated.

The basis for this monograph is information on file with the manufacturer. Published clinical data are needed to further assess this interaction. Because of the seriousness of the cardiac problem, clinical evaluation of the interaction in humans is not likely to be forthcoming.

[1] *Victrelis* [package insert]. Whitehouse Station, NJ: Schering Corporation; May 2011.

[2] *Incivek* [package insert]. Cambridge, MA: Vertex Pharmaceuticals Incorporated; May 2011.

* Asterisk indicates drugs cited in interaction reports.
† Available from the manufacturer on a limited-access protocol.

Cisapride — *Histamine H_2 Antagonists*

Cisapride*† (*Propulsid*)	Cimetidine* (eg, *Tagamet*)	Ranitidine* (eg, *Zantac*)

Significance	Onset	Severity	Documentation
2	☐ Rapid	☐ Major	☐ Established
	■ **Delayed**	■ **Moderate**	☐ Probable
		☐ Minor	■ **Suspected**
			☐ Possible
			☐ Unlikely

Effects The H_2 ANTAGONIST may have a faster onset of action. CIMETIDINE increases serum CISAPRIDE concentrations.

Mechanism CISAPRIDE may accelerate the absorption of the H_2 ANTAGONIST, while CIMETIDINE may inhibit the metabolism of CISAPRIDE.

Management No action is needed. If an interaction is suspected based on patient response, adjust the dosages of the drugs accordingly.

Discussion

The effects of oral administration of cisapride and cimetidine on the pharmacokinetics of each other were investigated in 8 healthy volunteers.[1] The study consisted of 3 phases in which each patient received: (1) c isapride 10 mg 3 times daily for 7 days, (2) cisapride 10 mg 3 times daily and cimetidine 400 mg 3 times daily for 7 days, and (3) cimetidine 400 mg 3 times daily for 7 days. Each phase was separated by a 3-week drug-free interval. During coadministration of cisapride and cimetidine, the cimetidine T_{max} concentrations decreased from 1.3 to 0.6 hours (54%), and the AUC was reduced 18%. In addition, the extent of cimetidine absorption may have been decreased because the residence time of cimetidine at absorption sites was reduced. The effects of single-dose oral administration of cisapride 10 mg and ranitidine 150 mg on the plasma concentrations of both drugs were studied in 12 healthy volunteers.[2] In a randomized, 3-way, crossover design, each subject received the following: (1) ranitidine 150 mg plus cisapride, (2) ranitidine alone, and (3) cisapride alone. Each treatment was separated by at least 1 week. The pharmacokinetics of ranitidine were altered by cisapride. The median C_{max} of ranitidine was reached 1 hour earlier, and the AUC was decreased 24% when ranitidine was administered with cisapride compared with ranitidine taken alone. In a study in 6 healthy men, pretreatment with cisapride reduced the ranitidine AUC 17%.[3]

Cimetidine,[1] but not ranitidine,[2] affected the pharmacokinetics of cisapride, increasing the C_{max} and the AUC of cisapride 45%. The effect of cimetidine on cisapride serum levels was not apparent during the first 2 days of coadministration of the drugs.

[1] Kirch W, et al. *Ther Drug Monit.* 1989;11(4):411.
[2] Rowbotham DJ, et al. *Br J Anaesth.* 1991;67(3):302.
[3] Lee HT, et al. *Res Commun Mol Pathol Pharmacol.* 2000;108(5-6):311.

* Asterisk indicates drugs cited in interaction reports.
† Available from the manufacturer on a limited-access protocol.

Cisapride — *HMG-CoA Reductase Inhibitors*

Cisapride*† (eg, *Propulsid*)	Simvastatin* (eg, *Zocor*)

Significance	Onset	Severity	Documentation
4	☐ Rapid	☐ Major	☐ Established
	■ **Delayed**	■ **Moderate**	☐ Probable
		☐ Minor	☐ Suspected
			■ **Possible**
			☐ Unlikely

Effects CISAPRIDE plasma levels may be elevated, increasing the risk of toxicity. Plasma concentrations of SIMVASTATIN may be reduced, decreasing the therapeutic effect.

Mechanism Unknown.

Management Monitor patients for a decrease in the cholesterol-lowering effect of SIMVASTATIN and for possible CISAPRIDE toxicity.

Discussion

The potential interaction between cisapride and simvastatin was studied in 11 healthy men.[1] Each subject received cisapride (10 mg every 8 hr) or simvastatin (20 mg every 12 hr) alone and in combination. Compared with administering cisapride alone, coadministration of simvastatin resulted in a 14% increase in the AUC of cisapride. In 1 subject, the mean plasma levels of cisapride increased 50%. Coadministration of cisapride and simvastatin caused a 28% decrease in the C_{max} of the active metabolite of simvastatin (ie, simvastatin acid) and a 33% decrease in the AUC, compared with giving simvastatin alone.

Additional studies are needed to determine the clinical importance of this interaction and to determine if other HMG-CoA reductase inhibitors interact with cisapride.

[1] Simard C, et al. *Eur J Clin Pharmacol.* 2001;57(3):229.

* Asterisk indicates drugs cited in interaction reports.
† Available from the manufacturer on a limited-access protocol.

Cisapride × *Loop Diuretics*

Cisapride	Loop Diuretics	
Cisapride*† (*Propulsid*)	Bumetanide*	Torsemide* (eg, *Demadex*)
	Ethacrynic Acid* (*Edecrin*)	
	Furosemide* (eg, *Lasix*)	

Significance	Onset	Severity	Documentation
1	☐ Rapid	■ **Major**	☐ Established
	■ **Delayed**	☐ Moderate	☐ Probable
		☐ Minor	■ **Suspected**
			☐ Possible
			☐ Unlikely

Effects The risk of life-threatening cardiac arrhythmias, including torsades de pointes, may be increased.

Mechanism Possible additive prolongation of the QT interval due to electrolyte loss.

Management CISAPRIDE is contraindicated in patients who may experience a rapid reduction in potassium, such as those receiving LOOP DIURETICS.

Discussion

Prolongation of the QT interval, torsades de pointes, cardiac arrest, and sudden death have occurred in patients receiving cisapride.[1] Frequently, patients had risk factors that may have predisposed them to arrhythmias (eg, uncorrected electrolyte disorders [eg, hypokalemia, hypomagnesemia]). Therefore, cisapride administration is contraindicated in patients who might experience a rapid reduction of plasma potassium, such as those receiving a potassium-wasting diuretic (eg, furosemide) in acute settings.[1]

The basis for this monograph is information on file with the manufacturer. Because of the seriousness of the cardiac problems, clinical evaluation of this interaction in humans is not likely to be forthcoming.

[1] *Propulsid* [package insert]. Titusville, NJ: Janssen Pharmaceutica; September 1998.

* Asterisk indicates drugs cited in interaction reports.
† Available from the manufacturer on a limited-access protocol.

Cisapride	*Macrolide & Related Antibiotics*	
Cisapride*†	Clarithromycin* (*Biaxin*)	Telithromycin* (*Ketek*)
	Erythromycin* (eg, *Ery-Tab*)	Troleandomycin*‡

Significance	Onset	Severity	Documentation
1	□ Rapid	■ **Major**	■ **Established**
	■ **Delayed**	□ Moderate	□ Probable
		□ Minor	□ Suspected
			□ Possible
			□ Unlikely

Effects Increased CISAPRIDE plasma concentrations with probable cardiotoxicity.

Mechanism Certain MACROLIDE AND RELATED ANTIBIOTICS may inhibit the hepatic metabolism (CYP3A4) of CISAPRIDE.

Management MACROLIDE AND RELATED ANTIBIOTICS are contraindicated in patients receiving CISAPRIDE.[1,2] Azithromycin (*Zithromax*) may be a safer alternative.[3]

Discussion

Cisapride is metabolized primarily by the CYP3A4 isozyme.[2,4] Drugs that inhibit this isozyme may lead to increased plasma cisapride concentrations. Life-threatening cardiac arrhythmias, including torsades de pointes, QT prolongation, ventricular tachycardia, and ventricular fibrillation, have been reported in patients taking cisapride with drugs that inhibit CYP3A4, including erythromycin[5,6] and clarithromycin.[3,7-9] In a summary of cases reported to the FDA, of the 57 patients taking cisapride in whom torsades de pointes or prolonged QT intervals developed, 32 of these patients were also taking an azole antifungal agent or macrolide antibiotic (clarithromycin, erythromycin).[10] Arrhythmias stopped in most patients after discontinuing cisapride, the azole antifungal agent, or the macrolide antibiotic. Other factors may have contributed to the increased risk of arrhythmia (eg, atrial fibrillation, abnormal electrolytes). Acute hypotension has also been reported during coadministration of cisapride and erythromycin.[11]

1 *Ketek* [package insert]. Kansas City, MO: Aventis Pharmaceuticals, Inc.; June 2004.
2 *Propulsid* [package insert]. Titusville, NJ: Janssen Pharmaceutica; February 1997.
3 Sekkarie MA. *Am J Kidney Dis.* 1997;30:437.
4 Communication from Janssen Pharmaceutica. October 14, 1995.
5 Jenkins IR, et al. *Anaesth Intensive Care.* 1996;24:728.
6 Kyrmizakis DE, et al. *Am J Otolaryngol.* 2002;23:303.
7 Gray VS. *Ann Pharmacother.* 1998;32:648.
8 van Haarst AD, et al. *Clin Pharmacol Ther.* 1998;64;542.
9 Piquette RK. *Ann Pharmacother.* 1999;33:22.
10 Wysowski DK, et al. *N Engl J Med.* 1996;335:290.
11 Mangoni AA, et al. *Br J Clin Pharmacol.* 2004;58:223.

* Asterisk indicates drugs cited in interaction reports.
† Available from the manufacturer on a limited-access protocol. ‡ Not available in the United States.

Cisapride — *Nefazodone*

Cisapride*† (*Propulsid*)	Nefazodone* (*Serzone*)

Significance	Onset	Severity	Documentation
1	☐ Rapid ■ **Delayed**	■ **Major** ☐ Moderate ☐ Minor	☐ Established ☐ Probable ■ **Suspected** ☐ Possible ☐ Unlikely

Effects Increased CISAPRIDE plasma concentrations with cardiotoxicity may occur.

Mechanism NEFAZODONE may inhibit the hepatic metabolism (CYP3A4) of CISAPRIDE.

Management Coadministration of CISAPRIDE and NEFAZODONE is contraindicated.

Discussion

Cisapride is metabolized primarily by the cytochrome P450 3A4 isozyme (CYP3A4).[1] Elevated serum concentrations of cisapride may cause QT prolongation and subsequent serious cardiac arrhythmias.[3] Drugs that inhibit this isozyme may lead to increased plasma cisapride concentrations. Life-threatening cardiac arrhythmias, including torsades de pointes, QT prolongation, ventricular tachycardia, and ventricular fibrillation have been reported in patients taking cisapride with drugs that inhibit CYP3A4.[1] In vitro studies have shown nefazodone to be an inhibitor of CYP3A4.[2] Therefore, coadministration of nefazodone with cisapride is contraindicated.[2]

The basis for this monograph is information on file with the manufacturer. However, because of the seriousness of the cardiac problems, clinical evaluation of this interaction in humans is not likely to be forthcoming.

[1] Product Information. Cisapride (*Propulsid*). Janssen Pharmaceutica. September 1995.

[2] Product information. Nefazodone (*Serzone*). Bristol-Myers Squibb Co. February 1996.

[3] Thomas M, et al. *Br J Clin Pharmacol.* 1996;41:77.

* Asterisk indicates drugs cited in interaction reports.

† Available from the manufacturer on a limited-access protocol.

Cisapride | *NNRT Inhibitors*

Cisapride*† (*Propulsid*)		Delavirdine* (*Rescriptor*)	Efavirenz* (*Sustiva*)

Significance	Onset	Severity	Documentation
1	□ Rapid	■ **Major**	□ Established
	■ **Delayed**	□ Moderate	□ Probable
		□ Minor	■ **Suspected**
			□ Possible
			□ Unlikely

Effects Elevated CISAPRIDE plasma concentrations with increased risk of adverse effects, including life-threatening cardiac arrhythmias (eg, torsades de pointes).

Mechanism NON-NUCLEOSIDE REVERSE TRANSCRIPTASE (NNRT) INHIBITORS may inhibit the hepatic metabolism (CYP3A4) of CISAPRIDE.

Management Do not administer CISAPRIDE with NNRT INHIBITORS.

Discussion

Cisapride is metabolized primarily by the cytochrome P450 3A4 (CYP3A4) isozyme.[4] Drugs that inhibit this isozyme may lead to increased plasma cisapride concentrations. Elevated serum concentrations of cisapride may cause QT prolongation and subsequent serious cardiac arrhythmias.[1] Life-threatening cardiac arrhythmias, including torsades de pointes, QT prolongation, ventricular tachycardia, and ventricular fibrillation have been reported in patients taking cisapride with drugs that inhibit CYP3A4. In vitro studies indicate that CYP3A4 is inhibited by delavirdine and efavirenz.[2,3] The manufacturers of both delavirdine and efavirenz warn that these antiviral agents should not be administered concurrently with cisapride because potentially serious and life-threatening adverse effects (eg, cardiac arrhythmias) could occur.[2,3]

The basis for this monograph is information on file with the manufacturer. Because of the seriousness of the cardiac problems, clinical evaluation of this interaction in humans is not likely to be forthcoming.

[1] Thomas M, et al. *Br J Clin Pharmacol.* 1996;41:77.
[2] Product Information. Delavirdine (*Rescriptor*). Upjohn Company. April 1997.
[3] Product Information. Efavirenz (*Sustiva*). DuPont Pharmaceuticals. September 1998.
[4] Product Information. Cisapride (*Propulsid*). Janssen Pharmaceutical. May 1999.

* Asterisk indicates drugs cited in interaction reports.
† Available from the manufacturer on a limited-access protocol.

Cisapride — *Phenothiazines*

Cisapride	Phenothiazines	
Cisapride*† (*Propulsid*)	Chlorpromazine	Promethazine (eg, *Phenergan*)
	Fluphenazine	Thioridazine
	Perphenazine	Trifluoperazine
	Prochlorperazine (eg, *Compro*)	

Significance	Onset	Severity	Documentation
1	☐ Rapid	■ **Major**	☐ Established
	■ **Delayed**	☐ Moderate	☐ Probable
		☐ Minor	■ **Suspected**
			☐ Possible
			☐ Unlikely

Effects The risk of life-threatening cardiac arrhythmias, including torsades de pointes, may be increased.

Mechanism Possible additive prolongation of the QT interval.

Management CISAPRIDE is contraindicated in patients receiving PHENOTHIAZINES.

Discussion

QT interval prolongation, torsades de pointes, cardiac arrest, and sudden death have occurred in patients receiving cisapride.[1] Frequently, patients had risk factors that may have predisposed them to arrhythmias (eg, concomitant medications known to prolong the QT interval). Thus, cisapride is contraindicated in those patients taking concurrent medications, such as phenothiazines (eg, chlorpromazine), known to prolong the QT interval and increase the risk of arrhythmia.[1,2]

The basis for this monograph is information on file with the manufacturer. Because of the seriousness of the cardiac problems, clinical evaluation of this interaction in humans is not likely to be forthcoming.

[1] *Propulsid* [package insert]. Titusville, NJ: Janssen Pharmaceutica; 1998.

[2] Thomas M, et al. *Br J Clin Pharmacol.* 1996;41(2):77.

* Asterisk indicates drugs cited in interaction reports. Based on pharmacologic and pharmacokinetic considerations, similar interactions may occur with other drugs that are listed.
† Available from the manufacturer on a limited-access protocol.

Cisapride ✕ *Protease Inhibitors*

Cisapride	Protease Inhibitors	
Cisapride*†	Amprenavir*††	Lopinavir/Ritonavir (*Kaletra*)
	Atazanavir* (*Reyataz*)	Nelfinavir (*Viracept*)
	Darunavir* (*Prezista*)	Ritonavir* (*Norvir*)
	Fosamprenavir* (*Lexiva*)	Saquinavir (*Invirase*)
	Indinavir* (*Crixivan*)	

Significance	Onset	Severity	Documentation
1	☐ Rapid ■ **Delayed**	■ **Major** ☐ Moderate ☐ Minor	☐ Established ☐ Probable ■ **Suspected** ☐ Possible ☐ Unlikely

Effects Increased CISAPRIDE plasma concentrations with cardiotoxicity may occur.

Mechanism PROTEASE INHIBITORS may inhibit the hepatic metabolism (CYP3A4) of CISAPRIDE.

Management AMPRENAVIR, ATAZANAVIR, DARUNAVIR, FOSAMPRENAVIR, INDINAVIR, and RITONAVIR are contraindicated in patients receiving CISAPRIDE.

Discussion

Cisapride is metabolized primarily by CYP3A4.[1] Drugs that inhibit this isozyme may lead to increased plasma cisapride concentrations. Elevated serum concentrations of cisapride may cause QT prolongation and subsequent serious cardiac arrhythmias.[2] Life-threatening cardiac arrhythmias, including torsades de pointes, QT prolongation, ventricular tachycardia, and ventricular fibrillation, have been reported in patients taking cisapride with drugs that inhibit CYP3A4. In vitro studies indicate that CYP3A4 is the major enzyme responsible for the metabolism of indinavir.[3] Coadministration of cisapride with amprenavir, atazanavir, darunavir, fosamprenavir, indinavir, or ritonavir is contraindicated.[3-8]

The basis for this monograph is information on file with the manufacturers. Published clinical data are needed to further assess this interaction. However, because of the seriousness of the cardiac problems, clinical evaluation of this interaction in humans is not likely to be forthcoming.

1 *Propulsid* [package insert]. Titusville, NJ: Janssen Pharmaceutica; January 2000.
2 Thomas M, et al. *Br J Clin Pharmacol.* 1996;41(2):77.
3 *Crixivan* [package insert]. Whitehouse Station, NJ: Merck & Co Inc; 1996.
4 *Norvir* [package insert]. Abbott Park, IL: Abbott Laboratories; 1996.
5 *Agenerase* [package insert]. Philadelphia, PA: GlaxoSmithKline; 1999.
6 *Reyataz* [package insert]. Princeton, NJ: Bristol-Myers Squibb; 2003.
7 *Prezista* [package insert]. Raritan, NJ: Tibotec Therapeutics; June 2006.
8 *Lexiva* [package insert]. Research Triangle Park, NC: GlaxoSmithKline; April 2010.

* Asterisk indicates drugs cited in interaction reports. Based on pharmacologic and pharmacokinetic considerations, similar interactions may occur with other drugs that are listed.
† Available from the manufacturer on a limited-access protocol.
†† Not available in the United States.

Cisapride — *Red Wine*

Cisapride*†
(*Propulsid*)

Red Wine*

Significance	Onset	Severity	Documentation
4	■ **Rapid**	□ Major	□ Established
	□ Delayed	■ **Moderate**	□ Probable
		□ Minor	□ Suspected
			■ **Possible**
			□ Unlikely

Effects CISAPRIDE plasma concentrations may be elevated, increasing the risk of side effects.

Mechanism Inhibition of CISAPRIDE metabolism (CYP3A4) in the GI tract by RED WINE is suspected.

Management Until more data are available, it may be prudent to advise patients to avoid ingestion of RED WINE while taking CISAPRIDE.

Discussion

The effects of red wine (eg, cabernet sauvignon) on the pharmacokinetics of cisapride were studied in 12 healthy men.[1] Using a randomized, crossover design, each subject received cisapride 10 mg with 250 mL of red wine or water. Compared with water, no statistically significant difference was noted when cisapride was taken with wine. However, the cisapride AUC and peak concentration were doubled in 1 subject, compared with values obtained when cisapride was taken with water. Additional studies are needed to determine if there is a subset of patients (eg, patients with high intestinal CYP3A4 content) who may be at risk of a clinically important interaction.

[1] Offman EM, et al. *Clin Pharmacol Ther.* 2001;70:17.

* Asterisk indicates drugs cited in interaction reports.
† Available from the manufacturer on a limited-access protocol.

Cisapride	*Tetracyclic Antidepressants*
Cisapride*† (*Propulsid*)	Maprotiline*

Significance	Onset	Severity	Documentation
1	☐ Rapid ■ **Delayed**	■ **Major** ☐ Moderate ☐ Minor	☐ Established ☐ Probable ■ **Suspected** ☐ Possible ☐ Unlikely

Effects The risk of life-threatening cardiac arrhythmias, including torsades de pointes, may be increased.

Mechanism Possible additive prolongation of the QT interval.

Management CISAPRIDE is contraindicated in patients receiving TETRACYCLIC ANTIDEPRESSANTS.

Discussion

Prolongation of the QT interval, torsades de pointes, cardiac arrest, and sudden death have occurred in patients receiving cisapride.[1] Frequently, patients had risk factors that may have predisposed them to arrhythmias (eg, concomitant medications known to prolong the QT interval). Thus, cisapride is contraindicated for those patients taking concurrent medications known to prolong the QT interval and increase the risk of arrhythmia, such as tetracyclic antidepressants.[1,2]

The basis for this monograph is information on file with the manufacturer. Because of the seriousness of the cardiac problems, clinical evaluation of this interaction in humans is not likely to be forthcoming.

[1] *Propulsid* [package insert]. Titusville, NJ:Janssen Pharmaceutica; September 1998.

[2] Thomas M, et al. *Br J Clin Pharmacol.* 1996;41:77.

* Asterisk indicates drugs cited in interaction reports.
† Available from the manufacturer on a limited-access protocol.

Cisapride — *Thiazide Diuretics*

Cisapride	Thiazide Diuretics	
Cisapride*† (*Propulsid*)	Bendroflumethiazide (*Naturetin*)	Indapamide (eg, *Lozol*)
	Chlorothiazide (eg, *Diuril*)	Methyclothiazide (eg, *Enduron*)
	Chlorthalidone (eg, *Hygroton*)	Metolazone (eg, *Zaroxolyn*)
	Hydrochlorothiazide (eg, *HydroDIURIL*)	

Significance	Onset	Severity	Documentation
1	☐ Rapid	■ **Major**	☐ Established
	■ **Delayed**	☐ Moderate	☐ Probable
		☐ Minor	■ **Suspected**
			☐ Possible
			☐ Unlikely

Effects The risk of life-threatening cardiac arrhythmias, including torsades de pointes, may be increased.

Mechanism Possible additive prolongation of the QT interval because of electrolyte loss.

Management CISAPRIDE is contraindicated in patients who may experience a rapid reduction in plasma potassium, such as those receiving THIAZIDE DIURETICS.

Discussion

Prolongation of the QT interval, torsades de pointes, cardiac arrest, and sudden death have occurred in patients receiving cisapride.[1] Frequently, patients had risk factors that may have predisposed them to arrhythmias such as uncorrected electrolyte disorders (eg, hypokalemia, hypomagnesemia). Thus, cisapride administration is contraindicated in patients who might experience a rapid reduction of plasma potassium, such as those patients receiving a potassium-wasting diuretic (eg, hydrochlorothiazide) in acute settings.[1]

The basis for this monograph is information on file with the manufacturer. Because of the seriousness of the cardiac problems, clinical evaluation of this interaction in humans is not likely to be forthcoming.

[1] *Propulsid* [package insert]. Titusville, NJ: Janssen Pharmaceutica; September 1998.

* Asterisk indicates drugs cited in interaction reports. Based on pharmacologic and pharmacokinetic considerations, similar interactions may occur with other drugs that are listed.
† Available from the manufacturer on a limited-access protocol.

Cisapride — *Tricyclic Antidepressants*

Cisapride	Tricyclic Antidepressants	
Cisapride*† (*Propulsid*)	Amitriptyline*	Imipramine* (eg, *Tofranil*)
	Amoxapine	Nortriptyline (eg, *Pamelor*)
	Clomipramine (eg, *Anafranil*)	Protriptyline (eg, *Vivactil*)
	Desipramine (eg, *Norpramin*)	Trimipramine (*Surmontil*)
	Doxepin (eg, *Sinequan*)	

Significance	Onset	Severity	Documentation
1	☐ Rapid	■ **Major**	☐ Established
	■ **Delayed**	☐ Moderate	☐ Probable
		☐ Minor	■ **Suspected**
			☐ Possible
			☐ Unlikely

Effects The risk of life-threatening cardiac arrhythmias, including torsades de pointes, may be increased.

Mechanism Possible additive prolongation of the QT interval.

Management CISAPRIDE is contraindicated in patients receiving TRICYCLIC ANTIDEPRESSANTS.

Discussion

Prolongation of the QT interval, torsades de pointes, cardiac arrest, and sudden death have occurred in patients receiving cisapride.[1] Frequently, patients had risk factors that may have predisposed them to arrhythmias, (eg, concomitant medications known to prolong the QT interval). Thus, cisapride is contraindicated for those patients taking concurrent medications known to prolong the QT interval and increase the risk of arrhythmia, such as tricyclic antidepressants.[1,2]

The basis for this monograph is information on file with the manufacturer. Because of the seriousness of the cardiac problems, clinical evaluation of this interaction in humans is not likely to be forthcoming.

[1] *Propulsid* [package insert]. Titusville, NJ: Janssen Pharmaceutica; September 1998.

[2] Thomas M, et al. *Br J Clin Pharmacol.* 1996;41:77.

* Asterisk indicates drugs cited in interaction reports. Based on pharmacologic and pharmacokinetic considerations, similar interactions may occur with other drugs that are listed.

† Available from the manufacturer on a limited-access protocol.

Cisplatin — *Ondansetron*

Cisplatin*	Ondansetron* (eg, *Zofran*)

Significance	Onset	Severity	Documentation
4	☐ Rapid ■ **Delayed**	☐ Major ■ **Moderate** ☐ Minor	☐ Established ☐ Probable ☐ Suspected ■ **Possible** ☐ Unlikely

Effects Plasma CISPLATIN concentrations may be decreased, reducing the therapeutic effect.

Mechanism Unknown.

Management Monitor the therapeutic response of the patient. If an interaction is suspected, it may be necessary to increase the dose of CISPLATIN.

Discussion

The effect of ondansetron 8 mg IV bolus on the pharmacokinetics of cisplatin was studied in a retrospective investigation involving 23 bone marrow transplant patients receiving high-dose cisplatin (165 mg/m^2/day as a 72-hour IV infusion), cyclophosphamide, and carmustine (eg, *BiCNU*).[1] The effect of ondansetron was compared with a control group of 129 patients who received the same chemotherapy but prochlorperazine (eg, *Compro*) was substituted for ondansetron. Compared with patients receiving prochlorperazine, ondansetron administration resulted in a 19% decrease in the AUC of cisplatin. See Cyclophosphamide-Ondansetron.

Additional studies are needed to determine the clinical importance of this drug interaction.

[1] Cagnoni PJ, et al. *Bone Marrow Transplant.* 1999;24(1):1.

* Asterisk indicates drugs cited in interaction reports.

Citalopram — *Fluconazole*

Citalopram* (eg, *Celexa*)	Fluconazole* (eg, *Diflucan*)

Significance	Onset	Severity	Documentation
4	☐ Rapid	☐ Major	☐ Established
	■ **Delayed**	■ **Moderate**	☐ Probable
		☐ Minor	☐ Suspected
			■ **Possible**
			☐ Unlikely

Effects Serotonin syndrome (eg, agitation, altered consciousness, ataxia, myoclonus, overactive reflexes, shivering) may occur.

Mechanism FLUCONAZOLE may inhibit the metabolism (CYP2C19, CYP3A4) of CITALOPRAM.

Management Closely monitor patients for adverse reactions. Serotonin syndrome requires immediate medical attention, including withdrawal of the serotonergic agent and supportive care. Administration of an antiserotonergic agent (eg, cyproheptadine) may be helpful.

Discussion

Serotonin syndrome was reported in 2 women during coadministration of citalopram and fluconazole.[1] A 46-year-old woman taking fluconazole 200 mg daily developed confusion and nonconvulsive seizures several weeks after starting citalopram 20 mg daily. Citalopram was stopped, and marked improvement was noted 24 hours later. A 73-year-old woman taking citalopram 40 mg daily and fluconazole 100 mg daily developed worsening delirium manifested by somnolence and disorientation. Citalopram was stopped, and within 72 hours, the patient's condition improved dramatically and she was alert and oriented.

[1] Levin TT, et al. *Gen Hosp Psychiatry*. 2008;30(4):372.

* Asterisk indicates drugs cited in interaction reports.

Clarithromycin — *Omeprazole*

Clarithromycin* (eg, *Biaxin*)	Omeprazole* (eg, *Prilosec*)

Significance	Onset	Severity	Documentation
3	□ Rapid ■ **Delayed**	□ Major □ Moderate ■ **Minor**	□ Established □ Probable ■ **Suspected** □ Possible □ Unlikely

Effects Serum concentrations of CLARITHROMYCIN and OMEPRAZOLE may be increased. In addition, the gastric mucus concentration of CLARITHROMYCIN may be increased.

Mechanism CLARITHROMYCIN may inhibit the metabolism (CYP3A4 and 2C19) of OMEPRAZOLE, while OMEPRAZOLE may increase the absorption of CLARITHROMYCIN.

Management Based on available clinical data, no special action is needed. Coadministration of these agents may be beneficial in the treatment of *Helicobacter pylori* infections.

Discussion

In a double-blind, placebo-controlled, randomized, crossover study, the effects of omeprazole 40 mg/day and clarithromycin 500 mg every 8 hours on the pharmacokinetics of each other, as well as the effects of omeprazole on clarithromycin plasma and gastric tissue concentrations, were assessed in 23 healthy men.[1] Clarithromycin administration increased the AUC of omeprazole 91%, increased the $t_{½}$ 33% (from 1.2 to 1.6 hours), and increased peak serum concentrations of omeprazole 27% (from 1.1 to 1.4 mcg/mL). However, clarithromycin did not alter the effect of omeprazole on gastric pH. Omeprazole administration increased the AUC of clarithromycin 15% and the minimum plasma concentrations 22% (from 1.8 to 2.2 mcg/mL). In addition, omeprazole administration increased clarithromycin tissue and gastric mucus concentrations. Omeprazole also increased the AUC, peak, and minimum concentrations of the 14-(R)-hydroxy metabolite of clarithromycin. In a study of 21 healthy volunteers, characterized as poor or extensive CYP2C19 metabolizers, administration of clarithromycin with omeprazole resulted in an increase in the AUC of both drugs.[2]

[1] Gustavson LE, et al. *Antimicrob Agents Chemother.* 1995;39(9):2078.

[2] Furuta T, et al. *Clin Pharmacol Ther.* 1999;66(3): 265.

* Asterisk indicates drugs cited in interaction reports.

Clofibrate — *Contraceptives, Hormonal*

Clofibrate* (*Atromid-S*)	Contraceptives, Oral* (eg, *Ortho-Novum*)

Significance	Onset	Severity	Documentation
5	☐ Rapid ■ **Delayed**	☐ Major ☐ Moderate ■ **Minor**	☐ Established ☐ Probable ☐ Suspected ■ **Possible** ☐ Unlikely

Effects The clearance of clofibric acid, the free acid form of CLOFIBRATE, increases and the plasma elimination half-life decreases, during concurrent use of ORAL CONTRACEPTIVES. Lower steady-state serum clofibric acid concentrations could result.

Mechanism ORAL CONTRACEPTIVE induction of clofibric acid metabolism has been suggested.

Management Observe for changes in serum lipoprotein concentrations during concurrent use of ORAL CONTRACEPTIVES. If control of serum lipoprotein concentrations is lost, consider discontinuing ORAL CONTRACEPTIVES or increasing CLOFIBRATE dose during concurrent administration.

Discussion

In a trial involving young, healthy volunteer subjects,[1] clofibric acid clearance was 49% greater in eight female subjects receiving oral contraceptives than in eight other female subjects not receiving oral contraceptives. Serum clofibric acid elimination half-life was correspondingly longer in the subjects receiving oral contraceptives; however, there was no difference in volume of distribution or percentage of free clofibric acid, suggesting that oral contraceptives induce clofibric acid metabolism.

The significance of this pharmacokinetic effect on serum lipoprotein concentrations remains to be determined.

[1] Miners JO, et al. *Br J Clin Pharmacol.* 1984;18:240.

* Asterisk indicates drugs cited in interaction reports.

Clofibrate — *Probenecid*

Clofibrate* (*Atromid-S*)	Probenecid*

Significance	Onset	Severity	Documentation
4	☐ Rapid	☐ Major	☐ Established
	■ **Delayed**	■ **Moderate**	☐ Probable
		☐ Minor	☐ Suspected
			■ **Possible**
			☐ Unlikely

Effects Accumulation of p-chlorophenoxyisobutyric acid (CPIB; clofibric acid) leading to higher steady-state serum concentrations.

Mechanism PROBENECID competitively inhibits renal tubular secretion of the ester glucuronide metabolite of clofibric acid. As clofibric acid glucuronide accumulates, it is hydrolyzed to active clofibric acid; therefore, net clearance of clofibric acid is reduced and steady-state serum concentrations increase.

Management Closely observe for signs of CLOFIBRATE toxicity during concomitant use of PROBENECID. Consider using lower doses of CLOFIBRATE and monitor for loss of serum lipoprotein control.

Discussion

In a study involving four healthy men,[1] total and percent-free clofibric acid serum concentrations approximately doubled and serum-free p-chlorophenoxyisobutyric acid (CPIB; clofibric acid) concentrations, the active metabolite of clofibrate, approximately quadrupled control values during concurrent probenecid use. In a later animal study,[2] it appeared that the increase in serum clofibric acid concentrations during probenecid use resulted from a decrease in clofibric acid clearance. The area under the plasma clofibric acid glucuronide concentration-time curve (AUC) increased, while renal clearance decreased. The clofibric acid glucuronide renal tubular secretion/plasma hydrolysis equilibrium is thus shifted to hydrolysis and consequently, a "net" decrease in clearance results.

The clinical consequences of this pharmacokinetic interaction remain to be assessed.

[1] Veenendaal JR, et al. *Clin Pharmacol Ther.* 1981;29:351.

[2] Meffin PJ, et al. *J Pharmacol Exp Ther.* 1983;227:739.

* Asterisk indicates drugs cited in interaction reports.

Clofibrate — *Rifampin*

Clofibrate* (*Atromid-S*)	Rifampin* (eg, *Rifadin*)

Significance	Onset	Severity	Documentation
5	☐ Rapid	☐ Major	☐ Established
	■ **Delayed**	☐ Moderate	☐ Probable
		■ **Minor**	☐ Suspected
			☐ Possible
			■ **Unlikely**

Effects Clearance of p-chlorophenoxyisobutyric acid (CPIB; clofibric acid) increases during concurrent RIFAMPIN therapy, thereby resulting in lower steady-state serum clofibric acid concentrations.

Mechanism RIFAMPIN induction of clofibric acid metabolism has been proposed but not established.

Management Observe for changes in serum lipoprotein concentrations during concurrent RIFAMPIN therapy. If control of serum lipoprotein concentrations is lost, consider discontinuing RIFAMPIN or increasing CLOFIBRATE dose during coadministration.

Discussion

Steady-state serum concentrations of p-chlorophenoxyisobutyric acid (CPIB; clofibric acid), the active metabolite of clofibrate, decreased in five volunteer subjects during concurrent rifampin administration and then returned to baseline after discontinuation of rifampin.[1]

The clinical significance of this pharmacokinetic effect on serum lipoprotein concentrations remains to be determined.

[1] Houin G, et al. *Int J Clin Pharmacol.* 1978;16:150.

* Asterisk indicates drugs cited in interaction reports.

Clomipramine — *Food*

Clomipramine* (eg, *Anafranil*)	Grapefruit Juice*

Significance	Onset	Severity	Documentation
4	☐ Rapid ■ **Delayed**	☐ Major ■ **Moderate** ☐ Minor	☐ Established ☐ Probable ☐ Suspected ■ **Possible** ☐ Unlikely

Effects Reduced desmethylclomipramine (DCMI) concentrations and increased clomipramine (CMI) levels, which may improve outcome in obsessive-compulsive disorders (OCD). Clinical improvement of OCD symptoms is related to CMI plasma concentrations and negatively correlated with DCMI levels.

Mechanism GRAPEFRUIT JUICE may inhibit intestinal cytochrome P450 3A3/4 (CYP3A3/4) and subsequent demethylation of CLOMIPRAMINE.

Management Observe the response to CLOMIPRAMINE if ingested with GRAPEFRUIT JUICE. Adjust the dose as needed.

Discussion

Coadministration of clomipramine and grapefruit juice has been utilized to improve symptom control of OCD.[1] Clomipramine metabolism involves demethylation of CMI to DCMI by several cytochromes, primarily CYP1A2 and 3A3/4, prior to hydroxylation to 8-hydroxyclomipramine. High ratios of DCMI/CMI may be associated with decreased efficacy of clomipramine treatment of OCD. Frozen grapefruit juice concentrate (250 mL) was given with each dose of clomipramine to two children with CMI-resistant OCD in an effort to inhibit demethylation of clomipramine, reduce the DCMI/CMI ratio and improve the therapeutic outcome.[1] The first child, an 8-year-old boy with Tourette's syndrome and OCD, was treated with clomipramine 25 mg three times daily. After 3 months of therapy, he had minimal improvement in his OCD symptoms (DCMI/CMI ratio of 2.4), and he started taking clomipramine with grapefruit juice. After 3 days, there was a 171% increase in clomipramine blood levels and a 62% increase in DCMI levels (DCMI/CMI ratio 1.1). The patient had sustained clinical improvement. The second patient, a 13-year-old girl with autistic spectrum disorder, received clomipramine 125 mg/day for 16 weeks (DCMI/CMI ratio of 4), after which she started taking clomipramine with grapefruit juice. After 3 days, CMI blood levels increased 44%, and DCMI levels decreased 13% (DCMI/CMI ratio of 2.4). There was no clinical improvement. The dose of clomipramine was increased to 150 mg, and grapefruit juice was continued. After 3 days, CMI and DCMI blood concentrations increased by 135% and 5%, respectively, over pregrapefruit juice levels (DCMI/CMI ratio of 1.8). However, there was no clinical improvement. See Tricyclic Antidepressants-Food.

[1] Oesterheld J, et al. *J Clin Psychopharmacol.* 1997;17:62.

* Asterisk indicates drugs cited in interaction reports.

Clonazepam — *Amiodarone*

Clonazepam* (*Klonopin*)	Amiodarone* (*Cordarone*)

Significance	Onset	Severity	Documentation
4	□ Rapid	□ Major	□ Established
	■ **Delayed**	■ **Moderate**	□ Probable
		□ Minor	□ Suspected
			■ **Possible**
			□ Unlikely

Effects The effects of CLONAZEPAM may be increased. The likelihood of CLONAZEPAM toxicity may be increased in the presence of AMIODARONE-induced hypothyroidism.

Mechanism Unknown.

Management Observe the patient for increased sensitivity to CLONAZEPAM. In addition, observe the patient for symptoms of hypothyroidism and measure TSH levels prior to starting AMIODARONE therapy and every 6 months therafter.

Discussion

Benzodiazepine toxicity occurred in a 78-year-old male patient during concurrent administration of amiodarone and clonazepam.[1] The patient had a history of congestive heart failure and coronary artery disease. He was hospitalized for ventricular tachycardia. After initiating therapy with amiodarone 600 mg/day, the arrhythmia was subsequently treated with amiodarone 200 mg/day with good results. Four months later, the patient developed restless leg syndrome, which was treated with clonazepam 0.5 mg at bedtime. After 2 months of concurrent therapy with amiodarone and clonazepam, the patient exhibited signs and symptoms of benzodiazepine toxicity including slurred speech, difficulty walking and confusion. Clonazepam was discontinued, and over the next 5 days, the patient's mental condition improved considerably. The patient was also receiving enalapril (*Vasotec*), furosemide (eg, *Lasix*), potassium and calcium supplements and a multivitamin preparation. Laboratory results revealed hypothyroidism for which the patient received levothyroxine (eg, *Synthroid*). Up to 11% of patients receiving amiodarone have been reported to experience hypothyroidism. Because some of the symptoms experienced by the patient (eg, slurred speech, confusion) may have been the result of hypothyroidism, thyroid assessment prior to administration of amiodarone and periodically thereafter is recommended.

[1] Witt DM, et al. *Ann Pharmacother.* 1993;27:1463.

* Asterisk indicates drugs cited in interaction reports.

Clonazepam — *Barbiturates*

Clonazepam	Barbiturates	
Clonazepam* (*Klonopin*)	Amobarbital (*Amytal*)	Pentobarbital (eg, *Nembutal*)
	Aprobarbital (*Alurate*)	Phenobarbital* (eg, *Solfoton*)
	Butabarbital (eg, *Butisol*)	Primidone (eg, *Mysoline*)
	Butalbital	Secobarbital (eg, *Seconal*)
	Mephobarbital (*Mebaral*)	

Significance	Onset	Severity	Documentation
4	□ Rapid	□ Major	□ Established
	■ **Delayed**	■ **Moderate**	□ Probable
		□ Minor	□ Suspected
			■ **Possible**
			□ Unlikely

Effects Increased CLONAZEPAM clearance, possibly leading to lower steady-state plasma concentrations and loss of effectiveness.

Mechanism Induction of CLONAZEPAM hepatic metabolism.

Management Observe the patient for loss of CLONAZEPAM effectiveness during concomitant BARBITURATE use. Increase CLONAZEPAM doses according to clinical requirements or plasma concentrations if necessary.

Discussion

The dose of clonazepam had to be increased to maintain seizure control in 4 of 36 patients receiving several antiseizure medications in one study,[2] but it is not known whether these patients were receiving a barbiturate at the same time. A correlation between higher plasma phenobarbital concentrations and lower plasma clonazepam concentrations was also noted, but a connection between this correlation and the clonazepam dosage increase required in some patients was not attempted. In eight volunteers,[4] clonazepam clearance increased 19% to 24% and elimination half-life decreased by approximately 10% after 3 weeks of phenobarbital ingestion. However, there was substantial interpatient variability.

Clonazepam does not appear to affect steady-state plasma barbiturate concentrations.[1,3]

[1] Huang CY, et al. *Med J Aust.* 1974;2:5.
[2] Nanda RN, et al. *J Neurol Neurosurg Psychiatry.* 1977;40:538.
[3] Johannessen SI, et al. *Acta Neurol Scand.* 1977;55:506.
[4] Khoo K-C, et al. *Clin Pharmacol Ther.* 1980;28:368.

* Asterisk indicates drugs cited in interaction reports. Based on pharmacologic and pharmacokinetic considerations, similar interactions may occur with other drugs that are listed.

Clonazepam — *Hydantoins*

Clonazepam* (eg, *Klonopin*)	Ethotoin (*Peganone*)	Phenytoin* (eg, *Dilantin*)

Significance	Onset	Severity	Documentation
4	□ Rapid ■ **Delayed**	□ Major ■ **Moderate** □ Minor	□ Established □ Probable □ Suspected ■ **Possible** □ Unlikely

Effects HYDANTOIN toxicity, or loss of HYDANTOIN or CLONAZEPAM effectiveness, could occur.

Mechanism Effects of HYDANTOINS on CLONAZEPAM are attributed to induction of its hepatic metabolism by HYDANTOINS. Effects of CLONAZEPAM on HYDANTOINS are thought to involve HYDANTOIN hepatic metabolism, but the precise mechanism is unknown.

Management Observe for loss of CLONAZEPAM or HYDANTOIN effectiveness, and for HYDANTOIN toxicity. Tailor doses of either agent according to clinical requirements or plasma concentrations.

Discussion

Conflicting information exists regarding the clinical consequences of combined treatment with clonazepam and hydantoins. Elevated plasma phenytoin concentrations with attendant signs of toxicity and decreases in plasma phenytoin concentrations with loss of seizure control have been reported after initiation of clonazepam.[1,2] However, in 2 clinical trials,[3,4] concomitant clonazepam administration did not affect plasma phenytoin concentrations.

Conversely, in a study involving 8 volunteers,[5] clonazepam clearance increased 46% to 58% and elimination $t_{1/2}$ decreased 31% after 3 weeks of phenobarbital ingestion. In another study,[6] substantial decreases in plasma clonazepam concentrations were recorded during phenytoin coadministration in 5 patients. Clonazepam doses had to be increased to maintain seizure control in 4 of 36 patients in 1 study,[4] but it is not known whether these patients were receiving phenytoin at the same time.

[1] Eeg-Olofsson O. *Acta Neurol Scand.* 1973;49 (suppl 53):29.
[2] Saavedra IN, et al. *Ther Drug Monit.* 1985;7:481.
[3] Johannesen SI, et al. *Acta Neurol Scand.* 1977;55:506.
[4] Nanda RN, et al. *J Neurol Neurosurg Psychiatry.* 1977;40:538.
[5] Khoo KC, et al. *Clin Pharmacol Ther.* 1980;28:368.
[6] Sjo O, et al. *Eur J Clin Pharmacol.* 1975;8:249.

* Asterisk indicates drugs cited in interaction reports. Based on pharmacologic and pharmacokinetic considerations, similar interactions may occur with other drugs that are listed.

Clonazepam — *Valproic Acid*

Clonazepam* (eg, *Klonopin*)	Valproic Acid* (eg, *Depakene*)

Significance	Onset	Severity	Documentation
4	☐ Rapid	■ **Major**	☐ Established
	■ **Delayed**	☐ Moderate	☐ Probable
		☐ Minor	☐ Suspected
			■ **Possible**
			☐ Unlikely

Effects Severe drowsiness and loss of seizure control.

Mechanism Unknown.

Management Observe for severe drowsiness and loss of seizure control during combined CLONAZEPAM and VALPROIC ACID use.

Discussion

Shortly after adding clonazepam to valproic acid in 12 patients, clonazepam was discontinued in 4 patients because of severe drowsiness and in 5 patients because of absence status.[1] These reactions were attributed to the combination of clonazepam and valproic acid. However, subsequent clinical investigations failed to demonstrate similar reactions or evidence suggesting that either clonazepam or valproic acid doses may require adjustment during combined use.[2-6] During coadministration of clonazepam and valproic acid, nonlinear mixed effects modeling was used to estimate blood level data from 317 pediatric and adult epileptic patients.[7] Coadministration of clonazepam and valproic acid increased clonazepam clearance 14% and decreased valproic acid clearance 17.9%.

[1] Jeavons PM, et al. *Dev Med Child Neurol.* 1977;19(1):9.
[2] Gram L, et al. *Epilepsia.* 1977;18(2):141.
[3] Wilder BJ, et al. *Neurology.* 1978;28(9, pt 1):892.
[4] Mihaly GW, et al. *Eur J Clin Pharmacol.* 1979;16(1):23.
[5] Flachs H, et al. *Epilepsia.* 1979;20(2):187.
[6] Hoffman F, et al. *Eur J Clin Pharmacol.* 1981;19(5):383.
[7] Yukawa E, et al. *J Clin Pharm Ther.* 2003;28(6):497.

* Asterisk indicates drugs cited in interaction reports.

Clonidine — *Beta-Blockers*

Clonidine	Beta-Blockers	
Clonidine* (eg, *Catapres*)	Acebutolol (eg, *Sectral*)	Nadolol (eg, *Corgard*)
	Atenolol* (eg, *Tenormin*)	Penbutolol (*Levatol*)
	Betaxolol (eg, *Kerlone*)	Pindolol
	Carteolol (*Cartrol*)	Propranolol* (eg, *Inderal*)
	Esmolol (eg, *Brevibloc*)	Timolol*
	Metoprolol (eg, *Lopressor*)	

Significance	Onset	Severity	Documentation
1	☐ Rapid	■ **Major**	☐ Established
	■ **Delayed**	☐ Moderate	☐ Probable
		☐ Minor	■ **Suspected**
			☐ Possible
			☐ Unlikely

Effects Potentially life-threatening increases in BP.

Mechanism BETA-BLOCKER inhibition of beta-2 receptor–mediated vasodilation leaves peripheral alpha-2 receptor–mediated vasoconstriction unopposed to CLONIDINE stimulation.

Management Closely monitor BP after initiation or discontinuation of CLONIDINE or a BETA-BLOCKER when they are given concurrently. Discontinue either agent gradually; preferably, discontinue the BETA-BLOCKER first.

Discussion

Life-threatening and fatal increases in BP after discontinuing clonidine in patients receiving a beta-blocker or after simultaneous discontinuation of clonidine and a beta-blocker have occurred.[1-4] However, it was not possible to determine whether increases in BP were caused by an interaction or the withdrawal syndrome associated with both agents.[5,6] BP increases were not observed in 11 patients given labetalol (eg, *Normodyne*) after clonidine discontinuation; however, plasma catecholamines increased, and tremor, insomnia, and apprehension were reported.[7] In contrast, BP increased in 4 patients after abrupt clonidine discontinuation and replacement with atenolol. Hypertension was observed in 2 of 14 patients with a more gradual discontinuation of clonidine and replacement with increasing atenolol or timolol doses.[8] A case report[9] suggests that propranolol attenuates or reverses the antihypertensive effects of clonidine.[10] However, addition of propranolol to clonidine therapy has added to the antihypertensive effects of clonidine.[6,11]

1 Bailey RR, et al. *Br Med J.* 1976;1(6015):942.
2 Strauss FG, et al. *JAMA.* 1977;238(16):1734.
3 Vernon C, et al. *Br J Clin Pract.* 1979;33(4):112.
4 Bruce DL, et al. *Anesthesiology.* 1979;51(1):90.
5 Cummings DM, et al. *Drug Intell Clin Pharm.* 1982;16(11):817.
6 Jounela AJ, et al. *Ann Clin Res.* 1984;16(4):181.
7 Rosenthal T, et al. *Eur J Clin Pharmacol.* 1981;20(4):237.
8 Lilja M, et al. *Acta Med Scand.* 1982;211(5):375.
9 Warren SE, et al. *Arch Intern Med.* 1979;139(2):253.
10 Lilja M. *Acta Med Scand.* 1983;214(2):119.
11 Lilja M, et al. *Acta Med Scand.* 1980;207(3):173.

* Asterisk indicates drugs cited in interaction reports. Based on pharmacologic and pharmacokinetic considerations, similar interactions may occur with other drugs that are listed.

Clonidine × **Mirtazapine**

Clonidine* (eg, *Catapres*)	Mirtazapine* (eg, *Remeron*)

Significance	Onset	Severity	Documentation
4	□ Rapid ■ **Delayed**	■ **Major** □ Moderate □ Minor	□ Established □ Probable □ Suspected ■ **Possible** □ Unlikely

Effects Attenuation of antihypertensive effects.

Mechanism Antagonism of the alpha-2 receptors at noradrenergic neurons by MIRTAZAPINE is suspected.

Management Carefully monitor BP if MIRTAZAPINE is started or stopped in patients receiving CLONIDINE.

Discussion

A possible interaction between clonidine and mirtazapine, resulting in hypertensive urgency, was reported in a 20-year-old man.[1] The patient had a history of Goodpasture syndrome for 2.5 years and end-stage renal disease. He had been receiving dialysis 3 days a week for 15 months. The patient was admitted to the hospital after being seen in the emergency room for progressive shortness of breath. His BP was 178/115 mm Hg and his chest radiograph showed increased pulmonary vascularity with overt edema. The patient had bilateral lower extremity edema. For the previous year, he had been maintained with metoprolol (eg, *Lopressor*), losartan (*Cozaar*), and clonidine with his BP in the range of 140 to 150/80 to 85 mm Hg. Two weeks before admission, the patient started taking mirtazapine for depression. Losartan was discontinued and minoxidil was started when it was noted that his BP had begun to increase. Upon admission, all previous medications were continued as well as a nitroglycerin drip that was started in the emergency room. Despite withholding metoprolol and administering IV labetalol (eg, *Normodyne*), the patient's BP remained elevated (187 to 208/113 to 131 mm Hg). In the medical intensive care unit, nitroprusside (eg, *Nitropress*) infusion and emergency dialysis were administered to control his BP at 160 to 180/95 to 105 mm Hg. Mirtazapine was discontinued and the patient was discharged with minoxidil, clonidine, and metoprolol. He did not experience any subsequent episodes of hypertensive urgency.

[1] Abo-Zena RA, et al. *Pharmacotherapy*. 2000;20(4):476.

* Asterisk indicates drugs cited in interaction reports.

Clonidine — *Prazosin*

Clonidine* (eg, *Catapres*)	Prazosin* (eg, *Minipress*)

Significance	Onset	Severity	Documentation
4	■ **Rapid**	□ Major	□ Established
	□ Delayed	■ **Moderate**	□ Probable
		□ Minor	□ Suspected
			■ **Possible**
			□ Unlikely

Effects The antihypertensive effectiveness of CLONIDINE may be decreased.

Mechanism Unknown.

Management May need a higher dose of CLONIDINE in patients pretreated with PRAZOSIN. Monitor BP and adjust the dose accordingly.

Discussion

In a study involving 18 patients with essential hypertension, the hypotensive action of IV clonidine was lower in patients pretreated with prazosin than in patients pretreated with chlorthalidone (eg, *Hygroton*) or placebo.[1]

[1] Kapocsi J, et al. *Eur J Clin Pharmacol.* 1987;32(4):331.

* Asterisk indicates drugs cited in interaction reports.

Clonidine — *Tricyclic Antidepressants*

Clonidine	Tricyclic Antidepressants	
Clonidine* (eg, *Catapres*)	Amitriptyline	Imipramine* (eg, *Tofranil*)
	Amoxapine	Nortriptyline (eg, *Pamelor*)
	Clomipramine (eg, *Anafranil*)	Protriptyline (eg, *Vivactil*)
	Desipramine* (eg, *Norpramin*)	Trimipramine (*Surmontil*)
	Doxepin (eg, *Sinequan*)	

Significance	Onset	Severity	Documentation
1	■ **Rapid** □ Delayed	■ **Major** □ Moderate □ Minor	□ Established ■ **Probable** □ Suspected □ Possible □ Unlikely

Effects Loss of BP control and possible life-threatening elevations in BP.

Mechanism TRICYCLIC ANTIDEPRESSANT inhibition of central alpha-2 adrenergic receptors has been postulated, but not conclusively established.

Management Avoid combination of CLONIDINE and TRICYCLIC ANTIDEPRESSANTS if possible by using other antihypertensive agents or nontricyclic antidepressants.

Discussion

Dangerous elevations in BP and hypertensive crisis have been reported in patients receiving clonidine and a tricyclic antidepressant concurrently.[1,2] Animal studies have confirmed that the antihypertensive effects of clonidine can be rapidly attenuated or reversed by tricyclic antidepressants and that the intensity of this effect is dependent on the dose of either agent.[3-6] In contrast, nontricyclic antidepressants such as maprotiline and bupropion (eg, *Wellbutrin*) do not affect the antihypertensive actions of clonidine.[7-10] Therefore, avoid the combination of clonidine and tricyclic antidepressants by using an alternative antihypertensive agent or antidepressant.

1 Briant RH, et al. *Br Med J.* 1973;1(5852):522.
2 Hui KK. *J Am Geriatr Soc.* 1983;31(3):164.
3 Briant RH, et al. *Br J Pharmacol.* 1972;46(3):563P.
4 van Spanning HW, et al. *Eur J Pharmacol.* 1973;24(3):402.
5 van Zwieten PA. *Arch Int Pharmacodyn Ther.* 1975;214(1):12.
6 van Zwieten PA. *Pharmacology.* 1976;14:227.
7 Elliott HL, et al. *Br J Clin Pharmacol.* 1983;15(suppl 2):323S.
8 Elliott HL, et al. *Eur J Clin Pharmacol.* 1983;24(1):15.
9 Gundert-Remy U, et al. *Eur J Clin Pharmacol.* 1983;25(5):595.
10 Cubeddu LX, et al. *Clin Pharmacol Ther.* 1984;35(5):576.

* Asterisk indicates drugs cited in interaction reports. Based on pharmacologic and pharmacokinetic considerations, similar interactions may occur with other drugs that are listed.

Clopidogrel | **Azole Antifungal Agents**

Clopidogrel* (eg, *Plavix*)	Ketoconazole* (eg, *Nizoral*)

Significance	Onset	Severity	Documentation
2	□ Rapid ■ **Delayed**	□ Major ■ **Moderate** □ Minor	□ Established □ Probable ■ **Suspected** □ Possible □ Unlikely

Effects The antiplatelet effect of CLOPIDOGREL may be inhibited by KETOCONAZOLE.

Mechanism CLOPIDOGREL is a prodrug that appears to be catalyzed to an active metabolite by CYP3A4 and CYP3A5. Because KETOCONAZOLE inhibits CYP3A4 and CYP3A5 isozymes, the metabolic conversion of CLOPIDOGREL to its active metabolite may be decreased.

Management If possible, avoid coadministration of these agents. It may be necessary to use alternative antiplatelet therapy.

Discussion

In a randomized, crossover study, the effects of ketoconazole on the pharmacokinetics of clopidogrel were investigated in 18 healthy subjects.[1] Each subject received a loading dose of clopidogrel 300 mg, followed by a maintenance dose of clopidogrel 75 mg daily for 5 days alone and with ketoconazole 400 mg daily. Compared with giving clopidogrel alone, coadministration of ketoconazole decreased the C_{max} of the active metabolite of clopidogrel 48% after the loading dose and 61% after maintenance dosing. In addition, ketoconazole reduced the clopidogrel active metabolite AUC after the clopidogrel loading and maintenance doses 22% and 29%, respectively, and reduced inhibition of platelet aggregation after the loading and maintenance doses 28% and 33%, respectively.

[1] Farid NA, et al. *Clin Pharmcol Ther.* 2007;81(5):735.

* Asterisk indicates drugs cited in interaction reports.

Clopidogrel — *Caffeine*

Clopidogrel* (eg, *Plavix*)	Caffeine*

Significance	Onset	Severity	Documentation
5	☐ Rapid	☐ Major	☐ Established
	■ **Delayed**	☐ Moderate	☐ Probable
		■ **Minor**	☐ Suspected
			■ **Possible**
			☐ Unlikely

Effects The antiplatelet effect of CLOPIDOGREL may be enhanced by CAFFEINE.

Mechanism CAFFEINE may increase platelet levels of cyclic adenosine monophosphate, which is important in inhibiting platelet activation and aggregation.

Management Based on available information, no special precautions are needed.

Discussion

The effect of acute caffeine administration on clopidogrel platelet inhibition was investigated in 12 healthy volunteers and 40 patients with coronary artery disease (CAD) who were receiving long-term clopidogrel treatment.[1] In a crossover design, healthy subjects took clopidogrel 300 mg alone and 30 minutes before receiving caffeine 300 mg. Patients with CAD received caffeine 300 mg approximately 150 minutes before their daily clopidogrel dose. In healthy volunteers, caffeine administration enhanced platelet inhibition 2 to 4 hours after clopidogrel administration. In patients with CAD, enhancement of platelet inhibition was less pronounced than in healthy subjects, but was associated with increased inhibition of platelet activation. Thus, caffeine augmented the antiplatelet effect of clopidogrel in healthy subjects and patients with CAD.

Additional studies are needed to determine the extent and clinical importance of the caffeine-augmented antiplatelet effect of clopidogrel.

[1] Lev EI, et al. *Am Heart J.* 2007;154(4):694.e1.

* Asterisk indicates drugs cited in interaction reports.

Clopidogrel | **HMG-CoA Reductase Inhibitors**

Clopidogrel* (eg, *Plavix*)	Atorvastatin* (eg, *Lipitor*)	Lovastatin (eg, *Mevacor*)
	Fluvastatin* (eg, *Lescol*)	Simvastatin* (eg, *Zocor*)

Significance	Onset	Severity	Documentation
5	□ Rapid	□ Major	□ Established
	■ **Delayed**	□ Moderate	□ Probable
		■ **Minor**	□ Suspected
			■ **Possible**
			□ Unlikely

Effects Certain HMG-CoA REDUCTASE INHIBITORS may interfere with CLOPIDOGREL platelet inhibition. One case of rhabdomyolysis has been reported.

Mechanism By competing for the same CYP3A4 isoform, certain HMG-CoA REDUCTASE INHIBITORS may inhibit the metabolic conversion of the prodrug CLOPIDOGREL to its active form.

Management Based on available data, no special precautions are needed.

Discussion

Data are conflicting. The effects of atorvastatin and simvastatin on the platelet inhibition activity of clopidogrel were studied in 47 patients.[1] Platelet inhibition activity of clopidogrel was assessed 5 hours (early loading phase) and 48 hours (maintenance phase) after administration of the loading dose. Atorvastatin and simvastatin impaired the platelet inhibitory effects of clopidogrel. The interference with clopidogrel platelet inhibition was more pronounced during the early loading phase than in the maintenance phase (relative reduction 29% compared with 17%, respectively). Another study found that atorvastatin interferes with clopidogrel platelet inhibition.[2] In contrast, a retrospective analysis of 25 patients receiving an HMG-CoA reductase inhibitor and clopidogrel concurrently found no evidence of an interaction.[3] Similarly, other studies found that HMG-CoA reductase inhibitors did not affect the ability of clopidogrel to inhibit platelet function.[1,4-12] In a sequential study of 20 healthy responders to clopidogrel, coadministration of clopidogrel and fluvastatin or simvastatin for 7 days attenuated the antiplatelet effect of clopidogrel, while atorvastatin, pravastatin (eg, *Pravachol*), and rosuvastatin (*Crestor*) had no effect.[13]

Rhabdomyolysis was reported in a 58-year-old woman on long-term, stable atorvastatin therapy within 4 weeks of starting clopidogrel.[14] Inhibition of atorvastatin metabolism (CYP3A4) was suspected.

1 Neubauer H, et al. *Eur Heart J.* 2003;24(19):1744.
2 Lau WC, et al. *Circulation.* 2003;107(1):32.
3 Serebruany VL, et al. *Atherosclerosis.* 2001;159(1):239.
4 Serebruany VL, et al. *Arch Intern Med.* 2004;164(18):2051.
5 Gorchakova O, et al. *Eur Heart J.* 2004;25(21):1898.
6 Ayalasomayajula SP, et al. *J Clin Pharmacol.* 2007;47(5):613.
7 Smith SM, et al. *Platelets.* 2004;15(8):465.
8 Trenk D, et al. *Thromb Haemost.* 2008;99(1):174.
9 Farid NA, et al. *Pharmacotherapy.* 2008;28(12):1483.
10 Riodino S, et al. *J Thrombolysis.* 2009;28(2):151.
11 Malmström RE, et al. *J Interm Med.* 2009;266(5):457.
12 Serrano CV Jr, et al. *Arg Bras Cardiol.* 2010;95(3):321.
13 Mach F, et al. *Eur J Clin Invest.* 2005;35(8):476.
14 Burton JR, et al. *Ann Pharmacother.* 2007;41(1):133.

* Asterisk indicates drugs cited in interaction reports. Based on pharmacologic and pharmacokinetic considerations, similar interactions may occur with other drugs that are listed.

Clopidogrel — *Macrolide & Related Antibiotics*

Clopidogrel	Macrolide & Related Antibiotics	
Clopidogrel* (eg, *Plavix*)	Clarithromycin (eg, *Biaxin*)	Telithromycin (*Ketek*)
	Erythromycin* (eg, *Ery-Tab*)	

Significance	Onset	Severity	Documentation
4	□ Rapid	□ Major	□ Established
	■ **Delayed**	■ **Moderate**	□ Probable
		□ Minor	□ Suspected
			■ **Possible**
			□ Unlikely

Effects The antiplatelet effect of CLOPIDOGREL may be inhibited by certain MACROLIDE AND RELATED ANTIBIOTICS.

Mechanism CLOPIDOGREL is a prodrug that appears to be catalyzed to its active metabolite by CYP3A4 and CYP3A5.[1] Because certain MACROLIDE AND RELATED ANTIBIOTICS are inhibitors of CYP3A4, they may decrease the metabolic conversion of CLOPIDOGREL to its active metabolite.

Management Carefully monitor platelet function when starting or stopping certain MACROLIDE AND RELATED ANTIBIOTICS. Adjust the CLOPIDOGREL dose as needed. Because azithromycin (eg, *Zithromax*) does not inhibit CYP3A4, it may be a safer alternative.

Discussion

The effects of erythromycin or troleandomycin† on clopidogrel inhibition of platelet aggregation were studied in healthy volunteers.[2] Nine subjects received erythromycin and clopidogrel while 8 received troleandomycin and clopidogrel. Both erythromycin and troleandomycin interfered with the ability of clopidogrel to inhibit platelet aggregation. Platelet aggregation was 42% with administration of clopidogrel alone compared with 55% when erythromycin was coadministered. Similarly, platelet aggregation was 45% with administration of clopidogrel alone, compared with 78% when troleandomycin was coadministered.[2]

[1] Clarke TA, et al. *Drug Metab Dispos.* 2003;31(1):53.
[2] Lau WC, et al. *Circulation.* 2003;107(1):32.

* Asterisk indicates drugs cited in interaction reports. Based on pharmacologic and pharmacokinetic considerations, similar interactions may occur with other drugs that are listed.
† Not available in the United States.

Clopidogrel — *NSAIDs*

Clopidogrel* (eg, *Plavix*)	Celecoxib* (*Celebrex*)

Significance	Onset	Severity	Documentation
4	☐ Rapid	■ **Major**	☐ Established
	■ **Delayed**	☐ Moderate	☐ Probable
		☐ Minor	☐ Suspected
			■ **Possible**
			☐ Unlikely

Effects Risk of hemorrhage may be increased.

Mechanism Unknown.

Management Carefully monitor patients when CLOPIDOGREL and CELECOXIB are coadministered.

Discussion

Intracerebral hemorrhage was reported in an 86-year-old woman during coadministration of clopidogrel 75 mg/day and celecoxib 200 mg/day.[1] The patient presented with headaches and left hemiparesis 3 weeks after starting both drugs. Intracerebral hemorrhage was found on a CT scan. Management included discontinuation of clopidogrel and celecoxib and rehabilitation. She was discharged after 10 days.

Additional documentation is needed to determine if the patient's reaction was caused by an interaction or an adverse reaction to either drug alone.

[1] Fisher AA, et al. *Ann Pharmacother.* 2001;35(12):1567.

* Asterisk indicates drugs cited in interaction reports.

Clopidogrel — *Proton Pump Inhibitors*

Clopidogrel	Proton Pump Inhibitors	
Clopidogrel* (eg, *Plavix*)	Dexlansoprazole (*Dexilant*)	Omeprazole* (eg, *Prilosec*)
	Esomeprazole* (*Nexium*)	Pantoprazole* (eg, *Protonix*)
	Lansoprazole* (eg, *Prevacid*)	Rabeprazole* (*Aciphex*)

Significance	Onset	Severity	Documentation
1	☐ Rapid ■ **Delayed**	■ **Major** ☐ Moderate ☐ Minor	☐ Established ☐ Probable ■ **Suspected** ☐ Possible ☐ Unlikely

Effects The antiplatelet activity of CLOPIDOGREL may be decreased by PROTON PUMP INHIBITORS.

Mechanism Interference with the metabolic (CYP2C19) conversion of CLOPIDOGREL to the active metabolite by certain PROTON PUMP INHIBITORS is suspected.

Management A histamine H_2 antagonist (eg, famotidine [eg, *Pepcid*], ranitidine [eg, *Zantac*], but not cimetidine [eg, *Tagamet*]) can be used safely in patients with low risk of GI bleeding on long-term CLOPIDOGREL therapy. Use a PROTON PUMP INHIBITOR in patients with a high risk of bleeding (eg, prior GI bleeding, advanced age, concurrent anticoagulant therapy, long-term steroid and/or NSAID therapy, *Helicobacter pylori* infection) or refractory gastroesophageal reflux disease on long-term CLOPIDOGREL therapy.[1] PANTOPRAZOLE may be a safer alternative in these situations.

Discussion

The interaction between proton pump inhibitors and clopidogrel has been widely reviewed, with conflicting findings and recommendations. Some retrospective studies assessed the outcome of patients taking clopidogrel with and without a proton pump inhibitor. Concurrent use of omeprazole,[2-6] lansoprazole, rabeprazole,[4,6,] esomeprazole,[7] or pantoprazole[8] with clopidogrel was associated with an increased risk of adverse cardiovascular outcomes (eg, MI, recurrent MI, death, target vessel failure) compared with clopidogrel therapy alone. Omeprazole has been reported to decrease the antiplatelet effect of clopidogrel.[2,9,10] Coadministration of clopidogrel and a proton pump inhibitor (including pantoprazole) was associated with rehospitalization for coronary stent placement or MI in 1 study[8] but not in another that included 20,500 patients.[11] In a study of 104 patients undergoing coronary stenting, omeprazole reduced the antiplatelet activity of clopidogrel to a greater extent than pantoprazole.[12] In another study, pantoprazole did not reduce the antiplatelet effectiveness of clopidogrel after coronary stenting.[13] Coadministration of pantoprazole and clopidogrel following an acute MI was not associated with an increased risk of recurrent MI.[4] A randomized study evaluated GI and cardiovascular end points in 3,761 patients receiving clopidogrel and aspirin with either omeprazole or placebo.[14] Patients receiving omeprazole had a 1.1% GI event rate compared with 2.9% event rate with placebo. The cardiovascular event rate was 4.9% with omeprazole compared with 5.7% with placebo. However, the findings could not rule out a clinically meaningful difference in cardiovascular events due to the use of omeprazole. A randomized, placebo-controlled study involving 282 healthy subjects concluded that a metabolic drug interaction occurs between clopidogrel and omeprazole but not pantoprazole.[13] Separating the administration times of the clopidogrel and omeprazole doses by 12 hours, or doubling the clopidogrel dose (150 g/day) did not diminish the clopidogrel-omeprazole interaction. In a study comparing post-MI patients receiving clopidogrel and esomeprazole, lansoprazole, omeprazole, or pantoprazole with post-MI patients receiving clopidogrel alone for 1 year, no increased risk of cardiovascular events or mortality was associated with coadministration of clopidogrel and a proton pump inhibitor.[16] The CYP2C19 genotype had no apparent influence on outcomes. In another study, clopidogrel increased omeprazole AUC 30% in CYP2C19-extensive metabolizers but had no effect on subjects genotyped as poor metabolizers.[17] However, the increase in omeprazole concentrations does not appear to be clinically important. A study from a Department of Veterans Affairs large database did not find any association between concomitant use of clopidogrel and proton pump inhibitors and cardiovascular events.[18] In a prospective, randomized, open-label study involving 87 patients with coronary artery disease, both omeprazole and rabeprazole decreased the antiplatelet effect of clopidogrel.[19] These agents resulted in a similar degree of interference on the action of clopidogrel as measured by adenosine 5-diphosphate–induced platelet aggregation. Esomeprazole reduced the antiplatelet effect of clopidogrel 75 mg, but increasing the clopidogrel dose to 150 mg compensated for the interaction.[20] The AUC of the active metabolite of clopidogrel and its antiplatelet activity were affected less by dexlansoprazole or lansoprazole compared with esomeprazole or omeprazole.[21] In an investigation of patients receiving clopidogrel in combination with aspirin, no association was found between concurrent proton pump inhibitor use and myocardial infarction compared with patients receiving clopidogrel with aspirin without proton pump inhibitors.[22] In 1,328 patients undergoing drug-eluting stent replacement treatment with clopidogrel plus either lansoprazole, omeprazole, or pantoprazole, the rate of major adverse events was the same as for patients receiving clopidogrel without a proton pump inhibitor.[23]

Additional studies are needed to determine the magnitude of this interaction with clopidogrel and each proton pump inhibitor.

1 Abrahams NS, et al. *Am J Gastroenterol.* 2010;105(12):2533.
2 Ho PM, et al. *JAMA.* 2009;301(9):937.
3 Juurlink DN, et al. *CMAJ.* 2009;180(7):713.
4 Siller-Matula JM, et al. *Am Heart J.* 2009;157(1):148.e1.
5 Gupta E, et al. *Dig Dis Sci.* 2010;55(7):1964.
6 Kreutz RP, et al. *Pharmacotherapy.* 2010;30(8):787.
7 Burkard T, et al. *J Intern Med.* 2012;271(3)257.
8 Stockl KM, et al. *Arch Intern Med.* 2010;170(8):704.
9 Gilard M, et al. *J Am Coll Cardiol.* 2008;51(3):256.
10 Yun KH, et al. *Int Heart J.* 2010;51(1):13.
11 Ray WA, et al. *Ann Intern Med.* 2010;152(6):337.
12 Cuisset T, et al. *J Am Coll Cardiol.* 2009;54(13):1149.
13 Neubauer H, et al. *J Cardiovasc Pharmacol.* 2010;56(1):91.
14 Bhatt DL, et al. *N Engl J Med.* 2010;363(20):1909.
15 Angiolillo DJ, et al. *Clin Pharmacol Ther.* 2011;89(1):65.
16 Simon T, et al. *Circulation.* 2011;123(5):474.
17 Chen BL, et al. *J Clin Pharmacol.* 2009;49(5):574.
18 Banerjee S, et al. *Am J Cardiol.* 2011;107(6):871.
19 Siriswangvat S, et al. *Circ J.* 2010;74(10):2187.
20 Moceri P, et al. *Thromb Res.* 2011;128(5):458.
21 Frelinger AL, et al. *J Am Coll Cardiol.* 2012;59(14):1304.
22 Douglas IJ, et al. *Br Med J.* 2012;345:(July 10):e4388.
23 Rossini R, et al. *Coron Artery Dis.* 2011;22(3):199.

* Asterisk indicates drugs cited in interaction reports. Based on pharmacologic and pharmacokinetic considerations, similar interactions may occur with other drugs that are listed.

Clopidogrel — *Rifamycins*

Clopidogrel* (*Plavix*)	Rifabutin (*Mycobutin*) Rifampin* (eg, *Rifadin*)	Rifapentine (*Priftin*)

Significance	Onset	Severity	Documentation
2	☐ Rapid ■ **Delayed**	☐ Major ■ **Moderate** ☐ Minor	☐ Established ☐ Probable ■ **Suspected** ☐ Possible ☐ Unlikely

Effects The antiplatelet effect of CLOPIDOGREL may be enhanced by RIFAMYCINS.

Mechanism CLOPIDOGREL is a prodrug that appears to be catalyzed to its active metabolite by CYP3A4 and CYP3A5.[1] Because RIFAMYCINS are inducers of CYP3A4, they may increase the metabolic conversion of CLOPIDOGREL to its active metabolite.

Management Carefully monitor platelet function when the RIFAMYCIN dose is started, stopped, or changed. Adjust the CLOPIDOGREL dose as needed.

Discussion

The effect of rifampin 300 mg twice daily on clopidogrel inhibition of platelet aggregation was studied in 10 healthy volunteers.[2] Coadministration of rifampin and clopidogrel increased the ability of clopidogrel to inhibit platelet aggregation. Platelet aggregation was 56% with clopidogrel alone, compared with 33% when rifampin was coadministered. In a study of 12 volunteers, administration of rifampin 300 mg twice daily with clopidogrel 75 mg daily for 7 days increased the concentration of the clopidogrel active metabolite approximately 3.75-fold.[3] This was correlated to greater blockade of platelet $P2Y_{12}$ receptors and enhanced inhibition of platelet aggregation.

[1] Clarke TA, et al. *Drug Metab Dispos.* 2003;31(1):53.
[2] Lau WC, et al. *Circulation.* 2003;107(1):32.
[3] Judge HM, et al. *J Thromb Haemost.* 2010;8(8):1820.

* Asterisk indicates drugs cited in interaction reports. Based on pharmacologic and pharmacokinetic considerations, similar interactions may occur with other drugs that are listed.

Clopidogrel — Salicylates

Clopidogrel	Salicylates
Clopidogrel* (*Plavix*)	Aspirin* (eg, *Bayer*)

Significance	Onset	Severity	Documentation
1	□ Rapid ■ **Delayed**	■ **Major** □ Moderate □ Minor	□ Established ■ **Probable** □ Suspected □ Possible □ Unlikely

Effects Risk of life-threatening bleeding (eg, intracranial and GI hemorrhage) may be increased in high-risk patients with transient ischemic attack or ischemic stroke.

Mechanism Unknown. However, the effects of ASPIRIN on the GI mucosa may be a risk factor.

Management Avoid ASPIRIN use in high-risk patients with recent ischemic stroke or transient ischemic attack who are receiving CLOPIDOGREL.

Discussion

The benefit and risk of adding aspirin to clopidogrel therapy in high-risk patients with ischemic stroke or transient ischemic attack were assessed in a randomized, double-blind, placebo-controlled study.[1] A total of 7,599 high-risk patients with recent ischemic stroke or transient ischemic attack plus at least 1 additional vascular risk factor who were receiving clopidogrel 75 mg/day were randomized to receive clopidogrel plus aspirin 75 mg/day (3,797 patients) or clopidogrel plus placebo (3,802 patients). Data were available for 7,276 patients at the 18-month follow-up. Compared with placebo, adding aspirin to clopidogrel therapy in high-risk patients with recent stroke or transient ischemic attack did not reduce major vascular events. However, life-threatening bleeding and major bleeding events were increased in the group receiving aspirin and clopidogrel compared with those receiving clopidogrel and placebo. Symptomatic intracranial hemorrhage and GI bleeding were the most common causes of the life-threatening and major bleeding episodes. There was no difference in recorded mortality between the groups. In 7 healthy men, the addition of clopidogrel (75 mg daily for 2 days) to aspirin (150 mg daily) therapy increased bleeding time from 7.6 to 17.5 minutes.[2] An epidemiological study of patients with GI bleeding reported an association between bleeding and the use of clopidogrel plus aspirin, compared with either drug alone.[3] In a large, observational study, the risk of nonfatal and fatal bleeding was estimated in more than 118,000 patients with atrial fibrillation and during their posthospital therapy with warfarin, aspirin, clopidogrel, and combinations of these drugs.[4] The incidence of bleeding with coadministration of clopidogrel and warfarin was 13.9% per patient-year and 15.7% per patient-year with concurrent use of clopidogrel, warfarin, and aspirin, compared with 3.9% per patient-year with warfarin monotherapy. See also Anticoagulants/Clopidogrel.

[1] Diener HC, et al. *Lancet.* 2004;364(9431):331.
[2] Payne DA, et al. *J Vasc Surg.* 2002;35(6):1204.
[3] Delaney JA, et al. *CMAJ.* 2007;177(4):347.
[4] Hansen ML, et al. *Arch Intern Med.* 2010;170(16):1433.

* Asterisk indicates drugs cited in interaction reports.

Clozapine — *ACE Inhibitors*

Clozapine* (eg, *Clozaril*)	Lisinopril* (eg, *Prinivil*)

Significance	Onset	Severity	Documentation
4	☐ Rapid ■ **Delayed**	☐ Major ■ **Moderate** ☐ Minor	☐ Established ☐ Probable ☐ Suspected ■ **Possible** ☐ Unlikely

Effects The pharmacologic and toxic effects of CLOZAPINE may be increased.

Mechanism Unknown.

Management Observe the clinical response, monitor CLOZAPINE plasma concentrations, and adjust the dose of CLOZAPINE as needed when the dose of LISINOPRIL is started, stopped, or changed.

Discussion

Elevated plasma levels of clozapine and one of its metabolites, norclozapine, were reported in a 39-year-old man during concurrent treatment with lisinopril.[1] The patient was receiving clozapine 300 mg/day (plasma level 490 ng/mL) for treatment-resistant schizophrenia and glipizide (eg, *Glucotrol*) for diabetes. After developing hypertension, lisinopril 5 mg/day was started. Shortly thereafter, clozapine and norclozapine plasma levels were 966 and 512 ng/mL, respectively. Six months later, the lisinopril dose was increased to 10 mg/day, and clozapine and norclozapine levels, measured on 2 occasions 1 month apart, were 1,092 and 380 ng/mL and 1,245 and 392 ng/mL, respectively. He experienced disorganization, episodes of irritability, angry outbursts, sleep disturbances, nightmares, awakenings, and excessive salivation. Six weeks after decreasing the clozapine dose to 200 mg/day, plasma levels of clozapine and norclozapine remained elevated. Six weeks after discontinuing lisinopril and starting diltiazem (eg, *Cardizem*), the clozapine and norclozapine levels decreased to 693 and 254 ng/mL, respectively. Sleep disturbances and irritability improved; however, the psychotic symptoms and salivation persisted.

[1] Abraham G, et al. *Am J Psychiatry*. 2001;158(6):969.

* Asterisk indicates drugs cited in interaction reports.

Clozapine — *Aripiprazole*

Clozapine* (eg, *Clozaril*)	Aripiprazole* (*Abilify*)

Significance	Onset	Severity	Documentation
4	☐ Rapid ■ **Delayed**	■ **Major** ☐ Moderate ☐ Minor	☐ Established ☐ Probable ☐ Suspected ■ **Possible** ☐ Unlikely

Effects The risk of neuroleptic malignant syndrome may be increased.

Mechanism Unknown.

Management Closely monitor the clinical response of the patient. If an interaction is suspected, adjust treatment as needed. If neuroleptic malignant syndrome is suspected, discontinue both drugs immediately and treat neuroleptic malignant syndrome appropriately.

Discussion

A 27-year-old man with paranoid schizophrenia had been receiving clozapine 300 mg daily when aripiprazole 15 mg daily was started.[1] The aripiprazole dose was titrated to 30 mg daily over a period of 15 days. Twelve days later, the patient developed symptoms consistent with neuroleptic malignant syndrome (eg, confusion, hyperthermia, slight extrapyramidal rigidity). Both drugs were stopped immediately. After 72 hours of intensive treatment, his symptoms improved.

[1] Dassa D, et al. *Prog Neuropsychopharmacol Biol Psychiatry*. 2010;34(2):427.

* Asterisk indicates drugs cited in interaction reports.

Clozapine — *Barbiturates*

Clozapine* (eg, *Clozaril*)	Phenobarbital* (eg, *Luminal*)

Significance	Onset	Severity	Documentation
2	☐ Rapid ■ **Delayed**	☐ Major ■ **Moderate** ☐ Minor	☐ Established ☐ Probable ■ **Suspected** ☐ Possible ☐ Unlikely

Effects CLOZAPINE plasma concentrations may be reduced, decreasing the pharmacologic effects.

Mechanism Induction of hepatic metabolism of CLOZAPINE.

Management Monitor CLOZAPINE therapy when PHENOBARBITAL is started or stopped. Observe the patient for CLOZAPINE toxicity when PHENOBARBITAL is stopped.

Discussion

The pharmacokinetics of clozapine and its 2 major metabolites, norclozapine and clozapine N-oxide, were evaluated in 22 schizophrenic outpatients treated with either clozapine alone (n = 15) or clozapine in combination with phenobarbital (n = 7).[1] All patients were stabilized on clozapine for at least 6 months. Patients had been receiving phenobarbital 100 to 150 mg/day for at least 6 months for the management of concurrent epilepsy. The 2 groups were comparable. Steady-state clozapine plasma concentrations were 35% lower in patients receiving concomitant phenobarbital compared with those receiving clozapine alone. While norclozapine plasma concentrations did not differ between the 2 groups, clozapine N-oxide levels were 117% higher in patients receiving phenobarbital. The plasma concentration ratios of the clozapine metabolites to the parent drug, clozapine, were higher in patients treated with phenobarbital than in those receiving clozapine alone.

[1] Facciolà G, et al. *Ther Drug Monit.* 1998;20(6):628.

* Asterisk indicates drugs cited in interaction reports.

Clozapine — *Caffeine*

Clozapine* (eg, *Clozaril*)	Caffeine*

Significance	Onset	Severity	Documentation
2	■ **Rapid** □ Delayed	□ Major ■ **Moderate** □ Minor	□ Established □ Probable ■ **Suspected** □ Possible □ Unlikely

Effects Elevation of CLOZAPINE concentrations and possible increase in adverse effects may occur.

Mechanism CAFFEINE may inhibit CLOZAPINE metabolism (CYP1A2).[1]

Management If an interaction is suspected, advise patients to avoid beverages and other products that contain CAFFEINE.

Discussion

A 39-year-old patient with a 20-year history of paranoid schizophrenia refractory to neuroleptics experienced acute exacerbation of psychotic episodes when clozapine was taken with caffeinated beverages.[2] At the time clozapine was started, the patient was being treated with haloperidol (eg, *Haldol*) and procyclidine.[†] He also ingested 5 to 10 cups of coffee daily. Clozapine was started because the patient had a long-standing refractoriness to neuroleptics. Procyclidine was gradually discontinued. While receiving clozapine, the patient experienced a progressive decrease in paranoid delusions and auditory hallucinations and tardive dyskinesia disappearance. However, each time the patient took clozapine with 2 cups of coffee, as he had done with his previous medication, he experienced acute psychotic exacerbation, consisting of anxiety, agitation, insomnia, weakness, headaches, stiffness, abdominal pain, and paranoid ideation. Similar reactions occurred when clozapine was ingested with *Diet Coke*. The patient was encouraged to avoid the intake of caffeinated beverages. No acute psychotic episode occurred when clozapine was taken with water or decaffeinated *Diet Coke*. A 31-year-old woman ingesting clozapine 550 mg/day, fluoxetine (eg, *Prozac*), diazepam (eg, *Valium*), caffeine tablets 200 mg/day, and approximately 1 liter of caffeinated iced tea (approximately caffeine 1,000 mg) per day had a clozapine level of 1,500 ng/mL and a norclozapine level of 630 ng/mL.[3] One week after being advised to discontinue caffeine tablets, caffeinated beverages, and chocolate, her clozapine and norclozapine levels were 630 and 330 ng/mL, respectively. In an open-label, randomized, crossover study involving 12 healthy volunteers, a 19% increase in the AUC of clozapine and a 14% decrease in clearance was noted during concomitant administration of clozapine and caffeine (mean dose, 550 mg/day) compared with taking clozapine alone.[4]

1 Carrillo JA, et al. *J Clin Psychopharmacol.* 1995;15(5):376.
2 Vainer JL, et al. *J Clin Psychopharmacol.* 1994;14(4):284.
3 Odom-White A, et al. *J Clin Psychiatry.* 1996;57(4):175.
4 Hägg S, et al. *Br J Clin Pharmacol.* 2000;49(1):59.

* Asterisk indicates drugs cited in interaction reports.

Clozapine — *Carbamazepine*

Clozapine*
(eg, *Clozaril*)

Carbamazepine*
(eg, *Tegretol*)

Significance	Onset	Severity	Documentation
4	☐ Rapid ■ **Delayed**	☐ Major ■ **Moderate** ☐ Minor	☐ Established ☐ Probable ☐ Suspected ■ **Possible** ☐ Unlikely

Effects The pharmacologic effects of CLOZAPINE may be decreased by coadministration of CARBAMAZEPINE. A single case of suspected neuroleptic malignant syndrome has been reported.

Mechanism Induction of hepatic microsomal enzymes by CARBAMAZEPINE is suspected.

Management Monitor serum clozapine levels when CARBAMAZEPINE therapy is started or stopped. When discontinuing CARBAMAZEPINE, observe the patient for signs of CLOZAPINE toxicity and adjust the dose accordingly. Administration of an alternate anticonvulsant agent, such as valproic acid (eg, *Depakene*) or valproic acid derivatives (eg, divalproex [*Depakote*]), may circumvent this interaction.

Discussion

In 2 patients, plasma clozapine concentrations increased after coadministration of carbamazepine was stopped.[1] A 25-year-old schizophrenic man had been receiving clozapine 800 mg/day and carbamazepine 600 mg/day for several months. After discontinuing carbamazepine, his plasma clozapine concentration increased from 1.4 to 2.4 mcmol/L (therapeutic level, 1.1 mcmol/L). The second patient, a 36-year-old schizophrenic man with epilepsy, had been taking clozapine 600 mg/day and carbamazepine 800 mg/day. When carbamazepine was discontinued, his serum clozapine concentration increased from 1.5 to 3 mcmol/L. In both patients, plasma clozapine concentrations increased within 2 weeks. A 76-year-old man with a history of bromperidol-induced neuroleptic malignant syndrome developed neuroleptic malignant syndrome 3 days after the addition of clozapine to a stable carbamazepine dose.[2]

[1] Raitasuo V, et al. *Am J Psychiatry*. 1993;150(1):169.
[2] Müller T, et al. *Lancet*. 1988;2(8626-8627):1500.

* Asterisk indicates drugs cited in interaction reports.

Clozapine — Cimetidine

Clozapine* (eg, *Clozaril*)	Cimetidine* (eg, *Tagamet*)

Significance	Onset	Severity	Documentation
4	□ Rapid ■ **Delayed**	□ Major ■ **Moderate** □ Minor	□ Established □ Probable □ Suspected ■ **Possible** □ Unlikely

Effects The pharmacologic and toxic effects of CLOZAPINE may be increased.

Mechanism Inhibition of the hepatic metabolism of CLOZAPINE is suspected.

Management Observe the patient for signs of CLOZAPINE toxicity and adjust the dose accordingly. Consider administering an H_2 antagonist that does not usually interact (eg, ranitidine [eg, *Zantac*]).

Discussion

A 24-year-old man developed dyspepsia and gastritis with GI reflux while taking clozapine 900 mg/day and atenolol (eg, *Tenormin*) 50 mg/day.[1] Atenolol was administered for clozapine-induced tachycardia. X-rays revealed a hiatal hernia, and treatment with oral cimetidine 400 mg twice daily was initiated. After 3 months, the patient's GI symptoms were only mildly relieved, and the dose of cimetidine was increased to 400 mg 3 times daily. Three days later, the patient complained of marked diaphoresis, dizziness, vomiting, generalized weakness, and severe light-headedness on standing. Over a 5-day period, after discontinuing cimetidine and decreasing the dose of clozapine to 200 mg/day, the symptoms of clozapine toxicity resolved. The dose of clozapine was increased over a 1-week period to 900 mg/day. When epigastric distress recurred, ranitidine 150 mg twice daily was started, and the symptoms were relieved. In this patient, elevated clozapine levels were measured during concurrent treatment with clozapine 900 mg/day and cimetidine 800 mg/day. Clozapine adverse effects occurred when the dose of cimetidine was increased to 1,200 mg/day. However, serum clozapine levels were not determined during administration of the higher cimetidine dose.

Controlled studies are needed to assess the importance of this possible interaction.

[1] Szymanski S, et al. *J Clin Psychiatry*. 1991;52(1):21.

* Asterisk indicates drugs cited in interaction reports.

Clozapine — *Contraceptives, Hormonal*

Clozapine* (eg, *Clozaril*)	Contraceptives, Oral* (eg, *Ortho-Novum*)

Significance	Onset	Severity	Documentation
4	☐ Rapid	☐ Major	☐ Established
	■ **Delayed**	■ **Moderate**	☐ Probable
		☐ Minor	☐ Suspected
			■ **Possible**
			☐ Unlikely

Effects CLOZAPINE plasma concentrations may be elevated, increasing the pharmacologic and adverse effects.

Mechanism Inhibition of CLOZAPINE metabolism by HORMONAL CONTRACEPTIVES is suspected.

Management Observe the clinical response of the patient and adjust the dose of CLOZAPINE as needed when HORMONAL CONTRACEPTIVES are started or stopped. Monitoring of CLOZAPINE plasma levels may assist in managing the patient.

Discussion

A possible drug interaction between clozapine and an oral contraceptive (ethinyl estradiol 35 mcg/norethindrone 0.5 mg) was reported in a 47-year-old woman with a 30-year history of paranoid schizophrenia.[1] The patient was hospitalized with severe psychosis. At the time of admission, she was taking oral contraceptives and smoking 1 pack of cigarettes daily. She was started on clozapine, and the dose was gradually increased to 550 mg/day. Most of her symptoms of psychosis resolved with clozapine therapy; however, she complained of drowsiness, weakness, and dizziness. Over the next 2 months, 3 clozapine plasma concentration determinations ranged between 736 to 792 ng/mL (therapeutic range, 300 to 700 ng/mL). The oral contraceptive was discontinued, and, within days, the patient reported resolution of clozapine adverse effects. One week after the oral contraceptive was stopped, the clozapine level was 401 ng/mL. The patient's smoking pattern did not change during the period of treatment.

[1] Gabbay V, et al. *J Clin Psychopharmacol.* 2002;22(6):621.

* Asterisk indicates drugs cited in interaction reports.

Clozapine — *Erythromycin*

Clozapine* (eg, *Clozaril*)	Erythromycin* (eg, *Ery-Tab*)

Significance	Onset	Severity	Documentation
4	□ Rapid ■ **Delayed**	□ Major ■ **Moderate** □ Minor	□ Established □ Probable □ Suspected ■ **Possible** □ Unlikely

Effects Serum CLOZAPINE concentrations may be elevated, increasing the pharmacologic and toxic effects of CLOZAPINE.

Mechanism ERYTHROMYCIN is suspected to inhibit the metabolism of CLOZAPINE.

Management Observe the clinical response of the patient and adjust the dose of CLOZAPINE as indicated when ERYTHROMYCIN is started or stopped.

Discussion

A seizure was reported in a schizophrenic patient maintained on a stable dose (800 mg/day) of clozapine 7 days after the addition of erythromycin 250 mg 4 times daily.[1] The serum clozapine concentration was 1,300 mcg/mL shortly after the seizure. Both drugs were stopped, and clozapine was restarted 2 days later at 400 mg/day. Over the following several weeks, the dose of clozapine was gradually increased back to 800 mg/day. After several weeks of this regimen, the serum clozapine concentration was 700 mcg/mL. A 34-year-old schizophrenic man experienced elevated clozapine levels of 1,150 mcg/L, leukocytosis, somnolence, incoordination, slurred speech, disorientation, and incontinence following addition of erythromycin 333 mg 3 times daily to his stable regimen, which included clozapine 600 mg/day.[2] His symptoms resolved after erythromycin and clozapine were discontinued. When clozapine was reinstated at the previous dose, he remained free of adverse effects. His clozapine level was 385 mcg/L.

Controlled studies are needed to determine the clinical importance of this drug interaction.

[1] Funderburg LG, et al. *Am J Psychiatry.* 1994;151(12):1840.

[2] Cohen LG, et al. *Arch Intern Med.* 1996;156(6):675.

* Asterisk indicates drugs cited in interaction reports.

Clozapine — *Hydantoins*

Clozapine	Hydantoins	
Clozapine* (eg, *Clozaril*)	Ethotoin (*Peganone*)	Phenytoin* (eg, *Dilantin*)
	Fosphenytoin	

Significance	Onset	Severity	Documentation
4	☐ Rapid	☐ Major	☐ Established
	■ **Delayed**	■ **Moderate**	☐ Probable
		☐ Minor	☐ Suspected
			■ **Possible**
			☐ Unlikely

Effects Possible reduction in the therapeutic response to CLOZAPINE. PHENYTOIN levels may be elevated, increasing the risk of toxicity.

Mechanism Altered hepatic metabolism of CLOZAPINE and PHENYTOIN is suspected.

Management Observe the patient's clinical response and adjust the dose of CLOZAPINE and PHENYTOIN accordingly.

Discussion

Two patients receiving clozapine experienced a decrease in serum clozapine levels and a loss of therapeutic effect following the addition of phenytoin to their treatment schedule.[1] Both patients were treated with clozapine because they had a history of nonresponsiveness to standard antipsychotic medications. The first patient was a 29-year-old man with a 12-year history of schizophrenia. Treatment was initiated with clozapine 50 mg/day, and the dose was gradually increased to 200 mg twice daily. On day 14 of treatment at this dosage, tonic-clonic seizures occurred. The clozapine dosage was decreased to 200 mg/day, and phenytoin 300 mg/day was started. Within 48 hours, acute worsening of psychotic symptoms was noted, and the dosage of clozapine was increased to 300 mg/day, then to 400 mg/day. Clozapine serum levels prior to phenytoin therapy were 282.2 and 295.9 ng/mL compared with 56.2 and 48.7 ng/mL during phenytoin coadministration. Psychotic symptoms persisted, and the dose of clozapine was increased to 500 mg/day. His plasma clozapine level was 92.6 ng/mL, and his clinical status improved somewhat. The second patient, a 29-year-old woman, had an 8-year history of psychotic illness. Clozapine therapy was started at 50 mg/day, and the dosage was slowly increased to 250 mg/day. Her serum clozapine level was 940.5 ng/mL. On day 8 of treatment at this dosage, tonic-clonic movements occurred, and the dosage of clozapine was reduced to 150 mg/day. A loading dose of phenytoin 1,200 mg was administered, followed by a maintenance dosage of 300 mg/day. She did not experience any further seizures; however, her psychosis worsened and clozapine was increased gradually to 250 mg/day. After 7 days of treatment at this dose, the plasma clozapine level was 334.7 ng/mL. Psychotic symptoms persisted, and the dosage of clozapine was increased to 400 mg/day, producing a decrease in psychosis. Serum clozapine levels decreased during phenytoin administration. A 40-year-old woman receiving clozapine developed a generalized tonic-clonic seizure and was hospitalized for evaluation.[2] Following a second seizure, the patient received IV phenytoin. The next evening, the patient experienced ataxia, dizziness, and nystagmus. The phenytoin level was 23.8 mcg/mL. Phenytoin levels slowly decreased to 15.9 mcg/mL on day 6, despite discontinuation of phenytoin on day 2.

[1] Miller DD. *J Clin Psychiatry*. 1991;52(1):23.

[2] Gandelman-Marton R, et al. *J Emerg Med*. 2008;35(4):407.

* Asterisk indicates drugs cited in interaction reports. Based on pharmacologic and pharmacokinetic considerations, similar interactions may occur with other drugs that are listed.

Clozapine — Isoniazid

Clozapine* (eg, *Clozaril*) | Isoniazid*

Significance	Onset	Severity	Documentation
4	□ Rapid	□ Major	□ Established
	■ **Delayed**	■ **Moderate**	□ Probable
		□ Minor	□ Suspected
			■ **Possible**
			□ Unlikely

Effects CLOZAPINE plasma concentrations may be elevated, increasing the pharmacologic effects and risk of adverse reactions.

Mechanism Inhibition of CLOZAPINE metabolism (CYP1A2) by ISONIAZID.

Management Monitor the clinical response of the patient and CLOZAPINE serum concentrations. Adjust the CLOZAPINE dose as needed.

Discussion

A 65-year-old man with schizophrenia was receiving clozapine 200 mg twice daily when a 9-month course of isoniazid 300 mg daily was started for tuberculosis.[1] Prior to starting isoniazid, clozapine and norclozapine concentrations were 397 and 384 ng/mL, respectively. Three days after the initiation of isoniazid, clozapine and norclozapine concentrations were 569 and 520 ng/mL, respectively. These values increased 6 days later to 756 and 725 ng/mL, respectively. The only sign of toxicity the patient displayed was sedation. The clozapine dose was reduced to 150 mg twice daily. The dose of clozapine was further reduced to 100 mg twice daily 11 days later. Another clozapine/norclozapine concentration was drawn 21 days later, and the results were 385 and 379 ng/mL, respectively. This clozapine dose was maintained for the duration of isoniazid therapy. Clozapine/norclozapine concentrations were drawn 54 days after completion of isoniazid therapy, and the results were 239 and 221 ng/mL, respectively. A month later, the patient became psychiatrically symptomatic, and the clozapine dose was titrated to 100 mg in the morning and 300 mg in the evening.

[1] Angelini MC, et al. *J Clin Psychopharmacol.* 2009;29(2):190.

* Asterisk indicates drugs cited in interaction reports.

Clozapine — *Lamotrigine*

Clozapine* (eg, *Clozaril*)	Lamotrigine* (eg, *Lamictal*)

Significance	Onset	Severity	Documentation
4	□ Rapid	□ Major	□ Established
	■ **Delayed**	■ **Moderate**	□ Probable
		□ Minor	□ Suspected
			■ **Possible**
			□ Unlikely

Effects CLOZAPINE plasma concentrations may be elevated, increasing the pharmacologic effects and adverse reactions.

Mechanism Unknown.

Management In patients receiving CLOZAPINE, closely monitor the clinical response when LAMOTRIGINE is started or stopped. CLOZAPINE plasma levels may be helpful in managing the patient.

Discussion

Lamotrigine was reported to increase clozapine plasma levels in a 35-year-old man.[1] The patient had been taking clozapine 400 mg/day for 3 years. During this time, his clozapine plasma concentrations were stable, measuring between 300 and 500 mcg/L. At the time lamotrigine was started, the patient's clozapine level was 350 mcg/L. The lamotrigine dose was titrated to 100 mg/day. After receiving lamotrigine 100 mg daily for 2 weeks, the patient complained of dizziness and sedation. His clozapine plasma concentration was 1,020 mcg/L. Over the next 2 weeks, the lamotrigine dose was tapered. At the end of this period, the plasma concentration of clozapine had decreased to 450 mcg/L. This interaction has been used for therapeutic benefit. Improvement was reported in 6 patients with treatment-resistant schizophrenia when lamotrigine (125 to 250 mg/day) was added to their clozapine (600 to 800 mg/day) regimen.[2] Eleven patients receiving clozapine 200 to 500 mg/day were studied at baseline and 6 or 10 weeks after the addition of lamotrigine (titrated to 200 mg/day).[3] No changes in clozapine plasma levels occurred.

[1] Kossen M, et al. *Am J Psychiatry*. 2001;158(11):1930.
[2] Dursun SM, et al. *Arch Gen Psychiatry*. 1999;56(10):950.
[3] Spina E, et al. *Ther Drug Monit*. 2006;28(5):599.

* Asterisk indicates drugs cited in interaction reports.

Clozapine — *Modafinil*

Clozapine* (eg, *Clozaril*)	Modafinil* (*Provigil*)

Significance	Onset	Severity	Documentation
4	☐ Rapid	☐ Major	☐ Established
	■ **Delayed**	■ **Moderate**	☐ Probable
		☐ Minor	☐ Suspected
			■ **Possible**
			☐ Unlikely

Effects CLOZAPINE serum levels may be elevated, increasing the pharmacologic and toxic effects.

Mechanism Inhibition of CLOZAPINE metabolism by MODAFINIL is suspected.

Management In patients receiving CLOZAPINE, closely observe the clinical response of the patient when starting or stopping MODAFINIL. Monitoring CLOZAPINE serum levels may be useful in managing the patient.

Discussion

Clozapine toxicity was reported in a 42-year-old man after modafinil was added to his treatment regimen.[1] Clozapine 25 mg at bedtime was started for the treatment of schizophrenia. The clozapine dose was titrated to 400 mg/day over a 13-day period. At this time, all other psychotropic drugs the patient was receiving were tapered and discontinued over an 8-week period. After 10 weeks of clozapine treatment, the serum level was 761 ng/mL. One week later, the clozapine dose was increased to 450 mg/day. To combat sedation associated with clozapine therapy, modafinil 100 mg/day was started and titrated to 300 mg/day over a 19-day period. Approximately 1 month after starting modafinil, the patient experienced dizziness, an unsteady gait, and fell twice. An ECG demonstrated sinus tachycardia. The clozapine serum concentration was 1400 ng/mL. Clozapine and modafinil were discontinued. The patient's gait disturbance resolved. Clozapine was restarted. Approximately 8 weeks after receiving 300 mg/day of clozapine, the serum level was 960 ng/mL.

[1] Dequardo JR. *Am J Psychiatry*. 2002;159:1243.

* Asterisk indicates drugs cited in interaction reports.

Clozapine — *Nefazodone*

Clozapine* (eg, *Clozaril*)	Nefazodone* (*Serzone*)

Significance	Onset	Severity	Documentation
4	☐ Rapid ■ **Delayed**	☐ Major ■ **Moderate** ☐ Minor	☐ Established ☐ Probable ☐ Suspected ■ **Possible** ☐ Unlikely

Effects CLOZAPINE plasma concentrations may be elevated, increasing the pharmacologic and adverse effects.

Mechanism Inhibition of CLOZAPINE metabolism (CYP3A4) by NEFAZODONE is suspected.

Management In patients receiving CLOZAPINE, closely monitor the clinical response when starting, stopping, or changing the dose of NEFAZODONE. Monitoring CLOZAPINE plasma levels may be useful in adjusting therapy.

Discussion

Increased clozapine plasma concentrations were reported in a 40-year-old man with schizophrenia after the addition of nefazodone to his treatment regimen.[1] The patient had been successfully treated with clozapine (425 to 475 mg/day) and risperidone (*Risperdal* [6 mg/day]) for several years. Nefazodone, 200 mg/day for 7 days then increased to 300 mg/day, was started for treatment of negative symptoms of schizophrenia. After 1 week of nefazodone treatment at the higher dose, the patient developed increased anxiety and dizziness as well as mild hypotension. Plasma levels of clozapine and norclozapine were found to be increased. The nefazodone dose was reduced to 200 mg/day and the symptoms resolved within 1 week. In addition, plasma levels of clozapine and norclozapine decreased. When nefazodone 300 mg/day was administered, clozapine and norclozapine levels were increased 75% and 89%, respectively, compared with 5% and 31%, respectively, when 200 mg/day of nefazodone was administered.

[1] Khan AY, et al. *J Clin Psychiatry*. 2001;62:375.

* Asterisk indicates drugs cited in interaction reports.

Clozapine — *Quinolones*

Clozapine* (eg, *Clozaril*)	Ciprofloxacin* (eg, *Cipro*)	Norfloxacin (*Noroxin*)

Significance	Onset	Severity	Documentation
2	☐ Rapid	☐ Major	☐ Established
	■ **Delayed**	■ **Moderate**	☐ Probable
		☐ Minor	■ **Suspected**
			☐ Possible
			☐ Unlikely

Effects CLOZAPINE plasma concentrations may be elevated, increasing the risk of adverse reactions.

Mechanism Inhibition of CLOZAPINE metabolism (CYP1A2) by certain QUINOLONE antibiotics is suspected.

Management Observe the clinical response of the patient and adjust the dose of CLOZAPINE as needed when certain QUINOLONES are started or stopped.

Discussion

A possible interaction between clozapine and ciprofloxacin was reported in a 72-year-old man with multiple infarct dementia, behavioral disturbances, and diabetes mellitus.[1] At the time of hospital admission to the behavioral intensive care unit, the patient was receiving clozapine 6.25 mg at 3 PM and 12.5 mg at 9 PM, and was on the last day of a 10-day course of ciprofloxacin 500 mg twice daily. The patient also was receiving glyburide (eg, *DiaBeta*), trazodone (eg, *Oleptro*), and melatonin. On admission, the clozapine plasma concentration was 90 ng/mL. At the time of discharge, and after the course of ciprofloxacin therapy had been completed, clozapine plasma concentrations were undetectable (lower limit of assay detection was 50 ng/mL). No other medication changes had been made. In 7 patients with schizophrenia on stable clozapine regimens, ciprofloxacin (250 mg twice daily for 7 days) increased mean clozapine and N-desmethylclozapine plasma levels 29% and 31%, respectively, compared with placebo.[2] No increase in adverse reactions was noted. Administration of ciprofloxacin 500 mg twice daily to a man taking clozapine 750 mg/day resulted in nearly a 5-fold increase in clozapine levels.[3] No adverse reactions were reported.

[1] Markowitz JS, et al. *Am J Psychiatry*. 1997;154(6):881.
[2] Raaska K, et al. *Eur J Clin Pharmacol*. 2000;56(8):585.
[3] Sambhi RS, et al. *Eur J Clin Pharmacol*. 2007;63(9):895.

* Asterisk indicates drugs cited in interaction reports. Based on pharmacologic and pharmacokinetic considerations, similar interactions may occur with other drugs that are listed.

Clozapine — *Rifamycins*

Clozapine	Rifamycins	
Clozapine* (eg, *Clozaril*)	Rifabutin (*Mycobutin*)	Rifapentine (*Priftin*)
	Rifampin* (eg, *Rifadin*)	

Significance	Onset	Severity	Documentation
4	☐ Rapid	☐ Major	☐ Established
	■ **Delayed**	■ **Moderate**	☐ Probable
		☐ Minor	☐ Suspected
			■ **Possible**
			☐ Unlikely

Effects RIFAMYCINS may decrease CLOZAPINE serum concentrations, decreasing the therapeutic effect.

Mechanism RIFAMYCINS may increase the metabolism of CLOZAPINE by enzyme induction.

Management Monitor serum CLOZAPINE concentrations and observe the clinical response of the patient when RIFAMYCINS are started or stopped. If the RIFAMYCIN is discontinued, observe the patient for signs of CLOZAPINE toxicity. Adjust the dose of CLOZAPINE as needed.

Discussion

Decreased serum clozapine concentrations were reported in a 33-year-old man with schizophrenia during coadministration of rifampin.[1] The patient was receiving clozapine 400 mg/day. His main symptoms consisted of paranoid thoughts, auditory hallucinations, and irritability. He was started on rifampin, isoniazid (eg, *Nydrazid*), and pyrazinamide when cavitary lesions were seen on a CT scan. Prior to this, the patient had complained of general malaise and a feeling of "having pus in his throat." Three and a half weeks later, clozapine serum concentrations were decreased, and the dose was increased from 400 to 600 mg/day. Microbiologic analysis of the patient's sputum and gastric fluid identified an atypical mycobacterial infection, *Mycobacterium xenopi*. Rifampin was replaced with ciprofloxacin (eg, *Cipro*), and within 3 days, clozapine serum concentrations increased to the therapeutic range with improvement in the patient's psychopathology. The clozapine dosage was decreased to 400 mg/day. Clozapine concentrations 40 to 60 days later appeared 60% higher than before antibiotic administration. A 30-year-old man with paranoid schizophrenia, nonresponsive to other antipsychotics, responded well to clozapine.[2] However, after starting rifampin for tuberculosis, the patient's psychotic symptoms worsened and clozapine adverse reactions disappeared. After discontinuing rifampin, clozapine adverse reactions reappeared, but his psychotic symptoms markedly improved.

[1] Joos AA, et al. *J Clin Psychopharmacol.* 1998;18(1):83.

[2] Peritogiannis V, et al. *Gen Hosp Psychiatry.* 2007;29(3):281.

* Asterisk indicates drugs cited in interaction reports. Based on pharmacologic and pharmacokinetic considerations, similar interactions may occur with other drugs that are listed.

Clozapine — *Risperidone*

Clozapine* (eg, *Clozaril*)	Risperidone* (eg, *Risperdal*)

Significance	Onset	Severity	Documentation
4	□ Rapid ■ **Delayed**	■ **Major** □ Moderate □ Minor	□ Established □ Probable □ Suspected ■ **Possible** □ Unlikely

Effects The pharmacologic effects and adverse reactions of CLOZAPINE may be increased. Neuroleptic malignant syndrome (NMS) has been reported.

Mechanism Unknown.

Management Observe the clinical response of the patient, monitor CLOZAPINE serum concentrations and adjust the dose of CLOZAPINE as indicated when RISPERIDONE is started or stopped.

Discussion

Elevated clozapine plasma concentrations were reported in a 32-year-old man with a 10-year history of schizoaffective disorder following the addition of risperidone to his stable clozapine regimen.[1] The patient experienced substantial, but not optimal, improvement while receiving clozapine 300 mg twice daily. Risperidone 0.5 mg twice daily increased to 1 mg twice daily after 1 week was added for augmentation. The clinical condition of the patient improved during concurrent treatment with both drugs. While receiving clozapine alone, the serum concentration was 344 ng/mL. Three weeks after starting risperidone, the clozapine concentration was 598 ng/mL. No adverse reactions were noted. However, in a prospective study, patients with schizophrenia or schizoaffective disorder received clozapine alone or with risperidone.[2] Pharmacokinetic analysis found no difference in clozapine clearance between the 2 treatment groups. A 20-year-old man, with first episode schizophrenia, was treated with risperidone (titrated to 16 mg/day) without clinical improvement.[3] Two days after the addition of clozapine (100 mg/day), he developed fever, muscle rigidity, tremor, dysphagia, diaphoresis, sialorrhea, tachycardia, tachypnea, and altered consciousness. A diagnosis of NMS was made and all antipsychotics were stopped. Subsequently, he was treated with clozapine alone without reappearance of NMS symptoms.

[1] Tyson SC, et al. *Am J Psychiatry*. 1995;152(9):1401.
[2] Chetty M, et al. *Br J Clin Pharmacol*. 2009;68(4):574.
[3] Kontaxakis VP, et al. *Prog Neuropsychopharmacol Biol Psychiatry*. 2002;26(2):407.

* Asterisk indicates drugs cited in interaction reports.

Clozapine ✕ Serotonin Reuptake Inhibitors

Clozapine	Serotonin Reuptake Inhibitors	
Clozapine* (eg, *Clozaril*)	Citalopram* (*Celexa*) Fluoxetine* (eg, *Prozac*)	Fluvoxamine* Sertraline* (*Zoloft*)

Significance	Onset	Severity	Documentation
1	☐ Rapid ■ **Delayed**	■ **Major** ☐ Moderate ☐ Minor	■ **Established** ☐ Probable ☐ Suspected ☐ Possible ☐ Unlikely

Effects Serum CLOZAPINE levels may be elevated, resulting in increased pharmacologic and toxic effects.

Mechanism Certain SSRIs inhibit CLOZAPINE hepatic metabolism.[1]

Management Monitor CLOZAPINE serum levels and observe the clinical response. Adjust the dose of CLOZAPINE as needed.

Discussion

Case reports and controlled clinical studies indicate that citalopram,[2] fluoxetine,[3] fluvoxamine,[4-10] and sertraline[7,11] can increase clozapine serum levels. Six patients experienced an average 76% increase in serum clozapine levels following the addition of fluoxetine to stable clozapine regimens.[3] No evidence of side effects or toxicity was noted. In a 35-year-old schizophrenic man, clozapine and norclozapine levels decreased 42% and 37%, respectively, 30 days after stopping sertraline.[11] A 26-year-old woman was started on sertraline 50 mg/day when her compulsive checking worsened while on clozapine 175 mg/day.[7] Four weeks later, her condition worsened, and her clozapine level increased 76% (from 395 to 695 ng/mL). Two weeks after stopping sertraline, her psychosis improved, and her clozapine level decreased to 460 ng/mL. Several case reports[4-8,10] and prospective studies[9,12-14] describe similar increases in serum clozapine during coadministration of fluvoxamine. In 1 of these studies, 16 schizophrenic patients on stable clozapine doses experienced a 3-fold increase in clozapine elimination $t_{½}$ and clozapine and norclozapine steady-state trough levels following introduction of fluvoxamine 50 mg/day.[9] The other studies showed a 2.58- and 2.3-fold increase in the AUC of clozapine.[12,13] In 1 study, clozapine 100 mg/day was given with fluvoxamine 50 or 100 mg/day to potentiate clozapine.[15] Therapeutic outcomes were improved. Clozapine levels were 327 and 478 ng/mL after 2 wk of fluvoxamine 50 mg/day and 6 wk of 100 mg/day, respectively. Paroxetine 20 mg/day did not alter clozapine pharmacokinetics in 14 patients when added to stable clozapine regimens.[9]

1 Olesen OV, et al. *J Clin Psychopharmacol.* 2000;20:35.
2 Borba CP, et al. *J Clin Psychiatry.* 2000;61:301.
3 Centorrino F, et al. *Am J Psychiatry.* 1994;151:123.
4 Hiemke C, et al. *J Clin Psychopharmacol.* 1994;14:279.
5 Jerling M, et al. *Ther Drug Monit.* 1994;16:368.
6 DuMortier G, et al. *Am J Psychiatry.* 1996;153:738.
7 Chong SA, et al. *J Clin Psychopharmacol.* 1997;17:68.
8 Armstrong SC, et al. *J Clin Psychiatry.* 1997;58:499.
9 Wetzel H, et al. *J Clin Psychopharmacol.* 1998;18:2.
10 Kuo FJ, et al. *J Clin Psychopharmacol.* 1998;18:483.
11 Pinninti NR, et al. *J Clin Psychopharmacol.* 1997;17:119.
12 Chang WH, et al. *Psychopharmacology.* 1999;145:91.
13 Lu ML, et al. *J Clin Psychiatry.* 2000;61:594.
14 Wang CY, et al. *J Clin Pharmacol.* 2004;44:785.
15 Lu ML, et al. *J Clin Psychopharmacol.* 2002;22:626.

* Asterisk indicates drugs cited in interaction reports.

Clozapine — *Valproic Acid*

Clozapine	Valproic Acid	
Clozapine* (eg, *Clozaril*)	Divalproex Sodium* (*Depakote*)	Valproic Acid* (eg, *Depakene*)
	Valproate Sodium (eg, *Depacon*)	

Significance	Onset	Severity	Documentation
4	☐ Rapid	☐ Major	☐ Established
	■ **Delayed**	■ **Moderate**	☐ Probable
		☐ Minor	☐ Suspected
			■ **Possible**
			☐ Unlikely

Effects Serum CLOZAPINE concentrations may be slightly elevated, increasing sedation and functional impairment.

Mechanism Unknown.

Management No precautions other than usual monitoring of the patient are needed. If an interaction is suspected, it may be necessary to discontinue VALPROIC ACID. VALPROATE is sometimes added to regimens containing high doses of CLOZAPINE to avoid CLOZAPINE-induced seizures.

Discussion

The effects of valproate on clozapine serum levels were assessed in 34 adults with schizophrenia or an affective psychotic disorder.[1] Participants were randomly selected from patients who had received clozapine alone; 17 patients were assigned to continue receiving clozapine alone, 11 patients received clozapine plus valproate, and 6 patients received clozapine with fluoxetine. When patients received clozapine alone, the mean daily dose was 300 mg. Serum clozapine levels increased 39% during coadministration of valproate. The effect of valproate on clozapine and its major metabolites virtually disappeared when corrections were made for individual dose and weight (6% above control values). There was no evidence of an increased risk of neurological or other side effects in any of the patients. Another study compared 15 patients on clozapine plus valproic acid with 22 matched controls receiving clozapine alone.[2] In addition, 6 other patients were compared before and after introduction of valproic acid to clozapine. In both instances, there was a small, statistically insignificant increase in clozapine levels while receiving combination therapy. In a case report, a 37-year-old man experienced sedation, confusion, and slurred speech following the addition of clozapine to a complex medication regimen containing valproic acid.[3] These symptoms resolved when valproic acid was discontinued. During a subsequent hospitalization, the same symptoms recurred within 4 days of restarting valproic acid for a seizure at a later date. These symptoms resolved when phenytoin (eg, *Dilantin*) was substituted for valproic acid.

[1] Centorrino F, et al. *Am J Psychiatry.* 1994;151:123.
[2] Facciola G, et al. *Ther Drug Monit.* 1999;21:341.
[3] Costello LE, et al. *J Clin Psychopharmacol.* 1995;15:139.

* Asterisk indicates drugs cited in interaction reports. Based on pharmacologic and pharmacokinetic considerations, similar interactions may occur with other drugs that are listed.

CNS Stimulants — *Furazolidone*

CNS Stimulants		Furazolidone
Amphetamine	Methamphetamine (*Desoxyn*)	Furazolidone*†
Benzphetamine (eg, *Didrex*)	Phendimetrazine (eg, *Prelu-2*)	
Dextroamphetamine* (eg, *Dexedrine*)	Phentermine (eg, *Ionamin*)	
Diethylpropion		
Lisdexamfetamine (*Vyvanse*)		

Significance	Onset	Severity	Documentation
1	☐ Rapid	■ **Major**	☐ Established
	■ **Delayed**	☐ Moderate	☐ Probable
		☐ Minor	■ **Suspected**
			☐ Possible
			☐ Unlikely

Effects Increased sensitivity to CNS STIMULANTS.

Mechanism Inhibition of monoamine oxidase by FURAZOLIDONE.

Management If an interaction is suspected, monitor patients for signs and symptoms of AMPHETAMINE toxicity, and reduce the dose of the CNS STIMULANT accordingly.

Discussion

Furazolidone, an MAOI, was administered daily (400 to 800 mg) to 9 patients for a total dose of 80 to 140 mg/kg.[1] A 2- to 4-fold increase in pressor sensitivity was measured with the coadministration of d-amphetamine and furazolidone after 5 days. D-amphetamine causes an increased release of norepinephrine from extragranular sites on the nerve terminal where norepinephrine concentrates during inhibition of monoamine oxidase.[2] Therefore, the coadministration of these agents may result in excessive norepinephrine responses.

[1] Pettinger WA, et al. *Clin Pharmacol Ther.* 1968;9(4):442.

[2] Pettinger WA, et al. *Clin Pharmacol Ther.* 1968;9(3):341.

* Asterisk indicates drugs cited in interaction reports. Based on pharmacologic and pharmacokinetic considerations, similar interactions may occur with other drugs that are listed.
† Not available in the United States.

CNS Stimulants — *MAOIs*

CNS Stimulants		MAOIs	
Amphetamine*	Methamphetamine* (eg, *Desoxyn*)	Isocarboxazid (*Marplan*)	Rasagiline (*Azilect*)
Benzphetamine (eg, *Didrex*)	Phendimetrazine (eg, *Prelu-2*)	Linezolid (*Zyvox*)	Selegiline (eg, *Eldepryl*)
Dextroamphetamine* (eg, *Dexedrine*)	Phentermine (eg, *Ionamin*)	Phenelzine* (*Nardil*)	Tranylcypromine* (eg, *Parnate*)
Diethylpropion			
Lisdexamfetamine (*Vyvanse*)			

Significance	Onset	Severity	Documentation
1	■ **Rapid**	■ **Major**	□ Established
	□ Delayed	□ Moderate	□ Probable
		□ Minor	■ **Suspected**
			□ Possible
			□ Unlikely

Effects Exaggerated pharmacologic effects caused by CNS STIMULANTS (amphetamines and related substances). Several deaths have been reported as a result of hypertensive crisis and ensuing cerebral hemorrhage. Hypotension, hyperpyrexia, and seizures occurred in 1 case report.

Mechanism Probably increased norepinephrine at synaptic cleft.[1]

Management Avoid coadministration. The hypertensive reaction may occur for up to several weeks after discontinuation of MAOIs. RASAGILINE is contraindicated in patients receiving CNS STIMULANTS.[2]

Discussion

Several case reports describe the very rapid onset of headache and severe hypertension when amphetamines are given to patients receiving MAOIs. Fatal cerebral hemorrhage has occurred.[3-5] In 1 illustrative case, a 38-year-old man was given IV methamphetamine 8 days after stopping phenelzine. An immediate increase in his BP from 120/80 mm Hg to 280/150 mm Hg was observed. BP and associated symptoms gradually decreased over the next 4 hours. This patient survived.[6] In another case, a 41-year-old woman took tranylcypromine 10 mg and a combination product containing dextroamphetamine 10 mg and amobarbital (*Amytal Sodium*) 65 mg. Over the next few hours, she became confused and agitated. Later, she developed opisthotonus, seizures, and elevated temperature (109.4°F). Paradoxically, hypotension requiring pressor support also developed.[7] See also Sympathomimetics-MAOIs.

[1] Pettinger WA, et al. *Clin Pharmacol Ther.* 1968;9(3):341.
[2] *Azilect* [package insert]. Kansas City, MO: Teva Neuroscience; May 2006.
[3] Zeck P. *Med J Aust.* 1961;2:607.
[4] Mason A. *Lancet.* 1962;1:1073.
[5] Lloyd JT, et al. *Br Med J.* 1965;2(5454):168.
[6] Dally PJ. *Lancet.* 1962;1:1235.
[7] KriskÓ I, et al. *Ann Intern Med.* 1969;70(3):559.

* Asterisk indicates drugs cited in interaction reports. Based on pharmacologic and pharmacokinetic considerations, similar interactions may occur with other drugs that are listed.

CNS Stimulants — *Phenothiazines*

CNS Stimulants		Phenothiazines	
Amphetamine	Methamphetamine (eg, *Desoxyn*)	Chlorpromazine* (eg, *Thorazine*)	Prochlorperazine (eg, *Compazine*)
Benzphetamine (*Didrex*)	Phendimetrazine (eg, *Prelu-2*)	Fluphenazine	Thioridazine*
Dextroamphetamine* (eg, *Dexedrine*)	Phentermine (eg, *Ionamin*)	Perphenazine	Trifluoperazine
Diethylpropion			
Lisdexamfetamine (*Vyvanse*)			

Significance	Onset	Severity	Documentation
4	☐ Rapid ■ **Delayed**	☐ Major ■ **Moderate** ☐ Minor	☐ Established ☐ Probable ☐ Suspected ■ **Possible** ☐ Unlikely

Effects The pharmacologic effects of AMPHETAMINES and congeners may be diminished. AMPHETAMINES may exacerbate psychotic symptoms.

Mechanism Unknown.

Management Do not use AMPHETAMINES or related substances for weight reduction in patients receiving PHENOTHIAZINES.

Discussion

A placebo-controlled study demonstrated a lack of effect of dextroamphetamine 5 mg 4 times daily on weight loss or sleep pattern when used in patients receiving chlorpromazine or thioridazine.[1] Two other studies have reported similar findings for patients on chlorpromazine when given phenmetrazine.[†,2,3] Additionally, a prospective, placebo-controlled, multicenter study of patients on chlorpromazine detected deterioration in hostile and paranoid belligerence and thinking disturbance following administration of dextroamphetamine 40 mg/day.[4] Whether this represents an antagonism of the phenothiazine or an independent effect of the amphetamine remains unknown. There are reports of amphetamines alone exacerbating psychotic symptoms in schizophrenic patients.[5] Conversely, one of the weight loss studies that recorded psychiatric symptoms did not report any changes in psychotic symptoms with chlorphentermine[†] or phenmetrazine.[3] Because amphetamines probably will not reduce weight and because they could cause psychiatric symptom exacerbation, it is not advisable to administer them to schizophrenic patients receiving phenothiazines.

[1] Modell W, et al. *JAMA*. 1965;193:275.
[2] Reid AA. *Med J Aust*. 1964;10:187.
[3] Sletten IW, et al. *Curr Ther Res Clin Exp*. 1967;9(11):570.
[4] Casey JF, et al. *Am J Psychiatry*. 1961;117:997.
[5] West AP. *Am J Psychiatry*. 1974;131(3):321.

* Asterisk indicates drugs cited in interaction reports. Based on pharmacologic and pharmacokinetic considerations, similar interactions may occur with other drugs that are listed.
† Not available in the US.

CNS Stimulants		*Urinary Acidifiers*	
Amphetamine* Dextroamphetamine* (eg, *Dexedrine*) Lisdexamfetamine (*Vyvanse*)	Methamphetamine* (eg, *Desoxyn*)	Ammonium Chloride* Potassium Acid Phosphate (*K-Phos*)	Sodium Acid Phosphate

Significance	Onset	Severity	Documentation
3	■ **Rapid** ☐ Delayed	☐ Major ☐ Moderate ■ **Minor**	■ **Established** ☐ Probable ☐ Suspected ☐ Possible ☐ Unlikely

Effects The elimination of CNS STIMULANTS (ie, AMPHETAMINES) is hastened with a concomitant reduction in their duration of action.

Mechanism ACIDIFICATION of the urine prevents AMPHETAMINE renal tubular reabsorption, thereby increasing AMPHETAMINE urinary elimination.

Management No special precautions necessary. This interaction has been exploited therapeutically in the management of AMPHETAMINE poisoning. See Discussion.

Discussion

Several pharmacokinetic studies have demonstrated an increase in amphetamine urinary excretion when the urine is acidified by administration of ammonium chloride.[1-4] One study[1] noted 54.5% of an amphetamine dose was eliminated unchanged in the acidic urine versus 2.9% when the urine is alkaline. Likewise, the plasma concentration of amphetamine and metabolites decrease faster when the urine is acidic.[3] With the urine acidified, the amphetamine $t_{1/2}$ has been measured as 8 to 10.5 hr versus 16 to 31 hr when the urine is alkaline.[5] Similar observations have been made with methylamphetamine[6] and ephedrine.[7] A proposed explanation for these changes is that amphetamines exist in an ionized form when the urine is acidic. Therefore, their renal tubular reabsorption is diminished.

Acidifying the urine has been used therapeutically for amphetamine[4] or methamphetamine[8] overdose. In one study, 11 amphetamine-intoxicated patients who had their urine acidified had a shorter amphetamine plasma $t_{1/2}$ (7 to 14 hr) and more rapid clearing of symptoms than patients who had alkaline urine.[4] See CNS Stimulants-Urinary Alkalinizers.

[1] Beckett AH, et al. *Lancet.* 1965;1:303.
[2] Beckett AH, et al. *J Pharm Pharmacol.* 1965;17(10):628.
[3] Beckett AH, et al. *J Pharm Pharmacol.* 1969;21(4):251.
[4] Anggard E, et al. *Clin Pharmacol Ther.* 1973;14(5):870.
[5] Davis JM, et al. *Ann NY Acad Sci.* 1971;179:493.
[6] Beckett AH, et al. *J Pharm Pharmacol.* 1965;17:109S.
[7] Wilkinson GR, et al. *J Pharmacol Exp Ther.* 1968;162(1):139.
[8] Gary NE, et al. *Am J Med.* 1978;64(3):537.

* Asterisk indicates drugs cited in interaction reports. Based on pharmacologic and pharmacokinetic considerations, similar interactions may occur with other drugs that are listed.

CNS Stimulants × *Urinary Alkalinizers*

CNS Stimulants		Urinary Alkalinizers	
Amphetamine*	Methamphetamine* (eg, *Desoxyn*)	Potassium Citrate (*Urocit-K*)	Sodium Citrate (*Citra pH*)
Dextroamphetamine* (eg, *Dexedrine*)		Sodium Acetate	Sodium Lactate
Lisdexamfetamine (*Vyvanse*)		Sodium Bicarbonate* (eg, *Neut*)	Tromethamine (*Tham*)

Significance	Onset	Severity	Documentation
2	■ **Rapid**	□ Major	■ **Established**
	□ Delayed	■ **Moderate**	□ Probable
		□ Minor	□ Suspected
			□ Possible
			□ Unlikely

Effects ALKALINIZED urine may prolong the effects of CNS STIMULANTS (eg, AMPHETAMINES). In the setting of AMPHETAMINE overdose, toxicity will be prolonged.

Mechanism Diminished urinary elimination of unchanged drug.

Management Avoid agents that may alkalinize the urine, particularly in overdose situations.

Discussion

Several pharmacokinetic studies of amphetamines have demonstrated a prolongation of the $t_{1/2}$ and a decrease in urinary elimination when the urine is alkaline. The unchanged amphetamine excretion fraction was diminished from 54.5% to 2.9% in 6 patients given sodium bicarbonate to maintain a urinary pH of around 8.[1] The excretion of both amphetamine isomers is equally affected.[2] As a result, higher plasma levels and a longer $t_{1/2}$ occur. When the urine is alkaline, the plasma $t_{1/2}$ is 16 to 31 hours, compared with 8 to 10.5 hours when urine is acidic. This reflects more of the drug is undergoing metabolic elimination.[3] Similar observations have been made with the closely related compounds methamphetamine[4] and ephedrine.[5]

One study has evaluated the clinical consequences of urinary alkalinization. Eleven patients with amphetamine psychosis had their urine acidified (n = 5) or alkalinized (n = 6).[6] Psychosis was measured and patients received radiolabeled amphetamine for a pharmacokinetic study. Psychosis was prolonged during urinary alkalinization and appeared to correlate with the formation of a hydroxyamphetamine metabolite.[7] See also CNS Stimulants-Urinary Acidifiers.

1 Beckett AH, et al. *Lancet.* 1965;1:303.
2 Beckett AH, et al. *J Pharm Pharmacol.* 1965;17(10):628.
3 Davis JM, et al. *Ann NY Acad Sci.* 1971;179:493.
4 Beckett AH, et al. *J Pharm Pharmacol.* 1965;17:109S.
5 Wilkinson GR, et al. *J Pharmacol Exp Ther.* 1968;162(1):139.
6 Beckett AH, et al. *J Pharm Pharmacol.* 1969;21(4):251.
7 Anggard E, et al. *Clin Pharmacol Ther.* 1973;14(5):870.

* Asterisk indicates drugs cited in interaction reports. Based on pharmacologic and pharmacokinetic considerations, similar interactions may occur with other drugs that are listed.

Cocaine — *Disulfiram*

Cocaine* | Disulfiram* (*Antabuse*)

Significance	Onset	Severity	Documentation
2	☐ Rapid	☐ Major	☐ Established
	■ **Delayed**	■ **Moderate**	☐ Probable
		☐ Minor	■ **Suspected**
			☐ Possible
			☐ Unlikely

Effects Cardiovascular adverse reactions of COCAINE may be increased.

Mechanism Unknown.

Management Avoid use of DISULFIRAM in COCAINE-dependent patients. Inform COCAINE abusers receiving DISULFIRAM of the increased risk of adverse reactions, especially cardiovascular responses.

Discussion

The safety and efficacy of disulfiram in the treatment of cocaine abuse was studied in 7 volunteers who abused cocaine.[1] In a randomized, double-blind, placebo-controlled study, subjects received disulfiram 250 or 500 mg or placebo once daily for 5 days. Following the third dose of disulfiram, subjects received intranasal cocaine 1 or 2 mg/kg or placebo. After treatment with either dose of disulfiram compared with placebo, the AUC of cocaine was increased 3- to 6-fold, and the peak plasma concentration was increased 2- to 3-fold. Disulfiram administration increased the heart rate response to cocaine. Systolic and diastolic BP also increased after pretreatment with disulfiram, but only with administration of cocaine 2 mg/kg. Disulfiram treatment had no effects on any behavioral response to cocaine.[1] A 31-year-old man who was being treated for alcohol and cocaine abuse with disulfiram 250 mg/day relapsed and used cocaine.[2] In addition to tremor and an increased pulse rate, the patient reported experiencing anxiety, delusions, and paranoia.

[1] McCance-Katz EF, et al. *Drug Alcohol Depend.* 1998;52(1):27.

[2] Mutschler J, et al. *J Clin Psychopharmacol.* 2009; 29(1):99.

* Asterisk indicates drugs cited in interaction reports.

Codeine — *Quinidine*

Codeine* | Quinidine*

Significance	Onset	Severity	Documentation
2	☐ Rapid	☐ Major	☐ Established
	■ **Delayed**	■ **Moderate**	■ **Probable**
		☐ Minor	☐ Suspected
			☐ Possible
			☐ Unlikely

Effects The analgesic effects of CODEINE may be decreased.

Mechanism Interference with metabolism of CODEINE to morphine.

Management Observe the patient's clinical response to CODEINE analgesia. If necessary, administer an alternative analgesic.

Discussion

The effect of quinidine on the analgesic activity of codeine has been studied in extensive and poor metabolizers of sparteine/debrisoquine.[1,2] CYP2D6 is the enzyme responsible for the metabolism of sparteine/debrisoquine and the metabolism of codeine to morphine. Hence, poor metabolizers of sparteine/debrisoquine are unable to metabolize codeine to morphine.[2-4] Quinidine also lowers cerebrospinal fluid morphine levels after codeine administration.[5] In 7 extensive metabolizers, a maximum serum morphine concentration of 5.1 ng/mL was measured after administration of codeine (100 mg) alone, compared with 0.43 ng/mL after quinidine (50 mg) administration.[1] In addition, the serum morphine level was 0.17 ng/mL in 1 poor metabolizer following administration of codeine. Patients experienced no analgesia with placebo administration or when codeine was preceded by quinidine. In a placebo-controlled investigation, the analgesic effect of oral codeine 100 mg following inhibition of metabolism to morphine by prior administration of quinidine 200 mg was studied in 16 extensive metabolizers of sparteine.[2] Patients received 1 of 4 treatment protocols: placebo/placebo, quinidine/placebo, placebo/codeine, quinidine/codeine. Following administration of placebo/codeine, the median C_{max} of morphine was 18 nmol/L. When patients were pretreated with quinidine, no morphine was detected (less than 4 nmol/L) after codeine was given. Pin-prick pain thresholds increased following placebo/codeine administration (but not after quinidine/codeine) compared with placebo/placebo. Pain tolerance increased following placebo/codeine and quinidine/codeine administration. Quinidine reduced the pharmacological effects of codeine in extensive metabolizers, as measured by respiratory dynamics, pupil response, psychomotor testing,[4] and feeling a psychological high.[6]

1 Desmeules J, et al. *Clin Pharmacol Ther.* 1989;45(2):122.

2 Sindrup SH, et al. *Eur J Clin Pharmacol.* 1992;42(6):587.

3 Sindrup SH, et al. *Clin Pharmacol Ther.* 1990;48(6):686.

4 Caraco Y, et al. *J Pharmacol Exp Ther.* 1996;278(3):1165.

5 Sindrup SH, et al. *Eur J Clin Pharmacol.* 1996;49(6):503.

6 Kathiramalainathan K, et al. *J Clin Psychopharmacol.* 2000;20(4):435.

* Asterisk indicates drugs cited in interaction reports.

Colchicine — Azole Antifungal Agents

Colchicine	Azole Antifungal Agents	
Colchicine* (eg, *Colcrys*)	Fluconazole* (eg, *Diflucan*)	Posaconazole (*Noxafil*)
	Itraconazole* (eg, *Sporanox*)	Voriconazole (eg, *Vfend*)
	Ketoconazole* (eg, *Nizoral*)	

Significance	Onset	Severity	Documentation
1	☐ Rapid ■ **Delayed**	■ **Major** ☐ Moderate ☐ Minor	☐ Established ☐ Probable ■ **Suspected** ☐ Possible ☐ Unlikely

Effects COLCHICINE plasma concentrations may be elevated, increasing the risk of toxicity.

Mechanism Inhibition of COLCHICINE metabolism (CYP3A4) and the P-gp efflux transporter by ITRACONAZOLE and KETOCONAZOLE, while FLUCONAZOLE, POSACONAZOLE, and VORICONAZOLE inhibit the metabolism (CYP3A4) of COLCHICINE.

Management If coadministration cannot be avoided, use with caution. For gout flares in patients receiving FLUCONAZOLE, administer a single dose of COLCHICINE 1.2 mg repeated no earlier than 3 days. For familial Mediterranean fever, a maximum daily dose of COLCHICINE 1.2 mg (0.6 mg twice daily) may be given concurrently with FLUCONAZOLE. For gout flares in patients receiving KETOCONAZOLE, administer a single dose of COLCHICINE 0.6 mg followed by 0.3 mg 1 hour later; repeat the dose no sooner than 3 days. For familial Mediterranean fever, a maximum daily dose of COLCHICINE 0.6 mg may be given concurrently with ITRACONAZOLE OR KETOCONAZOLE.

Discussion

The effect of ketoconazole on the pharmacokinetics of colchicine was studied in 24 healthy subjects.[2] Using an open-label, nonrandomized, 2-period design, colchicine 0.6 mg was administered alone and after pretreatment with ketoconazole 200 mg twice daily for 5 days. Coadministration of ketoconazole increased the colchicine AUC approximately 210% compared with giving colchicine alone. The total apparent oral clearance of colchicine decreased approximately 70%, and the terminal elimination $t_{1/2}$ increased from about 6.3 to 26 hours. The intersubject variability for the C_{max} ranged from an increase of 19.6% to 219% (mean, 101.7%), while the increase in the AUC ranged from 76.7% to 419.6% (mean, 212.2%).[1]

[1] *Colcrys* [package insert]. Philadelphia, PA: Mutual Pharmaceutical Company; July 2009.

[2] Terkeltaub RA, et al. *Arthritis Rheum.* 2011;63(8):2226.

* Asterisk indicates drugs cited in interaction reports. Based on pharmacologic and pharmacokinetic considerations, similar interactions may occur with other drugs that are listed.

Colchicine — *Diltiazem*

Colchicine* (eg, *Colcrys*)	Diltiazem* (eg, *Cardizem*)

Significance	Onset	Severity	Documentation
1	☐ Rapid ■ **Delayed**	■ **Major** ☐ Moderate ☐ Minor	☐ Established ☐ Probable ■ **Suspected** ☐ Possible ☐ Unlikely

Effects COLCHICINE plasma concentrations may be elevated, increasing the risk of toxicity.

Mechanism Inhibition of COLCHICINE metabolism (CYP3A4) and the P-gp efflux transporter by DILTIAZEM.

Management If coadministration cannot be avoided, use with caution. For gout flares in patients receiving DILTIAZEM, administer a single dose of COLCHICINE 1.2 mg repeated no earlier than 3 days. For familial Mediterranean fever, a maximum daily dose of COLCHICINE 1.2 mg (0.6 mg twice daily) may be given concurrently with DILTIAZEM.[1]

Discussion

The effect of diltiazem on the pharmacokinetics of colchicine was studied in 20 healthy subjects.[2] Using an open-label, nonrandomized, 2-period design, colchicine 0.6 mg was administered alone and after pretreatment with diltiazem 240 mg daily for 7 days. Coadministration of diltiazem increased the colchicine AUC approximately 93% compared with giving colchicine alone. The total apparent oral clearance of colchicine decreased approximately 40%, and the terminal elimination $t_{1/2}$ increased from about 6 to 12 hours. The intersubject variability for the C_{max} ranged from a 46% decrease to a 318.3% increase (mean, 44.2%), while the AUC ranged from a 30.2% decrease to a 338.6% increase (mean, 93.4%).[1]

[1] *Colcrys* [package insert]. Philadelphia, PA: Mutual Pharmaceutical Company; July 2009.

[2] Terkeltaub RA, et al. *Arthritis Rheum.* 2011;63(8):2226.

* Asterisk indicates drugs cited in interaction reports.

Colchicine — *Food*

Colchicine* (eg, *Colcrys*)	Grapefruit Juice*

Significance	Onset	Severity	Documentation
4	☐ Rapid ■ **Delayed**	■ **Major** ☐ Moderate ☐ Minor	☐ Established ☐ Probable ☐ Suspected ■ **Possible** ☐ Unlikely

Effects COLCHICINE serum concentrations may be elevated, increasing the risk of toxicity.

Mechanism Inhibition of COLCHICINE metabolism (CYP3A4) is suspected.

Management If possible, avoid coadministration. If GRAPEFRUIT JUICE is ingested in patients receiving COLCHICINE, give COLCHICINE with caution at reduced starting doses and lower maximum doses.[1] Monitor for adverse reactions.

Discussion

An 8-year-old girl with familial Mediterranean fever was admitted to the hospital with colchicine toxicity (eg, fever, recurrent vomiting, severe abdominal pain).[2] To control her disease, the patient had been receiving colchicine 2 mg/day. During the 2 months prior to hospital admission, the patient drank about 1 L of grapefruit juice daily. During her hospitalization, she experienced GI, CNS, cardiovascular, and hematologic disturbances. The patient was discharged from the hospital after 24 days in good medical condition and with a normal, complete blood cell count. It was recommended that she resume colchicine 1 mg/day and not drink grapefruit juice.

[1] *Colcrys* [package insert]. Philadelphia, PA: Mutual Pharmaceutical Company Inc; July 2009.

[2] Goldbart A, et al. *Eur J Pediatr.* 2000;159(12):895.

* Asterisk indicates drugs cited in interaction reports.

Colchicine — Macrolide & Related Antibiotics

Colchicine* (eg, *Colcrys*)	Clarithromycin* (eg, *Biaxin*)	Telithromycin* (*Ketek*)
	Erythromycin* (eg, *Ery-Tab*)	

Significance	Onset	Severity	Documentation
1	☐ Rapid	■ **Major**	■ **Established**
	■ **Delayed**	☐ Moderate	☐ Probable
		☐ Minor	☐ Suspected
			☐ Possible
			☐ Unlikely

Effects Increased COLCHICINE serum concentrations with toxicity (including death) may occur.

Mechanism Possible inhibition of COLCHICINE metabolism (CYP3A4).

Management Coadministration of COLCHICINE and CLARITHROMYCIN or TELITHROMYCIN is contraindicated in patients with hepatic or renal function impairment. In patients with normal hepatic and renal function, use caution and administer at a maximum dosage of COLCHICINE 0.3 mg twice daily. Coadminister COLCHICINE and ERYTHROMYCIN with caution at reduced starting and lower maximum doses of COLCHICINE. Monitor for adverse reactions.[1]

Discussion

In a retrospective review, the risk of death was increased in hospitalized patients receiving colchicine and clarithromycin.[2] Nine of 88 patients died after receiving the drugs concomitantly, and 1 of 28 patients died after the drugs were given sequentially. When erythromycin was added to the treatment regimen, severe colchicine toxicity developed in a 29-year-old patient with familial Mediterranean fever and amyloidosis involving the kidney, liver, and GI tract.[3] The patient had been receiving long-term treatment with colchicine 1 mg/day. After 2 weeks of concurrent erythromycin treatment, the patient was hospitalized with acute, life-threatening colchicine toxicity. Initial signs and symptoms included fever, diarrhea, abdominal pain, myalgia, and abnormal sensations in the lower extremities, followed by convulsions and hair loss. Serum colchicine concentrations of 22 ng/mL confirmed the diagnosis of colchicine toxicity. The patient had hepatic and renal function impairment, both of which predispose to colchicine toxicity. A 76-year-old man with familial Mediterranean fever taking colchicine experienced fever, abdominal pain, and diarrhea 3 days after starting clarithromycin.[4] His condition progressed to metabolic acidosis, dehydration, and pancytopenia by day 7. The patient had chronic renal failure. He recovered with supportive care and a reduced colchicine dose. Two cases of fatal agranulocytosis presumed to be caused by coadministration of colchicine and clarithromycin have been reported.[5] In 23 healthy volunteers who received a single dose of colchicine 0.6 mg after pretreatment with clarithromycin 250 mg twice daily for 7 days, there was a 197% and 239% increase in the colchicine C_{max} and AUC, respectively.[6] In contrast, azithromycin (eg, *Zithromax*) pharmacokinetics were not affected.

[1] *Colcrys* [package insert]. Philadelphia, PA: Mutual Pharmaceutical Company Inc; July 2009.
[2] Hung IF, et al. *Clin Infect Dis.* 2005;41(3):291.
[3] Caraco Y, et al. *J Rheumatol.* 1992;19(3):494.
[4] Rollot F, et al. *Ann Pharmacother.* 2004;38(12):2074.
[5] Cheng VC, et al. *South Med J.* 2005;98(8):811.
[6] Terketaub RA, et al. *Arthritis Rheum.* 2011;63(8):2226.

* Asterisk indicates drugs cited in interaction reports.

Colchicine		*Nefazodone*
Colchicine* (eg, *Colcrys*)		Nefazodone*

Significance	Onset	Severity	Documentation
1	□ Rapid ■ **Delayed**	■ **Major** □ Moderate □ Minor	□ Established □ Probable ■ **Suspected** □ Possible □ Unlikely

Effects COLCHICINE plasma concentrations may be elevated, increasing the risk of toxicity.

Mechanism Inhibition of COLCHICINE metabolism (CYP3A4) by NEFAZODONE.

Management Coadministration of COLCHICINE and NEFAZODONE is contraindicated in patients with hepatic or renal function impairment. In patients with normal hepatic and renal function, give COLCHICINE with NEFAZODONE with caution at a maximum dose of COLCHICINE 0.3 mg twice daily.[1] Monitor for adverse reactions.

Discussion

Life-threatening and fatal drug interactions have been reported in patients treated with colchicine and receiving a strong CYP3A4 inhibitor (eg, nefazodone). If coadministration of a strong CYP3A4 inhibitor and colchicine is required in patients with normal renal or hepatic function, the dose of colchicine needs to be reduced or withheld.[1] In patients with renal or hepatic function impairment, do not administer a strong CYP3A4 inhibitor with colchicine.

The basis for this monograph is information on file with the manufacturer. Published clinical data are needed to further assess this interaction. However, because of the seriousness of the adverse reactions, clinical evaluation of this interaction in humans is not likely to be forthcoming.

[1] *Colcrys* [package insert]. Philadelphia, PA: Mutual Pharmaceutical Company Inc; July 2009.

* Asterisk indicates drugs cited in interaction reports.

Colchicine — *Protease Inhibitors*

Colchicine	Protease Inhibitors	
Colchicine* (eg, *Colcrys*)	Atazanavir* (*Reyataz*)	Nelfinavir* (*Viracept*)
	Darunavir* (*Prezista*)	Ritonavir* (*Norvir*)
	Fosamprenavir (*Lexiva*)	Saquinavir* (*Invirase*)
	Indinavir* (*Crixivan*)	Tipranavir (*Aptivus*)
	Lopinavir/Ritonavir* (*Kaletra*)	

Significance	Onset	Severity	Documentation
1	☐ Rapid ■ **Delayed**	■ **Major** ☐ Moderate ☐ Minor	☐ Established ■ **Probable** ☐ Suspected ☐ Possible ☐ Unlikely

Effects COLCHICINE plasma concentrations may be elevated, increasing the risk of toxicity.

Mechanism Inhibition of COLCHICINE metabolism (CYP3A4) by PROTEASE INHIBITORS.

Management Coadministration of COLCHICINE and PROTEASE INHIBITORS is contraindicated in patients with hepatic or renal function impairment. In patients with normal hepatic and renal function, use caution when giving COLCHICINE with PROTEASE INHIBITORS and administer COLCHICINE at a maximum dosage of 0.3 mg twice daily.[1] Monitor for adverse reactions.

Discussion

Life-threatening and fatal drug interactions have been reported in patients treated with colchicine and receiving a strong CYP3A4 inhibitor (eg, ritonavir). If coadministration of a strong CYP3A4 inhibitor and colchicine is required in patients with normal renal or hepatic function, the dose of colchicine needs to be reduced or withheld.[1] In patients with renal or hepatic function impairment, do not administer a strong CYP3A4 inhibitor with colchicine. Seventeen healthy volunteers received ritonavir 100 mg twice daily for 5 days followed by a single dose of colchicine 0.6 mg.[2] The colchicine C_{max} and AUC increased 2.7- and 3.4-fold, respectively, suggesting a colchicine dosage reduction is needed.

[1] *Colcrys* [package insert]. Philadelphia, PA: Mutual Pharmaceutical Company; July 2009.

[2] Terkeltaub RA, et al. *Arthritis Rheum.* 2011;63(8):2226.

* Asterisk indicates drugs cited in interaction reports. Based on pharmacologic and pharmacokinetic considerations, similar interactions may occur with other drugs that are listed.

Colchicine — *Verapamil*

Colchicine*
(eg, *Colcrys*)

Verapamil*
(eg, *Calan*)

Significance	Onset	Severity	Documentation
1	☐ Rapid	■ **Major**	☐ Established
	■ **Delayed**	☐ Moderate	☐ Probable
		☐ Minor	■ **Suspected**
			☐ Possible
			☐ Unlikely

Effects Elevated COLCHICINE serum and cerebrospinal concentrations with toxicity may occur.

Mechanism VERAPAMIL may inhibit the P-gp transporter, which acts as a blood-brain barrier drug efflux pump. In addition, VERAPAMIL may inhibit COLCHICINE hepatic metabolism (CYP3A4).

Management Coadminister with caution and closely monitor for COLCHICINE toxicity. The recommended COLCHICINE dose for gout flares in patients receiving VERAPAMIL is 1.2 mg for 1 dose repeated no earlier than 3 days.[1] The recommended maximum COLCHICINE dose for familial Mediterranean fever in patients receiving VERAPAMIL is 1.2 mg daily.

Discussion

An 83-year-old man treated himself for an acute attack of gout with colchicine 2 mg for 2 days.[2] He was also taking slow-release verapamil 120 mg/day for tachyarrhythmia. Concurrently, he had muscle weakness in his limbs. Four days later, he became immobile and was admitted to the hospital with flaccid tetraparesis. When it was determined that he had excessive colchicine serum and cerebrospinal concentrations, he was diagnosed with colchicine-induced neuromyopathy. The ratio of colchicine cerebrospinal fluid to serum concentration was approximately 50% compared with a normal ratio of less than 10%. Twenty-four healthy volunteers received verapamil 240 mg daily for 5 days followed by a single dose of colchicine 0.6 mg. The colchicine C_{max} and AUC increased approximately 29.6% and 88.2%, respectively.[3]

[1] *Colcrys* [package insert]. Philadelphia, PA: Mutual Pharmaceutical Company; July 2009.
[2] Tröger U, et al. *BMJ.* 2005;331(7517):613.
[3] Terkeltaub RA, et al. *Arthritis Rheum.* 2011;63(8):2226.

* Asterisk indicates drugs cited in interaction reports.

Conivaptan — *Azole Antifungal Agents*

Conivaptan* (*Vaprisol*)	Itraconazole* (eg, *Sporanox*)	Ketoconazole* (eg, *Nizoral*)

Significance	Onset	Severity	Documentation
1	☐ Rapid ■ **Delayed**	■ **Major** ☐ Moderate ☐ Minor	☐ Established ☐ Probable ■ **Suspected** ☐ Possible ☐ Unlikely

Effects CONIVAPTAN plasma concentrations may be elevated, increasing the risk of adverse reactions.

Mechanism AZOLE ANTIFUNGAL AGENTS may inhibit the metabolism (CYP3A4) of CONIVAPTAN.

Management Coadministration of CONIVAPTAN and ITRACONAZOLE or KETOCONAZOLE is contraindicated.

Discussion

Because conivaptan is a substrate of CYP3A4, coadministration of itraconazole or ketoconazole may increase conivaptan plasma concentrations. The effect of ketoconazole or itraconazole on the pharmacokinetics of IV conivaptan has not been studied. However, coadministration of oral conivaptan 10 mg with ketoconazole 200 mg increased the C_{max} and AUC of conivaptan 4- and 11-fold, respectively. The consequences of increased conivaptan levels are unknown. Therefore, coadministration of conivaptan and itraconazole or ketoconazole is contraindicated.[1]

The basis for this monograph is information on file with the manufacturer. Clinical evaluation of this interaction is needed to determine the consequences of coadministration of conivaptan and azole antifungal agents.

[1] *Vaprisol* [package insert]. Deerfield, IL: Astellas Pharma US Inc; December 2005.

* Asterisk indicates drugs cited in interaction reports.

Conivaptan | *Macrolide Antibiotics*

Conivaptan* (*Vaprisol*)	Clarithromycin* (eg, *Biaxin*)

Significance	Onset	Severity	Documentation
1	☐ Rapid ■ **Delayed**	■ **Major** ☐ Moderate ☐ Minor	☐ Established ☐ Probable ■ **Suspected** ☐ Possible ☐ Unlikely

Effects CONIVAPTAN plasma concentrations may be elevated, increasing the risk of adverse reactions.

Mechanism MACROLIDE ANTIBIOTICS may inhibit the metabolism (CYP3A4) of CONIVAPTAN.

Management Coadministration of CONIVAPTAN and CLARITHROMYCIN is contraindicated.

Discussion

Because conivaptan is a substrate of CYP3A4, coadministration of clarithromycin may increase the conivaptan plasma concentrations. The consequences of increased conivaptan levels are unknown. Therefore, coadministration of conivaptan and clarithromycin is contraindicated.[1]

The basis for this monograph is information on file with the manufacturer. Clinical evaluation of this interaction is needed to determine the consequences of coadministration of conivaptan and macrolide antibiotics.

[1] *Vaprisol* [package insert]. Deerfield, IL: Astellas Pharma US Inc; December 2005.

* Asterisk indicates drugs cited in interaction reports.

Conivaptan — *Protease Inhibitors*

Conivaptan* (*Vaprisol*)	Indinavir* (*Crixivan*)	Ritonavir* (*Norvir*)

Significance	Onset	Severity	Documentation
1	□ Rapid ■ **Delayed**	■ **Major** □ Moderate □ Minor	□ Established □ Probable ■ **Suspected** □ Possible □ Unlikely

Effects CONIVAPTAN plasma concentrations may be elevated, increasing the risk of adverse reactions.

Mechanism PROTEASE INHIBITORS may inhibit the metabolism (CYP3A4) of CONIVAPTAN.

Management Coadministration of CONIVAPTAN and INDINAVIR or RITONAVIR is contraindicated.

Discussion

Because conivaptan is a substrate of CYP3A4, coadministration of indinavir or ritonavir may increase conivaptan plasma concentrations. The consequences of increased conivaptan levels are unknown. Therefore, coadministration of conivaptan and indinavir or ritonavir is contraindicated.[1]

The basis for this monograph is information on file with the manufacturer. Clinical evaluation of this interaction is needed to determine the consequences of coadministration of conivaptan and protease inhibitors.

[1] *Vaprisol* [package insert]. Deerfield, IL: Astellas Pharma US Inc; December 2005.

* Asterisk indicates drugs cited in interaction reports.

Contraceptives, Hormonal — *Ascorbic Acid*

Contraceptives, Oral* (eg, *Ortho-Novum*)	Ascorbic Acid* (eg, *Cevi-Bid*)

Significance	Onset	Severity	Documentation
5	□ Rapid ■ **Delayed**	□ Major □ Moderate ■ **Minor**	□ Established □ Probable □ Suspected ■ **Possible** □ Unlikely

Effects ASCORBIC ACID increases the serum levels of estrogen contained in ORAL CONTRACEPTIVES, possibly resulting in adverse reactions.

Mechanism Increased bioavailability of ORAL CONTRACEPTIVES due to impaired metabolism by ASCORBIC ACID is suspected.

Management If estrogen-related side effects appear, consider coadministration of ASCORBIC ACID as a possible cause.

Discussion

Five women taking an oral contraceptive preparation containing ethinyl estradiol participated in a randomized, controlled study.[1] After dosing with ascorbic acid 1 g, the mean plasma concentrations of ethinyl estradiol increased 47.6% after 24 hours (range, 22% to 100%). No adverse reactions were noted. However, 1 case report associated withdrawal of vitamin C therapy with breakthrough bleeding.[2] Another investigator concluded, after examining the effects of ascorbic acid on physiologic parameters, that administration of vitamin C effectively converted a low-dose estrogen preparation into a high-dose product.[3]

[1] Back DJ, et al. *Br Med J.* 1981;282(6275):1516.
[2] Morris JC, et al. *Br Med J.* 1981;283(6289):503.
[3] Briggs MH. *Br Med J.* 1981;283(6305):1547.

* Asterisk indicates drugs cited in interaction reports.

Contraceptives, Hormonal — *Azole Antifungal Agents*

Contraceptives, Hormonal	Azole Antifungal Agents	
Contraceptives, Oral* (eg, *Ortho-Novum*)	Fluconazole* (eg, *Diflucan*)	Ketoconazole* (eg, *Nizoral*)
	Itraconazole* (eg, *Sporanox*)	Voriconazole* (*Vfend*)

Significance	Onset	Severity	Documentation
2	☐ Rapid	☐ Major	☐ Established
	■ **Delayed**	■ **Moderate**	☐ Probable
		☐ Minor	■ **Suspected**
			☐ Possible
			☐ Unlikely

Effects The therapeutic efficacy of HORMONAL CONTRACEPTIVES may be reduced. In addition, elevated ethinyl estradiol blood levels may occur.

Mechanism Unknown.

Management Inform women of the possible increased risk of HORMONAL CONTRACEPTIVE failure. Consider an alternative method of contraception. Monitor for increased HORMONAL CONTRACEPTIVE adverse reactions.

Discussion

Data are unclear. Both unintended pregnancy and elevated estrogen/progestin have been reported. A case of unintended pregnancy in a 25-year-old woman was reported during concurrent use of itraconazole 200 mg/day and an oral contraceptive containing ethinyl estradiol 30 mcg and levonorgestrel 0.15 mg.[1] Reportedly, the patient did not miss any doses of the oral contraceptive. As of 1993, the World Health Organization reported 3 instances of unintended pregnancy in patients taking fluconazole, and 1 in a patient receiving ketoconazole while taking oral contraceptives.[1] In contrast, low doses of fluconazole 50 mg/day did not interfere with the effects of oral contraceptives,[2,3] while single-dose therapy with fluconazole 150 mg increased ethinyl estradiol serum concentrations.[4] The C_{max} and AUC of ethinyl estradiol were increased (125% and 126%, respectively) following a single dose of fluconazole 150 mg taken on oral contraceptive day 6 in 19 healthy women taking oral contraceptives containing ethinyl estradiol 30 to 35 mcg per tablet. In a randomized, double-blind, crossover study conducted over 3 menstrual cycles, 21 healthy women received a daily triphasic contraceptive alone for the first cycle.[5] During the second and third cycles, the contraceptive was given with either fluconazole 300 mg once a week or placebo. The AUC of estradiol and norethindrone were increased 21% and 13%, respectively, during fluconazole administration compared with placebo. In a study of 15 women taking ethinyl estradiol and norethindrone, voriconazole AUC increased 46%.[6] Also, voriconazole increased the AUC of ethinyl estradiol and norethindrone 61% and 33%, respectively.

1 Pillans PI, et al. *N Z Med J.* 1993;106(965):436.
2 Devenport MH, et al. *Br J Clin Pharmacol.* 1989;27(6):851.
3 Lazar JD, et al. *Rev Infect Dis.* 1990;12(suppl 3):S327.
4 Sinofsky FE, et al. *Am J Obstet Gynecol.* 1998;178(2):300.
5 Hilbert J, et al. *Obstet Gynecol.* 2001;98(2):218.
6 Andrews E, et al. *Br J Clin Pharmacol.* 2008;65(4):531.

* Asterisk indicates drugs cited in interaction reports.

Contraceptives, Hormonal — *Barbiturates*

Contraceptives, Hormonal	Barbiturates	
Contraceptives, Oral* (eg, *Ortho-Novum*)	Amobarbital (*Amytal*)	Pentobarbital
	Butabarbital (eg, *Butisol*)	Phenobarbital* (eg, *Solfoton*)
	Butalbital	Primidone* (eg, *Mysoline*)
	Mephobarbital (*Mebaral*)	Secobarbital (*Seconal*)

Significance	Onset	Severity	Documentation
1	□ Rapid	■ **Major**	□ Established
	■ **Delayed**	□ Moderate	□ Probable
		□ Minor	■ **Suspected**
			□ Possible
			□ Unlikely

Effects Loss of ORAL CONTRACEPTIVE efficacy, possibly leading to unintended pregnancy.

Mechanism BARBITURATE induction of CONTRACEPTIVE-steroid hepatic metabolism and sex hormone–binding globulin synthesis combine to reduce effective concentrations of ORAL CONTRACEPTIVES.

Management Use alternative methods of contraception altogether or while titrating ORAL CONTRACEPTIVE doses against breakthrough bleeding during BARBITURATE therapy.

Discussion

Several cases of unintended pregnancy in women who were receiving oral contraceptives and barbiturates concurrently have been reported.[1,2] The barbiturates were either administered alone or with other antiseizure medications. In a retrospective analysis of 82 women with seizure disorders receiving oral contraceptives,[2] the risk of pregnancy was 25 times greater in those patients also receiving antiseizure medications (including barbiturates) than in those patients who were not. Oral contraceptive failure during concurrent barbiturate use has been attributed to lower effective concentrations caused by barbiturate induction of contraceptive-steroid hepatic metabolism and sex hormone–binding globulin synthesis.[2-5]

[1] Janz D, et al. *Lancet.* 1974;1:1113.
[2] Coulam CB, et al. *Epilepsia.* 1979;20:519.
[3] Laengner H, et al. *Lancet.* 1974;2:600.
[4] Roberton YR, et al. *Curr Med Res Opin.* 1976;3:647.
[5] Back DJ, et al. *Contraception.* 1980;22:495.

* Asterisk indicates drugs cited in interaction reports. Based on pharmacologic and pharmacokinetic considerations, similar interactions may occur with other drugs that are listed.

Contraceptives, Hormonal — *Bosentan*

Ethinyl Estradiol* (eg, *Ortho-Novum*)	Bosentan* (*Tracleer*)

Significance	Onset	Severity	Documentation
1	□ Rapid	■ **Major**	□ Established
	■ **Delayed**	□ Moderate	□ Probable
		□ Minor	■ **Suspected**
			□ Possible
			□ Unlikely

Effects Loss of ORAL CONTRACEPTIVE efficacy, possibly leading to unintended pregnancy.

Mechanism Increased hepatic metabolism (CYP3A4) of the ORAL CONTRACEPTIVE is suspected.

Management Inform women of the increased risk of ORAL CONTRACEPTIVE failure. Consider an alternative nonhormonal or additional method of contraception.

Discussion

The effect of bosentan on the pharmacokinetics of an oral contraceptive containing ethinyl estradiol 35 mcg plus norethindrone 1 mg was evaluated in 19 healthy women.[1] Using a randomized, crossover design, each woman received a single dose of the oral contraceptive alone and after 7 days of pretreatment with bosentan 125 mg twice daily. Compared with taking the oral contraceptive alone, bosentan administration reduced the AUC of norethindrone nearly 14% and ethinyl estradiol 31%, respectively. The maximum decreases in AUC of norethindrone and ethinyl estradiol in an individual subject were 56% and 66%, respectively. In the subject with the largest decrease in norethindrone AUC, ethinyl estradiol levels could not be measured. The C_{max} of the oral contraceptive components was not affected by bosentan.

[1] van Giersbergen PL, et al. *Int J Clin Pharmacol Ther.* 2006;44:113.

* Asterisk indicates drugs cited in interaction reports.

Contraceptives, Hormonal — *Carbamazepine*

Contraceptives, Oral* (eg, *Ortho-Novum*)	Carbamazepine* (eg, *Tegretol*)

Significance	Onset	Severity	Documentation
1	☐ Rapid ■ **Delayed**	■ **Major** ☐ Moderate ☐ Minor	☐ Established ☐ Probable ■ **Suspected** ☐ Possible ☐ Unlikely

Effects Loss of HORMONAL CONTRACEPTIVE efficacy, possibly leading to unintended pregnancy.

Mechanism CARBAMAZEPINE may increase hepatic metabolism of HORMONAL CONTRACEPTIVES.

Management To help avoid unintended pregnancy, patients should use an alternative method of contraception. If larger doses of the HORMONAL CONTRACEPTIVE are being considered, titrate the HORMONAL CONTRACEPTIVE dose against breakthrough bleeding.

Discussion

The effects of carbamazepine 300 to 600 mg daily on the kinetics of an oral contraceptive containing ethinyl estradiol 50 mg plus levonorgestrel 0.25 mg were studied in 4 epileptic patients.[1] Carbamazepine reduced the AUC of ethinyl estradiol 42% and the AUC of levonorgestrel 40%. In 10 women, carbamazepine 600 mg daily decreased the AUC of norethindrone and ethinyl estradiol 58% and 42%, respectively.[2] In a case report, a 27-year-old woman with manic-depressive disorder became pregnant 6 weeks after starting treatment with carbamazepine while receiving a low-dose oral contraceptive.[3]

[1] Crawford P, et al. *Br J Clin Pharmacol.* 1990;30(6):892.

[2] Doose DR, et al. *Epilepsia.* 2003;44(4):540.

[3] Rapport DJ, et al. *Psychosomatics.* 1989;30(4):462.

* Asterisk indicates drugs cited in interaction reports.

Contraceptives, Oral — *Colesevelam*

Contraceptives, Oral* (eg, *Nortrel*)	Colesevelam* (*Welchol*)

Significance	Onset	Severity	Documentation
1	□ Rapid ■ **Delayed**	■ **Major** □ Moderate □ Minor	□ Established □ Probable ■ **Suspected** □ Possible □ Unlikely

Effects The therapeutic efficacy of ORAL CONTRACEPTIVES may be reduced.

Mechanism COLESEVELAM may bind with ETHINYL ESTRADIOL in the GI tract, decreasing ETHINYL ESTRADIOL absorption.

Management Administer ORAL CONTRACEPTIVES at least 4 hours prior to COLESEVELAM.[1]

Discussion

Using an open-label, randomized design, the effects of colesevelam on the pharmacokinetics of an oral contraceptive containing ethinyl estradiol 0.035 mg plus norethindrone 1 mg were evaluated in healthy women.[2] Thirty-five subjects received the oral contraceptive alone, simultaneously with colesevelam 3,750 mg, and 1 hour before colesevelam. Thirty-two subjects received the oral contraceptive alone and 4 hours before colesevelam. Simultaneous administration of colesevelam decreased the AUC and C_{max} of ethinyl estradiol and the C_{max} of norethindrone. The AUC and C_{max} of ethinyl estradiol, but not norethindrone, were decreased when the oral contraceptive was given 1 hour prior to colesevelam. When the oral contraceptive was given 4 hours before colesevelam, there was no interaction.

[1] *Welchol* [package insert]. Parsippany, NJ: Daiichi Sakyo Inc; February 2010.

[2] Brown KS, et al. *J Clin Pharmacol.* 2010;50(5):554.

* Asterisk indicates drugs cited in interaction reports.

Contraceptives, Hormonal — *Dirithromycin*

Contraceptives, Oral* (eg, *Ortho-Novum*)	Dirithromycin*†

Significance	Onset	Severity	Documentation
5	☐ Rapid	☐ Major	☐ Established
	■ **Delayed**	■ **Moderate**	☐ Probable
		☐ Minor	☐ Suspected
			☐ Possible
			■ **Unlikely**

Effects The therapeutic efficacy of HORMONAL CONTRACEPTIVES may be reduced.

Mechanism Unknown.

Management Inform women of the possible increased risk of HORMONAL CONTRACEPTIVE failure. Consider an alternative method of contraception.

Discussion

In a nonblinded, nonrandomized, fixed-dose study, the effects of dirithromycin on the pharmacokinetics of an oral contraceptive containing norethindrone and ethinyl estradiol were studied in 20 healthy women.[1] Fifteen women were compliant with medication assessment and completed the study. Breakthrough bleeding occurred in 2 subjects during the baseline phase but not during the dirithromycin phase, while minor bleeding occurred in 1 subject during the dirithromycin phase but not during baseline evaluation. A statistically significant decrease (7.6%) in the mean 24-hour ethinyl estradiol AUC and an increase in apparent oral clearance occurred. However, 1 subject had a 36% decrease in the AUC. No women became pregnant, displayed any evidence of ovulation, or demonstrated a decrease in oral contraceptive efficacy.

See also Contraceptives, Hormonal-Troleandomycin.

[1] Wermeling DP, et al. *Obstet Gynecol.* 1995;86(1):78.

* Asterisk indicates drugs cited in interaction reports.
† Not available in the United States.

Contraceptives, Hormonal — *Felbamate*

Contraceptives, Oral* (eg, *Ortho-Novum*)	Felbamate* (eg, *Felbatol*)

Significance	Onset	Severity	Documentation
4	☐ Rapid ■ **Delayed**	■ **Major** ☐ Moderate ☐ Minor	☐ Established ☐ Probable ☐ Suspected ■ **Possible** ☐ Unlikely

Effects The therapeutic efficacy of HORMONAL CONTRACEPTIVES may be reduced.

Mechanism Induction of the enzyme responsible for metabolism of the progestational component is suspected.

Management Inform women of the possible increased risk of HORMONAL CONTRACEPTIVE failure. Consider an alternative method of contraception.

Discussion

In a randomized, double-blind, placebo-controlled investigation, the effects of felbamate on the pharmacokinetics of an oral contraceptive containing ethinyl estradiol 30 mcg and gestodene† 75 mcg were studied in healthy women.[1] To determine whether ovulation occurred, plasma progesterone and urinary luteinizing hormone levels were measured. In addition, diaries recording vaginal bleeding were maintained. Felbamate 240 mg/day was taken from midcycle of 2 consecutive oral contraceptive cycles (months 1 and 2). Felbamate administration resulted in a 37% decrease in gestodene AUC and a 16% decrease in C_{max}. During the study, felbamate administration also resulted in a 13% decrease in the AUC of ethinyl estradiol and a 10% increase in the C_{max}. There was no pharmacokinetic evidence of ovulation during coadministration of felbamate; however, 1 subject reported an episode of menstrual irregularity.

Additional controlled studies are needed to assess the clinical importance of this drug interaction. Other anticonvulsants may decrease the action of oral contraceptives. Valproate sodium (eg, *Depakene*) does not appear to interfere with oral contraceptive therapy.[2] See also Contraceptives, Hormonal-Barbiturates; Contraceptives, Hormonal-Carbamazepine; and Contraceptives, Hormonal-Hydantoins.

[1] Saano V, et al. *Clin Pharmacol Ther.* 1995;58(5):523. [2] Crawford P, et al. *Contraception.* 1986;33(1):23.

* Asterisk indicates drugs cited in interaction reports.
† Not available in the United States.

Contraceptives, Hormonal — *Griseofulvin*

Contraceptives, Oral* (eg, *Ortho-Novum*)	Griseofulvin* (eg, *Grifulvin*)

Significance	Onset	Severity	Documentation
1	□ Rapid	■ **Major**	□ Established
	■ **Delayed**	□ Moderate	□ Probable
		□ Minor	■ **Suspected**
			□ Possible
			□ Unlikely

Effects Loss of HORMONAL CONTRACEPTIVE efficacy, possibly leading to breakthrough bleeding, amenorrhea, or unintended pregnancy.

Mechanism GRISEOFULVIN induction of HORMONAL CONTRACEPTIVE hepatic metabolism is suspected.

Management Use alternative or additional nonhormonal contraception methods during GRISEOFULVIN therapy.

Discussion

The Committee on Safety of Medicines in the United Kingdom and the Netherlands Centre for Monitoring of Adverse Reactions to Drugs jointly reported 22 cases in which the loss of oral contraceptive effectiveness was associated with griseofulvin treatment.[1] Within the first 2 cycles after initiation of griseofulvin treatment, breakthrough bleeding occurred in 15 women and amenorrhea in 5 women. Unintended pregnancy occurred in 2 women. Breakthrough bleeding and amenorrhea recurred upon rechallenge in 4 women. In addition, an individual case of oligomenorrhea after initiation of griseofulvin has been reported.[2] Regular menses returned after increasing the estrogen component of the oral contraceptive. A case of oral contraceptive failure has also been reported after initiation of griseofulvin therapy for onychomycosis.[3]

[1] van Dijke CP, et al. *Br Med J (Clin Res Ed).* 1984;288(6424):1125.

[2] McDaniel PA, et al. *Drug Intell Clin Pharm.* 1986;20(5):384.

[3] Côté J. *J Am Acad Dermatol.* 1990;22(1):124.

* Asterisk indicates drugs cited in interaction reports.

Contraceptives, Hormonal		*HCV Protease Inhibitors*	
Contraceptives, Oral* (eg, *Yasmin*)		Boceprevir* (*Victrelis*)	Telaprevir* (*Incivek*)

Significance	Onset	Severity	Documentation
1	☐ Rapid ■ **Delayed**	■ **Major** ☐ Moderate ☐ Minor	☐ Established ☐ Probable ■ **Suspected** ☐ Possible ☐ Unlikely

Effects Concentrations of certain PROGESTINS (eg, DROSPIRENONE) may be elevated, increasing the risk of hyperkalemia. ESTROGEN concentrations may be reduced, increasing the risk of unintended pregnancy.

Mechanism Unknown. However, HEPATITIS C VIRUS (HCV) PROTEASE INHIBITORS may increase ESTROGEN metabolism.

Management Coadministration of DROSPIRENONE and BOCEPREVIR is contraindicated.[1] Patients should use 2 effective nonhormonal methods of contraception during treatment with an HCV PROTEASE INHIBITOR.[1,2]

Discussion

Concurrent use of boceprevir with ethinyl estradiol/drospirenone increased the drospirenone C_{max} and AUC 57% and 99%, respectively, compared with giving ethinyl estradiol/drospirenone alone.[1] Ethinyl estradiol concentrations were decreased 24%. Elevated drospirenone concentrations may increase the risk of hyperkalemia. Coadministration of drospirenone and boceprevir is contraindicated.[1] Concomitant use of telaprevir with ethinyl estradiol/norethindrone decreased ethinyl estradiol concentrations 28% without a clinically important change in norethindrone concentrations.[2]

The basis for this monograph is information on file with the manufacturer. Published clinical data are needed to further assess this interaction. Because of the seriousness of the interaction, clinical evaluation in humans is not likely to be forthcoming.

1 *Victrelis* [package insert]. Whitehouse Station, NJ: Schering Corporation; May 2011.

2 *Incivek* [package insert]. Cambridge, MA: Vertex Pharmaceuticals Incorporated; May 2011.

* Asterisk indicates drugs cited in interaction reports.

Contraceptives, Hormonal — *Hydantoins*

Contraceptives, Hormonal	Hydantoins	
Contraceptives, Oral* (eg, *Ortho-Novum*)	Ethotoin (*Peganone*) Fosphenytoin	Mephenytoin*† Phenytoin* (eg, *Dilantin*)

Significance	Onset	Severity	Documentation
1	□ Rapid ■ **Delayed**	■ **Major** □ Moderate □ Minor	□ Established □ Probable ■ **Suspected** □ Possible □ Unlikely

Effects Loss of ORAL CONTRACEPTIVE efficacy, possibly leading to unintended pregnancy. HYDANTOIN levels may be elevated by ORAL CONTRACEPTIVES.

Mechanism HYDANTOIN induction of contraceptive-steroid hepatic metabolism and sex hormone–binding globulin synthesis combine to reduce effective concentrations of ORAL CONTRACEPTIVES. Inhibition of HYDANTOIN metabolism (CYP2C19) by ORAL CONTRACEPTIVES.[1]

Management Use alternative or nonhormonal methods of contraception during HYDANTOIN therapy.

Discussion

Several cases of unintended pregnancy in women who were receiving oral contraceptives and hydantoins have been reported.[2-4] The hydantoins were administered alone or with other anticonvulsants. In a retrospective analysis of 82 women with seizure disorders receiving oral contraceptives,[4] the risk of pregnancy was 25 times greater in patients also receiving anticonvulsants (including hydantoins) than in patients who were not. Oral contraceptive failure during concurrent hydantoin use has been attributed to lower hormone concentrations caused by hydantoin induction of contraceptive-steroid hepatic metabolism and sex hormone–binding globulin synthesis.[4-6] In a study involving 6 patients, the AUC of ethinyl estradiol and levonorgestrel decreased 49% and 42%, respectively, 8 to 12 weeks after phenytoin was started.[7]

In one study, phenytoin plasma concentrations were higher in patients receiving oral contraceptives than in patients receiving phenytoin alone.[8] Neurotoxicity occurred after initiation of oral contraceptive use in a patient receiving mephenytoin, primidone (eg, *Mysoline*), and ethosuximide (eg, *Zarontin*).[9]

[1] Laine K, et al. *Clin Pharmacol Ther.* 2000;68(2):151.
[2] Kenyon IE. *Br Med J.* 1972;1(5801):686.
[3] Janz D, et al. *Lancet.* 1974;1(7866):1113.
[4] Coulam CB, et al. *Epilepsia.* 1979;20(5):519.
[5] Laengner H, et al. *Lancet.* 1974;2(7880):600.
[6] Odlind V, et al. *Contraception.* 1986;33(3):257.
[7] Crawford P, et al. *Br J Clin Pharmacol.* 1990;30(6):892.
[8] De Leacy EA, et al. *Br J Clin Pharmacol.* 1979;8(1):33.
[9] Espir M, et al. *Br Med J.* 1969;1(5639):294.

* Asterisk indicates drugs cited in interaction reports. Based on pharmacologic and pharmacokinetic considerations, similar interactions may occur with other drugs that are listed.
† Not available in the United States.

Contraceptives, Hormonal — *Modafinil*

Contraceptives, Oral*
(eg, *Ortho-Novum*)

Modafinil*
(*Provigil*)

Significance	Onset	Severity	Documentation
2	☐ Rapid ■ **Delayed**	☐ Major ■ **Moderate** ☐ Minor	☐ Established ☐ Probable ■ **Suspected** ☐ Possible ☐ Unlikely

Effects Loss of HORMONAL CONTRACEPTIVE effectiveness, possibly leading to unintended pregnancy.

Mechanism Induction of GI (major) and hepatic (minor) metabolism (CYP3A4/5) of HORMONAL CONTRACEPTIVES by MODAFINIL is suspected.

Management Inform women of the increased risk of HORMONAL CONTRACEPTIVE failure. Patients taking HORMONAL CONTRACEPTIVES and MODAFINIL concomitantly should consider alternative or concurrent means of contraception, and continue these for at least 1 month after discontinuing MODAFINIL.

Discussion

The effects of daily administration of modafinil on the pharmacokinetics of steady-state ethinyl estradiol were studied in 41 healthy women.[1] In a randomized, placebo-controlled, single-blind, single-period study, each subject was randomized to 1 of 2 treatment groups. The treatment spanned 2 consecutive 28-day menstrual cycles plus the first week of the third cycle (ie, 9 weeks). During this time, all subjects received a daily dose of an oral contraceptive containing ethinyl estradiol plus norgestimate. Starting on day 6, 7, or 8 of the second cycle, subjects received modafinil 200 mg/day for 7 days, followed by 400 mg/day for 21 days, taken with the subject's daily dose of the oral contraceptive. The protocol for the second group was the same as for the first, except subjects received matching placebo in place of modafinil for 28 days. Thirty-nine subjects completed the study. Modafinil administration decreased the mean AUC of ethinyl estradiol 18% compared with a 4% decrease with placebo and decreased the mean peak plasma concentration 11% compared with 5% with placebo. See Estrogens-Modafinil.

[1] Robertson P Jr, et al. *Clin Pharmacol Ther.* 2002;71(1):46.

* Asterisk indicates drugs cited in interaction reports.

Contraceptives, Hormonal — *NNRT Inhibitors*

Contraceptives, Hormonal	NNRT Inhibitors	
Contraceptives, Oral* (eg, *Ortho-Novum*)	Delavirdine (*Rescriptor*) Efavirenz (*Sustiva*)	Nevirapine* (*Viramune*)

Significance	Onset	Severity	Documentation
4	☐ Rapid ■ **Delayed**	■ **Major** ☐ Moderate ☐ Minor	☐ Established ☐ Probable ☐ Suspected ■ **Possible** ☐ Unlikely

Effects Reduced HORMONAL CONTRACEPTIVE efficacy and increased incidence of menstrual abnormalities may occur.

Mechanism Increased hepatic metabolism of the estrogenic and progestational components of HORMONAL CONTRACEPTIVES by NNRT INHIBITORS is suspected.

Management Inform women of the increased risk of HORMONAL CONTRACEPTIVE failure. Advise them to use an alternative nonhormonal or additional method of contraception.

Discussion

The effects of nevirapine on the pharmacokinetics of ethinyl estradiol 1 mg plus norethindrone 35 mcg (*Ortho-Novum 1/35*) were evaluated in 10 HIV-1–infected women.[1] Each patient received nevirapine 200 mg once daily on days 2 to 15, followed by 200 mg twice daily on days 16 through 29. On days 0 and 30, single doses of ethinyl estradiol/norethindrone were administered. Coadministration of nevirapine with estradiol/norethindrone reduced the median AUC of ethinyl estradiol 29%, decreased the terminal $t_{½}$ (15.7 to 11.6 hours), and reduced the mean residence time (16.1 to 11.7 hours). In addition, nevirapine decreased the AUC of norethindrone 18%. The steady-state pharmacokinetics of nevirapine were not altered by estradiol/norethindrone administration. The effect of etravirine on the pharmacokinetics and pharmacodynamics of estradiol/norethindrone were assessed in female volunteers.[2] Each subject received estradiol/norethindrone for 3 cycles. On the first 15 days of the third cycle, etravirine was coadministered with estradiol/norethindrone. Etravirine increased the ethinyl estradiol AUC 22% but did not change the norethindrone AUC. Measurements of leutinizing hormone and follicle-stimulating hormone at day 1 and 14 were the same for giving estradiol/norethindrone alone or with etravirine, indicating a lack of effect of etravirine on estradiol/norethindrone efficacy. In 13 women, depomedroxyprogesterone acetate (eg, *Depo-Provera*) caused a 17% increase in nevirapine AUC.[3] Medroxyprogesterone acetate levels were not affected, indicating that this may be a suitable alternative to oral contraceptives in women taking nevirapine.

[1] Mildvan D, et al. *J Acquir Immune Defic Syndr.* 2002;29(5):471.
[2] Schöller-Gyüre M, et al. *Contraception.* 2009;80(1):44.
[3] Cohn SE, et al. *Clin Pharmacol Ther.* 2007;81(2):222.

* Asterisk indicates drugs cited in interaction reports. Based on pharmacologic and pharmacokinetic considerations, similar interactions may occur with other drugs that are listed.

Contraceptives, Hormonal — *Oxcarbazepine*

Contraceptives, Oral* (eg, *Ortho-Novum*)	Oxcarbazepine* (*Trileptal*)

Significance	Onset	Severity	Documentation
2	□ Rapid	□ Major	□ Established
	■ **Delayed**	■ **Moderate**	□ Probable
		□ Minor	■ **Suspected**
			□ Possible
			□ Unlikely

Effects Decrease in ORAL CONTRACEPTIVE effectiveness, possibly leading to unintended pregnancy.

Mechanism OXCARBAZEPINE may increase the hepatic metabolism of ORAL CONTRACEPTIVES.

Management Inform women of the possible increased risk of ORAL CONTRACEPTIVE failure and to consider using an alternative nonhormonal contraceptive or an additional method of contraception.

Discussion

The effect of oxcarbazepine on the pharmacokinetics of an oral contraceptive containing ethinyl estradiol and levonorgestrel was studied in 10 healthy women who were previously receiving the oral contraceptive for 3 months.[1] In addition to the oral contraceptive, each subject received oxcarbazepine 300 mg on day 16 of the first study cycle, 300 mg twice daily on day 17, and 300 mg 3 times daily from day 18 of the first cycle to day 18 of the next menstrual cycle. Coadministration of oxcarbazepine and the oral contraceptive decreased the AUCs of ethinyl estradiol 48% and levonorgestrel 32%. The incidence of breakthrough bleeding was 15% compared with an expected rate of 0.48% with the oral contraceptive alone. See also Contraceptives, Oral-Carbamazepine.

[1] Klosterskov Jensen P, et al. *Epilepsia.* 1992;33:1149.

* Asterisk indicates drugs cited in interaction reports.

Contraceptives, Hormonal		*Penicillins*	
Contraceptives, Oral* (eg, *Ortho-Novum*)		Amoxicillin* (eg, *Moxatag*) Ampicillin* Dicloxacillin Nafcillin	Oxacillin* Penicillin G (eg, *Pfizerpen*) Penicillin V* Ticarcillin

Significance	Onset	Severity	Documentation
4	☐ Rapid ■ **Delayed**	■ **Major** ☐ Moderate ☐ Minor	☐ Established ☐ Probable ☐ Suspected ■ **Possible** ☐ Unlikely

Effects The efficacy of ORAL CONTRACEPTIVES (OCs) may be reduced.

Mechanism PENICILLINS may suppress intestinal flora that provide hydrolytic enzymes essential for enterohepatic recirculation of certain contraceptive steroid conjugates.

Management Although infrequently reported, contraceptive failure is possible. For patients who wish to avoid even a slight increase in risk of pregnancy, the use of an additional form of contraception during PENICILLIN therapy is advisable.

Discussion

OC failure resulting in pregnancy has been reported during concurrent penicillin therapy.[1-5] These reports are rare, considering the large population of women who use OCs. Although most investigators agree that penicillins may interrupt the enterohepatic circulation of OCs, resulting in decreased plasma concentrations, several studies document no change in plasma concentration and no diminished efficacy, suggesting that an increased risk of pregnancy does not occur.[6-13] A review of all published reports of adverse drug reactions secondary to a penicillin-oral contraceptive interaction through 1987 did not document any greater risk of contraceptive failure in patients on low-dose OCs.[5] Therefore, breakthrough bleeding should not be used as an early indicator of contraceptive failure, as previously suggested by some authors. In an investigation of antibiotic use (eg, oral cephalosporins, penicillins, tetracyclines) in dermatological practice, no differences in OC failure rate were seen in a case-control study involving 311 woman-years of combined antibiotic/OC exposure compared with 1,245 woman-years of OC use alone.[14]

1 Dossetor J. *Br Med J.* 1975;4(5994):467.
2 DeSano EA Jr, et al. *Fertil Steril.* 1982;37(6):853.
3 Silber TJ. *J Adolesc Health Care.* 1983;4(4):287.
4 Baciewicz AM. *Ther Drug Monit.* 1985;7(1):26.
5 Szoka PR, et al. *Fertil Steril.* 1988;49(5)(suppl 2):31s.
6 Adlercreutz H, et al. *Am J Obstet Gynecol.* 1977;128(3):266.
7 Philipson A. *Acta Obstet Gynecol Scand.* 1979;58(1):69.
8 Friedman CI, et al. *Obstet Gynecol.* 1980;55(1):33.
9 Swenson L, et al. *Gastroenterology.* 1980;78(5):1332.
10 Bint AJ, et al. *Drugs.* 1980;20(1):57.
11 Joshi JV, et al. *Contraception.* 1980;22(6):643.
12 Back DJ, et al. *Drugs.* 1981;21(1):46.
13 Back DJ, et al. *Br J Clin Pharmacol.* 1982;14(1):43.
14 Helms SE, et al. *J Am Acad Dermatol.* 1997;36(5, pt 1):705.

* Asterisk indicates drugs cited in interaction reports. Based on pharmacologic and pharmacokinetic considerations, similar interactions may occur with other drugs that are listed.

Contraceptives, Hormonal ✕ *Protease Inhibitors*

Contraceptives, Hormonal	Protease Inhibitors	
Ethinyl Estradiol* (eg, *Ortho-Novum*)	Atazanavir (*Reyataz*)	Nelfinavir* (*Viracept*)
	Darunavir (*Prezista*)	Ritonavir* (*Norvir*)
	Fosamprenavir (*Lexiva*)	Saquinavir (*Invirase*)
	Lopinavir/Ritonavir* (*Kaletra*)	Tipranavir (*Aptivus*)

Significance	Onset	Severity	Documentation
1	☐ Rapid	■ **Major**	☐ Established
	■ **Delayed**	☐ Moderate	■ **Probable**
		☐ Minor	☐ Suspected
			☐ Possible
			☐ Unlikely

Effects Loss of HORMONAL CONTRACEPTIVE effectiveness, possibly leading to unintended pregnancy.

Mechanism Increased hepatic metabolism of the HORMONAL CONTRACEPTIVE is suspected.

Management Inform women of the increased risk of HORMONAL CONTRACEPTIVE failure. Consider use of an alternative nonhormonal or additional method of contraception, such as injectable medroxyprogesterone acetate (eg, *Depo-Provera*).[1] INDINAVIR (*Crixivan*) may be a suitable alternative.[2]

Discussion

The effects of ritonavir on the pharmacokinetics of ethinyl estradiol were investigated in 23 healthy women.[3] On days 1 and 29 of the study, subjects received a dose of an oral contraceptive (OC) containing ethinyl estradiol 50 mcg plus ethynodiol diacetate 1 mg. From days 15 through 30, subjects received ritonavir (300 mg every 12 hr on day 15, 400 mg every 12 hr on day 16, and 500 mg every 12 hr on the remaining 14 days). Compared with taking the OC alone, ritonavir decreased the ethinyl estradiol C_{max} and AUC 32% and 41%, respectively, and increased the elimination rate constant 31%. The mean $t_{½}$ of ethinyl estradiol decreased from 17 to 13 hr. All subjects except one demonstrated a decrease in the AUC of ethinyl estradiol with ritonavir administration. A similar interaction may occur with nelfinavir.[4] In 12 subjects, nelfinavir 750 mg every 8 hr for 7 days reduced the AUC and C_{max} of ethinyl estradiol (35 mcg/day for 15 days) 47% and 28%, respectively, while reducing the AUC of norethindrone (0.4 mg/day for 15 days) 18%.

Administration of indinavir 800 mg every 8 hr with ethinyl estradiol 35 mcg in combination with norethindrone 1 mg for 7 days increased the AUC of ethinyl estradiol and norethindrone 24% and 26%, respectively.[2] Thus, indinavir can be given with ethinyl estradiol 35 mcg plus norethindrone 1 mg. The effects of protease inhibitors on other estrogens (eg, mestranol) have not been determined. Injectable depot medroxyprogesterone acetate was given to 20 women taking nelfinavir.[1] After 4 weeks, nelfinavir AUC was reduced 18% with no effect on antiretroviral activity as measured by HIV-1 RNA copies or CD4 counts. Medroxyprogesterone levels were not changed. In 8 HIV-infected women treated with a contraceptive patch containing ethinyl estradiol plus norelgestromin (*Ortho Evra*) and an HIV regimen that included lopinavir/ritonavir, the ethinyl estradiol AUC was decreased 45% and the norelgestromin AUC was increased 83% compared with controls.[5] Hormonal analysis indicated that progesterone concentrations were suppressed, suggesting that contraceptive efficacy was unaffected.

[1] Cohn SE, et al. *Clin Pharmacol Ther.* 2007;81(2):222.
[2] *Crixivan* [package insert]. Whitehouse Station, NJ: Merck & Co Inc; March 1996.
[3] Ouellet D, et al. *Br J Clin Pharmacol.* 1998;46(2):111.
[4] *Viracept* [package insert]. La Jolla, CA: Agouron Pharmaceuticals Inc; March 1997.
[5] Vogler MA, et al. *J Acquir Immune Defic Syndr.* 2010;55(4):473.

* Asterisk indicates drugs cited in interaction reports. Based on pharmacologic and pharmacokinetic considerations, similar interactions may occur with other drugs that are listed.

Contraceptives, Hormonal — *Rifamycins*

Contraceptives, Hormonal	Rifamycins
Contraceptives, Oral* (eg, *Ortho-Novum*)	Rifabutin* (*Mycobutin*) Rifampin* (eg, *Rifadin*) Rifapentine (*Priftin*)

Significance	Onset	Severity	Documentation
1	□ Rapid ■ **Delayed**	■ **Major** □ Moderate □ Minor	■ **Established** □ Probable □ Suspected □ Possible □ Unlikely

Effects Reduced HORMONAL CONTRACEPTIVE efficacy that may result in pregnancy and menstrual abnormalities.

Mechanism RIFAMPIN induces hepatic microsomal enzymes that result in more rapid elimination of the estrogenic and progestational components of HORMONAL CONTRACEPTIVES.[1,2] In addition, sex hormone binding globulin capacity is increased, resulting in a decreased amount of free hormone.

Management Advise patients to use an additional form of contraception while receiving RIFAMPIN therapy.

Discussion

This drug combination is associated with pregnancy and menstrual abnormalities.[3-13] A review of the reported cases indicated that approximately 70% of women taking oral contraceptives may experience menstrual abnormalities and 6% may become pregnant when rifampin is coadministered.[9] Breakthrough bleeding was the most frequently reported menstrual abnormality, with amenorrhea and irregular menses reported less frequently.[12] These effects are secondary to a decrease in the estrogenic and progestational components of oral contraceptives resulting from rifampin-induced increases in metabolism and protein-bound fractions.[5,14-17] There is no indication that the use of low-dose oral contraceptives places the patient at greater risk, that increasing the estrogen dose will protect against pregnancy, or that patients who do not experience menstrual abnormalities are unlikely to become pregnant.[12] While rifampin and rifabutin affect the pharmacokinetics of oral contraceptives, the magnitude of the effects is greater with rifampin.[1,2]

[1] LeBel M, et al. *J Clin Pharmacol.* 1998;38(11):1042.
[2] Barditch-Crovo P, et al. *Clin Pharmacol Ther.* 1999;65(4):428.
[3] Altschuler SL, et al. *Obstet Gynecol.* 1974;44(5):771.
[4] Skolnick JL, et al. *JAMA.* 1976;236(12):1382.
[5] Joshi JV, et al. *Contraception.* 1980;21(6):617.
[6] Bint AJ, et al. *Drugs.* 1980;20(1):57.
[7] Gupta KC, et al. *Med J Zambia.* 1981;15(1):23.
[8] Back DJ, et al. *Drugs.* 1981;21(1):46.
[9] Baciewicz AM, et al. *Arch Intern Med.* 1984;144(8):1667.
[10] Barnett ML. *J Periodontol.* 1985;56(1):18.
[11] Baciewicz AM. *Ther Drug Monit.* 1985;7(1):26.
[12] Szoka PR, et al. *Fertil Steril.* 1988;49(5)(suppl 2):31S.
[13] Wibaux C, et al. *Joint Bone Spine.* 2010;77(3):268.
[14] Bolt HM, et al. *Eur J Clin Pharmacol.* 1975;8(5):301.
[15] Bolt HM, et al. *Acta Endocrinol (Copenh).* 1977;85(1):189.
[16] Back DJ, et al. *Eur J Clin Pharmacol.* 1979;15(3):193.
[17] Back DJ, et al. *Contraception.* 1980;21(2):135.

* Asterisk indicates drugs cited in interaction reports. Based on pharmacologic and pharmacokinetic considerations, similar interactions may occur with other drugs that are listed.

Contraceptives, Hormonal — *Serotonin Reuptake Inhibitors*

Contraceptives, Hormonal	Serotonin Reuptake Inhibitors	
Contraceptives, Oral* (eg, *Ortho-Novum*)	Fluoxetine (eg, *Prozac*)	Nefazodone*
	Fluvoxamine (eg, *Luvox*)	Sertraline (eg, *Zoloft*)

Significance	Onset	Severity	Documentation
4	☐ Rapid	☐ Major	☐ Established
	■ **Delayed**	■ **Moderate**	☐ Probable
		☐ Minor	☐ Suspected
			■ **Possible**
			☐ Unlikely

Effects Plasma concentrations of the estrogen component in HORMONAL CONTRACEPTIVES may be increased, resulting in adverse reactions.

Mechanism Inhibition of metabolism (CYP3A4) of the estrogen contained in the HORMONAL CONTRACEPTIVE by certain SRIs is suspected.

Management If estrogen-related adverse reactions occur, consider coadministration of the SRI as a possible cause. Consider use of a noninteracting SRI (eg, citalopram [eg, *Celexa*]).

Discussion

A possible interaction between a low-dose oral contraceptive, desogestrel plus ethinyl estradiol, and nefazodone was reported in a 27-year-old woman.[1] The patient was started on a low-dose contraceptive for birth control after previously receiving an oral contraceptive with a higher estrogen dose. The high-dose contraceptive was discontinued because of adverse reactions (eg, breast tenderness, bloating, weight gain, increased irritability). The patient was started on nefazodone 50 mg twice daily, which was increased incrementally to 100 mg at bedtime and 50 mg in the morning (higher doses were not tolerated), for periodic depressive symptoms. One week after starting nefazodone treatment, the patient experienced breast tenderness, bloating, weight gain, and increased premenstrual irritability. In addition, her menstrual cycle was delayed by 5 days. Nefazodone was continued for approximately 6 weeks, at which time it was discontinued because of intolerance. Within 24 hours of stopping nefazodone and starting citalopram, the adverse reactions resolved and the patient's menstrual cycle became regular.

[1] Adson DE, et al. *J Clin Psychopharmacol.* 2001;21(6):618.

* Asterisk indicates drugs cited in interaction reports. Based on pharmacologic and pharmacokinetic considerations, similar interactions may occur with other drugs that are listed.

Contraceptives, Hormonal — *St. John's Wort*

Contraceptives, Oral* (eg, *Ortho-Novum*)	St. John's Wort*

Significance	Onset	Severity	Documentation
1	☐ Rapid	■ **Major**	☐ Established
	■ **Delayed**	☐ Moderate	■ **Probable**
		☐ Minor	☐ Suspected
			☐ Possible
			☐ Unlikely

Effects The efficacy of HORMONAL CONTRACEPTIVES may be reduced.

Mechanism Increased hepatic metabolism (CYP3A4) of the HORMONAL CONTRACEPTIVE is suspected.

Management Caution patients to consult their health care provider or pharmacist before using nonprescription or herbal products. If use of ST. JOHN'S WORT (SJW) cannot be avoided, inform women of the increased risk of HORMONAL CONTRACEPTIVE failure. Consider an alternative nonhormonal contraceptive or an additional method of contraception.

Discussion

At least 9 cases of changes in menstrual bleeding (primarily intermenstrual bleeding) in women taking oral contraceptives (OCs) during ingestion of SJW have been reported to the Medical Products Agency in Uppsala, Sweden.[1] Most women had been taking OCs for many years prior to receiving SJW. In 5 women, the onset of menstrual disorders occurred approximately 7 days after starting SJW. After stopping SJW, menstrual disorders resolved in 3 women in whom the outcome was known. The effect of SJW on the efficacy of an OC containing ethinyl estradiol plus norethindrone (eg, *Norinyl*) was studied in 12 healthy women.[2] Each woman received the OC for 3 months. SJW was taken during months 2 and 3. The oral clearance of norethindrone was increased 16% by SJW. Breakthrough bleeding occurred in 7 of 12 women during month 3, compared with 2 of 12 during the first month. In women taking low-dose contraception (ethinyl estradiol 20 mcg plus norethindrone 1 mg [eg, *Loestrin*]), SJW 300 mg 3 times daily decreased dose exposure from the OC 13% to 15%, and increased breakthrough bleeding, follicle growth, and ovulation.[3] In another report, an unwanted pregnancy occurred in a 36-year-old woman using an oral contraceptive (ethinyl estradiol plus dienogest[†]) after starting SJW 1,700 mg/day.[4] Breakthrough bleeding has been reported in healthy women receiving low-dose OCs (ethinyl estradiol 0.2 mg plus desogestrel 0.15 mg) and SJW extract 300 mg twice daily.[5] SJW does not appear to interfere with the antiandrogenic effect of OCs.[6] The effects of SJW extract on a low-dose OC (ethinyl-estradiol 0.02 mg plus desogestrol 0.15 mg) were studied in 16 healthy women.[7] The subjects had been taking the OC for at least 3 months when a 14-day course of SJW extract 250 mg twice daily was started. SJW with low hypericum content did not interfere with the pharmacokinetics of the low-dose contraceptive.

[1] Yue QY, et al. *Lancet.* 2000;355(9203):576.
[2] Hall SD, et al. *Clin Pharmacol Ther.* 2003;74(6):525.
[3] Murphy PA, et al. *Contraception.* 2005;71(6):402.
[4] Schwarz UI, et al. *Eur J Clin Pharmacol.* 2001;57:A25.
[5] Pfrunder A, et al. *Br J Clin Pharmacol.* 2003;56(6):683.
[6] Fogle RH, et al. *Contraception.* 2006;74(3):245.
[7] Will-Shahab L, et al. *Eur J Clin Pharmacol.* 2009; 65(3):287.

* Asterisk indicates drugs cited in interaction reports.
† Not available in the United States.

Contraceptives, Hormonal — *Tetracyclines*

Contraceptives, Hormonal	Tetracyclines	
Contraceptives, Oral* (eg, *Ortho-Novum*)	Demeclocycline (eg, *Declomycin*)	Oxytetracycline*
	Doxycycline (eg, *Vibramycin*)	Tetracycline* (eg, *Sumycin*)
	Minocycline (eg, *Minocin*)	

Significance	Onset	Severity	Documentation
4	☐ Rapid	☐ Major	☐ Established
	■ **Delayed**	■ **Moderate**	☐ Probable
		☐ Minor	☐ Suspected
			■ **Possible**
			☐ Unlikely

Effects The efficacy of HORMONAL CONTRACEPTIVES may be reduced.

Mechanism TETRACYCLINES may suppress intestinal flora that normally provide hydrolytic enzymes essential for enterohepatic recirculation of certain CONTRACEPTIVE steroid conjugates. This may lead to decreased CONTRACEPTIVE plasma levels.

Management Although infrequently reported, CONTRACEPTIVE failure is possible. Patients who wish to avoid even a slight increase in the risk of pregnancy should use an additional nonhormonal form of contraception during TETRACYCLINE therapy.

Discussion

Fewer than 10 instances of pregnancy possibly linked to the coadministration of oral contraceptives and tetracycline or oxytetracycline have been reported.[1-5] A review of all published reports of adverse drug reactions secondary to a tetracycline oral contraceptive interaction through 1987 did not document any greater risk of contraceptive failure in patients on low-dose oral contraceptives. Pregnancy was the only documented reaction.[5] Therefore, breakthrough bleeding should not be used, as previously suggested by some authors, as an early indicator of contraceptive failure. In an investigation of antibiotic use (eg, oral cephalosporins, penicillins, tetracyclines) in dermatological practice, no differences in oral contraceptive failure rate were seen in a case-control study involving 311 women-years of combined antibiotic/oral contraceptive exposure, compared with 1,245 women-years of oral contraceptive use alone.[6]

1 Swenson L, et al. *Gastroenterology*. 1980;78(5, pt 2):1332.
2 Bacon JF, et al. *Br Med J*. 1980;280(6210):293.
3 Back DJ, et al. *Drugs*. 1981;21(1):46.
4 Barnett ML. *J Periodontol*. 1985;56(1):18.
5 Szoka PR, et al. *Fertil Steril*. 1988;49(5)(suppl 2):31S.
6 Helms SE, et al. *J Am Acad Dermatol*. 1997;36(5, pt 1):705.

* Asterisk indicates drugs cited in interaction reports. Based on pharmacologic and pharmacokinetic considerations, similar interactions may occur with other drugs that are listed.

Contraceptives, Hormonal — *Troglitazone*

Contraceptives, Oral* (eg, *Ortho-Novum*)	Troglitazone*† (*Rezulin*)

Significance	Onset	Severity	Documentation
2	☐ Rapid ■ **Delayed**	☐ Major ■ **Moderate** ☐ Minor	☐ Established ☐ Probable ■ **Suspected** ☐ Possible ☐ Unlikely

Effects Loss of ORAL CONTRACEPTIVE effectiveness, possibly leading to unintended pregnancy.

Mechanism Increased hepatic metabolism (CYP3A4) of the ORAL CONTRACEPTIVE is suspected. Plasma protein binding of norethindrone may be increased.

Management Inform women of the increased risk of ORAL CONTRACEPTIVE failure. Consider a higher dose of ORAL CONTRACEPTIVE, an alternative nonhormonal contraceptive, or an additional method of contraception.

Discussion

The effect of troglitazone on the pharmacokinetics of an oral contraceptive agent containing ethinyl estradiol 35 mcg plus norethindrone 1 mg (*Ortho-Novum*) was studied in healthy, nonsmoking women.[1] Of the 16 women participating in the study, 15 completed the investigation. All subjects received the oral contraceptive for 3 cycles (21 days of active drug followed by 7 days without drug). During the third cycle, troglitazone 600 mg/day was taken for 22 days with the oral contraceptive. Blood samples were collected on day 21 of cycles 2 and 3. The mean peak concentration and area under the plasma concentration-time curve (AUC) of ethinyl estradiol were 33% and 32% lower, respectively, during troglitazone administration compared with taking the oral contraceptive alone. Similarly, concurrent administration of troglitazone decreased the peak concentrations of norethindrone 31% and the AUC 29%. In addition, the unbound fraction of norethindrone decreased 29%. The mean plasma sex hormone binding globulin was increased 95% during concurrent troglitazone administration compared with taking the oral contraceptive alone.

[1] Loi CM, et al. *J Clin Pharmacol.* 1999 Apr;39:410.

* Asterisk indicates drugs cited in interaction reports.
† Not available in the United States.

Contraceptives, Hormonal — *Troleandomycin*

Contraceptives, Oral* (eg, *Ortho-Novum*)	Troleandomycin*† (*Tao*)

Significance	Onset	Severity	Documentation
2	☐ Rapid	☐ Major	☐ Established
	■ **Delayed**	■ **Moderate**	☐ Probable
		☐ Minor	■ **Suspected**
			☐ Possible
			☐ Unlikely

Effects The concurrent use of these agents may result in an increased risk of intrahepatic cholestasis.

Mechanism TROLEANDOMYCIN may slow the metabolism of ORAL CONTRACEPTIVES, leading to accumulation that appears to have a direct toxic effect on the secretory mechanisms of conjugated bilirubin and bile acids.

Management Avoid administering TROLEANDOMYCIN to women taking ORAL CONTRACEPTIVES.

Discussion

A study describing 12 patients receiving oral contraceptives documented the occurrence of intrahepatic cholestasis 2 to 20 days after the initiation of troleandomycin therapy. Eight of the 12 patients experienced clinical symptoms (eg, fatigue, anorexia, itching, jaundice) 2 to 5 days after initiation of troleandomycin therapy.[3] Most patients recovered completely 11 to 20 weeks after withdrawal of the offending agents. At least 39 cases of this interaction are documented in the literature.[1-4] Review of these cases suggests that oral contraceptives can be safely administered after the patient has recovered.[1-4]

[1] Rollux R, et al. *Nouv Presse Med.* 1979;8:1694.
[2] Miguet JP, et al. *Gastroenterol Clin Biol.* 1980;4:420.
[3] Fevery J, et al. *Acta Clin Belg.* 1983;38:242.
[4] Ludden TM, et al. *Clin Pharmacokinet.* 1985;10:63.

* Asterisk indicates drugs cited in interaction reports.
† Not available in the United States.

Corticosteroids ✕ *Aminoglutethimide*

Corticosteroids	Aminoglutethimide
Dexamethasone* (eg, *Decadron*)	Aminoglutethimide* (*Cytadren*)

Significance	Onset	Severity	Documentation
2	☐ Rapid	☐ Major	☐ Established
	■ **Delayed**	■ **Moderate**	☐ Probable
		☐ Minor	■ **Suspected**
			☐ Possible
			☐ Unlikely

Effects Possible loss of DEXAMETHASONE-induced adrenal suppression. This may result in an unsuccessful chemical adrenalectomy with AMINOGLUTETHIMIDE. Anti-inflammatory activity may also be reduced.

Mechanism Unknown.

Management Increased doses of DEXAMETHASONE, above those usually required for adrenal suppression, may be required. If possible, substitute hydrocortisone for DEXAMETHASONE.

Discussion

Two uncontrolled clinical studies of patients with metastatic breast cancer treated with dexamethasone and aminoglutethimide revealed the loss of successful chemical adrenalectomy secondary to increased ACTH production.[1-3] In both trials, the desired effect could be achieved by increasing the dexamethasone dose two to three times above that which is usually required for successful adrenal suppression. Both investigations documented a marked decrease in dexamethasone half-life in one or more patients when used with aminoglutethimide. In an additional case, the dose of dexamethasone had to be increased from 6 to 16 mg daily to control brain edema after aminoglutethimide therapy was started.[4]

In a separate trial of 15 metastatic breast cancer patients, successful chemical adrenalectomy without subsequent loss of adrenal suppression was achieved by combining hydrocortisone, rather than dexamethasone, with aminoglutethimide. These investigators also demonstrated marked changes in dexamethasone clearance but no alterations with hydrocortisone.

[1] Lipton A, et al. *Cancer.* 1974;33:503.
[2] Santen RJ, et al. *JAMA.* 1974;230:1661.
[3] Santen RJ, et al. *J Clin Endocrinol Metab.* 1977;45:469.
[4] Halpern J, et al. *J Med.* 1984;15:59.

* Asterisk indicates drugs cited in interaction reports.

Corticosteroids — *Antacids*

Corticosteroids		Antacids	
Betamethasone (eg, *Celestone*)	Hydrocortisone (eg, *Cortef*)	Aluminum Hydroxide* (eg, *Amphojel*)	Magnesium Hydroxide* (eg, *Milk of Magnesia*)
Cortisone (eg, *Cortone*)	Prednisone* (eg, *Deltasone*)	Aluminum/Magnesium Hydroxide* (eg, *Maalox*)	
Dexamethasone* (eg, *Decadron*)	Triamcinolone (eg, *Kenalog*)		

Significance	Onset	Severity	Documentation
5	☐ Rapid ■ **Delayed**	☐ Major ☐ Moderate ■ **Minor**	☐ Established ☐ Probable ☐ Suspected ■ **Possible** ☐ Unlikely

Effects A decrease in the pharmacologic effect of DEXAMETHASONE may occur.

Mechanism Unknown.

Management Follow standard monitoring procedures. Close monitoring of the pharmacologic effects of DEXAMETHASONE is advisable. An H_2 antagonist, such as cimetidine, may be considered as an alternative to antacid therapy.

Discussion

Four well controlled pharmacokinetic trials found no significant alterations in prednisolone pharmacokinetics when administered with either aluminum, magnesium or a combination aluminum/magnesium antacid.[2-4,6] One study of five healthy volunteers and 12 patients with chronic liver disease observed significant decreases in prednisolone maximum plasma concentrations and in the area under the curve after administration of prednisone with different aluminum/magnesium antacid combinations, irrespective of liver disease.[5] An additional study found an increase in the 24-hour urinary cortisol when dexamethasone was administered with a magnesium trisilicate antacid.[1] This change was most likely the result of a decrease in dexamethasone absorption secondary to the antacid. A single trial examined the effect of both cimetidine (eg, *Tagamet*) and ranitidine (eg, *Zantac*) on the conversion of prednisone to prednisolone.[8] No significant changes in this conversion occurred with either agent. Cimetidine also had no influence on the bioavailability or plasma clearance of methylprednisolone in a single case report.[7] Evidence suggests that corticosteroids may be administered with either cimetidine, ranitidine or antacids without alterations in their bioavailability.

1 Naggar VF, et al. *J Pharm Sci.* 1978;67:1029.
2 Tanner AR, et al. *Br J Clin Pharmacol.* 1979;7:397.
3 Lee DAH, et al. *Br J Clin Pharmacol.* 1979;8:92.
4 Bergrem H, et al. *Scand J Urol Nephrol.* 1981;64 (Suppl):167.
5 Uribe M, et al. *Gastroenterology.* 1981;80:661.
6 Albin H, et al. *Eur J Clin Pharmacol.* 1984;26:271.
7 Green A, et al. *Am J Med.* 1984;77:1115.
8 Sirgo MA, et al. *Clin Pharmacol Ther.* 1985;37:534.

* Asterisk indicates drugs cited in interaction reports. Based on pharmacologic and pharmacokinetic considerations, similar interactions may occur with other drugs that are listed.

Corticosteroids — Aprepitant

Corticosteroids		Aprepitant
Dexamethasone* (eg, *Baycadron*)	Methylprednisolone* (eg, *Medrol*)	Aprepitant* (*Emend*)
Hydrocortisone (eg, *Cortef*)		

Significance	Onset	Severity	Documentation
2	☐ Rapid	☐ Major	☐ Established
	■ **Delayed**	■ **Moderate**	☐ Probable
		☐ Minor	■ **Suspected**
			☐ Possible
			☐ Unlikely

Effects CORTICOSTEROID plasma concentrations may be increased and the t½ prolonged.

Mechanism Inhibition of first-pass and systemic metabolism (CYP3A4) by APREPITANT is suspected.

Management In patients receiving certain CORTICOSTEROIDS, adjustments in the dosage may be needed when APREPITANT is started or stopped.

Discussion

The effects of aprepitant on the pharmacokinetics of dexamethasone and methylprednisolone were evaluated in 2 studies.[1] The first study, an open-label, randomized, crossover investigation, included 20 healthy subjects. Each subject received: 1) a standard oral dexamethasone regimen for treatment of chemotherapy-induced nausea and vomiting (dexamethasone 20 mg on day 1, 8 mg on days 2 to 5); 2) aprepitant (125 mg on day 1, 80 mg once daily on days 2 to 5) and the above dexamethasone regimen; and 3) aprepitant with a modified oral dexamethasone regimen (dexamethasone 12 mg on day 1 and 4 mg on days 2 to 5). All subjects also received IV ondansetron (eg, *Zofran*) 32 mg on day 1. Two other treatment regimens were administered, but the data were not relevant for the purposes of this investigation. Aprepitant increased the AUC 2.2-fold compared with the other treatment regimens. In addition, aprepitant increased the peak plasma levels and prolonged the t½ of dexamethasone. The second study, a randomized, double-blind, placebo-controlled, 2-period crossover design, included 10 healthy subjects. Subjects received a regimen of IV methylprednisolone 125 mg on day 1 and 40 mg orally on days 2 to 3 with a placebo or aprepitant (125 mg on day 1 and 80 mg on days 2 to 3). Aprepitant increased the AUC of IV methylprednisolone 1.3-fold on day 1 and the AUC of oral methylprednisolone 2.5-fold on day 3. In addition, aprepitant increased the C_{max} and prolonged the t½ of oral methylprednisolone.

[1] McCrea JB, et al. *Clin Pharmacol Ther.* 2003;74(1):17.

* Asterisk indicates drugs cited in interaction reports. Based on pharmacologic and pharmacokinetic considerations, similar interactions may occur with other drugs that are listed.

Corticosteroids — *Azole Antifungal Agents*

Corticosteroids		Azole Antifungal Agents	
Betamethasone (eg, *Celestone*)	Methylprednisolone* (eg, *Medrol*)	Fluconazole (eg, *Diflucan*)	Posaconazole (*Noxafil*)
Budesonide* (eg, *Pulmicort*)	Prednisolone* (eg, *Orapred*)	Itraconazole* (eg, *Sporanox*)	Voriconazole (eg, *Vfend*)
Dexamethasone* (eg, *Baycadron*)	Prednisone* (eg, *Sterapred*)	Ketoconazole* (eg, *Nizoral*)	
Fluticasone* (eg, *Flovent*)			

Significance	Onset	Severity	Documentation
2	☐ Rapid	☐ Major	☐ Established
	■ **Delayed**	■ **Moderate**	☐ Probable
		☐ Minor	■ **Suspected**
			☐ Possible
			☐ Unlikely

Effects CORTICOSTEROID effects and toxicity may be increased.

Mechanism Possible inhibition of CORTICOSTEROID metabolism (CYP3A4) and decrease in elimination.

Management Closely monitor patients for CORTICOSTEROID adverse reactions. Adjust dose as needed.

Discussion

In 6 subjects, ketoconazole more than doubled methylprednisolone AUC and reduced clearance more than 50%.[1] Serum cortisol suppression was more marked and persisted longer during ketoconazole treatment. Another study recommended a 50% decrease in methylprednisolone dosage when given with ketoconazole.[2] Ketoconazole decreased prednisone elimination (40%) and volume of distribution while increasing systemic bioavailability and unbound prednisolone levels.[3] A critical reply and response to this study were published.[4,5] In 10 healthy subjects, itraconazole increased the single-dose methylprednisolone AUC 3.9-fold, C_{max} 1.9-fold, and elimination $t_{½}$ 2.4-fold compared with placebo.[6] Mean plasma cortisol levels were 87% lower. Another study found itraconazole markedly increases methylprednisolone levels.[7] Similar results occurred with oral itraconazole and IV methylprednisolone[8] and oral or IV dexamethasone.[9] Itraconazole increased the AUC and $t_{½}$ of prednisolone 24% and 29%, respectively.[10] Itraconazole therapy has resulted in Cushing syndrome in patients receiving fluticasone[11] or budesonide[12,13] by inhalation. A 4.2-fold increase in inhaled budesonide plasma levels was reported in 10 healthy subjects receiving itraconazole.[14] Others found no interaction between itraconazole and prednisolone,[7] or ketoconazole and budesonide[15] or prednisone.[16]

1 Glynn AM, et al. *Clin Pharmacol Ther.* 1986;39(6):654.
2 Kandrotas RJ, et al. *Clin Pharmacol Ther.* 1987;42(4):465.
3 Zürcher RM, et al. *Clin Pharmacol Ther.* 1989;45(4):366.
4 Jasko WJ. *Clin Pharmacol Ther.* 1990;47(3):418.
5 Zürcher RM, et al. *Clin Pharmacol Ther.* 1990;47(3):419.
6 Varis T, et al. *Clin Pharmacol Ther.* 1998;64(4):363.
7 Lebrun-Vignes B, et al. *Br J Clin Pharmacol.* 2001;51(5):443.
8 Varis T, et al. *Pharmacol Toxicol.* 1999;85(1):29.
9 Varis T, et al. *Clin Pharmacol Ther.* 2000;68(5):487.
10 Varis T, et al. *Eur J Clin Pharmacol.* 2000;56(1):57.
11 Parmar JS, et al. *Thorax.* 2002;57(8):749.
12 Main KM, et al. *Acta Paediatr.* 2002;91(9):1008.
13 Bolland MJ, et al. *Ann Pharmacother.* 2004;38(1):46.
14 Raaska K, et al. *Clin Pharmacol Ther.* 2002;72(4):362.
15 Seidegård J. *Clin Pharmacol Ther.* 2000;68(1):13.
16 Yamashita SK, et al. *Clin Pharmacol Ther.* 1991;49(5):558.

* Asterisk indicates drugs cited in interaction reports. Based on pharmacologic and pharmacokinetic considerations, similar interactions may occur with other drugs that are listed.

Corticosteroids — Barbiturates

Corticosteroids		Barbiturates	
Betamethasone (*Celestone*)	Fludrocortisone	Amobarbital (*Amytal*)	Phenobarbital* (eg, *Luminal*)
Budesonide (eg, *Pulmicort*)	Hydrocortisone* (eg, *Cortef*)	Butabarbital (*Butisol*)	Primidone* (eg, *Mysoline*)
Corticotropin (ACTH)	Methylprednisolone* (eg, *Medrol*)	Butalbital	Secobarbital (*Seconal*)
Cortisone	Prednisolone* (eg, *Prelone*)	Mephobarbital (eg, *Mebaral*)	
Cosyntropin (eg, *Cortrosyn*)	Prednisone*	Pentobarbital* (*Nembutal*)	
Dexamethasone* (eg, *Baycadron*)	Triamcinolone (eg, *Kenalog*)		

Significance	Onset	Severity	Documentation
2	☐ Rapid ■ **Delayed**	☐ Major ■ **Moderate** ☐ Minor	■ **Established** ☐ Probable ☐ Suspected ☐ Possible ☐ Unlikely

Effects Decreased pharmacologic effects of the CORTICOSTEROID may be observed.

Mechanism Stimulated CORTICOSTEROID metabolism (6-beta-hydroxylation) secondary to BARBITURATE induction of liver enzymes.

Management If possible, avoid this combination. Carefully monitor patients receiving CORTICOSTEROIDS when a BARBITURATE is added or discontinued. Increases in the CORTICOSTEROID dosage may be required to maintain the desired effect.[1,2]

Discussion

Phenobarbital dosing for 3 weeks in a group of 16 asthmatic patients resulted in a 44% decrease in dexamethasone t½ and an 88% increase in the mean clearance rate.[3] In the 3 patients in this trial who were steroid-dependent, a marked worsening of asthma symptoms occurred within days of phenobarbital initiation. Similar results were noted in 8 of 9 prednisone-treated rheumatoid arthritis patients in whom 2 weeks of phenobarbital treatment produced worsening symptoms.[4] In addition, a decrease in prednisone t½ was noted. Also, a 100% decrease in the t½ along with a 90% increase in mean clearance rate was observed with methylprednisolone following a 3-week course of phenobarbital.[5] Decreases in methylprednisolone t½ (versus historical controls) also have been noted during phenobarbital infusion to a group of 6 neurosurgical patients.[6] A patient receiving dexamethasone for congenital adrenal hyperplasia converted from undertreatment to overtreatment when primidone therapy was withdrawn.[7]

1 Kuntzman R, et al. *Biochem Pharmacol.* 1968;17(4):565.
2 Hancock KW, et al. *Lancet.* 1978;2(8080):97.
3 Brooks SM, et al. *N Engl J Med.* 1972;286(21):1125.
4 Brooks PM, et al. *Ann Rheum Dis.* 1976;35(4):339.
5 Stjernholm MR, et al. *J Clin Endocrinol Metab.* 1975;41(5):887.
6 Gabrielsen J, et al. *J Neurosurg.* 1985;62(2):182.
7 Young MC, et al. *Acta Paediatr Scand.* 1991;80(1):120.

* Asterisk indicates drugs cited in interaction reports. Based on pharmacologic and pharmacokinetic considerations, similar interactions may occur with other drugs that are listed.

Corticosteroids — *Bile Acid Sequestrants*

Hydrocortisone* (eg, *Cortef*)	Cholestyramine* (eg, *Questran*)	Colestipol* (eg, *Colestid*)

Significance	Onset	Severity	Documentation
2	☐ Rapid ■ **Delayed**	☐ Major ■ **Moderate** ☐ Minor	☐ Established ☐ Probable ■ **Suspected** ☐ Possible ☐ Unlikely

Effects A decrease in the therapeutic effect of HYDROCORTISONE may occur.

Mechanism CHOLESTYRAMINE and COLESTIPOL appear to interfere with the GI absorption of HYDROCORTISONE.

Management While separate administration of these 2 agents may improve the absorption of HYDROCORTISONE, no data currently exist to support this. Patients may require larger HYDROCORTISONE doses to achieve the desired effect when these agents are coadministered. Consider alternative cholesterol-lowering therapy.

Discussion

Ten healthy subjects were studied after receiving doses of oral hydrocortisone 50 mg with and without prior administration of cholestyramine 4 g.[1] Two additional subjects were evaluated after a dose of cholestyramine 8 g. The results revealed a mean 35% decrease in hydrocortisone AUC following concomitant cholestyramine. The hydrocortisone C_{max} also was reduced and the time to C_{max} was delayed after cholestyramine. Further reductions in the oral bioavailability of hydrocortisone were observed after the dose of cholestyramine 8 g. Colestipol, a bile acid–binding resin similar to cholestyramine, decreased the efficacy of oral hydrocortisone in a patient with hypopituitarism.[2]

Five other subjects exhibited a reduction in gastric emptying time following cholestyramine. An in vitro binding study demonstrated decreasing quantities of hydrocortisone in solution with increasing concentrations of cholestyramine.[1] This finding is supported by a similar in vitro study.[3] This second group, however, failed to document that concomitant cholestyramine inhibited the absorption of hydrocortisone in rats.

[1] Johansson C, et al. *Acta Med Scand.* 1978;204(6):509.
[2] Nekl KE, et al. *Ann Pharmacother.* 1993;27(7-8):980.
[3] Ware AJ, et al. *Gastroenterology.* 1973;64(6):1150.

* Asterisk indicates drugs cited in interaction reports.

Corticosteroids — *Contraceptives, Hormonal*

Corticosteroids		Contraceptives, Hormonal
Budesonide (eg, *Pulmicort*)	Prednisolone* (eg, *Prelone*)	Contraceptives, Hormonal* (eg, *Ortho-Novum*)
Dexamethasone (eg, *Baycadron*)	Prednisone* (eg, *Sterapred*)	
Hydrocortisone* (eg, *Cortef*)	Triamcinolone (eg, *Kenalog*)	
Methylprednisolone* (eg, *Medrol*)		

Significance	Onset	Severity	Documentation
3	☐ Rapid	☐ Major	☐ Established
	■ **Delayed**	☐ Moderate	☐ Probable
		■ **Minor**	■ **Suspected**
			☐ Possible
			☐ Unlikely

Effects Therapeutic and adverse actions of certain CORTICOSTEROIDS could be enhanced.

Mechanism Reduced metabolism and increased systemic availability of certain CORTICOSTEROIDS by ORAL CONTRACEPTIVES.

Management A reduction in CORTICOSTEROID dose may be required if an ORAL CONTRACEPTIVE is added to the regimen.

Discussion

It has been demonstrated that combination oral contraceptives alter prednisolone pharmacokinetics.[1-7] The plasma t½ was approximately doubled, the free prednisolone plasma concentration was doubled, the apparent volume of distribution was decreased approximately 50%, plasma clearance was decreased 2- to 5-fold, and the AUC was increased 2- to 5-fold.[1-4] This increase in AUC may result from decreased metabolism by the liver related to estrogen-induced decreased enzyme activity or oral contraceptive competition at the site of prednisolone metabolism, as well as increased protein binding secondary to oral contraceptive–induced increased transcortin concentration.[2] Similar kinetic alterations will occur with prednisone, which is converted to prednisolone,[3] and methylprednisolone.[8] Despite the magnitude of these reported kinetic changes, no cases of steroid excess have been documented.[9] A study involving coadministration of oral contraceptives and fluocortolone† reported no interaction, supporting the theory that this interaction is specific to certain corticosteroids.[10]

1 Legler UF, et al. *Clin Pharmacol Ther.* 1982;31(2):243.
2 Boekenoogen SJ, et al. *J Clin Endocrinol Metab.* 1983;56(4):702.
3 Frey BM, et al. *Eur J Clin Pharmacol.* 1984;26(4):505.
4 Meffin PJ, et al. *Br J Clin Pharmacol.* 1984;17(6):655.
5 Frey BM, et al. *J Clin Endocrinol Metab.* 1985;60(2):361.
6 Baciewicz AM, et al. *Ther Drug Monit.* 1985;7(1):26.
7 Legler UF, et al. *Clin Pharmacol Ther.* 1986;39(4):425.
8 Slayter KL, et al. *Clin Pharmacol Ther.* 1996;59(3):312.
9 Szoka PR, et al. *Fertil Steril.* 1988;49(5)(suppl 2):31S.
10 Legler UF. *Eur J Clin Pharmacol.* 1988;35(1):101.

* Asterisk indicates drugs cited in interaction reports. Based on pharmacologic and pharmacokinetic considerations, similar interactions may occur with other drugs that are listed.

† Not available in the United States.

Corticosteroids — *Diltiazem*

Methylprednisolone* (eg, *Medrol*)	Diltiazem* (eg, *Cardizem*)

Significance	Onset	Severity	Documentation
2	☐ Rapid ■ **Delayed**	☐ Major ■ **Moderate** ☐ Minor	☐ Established ☐ Probable ■ **Suspected** ☐ Possible ☐ Unlikely

Effects The pharmacologic and toxic effects of METHYLPREDNISOLONE may be increased.

Mechanism Inhibition of METHYLPREDNISOLONE metabolism (CYP3A4) is suspected. In addition, inhibition of P-glycoprotein may contribute to the interaction.

Management Carefully observe the patient response to METHYLPREDNISOLONE when DILTIAZEM is coadministered. Adjust the dose of METHYLPREDNISOLONE as needed.

Discussion

In a randomized, double-blind, placebo-controlled, crossover study, the effect of diltiazem on the pharmacokinetics of methylprednisolone was assessed in 9 healthy volunteers.[1] Each subject received oral diltiazem 60 mg 3 times/day or placebo orally for 3 days. On the third day, oral methylprednisolone 16 mg was given. Compared with placebo, diltiazem administration increased the total AUC of methylprednisolone 2.6-fold, the C_{max} 1.6-fold, and the elimination $t_{½}$ 1.9-fold. In addition, diltiazem increased the nighttime exposure to methylprednisolone 28.2-fold and correlated negatively with the morning plasma cortisol level, which was 12% of the placebo phase. In a similar study, 5 volunteers were given IV methylprednisolone (0.3 mg/kg) with and without diltiazem (180 mg sustained release).[2] During coadministration of both drugs, the $t_{½}$ of methylprednisolone increased from 2.28 to 3.12 hours. No changes in cortisol levels or T-lymphocyte activity were detected.

[1] Varis T, et al. *Clin Pharmacol Ther.* 2000;67(3):215.

[2] Booker BM, et al. *Clin Pharmacol Ther.* 2002;72(4):370.

* Asterisk indicates drugs cited in interaction reports.

Corticosteroids — *Ephedrine*

Dexamethasone* (eg, *Decadron*)	Ephedrine*

Significance	Onset	Severity	Documentation
5	☐ Rapid ■ **Delayed**	☐ Major ☐ Moderate ■ **Minor**	☐ Established ☐ Probable ☐ Suspected ■ **Possible** ☐ Unlikely

Effects A decrease in the effects of DEXAMETHASONE may occur.

Mechanism Unknown.

Management Based on current information, no special precautions are needed.

Discussion

In a trial of 9 patients, a pharmacokinetic study of dexamethasone was performed prior to and following 4 weeks of ephedrine therapy.[1] A 36% decrease in dexamethasone half-life and a 43% increase in clearance were observed when dexamethasone was administered with ephedrine. No reports of a loss of dexamethasone efficacy during concomitant ephedrine therapy have been documented.

[1] Brooks SM, et al. *J Clin Pharmacol.* 1977;17:308.

* Asterisk indicates drugs cited in interaction reports.

Corticosteroids — *Estrogens*

Corticosteroids		Estrogens	
Hydrocortisone (eg, *Cortef*) Prednisolone*	Prednisone* (eg, *Deltasone*)	Chlorotrianisene*† Conjugated Estrogens* (*Premarin*) Diethylstilbestrol*† Esterified Estrogens* (eg, *Estratab*) Estradiol* (eg, *Estrace*)	Estrone* (eg, *Kestrone 5*) Estropipate* (eg, *Ogen*) Ethinyl Estradiol* (*Estinyl*)

Significance	Onset	Severity	Documentation
2	☐ Rapid ■ **Delayed**	☐ Major ■ **Moderate** ☐ Minor	☐ Established ☐ Probable ■ **Suspected** ☐ Possible ☐ Unlikely

Effects May result in an increase in the pharmacologic and toxicologic effects of CORTICOSTEROIDS. It is not known how rapidly this effect may reverse after ESTROGEN therapy is discontinued.

Mechanism Inactivation of hepatic cytochrome P450, which may result in decreased formation of the 6-betahydroxy metabolite of PREDNISOLONE.

Management Monitor patients for the therapeutic and toxic effects of CORTICOSTEROIDS to aid in appropriate dosage adjustment.

Discussion

In a single pharmacokinetic trial, women treated with estrogen-containing oral contraceptives displayed a 3-fold decrease in total and unbound prednisolone clearance vs age-matched control subjects.[2] In this same study, women receiving conjugated estrogen therapy had a 25% decrease in unbound prednisolone clearance vs a group of age-matched controls. For this latter group, this effect was independent of the estrogen dosage. Norethisterone, an ethinyl sterol similar to agents present in almost all oral contraceptives, was shown to bind irreversibly to rat hepatic cytochrome P450, destroying its metabolic activity.[1]

[1] Ortiz de Montellano PR, et al. *Proc Natl Acad Sci U S A*. 1979;76:746.

[2] Gustavson LE, et al. *J Clin Endocrinol Metab*. 1986;62:234.

* Asterisk indicates drugs cited in interaction reports. Based on pharmacologic and pharmacokinetic considerations, similar interactions may occur with other drugs that are listed.

† Not available in the US.

Corticosteroids — *Food*

Budesonide* (eg, *Entocort EC*)	Methylprednisolone* (eg, *Medrol*)	Grapefruit Juice*

Significance	Onset	Severity	Documentation
3	□ Rapid ■ **Delayed**	□ Major □ Moderate ■ **Minor**	□ Established □ Probable ■ **Suspected** □ Possible □ Unlikely

Effects The effect of the CORTICOSTEROID may be enhanced, increasing the risk of adverse reactions.

Mechanism Inhibition of intestinal first-pass metabolism (CYP3A4) of the CORTICOSTEROID is suspected.

Management Observe patients for an increase in CORTICOSTEROID adverse reactions and adjust the dose as needed.

Discussion

The effects of administration of methylprednisolone with grapefruit juice on the pharmacokinetics and plasma cortisol concentrations were evaluated in 10 healthy volunteers.[1] Using a randomized, 2-phase, crossover design, each subject received 200 mL of double-strength grapefruit juice or water 3 times daily for 2 days. On day 3, methylprednisolone 16 mg was given with 200 mL of grapefruit juice or water. In addition, 200 mL of grapefruit juice or water was ingested 0.5 and 1.5 hours after administration of methylprednisolone. Compared with water, grapefruit juice delayed the absorption and increased plasma concentrations of methylprednisolone from 2 hours onward. Grapefruit juice increased the AUC of methylprednisolone 75%, the peak concentration 27%, and the $t_{½}$ 35%. There was no difference in the plasma cortisol concentrations after methylprednisolone administration when taken with grapefruit juice or water. The effect of regular-strength grapefruit juice on the systemic availability of budesonide was evaluated in 8 healthy men.[2] Using an open-label, crossover design, each subject received budesonide 3 mg extended-release or immediate-release capsules alone or after 4 days of pretreatment with 200 mL of grapefruit juice 3 times daily. Compared with taking budesonide alone, pretreatment with grapefruit juice approximately doubled the bioavailability of extended- and immediate-release budesonide.

[1] Varis T, et al. *Eur J Clin Pharmacol.* 2000;56(6-7):489.

[2] Seidegard J, et al. *Pharmazie.* 2009;64(7):461.

* Asterisk indicates drugs cited in interaction reports.

Corticosteroids — Hydantoins

Corticosteroids		Hydantoins	
Betamethasone (*Celestone*)	Hydrocortisone* (eg, *Cortef*)	Ethotoin (*Peganone*)	Phenytoin* (eg, *Dilantin*)
Budesonide (eg, *Pulmicort*)	Methylprednisolone* (eg, *Medrol*)	Fosphenytoin (eg, *Cerebyx*)	
Cortisone	Prednisolone* (eg, *Prelone*)		
Cosyntropin (eg, *Cortrosyn*)	Prednisone (eg, *Sterapred*)		
Dexamethasone* (eg, *Baycadron*)	Triamcinolone (eg, *Kenalog*)		
Fludrocortisone*			

Significance	Onset	Severity	Documentation
2	☐ Rapid	☐ Major	■ **Established**
	■ **Delayed**	■ **Moderate**	☐ Probable
		☐ Minor	☐ Suspected
			☐ Possible
			☐ Unlikely

Effects Decreased STEROID effects may occur within days of PHENYTOIN initiation and persist for 3 weeks after discontinuation. DEXAMETHASONE may reduce PHENYTOIN levels.

Mechanism Increased STEROID metabolism via 6-beta-hydroxylation because of enzyme induction by PHENYTOIN. DEXAMETHASONE may enhance hepatic clearance of PHENYTOIN.

Management A 2-fold or more increase in the STEROID dose may be needed. Greater than expected PHENYTOIN doses may also be required. If unable to avoid this combination, monitor PHENYTOIN levels and adjust the dose of either agent.

Discussion

Pharmacokinetic data support this interaction.[1-7] When phenytoin was used with prednisolone, increases of approximately 30% in total body clearance of total and free prednisolone were observed.[7] Methylprednisolone clearance may increase with concomitant phenytoin.[3] Phenytoin markedly increased dexamethasone clearance[2,6] and decreased fludrocortisone efficacy.[8] This interaction decreases the dexamethasone effect on serum cortisol suppression[1,9] and its efficacy in disease states.[10,11] Whether dexamethasone increases[12] or decreases[13,14] phenytoin levels is controversial. The effect of phenytoin appears to be more pronounced when given with corticosteroids with a long $t_{1/2}$.

[1] Jubiz W, et al. *N Engl J Med.* 1970;283(1):11.
[2] Haque N, et al. *J Clin Endocrinol Metab.* 1972;34(1):44.
[3] Stjernholm MR, et al. *J Clin Endocrinol Metab.* 1975;41(5):887.
[4] Petereit LB, et al. *Clin Pharmacol Ther.* 1977;22(6):912.
[5] Frey FJ, et al. *J Lab Clin Med.* 1983;101(4):593.
[6] Chalk JB, et al. *J Neurol Neurosurg Psychiatry.* 1984;47(10):1087.
[7] Frey BM, et al. *Eur J Clin Invest.* 1984;14(1):1.
[8] Keilholz U, et al. *Am J Med Sci.* 1986;291(4):280.
[9] Werk EE Jr, et al. *N Engl J Med.* 1969;281(1):32.
[10] Boylan JJ, et al. *JAMA.* 1976;235(8):803.
[11] McLelland J, et al. *Lancet.* 1978;1(8073):1096.
[12] Lawson LA, et al. *Surg Neurol.* 1981;16(1):23.
[13] Wong DD, et al. *JAMA.* 1985;254(15):2062.
[14] Lackner TE. *Pharmacotherapy.* 1991;11(4):344.

* Asterisk indicates drugs cited in interaction reports. Based on pharmacologic and pharmacokinetic considerations, similar interactions may occur with other drugs that are listed.

Corticosteroids — *Macrolide Antibiotics*

Corticosteroids	Macrolide Antibiotics	
Methylprednisolone* (eg, *Medrol*)	Clarithromycin* (eg, *Biaxin*)	Troleandomycin*†
	Erythromycin* (eg, *Ery-Tab*)	

Significance	Onset	Severity	Documentation
2	☐ Rapid	☐ Major	☐ Established
	■ **Delayed**	■ **Moderate**	■ **Probable**
		☐ Minor	☐ Suspected
			☐ Possible
			☐ Unlikely

Effects The pharmacologic and toxic effects of METHYLPREDNISOLONE may be increased.

Mechanism Although this interaction results in an increase in plasma concentrations of METHYLPREDNISOLONE, it is unclear if this alone is responsible for the marked increase in METHYLPREDNISOLONE's effect.

Management It may be necessary to decrease the METHYLPREDNISOLONE dose and the dosing interval in patients treated concomitantly with MACROLIDE ANTIBIOTICS.

Discussion

Troleandomycin results in a more than a 100% decrease in the total body clearance of methylprednisolone.[1] This effect of troleandomycin appears to be immediate, more pronounced when it is administered on the same day as methylprednisolone, and independent of the methylprednisolone dose.[2] Because similar changes are not observed with prednisolone, it appears that the effect of troleandomycin is steroid specific.[3] This effect of troleandomycin has been used to therapeutic advantage, allowing a methylprednisolone dose reduction in many steroid-dependent asthma patients.[4-6] A pharmacokinetic study documented a 46% decrease in methylprednisolone clearance during concomitant therapy with erythromycin base.[7] In a separate report, erythromycin estolate was associated with a decrease in steroid dosage and improved efficacy in chronic asthma patients.[8] It is not known whether erythromycin may allow for increased efficacy and reduced toxicity of methylprednisolone in chronic asthma. In another pharmacokinetic study, clarithromycin produced a 65% decrease in methylprednisolone clearance but had no effect on prednisone pharmacokinetics.[9] A study using an ex vivo lymphocyte proliferation assay suggests that clarithromycin may have inherent immunomodulatory properties.[10]

1 Szefler SJ, et al. *J Allergy Clin Immunol.* 1980;66(6):447.
2 Szefler SJ, et al. *Clin Pharmacol Ther.* 1982;32(2):166.
3 Szefler SJ, et al. *J Allergy Clin Immunol.* 1982;69(5):455.
4 Spector SL, et al. *J Allergy Clin Immunol.* 1974;54:367.
5 Schatz M, et al. *Am Rev Respir Dis.* 1979;119(suppl):167.
6 Zeiger RS, et al. *J Allergy Clin Immunol.* 1980;66(6):438.
7 LaForce CF, et al. *J Allergy Clin Immunol.* 1983;72(1):34.
8 Itkin IH, et al. *J Allergy.* 1970;45(3):146.
9 Fost DA, et al. *J Allergy Clin Immunol.* 1999;103(6):1031.
10 Spahn JD, et al. *Ann Allergy Asthma Immunol.* 2001;87(6):501.

* Asterisk indicates drugs cited in interaction reports.
† Not available in the United States.

Corticosteroids — *Mifepristone*

Corticosteroids		Mifepristone
Betamethasone* (eg, *Celestone*)	Fludrocortisone*	Mifepristone* (eg, *Korlym*)
Budesonide* (eg, *Pulmicort*)	Hydrocortisone* (eg, *Cortef*)	
Corticotropin* (eg, *Acthar*)	Methylprednisolone* (eg, *Medrol*)	
Cortisone*	Prednisolone* (eg, *Prelone*)	
Cosyntropin* (eg, *Cortrosyn*)	Prednisone*	
Dexamethasone* (eg, *Baycadron*)	Triamcinolone* (eg, *Kenolog*)	

Significance	Onset	Severity	Documentation
2	☐ Rapid	☐ Major	☐ Established
	■ **Delayed**	■ **Moderate**	☐ Probable
		☐ Minor	■ **Suspected**
			☐ Possible
			☐ Unlikely

Effects The pharmacologic effects of CORTICOSTEROIDS may be reduced.

Mechanism MIFEPRISTONE antagonizes the pharmacologic effects of CORTICOSTEROIDS.

Management Coadministration of CORTICOSTEROIDS with MIFEPRISTONE is contraindicated.[1]

Discussion

Mifepristone is contraindicated in patients concurrently being treated with systemic corticosteroids for serious medical conditions or illness (eg, immunosuppression after organ transplantation) because mifepristone antagonizes the effect of corticosteroids.[1]

[1] *Korlym* [package insert]. Menlo Park, CA: Corcept Therapeutics Incorporated; February 2012.

* Asterisk indicates drugs cited in interaction reports.

Corticosteroids — *Montelukast*

Corticosteroids	Montelukast
Prednisone*	Montelukast* (*Singulair*)

Significance	Onset	Severity	Documentation
4	□ Rapid ■ **Delayed**	□ Major ■ **Moderate** □ Minor	□ Established □ Probable □ Suspected ■ **Possible** □ Unlikely

Effects Adverse reactions of PREDNISONE (eg, edema) may be increased.

Mechanism Unknown.

Management If an interaction is suspected, consider discontinuing one of the agents.

Discussion

Severe peripheral edema was reported in a 23-year-old man with persistent severe perennial allergic asthma and rhinoconjunctivitis during coadministration of oral prednisone and montelukast.[1] The patient had exercise-induced asthma and sensitivity to house dust mites, as well as a history (from 1 to 7 years of age) of minimal-change nephrotic syndrome that had completely resolved. He was receiving salmeterol (*Serevent*), fluticasone (eg, *Flovent*), and cetirizine (eg, *Zyrtec*). For 1 week, the patient was being treated with prednisone 40 mg/day in divided doses, followed by 20 mg in the morning for another week. Upon stopping oral prednisone therapy, severe asthma returned and the patient received prednisone 60 mg/day in divided doses for 1 week, followed by 40 mg/day for 1 week. He was also given oral montelukast 10 mg/day at night. On the tenth day of prednisone therapy, he developed severe peripheral edema without dyspnea and had gained 13 kg. Prednisone therapy was stopped. The patient's asthma was controlled and his edema resolved. Because of the lack of rechallenge, it is difficult to determine adverse reactions from high-dose prednisone therapy versus a drug interaction. Additional clinical data are needed to determine the importance of this possible interaction.

[1] Geller M. *Ann Intern Med.* 2000;132(11):924.

* Asterisk indicates drugs cited in interaction reports.

Corticosteroids — *Nefazodone*

Dexamethasone (eg, *Baycadron*)	Methylprednisolone* (eg, *Medrol*)	Nefazodone*
Hydrocortisone (eg, *Cortef*)	Triamcinolone* (eg, *Kenalog*)	

Significance	Onset	Severity	Documentation
2	☐ Rapid ■ **Delayed**	☐ Major ■ **Moderate** ☐ Minor	☐ Established ☐ Probable ■ **Suspected** ☐ Possible ☐ Unlikely

Effects The pharmacologic effects and adverse reactions of certain CORTICOSTEROIDS may be enhanced.

Mechanism Inhibition of CORTICOSTEROID metabolism (CYP3A4) and increased duration of cortisol suppression is suspected.

Management A reduction in the dosage of certain CORTICOSTEROIDS may be warranted when NEFAZODONE is started and an increase may be warranted when NEFAZODONE is discontinued.

Discussion

The effects of nefazodone on the pharmacokinetics and cortisol suppressant effects of methylprednisolone were studied in 8 healthy volunteers.[1] Using a sequential, 2-phase, open-label design, each subject received nefazodone every 12 hours for 9 days (100 mg/dose for the first 3 doses, 150 mg/dose for the next 4 doses, and 200 mg/dose for the remainder of the doses). Each subject received a single IV bolus of methylprednisolone 0.6 mg/kg before and after nefazodone administration. Nefazodone administration increased the AUC of methylprednisolone 113%, prolonged the $t_{½}$ from 2.28 to 3.32 hours, and decreased the clearance 49% and the volume of distribution 30%. In addition, the length of cortisol suppression was longer (more than 32 hours compared with 23.3 hours) in subjects after they received nefazodone. A 43-year-old woman taking nefazodone 600 mg daily received 2 sacroiliac injections of triamcinolone 20 mg for low back pain.[2] She experienced symptoms consistent with Cushing syndrome, including face and neck swelling. Endocrinologic evaluation confirmed secondary adrenal insufficiency. Triamcinolone blood levels were detectable 2.5 months after the last injection.

[1] Kotlyar M, et al. *J Clin Psychopharmacol.* 2003;23(6):652.

[2] Hagan JB, et al. *Pain Med.* 2010;11(7):1132.

* Asterisk indicates drugs cited in interaction reports. Based on pharmacologic and pharmacokinetic considerations, similar interactions may occur with other drugs that are listed.

Corticosteroids — *Protease Inhibitors*

Corticosteroids		Protease Inhibitors	
Budesonide* (eg, *Entocort EC*)	Prednisone* (eg, *Sterapred*)	Atazanavir (*Reyataz*)	Nelfinavir (*Viracept*)
Fluticasone* (eg, *Flonase*)		Darunavir (*Prezista*)	Ritonavir* (*Norvir*)
		Fosamprenavir (*Lexiva*)	Saquinavir (*Invirase*)
		Indinavir (*Crixivan*)	Tipranavir (*Aptivus*)
		Lopinavir/Ritonavir* (*Kaletra*)	

Significance	Onset	Severity	Documentation
1	□ Rapid	■ **Major**	□ Established
	■ **Delayed**	□ Moderate	■ **Probable**
		□ Minor	□ Suspected
			□ Possible
			□ Unlikely

Effects CORTICOSTEROID plasma concentrations may be elevated, increasing the pharmacologic and toxic effects (ie, Cushing syndrome with secondary adrenal insufficiency).

Mechanism PROTEASE INHIBITORS may inhibit CORTICOSTEROID metabolism (CYP3A4), increasing systemic availability.

Management If coadministration of these agents cannot be avoided, closely monitor patients for signs of adrenal insufficiency. When an inhaled or intranasal steroid is needed, give the lowest effective dose and a less systemically available agent (eg, beclomethasone [*QVAR*], budesonide [eg, *Pulmicort*]).[1]

Discussion

Cushing syndrome with secondary adrenal insufficiency occurred during coadministration of fluticasone and ritonavir in a 12-year-old girl and 15-year-old girl both with HIV and asthma.[2] Neither the maximum dose of fluticasone nor ritonavir exceeded the recommended dosage range. Both patients were receiving other medications, including a short course of systemic corticosteroid therapy. Both patients exhibited weight gain 4 to 13 weeks after receiving concurrent fluticasone and ritonavir and became increasingly cushingoid, with cushingoid facies, multiple striae, central adiposity, and hirsutism. Cushing syndrome with overt adrenal suppression was diagnosed. At least 19 other cases of Cushing syndrome with secondary adrenal suppression have been reported in adults treated with fluticasone and ritonavir.[3-11] Coadministration of ritonavir and budesonide in 3 children with perinatally acquired HIV infection resulted in Cushing syndrome.[12] A study in 10 HIV-infected patients demonstrated that ritonavir increased the AUC and reduced the clearance of prednisone.[13]

1 Li AM. *J Pediatr.* 2006;148(3):294.
2 Johnson SR, et al. *J Pediatr.* 2006;148(3):386.
3 Chen F, et al. *Sex Transm Infect.* 1999;75(4):274.
4 Hillebrand-Haverkort ME, et al. *AIDS.* 1999;13(13):1803.
5 Clevenbergh P, et al. *J Infect.* 2002;44(3):194.
6 Rouanet I, et al. *HIV Med.* 2003;4(2):149.
7 Samaras K, et al. *J Clin Endocrinol Metab.* 2005;90(7):4394.
8 Gillett MJ, et al. *AIDS.* 2005;19(7):740.
9 Soldatos G, et al. *Intern Med J.* 2005;35(1):67.
10 Arrington-Sanders R, et al. *Pediatr Infect Dis J.* 2006;25(11):1044.
11 St. Germain RM, et al. *AIDS Patient Care STDS.* 2007;21(6):373.
12 Gray D, et al. *S Afr Med J.* 2010;100(5):296.
13 Penzak SR, et al. *J Acquir Immune Defic Syndr.* 2005;40(5):573.

* Asterisk indicates drugs cited in interaction reports. Based on pharmacologic and pharmacokinetic considerations, similar interactions may occur with other drugs that are listed.

Corticosteroids — *Rifamycins*

Corticosteroids		Rifamycins	
Betamethasone (*Celestone*)	Methylprednisolone* (eg, *Medrol*)	Rifabutin (*Mycobutin*)	Rifapentine (*Priftin*)
Budesonide (eg, *Pulmicort*)	Prednisolone* (eg, *Prelone*)	Rifampin* (eg, *Rifadin*)	
Cortisone*	Prednisone*		
Dexamethasone (eg, *Baycadron*)	Triamcinolone (eg, *Kenalog*)		
Fludrocortisone*			
Hydrocortisone* (eg, *Cortef*)			

Significance	Onset	Severity	Documentation
2	☐ Rapid	☐ Major	■ **Established**
	■ **Delayed**	■ **Moderate**	☐ Probable
		☐ Minor	☐ Suspected
			☐ Possible
			☐ Unlikely

Effects The pharmacologic effects of CORTICOSTEROIDS may be decreased. Loss of disease control has been reported. This may occur within a few days of adding RIFAMPIN and reverse 2 to 3 weeks following its discontinuation.

Mechanism RIFAMYCINS may increase hepatic CORTICOSTEROID metabolism.

Management Avoid this combination if possible. If combined use cannot be avoided, monitor the patient closely and be prepared to at least double the CORTICOSTEROID dosage following addition of RIFAMPIN 300 mg/day.

Discussion

Pharmacokinetic studies have demonstrated marked increases in prednisolone clearance during rifampin therapy. At least a doubling of prednisolone dosage may be necessary to restore levels to their pretreatment values.[1-4] This interaction has been associated with a loss of disease control in patients with Addison disease[5-7] and nephrotic syndrome.[8] It also has been related to a decrease in renal allograft function,[9] allograft loss,[10] and giant cell arteritis.[4] A steroid-dependent asthmatic patient stable on methylprednisolone experienced deterioration in control of their asthma after starting rifampin.[11] Neither increasing the methylprednisolone dose nor switching to prednisone controlled his condition. Subsequent discontinuation of rifampin restored control of the patient's asthma. It appears that effective corticosteroid therapy is difficult during rifampin coadministration.

[1] McAllister WA, et al. *Br Med J (Clin Res Ed)*. 1983;286(6369):923.
[2] Powell-Jackson PR, et al. *Am Rev Respir Dis*. 1983;128(2):307.
[3] Bergrem H, et al. *Acta Med Scand*. 1983;213(5):339.
[4] Carrie F, et al. *Arch Intern Med*. 1994;154(13):1521.
[5] Edwards OM, et al. *Lancet*. 1974;2(7880):548.
[6] Maisey DN, et al. *Lancet*. 1974;2(7885):896.
[7] Kyriazopoulou V, et al. *J Clin Endocrinol Metab*. 1984;59(6):1204.
[8] Hendrickse W, et al. *Br Med J*. 1979;1(6159):306.
[9] Buffington GA, et al. *JAMA*. 1976;236(17):1958.
[10] Langhoff E, et al. *Lancet*. 1983;2(8357):1031.
[11] Lin FL. *J Allergy Clin Immunol*. 1996;98(6, pt 1):1125.

* Asterisk indicates drugs cited in interaction reports. Based on pharmacologic and pharmacokinetic considerations, similar interactions may occur with other drugs that are listed.

Corticosteroids | *Topiramate*

Corticosteroids		Topiramate
Dexamethasone* (eg, *Baycadron*)	Fludrocortisone*	Topiramate* (eg, *Topamax*)

Significance	Onset	Severity	Documentation
4	☐ Rapid	☐ Major	☐ Established
	■ **Delayed**	■ **Moderate**	☐ Probable
		☐ Minor	☐ Suspected
			■ **Possible**
			☐ Unlikely

Effects DEXAMETHASONE plasma concentrations may be reduced, decreasing the pharmacologic effects.

Mechanism TOPIRAMATE may induce the metabolism (CYP3A4) of the CORTICOSTEROID.

Management Monitor clinical response and adjust the CORTICOSTEROID dose as needed.

Discussion

A 35-year-old woman taking dexamethasone 0.25 mg daily and fludrocortisone 100 mcg daily complained of muscle aches, nausea, tiredness, and weight loss within a few weeks of starting topiramate (titrated to 100 mg daily).[1] She was diagnosed with hypoadrenalism, which was supported by biochemical tests. Increasing the daily doses of dexamethasone to 0.75 mg and fludrocortisone to 150 mcg resulted in biochemical improvement.

[1] Jacob K, et al. *BMJ.* 2009;338:a1788.

* Asterisk indicates drugs cited in interaction reports.

Crizotinib — *Food*

Crizotinib* (*Xalkori*)	Grapefruit Juice*

Significance	Onset	Severity	Documentation
2	☐ Rapid ■ **Delayed**	☐ Major ■ **Moderate** ☐ Minor	☐ Established ☐ Probable ■ **Suspected** ☐ Possible ☐ Unlikely

Effects CRIZOTINIB plasma concentrations may be elevated, increasing the risk of adverse reactions.

Mechanism CRIZOTINIB metabolism (CYP3A4) may be inhibited by GRAPEFRUIT PRODUCTS.

Management Avoid coadministration of CRIZOTINIB and GRAPEFRUIT PRODUCTS.[1] Patients should take CRIZOTINIB with a liquid other than GRAPEFRUIT JUICE.

Discussion

Concurrent use of CYP3A4 inhibitors, such as grapefruit or grapefruit juice, may elevate crizotinib plasma concentrations increasing the risk of adverse reactions.[1] Concomitant use of crizotinib and grapefruit or grapefruit juice should be avoided.

The basis for this monograph is information on file with the manufacturer. Studies are needed to determine the clinical importance of this interaction.

[1] *Xalkori* [package insert]. New York, NY: Pfizer Labs; August 2011.

* Asterisk indicates drugs cited in interaction reports.

Crizotinib — *St. John's Wort*

Crizotinib* (*Xalkori*)	St. John's Wort*

Significance	Onset	Severity	Documentation
1	☐ Rapid ■ **Delayed**	■ **Major** ☐ Moderate ☐ Minor	☐ Established ☐ Probable ■ **Suspected** ☐ Possible ☐ Unlikely

Effects CRIZOTINIB plasma concentrations may be reduced, resulting in a decrease in the pharmacologic effects.

Mechanism CRIZOTINIB metabolism (CYP3A4) may be increased by ST. JOHN'S WORT.

Management Avoid coadministration of CRIZOTINIB and ST. JOHN'S WORT.[1]

Discussion

Strong CYP3A4 inducers, such as St. John's wort, may reduce crizotinib plasma concentrations, which may result in decrease in the crizotinib pharmacologic effects.[1] Concomitant use of crizotinib with St. John's wort should be avoided.

The basis for this monograph is information on file with the manufacturer. Published clinical data are needed to further assess this interaction. Because of the seriousness of this interaction, clinical evaluation in humans is not likely to be forthcoming.

[1] *Xalkori* [package insert]. New York, NY: Pfizer Labs; August 2011.

* Asterisk indicates drugs cited in interaction reports.

Cyclophosphamide — *Allopurinol*

Cyclophosphamide*	Allopurinol* (eg, *Zyloprim*)

Significance	Onset	Severity	Documentation
4	☐ Rapid	☐ Major	☐ Established
	■ **Delayed**	■ **Moderate**	☐ Probable
		☐ Minor	☐ Suspected
			■ **Possible**
			☐ Unlikely

Effects The myelosuppressive effects of CYCLOPHOSPHAMIDE may be enhanced, possibly increasing risk of bleeding or infection. Currently, no information exists regarding duration of this interaction once ALLOPURINOL is discontinued.

Mechanism Not known.

Management Frequent monitoring with a CBC may be required.

Discussion

In a retrospective study of patients receiving various chemotherapy agents, an increase in myelosuppression was noted in patients receiving cyclophosphamide with allopurinol versus without allopurinol.[1] Myelosuppression also appeared to have an earlier onset in these allopurinol-treated patients. No information was available regarding the dose of allopurinol in this trial. A further controlled trial reported data on 81 patients randomized to receive allopurinol 200 mg/m^2 with either the first 3 or the first 6 chemotherapy courses, the majority of which contained cyclophosphamide.[2] Using weekly blood cell counts, no differences were found in WBC or platelet nadirs between the 2 groups. It is unclear if the weekly monitoring of blood cell counts or the allopurinol dosing schema may have obscured a difference. Whether a pharmacokinetic interaction exists between these 2 drugs is also controversial. One report revealed an increase in cyclophosphamide $t_{1/2}$ in 4 patients receiving concurrent allopurinol, but found no change in the concentration of alkylating metabolites in the plasma or urine or of intact cyclophosphamide in the urine.[3] A second trial found no change in cyclophosphamide $t_{1/2}$ but did observe an increase in the concentration of alkylating metabolites with concurrent allopurinol.[4] No direct relationship has been established between the concentration of cyclophosphamide metabolites and myelosuppression.[5]

[1] Boston Collaborative Drug Surveillance Program. *JAMA*. 1974;227(9):1036.
[2] Stolbach L, et al. *JAMA*. 1982;247(3):334.
[3] Bagley CM Jr, et al. *Cancer Res*. 1973;33(2):226.
[4] Witten J, et al. *Acta Pharmacol Toxicol (Copenh)*. 1980;46(5):392.
[5] Mouridsen HT, et al. *Acta Pharmacol Toxicol (Copenh)*. 1978;43(4):328.

* Asterisk indicates drugs cited in interaction reports.

Cyclophosphamide — *Azole Antifungal Agents*

Cyclophosphamide*	Fluconazole* (eg, *Diflucan*)	Ketoconazole (eg, *Nizoral*)
	Itraconazole* (eg, *Sporanox*)	Posaconazole (eg, *Noxafil*)

Significance	Onset	Severity	Documentation
2	□ Rapid	□ Major	□ Established
	■ **Delayed**	■ **Moderate**	□ Probable
		□ Minor	■ **Suspected**
			□ Possible
			□ Unlikely

Effects Exposure to CYCLOPHOSPHAMIDE and its metabolites may be increased, increasing the risk of adverse reactions.

Mechanism Inhibition of CYCLOPHOSPHAMIDE hepatic metabolism is suspected.

Management Closely monitor patient for CYCLOPHOSPHAMIDE adverse reactions during coadministration of AZOLE ANTIFUNGAL AGENTS.

Discussion

The effects of fluconazole or itraconazole on cyclophosphamide metabolism were investigated in a randomized study in 209 patients undergoing allogeneic stem cell transplantation.[1] Each patient received cyclophosphamide (most common conditioning regimen was 60 mg/kg plus total body irradiation) and fluconazole (400 mg/day IV or oral) or itraconazole (200 mg/day IV or oral solution 2.5 mg/kg 3 times daily). There was a trend to higher average serum bilirubin levels before day 20 in patients receiving itraconazole compared with fluconazole. Baseline creatinine levels increased at least 2-fold within 20 days of undergoing allogeneic stem cell transplantation in 34% of patients receiving itraconazole plus cyclophosphamide compared with 20% of patients receiving cyclophosphamide plus fluconazole. Patients receiving fluconazole had increased exposure to cyclophosphamide and the deschloroethyl metabolite of cyclophosphamide, while patients receiving itraconazole had increased exposure to the 4-hydroxy and 4-ketocyclophosphamide metabolites.

[1] Marr KA, et al. *Blood.* 2004;103(4):1557.

* Asterisk indicates drugs cited in interaction reports. Based on pharmacologic and pharmacokinetic considerations, similar interactions may occur with other drugs that are listed.

Cyclophosphamide — *Carbamazepine*

Cyclophosphamide*	Carbamazepine* (eg, *Tegretol*)

Significance	Onset	Severity	Documentation
4	■ **Rapid**	□ Major	□ Established
	□ Delayed	■ **Moderate**	□ Probable
		□ Minor	□ Suspected
			■ **Possible**
			□ Unlikely

Effects Exposure to the active metabolite of CYCLOPHOSPHAMIDE, 4-hydroxycyclophosphamide, may be increased, increasing the risk of toxicity.

Mechanism CARBAMAZEPINE may increase the metabolism (CYP3A4) of CYCLOPHOSPHAMIDE.

Management Consider reducing the initial dose of CYCLOPHOSPHAMIDE and monitoring the concentrations of the 4-hydroxycyclophosphamide metabolite as a guide to CYCLOPHOSPHAMIDE dosing. Gabapentin (eg, *Neurontin*) or valproic acid derivatives (eg, *Depakote*) may be safer alternative anticonvulsant agents.

Discussion

A 52-year-old woman with metastatic breast cancer received a chemotherapy regimen that included cyclophosphamide with and without coadministration of carbamazepine.[1] Each chemotherapy cycle lasted 4 days. On the first day of the cycles when cyclophosphamide was given with carbamazepine, exposure to the active metabolite of cyclophosphamide, 4-hydroxycyclophosphamide, was increased 58%, while exposure to cyclophosphamide was reduced 40%, compared with not administering carbamazepine. The effect of carbamazepine diminished over the 4-day course of treatment, being most pronounced during the first day of the cycle. Therefore, the clinical importance of this interaction appears to be of greatest consequences with single-dose administration of cyclophosphamide.

[1] Ekhart C, et al. *Cancer Chemother Pharmacol.* 2009;63(3):543.

* Asterisk indicates drugs cited in interaction reports.

Cyclophosphamide — *Chloramphenicol*

Cyclophosphamide* (eg, *Cytoxan*)	Chloramphenicol*

Significance	Onset	Severity	Documentation
4	☐ Rapid ■ **Delayed**	☐ Major ■ **Moderate** ☐ Minor	☐ Established ☐ Probable ☐ Suspected ■ **Possible** ☐ Unlikely

Effects The interaction may result in a decreased or delayed activation of CYCLOPHOSPHAMIDE. It is currently unclear if a clinically important decrease in the effect of CYCLOPHOSPHAMIDE would result from this interaction.

Mechanism Inhibition of the hepatic microsomal enzyme system by CHLORAMPHENICOL is suspected.

Management None, other than standard monitoring procedures for both drugs.

Discussion

Only 1 study exists to support this interaction. In this trial, cyclophosphamide pharmacokinetics were determined in 4 patients prior to and 12 days into oral dosing of chloramphenicol 1 g twice daily.[1] The t½ of cyclophosphamide increased in all patients by a mean of 50%. In addition, decreases in the cyclophosphamide metabolite concentrations were observed in these patients. Also, an immediate prolongation in cyclophosphamide t½ was evident in a single patient receiving a dose of chloramphenicol 3 g IV shortly after cyclophosphamide administration. In a trial examining the relationship between cyclophosphamide metabolite concentration and hematologic toxicity, no direct correlation was found.[2] This latter trial reveals the inadequacy of attempting to relate cyclophosphamide metabolite concentration to pharmacologic effect and questions the overall importance of this measurement.

[1] Faber OK, et al. *Br J Clin Pharmacol.* 1975;2:281.

[2] Mouridsen HT, et al. *Acta Pharmacol Toxicol.* 1978;43:328.

* Asterisk indicates drugs cited in interaction reports.

Cyclophosphamide — *Corticosteroids*

Cyclophosphamide* (eg, *Cytoxan*)	Prednisolone (eg, *Prelone*)	Prednisone* (eg, *Deltasone*)

Significance	Onset	Severity	Documentation
5	☐ Rapid ■ **Delayed**	☐ Major ■ **Moderate** ☐ Minor	☐ Established ☐ Probable ☐ Suspected ☐ Possible ■ **Unlikely**

Effects A change in the pharmacologic effect of CYCLOPHOSPHAMIDE is unlikely, based on the limited evidence available.

Mechanism Unknown.

Management No special precautions other than standard monitoring procedures for both drugs.

Discussion

In a trial of 6 patients, cyclophosphamide pharmacokinetics were determined prior to and following 12 days of prednisone 50 mg/day.[1] This trial reported a mean 19% reduction in cyclophosphamide $t_{½}$ following prednisone. No changes were observed in cyclophosphamide metabolite pharmacokinetics in plasma or urine, nor in urinary excretion of the parent drug. In 1 patient, there was an increase in cyclophosphamide $t_{½}$ immediately following an IV bolus dose of prednisolone. In a separate trial of 5 patients receiving prednisolone 1,000 mg, just prior to a dose of cyclophosphamide 400 mg/m^{2}, decreases in cyclophosphamide $t_{½}$, and increases in the concentrations of its metabolites were observed.[2] However, these changes were not different than what was observed in the control patients in this trial. While the toxicity (LD50) of cyclophosphamide increases in rats when combined with prednisone,[3] no human data exist to support this, despite widespread use of this combination.

[1] Faber OK, et al. *Acta Pharmacol Toxicol.* 1974;35:195.
[2] Bagley CM Jr, et al. *Cancer Res.* 1973;33:226.
[3] Shepherd R, et al. *Br J Cancer.* 1982;45:413.

* Asterisk indicates drugs cited in interaction reports. Based on pharmacologic and pharmacokinetic considerations, similar interactions may occur with other drugs that are listed.

Cyclophosphamide — *Hydantoins*

Cyclophosphamide* (eg, *Cytoxan*)	Phenytoin* (eg, *Dilantin*)

Significance	Onset	Severity	Documentation
4	☐ Rapid	☐ Major	☐ Established
	■ **Delayed**	■ **Moderate**	☐ Probable
		☐ Minor	☐ Suspected
			■ **Possible**
			☐ Unlikely

Effects Exposure to the active CYCLOPHOSPHAMIDE metabolite may be increased, increasing the risk of toxicity.

Mechanism Induction of CYCLOPHOSPHAMIDE metabolism (CYP2B6) by PHENYTOIN is suspected.

Management If PHENYTOIN administration cannot be avoided, consider reducing the initial dose of CYCLOPHOSPHAMIDE and monitoring the concentration of the 4-hydroxycyclophosphamide metabolite as a guide to CYCLOPHOSPHAMIDE dosing. Valproic acid derivatives (eg, *Depakote*) or gabapentin (eg, *Neurontin*) may be safer anticonvulsant agents.

Discussion

The effect of phenytoin on the metabolism of cyclophosphamide was assessed during high-dose chemotherapy with cyclophosphamide 1,500 mg/m^2 daily, thiotepa (eg, *Thioplex*), and carboplatin (eg, *Paraplatin*) in a 42-year-old man with relapsing germ-cell cancer.[1] Five days before the start of the second course of chemotherapy, the patient received phenytoin for generalized epileptic seizures, which developed 3 weeks after the first course of chemotherapy. Blood samples were analyzed for cyclophosphamide and the main active metabolite, 4-hydroxycyclophosphamide. Compared with the first course of chemotherapy, the AUC of 4-hydroxycyclophosphamide during the second course of chemotherapy was increased 51%. The AUC of cyclophosphamide was reduced 67%. Because increased exposure to the active metabolite correlates with higher toxicity, the dose of cyclophosphamide was reduced on the third day of the second course of chemotherapy.

[1] de Jonge ME, et al. *Cancer Chemother Pharmacol.* 2005;55:507.

* Asterisk indicates drugs cited in interaction reports.

Cyclophosphamide — *Methotrexate*

Cyclophosphamide* (eg, *Cytoxan*)	Methotrexate* (eg, *Rheumatrex*)

Significance	Onset	Severity	Documentation
4	☐ Rapid ■ **Delayed**	☐ Major ■ **Moderate** ☐ Minor	☐ Established ☐ Probable ☐ Suspected ■ **Possible** ☐ Unlikely

Effects Based on the available data, an alteration in the effect of either drug is unlikely.

Mechanism Unknown.

Management No special precautions other than standard monitoring procedures for both drugs.

Discussion

The majority of data supporting an interaction between these 2 agents has been obtained from experiments in animals. In rats, methotrexate inhibits and cyclophosphamide stimulates O-demethylation and parahydroxylation pathways.[1] However, in a separate report using a different dosing schedule, cyclophosphamide exhibited an inhibitory effect on hepatic mixed-function oxidase in the rat.[2] In a pharmacokinetic study in rats, methotrexate combined with 5-fluorouracil and cyclophosphamide resulted in a 40% increase in methotrexate clearance versus methotrexate alone.[3] Use of an inaccurate estimate of AUC in this trial may have resulted in an erroneous conclusion. In a human trial, 7 patients were studied for changes in cyclophosphamide pharmacokinetics prior to and following 9 days of low-dose daily oral methotrexate.[1] Two of these patients developed an increase in cyclophosphamide $t_{1/2}$, a decrease in metabolite concentrations and an increase in the ratio of parent drug/metabolites in urine. Because changes were not observed in the majority of patients and alterations in metabolite concentration do not appear to be directly related to effect,[5] it is questionable if this interaction would result in any loss of cyclophosphamide activity.

1 Donelli MG, et al. *Eur J Cancer.* 1971;7:361.
2 Gurtoo HL, et al. *Br J Cancer.* 1985;51:67.
3 de Bruijn EA, et al. *Cancer Treat Rep.* 1986;70:1159.
4 Mouridsen HT, et al. *Acta Pharmacol Toxicol.* 1976;38:508.
5 Mouridsen HT, et al. *Acta Pharmacol Toxicol.* 1978;43:328.

* Asterisk indicates drugs cited in interaction reports.

Cyclophosphamide — *Ondansetron*

Cyclophosphamide* (eg, *Cytoxan*)	Ondansetron* (*Zofran*)

Significance	Onset	Severity	Documentation
4	☐ Rapid ■ **Delayed**	☐ Major ■ **Moderate** ☐ Minor	☐ Established ☐ Probable ☐ Suspected ■ **Possible** ☐ Unlikely

Effects Plasma CYCLOPHOSPHAMIDE concentrations may be decreased, reducing the therapeutic effect.

Mechanism Unknown.

Management Monitor the therapeutic response of the patient. If an interaction is suspected, it may be necessary to increase the dose of CYCLOPHOSPHAMIDE.

Discussion

The effect of ondansetron 8 mg IV bolus on the pharmacokinetics of cyclophosphamide was studied in a retrospective investigation involving 23 bone marrow transplant patients receiving high dose cyclophosphamide (1875 mg/m^2/day IV on 3 consecutive days), cisplatin (eg, *Platinol-AQ*), and BCNU (eg, *BiCNU*).[1] The effect of ondansetron was compared with a control group of 129 patients who received the same chemotherapy but prochlorperazine (eg, *Compazine*) was substituted for ondansetron. Compared with patients receiving prochlorperazine, ondansetron administration resulted in a 15% decrease in the area under the plasma concentration-time curve of cyclophosphamide. See Cisplatin-Ondansetron.

Additional studies are needed to determine the clinical importance of this drug interaction.

[1] Cagnoni PJ, et al. *Bone Marrow Transplant.* 1999;24:1.

* Asterisk indicates drugs cited in interaction reports.

Cyclophosphamide — *Sulfonamides*

Cyclophosphamide	Sulfonamides
Cyclophosphamide*	Sulfadiazine
	Sulfisoxazole (*Gantrisin Pediatric*)

Significance	Onset	Severity	Documentation
5	☐ Rapid	☐ Major	☐ Established
	■ **Delayed**	☐ Moderate	☐ Probable
		■ **Minor**	☐ Suspected
			☐ Possible
			■ **Unlikely**

Effects It currently appears unlikely that a clinically important interaction occurs.

Mechanism Unknown.

Management No special precautions other than standard monitoring for both drugs.

Discussion

In a study of 7 subjects, cyclophosphamide pharmacokinetics were determined prior to and after 9 to 14 days of oral sulphaphenazole† 1 g twice daily.[1] Cyclophosphamide $t_{1/2}$ was unchanged in 3 subjects, prolonged in 2 subjects, and decreased in 2 subjects. Changes in cyclophosphamide metabolite pharmacokinetics also were observed in 1 of the subjects with a reduced $t_{1/2}$. However, there are no reports supporting a change in the effect of cyclophosphamide when it is administered in conjunction with sulfonamides. In addition, a trial examining the efficacy of trimethoprim/sulfamethoxazole (eg, *Septra DS*) versus placebo for infection prophylaxis in patients treated with a regimen containing cyclophosphamide found no differences in granulocytopenia between the 2 groups.[2]

[1] Faber OK, et al. *Br J Clin Pharmacol.* 1975;2(3):281.

[2] de Jongh CA, et al. *J Clin Oncol.* 1983;1(5):302.

* Asterisk indicates drugs cited in interaction reports. Based on pharmacologic and pharmacokinetic considerations, similar interactions may occur with other drugs that are listed.

† Not available in the United States.

Cycloserine — *Isoniazid*

Cycloserine* (*Seromycin*)	Isoniazid* (eg, *Nydrazid*)

Significance	Onset	Severity	Documentation
5	□ Rapid ■ **Delayed**	□ Major □ Moderate ■ **Minor**	□ Established □ Probable □ Suspected ■ **Possible** □ Unlikely

Effects Coadministration results in an increased incidence of CYCLOSERINE CNS adverse reactions, most notably dizziness.

Mechanism Unknown.

Management No special precautions appear necessary. Because of a lack of evidence for a dose or serum-concentration relationship, dosage reduction would not be expected to reduce the severity of the reaction.

Discussion

Cycloserine and isoniazid may be coadministered in the treatment of tuberculosis. In an attempt to determine whether the cause of the observed increased incidence of adverse reactions with combination therapy could be attributed to elevated cycloserine levels, 6 patients and 5 controls received 2 days of cycloserine therapy alone and in combination with INH.[1] Nine of the 11 subjects experienced dizziness and unstable gait, in some cases severe enough to require bedrest, with the combination therapy; 1 patient experienced similar symptoms on cycloserine alone. Cycloserine $t_{1/2}$, serum levels or urinary clearance were not affected by this drug combination.

Additional studies are necessary to verify this possible interaction.

[1] Mattila MJ, et al. *Scand J Respir Dis.* 1969;50(4):291.

* Asterisk indicates drugs cited in interaction reports.

Cyclosporine — *Acetazolamide*

Cyclosporine* (eg, *Neoral*)	Acetazolamide* (eg, *Diamox*)

Significance	Onset	Severity	Documentation
4	☐ Rapid ■ **Delayed**	☐ Major ■ **Moderate** ☐ Minor	☐ Established ☐ Probable ☐ Suspected ■ **Possible** ☐ Unlikely

Effects The pharmacologic effects of CYCLOSPORINE may be increased. Increased trough CYCLOSPORINE levels with possible nephrotoxicity and neurotoxicity may occur.

Mechanism Unknown.

Management Monitor serum creatinine and CYCLOSPORINE levels; adjust the dose of CYCLOSPORINE accordingly.

Discussion

A 50-year-old male cardiac transplant recipient had maintained stable creatinine levels of 1.7 mg/dL and trough serum cyclosporine levels of 290 ng/L (using radioimmunoassay, RIA) while receiving cyclosporine 5.2 mg/kg/day and azathioprine (eg, *Imuran*) 1.1 mg/kg/day.[1] In addition, the patient's treatment regimen included furosemide (eg, *Lasix*), enalapril (*Vasotec*), and aspirin (eg, *Bayer*). Ocular examination revealed moderate anterior uveitis and increased intraocular pressure in the right eye only. Treatment with acetazolamide 250 mg 4 times daily, timolol (eg, *Timoptic*) 0.5%, and prednisolone (eg, *Pred Forte*) 1% drops was instituted. Shortly after starting treatment for uveitis, the patient experienced increased drowsiness, anorexia, and diarrhea. After 1 month, dehydration and elevated whole blood trough cyclosporine levels (1736 ng/mL, using RIA) ensued, resulting in marked renal impairment and neurotoxicity. Serum creatinine was 2.9 mg/dL. Acetazolamide was discontinued, and cyclosporine therapy was suspended for 36 hours, then reinstated at 3.4 mg/kg/day. Four days later, the whole blood cyclosporine level was 999 ng/mL, and creatinine was 2.3 mg/dL. Neurologic signs reversed within 5 days. The serum cyclosporine level was 150 ng/L, and creatinine returned to 1.7 mg/dL 10 days later. The cyclosporine dose was reestablished at 5.2 mg/kg/day. In a small-case series, 3 patients receiving cyclosporine were given acetazolamide.[2] Three days after coadministration of the drugs, cyclosporine levels increased from a mean of 170 ng/mL to 1130 ng/mL. Details of drug doses or other treatments were not provided.

[1] Keogh A, et al. *Transplantation.* 1988;46:478.

[2] Tabbara KF, et al. *Arch Ophthalmol.* 1998;116:832.

* Asterisk indicates drugs cited in interaction reports.

Cyclosporine — *Aminoquinolines*

Cyclosporine* (eg, *Neoral*)

Chloroquine* (eg, *Aralen*)

Significance	Onset	Severity	Documentation
4	☐ Rapid ■ **Delayed**	☐ Major ■ **Moderate** ☐ Minor	☐ Established ☐ Probable ☐ Suspected ■ **Possible** ☐ Unlikely

Effects Elevated CYCLOSPORINE concentrations may occur, increasing the risk of toxicity (eg, nephrotoxicity).

Mechanism Possibly due to inhibition of CYCLOSPORINE metabolism.

Management Consider monitoring CYCLOSPORINE concentrations and serum creatinine levels. Adjust the dose of CYCLOSPORINE accordingly.

Discussion

In a 51-year-old male kidney transplant recipient, cyclosporine blood concentrations and serum creatinine levels increased after chloroquine was added to his treatment schedule.[1] The patient was receiving immunosuppression with prednisolone (eg, *Prelone*) 17.5 mg, cyclosporine 3.4 mg/kg, and azathioprine (eg, *Imuran*) 0.5 mg/kg/day. For 10 days, he experienced a fever occurring every 48 to 72 hours and lasting 3 to 4 hours. The fever terminated with marked sweating. Physical examination and laboratory tests failed to identify the source of the fever. Because of the pattern of the fever, and because the patient had recently returned from a malaria-endemic country, he was started on chloroquine. The dose of cyclosporine was not changed, but blood levels were measured daily by radioimmunoassay. Within 48 hours of starting chloroquine, cyclosporine concentrations rose nearly 3-fold (from 148 to 420 ng/mL). The increase in cyclosporine blood concentration was associated with an increase in serum creatinine level from 95 to 140 mcmol/L. The course of chloroquine treatment was continued for 3 days, and cyclosporine concentrations remained elevated during that time. Seven days after stopping chloroquine, the cyclosporine concentration, as well as the serum creatinine level, returned to baseline values.

[1] Nampoory MRN, et al. *Nephron*. 1992;62:108.

* Asterisk indicates drugs cited in interaction reports.

Cyclosporine — *Amiodarone*

Cyclosporine* (eg, *Neoral*)	Amiodarone* (eg, *Cordarone*)

Significance	Onset	Severity	Documentation
2	☐ Rapid ■ **Delayed**	☐ Major ■ **Moderate** ☐ Minor	☐ Established ☐ Probable ■ **Suspected** ☐ Possible ☐ Unlikely

Effects AMIODARONE may increase CYCLOSPORINE blood concentrations, possibly increasing the risk of nephrotoxicity.

Mechanism Unknown. Inhibition of CYCLOSPORINE metabolism by AMIODARONE is suspected.

Management Monitor CYCLOSPORINE concentrations closely when AMIODARONE is started, stopped, or the dose is altered. In order to minimize nephrotoxicity, it may be necessary to decrease the dose of CYCLOSPORINE. Because AMIODARONE has a long $t_{1/2}$, closely monitor CYCLOSPORINE concentrations for several weeks after the dose of AMIODARONE is changed.

Discussion

Eight patients undergoing heart or heart-lung transplantation experienced prolonged atrial tachycardia and received treatment with oral amiodarone.[1] All patients had been taking cyclosporine prior to initiation of amiodarone. After the start of amiodarone therapy, cyclosporine concentrations increased 31% (from 248 to 325 ng/mL; not statistically significant). Despite a 44% decrease in cyclosporine dose (from 6.2 to 3.5 mg/kg/day; $P < 0.01$), serum creatinine increased (from 158 to 219 mcmol/L; $P < 0.06$). In 2 additional transplant patients, the addition of amiodarone to the treatment schedule resulted in marked increases in cyclosporine blood concentrations.[2,3] Substantial decreases in the cyclosporine dosage (28% to 50% reduction) were necessary to maintain cyclosporine concentrations within the desired range. Cyclosporine toxicity was not mentioned in either patient. See Sirolimus-Amiodarone and Tacrolimus-Amiodarone.

[1] Mamprin F, et al. *Am Heart J.* 1992;123(6):1725.
[2] Nicolau DP, et al. *J Heart Lung Transplant.* 1992;11(3, pt 1):564.
[3] Chitwood KK, et al. *Ann Pharmacother.* 1993;27(5):569.

* Asterisk indicates drugs cited in interaction reports.

Cyclosporine — *Amphotericin B*

Cyclosporine* (eg, *Neoral*)	Amphotericin B* (eg, *Amphotec*)

Significance	Onset	Severity	Documentation
4	☐ Rapid	☐ Major	☐ Established
	■ **Delayed**	■ **Moderate**	☐ Probable
		☐ Minor	☐ Suspected
			■ **Possible**
			☐ Unlikely

Effects The nephrotoxic effects of CYCLOSPORINE appear to be increased. The interaction appears to occur in a few days following the addition of AMPHOTERICIN B to CYCLOSPORINE therapy. It is currently unknown how soon renal dysfunction will resolve once AMPHOTERICIN B is discontinued.

Mechanism Unknown.

Management If AMPHOTERICIN B therapy is required, consider alternative immunosuppressive therapy (eg, steroids, methotrexate). Frequent serum creatinine determinations are required if these agents are used concurrently. Patients who develop renal impairment will require either temporary CYCLOSPORINE dosage reduction or replacement with another immunosuppressive agent.

Discussion

Only one study exists to support the toxic interaction between cyclosporine and amphotericin B.[1] In this trial of bone marrow transplant patients, 8 of 10 patients receiving cyclosporine developed either a doubling or tripling in their serum creatinine within 5 days of starting amphotericin B. In contrast, only 8 of 21 patients receiving cyclosporine alone and only 3 of 16 patients receiving amphotericin B alone doubled their serum creatinine. However, with one exception, all patients who received cyclosporine and amphotericin B also received aminoglycosides. It is therefore possible that the aminoglycosides also contributed significantly to the nephrotoxicity these patients experienced.

[1] Kennedy MS, et al. *Transplantation.* 1983;35(3):211.

* Asterisk indicates drugs cited in interaction reports.

Cyclosporine — *Androgens*

Cyclosporine* (eg, *Neoral*)	Danazol* (*Danocrine*)	Methyltestosterone* (eg, *Testred*)

Significance	Onset	Severity	Documentation
2	☐ Rapid ■ **Delayed**	☐ Major ■ **Moderate** ☐ Minor	☐ Established ☐ Probable ■ **Suspected** ☐ Possible ☐ Unlikely

Effects Increased CYCLOSPORINE blood concentrations with possible toxicity (eg, nephrotoxicity).

Mechanism Possible inhibition of CYCLOSPORINE metabolism.

Management Consider monitoring serum bilirubin, serum creatinine, and CYCLOSPORINE concentrations in patients receiving CYCLOSPORINE and an ANDROGEN concurrently. Adjust the dose of CYCLOSPORINE or ANDROGEN as needed.

Discussion

Three patients who received cadaveric renal transplants experienced increased cyclosporine concentrations and changes in hepatic or renal function during coadministration of cyclosporine and methyltestosterone[1,3] or danazol.[2] A cause-and-effect relationship was not established in these patients; however, the temporal association between androgen administration and the observed changes in renal and hepatic function as well as the increase in cyclosporine concentrations strongly suggested a drug interaction. Cyclosporine pharmacokinetics were studied in a renal transplant patient receiving danazol for immune thrombocytopenia.[4] Cyclosporine area under the plasma concentration-time curve increased 65% (in spite of a 20% reduction in cyclosporine dose), half-life increased 60%, and clearance decreased 50% during coadministration of danazol. A 28-year-old man receiving cyclosporine 250 mg/day was started on danazol 200 mg every 8 hours.[5] Cyclosporine blood levels increased 38% after starting danazol. The cyclosporine dose was reduced to 200 mg/day while continuing danazol and cyclosporine levels returned to normal. No signs of cyclosporine toxicity were noted.

Controlled studies are needed to assess the importance of this drug interaction and to determine whether other 17-alkyl androgens can interact similarly.

1 Møller BB, et al. *N Engl J Med.* 1985;313:1416.
2 Ross WB, et al. *Lancet.* 1986;1:330.
3 Goffin E, et al. *Nephron.* 1991;59:174.
4 Passfall J, et al. *Nephrol Dial Transplant.* 1994;9:1807.
5 Borrás-Blasco J, et al. *Am J Hematol.* 1999;62:63.

* Asterisk indicates drugs cited in interaction reports.

Cyclosporine — *Azathioprine*

Cyclosporine* (eg, *Neoral*)	Azathioprine* (eg, *Imuran*)

Significance	Onset	Severity	Documentation
4	☐ Rapid	☐ Major	☐ Established
	■ **Delayed**	■ **Moderate**	☐ Probable
		☐ Minor	☐ Suspected
			■ **Possible**
			☐ Unlikely

Effects Plasma CYCLOSPORINE concentrations may be reduced, resulting in a decrease in pharmacologic effects.

Mechanism Unknown.

Management Consider regular monitoring of CYCLOSPORINE blood levels and observing the patient for signs of rejection or toxicity when AZATHIOPRINE therapy is initiated or discontinued, respectively.

Discussion

The effects of azathioprine on the pharmacokinetics of cyclosporine were studied in renal transplant recipients.[1] The pharmacokinetics of cyclosporine were investigated in 5 patients receiving cyclosporine 4 mg/kg and methylprednisolone (eg, *Medrol*) 8 mg as well as in 5 patients being given azathioprine 2 mg/kg in addition to cyclosporine 4 mg/kg and methylprednisolone 8 mg. Three to 6 months after transplantation, each patient received single oral doses of cyclosporine 600 mg, methylprednisolone 8 mg, and azathioprine 50 mg. The drugs were given concurrently, following an overnight fast. In both groups of patients, cyclosporine levels increased progressively with time, but the mean peak cyclosporine levels were achieved within 2 hours by the patients who had received cyclosporine and methylprednisolone vs 3 hours in the group that had received azathioprine in addition to cyclosporine and methylprednisolone. The area under the cyclosporine concentration-time curve was significantly different ($p < 0.001$) for the 2 groups, 7533 and 3635 ng•hr/mL, respectively.

[1] Grekas D, et al. *Nephron.* 1992;60:489.

* Asterisk indicates drugs cited in interaction reports.

Cyclosporine — *Azole Antifungal Agents*

Cyclosporine* (eg, *Neoral*)	Fluconazole* (eg, *Diflucan*)	Posaconazole* (*Noxafil*)
	Itraconazole* (eg, *Sporanox*)	Voriconazole* (*Vfend*)
	Ketoconazole* (eg, *Nizoral*)	

Significance	Onset	Severity	Documentation
1	□ Rapid	■ **Major**	■ **Established**
	■ **Delayed**	□ Moderate	□ Probable
		□ Minor	□ Suspected
			□ Possible
			□ Unlikely

Effects CYCLOSPORINE (CSA) levels and toxicity may increase 1 to 3 days after starting and persist more than 1 week after stopping antifungal therapy.

Mechanism Inhibition of hepatic and gut metabolism (CYP3A4) of CSA.[1-6]

Management Monitor CSA levels and serum creatinine and be prepared to adjust the CSA dose. When coadministering POSACONAZOLE, reduce the CSA dose 25%.[7] Perform frequent monitoring of whole blood trough levels of CSA during and after POSACONAZOLE discontinuation.

Discussion

Case reports document interactions between CSA and ketoconazole,[8-16] fluconazole,[8,16-20] itraconazole,[21-23] and voriconazole.[24] CSA dosage reductions of 68% to 97% were needed to prevent CSA toxicity during ketoconazole therapy.[25] In 95 transplant patients receiving CSA and ketoconazole, markedly lower CSA dosages were needed to achieve CSA levels similar to those in patients taking CSA alone.[26,27] Rhabdomyolysis has been reported.[28] Ketoconazole may reduce CSA dose and cost in renal[26,29-31] and cardiac[32] transplant patients and children with nephrotic syndrome[33,34]; however, the risk of rejection may be increased.[35] Ketoconazole inhibits CSA metabolism the most and fluconazole the least.[3] No alterations in CSA levels or dose were necessary in patients taking low-dose ketoconazole 50 mg/day.[36] Compared with placebo, voriconazole increased the AUC of CSA 1.7-fold, and CSA plasma trough levels were higher.[37] In a cohort of 10 patients, the median cyclosporine concentration to dose ratio increased from 86 to 120.2 (ng/mL)/(mg/kg) after starting voriconazole.[38]

1 Shaw MA, et al. *Lancet.* 1987;2(8559):637.
2 Ah-Sing E, et al. *Arch Toxicol.* 1990;64(6):511.
3 Back DJ, et al. *Br J Clin Pharmacol.* 1991;32(5):624.
4 Albengres E, et al. *Int J Clin Pharmacol Ther Toxicol.* 1992;30(12):555.
5 Gomez DY, et al. *Clin Pharmacol Ther.* 1995;58(1):15.
6 Omar G, et al. *Ther Drug Monit.* 1997;19(4):436.
7 *Noxafil* [package insert]. Kenilworth, NJ: Schering Corporation; October 2006.
8 Ferguson RM, et al. *Lancet.* 1982;2(8303):882.
9 Dieperink H, et al. *Lancet.* 1982;2(8309):1217.
10 Morgenstern GR, et al. *Lancet.* 1982;2(8311):1342.
11 Daneshmend TK. *Lancet.* 1982;2(8311):1342.
12 Smith JM, et al. *Clin Sci.* 1983;64(2):67P.
13 Shepard JH, et al. *Clin Pharm.* 1986;5(6):468.
14 Sugar AM, et al. *Ann Intern Med.* 1989;110(10):844.
15 Charles BG, et al. *Aust N Z J Med.* 1989;19(3):292.
16 Koselj M, et al. *Transplant Proc.* 1994;26(5):2823.
17 Collignon P, et al. *Lancet.* 1989;1(8649):1262.
18 Lazar JD, et al. *Rev Infect Dis.* 1990;12(suppl 3):S327.
19 Canafax DM, et al. *Transplant Proc.* 1991;23(1, pt 2):1041.
20 Osowski CL, et al. *Transplantation.* 1996;61(8):1268.
21 Kwan JT, et al. *Lancet.* 1987;2(8553):282.
22 Trenk D, et al. *Lancet.* 1987;2(8571):1335.
23 Kramer MR, et al. *Ann Intern Med.* 1990;113(4):327.
24 Groll AH, et al. *J Antimicrob Chemother.* 2004;53(1):113.
25 First MR, et al. *Lancet.* 1989;2(8673):1198.
26 First MR, et al. *Transplantation.* 1993;55(5):1000.
27 Patton PR, et al. *Transplantation.* 1994;57(6):889.
28 Cohen E, et al. *Transplantation.* 2000;70(1):119.
29 Florea NR, et al. *Transplant Proc.* 2003;35(8):2873.
30 Gerntholtz T, et al. *Eur J Clin Pharmacol.* 2004;60(3):143.
31 Carbajal H, et al. *Transplantation.* 2004;77(7):1038.
32 Keogh A, et al. *N Eng J Med.* 1995;333(10):628.
33 El-Husseini A, et al. *Pediatr Nephrol.* 2004;19(9):976.
34 El-Husseini A, et al. *Eur J Clin Pharmacol.* 2006;62(1):3.
35 Dominguez J, et al. *Transplant Proc.* 2003;35(7):2522.
36 Smith L, et al. *Pharmacotherapy.* 2000;20:359.
37 Romero AJ, et al. *Clin Pharmacol Ther.* 2002;71(4):226.
38 Mori T, et al. *Bone Marrow Transplant.* 2009;44(6):371.

* Asterisk indicates drugs cited in interaction reports.

Cyclosporine — Barbiturates

Cyclosporine		Barbiturates	
Cyclosporine* (eg, *Neoral*)		Amobarbital (*Amytal*)	Phenobarbital* (eg, *Luminal*)
		Butabarbital (eg, *Butisol*)	Primidone (eg, *Mysoline*)
		Mephobarbital (*Mebaral*)	Secobarbital (*Seconal*)

Significance	Onset	Severity	Documentation
4	☐ Rapid	☐ Major	☐ Established
	■ **Delayed**	■ **Moderate**	☐ Probable
		☐ Minor	☐ Suspected
			■ **Possible**
			☐ Unlikely

Effects BARBITURATES may reduce CYCLOSPORINE concentrations, decreasing the efficacy of CYCLOSPORINE.

Mechanism Induction of the hepatic microsomal enzyme system, leading to increased biotransformation and elimination of CYCLOSPORINE by BARBITURATES, is suspected.

Management Frequently monitor serum CYCLOSPORINE concentrations when a BARBITURATE is started or stopped. Increases in CYCLOSPORINE dosage may be required to maintain adequate concentrations for immunosuppressive efficacy.

Discussion

Documented support for this interaction is limited. A case report documented difficulty achieving therapeutic cyclosporine concentrations despite high doses in a patient receiving phenobarbital.[1] Upon reduction of the phenobarbital dose, cyclosporine concentrations increased. In another patient receiving cyclosporine 4 mg/kg IV twice daily, the average cyclosporine concentration increased from 522 to 810 ng/mL following discontinuation of phenobarbital and phenytoin (eg, *Dilantin*).[2] Because phenytoin is known to enhance cyclosporine metabolism, the role played by phenobarbital in this case cannot be determined (see Cyclosporine-Hydantoins). Another report of this interaction provided no data for evaluation.[3]

[1] Carstensen H, et al. *Br J Clin Pharmacol.* 1986;21(5):550.

[2] Noguchi M, et al. *Bone Marrow Transplant.* 1992;9(5):391.

[3] Ptachcinski RJ, et al. *Clin Pharmacol Ther.* 1985;38(3):296.

* Asterisk indicates drugs cited in interaction reports. Based on pharmacologic and pharmacokinetic considerations, similar interactions may occur with other drugs that are listed.

Cyclosporine — *Berberine*

Cyclosporine* (eg, *Neoral*)	Berberine*†

Significance	Onset	Severity	Documentation
4	□ Rapid ■ **Delayed**	□ Major ■ **Moderate** □ Minor	□ Established □ Probable □ Suspected ■ **Possible** □ Unlikely

Effects CYCLOSPORINE blood levels may be elevated, increasing the risk of toxicity.

Mechanism Inhibition of CYCLOSPORINE metabolism (CYP3A4) in the liver and/or small intestine by BERBERINE is suspected.

Management Advise patients taking CYCLOSPORINE to avoid BERBERINE. Caution patients not to use herbal products and CYCLOSPORINE without consulting their health care provider.

Discussion

The effects of berberine on cyclosporine blood concentrations and pharmacokinetics were studied in renal transplant recipients.[1] To assess the effects of berberine on cyclosporine blood concentrations, 52 patients received cyclosporine with berberine 0.2 g 3 times daily for 3 months, and another 52 patients received cyclosporine without berberine. The effects of berberine on cyclosporine pharmacokinetics were studied in 6 renal transplant recipients who received cyclosporine 3 mg/kg twice daily before and after coadministration of berberine 0.2 g 3 times daily for 12 days. Compared with baseline, berberine ingestion increased the cyclosporine trough blood concentrations and ratios of concentration to dose of cyclosporine 88.9% and 98.4%, respectively. In patients receiving cyclosporine alone, these values increased 64.5% and 69.4%, respectively, compared with baseline. In the pharmacokinetic study, berberine ingestion increased cyclosporine AUC 34.5% and mean time to reach C_{max} and $t_{½}$ 1.7 and 2.7 hours, respectively. The average percentage increases in the steady-state cyclosporine concentration and minimum blood concentration were 34.5% and 88.3%, respectively.

[1] Wu X, et al. *Eur J Clin Pharmacol.* 2005;61(8):567.

* Asterisk indicates drugs cited in interaction reports.
† Not available in the US.

Cyclosporine — *Beta-Blockers*

Cyclosporine* (eg, *Neoral*)	Carvedilol* (*Coreg*)

Significance	Onset	Severity	Documentation
2	☐ Rapid ■ **Delayed**	☐ Major ■ **Moderate** ☐ Minor	☐ Established ☐ Probable ■ **Suspected** ☐ Possible ☐ Unlikely

Effects Elevated CYCLOSPORINE concentrations with an increased risk of toxicity (nephrotoxicity, neurotoxicity) may occur.

Mechanism Certain BETA-BLOCKERS may interfere with CYCLOSPORINE metabolism or P-glycoprotein transport.

Management Monitor CYCLOSPORINE concentrations and serum creatinine and observe patients for toxicity. Adjust the CYCLOSPORINE dose as needed.

Discussion

The effects of carvedilol on the pharmacokinetics of cyclosporine were assessed in 21 renal transplant patients with chronic vascular rejection.[1] Carvedilol 6.25 or 12.5 mg/day was added to each patient's daily drug regimen, which consisted of multiple drugs (including other beta-blockers) in addition to cyclosporine 3.7 mg/kg. The dose of carvedilol was increased in increments to 50 mg/day as the doses of other beta-blockers were decreased. When carvedilol treatment was started, cyclosporine trough blood concentrations increased. It was necessary to decrease the dose of cyclosporine to maintain blood levels that were within the therapeutic range. By day 90 of concurrent treatment, the daily cyclosporine dose had been decreased from 3.7 to 3 mg/kg (19%) in some patients. However, there was a high degree of interindividual variation in the need for cyclosporine dosage reduction. Most of the dosage decreases occurred in 7 patients; cyclosporine levels were stable in the remaining patients. No correlation was found between the doses of carvedilol and the doses of cyclosporine. In cardiac transplant recipients, administration of carvedilol to 12 patients receiving cyclosporine resulted in an increase in the mean cyclosporine level from 257 to 380 ng/mL.[2] To maintain therapeutic cyclosporine levels, the mean cyclosporine dose was reduced 10%.

[1] Kaijser M, et al. *Clin Transplant.* 1997;11(6):577.

[2] Bader FM, et al. *J Heart Lung Transplant.* 2005; 24(12):2144.

* Asterisk indicates drugs cited in interaction reports.

Cyclosporine — *Bupropion*

Cyclosporine* (eg, *Neoral*)	Bupropion* (eg, *Wellbutrin*)

Significance	Onset	Severity	Documentation
4	☐ Rapid	■ **Major**	☐ Established
	■ **Delayed**	☐ Moderate	☐ Probable
		☐ Minor	☐ Suspected
			■ **Possible**
			☐ Unlikely

Effects CYCLOSPORINE concentrations may be reduced, decreasing the pharmacologic effects.

Mechanism Unknown.

Management Monitor CYCLOSPORINE blood levels and observe the patient for signs of rejection or toxicity when BUPROPION therapy is started or stopped, respectively. Be prepared to adjust therapy as needed.

Discussion

A possible drug interaction between cyclosporine and bupropion was reported in a 10-year-old boy with a heart transplant, attention deficit hyperactivity disorder, and oppositional defiant disorder.[1] Two months prior to the start of bupropion therapy, the patient's cyclosporine level was 197 mcg/L. His other medications consisted of aluminum-magnesium hydroxide, azathioprine (eg, *Imuran*), calcium carbonate, dipyridamole (eg, *Persantine*), nifedipine (eg, *Procardia*), prednisone (eg, *Deltasone*), and trimethoprim/sulfamethoxazole (eg, *Bactrim*). At the time bupropion 75 mg twice daily was started, the patient was receiving cyclosporine 420 mg/day. The cyclosporine level decreased to 39 mcg/L 23 days after starting bupropion. The cyclosporine dose was increased to 500 mg/day, and 12 days later the cyclosporine level was 27 mcg/L. The cyclosporine dose was increased to 550 mg/day, and bupropion was discontinued. The cyclosporine level increased to 224 mcg/L 4 days later.

[1] Lewis BR, et al. *J Child Adolesc Psychopharmacol.* 2001;11:193.

* Asterisk indicates drugs cited in interaction reports.

Cyclosporine			*Carbamazepine*
Cyclosporine* (eg, *Neoral*)		Carbamazepine* (eg, *Tegretol*)	
Significance	Onset	Severity	Documentation
2	☐ Rapid ■ **Delayed**	☐ Major ■ **Moderate** ☐ Minor	☐ Established ☐ Probable ■ **Suspected** ☐ Possible ☐ Unlikely

Effects CYCLOSPORINE levels may be decreased, resulting in a reduction of pharmacologic effects.

Mechanism CARBAMAZEPINE may induce the hepatic microsomal enzyme metabolism of CYCLOSPORINE.

Management Monitor CYCLOSPORINE levels; observe patient for signs of rejection or toxicity if CARBAMAZEPINE is added to or discontinued from the treatment regimen. Adjust the CYCLOSPORINE dose as needed.

Discussion

Dramatically reduced cyclosporine levels occurred in 3 patients during carbamazepine coadministration.[1-3] A 44-yr-old man with an 18-yr history of severe erythrodermic psoriasis was receiving chronic treatment with methotrexate (eg, *Rheumatrex*), razoxane,† etretinate, chlorambucil (*Leukeran*), and carbamazepine 200 mg twice daily.[2] On hospital admission, he received cyclosporine for psoriasis. All medications except carbamazepine were discontinued. Despite high cyclosporine doses (1,200 mg/day), trough cyclosporine whole blood levels (by radioimmunoassay [RIA]) remained subtherapeutic, and no clinical improvement was seen. Within days of discontinuing carbamazepine and starting sodium valproate (eg, *Depakene*), cyclosporine blood levels increased, and his psoriasis improved. The second patient was a 55-yr-old cadaver kidney recipient.[2] Four months after the transplant, cyclosporine serum levels were 346 ng/mL (by RIA). Within 3 days of starting carbamazepine 200 mg 3 times daily for severe eye pain, cyclosporine levels decreased to 64 ng/mL and, 1 wk later, declined to 37 ng/mL. Carbamazepine was discontinued, and cyclosporine levels increased to 100 to 200 ng/mL. During coadministration, it was necessary to increase the cyclosporine dose to maintain the therapeutic level. A 53-yr-old renal transplant patient stabilized on cyclosporine for 8 mo was started on carbamazepine 400 mg twice daily for seizures.[3] Within 3 days, cyclosporine levels became subtherapeutic but returned to the therapeutic range when carbamazepine was discontinued. Cyclosporine pharmacokinetics were compared in 3 pediatric renal transplant patients taking cyclosporine and carbamazepine vs a matched control group receiving cyclosporine alone.[4] The mean daily cyclosporine dose was higher in the carbamazepine group (16.2 vs 10.8 mg/kg/day), but predose trough cyclosporine blood levels were 65% lower.

[1] Lele P, et al. *Kidney Int.* 1985;27:344.
[2] Schofield OM, et al. *Br J Dermatol.* 1990;122:425.
[3] Soto Alvarez J, et al. *Nephron.* 1991;58:235.
[4] Cooney GF, et al. *Pharmacotherapy.* 1995;15:353.

* Asterisk indicates drugs cited in interaction reports.
† Not available in the US.

Cyclosporine — *Ceftriaxone*

Cyclosporine* (eg, *Neoral*)	Ceftriaxone* (*Rocephin*)

Significance	Onset	Severity	Documentation
4	☐ Rapid	☐ Major	☐ Established
	■ **Delayed**	■ **Moderate**	☐ Probable
		☐ Minor	☐ Suspected
			■ **Possible**
			☐ Unlikely

Effects Elevated CYCLOSPORINE levels with increased risk of toxicity may occur.

Mechanism Unknown.

Management Consider monitoring serum CYCLOSPORINE and creatinine levels. Adjust the dose of CYCLOSPORINE accordingly.

Discussion

Increased plasma cyclosporine levels were reported in 2 renal transplant patients following the addition of ceftriaxone to their treatment regimens.[1] The first patient was a 30-year-old woman diagnosed with pneumonia 12 weeks after transplantation. She was receiving cyclosporine 125 mg twice daily, azathioprine (eg, *Imuran*) 100 mg/day, and prednisone (eg, *Deltasone*) 10 mg twice daily. Treatment with ceftriaxone 1 g twice daily was started. Two days later, serum cyclosporine and cyclosporine metabolite concentrations were elevated. Plasma cyclosporine levels reached potentially toxic concentrations and remained elevated while ceftriaxone was administered concurrently. Ceftriaxone was discontinued, and, 9 days later, serum cyclosporine levels decreased to within the therapeutic range. The second case was a 64-year-old woman who was receiving cyclosporine 250 mg twice daily, azathioprine 75 mg/day, and prednisone 10 mg twice daily. Three weeks after transplantation, *Streptococcus faecalis* bacteremia was diagnosed and the patient was treated with gentamicin (eg, *Garamycin*) 40 mg twice daily and ceftriaxone 1 g twice daily. Three days after the antibiotics were started, cyclosporine levels increased, reaching toxic concentrations during coadministration of ceftriaxone. Twelve days after discontinuing ceftriaxone, serum cyclosporine levels returned to within the therapeutic range.

[1] Soto Alvarez J, et al. *Nephron*. 1991;59:681.

* Asterisk indicates drugs cited in interaction reports.

Cyclosporine — *Chloramphenicol*

Cyclosporine* (eg, *Neoral*)	Chloramphenicol* (eg, *Chloromycetin*)

Significance	Onset	Severity	Documentation
4	□ Rapid	□ Major	□ Established
	■ **Delayed**	■ **Moderate**	□ Probable
		□ Minor	□ Suspected
			■ **Possible**
			□ Unlikely

Effects Trough plasma concentrations of CYCLOSPORINE may be elevated, increasing the likelihood of adverse effects (eg, nephrotoxicity).

Mechanism Unknown.

Management Closely monitor CYCLOSPORINE trough concentrations and observe the patient for signs of toxicity. Be prepared to adjust the dose of CYCLOSPORINE as needed.

Discussion

Increased cyclosporine trough concentrations have been reported in transplant patients receiving chloramphenicol. A 17-year-old morbidly obese girl had received a cadaveric renal transplant 5 years earlier and was stabilized on cyclosporine and prednisone (eg, *Deltasone*).[2] Other medications she was receiving included epoetin alfa (eg, *Epogen*) and gabapentin (*Neurontin*). She was admitted to the hospital for a partial gastrectomy with feeding jejunostomy. Before hospital admission, the patient required cyclosporine 50 to 75 mg (microemulsion formulation) via the jejunostomy tube (JT) twice daily to maintain trough concentrations of 100 to 150 mcg/L. Prior to receiving chloramphenicol, the patient successfully completed a course of treatment with rifampin (eg, *Rifadin*) and vancomycin (eg, *Vancocin*) for line sepsis. At that time, her cyclosporine dosage requirement was 300 mg via JT twice daily to maintain trough concentrations of 100 to 150 mcg/L. The need for the increase in cyclosporine dose was attributed to concurrent rifampin therapy. The patient was started on ceftazidime (eg, *Fortaz*), which was changed to ciprofloxacin (*Cipro*) after 2 days, for a UTI and chloramphenicol 875 mg IV every 6 hours for vancomycin-resistant *Enterococcus* sinusitis. At this time, the cyclosporine trough level was 70 mcg/L. Cyclosporine 250 mg via JT twice daily was ordered. By the following day, there was a 4-fold increase in the trough concentration (280 mcg/L). The dose of cyclosporine was tapered to 50 to 100 mg/day; however, cyclosporine concentrations continued to rise, reaching 600 mcg/L within 2 weeks. After 21 days of treatment, chloramphenicol was discontinued and, within 4 days, cyclosporine trough concentrations decreased to 100 to 150 mcg/L. At this time, the cyclosporine dosage requirement was 50 mg JT twice daily. In a 47-year-old woman with a heart-lung transplant, the cyclosporine trough level increased approximately 3-fold 1 day after starting chloramphenicol.[1] Within 8 days of reducing the chloramphenicol dose from 300 to 225 mg/day, cyclosporine levels decreased to the therapeutic range.

[1] Steinfort CL, et al. *Med J Aust.* 1994;161:455.
[2] Bui L, et al. *Ann Pharmacother.* 1999;33:252.

* Asterisk indicates drugs cited in interaction reports.

Cyclosporine — *Clindamycin*

Cyclosporine* (eg, *Neoral*)	Clindamycin* (eg, *Cleocin*)

Significance	Onset	Severity	Documentation
4	□ Rapid ■ **Delayed**	□ Major ■ **Moderate** □ Minor	□ Established □ Probable □ Suspected ■ **Possible** □ Unlikely

Effects CYCLOSPORINE concentrations may be reduced, decreasing the pharmacologic effects.

Mechanism Unknown.

Management Closely monitor CYCLOSPORINE concentrations when CLINDAMYCIN is started, stopped, or changed in dosage. Adjust the CYCLOSPORINE dose as needed.

Discussion

A possible drug interaction between clindamycin and cyclosporine was reported in 2 patients receiving lung transplants.[1] The target cyclosporine concentration in 1 patient was 100 to 150 mcg/L, while in the second patient, the goal was to maintain cyclosporine levels at approximately 200 mcg/L. Both patients were treated with oral clindamycin 600 mg 3 times daily for a *Staphylococcus aureus* infection that developed following transplantation and while receiving cyclosporine. During clindamycin administration, it was necessary to continually increase the dose of cyclosporine (eg, from 325 to 1100 mg/day in 1 patient) to maintain target cyclosporine concentrations. When clindamycin therapy was stopped, the dose of cyclosporine was reduced to the dosage needed before clindamycin treatment.

[1] Thurnheer R, et al. *BMJ.* 1999;319:163.

* Asterisk indicates drugs cited in interaction reports.

Cyclosporine — *Clonidine*

Cyclosporine* (eg, *Neoral*)	Clonidine* (eg, *Catapres*)

Significance	Onset	Severity	Documentation
4	☐ Rapid ■ **Delayed**	☐ Major ■ **Moderate** ☐ Minor	☐ Established ☐ Probable ☐ Suspected ■ **Possible** ☐ Unlikely

Effects CLONIDINE may increase CYCLOSPORINE concentrations and side effects.

Mechanism Unknown.

Management Monitor whole-blood CYCLOSPORINE concentrations when starting or stopping CLONIDINE. Adjust the dose of CYCLOSPORINE as needed.

Discussion

In a study comparing nephrotoxicity in allogenic bone marrow transplant patients who received cyclosporine with and without clonidine, cyclosporine concentrations and dosages were higher (by 111% and 55%, respectively) in patients who received clonidine concurrently.[1] In a 3-year-old boy, whole-blood cyclosporine concentration increased dramatically (to 927 mcg/L) after clonidine was added to his treatment regimen, in spite of a reduction in cyclosporine dosage.[2] When clonidine was discontinued, the cyclosporine concentration decreased.

Controlled studies are needed to assess this possible drug interaction.

[1] Luke J, et al. *Clin Pharm.* 1990;9:49.

[2] Gilbert RD, et al. *Nephron.* 1995;71:105.

* Asterisk indicates drugs cited in interaction reports.

Cyclosporine — *Colchicine*

Cyclosporine* (eg, *Neoral*)	Colchicine* (eg, *Colcrys*)

Significance	Onset	Severity	Documentation
1	☐ Rapid ■ **Delayed**	■ **Major** ☐ Moderate ☐ Minor	☐ Established ■ **Probable** ☐ Suspected ☐ Possible ☐ Unlikely

Effects Severe adverse reactions, including GI, hepatic, renal, and neuromuscular toxicity, may occur during coadministration of CYCLOSPORINE and COLCHICINE.

Mechanism Unknown.

Management Coadministration of COLCHICINE and CYCLOSPORINE is contraindicated in patients with hepatic or renal function impairment. In patients with normal hepatic or renal function, the recommended colchicine dose for gout flares in patients receiving cyclosporine is 0.6 mg for 1 dose repeated no earlier than 3 days.[1] The recommended maximum colchicine dose for familial Mediterranean fever in patients receiving cyclosporine is 0.6 mg daily. Monitor for adverse reactions.

Discussion

During conversion of 4 renal transplant patients from azathioprine (eg, *Imuran*) to cyclosporine, a syndrome of severe renal, hepatic, and neuromuscular toxicity occurred.[2] The patients, immunosuppressed with azathioprine and prednisone while also receiving colchicine 1 to 2 mg daily, were scheduled to be converted from azathioprine therapy to cyclosporine. The conversion protocol involved the gradual addition of cyclosporine, starting with 3 mg/kg/day, to the unchanged azathioprine dosage. The protocol specified cessation of azathioprine when therapeutic cyclosporine concentrations were obtained. Prior to achieving therapeutic levels of cyclosporine, all patients experienced pronounced adverse reactions, including diarrhea and elevated serum lactic dehydrogenase. In addition, 3 patients demonstrated clinically important increases in serum ALT and bilirubin, while 2 patients experienced elevated serum creatinine. One patient was hospitalized for severe myalgia and general muscular weakness. The conversion of the patients from azathioprine to cyclosporine was terminated; upon discontinuing cyclosporine, the adverse reactions rapidly reversed. Hepatic and renal functions returned to baseline values. At least 2 additional case histories of a possible drug interaction have been reported.[3,4] A renal transplant patient developed severe neuromyopathy and liver impairment during coadministration of cyclosporine and colchicine, which persisted until colchicine was discontinued.[4] A second renal transplant patient developed increased serum cyclosporine concentrations and nephrotoxicity after colchicine was added to the cyclosporine regimen.[3] Cyclosporine levels returned to baseline values, and the symptoms of nephrotoxicity rapidly resolved after colchicine was discontinued. In a study of 23 healthy volunteers, coadministration of single doses of colchicine 0.6 mg with cyclosporine 100 mg increased the colchicine C_{max} and AUC 224% and 217%, respectively.[5]

[1] *Colcrys* [package insert]. Philadelphia, PA: Mutual Pharmaceutical Company Inc; July 2009.
[2] Yussim A, et al. *Transplant Proc.* 1994;26(5):2825.
[3] Menta R, et al. *Nephrol Dial Transplant.* 1987;2(5):380.
[4] Rieger EH, et al. *Transplantation.* 1990;49(6):1196.
[5] Terkeltaub RA, et al. *Arthritis Rheum.* 2011;63(8):2226.

* Asterisk indicates drugs cited in interaction reports.

Cyclosporine — *Colesevelam*

Cyclosporine* (eg, *Neoral*)	Colesevelam* (*Welchol*)

Significance	Onset	Severity	Documentation
2	☐ Rapid ■ **Delayed**	☐ Major ■ **Moderate** ☐ Minor	☐ Established ☐ Probable ■ **Suspected** ☐ Possible ☐ Unlikely

Effects Whole blood concentrations and efficacy of CYCLOSPORINE may be reduced.

Mechanism COLESEVELAM may bind with CYCLOSPORINE in the GI tract, decreasing CYCLOSPORINE absorption.

Management Administer CYCLOSPORINE at least 4 hours prior to COLESEVELAM.[1] Monitor CYCLOSPORINE concentrations.

Discussion

Simultaneous administration of cyclosporine 200 mg and colesevelam 3,750 mg reduced the cyclosporine AUC and C_{max} 34% and 44%, respectively.[1] No data are available for the effects of colesevelam on cyclosporine pharmacokinetics when the administration times are separated.

[1] *Welchol* [package insert]. Parsippany, NJ: Daiichi Sakyo Inc; February 2010.

* Asterisk indicates drugs cited in interaction reports.

Cyclosporine × *Contraceptives, Hormonal*

Cyclosporine* (eg, *Neoral*)	Contraceptives, Oral* (eg, *Ortho-Novum*)

Significance	Onset	Severity	Documentation
4	☐ Rapid	☐ Major	☐ Established
	■ **Delayed**	■ **Moderate**	☐ Probable
		☐ Minor	☐ Suspected
			■ **Possible**
			☐ Unlikely

Effects Elevated CYCLOSPORINE concentrations, increasing the risk of toxicity.

Mechanism Possible inhibition of CYCLOSPORINE metabolism.

Management Avoid this combination if possible. If given together, monitor CYCLOSPORINE concentrations, as well as renal and hepatic function. Adjust the CYCLOSPORINE dose as indicated. Cyclic adjustments may be necessary.

Discussion

Severe hepatotoxicity was reported in a 32-year-old woman receiving cyclosporine 5 mg/kg/day for idiopathic uveitis after starting an oral contraceptive containing levonorgestrel 0.15 mg and ethinyl estradiol 30 mcg.[1] On 2 separate cycles, during concurrent treatment with cyclosporine and the oral contraceptive, there were increases in plasma trough concentrations of cyclosporine, serum creatinine, aminotransferases, serum bilirubin, and alkaline phosphatase. In addition, the patient experienced nausea, vomiting, and hepatalgia. Others have reported an increase and then a return to therapeutic cyclosporine plasma concentrations when an oral contraceptive containing desogestrel 0.15 mg and ethinyl estradiol 30 mcg was started and stopped, respectively.[2]

[1] Deray G, et al. *Lancet.* 1987;1(8525):158.

[2] Maurer G. *Transplant Proc.* 1985;17(4) (suppl):19.

* Asterisk indicates drugs cited in interaction reports.

Cyclosporine		Corticosteroids	
Cyclosporine* (eg, *Neoral*)		Methylprednisolone* (eg, *Medrol*) Prednisolone* (eg, *Prelone*)	Prednisone* (eg, *Deltasone*)

Significance	Onset	Severity	Documentation
4	□ Rapid ■ **Delayed**	□ Major ■ **Moderate** □ Minor	□ Established □ Probable □ Suspected ■ **Possible** □ Unlikely

Effects Although this combination is therapeutically beneficial for organ transplants, toxicity may be enhanced.

Mechanism Reduced liver degradation of one or both of the drugs.

Management Tailor the dosage of one or both of the drugs if signs of toxicity or rejection occur.

Discussion

In a retrospective analysis of 33 consecutive patients treated for rejection, cyclosporine (CSA) trough plasma levels measured by radioimmunoassay (RIA) increased in 22 patients by an average of 58% (205 to 482 ng/mL) following methylprednisolone.[1] Reduction of CSA doses was necessary in 6 patients; CSA levels restabilized following methylprednisolone in 14 patients. Five bone marrow transplant patients experienced convulsions, possibly caused by the CSA high-dose methylprednisolone combination; however, a causal relationship was not established.[2,3] Conflicting data, possibly because of the method of measuring CSA blood levels, are presented in a prospective study.[4] Cyclosporine levels were higher in 37 patients receiving CSA and azathioprine (eg, *Imuran*) compared with 35 patients receiving CSA, azathioprine, and prednisone. Because RIA measures the parent compound plus metabolites, while high-performance liquid chromatography (HPLC) measures only the parent compound, steroids may enhance CSA degradation, producing higher levels of metabolites (RIA) and low levels of CSA (HPLC).

Symptoms of corticosteroid excess were observed in transplant patients on CSA and prednisolone.[5] Prednisolone clearance was 29% lower in the CSA group (n = 39) than in the azathioprine group (n = 38).[6,7] Eleven patients were changed from azathioprine to CSA, and prednisolone clearance decreased. Two patients were changed in the opposite direction, and prednisolone clearance increased.[8] Also, 2 groups of 8 patients received either CSA and prednisone or azathioprine and prednisone after renal transplants.[9] The CSA group showed an average decrease of 22% in the total body clearance of prednisone. These 2 studies were not well controlled. However, another trial did not demonstrate an effect of CSA on prednisolone clearance or volume of distribution.[10]

[1] Klintmalm G, et al. *Lancet.* 1984;1:731.
[2] Durrant S, et al. *Lancet.* 1982;2:829.
[3] Boogaerts MA, et al. *Lancet.* 1982;2:1216.
[4] Hricik DE, et al. *Transplantation.* 1990;49:221.
[5] Ost L. *Lancet.* 1984;1:451.
[6] Frey FJ, et al. *Eur J Clin Pharmacol.* 1981;19:209.
[7] Gambertoglio JG, et al. *Am J Kidney Dis.* 1984;3:425.
[8] Ost L. *Transplantation.* 1987;44:533.
[9] Langhoff E, et al. *Transplantation.* 1985;39:107.
[10] Rocci ML, et al. *Clin Pharmacol Ther.* 1987;41:235.

* Asterisk indicates drugs cited in interaction reports.

Cyclosporine — *Diltiazem*

Cyclosporine*
(eg, *Neoral*)

Diltiazem*
(eg, *Cardizem*)

Significance	Onset	Severity	Documentation
2	☐ Rapid	☐ Major	■ **Established**
	■ **Delayed**	■ **Moderate**	☐ Probable
		☐ Minor	☐ Suspected
			☐ Possible
			☐ Unlikely

Effects CYCLOSPORINE levels and toxicity may be increased.

Mechanism DILTIAZEM is believed to inhibit the hepatic microsomal enzyme metabolism of CYCLOSPORINE.

Management Monitor CYCLOSPORINE levels when adding or discontinuing DILTIAZEM. Adjust the CYCLOSPORINE dose as needed.

Discussion

Cyclosporine (CSA) levels are higher in transplant patients receiving CSA and diltiazem.[1-9] One patient experienced elevated CSA trough serum levels and renal toxicity twice following the addition of diltiazem, which returned to pre-diltiazem levels when diltiazem was discontinued.[2] Cyclosporine whole blood levels increased 314% following the initiation of diltiazem in another patient.[3] Arthralgia[10] and encephalopathy[11] have been associated with elevated CSA levels during coadministration of diltiazem.[10] Diltiazem decreased CSA clearance 50% to 70%.[1,5] Similar results were noted with the microemulsion formulation of CSA.[12,13] A 20% to 50% reduction in CSA dosage may be necessary during diltiazem treatment.[14-16] In patients receiving diltiazem, switching from *Sandimmune* to *Neoral* increased the CSA AUC 37.5%, suggesting a need to lower the CSA dosage.[17] Trough levels were not affected. Diltiazem may protect the kidney during the immediate postoperative period.[18] In 19 of 22 renal transplant patients, diltiazem increased CSA levels 45%.[19,20] However, a single diltiazem dose does not appear to affect CSA kinetics,[21] but a single daily dose has effects similar to those of multiple daily doses.[22] Discontinuing diltiazem may decrease CSA levels, increasing rejection episodes.[5]

1 Wagner K, et al. *Lancet.* 1985;2:1355.
2 Pochet JM, et al. *Lancet.* 1986;1:979.
3 Grino JM, et al. *Lancet.* 1986;1:1387.
4 Neumayer HH, et al. *Lancet.* 1986;2:523.
5 Wagner K, et al. *Transplant Proc.* 1988;20;(2 suppl 2):561.
6 Kelly JJ, et al. *Transplant Proc.* 1990;22:2127.
7 Dy GR, et al. *Transplant Proc.* 1991;23:1258.
8 Bourge RC, et al. *Am J Med.* 1991;90:402.
9 Patton PR, et al. *Transplantation.* 1994;57:889.
10 Bailie GR, et al. *Clin Nephrol.* 1990;33:256.
11 Jiang TT, et al. *Ann Pharmacother.* 1999;33:750.
12 Mezzano S, et al. *Transplant Proc.* 1998;30:1660.
13 Asberg A, et al. *Eur J Clin Pharmacol.* 1999;55:383.
14 Kohlhaw K, et al. *Transplant Proc.* 1988;20;(2 suppl 2):572.
15 McCauley J, et al. *Transplant Proc.* 1989;21:3955.
16 Leibbrandt DM, et al. *Med J Aust.* 1992;157:296.
17 Akhlaghi F, et al. *J Heart Lung Transplant.* 2001;20:431.
18 Tenschert W, et al. *Transplant Proc.* 1991;23;(1 pt 2):1334.
19 Brockmöller J, et al. *Eur J Clin Pharmacol.* 1990; 38:237.
20 Kunzendorf U, et al. *Transplantation.* 1991;52:280.
21 Roy LF, et al. *Clin Pharmacol Ther.* 1989;46:657.
22 Morris RG, et al. *Ther Drug Monit.* 1999;21:437.

* Asterisk indicates drugs cited in interaction reports.

Cyclosporine — *Ezetimibe*

Cyclosporine* (eg, *Neoral*)	Ezetimibe* (*Zetia*)

Significance	Onset	Severity	Documentation
2	☐ Rapid ■ **Delayed**	☐ Major ■ **Moderate** ☐ Minor	☐ Established ☐ Probable ■ **Suspected** ☐ Possible ☐ Unlikely

Effects CYCLOSPORINE and EZETIMIBE exposure may be increased, increasing the pharmacologic effects and adverse reactions.

Mechanism Unknown.

Management Monitor CYCLOSPORINE concentrations when EZETIMIBE is coadministered. Adjust the CYCLOSPORINE dose as needed. In addition, monitor patients for CYCLOSPORINE or EZETIMIBE adverse reactions.

Discussion

The effects of multiple-dose administration of ezetimibe on the pharmacokinetics of cyclosporine were evaluated in 12 healthy subjects.[1] Using an open-label, crossover design, each subject received a single oral dose of cyclosporine 100 mg (treatment A) or ezetimibe 20 mg daily for 8 days and a single dose of cyclosporine 100 mg on day 7 (treatment B). Compared with taking cyclosporine alone, pretreatment with ezetimibe increased cyclosporine exposure 15%. In another study, the effects of cyclosporine at steady state (75 to 150 mg twice daily) on the single-dose pharmacokinetics of ezetimibe 10 mg were evaluated in 8 postrenal transplant patients with CrCl greater than 50 mL/min.[2] Compared with healthy controls derived from a prespecified database, cyclosporine increased ezetimibe-total AUC 3.4-fold in the transplant patients. Additional studies are needed to determine the clinical importance of this interaction. Supratherapeutic LDL reductions were reported in a 64-year-old man when ezetimibe 10 mg/day was administered with cyclosporine 100 mg twice daily.[3] Subsequently, the ezetimibe dosage was reduced to 5 mg/day.

[1] Bergman AJ, et al. *J Clin Pharmacol.* 2006;46(3):321.
[2] Bergman AJ, et al. *J Clin Pharmacol.* 2006;46(3):328.
[3] Koshman SL, et al. *Ann Pharmacother.* 2005;39(9):1561.

* Asterisk indicates drugs cited in interaction reports.

Cyclosporine — *Food*

Cyclosporine* (eg, *Neoral*)	Grapefruit Juice*	High-Fat Diet*

Significance	Onset	Severity	Documentation
2	■ **Rapid** □ Delayed	□ Major ■ **Moderate** □ Minor	□ Established ■ **Probable** □ Suspected □ Possible □ Unlikely

Effects CYCLOSPORINE concentrations may be increased.

Mechanism Inhibition of CYP-450 (CYP3A) in the intestinal mucosa.

Management Caution patients to avoid fluctuations in the ingestion of GRAPEFRUIT JUICE while taking CYCLOSPORINE.

Discussion

Several studies documented an increase in the cyclosporine C_{max} and AUC when cyclosporine capsules,[1-11] solution,[12] or microemulsion[13,14] were taken with grapefruit juice. When 11 renal transplant patients on stable doses of cyclosporine (mean, 250 mg/day) ingested their cyclosporine dose with grapefruit juice, the mean trough concentrations increased about 25% compared with water.[2] Cyclosporine levels increased in 8 of 11 patients when they ingested the medication with grapefruit juice and decreased in 10 of 11 patients when subjects resumed taking the drug with water. In 14 healthy adults, administration of cyclosporine with grapefruit juice, orange juice, or water was evaluated.[4] Grapefruit juice resulted in a 16% to 200% increase in the AUC of cyclosporine in 12 subjects compared with orange juice or water. Comparison of the effects of grapefruit juice after IV or oral cyclosporine demonstrate increased bioavailability.[7] In 4 patients with resistant, cyclosporine-dependent hematologic disorders, simultaneous administration of cyclosporine with grapefruit juice resulted in elevation of cyclosporine levels in spite of dosage reduction and hematologic improvement.[15] One study found that grapefruit juice increased the bioavailability of cyclosporine in black subjects to a higher magnitude than in white subjects.[16] Cyclosporine AUC increased with grapefruit juice ingestion but not with ingestion of grapefruit juice free of furanocoumarins, indicating these compounds are involved, at least partially, in CYP3A inhibition.[17] Administration of cyclosporine with trace- or moderate-fat content meals (21 g) did not alter cyclosporine pharmacokinetics, while high-fat content meals (45 g) increased cyclosporine bioavailability and clearance.[6] This effect is probably not clinically important.

[1] Honcharik N, et al. *Transplantation.* 1991;52(6):1087.
[2] Ducharme MP, et al. *Br J Clin Pharmacol.* 1993;36(5):457.
[3] Herlitz H, et al. *Nephrol Dial Transplant.* 1993;8(4):375.
[4] Yee GC, et al. *Lancet.* 1995;345(8955):955.
[5] Hollander AA, et al. *Clin Pharmacol Ther.* 1995;57(3):318.
[6] Tan KK, et al. *Clin Pharmacol Ther.* 1995;57(4):425.
[7] Ducharme MP, et al. *Clin Pharmacol Ther.* 1995;57(5):485.
[8] Proppe DG, et al. *Br J Clin Pharmacol.* 1995;39(3):337.
[9] Min DI, et al. *Transplantation.* 1996;62(1):123.
[10] Ioannides-Demos LL, et al. *J Rheumatol.* 1997;24(1):49.
[11] Edwards DJ, et al. *Clin Pharmacol Ther.* 1999;65(3):237.
[12] Brunner LJ, et al. *Pharmacotherapy.* 1998;18(1):23.
[13] Ku YM, et al. *J Clin Pharmacol.* 1998;38(10):959.
[14] Hermann M, et al. *Int J Clin Pharmacol Ther.* 2002;40(10):451.
[15] Emilia G, et al. *Blood.* 1998;91(1):362.
[16] Lee M, et al. *J Clin Pharmacol.* 2001;41(3):317.
[17] Paine MF, et al. *Am J Clin Nutr.* 2008;87(4):863.

* Asterisk indicates drugs cited in interaction reports.

Cyclosporine — *Gemfibrozil*

Cyclosporine* (eg, *Neoral*)	Gemfibrozil* (eg, *Lopid*)

Significance	Onset	Severity	Documentation
4	□ Rapid	□ Major	□ Established
	■ **Delayed**	■ **Moderate**	□ Probable
		□ Minor	□ Suspected
			■ **Possible**
			□ Unlikely

Effects CYCLOSPORINE concentrations may be reduced, decreasing the pharmacologic effects.

Mechanism Unknown.

Management Monitor CYCLOSPORINE trough whole blood concentrations, adjust the CYCLOSPORINE dose as indicated, and observe the patient for signs of rejection or toxicity when GEMFIBROZIL therapy is started or stopped, respectively.

Discussion

In a placebo controlled study, the effects of gemfibrozil on atherosclerosis were investigated in kidney transplant patients with severe hyperlipidemia.[1] All patients were receiving cyclosporine therapy. The investigation included patients with serum cholesterol levels of more than 6.5 mmol/L (251 mg/dL) after at least 3 months of diet modification. The dose of gemfibrozil was 450 mg once daily when serum creatinine was at least 200 mcmol/L and 450 mg twice daily when the levels were less than 200 mcmol/L (2.3 mg/dL). Seven patients received gemfibrozil and 8 were given placebo. After 6 weeks of treatment, a significant decline in 12-hour cyclosporine trough whole blood concentrations from 93 ng/mL to 76 ng/mL ($P < 0.05$) was measured compared with 99 ng/mL and 98 ng/mL, respectively, in the patients who received placebo. After 3 months of treatment, the study was stopped because of a suspected interaction between cyclosporine and gemfibrozil.

[1] Fehrman-Ekholm I, et al. *Nephron*. 1996;72(3):483.

* Asterisk indicates drugs cited in interaction reports.

Cyclosporine — *Griseofulvin*

Cyclosporine* (eg, *Neoral*)	Griseofulvin* (eg, *Grifulvin*)

Significance	Onset	Severity	Documentation
4	☐ Rapid ■ **Delayed**	☐ Major ■ **Moderate** ☐ Minor	☐ Established ☐ Probable ☐ Suspected ■ **Possible** ☐ Unlikely

Effects CYCLOSPORINE levels may be reduced, resulting in a decrease in the pharmacologic effects.

Mechanism Unknown.

Management Monitor CYCLOSPORINE blood levels and observe the patient for signs of rejection or toxicity when GRISEOFULVIN therapy is started or stopped, respectively.

Discussion

A case of a possible drug interaction between cyclosporine and griseofulvin has been reported.[1] The patient, a 57-year-old man with hypertensive nephrosclerosis and diabetes mellitus, received a histocompatibility locus (HLA)–identical renal allograft. He received cyclosporine 2.8 mg/kg/day, azathioprine (eg, *Imuran*) 75 mg/day, and prednisone (eg, *Sterapred*) for immunosuppressive therapy. In addition, the patient was given sustained-release nifedipine (eg, *Procardia*) for mild systolic hypertension and isoniazid as prophylaxis for a history of tuberculosis. His trough cyclosporine blood level, as measured by monoclonal whole blood radioimmunoassay, was maintained at approximately 90 ng/mL. He was administered griseofulvin 500 mg/day for the treatment of onychomycosis. Two weeks after the start of griseofulvin therapy, his cyclosporine level decreased to 50 ng/mL. The cyclosporine dosage was increased to 4.8 mg/kg; however, the cyclosporine level did not increase. After 16 weeks, griseofulvin was stopped and cyclosporine blood levels increased to more than 200 ng/mL.

Controlled studies are needed to assess the clinical importance of this possible drug interaction.

[1] Abu-Romeh SH, et al. *Nephron.* 1991;58(2):237.

* Asterisk indicates drugs cited in interaction reports.

Cyclosporine — *HCV Protease Inhibitors*

Cyclosporine* (eg, *Neoral*)	Boceprevir* (*Victrelis*)	Telaprevir* (*Incivek*)

Significance	Onset	Severity	Documentation
1	☐ Rapid ■ **Delayed**	■ **Major** ☐ Moderate ☐ Minor	☐ Established ☐ Probable ■ **Suspected** ☐ Possible ☐ Unlikely

Effects CYCLOSPORINE plasma concentrations may be elevated, increasing the pharmacologic effects and risk of adverse reactions.

Mechanism CYCLOSPORINE metabolism (CYP3A) may be inhibited by HEPATITIS C VIRUS (HCV) PROTEASE INHIBITORS.

Management Closely monitor CYCLOSPORINE blood concentrations as well as renal function and CYCLOSPORINE-related adverse reactions when an HCV PROTEASE INHIBITOR is coadministered.[1,2] Adjust the CYCLOSPORINE dose and dosing interval as needed. CYCLOSPORINE blood concentration monitoring may be needed for approximately 2 weeks after stopping TELAPREVIR.[3]

Discussion

The effects of telaprevir on the pharmacokinetics of a single oral dose of cyclosporine were evaluated in 9 healthy volunteers.[3] Using an open-label, randomized design, each subject received a single dose of cyclosporine 100 mg, followed by a minimum 8-day washout period, and subsequent administration of a single dose of cyclosporine 10 mg with either a single dose of telaprevir 750 mg or with steady-state telaprevir (750 mg every 8 hours). Steady-state telaprevir increased the cyclosporine dose-normalized AUC approximately 4.6-fold and prolonged the terminal elimination $t_{1/2}$ from a mean of 12 hours to 42.1 hours compared with giving cyclosporine alone.

[1] *Victrelis* [package insert]. Whitehouse Station, NJ: Schering Corporation; May 2011.

[2] *Incivek* [package insert]. Cambridge, MA: Vertex Pharmaceuticals Incorporated; May 2011.

[3] Garg V, et al. *Hepatology*. 2011;54(1):20.

* Asterisk indicates drugs cited in interaction reports.

Cyclosporine — *Hydantoins*

Cyclosporine* (eg, *Neoral*)	Ethotoin (*Peganone*)	Mephenytoin† (*Mesantoin*)
	Fosphenytoin (*Cerebyx*)	Phenytoin* (eg, *Dilantin*)

Significance	Onset	Severity	Documentation
1	☐ Rapid ■ **Delayed**	■ **Major** ☐ Moderate ☐ Minor	☐ Established ■ **Probable** ☐ Suspected ☐ Possible ☐ Unlikely

Effects CYCLOSPORINE concentrations are decreased by PHENYTOIN, resulting in a decrease in the immunosuppressive activity of CYCLOSPORINE, which may predispose patients to transplant rejection. This appears to occur within 48 hours of PHENYTOIN therapy and abates within 1 week of PHENYTOIN discontinuation.

Mechanism Possibly decreased CYCLOSPORINE absorption or increased metabolism.

Management Closely monitor CYCLOSPORINE concentrations during concurrent PHENYTOIN administration; tailor CYCLOSPORINE dosage to maintain concentrations in the therapeutic range.

Discussion

In a controlled study of six subjects, the mean cyclosporine area under the plasma concentration-time curve (AUC) was reduced approximately 50% after 9 days of phenytoin dosing.[2] These reductions were observed regardless of the assay (RIA polyclonal or HPLC) or sample matrix (serum or whole blood) utilized. Similar reductions were also observed in the concentrations of two of the cyclosporine metabolites. Little change was observed in the cyclosporine/metabolite ratios or in the terminal slope following phenytoin therapy compared with cyclosporine alone, suggesting that the observed decrease in cyclosporine concentrations with phenytoin is most likely the result of a decrease in absorption.[4] However, in a separate report, a similar decrease in cyclosporine concentrations was observed in one patient receiving IV cyclosporine.[3] A 50% reduction in cyclosporine AUC occurred in five patients following phenytoin therapy; the interaction was not present within 72 hours of phenytoin discontinuation.[1] There was no evidence of graft rejection. It does not appear that separation of the administration times of cyclosporine and phenytoin will circumvent this interaction.

[1] Keown PA, et al. *Transplant Proc.* 1982;14:659.
[2] Freeman DJ, et al. *Br J Clin Pharmacol.* 1984;18:887.
[3] Keown PA, et al. *Transplantation.* 1984;38:304.
[4] Rowland M, et al. *Br J Clin Pharmacol.* 1987;24:329.

* Asterisk indicates drugs cited in interaction reports. Based on pharmacologic and pharmacokinetic considerations, similar interactions may occur with other drugs that are listed.
† Not available in the United States.

Cyclosporine — *Imipenem/Cilastatin*

Cyclosporine* (eg, *Neoral*)	Imipenem/Cilastatin* (*Primaxin*)

Significance	Onset	Severity	Documentation
2	■ **Rapid**	□ Major	□ Established
	□ Delayed	■ **Moderate**	□ Probable
		□ Minor	■ **Suspected**
			□ Possible
			□ Unlikely

Effects The CNS side effects of both agents may be increased.

Mechanism This interaction may be the result of additive or synergistic toxicity.

Management If an interaction is suspected, consider administering an alternative antibiotic.

Discussion

A 62-year-old renal transplant patient developed severe CNS disturbances during concurrent administration of imipenem/cilastatin and cyclosporine.[1] Cyclosporine was given as prophylaxis against kidney rejection. Because the patient was allergic to penicillin, IV imipenem/cilastatin 500 mg every 12 hours was administered for a *Streptococcus faecalis* urinary tract infection. Approximately 20 minutes after the second dose of the antibiotic, CNS effects developed including confusion, agitation and intense tremor. A neurologic examination revealed personal and temporal disorientation, agitation, motor aphasia and arm tremors. Antibiotic therapy was discontinued, and the patient's condition improved. In five additional recipients of various allografts who were receiving cyclosporine, the addition of imipenem/cilastatin 500 mg every 12 hours resulted in seizures (four patients) and myoclonia (one patient).[2] Symptoms developed in four patients within 1 day of starting the antibiotic. Seizures did not recur after discontinuing the antibiotic (three patients) or decreasing the dose or discontinuing the cyclosporine (two patients).

Because both drugs can cause CNS disturbances, additional controlled studies are needed to confirm the clinical importance of this interaction.

[1] Zazgornik J, et al. *Clin Nephrol.* 1986;26:265.
[2] Bosmuller C, et al. *Nephron.* 1991;58:362.

* Asterisk indicates drugs cited in interaction reports.

Cyclosporine — *Macrolide Antibiotics*

Cyclosporine	Macrolide Antibiotics	
Cyclosporine* (eg, *Neoral*)	Azithromycin* (*Zithromax*)	Erythromycin* (eg, *Ery-Tab*)
	Clarithromycin* (eg, *Biaxin*)	Troleandomycin*† (*Tao*)

Significance	Onset	Severity	Documentation
2	□ Rapid	□ Major	■ **Established**
	■ **Delayed**	■ **Moderate**	□ Probable
		□ Minor	□ Suspected
			□ Possible
			□ Unlikely

Effects Elevated CYCLOSPORINE (CSA) levels, increasing the risk of toxicity (nephrotoxicity, neurotoxicity), may occur.

Mechanism MACROLIDE ANTIBIOTICS may interfere with CSA metabolism and may increase rate and extent of absorption or reduce volume of distribution.[1-8]

Management Monitor CSA levels and serum creatinine and observe for toxicity; adjust CSA dose as needed.

Discussion

Erythromycin administration can increase CSA levels.[2-6,9-23] Peak CSA serum concentration occurred 4 hr after administration in 8 subjects receiving erythromycin.[5] Elevated serum CSA levels occurred with both oral and IV erythromycin,[2,17] with erythromycin base[16] with the ethylsuccinate and estolate,[5,15,18] and with doses as low as 250 mg twice daily. Increases in BUN, serum creatinine, or a decrease in Ccr indicated renal dysfunction.[2,4,11,15,18] Neurotoxicity has also been reported.[2] Similar effects have been reported with josamycin, rokitamycin, roxithromycin (none available in the US), clarithromycin, and troleandomycin; however, spiramycin (not available in the US) does not appear to interact.[7,24-28] Two case reports imply that azithromycin may interact with CSA.[29,30] However, a subsequent report in 6 patients noted no effect on CSA levels.[31]

1 Danan G, et al. *J Pharmacol Exper Ther.* 1981;218:509.
2 Gonwa TA, et al. *Transplantation.* 1986;41:797.
3 Aoki FY, et al. *Clin Pharmacol Ther.* 1987;41:221.
4 Wadhwa NK, et al. *Ther Drug Monit.* 1987;9:123.
5 Vereerstraeten P, et al. *Transplantation.* 1987;44:155.
6 Gupta SK, et al. *Br J Clin Pharmacol.* 1988;25:401.
7 Marre F, et al. *Br J Clin Pharmacol.* 1993;35:447.
8 Sketris IS, et al. *Pharmacotherapy.* 1996;16:301.
9 Ptachcinski RJ, et al. *N Engl J Med.* 1985;313:1416.
10 Kohan DE, et al. *N Engl J Med.* 1986;314:448.
11 Godin JR, et al. *Drug Intell Clin Pharm.* 1986;20:504-505.
12 Freeman DJ, et al. *Clin Pharmacol Ther.* 1986;39:193.
13 Grino JM, et al. *Ann Intern Med.* 1986;105:467.
14 Kessler M, et al. *Eur J Clin Pharmacol.* 1986;30:633.
15 Martell R, et al. *Ann Intern Med.* 1986;104:660.
16 Freeman DJ, et al. *Br J Clin Pharmacol.* 1987;23:776.
17 Harnett JD, et al. *Transplantation.* 1987;43:316.
18 Jensen CW, et al. *Transplantation.* 1987;43:263.
19 Murray BM, et al. *Transplantation.* 1987;43:602.
20 Ben-Ari J, et al. *J Pediatr.* 1988;112:992.
21 Lysz K, et al. *Transplant Proc.* 1988;20(suppl 2):543.
22 Gupta SK, et al. *Br J Clin Pharmacol.* 1989;27:475.
23 Koselj M, et al. *Transplant Proc.* 1994;26:2823.
24 Guillemain R, et al. *Eur J Clin Pharmacol.* 1989;36:97.
25 Vernillet L, et al. *Br J Clin Pharmacol.* 1989;27:789.
26 Ferrari SL, et al. *Transplantation.* 1994;58:725.
27 Treille S, et al. *Nephrol Dial Transplant.* 1996;11:1192.
28 Sádaba B, et al. *J Antimicrobial Chemother.* 1998;42:393.
29 Ljutic D, et al. *Nephron.* 1995;70:130.
30 Page RL, et al. *Pharmacotherapy.* 2001;21:1436.
31 Gomez E, et al. *Nephron.* 1996;73:724.

* Asterisk indicates drugs cited in interaction reports.
†Not available in the United States.

Cyclosporine — *Melphalan*

Cyclosporine*
(eg, *Neoral*)

Melphalan*
(*Alkeran*)

Significance	Onset	Severity	Documentation
4	□ Rapid	□ Major	□ Established
	■ **Delayed**	■ **Moderate**	□ Probable
		□ Minor	□ Suspected
			■ **Possible**
			□ Unlikely

Effects An increase in the toxicity of CYCLOSPORINE, particularly nephrotoxicity, has been observed following ANTINEOPLASTIC coadministration. The onset and duration of this interaction following addition of the ANTINEOPLASTIC agent has not been determined.

Mechanism Unknown.

Management When CYCLOSPORINE is to be used with ETOPOSIDE or following high-dose MELPHALAN, a lower CYCLOSPORINE dose may be necessary to avoid excessive toxicity. Plasma concentration monitoring and serum creatinine determinations may be helpful in aiding CYCLOSPORINE dosage adjustment.

Discussion

Only 2 brief reports exist to support these interactions. In 1 case report, a patient treated with cyclosporine and etoposide had a good response to his T-cell leukemia but developed severe CNS, renal, and hepatic toxicity.[1] In the second report of bone marrow transplant patients treated with high-dose melphalan followed by cyclosporine, 13 of 17 patients developed severe renal failure vs none of 7 patients not receiving this combination.[2]

[1] Kloke O, et al. *Klin Wochenschr.* 1985;63:1081.

[2] Morgenstern GR, et al. *Lancet.* 1982;2:1342.

* Asterisk indicates drugs cited in interaction reports.

Cyclosporine — *Methoxsalen*

Cyclosporine*
(eg, *Neoral*)

Methoxsalen*
(eg, *Oxsoralen-Ultra*)

Significance	Onset	Severity	Documentation
2	☐ Rapid	☐ Major	☐ Established
	■ **Delayed**	■ **Moderate**	☐ Probable
		☐ Minor	■ **Suspected**
			☐ Possible
			☐ Unlikely

Effects CYCLOSPORINE bioavailability may be elevated, increasing the risk of toxicity (eg, nephrotoxicity).

Mechanism Inhibition of CYCLOSPORINE intestinal metabolism (CYP3A4) by METHOXSALEN is suspected.

Management Monitor CYCLOSPORINE concentrations and for adverse reactions when METHOXSALEN is coadministered. Adjust the dose of CYCLOSPORINE as needed.

Discussion

The effects of methoxsalen on the pharmacokinetics of cyclosporine were studied in 12 healthy men.[1] In a randomized, crossover study, each subject received a single dose of cyclosporine microemulsion 200 mg, methoxsalen 40 mg, or coadministration of both drugs. Compared with receiving cyclosporine alone, coadministration of methoxsalen increased the mean AUC and mean C_{max} of cyclosporine 29% and 8%, respectively. In 2 subjects, the cyclosporine AUC increased 1.8- and 2.7-fold, respectively. Cyclosporine $t_{1/2}$ and time to reach peak concentrations were not affected. Cyclosporine did not affect the pharmacokinetics of methoxsalen.

Additional studies are needed to determine if more prolonged administration of these agents would affect cyclosporine hepatic metabolism.

[1] Rheeders M, et al. *J Clin Pharmacol.* 2006;46:768.

* Asterisk indicates drugs cited in interaction reports.

Cyclosporine — *Methylphenidate*

Cyclosporine* (eg, *Neoral*)	Methylphenidate* (eg, *Ritalin*)

Significance	Onset	Severity	Documentation
4	□ Rapid ■ **Delayed**	■ **Major** □ Moderate □ Minor	□ Established □ Probable □ Suspected ■ **Possible** □ Unlikely

Effects CYCLOSPORINE concentrations may be elevated, increasing the risk of toxicity.

Mechanism Unknown.

Management Monitor CYCLOSPORINE blood levels and serum creatinine. Observe the patient for toxicity. Be prepared to adjust the CYCLOSPORINE dose as needed.

Discussion

A possible drug interaction between cyclosporine and methylphenidate was reported in a 10-year-old boy with a heart transplant, attention deficit hyperactivity disorder, and oppositional defiant disorder.[1] His other medications consisted of azathioprine (eg, *Imuran*), prednisone (eg, *Deltasone*), dipyridamole (eg, *Persantine*), trimethoprim/sulfamethoxazole (eg, *Bactrim*), nifedipine (eg, *Procardia*), calcium carbonate, and aluminum-magnesium hydroxide. Prior to starting methylphenidate 5 mg twice daily, the cyclosporine dose was 550 mg/day (cyclosporine level 195 mcg/L). Four days after starting methylphenidate, the cyclosporine level increased to 302 mcg/L. The dose of cyclosporine was reduced to 500 mg/day and the dose of methylphenidate was increased to 7.5 mg twice daily. The cyclosporine level continued to be elevated, necessitating a dose reduction to 450 mg daily. Later, the methylphenidate dose was gradually increased to 20 mg twice daily without producing major changes in the cyclosporine level.

[1] Lewis BR, et al. *J Child Adolesc Psychopharmacol.* 2001;11:193.

* Asterisk indicates drugs cited in interaction reports.

Cyclosporine | *Metoclopramide*

Cyclosporine* (eg, *Neoral*)	Metoclopramide* (eg, *Reglan*)

Significance	Onset	Severity	Documentation
2	☐ Rapid ■ **Delayed**	☐ Major ■ **Moderate** ☐ Minor	☐ Established ☐ Probable ■ **Suspected** ☐ Possible ☐ Unlikely

Effects An increase in the immunosuppressive and toxic effects of CYCLOSPORINE may result with METOCLOPRAMIDE coadministration. The duration of this interaction once METOCLOPRAMIDE is withdrawn is currently unknown.

Mechanism It is postulated that the increase in gastric emptying time secondary to METOCLOPRAMIDE may allow for an increase in CYCLOSPORINE absorption.

Management When METOCLOPRAMIDE is added to or discontinued from CYCLOSPORINE therapy, frequent monitoring of the CYCLOSPORINE concentration is necessary.

Discussion

Only 1 well-controlled study supports this interaction. This trial studied 14 patients receiving cyclosporine before and after receiving concurrent metoclopramide.[1] A cyclosporine assay specific for the parent drug was used. The results revealed a 29% increase in the cyclosporine area under the curve when given with metoclopramide. It is currently unclear if this interaction would be reproducible with time. It is also unknown what degree of interaction would be observed with different doses or dosing schedules of metoclopramide. A separate study examining changes in cyclosporine bioavailability over time found a similar result in 1 patient receiving a different metoclopramide schedule.[2] This interaction has been proposed as a "positive" interaction, because it may allow a cyclosporine dosage reduction.

[1] Wadhwa NK, et al. *Transplant Proc.* 1987;19:1730.

[2] Morse GD, et al. *Clin Pharmacol Ther.* 1988;44:654.

* Asterisk indicates drugs cited in interaction reports.

Cyclosporine	***Metronidazole***
Cyclosporine* (eg, *Neoral*)	Metronidazole* (eg, *Flagyl*)

Significance	Onset	Severity	Documentation
4	□ Rapid ■ **Delayed**	□ Major ■ **Moderate** □ Minor	□ Established □ Probable □ Suspected ■ **Possible** □ Unlikely

Effects CYCLOSPORINE blood concentrations and the risk of toxicity may be increased.

Mechanism Possible inhibition of CYCLOSPORINE metabolism.

Management It may be necessary to adjust the dose of CYCLOSPORINE when starting, stopping, or changing the dose of METRONIDAZOLE. Monitor CYCLOSPORINE blood levels, and adjust the dose as needed.

Discussion

In a 43-year-old woman with a renal transplant, cyclosporine trough blood concentrations increased from 850 to 1930 ng/mL within 2 weeks of starting metronidazole 1500 mg/day and cimetidine (eg, *Tagamet*).[1] When cimetidine was discontinued and the dose of metronidazole was decreased to 1200 mg/day, cyclosporine blood levels ranged between 1200 to 1380 ng/mL. After stopping metronidazole treatment, cyclosporine trough whole blood concentrations ranged from 501 to 885 ng/mL. The temporal association indicates that metronidazole administration may have been responsible for the increase in cyclosporine trough whole blood concentrations. A 50-year-old man with a renal transplant was stable on an immunosuppressive regimen of azathioprine (eg, *Imuran*), prednisolone (eg, *Prelone*), and cyclosporine (125 mg twice daily).[2] He received metronidazole (400 mg 3 times daily) for terminal ileitis. Cyclosporine levels increased over 3 days from 134 to 264 mcg/L and serum creatinine increased to 0.19 mmol/L. When metronidazole was stopped, cyclosporine levels decreased to 120 mcg/L.

Controlled studies are needed to determine the clinical importance of this possible interaction.

[1] Zylber-Katz E, et al. *DICP*. 1988;22:504.

[2] Herzig K, et al. *Nephrol Dial Transplant*. 1999;14:521.

* Asterisk indicates drugs cited in interaction reports.

Cyclosporine — *Micafungin*

Cyclosporine* (eg, *Neoral*)	Micafungin* (*Mycamine*)

Significance	Onset	Severity	Documentation
2	☐ Rapid	☐ Major	☐ Established
	■ **Delayed**	■ **Moderate**	☐ Probable
		☐ Minor	■ **Suspected**
			☐ Possible
			☐ Unlikely

Effects CYCLOSPORINE whole-blood concentrations may be elevated, increasing the pharmacologic effects and adverse reactions.

Mechanism Suspected inhibition of CYCLOSPORINE metabolism (CYP3A) by MICAFUNGIN.

Management Monitor CYCLOSPORINE whole-blood concentrations and adjust the dosage as needed when MICAFUNGIN therapy is started or stopped.

Discussion

The effect of single-dose and steady-state administration of micafungin on the pharmacokinetics of cyclosporine was evaluated in 27 healthy volunteers.[1] Each subject received 3 oral doses of cyclosporine 5 mg/kg on study days 1, 9, and 15. A single 1-hour IV infusion of micafungin 100 mg was administered on study days 7, 9, and 11 through 15. Compared with administration of cyclosporine alone (study day 1), the apparent oral cyclosporine clearance was decreased 10.1% with single-dose administration of micafungin (study day 9) and 10.3% at steady-state micafungin administration (study day 15). In approximately 20% of the subjects, there was a clinically important increase in cyclosporine plasma whole-blood concentrations.

[1] Hebert MF, et al. *J Clin Pharmacol.* 2005;45(8):954.

* Asterisk indicates drugs cited in interaction reports.

Cyclosporine — *Mifepristone*

Cyclosporine*
(eg, *Neoral*)

Mifepristone*
(eg, *Korlym*)

Significance	Onset	Severity	Documentation
1	☐ Rapid ■ **Delayed**	■ **Major** ☐ Moderate ☐ Minor	☐ Established ☐ Probable ■ **Suspected** ☐ Possible ☐ Unlikely

Effects CYCLOSPORINE plasma concentrations may be elevated, increasing the pharmacologic effects and risk of adverse reactions.

Mechanism MIFEPRISTONE may inhibit CYCLOSPORINE metabolism (CYP3A4).

Management Coadministration of CYCLOSPORINE with MIFEPRISTONE is contraindicated.[1]

Discussion

Because mifepristone inhibits CYP3A4, coadministration of mifepristone with a drug that is metabolized mainly or solely by CYP3A4 (eg, cyclosporine) is likely to increase plasma concentrations of the drug.[1] Therefore, the concurrent use of drugs with a narrow therapeutic index that are CYP3A4 substrates, such as cyclosporine, is contraindicated. The risk of cyclosporine adverse reactions (eg, renal toxicity) may be increased.

[1] *Korlym* [package insert]. Menlo Park, CA: Corcept Therapeutics Incorporated; February 2012.

* Asterisk indicates drugs cited in interaction reports.

Cyclosporine — *Nefazodone*

Cyclosporine* (eg, *Neoral*)	Nefazodone*

Significance	Onset	Severity	Documentation
2	☐ Rapid ■ **Delayed**	☐ Major ■ **Moderate** ☐ Minor	☐ Established ■ **Probable** ☐ Suspected ☐ Possible ☐ Unlikely

Effects CYCLOSPORINE concentrations and toxicity may be increased.

Mechanism NEFAZODONE may inhibit the metabolism (CYP3A4) of CYCLOSPORINE.

Management Closely monitor CYCLOSPORINE trough whole-blood concentrations when NEFAZODONE is started or stopped. Adjust the dose of CYCLOSPORINE as needed.

Discussion

A 23-year-old male renal transplant patient was being treated for depression following a suicide attempt.[1] On admission to the inpatient psychiatry service, he was receiving cyclosporine 225 mg twice daily. Treatment with nefazodone 25 mg twice daily was initiated. Prior to nefazodone administration, the cyclosporine trough concentration was 122 ng/mL. Three days after starting nefazodone, the cyclosporine trough concentration increased to 204 ng/mL. Nefazodone was discontinued, and the cyclosporine concentration decreased to 123 ng/mL over the next 4 days. In a 50-year-old male renal transplant patient with stable renal function and a medication regimen that included cyclosporine 200 mg twice daily, the cyclosporine trough blood level increased from a baseline of 250 to 300 to 802 ng/mL after starting nefazodone 100 mg twice daily.[2] He experienced shakiness, headaches, tremor, and hypertension. In addition, his serum creatinine increased from 1.6 to 2.3 mg/dL. The dose of cyclosporine was reduced 50%, which resulted in normalization of his cyclosporine blood levels and renal function. A 58-year old woman on a stable cyclosporine dose was started on nefazodone 150 mg twice daily.[3] Thirteen days later, her cyclosporine levels increased from 78 ng/mL (before nefazodone administration) to 775 ng/mL. The patient experienced headache and fatigue.

[1] Helms-Smith KM, et al. *Ann Intern Med.* 1996;125(5):424.
[2] Vella JP, et al. *Am J Kidney Dis.* 1998;31(2):320.
[3] Wright DH, et al. *J Heart Lung Transplant.* 1999;18(9):913.

* Asterisk indicates drugs cited in interaction reports.

Cyclosporine — *Nicardipine*

Cyclosporine* (eg, *Neoral*)	Nicardipine* (eg, *Cardene*)

Significance	Onset	Severity	Documentation
2	□ Rapid	□ Major	□ Established
	■ **Delayed**	■ **Moderate**	□ Probable
		□ Minor	■ **Suspected**
			□ Possible
			□ Unlikely

Effects Increased CYCLOSPORINE trough blood levels, possibly associated with renal toxicity, may occur.

Mechanism NICARDIPINE is suspected to inhibit the hepatic metabolism of CYCLOSPORINE.

Management If coadministration of these drugs is necessary, monitor CYCLOSPORINE levels and renal function and observe the patient for evidence of toxicity. Adjust the dose of CYCLOSPORINE accordingly. Upon discontinuation of NICARDIPINE, the dose of CYCLOSPORINE may need to be increased to prevent rejection.

Discussion

After an observed rise in cyclosporine blood levels in a patient treated with nicardipine concomitantly, the data from 9 patients receiving both drugs were reviewed.[1] Cyclosporine trough levels increased 110% following the addition of nicardipine 20 mg 3 times daily to their treatment regimens. Before nicardipine administration, patients were receiving cyclosporine 254 mg/day, and trough cyclosporine blood levels were 226 ng/mL. During administration of nicardipine, patients received cyclosporine 243 mg/day. Trough cyclosporine blood levels were 430 ng/mL. Because patients had been receiving cyclosporine for 0.5 to 14 months, the difference could not be explained by the increase in cyclosporine bioavailability observed upon initiation of immunosuppressive therapy. In a study of 8 patients, cyclosporine C_{max} increased from 94 to 341 ng/mL on days 1 to 30 after the initiation of nicardipine treatment.[2] Nicardipine therapy was started 3 to 36 weeks after transplantation. Serum creatinine increased in 1 patient. In a retrospective study, the mean daily dose of cyclosporine decreased from 5.1 to 3.9 mg/kg, and the trough plasma cyclosporine concentration increased from 53.4 to 70.3 ng/mL in 21 renal transplant patients 10 weeks after the start of nicardipine therapy.[3] No change was observed in renal function. In 20 of 21 patients, there was a mean increase of 77% in cyclosporine plasma levels following the addition of nicardipine to their previously stable regimen.[4] There was no evidence of renal toxicity.

1 Bourbigot B, et al. *Lancet*. 1986;1(8495):1447.
2 Cantarovich M, et al. *Clin Nephrol*. 1987;28(4):190.
3 Kessler M, et al. *Eur J Clin Pharmacol*. 1989;36(6):637.
4 Guan D, et al. *Transplant Proc*. 1996;28(3):1311.

* Asterisk indicates drugs cited in interaction reports.

Cyclosporine — *NNRT Inhibitors*

Cyclosporine* (eg, *Neoral*)	Efavirenz* (*Sustiva*)	Nevirapine (*Viramune*)

Significance	Onset	Severity	Documentation
4	☐ Rapid ■ **Delayed**	☐ Major ■ **Moderate** ☐ Minor	☐ Established ☐ Probable ☐ Suspected ■ **Possible** ☐ Unlikely

Effects CYCLOSPORINE concentrations may be reduced, decreasing the pharmacologic effect.

Mechanism Induction of CYCLOSPORINE metabolism (CYP3A4) by NON-NUCLEOSIDE TRANSCRIPTASE (NNRT) INHIBITORS is suspected.

Management In patients receiving CYCLOSPORINE, closely monitor CYCLOSPORINE concentrations and serum creatinine when NNRT INHIBITORS are started or stopped. Be prepared to adjust the CYCLOSPORINE dose as needed.

Discussion

A 39-year-old male renal transplant patient, newly diagnosed as HIV-positive, experienced a decrease in cyclosporine levels after starting efavirenz.[1] The patient had a past history of depression and hypertension. He was receiving nefazodone, nifedipine (eg, *Procardia XL*), and metoprolol (eg, *Lopressor*). After receiving a living-related kidney transplant for end-stage renal disease, the patient was given prednisone and cyclosporine (200 mg twice daily) for rejection prophylaxis. At this dose, the mean cyclosporine level was 328 mcg/L. The patient was admitted to the hospital for fever of unknown cause, weight loss, general malaise, and worsening fatigue (cyclosporine level 307 mcg/L). Treatment with IV ciprofloxacin (eg, *Cipro*) was started. Three days after admission, the cyclosporine levels increased to 372 mcg/L. The cyclosporine dose was reduced to 175 mg twice daily. The cyclosporine concentrations gradually decreased to 203 mcg/L. Nefazodone was discontinued and efavirenz (600 mg at bedtime), zidovudine (eg, *Retrovir*), and lamivudine (*Epivir*) were started. Approximately 7 days after starting efavirenz, cyclosporine levels decreased to 80 mcg/L. The cyclosporine dose was increased to 200 mg twice daily, and then changed to a maintenance dose of 175 mg twice daily. One month later, the cyclosporine level reached a nadir of 50 mcg/L. Two years later, the patient was doing extremely well on the same dose of medications.

[1] Tseng A, et al. *AIDS*. 2002;16(3):505.

* Asterisk indicates drugs cited in interaction reports. Based on pharmacologic and pharmacokinetic considerations, similar interactions may occur with other drugs that are listed.

Cyclosporine — *NSAIDs*

Cyclosporine	NSAIDs	
Cyclosporine* (eg, *Neoral*)	Diclofenac* (eg, *Cataflam*)	Mefenamic Acid (eg, *Ponstel*)
	Etodolac (eg, *Lodine*)	Meloxicam (*Mobic*)
	Fenoprofen (eg, *Nalfon*)	Nabumetone (eg, *Relafen*)
	Flurbiprofen (eg, *Ansaid*)	Naproxen (eg, *Naprosyn*)
	Ibuprofen (eg, *Motrin*)	Oxaprozin (eg, *Daypro*)
	Indomethacin (eg, *Indocin*)	Piroxicam (eg, *Feldene*)
	Ketoprofen (eg, *Orudis*)	Sulindac* (eg, *Clinoril*)
	Ketorolac (eg, *Toradol*)	Tolmetin (eg, *Tolectin*)
	Meclofenamate	

Significance	Onset	Severity	Documentation
4	■ **Rapid**	□ Major	□ Established
	□ Delayed	■ **Moderate**	□ Probable
		□ Minor	□ Suspected
			■ **Possible**
			□ Unlikely

Effects The nephrotoxicity of both agents may be increased.

Mechanism Unknown (see Discussion).

Management Frequent monitoring of renal function may be necessary.

Discussion

Two patients experienced decreased renal function during coadministration of cyclosporine (CSA) with either diclofenac or sulindac.[1] Renal impairment was independent of CSA whole blood levels and appeared to be caused by an increase in pharmacological effects associated with administration of both drugs. In 32 patients with rheumatoid arthritis, after CSA levels were stabilized, patients received acetaminophen (eg, *Tylenol*) and at least 1 NSAID (eg, indomethacin, ketoprofen, sulindac) during subsequent 4-week treatment periods.[5] No changes in renal function were detected. In a report of CSA and diclofenac use in 20 patients with severe rheumatoid arthritis, 7 patients appeared to experience renal function impairment.[2] Discontinuing diclofenac corrected renal function. The interaction was suspected in 9 other patients. In 24 healthy volunteers, the pharmacokinetics of CSA were not changed during concurrent use of diclofenac.[3] Decreases in renal function appear to be independent of changes in whole blood CSA levels. If the decrease is related to CSA, causing renal function to become prostaglandin-dependent, inhibition of prostaglandin by any NSAID could decrease renal function. Additional studies have documented increases in diclofenac bioavailability by CSA.[4] Whether this is responsible for the decrease in renal function has not been determined.

[1] Harris KP, et al. *Transplantation.* 1988;46:598.
[2] Branthwaite JP, et al. *Lancet.* 1991;337:252.
[3] Mueller EA, et al. *J Clin Pharmacol.* 1993;33:936.
[4] Kovarik JM, et al. *J Clin Pharmacol.* 1997;37:336.
[5] Tugwell P, et al. *J Rheumatol.* 1997;24:1122.

* Asterisk indicates drugs cited in interaction reports. Based on pharmacologic and pharmacokinetic considerations, similar interactions may occur with other drugs that are listed.

Cyclosporine — *Omeprazole*

Cyclosporine* (eg, *Neoral*)	Omeprazole* (*Prilosec*)

Significance	Onset	Severity	Documentation
4	☐ Rapid ■ **Delayed**	☐ Major ■ **Moderate** ☐ Minor	☐ Established ☐ Probable ☐ Suspected ■ **Possible** ☐ Unlikely

Effects Increased, decreased, and unchanged CYCLOSPORINE levels have been reported.

Mechanism Inhibition of CYCLOSPORINE metabolism by OMEPRAZOLE is suspected.

Management If the combination cannot be avoided, monitor CYCLOSPORINE levels frequently when starting or stopping OMEPRAZOLE. Adjust the dose of CYCLOSPORINE accordingly.

Discussion

A possible drug interaction between cyclosporine and omeprazole was reported in a 44-year-old liver transplant patient.[1] After transplantation, the patient was treated with cyclosporine 130 mg twice daily and prednisolone (eg, *Prelone*) 10 mg/day. Whole-blood cyclosporine concentrations ranged between 187 and 261 ng/mL for 6 months. The patient was diagnosed with stage III erosive esophagitis, and omeprazole 40 mg/day was administered. Two weeks later, the cyclosporine level increased to 510 ng/mL. The dose of cyclosporine was decreased to 80 mg twice daily. The cyclosporine levels decreased to 171 ng/mL and remained constant during the 4 months of omeprazole administration. In a 32-year-old bone marrow transplant patient receiving cyclosporine 1.5 mg/kg IV twice daily, the addition of omeprazole 400 mg/day IV produced a progressive decline in cyclosporine concentrations (from 254 to 81 ng/mL).[2] Cyclosporine levels increased to 270 ng/mL within 4 days of stopping omeprazole. In a blinded, crossover study of 10 renal transplant patients stabilized on cyclosporine, addition of omeprazole 20 mg/day for 2 weeks did not alter cyclosporine blood levels.[3] Pantoprazole (*Protonix*) did not affect cyclosporine levels in transplant patients.[4,5]

Controlled studies are needed to clarify this possible interaction.

[1] Schouler L, et al. *Am J Gastroenterol.* 1991;86:1097.
[2] Arranz R, et al. *Am J Gastroenterol.* 1993;88:154.
[3] Blohmé I, et al. *Br J Clin Pharmacol.* 1993;35:156.
[4] Lorf T, et al. *Eur J Clin Pharmacol.* 2000;56:439.
[5] Lorf T, et al. *Eur J Clin Pharmacol.* 2000;55:733.

* Asterisk indicates drugs cited in interaction reports.

Cyclosporine — *Orlistat*

Cyclosporine* (eg, *Neoral*)	Orlistat* (*Xenical*)

Significance	Onset	Severity	Documentation
1	☐ Rapid ■ **Delayed**	■ **Major** ☐ Moderate ☐ Minor	☐ Established ■ **Probable** ☐ Suspected ☐ Possible ☐ Unlikely

Effects Whole blood CYCLOSPORINE concentrations may be decreased, possibly resulting in a decrease in the immunosuppressive action of CYCLOSPORINE.

Mechanism ORLISTAT may decrease absorption of CYCLOSPORINE.

Management Avoid ORLISTAT in patients receiving CYCLOSPORINE.

Discussion

In several case reports, cyclosporine levels have decreased after the introduction of orlistat.[1-5] The effect of orlistat on a nonmicroemulsion formulation of cyclosporine was studied in an obese patient who received a heart transplant because of ischemic cardiomyopathy.[1] Following his transplant, the patient was treated with cyclosporine 100 mg twice daily, azathioprine (eg, *Imuran*), and prednisone (eg, *Deltasone*). In addition, the patient was being treated for hyperlipidemia, hypertension, and hyperuricemia. His medication regimen had remained stable over the preceding 6 months. The patient also experienced weight gain (from 79.8 to 97 kg) and, because he felt depressed about his weight gain, his general practitioner started him on orlistat 120 mg 3 times daily without notifying the transplant center. Routine cyclosporine monitoring 2 weeks after starting orlistat indicated that cyclosporine whole blood levels had decreased 50% (from 101 to 50 ng/mL). The dose of cyclosporine was increased to 110 mg twice daily, but cyclosporine blood levels did not increase when measured 1 week later. Orlistat was discontinued and the cyclosporine level increased to 104 ng/mL. Plasma concentration-time kinetics of cyclosporine were measured following withdrawal of orlistat and 24 hours after its reinitiation. Subsequently, cyclosporine trough levels decreased 47% (from 98 to 52 ng/mL), the peak concentration decreased 86% (from 532 to 74 ng/mL), and the AUC decreased 75%. In 30 healthy volunteers, orlistat decreased the AUC of cyclosporine 34% but had no effect on the $t_{1/2}$.[6] The FDA has received at least 6 reports of transplant patients who had subtherapeutic cyclosporine blood levels shortly after starting orlistat therapy.[2]

[1] Nägele H, et al. *Eur J Clin Pharmacol.* 1999;55:667.
[2] Colman E, et al. *N Engl J Med.* 2000;342:1141.
[3] Le Beller C, et al. *Transplantation.* 2000;70:1541.
[4] Schnetzler B, et al. *Transplantation.* 2000;70:1540.
[5] Evans S, et al. *Am J Kidney Dis.* 2003;41:493.
[6] Zhi J, et al. *J Clin Pharmacol.* 2002;42:1011.

* Asterisk indicates drugs cited in interaction reports.

Cyclosporine — *Oxcarbazepine*

Cyclosporine* (eg, *Neoral*)	Oxcarbazepine* (*Trileptal*)

Significance	Onset	Severity	Documentation
4	☐ Rapid	☐ Major	☐ Established
	■ **Delayed**	■ **Moderate**	☐ Probable
		☐ Minor	☐ Suspected
			■ **Possible**
			☐ Unlikely

Effects CYCLOSPORINE concentrations may be decreased, reducing the pharmacologic effect.

Mechanism Induction of hepatic microsomal enzyme metabolism (CYP3A) of CYCLOSPORINE by OXCARBAZEPINE is suspected.

Management Monitor CYCLOSPORINE trough levels and observe patient's clinical response when starting or stopping OXCARBAZEPINE. Adjust the CYCLOSPORINE dose as needed.

Discussion

The influence of oxcarbazepine on cyclosporine trough concentrations was studied in a renal transplant recipient with epilepsy.[1] The patient was a 32-year-old man with a history of drug-resistant epilepsy. When oxcarbazepine was added to the patient's drug regimen, he was receiving allopurinol (eg, *Zyloprim*), cyclosporine (270 mg/day), doxepin (eg, *Sinequan*), gabapentin (*Neurontin*), levothyroxine (eg, *Synthroid*), pravastatin (*Pravachol*), prednisone (eg, *Deltasone*), and valproate (eg, *Depakote*). Also, mycophenolate mofetil (*CellCept*) was added to ensure effective immunosuppression in the event of a sudden decrease in cyclosporine trough concentration. Cyclosporine trough levels decreased to below the lower limit of the therapeutic range (100 ng/L) 14 days after starting oxcarbazepine. Two days later, the cyclosporine trough concentration was 87 ng/L, and the dose of cyclosporine was increased to 290 mg/day. Because of a decrease in serum sodium levels, the dose of oxcarbazepine was reduced from 750 to 600 mg/day. At this time, cyclosporine trough concentrations remained stable.

Additional studies are needed to determine the clinical importance of this interaction.

[1] Rösche J, et al. *Clin Neuropharmacol.* 2001;24:113.

* Asterisk indicates drugs cited in interaction reports.

Cyclosporine — *Penicillins*

Cyclosporine* (eg, *Neoral*)	Nafcillin*

Significance	Onset	Severity	Documentation
4	☐ Rapid ■ **Delayed**	■ **Major** ☐ Moderate ☐ Minor	☐ Established ☐ Probable ☐ Suspected ■ **Possible** ☐ Unlikely

Effects Increased and decreased whole-blood CYCLOSPORINE concentrations have been reported during coadministration of NAFCILLIN.

Mechanism See discussion.

Management Consider giving an alternative antibiotic for NAFCILLIN in the treatment of, or prophylaxis against, staphylococcal infection in patients receiving CYCLOSPORINE.

Discussion

Reports of an interaction between cyclosporine and nafcillin are conflicting. A retrospective investigation was conducted as a result of observing renal function deterioration in patients with lung transplants receiving cyclosporine and a prophylactic triple-antibiotic regimen consisting of nafcillin, cefuroxime (eg, *Zinacef*), and erythromycin (eg, *Ery-Tab*).[1] All patients received immunosuppressive therapy with azathioprine (eg, *Imuran*), prednisone (eg, *Deltasone*), and cyclosporine 10 mg/kg twice daily. The dose was adjusted to keep whole-blood monoclonal radioimmunoassay between 400 and 500 ng/mL. In addition, 9 patients received prophylactic nafcillin, while 10 patients did not. Patients receiving nafcillin experienced a progressive increase in serum creatinine. No change was seen in patients who did not receive nafcillin. Three patients in the nafcillin group required hemodialysis compared with none of the patients who did not receive nafcillin. There were no differences in cyclosporine concentrations between the 2 groups of patients, except on posttransplant day 5 when cyclosporine levels were lower in the nafcillin group. Nafcillin-induced interstitial nephritis or true renal insufficiency, rather than cyclosporine nephrotoxicity resulting from a drug interaction, was not ruled out as a cause of the reaction in this study. Although serum creatinine was measured, it is not possible to determine the cause of the reactions because renal biopsy results, serum blood urea levels, and creatinine clearance were not reported. The finding of this study is in contrast to that reported in a 34-year-old woman who underwent a successful living-related donor renal transplant.[2] Immunosuppression consisted of cyclosporine and prednisone. On 2 separate occasions, whole-blood cyclosporine levels decreased after the patient received nafcillin, then increased again when the antibiotic was discontinued. In the first instance, the cyclosporine trough level decreased from 229 to 68 ng/mL after 7 days of nafcillin treatment. On the second occurrence, the cyclosporine trough concentration decreased from 272 to 42 ng/mL by day 9 of nafcillin treatment.

[1] Jahansouz F, et al. *Transplantation.* 1993;55:1045.

[2] Veremis SA, et al. *Transplantation.* 1987;43:913.

* Asterisk indicates drugs cited in interaction reports.

Cyclosporine — *Pomelo Juice*

Cyclosporine* (eg, *Neoral*)	Pomelo Juice*

Significance	Onset	Severity	Documentation
4	☐ Rapid ■ **Delayed**	☐ Major ■ **Moderate** ☐ Minor	☐ Established ☐ Probable ☐ Suspected ■ **Possible** ☐ Unlikely

Effects CYCLOSPORINE bioavailability may be increased, increasing the pharmacologic and adverse effects.

Mechanism POMELO JUICE may inhibit CYCLOSPORINE metabolism (CYP3A4 and/or P-glycoprotein) in the gut wall.

Management Until more data are available, advise patients taking CYCLOSPORINE to avoid POMELO JUICE.

Discussion

In an open-label, randomized, crossover study, 12 healthy men received a single oral dose of cyclosporine 200 mg with 240 mL of pomelo juice, cranberry juice, or water under fasting conditions.[1] Compared with water, pomelo juice increased the AUC and C_{max} of cyclosporine 18.9% and 12.1%, respectively. In contrast, cranberry juice did not affect the pharmacokinetics of cyclosporine.

[1] Grenier J, et al. *Clin Pharmacol Ther.* 2006;79:255.

* Asterisk indicates drugs cited in interaction reports.

Cyclosporine — *Probucol*

Cyclosporine* (eg, *Neoral*)	Probucol*†

Significance	Onset	Severity	Documentation
2	□ Rapid ■ **Delayed**	□ Major ■ **Moderate** □ Minor	□ Established □ Probable ■ **Suspected** □ Possible □ Unlikely

Effects Whole blood CYCLOSPORINE concentrations may be reduced, producing a decrease in clinical effect.

Mechanism Reduced bioavailability is suspected.

Management Monitor CYCLOSPORINE concentrations and observe the clinical response of the patient when PROBUCOL is started or stopped in patients receiving CYCLOSPORINE.

Discussion

The effects of probucol on cyclosporine concentrations were investigated in two studies involving 10 renal and 6 heart transplant patients.[1,2] The renal transplant patients had been treated with cyclosporine for at least 6 months.[2] To be included in the study, it was necessary for patients to have been receiving probucol for at least 8 weeks because of the slow distribution of probucol. Other immunosuppressive therapy included azathioprine (eg, *Imuran*) and prednisone (eg, *Deltasone*). During the investigation, patients continued to receive probucol for the first 5 weeks of a 15-week trial and blood samples were collected. Probucol was then discontinued until the end of the study. After stopping probucol, no blood samples were obtained for 5 weeks to allow elimination of the drug. Blood samples were again collected during the last 5 weeks of cyclosporine administration in the absence of probucol. A significant increase in the whole blood cyclosporine concentrations was observed when cyclosporine was taken without probucol ($p = 0.02$) compared with when probucol was administered concurrently. These findings are in agreement with an earlier evaluation of the effects of probucol on cyclosporine concentrations.[1] In six heart transplant patients, there was a 40% decrease in the availability of cyclosporine during administration of probucol compared with giving cyclosporine alone.

1 Sundararajan V, et al. *Transplant Proc.* 1991;23:2028.

2 Gallego C, et al. *Ann Pharmacother.* 1994;28:940.

* Asterisk indicates drugs cited in interaction reports.
† Not available in the US.

Cyclosporine — *Propafenone*

Cyclosporine* (eg, *Neoral*)	Propafenone* (*Rythmol*)

Significance	Onset	Severity	Documentation
4	■ **Rapid**	□ Major	□ Established
	□ Delayed	■ **Moderate**	□ Probable
		□ Minor	□ Suspected
			■ **Possible**
			□ Unlikely

Effects Increased whole blood CYCLOSPORINE trough levels and decreased renal function may occur.

Mechanism Unknown. However, interference with CYCLOSPORINE metabolism or increased CYCLOSPORINE absorption produced by PROPAFENONE may be involved.

Management Consider monitoring renal function and CYCLOSPORINE levels during coadministration of PROPAFENONE.

Discussion

Increased cyclosporine levels and decreased renal function occurred in a 51-year-old cardiac transplant recipient during coadministration of cyclosporine and propafenone. The patient was receiving cyclosporine 240 mg/day, prednisone (eg, *Deltasone*) 7.5 mg/day and azathioprine (eg, *Imuran*) 75 mg/day. Stable whole blood cyclosporine trough levels were 450 ng/mL. Nine months after transplantation, the patient developed nonsustained ventricular tachycardia; treatment with propafenone 750 mg/day was initiated. Therapy successfully suppressed the arrhythmia; however, within 24 hours whole blood cyclosporine trough levels increased dramatically (to approximately 750 ng/mL). Simultaneously with the increases in cyclosporine levels, serum creatinine increased from 1.9 to 2.4 mg/dL. Reducing the cyclosporine dosage to 160 mg/day resulted in a decrease in both the cyclosporine and the serum creatinine levels. Whole blood cyclosporine trough levels of 400 to 450 ng/mL were maintained with 200 mg/day of cyclosporine during coadministration of 600 mg/day of propafenone. Additional studies are needed to determine the clinical significance of this possible interaction.[1]

[1] Spes CH, et al. *Klin Wochenschr.* 1990;68:872.

* Asterisk indicates drugs cited in interaction reports.

Cyclosporine — *Protease Inhibitors*

Cyclosporine	Protease Inhibitors	
Cyclosporine* (eg, *Neoral*)	Amprenavir* (*Agenerase*)	Nelfinavir (*Viracept*)
	Fosamprenavir* (*Lexiva*)	Ritonavir* (*Norvir*)
	Indinavir (*Crixivan*)	Saquinavir* (*Invirase*)

Significance	Onset	Severity	Documentation
4	☐ Rapid	☐ Major	☐ Established
	■ **Delayed**	■ **Moderate**	☐ Probable
		☐ Minor	☐ Suspected
			■ **Possible**
			☐ Unlikely

Effects Elevated concentrations of CYCLOSPORINE with increased risk of toxicity may occur. It is also possible that PROTEASE INHIBITOR concentrations may be increased. Increased concentrations of these agents may occur within 3 days of concurrent therapy.

Mechanism Possible inhibition of metabolism (CYP3A4) of either agent.

Management Monitor CYCLOSPORINE concentrations and serum creatinine when a PROTEASE INHIBITOR is started or stopped. Monitor the clinical response to the PROTEASE INHIBITOR. It may be necessary to reduce the dose of one or both drugs during coadministration.

Discussion

Cyclosporine and saquinavir concentrations were measured in an HIV-positive renal transplant patient.[1] The patient had been receiving cyclosporine, prednisone (eg, *Deltasone*), zidovudine (eg, *Retrovir*), and lamivudine (*Epivir*). At a dose of cyclosporine 150 mg twice daily, trough cyclosporine concentrations were stable at 150 to 200 mcg/L. Saquinavir 1,200 mg 3 times daily was added to the patient's drug regimen. Within 3 days of starting saquinavir, the patient reported fatigue, headache, and GI discomfort. At this time, the cyclosporine trough concentration increased to 580 mcg/L. The dose of cyclosporine was decreased to 75 mg twice daily, and the dose of saquinavir was decreased to 600 mg 3 times daily. The patient's symptoms subsided. The AUC of cyclosporine 75 mg twice daily during saquinavir administration was 90% of the AUC value measured when cyclosporine 150 mg twice daily was given alone. The AUC of saquinavir was 4.3 times greater than the average value observed in 5 control patients who were receiving saquinavir 600 mg twice daily without cyclosporine and 11.1 times greater than the value reported in the literature. In 2 patients receiving cyclosporine for orthotopic liver transplantation, marked elevations in cyclosporine concentration occurred when the patients were given amprenavir/ritonavir or fosamprenavir.[2] In both cases, it was necessary to reduce the cyclosporine dose.

[1] Brinkman K, et al. *Ann Intern Med.* 1998;129:914.
[2] Guaraldi G, et al. *Transplant Proc.* 2006;38:1138.

* Asterisk indicates drugs cited in interaction reports. Based on pharmacologic and pharmacokinetic considerations, similar interactions may occur with other drugs that are listed.

Cyclosporine — *Pyrazinamide*

Cyclosporine* (eg, *Neoral*)	Pyrazinamide*

Significance	Onset	Severity	Documentation
4	□ Rapid ■ **Delayed**	■ **Major** □ Moderate □ Minor	□ Established □ Probable □ Suspected ■ **Possible** □ Unlikely

Effects Whole blood CYCLOSPORINE concentrations may be decreased, possibly resulting in a decrease in the immunosuppressive action of CYCLOSPORINE.

Mechanism Unknown.

Management Consider monitoring CYCLOSPORINE concentrations during PYRAZINAMIDE coadministration and observing the patient for signs of reduced immunosuppression. If an interaction is suspected, adjust the dose of CYCLOSPORINE as needed.

Discussion

A case report indicates that pyrazinamide administration may decrease cyclosporine levels.[1] A 28-year-old man with renal failure due to interstitial nephritis underwent cadaveric renal transplantation. His immunosuppression therapy included prednisone (eg, *Deltasone*), azathioprine (eg, *Imuran*), and low-dose cyclosporine 5 mg/kg/day. The patient was well until 13 months after the transplant when miliary tuberculosis was diagnosed. The patient was treated with isoniazid (eg, *Nydrazid*) 300 mg/day, rifampin (eg, *Rimactane*) 600 mg/day, and ethambutol (*Myambutol*) 1,200 mg/day. The cyclosporine dose was increased to 8.3 mg/kg/day after starting treatment for tuberculosis. The patient did not improve, and pyrazinamide was started at a dose of 15 mg/kg/day (cyclosporine whole blood level, 90 ng/mL). Within 2 days, cyclosporine levels decreased to 53 ng/mL. After the daily dose of cyclosporine was increased to 9.3 mg/kg, the cyclosporine concentration increased to 94 ng/mL. The dose of pyrazinamide was gradually increased to 30 mg/kg/day, and the dose of cyclosporine was increased to 11.5 mg/kg/day. The patient completed a 14-week course of treatment with pyrazinamide. Pyrazinamide was discontinued, and the cyclosporine dose was reduced to 8.2 mg/kg/day. At that time, the patient was receiving cyclosporine 10 mg/kg/day (mean whole blood cyclosporine level, 322 ng/mL). Four days later, the trough cyclosporine blood concentration was 159 ng/mL. Although isoniazid may decrease cyclosporine concentrations by decreasing absorption of the immunosuppressive agent and rifampin may decrease cyclosporine levels by increasing metabolism, pyrazinamide appears to further decrease cyclosporine concentrations. See also Cyclosporine-Rifamycins.

[1] Jiménez del Cerro LA, et al. *Nephron*. 1992;62:113.

* Asterisk indicates drugs cited in interaction reports.

Cyclosporine — *Quercetin*

Cyclosporine* (eg, *Sandimmune*)	Quercetin*

Significance	Onset	Severity	Documentation
4	☐ Rapid ■ **Delayed**	☐ Major ■ **Moderate** ☐ Minor	☐ Established ☐ Probable ☐ Suspected ■ **Possible** ☐ Unlikely

Effects CYCLOSPORINE concentrations may be elevated, increasing the risk of adverse effects.

Mechanism Unknown.

Management Patients taking CYCLOSPORINE should avoid QUERCETIN. If QUERCETIN administration cannot be avoided, closely monitor CYCLOSPORINE concentrations when QUERCETIN is started or stopped. Adjust the CYCLOSPORINE dosage as needed.

Discussion

The effects of the bioflavonoids in quercetin on the pharmacokinetics of oral cyclosporine were studied in 8 healthy men.[1] Quercetin is present as glycosides in apples, berries, ginkgo, grapefruit, onions, red wine, and tea. In the United States, one preparation is derived from eucalyptus and is available without a prescription. The absolute bioavailability of cyclosporine was determined after giving a 100 mg IV infusion. Subjects received an oral dose of cyclosporine 300 mg (1) alone (control group), (2) simultaneously with quercetin 5 mg/kg, (3) 30 minutes after taking quercetin 5 mg/kg, and (4) after receiving quercetin 5 mg/kg twice daily for 3 days. Administration of cyclosporine 30 minutes after taking quercetin and after receiving quercetin for 3 days increased cyclosporine whole blood concentrations compared with taking cyclosporine alone. The AUC and the C_{max} of cyclosporine were also higher in these treatment groups compared with taking cyclosporine alone. Compared with the control group, the $t_{1/2}$ of cyclosporine was longer in subjects pretreated with quercetin for 3 days. The bioavailability of cyclosporine was approximately 36% in the control group, compared with 49% in subjects receiving cyclosporine and quercetin together, and 54% after 3 days of pretreatment with quercetin.

[1] Choi JS, et al. *Am J Health Syst Pharm.* 2004;61(22):2406.

* Asterisk indicates drugs cited in interaction reports.

Cyclosporine | *Quinolones*

Cyclosporine*	Quinolones	
Cyclosporine* (eg, *Neoral*)	Ciprofloxacin* (eg, *Cipro*)	Norfloxacin* (*Noroxin*)
	Levofloxacin* (*Levaquin*)	

Significance	Onset	Severity	Documentation
4	☐ Rapid	☐ Major	☐ Established
	■ **Delayed**	■ **Moderate**	☐ Probable
		☐ Minor	☐ Suspected
			■ **Possible**
			☐ Unlikely

Effects Possible increased CYCLOSPORINE (CSA) toxicity.[1,2]

Mechanism Inhibition of CSA metabolism (CYP3A4) is suspected.[3]

Management If renal function decreases or CSA concentrations increase, consider an alternative antimicrobial.

Discussion

Case reports have been equivocal.[4] Increased renal function impairment occurred in a 52-year-old renal transplant patient during administration of CSA and ciprofloxacin.[5] On day 6 of therapy, serum creatinine rose from a baseline of 1.6 to 2.1 mg/dL and to 2.3 mg/dL after 2 wk. Ciprofloxacin was stopped; 2 days later, creatinine fell to 1.6 mg/dL. There was no sign of infection and CSA whole-blood trough levels were satisfactory. Serum creatinine increased from 1.4 to 2.2 mg/dL 4 days after starting ciprofloxacin in a 58-year-old patient stabilized on CSA therapy.[6] Ciprofloxacin was discontinued, and, by day 8, the serum creatinine peaked at 14.1 mg/dL without increased CSA levels. Trough serum CSA levels increased from approximately 200 to approximately 400 ng/mL 2 days after the addition of norfloxacin to the drug regimen of a 57-year-old cardiac transplant patient.[7] In pediatric renal transplant patients, 5 children given CSA and norfloxacin required lower doses of CSA at discharge than 6 children not given norfloxacin.[3] In 2 patients, CSA levels markedly increased after therapy when ciprofloxacin was started.[8] Renal function deteriorated in 1 patient. Compared with patients receiving CSA alone, an increased incidence of rejection occurred in patients receiving ciprofloxacin in the 6 mo following renal transplantation.[9] Conversely, in 6 patients receiving norfloxacin[1] and 10 patients receiving ciprofloxacin,[10] neither drug affected CSA levels or renal function. In 39 renal transplant recipients, ofloxacin oral therapy did not impair renal graft function or interact with CSA.[11] In a study in 14 healthy volunteers, levofloxacin did not affect CSA pharmacokinetics[12]; however, in transplant patients receiving CSA microemulsion, levofloxacin inhibited CSA metabolism.[13] Moxifloxacin did not affect cyclosporine levels in 11 kidney transplant patients.[14]

[1] Jadoul M, et al. *Transplantation.* 1989;47(4):747.
[2] Tan KK, et al. *Br J Clin Pharmacol.* 1989;28(2):185.
[3] McLellan RA, et al. *Clin Pharmacol Ther.* 1995;58(3):322.
[4] Hoey LL, et al. *Ann Pharmacother.* 1994;28(1):93.
[5] Elston RA, et al. *J Antimicrob Chemother.* 1988;21(5):679.
[6] Avent CK, et al. *Am J Med.* 1988;85(3):452.
[7] Thomson DJ, et al. *Transplantation.* 1988;46(2):312.
[8] Nasir M, et al. *Nephron.* 1991;57(2):245.
[9] Wrishko RE, et al. *Transplantation.* 1997;64(7):996.
[10] Krüger HU, et al. *Antimicrob Agents Chemother.* 1990;34(6):1048.
[11] Vogt P, et al. *Infection.* 1988;16(3):175.
[12] Doose DR, et al. *J Clin Pharmacol.* 1998;38(1):90.
[13] Federico S, et al. *Clin Pharmacokinet.* 2006;45(2):169.
[14] Capone D, et al. *J Clin Pharmacol.* 2010;50(5):576.

* Asterisk indicates drugs cited in interaction reports.

Cyclosporine — *Red Wine*

Cyclosporine* (eg, *Sandimmune*)	Red Wine*

Significance	Onset	Severity	Documentation
4	☐ Rapid ■ **Delayed**	☐ Major ■ **Moderate** ☐ Minor	☐ Established ☐ Probable ☐ Suspected ■ **Possible** ☐ Unlikely

Effects CYCLOSPORINE concentrations may be reduced, decreasing the pharmacologic effect and increasing the risk of rejection of organ transplants.

Mechanism Unknown.

Management Until more information is available, patients taking CYCLOSPORINE should avoid ingestion of RED WINE. If a patient does ingest RED WINE, monitor CYCLOSPORINE levels and be prepared to adjust the CYCLOSPORINE dose.

Discussion

The effects of red wine (a merlot) on the pharmacokinetics of cyclosporine were investigated in 12 healthy subjects.[1] In a 2-way crossover study, each subject received a single dose of cyclosporine 8 mg/kg with water or 12 oz of red wine. The red wine was consumed as two 6 oz portions, the first portion 15 minutes prior to cyclosporine administration and the second portion with the cyclosporine and during the 15 minutes after dosing. Compared with water, red wine increased the oral clearance of cyclosporine 50%, decreased the AUC approximately 30%, and decreased the peak concentration 38% (from 1,258 to 779 mcg/L). The majority of the decrease in the AUC occurred in the initial portion of the AUC. Also, red wine ingestion doubled the time for cyclosporine to reach the peak concentration, compared with water. There was no change in the elimination $t_{1/2}$.

Because white wine does not affect cyclosporine pharmacokinetics, the mechanism does not appear to involve the alcohol contained in red wine. Also, this study involved administration of the standard formulation of cyclosporine (eg, *Sandimmune*); therefore, the results should not be extrapolated to other formulations of cyclosporine (eg, *Neoral*).

[1] Tsunoda SM, et al. *Clin Pharmacol Ther.* 2001;70:462.

* Asterisk indicates drugs cited in interaction reports.

Cyclosporine — *Rifamycins*

Cyclosporine	Rifamycins	
Cyclosporine* (eg, *Neoral*)	Rifabutin* (*Mycobutin*)	Rifapentine (*Priftin*)
	Rifampin* (eg, *Rifadin*)	

Significance	Onset	Severity	Documentation
1	☐ Rapid	■ **Major**	☐ Established
	■ **Delayed**	☐ Moderate	■ **Probable**
		☐ Minor	☐ Suspected
			☐ Possible
			☐ Unlikely

Effects The immunosuppressive effects of CYCLOSPORINE may be reduced. This appears to occur as early as 2 days following the initiation of RIFAMYCINS and may persist for 1 to 3 weeks after discontinuation.

Mechanism Increased hepatic and intestinal metabolism (CYP3A4) of CYCLOSPORINE induced by RIFAMYCINS.[1]

Management Increased doses of CYCLOSPORINE may be necessary during concomitant RIFAMYCIN therapy. Frequent monitoring of CYCLOSPORINE concentrations and serum creatinine is required during RIFAMYCIN therapy and following its discontinuation. Avoid this combination if possible.

Discussion

In many of the patients receiving rifampin, cyclosporine concentrations decreased to below the detection limit of the assay.[2-6] Despite large dosage increases, it was difficult to maintain therapeutic cyclosporine concentrations in many of these patients while they were receiving rifampin.[2,6-12] The majority of case reports documenting this interaction also report rejection episodes, 1 resulting in fatality, associated with these marked decreases in cyclosporine concentrations.[2,4,5,7,9,13,14] In a 10-year-old bone marrow transplant patient, it was necessary to increase the IV cyclosporin dose 2.5-fold (from 90 to 225 mg every 12 hr) in order to maintain therapeutic levels during coadministration of IV rifampin.[6] However, successful coadministration of cyclosporine and rifampin can be achieved by careful monitoring of the patient and by adjusting the cyclosporine dosage.[14-16] Rifabutin, chemically related to rifampin, may affect cyclosporine disposition to a lesser extent.[16]

1 Hebert MF, et al. *Clin Pharmacol Ther.* 1992;52:453.
2 Langhoff E, et al. *Lancet.* 1983;2:1031.
3 Daniels NJ, et al. *Lancet.* 1984;2:639.
4 *Lancet.* 1985;1:1342.
5 Allen RD, et al. *Lancet.* 1985;1:980.
6 Zelunka EJ. *Pharmacotherapy.* 2002;22:387.
7 Howard P, et al. *Drug Intell Clin Pharm.* 1985;19:763.
8 Cassidy MJ, et al. *Nephron.* 1985;41:207.
9 Offermann G, et al. *Am J Nephrol.* 1985;5:385.
10 Wandel C, et al. *J Cardiothorac Vasc Anesth.* 1995;9:621.
11 Capone D, et al. *Int J Clin Pharmacol Res.* 1996;16:73.
12 Freitag VL, et al. *Ann Pharmacother.* 1999;33:871.
13 Van Buren D, et al. *Transplant Proc.* 1984;16:1642.
14 Koselj M, et al. *Transplant Proc.* 1994;26:2823
15 al-Sulaiman MH, et al. *Transplantation.* 1990;50:597.
16 Vandevelde C, et al. *Pharmacotherapy.* 1991;11:88.

* Asterisk indicates drugs cited in interaction reports. Based on pharmacologic and pharmacokinetic considerations, similar interactions may occur with other drugs that are listed.

Cyclosporine — *Serotonin Reuptake Inhibitors*

Cyclosporine	Serotonin Reuptake Inhibitors	
Cyclosporine* (eg, *Neoral*)	Fluoxetine* (eg, *Prozac*)	Paroxetine (*Paxil*)
	Fluvoxamine* (eg, *Luvox*)	Sertraline (*Zoloft*)

Significance	Onset	Severity	Documentation
2	□ Rapid	□ Major	□ Established
	■ **Delayed**	■ **Moderate**	□ Probable
		□ Minor	■ **Suspected**
			□ Possible
			□ Unlikely

Effects SEROTONIN REUPTAKE INHIBITORS may increase CYCLOSPORINE concentrations and toxicity.

Mechanism Inhibition of CYCLOSPORINE metabolism (CYP3A4).

Management Monitor CYCLOSPORINE trough whole blood concentrations when adding or discontinuing a SEROTONIN REUPTAKE INHIBITOR. Adjust the dose of CYCLOSPORINE as needed. Citalopram (*Celexa*) may be a safer alternative.[1]

Discussion

Increased cyclosporine concentrations were reported following addition of fluoxetine to the treatment regimen of a 59-year-old male cardiac transplant patient.[2] Following cardiac transplantation for end-stage heart failure, the patient was maintained on cyclosporine 225 mg twice daily. At this dose, trough whole blood cyclosporine concentrations were stable at 300 mcg/L. The patient developed acute depression 17 days postoperatively and was started on fluoxetine 20 mg/day. After 10 days, the cyclosporine concentration increased to 588 mcg/L, and it was necessary to decrease the dose of cyclosporine to 75 mg twice daily, resulting in a blood cyclosporine concentration of 250 mcg/mL. Because the patient did not respond to fluoxetine, the drug was discontinued. After 1 week, his cyclosporine concentration decreased to 95 mcg/L, and it was necessary to increase the dose of cyclosporine to 200 mg twice daily. This resulted in a cyclosporine concentration of 300 mcg/L. Fluvoxamine 100 mg twice daily increased cyclosporine levels in a 62-year-old woman receiving cyclosporine 300 mg/day after a renal transplant.[3] Baseline trough cyclosporine blood levels of 200 to 250 ng/mL increased to 380 ng/mL, while serum creatinine increased from 1.5 to 1.9 mg/dL. The cyclosporine dose was reduced 33%, resulting in a return of cyclosporine level and renal function to baseline. No pharmacokinetic interaction occurred with coadministration of cyclosporine and citalopram.[1]

[1] Liston HL, et al. *Psychosomatics.* 2001;42:370.
[2] Horton RC, et al. *BMJ.* 1995;311:422.
[3] Vella JP, et al. *Am J Kidney Dis.* 1998;31:320.

* Asterisk indicates drugs cited in interaction reports. Based on pharmacologic and pharmacokinetic considerations, similar interactions may occur with other drugs that are listed.

Cyclosporine — *Sevelamer*

Cyclosporine* (eg, *Neoral*)	Sevelamer* (*Renagel*)

Significance	Onset	Severity	Documentation
4	□ Rapid ■ **Delayed**	□ Major ■ **Moderate** □ Minor	□ Established □ Probable □ Suspected ■ **Possible** □ Unlikely

Effects CYCLOSPORINE concentrations may be reduced, decreasing the immunosuppressive effect and increasing the risk of transplant rejection.

Mechanism SEVELAMER binds bile acids; thus, CYCLOSPORINE absorption may be decreased as a result of the effect of SEVELAMER on the enterohepatic cycle of bile acids.

Management Closely monitor CYCLOSPORINE concentrations when starting or stopping SEVELAMER. Adjust CYCLOSPORINE dosage as needed.

Discussion

A potential interaction between cyclosporine and sevelamer was reported in a 70-year-old woman on maintenance hemodialysis.[1] The patient had a history of type 2 diabetes mellitus and orthotopic liver transplantation for cirrhotic hepatitis C. She was receiving cyclosporine 60 mg daily when sevelamer 806 mg 3 times daily was started for hyperphosphatemia (phosphate level 7.1 mg/dL). After starting sevelamer, the cyclosporine trough concentration markedly decreased, necessitating an increase in the daily cyclosporine dose to 85 mg. The patient experienced GI intolerance to sevelamer, and the drug was stopped. Subsequently, the cyclosporine concentration increased and then decreased when sevelamer was restarted. In a study in 10 adults and 8 children with stable renal graft function and stable cyclosporine trough levels, sevelamer administration for 4 days did not affect the pharmacokinetics of cyclosporine.[2]

[1] Guillen-Anaya MA, et al. *Nephrol Dial Transplant.* 2004;19:515.

[2] Piper AK, et al. *Nephrol Dial Transplant.* 2004;19:2630.

* Asterisk indicates drugs cited in interaction reports.

Cyclosporine — *Sibutramine*

Cyclosporine* (eg, *Neoral*)	Sibutramine*†

Significance	Onset	Severity	Documentation
4	□ Rapid ■ **Delayed**	□ Major ■ **Moderate** □ Minor	□ Established □ Probable □ Suspected ■ **Possible** □ Unlikely

Effects CYCLOSPORINE plasma concentrations may be elevated, increasing the pharmacologic effects and risk of adverse reactions.

Mechanism Inhibition of CYCLOSPORINE metabolism (CYP3A4) by SIBUTRAMINE is suspected.

Management Closely monitor CYCLOSPORINE serum trough concentrations when SIBUTRAMINE is started or stopped. Adjust the CYCLOSPORINE dose as needed.

Discussion

A sharp increase in cyclosporine trough concentrations following the start of sibutramine therapy was reported in a 26-year-old woman who received a living-related kidney transplant.[1] The patient was receiving cyclosporine 100 mg twice daily when sibutramine 10 mg/daily was started. The cyclosporine serum trough concentration increased from 79 to 152 ng/mL one week after sibutramine was started, necessitating a decrease of 25 mg/ day in the cyclosporine dose. One week later, the cyclosporine serum trough concentration was 162 ng/mL and the daily dose of cyclosporine was further reduced by 25 mg. After 10 months of concurrent treatment of sibutramine and cyclosporine at the reduced dose, cyclosporine serum trough concentrations remained stable and similar to those before the start of sibutramine.

[1] Clerbaux G, et al. *Am J Transplant.* 2003;3(7):906.

* Asterisk indicates drugs cited in interaction reports.
† Not available in the United States.

Cyclosporine — *St. John's Wort*

Cyclosporine* (eg, *Neoral*)	St. John's Wort*

Significance	Onset	Severity	Documentation
1	☐ Rapid ■ **Delayed**	■ **Major** ☐ Moderate ☐ Minor	☐ Established ■ **Probable** ☐ Suspected ☐ Possible ☐ Unlikely

Effects Decreased CYCLOSPORINE (CSA) levels and efficacy.

Mechanism Increased hepatic metabolism (CYP3A4) of CSA and possibly increased intestinal P-gp efflux pump activity. ST. JOHN'S WORT hyperforin content is a major factor in the extent of the interaction.[1]

Management Because CSA has a narrow therapeutic index, caution patients to consult a health care provider before using nonprescription or herbal products. If use of ST. JOHN'S WORT cannot be avoided, monitor CSA whole blood levels frequently when ST. JOHN'S WORT is started or stopped. Be prepared to adjust the CSA dose soon after starting ST. JOHN'S WORT and for at least 2 weeks after discontinuation of ST. JOHN'S WORT.

Discussion

Subtherapeutic CSA levels have been reported in organ transplant patients ingesting St. John's wort (*Hypericum perforatum*).[2-6] Heart,[2] kidney,[4,6] liver,[5] and kidney-pancreas[6] transplant rejection episodes with decreased CSA levels have been reported after patients started St. John's wort. CSA levels increased after St. John's wort was stopped.[2,3,5,6] At least 46 kidney or liver transplant patients have had CSA blood levels decreased 49% after starting St. John's wort.[3] Two patients experienced rejection episodes. In an open-label study of 11 renal transplant patients on stable CSA regimens, AUC, C_{max}, and trough plasma levels decreased 46%, 42%, and 41%, respectively, during coadministration of St. John's wort extract 600 mg/day for 14 days.[7] To maintain therapeutic CSA levels, the CSA dose was increased 60%. The effects of 2 St. John's wort preparations (300 mg 3 times/day for 14 days) with high (commercially available preparation) and very low hyperforin content on the pharmacokinetics of CSA were studied in 10 renal transplant patients.[1] In the very low hyperforin, hyperforin was removed from the commercially available preparation. The high hyperforin preparation reduced the CSA AUC 45% and the C_{max} 43%. It was necessary to increase the daily dose of CSA 65%. Low-content hyperforin did not affect CSA pharmacokinetics or necessitate dose adjustments.

[1] Mai I, et al. *Clin Pharmacol Ther.* 2004;76(4):330.
[2] Ruschitzka F, et al. *Lancet.* 2000;355(9203):548.
[3] Breidenbach T, et al. *Lancet.* 2000;355(9218):1912.
[4] Mai I, et al. *Int J Clin Pharmacol Ther.* 2000;38(10):500.
[5] Karliova M, et al. *J Hepatol.* 2000;33(5):853.
[6] Barone GW, et al. *Transplantation.* 2001;71(2):239.
[7] Bauer S, et al. *Br J Clin Pharmacol.* 2003;55(2):203.

* Asterisk indicates drugs cited in interaction reports.

Cyclosporine — *Sulfonamides*

Cyclosporine	Sulfonamides	
Cyclosporine* (eg, *Neoral*)	Sulfadiazine* Sulfamethoxazole*† Sulfasalazine (eg, *Azulfidine*)	Trimethoprim/ Sulfamethoxazole*

Significance	Onset	Severity	Documentation
1	☐ Rapid ■ **Delayed**	■ **Major** ☐ Moderate ☐ Minor	☐ Established ☐ Probable ■ **Suspected** ☐ Possible ☐ Unlikely

Effects The action of CYCLOSPORINE (CSA) may be reduced. Oral SULFONAMIDES may increase the risk of nephrotoxicity.

Mechanism Unknown.

Management If coadministration cannot be avoided, frequently monitor serum creatinine and CSA levels and adjust the CSA dose as needed.

Discussion

Serum CSA levels decreased in 5 cardiac transplant patients treated with IV sulfamethazine† and IV trimethoprim/sulfamethoxazole (TMP/SMZ).[1] The patients had been stable on CSA for 3 to 6 months, with trough serum CSA levels at least 100 ng/mL. After 5 to 24 days of IV therapy, oral TMP/SMZ was started. CSA levels became undetectable in 4 patients after initiation of IV antibiotics. Despite dose increases, CSA serum levels did not increase until IV sulfamethazine was stopped. Elevated serum creatinine levels were observed in 6 of 56 renal transplant patients receiving TMP or TMP/SMZ with CSA.[2] In a retrospective study, 73% of those treated with CSA had increases in serum creatinine during TMP/SMZ treatment, compared with 13% treated with azathioprine (eg, *Imuran*).[3] In a prospective, randomized, double-blind study of 132 patients, there was a 15% increase in serum creatinine with oral TMP/SMZ prophylaxis.[4] However, no rejection episodes were documented. In a 46-year-old heart transplant patient receiving CSA and oral prednisolone, serum CSA trough levels ranged from 250 to 700 ng/mL.[5] Seven months later, he was treated with IV sulfamethazine and TMP. CSA levels became unmeasurable after 7 days of treatment; after 15 days, he had a rejection episode. After controlling the rejection episode, the antibiotics were switched to the oral route with adequate response. A cause-and-effect relationship among any of these events is not clear. Many patients developed rejection episodes.[1,5] Three cardiac transplant recipients experienced dramatic, reversible reductions in CSA levels after introduction of sulfadiazine.[6] An increase in CSA dose was necessary to maintain therapeutic levels. Increased CSA levels occurred in a renal transplant patient after discontinuing sulfasalazine, necessitating a dosage reduction from 9.6 to 5.6 mg/kg/day.[7] See Cyclosporine-Trimethoprim.

[1] Jones DK, et al. *Br Med J (Clin Res Ed)*. 1986;292(6522):728.
[2] Thompson JF, et al. *Transplantation*. 1983;36(2):204.
[3] Ringdén O, et al. *Lancet*. 1984;1(8384):1016.
[4] Maki DG, et al. *J Lab Clin Med*. 1992;119(1):11.
[5] Wallwork J, et al. *Lancet*. 1983;1(8320):366.
[6] Spes CH, et al. *Clin Investig*. 1992;70(9):752.
[7] Du Cheyron D, et al. *Eur J Clin Pharmacol*. 1999;55(3):227.

* Asterisk indicates drugs cited in interaction reports. Based on pharmacologic and pharmacokinetic considerations, similar interactions may occur with other drugs that are listed.
† Not available in the United States.

Cyclosporine — *Sulfonylureas*

Cyclosporine	Sulfonylureas	
Cyclosporine* (eg, *Neoral*)	Glimepiride (*Amaryl*)	Glyburide* (eg, *Micronase*)
	Glipizide* (eg, *Glucotrol*)	

Significance	Onset	Severity	Documentation
4	□ Rapid	□ Major	□ Established
	■ **Delayed**	■ **Moderate**	□ Probable
		□ Minor	□ Suspected
			■ **Possible**
			□ Unlikely

Effects Elevated whole blood CYCLOSPORINE concentrations with an increased risk of toxicity may occur. It is also possible that GLIPIZIDE levels may increase, producing hypoglycemia.

Mechanism Unknown; possibly enzyme inhibition, resulting in delayed metabolism of either agent.

Management Consider monitoring serum creatinine and CYCLOSPORINE concentrations as well as blood glucose levels. Adjust the dose of CYCLOSPORINE or SULFONYLUREA accordingly.

Discussion

Glipizide has been reported to increase whole blood cyclosporine concentrations in two patients.[1] Both patients had received cadaveric kidney transplants for end-stage renal failure and glipizide for diabetes mellitus. The patients were maintained on immunosuppressant regimens of azathioprine (eg, *Imuran*), cyclosporine and prednisone (eg, *Deltasone*). Concurrent administration of cyclosporine and glipizide produced a 1.5- to 3-fold increase in cyclosporine concentrations. A 20% to 30% reduction in cyclosporine dose was required to achieve therapeutic cyclosporine concentrations. A report reviewing data in six renal transplant patients treated with cyclosporine and glyburide concurrently indicates that glyburide may also inhibit cyclosporine metabolism.[2] Cyclosporine plasma concentrations increased by 57% following addition of glyburide to a stable cyclosporine, azathioprine and prednisolone regimen.

Controlled studies are needed to evaluate the importance of this interaction and to determine whether other sulfonylurea hypoglycemic agents can cause a similar interaction.

[1] Chidester PD, et al. *Transplant Proc.* 1993;25:2136.
[2] Islam SI, et al. *Ther Drug Monit.* 1996;18;624.

* Asterisk indicates drugs cited in interaction reports. Based on pharmacologic and pharmacokinetic considerations, similar interactions may occur with other drugs that are listed.

Cyclosporine — *Terbinafine*

Cyclosporine* (eg, *Neoral*)	Terbinafine* (*Lamisil*)

Significance	Onset	Severity	Documentation
2	□ Rapid ■ **Delayed**	□ Major ■ **Moderate** □ Minor	□ Established □ Probable ■ **Suspected** □ Possible □ Unlikely

Effects TERBINAFINE administration may decrease CYCLOSPORINE concentrations.

Mechanism TERBINAFINE may increase CYCLOSPORINE metabolism.

Management Monitor CYCLOSPORINE concentrations, and observe the clinical response of the patient when TERBINAFINE is started or stopped. Adjust the dose of CYCLOSPORINE as needed.

Discussion

The effects of terbinafine on cyclosporine blood concentrations were reported in four renal transplant patients.[1] Terbinafine 250 mg/day was administered to each patient for the treatment of fungal infections of the skin or nails. In addition, each patient was receiving between 2.2 and 5.2 mg/kg/day of cyclosporine. Cyclosporine blood concentrations decreased in all four patients. However, in three of the patients, the drop in cyclosporine concentrations was small and remained within the therapeutic range (70 to 250 ng/mL). No change in cyclosporine dosage was necessary. In the remaining patient, who had been receiving 3.6 mg/kg/day of cyclosporine, the cyclosporine concentration decreased from 71 ng/mL at baseline to 50 ng/mL when measured 8 weeks later while receiving terbinafine concomitantly. The dose of cyclosporine was increased in increments to 6.5 mg/kg/day. One week after discontinuing terbinafine, cyclosporine blood concentrations increased from 93 to 173 ng/mL, and the dose of cyclosporine was decreased. Renal function remained stable in all patients.

[1] Lo ACY, et al. *Br J Clin Pharmacol*. 1997;43:340.

* Asterisk indicates drugs cited in interaction reports.

Cyclosporine — *Ticlopidine*

Cyclosporine* (eg, *Neoral*)	Ticlopidine* (eg, *Ticlid*)

Significance	Onset	Severity	Documentation
2	□ Rapid ■ **Delayed**	□ Major ■ **Moderate** □ Minor	□ Established □ Probable ■ **Suspected** □ Possible □ Unlikely

Effects CYCLOSPORINE whole blood concentrations may decrease, producing a decrease in pharmacologic effects.

Mechanism Unknown.

Management Consider frequent monitoring of CYCLOSPORINE blood concentrations if TICLOPIDINE therapy is started or discontinued. Adjust the dose of CYCLOSPORINE or discontinue TICLOPIDINE as indicated.

Discussion

Addition of ticlopidine to the cyclosporine treatment schedule of an 18-year-old patient with nephrotic syndrome resulted in a decrease in cyclosporine whole blood levels.[1] This decrease was associated with a loss of cyclosporine efficacy that persisted throughout the course of ticlopidine administration despite an increase in cyclosporine dosage. Cyclosporine levels increased and efficacy returned when ticlopidine was discontinued. When the patient was rechallenged with ticlopidine, cyclosporine concentrations decreased. In a 64-year-old renal transplant patient, cyclosporine levels rapidly declined during coadministration of ticlopidine and rapidly returned to pre-ticlopidine concentrations following discontinuation of ticlopidine.[2] Another patient experienced a decrease in cyclosporine blood trough levels during the month after starting ticlopidine despite an increase in the cyclosporine dose.[3] Conversely, a study in 20 heart transplant patients did not detect differences in cyclosporine pharmacokinetics when ticlopidine 250 mg/day was given concurrently.[4]

[1] Birmelé B, et al. *Nephrol Dial Transplant.* 1991;6(2):150.
[2] Verdejo A, et al. *BMJ.* 2000;320(7241):1037.
[3] Feriozzi S, et al. *Nephron.* 2002;92(1):249.
[4] Boissonnat P, et al. *Eur J Clin Pharmacol.* 1997;53(1):39.

* Asterisk indicates drugs cited in interaction reports.

Cyclosporine — *Tigecycline*

Cyclosporine* (eg, *Neoral*)	Tigecycline* (*Tygacil*)

Significance	Onset	Severity	Documentation
4	☐ Rapid	☐ Major	☐ Established
	■ **Delayed**	■ **Moderate**	☐ Probable
		☐ Minor	☐ Suspected
			■ **Possible**
			☐ Unlikely

Effects CYCLOSPORINE concentrations and risk of toxicity may be increased.

Mechanism Unknown.

Management Closely monitor CYCLOSPORINE trough whole blood concentrations when TIGECYCLINE is started or stopped. Adjust the CYCLOSPORINE dose as needed.

Discussion

A 61-year-old female renal transplant patient receiving cyclosporine 120 mg daily experienced increased cyclosporine concentrations and creatine levels after IV tigecycline was added to her treatment regimen.[1] To maintain acceptable cyclosporine concentrations, it was necessary to withhold cyclosporine treatment for 1 day and reduce the dose 50%. Three days after discontinuing tigecycline, it was necessary to increase the dosage of cyclosporine to 120 mg daily to maintain therapeutic concentrations.

[1] Stumpf AN, et al. *Eur J Clin Pharmacol.* 2009;65(1):101.

* Asterisk indicates drugs cited in interaction reports.

Cyclosporine — *Trimethoprim*

Cyclosporine*
(eg, *Neoral*)

Trimethoprim*
(eg, *Proloprim*)

Significance	Onset	Severity	Documentation
4	☐ Rapid ■ **Delayed**	■ **Major** ☐ Moderate ☐ Minor	☐ Established ☐ Probable ☐ Suspected ■ **Possible** ☐ Unlikely

Effects The actions of CYCLOSPORINE may be altered by TRIMETHOPRIM; decreased effectiveness and increased nephrotoxicity have been reported.

Mechanism Unknown.

Management No clinical interventions, other than usual monitoring, are needed.

Discussion

Elevated serum creatinine levels were observed in 6 of 56 renal transplant patients receiving trimethoprim or trimethoprim-sulfamethoxazole (eg, *Septra*) concurrently with cyclosporine.[1] In a retrospectively analyzed group, 73% (30/41) of those treated with cyclosporine had increases in serum creatinine during treatment with trimethoprim-sulfamethoxazole compared with 13% (6/46) of those treated with azathioprine (eg, *Imuran*).[2] A reversible increase in serum creatinine and decreased CrCl were reported in 8 patients following the addition of oral trimethoprim 160 mg twice daily.[3] It is not clear whether sulfamethoxazole, trimethoprim, the combination, or the route of administration was responsible for these findings.

Decreased cyclosporine concentrations and rejection episodes also have occurred with trimethoprim IV† and sulfamethazine IV.†,[1,2,4,5] See also Cyclosporine-Sulfonamides.

1 Thompson JF, et al. *Transplantation.* 1983;36(2):204.
2 Ringdén O, et al. *Lancet.* 1984;1(8384):1016.
3 Berg KJ, et al. *Transplant Proc.* 1988;20(3):413.
4 Wallwork J, et al. *Lancet.* 1983;1(8320):366.
5 Jones DK, et al. *Br Med J (Clin Res Ed).* 1986;292(6522):728.

* Asterisk indicates drugs cited in interaction reports.
† Not available in the United States.

Cyclosporine — *Verapamil*

Cyclosporine* (eg, *Neoral*)	Verapamil* (eg, *Calan*)

Significance	Onset	Severity	Documentation
2	☐ Rapid ■ **Delayed**	☐ Major ■ **Moderate** ☐ Minor	■ **Established** ☐ Probable ☐ Suspected ☐ Possible ☐ Unlikely

Effects Increased CYCLOSPORINE levels with possible toxicity (eg, nephrotoxicity). However, giving VERAPAMIL before CYCLOSPORINE may be nephroprotective. The interaction is typically observed within 7 days of starting VERAPAMIL and may abate within 1 week after discontinuation.

Mechanism Inhibition of CYCLOSPORINE metabolism mediated by hepatic microsomal and gut wall enzymes is suspected.

Management Monitor CYCLOSPORINE levels when altering the dose of VERAPAMIL. Adjust the CYCLOSPORINE dose accordingly.

Discussion

In a retrospective study of 5 patients receiving cyclosporine and verapamil, cyclosporine trough levels increased in all.[1] In 22 patients, average cyclosporine levels were 130.5 ng/mL while patients were receiving verapamil, compared with 83 ng/mL after verapamil washout.[2] A similar interaction occurred in a patient after an increase in verapamil dose, suggesting that this interaction may be dose-related.[3] In a prospective study of 11 renal transplant patients, verapamil produced a 45% increase in cyclosporine AUC, peak level, trough level, and steady-state level.[4] In a retrospective study of 70 renal transplant patients receiving IV cyclosporine for 5 days followed by oral cyclosporine, verapamil had no effect on clearance of IV cyclosporine.[5] Cyclosporine clearance and dosage requirements were reduced when the oral doseform was given. Verapamil 240 to 360 mg/day, given before cyclosporine to renal transplant patients, prevented cyclosporine-induced inhibition of renal blood flow, ameliorated cyclosporine-induced acute nephrotoxicity, improved immunosuppression, and reduced the incidence of early rejection.[6,7] In 27 renal transplant patients, verapamil, initially injected into the renal artery and then continued orally, produced similar beneficial effects.[8] Studies suggest that nifedipine (eg, *Procardia*) lacks this interactive potential.[4,9-11] There are conflicting data as to whether nifedipine decreases the risk of cyclosporine nephrotoxicity.[12,13] See also Cyclosporine-Diltiazem, Cyclosporine-Nicardipine, and Nifedipine-Cyclosporine.

1 Lindholm A, et al. *Lancet.* 1987;1(8544):1262.
2 Yildiz A, et al. *Nephron.* 1999;81(1):117.
3 Maggio TG, et al. *Drug Intell Clin Pharm.* 1988;22(9):705.
4 Tortorice KL, et al. *Ther Drug Monit.* 1990;12(4):321.
5 Sketris IS, et al. *Ann Pharmacother.* 1994;28(11):1227.
6 Dawidson I, et al. *Transplant Proc.* 1989;21(1, pt 2):1511.
7 Dawidson I, et al. *Transplantation.* 1989;48(4):575.
8 Dawidson I, et al. *Transplant Proc.* 1990;22(4):1379.
9 Wagner K, et al. *Transplant Proc.* 1988;20(2)(suppl 2):561.
10 Howard RL, et al. *Ren Fail.* 1990;12(2):89.
11 Dy GR, et al. *Transplant Proc.* 1991;23(1, p t 2):1258.
12 Feehally J, et al. *Br Med J (Clin Res Ed).* 1987;295(6593):310.
13 Kwan JT, et al. *Br Med J (Clin Res Ed).* 1987;295(6602):851.

* Asterisk indicates drugs cited in interaction reports.

Cyproheptadine — *MAOIs*

Cyproheptadine	MAOIs	
Cyproheptadine*	Isocarboxazid (*Marplan*)	Tranylcypromine (eg, *Parnate*)
	Phenelzine* (*Nardil*)	

Significance	Onset	Severity	Documentation
5	☐ Rapid	☐ Major	☐ Established
	■ **Delayed**	■ **Moderate**	☐ Probable
		☐ Minor	☐ Suspected
			☐ Possible
			■ **Unlikely**

Effects This drug combination may produce an effect (eg, hallucinations) that is not expected with either drug alone.

Mechanism Unknown.

Management Based on present evidence, no specific recommendations can be made. If an interaction is suspected, discontinue this drug combination.

Discussion

Visual hallucinations occurred in a 30-year-old woman after coadministration of cyproheptadine and the MAOI phenelzine.[1] The patient had a history of bulimia and recurrent unipolar depression. She responded to phenelzine 30 mg/day but experienced adverse reactions of anorgasmia, insomnia, and orthostatic hypotension. Four months later, the patient was started on cyproheptadine 2 mg at bedtime, which successfully relieved her anorgasmia. However, after 2 months of receiving both drugs, she became irritable and suddenly developed visual hallucinations. Her medications were discontinued, and over the next 48 hours, the hallucinations disappeared. It is difficult to explain the 2-month delay in the onset of this reported interaction. The clinical importance of these findings remains to be determined.

[1] Kahn DA. *Am J Psychiatry.* 1987;144(9):1242.

* Asterisk indicates drugs cited in interaction reports. Based on pharmacologic and pharmacokinetic considerations, similar interactions may occur with other drugs that are listed.

Dapsone — *Didanosine*

Dapsone	Didanosine
Dapsone*	Didanosine* (eg, *Videx*)

Significance	Onset	Severity	Documentation
4	■ **Rapid**	■ **Major**	□ Established
	□ Delayed	□ Moderate	□ Probable
		□ Minor	□ Suspected
			■ **Possible**
			□ Unlikely

Effects Possible therapeutic failure of DAPSONE, leading to an increase in infection (eg, *Pneumocystis carinii* pneumonia [PCP]).

Mechanism DAPSONE is very insoluble at neutral pH. The citrate-phosphate buffer in DIDANOSINE may interfere with the dissolution of DAPSONE, decreasing absorption.

Management Administer DAPSONE at least 2 hours before DIDANOSINE.

Discussion

In a report of 57 patients infected with HIV and receiving didanosine, all patients were also given prophylactic treatment against PCP.[1] Twenty-eight patients received dapsone, 17 received trimethoprim-sulfamethoxazole (eg, *Bactrim*), and 12 received aerosolized pentamidine (eg, *NebuPent*). Prophylaxis failed in 11 patients taking dapsone (4 died of respiratory failure), in 1 patient receiving pentamidine (patient died of respiratory failure), and in none of the patients treated with trimethoprim-sulfamethoxazole. The remaining 17 patients who received didanosine plus dapsone took both drugs for at least 14 months without developing PCP. In a previously unpublished study by the same author, only 2 of 162 patients became infected with pneumocystis while taking dapsone alone. Based on this report, the increase in pneumocystis infection in patients receiving didanosine and dapsone concurrently compared with those patients given dapsone alone appears to be clinically important. However, in a study of 6 healthy subjects and 6 patients who were HIV-positive, neither didanosine tablets nor didanosine-placebo tablets (containing the aluminum-magnesium buffer) altered the kinetics of dapsone.[2] Likewise, a study of 9 healthy volunteers given antacids to raise gastric pH failed to show any alteration in didanosine pharmacokinetics.[3]

This interaction may also occur if didanosine is coadministered with other drugs. The dissolution of ketoconazole (eg, *Nizoral*) may be decreased by an increase in gastric pH.[4] See also Ketoconazole-Antacids.

[1] Metroka CE, et al. *N Engl J Med.* 1991;325(10):737.
[2] Sahai J, et al. *Ann Intern Med.* 1995;123(8):584.
[3] Breen GA, et al. *Antimicrob Agents Chemother.* 1994;38(9):2227.
[4] Knupp CA, et al. *Clin Pharmacol Ther.* 1992;51(2):155.

* Asterisk indicates drugs cited in interaction reports.

Darifenacin — *Azole Antifungal Agents*

Darifenacin* (*Enablex*)	Itraconazole* (eg, *Sporanox*)	Ketoconazole* (eg, *Neoral*)

Significance	Onset	Severity	Documentation
2	☐ Rapid ■ **Delayed**	☐ Major ■ **Moderate** ☐ Minor	☐ Established ☐ Probable ■ **Suspected** ☐ Possible ☐ Unlikely

Effects DARIFENACIN plasma concentrations may be elevated, increasing the pharmacologic effects and adverse reactions.

Mechanism AZOLE ANTIFUNGAL AGENTS may inhibit DARIFENACIN metabolism (CYP3A4).

Management When administered with ITRACONAZOLE or KETOCONAZOLE, it is recommended that the dose of DARIFENACIN not exceed 7.5 mg daily.[1]

Discussion

When darifenacin 7.5 mg once daily (administered to steady state) was coadministered with ketoconazole 400 mg, the mean darifenacin C_{max} increased to 11.2 ng/mL in 10 extensive metabolizers (EMs) and 55.4 ng/mL in 1 poor metabolizer (PM).[1] The mean AUC increased to 143 and 939 ng•hr/mL for the EMs and PM, respectively. When darifenacin 15 mg daily was given with ketoconazole, the mean darifenacin C_{max} increased to 67.6 and 58.9 ng/mL for 3 EMs and 1 PM, respectively. The mean AUC increased to 1,110 and 931 ng•hr/mL for the EMs and PM, respectively. The darifenacin dose should not exceed 7.5 mg daily when administered with potent CYP3A4 inhibitors (eg, itraconazole, ketoconazole).[1]

The basis for this monograph is information on file with the manufacturer. Published clinical data are needed to further assess this interaction.

[1] *Enablex* [package insert]. East Hanover, NJ: Novartis Pharmaceutical Company; April 2008.

* Asterisk indicates drugs cited in interaction reports.

Darifenacin		Macrolide & Related Antibiotics	
Darifenacin* (*Enablex*)		Clarithromycin* (eg, *Biaxin*)	Telithromycin (*Ketek*)

Significance	Onset	Severity	Documentation
2	☐ Rapid ■ **Delayed**	☐ Major ■ **Moderate** ☐ Minor	☐ Established ☐ Probable ■ **Suspected** ☐ Possible ☐ Unlikely

Effects DARIFENACIN plasma concentrations may be elevated, increasing the pharmacologic effects and adverse reactions.

Mechanism MACROLIDE & RELATED ANTIBIOTICS may inhibit DARIFENACIN metabolism (CYP3A4).

Management When administered with CLARITHROMYCIN, it is recommended that the dose of DARIFENACIN not exceed 7.5 mg daily.[1]

Discussion

When darifenacin 7.5 mg once daily (administered to steady state) was coadministered with the potent CYP3A4 inhibitor ketoconazole 400 mg, the mean darifenacin C_{max} in 10 extensive metabolizers (EMs) increased to 11.2 ng/mL and 55.4 ng/mL in 1 poor metabolizer (PM).[1] The mean AUC increased to 143 and 939 ng•h/mL for the EMs and PM, respectively. When darifenacin 15 mg daily was given with ketoconazole, the mean darifenacin C_{max} increased to 67.6 and 58.9 ng/mL for 3 EMs and 1 PM, respectively. The mean AUC increased to 1,110 and 931 ng•h/mL for the EMs and PM, respectively. The darifenacin dose should not exceed 7.5 mg daily when administered with potent CYP3A4 inhibitors (eg, clarithromycin).

The basis for this monograph is information on file with the manufacturer. Published clinical data are needed to further assess this interaction.

[1] *Enablex* [package insert]. East Hanover, NJ: Novartis Pharmaceutical Co; April 2008.

* Asterisk indicates drugs cited in interaction reports. Based on pharmacologic and pharmacokinetic considerations, similar interactions may occur with other drugs that are listed.

Darifenacin — *Nefazodone*

Darifenacin* (*Enablex*)	Nefazodone*

Significance	Onset	Severity	Documentation
2	☐ Rapid ■ **Delayed**	☐ Major ■ **Moderate** ☐ Minor	☐ Established ☐ Probable ■ **Suspected** ☐ Possible ☐ Unlikely

Effects DARIFENACIN plasma concentrations may be elevated, increasing the pharmacologic effects and adverse reactions.

Mechanism NEFAZODONE may inhibit DARIFENACIN metabolism (CYP3A4).

Management When administered with NEFAZODONE, it is recommended that the dose of DARIFENACIN not exceed 7.5 mg daily.[1]

Discussion

When darifenacin 7.5 mg once daily (administered to steady state) was coadministered with the potent CYP3A4 inhibitor ketoconazole 400 mg, the mean darifenacin C_{max} increased to 11.2 ng/mL in 10 extensive metabolizers (EMs) and 55.4 ng/mL in 1 poor metabolizer (PM).[1] The mean AUC increased to 143 and 939 ng•hr/mL for the EMs and PM, respectively. When darifenacin 15 mg daily was given with ketoconazole, the mean darifenacin C_{max} increased to 67.6 and 58.9 ng/mL for 3 EMs and 1 PM, respectively. The mean AUC increased to 1,110 and 931 ng•hr/mL for the EMs and PM, respectively. The darifenacin dose should not exceed 7.5 mg daily when administered with potent CYP3A4 inhibitors (eg, nefazodone).

The basis for this monograph is information on file with the manufacturer. Published clinical data are needed to further assess this interaction.

[1] *Enablex* [package insert]. East Hanover, NJ: Novartis Pharmaceutical Company; April 2008.

* Asterisk indicates drugs cited in interaction reports.

Darifenacin / *Protease Inhibitors*

Darifenacin* (*Enablex*)	Atazanavir (*Reyataz*)	Nelfinavir* (*Viracept*)
	Fosamprenavir (*Lexiva*)	Ritonavir* (*Norvir*)
	Indinavir (*Crixivan*)	Saquinavir (*Invirase*)
	Lopinavir/Ritonavir (*Kaletra*)	Tipranavir (*Aptivus*)

Significance	Onset	Severity	Documentation
2	☐ Rapid	☐ Major	☐ Established
	■ **Delayed**	■ **Moderate**	☐ Probable
		☐ Minor	■ **Suspected**
			☐ Possible
			☐ Unlikely

Effects DARIFENACIN plasma concentrations may be elevated, increasing the pharmacologic effects and adverse reactions.

Mechanism PROTEASE INHIBITORS may inhibit DARIFENACIN metabolism (CYP3A4).

Management When administered with NELFINAVIR or RITONAVIR, it is recommended that the dose of DARIFENACIN not exceed 7.5 mg daily.[1]

Discussion

When darifenacin 7.5 mg once daily (administered to steady state) was coadministered with the potent CYP3A4 inhibitor ketoconazole 400 mg, the mean darifenacin C_{max} increased to 11.2 in 10 extensive metabolizers (EMs) and 55.4 ng/mL in 1 poor metabolizer (PM).[1] The mean AUC increased to 143 and 939 ng•h/mL for the EMs and PM, respectively. When darifenacin 15 mg daily was given with ketoconazole, the mean darifenacin C_{max} increased to 67.6 and 58.9 ng/mL for 3 EMs and 1 PM, respectively. The mean AUC increased to 1,110 and 931 ng•h/mL for the EMs and PM, respectively. The darifenacin dose should not exceed 7.5 mg daily when administered with potent CYP3A4 inhibitors (eg, nelfinavir, ritonavir).

The basis for this monograph is information on file with the manufacturer. Published clinical data are needed to further assess this interaction.

[1] *Enablex* [package insert]. East Hanover, NJ: Novartis Pharmaceutical Co; April 2008.

* Asterisk indicates drugs cited in interaction reports. Based on pharmacologic and pharmacokinetic considerations, similar interactions may occur with other drugs that are listed.

Darunavir — *Echinacea*

Darunavir* (*Prezista*)	Echinacea*

Significance	Onset	Severity	Documentation
4	☐ Rapid	☐ Major	☐ Established
	■ **Delayed**	■ **Moderate**	☐ Probable
		☐ Minor	☐ Suspected
			■ **Possible**
			☐ Unlikely

Effects DARUNAVIR concentrations may be reduced, decreasing the pharmacologic effect.

Mechanism ECHINACEA may increase DARUNAVIR metabolism (CYP3A4). However, it is possible that the pharmacokinetics of DARUNAVIR may be altered only slightly because of the presence of ritonavir, a potent CYP3A inhibitor.

Management No routine adjustment in DARUNAVIR dosage appears to be necessary. However, monitor DARUNAVIR concentrations on an individual patient basis.

Discussion

In an open-label, fixed-sequence study, the effects of echinacea on the pharmacokinetics of darunavir were studied in 15 HIV-infected patients.[1] Each patient had been receiving darunavir 600 mg plus ritonavir 100 mg (*Norvir*) for at least 4 weeks. *Echinacea purpura* root extract 500 mg every 6 hours was added to the antiretroviral regimen from days 1 to 14. Coadministration of echinacea decreased the darunavir concentration at the end of the dosing interval and AUC by an average of 16% and 10%, respectively. However, the changes were as much as 40% and 30%, respectively, in some patients. Although individual patients demonstrated a decrease in darunavir concentrations, there was no affect on the overall darunavir or ritonavir pharmacokinetics. No darunavir dosage adjustment was required.

[1] Moltó J, et al. *Antimicrob Agents Chemother.* 2011;55(1):326.

* Asterisk indicates drugs cited in interaction reports.

Darunavir — *Saquinavir*

Darunavir*	Saquinavir*
(*Prezista*)	(*Invirase*)

Significance	Onset	Severity	Documentation
4	☐ Rapid	☐ Major	☐ Established
	■ **Delayed**	■ **Moderate**	☐ Probable
		☐ Minor	☐ Suspected
			■ **Possible**
			☐ Unlikely

Effects DARUNAVIR plasma concentrations may be reduced, decreasing the clinical efficacy.

Mechanism Unknown.

Management Based on available information, avoid coadministration of SAQUINAVIR and DARUNAVIR.

Discussion

The effects of saquinavir on the pharmacokinetics of darunavir administered with low-dose ritonavir were studied in 32 HIV-negative healthy volunteers.[1] Subjects were randomized into 2 cohorts (panels 1 and 2). During different sessions separated by a 14-day washout period, subjects in panel 1 received darunavir 400 mg/ritonavir 100 mg or darunavir 400 mg/saquinavir 1,000 mg/ritonavir 100 mg, while subjects in panel 2 received saquinavir 1,000 mg/ritonavir 100 mg or darunavir 400 mg/saquinavir 1,000 mg/ ritonavir 100 mg twice daily for 13 days with a single morning dose on day 14. Six subjects discontinued the study because of adverse reactions. Coadministration of saquinavir with darunavir/ritonavir decreased darunavir AUC, C_{max}, and C_{min} 26%, 17%, and 42%, respectively, compared with giving darunavir/ritonavir without saquinavir. In addition, ritonavir AUC increased 34% when saquinavir was coadministered with darunavir/ ritonavir compared with administration of darunavir/ritonavir alone. See also Saquinavir-Ritonavir.

[1] Sekar VJ, et al. *Ther Drug Monit.* 2007;29(6):795.

* Asterisk indicates drugs cited in interaction reports.

Dasatinib — *Antacids*

Dasatinib	Antacids	
Dasatinib* (*Sprycel*)	Aluminum Hydroxide (eg, *Alternagel*)	Magnesium Hydroxide (eg, *Milk of Magnesia*)
	Aluminum Hydroxide/ Magnesium Hydroxide* (eg, *Maalox*)	

Significance	Onset	Severity	Documentation
2	■ **Rapid**	□ Major	□ Established
	□ Delayed	■ **Moderate**	□ Probable
		□ Minor	■ **Suspected**
			□ Possible
			□ Unlikely

Effects DASATINIB plasma concentrations may be reduced, decreasing the therapeutic effect.

Mechanism The pH-dependent solubility of DASATINIB may be reduced, decreasing absorption.

Management Avoid simultaneous administration of DASATINIB and ANTACIDS. If ANTACID therapy is needed, administer the ANTACID at least 2 hours before or after giving DASATINIB.

Discussion

The effects of an aluminum hydroxide/magnesium hydroxide–containing antacid on the pharmacokinetics of dasatinib were studied in 24 healthy subjects.[1] In an open-label, randomized, crossover study, each subject received either 2 doses of dasatinib 50 mg 12 hours apart or 30 mL of aluminum hydroxide/magnesium hydroxide 2 hours before administering dasatinib 50 mg and concurrently with dasatinib 50 mg 12 hours after the initial dose of dasatinib. Compared with giving dasatinib alone, simultaneous administration of the antacid reduced the dasatinib C_{max} and AUC 58% and 55%, respectively. Separating the administration times of the antacid and dasatinib by 2 hours increased the dasatinib C_{max} approximately 26% and had no effect on the AUC.

[1] Eley T, et al. *J Clin Pharmacol.* 2009;49(6):700.

* Asterisk indicates drugs cited in interaction reports. Based on pharmacologic and pharmacokinetic considerations, similar interactions may occur with other drugs that are listed.

Dasatinib | **Azole Antifungal Agents**

Dasatinib* (*Sprycel*)	Itraconazole (eg, *Sporanox*)	Posaconazole (*Noxafil*)
	Ketoconazole* (eg, *Nizoral*)	Voriconazole (eg, *Vfend*)

Significance	Onset	Severity	Documentation
2	□ Rapid	□ Major	□ Established
	■ **Delayed**	■ **Moderate**	□ Probable
		□ Minor	■ **Suspected**
			□ Possible
			□ Unlikely

Effects DASATINIB plasma concentrations may be elevated, increasing the pharmacologic effects and risk of adverse reactions, including increased QT interval prolongation and risk of life-threatening cardiac arrhythmias.

Mechanism Inhibition of DASATINIB metabolism (CYP3A4) by AZOLE ANTIFUNGAL AGENTS.

Management If coadministration cannot be avoided, closely monitor for toxicity and QTc interval prolongation. Be prepared to reduce the DASATINIB dose as needed.

Discussion

The effects of ketoconazole on the pharmacokinetics of dasatinib were evaluated in 28 patients with advanced solid tumors.[1] Coadministration of dasatinib and ketoconazole 400 mg markedly increased dasatinib C_{max} and AUC 4- and 5-fold, respectively, which correlated with an increase in the QTc interval of approximately 6 msec. No adverse cardiac reactions occurred.

[1] Johnson FM, et al. *Cancer.* 2010;116(6):1582.

* Asterisk indicates drugs cited in interaction reports. Based on pharmacologic and pharmacokinetic considerations, similar interactions may occur with other drugs that are listed.

Dasatinib — *Food*

Dasatinib*
(*Sprycel*)

Grapefruit Juice*

Significance	Onset	Severity	Documentation
2	□ Rapid ■ **Delayed**	□ Major ■ **Moderate** □ Minor	□ Established □ Probable ■ **Suspected** □ Possible □ Unlikely

Effects DASATINIB plasma concentrations may be elevated, increasing the risk of DASATINIB toxicity.

Mechanism Inhibition of DASATINIB metabolism (CYP3A4) in the small intestine by GRAPEFRUIT.

Management Avoid coadministration of DASATINIB and GRAPEFRUIT. Administer DASATINIB with a liquid other than GRAPEFRUIT JUICE.

Discussion

Because dasatinib undergoes extensive metabolism by CYP3A4, ingestion of dasatinib and grapefruit juice, an inhibitor of CYP3A4, is expected to increase dasatinib plasma concentrations. Therefore, patients taking dasatinib should avoid grapefruit.[1]

The basis for this monograph is information on file with the manufacturer. There are no clinical data with dose adjustments in patients receiving dasatinib and grapefruit. Studies are needed to determine the clinical importance of this interaction.

[1] *Sprycel* [package insert]. Princeton, NJ: Bristol-Myers Squibb Company; May 2009.

* Asterisk indicates drugs cited in interaction reports.

Dasatinib		*Histamine H_2 Antagonists*	
Dasatinib* (*Sprycel*)		Cimetidine (eg, *Tagamet*)	Nizatidine (eg, *Axid*)
		Famotidine* (eg, *Pepcid*)	Ranitidine (eg, *Zantac*)

Significance	Onset	Severity	Documentation
2	■ **Rapid**	□ Major	□ Established
	□ Delayed	■ **Moderate**	□ Probable
		□ Minor	■ **Suspected**
			□ Possible
			□ Unlikely

Effects DASATINIB plasma concentrations may be reduced, decreasing the therapeutic effect.

Mechanism The pH-dependent solubility of DASATINIB may be reduced, decreasing absorption.

Management Avoid coadministration of HISTAMINE H_2 ANTAGONISTS with oral DASATINIB.

Discussion

The effects of famotidine on the pharmacokinetics of dasatinib were studied in 24 healthy subjects.[1] In an open-label, randomized, crossover study, each subject received either 2 doses of dasatinib 50 mg 12 hours apart or a single dose of famotidine 40 mg administered in the evening 2 hours after the first dose of dasatinib 50 mg, which was also 10 hours before the second dasatinib dose. Compared with giving dasatinib alone, famotidine reduced the dasatinib C_{max} and AUC 63% and 61%, respectively.

[1] Eley T, et al. *J Clin Pharmacol.* 2009;49(6):700.

* Asterisk indicates drugs cited in interaction reports. Based on pharmacologic and pharmacokinetic considerations, similar interactions may occur with other drugs that are listed.

Dasatinib — *St. John's Wort*

Dasatinib* (*Sprycel*)	St. John's Wort*

Significance	Onset	Severity	Documentation
2	☐ Rapid	☐ Major	☐ Established
	■ **Delayed**	■ **Moderate**	☐ Probable
		☐ Minor	■ **Suspected**
			☐ Possible
			☐ Unlikely

Effects DASATINIB plasma concentrations may be reduced, decreasing the efficacy.

Mechanism Increased DASATINIB metabolism (CYP3A4) by ST. JOHN'S WORT is suspected.

Management Advise patients to avoid coadministration of DASATINIB and ST. JOHN'S WORT.[1] Caution patients receiving DASATINIB to consult their health care provider before using nonprescription or herbal products.

Discussion

St. John's wort may cause unpredictable decreases in dasatinib plasma concentration. The manufacturer of dasatinib cautions patients to avoid concurrent ingestion of St. John's wort.[1]

[1] *Sprycel* [package insert]. Princeton, NJ: Bristol-Myers Squibb Co; May 2009.

* Asterisk indicates drugs cited in interaction reports.

Deferasirox — *Cholestyramine*

Deferasirox* (*Exjade*)	Cholestyramine* (eg, *Questran*)

Significance	Onset	Severity	Documentation
2	■ **Rapid**	□ Major	□ Established
	□ Delayed	■ **Moderate**	□ Probable
		□ Minor	■ **Suspected**
			□ Possible
			□ Unlikely

Effects DEFERASIROX plasma concentrations may be reduced, decreasing the pharmacologic effects.

Mechanism DEFERASIROX may form a complex with CHOLESTYRAMINE, decreasing GI absorption and enterohepatic recirculation.

Management If coadministration of DEFERASIROX and CHOLESTYRAMINE cannot be avoided, initiate treatment with DEFERASIROX 30 mg/kg daily.[1] Carefully monitor serum ferritin concentrations and the clinical response of the patient for further DEFERASIROX dosage adjustments.

Discussion

Coadministration of deferasirox and cholestyramine decreases deferasirox systemic exposure (AUC).[1] In healthy volunteers, administration of cholestyramine after a singe dose of deferasirox decreased the deferasirox AUC 45%. If coadministration of deferasirox and cholestyramine cannot be avoided, initiate treatment with deferasirox 30 mg/kg daily. Carefully monitor serum ferritin concentrations and the clinical response of the patient for further deferasirox dosage adjustments. Doses above deferasirox 40 mg daily are not recommended.

The basis for this monograph is information on file with the manufacturer. Additional clinical studies are needed to assess the clinical importance of this interaction.

[1] *Exjade* [package insert]. East Hanover, NJ: Novartis Pharmaceuticals Corporation; January 2010.

* Asterisk indicates drugs cited in interaction reports.

Deferasirox — *Rifamycins*

Deferasirox* (*Exjade*)	Rifampin* (eg, *Rifadin*)

Significance	Onset	Severity	Documentation
2	□ Rapid	□ Major	□ Established
	■ **Delayed**	■ **Moderate**	□ Probable
		□ Minor	■ **Suspected**
			□ Possible
			□ Unlikely

Effects DEFERASIROX plasma concentrations may be reduced, decreasing the pharmacologic effects.

Mechanism RIFAMPIN may increase the metabolism (glucuronidation) of DEFERASIROX.

Management If coadministration of DEFERASIROX and RIFAMPIN cannot be avoided, initiate treatment with DEFERASIROX 30 mg/kg daily.[1] Carefully monitor serum ferritin concentrations and the clinical response of the patient for further DEFERASIROX dosage adjustments.

Discussion

The effects of rifampin on the pharmacokinetics of deferasirox were studied in 20 healthy men.[2] Each subject received a single dose of deferasirox 30 mg/kg alone and after 9 days of receiving rifampin 600 mg once daily. Compared with receiving deferasirox alone, pretreatment with rifampin decreased deferasirox exposure (AUC) 45% and reduced the $t_{½}$ from 9.8 to 8.1 hours. The deferasirox C_{max} was not affected.

1 *Exjade* [package insert]. East Hanover, NJ: Novartis Pharmaceuticals Corporation; January 2010.

2 Skerjanec A, et al. *J Clin Pharmacol.* 2010;50(2):205.

* Asterisk indicates drugs cited in interaction reports.

Delavirdine — *Fosamprenavir*

Delavirdine*
(*Rescriptor*)

Fosamprenavir*
(*Lexiva*)

Significance	Onset	Severity	Documentation
1	☐ Rapid	■ **Major**	☐ Established
	■ **Delayed**	☐ Moderate	☐ Probable
		☐ Minor	■ **Suspected**
			☐ Possible
			☐ Unlikely

Effects DELAVIRDINE plasma levels may be decreased, while FOSAMPRENAVIR concentrations may be elevated. This may lead to loss of virologic response and possible resistance to DELAVIRDINE.

Mechanism FOSAMPRENAVIR may induce the metabolism (CYP3A4) of DELAVIRDINE, while DELAVIRDINE may inhibit the metabolism (CYP3A4) of FOSAMPRENAVIR.

Management Coadministration of FOSAMPRENAVIR and DELAVIRDINE is contraindicated.

Discussion

After oral administration, fosamprenavir is rapidly and almost completely hydrolyzed to amprenavir and inorganic phosphate in the gut epithelium during absorption.[1] The effects of administration of amprenavir and delavirdine on the pharmacokinetics of each other were investigated in a prospective, open-label, randomized, 2-period, multiple-dose study involving 18 healthy subjects.[2] Each subject received amprenavir 600 mg twice daily or delavirdine 600 mg twice daily for 10 days, followed by both drugs concurrently for another 10 days. Compared with administration of delavirdine alone, amprenavir administration decreased the plasma concentration of delavirdine at 12 hours by 88% (from 7,916 to 933 ng/mL) and the median AUC and C_{max} 61% and 47%, respectively. Compared with administration of amprenavir alone, delavirdine administration increased the median concentration of amprenavir at 12 hours by 125%, the C_{max} 40%, and the AUC 130%, while decreasing the $t_{1/2}$ 31% (from 7 to 4.8 hours). The most frequently reported adverse reactions were GI symptoms, headache, fatigue, and rash. See also Protease Inhibitors-Nevirapine.

[1] *Lexiva* [package insert]. Research Triangle Park, NY: GlaxoSmithKline; May 2011.

[2] Justesen US, et al. *Br J Clin Pharmacol.* 2003;55(1):100.

* Asterisk indicates drugs cited in interaction reports.

Delavirdine — *Rifamycins*

Delavirdine* (*Rescriptor*)	Rifabutin* (*Mycobutin*)	Rifapentine (*Priftin*)
	Rifampin* (eg, *Rifadin*)	

Significance	Onset	Severity	Documentation
2	☐ Rapid	☐ Major	☐ Established
	■ **Delayed**	■ **Moderate**	☐ Probable
		☐ Minor	■ **Suspected**
			☐ Possible
			☐ Unlikely

Effects RIFAMYCINS may decrease DELAVIRDINE plasma concentrations.

Mechanism RIFAMYCINS may increase the metabolism of DELAVIRDINE by enzyme induction (CYP3A4).

Management Avoid concurrent use of DELAVIRDINE and RIFAMYCINS.

Discussion

The effects of rifabutin on the pharmacokinetics of the antiviral agent delavirdine were studied in 12 HIV-positive patients. The study design was an open-label, parallel-group, multidose investigation. Each subject received an oral dose of delavirdine 400 mg 3 times daily for 30 days. In addition to delavirdine, the 7 subjects in the rifabutin group were given rifabutin 300 mg once daily on days 16 to 30. Coadministration of rifabutin and delavirdine produced a 5-fold increase in the clearance of delavirdine, resulting in an 84% decrease in steady-state delavirdine plasma concentrations, a 95% decrease in the trough plasma concentration, and a 75% decrease in C_{max}. Rifabutin had no effect on delavirdine plasma concentrations during the first 2 days of coadministration; however, mean plasma delavirdine concentrations were much lower on day 30 (after 2 weeks of concurrent rifabutin) than on day 15.[1] In a similar study, after 2 weeks of coadministration of delavirdine and rifampin, the oral clearance of delavirdine increased approximately 27-fold, resulting in negligible steady-state trough concentrations of delavirdine in all 12 patients.[2] In addition, the delavirdine elimination $t_{½}$ decreased from 4.3 to 1.7 hours.

[1] Borin MT, et al. *Antiviral Res.* 1997;35(1):53.

[2] Borin MT, et al. *Clin Pharmacol Ther.* 1997;61(5):544.

* Asterisk indicates drugs cited in interaction reports. Based on pharmacologic and pharmacokinetic considerations, similar interactions may occur with other drugs that are listed.

Desmopressin — *Loperamide*

Desmopressin* (eg, *DDAVP*)	Loperamide* (eg, *Imodium A-D*)

Significance	Onset	Severity	Documentation
5	☐ Rapid ■ **Delayed**	☐ Major ☐ Moderate ■ **Minor**	☐ Established ☐ Probable ☐ Suspected ■ **Possible** ☐ Unlikely

Effects DESMOPRESSIN plasma concentrations may be elevated, increasing the pharmacologic and adverse effects.

Mechanism LOPERAMIDE may slow GI motility, increasing the absorption of DESMOPRESSIN.

Management Based on available information, no special precautions are necessary.

Discussion

The effect of loperamide administration on the pharmacokinetics of oral desmopressin was assessed in 18 healthy subjects.[1] In an open-label, randomized study, each subject received a single oral dose of desmopressin 400 mcg alone or after pretreatment with 3 doses of loperamide 4 mg. Compared with administration of desmopressin alone, pretreatment with loperamide increased the AUC of desmopressin 3.1-fold and the C_{max} 2.3-fold. In addition, the T_{max} was longer after pretreatment with loperamide. No serious adverse reactions were attributed to the study treatments or procedures.

[1] Callréus T, et al. *Eur J Clin Pharmacol.* 1999;55(4):305.

* Asterisk indicates drugs cited in interaction reports.

Dextromethorphan — *Berberine*

Dextromethorphan* (eg, *Robitussin*)	Berberine*

Significance	Onset	Severity	Documentation
5	☐ Rapid ■ **Delayed**	☐ Major ☐ Moderate ■ **Minor**	☐ Established ☐ Probable ☐ Suspected ■ **Possible** ☐ Unlikely

Effects DEXTROMETHORPHAN plasma concentrations may be elevated, increasing the pharmacologic effects and risk of adverse reactions.

Mechanism Inhibition of DEXTROMETHORPHAN metabolism (CYP2D6) by BERBERINE is suspected.

Management Patients may require a lower dose of DEXTROMETHORPHAN when taking BERBERINE.

Discussion

The effects of berberine (a plant alkaloid found in herbs such as goldenseal) on the pharmacokinetics of dextromethorphan were evaluated in 17 healthy men.[1] Using a randomized, crossover design, each subject received either placebo or berberine 300 mg 3 times daily for 14 days. Dextromethorphan 30 mg was administered before and at the end of the 14 days. Compared with placebo, berberine ingestion increased the ratio of dextromethorphan to its metabolite, dextrorphan, 9-fold.

[1] Guo Y, et al. *Eur J Clin Pharmacol.* 2012;68(2):213.

* Asterisk indicates drugs cited in interaction reports.

Dextromethorphan — *Cinacalcet*

Dextromethorphan* (eg, *Robitussin CoughGels*)	Cinacalcet* (*Sensipar*)

Significance	Onset	Severity	Documentation
3	□ Rapid	□ Major	□ Established
	■ **Delayed**	□ Moderate	□ Probable
		■ **Minor**	■ **Suspected**
			□ Possible
			□ Unlikely

Effects DEXTROMETHORPHAN plasma concentrations may be elevated, increasing the pharmacologic effects and adverse reactions.

Mechanism Inhibition of DEXTROMETHORPHAN metabolism (CYP2D6) by CINACALCET.

Management Monitor patients for DEXTROMETHORPHAN-induced adverse reactions when starting CINACALCET. Adjust the DEXTROMETHORPHAN dose as needed.

Discussion

The effects of cinacalcet on the pharmacokinetics of dextromethorphan were studied in 24 healthy men.[1] Using a double-blind, randomized, crossover design, each subject received cinacalcet 50 mg or a matching placebo once daily for 8 days. On day 8, dextromethorphan 30 mg was administered. Compared with placebo, pretreatment with cinacalcet increased the mean AUC and C_{max} of dextromethorphan 11- and 7-fold, respectively. All adverse reactions were of mild intensity with stomach discomfort, increased alanine aminotransferase, and epistaxis occurring more frequently when dextromethorphan and cinacalcet were coadministered.

[1] Nakashima D, et al. *J Clin Pharmacol.* 2007;47(10):1311.

* Asterisk indicates drugs cited in interaction reports.

Dextromethorphan — *Food*

Dextromethorphan* (eg, *Robitussin*)	Grapefruit Juice*	Seville Orange Juice*

Significance	Onset	Severity	Documentation
5	■ **Rapid**	□ Major	□ Established
	□ Delayed	□ Moderate	□ Probable
		■ **Minor**	□ Suspected
			■ **Possible**
			□ Unlikely

Effects DEXTROMETHORPHAN plasma concentrations may be elevated, increasing the pharmacologic and adverse effects. The effect may last for several days.

Mechanism Inhibition of DEXTROMETHORPHAN metabolism (CYP3A4) and intestinal efflux (P-glycoprotein) in the small intestine by GRAPEFRUIT JUICE or SEVILLE ORANGE JUICE is suspected.

Management Based on available data, no special precautions are needed.

Discussion

The effects of grapefruit juice and Seville orange juice on dextromethorphan pharmacokinetics were studied in 11 healthy volunteers.[1] Each subject received dextromethorphan 30 mg with water 200 mL, grapefruit juice 200 mL, and Seville orange juice 200 mL. Compared with water, grapefruit juice, and Seville orange juice significantly increased the bioavailability of dextromethorphan from 0.1 to 0.54 and 0.46 ($P < 0.05$), respectively. After 3 days of washout, the bioavailability of dextromethorphan returned to 50% of its baseline value. It is not known if the confectioneries that contain Seville oranges (eg, marmalade) include a sufficient amount to produce an interaction with dextromethorphan.

[1] Di Marco MP, et al. *Life Sci.* 2002;71(10):1149.

* Asterisk indicates drugs cited in interaction reports.

Dextromethorphan — MAOIs

Dextromethorphan	MAOIs	
Dextromethorphan* (eg, *Robitussin Cough*)	Isocarboxazid* (*Marplan*)	Selegiline* (eg, *Zelapar*)
	Phenelzine* (*Nardil*)	Tranylcypromine (eg, *Parnate*)
	Rasagiline* (*Azilect*)	

Significance	Onset	Severity	Documentation
1	■ **Rapid**	■ **Major**	□ Established
	□ Delayed	□ Moderate	□ Probable
		□ Minor	■ **Suspected**
			□ Possible
			□ Unlikely

Effects Hyperpyrexia, abnormal muscle movement, hypotension, coma, and death have been associated with coadministration of these agents.

Mechanism Serotonin syndrome resulting from decreased serotonin metabolism (MAOI) and decreased synaptic reuptake of serotonin (DEXTROMETHORPHAN).

Management Because of potential severity of reaction, avoid coadministration of these agents. Coadministration of DEXTROMETHORPHAN and RASAGILINE or SELEGILINE is contraindicated.[1,2]

Discussion

A possible serious interaction between MAOIs and dextromethorphan has been reported.[3-5] A 26-yr-old woman who had been taking phenelzine 60 mg/day for several months developed nausea and dizziness, then collapsed approximately 30 min after ingesting dextromethorphan.[3] She was severely hypotensive and her temperature was 42°C. Approximately 4 hr after admission to the hospital, she experienced cardiac arrest and died. The autopsy did not disclose a specific cause of death. A 32-yr-old woman taking isocarboxazid 30 mg/day for 8 wk experienced nausea and dizziness 20 min following ingestion of diazepam (eg, *Valium*) and 10 mL of a preparation containing dextromethorphan and guaifenesin (eg, *Robitussin DM*).[4] Within 45 min, fine bilateral leg tremors, muscle spasms of the abdomen and lower back, bilateral persistent myoclonic leg jerks, occasional choreoathetoid feet movements, and marked urinary retention occurred. The patient was greatly improved 19 hr later. Occasional myoclonic jerks persisted for 2 months. A 28-yr-old woman taking phenelzine 45 mg/day developed dizziness, nausea, severe headache, and a dazed feeling 1 hr after ingesting 10 to 20 mg of dextromethorphan.[5] She became unresponsive and was admitted with obtundation, myoclonus, rigidity, opisthotonos, and apneic periods. She required mechanical ventilation and skeletal muscle paralysis. She was discharged after 6 days with resistant ankle clonus and increased deep tendon leg reflexes.

1 *Zelapar* [package insert]. Costa Mesa, CA: Valeant Pharmaceutical International; June 2006.
2 *Azilect* [package insert]. Kansas City, MO: Teva Neuroscience, Inc; May 2006.
3 Rivers N, et al. *CMAJ*. 1970;103:85.
4 Sovner R, et al. *N Engl J Med*. 1988;319(25):1671.
5 Nierenberg DW, et al. *Clin Pharmacol Ther*. 1993;53(1):84.

* Asterisk indicates drugs cited in interaction reports. Based on pharmacologic and pharmacokinetic considerations, similar interactions may occur with other drugs that are listed.

Dextromethorphan — *Quinidine*

Dextromethorphan* (eg, *Robitussin Cough*)	Quinidine*

Significance	Onset	Severity	Documentation
3	☐ Rapid ■ **Delayed**	☐ Major ☐ Moderate ■ **Minor**	☐ Established ■ **Probable** ☐ Suspected ☐ Possible ☐ Unlikely

Effects Plasma DEXTROMETHORPHAN concentrations may be elevated, increasing the pharmacologic and toxic effects.

Mechanism QUINIDINE inhibits DEXTROMETHORPHAN metabolism via the CYP-450 2D6 enzyme.[1]

Management Monitor patients for DEXTROMETHORPHAN-induced adverse reactions and reduce the dose if needed.

Discussion

A study was conducted in 14 patients with amyotrophic lateral sclerosis to determine if quinidine improves the systemic delivery of dextromethorphan.[2] In the first phase of the study, steady-state plasma dextromethorphan levels were evaluated in 6 efficient metabolizers receiving dextromethorphan 60 mg twice daily. In the second phase, 7 efficient metabolizers and 1 poor metabolizer stabilized on quinidine 75 mg twice daily received escalating doses of dextromethorphan (15, 30, 45, 60, 90, and 120 mg/day) added at 1-week intervals. In patients receiving only dextromethorphan, plasma levels ranged from 5 to 40 ng/mL. None of these patients reported any adverse reactions. In contrast, dextromethorphan 60 mg twice daily in patients receiving quinidine 75 mg every 12 hours produced mean plasma dextromethorphan levels ranging from 157 to 402 ng/mL. In addition, the higher levels of dextromethorphan were associated with an increase in adverse reactions (eg, nervousness, fatigue, unsteady gait, dizziness, insomnia, confusion, shortness of breath). When the dose of dextromethorphan was reduced, many adverse reactions disappeared or became less severe. Because of adverse reactions, only 5 patients in phase 2 of the study were able to tolerate the entire range of dextromethorphan dosage. All patients completed the trial with dextromethorphan up to 60 mg/day given with quinidine. In a study with 5 extensive and 4 poor metabolizers of dextromethorphan, coadministration of quinidine 100 mg increased plasma dextromethorphan levels and prolonged the $t_{½}$.[1] Similar findings were reported in another study of 6 extensive and 6 poor metabolizers.[3]

The increased systemic delivery of dextromethorphan occurring as a result of this interaction may be useful in treating certain neurologic conditions. However, awareness of the adverse reactions associated with this interaction may be important with respect to patients who take quinidine for arrhythmia control and require a cough suppressant.

[1] Schadel M, et al. *J Clin Psychopharmacol.* 1995;15(4):263.
[2] Zhang Y, et al. *Clin Pharmacol Ther.* 1992;51(6):647.
[3] Capon DA, et al. *Clin Pharmacol Ther.* 1996;60(3):295.

* Asterisk indicates drugs cited in interaction reports.

Dextromethorphan — *Terbinafine*

Dextromethorphan* (eg, *Robitussin DM*)	Terbinafine* (eg, *Lamisil*)

Significance	Onset	Severity	Documentation
3	☐ Rapid ■ **Delayed**	☐ Major ☐ Moderate ■ **Minor**	☐ Established ■ **Probable** ☐ Suspected ☐ Possible ☐ Unlikely

Effects Plasma DEXTROMETHORPHAN concentrations may be elevated, increasing the pharmacologic and adverse effects.

Mechanism TERBINAFINE inhibits DEXTROMETHORPHAN metabolism via the CYP2D6 enzyme.

Management Monitor the patient for DEXTROMETHORPHAN-induced adverse effects when starting TERBINAFINE. Reduce the dose of DEXTROMETHORPHAN as needed.

Discussion

The effect of terbinafine on CYP2D6 inhibition was studied in 9 healthy volunteers using the metabolism of dextromethorphan to dextrorphan as a marker of enzyme activity.[1] Six subjects were genotypically consistent with an extensive-metabolizer phenotype, and 3 were consistent with a poor-metabolizer phenotype. The change in CYP2D6 enzyme activity was assessed after the administration of terbinafine 250 mg/day for 14 days. Each subject received dextromethorphan 0.3 mg/kg before terbinafine, after the last dose of terbinafine, and then monthly for 6 months. In all extensive metabolizers, terbinafine administration resulted, on average, in a 97-fold increase in the dextromethorphan/dextrorphan urinary ratio, converting 4 of the 6 extensive metabolizers into phenotypic poor metabolizers. No change in the dextromethorphan/dextrorphan ratio was detected in the poor metabolizers. The CYP2D6 activity returned to baseline values within 3 months after the 14-day course of terbinafine.

The results of this study indicate that the inhibition of CYP2D6 by terbinafine is of sufficient magnitude to warrant further investigation of the effects of terbinafine on other drugs metabolized by CYP2D6 (see Inhibitors, Inducers, and Substrates of Cytochrome P450 Enzymes table).

[1] Abdel-Rahman SM, et al. *Clin Pharmacol Ther.* 1999;65(5):465.

* Asterisk indicates drugs cited in interaction reports.

Diazoxide ╳ *Phenothiazines*

Diazoxide* (*Proglycem*)	Chlorpromazine*

Significance	Onset	Severity	Documentation
4	■ **Rapid**	□ Major	□ Established
	□ Delayed	■ **Moderate**	□ Probable
		□ Minor	□ Suspected
			■ **Possible**
			□ Unlikely

Effects An increase in the hyperglycemic effect of DIAZOXIDE may occur. It is unclear how long this effect may persist once CHLORPROMAZINE is discontinued.

Mechanism Unknown.

Management It is advisable to frequently monitor blood glucose concentrations if these 2 agents are used in combination. If possible, use a PHENOTHIAZINE with a lower potential for producing hyperglycemia in place of CHLORPROMAZINE.

Discussion

Several reports support the occasional occurrence of hyperglycemia secondary to chlorpromazine.[1-4] In addition, hyperglycemia is a well known effect of diazoxide.[5] However, only one case report exists to support this interaction.[6] In the report, a child treated with diazoxide maintenance therapy for hypoglycemia became profoundly hyperglycemic after a single dose of chlorpromazine. The patient's blood glucose continued to increase for 21 hours after the chlorpromazine dose. The patient's condition resolved on the second day following the chlorpromazine. The mechanism by which either agent induces hyperglycemia remains obscure.

[1] Hiles BW. *JAMA*. 1955;162:1651.
[2] Arneson GA. *J Neuropsychiatr*. 1964;5:181.
[3] Schwarz L, et al. *Am J Psychiatry*. 1968;125(2):253.
[4] Korenyi C, et al. *Dis Nerv Syst*. 1968;29(12):827.
[5] Altszuler N, et al. *Diabetes*. 1977;26(10):931.
[6] Aynsley-Green A, et al. *Lancet*. 1975;2(7936):658.

* Asterisk indicates drugs cited in interaction reports.

Diazoxide — **Thiazide Diuretics**

Diazoxide	Thiazide Diuretics	
Diazoxide* (*Proglycem*)	Bendroflumethiazide* (*Naturetin*)	Indapamide
	Benzthiazide (eg, *Aquatag*)	Methyclothiazide*
	Chlorothiazide (eg, *Diuril*)	Metolazone (eg, *Zaroxolyn*)
	Chlorthalidone (eg, *Thalitone*)	Polythiazide (*Renese*)
	Cyclothiazide (*Anhydron*)	Quinethazone (*Hydromox*)
	Hydrochlorothiazide* (eg, *HydroDiuril*)	Trichlormethiazide* (eg, *Naqua*)
	Hydroflumethiazide (eg, *Saluron*)	

Significance	Onset	Severity	Documentation
2	□ Rapid ■ **Delayed**	□ Major ■ **Moderate** □ Minor	■ **Established** □ Probable □ Suspected □ Possible □ Unlikely

Effects Hyperglycemia, often with symptoms similar to frank diabetes, may occur. The effect appears to return to pretreatment values approximately 2 weeks after these medications are discontinued.

Mechanism Unknown.

Management Decreased dosage of 1 or both agents may be required. Frequent monitoring of blood and urine glucose levels is essential. If possible, avoid this combination.

Discussion

This interaction is well established. In 8 normal males, diazoxide 400 to 645 mg/day in 3 divided doses in combination with trichlormethiazide 4 mg twice daily for 4 to 7 days revealed a marked blunting of insulin secretion in response to a glycemic stimulus.[1] All subjects developed symptomatic hyperglycemia by day 3. In a separate study, 45 hypertensive patients were randomly allocated to treatment with trichlormethiazide 4 mg twice daily either alone or in combination with diazoxide 200 or 400 mg/day for 4 weeks following a 3-week control period of trichlormethiazide alone.[2] Five patients receiving the higher dose diazoxide combination did not complete the study because of hyperglycemia and acidosis. In all, 15 patients treated with one of the diazoxide combinations developed hyperglycemia, and both combinations resulted in large increases in postprandial blood glucose. Similar effects have also been observed in case reports of patients receiving diazoxide in combination with hydrochlorothiazide[3] and bendroflumethiazide, but not with methyclothiazide.[4]

[1] Seltzer HS, et al. *Diabetes.* 1969;18(1):19.
[2] Okun R, et al. *Arch Intern Med.* 1963;112:120.
[3] Dollery CT, et al. *Lancet.* 1962;2(7259):735.
[4] Ernesti M, et al. *Lancet.* 1965;1(7386):628.

* Asterisk indicates drugs cited in interaction reports. Based on pharmacologic and pharmacokinetic considerations, similar interactions may occur with other drugs that are listed.

Didanosine — *Food*

Didanosine*
(eg, *Videx*)

Food*

Significance	Onset	Severity	Documentation
2	■ **Rapid**	□ Major	□ Established
	□ Delayed	■ **Moderate**	□ Probable
		□ Minor	■ **Suspected**
			□ Possible
			□ Unlikely

Effects FOOD may decrease the absorption of DIDANOSINE by as much as 50%. Serum DIDANOSINE concentrations may be reduced, producing a decrease in the therapeutic effects of DIDANOSINE.

Mechanism Because DIDANOSINE is acid labile, administration with FOOD may decrease the bioavailability of DIDANOSINE by increasing the contact time with gastric acid.

Management Administer DIDANOSINE under fasting conditions, not less than 30 minutes before or 2 hours after a meal.[1]

Discussion

The effect of food on the pharmacokinetics of didanosine was studied in 8 men who were seropositive for HIV using a 2-way crossover design.[2] Each patient was given a single oral dose of didanosine 375 mg (three 125 mg tablets) after an overnight fast or after a standardized breakfast consisting of 2 eggs, 1 slice of toast with a pat of butter and jelly, 2 strips of bacon, 4 ounces of hash brown potatoes, and 8 ounces of whole milk. In the fasted state, the mean values for the didanosine C_{max} and AUC were 2,789 ng/mL and 3,902 ng•h/mL, respectively, while urinary excretion accounted for 21% of the intact didanosine. After eating the standard breakfast, the mean values for the didanosine C_{max} and the AUC were 1,291 ng/mL and 2,083 ng•h/mL, respectively, while urinary excretion accounted for 11% of the intact didanosine. The T_{max}, mean residence time, elimination $t_{½}$, and renal clearance were not different for the fed and fasted treatments. These results indicate that the rates of absorption and elimination were not affected by food. However, the extent of absorption was reduced by food. In a second report involving 3 patients, administration of sachets containing didanosine 375 mg, citrate phosphate buffer 5 g, and sucrose with meals decreased the bioavailability of didanosine from 31% to 17% when compared with taking the drug in a fasted state.[3]

[1] Knupp CA, et al. *J Clin Pharmacol.* 1993;33(6):568.
[2] Shyu WC, et al. *Clin Pharmacol Ther.* 1991;50(5, pt 1):503.
[3] Hartman NR, et al. *Clin Pharmacol Ther.* 1991;50(3):278.

* Asterisk indicates drugs cited in interaction reports.

Didanosine — *Ganciclovir*

Didanosine* (eg, *Videx*)	Ganciclovir (eg, *Cytovene*)	Valganciclovir* (*Valcyte*)

Significance	Onset	Severity	Documentation
2	□ Rapid ■ **Delayed**	□ Major ■ **Moderate** □ Minor	□ Established ■ **Probable** □ Suspected □ Possible □ Unlikely

Effects Risk of DIDANOSINE toxicity and CD4+ cell loss or failure of CD4+ cell recovery may be increased.

Mechanism Unknown.

Management Monitor patients for DIDANOSINE toxicity and unexpected CD4+ cell loss or failure of CD4+ cell recovery. DIDANOSINE dosage reduction or alternative antiretroviral therapy may be needed.

Discussion

A 68-year-old woman with HIV and cytomegalovirus enteritis was treated with valganciclovir 900 mg twice daily and an HIV treatment regimen that included didanosine 200 mg twice daily.[1] After 3 months of treatment, her viral load was less than 50 copies/mL and her CD4+ cell count was 317 cells/mm^3. Her viral load remained suppressed over the next 9 months; however, the CD4+ cell count decreased to 83 cells/mm^3 and she experienced didanosine toxicity. Abacavir (eg, *Ziagen*) was substituted for didanosine, resulting in complete CD4+ cell recovery and resolution of didanosine toxicity. The effects of high-dose oral ganciclovir (6,000 mg/day) on steady-state didanosine pharmacokinetics were evaluated in 15 patients who were seropositive for HIV and cytomegalovirus.[2] When ganciclovir was administered either before or 3 hours after didanosine, the mean increases in C_{max}, AUC, and percent excreted in urine were approximately 59% and 87%, 87% and 124%, and 100% and 153%, respectively. In a study of subjects who where HIV- and cytomegalovirus-seropositive, subjects received didanosine alone, simultaneously with ganciclovir, and 2 hours before ganciclovir.[3] Compared with giving didanosine alone, simultaneous administration of ganciclovir and administration of ganciclovir 2 hours after didanosine increased didanosine AUC 107.1% and 114.6%, respectively. Similar increases occurred for didanosine C_{max} (ie, 107.9% and 116%, respectively). In addition, ganciclovir AUC and C_{max} decreased 22.7% and 22.1%, respectively, when ganciclovir was administered 2 hours after didanosine compared with administration of ganciclovir alone.

[1] Tseng AL, et al. *Ann Pharmacother.* 2007;41(3):512.
[2] Jung D, et al. *J Clin Phamacol.* 1998;38(11):1057.
[3] Cimoch PJ, et al. *J Acquir Immune Defic Syndr Hum Retrovirol.* 1998;17(3):227.

* Asterisk indicates drugs cited in interaction reports. Based on pharmacologic and pharmacokinetic considerations, similar interactions may occur with other drugs that are listed.

Didanosine — *Metformin*

Didanosine* (eg, *Videx*)	Metformin* (eg, *Glucophage*)

Significance	Onset	Severity	Documentation
4	☐ Rapid ■ **Delayed**	■ **Major** ☐ Moderate ☐ Minor	☐ Established ☐ Probable ☐ Suspected ■ **Possible** ☐ Unlikely

Effects Risk of life-threatening lactic acidosis may be increased.

Mechanism Unknown.

Management Consider avoiding METFORMIN use in patients receiving DIDANOSINE who have evidence of mitochondrial toxicity (as suggested by fatty liver and elevated liver transaminases).

Discussion

Fatal lactic acidosis was reported in a 53-year-old man with advanced HIV infection during concurrent treatment with didanosine and metformin.[1] Ten days prior to hospital admission, the patient developed polyuria and polydypsia and had a fasting blood glucose of 11 mmol/L (normal range, 3.6 to 6.3 mmol/L). Metformin 500 mg twice daily was started. At that time, he was receiving didanosine 300 mg daily in addition to other antiretroviral and antibiotic agents. Three days before admission, the patient experienced persistent nausea, vomiting, abdominal pain, lethargy, and jaundice. On admission, the patient was afebrile, normotensive, and tachycardic. In addition to a number of abnormal laboratory values, his venous lactic acid level was 14.6 mmol/L (normal range 0.2 to 1.8 mmol/L). Antiretroviral therapy and metformin were discontinued and IV therapy was administered to correct the lactic acidosis and abnormal blood chemistry values. The patient developed cardiac failure and electromechanical dissociation and died 30 hours after hospitalization.

Because lactic acidosis has been reported with use of nucleoside analogs alone, additional documentation is needed to determine if the risk of lactic acidosis is increased with coadministration of metformin and other nucleoside analogs.

[1] Worth L, et al. *Clin Infect Dis.* 2003;37(2):315.

* Asterisk indicates drugs cited in interaction reports.

Didanosine — Ranitidine

Didanosine* (eg, *Videx*)	Ranitidine* (eg, *Zantac*)

Significance	Onset	Severity	Documentation
5	■ **Rapid** □ Delayed	□ Major □ Moderate ■ **Minor**	□ Established □ Probable □ Suspected ■ **Possible** □ Unlikely

Effects The pharmacologic effects of DIDANOSINE may be increased, while those of RANITIDINE may be decreased.

Mechanism Inhibition of gastric acid production by RANITIDINE may increase the bioavailability of DIDANOSINE.

Management No adjustments in therapy appear necessary.

Discussion

The effects of ranitidine administration on the pharmacokinetics and bioavailability of didanosine were studied in 12 men who were seropositive for HIV.[1] In addition, the effect of didanosine on the pharmacokinetics of ranitidine was studied. In an open, randomized, 3-way, crossover trial with each treatment session separated by 1 week, patients received a single dose of didanosine 375 mg, a single oral dose of ranitidine 150 mg, or a single dose of ranitidine 150 mg followed 2 hours later by didanosine 375 mg. Didanosine was administered as a sachet containing didanosine 375 mg, buffering agents (sodium citrate dihydrate, dibasic sodium phosphate anhydrous, and citric acid), and sucrose. The contents of the packet were reconstituted with 120 mL of drinking water. Didanosine AUC increased from 2,953 to 3,359 ng•hr/mL when given with ranitidine versus administration alone. Conversely, the AUC for ranitidine when administered with didanosine was less than when ranitidine was given alone, 1,483 versus 1,771 ng•hr/mL, respectively.

[1] Knupp CA, et al. *Antimicrob Agents Chemother.* 1992;36(10):2075.

* Asterisk indicates drugs cited in interaction reports.

Didanosine — *Ribavirin*

Didanosine* (eg, *Videx*)	Ribavirin* (eg, *Rebetol*)

Significance	Onset	Severity	Documentation
1	☐ Rapid ■ **Delayed**	■ **Major** ☐ Moderate ☐ Minor	☐ Established ☐ Probable ■ **Suspected** ☐ Possible ☐ Unlikely

Effects Systemic exposure to the active metabolite of DIDANOSINE increased, raising the risk of toxicity. Fatal hepatic failure has been reported.

Mechanism Unknown.

Management Concurrent use of RIBAVIRIN and DIDANOSINE is contraindicated.

Discussion

Concurrent use of didanosine with ribavirin is contraindicated because exposure to the active metabolite of didanosine, dideoxyadenosine 5'-triphosphate, is increased. Fatal hepatic failure, peripheral neuropathy, pancreatitis, and symptomatic hyperlactatemia/lactic acidosis have been reported in patients taking both didanosine and ribavirin.[1,2]

The basis for this monograph is information on file with the manufacturer. Published clinical data are needed to further assess this interaction. Because of the seriousness of the adverse reactions, clinical evaluation of the interaction in humans is not likely to be forthcoming.

[1] *Videx* [package insert]. Princeton, NJ: Bristol-Myers Squibb; July 2010.

[2] *Rebetol* [package insert]. Kenilworth, NJ: Schering Corporation; November 2009.

* Asterisk indicates drugs cited in interaction reports.

Didanosine — *Tenofovir*

Didanosine* (eg, *Videx*)	Tenofovir* (*Viread*)

Significance	Onset	Severity	Documentation
1	☐ Rapid ■ **Delayed**	■ **Major** ☐ Moderate ☐ Minor	☐ Established ☐ Probable ■ **Suspected** ☐ Possible ☐ Unlikely

Effects DIDANOSINE plasma levels may be elevated, increasing the risk of life-threatening adverse reactions (eg, lactic acidosis, pancreatitis).

Mechanism Unknown. Lactic acidosis may result from DIDANOSINE-induced mitochondrial toxicity.

Management Coadminister DIDANOSINE and TENOFOVIR with caution and monitor closely for adverse reactions (eg, lactic acidosis, pancreatitis, neuropathy), especially in patients with renal insufficiency. Adjust the DIDANOSINE dosage as needed.

Discussion

A possible drug interaction between didanosine and tenofovir was reported in a 49-year-old man with HIV infection and stable chronic renal insufficiency.[1] Seven weeks after tenofovir was added to the patient's HIV regimen, which included didanosine, he was seen in the emergency department with a 4-day history of progressive fatigue, weakness, confusion, oliguria, and myalgia. After admission, the patient was diagnosed with acute oliguric renal failure and lactic acidosis. Therapy was withdrawn per instructions in the patient's living will. The patient died after discharge to home with hospice. At least 10 cases of pancreatitis were reported during coadministration of didanosine and tenofovir.[2-4] Lactic acidosis and pancreatitis have been reported in patients receiving didanosine alone and in combination with other antiretroviral agents.[5] Didanosine-induced pancreatitis is dose-related.[5] However, there have been cases reported with tenofovir and low-dose didanosine.[3,4] Coadministration of didanosine and tenofovir may increase the C_{max} and AUC of didanosine, which could potentiate didanosine adverse reactions.[6,7] Five of 185 patients receiving didanosine and tenofovir developed pancreatitis.[3] A 63-year-old man who tolerated several didanosine-containing antiretroviral regimens developed lactic acidosis 1.5 years after tenofovir was added to the regimen.[8] In an observational cohort study of patients with HIV, patients receiving didanosine with tenofovir were 3 times more likely to develop decreased renal function than patients receiving lamivudine with tenofovir.[9]

1 Murphy MD, et al. *Clin Infect Dis.* 2003;36(8):1082.
2 Blanchard JN, et al. *Clin Infect Dis.* 2003;37(5):e57.
3 Martínez E, et al. *Lancet.* 2004;364(9428):65.
4 Kirian MA, et al. *Ann Pharmacother.* 2004;38(10):1660.
5 *Videx* [package insert]. Princeton, NJ: Bristol-Myers Squibb Company; December 2000.
6 *Viread* [package insert]. Foster City, CA: Gilead Sciences Inc; October 2003.
7 Kearney BP, et al. *J Clin Pharmacol.* 2005;45(12):1360.
8 Guo Y, et al. *Pharmacotherapy.* 2004;24(8):1089.
9 Crane HM, et al. *AIDS.* 2007;21(11):1431.

* Asterisk indicates drugs cited in interaction reports.

Didanosine — *Xanthine Oxidase Inhibitors*

Didanosine* (eg, *Videx*)	Allopurinol* (eg, *Zyloprim*)	Febuxostat (*Uloric*)

Significance	Onset	Severity	Documentation
2	☐ Rapid	☐ Major	☐ Established
	■ **Delayed**	■ **Moderate**	☐ Probable
		☐ Minor	■ **Suspected**
			☐ Possible
			☐ Unlikely

Effects DIDANOSINE plasma concentration may be elevated, increasing the risk of toxicity.

Mechanism XANTHINE OXIDASE INHIBITORS decrease the metabolism (inhibit purine nucleoside phosphorylase) of DIDANOSINE.

Management Concurrent use of XANTHINE OXIDASE INHIBITORS and DIDANOSINE is contraindicated.

Discussion

In renally impaired patients, coadministration of didanosine with allopurinol increased the didanosine AUC and C_{max} 312% and 232%, respectively. In healthy volunteers, concomitant use of didanosine with allopurinol increased the didanosine AUC and C_{max} 113% and 69%, respectively. Coadministration of didanosine and allopurinol is contraindicated because systemic exposure of didanosine is increased, which may increase didanosine toxicity.[1]

The basis for this monograph is information on file with the manufacturer. Published clinical data are needed to further assess this interaction.

[1] *Videx* [package insert]. Princeton, NJ: Bristol-Myers Squibb; July 2010.

* Asterisk indicates drugs cited in interaction reports. Based on pharmacologic and pharmacokinetic considerations, similar interactions may occur with other drugs that are listed.

Didanosine — Zidovudine

Didanosine*
(eg, *Videx*)

Zidovudine*
(eg, *Retrovir*)

Significance	Onset	Severity	Documentation
4	□ Rapid	□ Major	□ Established
	■ **Delayed**	■ **Moderate**	□ Probable
		□ Minor	□ Suspected
			■ **Possible**
			□ Unlikely

Effects The area under the plasma concentration-time curve of DIDANOSINE may be decreased, while the plasma concentration of ZIDOVUDINE may be increased.

Mechanism Unknown.

Management Based on available clinical data, no special precautions are needed. Monitor the response of the patient and adjust therapy as needed.

Discussion

Didanosine and zidovudine are used concurrently with beneficial clinical effects. In a study involving 8 pediatric patients with HIV infection, zidovudine administration decreased the AUC of didanosine 19%.[3] Didanosine did not alter the pharmacokinetics of zidovudine. In a study of 8 adults with HIV infection, zidovudine plasma concentrations increased 30% during concurrent administration of didanosine compared with giving zidovudine alone.[2] Zidovudine did not alter the pharmacokinetics of didanosine. The pharmacokinetics of zidovudine (60 to 180 mg/m^2/dose) and didanosine (60 to 180 mg/m^2/dose), administered alone and in combination, were studied in HIV-infected patients between the ages of 3 months and 21 years.[1] There was no change in the AUC of either drug during coadministration.

[1] Mueller BU, et al. *J Pediatr.* 1994;125:142.
[2] Barry M, et al. *Br J Clin Pharmacol.* 1994;37:421.
[3] Gibb I, et al. *Br J Clin Pharmacol.* 1994;39:527.

* Asterisk indicates drugs cited in interaction reports.

Diflunisal — *Aluminum Salts*

Diflunisal*
(eg, *Dolobid*)

Aluminum Carbonate (*Basaljel*)
Aluminum Hydroxide* (eg, *Amphojel*)
Attapulgite (eg, *Kaopectate*)
Kaolin
Magaldrate (eg, *Losopan*)

Significance	Onset	Severity	Documentation
4	☐ Rapid ■ **Delayed**	☐ Major ■ **Moderate** ☐ Minor	☐ Established ☐ Probable ☐ Suspected ■ **Possible** ☐ Unlikely

Effects Serum levels of DIFLUNISAL may be decreased, reducing the therapeutic effect.

Mechanism Unknown. However, decreased GI absorption is presumed, because DIFLUNISAL plasma concentrations are not affected by urinary alkalinization.

Management Occasional administration of aluminum-containing antacids probably require no dosage adjustments. However, regular ingestion may require increased doses of DIFLUNISAL or separation of the doses of DIFLUNISAL and antacid by 2 to 3 hours.[4]

Discussion

Administration of aluminum-containing antacids has decreased the bioavailability of diflunisal by up to 40%.[1-3] This reduction in absorption was only evident when the drugs were administered in the fasting state.[3] In patients who were fed, neither aluminum hydroxide nor aluminum/magnesium hydroxide had any detectable effects.[3]

Antacids are frequently administered with nonsteroidal anti-inflammatory drugs to reduce GI irritation. A reduction in absorption may require increased doses, which could increase the risk of GI bleeding.

[1] Verbeeck R, et al. *Br J Clin Pharmacol.* 1979;7:519.
[2] Holmes GI, et al. *Clin Pharmacol Ther.* 1979;25:229.
[3] Tobert JA, et al. *Clin Pharmacol Ther.* 1981;30:385.
[4] D'Arcy PF, et al. *Drug Intell Clin Pharm.* 1987;21:607.

* Asterisk indicates drugs cited in interaction reports. Based on pharmacologic and pharmacokinetic considerations, similar interactions may occur with other drugs that are listed.

Diflunisal — *Probenecid*

Diflunisal*	Probenecid*

Significance	Onset	Severity	Documentation
2	☐ Rapid ■ **Delayed**	☐ Major ■ **Moderate** ☐ Minor	☐ Established ☐ Probable ■ **Suspected** ☐ Possible ☐ Unlikely

Effects The pharmacologic and toxic effects of DIFLUNISAL may be increased.

Mechanism PROBENECID inhibits the metabolism of DIFLUNISAL and displaces DIFLUNISAL from plasma protein-binding sites.

Management Observe patients for DIFLUNISAL toxicity or a decrease in effectiveness if PROBENECID is added to or discontinued from the treatment regimen, respectively.

Discussion

The effects of probenecid on the pharmacokinetics of diflunisal were studied in a multiple-dose investigation involving 8 men.[1] Each subject received oral diflunisal 250 mg twice daily alone (controls) or with probenecid 500 mg every 12 hours. Each study period was 16 days, separated by a 2-week washout period. During coadministration of probenecid, diflunisal plasma clearance was significantly decreased from 5.8 to 3.4 mL/min ($P < 0.001$). The decrease was caused by a reduction in the metabolic clearance of diflunisal to acyl and phenolic glucuronide metabolites, which resulted in a 65% increase in steady-state plasma diflunisal concentrations from 63.1 to 104 mcg/mL ($P < 0.001$). In addition, probenecid increased the unbound fraction of diflunisal 30% to 40%.

[1] Macdonald JI, et al. *Eur J Clin Pharmacol.* 1995;47(6):519.

* Asterisk indicates drugs cited in interaction reports.

Digitalis Glycosides — *Hydantoins*

Digitalis Glycosides	Hydantoins	
Digitoxin*†	Fosphenytoin (*Cerebyx*)	Phenytoin* (eg, *Dilantin*)
Digoxin* (eg, *Lanoxin*)		

Significance	Onset	Severity	Documentation
4	☐ Rapid	☐ Major	☐ Established
	■ **Delayed**	■ **Moderate**	☐ Probable
		☐ Minor	☐ Suspected
			■ **Possible**
			☐ Unlikely

Effects DIGITALIS GLYCOSIDE serum levels may be decreased and actions may be reduced.

Mechanism Unknown.

Management If an interaction is suspected, monitor serum levels and monitor patients for a loss of therapeutic effect. Increase the DIGITALIS GLYCOSIDE dosage as needed.

Discussion

Six healthy volunteers received digitalis glycosides (as digoxin 1 mg IV followed by beta-acetyldigoxin 0.4 mg orally), phenytoin (400 mg/day), or both for 7 days. Steady-state serum concentrations of digoxin were reduced, and AUC and elimination $t_{1/2}$ were reduced 22% and 30%, respectively. Total digoxin clearance was increased 27%; there was no change in renal clearance of digoxin.[1] One patient experienced reductions in digitoxin serum levels during 3 separate courses of phenytoin therapy.[2]

Recommendations for the use of phenytoin in the management of digitalis induced arrhythmias are based on electrophysiologic, not pharmacokinetic, considerations. Therefore, the clinical importance of this interaction remains to be established.

[1] Rameis H. *Eur J Clin Pharmacol.* 1985;29(1):49. [2] Solomon HM, et al. *Ann N Y Acad Sci.* 1971;179:362.

* Asterisk indicates drugs cited in interaction reports. Based on pharmacologic and pharmacokinetic considerations, similar interactions may occur with other drugs that are listed.
† Not available in the United States.

Digitalis Glycosides — *Loop Diuretics*

Digitalis*†	Digoxin* (eg, *Lanoxin*)	Bumetanide*	Furosemide* (eg, *Lasix*)
Digitoxin*†		Ethacrynic Acid* (eg, *Edecrin*)	

Significance	Onset	Severity	Documentation
1	□ Rapid	■ **Major**	□ Established
	■ **Delayed**	□ Moderate	■ **Probable**
		□ Minor	□ Suspected
			□ Possible
			□ Unlikely

Effects Diuretic-induced electrolyte disturbances may predispose patients to DIGITALIS-induced arrhythmias.

Mechanism Increased urinary excretion of potassium and magnesium affecting cardiac muscle action. Other factors may also be involved.

Management Measure plasma levels of potassium and magnesium when using these drugs in combination. Supplement patients with low levels. Prevent further losses with dietary sodium restriction or addition of potassium-sparing diuretics.

Discussion

A dose-dependent reduction in serum potassium and magnesium may occur during therapy with loop diuretics.[1-4] Although other factors may contribute, these electrolyte abnormalities may precipitate or contribute to the development of arrhythmias, especially in patients with preexisting cardiac abnormalities who are receiving digitalis glycosides.[5-9] Magnesium therapy has been used to treat arrhythmias occurring in the setting of "normal" digoxin levels, even when serum levels of magnesium were within the normal range.[9] The benefit may be due to repletion of cellular magnesium losses not reflected by the serum level or the ability of magnesium to facilitate intracellular potassium repletion.[9,10] A case-control study of patients hospitalized for digoxin toxicity found an odds ratio of 2.97 for loop diuretic exposure in the 30 days preceding hospitalization.[11] The risk of hospitalization was even higher when taking digoxin in combination with loop diuretics plus thiazides (odds ratio, 4.06) or digoxin in combination with loop diuretics plus thiazides and potassium-sparing diuretics (odds ratio, 6.85).

Although the relationship between electrolyte depletion and digitalis-induced arrhythmias is well accepted, a clear cause and effect relationship has not been established.[7] Despite this, avoid hypokalemia and hypomagnesemia in digitalis-treated patients by using dietary sodium restriction, supplementation, or potassium/magnesium-sparing diuretics; monitoring plasma levels may be useful.

[1] Lim P, et al. *Br Med J.* 1972;3(5827):620.
[2] Leary WP, et al. *Drugs.* 1984;28(suppl 1):182.
[3] Knochel JP. *Am J Med.* 1984;77(5A):18.
[4] Whang R, et al. *Arch Intern Med.* 1985;145(4):655.
[5] Seller RH, et al. *Am Heart J.* 1970;79(1):57.
[6] Beller GA, et al. *Am J Cardiol.* 1974;33(2):225.
[7] Steiness E, et al. *Br Heart J.* 1976;38(2):167.
[8] Multiple Risk Factor Intervention Trial Research Group. *JAMA.* 1982;248(12):1465.
[9] Cohen L, et al. *JAMA.* 1983;249(20):2808.
[10] Wester PO, et al. *Acta Med Scand Suppl.* 1981;647:145.
[11] Wang MT, et al. *Br J Clin Pharmacol.* 2010;70(2):258.

* Asterisk indicates drugs cited in interaction reports.
† Not available in the United States.

Digitalis Glycosides | **Nondepol. Muscle Relaxants**

Digitoxin†
Digoxin*
(eg, *Lanoxin*)

Pancuronium*

Significance	Onset	Severity	Documentation
4	■ **Rapid** □ Delayed	□ Major ■ **Moderate** □ Minor	□ Established □ Probable □ Suspected ■ **Possible** □ Unlikely

Effects The ability of either drug to precipitate new arrhythmias or potentiate existing rhythm disturbances may be increased when PANCURONIUM is administered to digitalized patients.

Mechanism Unknown.

Management Routine cardiac monitoring is indicated in patients receiving NONDEPOLARIZING MUSCLE RELAXANTS and is sufficient to detect clinically important arrhythmias, which might occur as the result of any interaction.

Discussion

In the only study to implicate an interaction between this class of drugs and digitalis glycosides, digitalized (digoxin) and nondigitalized patients were randomly assigned to receive succinylcholine or pancuronium.[1] The muscle relaxants were given by IV push over 30 seconds to facilitate rapid sequence induction of anesthesia and endotracheal intubation. While both relaxants produced dysrhythmias in the digitalized and nondigitalized groups, the group receiving the combination of pancuronium and digoxin had more arrhythmias than the group receiving succinylcholine and digoxin. Differences among other groups were not statistically significant. Of the patients who developed arrhythmias in the pancuronium-digoxin treated group (6 of 18), 4 demonstrated sinus tachycardia of at least 150 beats/min, while the other 2 patients demonstrated atrial flutter.

If the indication for digoxin in these patients was control of atrial flutter, then this occurrence of the arrhythmia may have represented spontaneous variation in control of this unstable rhythm; therefore, the incidence would not have achieved statistical significance. Additional studies are necessary to confirm the presence of an interaction between these 2 drugs.

[1] Bartolone RS, et al. *Anesthesiology*. 1983;58(6):567.

* Asterisk indicates drugs cited in interaction reports. Based on pharmacologic and pharmacokinetic considerations, similar interactions may occur with other drugs that are listed.
† Not available in the United States.

Digitalis Glycosides — *Succinylcholine*

Digitalis Glycosides	Succinylcholine
Digitoxin†	Succinylcholine* (eg, *Anectine*)
Digoxin* (eg, *Lanoxin*)	

Significance	Onset	Severity	Documentation
4	■ **Rapid**	□ Major	□ Established
	□ Delayed	■ **Moderate**	□ Probable
		□ Minor	□ Suspected
			■ **Possible**
			□ Unlikely

Effects The ability of either drug to precipitate new arrhythmias or potentiate existing rhythm disturbances may be increased when SUCCINYLCHOLINE is given to digitalized patients.

Mechanism Unknown.

Management Routine cardiac monitoring is indicated in patients receiving SUCCINYLCHOLINE and is sufficient to detect any clinically important arrhythmias. D-tubocurarine has been reported to abolish arrhythmias caused by digitalis, succinylcholine, and the combination. However, additional documentation is needed to support its use over conventional arrhythmia treatment protocols.

Discussion

Early reports of succinylcholine administration to digitalized patients, intact animals, and in isolated animal hearts led investigators to conclude that the combination was associated with a high frequency of arrhythmias, including life-threatening ventricular arrhythmias.[1,2,5] However, these reports predate the availability of digitalis glycoside blood levels, so the possibility of digitalis toxicity as a contributing factor cannot be excluded. It is likely that this was a factor in at least 1 report in which the patient was hypercalcemic and had quinidine added to a stable digoxin regimen 48 hours prior to receiving succinylcholine[4] (see also Digoxin-Quinidine).

Additional studies of larger groups of digitalized and nondigitalized patients have concluded that succinylcholine alone is able to induce a variety of arrhythmias, and that the incidence of succinylcholine-induced arrhythmias is no greater in patients receiving digitalis glycosides.[3,4,6] In the one study for which levels were available, all patients were receiving digoxin, with a mean serum level of 1.81 ng/mL.[6] Further studies are required to evaluate this interaction. Whether nondepolarizing muscle relaxants (eg, pancuronium) are alternatives to succinylcholine in digitalized patients also requires additional study. See also Digitalis Glycosides-Nondepolarizing Muscle Relaxants.

[1] Dowdy EG, et al. *Anesth Analg.* 1963;42:501.
[2] Dowdy EG, et al. *Anesth Analg.* 1965;44:608.
[3] Akdikmen SA, et al. *N Y State J Med.* 1965;65:2902.
[4] Perez HR. *Anesth Analg.* 1970;49:33.
[5] Smith RB, et al. *Anesth Analg.* 1972;51:202.
[6] Bartolone RS, et al. *Anesthesiology.* 1983;58:567.

* Asterisk indicates drugs cited in interaction reports. Based on pharmacologic and pharmacokinetic considerations, similar interactions may occur with other drugs that are listed.
† Not available in the United States.

Digitalis Glycosides — *Sulfonylureas*

Digitalis Glycosides	Sulfonylureas	
Digitoxin†	Glyburide* (eg, *DiaBeta*)	Tolbutamide* (eg, *Orinase*)
Digoxin* (eg, *Lanoxin*)		

Significance	Onset	Severity	Documentation
4	☐ Rapid	☐ Major	☐ Established
	■ **Delayed**	■ **Moderate**	☐ Probable
		☐ Minor	☐ Suspected
			■ **Possible**
			☐ Unlikely

Effects DIGITALIS serum levels may rise with coadministration of TOLBUTAMIDE.

Mechanism TOLBUTAMIDE can displace DIGITOXIN from albumin binding sites, temporarily increasing the serum concentration of free DIGITOXIN.[3]

Management Monitor patients receiving DIGITALIS and TOLBUTAMIDE concurrently to assure that DIGITALIS intoxication does not occur. Tailor dosages as needed.

Discussion

One retrospective study of digitalized noninsulin-dependent diabetics reported multifocal ectopic ventricular beats in 12 of 71 patients when tolbutamide was added to the regimen and in none of 80 patients when glyburide was added to the regimen. The same study also reported digitalis intoxication more often in patients who received tolbutamide compared with patients treated with glyburide or diet alone.[1,2]

Further studies are necessary to clarify this interaction and identify whether certain sulfonylureas are preferable in digitalized patients.

[1] Pogatsa G, et al. *Eur J Clin Pharmacol.* 1985;28:367.
[2] Pogatsa G, et al. *Acta Physiol Hung.* 1988;71:243.
[3] Mooradian AD. *Clin Pharmacokinet.* 1988;15:165.

* Asterisk indicates drugs cited in interaction reports. Based on pharmacologic and pharmacokinetic considerations, similar interactions may occur with other drugs that are listed.
† Not available in the United States.

Digitalis Glycosides — Thiazide Diuretics

Digitalis Glycosides	Thiazide Diuretics	
Digitoxin*†	Chlorothiazide* (eg, *Diuril*)	Indapamide
Digoxin* (eg, *Lanoxin*)	Chlorthalidone (eg, *Thalitone*)	Methyclothiazide
	Hydrochlorothiazide* (eg, *Microzide*)	Metolazone (eg, *Zaroxolyn*)
		Trichlormethiazide*

Significance	Onset	Severity	Documentation
1	☐ Rapid	■ **Major**	☐ Established
	■ **Delayed**	☐ Moderate	■ **Probable**
		☐ Minor	☐ Suspected
			☐ Possible
			☐ Unlikely

Effects THIAZIDE-induced electrolyte disturbances may predispose to DIGITALIS-induced arrhythmias.

Mechanism Increased urinary excretion of potassium and magnesium affecting cardiac muscle; other factors may be involved.

Management Measure plasma levels of potassium and magnesium; supplement low levels. Prevent further losses with dietary sodium restriction or potassium-sparing diuretics.

Discussion

A dose-dependent reduction in serum potassium and magnesium may occur with thiazide diuretics.[1-5] These electrolyte abnormalities may contribute to development of arrhythmias, especially in patients with cardiac abnormalities receiving digitalis glycosides.[5-10] Magnesium has been used to treat arrhythmias occurring with "normal" digoxin levels, even when magnesium serum levels were normal.[3] The benefit may be because of repletion of cellular magnesium losses not reflected by the serum level, or to the ability of magnesium to facilitate intracellular potassium repletion.[10,11] A case-control study of patients hospitalized for digoxin toxicity found an association with the use of thiazide diuretics in the 30 days prior to hospitalization (odds ratio, 2.36).[12] The risk was highest with digoxin plus hydrochlorothiazide exposure (odds ratio, 4.63). Although the relationship between electrolyte depletion and digitalis-induced arrhythmias is well accepted, a clear cause-and-effect relationship has not been established.[8] Despite this, avoid hypokalemia and hypomagnesemia in digitalis-treated patients.

1 Lim P, et al. *Br Med J.* 1972;3(5827):620.
2 Leary WP, et al. *Drugs.* 1984;28(suppl 1):182.
3 Knochel JP. *Am J Med.* 1984;77(5A):18.
4 Whang R, et al. *Arch Intern Med.* 1985;145(4):655.
5 Hollifield JW. *Am J Med.* 1986;80(4A):8.
6 Seller RH, et al. *Am Heart J.* 1970;79(1):57.
7 Beller GA, et al. *Am J Cardiol.* 1974;33(2):225.
8 Steiness E, et al. *Br Heart J.* 1976;38(2):167.
9 Multiple Risk Factor Intervention Trial Research Group. *JAMA.* 1982;248(12):1465.
10 Cohen L, et al. *JAMA.* 1983;249(20):2808.
11 Wester PO, et al. *Acta Med Scand Suppl.* 1981;647:145.
12 Wang MT, et al. *Br J Clin Pharmacol.* 2010;70(2):258.

* Asterisk indicates drugs cited in interaction reports. Based on pharmacologic and pharmacokinetic considerations, similar interactions may occur with other drugs that are listed.
† Not available in the United States.

Digitalis Glycosides — *Thioamines*

Digitoxin*†
Digoxin*
(eg, *Lanoxin*)

Methimazole
(eg, *Tapazole*)

Propylthiouracil*
(PTU)

Significance	Onset	Severity	Documentation
2	☐ Rapid ■ **Delayed**	☐ Major ■ **Moderate** ☐ Minor	■ **Established** ☐ Probable ☐ Suspected ☐ Possible ☐ Unlikely

Effects Serum levels of DIGITALIS GLYCOSIDES are increased in hypothyroidism or when hyperthyroid patients on a stable DIGITALIS GLYCOSIDE regimen are rendered euthyroid by THIOAMINES. The therapeutic effect of DIGITALIS GLYCOSIDES may be increased; toxicity may occur.

Mechanism Unknown.

Management Patients maintained in the euthyroid state by THIOAMINES who are started on a DIGITALIS GLYCOSIDE require no special management. However, hyperthyroid patients may require a reduced dose of DIGITALIS GLYCOSIDES if they become euthyroid.

Discussion

A number of studies have confirmed the observations that thyrotoxic patients are resistant to digitalis preparations, while hypothyroid patients are particularly sensitive.[1-8] One investigator found that euthyroid patients with atrial fibrillation required 25% of the daily digoxin dose of mild thyrotoxic patients to maintain the ventricular rate at the control level.[1] Another study showed that hyperthyroid patients had lower serum levels of digoxin, while hypothyroid patients had higher levels, regardless of the route of administration (IV vs oral).[2] The mechanism for this variable response is controversial. Changes in absorption,[1] renal clearance,[3,4,7,8] volume of distribution,[2,7,8] and serum $t_{½}$[4,8] have been invoked, as have changes in myocardial responsiveness. Similar effects have been observed with digitoxin.[3]

1 Frye RL, et al. *Circulation.* 1961;23:376.
2 Doherty JE, et al. *Ann Intern Med.* 1966;64(3):489.
3 Eickenbusch W, et al. *Klin Wochenschr.* 1970;48(5):270.
4 Croxson MS, et al. *Br Med J.* 1975;3(5983):566.
5 Lawrence JR, et al. *Clin Pharmacol Ther.* 1977;22(1):7.
6 Huffman DH, et al. *Clin Pharmacol Ther.* 1977;22(5, pt 1):533.
7 Shenfield GM, et al. *Eur J Clin Pharmacol.* 1977;12(6):437.
8 Bonelli J, et al. *Int J Clin Pharmacol Biopharm.* 1978;16(7):302.

* Asterisk indicates drugs cited in interaction reports. Based on pharmacologic and pharmacokinetic considerations, similar interactions may occur with other drugs that are listed.
† Not available in the United States.

Digitalis Glycosides — Thyroid Hormones

Digitalis Glycosides	Thyroid Hormones	
Digitoxin*†	Levothyroxine* (eg, *Synthroid*)	Liotrix (*Thyrolar*)
Digoxin* (eg, *Lanoxin*)	Liothyronine* (eg, *Cytomel*)	Thyroid (eg, *Armour Thyroid*)

Significance	Onset	Severity	Documentation
2	□ Rapid	□ Major	■ **Established**
	■ **Delayed**	■ **Moderate**	□ Probable
		□ Minor	□ Suspected
			□ Possible
			□ Unlikely

Effects Serum levels of DIGITALIS GLYCOSIDES are reduced in hyperthyroidism or when hypothyroid patients on a stable DIGITALIS GLYCOSIDE regimen are rendered euthyroid by THYROID HORMONE therapy. The therapeutic effect of DIGITALIS GLYCOSIDES may be reduced.

Mechanism Unknown.

Management Patients maintained in the euthyroid state by THYROID HORMONE therapy who are started on a DIGITALIS GLYCOSIDE require no special management. However, hypothyroid patients may require increased dosage of DIGITALIS GLYCOSIDES if they become euthyroid.

Discussion

A number of studies have confirmed the observations that thyrotoxic patients are resistant to digitalis preparations while hypothyroid patients are particularly sensitive.[1-8] One investigator found that induction of mild thyrotoxicosis in 3 euthyroid patients with atrial fibrillation required up to 4 times more daily digoxin to control ventricular rate.[1] Another study showed that hyperthyroid patients had lower serum levels of digoxin, while hypothyroid patients had higher levels, regardless of the route of administration (IV vs oral).[2] The mechanism for this variable response is controversial. Changes in absorption,[1] renal clearance,[3,4,7,8] volume of distribution,[2,7,8] and serum half-life[4,8] have been invoked, as have changes in myocardial responsiveness. Similar effects have been observed with digitoxin.[3]

1 Frye RL, et al. *Circulation*. 1961;23;376.
2 Doherty JE, et al. *Ann Intern Med*. 1966;64:489.
3 Eickenbusch W, et al. *Klin Wochenschr*. 1970;48:270.
4 Croxson MS, et al. *Br Med J*. 1975;3:566.
5 Lawrence JR, et al. *Clin Pharmacol Ther*. 1977;22:7.
6 Huffman DH, et al. *Clin Pharmacol Ther*. 1977;22:533.
7 Shenfield GM, et al. *Eur J Clin Pharmacol*. 1977;12:437.
8 Bonelli J, et al. *Int J Clin Pharmacol Biopharm*. 1978;16:302.

* Asterisk indicates drugs cited in interaction reports. Based on pharmacologic and pharmacokinetic considerations, similar interactions may occur with other drugs that are listed.

† Not available in the United States.

Digoxin — *Acarbose*

Digoxin*
(eg, *Lanoxin*)

Acarbose*
(*Precose*)

Significance	Onset	Severity	Documentation
2	☐ Rapid ■ **Delayed**	☐ Major ■ **Moderate** ☐ Minor	☐ Established ■ **Probable** ☐ Suspected ☐ Possible ☐ Unlikely

Effects Serum DIGOXIN concentrations may be reduced, decreasing the therapeutic effects.

Mechanism Impaired DIGOXIN absorption is suspected.

Management Monitor the patient for a decreased therapeutic response to DIGOXIN. If an interaction is suspected, it may be necessary to increase the dose of DIGOXIN or discontinue ACARBOSE. Giving ACARBOSE 6 hr after the DIGOXIN dose may circumvent this interaction.[3]

Discussion

Subtherapeutic digoxin plasma concentrations were reported in a 69-year-old woman following addition of acarbose to her drug regimen.[1] The patient had a history of unstable angina, congestive heart failure, and type 1 diabetes. She had been treated for years with insulin, nifedipine (eg, *Procardia*), isosorbide dinitrate (eg, *Isordil*), clorazepate (eg, *Tranxene*), nabumetone (*Relafen*), and digoxin 0.25 mg/day. Acarbose was added to her therapeutic regimen, and 13 months later, the plasma digoxin concentration was 0.48 ng/mL, which was below the therapeutic range for the hospital (0.8 to 2.1 ng/mL). Despite supplementing the digoxin dose with 0.125 mg digoxin twice weekly, subtherapeutic digoxin levels persisted (0.64 ng/mL). Acarbose treatment was discontinued, the digoxin dose returned to 0.25 mg/day, and the serum digoxin concentration increased to 1.9 ng/mL. Because the clinical condition of the patient did not deteriorate when the concentrations of digoxin were subtherapeutic, administration of digoxin was discontinued. Subtherapeutic digoxin levels occurred in 2 patients after acarbose therapy was started.[3] In 1 patient, atrial fibrillation developed. In both patients, acarbose discontinuation increased digoxin levels and rechallenge with acarbose again resulted in decreased digoxin levels. In 1 study, 7 volunteers received 0.5 mg digoxin alone, 30 minutes after a single 200 mg dose of acarbose, or after 3 days of 100 mg acarbose 3 times daily.[2] Peak digoxin concentrations were reduced. The single dose of acarbose decreased the AUC of digoxin 39%, while 100 mg 3 times daily decreased the AUC 43%.

[1] Serrano JS, et al. *Clin Pharmacol Ther.* 1996;60:589.
[2] Miura T, et al. *J Clin Pharmacol.* 1998;38:654.
[3] Ben-Ami H, et al. *Diabetes Care.* 1999;22:860.

* Asterisk indicates drugs cited in interaction reports.

Digoxin — ACE Inhibitors

Digoxin*
(eg, *Lanoxin*)

Benazepril (eg, *Lotensin*)	Moexipril (eg, *Univasc*)
Captopril* (eg, *Capoten*)	Perindopril (*Aceon*)
Enalapril* (eg, *Vasotec*)	Quinapril (eg, *Accupril*)
Fosinopril (eg, *Monopril*)	Ramipril (*Altace*)
Lisinopril* (eg, *Prinivil*)	Trandolapril (eg, *Mavik*)

Significance	Onset	Severity	Documentation
4	☐ Rapid ■ **Delayed**	☐ Major ■ **Moderate** ☐ Minor	☐ Established ☐ Probable ☐ Suspected ■ **Possible** ☐ Unlikely

Effects Plasma levels of DIGOXIN may be increased or decreased.

Mechanism Unknown. Renal clearance of DIGOXIN may be altered.

Management No additional precautions appear necessary other than routine monitoring for DIGOXIN toxicity. Monitoring DIGOXIN plasma levels may be useful in managing patients.

Discussion

In a double-blind study of 20 patients with CHF, the addition of captopril 37.5 to 150 mg/day (mean, 93.75 mg) to a regimen of digoxin and furosemide (eg, *Lasix*) resulted in a statistically significant increase in digoxin serum levels from a mean of 1.4 to 1.7 mmol/L.[1,2] Renal digoxin clearance also decreased.[2] Captopril 12.5 mg 3 times daily for 7 days was given to 8 patients with heart failure who were receiving digoxin.[3] Peak digoxin levels increased from 1.7 to 2.7 ng/mL. No symptoms of digoxin toxicity were observed. In contrast, no difference in digoxin levels was observed in 67 patients maintained for 6 months on both drugs.[4] A study of this interaction in patients receiving enalapril 20 mg/day failed to demonstrate a change in digoxin serum levels after 30 days.[5] However, a trial evaluating the effect of enalapril on ventricular arrhythmias noted a slight decrease in digoxin serum levels.[6] Plasma digoxin concentrations were slightly lower, while urinary excretion of digoxin was slightly higher (20%) during lisinopril and digoxin coadministration to healthy volunteers.[7] No pharmacokinetic interaction was observed during administration of ramipril (*Altace*) and digoxin.[8]

1 Cleland JG, et al. *Br J Clin Pharmacol.* 1984;17:214.
2 Cleland JG, et al. *Am Heart J.* 1986;112(1):130.
3 Kirimli O, et al. *Int J Clin Pharmacol Ther.* 2001;39(7):311.
4 Magelli C, et al. *Eur J Clin Pharmacol.* 1989;36(1):99.
5 Douste-Blazy P, et al. *Br J Clin Pharmacol.* 1986;22(6):752.
6 Webster MW, et al. *Am J Cardiol.* 1985;56(8):566.
7 Vandenburg MJ, et al. *Xenobiotica.* 1988;18(10):1179.
8 Doering W, et al. *Am J Cardiol.* 1987;59(10):60D.

* Asterisk indicates drugs cited in interaction reports. Based on pharmacologic and pharmacokinetic considerations, similar interactions may occur with other drugs that are listed.

Digoxin — *Albuterol*

Digoxin	Albuterol
Digoxin* (eg, *Lanoxin*)	Albuterol* (eg, *Proventil*)

Significance	Onset	Severity	Documentation
4	■ **Rapid**	□ Major	□ Established
	□ Delayed	■ **Moderate**	□ Probable
		□ Minor	□ Suspected
			■ **Possible**
			□ Unlikely

Effects ALBUTEROL may decrease serum DIGOXIN levels, possibly decreasing the therapeutic effects of DIGOXIN.

Mechanism Unknown. Possible $beta_2$-agonist enhanced skeletal muscle binding of DIGOXIN.

Management Consider monitoring serum DIGOXIN levels and clinical effectiveness in patients receiving ALBUTEROL concurrently. Adjust the DIGOXIN dose as needed.

Discussion

In a study involving 10 healthy male volunteers, coadministration of digoxin and a single dose of albuterol decreased serum digoxin and potassium concentrations.[1] Following oral administration of digoxin 0.5 mg daily for 10 days, each subject was studied on 2 different occasions separated by 2 to 3 days. After serum digoxin levels stabilized, each subject received a single oral dose of albuterol 3 mg (4 mg if their body weight was greater than 80 kg). Subsequent to the administration of albuterol, both serum digoxin levels and serum potassium concentrations decreased significantly ($P < 0.05$ and $P < 0.001$, respectively) compared with the control period. Blood samples were drawn up to 3 hours after the administration of albuterol. The greatest difference was a 22% decrease (0.3 nmol/L) in the digoxin level and a 14% decrease (0.58 mmol/L) in potassium concentration. There was no change in skeletal muscle digoxin concentration. In 9 healthy volunteers, oral pretreatment, 10-hour infusion, and oral posttreatment with albuterol produced a reduction in the area under the concentration-time curve of digoxin by 15% with no change in volume of distribution and clearance following a single IV digoxin dose.[2] Skeletal muscle digoxin concentration was 48% higher after the albuterol infusion.

Additional studies are needed to determine the effect of chronic or intermittent albuterol treatment on the pharmacokinetics, pharmacodynamics, and clinical effectiveness of digoxin.

[1] Edner M, et al. *Eur J Clin Pharmacol.* 1990;38:195. [2] Edner M, et al. *Eur J Clin Pharmacol.* 1992;42:197.

* Asterisk indicates drugs cited in interaction reports.

Digoxin — Aluminum Salts

Digoxin*
(eg, *Lanoxin*)

Aluminum Carbonate (*Basaljel*)
Aluminum Hydroxide* (eg, *Amphojel*)
Attapulgite (eg, *Donnagel*)
Kaolin*
Magaldrate (eg, *Riopan*)

Significance	Onset	Severity	Documentation
4	☐ Rapid	☐ Major	☐ Established
	■ **Delayed**	■ **Moderate**	☐ Probable
		☐ Minor	☐ Suspected
			■ **Possible**
			☐ Unlikely

Effects DIGOXIN serum levels may be reduced; therapeutic effects may be decreased.

Mechanism Unknown. Probably caused by adsorption of DIGOXIN by ALUMINUM SALTS.

Management Occasional use of ALUMINUM SALTS appears acceptable. However, if regular administration is required, give ALUMINUM SALTS several hours following DIGOXIN.

Discussion

In vitro and volunteer studies indicate that aluminum hydroxide gel can reduce the absorption of digoxin 11% to 15%, presumably by adsorption.[1-4,7] One study reported that the administration of 60 mL of 4% aluminum hydroxide gel or kaolin (aluminum silicate)-pectin suspension (*Kaopectate* [formulation no longer available in the US]) in 10 volunteers reduced digoxin oral bioavailability 23% and 42%, respectively.[2] Another study examined the effects of administration of 90 mL of a concentrated kaolin-pectin suspension 2 hours prior to, along with, and 2 hours after 0.5 mg of digoxin tablets. Coadministration reduced digoxin bioavailability 62%. Prior administration reduced absorption 20%. Administering the antidiarrheal 2 hours after digoxin did not affect the extent of absorption.[3] Other studies have failed to support the interaction. A 15% reduction in oral absorption in volunteers with steady-state levels of digoxin receiving *Maalox* (aluminum/magnesium hydroxide gel) or *Kaopectate* was of little clinical importance.[5] Similarly, a 15% reduction in absorption after 90 mL of kaolin-pectin was not significant and could be completely abolished by separating the administration by 2 hours.[6]

1 Khalil SA. *J Pharm Pharmacol.* 1974;26:961.
2 Brown DD, et al. *N Engl J Med.* 1976;295:1034.
3 Albert KS, et al. *J Pharm Sci.* 1978;67:1582.
4 McElnay JC, et al. *BMJ.* 1978;1:1554.
5 Allen MD, et al. *J Clin Pharmacol.* 1981;21:26.
6 Albert KS, et al. *J Clin Pharmacol.* 1981;21:449.
7 Saris SD, et al. *Curr Ther Res.* 1983;34:662.

* Asterisk indicates drugs cited in interaction reports. Based on pharmacologic and pharmacokinetic considerations, similar interactions may occur with other drugs that are listed.

Digoxin — *Ambrisentan*

Digoxin* (eg, *Lanoxin*)	Ambrisentan* (*Letairis*)

Significance	Onset	Severity	Documentation
4	☐ Rapid	☐ Major	☐ Established
	■ **Delayed**	■ **Moderate**	☐ Probable
		☐ Minor	☐ Suspected
			■ **Possible**
			☐ Unlikely

Effects DIGOXIN plasma concentrations may be elevated slightly, possibly increasing the risk of adverse reactions.

Mechanism Unknown.

Management Based on the magnitude of the change in the DIGOXIN plasma concentration, it is unlikely that a clinically important drug interaction will occur. However, because DIGOXIN has a narrow therapeutic index, routine monitoring of the patient for clinical and ECG evidence of toxicity as well as monitoring of DIGOXIN plasma concentrations during AMBRISENTAN administration is warranted.

Discussion

In an open-label, nonrandomized study, the effects of ambrisentan on the pharmacokinetics of digoxin were evaluated in 15 healthy men.[1] Each subject received a single dose of digoxin 0.5 mg alone and after 5 days of administration of ambrisentan 10 mg daily. Compared with giving digoxin alone, pretreatment with ambrisentan increased the digoxin C_{max} and AUC 29% and 9%, respectively.

[1] Richards DB, et al. *J Clin Pharmacol.* 2011;51(1):102.

* Asterisk indicates drugs cited in interaction reports.

Digoxin — *Amiloride*

Digoxin* (eg, *Lanoxin*)	Amiloride* (eg, *Midamor*)

Significance	Onset	Severity	Documentation
4	■ **Rapid**	□ Major	□ Established
	□ Delayed	■ **Moderate**	□ Probable
		□ Minor	□ Suspected
			■ **Possible**
			□ Unlikely

Effects Pharmacologic effects of DIGOXIN may be reduced.

Mechanism Unknown.

Management Monitor patients on this combination for reduced pharmacologic effects of DIGOXIN. Serum level monitoring is probably not useful, since the effect appears to be independent of DIGOXIN levels.

Discussion

Amiloride has been shown to modify digoxin clearance and attenuate digoxin-induced positive inotropism.[1,2] In 6 healthy volunteers, amiloride was shown to increase mean renal digoxin clearance from 1.3 to 2.4 mL/kg/min while nonrenal clearance declined greater than 90%. The net effect on total body clearance was not statistically significant. Pretreatment with amiloride was also shown to abolish the concentration-dependent increase in contractility induced by digoxin.[1] In vitro studies support the ability of amiloride to decrease the maximum positive inotropic and toxic effect of dihydrodigoxin.[2] Possible mechanisms for the antagonism include inhibition of sarcolemmal cation exchange.[2]

Additional studies are necessary to establish the importance of this possible interaction on the inotropic and electrophysiologic effects of digoxin. See also Digoxin-Spironolactone and Digoxin-Triamterene.

[1] Waldorff S, et al. *Clin Pharmacol Ther.* 1981;30:172. [2] Kennedy RH, et al. *Eur J Pharmacol.* 1985;115:199.

* Asterisk indicates drugs cited in interaction reports.

Digoxin — **Aminoglycosides**

Digoxin	Aminoglycosides	
Digoxin* (eg, *Lanoxin*)	Kanamycin (*Kantrex*)	Paromomycin (eg, *Humatin*)
	Neomycin* (eg, *Neo-fradin*)	

Significance	Onset	Severity	Documentation
2	☐ Rapid ■ **Delayed**	☐ Major ■ **Moderate** ☐ Minor	☐ Established ☐ Probable ■ **Suspected** ☐ Possible ☐ Unlikely

Effects

The rate and extent of DIGOXIN absorption may be reduced, which could reduce the pharmacologic effect of the drug. However, in a small number of patients (< 10%), this may be offset by a NEOMYCIN-induced reduction in metabolism of the drug.

Mechanism

The mechanism for the reduction in rate and extent of absorption is unknown. The potential for decreased metabolism is presumed to be caused by NEOMYCIN's killing of intestinal bacteria that contribute to the formation of DIGOXIN-reduction products (DRPs).

Management

Most patients on maintenance DIGOXIN who receive a single dose of NEOMYCIN probably require no special monitoring. However, monitor poorly controlled patients or those who require repeated or prolonged administration of NEOMYCIN for change in clinical status or DIGOXIN levels, with appropriate dosage modification.

Discussion

A single, well-designed study in healthy volunteers has demonstrated that oral neomycin in doses of 1 to 3 g depresses peak serum digoxin concentrations, the time to reach peak, and the area under the concentration-time curve. The inhibition of digoxin absorption was evident after single and multiple doses of neomycin, but most pronounced after the single dose studies (mean decrease of 60% in serum digoxin concentrations vs 28% reduction after 9 days of coadministration).[1]

A subsequent study of DRPs from the same investigator suggested that the small percentage of patients (less than 10%) who inactivate significant amounts of digoxin by the GI flora may have enhanced bioavailability, presumably because of neomycin-induced reduction in intestinal bacteria.[2] However, this effect was not directly observed in the 6 patients studied.

[1] Lindenbaum J, et al. *Gastroenterology*. 1976;71:399.

[2] Lindenbaum J, et al. *Am J Med*. 1981;71:67.

* Asterisk indicates drugs cited in interaction reports. Based on pharmacologic and pharmacokinetic considerations, similar interactions may occur with other drugs that are listed.

Digoxin — *Aminoquinolines*

Digoxin*
(eg, *Lanoxin*)

Hydroxychloroquine*
(eg, *Plaquenil*)

Significance	Onset	Severity	Documentation
4	□ Rapid ■ **Delayed**	■ **Major** □ Moderate □ Minor	□ Established □ Probable □ Suspected ■ **Possible** □ Unlikely

Effects Serum levels of DIGOXIN may be increased. The actions of DIGOXIN may be enhanced or toxicity may develop.

Mechanism Unknown.

Management Monitor patients on combined therapy for signs and symptoms of DIGOXIN toxicity; reduce the dose if necessary. Serum level monitoring may facilitate tailoring of dosage.

Discussion

Two patients experienced increases in serum digoxin levels when hydroxychloroquine was added to their stable digoxin regimens.[2] During therapy with hydroxychloroquine 250 mg twice daily for rheumatoid arthritis, digoxin serum levels were 3.1 nmol/L (2.4 ng/mL) and 3 nmol/L (2.3 ng/mL) in the 2 patients. Following discontinuation of hydroxychloroquine, the levels on the same dose of digoxin were 0.9 nmol/L (7 ng/mL) and 0.7 nmol/L (5.5 ng/mL), respectively. No pretreatment levels were available, and no signs and symptoms of digoxin toxicity were reported.

An interaction between digoxin and hydroxychloroquine, a semisynthetic derivative of quinine, could be anticipated on the basis of the confirmed interaction between digoxin, the cinchona alkaloid quinine and its optical isomer, quinidine.[1] See also Digoxin-Quinidine and Digoxin-Quinine. However, additional studies are necessary to establish the incidence and clinical importance of this likely interaction.

[1] Bigger JT, et al. *Drugs*. 1982;24:229. Review.

[2] Leden I. *Acta Med Scand*. 1982;211:411.

* Asterisk indicates drugs cited in interaction reports.

Digoxin — *Aminosalicylic Acid*

Digoxin* (eg, *Lanoxin*)	Aminosalicylic Acid (*Paser*)*

Significance	Onset	Severity	Documentation
4	☐ Rapid	☐ Major	☐ Established
	■ **Delayed**	■ **Moderate**	☐ Probable
		☐ Minor	☐ Suspected
			■ **Possible**
			☐ Unlikely

Effects Oral absorption of DIGOXIN may be reduced with a subsequent reduction in serum levels. The actions of DIGOXIN may be reduced.

Mechanism Unknown. Available data suggest that PAS induces changes in the function of the intestinal wall.

Management Monitor patients on a stable digoxin regimen who are started on PAS for a reduction in digoxin effect. The addition of DIGOXIN to a PAS regimen may require higher than anticipated DIGOXIN doses. DIGOXIN serum level monitoring may be advisable whenever PAS is added or withdrawn to determine if any tailoring of dosage is necessary.

Discussion

A study in 10 healthy volunteers showed that the absorption of single doses of 0.75 mg of digoxin tablets was reduced approximately 20% after 2 weeks of treatment with para-aminosalicylic acid (PAS) 2 g/day.[1]

Additional studies are necessary in patients who have achieved digoxin steady-state to determine the importance of this interaction in maintenance digoxin therapy.

[1] Brown DD, et al. *Circulation.* 1978;58:164.

* Asterisk indicates drugs cited in interaction reports.

Digoxin — Amiodarone

Digoxin*
(eg, *Lanoxin*)

Amiodarone*
(eg, *Cordarone*)

Significance	Onset	Severity	Documentation
1	☐ Rapid	■ **Major**	☐ Established
	■ **Delayed**	☐ Moderate	■ **Probable**
		☐ Minor	☐ Suspected
			☐ Possible
			☐ Unlikely

Effects Serum DIGOXIN levels may be increased, resulting in an increase in the pharmacologic and toxic effects of DIGOXIN.

Mechanism Unknown. Multiple mechanisms are probably involved.

Management Monitor patients for signs and symptoms of DIGOXIN toxicity, and adjust the dose accordingly. Consider empiric reduction of the DIGOXIN dose during AMIODARONE therapy. Serum DIGOXIN levels may aid in dose adjustment.

Discussion

Administration of amiodarone to patients on stable doses of digoxin results in increased digoxin serum levels.[1-6] Digoxin toxicity has been observed in some patients.[1,2,4] The increase in serum digoxin levels has been between 69% and 800%, with most studies reporting an approximate doubling of the digoxin level.[4,5] The increase appears to be dose-related, with higher doses of amiodarone (such as those used during loading regimens) associated with the greatest increase in digoxin levels. Digoxin levels usually start to increase within the first few days after addition of amiodarone and may not reach steady state even after 2 weeks of combined therapy.[5] Because of the long t½ of amiodarone, the effects of the interaction may persist long after the drug is discontinued.[5,7]

The exact mechanism of the interaction is unknown and is probably multifactorial. Reductions in the volume of distribution of digoxin and its renal and nonrenal clearance have been measured.[2,3,5,6] Displacement of digoxin from tissue binding sites may also occur.[3,5] One study of 5 patients receiving the combination failed to demonstrate any change in serum digoxin levels.[8]

Because patients who receive amiodarone therapy frequently have underlying heart disease and are often at greater risk of arrhythmic complications, monitor use of this combination carefully.

1 Moysey JO, et al. *Br Med J.* 1981;282(6260):272.
2 Koren G, et al. *J Pediatr.* 1984;104(3):467.
3 Douste-Blazy P, et al. *Lancet.* 1984;1(8382):905.
4 Oetgen WJ, et al. *Chest.* 1984;86(1):75.
5 Nademanee K, et al. *J Am Coll Cardiol.* 1984;4(1):111.
6 Fenster PE, et al. *J Am Coll Cardiol.* 1985;5(1):108.
7 DeVore KJ, et al. *Pharmacotherapy.* 2007;27(3):472.
8 Achilli A, et al. *Br Med J.* 1981;282(6276):1630.

* Asterisk indicates drugs cited in interaction reports.

Digoxin — *Anticholinergics*

Digoxin* (eg, *Lanoxin*)

Anticholinergics	
Atropine (eg, *Sal-Tropine*)	Orphenadrine (eg, *Norflex*)
Belladonna	Oxybutynin (eg, *Ditropan*)
Benztropine (eg, *Cogentin*)	Procyclidine (*Kemadrin*)
Biperiden (*Akineton*)	Propantheline* (eg, *Pro-Banthine*)
Clidinium (*Quarzan*)	Scopolamine (eg, *Scopace*)
Dicyclomine (eg, *Bentyl*)	Trihexyphenidyl (eg, *Artane*)
Glycopyrrolate (eg, *Robinul*)	
Hyoscyamine (eg, *Anaspaz*)	
Mepenzolate (*Cantil*)	
Methscopolamine (*Pamine*)	

Significance	Onset	Severity	Documentation
4	☐ Rapid	☐ Major	☐ Established
	■ **Delayed**	■ **Moderate**	☐ Probable
		☐ Minor	☐ Suspected
			■ **Possible**
			☐ Unlikely

Effects Serum levels of DIGOXIN administered as slow dissolution oral tablets may be increased and actions enhanced.

Mechanism Unknown. ANTICHOLINERGICS probably reduce GI motility with resultant increased time for absorption.

Management Monitor patients receiving slow dissolution DIGOXIN for increased action if ANTICHOLINERGICS are coadministered regularly. Serum level monitoring may assist in tailoring dosage. Problems may be avoided with use of DIGOXIN elixir or capsules.

Discussion

Studies in patients and healthy volunteers demonstrate an increase in digoxin bioavailability after coadministration of propantheline.[1,2,4,5] In 1 trial, propantheline 15 mg was administered 3 times daily to elderly women on maintenance digoxin therapy.[1] After 10 days, serum digoxin levels rose from a mean of 1.02 to 1.33 ng/mL in 9 of the 13; the digoxin formulation used (*Orion*) had a very low rate of dissolution.[3] The rate of dissolution of the formula seems critical since no effect is seen when propantheline is administered with digoxin elixir, rapid-dissolution tablets (eg, *Lanoxin*), micronized formulations, or solution in capsules (*Lanoxicaps*).[1,2,4,5] Most of these studies with slow dissolution tablets predate USP revisions.

1 Manninen V, et al. *Lancet*. 1973;1:398.
2 Manninen V, et al. *Lancet*. 1973;1:1118.
3 Medin S, et al. *Lancet*. 1973;1:1393.
4 Johnson BF, et al. *Br J Clin Pharmacol*. 1978;5:465.
5 Brown DD, et al. *J Clin Pharmacol*. 1985;25:360.

* Asterisk indicates drugs cited in interaction reports. Based on pharmacologic and pharmacokinetic considerations, similar interactions may occur with other drugs that are listed.

Digoxin — Antineoplastic Agents

Digoxin	Antineoplastic Agents	
Digoxin* (eg, *Lanoxin*)	Bleomycin* (eg, *Blenoxane*)	Doxorubicin* (eg, *Adriamycin*)
	Carmustine* (eg, *BiCNU*)	Methotrexate* (eg, *Rheumatrex*)
	Cyclophosphamide* (eg, *Cytoxan*)	Vincristine* (eg, *Oncovin*)
	Cytarabine* (eg, *Cytosar-U*)	

Significance	Onset	Severity	Documentation
2	☐ Rapid	☐ Major	☐ Established
	■ **Delayed**	■ **Moderate**	☐ Probable
		☐ Minor	■ **Suspected**
			☐ Possible
			☐ Unlikely

Effects Serum levels of DIGOXIN may be reduced and actions may be decreased. Some agents or combinations may not be involved.

Mechanism Drug-induced alterations of the intestinal mucosa may be involved in reduced GI absorption of DIGOXIN.

Management Monitor patients for signs of reduction in pharmacologic effect (eg, deteriorating heart failure, loss of control of ventricular rate). Increase dose of DIGOXIN if necessary; serum level monitoring may facilitate tailoring dosage.

Discussion

The rate and extent of oral absorption of beta-acetyldigoxin was reduced in patients on the following chemotherapy regimens: COPP (cyclophosphamide, *Oncovin*, procarbazine, prednisone), COP (cyclophosphamide, *Oncovin*, prednisone), ABP (*Adriamycin*, bleomycin, prednisone), and COAP (cyclophosphamide, *Oncovin*, cytosine-arabinoside, prednisone).[1] Mean maximal digoxin plasma levels were reduced from 3.4 to 2.6 ng/mL. Mean steady-state plasma levels were 50% lower than control during cytostatic therapy. Area under the plasma concentration-time curve was reduced 20% to 30% in all patients. High-dose antineoplastic regimens reduced the absorption of *Lanoxin* tablets 46%; absorption of *Lanoxicaps* was not reduced.[2] Further studies are necessary to characterize this interaction. However, available data suggest that the use of digitoxin or digoxin capsules can eliminate alteration of absorption by chemotherapy.

[1] Kuhlmann J, et al. *Clin Pharmacol Ther.* 1981;30:518. [2] Bjornsson TD, et al. *Clin Pharmacol Ther.* 1986;39:25.

* Asterisk indicates drugs cited in interaction reports.

Digoxin | **Azole Antifungal Agents**

Digoxin*
(eg, *Lanoxin*)

Itraconazole*
(eg, *Sporanox*)

Significance	Onset	Severity	Documentation
2	□ Rapid ■ **Delayed**	□ Major ■ **Moderate** □ Minor	■ **Established** □ Probable □ Suspected □ Possible □ Unlikely

Effects Serum DIGOXIN concentrations may be increased, enhancing its pharmacologic and adverse reactions.

Mechanism Reduced renal clearance because of inhibition of the P-glycoprotein transport of DIGOXIN[1,2] and increased absorption[2] may be involved.

Management Monitor plasma DIGOXIN concentrations and observe the patient for signs of DIGOXIN toxicity. Adjust the dose of DIGOXIN accordingly.

Discussion

A 68-year-old man with right elbow swelling caused by *Sporothrix schenckii* osteoarthritis was started on itraconazole 400 mg/day.[3] The patient had a history of atrial fibrillation and was receiving digoxin 0.25 mg twice daily as well as ibuprofen (eg, *Motrin*) 400 mg as needed. While taking the same dose 1 year prior, his plasma digoxin concentration was 1.6 ng/mL. On 2 occasions, while receiving digoxin and itraconazole, the patient developed nausea and fatigue. During cotreatment with digoxin and itraconazole, he had a digoxin serum concentration of 3.2 ng/mL and an irregular heart rate of 40 bpm. After stopping all drugs, digoxin and itraconazole were gradually restarted. The doses of digoxin and itraconazole were stabilized at 0.125 mg/day and 400 mg/day, respectively. On this schedule, digoxin concentrations ranged from 0.8 to 1.8 ng/mL. Additional cases of itraconazole-induced elevations in digoxin levels, with[4,5] and without toxicity,[6] have been reported. In a randomized, crossover study in 10 healthy volunteers, digoxin 0.25 mg was administered with placebo or itraconazole 200 mg/day for 10 days.[7] Compared with placebo, itraconazole produced a 56% increase in serum digoxin concentrations.

[1] Ito S, et al. *Ann Pharmacother.* 1997;31:1091.
[2] Jalava KM, et al. *Ther Drug Monit.* 1997;19:609.
[3] Rex J. *Ann Intern Med.* 1992;116:525.
[4] Cone LA, et al. *West J Med.* 1996;165:322.
[5] Mathis AS, et al. *Am J Kidney Dis.* 2001;37:E18.
[6] Alderman CP, et al. *Ann Pharmacother.* 1997;31:438.
[7] Partanen J, et al. *Pharmacol Toxicol.* 1996;79:274.

* Asterisk indicates drugs cited in interaction reports.

Digoxin — *Benzodiazepines*

Digoxin	Benzodiazepines	
Digoxin* (eg, *Lanoxin*)	Alprazolam* (eg, *Xanax*)	Lorazepam (eg, *Ativan*)
	Chlordiazepoxide (eg, *Librium*)	Midazolam
	Clonazepam (eg, *Klonopin*)	Oxazepam (eg, *Serax*)
	Clorazepate (eg, *Tranxene*)	Quazepam (*Doral*)
	Diazepam* (eg, *Valium*)	Temazepam (eg, *Restoril*)
	Estazolam (*ProSom*)	Triazolam (eg, *Halcion*)
	Flurazepam (eg, *Dalmane*)	

Significance	Onset	Severity	Documentation
4	☐ Rapid	☐ Major	☐ Established
	■ **Delayed**	■ **Moderate**	☐ Probable
		☐ Minor	☐ Suspected
			■ **Possible**
			☐ Unlikely

Effects DIGOXIN serum concentrations and toxicity may increase.

Mechanism Unknown.

Management Consider monitoring DIGOXIN concentrations and the patient's clinical status during BENZODIAZEPINE coadministration. Adjust the dose accordingly.

Discussion

Increased digoxin levels occurred in 3 patients receiving diazepam, prompting in vitro and dog studies that suggested increased digoxin binding to plasma proteins and decreased tissue concentration by benzodiazepines.[1,2] Seven subjects received a single dose of digoxin 0.5 mg and diazepam 5 mg;[1] 5 of 7 had moderate increases in digoxin half-life, and all had a decrease in urinary digoxin excretion. A 72-year-old woman receiving digoxin 0.25 mg/day and several other drugs was administered alprazolam 1 mg at bedtime.[3] During the second week of alprazolam, she developed fatigue, "head pressure," and GI discomfort. The digoxin serum concentration increased to 4.3 ng/mL (baseline, 1.6 to 1.8 ng/mL), and the apparent oral clearance of digoxin was reduced approximately 39%. Alprazolam and digoxin were discontinued, and cardiac arrhythmias developed. The digoxin concentration was 1.5 ng/mL following reinitiation of digoxin 0.125 mg/day; 6 months later it was 1.1 ng/mL. Twelve patients on stable digoxin doses received alprazolam 0.5 or 1 mg for 7 days.[4] Digoxin AUC increased in patients receiving alprazolam 1 mg but not 0.5 mg. In contrast, the renal clearance and $t_{1/2}$ of digoxin were not affected by alprazolam 1.5 mg/day for 5 days following a single dose of digoxin in 8 healthy subjects.[5]

1 Castillo-Ferrando JR, et al. *Lancet.* 1980;2:368.
2 Castillo-Ferrando JR, et al. *J Pharm Pharmacol.* 1983;35:462.
3 Tollefson G, et al. *Am J Psychiatry.* 1984;141:1612.
4 Guven H, et al. *Clin Pharmacol Ther.* 1993;54:42.
5 Ochs HR, et al. *Clin Pharmacol Ther.* 1985;38:595.

* Asterisk indicates drugs cited in interaction reports. Based on pharmacologic and pharmacokinetic considerations, similar interactions may occur with other drugs that are listed.

Digoxin ✕ **Beta-Blockers**

Digoxin	Beta-Blockers	
Digoxin* (eg, *Lanoxin*)	Carvedilol* (eg, *Coreg*)	Propranolol* (eg, *Inderal*)
	Nebivolol (*Bystolic*)	

Significance	Onset	Severity	Documentation
2	■ **Rapid**	□ Major	□ Established
	□ Delayed	■ **Moderate**	■ **Probable**
		□ Minor	□ Suspected
			□ Possible
			□ Unlikely

Effects Serum DIGOXIN concentrations may be increased by coadministration of CARVEDILOL. Synergistic bradycardia may occur in some patients.

Mechanism CARVEDILOL may increase DIGOXIN bioavailability. Possible additive depression of myocardial conduction and decreased renal tubular DIGOXIN secretion may occur.

Management Monitor heart rate and serum DIGOXIN concentrations and observe for digitalis toxicity when initiating CARVEDILOL in patients receiving DIGOXIN.

Discussion

Coadministration of digoxin and propranolol is useful in treating angina pectoris in patients who have abnormal ventricular function or enlarged hearts,[1] and in treating atrioventricular reentrant tachycardia in patients with Wolff-Parkinson-White syndrome.[2] Coadministration of digoxin and propranolol has resulted in synergistic action and progressive bradycardia.[3] In 8 healthy subjects, single-dose oral administration of carvedilol 25 mg and oral digoxin 0.5 mg increased serum digoxin concentrations approximately 60% and the AUC 20%.[4] No change occurred in digoxin concentration when digoxin 0.5 mg was given IV. A study in 8 children receiving digoxin found a 47% decrease in digoxin clearance after carvedilol was started.[5] Two children experienced digoxin toxicity (eg, anorexia, high digoxin levels, vomiting). Digoxin dosage reduction may be necessary to avoid toxicity. In a study in patients with mild to moderate heart failure, carvedilol produced a 26% increase in trough serum digoxin concentrations (drawn at 20 to 24 hours after the last dose) when compared with placebo administration.[6] It was not necessary to adjust the digoxin dosage, and no patient demonstrated adverse reactions attributable to the increase in serum digoxin concentration.[6] However, the risk of digoxin toxicity is increased in patients maintained with higher serum digoxin concentrations. A study found carvedilol increased the AUC and plasma levels of digoxin in men but not in women.[7]

1 Crawford MH, et al. *Ann Intern Med.* 1975;83(4):449.
2 Hung JS, et al. *Ann Intern Med.* 1982;97(2):175.
3 Watt DA. *Br Med J.* 1968;3(5615):413.
4 De Mey C, et al. *Br J Clin Pharmacol.* 1990;29(4):486.
5 Ratnapalan S, et al. *J Pediatr.* 2003;142(5):572.
6 Grunden JW, et al. *Am J Ther.* 1994;1(2):157.
7 Baris N, et al. *Eur J Clin Pharmacol.* 2006;62(7):535.

* Asterisk indicates drugs cited in interaction reports. Based on pharmacologic and pharmacokinetic considerations, similar interactions may occur with other drugs that are listed.

Digoxin — Cholestyramine

Digoxin* (eg, *Lanoxin*)	Cholestyramine* (eg, *Questran*)

Significance	Onset	Severity	Documentation
2	☐ Rapid ■ **Delayed**	☐ Major ■ **Moderate** ☐ Minor	☐ Established ■ **Probable** ☐ Suspected ☐ Possible ☐ Unlikely

Effects CHOLESTYRAMINE coadministration may reduce DIGOXIN bioavailability. Although this may be useful in DIGOXIN toxicity,[7] decreased DIGOXIN effects may occur in patients taking CHOLESTYRAMINE regularly.

Mechanism CHOLESTYRAMINE may decrease the GI absorption of DIGOXIN by physically binding to it. CHOLESTYRAMINE may also interrupt the enterohepatic recycling of DIGOXIN.

Management Monitor patients for decreased DIGOXIN serum levels or a decreased therapeutic effect. Separating administration times or the use of the DIGOXIN capsule may minimize this interaction. Tailor the DIGOXIN dose if needed.

Discussion

Cholestyramine appears to reduce bioavailability of coadministered digoxin; this may be useful in treating digoxin intoxication. In 1 study, 18 volunteers received either 0.5 mg/day digoxin tablets or 0.4 mg/day digoxin capsules (*Lanoxicaps*) daily with 8 g cholestyramine simultaneously for 2 weeks.[5] The digoxin AUC decreased 32% following coadministration of digoxin tablets and cholestyramine; a 22% decrease in digoxin AUC occurred with coadministration of digoxin capsules and cholestyramine; this was not statistically significant. Mean trough digoxin concentration after the tablets was markedly reduced (31%) by cholestyramine; there was no reduction after the capsules. In a study of 12 volunteers, simultaneous administration of digoxin 0.75 mg and cholestyramine 4 g resulted in a 25% decrease in digoxin AUC and a 17% decrease in its cumulative 6-day urinary excretion.[4] As the cholestyramine dose was increased, digoxin serum levels decreased, and daily urinary digoxin excretion increased. Administering cholestyramine 8 hours before or after digoxin appeared to minimize the effects of the interaction. In 6 healthy subjects, a single 8 g cholestyramine dose given immediately after a single 0.25 mg digoxin dose reduced digoxin absorption 30% to 40%.[6] Other reports conflict.[2,3]

Although an in vitro study indicated the binding capacity of cholestyramine to digoxin is greater than that of colestipol (*Colestid*), the presence of duodenal juice decreases the binding capacity of cholestyramine but not colestipol.[1] See Digoxin-Colestipol.

[1] Bazzano G, et al. *JAMA.* 1972;220:828.
[2] Hall WH, et al. *Am J Cardiol.* 1977;39:213.
[3] Klotz U, et al. *Int J Clin Pharmacol Biopharm.* 1977;15:332.
[4] Brown DD, et al. *Circulation.* 1978;58:164.
[5] Brown DD, et al. *J Clin Pharmacol.* 1985;25:360.
[6] Neuvonen PJ, et al. *Br J Clin Pharmacol.* 1988;25:229.
[7] Henderson RP, et al. *Arch Intern Med.* 1988;148:745.

* Asterisk indicates drugs cited in interaction reports.

Digoxin — *Cimetidine*

Digoxin* (eg, *Lanoxin*)	Cimetidine* (eg, *Tagamet*)

Significance	Onset	Severity	Documentation
5	☐ Rapid	☐ Major	☐ Established
	■ **Delayed**	☐ Moderate	☐ Probable
		■ **Minor**	☐ Suspected
			■ **Possible**
			☐ Unlikely

Effects CIMETIDINE may either decrease or increase the plasma concentrations of DIGOXIN.

Mechanism Unknown.

Management Although a clinically important interaction in patients appears unlikely, routinely monitor plasma DIGOXIN concentrations and clinical response. Tailor the dose as needed.

Discussion

Eleven patients receiving digoxin 0.125 to 0.25 mg/day for greater than or equal to 2 weeks were coadministered cimetidine 600 to 1200 mg/day (oral or IV) for 7 to 14 days.[2] The mean serum digoxin concentration decreased from 2 to 1.5 ng/mL; however, no patient had signs of worsening congestive heart failure (CHF). In contrast, a series of studies in 17 healthy subjects resulted in increased digoxin levels.[4] Six individuals received a single dose of cimetidine 400 mg and digoxin 0.5 mg; cimetidine increased digoxin area under the concentration-time curve 23.3% and peak plasma digoxin concentration 50.5%. Five subjects received digoxin 0.25 mg/day for 16 days and cimetidine 1600 mg/day for 8 days; the average increase in digoxin concentration was 0.12 ng/mL. Six subjects received digoxin 0.5 mg/day for 12 days and cimetidine 1600 mg/day for 5 days; the average increase in digoxin concentration was 0.19 ng/mL.

Others report no observable changes. In 11 patients receiving digoxin 0.0625 to 0.25 mg/day for greater than 3 months, coadministration of cimetidine 1600 mg/day for 2 weeks did not affect digoxin concentrations.[4] Addition of oral cimetidine 300 mg every 6 hours for 6 days to the treatment regimen of 4 patients with stable CHF receiving digoxin 0.125 mg to 0.25 mg daily did not alter digoxin pharmacokinetics.[6] Similarily, in 3 single-dose studies, the coadministration of cimetidine and digoxin (oral or IV) did not affect the clearance or serum concentrations of digoxin.[1,3,5]

[1] Jordaens L, et al. *Acta Clin Belg.* 1981;36:109.
[2] Fraley DS, et al. *Clin Pharm.* 1983;2:163.
[3] Ochs HR, et al. *Am Heart J.* 1984;107:170.
[4] Crome P, et al. *Hum Toxicol.* 1985;4:391.
[5] Garty M, et al. *Eur J Clin Pharmacol.* 1986;30:489.
[6] Mouser B, et al. *DICP.* 1990;24:286.

* Asterisk indicates drugs cited in interaction reports.

Digoxin — *Colestipol*

Digoxin* (eg, *Lanoxin*)	Colestipol* (*Colestid*)

Significance	Onset	Severity	Documentation
2	■ **Rapid** ☐ Delayed	☐ Major ■ **Moderate** ☐ Minor	☐ Established ☐ Probable ■ **Suspected** ☐ Possible ☐ Unlikely

Effects COLESTIPOL may decrease the half-life of DIGOXIN, possibly reducing its therapeutic effect. COLESTIPOL may also be useful in the treatment of DIGOXIN toxicity.

Mechanism COLESTIPOL may physically bind with DIGOXIN. This may decrease its GI absorption and normal enterohepatic recycling.

Management If a patient maintained on DIGOXIN will be receiving COLESTIPOL on a routine basis, monitor DIGOXIN serum concentrations. If the concentration or clinical response decreases, tailor the dose of DIGOXIN as needed.

Discussion

Several case reports suggest digoxin absorption may be decreased by coadministration of colestipol.[1-3] In each case, the patients were being treated for digoxin toxicity. The digoxin half-life in 1 patient treated with colestipol was 16 hours; 2 patients who did not receive colestipol who also had digoxin toxicity had half-lives of 1.8 and 2 days, respectively.[1] In 2 other patients, colestipol decreased the digoxin half-life from 3.5 to 2.3 days and from 4.2 to 2 days.[2,3] The enterohepatic cycling of digoxin may also be decreased by colestipol. An in vitro study suggested that colestipol may have a greater binding capacity to digoxin than cholestyramine in the presence of duodenal juice.[1] In a single-dose study, coadministration of digoxin 0.25 mg and colestipol 10 g did not affect the GI absorption of digoxin; however, colestipol was administered immediately after digoxin.[4]

Although these reports were based on the treatment of digoxin toxicity, a similar interaction may be expected during routine use of colestipol in patients receiving digoxin.

[1] Bazzano G, et al. *JAMA*. 1972;220:828.
[2] Payne VW, et al. *DICP*. 1981;15:902.
[3] Kilgore TL, et al. *South Med J*. 1982;75:1259.
[4] Neuvonen PJ, et al. *Br J Clin Pharmacol*. 1988;25:229.

* Asterisk indicates drugs cited in interaction reports.

Digoxin — *Cyclosporine*

Digoxin* (eg, *Lanoxin*)	Cyclosporine* (eg, *Neoral*)

Significance	Onset	Severity	Documentation
1	☐ Rapid ■ **Delayed**	■ **Major** ☐ Moderate ☐ Minor	☐ Established ☐ Probable ■ **Suspected** ☐ Possible ☐ Unlikely

Effects The pharmacologic effects of DIGOXIN may be increased. Elevated DIGOXIN levels with toxicity may occur.

Mechanism Unknown; most likely pharmacokinetic in origin.

Management Monitor patients for elevated DIGOXIN concentrations and signs of DIGOXIN toxicity when CYCLOSPORINE is given concomitantly. If evidence of DIGOXIN toxicity occurs, discontinue DIGOXIN and lower the dose when resuming treatment. Readjust DIGOXIN dose after cardiac transplantation.

Discussion

Severe digoxin toxicity occurred following the initiation of cyclosporine therapy in 2 patients awaiting cardiac transplantation.[1] One patient was a 50-year-old man with ischemic cardiomyopathy and atrial fibrillation. The second patient was a 47-year-old man with idiopathic congestive cardiomyopathy and refractory CHF. Both patients were receiving digoxin 0.375 mg/day. Within 2 and 3 days of starting cyclosporine (750 and 800 mg/day, respectively), both patients developed increased serum digoxin concentrations (8.3 and 4.5 ng/mL, respectively), GI symptoms (eg, nausea, vomiting, diarrhea), and arrhythmias consistent with digoxin toxicity. An interaction was suspected, leading to the prospective study of digoxin pharmacokinetics in 2 additional patients before and after cyclosporine administration (10 mg/kg/day orally) prior to cardiac transplantation. The apparent volume of distribution of digoxin was decreased from 9.2 to 2.6 and 6.2 to 1.9 L/kg (by 72% and 69%, respectively) and plasma clearance was decreased from 11.4 to 4.8 and 3 to 1.6 L/hr (by 58% and 47%, respectively) following cyclosporine administration. The elimination half-life of digoxin was decreased from 53 to 35 and 111 to 65 hours (a decrease of 34% and 41%, respectively), indicating a greater decrease in apparent volume of distribution than in plasma clearance. Creatinine clearance decreased from 55.2 to 24 and 52.9 to 17.6 mL/min (by 57% and 67%, respectively). This interaction may be reversed or counterbalanced by successful cardiac transplantation.[2] In 7 patients continued on digoxin and cyclosporine after cardiac transplantation, volume of distribution of digoxin increased from 5.1 to 8 L/kg while clearance was unchanged.

[1] Dorian P, et al. *Clin Invest Med.* 1988;11:108.

[2] Robieux I, et al. *J Clin Pharmacol.* 1992;32:338.

* Asterisk indicates drugs cited in interaction reports.

Digoxin — **Diltiazem**

Digoxin* (eg, *Lanoxin*)	Diltiazem* (eg, *Cardizem*)

Significance	Onset	Severity	Documentation
2	☐ Rapid ■ **Delayed**	☐ Major ■ **Moderate** ☐ Minor	☐ Established ☐ Probable ■ **Suspected** ☐ Possible ☐ Unlikely

Effects DILTIAZEM may increase DIGOXIN concentrations, possibly resulting in DIGOXIN toxicity.

Mechanism DILTIAZEM appears to decrease the renal or extra-renal clearance of DIGOXIN.

Management Monitor DIGOXIN levels and clinical status in patients receiving concurrent DILTIAZEM. If increased DIGOXIN levels or signs of toxicity develop, the DIGOXIN dose may need to be decreased.

Discussion

Reports are conflicting. Many studies have shown that diltiazem increases digoxin serum levels,[1-8] while other studies report no effect on digoxin concentrations.[9-13] In several studies, subjects receiving digoxin or beta-acetyldigoxin† and diltiazem had increases in digoxin concentrations of 22% to 70%.[1-6,8] Renal clearance of digoxin decreased 26% to 31%[1,2,6]; however, in 1 study the renal clearance of digoxin was not affected, but total body clearance decreased 28% and extra-renal clearance decreased 44%.[4] In 1 study, the t½ of digoxin increased 23% (36.2 to 44.5 hours).[2] Digoxin toxicity was not reported in any of the studies. In a case report, a patient receiving nifedipine was started on digoxin 0.125 mg/day.[7] Two weeks later, diltiazem 30 mg every 8 hours was added to the therapy. By day 4, serum digoxin concentrations increased from 1.7 to 3.5 ng/mL, and the patient developed nausea and vomiting. Both drugs were discontinued, and within 24 hours, symptoms resolved. The digoxin level was 1.3 ng/mL.

In contrast, coadministration of digoxin and diltiazem for several weeks did not change serum levels, renal clearance, t½, or volume of distribution of digoxin.[9-13] Diltiazem did not alter digoxin plasma levels and counteracted digoxin-induced splanchnic vasoconstriction without affecting the positive inotropic effects of digoxin.[14]

1 Yoshida A, et al. *Clin Pharmacol Ther.* 1984;35(5):681.
2 Rameis H, et al. *Clin Pharmacol Ther.* 1984;36(2):183.
3 Oyama Y, et al. *Am J Cardiol.* 1984;53(10):1480.
4 Kuhlmann J. *Clin Pharmacol Ther.* 1985;37(2):150.
5 De Vito JM, et al. *Pharmacotherapy.* 1986;6(2):73.
6 North DS, et al. *Drug Intell Clin Pharm.* 1986;20(6):500.
7 Kasmer RJ, et al. *Drug Intell Clin Pharm.* 1986;20(12):985.
8 Andrejak M, et al. *J Clin Pharmacol.* 1987;27(12):967.
9 Schrager BR, et al. *Circulation.* 1983;68(suppl 3):368.
10 Beltrami TR, et al. *J Clin Pharmacol.* 1985;25(5):390.
11 Elkayam U, et al. *Am J Cardiol.* 1985;55(11):1393.
12 Jones WN, et al. *Eur J Clin Pharmacol.* 1986;31(3):351.
13 Boden WE, et al. *Am J Med.* 1986;81(3):425.
14 Gasic S, et al. *Int J Clin Pharmacol Ther Toxicol.* 1987;25(10):553.

* Asterisk indicates drugs cited in interaction reports.
† Not available in the United States.

Digoxin — *Dipyridamole*

Digoxin* (eg, *Lanoxin*)	Dipyridamole* (eg, *Persantine*)

Significance	Onset	Severity	Documentation
5	■ **Rapid**	□ Major	□ Established
	□ Delayed	□ Moderate	□ Probable
		■ **Minor**	□ Suspected
			■ **Possible**
			□ Unlikely

Effects DIGOXIN bioavailability may be increased.

Mechanism Increased GI absorption of DIGOXIN, resulting from inhibition of P-glycoprotein expression by DIPYRIDAMOLE, is suspected.

Management Based on the magnitude of the interaction, no special precautions other than routine monitoring are needed.

Discussion

The effect of dipyridamole on the bioavailability of digoxin was studied in 12 healthy volunteers.[1] Using an open-label, randomized, 2-period crossover design, each subject received 1) digoxin 0.5 mg alone and 2) dipyridamole 75 mg at 9 AM and 12 PM and 150 mg at 9 PM for 2 days. On the third day, after an overnight fast, dipyridamole 150 mg and digoxin 0.5 mg were administered simultaneously. Coadministration of dipyridamole and digoxin increased the digoxin AUC from 0 to 4 hours and 0 to 24 hours 20% and 13%, respectively, compared with administration of digoxin alone. The effect of dipyridamole on digoxin pharmacokinetics was noted primarily during the first hours after dosing, indicating that the interaction involved the absorption process. However, the magnitude of the increase in digoxin bioavailability does not appear to be clinically important.

[1] Verstuyft C, et al. *Clin Pharmacol Ther.* 2003;73(1):51.

* Asterisk indicates drugs cited in interaction reports.

Digoxin — *Disopyramide*

Digoxin* (eg, *Lanoxin*)	Disopyramide* (eg, *Norpace*)

Significance	Onset	Severity	Documentation
5	☐ Rapid	☐ Major	☐ Established
	■ **Delayed**	☐ Moderate	☐ Probable
		■ **Minor**	☐ Suspected
			☐ Possible
			■ **Unlikely**

Effects Although DIGOXIN serum levels may be increased by DISOPYRAMIDE, a clinically important interaction appears unlikely. Left ventricular dysfunction may occur; however, a beneficial interaction has also been suggested.

Mechanism Unknown.

Management No special precautions appear necessary. However, routinely monitor patients, especially those with preexisting cardiac decompensation.

Discussion

Coadministration of digoxin and disopyramide does not appear to significantly affect digoxin. In 1 study, 9 patients receiving maintenance digoxin therapy were given disopyramide 200 mg 3 times daily for 2 weeks.[1] Although serum digoxin concentrations increased from 1.3 to 1.5 nmol/L, it was considered small and clinically insignificant. In another study, 9 subjects received digoxin 0.375 mg/day.[2] Digoxin serum concentrations did not change after disopyramide 300 mg/day; however, the digoxin levels increased from 0.6 to 0.8 ng/mL following disopyramide doses of 600 mg/day. In 5 other subjects, disopyramide doses of 600 mg/day decreased the t½ of digoxin from 40.2 to 22 hours and reduced the volume of distribution 40% following a single IV dose of digoxin 0.8 mg. Digoxin clearance was not affected. Another study reported evidence of left ventricular dysfunction in 11 patients with CHF who were given disopyramide while receiving digitalis (agent not specified) and diuretics.[3]

Other studies have reported no effect of disopyramide on digoxin pharmacokinetics.[1,4-7] However, 1 study suggested that digoxin may enhance the antiarrhythmic effect of disopyramide by preventing disopyramide's negative inotropic changes.

1 Manolas EG, et al. *Aust N Z J Med.* 1980;10(4):426.
2 Risler T, et al. *Clin Pharmacol Ther.* 1983;34(2):176.
3 Podrid PJ, et al. *N Engl J Med.* 1980;302(11):614.
4 Wellens HJ, et al. *Am Heart J.* 1980;100(6, pt 1):934.
5 Leahey EB Jr, et al. *Ann Intern Med.* 1980;92(5):605.
6 García-Barreto D, et al. *J Cardiovasc Pharmacol.* 1981;3(6):1236.
7 Elliott HL, et al. *Br J Clin Pharmacol.* 1982;14:141p.

* Asterisk indicates drugs cited in interaction reports.

Digoxin — *Dronedarone*

Digoxin* (eg, *Lanoxin*)	Dronedarone* (*Multaq*)

Significance	Onset	Severity	Documentation
2	☐ Rapid ■ **Delayed**	☐ Major ■ **Moderate** ☐ Minor	☐ Established ☐ Probable ■ **Suspected** ☐ Possible ☐ Unlikely

Effects DIGOXIN plasma concentrations may be elevated, increasing the pharmacologic effects and risk of adverse reactions.

Mechanism Inhibition of P-glycoprotein efflux transport may increase DIGOXIN GI absorption. In addition, DIGOXIN and DRONEDARONE have additive electrophysiological effects (eg, decreased atrioventricular-node conduction).[1]

Management If coadministration cannot be avoided, reduce the DIGOXIN dose by 50%. Monitor DIGOXIN plasma concentrations and observe for toxicity.[1] Adjust the DIGOXIN dose further as needed.

Discussion

In a randomized, double-blind, placebo-controlled study in 34 patients with symptomatic permanent atrial fibrillation, addition of dronedarone to stable digoxin therapy increased digoxin concentration 41.4% and decreased the heart rate 11.5 bpm.[2] Dronedarone has been reported to increase digoxin exposure 2.5-fold.[1]

[1] *Multaq* [package insert]. Bridgewater, NJ: Sanofi-Aventis US LLC; July 2009.

[2] Davy JM, et al. *Am Heart J.* 2008;156(3):527.e1.

* Asterisk indicates drugs cited in interaction reports.

Digoxin — Esmolol

Digoxin* (eg, *Lanoxin*)	Esmolol* (*Brevibloc*)

Significance	Onset	Severity	Documentation
4	■ **Rapid**	□ Major	□ Established
	□ Delayed	■ **Moderate**	□ Probable
		□ Minor	□ Suspected
			■ **Possible**
			□ Unlikely

Effects The pharmacologic effects of DIGOXIN may be increased.

Mechanism Unknown.

Management If signs of DIGOXIN toxicity occur, a lower dose of DIGOXIN during coadministration of ESMOLOL may be needed. Monitor DIGOXIN concentrations and the patient for symptoms of DIGOXIN toxicity; adjust the dose accordingly.

Discussion

In healthy male subjects, steady-state serum digoxin concentrations obtained during administration of digoxin alone, were compared with those resulting from coadministration of esmolol (6 hour infusion of 300 mcg/kg/min).[1,2] No changes in the pharmacokinetics of esmolol were observed; however, serum digoxin concentrations increased by 9.6% to 19.2% during combined drug administration compared with treatment with digoxin alone. In addition, the total area under the serum digoxin concentration-time curve was higher during administration of both drugs. The clinical importance of this increase has not been evaluated.

Although a pharmacokinetic interaction appears to occur, it has not been determined if an altered clinical response occurs.

[1] Lowenthal DT, et al. *Am J Cardiol.* 1985;56:14F.
[2] Lowenthal DT, et al. *J Clin Pharmacol.* 1987;27:561.

* Asterisk indicates drugs cited in interaction reports.

Digoxin — *Felodipine*

Digoxin* (eg, *Lanoxin*)	Felodipine* (*Plendil*)

Significance	Onset	Severity	Documentation
5	■ **Rapid** ☐ Delayed	☐ Major ☐ Moderate ■ **Minor**	☐ Established ☐ Probable ☐ Suspected ☐ Possible ■ **Unlikely**

Effects Serum DIGOXIN levels may be increased (see discussion).

Mechanism Unknown.

Management Based on currently available documentation, no special precautions appear necessary.

Discussion

The effect of felodipine on the serum concentration of digoxin was studied in 23 patients with congestive heart failure.[1] The investigation was a prospective, double-blind, placebo controlled, parallel study. All patients were maintained on digoxin 0.25 to 0.375 mg/day and hydrochlorothiazide (eg, *HydroDIURIL*) 50 mg/day with potassium supplementation if necessary. Patients were randomized to receive either felodipine 10 mg twice daily or placebo. After 8 weeks of treatment, there was no statistically significant difference between the felodipine and placebo subgroups. There was no change in the trough digoxin levels or digoxin levels 6 hours after the administration of digoxin in the felodipine group compared with the placebo group. A 15% increase ($P = 0.13$) in the serum digoxin levels 2 hours after administration of digoxin occurred in the felodipine group compared with the placebo group. In addition, a bimodal distribution pattern in serum digoxin levels was noted in patients receiving felodipine concurrently. A significant increase ($P < 0.001$) in the 2-hour post-digoxin level was observed only in those patients with high serum felodipine levels (30.3 nmol/L). In patients with low serum felodipine levels (11.8 nmol/L), serum digoxin levels were not changed or were slightly lower than those occurring with placebo administration. Analysis of the clinical characteristics of the felodipine and placebo groups did not reveal any difference between the populations.

The present data do not indicate the occurrence of an either clinically or statistically significant drug interaction.

[1] Dunselman PHJM, et al. *Eur J Clin Pharmacol.* 1988;35:461.

* Asterisk indicates drugs cited in interaction reports.

Digoxin — *Flecainide*

Digoxin* (eg, *Lanoxin*)	Flecainide* (eg, *Tambocor*)

Significance	Onset	Severity	Documentation
4	☐ Rapid ■ **Delayed**	☐ Major ■ **Moderate** ☐ Minor	☐ Established ☐ Probable ☐ Suspected ■ **Possible** ☐ Unlikely

Effects The pharmacologic effects of DIGOXIN may be increased.

Mechanism Unknown.

Management If DIGOXIN toxicity develops and an interaction is suspected, consider decreasing the dose of DIGOXIN during coadministration of FLECAINIDE. Serum DIGOXIN levels may provide useful information.

Discussion

The effects of flecainide 200 mg twice daily on the pharmacokinetics of digoxin have been studied in healthy volunteers.[1,2] In 1 investigation, a single oral dose of digoxin 1 mg was administered on 3 occasions (1 week prior to the initiation of flecainide therapy, on the first day of concurrent flecainide treatment, and on the eighth day of coadministration of the drugs).[1] During concurrent therapy, digoxin absorption was more rapid, peak plasma concentrations were 80% to 100% higher, time to reach peak concentration decreased 34%, and the AUC for the single dose of digoxin was increased 25% to 40%. In addition, the mean plasma $t_{½}$ was 20% to 35% shorter, the apparent volume of distribution decreased 22% to 37%, and renal clearance decreased 20% to 25%. Digoxin bioavailability did not appear to be altered. In patients receiving digoxin 0.25 mg daily for 22 days, coadministration of flecainide produced a predose and a 6-hour postdose increase in digoxin levels of 24% and 13%, respectively.[2] These increases in digoxin levels are expected to be of clinical significance only in patients with levels in the upper portion of the therapeutic range.

[1] Tjandramaga TB, et al. *Arch Int Pharmacodyn.* 1982;260:302.

[2] Lewis GP, et al. *Am J Cardiol.* 1984;53:52B.

* Asterisk indicates drugs cited in interaction reports.

Digoxin — *Food*

Digoxin* (eg, *Lanoxin*)	Grapefruit Juice*

Significance	Onset	Severity	Documentation
5	☐ Rapid ■ **Delayed**	☐ Major ☐ Moderate ■ **Minor**	☐ Established ☐ Probable ☐ Suspected ■ **Possible** ☐ Unlikely

Effects DIGOXIN plasma levels may be slightly elevated.

Mechanism Unknown.

Management Based on available data, no special precautions are warranted.

Discussion

The effect of grapefruit juice on the bioavailability of digoxin was evaluated in 2 studies.[1,2] In the first study, 12 healthy subjects received a single dose of digoxin 0.5 mg with 220 mL of water or grapefruit juice.[1] Each subject received 50 mL of water or grapefruit juice 30 minutes before digoxin administration and 3.5, 7.5, and 11.5 hours after digoxin. Compared with water, grapefruit juice increased the digoxin AUC 9% from 0 to 4 hours and from 0 to 24 hours. Grapefruit juice did not affect the C_{max}, AUC (from 0 to 48 hours), or renal clearance of digoxin. In the second study, 7 healthy subjects received digoxin 1 mg with water or following ingestion of 240 mL of single-strength grapefruit juice 3 times daily for 5 days.[2] Compared with water, grapefruit juice had no effect on digoxin C_{max}, AUC, $t_{½}$, or renal clearance.

[1] Becquemont L, et al. *Clin Pharmacol Ther.* 2001;70:311.

[2] Parker RB, et al. *Pharmacotherapy.* 2003;23:979.

* Asterisk indicates drugs cited in interaction reports.

Digoxin / Ginseng

Digoxin	Ginseng	
Digoxin* (eg, *Lanoxin*)	Asian Ginseng* Indian Ginseng* North American Ginseng*	Siberian Ginseng*

Significance	Onset	Severity	Documentation
4	☐ Rapid ■ **Delayed**	☐ Major ■ **Moderate** ☐ Minor	☐ Established ☐ Probable ☐ Suspected ■ **Possible** ☐ Unlikely

Effects Serum DIGOXIN levels falsely increased or decreased.

Mechanism Possibly caused by laboratory test interference of DIGOXIN-like immunoreactive components of GINSENG with polyclonal antibody–based DIGOXIN immunoassays.

Management Because of DIGOXIN's narrow therapeutic index, caution patients about using nonprescription or herbal products. Advise patients taking DIGOXIN to avoid GINSENG. Monitor DIGOXIN serum levels routinely when herbal products are started or stopped. If an interaction is suspected, discontinue GINSENG and monitor serum DIGOXIN levels.

Discussion

Elevated serum digoxin levels were reported in a 74-yr-old man taking a constant digoxin dose (0.25 mg/day) for several years to control atrial fibrillation.[1] His serum digoxin levels ranged from 0.9 to 2.2 nmol/L for more than 10 yr. A routine serum digoxin measurement reported a level of 5.2 nmol/L with no signs of digoxin toxicity. Digoxin therapy was withheld, then resumed at a reduced dose, and finally discontinued 10 days after the high serum digoxin level was reported. The serum digoxin level remained high for 2 wk but decreased to 2.2 nmol/L 5 days after he stopped Siberian ginseng. Digoxin 0.125 and 0.25 mg on alternate days was started, and serum digoxin levels remained between 0.8 and 1.1 nmol/L. Nearly 9 mo later, he resumed taking ginseng; serum digoxin levels increased again (3.2 nmol/L). Ginseng was stopped, and serum digoxin levels decreased to the therapeutic range (1.2 nmol/L). An in vitro study on the effects of Asian, Brazilian, Indian, North American, and Siberian ginseng on serum digoxin immunoassays reported all ginsengs, except Brazilian, display digoxin-like immunoreactivity with a fluorescence polarization immunoassay (FPIA), modest immunoreactivity with microparticle enzyme immunoassay (MEIA), and no apparent activity with a monoclonal-based digoxin immunoassay (*Tina-quant*).[2] Brazilian ginseng produced no immunoreactivity with any assay. When aliquot serum pools prepared from patients receiving digoxin were supplemented with ginseng, digoxin values were falsely elevated with FPIA and falsely reduced with MEIA, but no interference with *Tina-quant* was observed. Also, digoxin immune fab (eg, *Digibind*) can bind ginseng's free digoxin-like immunoreactive components.

[1] McRae S. *CMAJ.* 1996;155(3):293.

[2] Dasgupta A, et al. *Am J Clin Pathol.* 2005;124(2):229.

* Asterisk indicates drugs cited in interaction reports.

Digoxin — *Goldenseal*

Digoxin* (eg, *Lanoxin*)	Goldenseal*

Significance	Onset	Severity	Documentation
5	☐ Rapid ■ **Delayed**	☐ Major ☐ Moderate ■ **Minor**	☐ Established ☐ Probable ☐ Suspected ■ **Possible** ☐ Unlikely

Effects DIGOXIN plasma concentration may be increased slightly.

Mechanism Increased DIGOXIN absorption resulting from inhibition of P-glycoprotein–mediated secretion of digoxin in the intestine by GOLDENSEAL is suspected.

Management Based on available data, no special precautions are necessary.

Discussion

The effects of goldenseal on the pharmacokinetics of digoxin were studied in 20 healthy subjects.[1] Using an open-label, randomized design, each subject received goldenseal root extract 1,070 mg (standardized to contain 24.1 mg of isoquinoline alkaloids per capsule) 3 times daily for 14 days. Digoxin 0.5 mg was administered 24 hours before the start of goldenseal and on the last day of goldenseal administration. Compared with administration of digoxin alone, goldenseal increased digoxin C_{max} 14%. No other digoxin pharmacokinetic measurements were altered by goldenseal.

[1] Gurley BJ, et al. *Drug Metab Dispos.* 2007;35(2):240.

* Asterisk indicates drugs cited in interaction reports.

Digoxin | ***HMG-CoA Reductase Inhibitors***

Digoxin* (eg, *Lanoxin*)	Atorvastatin* (*Lipitor*)	Fluvastatin* (*Lescol*)

Significance	Onset	Severity	Documentation
4	□ Rapid	□ Major	□ Established
	■ **Delayed**	■ **Moderate**	□ Probable
		□ Minor	□ Suspected
			■ **Possible**
			□ Unlikely

Effects DIGOXIN plasma concentrations may be elevated, increasing the risk of toxicity.

Mechanism Increased absorption of DIGOXIN resulting from inhibition of P-glycoprotein–mediated secretion of DIGOXIN in the intestine by the HMG-CoA REDUCTASE INHIBITOR is suspected.

Management Monitor DIGOXIN concentrations and observe the patient's clinical response. If an interaction is suspected, adjust the DIGOXIN dose as needed.

Discussion

The effect of atorvastatin on the pharmacokinetics of digoxin was studied in 2 groups of 12 healthy volunteers.[1] Each subject received digoxin 0.25 mg/day for 20 days. Digoxin was administered alone for the first 10 days, then 12 subjects in each group received atorvastatin 10 or 80 mg concurrently for the next 10 days. During coadministration of atorvastatin 10 mg and digoxin, concentrations of digoxin were unchanged. However, coadministration of atorvastatin 80 mg and digoxin increased the C_{max} of digoxin 20% (from 1.3 to 1.56 ng/mL), the plasma concentration at 24 hours 22% (from 0.45 to 0.55 ng/mL), and the AUC 15%. The effects of a single dose of fluvastatin 40 mg on the steady-state pharmacokinetics of digoxin (doses of 0.25 to 0.5 mg/day) were evaluated in a double-blind, randomized, crossover study involving 18 patients.[2] Fluvastatin administration increased digoxin C_{max} 11% (from 2.14 to 2.38 ng/mL) and renal clearance 15%. In 18 healthy men, coadministration of pravastatin (eg, *Pravachol*) and digoxin did not change the pharmacokinetics of either drug.[3]

[1] Boyd RA, et al. *J Clin Pharmacol.* 2000;40(1):91.
[2] Garnett WR, et al. *Am J Med.* 1994;96(6A):84S.
[3] Triscari J, et al. *Br J Clin Pharmacol.* 1993;36(3):263.

* Asterisk indicates drugs cited in interaction reports.

Digoxin — *Ibuprofen*

Digoxin* (eg, *Lanoxin*)	Ibuprofen* (eg, *Motrin*)

Significance	Onset	Severity	Documentation
5	☐ Rapid ■ **Delayed**	☐ Major ☐ Moderate ■ **Minor**	☐ Established ☐ Probable ☐ Suspected ■ **Possible** ☐ Unlikely

Effects IBUPROFEN coadministration may increase DIGOXIN serum levels, although the effect appears to be transient.

Mechanism Unknown; possibly decreased DIGOXIN renal excretion.

Management Routinely monitor DIGOXIN serum concentrations during coadministration of IBUPROFEN. A decrease in the DIGOXIN dose may be necessary; however, continue to monitor DIGOXIN levels because the effect appears transient.

Discussion

Digoxin therapy was stabilized in 12 patients (range, 0.125 to 0.25 mg/day) for greater than 2 months before they received 1600 mg/day of ibuprofen.[1] Following 7 days of ibuprofen, the mean digoxin serum concentration increased 59.6% (10.7% to 325%), a statistically significant increase ($P < 0.05$). Interestingly, digoxin levels after 28 days of ibuprofen did not differ significantly from the 7-day level or from baseline. No signs or symptoms of digoxin toxicity were noted. Serum creatinine concentrations did not differ between baseline 7-day or 28-day concentrations.

The study design and choice of statistical test have been questioned.[2] Further study is needed to better assess the importance of this interaction.

[1] Quattrocchi FP, et al. *DICP.* 1983;17:286.

[2] Miller BS. *DICP.* 1984;18:254.

* Asterisk indicates drugs cited in interaction reports.

Digoxin		*Indomethacin*	
Digoxin* (eg, *Lanoxin*)		Indomethacin* (eg, *Indocin*)	
Significance	Onset	Severity	Documentation
2	☐ Rapid ■ **Delayed**	☐ Major ■ **Moderate** ☐ Minor	☐ Established ☐ Probable ■ **Suspected** ☐ Possible ☐ Unlikely

Effects INDOMETHACIN may increase the serum levels of DIGOXIN in premature infants, possibly resulting in increased pharmacologic effects or toxicity. This may not occur in patients with healthy renal function.

Mechanism Because of reduced renal function, INDOMETHACIN may decrease DIGOXIN renal elimination.

Management Caution is warranted in preterm infants with reduced renal function. Until urine output and serum DIGOXIN levels are assessed, consider decreasing the DIGOXIN dose 50% when INDOMETHACIN is added to DIGOXIN therapy in preterm infants.

Discussion

Observations of preterm infants indicate that the coadministration of digoxin and indomethacin results in elevated serum digoxin levels with possible toxicity.[1-3] Three infants receiving digoxin for 3 days (loading dose, 40 mcg/kg; maintenance dose, 10 mcg/kg/day) developed prolonged periods of sinus bradycardia and ECG wave segment elevation, and 1 infant had intermittent nodal rhythm following administration of indomethacin 0.2 mg/kg.[1] Another infant receiving indomethacin 0.2 mg/kg every 8 hours was given a digoxin 40 mcg/kg loading dose, followed by 2.5 mcg/kg every 12 hours.[2] Within 3 days, the digoxin serum level was 8.5 ng/mL, and the $t_{½}$ was 96 hours. Eleven other preterm infants received indomethacin 0.32 mg/kg at least 4 days after initiation of digoxin 4.4 mcg/kg twice daily.[3] The mean serum digoxin level increased from 2.24 to 3.15 ng/mL (41%), and urine output was decreased. The $t_{½}$ in 5 patients was 97 hours, compared with an age-matched control group value of 43 hours.

Studies in adults are conflicting. Coadministration of indomethacin 150 mg/day and digoxin to 10 patients resulted in a 40% increase (range, 0% to 100%) in digoxin levels.[4] Coadministration of ibuprofen (eg, *Motrin*) and digoxin did not change the steady-state serum digoxin levels. In contrast, in 6 healthy adults, indomethacin 150 mg/day for 3 days did not affect the elimination $t_{½}$, systemic clearance, or distribution of digoxin following a 0.75 mg IV dose.[5]

[1] Mayes LC, et al. *Pediatr Res.* 1980;14:469.
[2] Schimmel MS, et al. *Clin Pediatr.* 1980;19(11):768.
[3] Koren G, et al. *Pediatr Pharmacol.* 1984;4(1):25.
[4] Jorgensen HS, et al. *Br J Clin Pharmacol.* 1991;31(1):108.
[5] Finch MB, et al. *Br J Clin Pharmacol.* 1984;17(3):353.

* Asterisk indicates drugs cited in interaction reports.

Digoxin — Macrolide & Related Antibiotics

Digoxin	Macrolide & Related Antibiotics	
Digoxin* (eg, *Lanoxin*)	Azithromycin* (eg, *Zithromax*)	Erythromycin* (eg, *EryPed*)
	Clarithromycin* (eg, *Biaxin*)	Telithromycin* (*Ketek*)

Significance	Onset	Severity	Documentation
1	☐ Rapid	■ **Major**	■ **Established**
	■ **Delayed**	☐ Moderate	☐ Probable
		☐ Minor	☐ Suspected
			☐ Possible
			☐ Unlikely

Effects Coadministration of MACROLIDE AND RELATED ANTIBIOTICS and DIGOXIN may increase DIGOXIN serum levels; toxicity may occur. The effects of this interaction may persist for several weeks following ERYTHROMYCIN administration.[1]

Mechanism MACROLIDE AND RELATED ANTIBIOTICS may inhibit renal tubular P-glycoprotein excretion of DIGOXIN.[2] Genetic variation in this effect is suspected.[3]

Management Monitor for increased DIGOXIN levels and symptoms of toxicity; a decreased DIGOXIN dose may be necessary. The capsule formulation may increase bioavailability, thereby decreasing the likelihood of an interaction.

Discussion

Digoxin toxicity has been reported in several cases after clarithromycin,[4-14] erythromycin,[1,15,16] or telithromycin[17] was started. Increases in digoxin concentration during coadministration of clarithromycin may be dose-dependent on clarithromycin.[18] Administration of clarithromycin 200 to 400 mg/day increased digoxin serum levels 1.8- to 4-fold.[13] Neither clarithromycin nor erythromycin affects digoxin concentrations despite an increase in renal digoxin clearance.[19] There are more than 100 spontaneous-event reports of a possible digoxin-azithromycin interaction.[20]

1 Morton MR, et al. *DICP.* 1989;23(9):668.
2 Wakasugi H, et al. *Clin Pharmacol Ther.* 1998;64(1):123.
3 Kurata Y, et al. *Clin Pharmacol Ther.* 2002;72(2):209.
4 Midoneck SR, et al. *N Engl J Med.* 1995;333(22):1505.
5 Ford A, et al. *Clin Infect Dis.* 1995;21(4):1051.
6 Nawarskas JJ, et al. *Ann Pharmacother.* 1997;31(7-8):864.
7 Guerriero SE, et al. *Pharmacotherapy.* 1997;17(5):1035.
8 Laberge P, et al. *Ann Pharmacother.* 1997;31(9):999.
9 Nordt SP, et al. *J Accid Emerg Med.* 1998;15(3):194.
10 Gooderham MJ, et al. *Ann Pharmacother.* 1999;33(7-8):796.
11 Xu H, et al. *Conn Med.* 2001;65(9):527.
12 Zapater P, et al. *J Antimicrob Chemother.* 2002;50(4):601.
13 Hirata S, et al. *Int J Clin Pharmacol Ther.* 2005;43(1):30.
14 Lee CY, et al. *Can J Cardiol.* 2011;27(6):870.e15.
15 Friedman HS, et al. *Chest.* 1982;82(2):202.
16 Maxwell DL, et al. *BMJ.* 1989;298(6673):572.
17 Nenciu LM, et al. *Pharmacotherapy.* 2006;26(6):872.
18 Tanaka H, et al. *Ann Pharmacother.* 2003;37(2):178.
19 Tsutsumi K, et al. *J Clin Pharmacol.* 2002;42(10):1159.
20 Ten Eick AP, et al. *Curr Ther Res.* 2001;62(2):178.

* Asterisk indicates drugs cited in interaction reports.

Digoxin — *Magnesium Salts*

Digoxin	Magnesium Salts	
Digoxin* (eg, *Lanoxin*)	Magnesium Carbonate (eg, *Marblen*)	Magnesium Oxide (eg, *Mag-Ox*)
	Magnesium Citrate	Magnesium Sulfate (eg, *Epsom Salts*)
	Magnesium Gluconate	Magnesium Trisilicate*
	Magnesium Hydroxide* (eg, *Milk of Magnesia*)	

Significance	Onset	Severity	Documentation
4	□ Rapid	□ Major	□ Established
	■ **Delayed**	■ **Moderate**	□ Probable
		□ Minor	□ Suspected
			■ **Possible**
			□ Unlikely

Effects Antacids containing MAGNESIUM SALTS, specifically MAGNESIUM TRISILICATE, may decrease the bioavailability of DIGOXIN; therapeutic effects may be decreased. However, the clinical significance has been questioned.

Mechanism The MAGNESIUM SALT may physically absorb DIGOXIN in the GI tract; however, other mechanisms may exist.

Management It is not known if separating administration times of these agents would avoid or lessen the interaction. Monitor patients for a decreased therapeutic response. An increased DIGOXIN dosage or a DIGOXIN capsule may be necessary.

Discussion

Antacids containing magnesium salts may decrease the bioavailability of digoxin. In one study, 10 healthy volunteers were given digoxin 0.75 mg with 60 mL of either 8% magnesium hydroxide or magnesium trisilicate.[3] Compared with controls, magnesium hydroxide and magnesium trisilicate decreased the area under the plasma concentration-time curve of digoxin by 25% and 38% and decreased the cumulative 6-day urinary digoxin excretion by 35% and 29%, respectively. In another study, 12 healthy volunteers received two 0.2 mg digoxin capsules or tablets with 60 mL of a combination antacid containing aluminum hydroxide and magnesium hydroxide.[5] The antacid reduced peak plasma concentrations of digoxin from both tablets and capsules; bioavailability was not significantly impaired. However, urinary excretion data suggested that the antacid impaired digoxin absorption from the tablet but not the capsule. In vitro studies indicate that magnesium trisilicate significantly absorbed digoxin; however, magnesium carbonate and magnesium oxide have weak absorptive effects.[1,2,4] One study found no effect of magnesium trisilicate on the absorption of digoxin.[6] The possibility of a clinically significant interaction has perhaps been overemphasized.

[1] Khalil SAH. *J Pharm Sci.* 1974;63:1641.
[2] Khalil SAH. *J Pharm Pharmacol.* 1974;26:961.
[3] Brown DD, et al. *N Engl J Med.* 1976;295;1034.
[4] McElnay JC, et al. *BMJ.* 1978;1:1554.
[5] Allen MD, et al. *J Clin Pharmacol.* 1981;21:26.
[6] D'Arcy PF, et al. *DICP.* 1987;21:607. Review.

* Asterisk indicates drugs cited in interaction reports. Based on pharmacologic and pharmacokinetic considerations, similar interactions may occur with other drugs that are listed.

Digoxin | **Metoclopramide**

Digoxin*
(eg, *Lanoxin*)

Metoclopramide*
(eg, *Reglan*)

Significance	Onset	Severity	Documentation
2	☐ Rapid ■ **Delayed**	☐ Major ■ **Moderate** ☐ Minor	☐ Established ■ **Probable** ☐ Suspected ☐ Possible ☐ Unlikely

Effects METOCLOPRAMIDE may decrease the plasma levels of DIGOXIN, decreasing therapeutic effects. This interaction may not occur with high-bioavailability DIGOXIN formulations.

Mechanism By increasing GI motility METOCLOPRAMIDE may decrease the absorption of DIGOXIN.

Management Monitor patients for decreased therapeutic response to DIGOXIN or for decreased DIGOXIN serum levels. The dose of DIGOXIN may need to be increased, or consider switching to a formulation with high bioavailability (eg, capsule, elixir, tablet with a high dissolution rate).

Discussion

The bioavailability of digoxin may be decreased by administration of metoclopramide because of increased GI motility.[1,3-5] However, this interaction may be dependent on the dissolution rate of the digoxin product.[1-5] In 1 study, 6 volunteers were given digoxin 0.25 mg twice daily for 1 week, plus metoclopramide 10 mg 3 times daily.[5] Peak plasma digoxin concentrations were decreased from 1.5 to 1.1 ng/mL by metoclopramide. The time to peak plasma concentration was also prolonged from 2 to 2.7 hours, and the area under the digoxin concentration-time curve (AUC) was decreased 10%. However, the dissolution rate of the tablets was only 30%.[3] In another study, 11 patients on maintenance digoxin therapy received metoclopramide 10 mg 3 times daily for 10 days.[1] Metoclopramide decreased mean serum digoxin concentrations from 0.72 to 0.46 ng/mL. Following metoclopramide discontinuation, mean digoxin levels increased to 0.75 ng/mL after 10 days. Sixteen healthy subjects were given metoclopramide with either digoxin 0.5 mg as tablets or digoxin 0.4 mg as capsules;[4] tablet dissolution rate was 79.4%. The AUC, when digoxin was administered as a tablet, was reduced 23.5% by metoclopramide. The AUC attained with the capsule was not affected by metoclopramide. In 10 healthy volunteers, metoclopramide decreased digoxin absorption from a tablet with a 34% dissolution rate but did not affect absorption from digoxin tablets with a 98% or 100% dissolution rate. It appears that this interaction is dependent on the dissolution rate of the digoxin formulation and that the digoxin capsule and elixir formulations are least affected by metoclopramide. Tablets with a high dissolution rate may also lessen this interaction.

[1] Manninen V, et al. *Lancet.* 1973;1:398.
[2] Medin S, et al. *Lancet.* 1973;1:1393.
[3] Johnson BF, et al. *Br J Clin Pharmacol.* 1978;5:465.
[4] Johnson BF, et al. *Clin Pharmacol Ther.* 1984;36:724.
[5] Kirch W, et al. *Eur J Drug Metab Pharmacokinet.* 1986;11:249.

* Asterisk indicates drugs cited in interaction reports.

Digoxin — *Nefazodone*

Digoxin* (eg, *Lanoxin*)	Nefazodone* (*Serzone*)

Significance	Onset	Severity	Documentation
4	☐ Rapid	☐ Major	☐ Established
	■ **Delayed**	■ **Moderate**	☐ Probable
		☐ Minor	☐ Suspected
			■ **Possible**
			☐ Unlikely

Effects NEFAZODONE may slightly increase serum DIGOXIN concentrations, possibly resulting in DIGOXIN toxicity.

Mechanism Unknown.

Management Monitor serum DIGOXIN concentrations and observe the patient for possible DIGOXIN toxicity during concurrent administration of NEFAZODONE. Adjust the DIGOXIN dose as indicated.

Discussion

Utilizing an open labeled, randomized, multiple-dose, three-way crossover design, the effects of nefazodone on the pharmacokinetics and pharmacodynamics of oral digoxin were evaluated in 18 healthy male volunteers.[1] During 8–day treatment periods, plus one dose on the morning of the ninth day, each subject received nefazodone 200 mg twice daily alone, digoxin 0.2 mg once daily alone or digoxin combined with nefazodone. Each treatment period was followed by a 10–day washout period. Concurrent administration of nefazodone and digoxin resulted in increased steady-state area under the plasma concentration-time-curve of digoxin by 15% (from 12.83 to 14.7 ng•hr/mL), as well as increases in serum digoxin peak concentrations by 29% (from 1.87 to 2.41 ng/mL) and trough concentrations by 27% (from 0.41 to 0.52 ng/mL). These changes were statistically significant ($P < 0.05$). Compared with when either drug was given alone, concomitant administration of nefazodone and digoxin did not affect the frequency or severity of side effects. In addition, compared with digoxin monotherapy, coadministration of nefazodone did not cause any clinically important changes in heart rate, vital signs or PR, QRS and QT intervals. Digoxin administration did not affect the pharmacokinetics of nefazodone or its metabolites.

[1] Dockens RC, et al. *J Clin Pharmacol.* 1996;36:160.

* Asterisk indicates drugs cited in interaction reports.

Digoxin ✕ Nifedipine

Digoxin* (eg, *Lanoxin*)	Nifedipine* (eg, *Procardia*)

Significance	Onset	Severity	Documentation
4	□ Rapid ■ **Delayed**	□ Major ■ **Moderate** □ Minor	□ Established □ Probable □ Suspected ■ **Possible** □ Unlikely

Effects Although NIFEDIPINE may increase DIGOXIN serum levels, possibly resulting in DIGOXIN toxicity, most studies indicate that no clinically important interaction occurs.

Mechanism NIFEDIPINE appears to decrease the renal or extrarenal clearance of DIGOXIN.

Management Consider monitoring DIGOXIN concentrations during NIFEDIPINE therapy. If increased DIGOXIN levels or toxicity develop, the DIGOXIN dose may need to be decreased.

Discussion

Results are controversial.[1,2] Although most studies indicate that nifedipine does not affect digoxin serum concentrations in patients or healthy subjects,[3-10] several studies demonstrated that the plasma concentrations of digoxin are increased by nifedipine.[11-15] One report concluded that the interaction probably has little clinical relevance.[14] In 1 trial, 12 healthy volunteers received digoxin 0.375 mg/day for 6 weeks and nifedipine 10 mg 3 times a day for 2 weeks.[11] The plasma digoxin level increased 45% in 9 of the 12 volunteers. In another investigation, nifedipine increased digoxin levels approximately 15% at nifedipine doses ranging from 5 to 20 mg 3 times daily, indicating the interaction is not dependent on the dose of nifedipine.[15] A 15% increase in digoxin serum levels following coadministration with a sustained-release tablet formulation of nifedipine has been reported.[14] Nifedipine had no overall effect on digoxin but increased the extrarenal clearance and decreased the total urinary recovery of digoxin.[12] In 1 study, nifedipine attenuated the positive inotropic action of digoxin,[6] while in another study the coadministration of these agents improved cardiac performance.[16] One study reported no effect on digitoxin plasma levels or renal excretion.[17]

1 Schwartz JB. *Am J Cardiol.* 1985;55:31E.
2 De Vito JM, et al. *Pharmacotherapy.* 1986;6:73.
3 Schwartz JB, et al. *Am Heart J.* 1984;107:669.
4 Kuhlmann J, et al. *Klin Wochenschr.* 1984;62:451.
5 Schwartz JB, et al. *Clin Pharmacol Ther.* 1984;36:19.
6 Hansen PB, et al. *Br J Clin Pharmacol.* 1984;18:817.
7 Kuhlmann J. *Clin Pharmacol Ther.* 1985;37:150.
8 Koren G, et al. *Int J Clin Pharmacol Ther Toxicol.* 1986;24:39.
9 Garty M, et al. *J Clin Pharmacol.* 1986;26:304.
10 Pedersen KE, et al. *Dan Med Bull.* 1986;33:109.
11 Belz GG, et al. *Lancet.* 1981;1:844.
12 Pedersen KE, et al. *Clin Pharmacol Ther.* 1982;32:562.
13 Belz GG, et al. *Clin Pharmacol Ther.* 1983;33:410
14 Kleinbloesem CH, et al. *Ther Drug Monit.* 1985;7:372.
15 Kirch W, et al. *Clin Pharmacol Ther.* 1986;39:35.
16 Cantelli I, et al. *Am Heart J.* 1983;106:308.
17 Kuhlmann J. *Clin Pharmacol Ther.* 1985;38:667.

* Asterisk indicates drugs cited in interaction reports.

Digoxin — *Paroxetine*

Digoxin* (eg, *Lanoxin*)	Paroxetine* (eg, *Paxil*)

Significance	Onset	Severity	Documentation
1	☐ Rapid ■ **Delayed**	■ **Major** ☐ Moderate ☐ Minor	☐ Established ☐ Probable ■ **Suspected** ☐ Possible ☐ Unlikely

Effects DIGOXIN serum concentrations may be elevated, increasing the pharmacologic and toxic effects.

Mechanism Inhibition of renal tubular P-glycoprotein excretion of DIGOXIN by PAROXETINE is suspected.

Management In patients receiving DIGOXIN, closely monitor DIGOXIN serum levels and observe the patient for signs of digitalis toxicity when PAROXETINE is coadministered. Adjust the DIGOXIN dose as needed. Because citalopram (eg, *Celexa*) and venlafaxine (*Effexor*) have less of an effect on P-glycoprotein, they may be less likely to interact with DIGOXIN.

Discussion

A 68-year-old woman receiving digoxin 0.25 mg/day and warfarin (eg, *Coumadin*) 1 mg daily for atrial fibrillation developed a major depressive disorder and was hospitalized.[1] On day 3 of her hospital admission, paroxetine 20 mg/day was started and, 2 days later, the patient experienced dizziness, nausea, and vomiting. On day 7, delirium with visual hallucinations and disorientation developed. By day 10, she was unable to eat or walk. On day 11, digitalis toxicity was suspected and all medications were discontinued. Her digoxin concentration was elevated (5.2 ng/mL), and the ECG indicated premature ventricular contractions and complete atrioventricular block. On day 21, digoxin and warfarin were reinstated. By day 28, the delirium with disorientation was no longer present. The patient subsequently died of pneumonia.

[1] Yasui-Furukori N, et al. *Lancet*. 2006;367:788.

* Asterisk indicates drugs cited in interaction reports.

Digoxin | *Penicillamine*

Digoxin* (eg, *Lanoxin*)	Penicillamine* (eg, *Cuprimine*)

Significance	Onset	Severity	Documentation
2	■ **Rapid** ☐ Delayed	☐ Major ■ **Moderate** ☐ Minor	☐ Established ☐ Probable ■ **Suspected** ☐ Possible ☐ Unlikely

Effects PENICILLAMINE may decrease the serum levels of DIGOXIN, possibly decreasing its therapeutic effect.

Mechanism Unknown.

Management Monitor plasma DIGOXIN levels. If decreased clinical response or decreased DIGOXIN levels occur, an increased DIGOXIN dose may be necessary.

Discussion

In 1 study, 33 patients maintained on digoxin received concurrent penicillamine 1 g.[1] When penicillamine was given 2 hours after digoxin (n = 10), the mean serum digoxin level decreased from 1.86 to 1.62 ng/mL (13%). When penicillamine was given 16 hours after digoxin (n = 13), the mean serum digoxin level decreased from 1.5 to 1.16 ng/mL (23%). Penicillamine also reduced digoxin levels in 10 patients who received IV digoxin for 5 days before the penicillamine dose. The effect was significant at 4 and 6 hours following the penicillamine dose but not at 2 hours. In another study, 10 children with CHF receiving digoxin 0.02 mg/kg/day for 6 days were given penicillamine 1 g.[2] Mean digoxin serum levels decreased from 1.87 to 1.14 ng/mL (39%).

[1] Moezzi B, et al. *Jpn Heart J.* 1978;19:366.

[2] Moezzi B, et al. *Jpn Heart J.* 1980;21:335.

* Asterisk indicates drugs cited in interaction reports.

Digoxin — *Propafenone*

Digoxin* (eg, *Lanoxin*)	Propafenone* (eg, *Rythmol*)

Significance	Onset	Severity	Documentation
1	□ Rapid	■ **Major**	■ **Established**
	■ **Delayed**	□ Moderate	□ Probable
		□ Minor	□ Suspected
			□ Possible
			□ Unlikely

Effects Serum DIGOXIN levels may be increased, resulting in toxicity.

Mechanism Unknown. However, decreased DIGOXIN volume of distribution and renal and nonrenal clearance appear to be involved.

Management Monitor serum DIGOXIN levels and observe patients for toxicity. Adjust the DIGOXIN dose if PROPAFENONE is added to or discontinued from the treatment regimen.

Discussion

Several studies have demonstrated an interaction between digoxin and propafenone.[1-5] Ten patients received oral digoxin 0.25 mg/day for at least 10 days prior to coadministration of propafenone 600 mg/day for 1 week.[3] In 3 patients the study was prolonged, with propafenone doses increased to 750 and 900 mg/day for periods of 1 week each. The mean serum digoxin concentration increased from 0.97 to 1.54 ng/mL with administration of propafenone 600 mg/day and was associated with a decrease in heart rate and shortening of the QTc interval. Propafenone produced a 31.1% and 31.7% decrease in total and renal digoxin clearance, respectively. Two patients experienced symptoms consistent with digoxin toxicity. In a second study, propafenone 300 mg every 8 h increased serum digoxin levels in all 5 patients receiving digoxin 0.125 to 0.25 mg/day.[2] During placebo coadministration, the mean digoxin level was 0.69 ng/mL, compared with 1.3 ng/mL after 3 days of propafenone therapy. Three patients receiving both drugs for 6 months demonstrated a mean increase of 63% in serum digoxin levels. No patient experienced toxicity. In 6 healthy volunteers receiving a single IV dose of digoxin 1 mg alone and after 7 days of propafenone at either 150 or 300 mg every 8 h, the volume of distribution of digoxin decreased from 9.43 to 9.33 and 8.02 L/kg, respectively, while nonrenal clearance decreased from 1.21 to 1.01 and 0.75 mL/min/kg, respectively.[4] A study in 9 patients demonstrated a better correlation between propafenone serum levels and increased digoxin levels than with the dose of propafenone.[6] In 6 children receiving digoxin, the addition of propafenone 250 to 500 mg/m^2/day produced a 6% to 254% increase in serum digoxin levels.[5] In 3 patients, the digoxin dosage was decreased 25% to 50% prior to giving propafenone, resulting in a stable digoxin level after propafenone was added. During administration of propafenone, total body clearance of digoxin decreased.

[1] Belz GG, et al. *Clin Pharmacol Ther.* 1983;33(4):410.
[2] Salerno DM, et al. *Am J Cardiol.* 1984:53(1):77.
[3] Calvo MV, et al. *Ther Drug Monit.* 1989;11(1):10.
[4] Nolan PE Jr, et al. *J Clin Pharmacol.* 1989;29(1):46.
[5] Zalzstein E, et al. *J Pediatr.* 1990:116(2):310.
[6] Bigot MC, et al. *J Clin Pharmacol.* 1991;31(6):521.

* Asterisk indicates drugs cited in interaction reports.

Digoxin | **Protease Inhibitors**

Digoxin	Protease Inhibitors	
Digoxin* (eg, *Lanoxin*)	Lopinavir/Ritonavir (*Kaletra*)	Saquinavir (*Invirase*)
	Ritonavir* (*Norvir*)	

Significance	Onset	Severity	Documentation
1	☐ Rapid ■ **Delayed**	■ **Major** ☐ Moderate ☐ Minor	☐ Established ☐ Probable ■ **Suspected** ☐ Possible ☐ Unlikely

Effects DIGOXIN plasma concentrations may be elevated, increasing the pharmacologic and toxic effects.

Mechanism Reduced renal clearance of DIGOXIN caused by inhibition of P-gp transport of DIGOXIN in the renal proximal tubules is suspected.

Management Monitor DIGOXIN plasma concentrations and observe patients for signs of DIGOXIN toxicity when certain PROTEASE INHIBITORS are started. Adjust the dose of DIGOXIN as needed.

Discussion

Digoxin toxicity was reported in a 61-year-old woman after ritonavir was added to her treatment regimen.[1] The patient had been receiving digoxin 0.25 mg daily for 8 years. In addition, she had been taking indinavir (*Crixivan*), lamivudine (eg, *Epivir*), and stavudine (eg, *Zerit*) for 3 years. The patient went to the emergency department with increasing nausea and vomiting 3 days after starting ritonavir 200 mg twice daily. Her digoxin level on admission was 7.2 nmol/L (normal range, 1 to 2.6 nmol/L). Her medications were discontinued and she improved clinically by the second hospital day. Digoxin was permanently discontinued and indinavir, lamivudine, and stavudine were restarted without important clinical adverse effects. The effects of ritonavir administration on digoxin pharmacokinetics were studied in 12 healthy men.[2] In a placebo-controlled, randomized, crossover study, each subject received oral ritonavir 300 mg or placebo twice daily for 11 days. On day 3, each subject received digoxin 0.5 mg IV. Compared with placebo administration, ritonavir increased the digoxin AUC 86%, volume of distribution 77%, and terminal $t_{½}$ 156%, and decreased nonrenal and renal clearance 48% and 35%, respectively. Additional studies are needed to determine if other protease inhibitors interact similarly with digoxin.

[1] Phillips EJ, et al. *AIDS*. 2003;17(10):1577.

[2] Ding R, et al. *Clin Pharmacol Ther*. 2004;76(1):73.

* Asterisk indicates drugs cited in interaction reports. Based on pharmacologic and pharmacokinetic considerations, similar interactions may occur with other drugs that are listed.

Digoxin ✕ Proton Pump Inhibitors

Digoxin	Proton Pump Inhibitors	
Digoxin* (eg, *Lanoxin*)	Esomeprazole (*Nexium*)	Pantoprazole (*Protonix*)
	Lansoprazole (*Prevacid*)	Rabeprazole* (*Aciphex*)
	Omeprazole* (eg, *Prilosec*)	

Significance	Onset	Severity	Documentation
4	☐ Rapid	☐ Major	☐ Established
	■ **Delayed**	■ **Moderate**	☐ Probable
		☐ Minor	☐ Suspected
			■ **Possible**
			☐ Unlikely

Effects Increased serum DIGOXIN levels may occur.

Mechanism Possible increased DIGOXIN absorption.

Management The magnitude of the change is not expected to be clinically important in most patients. However, because DIGOXIN has a narrow therapeutic index, the increase in serum level may be important if DIGOXIN concentrations are in the upper range when PROTON PUMP INHIBITOR therapy is started.

Discussion

In a randomized, 2-way, crossover study, the effects of omeprazole on the pharmacokinetics of a single oral dose of digoxin were studied in 10 healthy men.[1] On 2 separate occasions, each subject received digoxin 1 mg alone or on day 8 of an 11-day course of omeprazole 20 mg once daily. The mean serum digoxin C_{max} was slightly higher (4.2 vs 3.98 mcg/L) and the time to reach the C_{max} tended to be faster (45 vs 60 minutes) during coadministration of digoxin and omeprazole. These differences were not statistically significant. However, digoxin AUC increased approximately 10%. This increase was statistically significant ($P < 0.05$). Two subjects had a 30% increase in the AUC. No serious adverse reactions were reported during the study. There were no pathological changes in the ECG recordings, and the BP, heart rate, and oral body temperature did not show changes that could be attributed to the medications. An observational study of patients receiving digoxin while being converted to rabeprazole from lansoprazole or omeprazole identified a change in digoxin levels of greater than 15% in a subset of patients.[2] It is not known if the effect would be greater if the patients were starting proton pump inhibitor therapy. After the initiation of omeprazole 20 mg/day, elevated digoxin serum levels and toxicity were reported in a 65-year-old woman who had been taking digoxin 0.625 mg/day for several years.[3] She was treated with digoxin immune fab and recovered uneventfully.

[1] Oosterhuis B, et al. *Br J Clin Pharmacol.* 1991;32(5):569.
[2] Le GH, et al. *Am J Health Syst Pharm.* 2003;60(13):1343.
[3] Kiley CA, et al. *South Med J.* 2007;100(4):400.

* Asterisk indicates drugs cited in interaction reports. Based on pharmacologic and pharmacokinetic considerations, similar interactions may occur with other drugs that are listed.

Digoxin — *Quinidine*

Digoxin* (eg, *Lanoxin*)	Quinidine*

Significance	Onset	Severity	Documentation
1	☐ Rapid	■ **Major**	■ **Established**
	■ **Delayed**	☐ Moderate	☐ Probable
		☐ Minor	☐ Suspected
			☐ Possible
			☐ Unlikely

Effects Increased serum DIGOXIN levels with possible toxicity.

Mechanism Reduced renal and biliary clearance and volume of distribution of DIGOXIN.

Management In patients receiving DIGOXIN and QUINIDINE for signs and symptoms of digoxin toxicity. It may be necessary to reduce the DIGOXIN dose 50% in some patients when QUINIDINE is initiated. Monitor serum DIGOXIN levels.

Discussion

The digoxin-quinidine interaction is well documented.[1-19] An increase in serum digoxin levels of at least 0.5 ng/mL occurs in approximately 90% of patients when given quinidine. The serum digoxin concentration will usually double, but the magnitude of the increase can vary significantly. The serum digoxin level will begin to rise on the first day of concomitant therapy, and a new steady-state level is usually achieved in 3 to 6 days. Quinidine increases the bioavailability of digoxin, reduces the volume of distribution 30% to 40%, and reduces the total clearance of digoxin 30% to 40%.

Cardiac and GI signs and symptoms of toxicity occur more commonly in patients receiving quinidine and digoxin than in those receiving digoxin alone. However, the adverse reaction profile of the combination is similar to that of quinidine alone. The increase in cardiac effects reflects an increase in serum digoxin concentration; thus, expect usual digoxin toxic or therapeutic effects at a given serum digoxin level in most patients. However, in some patients, digitalis toxicity can occur within the therapeutic range of serum digoxin concentrations.[20]

[1] Doering W. *N Engl J Med.* 1979:301(8):400.
[2] Bigger JT Jr, et al. *Drugs.* 1982;24(3):229.
[3] Bigger JT Jr. *Mod Concepts Cardiovasc Dis.* 1982;51(1):73.
[4] Bussey HI. *Am Heart J.* 1982;104(2, pt 1):289.
[5] Belz GG, et al. *Clin Pharmacol Ther.* 1982;31(5):548.
[6] Fichtl B, et al. *Clin Pharmacokinet.* 1983;8(2):137.
[7] Pedersen KE, et al. *Eur J Clin Pharmacol.* 1983;24(1):41.
[8] Walker AM, et al. *Am Heart J.* 1983;105(6):1025.
[9] Schenck-Gustafsson K, et al. *Am J Cardiol.* 1983;51(5):777.
[10] Doering W. *Eur J Clin Pharmacol.* 1983;25(4):517.
[11] Bussey HI. *Am Heart J.* 1984;107(1):143.
[12] Jogestrand T, et al. *Eur J Clin Pharmacol.* 1984;27(5):571.
[13] Das G, et al. *Clin Pharmacol Ther.* 1984;35(3):317.
[14] Fenster PE, et al. *Clin Pharmacol Ther.* 1984;36(1):70.
[15] Angelin B, et al. *Eur J Clin Invest.* 1987;17(3):262.
[16] Hedman A, et al. *Clin Pharmacol Ther.* 1990;47(1):20.
[17] Hedman A. *Eur J Clin Pharmacol.* 1992;42(4):457.
[18] Williams PJ, et al. *Clin Pharmacokinet.* 1992; 22(1):66.
[19] Bauer LA, et al. *Ther Drug Monit.* 1996;18(1):46.
[20] Mordel A, et al. *Clin Pharmacol Ther.* 1993;53(4):457.

* Asterisk indicates drugs cited in interaction reports.

Digoxin | **Quinine**

Digoxin*
(eg, *Lanoxin*)

Quinine*
(*Qualaquin*)

Significance	Onset	Severity	Documentation
2	☐ Rapid ■ **Delayed**	☐ Major ■ **Moderate** ☐ Minor	☐ Established ■ **Probable** ☐ Suspected ☐ Possible ☐ Unlikely

Effects Increased serum DIGOXIN levels with possible toxicity.

Mechanism QUININE appears to decrease the biliary clearance of DIGOXIN.

Management Monitor patients for signs of DIGOXIN toxicity or increased DIGOXIN serum levels. A decreased dose of DIGOXIN may be necessary.

Discussion

Several studies support an interaction between digoxin and quinine.[1-5] In a study of 7 healthy subjects, digoxin 0.1875 mg twice daily was administered; after 2 weeks, quinine 250 mg/day was started, followed 1 week later by quinine 250 mg 3 times daily for an additional week. During coadministration of quinine 250 mg/day, mean serum digoxin concentrations increased from 0.64 to 0.8 ng/mL (25%); when quinine 750 mg/day was administered, digoxin levels increased to 0.85 ng/mL (33%) in 6 of the subjects. Renal digoxin clearance increased slightly but insignificantly, and mean urinary digoxin recovery increased. In another study, 4 volunteers received digoxin 0.25 mg/day and concurrent quinine 300 mg 4 times daily.[2] Plasma digoxin concentration increased from 0.63 to 1.03 nmol/L (63%) on day 1 of quinine and to 1.1 nmol/L (75%) on day 4. Digoxin renal clearance decreased 20%. Six subjects received quinine 200 mg every 8 hours for 4 days before and 4 days after a single 1 mg IV dose of digoxin.[1] Total body clearance of digoxin decreased 26%, and the mean digoxin elimination $t_{½}$ increased from 34.2 to 51.8 hours. Nonrenal digoxin clearance decreased 55%. Digoxin toxicity was not reported in any of these studies.

[1] Wandell M, et al. *Clin Pharmacol Ther.* 1980;28(4):425.
[2] Aronson JK, et al. *Lancet.* 1981;1(8235):1418.
[3] Pedersen KE, et al. *Acta Med Scand.* 1985;218(2):229.
[4] Hedman A, et al. *Clin Pharmacol Ther.* 1990;47(1):20.
[5] Hedman A. *Eur J Clin Pharmacol.* 1992;42(4):457.

* Asterisk indicates drugs cited in interaction reports.

Digoxin — *Ranolazine*

Digoxin* (eg, *Lanoxin*)	Ranolazine* (*Ranexa*)

Significance	Onset	Severity	Documentation
4	□ Rapid ■ **Delayed**	□ Major ■ **Moderate** □ Minor	□ Established □ Probable □ Suspected ■ **Possible** □ Unlikely

Effects DIGOXIN plasma concentrations may be elevated, increasing the pharmacologic effects and adverse reactions.

Mechanism Increased absorption and decreased elimination of DIGOXIN due to P-glycoprotein inhibition by RANOLAZINE is suspected.

Management Closely monitor DIGOXIN plasma concentrations and observe the patient for signs of DIGOXIN toxicity. Digoxin dosage adjustments may be needed when RANOLAZINE is started or stopped.

Discussion

The effects of ranolazine on the pharmacokinetics of digoxin were studied in 16 healthy men.[1] In a double-blind, placebo-controlled, parallel-group study, each subject received digoxin 0.125 mg daily for 14 days. During the last 7 days of digoxin administration, ranolazine 1,000 mg twice daily or placebo were given. Compared with placebo, ranolazine increased the digoxin C_{max} and AUC 1.46- and 1.6-fold, respectively.[1]

[1] Jerling M. *Clin Pharmacokinet.* 2006;45(5):469.

* Asterisk indicates drugs cited in interaction reports.

Digoxin — *Rifampin*

Digoxin* (eg, *Lanoxin*)	Rifampin* (eg, *Rifadin*)

Significance	Onset	Severity	Documentation
4	□ Rapid ■ **Delayed**	□ Major ■ **Moderate** □ Minor	□ Established □ Probable □ Suspected ■ **Possible** □ Unlikely

Effects RIFAMPIN may reduce DIGOXIN serum concentrations, decreasing the therapeutic effect.

Mechanism Unknown.

Management An increased DIGOXIN dosage may be necessary. Monitor serum DIGOXIN concentration and tailor the dose as needed. A decreased dose may be required upon RIFAMPIN discontinuation to avoid toxicity.

Discussion

In several case reports, coadministration of rifampin and digoxin resulted in decreased digoxin concentrations.[1-3] Two patients on dialysis receiving digoxin elixir 0.08 mg/day or tablets 0.125 to 0.25 mg/day were given rifampin 300 to 600 mg/day.[3] Serum digoxin concentrations decreased to 0.2 to 0.3 ng/mL; digoxin dose requirements increased 34% in 1 patient and approximately 100% in the other patient. When rifampin was discontinued, the digoxin doses required to maintain a digoxin serum concentration of 0.7 to 2 ng/mL were 50% of those during concomitant rifampin. A similar decrease in digoxin concentration was reported in another patient; digoxin levels increased when rifampin was discontinued.[1] Another patient was receiving digoxin 0.25 mg/day, with a serum digoxin concentration of 2.9 ng/mL.[4] After 4 days of rifampin 600 mg/day, the digoxin level decreased to 1.7 ng/mL. The digoxin dose was increased to 0.25 mg/day alternating with 0.375 mg/day, but the digoxin level decreased to 0.6 ng/mL. Rifampin was discontinued, digoxin was reduced to 0.25 mg/day, and the digoxin levels increased to 1.6 ng/mL after 8 days and 2.6 ng/mL after 15 days.

[1] Novi C, et al. *JAMA*. 1980;244:2521.
[2] Bussey HI, et al. *Arch Intern Med*. 1984;144:1021.
[3] Gault H, et al. *Clin Pharmacol Ther*. 1984;35:750.
[4] Baciewicz AM, et al. *Arch Intern Med*. 1987;147:565.

* Asterisk indicates drugs cited in interaction reports.

Digoxin — *Serotonin Reuptake Inhibitors*

Digoxin	Serotonin Reuptake Inhibitors	
Digoxin* (eg, *Lanoxin*)	Fluoxetine* (eg, *Prozac*)	Sertraline* (*Zoloft*)
	Fluvoxamine*	

Significance	Onset	Severity	Documentation
4	□ Rapid	□ Major	□ Established
	■ **Delayed**	■ **Moderate**	□ Probable
		□ Minor	□ Suspected
			■ **Possible**
			□ Unlikely

Effects DIGOXIN serum concentrations may be elevated, increasing the pharmacologic and toxic effects.

Mechanism Unknown.

Management If there is no suitable alternative therapy, closely monitor DIGOXIN serum concentrations when SRIs are coadministered. Adjust the DIGOXIN dose as needed.

Discussion

Increased serum digoxin concentrations associated with anorexia were reported in a 93-year-old woman following the addition of fluoxetine to her treatment regimen.[1] The patient, a nursing home resident, had a history of CHF, paroxysmal atrial fibrillation, hypertension, and diverticulosis. The medications she had been taking for several months consisted of digoxin 0.125 mg/day, captopril (eg, *Capoten*), furosemide (eg, *Lasix*), and ranitidine (eg, *Zantac*). During this time, her digoxin concentrations ranged from 1 to 1.4 nmol/L. The patient was started on fluoxetine 10 mg/day for depression. One week later, anorexia developed, and her digoxin level had increased to 4.2 nmol/L. Renal function was unchanged. Digoxin and fluoxetine were discontinued. After 5 days, the anorexia subsided, and her digoxin concentration returned to baseline. Treatment with digoxin 0.125 mg/day was resumed, and, over the next 3 weeks, serum digoxin concentrations ranged from 0.9 to 1.4 nmol/L. A second attempt to treat the patient's depression with fluoxetine 10 mg/day resulted in an increase in digoxin levels to 2 nmol/L after 2 days and 2.8 nmol/L after 4 days. Anorexia was present. Digoxin and fluoxetine were discontinued. In a retrospective study, an increased risk of hospital admission for digoxin toxicity was seen with several SSRIs.[2] However, an increased risk was also seen with benzodiazepines and tricyclic antidepressants, which are drug classes with no known pharmacokinetic interaction with digoxin.

[1] Leibovitz A, et al. *Arch Intern Med.* 1998;158:1152.

[2] Juurlink DN, et al. *Br J Clin Pharmacol.* 2005;59:102.

* Asterisk indicates drugs cited in interaction reports.

Digoxin | **Spironolactone**

Digoxin* (eg, *Lanoxin*)	Spironolactone* (eg, *Aldactone*)

Significance	Onset	Severity	Documentation
2	■ **Rapid** □ Delayed	□ Major ■ **Moderate** □ Minor	□ Established □ Probable ■ **Suspected** □ Possible □ Unlikely

Effects SPIRONOLACTONE may attenuate the positive inotropic effect of DIGOXIN. Serum levels of DIGOXIN also may be increased. Additionally, SPIRONOLACTONE may interfere with the DIGOXIN radioimmunoassay, resulting in falsely elevated DIGOXIN levels.

Mechanism DIGOXIN'S positive inotropic effect may be attenuated by SPIRONOLACTONE'S negative inotropic effect. Also, SPIRONOLACTONE may block tubular secretion of DIGOXIN, reducing its clearance and increasing plasma levels.[1]

Management The dose of DIGOXIN may need to be adjusted during SPIRONOLACTONE coadministration; monitor patients closely. Also, be aware of the falsely elevated DIGOXIN levels that may occur because of interference with the radioimmunoassay. Unnecessary DIGOXIN dosage adjustments may be made in response to the false levels.

Discussion

In 2 studies involving patients and healthy subjects, spironolactone caused a negative inotropic effect that attenuated the positive inotropic effect of concurrent digoxin.[2,3] Spironolactone also decreased renal tubular secretion of digoxin. Spironolactone has decreased clearance and increased plasma levels of digoxin.[1,4-6] In contrast, when patients receiving digoxin were given a combination diuretic (spironolactone/hydrochlorothiazide), the diuretic had no effect on digoxin concentrations.[7]

Additionally, spironolactone and its metabolites (eg, potassium canrenoate) may interfere with digoxin radioimmunoassay, resulting in falsely elevated digoxin levels.[8,9] This effect can be eliminated with adequate laboratory controls; however, it is important to be aware of this potential effect. Potassium canrenoate (not available in the US) also has been used to treat the ventricular arrhythmias that may occur with digoxin toxicity.[10]

1 Hedman A, et al. *Eur J Clin Pharmacol.* 1992;42:481.
2 Waldorff S, et al. *Eur J Clin Pharmacol.* 1982;21:269.
3 Waldorff S, et al. *Clin Pharmacol Ther.* 1983;33:418.
4 Steiness E. *Circulation.* 1974;50:103.
5 Waldorff S, et al. *Clin Pharmacol Ther.* 1978;24:162.
6 Paladino JA, et al. *JAMA.* 1984;251:470.
7 Finnegan TP, et al. *J Am Geriatr Soc.* 1984;32:129.
8 Thomas RW, et al. *Ther Drug Monit.* 1981;3:117.
9 Morris RG, et al. *Eur J Clin Pharmacol.* 1988;34:233.
10 Yeh BK, et al. *Am Heart J.* 1976;92:308.

* Asterisk indicates drugs cited in interaction reports.

Digoxin — *St. John's Wort*

Digoxin* (eg, *Lanoxin*)	St. John's Wort*

Significance	Onset	Severity	Documentation
2	□ Rapid	□ Major	□ Established
	■ **Delayed**	■ **Moderate**	□ Probable
		□ Minor	■ **Suspected**
			□ Possible
			□ Unlikely

Effects Decreased DIGOXIN plasma levels and clinical efficacy.

Mechanism Induction of intestinal P-glycoprotein transporter as well as intestinal and hepatic CYP3A4 metabolism of DIGOXIN by ST. JOHN'S WORT.[1]

Management Because DIGOXIN has a narrow therapeutic index, caution patients to consult their health care provider before use of nonprescription or herbal products. If ST. JOHN'S WORT cannot be avoided, assess the patient's response to DIGOXIN when ST. JOHN'S WORT is started or stopped. Monitoring DIGOXIN plasma levels may be useful in adjusting the dose.

Discussion

The effect of single- and multiple-dose administration of an extract of St. John's wort (hypericum extract) on the pharmacokinetics of steady-state digoxin plasma concentrations was studied in 25 healthy volunteers.[2] Using a single-blind, placebo-controlled parallel design, 1 group received digoxin 0.25 mg/day with St. John's wort extract 900 mg/day, while the other group received digoxin 0.25 mg/day with placebo. Single-dose administration of hypericum extract did not affect the pharmacokinetics of digoxin. However, multiple dosing of digoxin and hypericum extract concurrently for 10 days decreased the AUC of digoxin 25%, the peak concentration 26% (from 1.9 to 1.4 mcg/L), and the trough concentration 33% (from 0.57 to 0.38 mcg/L). Administration of St. John's wort extract to 8 healthy men resulted in an 18% decrease in digoxin exposure after a single 0.5 mg dose of digoxin and a 1.5-fold increase in expression of duodenal P-glycoprotein and CYP3A4.[1] There was also a 1.4-fold increase in functional activity of hepatic CYP3A4. The magnitude of the interaction between St. John's wort and digoxin appears to be related to the hyperforin (a constituent of St. John's wort) dose.[3]

The ingredients of many herbal products are not standardized. It is unclear if herbal products contain ingredients other than those listed on the label or purported to be present that could interact with digoxin.

[1] Dürr D, et al. *Clin Pharmacol Ther.* 2000;68:598.
[2] Johne A, et al. *Clin Pharmacol Ther.* 1999;66:338.
[3] Mueller SC, et al. *Clin Pharmacol Ther.* 2004;75:546.

* Asterisk indicates drugs cited in interaction reports.

Digoxin — *Sucralfate*

Digoxin* (eg, *Lanoxin*)	Sucralfate* (eg, *Carafate*)

Significance	Onset	Severity	Documentation
4	☐ Rapid ■ **Delayed**	☐ Major ■ **Moderate** ☐ Minor	☐ Established ☐ Probable ☐ Suspected ■ **Possible** ☐ Unlikely

Effects Serum DIGOXIN levels may be reduced, decreasing the therapeutic effects.

Mechanism Unknown. However, DIGOXIN possibly binds to SUCRALFATE, decreasing GI absorption.

Management Monitor DIGOXIN levels. If a decrease in clinical response occurs, consider discontinuing SUCRALFATE.

Discussion

In a preliminary report, the pharmacokinetics of digoxin were studied in 12 healthy male subjects receiving digoxin alone, in combination with sucralfate, and 2 hours before sucralfate administration.[1] Digoxin was given as a single 0.75 mg dose while sucralfate was administered in 1 g doses four times daily for 2 days before and during digoxin dosing. The mean area under the digoxin concentration-time curve was reduced by 19% during concurrent administration of both drugs compared to digoxin alone. This difference was not seen when the dosing was separated by 2 hours. In a subsequent report, concurrent administration of sucralfate produced subtherapeutic levels of digoxin.[2] A 71-year-old woman with a 3-day history of intermittent chest pain, shortness of breath and fatigue was admitted to the hospital to rule out myocardial infarction. She was receiving digoxin 0.125 mg/day, sustained release quinidine (eg, *Quinidex Extentabs*) 300 mg twice daily, warfarin (*Coumadin*) 7.5 mg/day and sucralfate 2 g twice daily. The sucralfate was separated from her other medications by 2 hours. Upon admission, the drug doses were not changed and they were administered concurrently with sucralfate. In addition, she was prescribed nitroglycerin paste (eg, *Nitrostat*), diltiazem (eg, *Cardizem*), subcutaneous heparin, meperidine (eg, *Demerol*) with promethazine (eg, *Phenergan*) for chest pain unrelieved by three sublingual nitroglycerin tablets, and acetaminophen (eg, *Tylenol*). On the evening of admission, the patient had an episode of atrial flutter with a rapid ventricular response, which was accompanied by chest pain and shortness of breath. The patient was given digoxin 0.25 mg IV on two consecutive days. Her symptoms resolved and the serum digoxin level increased from 0.13 to 1.9 nmol/L. On the same day, sucralfate administration was changed to be given 4 hours apart from her other medication. On the next day, sucralfate was discontinued. One day later, the patient's digoxin level was 1.15 nmol/L. Except for sucralfate, the patient was maintained on her initial drug regimen and 2 weeks after hospitalization, her serum digoxin level remained therapeutic (ie, 0.9 nmol/L).

[1] Giesing DH, et al. *Gastroenterology*. 1983;84:1165. (Abstract)

[2] Rey AM, et al. *DICP, Ann Pharmacother*. 1991;25:745.

* Asterisk indicates drugs cited in interaction reports.

Digoxin — *Sulfasalazine*

Digoxin* (eg, *Lanoxin*)	Sulfasalazine* (eg, *Azulfidine*)

Significance	Onset	Severity	Documentation
4	■ **Rapid**	□ Major	□ Established
	□ Delayed	■ **Moderate**	□ Probable
		□ Minor	□ Suspected
			■ **Possible**
			□ Unlikely

Effects SULFASALAZINE may decrease DIGOXIN's bioavailability, possibly resulting in a reduced therapeutic effect.

Mechanism Impaired absorption of DIGOXIN by an unknown mechanism.

Management Monitor DIGOXIN levels during concurrent SULFASALAZINE therapy. If reduced levels or clinical response occur, SULFASALAZINE may need to be discontinued.

Discussion

In a case report, a patient receiving digoxin 0.25 mg/day and sulfasalazine 8 g/day for 3 months had a digoxin serum level of less than 0.4 ng/mL.[1] Increasing the digoxin dose to 0.5 mg/day, switching from digoxin tablets to the elixir, or separating administration times did not increase the serum levels. However, when sulfasalazine was discontinued, the digoxin levels rose to 0.9 to 1.1 ng/mL. To determine if sulfasalazine was affecting the absorption of digoxin, a study was done in 10 healthy subjects.[1] The subjects received a single 0.5 mg dose of digoxin elixir after 6 days of sulfasalazine 2 g/day in 4 subjects or increasing doses in 6 subjects. With sulfasalazine coadministration, the digoxin area under the curve (AUC) decreased from 8.79 to 6.66 ng/hr•mL (24.2%). Total urinary excretion also decreased from 278 to 228 mcg/10 days. The decrease in the AUC was statistically significant.

[1] Juhl RP, et al. *Clin Pharmacol Ther.* 1976;20:387.

* Asterisk indicates drugs cited in interaction reports.

Digoxin — *Telmisartan*

Digoxin* (eg, *Lanoxin*)	Telmisartan* (*Micardis*)

Significance	Onset	Severity	Documentation
4	☐ Rapid ■ **Delayed**	☐ Major ■ **Moderate** ☐ Minor	☐ Established ☐ Probable ☐ Suspected ■ **Possible** ☐ Unlikely

Effects DIGOXIN peak serum concentrations may be elevated, increasing the risk of toxicity.

Mechanism Increased rate of DIGOXIN absorption is suspected.

Management Observe the patient for DIGOXIN adverse reactions and monitor DIGOXIN serum concentrations when starting, stopping, or changing the dose of TELMISARTAN.

Discussion

The effect of telmisartan on the steady-state pharmacokinetics of digoxin was studied in 12 healthy male volunteers.[1] The study was an open-label, randomized, 2-period, cross-over design in which each subject received digoxin alone for 7 days and with telmisartan for 7 days. On the first day of each phase, a loading dose of digoxin 0.5 mg was administered in the morning followed by a 0.25 mg evening dose. For the next 6 days, subjects received digoxin 0.25 mg in the morning. During the first period of the study, subjects received digoxin alone; in the second period, subjects received telmisartan 120 mg with the morning dose of digoxin. Compared with giving digoxin alone, telmisartan coadministration resulted in higher digoxin serum concentrations, which were most pronounced during the first 3 to 4 hours of the dosing interval. The AUC, peak concentration, and trough concentration for digoxin were elevated 22%, 50%, and 13%, respectively. Telmisartan did not affect digoxin steady-state trough levels, and digoxin did not affect the steady-state pharmacokinetics of telmisartan. Adverse reactions were mild to moderate in severity and were similar when digoxin was administered alone or with telmisartan.

[1] Stangier J, et al. *J Clin Pharmacol.* 2000;40(12 Pt 1):1373.

* Asterisk indicates drugs cited in interaction reports.

Digoxin		***Tetracyclines***
Digoxin* (eg, *Lanoxin*)	Demeclocycline Doxycycline (eg, *Vibramycin*)	Minocycline (eg, *Minocin*) Tetracycline*

Significance	Onset	Severity	Documentation
1	☐ Rapid ■ **Delayed**	■ **Major** ☐ Moderate ☐ Minor	☐ Established ☐ Probable ■ **Suspected** ☐ Possible ☐ Unlikely

Effects

Coadministration of TETRACYCLINE and DIGOXIN may result in increased serum levels of DIGOXIN in a small subset of patients (approximately 10%); DIGOXIN toxicity may occur. The effects may persist for months after stopping TETRACYCLINE.

Mechanism

In approximately 10% of patients, a large amount of DIGOXIN is metabolized by bacteria in the GI tract to digoxin reduction products (DRPs), inactive metabolites. TETRACYCLINE may reverse the process by altering GI flora, allowing for more DIGOXIN to be absorbed and increasing DIGOXIN serum levels.

Management

Monitor patients for increased DIGOXIN levels and signs of DIGOXIN excess. A decreased DIGOXIN dose may be necessary. The use of the capsule formulation may minimize DRP production because of increased bioavailability.

Discussion

Approximately 10% of patients receiving digoxin convert 30% to 40% or more of the parent drug to DRPs, which are inactive by-products.[1,2] When poorly absorbed digoxin preparations were taken, there appeared to be an increase in the excretion of DRPs. When large amounts of DRPs are excreted, patients have required an increased digoxin dose. Antibiotic therapy may reverse the tendency for these patients to metabolize digoxin in the GI tract to DRPs, resulting in increased digoxin levels. One subject who excreted 17% to 40% DRPs after a single digoxin dose in previous studies received digoxin 0.5 mg/day for 22 to 29 days.[2] After 17 days, the subject was given tetracycline 500 mg every 6 hours for 5 days. Urinary DRP excretion decreased markedly within 48 hours of tetracycline administration (from 39% to 4%). Following antibiotic treatment, steady-state digoxin serum levels increased (compared with baseline levels) from 0.72 to 1.03 ng/mL. When subjects were given digoxin 9 weeks after the study, less than 2% urinary DRPs were excreted, indicating that the effects of the interaction occurred for several months. See also Digoxin-Aminoglycosides and Digoxin-Erythromycin.

[1] Lindenbaum J, et al. *Am J Med.* 1981;71(1):67.

[2] Lindenbaum J, et al. *N Engl J Med.* 1981;305(14):789.

* Asterisk indicates drugs cited in interaction reports. Based on pharmacologic and pharmacokinetic considerations, similar interactions may occur with other drugs that are listed.

Digoxin — *Tolvaptan*

Digoxin* (eg, *Lanoxin*)	Tolvaptan* (*Samsca*)

Significance	Onset	Severity	Documentation
4	☐ Rapid ■ **Delayed**	☐ Major ■ **Moderate** ☐ Minor	☐ Established ☐ Probable ☐ Suspected ■ **Possible** ☐ Unlikely

Effects DIGOXIN plasma concentrations may be elevated, increasing the risk of toxicity.

Mechanism Increased GI absorption of DIGOXIN, resulting from inhibition of P-gp expression by TOLVAPTAN, is suspected.

Management Monitor DIGOXIN concentrations and observe the clinical response. If an interaction is suspected, adjust the DIGOXIN dose as needed.

Discussion

The potential for an interaction between digoxin and tolvaptan was evaluated in 14 healthy subjects.[1] Using an open-label, sequential design, each subject received tolvaptan 60 mg once daily on days 1 and 12 to 16 and digoxin 0.25 mg once daily on days 5 to 16. The digoxin C_{max} and AUC with tolvaptan (day 16) were increased 1.27- and 1.18-fold, respectively, compared with digoxin alone (day 11). The mean renal clearance of digoxin was decreased 59%. The single-dose tolvaptan C_{max} and AUC with digoxin (day 12) were increased approximately 10% compared with tolvaptan alone (day 1). Tolvaptan did not accumulate with multiple dosing. No serious adverse events were reported, and no subjects were withdrawn from the study due to adverse events.

[1] Shoaf SE, et al. *J Clin Pharmacol.* 2011;51(5):761.

* Asterisk indicates drugs cited in interaction reports.

Digoxin — *Triamterene*

Digoxin* (eg, *Lanoxin*)	Triamterene* (*Dyrenium*)

Significance	Onset	Severity	Documentation
5	☐ Rapid ■ **Delayed**	☐ Major ☐ Moderate ■ **Minor**	☐ Established ☐ Probable ☐ Suspected ☐ Possible ■ **Unlikely**

Effects Although TRIAMTERENE may decrease the elimination of DIGOXIN in some patients, a clinically important interaction appears unlikely.

Mechanism TRIAMTERENE may reduce the extrarenal elimination of DIGOXIN.

Management No special precautions appear necessary. However, routinely monitor patients. If signs of DIGOXIN toxicity occur or if serum DIGOXIN levels increase, a decreased DIGOXIN dose may be necessary.

Discussion

In 1 study, 6 healthy volunteers were given triamterene 50 mg 3 times daily for 1 week before and 4 days after a single IV digoxin dose (15 mcg/kg).[1] Total digoxin elimination was reduced 20%, extrarenal clearance was reduced, and renal elimination was unchanged. The distribution of digoxin was not affected. Triamterene did not appear to affect the inotropic action of digoxin. In another study, 81 patients receiving digoxin and concurrent triamterene with either a thiazide or a loop diuretic had a higher serum digoxin concentration than patients on digoxin receiving no diuretic, a thiazide or loop diuretic, or amiloride (eg, *Midamor*) with a thiazide or loop diuretic.[2] Digoxin toxicity was not reported in either of these studies.

In 1 study, 9 patients receiving digoxin were given a combination of triamterene and hydrochlorothiazide (eg, *HydroDiuril*).[3] There was no increase in serum digoxin levels compared with digoxin with concurrent spironolactone (eg, *Aldactone*) plus hydrochlorothiazide, furosemide (eg, *Lasix*) alone, or hydrochlorothiazide alone.

[1] Waldorff S, et al. *Clin Pharmacol Ther.* 1983;33(4):418.
[2] Impivaara O, et al. *Eur J Clin Pharmacol.* 1985;27(6):627.
[3] Finnegan TP, et al. *J Am Geriatr Soc.* 1984;32(2):129.

* Asterisk indicates drugs cited in interaction reports.

Digoxin — *Verapamil*

Digoxin* (eg, *Lanoxin*)	Verapamil* (eg, *Calan*)

Significance	Onset	Severity	Documentation
1	☐ Rapid	■ **Major**	■ **Established**
	■ **Delayed**	☐ Moderate	☐ Probable
		☐ Minor	☐ Suspected
			☐ Possible
			☐ Unlikely

Effects DIGOXIN effects may be enhanced. Increased DIGOXIN levels and toxicity could occur.

Mechanism Complex. See discussion.

Management Monitor DIGOXIN plasma concentrations and observe patients for signs of toxicity. Adjust the dose as needed. It may be necessary to decrease the DIGOXIN dosage.

Discussion

Verapamil and digoxin have additive effects to slow atrioventricular conduction; investigations in healthy volunteers and cardiac patients indicate that verapamil raises plasma digoxin concentrations 60% to 75%.[1-7] In addition, verapamil decreases digoxin elimination;[1-3] total body digoxin clearance is reduced approximately 35%.[1,6-11] Impaired biliary digoxin clearance is suggested in 2 studies as the explanation for increased digoxin levels.[12,13] Decreased volume of distribution data are controversial.[1,6] Cirrhotic patients receiving this drug combination experienced greater increases in peak digoxin serum levels and total AUC compared with healthy volunteers.[14] Verapamil affects digitoxin serum levels similarly.[15]

It is unclear if an increased risk of digoxin-induced arrhythmias exists; investigators document both adverse effects[3-6,16,17] and lack thereof.[18] There was an increase in premature ventricular contraction frequency in 1 of 10 patients on the combination.[4] Another study reported digoxin toxicity in 7 of 49 patients treated with verapamil, while an average 42% increase in serum digoxin levels occurred.[3] An apparent rise in digoxin serum level caused by verapamil is associated with increased digoxin activity.[3,5,16] Intraerythrocytic sodium concentration also has been noted to rise, which may correlate with the risk of digoxin toxicity.[6] The inotropic effect of digoxin apparently is not negated by verapamil.[8]

1 Pedersen KE, et al. *Clin Pharmacol Ther.* 1981;30:311.
2 Pedersen KE, et al. *Eur J Clin Pharmacol.* 1982;22:123.
3 Klein HO, et al. *Circulation.* 1982;65:998.
4 Schwartz JB, et al. *Circulation.* 1982;65:1163.
5 Belz GG, et al. *Clin Pharmacol Ther.* 1983;33:410.
6 Pedersen KE, et al. *Clin Pharmacol Ther.* 1983;34:8.
7 Gordon M, et al. *J Am Geriatr Soc.* 1986;34:659.
8 Pedersen KE, et al. *Eur J Clin Pharmacol.* 1983;25:199.
9 Johnson BF, et al. *Clin Pharmacol Ther.* 1987;42:66.
10 Rodin SM, et al. *Clin Pharmacol Ther.* 1988;43:668.
11 Bauer LA, et al. *Ther Drug Monit.* 1996;18:46.
12 Rendtorff C, et al. *Scand J Urol Nephrol.* 1990;24:137.
13 Hedman A, et al. *Clin Pharmacol Ther.* 1991;49:256.
14 Maragno I, et al. *Eur J Clin Pharmacol.* 1987;32:309.
15 Kuhlmann J. *Clin Pharmacol Ther.* 1985;38:667.
16 Doering W. *Eur J Clin Pharmacol.* 1983;25:517.
17 Zatuchni J. *Am Heart J.* 1984;108:412.
18 Panidis JP, et al. *Am J Cardiol.* 1983;52:1197.

* Asterisk indicates drugs cited in interaction reports.

Diltiazem — **Bile Acid Sequestrants**

Diltiazem* (eg, *Cardizem*)	Colestipol* (*Colestid*)

Significance	Onset	Severity	Documentation
4	☐ Rapid ■ **Delayed**	☐ Major ■ **Moderate** ☐ Minor	☐ Established ☐ Probable ☐ Suspected ■ **Possible** ☐ Unlikely

Effects DILTIAZEM plasma concentrations may be reduced, decreasing the pharmacologic effects.

Mechanism Unknown; however, the rate and extent of DILTIAZEM absorption appear to be decreased.

Management Until more clinical data are available, it would be prudent to coadminister these agents with caution and to monitor the clinical response of the patient to DILTIAZEM. Be prepared to adjust the dose of DILTIAZEM as needed.

Discussion

The effects of colestipol on the bioavailability of sustained-release (SR) and immediate-release (IR) diltiazem were studied in 12 healthy subjects.[1] In addition, the effect of the time of colestipol administration on the absorption of diltiazem SR was assessed. Both studies utilized a 2-way, crossover design. In the first study, each subject received 120 mg diltiazem SR or IR alone and in combination with colestipol 15 g. Following coadministration of diltiazem SR with colestipol, the AUC and C_{max} of diltiazem were reduced 22% and 36%, respectively, compared with taking diltiazem alone. Similarly, when diltiazem IR was studied, the AUC and C_{max} were decreased 27% and 33%, respectively. Coadministration of diltiazem and colestipol caused a 58% increase in the time to reach diltiazem peak plasma concentrations and a 13% shorter $t_{½}$. The AUC and C_{max} of the desacetyldiltiazem metabolite of diltiazem were 14% and 27% lower, respectively, while the time to reach the peak concentration was 32% longer. In the second study, 120 mg of diltiazem SR was administered alone, 1 hr prior to, and 4 hr after colestipol 5 g. Compared with giving diltiazem alone, when diltiazem was taken 1 hr prior to colestipol, there was a 17% decrease in the AUC of diltiazem and a 22% decrease when diltiazem was taken 4 hr after colestipol. The C_{max} of diltiazem, when given 1 hr before or 4 hr after colestipol, decreased 29% and 34%, respectively.

[1] Turner SW, et al. *Biopharm Drug Dispos.* 2002;23:369.

* Asterisk indicates drugs cited in interaction reports.

Diltiazem — *Food*

Diltiazem* (eg, *Cardizem*)	Grapefruit Juice*

Significance	Onset	Severity	Documentation
5	■ **Rapid** □ Delayed	□ Major □ Moderate ■ **Minor**	□ Established □ Probable □ Suspected ■ **Possible** □ Unlikely

Effects DILTIAZEM plasma concentrations may be slightly elevated, increasing the therapeutic and adverse effects.

Mechanism GRAPEFRUIT JUICE may inhibit DILTIAZEM metabolism (CYP3A4) in the small intestine.

Management Based on available data, no special precautions are needed.

Discussion

The effects of grapefruit juice on the pharmacokinetics of diltiazem were studied in 10 healthy men.[1] In a randomized, open-label, crossover study, each subject received nonsustained-release diltiazem 120 mg with 250 mL of grapefruit juice or water. Compared with water, grapefruit juice increased the AUC of diltiazem 20%. The effects of grapefruit juice on other pharmacokinetic parameters, heart rate, and BP were not statistically significant compared with water.

[1] Christensen H, et al. *Eur J Clin Pharmacol.* 2002;58:515.

* Asterisk indicates drugs cited in interaction reports.

Diltiazem — *Histamine H_2 Antagonists*

Diltiazem* (eg, *Cardizem*)	Cimetidine* (eg, *Tagamet*)	Ranitidine* (eg, *Zantac*)

Significance	Onset	Severity	Documentation
4	■ **Rapid** ☐ Delayed	☐ Major ■ **Moderate** ☐ Minor	☐ Established ☐ Probable ☐ Suspected ■ **Possible** ☐ Unlikely

Effects The therapeutic and toxic effects of DILTIAZEM may be increased by HISTAMINE H_2 ANTAGONISTS.

Mechanism The bioavailability of DILTIAZEM may be increased as a result of reduced first-pass hepatic degradation.

Management Reduce the DILTIAZEM dose if signs of toxicity appear.

Discussion

In a controlled study of 6 volunteers, the effects of cimetidine 1,200 mg/day for 7 days and ranitidine 300 mg/day for 7 days on the single-dose pharmacokinetics of diltiazem 60 mg were determined.[1] Although both drugs affected diltiazem similarly, the only parameters affected were cimetidine-induced increases in diltiazem AUC (35%) and peak plasma concentration (37%). Diltiazem $t_{½}$ and levels of deacetyldiltiazem, an active metabolite, also were increased by cimetidine and ranitidine. Another calcium channel blocker, nisoldipine, also is affected by cimetidine, but hemodynamic parameters appear unaffected.[2]

Ranitidine and cimetidine may stimulate a rise in the serum levels of diltiazem and its active metabolite deacetyldiltiazem. However, this study is not definitive; more data are needed.

[1] Winship LC, et al. *Pharmacotherapy*. 1985;5:16.

[2] van Harten J, et al. *Clin Pharmacol Ther*. 1988;43:332.

* Asterisk indicates drugs cited in interaction reports.

Diltiazem — **Moricizine**

Diltiazem* (eg, *Cardizem*)	Moricizine* (*Ethmozine*)

Significance	Onset	Severity	Documentation
2	□ Rapid ■ **Delayed**	□ Major ■ **Moderate** □ Minor	□ Established □ Probable ■ **Suspected** □ Possible □ Unlikely

Effects DILTIAZEM may elevate MORICIZINE concentrations, increasing the pharmacologic and adverse reactions, while MORICIZINE may reduce DILTIAZEM concentrations, decreasing the pharmacologic effects.

Mechanism DILTIAZEM may decrease the metabolism of MORICIZINE, while MORICIZINE may increase the metabolism of DILTIAZEM.

Management If both drugs are given concurrently, carefully monitor the patient's clinical response when either drug is started, stopped, or changed in dosage. Adjust therapy as needed.

Discussion

The steady-state pharmacokinetics of coadministered moricizine and diltiazem were evaluated in 16 healthy men.[1] Using an open-labeled, nonrandomized design, each subject received sequential administration of the following: 1) moricizine 250 mg every 8 hours for 7 days, 2) diltiazem 60 mg every 8 hours for 7 days, and 3) coadministration of moricizine 250 mg and diltiazem 60 mg every 8 hours for 7 days. Coadministration of both drugs resulted in an increase in the peak plasma concentration of moricizine from 0.788 to 1.488 mcg/mL, an increase in the AUC of moricizine by 122%, and a decrease in the oral clearance by 54%. In contrast, coadministration of the drugs had the opposite effects on the pharmacokinetics of diltiazem. The peak concentration of diltiazem decreased from 205.6 to 132.5 ng/mL, the $t_{1/2}$ decreased from 4.6 to 3.6 hours, and the oral clearance increased 52%. The frequencies of adverse reactions were 54% and 45% for moricizine and diltiazem alone, respectively, and 76% with coadministration of both drugs. The most frequent adverse reactions were dizziness, headache, and paresthesia.

[1] Shum L, et al. *J Clin Pharmacol.* 1996;36:1161.

* Asterisk indicates drugs cited in interaction reports.

Diltiazem — *Protease Inhibitors*

Diltiazem	Protease Inhibitors	
Diltiazem* (eg, *Cardizem*)	Amprenavir (*Agenerase*)	Nelfinavir (*Viracept*)
	Atazanavir (*Reyataz*)	Ritonavir* (*Norvir*)
	Fosamprenavir (*Lexiva*)	Saquinavir (*Invirase*)
	Indinavir* (*Crixivan*)	Tipranavir (*Aptivus*)
	Lopinavir/Ritonavir (*Kaletra*)	

Significance	Onset	Severity	Documentation
4	□ Rapid	□ Major	□ Established
	■ **Delayed**	■ **Moderate**	□ Probable
		□ Minor	□ Suspected
			■ **Possible**
			□ Unlikely

Effects DILTIAZEM plasma concentrations may be elevated, increasing the pharmacologic, pharmacodynamic, and adverse effects.

Mechanism Inhibition of DILTIAZEM metabolism (CYP3A) by the PROTEASE INHIBITOR.

Management Monitor DILTIAZEM clinical response and adverse reactions when PROTEASE INHIBITORS are started or stopped. Adjust the dose as needed.

Discussion

The potential for a 2-way pharmacokinetic drug interaction between indinavir plus ritonavir and diltiazem was evaluated in 13 healthy HIV-seronegative subjects.[1] Each subject received diltiazem 120 mg daily for days 1 through 7 and 20 through 26. In addition, each subject received indinavir 800 mg and ritonavir 100 mg every 12 hours on days 8 through 26. Indinavir plus ritonavir increased the median diltiazem AUC 26%. Two of 13 diltiazem subjects had more than a 4-fold increase in diltiazem AUC. The AUC of the diltiazem metabolite desacetyldiltiazem increased 102%, while the AUC of desmethyldiltiazem decreased 27%. The steady-state AUCs of indinavir and ritonavir were not affected by diltiazem.

[1] Glesby MJ, et al. *Clin Pharmacol Ther.* 2005;78:143.

* Asterisk indicates drugs cited in interaction reports. Based on pharmacologic and pharmacokinetic considerations, similar interactions may occur with other drugs that are listed.

Dipyridamole — *Indomethacin*

Dipyridamole* (eg, *Persantine*)	Indomethacin* (eg, *Indocin*)

Significance	Onset	Severity	Documentation
4	□ Rapid ■ **Delayed**	□ Major ■ **Moderate** □ Minor	□ Established □ Probable □ Suspected ■ **Possible** □ Unlikely

Effects This combination may cause augmented water retention.

Mechanism Probable additive or synergistic toxicity.

Management During coadministration of DIPYRIDAMOLE and INDOMETHACIN, consider monitoring glomerular filtration rate and sodium excretion.

Discussion

In water-loaded subjects with normal renal function, coadministration of dipyridamole and indomethacin produced marked water retention.[1] The study indicated that dipyridamole and indomethacin affected renal function when administered separately, and these effects were increased with combination therapy. When administered alone, dipyridamole or indomethacin decreased diuresis 25% to 50%. When given concurrently, the decrease was approximately 80%. These effects appear to be partially related to a reduction in glomerular filtration rate (GFR). Sodium excretion was decreased parallel to the fall in GFR. Free water clearance was reduced by both drugs.

[1] Seideman P, et al. *Br J Clin Pharmacol.* 1987;23:323.

* Asterisk indicates drugs cited in interaction reports.

Disopyramide — Beta Blockers

Disopyramide* (eg, *Norpace*)

Acebutolol (eg, *Sectral*)	Metoprolol* (eg, *Lopressor*)
Atenolol* (eg, *Tenormin*)	Nadolol (eg, *Corgard*)
Betaxolol (*Kerlone*)	Penbutolol (*Levatol*)
Bisoprolol (*Zebeta*)	Pindolol (eg, *Visken*)
Carteolol (*Cartrol*)	Propranolol (eg, *Inderal*)
Carvedilol (*Coreg*)	Sotalol (eg, *Betapace*)
Esmolol (*Brevibloc*)	Timolol (eg, *Blocadren*)
Labetalol (eg, *Normodyne*)	

Significance	Onset	Severity	Documentation
4	■ **Rapid**	□ Major	□ Established
	□ Delayed	■ **Moderate**	□ Probable
		□ Minor	□ Suspected
			■ **Possible**
			□ Unlikely

Effects The clearance of DISOPYRAMIDE may be decreased by BETA BLOCKERS; adverse effects (eg, sinus bradycardia, hypotension) may occur.

Mechanism Both agents may depress cardiac output.

Management If concurrent use cannot be avoided, use DISOPYRAMIDE and BETA BLOCKERS with caution, and closely monitor patients.

Discussion

In 1 study, 6 patients and 3 healthy volunteers received a single IV dose of disopyramide following administration of atenolol 50 mg twice daily.[5] Disopyramide clearance decreased approximately 20% compared with disopyramide alone; volume of distribution and half-life were unchanged. Heart failure or adverse reactions did not occur in any subject. In 2 case reports, patients developed sinus bradycardia and profound hypotension following the coadministration of single doses of practotol (not available in the US) and disopyramide.[1] In another case report, a 54-year-old man developed hypotension, bradycardia, and conduction disturbances 5 days after metoprolol 25 mg twice daily was added to his disopyramide regimen.[8] In contrast, the coadministration of disopyramide 200 mg every 6 hours for 10 days and propranolol 80 mg every 8 hours for 6 days did not affect the steady-state concentrations or area under the curve of disopyramide.[4] While it has been suggested that coadministration of propranolol and disopyramide causes a pronounced decrease in cardiac output, investigators report no synergistic or additive effect of the negative inotropic effects of these agents.[2,3,6] Another study reported that this combination may be useful in the treatment of hypertrophic cardiomyopathy.[7]

1 Cumming AD, et al. *BMJ*. 1979;3:1264.
2 Cathcart-Rake WF, et al. *Clin Pharmacol Ther*. 1979;25:217.
3 Cathcart-Rake WF, et al. *Circulation*. 1980;61:938.
4 Karim A, et al. *J Pharmacokinet Biopharm*. 1982;10:465.
5 Bonde J, et al. *Eur J Clin Pharmacol*. 1985;28:41.
6 Bonde J, et al. *Eur J Clin Pharmacol*. 1986;30:161.
7 Cokkinos DV, et al. *Can J Cardiol*. 1989;5:33.
8 Pernat A, et al. *J Electrocardiol*. 1997;30:341.

* Asterisk indicates drugs cited in interaction reports. Based on pharmacologic and pharmacokinetic considerations, similar interactions may occur with other drugs that are listed.

Disopyramide	*Histamine H_2 Antagonists*
Disopyramide* (eg, *Norpace*)	Cimetidine* (eg, *Tagamet*)

Significance	Onset	Severity	Documentation
4	■ **Rapid**	□ Major	□ Established
	□ Delayed	■ **Moderate**	□ Probable
		□ Minor	□ Suspected
			■ **Possible**
			□ Unlikely

Effects Plasma DISOPYRAMIDE concentrations may be elevated, increasing the pharmacologic and adverse effects.

Mechanism CIMETIDINE may increase the absorption of DISOPYRAMIDE.

Management If an interaction is suspected, it may be necessary to decrease the dose of DISOPYRAMIDE.

Discussion

The effects of a single oral dose of cimetidine 400 mg or ranitidine (eg, *Zantac*) 150 mg on the pharmacokinetics of disopyramide 300 mg and its major metabolite (mono-N-dealkyldisopyramide) were investigated in a randomized, crossover study.[2] Six healthy subjects received disopyramide alone or in combination with the H^2 antagonist. Ranitidine did not alter the pharmacokinetics of disopyramide or the major metabolite. However, compared with giving disopyramide alone, concurrent administration of cimetidine resulted in an increase in the peak plasma concentration (19%) of disopyramide, the area under the plasma concentration-time curve (9%), and the total amount of disopyramide excreted unchanged in the urine (20%). The pharmacokinetics of the major metabolite were not affected. In 7 healthy volunteers, oral administration of cimetidine 400 mg twice daily for 2 weeks did not alter the pharmacokinetics of a single 150 mg dose of disopyramide given as an IV bolus.[1]

[1] Bonde J, et al. *Br J Clin Pharmacol.* 1991;31:708. [2] Jou M-J, et al. *J Pharm Pharmacol.* 1997;49:1072.

* Asterisk indicates drugs cited in interaction reports.

Disopyramide — *Hydantoins*

Disopyramide		Hydantoins	
Disopyramide* (eg, *Norpace*)		Ethotoin (*Peganone*) Fosphenytoin (*Cerebyx*)	Phenytoin* (eg, *Dilantin*)

Significance	Onset	Severity	Documentation
2	☐ Rapid ■ **Delayed**	☐ Major ■ **Moderate** ☐ Minor	☐ Established ☐ Probable ■ **Suspected** ☐ Possible ☐ Unlikely

Effects PHENYTOIN coadministration may decrease the serum levels, $t_{½}$, and bioavailability of DISOPYRAMIDE while increasing mono-N-dealkyldisopyramide (MND), a metabolite of DISOPYRAMIDE, serum levels. Anticholinergic actions may be enhanced. The effects of this interaction may persist for several days following PHENYTOIN discontinuation.

Mechanism PHENYTOIN appears to increase the hepatic metabolism of DISOPYRAMIDE via stimulation of microsomal enzymes.

Management The dose of DISOPYRAMIDE may need to be increased during concurrent PHENYTOIN therapy. If increased anticholinergic effects occur, consider an alternative to DISOPYRAMIDE.

Discussion

Several studies and case reports have shown that the coadministration of disopyramide and phenytoin results in decreased disopyramide serum concentrations.[1-6] Increased anticholinergic effects have also occurred.[6] Phenytoin was used in doses of 200 to 600 mg/day, and disopyramide was given as a single dose or long-term therapy (300 mg to 2 g/day). The disopyramide plasma concentration decreased 19.6% to 76%, the AUC decreased 30% to 53%, and the $t_{½}$ decreased 51% to 69.5%. In 1 patient, the disopyramide dose had to be doubled to maintain a therapeutic serum level. At the same time, plasma levels and AUC of MND (having some antiarrhythmic activity) increased. The effects of this interaction generally occurred after a week of concurrent therapy or a week of phenytoin in the single-dose studies. When phenytoin was discontinued, disopyramide levels gradually increased. Although MND has some antiarrhythmic activity and, therefore, may aid in the prevention of a decreased therapeutic response, it has more anticholinergic activity than the parent compound and may contribute to increased anticholinergic adverse reactions.[6]

[1] Aitio ML, et al. *Br J Clin Pharmacol.* 1980;9(2):149.
[2] Aitio ML, et al. *Br J Clin Pharmacol.* 1981;11(3):279.
[3] Aitio ML. *Br J Clin Pharmacol.* 1981;11(4):369.
[4] Matos JA, et al. *Clin Res.* 1981;29:655A.
[5] Kessler JM, et al. *Clin Pharm.* 1982;1(3):263.
[6] Nightingale J, et al. *Clin Pharm.* 1987;6(1):46.

* Asterisk indicates drugs cited in interaction reports. Based on pharmacologic and pharmacokinetic considerations, similar interactions may occur with other drugs that are listed.

Disopyramide — *Quinidine*

Disopyramide* (eg, *Norpace*)	Quinidine*

Significance	Onset	Severity	Documentation
4	■ **Rapid**	□ Major	□ Established
	□ Delayed	■ **Moderate**	□ Probable
		□ Minor	□ Suspected
			■ **Possible**
			□ Unlikely

Effects Coadministration may result in increased DISOPYRAMIDE serum levels or decreased QUINIDINE serum levels. This may result in DISOPYRAMIDE toxicity in some patients, or a decreased therapeutic response to QUINIDINE.

Mechanism Unknown.

Management Monitor patients for DISOPYRAMIDE toxicity when QUINIDINE is added to their therapy, especially patients receiving high-dose DISOPYRAMIDE therapy. The dose of DISOPYRAMIDE may need to be decreased.

Discussion

Sixteen healthy subjects were given concurrent quinidine and disopyramide.[1] Group 1 received quinidine 200 mg 4 times daily for 6 days and disopyramide (single 150 mg dose on day 4, 150 mg 4 times daily on days 5 and 6). Group 2 received disopyramide 150 mg 4 times daily for 6 days and quinidine (single 200 mg dose on day 4, 200 mg 4 times daily on days 5 and 6). During coadministration, a small but significant increase (14% to 20.5%) occurred in the peak serum concentration of disopyramide, and a significant decrease (21%) occurred in the peak serum quinidine concentration. The half-lives did not change for either drug administered. The clinical significance was not determined. There was no significant change in heart rate, blood pressure, PR interval, or QRS duration on any of the drug regimens. Additional lengthening of the corrected QT interval occurred with coadministration, although either agent alone prolongs the QT interval.

[1] Baker BJ, et al. *Am Heart J.* 1983;105:12.

* Asterisk indicates drugs cited in interaction reports.

Disopyramide — *Rifampin*

Disopyramide* (eg, *Norpace*)	Rifampin* (eg, *Rifadin*)

Significance	Onset	Severity	Documentation
2	□ Rapid ■ **Delayed**	□ Major ■ **Moderate** □ Minor	□ Established □ Probable ■ **Suspected** □ Possible □ Unlikely

Effects RIFAMPIN may decrease the serum levels of DISOPYRAMIDE. However, since the levels of an active metabolite may increase, it is difficult to predict if a decreased therapeutic response would occur.

Mechanism Hepatic metabolism of DISOPYRAMIDE is increased.

Management Monitor DISOPYRAMIDE concentrations and the patient's electrocardiogram during concurrent RIFAMPIN therapy. An increased DISOPYRAMIDE dose may be necessary.

Discussion

Eleven patients with tuberculosis were given a single dose of disopyramide 200 to 300 mg before and after 2 weeks of rifampin therapy plus 1 or 2 other agents (isoniazid, pyrazinamide, or ethambutol).[1] Compared with disopyramide alone, rifampin decreased disopyramide's elimination half-life 44.5%, its area under the plasma concentration-time curve (AUC) 59.5%, and its renal clearance 26%. The AUC of mono-N-dealkyldisopyramide (MND, an active metabolite of disopyramide) increased 91.8%, while the renal clearance of MND was not significantly increased. The amount of unchanged disopyramide excreted in urine in 24 hours decreased 76.5%, while that of MND increased 58.5%. The ratio of MND/disopyramide in 24-hour urine increased 6.9 fold. These parameters indicate the increased metabolism of disopyramide by rifampin. However, since MND has some antiarrhythmic activity, it is not known if the interaction would result in reduced therapeutic efficacy of disopyramide. Administration of disopyramide to a 62-year-old patient receiving rifampin 600 mg/day resulted in subtherapeutic disopyramide levels and failure to correct the arrhythmia in spite of escalating doses of disopyramide up to 900 mg/day. Within 5 days of discontinuing rifampin, disopyramide serum levels increased and the arrhythmia was abolished.[2]

[1] Aitio ML, et al. *Br J Clin Pharmacol.* 1981;11:279.

[2] Staum JM. *DICP, Ann Pharmacother.* 1990;24:701.

* Asterisk indicates drugs cited in interaction reports.

Disulfiram — *Isoniazid*

Disulfiram*
(eg, *Antabuse*)

Isoniazid*
(eg, *Nydrazid*)

Significance	Onset	Severity	Documentation
4	☐ Rapid	☐ Major	☐ Established
	■ **Delayed**	■ **Moderate**	☐ Probable
		☐ Minor	☐ Suspected
			■ **Possible**
			☐ Unlikely

Effects The coadministration of DISULFIRAM and ISONIAZID may result in acute behavioral and coordination changes. Acute encephalopathy has occurred with DISULFIRAM alone.

Mechanism Unknown; possible excess dopaminergic activity.

Management If acute behavioral or coordination changes develop during concurrent administration of DISULFIRAM and ISONIAZID, the DISULFIRAM dose may need to be decreased or the drug discontinued.

Discussion

In case reports involving seven patients, the concurrent administration of isoniazid (600 mg 1 to 4 times a day or 600 mg to 1 g twice weekly) and disulfiram 500 mg/day resulted in acute behavioral and coordination changes characterized by irritability, poor coordination, aggressiveness, staggering gait, confusion and disorientation.[2] The effects appeared within a few days of combined therapy and decreased or disappeared following a decrease in the dosage or discontinuation of disulfiram.

Disulfiram alone has been reported to result in encephalopathy and acute organic brain syndrome; symptoms include paranoid ideas, disorientation, impaired memory, ataxia and confusion.[1,3,4] This may be related to excess dopaminergic activity.

[1] Liddon SC, et al. *Am J Psychiatry.* 1967;123:1284.
[2] Whittington HG, et al. *Am J Psychiatry.* 1969;125:139.
[3] Knee ST, et al. *Am J Psychiatry.* 1974;131:1281.
[4] Hotson JR, et al. *Arch Neurol.* 1976;33:141.

* Asterisk indicates drugs cited in interaction reports.

Disulfiram — *MAOIs*

Disulfiram* (eg, *Antabuse*)	Phenelzine (*Nardil*)	Tranylcypromine* (*Parnate*)

Significance	Onset	Severity	Documentation
4	■ **Rapid**	□ Major	□ Established
	□ Delayed	■ **Moderate**	□ Probable
		□ Minor	□ Suspected
			■ **Possible**
			□ Unlikely

Effects CNS delirium including agitation, disorientation and visual hallucinations.

Mechanism Unknown.

Management Observe the patient for signs and symptoms of delirium. Adjust therapy as needed.

Discussion

A case of delirium has been reported in a 48-year-old male patient after adding tranylcypromine to his disulfiram and lithium (eg, *Eskalith*; 200 mg 3 times daily), treatment regimen.[1] Two days after starting treatment with tranylcypromine 10 mg twice daily the patient became delirious. He became agitated, disoriented, incoherent and suffered from vivid visual hallucinations. Later he became subcomatose and developed a nystagmus. He was well within 24 hours. It was not determined whether lithium contributed to this possible drug interaction.

Additional documentation is needed to clarify this possible drug interaction.

[1] Blansjaar BA, et al. *Am J Psychiatry*. 1995;152:296.

* Asterisk indicates drugs cited in interaction reports. Based on pharmacologic and pharmacokinetic considerations, similar interactions may occur with other drugs that are listed.

Disulfiram — Metronidazole

Disulfiram* (eg, *Antabuse*)	Metronidazole* (eg, *Flagyl*)

Significance	Onset	Severity	Documentation
2	☐ Rapid ■ **Delayed**	☐ Major ■ **Moderate** ☐ Minor	☐ Established ☐ Probable ■ **Suspected** ☐ Possible ☐ Unlikely

Effects The coadministration of DISULFIRAM and METRONIDAZOLE may result in acute psychosis or a confusional state. Acute encephalopathy has occurred with DISULFIRAM alone.

Mechanism Possibly excess dopaminergic activity.

Management If acute psychosis or a confusional state develops during coadministration of DISULFIRAM and METRONIDAZOLE, one or both agents may need to be discontinued; monitor patients closely. Avoid coadministration.

Discussion

In one study, 58 patients received disulfiram 500 mg/day for 1 month, then 250 mg/day.[1] Metronidazole 750 mg/day for 1 month, then 250 mg/day, was given concurrently to 29 of the patients. Six of the 29 patients developed acute psychosis or a confusional state compared with none of the patients receiving disulfiram alone. The symptoms developed at days 10 to 14 of coadministration and included paranoid delusions and visual and auditory hallucinations. Symptoms persisted and increased for a few days following discontinuation of the drugs; each patient recovered within 2 weeks. Disulfiram alone was restarted with no recurrence of symptoms. An acute psychotic paranoid reaction with hallucinations also occurred in 1 patient when metronidazole was added to his disulfiram therapy.[2]

Disulfiram alone has been reported to result in encephalopathy and acute organic brain syndrome; symptoms include ataxia, confusion, disorientation, impaired memory, and paranoid ideas.[3-5] This may be related to excess dopaminergic activity.

1 Rothstein E, et al. *N Engl J Med.* 1969;280(18):1006.
2 Scher JM. *JAMA.* 1967;201(13):1051.
3 Liddon SC, et al. *Am J Psychiatry.* 1967;123(10):1284.
4 Knee ST, et al. *Am J Psychiatry.* 1974;131(11):1281.
5 Hotson JR, et al. *Arch Neurol.* 1976;33(2):141.

* Asterisk indicates drugs cited in interaction reports.

Disulfiram — *Tricyclic Antidepressants*

Disulfiram*
(*Antabuse*)

Amitriptyline*
Amoxapine
Desipramine*
(eg, *Norpramin*)
Doxepin
(eg, *Sinequan*)
Imipramine*
(eg, *Tofranil*)
Nortriptyline
(eg, *Aventyl*)
Protriptyline
(eg, *Vivactil*)
Trimipramine
(*Surmontil*)

Significance	Onset	Severity	Documentation
4	☐ Rapid	☐ Major	☐ Established
	■ **Delayed**	■ **Moderate**	☐ Probable
		☐ Minor	☐ Suspected
			■ **Possible**
			☐ Unlikely

Effects The coadministration of DISULFIRAM and a TRICYCLIC ANTIDEPRESSANT may result in acute organic brain syndrome. The bioavailability of the TRICYCLIC ANTIDEPRESSANT also may be increased by DISULFIRAM.

Mechanism Both agents may increase dopamine levels, which may result in organic brain syndrome and psychosis. Also, DISULFIRAM may inhibit the hepatic metabolism of the TRICYCLIC ANTIDEPRESSANT.

Management Monitor patients for acute organic brain syndrome or for TRICYCLIC ANTIDEPRESSANT toxicity. It may be necessary to discontinue one or both agents.

Discussion

In 2 patients, amitriptyline 25 mg/day (increased to 150 mg/day in 1 patient) added to their disulfiram therapy resulted in acute organic brain syndrome.[1] These effects occurred within 1 to 4 weeks of amitriptyline therapy. Both drugs were discontinued in 1 patient, and amitriptyline was discontinued in the other. Both patients improved within a few days. In 2 other patients, a single IV dose of imipramine 12.5 mg was administered following 14 days of disulfiram therapy.[2] In each patient, the imipramine AUC increased 26.8% and 32.5%, respectively, the $t_{½}$ increased 13.6% and 18.3%, and total body clearance decreased 21.3% and 24.5%. One patient received a single IV dose of desipramine 12.5 mg following an additional 4 weeks of disulfiram. The desipramine AUC increased 32.3%, the $t_{½}$ increased 19.8%, and total body clearance decreased 24.3%. Amitriptyline may potentiate the effect of disulfiram, allowing a decreased disulfiram dose and minimizing adverse reactions.[3] However, this has been questioned.[4]

[1] Maany I, et al. *Arch Gen Psychiatry*. 1982;39(6):743.
[2] Ciraulo DA, et al. *Am J Psychiatry*. 1985;142(11):1373.
[3] MacCallum WA. *Lancet*. 1969;1(7589):313.
[4] Ciraulo DA, et al. *Am J Psychiatry*. 1986;143(10):1327.

* Asterisk indicates drugs cited in interaction reports. Based on pharmacologic and pharmacokinetic considerations, similar interactions may occur with other drugs that are listed.

Docetaxel — Protease Inhibitors

Docetaxel	Protease Inhibitors	
Docetaxel* (*Taxotere*)	Atazanavir* (*Reyataz*)	Nelfinavir* (*Viracept*)
	Fosamprenavir (*Lexiva*)	Ritonavir* (*Norvir*)
	Indinavir* (*Crixivan*)	Saquinavir* (*Invirase*)
	Lopinavir/Ritonavir* (*Kaletra*)	

Significance	Onset	Severity	Documentation
1	□ Rapid ■ **Delayed**	■ **Major** □ Moderate □ Minor	□ Established □ Probable ■ **Suspected** □ Possible □ Unlikely

Effects DOCETAXEL plasma concentrations may be elevated, increasing the pharmacologic effects and adverse reactions.

Mechanism Inhibition of DOCETAXEL metabolism (CYP3A4) by RITONAVIR is suspected.

Management Avoid this combination.[1] If DOCETAXEL and RITONAVIR must be given concurrently, closely monitor patients for DOCETAXEL adverse reactions. A reduction of the DOCETAXEL dosage may be necessary. Paclitaxel may be a safer alternative.

Discussion

A 40-year-old man infected with HIV was receiving ritonavir-boosted lopinavir as part of his antiretroviral therapy.[2] He was started on docetaxel 25 mg/m^2 weekly for possible Kaposi sarcoma of the eyelid. Eight days after the first docetaxel infusion, he developed neutropenic fever. An interaction with ritonavir was suspected and docetaxel was discontinued. The patient was hospitalized and treated with IV antibiotics. The neutropenia resolved the following week. Three patients receiving docetaxel plus ritonavir-boosted antiretroviral regimens developed febrile neutropenia, grade 3 mucositis, skin rash, and hand-foot syndrome.[3] A pharmacokinetic model was developed using data from 2 clinical trials in which oral or IV docetaxel was administered with or without ritonavir 100 mg.[4] The bioavailability of docetaxel was increased from 19% to 39%, while docetaxel clearance was inhibited in a concentration-dependent manner, reaching a maximum inhibition of 90%.

1 *Taxotere* [package insert]. Bridgewater, NJ: Sanofi-Aventis; May 2010.
2 Loulergue P, et al. *AIDS*. 2008;22(10):1237.
3 Mir O, et al. *Br J Clin Pharmacol*. 2010;69(1):99.
4 Koolen SL, et al. *Br J Clin Pharmacol*. 2010;69(5): 465.

* Asterisk indicates drugs cited in interaction reports. Based on pharmacologic and pharmacokinetic considerations, similar interactions may occur with other drugs that are listed.

Dofetilide — *Azole Antifungal Agents*

Dofetilide* (*Tikosyn*)	Itraconazole* (*Sporanox*)	Ketoconazole* (eg, *Nizoral*)

Significance	Onset	Severity	Documentation
1	☐ Rapid ■ **Delayed**	■ **Major** ☐ Moderate ☐ Minor	☐ Established ☐ Probable ■ **Suspected** ☐ Possible ☐ Unlikely

Effects Elevated DOFETILIDE plasma concentrations may occur with increased risk of ventricular arrhythmias, including torsades de pointes.

Mechanism KETOCONAZOLE may inhibit the renal cation transport system, which is responsible for DOFETILIDE elimination. Also, ITRACONAZOLE and KETOCONAZOLE may inhibit metabolism (CYP3A4) of DOFETILIDE.

Management Coadministration of DOFETILIDE and ITRACONAZOLE or KETOCONAZOLE is contraindicated.

Discussion

Coadministration of ketoconazole 400 mg/day and dofetilide 500 mcg twice daily for 7 days increased dofetilide peak plasma concentrations 53% in men and 97% in women, and increased the AUC 41% in men and 69% in women.[1] Because itraconazole administration may result in increased plasma levels of dofetilide, which could lead to potentially life-threatening arrhythmias, coadministration of itraconazole and dofetilide is contraindicated.[2]

The basis for this monograph is information on file with the manufacturer. Published data are needed to further assess this interaction. However, because of the seriousness of the cardiac problems, clinical evaluation of this interaction in humans is not likely to be forthcoming.

[1] *Tikosyn* [package insert]. New York, NY: Pfizer Labs; December 1999.

[2] *Sporanox* [package insert]. Titusville, NJ: Janssen Pharmaceutia Products, LP; January 2004.

* Asterisk indicates drugs cited in interaction reports.

Dofetilide — *Cimetidine*

Dofetilide* (*Tikosyn*)	Cimetidine* (eg, *Tagamet*)

Significance	Onset	Severity	Documentation
1	☐ Rapid ■ **Delayed**	■ **Major** ☐ Moderate ☐ Minor	☐ Established ☐ Probable ■ **Suspected** ☐ Possible ☐ Unlikely

Effects Elevated DOFETILIDE plasma concentrations may occur with increased risk of ventricular arrhythmias, including torsades de pointes.

Mechanism Inhibition of the renal cation transport system responsible for DOFETILIDE elimination.

Management Coadministration of DOFETILIDE and CIMETIDINE is contraindicated. Omeprazole (*Prilosec*), ranitidine (eg, *Zantac*), and antacids (aluminum and magnesium hydroxides) do not affect DOFETILIDE pharmacokinetics and may be suitable alternatives to CIMETIDINE.

Discussion

Coadministration of cimetidine 400 mg twice daily and dofetilide 500 mcg twice daily for 7 days increased dofetilide plasma concentrations 58%.[1] OTC doses of cimetidine (100 mg twice daily) increased dofetilide plasma levels 13%. Studies have not been conducted on intermediate doses of cimetidine. Using an open-label, placebo-controlled, randomized, crossover design, the effects of cimetidine and ranitidine on the pharmacokinetics and pharmacodynamics of dofetilide were studied in 20 healthy men.[2] Each subject received cimetidine 100 or 400 mg twice daily, ranitidine 150 mg twice daily, or placebo for 4 days. On the second day, dofetilide 500 mcg was administered immediately after the morning dose of cimetidine, ranitidine, or placebo. Coadministration of dofetilide and cimetidine 100 and 400 mg increased the AUC of dofetilide 11% and 48%, respectively, and the peak plasma concentration 11% and 29%, respectively. The renal clearance of dofetilide was reduced 13% and 33%, while the nonrenal clearance was reduced 5% and 21% by cimetidine 100 and 400 mg, respectively. Compared with baseline values, cimetidine 100 and 400 mg increased the dofetilide-induced prolongation of the QTc interval 22% and 33%, respectively. However, the QTc interval did not exceed 450 ms in any subject. Ranitidine had no significant effect on the pharmacokinetics or pharmacodynamics of dofetilide.

[1] *Tikosyn* [package insert]. New York, NY: Pfizer; December 1999.

[2] Abel, S. et al. *Br J Clin Pharmacol.* 2000;49:64.

* Asterisk indicates drugs cited in interaction reports.

Dofetilide — *Megestrol*

Dofetilide* (*Tikosyn*)	Megestrol* (eg, *Megace*)

Significance	Onset	Severity	Documentation
1	☐ Rapid ■ **Delayed**	■ **Major** ☐ Moderate ☐ Minor	☐ Established ☐ Probable ■ **Suspected** ☐ Possible ☐ Unlikely

Effects Elevated DOFETILIDE plasma concentrations may occur, with increased risk of ventricular arrhythmias, including torsades de pointes.

Mechanism Inhibition of the renal cation transport system responsible for DOFETILIDE elimination.

Management Do not use MEGESTROL in patients receiving DOFETILIDE.

Discussion

Dofetilide is eliminated from the body by cationic renal secretion. Drugs that inhibit this process have been shown to elevate dofetilide plasma levels.[1] Because megestrol inhibits the renal cation transport system, it should not be administered to patients receiving dofetilide.

The basis for this monograph is an extrapolation of information on file with the manufacturer. Published data are needed to further assess this interaction. However, because of the seriousness of the cardiac problems, clinical evaluation of this interaction in humans is not likely to be forthcoming.

[1] *Tikosyn* [package insert]. New York, NY: Pfizer Labs; December 1999.

* Asterisk indicates drugs cited in interaction reports.

Dofetilide — *Phenothiazines*

Dofetilide* (*Tikosyn*)	Prochlorperazine* (eg, *Compazine*)	Thioridazine*

Significance	Onset	Severity	Documentation
1	■ **Rapid** □ Delayed	■ **Major** □ Moderate □ Minor	□ Established □ Probable ■ **Suspected** □ Possible □ Unlikely

Effects The risk of life-threatening cardiac arrhythmias, including torsades de pointes, may be increased.

Mechanism PROCHLORPERAZINE inhibits the renal cation transport system responsible for DOFETILIDE elimination. Possible prolongation of the QTc interval with coadministration of DOFETILIDE and THIORIDAZINE.

Management THIORIDAZINE is contraindicated in patients receiving DOFETILIDE.[1] Do not use PROCHLORPERAZINE in patients receiving DOFETILIDE.[2]

Discussion

Sudden, unexplained deaths have been reported in patients receiving drugs that prolong the QTc interval. Do not use thioridazine with other drugs that prolong the QTc interval. Thioridazine causes dose-related prolongation of the QTc interval, and other drugs that prolong the QTc interval (eg, dofetilide) have been associated with fatal arrhythmias.[1] Dofetilide is eliminated from the body by cationic renal secretion. Drugs that inhibit this process have been shown to elevate dofetilide plasma levels.[2] Because prochlorperazine inhibits the renal cation transport system, do not administer it to patients receiving dofetilide.

The basis for this monograph is information on file with the manufacturer. Because of the seriousness of the cardiac problems, clinical evaluation of this interaction in humans is not likely to be forthcoming.

1 *Mellaril* [package insert]. East Hanover, NJ: Novartis Pharmaceutical Corporation; June 2000.

2 *Tikosyn* [package insert]. New York, NY: Pfizer Labs; March 2004.

* Asterisk indicates drugs cited in interaction reports.

Dofetilide — *Thiazide Diuretics*

Dofetilide*
(*Tikosyn*)

Bendroflumethiazide (*Naturetin*)
Chlorothiazide (eg, *Diuril*)
Chlorthalidone (eg, *Hygroton*)
Hydrochlorothiazide* (eg, *HydroDiuril*)
Hydroflumethiazide
Indapamide (eg, *Lozol*)
Methyclothiazide (eg, *Enduron*)
Metolazone (eg, *Zaroxolyn*)
Polythiazide
Quinethazone

Significance	Onset	Severity	Documentation
1	☐ Rapid	■ **Major**	☐ Established
	■ **Delayed**	☐ Moderate	☐ Probable
		☐ Minor	■ **Suspected**
			☐ Possible
			☐ Unlikely

Effects Hypokalemia may occur, increasing the risk of torsades de pointes.

Mechanism Increased potassium excretion caused by THIAZIDE DIURETIC administration.

Management Coadministration of DOFETILIDE and THIAZIDE DIURETICS, alone and in combination with potassium-sparing diuretics such as triamterene (eg, *Dyrenium*), is contraindicated.

Discussion

Hypokalemia may occur in patients receiving thiazide diuretics (alone and in combination with potassium-sparing diuretics), which could increase the potential for torsades de pointes.[1-3] Potassium concentrations should be within the normal range prior to dofetilide administration and maintained in the normal range during dofetilide therapy.[3] In addition, dofetilide mean clearance was 16% lower in patients receiving concurrent thiazide diuretics compared with dofetilide alone.[3] Because administration of loop diuretics (eg, furosemide [eg, *Lasix*]) may result in hypokalemia and hypomagnesemia, a similar interaction may occur with coadministration of dofetilide and loop diuretics.

The basis for this monograph is information on file with the manufacturer. Because of the seriousness of the cardiac problems, clinical evaluation in humans is not likely to be forthcoming.

1 Pfizer Pharmaceuticals (written communication, December 30, 2003).
2 http://www.tikosyn.com. Accessed January 20, 2004.
3 *Tikosyn* [package insert]. New York, NY: Pfizer, Inc; December 1999.

* Asterisk indicates drugs cited in interaction reports. Based on pharmacologic and pharmacokinetic considerations, similar interactions may occur with other drugs that are listed.

Dofetilide — *Trimethoprim*

Dofetilide* (*Tikosyn*)	Trimethoprim* (eg, *Proloprim*)	Trimethoprim/ Sulfamethoxazole* (eg, *Septra*)

Significance	Onset	Severity	Documentation
1	☐ Rapid ■ **Delayed**	■ **Major** ☐ Moderate ☐ Minor	☐ Established ☐ Probable ■ **Suspected** ☐ Possible ☐ Unlikely

Effects Elevated DOFETILIDE plasma concentrations may occur with increased risk of ventricular arrhythmias, including torsades de pointes.

Mechanism Inhibition of the renal cation transport system responsible for DOFETILIDE elimination.

Management Coadministration of DOFETILIDE and TRIMETHOPRIM alone or in combination with SULFAMETHOXAZOLE is contraindicated.

Discussion

Trimethoprim 160 mg in combination with sulfamethoxazole 800 mg given twice daily concurrently with dofetilide 500 mcg twice daily for 4 days increased dofetilide peak plasma concentrations 93% and the AUC 103%.[1]

The basis for this monograph is information on file with the manufacturer. Published data are needed to further assess this interaction. However, because of the seriousness of the cardiac problems, clinical evaluation of this interaction in humans is not likely to be forthcoming.

[1] Product Information. Dofetilide (*Tikosyn*). Pfizer Laboratories. December 1999.

* Asterisk indicates drugs cited in interaction reports.

Dofetilide — *Verapamil*

Dofetilide* (*Tikosyn*)	Verapamil* (eg, *Calan*)

Significance	Onset	Severity	Documentation
1	☐ Rapid	■ **Major**	☐ Established
	■ **Delayed**	☐ Moderate	☐ Probable
		☐ Minor	■ **Suspected**
			☐ Possible
			☐ Unlikely

Effects Elevated DOFETILIDE plasma concentrations may occur with increased risk of ventricular arrhythmias, including torsades de pointes.

Mechanism VERAPAMIL may increase portal blood flow, increasing the rate of DOFETILIDE absorption.

Management Coadministration of DOFETILIDE and VERAPAMIL is contraindicated.

Discussion

Coadministration of verapamil and dofetilide increased dofetilide peak plasma concentrations 42%; however, overall exposure to dofetilide was not increased.[1] In an analysis of supraventricular arrhythmia and the Danish investigations of arrhythmia and mortality on dofetilide (DIAMOND) patient populations, coadministration of verapamil and dofetilide was associated with a higher incidence of torsades de pointes.[1] Twelve healthy young volunteers were given verapamil 80 mg 3 times/day, dofetilide 0.5 mg twice/day, or both drugs concurrently for 3 days.[2] Verapamil increased the peak level of dofetilide 43% (from 2.4 to 3.43 ng/mL) and the AUC 24%. Associated with the increased peak levels was an increase in the QTc interval (from 20 to 26 msec). These changes were attributed to a faster rate of dofetilide absorption.

[1] Product Information. Dofetilide (*Tikosyn*). Pfizer Laboratories. December 1999.

[2] Johnson BF, et al. *J Clin Pharmacol.* 2001;41:1248.

* Asterisk indicates drugs cited in interaction reports.

Donepezil — Azole Antifungal Agents

Donepezil		Azole Antifungal Agents	
Donepezil* (*Aricept*)		Fluconazole (*Diflucan*)	Ketoconazole* (*Nizoral*)
		Itraconazole (*Sporanox*)	Miconazole

Significance	Onset	Severity	Documentation
5	■ **Rapid**	□ Major	□ Established
	□ Delayed	□ Moderate	□ Probable
		■ **Minor**	□ Suspected
			■ **Possible**
			□ Unlikely

Effects DONEPEZIL plasma concentration and side effects may be increased.

Mechanism AZOLE ANTIFUNGAL AGENTS may inhibit the metabolism (CYP3A4) of DONEPEZIL. FLUCONAZOLE, especially greater than or equal to 200 mg/day, may inhibit CYP3A4.

Management If an interaction is suspected, it may be necessary to reduce the dose of DONEPEZIL.

Discussion

The effects of ketoconazole administration on the pharmacokinetics of donepezil were studied in 18 healthy volunteers.[1] During each 7-day study period in this open-labeled, randomized, 3-period crossover investigation, the subjects received donepezil 5 mg alone, ketoconazole 200 mg alone, or donepezil 5 mg plus ketoconazole 200 mg. Pharmacokinetic comparisons were determined for day 1 and day 7 of each treatment period. On day 1 of concomitant administration, there was an increase in the peak plasma concentration of donepezil from 8.4 to 9.5 ng/mL (13%) and area under the plasma concentration-time curve (AUC) from 118.7 to 135.2 ng•hr/mL (14%) compared with giving donepezil alone. These differences were statistically significant ($P = 0.01$ and 0.001, respectively). On day 7 of concurrent administration of donepezil and ketoconazole, there was an increase in peak donepezil concentration from 27.6 to 37.7 ng/ml (37%) and AUC from 501.1 to 680.9 ng•hr/mL (36%) compared with giving donepezil alone. These differences were also statistically significant ($P = 0.0001$). Donepezil did not affect the pharmacokinetics of ketoconazole. Side effects were mild to moderate in severity and were similar whether donepezil was administered alone or in combination with ketoconazole.

[1] Tiseo PJ, et al. *Br J Clin Pharmacol.* 1998;46 (Suppl 1):30.

* Asterisk indicates drugs cited in interaction reports. Based on pharmacologic and pharmacokinetic considerations, similar interactions may occur with other drugs that are listed.

Doxorubicin — *Barbiturates*

Doxorubicin	Barbiturates	
Doxorubicin* (eg, *Adriamycin RDF*)	Amobarbital (*Amytal*)	Pentobarbital
	Butabarbital (eg, *Butisol*)	Phenobarbital*
	Butalbital	Primidone (eg, *Mysoline*)
	Mephobarbital (*Mebaral*)	Secobarbital (*Seconal*)

Significance	Onset	Severity	Documentation
4	☐ Rapid ■ **Delayed**	☐ Major ■ **Moderate** ☐ Minor	☐ Established ☐ Probable ☐ Suspected ■ **Possible** ☐ Unlikely

Effects The total plasma clearance of DOXORUBICIN may be increased by BARBITURATES, possibly decreasing its therapeutic effect.

Mechanism The hepatic metabolism of DOXORUBICIN is probably increased by BARBITURATES via hepatic microsomal enzyme induction.

Management Monitor patients receiving these agents concurrently. Adjust the dose of DOXORUBICIN upward as needed.

Discussion

Barbiturates appear to increase the clearance of doxorubicin.[1,2] In 8 patients, the coadministration of doxorubicin and a barbiturate (specific agent not stated) resulted in a median plasma clearance of 318 mL/min compared with 202 mL/min in 97 control patients receiving doxorubicin and no other hepatic-active drugs.[1] In rats, phenobarbital increased the cumulative excretion of doxorubicin by approximately 27%.[2] In another study involving mice, the half-life of doxorubicin was also decreased by 38% with concurrent phenobarbital.[3]

[1] Reich SD, et al. *Cancer.* 1976;36:3803.
[2] Riggs CE Jr, et al. *Clin Pharmacol Ther.* 1982;31:263.
[3] Wosilait WD, et al. *Res Comm Chem Path Pharmacol.* 1987;56:335.

* Asterisk indicates drugs cited in interaction reports. Based on pharmacologic and pharmacokinetic considerations, similar interactions may occur with other drugs that are listed.

Doxycycline — *Barbiturates*

Doxycycline	Barbiturates	
Doxycycline* (eg, *Vibramycin*)	Amobarbital (eg, *Amytal*)	Pentobarbital*
	Butabarbital (eg, *Butisol*)	Phenobarbital*
	Butalbital	Primidone* (eg, *Mysoline*)
	Mephobarbital (*Mebaral*)	Secobarbital (*Seconal*)
	Metharbital (*Gemonil*)	Talbutal (*Lotusate*)

Significance	Onset	Severity	Documentation
2	☐ Rapid	☐ Major	☐ Established
	■ **Delayed**	■ **Moderate**	☐ Probable
		☐ Minor	■ **Suspected**
			☐ Possible
			☐ Unlikely

Effects The coadministration of a BARBITURATE with DOXYCYCLINE may decrease DOXYCYCLINE'S half-life and serum levels, possibly resulting in a decreased therapeutic effect. These effects may persist for weeks following the discontinuation of the BARBITURATE.

Mechanism BARBITURATES may increase the hepatic metabolism of DOXYCYCLINE via stimulation of microsomal enzymes.

Management The dose of DOXYCYCLINE may need to be increased during BARBITURATE coadministration. Consider an alternative TETRACYCLINE.

Discussion

In 1 study, 5 patients were given a single 100 mg IV dose of doxycycline following phenobarbital 50 mg 3 times daily for 10 days; 5 patients taking phenobarbital (one patient was taking pentobarbital) for several weeks to several years were given the same single IV dose of doxycycline.[2] In the first group of patients, phenobarbital reduced the mean half-life of doxycycline 27% (15.3 to 11.1 hours) compared with doxycycline alone. The half-life did not return to baseline for 2 weeks after the discontinuation of phenobarbital. The patients receiving the long-term barbiturates had a mean doxycycline half-life of 7.7 hours. Four patients taking multiple antiepileptic agents, including primidone or phenobarbital, received doxycycline 200 mg followed by a 100 mg dose on the following 2 days.[3] Compared with controls, the half-life and serum levels of doxycycline were significantly lower. The elimination of tetracycline (eg, *Achromycin V*), oxytetracycline (eg, *Terramycin*), demeclocycline (*Declomycin*), and methacycline (*Rondomycin*) was not affected by antiepileptic therapy.

In contrast, phenobarbital administration for 6 to 8 days did not affect the half-life or serum levels of a single dose of doxycycline 200 or 300 mg.[1]

[1] Alestig K. *Scand J Infect Dis.* 1974;6:265.
[2] Neuvonen PJ, et al. *Br Med J.* 1974;1:535.
[3] Neuvonen PJ, et al. *Eur J Clin Pharmacol.* 1975;9:147.

* Asterisk indicates drugs cited in interaction reports. Based on pharmacologic and pharmacokinetic considerations, similar interactions may occur with other drugs that are listed.

Doxycycline — *Carbamazepine*

Doxycycline* (eg, *Vibramycin*)	Carbamazepine* (eg, *Tegretol*)

Significance	Onset	Severity	Documentation
2	☐ Rapid	☐ Major	☐ Established
	■ **Delayed**	■ **Moderate**	☐ Probable
		☐ Minor	■ **Suspected**
			☐ Possible
			☐ Unlikely

Effects CARBAMAZEPINE may decrease the half-life and serum levels of DOXYCYCLINE, possibly reducing its therapeutic efficacy.

Mechanism CARBAMAZEPINE may increase the hepatic metabolism of DOXYCYCLINE.

Management The dose of DOXYCYCLINE may need to be increased during CARBAMAZEPINE coadministration. Consider the use of another tetracycline.

Discussion

In 1 study, 5 patients taking carbamazepine 300 to 1,000 mg/day were given a single IV dose of doxycycline HCl 100 mg.[1] Compared with controls, the half-life of doxycycline was significantly shorter (15.1 vs 8.4 hours). The half-life of doxycycline in patients taking both carbamazepine and phenytoin was 7.4 hours. In another study, 6 patients taking carbamazepine 400 to 1,000 mg/day alone or with other anticonvulsants who were given doxycycline chloride 200 mg followed by a 100 mg dose on the next 2 days.[2] The half-life of doxycycline was 7.1 hours, compared with 13.0 hours in controls, and serum concentrations were significantly lower during the 6 to 24 hours after its administration. In 10 other subjects, the elimination of tetracycline, oxytetracycline, methacycline, and demeclocycline was not affected by concurrent anticonvulsant therapy, including carbamazepine.

[1] Penttila O, et al. *BMJ.* 1974;2:470.

[2] Neuvonen PJ, et al. *Eur J Clin Pharmacol.* 1975;9:147.

* Asterisk indicates drugs cited in interaction reports.

Doxycycline — *Hydantoins*

Doxycycline	Hydantoins	
Doxycycline* (eg, *Vibramycin*)	Ethotoin (*Peganone*)	Phenytoin* (eg, *Dilantin*)
	Fosphenytoin (eg, *Cerebyx*)	

Significance	Onset	Severity	Documentation
2	☐ Rapid	☐ Major	☐ Established
	■ **Delayed**	■ **Moderate**	■ **Probable**
		☐ Minor	☐ Suspected
			☐ Possible
			☐ Unlikely

Effects The $t_{½}$ of DOXYCYCLINE is decreased by the coadministration of PHENYTOIN.

Mechanism Stimulation of hepatic microsomal enzymes by PHENYTOIN induces metabolism of DOXYCYCLINE; displacement of DOXYCYCLINE from plasma proteins may contribute to this phenomenon.

Management Monitor clinical response closely when PHENYTOIN is used concomitantly. Some researchers recommend doubling the daily dose of DOXYCYCLINE to maintain adequate serum levels.

Discussion

A study evaluating the effects of phenytoin and carbamazepine (eg, *Tegretol*) on doxycycline pharmacokinetics included 16 patients taking phenytoin, carbamazepine, or a combination who were given doxycycline 100 mg IV. In comparison with 9 control patients, patients receiving antiepileptic agents and doxycycline exhibited an approximately 50% shorter $t_{½}$.[1]

A subsequent trial[2] compared the serum $t_{½}$ and urinary excretion of 6 different tetracycline derivatives in patients on long-term antiepileptic therapy. Six patients received doxycycline for 3 days. The serum $t_{½}$ of doxycycline was significantly shorter in those on antiepileptic therapy versus controls (7.1 vs 13.3 hours, respectively). Differences were noted in AUC and possibly volume of distribution; however, these were not studied. Alteration in the elimination of other tetracycline derivatives was not detected. Based on this data, the authors recommend that daily dosages of doxycycline be doubled.

[1] Penttila O, et al. *Br Med J.* 1974;2(5917):470.

[2] Neuvonen PJ, et al. *Eur J Clin Pharmacol.* 1975;9(2-3):147.

* Asterisk indicates drugs cited in interaction reports. Based on pharmacologic and pharmacokinetic considerations, similar interactions may occur with other drugs that are listed.

Doxycycline — *Rifamycins*

Doxycycline* (eg, *Vibramycin*)	Rifabutin (*Mycobutin*)	Rifampin* (eg, *Rifadin*)

Significance	Onset	Severity	Documentation
2	□ Rapid ■ **Delayed**	□ Major ■ **Moderate** □ Minor	□ Established □ Probable ■ **Suspected** □ Possible □ Unlikely

Effects RIFAMYCINS may decrease the serum concentration and $t_{1/2}$ of DOXYCYCLINE, possibly reducing the therapeutic effect.

Mechanism RIFAMYCINS may increase the hepatic metabolism of DOXYCYCLINE.

Management Monitor the clinical response of the patient. It may be necessary to increase the dose of DOXYCYCLINE. Streptomycin does not appear to decrease DOXYCYCLINE concentrations.

Discussion

The effect of rifampin on plasma doxycycline concentrations was investigated in 20 patients with brucellosis randomly treated with doxycycline 100 mg twice daily plus rifampin 600 to 1,200 mg/day or streptomycin 1 g/day.[1] When compared with streptomycin plus doxycycline therapy, coadministration of rifampin resulted in decreases in doxycycline plasma concentrations, $t_{1/2}$, and AUC. Rifampin increased the clearance of doxycycline. In addition, in 2 of the 10 patients treated with doxycycline plus rifampin, there was a therapeutic failure or a relapse, whereas there was no therapeutic failure or relapse in any of the 10 patients receiving doxycycline plus streptomycin. In patients receiving rifampin and doxycycline concomitantly, doxycycline concentrations were lower in rapid acetylators of doxycycline than in slow acetylators. These results may support those of a previous clinical trial that found a lower degree of clinical efficacy in patients with brucellosis treated with doxycycline plus rifampin than in patients receiving doxycycline plus streptomycin.[2]

[1] Colmenero JD, et al. *Antimicrob Agents Chemother.* 1994;38(12):2798.

[2] Ariza J, et al. *Ann Intern Med.* 1992;117(1):25.

* Asterisk indicates drugs cited in interaction reports. Based on pharmacologic and pharmacokinetic considerations, similar interactions may occur with other drugs that are listed.

Dronedarone — *Antiarrhythmic Agents*

Dronedarone	Antiarrhythmic Agents	
Dronedarone* (*Multaq*)	Amiodarone* (eg, *Cordarone*)	Procainamide*
	Disopyramide* (eg, *Norpace*)	Propafenone* (eg, *Rythmol*)
	Dofetilide* (*Tikosyn*)	Quinidine*
	Flecainide* (eg, *Tambocor*)	Sotalol* (eg, *Betapace*)
	Ibutilide* (eg, *Corvert*)	

Significance	Onset	Severity	Documentation
1	☐ Rapid ■ **Delayed**	■ **Major** ☐ Moderate ☐ Minor	☐ Established ☐ Probable ■ **Suspected** ☐ Possible ☐ Unlikely

Effects The risk of life-threatening cardiac arrhythmias, including torsades de pointes, may be increased.

Mechanism Possible additive or synergistic prolongation of the QT interval.

Management DRONEDARONE is contraindicated in patients receiving class I or class III ANTIARRHYTHMIC AGENTS. Treatment with class I or class III ANTIARRHYTHMIC AGENTS must be stopped before starting DRONEDARONE.[1]

Discussion

Concurrent use of dronedarone and drugs or herbal products that prolong the QT interval and might increase the risk of torsades de pointes–type ventricular tachycardia, such as class I or class III antiarrhythmic agents, is contraindicated.[1]

The basis for this monograph is information on file with the manufacturer. Published clinical data are needed to further assess this interaction. Because of the seriousness of the cardiac problem, clinical evaluation of the interaction in humans is not likely to be forthcoming.

[1] *Multaq* [package insert]. Bridgewater, NJ: Sanofi-Aventis; July 2009.

* Asterisk indicates drugs cited in interaction reports.

Dronedarone | *Azole Antifungal Agents*

Dronedarone*	Itraconazole*	Posaconazole
(*Multaq*)	(eg, *Sporanox*)	(*Noxafil*)
	Ketoconazole*	Voriconazole*
	(eg, *Nizoral*)	(*Vfend*)

Significance	Onset	Severity	Documentation
1	☐ Rapid	■ **Major**	☐ Established
	■ **Delayed**	☐ Moderate	☐ Probable
		☐ Minor	■ **Suspected**
			☐ Possible
			☐ Unlikely

Effects DRONEDARONE plasma concentrations may be elevated, increasing the risk of toxicity, including life-threatening cardiotoxicity.

Mechanism DRONEDARONE metabolism (CYP3A) may be inhibited by certain AZOLE ANTIFUNGAL AGENTS.

Management Coadministration of DRONEDARONE and certain AZOLE ANTIFUNGAL AGENTS is contraindicated.[1]

Discussion

Concurrent use of strong CYP3A inhibitors, such as ketoconazole, may elevate dronedarone plasma concentrations increasing the risk of life-threatening cardiotoxicity, including torsades de pointes–type ventricular tachycardia.[1] Repeated doses of ketoconazole, a strong CYP3A inhibitor, increased the dronedarone C_{max} and AUC 9- and 17-fold, respectively. Concomitant use of dronedarone and itraconazole, ketoconazole, and voriconazole, strong CYP3A inhibitors, is contraindicated.

The basis for this monograph is information on file with the manufacturer. Published clinical data are needed to further assess this interaction. Because of the seriousness of the cardiac problem, clinical evaluation of the interaction in humans is not likely to be forthcoming.

[1] *Multaq* [package insert]. Bridgewater, NJ: Sanofi-Aventis; July 2009.

* Asterisk indicates drugs cited in interaction reports. Based on pharmacologic and pharmacokinetic considerations, similar interactions may occur with other drugs that are listed.

Dronedarone — *Cyclosporine*

Dronedarone*	Cyclosporine*
(*Multaq*)	(eg, *Neoral*)

Significance	Onset	Severity	Documentation
1	☐ Rapid	■ **Major**	☐ Established
	■ **Delayed**	☐ Moderate	☐ Probable
		☐ Minor	■ **Suspected**
			☐ Possible
			☐ Unlikely

Effects DRONEDARONE plasma concentrations may be elevated, increasing the risk of toxicity, including life-threatening cardiotoxicity.

Mechanism DRONEDARONE metabolism (CYP3A) may be inhibited by CYCLOSPORINE.

Management Coadministration of DRONEDARONE and CYCLOSPORINE is contraindicated.[1]

Discussion

Concurrent use of ketoconazole, a strong CYP3A inhibitors, may elevate dronedarone plasma concentrations, increasing the risk of life-threading cardiotoxicity, including torsades de pointes-type ventricular tachycardia. Repeated doses of ketoconazole increased the dronedarone C_{max} and AUC 9- and 17-fold, respectively. Concomitant use of dronedarone and cyclosporine, a CYP3A inhibitor, is contraindicated.[1]

The basis for this monograph is information on file with the manufacturer. Published clinical data are needed to further assess this interaction. Because of the seriousness of the cardiac problem, clinical evaluation of the interaction in humans is not likely to be forthcoming.

[1] *Multaq* [package insert]. Bridgewater, NJ: Sanofi-Aventis; January 2012.

* Asterisk indicates drugs cited in interaction reports.

Dronedarone — *Food*

Dronedarone* (*Multaq*)	Grapefruit Juice*

Significance	Onset	Severity	Documentation
2	☐ Rapid	☐ Major	☐ Established
	■ **Delayed**	■ **Moderate**	☐ Probable
		☐ Minor	■ **Suspected**
			☐ Possible
			☐ Unlikely

Effects DRONEDARONE plasma concentrations may be elevated, increasing the pharmacologic effects and risk of adverse reactions (eg, cardiac arrhythmias).

Mechanism Inhibition of DRONEDARONE metabolism (CYP3A4) by GRAPEFRUIT JUICE.

Management GRAPEFRUIT JUICE should be avoided in patients taking DRONEDARONE.[1] DRONEDARONE should be taken with a liquid other than GRAPEFRUIT JUICE.

Discussion

Coadministration of dronedarone and grapefruit juice increased dronedarone exposure (AUC) and C_{max} 3- and 2.5-fold, respectively.[1] Therefore, avoid grapefruit juice while taking dronedarone. Because dronedarone shows a moderate dose-related effect on the QTc interval, an increase in dronedarone exposure may increase the risk of QT prolongation and cardiac arrhythmias.

The basis for this monograph is information on file with the manufacturer. Published clinical data are needed to further assess this interaction.

[1] *Multaq* [package insert]. Bridgewater, NJ: Sanofi-Aventis; July 2009.

* Asterisk indicates drugs cited in interaction reports.

Dronedarone / Macrolide & Related Antibiotics

Dronedarone	Macrolide & Related Antibiotics	
Dronedarone* (*Multaq*)	Azithromycin (eg, *Zithromax*)	Erythromycin (eg, *Ery-Tab*)
	Clarithromycin* (eg, *Biaxin*)	Telithromycin* (*Ketek*)

Significance	Onset	Severity	Documentation
1	□ Rapid	■ **Major**	□ Established
	■ **Delayed**	□ Moderate	□ Probable
		□ Minor	■ **Suspected**
			□ Possible
			□ Unlikely

Effects The risk of life-threatening cardiac arrhythmias, including torsades de pointes, may be increased.

Mechanism Possible additive or synergistic prolongation of the QT interval. In addition, the metabolism (CYP3A) of DRONEDARONE may be inhibited.

Management DRONEDARONE is contraindicated in patients receiving certain MACROLIDE AND RELATED ANTIBIOTICS.[1]

Discussion

Concurrent use of dronedarone and drugs or herbal products that prolong the QT interval and might increase the risk of torsades de pointes–type ventricular tachycardia, such as clarithromycin,[2] is contraindicated.[1] In addition, because dronedarone is associated with a dose-related increase in the QT interval, coadministration of dronedarone and strong CYP3A inhibitors, such as clarithromycin or telithromycin, is contraindicated.[1]

The basis for this monograph is information on file with the manufacturer. Published clinical data are needed to further assess this interaction. Because of the seriousness of the cardiac problem, clinical evaluation of the interaction in humans is not likely to be forthcoming.

[1] *Multaq* [package insert]. Bridgewater, NJ: Sanofi-Aventis; July 2009.

[2] Raschi E, et al. *Br J Clin Pharmacol.* 2009;67(1):88.

* Asterisk indicates drugs cited in interaction reports. Based on pharmacologic and pharmacokinetic considerations, similar interactions may occur with other drugs that are listed.

Dronedarone — *Nefazodone*

Dronedarone* (*Multaq*)	Nefazodone*

Significance	Onset	Severity	Documentation
1	☐ Rapid ■ **Delayed**	■ **Major** ☐ Moderate ☐ Minor	☐ Established ☐ Probable ■ **Suspected** ☐ Possible ☐ Unlikely

Effects DRONEDARONE plasma concentrations may be elevated, increasing the risk of toxicity, including life-threatening cardiotoxicity.

Mechanism DRONEDARONE metabolism (CYP3A) may be inhibited by NEFAZODONE.

Management Coadministration of DRONEDARONE and NEFAZODONE is contraindicated.[1]

Discussion

Concurrent use of strong CYP3A inhibitors, such as nefazodone, may elevate dronedarone plasma concentrations, increasing the risk of life-threatening cardiotoxicity, including torsades de pointes–type ventricular tachycardia.[1] Repeated doses of ketoconazole, a strong CYP3A inhibitor, increased the dronedarone C_{max} and AUC 9- and 17-fold, respectively. Concomitant use of dronedarone and nefazodone, a strong CYP3A inhibitor, is contraindicated.

The basis for this monograph is information on file with the manufacturer. Published clinical data are needed to further assess this interaction. Because of the seriousness of the cardiac problem, clinical evaluation of the interaction in humans is not likely to be forthcoming.

[1] *Multaq* [package insert]. Bridgewater, NJ: Sanofi-Aventis; July 2009.

* Asterisk indicates drugs cited in interaction reports.

Dronedarone — *Phenothiazines*

Dronedarone* (*Multaq*)	Chlorpromazine*	Thioridazine*

Significance	Onset	Severity	Documentation
1	☐ Rapid ■ **Delayed**	■ **Major** ☐ Moderate ☐ Minor	☐ Established ☐ Probable ■ **Suspected** ☐ Possible ☐ Unlikely

Effects The risk of life-threatening cardiac arrhythmias, including torsades de pointes, may be increased.

Mechanism Possible additive or synergistic prolongation of the QT interval.

Management DRONEDARONE is contraindicated in patients receiving certain PHENOTHIAZINES.[1]

Discussion

Concurrent use of dronedarone and drugs or herbal products that prolong the QT interval and might increase the risk of torsades de pointes–type ventricular tachycardia, such as thioridazine, is contraindicated.[1]

The basis for this monograph is information on file with the manufacturer. Published clinical data are needed to further assess this interaction. Because of the seriousness of the cardiac problem, clinical evaluation of the interaction in humans is not likely to be forthcoming.

[1] *Multaq* [package insert]. Bridgewater, NJ: Sanofi-Aventis; July 2009.

* Asterisk indicates drugs cited in interaction reports.

Dronedarone — *Protease Inhibitors*

Dronedarone	Protease Inhibitors	
Dronedarone* (*Multaq*)	Atazanavir (*Reyataz*)	Nelfinavir (*Viracept*)
	Darunavir (*Prezista*)	Ritonavir* (*Norvir*)
	Fosamprenavir (*Lexiva*)	Saquinavir (*Invirase*)
	Indinavir (*Crixivan*)	Tipranavir (*Aptivus*)
	Lopinavir/Ritonavir (*Kaletra*)	

Significance	Onset	Severity	Documentation
1	☐ Rapid	■ **Major**	☐ Established
	■ **Delayed**	☐ Moderate	☐ Probable
		☐ Minor	■ **Suspected**
			☐ Possible
			☐ Unlikely

Effects DRONEDARONE plasma concentrations may be elevated, increasing the risk of toxicity, including life-threatening cardiotoxicity.

Mechanism DRONEDARONE metabolism (CYP3A) may be inhibited by PROTEASE INHIBITORS.

Management Coadministration of DRONEDARONE and PROTEASE INHIBITORS is contraindicated.[1]

Discussion

Concurrent use of strong CYP3A inhibitors, such as ritonavir, may elevate dronedarone plasma concentrations increasing the risk of life-threatening cardiotoxicity, including torsades de pointes–type ventricular tachycardia.[1] Repeated doses of ketoconazole, a strong CYP3A inhibitor, increased the dronedarone C_{max} and AUC 9- and 17-fold, respectively. Concomitant use of dronedarone and ritonavir is contraindicated.

The basis for this monograph is information on file with the manufacturer. Published clinical data are needed to further assess this interaction. Because of the seriousness of the cardiac problem, clinical evaluation of the interaction in humans is not likely to be forthcoming.

[1] *Multaq* [package insert]. Bridgewater, NJ: Sanofi-Aventis; July 2009.

* Asterisk indicates drugs cited in interaction reports. Based on pharmacologic and pharmacokinetic considerations, similar interactions may occur with other drugs that are listed.

Dronedarone — *St. John's Wort*

Dronedarone* (*Multaq*)	St. John's Wort*

Significance

2

Onset	Severity	Documentation
□ Rapid	□ Major	□ Established
■ **Delayed**	■ **Moderate**	□ Probable
	□ Minor	■ **Suspected**
		□ Possible
		□ Unlikely

Effects DRONEDARONE plasma concentrations may be reduced, decreasing the pharmacologic effects.

Mechanism ST. JOHN'S WORT increases the metabolism (CYP3A4) of DRONEDARONE.

Management Caution patients receiving DRONEDARONE to consult a health care provider before using nonprescription or herbal products. Advise patients to avoid coadministration of DRONEDARONE and ST. JOHN'S WORT.[1]

Discussion

Dronedarone is a CYP3A substrate. The manufacturer of dronedarone states that coadministration of CYP3A inducers (eg, St. John's wort) and dronedarone results in an important decrease in dronedarone exposure.[1] Patients receiving dronedarone should avoid taking St. John's wort concurrently.

The basis for this monograph is information on file with the manufacturer. Published clinical data are needed to further assess this interaction.

[1] *Multaq* [package insert]. Bridgewater, NJ: Sanofi-Aventis; July 2009.

* Asterisk indicates drugs cited in interaction reports.

Dronedarone — *Tricyclic Antidepressants*

Dronedarone* (*Multaq*)	Doxepin* (eg, *Silenor*)	Nortriptyline* (eg, *Pamelor*)

Significance	Onset	Severity	Documentation
1	☐ Rapid ■ **Delayed**	■ **Major** ☐ Moderate ☐ Minor	☐ Established ☐ Probable ■ **Suspected** ☐ Possible ☐ Unlikely

Effects The risk of life-threatening cardiac arrhythmias, including torsades de pointes, may be increased.

Mechanism Possible additive or synergistic prolongation of the QT interval.

Management DRONEDARONE is contraindicated in patients receiving certain TRICYCLIC ANTIDEPRESSANTS.[1]

Discussion

Concurrent use of dronedarone and drugs or herbal products that prolong the QT interval and might increase the risk of torsades de pointes–type ventricular tachycardia, such as nortriptyline, is contraindicated.[1]

The basis for this monograph is information on file with the manufacturer. Published clinical data are needed to further assess this interaction. Because of the seriousness of the cardiac problem, clinical evaluation of the interaction in humans is not likely to be forthcoming.

[1] *Multaq* [package insert]. Bridgewater, NJ: Sanofi-Aventis; July 2009.

* Asterisk indicates drugs cited in interaction reports.

Dyphylline — *Probenecid*

Dyphylline* (eg, *Lufyllin*)	Probenecid*

Significance	Onset	Severity	Documentation
2	□ Rapid	□ Major	□ Established
	■ **Delayed**	■ **Moderate**	■ **Probable**
		□ Minor	□ Suspected
			□ Possible
			□ Unlikely

Effects PROBENECID increases the $t_{½}$ and decreases the total body clearance of DYPHYLLINE.[1-3]

Mechanism PROBENECID, through its direct effects on the kidney, affects the active tubular secretion of DYPHYLLINE, thus decreasing clearance and prolonging the $t_{½}$.[1,2]

Management It has been postulated that this interaction may prove to be beneficial in extending the DYPHYLLINE dosing interval. Although studied in few patients, adverse reactions were less frequent with combination therapy.

Discussion

A preliminary report involving 5 healthy volunteers showed that dyphylline total body clearance was decreased by probenecid.[1] A subsequent investigation in 12 patients confirmed the preliminary report, indicating a prolonged $t_{½}$ (2.57 to 4.8 hours), decreased total body clearance (73 to 95 mL/kg), and decreased elimination rate constant (0.276 to 0.15 h^{-1}). There was no significant difference in volume of distribution between treatment and control groups.[2] A reported 150% decrease in rate of elimination and an increase in $t_{½}$ occurred from 2.05 to 5.01 hours. Although urine volume was increased, clearance of dyphylline was prolonged.[3] Probenecid does not influence the pharmacokinetics of aminophylline or theophylline.[4,5]

1 May DC, et al. *N Engl J Med.* 1981;304(13):791.
2 May DC, et al. *Clin Pharmacol Ther.* 1983;33(6):822.
3 Acara M, et al. *J Pharm Pharmacol.* 1987;39(7):526.
4 Chen TW, et al. *Drug Intell Clin Pharm.* 1983;17(6):465.
5 Marquardt ED, et al. *Drug Intell Clin Pharm.* 1985;19(11):840.

* Asterisk indicates drugs cited in interaction reports.

Efavirenz — *Ginkgo biloba*

Efavirenz* (*Sustiva*)	Ginkgo biloba*

Significance	Onset	Severity	Documentation
4	☐ Rapid	☐ Major	☐ Established
	■ **Delayed**	■ **Moderate**	☐ Probable
		☐ Minor	☐ Suspected
			■ **Possible**
			☐ Unlikely

Effects EFAVIRENZ plasma concentrations may be reduced, decreasing the efficacy.

Mechanism Unknown.

Management Caution patients taking EFAVIRENZ to avoid GINKGO BILOBA.

Discussion

Virologic failure was reported in a 47-year-old patient infected with HIV who received antiretroviral therapy for 10 years.[1] The patient had been receiving efavirenz for 2 years in combination with emtricitabine (*Emtriva*) and tenofovir disoproxil fumarate (*Viread*). When virologic failure developed, mutation in the reverse transcriptase gene was found. The patient history revealed he had been using *Ginkgo biloba* for a number of months. Retrospective analysis of plasma samples dating back 2 years indicated that efavirenz concentrations had decreased over time, coinciding with an increase in viral load.

[1] Wiegman DJ, et al. *AIDS*. 2009;23(9):1184.

* Asterisk indicates drugs cited in interaction reports.

Efavirenz — *Nevirapine*

Efavirenz*
(*Sustiva*)

Nevirapine*
(*Viramune*)

Significance	Onset	Severity	Documentation
2	☐ Rapid ■ **Delayed**	☐ Major ■ **Moderate** ☐ Minor	☐ Established ☐ Probable ■ **Suspected** ☐ Possible ☐ Unlikely

Effects EFAVIRENZ plasma concentrations may be reduced; however, the risk of adverse reactions may be increased.

Mechanism Induction of EFAVIRENZ metabolism by NEVIRAPINE is suspected. However, this does not account for the increased incidence of adverse reactions observed when both agents are coadministered.

Management Closely monitor patients when EFAVIRENZ and NEVIRAPINE are coadministered.

Discussion

The effects of nevirapine on the pharmacokinetics of efavirenz were studied in 14 patients infected with HIV-1 who had been taking efavirenz 600 mg once daily for at least 2 weeks.[1] Patients were instructed to continue taking efavirenz for 43 days. On study day 14, the pharmacokinetics of efavirenz were assessed. On study day 15, nevirapine 200 mg once daily was added to their regimen. On study day 29, the nevirapine dosage was increased to 400 mg once daily. On study day 43, the pharmacokinetics of efavirenz and nevirapine were assessed. Compared with taking efavirenz without nevirapine, coadministration of the 2 agents decreased the efavirenz AUC 22%, C_{max} 17%, and C_{min} 36%. Compared with data from historical controls, efavirenz did not affect the pharmacokinetics of nevirapine. In a randomized trial involving 1,216 antiretroviral therapy naive-patients, therapeutic outcomes and adverse reactions were compared in patients receiving regimens that included lamivudine (*Epivir*) and stavudine (eg, *Zerit*) plus either nevirapine or efavirenz or both nevirapine and efavirenz.[2] After 48 weeks, treatment failure was highest in patients receiving the regimen containing nevirapine and efavirenz, compared with either drug alone. In addition, adverse reactions, including grade 3 or 4 toxicity, were greatest in the regimen that included nevirapine and efavirenz.

[1] Veldkamp AI, et al. *J Infect Dis.* 2001;184(1):37.
[2] van Leth F, et al. *Lancet.* 2004;363(9417):1253.

* Asterisk indicates drugs cited in interaction reports.

Eltrombopag | *Aluminum Salts*

Eltrombopag* (*Promacta*)	Aluminum Carbonate† Aluminum Hydroxide* (eg, *Amphojel*)

Significance	Onset	Severity	Documentation
2	☐ Rapid	☐ Major	☐ Established
	■ **Delayed**	■ **Moderate**	☐ Probable
		☐ Minor	■ **Suspected**
			☐ Possible
			☐ Unlikely

Effects ELTROMBOPAG plasma concentrations may be reduced, decreasing the pharmacologic effect.

Mechanism Decreased ELTROMBOPAG GI absorption due to formation of chelates with ALUMINUM SALTS.

Management Separate the administration times of ELTROMBOPAG and ALUMINUM SALTS or mineral supplements by at least 4 hours.

Discussion

The effects of an antacid on the pharmacokinetics of eltrombopag were studied in healthy volunteers.[1] Each subject received a single dose of eltrombopag 75 mg 1 hour before receiving 30 mL of an antacid containing aluminum hydroxide 1,524 mg and magnesium carbonate 1,425 mg. Compared with administration of eltrombopag with a low-calcium meal, the antacid decreased the eltrombopag AUC and C_{max} approximately 70%. The manufacturer of eltrombopag states that eltrombopag chelates polyvalent cations (eg, aluminum, calcium, iron, magnesium, selenium, zinc), decreasing eltrombopag systemic exposure approximately 70%. Eltrombopag must not be taken within 4 hours of any medication or product containing polyvalent cations, such as antacids, dairy products, and mineral supplements.[2]

[1] Williams DD, et al. *Clin Ther*. 2009;31(4):764.

[2] *Promacta* [package insert]. Research Triangle Park, NC: GlaxoSmithKline; October 2008.

* Asterisk indicates drugs cited in interaction reports. Based on pharmacologic and pharmacokinetic considerations, similar interactions may occur with other drugs that are listed.

† Not available in the United States.

Eltrombopag | **_Antacids_**

Eltrombopag*
(*Promacta*)

Aluminum Hydroxide/ Magnesium Carbonate* (eg, *Gaviscon*)

Aluminum Hydroxide/ Magnesium Hydroxide (eg, *Riopan*)

Significance	Onset	Severity	Documentation
2	☐ Rapid ■ **Delayed**	☐ Major ■ **Moderate** ☐ Minor	☐ Established ☐ Probable ■ **Suspected** ☐ Possible ☐ Unlikely

Effects ELTROMBOPAG plasma concentrations may be reduced, decreasing the pharmacologic effect.

Mechanism Decreased ELTROMBOPAG GI absorption due to formation of chelates with ALUMINUM and/or MAGNESIUM.

Management Separate the administration times of ELTROMBOPAG and ANTACIDS or other ALUMINUM- or MAGNESIUM-containing substances by at least 4 hours.

Discussion

The effects of an antacid on the pharmacokinetics of eltrombopag were studied in healthy volunteers.[1] Each subject received a single dose of eltrombopag 75 mg 1 hour before receiving 30 mL of an antacid containing aluminum hydroxide 1,524 mg and magnesium carbonate 1,425 mg. Compared with administration of eltrombopag with a low-calcium meal, the antacid decreased the eltrombopag AUC and C_{max} approximately 70%. The manufacturer of eltrombopag states that eltrombopag chelates polyvalent cations (eg, aluminum, calcium, iron, magnesium, selenium, zinc), decreasing eltrombopag systemic exposure approximately 70%. Eltrombopag must not be taken within 4 hours of any medication or product containing polyvalent cations, such as antacids, dairy products, and mineral supplements.[2]

[1] Williams DD, et al. *Clin Ther*. 2009;31(4):764.

[2] *Promacta* [package insert]. Research Triangle Park, NC: GlaxoSmithKline; October 2008.

* Asterisk indicates drugs cited in interaction reports. Based on pharmacologic and pharmacokinetic considerations, similar interactions may occur with other drugs that are listed.

Eltrombopag — *Calcium Salts*

Eltrombopag	Calcium Salts	
Eltrombopag* (*Promacta*)	Calcium Carbonate* (eg, *Os-Cal 500*)	Calcium Lactate* (eg, *Cal-Lac*)
	Calcium Citrate* (eg, *Citracal*)	Tricalcium Phosphate* (*Posture*)
	Calcium Glubionate* (eg, *Calcionate*)	
	Calcium Gluconate* (eg, *Cal-G*)	

Significance	Onset	Severity	Documentation
2	☐ Rapid ■ **Delayed**	☐ Major ■ **Moderate** ☐ Minor	☐ Established ☐ Probable ■ **Suspected** ☐ Possible ☐ Unlikely

Effects ELTROMBOPAG absorption and plasma concentrations may be reduced, decreasing the pharmacologic effects.

Mechanism Decreased ELTROMBOPAG GI absorption due to formation of chelates with CALCIUM SALTS.

Management Separate the administration times of ELTROMBOPAG and CALCIUM SALTS, high-calcium foods (eg, dairy products), or mineral supplements by at least 4 hours.

Discussion

In a study in healthy volunteers, each subject received a single dose of eltrombopag 50 mg immediately after a high-fat, high-calcium (427 mg) breakfast.[1] Compared with subjects in a fasted state, taking eltrombopag with a high-fat, high-calcium meal reduced the eltrombopag AUC and C_{max} 59% and 65%, respectively. Regardless of the fat content, food that was low in calcium did not affect eltrombopag bioavailability. The manufacturer of eltrombopag states that eltrombopag chelates polyvalent cations (eg, aluminum, calcium, iron, magnesium, selenium, zinc), decreasing eltrombopag systemic exposure. Eltrombopag must not be taken within 4 hours of any medication or product containing polyvalent cations, such as antacids, dairy products, and mineral supplements.[2]

[1] Williams DD, et al. *Clin Ther*. 2009;31(4):764.

[2] *Promacta* [package insert]. Research Triangle Park, NC: GlaxoSmithKline; October 2008.

* Asterisk indicates drugs cited in interaction reports.

Eltrombopag — *Iron Salts*

Eltrombopag	Iron Salts	
Eltrombopag* (*Promacta*)	Ferrous Fumarate* (eg, *Hemocyte*)	Ferrous Sulfate* (eg, *Feosol*)
	Ferrous Gluconate* (eg, *Fergon*)	Iron Polysaccharide* (eg, *Niferex*)

Significance	Onset	Severity	Documentation
2	☐ Rapid	☐ Major	☐ Established
	■ **Delayed**	■ **Moderate**	☐ Probable
		☐ Minor	■ **Suspected**
			☐ Possible
			☐ Unlikely

Effects ELTROMBOPAG absorption and plasma concentrations may be reduced, decreasing the pharmacologic effects.

Mechanism Decreased ELTROMBOPAG GI absorption due to formation of chelates with IRON SALTS.

Management Separate the administration times of ELTROMBOPAG and IRON SALTS or mineral supplements by at least 4 hours.

Discussion

Administration of eltrombopag with high-calcium food or an antacid containing aluminum and magnesium was associated with reduced eltrombopag systemic exposure.[1] The manufacturer of eltrombopag states that eltrombopag chelates polyvalent cations (eg, aluminum, calcium, iron, magnesium, selenium, zinc), decreasing eltrombopag systemic exposure. Eltrombopag must not be taken within 4 hours of any medication or product containing polyvalent cations, such as antacids, dairy products, and mineral supplements.[2]

[1] Williams DD, et al. *Clin Ther.* 2009;31(4):764.

[2] *Promacta* [package insert]. Research Triangle Park, NC: GlaxoSmithKline; October 2008.

* Asterisk indicates drugs cited in interaction reports.

Eltrombopag — *Magnesium Salts*

Eltrombopag	Magnesium Salts	
Eltrombopag* (*Promacta*)	Magaldrate (eg, *Riopan*)	Magnesium Hydroxide (eg, *Milk of Magnesia*)
	Magnesium Carbonate*	Magnesium Oxide
	Magnesium Citrate	Magnesium Sulfate
	Magnesium Gluconate (eg, *Magtrate*)	

Significance	Onset	Severity	Documentation
2	☐ Rapid	☐ Major	☐ Established
	■ **Delayed**	■ **Moderate**	☐ Probable
		☐ Minor	■ **Suspected**
			☐ Possible
			☐ Unlikely

Effects ELTROMBOPAG plasma concentrations may be reduced, decreasing the pharmacologic effect.

Mechanism Decreased ELTROMBOPAG GI absorption due to formation of chelates with MAGNESIUM SALTS.

Management Separate the administration times of ELTROMBOPAG and MAGNESIUM SALTS or mineral supplements by at least 4 hours.

Discussion

The effects of an antacid on the pharmacokinetics of eltrombopag were studied in healthy volunteers.[1] Each subject received a single dose of eltrombopag 75 mg 1 hour before receiving 30 mL of an antacid containing aluminum hydroxide 1,524 mg and magnesium carbonate 1,425 mg. Compared with administration of eltrombopag with a low-calcium meal, the antacid decreased the eltrombopag AUC and C_{max} approximately 70%. The manufacturer of eltrombopag states that eltrombopag chelates polyvalent cations (eg, aluminum, calcium, iron, magnesium, selenium, zinc), decreasing eltrombopag systemic exposure approximately 70%. Eltrombopag must not be taken within 4 hours of any medication or product containing polyvalent cations such as antacids, dairy products, and mineral supplements.[2]

[1] Williams DD, et al. *Clin Ther.* 2009;31(4):764.

[2] *Promacta* [package insert]. Research Triangle Park, NC: GlaxoSmithKline; October 2008.

* Asterisk indicates drugs cited in interaction reports. Based on pharmacologic and pharmacokinetic considerations, similar interactions may occur with other drugs that are listed.

Eltrombopag	**Zinc Salts**
Eltrombopag* (*Promacta*)	Zinc Gluconate* Zinc Sulfate* (eg, *Orazinc*)

Significance	Onset	Severity	Documentation
2	□ Rapid ■ **Delayed**	□ Major ■ **Moderate** □ Minor	□ Established □ Probable ■ **Suspected** □ Possible □ Unlikely

Effects ELTROMBOPAG absorption and plasma concentrations may be reduced, decreasing the pharmacologic effects.

Mechanism Decreased ELTROMBOPAG GI absorption due to formation of chelates with ZINC SALTS.

Management Separate the administration times of ELTROMBOPAG and ZINC SALTS or mineral supplements by at least 4 hours.

Discussion

Administration of eltrombopag with high-calcium food or an antacid-containing aluminum and magnesium was associated with reduced eltrombopag systemic exposure.[1] The manufacturer of eltrombopag states that eltrombopag chelates polyvalent cations (eg, aluminum, calcium, iron, magnesium, selenium, zinc), decreasing eltrombopag systemic exposure. Eltrombopag must not be taken within 4 hours of any medication or product containing polyvalent cations, such as antacids, dairy products, and mineral supplements.[2]

¹ Williams DD, et al. *Clin Ther*. 2009;31(4):764.

² *Promacta* [package insert]. Research Triangle Park, NC: GlaxoSmithKline; October 2008.

* Asterisk indicates drugs cited in interaction reports.

Encainide — *Diltiazem*

Encainide*†

Diltiazem*
(eg, *Cardizem*)

Significance	Onset	Severity	Documentation
3	■ **Rapid**	□ Major	□ Established
	□ Delayed	□ Moderate	□ Probable
		■ **Minor**	■ **Suspected**
			□ Possible
			□ Unlikely

Effects Serum ENCAINIDE levels may be increased without any change in the levels of the active metabolites of ENCAINIDE.

Mechanism DILTIAZEM appears to decrease the metabolism of ENCAINIDE, thereby increasing its bioavailability and decreasing its clearance, possibly by enzyme inhibition.

Management Based on available data, no special precautions are necessary, other than the usual monitoring of cardiac function.

Discussion

In a randomized, crossover study, the disposition of encainide and its active metabolites was investigated in 8 extensive and 1 poor metabolizer before and after the administration of diltiazem.[1] Subjects received oral encainide 25 mg every 8 hours for 7 days and oral diltiazem 90 mg every 8 hours for 10 days. In the extensive metabolizers of encainide, diltiazem administration increased the encainide AUC from 178 to 283 ng•h/mL (59%) and the percent recovered in the urine from 1.3% to 2.2% (69%), compared with administration of encainide alone. These increases were statistically significant. In the poor metabolizer, diltiazem increased the encainide AUC 33% and the $t_{1/2}$ 50% (from 8 to 12 hours). There was no significant change in the AUC or the $t_{1/2}$ of the active metabolites of encainide in the extensive metabolizers, implying not only a decrease in metabolite formation, but also a decrease in metabolite clearance. No patient exhibited pharmacodynamic changes, measured by effects on ECG intervals, which would be expected based on no change in levels of the active metabolites O-desmethylencainide and 3-methoxy-O-desmethylencainide.

[1] Kazierad DJ, et al. *Clin Pharmacol Ther.* 1989;46(6):668.

* Asterisk indicates drugs cited in interaction reports.
† Voluntarily withdrawn by the manufacturer. Still available on a limited basis.

Encainide — *Quinidine*

Encainide*†	Quinidine*

Significance	Onset	Severity	Documentation
5	☐ Rapid ■ **Delayed**	☐ Major ☐ Moderate ■ **Minor**	☐ Established ☐ Probable ☐ Suspected ■ **Possible** ☐ Unlikely

Effects QUINIDINE reduces the level of active metabolites of ENCAINIDE in extensive metabolizers of the drug.

Mechanism QUINIDINE inhibition of a specific CYP-450 enzyme type in genetically- determined extensive metabolizers of ENCAINIDE to O-desmethyl and 3-methoxy-O-desmethyl ENCAINIDE. Both metabolites have antiarrhythmic activity and may account for most of the antiarrhythmic effect in extensive metabolizers.

Management Based on available information, no precautions are warranted at this time.

Discussion

A detailed pharmacokinetic and pharmacodynamic study was conducted in 11 healthy volunteers.[1] In this study, low quinidine doses, chosen to avoid the antiarrhythmic effects, prolonged the $t_{1/2}$ of encainide and substantially decreased the production of the metabolites in extensive metabolizers. Clearance of the drug was decreased after oral and IV administration. Accompanying these pharmacokinetic changes, quinidine blunted the prolongation in QRS and PR intervals in the ECG. By contrast, poor metabolizers had no pharmacokinetic, pharmacodynamic, or ECG changes. Whether the overall therapeutic efficacy of encainide is affected by quinidine is unknown. Clinical trials are needed.

[1] Funck-Brentano C, et al. *J Pharmacol Exp Ther.* 1989;249(1):134.

* Asterisk indicates drugs cited in interaction reports.
† Voluntarily withdrawn by the manufacturer. Still available on a limited basis.

Encainide — *Ritonavir*

Encainide*†	Ritonavir* (*Norvir*)

Significance	Onset	Severity	Documentation
1	☐ Rapid ■ **Delayed**	■ **Major** ☐ Moderate ☐ Minor	☐ Established ☐ Probable ■ **Suspected** ☐ Possible ☐ Unlikely

Effects Large increases in serum ENCAINIDE concentrations may occur, increasing the risk of ENCAINIDE toxicity.

Mechanism RITONAVIR may inhibit the metabolism (CYP2D6) of ENCAINIDE.

Management RITONAVIR is contraindicated in patients receiving ENCAINIDE.

Discussion

Encainide administration produces dose-related changes in the PR and QRS intervals. Ritonavir is expected to produce large increases in encainide plasma concentrations, increasing the risk of toxicity.[1] Cardiovascular adverse reactions reported with encainide include new or worsened arrhythmias, new or worsened congestive heart failure, and sick sinus syndrome.

The basis for this monograph is information on file with the manufacturer.

[1] *Norvir* [package insert]. North Chicago, IL: Abbott Laboratories; February 1996.

* Asterisk indicates drugs cited in interaction reports.
† Voluntarily withdrawn by the manufacturer. Still available on a limited basis.

Enflurane — *Isoniazid*

Enflurane* (eg, *Ethrane*)	Isoniazid*

Significance	Onset	Severity	Documentation
2	■ **Rapid** □ Delayed	□ Major ■ **Moderate** □ Minor	□ Established □ Probable ■ **Suspected** □ Possible □ Unlikely

Effects In rapid ISONIAZID acetylators, high-output renal failure may occur due to nephrotoxic concentrations of inorganic fluoride (greater than 50 mcmol).

Mechanism Rapid acetylation of ISONIAZID produces high concentrations of hydrazine that facilitates defluorination of ENFLURANE.

Management Monitor renal function in patients receiving this combination, particularly those who are rapid acetylators.

Discussion

A healthy subject exhibited a peak serum inorganic fluoride level of 106 mcmol.[1] This subject was concurrently taking chlorpromazine, diazepam (eg, *Valium*), and isoniazid. Transient postanesthesia impairment of renal function was noted. Defluorination of enflurane has been demonstrated in vitro[2,3] and in Fischer rats.[4,5] In a study of enflurane defluorination in 20 patients receiving isoniazid, 9 patients exhibited fluoride levels that were significantly higher than those in the other 11 patients and 36 control patients.[6] The difference was attributed to variations in isoniazid acetylation. Other classical enzyme inducers have not produced this effect on enflurane.[4] isoniazid affects methoxyflurane† and isoflurane (eg, *Forane*) in a similar fashion in vitro.[5,6] Although no adverse consequences occurred, 1 of 2 patients receiving isoniazid exhibited elevated fluoride concentration (30 mcmol) following isoflurane administration.[7]

1 Cousins MJ, et al. *Anesthesiology.* 1976;44(1):44.
2 Rice SA, et al. *Pharmacologist.* 1978;20;258.
3 Rice SA, et al. *Drug Metab Dispos.* 1979;7(5):260.
4 Fish MP, et al. *Anesthesiology.* 1979;51(suppl 3):S257.
5 Rice SA, et al. *Anesthesiology.* 1980;53(6):489.
6 Mazze RI, et al. *Anesthesiology.* 1982;57(1):5.
7 Gauntlett IS, et al. *Anesth Analg.* 1989;69(2):245.

* Asterisk indicates drugs cited in interaction reports.
† Not available in the United States.

Enfuvirtide — *Niacin*

Enfuvirtide* (*Fuzeon*)	Niacin* (Nicotinic Acid; eg, *Niaspan*)

Significance	Onset	Severity	Documentation
4	☐ Rapid ■ **Delayed**	☐ Major ■ **Moderate** ☐ Minor	☐ Established ☐ Probable ☐ Suspected ■ **Possible** ☐ Unlikely

Effects The risk of an exaggerated reaction at the ENFUVIRTIDE injection site may be increased.

Mechanism Unknown.

Management Coadminister with caution. Closely monitor the injection site. If coadministration of ENFUVIRTIDE and NIACIN is associated with an exaggerated injection site reaction, consider an alternative agent for NIACIN.

Discussion

A possible interaction between enfuvirtide and niacin was reported in a 47-year-old HIV-infected man receiving subcutaneous enfuvirtide 90 mg twice daily as part of his antiretroviral regimen and oral extended-release niacin 500 mg daily for HDL.[1] One week after concurrent therapy, the patient experienced extreme redness, edema, and swelling at the enfuvirtide injection site that corresponded with the flushing sensation caused by niacin. The patient discontinued both drugs. Because the patient had tolerated enfuvirtide therapy before the start of niacin, enfuvirtide was restarted and niacin was replaced with atorvastatin (*Lipitor*) 20 mg daily. Coadministration of enfuvirtide and atorvastatin was well tolerated.

[1] Oates E, et al. *Ann Pharmacother.* 2010;44(12):2014.

* Asterisk indicates drugs cited in interaction reports.

Epinephrine — *Beta-Blockers*

Epinephrine	Beta-Blockers	
Epinephrine* (eg, *Adrenalin*)	Carteolol (*Cartrol*)	Pindolol
	Nadolol* (eg, *Corgard*)	Propranolol* (eg, *Inderal LA*)
	Penbutolol (*Levatol*)	Timolol

Significance	Onset	Severity	Documentation
1	■ **Rapid**	■ **Major**	■ **Established**
	□ Delayed	□ Moderate	□ Probable
		□ Minor	□ Suspected
			□ Possible
			□ Unlikely

Effects Initial hypertensive episode followed by bradycardia.

Mechanism Nonselective beta-blockade allows alpha-receptor effects of EPINEPHRINE to predominate. Increasing vascular resistance leads to a rise in blood pressure and reflex bradycardia.

Management When EPINEPHRINE exposure is anticipated, discontinue the BETA-BLOCKER 3 days prior or, if possible, do not use EPINEPHRINE. Closely monitor the patient's vital signs. If a cardiovascular reaction occurs, pharmacologic interventions include IV chlorpromazine, IV hydralazine, IV aminophylline, or atropine (eg, *Sal-Tropine*).[1]

Discussion

Patients on propranolol exhibit marked hypertension followed by bradycardia when epinephrine is given.[2-9] The severity of response may be due to beta-2 blockade that accompanies nonselective beta-blocker use. Single dose[4] and steady-state trials[5,6,10] comparing the effects of epinephrine on metoprolol (eg, *Lopressor*) versus propranolol have substantiated this mechanism. The epinephrine-propranolol combination increases systolic and diastolic pressures and vascular resistance with a subsequent reduction in heart rate.[1,3,5-7,10,11] Diuretics and vasodilators do not alter this effect.[6] Low doses of epinephrine have also been implicated, causing speculation into the effect of endogenous catecholamine release in patients under stress.[10] Hypertension in a patient receiving methyldopa, oxprenolol,† and phenylpropanolamine† has been reported.[12] In 2 instances, propranolol has been implicated in causing epinephrine resistance in anaphylaxis.[13,14] Selective beta blockers may be less likely to interact.

1 Foster CA, et al. *Plast Reconstr Surg.* 1983;72(1):74.
2 Harris WS, et al. *Am J Cardiol.* 1966;17(4):484.
3 Kram J, et al. *Ann Intern Med.* 1974;80(2):282.
4 Johnsson G. *Acta Pharmacol Toxicol (Copenh).* 1975;36(suppl 5):59.
5 van Herwaarden CL, et al. *Eur J Clin Pharmacol.* 1977;12(6):397.
6 Houben H, et al. *Clin Sci (Lond).* 1979;57(suppl 5):397s.
7 Hansbrough JF, et al. *Ann Intern Med.* 1980;92(5):717.
8 Lampman RM, et al. *Diabetes.* 1981;30(7):618.
9 Gandy W. *Ann Emerg Med.* 1989;18(1):98.
10 Houben H, et al. *Clin Pharmacol Ther.* 1982;31(6):685.
11 Whelan TV. *Ann Intern Med.* 1987;106(2):327.
12 McLaren EH. *Br Med J.* 1976;2(6030):283.
13 Newman BR, et al. *Ann Allergy.* 1981;47(1):35.
14 Awai LE, et al. *Ann Allergy.* 1984;53(1):48.

* Asterisk indicates drugs cited in interaction reports. Based on pharmacologic and pharmacokinetic considerations, similar interactions may occur with other drugs that are listed.
† Not available in the United States.

Epinephrine | **Phenothiazines**

Epinephrine* (eg, *Adrenalin*)	Norepinephrine* (eg, *Levophed*)	Chlorpromazine* (eg, *Thorazine*)

Significance	Onset	Severity	Documentation
3	■ **Rapid**	□ Major	□ Established
	□ Delayed	□ Moderate	□ Probable
		■ **Minor**	■ **Suspected**
			□ Possible
			□ Unlikely

Effects CHLORPROMAZINE decreases the pressor effect of NOREPINEPHRINE and eliminates bradycardia. CHLORPROMAZINE has been noted to antagonize the peripheral vasoconstrictive effects of EPINEPHRINE and, in some instances, reverse the action of EPINEPHRINE.

Mechanism Based upon clinical observation, the mechanism probably involves pharmacologic antagonism, decreasing the overall effects of adrenergic agents, NOREPINEPHRINE and EPINEPHRINE.

Management Monitor patient's vital signs when these agents are used concomitantly. In acute situations, employ supportive measures.

Discussion

From interest in the effects of chlorpromazine on circulation, researchers noted that chlorpromazine decreased BP and increased pulse rate and peripheral blood flow. Studies using chlorpromazine in conjunction with epinephrine or norepinephrine illustrated that chlorpromazine decreased the pressor effect of norepinephrine, eliminating bradycardia, and antagonized the peripheral vasoconstrictive properties of epinephrine.[1-4] Some studies have illustrated that chlorpromazine reversed the action of epinephrine,[1,4] although other trials were either inconclusive[2] or failed to document this effect.[3] Researchers also described a paradoxical effect of epinephrine in the presence of chlorpromazine that clinically manifested as vasodilatation and hypotension.[5] Conclusive clinical evidence of the effects of this interaction is needed in order to assess the clinical importance.

[1] Foster CA, et al. *Lancet.* 1954;2:614.
[2] Ginsburg J, et al. *Br J Pharmacol.* 1956;11:180.
[3] Chiron AE, et al. *JAMA.* 1957;163:30.
[4] Sletten IW, et al. *Clin Pharmacol Ther.* 1965;6:575.
[5] Cancro R, et al. *Am J Psychiatry.* 1970;127:368.

* Asterisk indicates drugs cited in interaction reports.

Epirubicin — *Paclitaxel*

Epirubicin* (*Ellence*)	Paclitaxel* (eg, *Taxol*)

Significance	Onset	Severity	Documentation
4	☐ Rapid ■ **Delayed**	☐ Major ■ **Moderate** ☐ Minor	☐ Established ☐ Probable ☐ Suspected ■ **Possible** ☐ Unlikely

Effects EPIRUBICIN plasma levels may be increased.

Mechanism Alteration in EPIRUBICIN P-glycoprotein-mediated excretion by PACLITAXEL or its vehicle is suspected.

Management Monitor the clinical response of patients receiving EPIRUBICIN and PACLITAXEL concurrently and adjust therapy as needed.

Discussion

The effects of paclitaxel on the disposition of epirubicin were studied in patients who received an IV bolus of epirubicin 90 mg/m^2 followed 10 minutes later by paclitaxel 175 mg/m^2 infused IV over 3 hours.[1] The effects were compared with patients who received epirubicin followed 24 hours later by paclitaxel (considered epirubicin alone). Coadministration of epirubicin and paclitaxel reduced the renal clearance of epirubicin and the metabolite, epirubicinol, and increased the AUC of epirubicin compared with giving epirubicin alone.

Additional studies are needed to determine the clinical relevance of elevated epirubicinol concentrations on antitumor efficacy.

[1] Fogli S, et al. *Ann Oncol.* 2002;13:919.

* Asterisk indicates drugs cited in interaction reports.

Eplerenone — *Azole Antifungal Agents*

Eplerenone* (*Inspra*)	Itraconazole* (eg, *Sporanox*)	Ketoconazole* (eg, *Nizoral*)

Significance	Onset	Severity	Documentation
1	☐ Rapid ■ **Delayed**	■ **Major** ☐ Moderate ☐ Minor	☐ Established ☐ Probable ■ **Suspected** ☐ Possible ☐ Unlikely

Effects Elevated EPLERENONE plasma concentrations, which may increase the risk of hyperkalemia and associated serious, sometimes fatal, arrhythmias.

Mechanism ITRACONAZOLE and KETOCONAZOLE inhibit the metabolism (CYP3A4) of EPLERENONE.

Management Coadministration of EPLERENONE and ITRACONAZOLE or KETOCONAZOLE is contraindicated.[1]

Discussion

The primary risk of eplerenone therapy is hyperkalemia, which can cause serious, sometimes fatal, arrhythmias.[1] Potent CYP3A4 inhibitors (eg, itraconazole, ketoconazole) can increase eplerenone plasma concentrations and the risk of hyperkalemia. The risk of hyperkalemia can be minimized by avoiding certain concurrent treatments (eg, itraconazole, ketoconazole). In a study of the effects of ketoconazole 200 mg twice daily on the pharmacokinetics of a single dose of eplerenone 100 mg, ketoconazole administration increased the peak plasma concentration and AUC of eplerenone 1.7- and 5.4-fold, respectively.[1]

The basis for this interaction is information on file with the manufacturer. Published clinical data are needed to further assess this interaction. Because of the seriousness of this interaction, clinical evaluation in humans is not likely to be forthcoming.

[1] *Inspra* [package insert]. New York, NY: Pfizer Inc.; October 2003.

* Asterisk indicates drugs cited in interaction reports.

Eplerenone	*Macrolide Antibiotics*	
Eplerenone* (*Inspra*)	Clarithromycin* (eg, *Biaxin*)	Troleandomycin*†

Significance	Onset	Severity	Documentation
1	☐ Rapid ■ **Delayed**	■ **Major** ☐ Moderate ☐ Minor	☐ Established ☐ Probable ■ **Suspected** ☐ Possible ☐ Unlikely

Effects Elevated EPLERENONE plasma concentrations, which may increase the risk of hyperkalemia and associated serious, sometimes fatal, arrhythmias.

Mechanism CLARITHROMYCIN and TROLEANDOMYCIN inhibit the metabolism (CYP3A4) of EPLERENONE.

Management Coadministration of EPLERENONE and CLARITHROMYCIN or TROLEANDOMYCIN is contraindicated.[1]

Discussion

The primary risk of eplerenone therapy is hyperkalemia, which can cause serious, sometimes fatal, arrhythmias.[1] Potent CYP3A4 inhibitors (eg, clarithromycin, troleandomycin) can increase eplerenone plasma concentrations and the risk of hyperkalemia. The risk of hyperkalemia can be minimized by avoiding certain concurrent treatments (eg, clarithromycin, troleandomycin).

The basis for this interaction is information on file with the manufacturer. Published clinical data are needed to further assess this interaction. Because of the seriousness of this interaction, clinical evaluation in humans is not likely to be forthcoming.

[1] *Inspra* [package insert]. New York, NY: Pfizer, Inc.; October 2003.

* Asterisk indicates drugs cited in interaction reports.
† Not available in the United States.

Eplerenone — *Nefazodone*

Eplerenone* (*Inspra*)	Nefazodone*

Significance	Onset	Severity	Documentation
1	☐ Rapid ■ **Delayed**	■ **Major** ☐ Moderate ☐ Minor	☐ Established ☐ Probable ■ **Suspected** ☐ Possible ☐ Unlikely

Effects Elevated EPLERENONE plasma concentrations, which may increase the risk of hyperkalemia and associated serious, sometimes fatal, arrhythmias.

Mechanism NEFAZODONE inhibits the metabolism (CYP3A4) of EPLERENONE.

Management Coadministration of EPLERENONE and NEFAZODONE is contraindicated.[1]

Discussion

The primary risk of eplerenone therapy is hyperkalemia, which can cause serious, sometimes fatal, arrhythmias.[1] Potent CYP3A4 inhibitors (eg, nefazodone) can increase eplerenone plasma concentrations and the risk of hyperkalemia. The risk of hyperkalemia can be minimized by avoiding certain concurrent treatments (eg, nefazodone).

The basis for this interaction is information on file with the manufacturer. Published clinical data are needed to further assess this interaction. Because of the seriousness of this interaction, clinical evaluation in humans is not likely to be forthcoming.

[1] *Inspra* [package insert]. New York, NY: Pfizer, Inc.; October 2003.

* Asterisk indicates drugs cited in interaction reports.

Eplerenone | Potassium-Sparing Diuretics

Eplerenone* (*Inspra*)	Amiloride* (*Midamor*)	Triamterene* (*Dyrenium*)
	Spironolactone* (eg, *Aldactone*)	

Significance	Onset	Severity	Documentation
1	☐ Rapid	■ **Major**	☐ Established
	■ **Delayed**	☐ Moderate	☐ Probable
		☐ Minor	■ **Suspected**
			☐ Possible
			☐ Unlikely

Effects POTASSIUM-SPARING DIURETICS will increase potassium retention, which may increase the risk of hyperkalemia and associated serious, sometimes fatal, arrhythmias.

Mechanism A reduction in renal elimination of potassium ions by POTASSIUM-SPARING DIURETICS in association with EPLERENONE-induced hyperkalemia.

Management Coadministration of EPLERENONE and POTASSIUM-SPARING DIURETICS is contraindicated.[1]

Discussion

The primary risk of eplerenone therapy is hyperkalemia, which can cause serious, sometimes fatal, arrhythmias.[1] Potassium-sparing diuretics (eg, spironolactone) can increase potassium retention and the risk of hyperkalemia. The risk of hyperkalemia can be minimized by avoiding eplerenone with certain concurrent treatments (eg, spironolactone).

The basis for this interaction is information on file with the manufacturer. Published clinical data are needed to further assess this interaction. Because of the seriousness of this interaction, clinical evaluation in humans is not likely to be forthcoming.

[1] *Inspra* [package insert]. New York, NY: Pfizer, Inc.; October 2003.

* Asterisk indicates drugs cited in interaction reports.

Eplerenone × *Potassium Supplements*

Eplerenone	Potassium Supplements	
Eplerenone* (*Inspra*)	Potassium Acetate*	Potassium Citrate* (eg, *Urocit-K*)
	Potassium Acid Phosphate* (eg, *K-Phos*)	Potassium Gluconate* (eg, *Kaon*)
	Potassium Bicarbonate* (eg, *K+ Care ET*)	Potassium Iodide* (eg, *SSKI*)
	Potassium Chloride* (eg, *Kaochlor*)	Potassium Phosphate*

Significance	Onset	Severity	Documentation
1	□ Rapid ■ **Delayed**	■ **Major** □ Moderate □ Minor	□ Established □ Probable ■ **Suspected** □ Possible □ Unlikely

Effects POTASSIUM SUPPLEMENTS will increase potassium serum concentrations, which may increase the risk of hyperkalemia and associated serious (sometimes fatal) arrhythmias.

Mechanism Elevated potassium serum concentrations caused by POTASSIUM SUPPLEMENTS in association with EPLERENONE-induced hyperkalemia.

Management Administration of EPLERENONE and POTASSIUM SUPPLEMENTS is contraindicated.[1]

Discussion

The primary risk of eplerenone therapy is hyperkalemia, which can cause serious, sometimes fatal, arrhythmias.[1] Potassium supplements (eg, potassium chloride) can increase potassium serum concentrations and the risk of hyperkalemia. The risk of hyperkalemia can be minimized by avoiding eplerenone with certain concurrent treatments (eg, potassium chloride).

The basis for this interaction is information on file with the manufacturer. Published clinical data are needed to further assess this interaction. Because of the seriousness of this interaction, clinical evaluation in humans is not likely to be forthcoming.

[1] *Inspra* [package insert]. New York, NY: Pfizer, Inc.; October 2003.

* Asterisk indicates drugs cited in interaction reports.

Eplerenone — *Protease Inhibitors*

Eplerenone	Protease Inhibitors	
Eplerenone* (eg, *Inspra*)	Atazanavir (*Reyataz*)	Nelfinavir* (*Viracept*)
	Fosamprenavir (*Lexiva*)	Ritonavir* (*Norvir*)
	Indinavir (*Crixivan*)	Saquinavir (*Invirase*)
	Lopinavir/Ritonavir (*Kaletra*)	Tipranavir (*Aptivus*)

Significance	Onset	Severity	Documentation
1	□ Rapid	■ **Major**	□ Established
	■ **Delayed**	□ Moderate	□ Probable
		□ Minor	■ **Suspected**
			□ Possible
			□ Unlikely

Effects Elevated EPLERENONE plasma concentrations, which may increase the risk of hyperkalemia and associated serious (sometimes fatal) arrhythmias.

Mechanism NELFINAVIR and RITONAVIR inhibit the metabolism (CYP3A4) of EPLERENONE.

Management Administration of EPLERENONE and NELFINAVIR or RITONAVIR is contraindicated.[1]

Discussion

The primary risk of eplerenone therapy is hyperkalemia, which can cause serious, sometimes fatal, arrhythmias.[1] Potent CYP3A4 inhibitors (eg, nelfinavir, ritonavir) can increase eplerenone plasma concentrations and the risk of hyperkalemia. The risk of hyperkalemia can be minimized by avoiding certain concurrent treatments (eg, nelfinavir, ritonavir).

The basis for this interaction is information on file with the manufacturer. Published clinical data are needed to further assess this interaction. Because of the seriousness of this interaction, clinical evaluation in humans is not likely to be forthcoming.

[1] *Inspra* [package insert]. New York, NY: Pfizer Inc; October 2003.

* Asterisk indicates drugs cited in interaction reports. Based on pharmacologic and pharmacokinetic considerations, similar interactions may occur with other drugs that are listed.

Eplerenone — *Voriconazole*

Eplerenone* (eg, *Inspra*)	Voriconazole* (*Vfend*)

Significance	Onset	Severity	Documentation
4	■ **Rapid**	□ Major	□ Established
	□ Delayed	■ **Moderate**	□ Probable
		□ Minor	□ Suspected
			■ **Possible**
			□ Unlikely

Effects EPLERENONE plasma concentrations may be elevated, increasing pharmacologic effects and adverse reactions.

Mechanism Inhibition of EPLERENONE metabolism (CYP3A4) by VORICONAZOLE is suspected.

Management Closely monitor blood pressure and serum potassium when VORICONAZOLE is started or stopped in patients receiving EPLERENONE. Adjust the EPLERENONE dose as needed.

Discussion

A 48-year-old bone marrow transplant recipient whose blood pressure had been adequately maintained while receiving a drug regimen that included eplerenone 50 mg daily, candesartan (*Atacand*), and nifedipine (eg, *Procardia*) developed hypotension 1 day after IV voriconazole was started.[1] All antihypertensive agents were discontinued immediately, and blood pressure control was restored. His antihypertensive regimen was restarted without eplerenone, which was no longer needed to control his hypertension. See also Eplerenone-Azole Antifungal Agents and Nifedipine-Azole Antifungal Agents.

[1] Kato J, et al. *Eur J Clin Pharmacol.* 2009;65(3):323.

* Asterisk indicates drugs cited in interaction reports.

Ergot Derivatives — *Azole Antifungal Agents*

Ergot Derivatives		Azole Antifungal Agents	
Dihydroergotamine* (eg, *D.H.E. 45*) Ergonovine* (*Ergotrate*)	Ergotamine*† Methylergonovine* (eg, *Methergine*)	Itraconazole* (eg, *Sporanox*) Ketoconazole* Posaconazole* (*Noxafil*)	Voriconazole* (eg, *Vfend*)

Significance	Onset	Severity	Documentation
1	□ Rapid ■ **Delayed**	■ **Major** □ Moderate □ Minor	□ Established □ Probable ■ **Suspected** □ Possible □ Unlikely

Effects The risk of ERGOT toxicity (eg, peripheral vasospasm, ischemia of the extremities) may be increased.

Mechanism AZOLE ANTIFUNGAL AGENTS inhibit the metabolism (CYP3A4) of ERGOT DERIVATIVES.

Management Coadministration of AZOLE ANTIFUNGAL AGENTS and ERGOT DERIVATIVES is contraindicated.

Discussion

Although not studied, coadministration of itraconazole,[1] ketoconazole,[2] posaconazole,[3] or voriconazole[4] with an ergot derivative may increase plasma concentrations of the ergot derivative, leading to ergotism. Do not coadminister ergot derivatives and these azole antifungal agents. In a study with 24 healthy volunteers, plasma levels of dihydroergotamine administered by inhalation† were the same when given alone or after receiving oral ketoconazole.[5]

The basis for this interaction is information on file with the manufacturers. Published clinical data are needed to further assess this interaction. Because of the seriousness of this interaction, clinical evaluation in humans is not likely to be forthcoming.

1 *Sporanox* [package insert]. Titusville, NJ: Janssen Pharmaceutica LP; January 2004.
2 *Methergine* [package insert]. East Hanover, NJ: Novartis Pharmaceuticals Corporation; 2006.
3 *Noxafil* [package insert]. Kenilworth, NJ: Schering Corporation; October 2006.
4 *Vfend* [package insert]. New York, NY: Pfizer Inc; November 2006.
5 Kellerman D, et al. *Cephalalgia*. 2012;32(2):150.

* Asterisk indicates drugs cited in interaction reports.
† Not available in the United States.

Ergot Derivatives — *Beta-Blockers*

Ergot Derivatives		Beta-Blockers	
Dihydroergotamine* (eg, *D.H.E. 45*) Ergotamine* (*Ergomar*)	Methysergide*†	Carteolol (eg, *Cartrol*) Nadolol (eg, *Corgard*) Penbutolol (*Levatol*)	Pindolol Propranolol* (eg, *Inderal LA*) Timolol

Significance	Onset	Severity	Documentation
2	☐ Rapid ■ **Delayed**	☐ Major ■ **Moderate** ☐ Minor	☐ Established ☐ Probable ■ **Suspected** ☐ Possible ☐ Unlikely

Effects Peripheral ischemia manifested by cold extremities; possible peripheral gangrene.

Mechanism ERGOT alkaloid-mediated vasoconstriction and BETA-BLOCKER–mediated blockade of peripheral beta-2 receptors allows for unopposed ERGOT action.

Management Monitor patients for signs of peripheral ischemia. Tailoring the ERGOT dosage and discontinuing the BETA-BLOCKER may be required.

Discussion

Propranolol produced a paradoxical response, exacerbating headaches in a 50-year-old man taking a combination of oral ergotamine-caffeine (eg, *Cafergot*) for migraine headaches. The headaches, which were refractory to ergot preparations, ceased after discontinuation of propranolol and returned upon rechallenge.[1] A 61-year-old man developed purple, painful feet with the use of *Cafergot* suppositories twice daily and propranolol 30 mg/day.[2] This resolved after discontinuation of propranolol. A subsequent letter to the editor[3] refuted the possibility of an interaction, reporting 50 instances in which the combination had been used with no problems. The dose of *Cafergot* used by the patients has also been questioned.[3] Two cases of peripheral ischemia resulting from combinations of ergot preparations and nonselective beta-blockers have been described.[4] While 1 case was successfully treated, the other required bilateral below-the-knee amputations. A 26-year-old woman taking propranolol for migraine prophylaxis developed hypertension and crushing substernal chest pain after receiving dihydroergotamine 0.75 mg IV.[5] The patient had hyperthyroidism without evidence of an MI and recovered uneventfully.

The data presented are not conclusive; however, caution is warranted.

[1] Blank NK, et al. *Lancet.* 1973;2(7841):1336.
[2] Baumrucker JF. *N Engl J Med.* 1973;288(17):916.
[3] Diamond S. *N Engl J Med.* 1973;289(3):159.
[4] Venter CP, et al. *Br Med J (Clin Res Ed).* 1984;289(6440):288.
[5] Gandy W. *Ann Emerg Med.* 1990;19(2):221.

* Asterisk indicates drugs cited in interaction reports. Based on pharmacologic and pharmacokinetic considerations, similar interactions may occur with other drugs that are listed.
† Not available in the United States.

Ergot Derivatives — *HCV Protease Inhibitors*

Ergot Derivatives		HCV Protease Inhibitors	
Dihydroergotamine* (eg, *D.H.E. 45*)	Methylergonovine* (eg, *Methergine*)	Boceprevir* (*Victrelis*)	Telaprevir* (*Incivek*)
Ergonovine*			
Ergotamine* (*Ergomar*)			

Significance	Onset	Severity	Documentation
1	□ Rapid	■ **Major**	□ Established
	■ **Delayed**	□ Moderate	□ Probable
		□ Minor	■ **Suspected**
			□ Possible
			□ Unlikely

Effects ERGOT DERIVATIVE plasma concentrations may be elevated, increasing the pharmacologic effects and risk of adverse reactions (eg, peripheral vasospasm, ischemia of the extremities).

Mechanism ERGOT DERIVATIVE metabolism (CYP3A) may be inhibited by HEPATITIS C VIRUS (HCV) PROTEASE INHIBITORS.

Management Coadministration of ERGOT DERIVATIVES and HCV PROTEASE INHIBITORS is contraindicated.[1,2]

Discussion

Concurrent use of strong CYP3A4 inhibitors, such as boceprevir, may elevate ergot derivative (eg, ergonovine) plasma concentrations, increasing the risk of serious adverse reactions (eg, acute ergot toxicity).[1,2] Concomitant use of ergot derivatives and boceprevir or telaprevir is contraindicated.

The basis for this monograph is information on file with the manufacturer. Published clinical data are needed to further assess this interaction. Because of the seriousness of the interaction, clinical evaluation in humans is not likely to be forthcoming.

[1] *Victrelis* [package insert]. Whitehouse Station, NJ: Schering Corporation; May 2011.

[2] *Incivek* [package insert]. Cambridge, MA: Vertex Pharmaceuticals Incorporated; May 2011.

* Asterisk indicates drugs cited in interaction reports.

Ergot Derivatives — *Macrolide & Related Antibiotics*

Ergot Derivatives		Macrolide & Related Antibiotics	
Dihydroergotamine* (eg, *D.H.E. 45*)	Ergotamine* (*Ergomar*)	Clarithromycin* (eg, *Biaxin*)	Telithromycin* (*Ketek*)
		Erythromycin* (eg, *Ery-Tab*)	Troleandomycin*†

Significance	Onset	Severity	Documentation
1	■ **Rapid**	■ **Major**	□ Established
	□ Delayed	□ Moderate	■ **Probable**
		□ Minor	□ Suspected
			□ Possible
			□ Unlikely

Effects Acute ergotism, manifesting as peripheral ischemia, has been reported with concomitant use of these agents.

Mechanism Interference of MACROLIDE AND RELATED ANTIBIOTICS with ERGOTAMINE hepatic metabolism is suspected.[1]

Management Monitor and counsel the patient to watch for signs of ergotism. The ERGOT preparation dosage may need to be decreased. One or both agents may require discontinuation. Sodium nitroprusside (*Nitropress*) has been beneficial in reducing MACROLIDE-ERGOT–induced vasospasm.[2]

Discussion

Ergotism associated with concomitant use of ergot preparations and the macrolide antibiotics troleandomycin,[1-6] erythromycin,[7-11] and clarithromycin[12,13] has been reported in 18 patients. These cases similarly report low ergot dosages and clinically severe vasospasm, regardless of the order in which they were ingested. The interaction has been reported with ergot dosages as low as 0.4 mg/day and as high as 30 mg/day. While most patients recover with treatment, including sodium nitroprusside, nitroglycerin IV (eg, *Nitro-Bid*), prazosin (eg, *Minipress*), nifedipine (eg, *Procardia*), or captopril, 1 patient required limb amputation, and 4 manifested continued paresthesia. Because of the low dosages implicated, it has been suggested that this interaction occurs more frequently than reported; however, it may be attributed to single doses of ergot preparation. Coadministration of telithromycin and an ergot derivative is not recommended.[14]

1 Hayton AC. *N Z Med J.* 1969;69(440):42.
2 Matthews NT, et al. *N Z Med J.* 1979;89(638):476.
3 Bigorie B, et al. *Nouv Presse Med.* 1975;4(38):2723.
4 Franco A, et al. *Nouv Presse Med.* 1978;7(3):205.
5 Vayssairat M, et al. *Nouv Presse Med.* 1978;7(23):2077.
6 Chignier E, et al. *Nouv Presse Med.* 1978;7(28):2478.
7 Boucharlat J, et al. *Ann Med Psychol (Paris).* 1980;138(3):292.
8 Neveux E, et al. *Nouv Presse Med.* 1981;10(34):2830.
9 Collet AM, et al. *Sem Hop.* 1982;58(26-27):1624.
10 Francis H, et al. *Clin Rheumatol.* 1984;3(2):243.
11 Ghali R, et al. *Ann Vasc Surg.* 1993;7(3):291.
12 Horowitz RS, et al. *Arch Intern Med.* 1996;156(4):456.
13 Ausband SC, et al. *J Emerg Med.* 2001;21(4):411.
14 *Ketek* [package insert]. Kansas City, MO: Aventis Pharmaceuticals Inc; June 2004.

* Asterisk indicates drugs cited in interaction reports.
† Not available in the United States.

Ergot Derivatives — *Mifepristone*

Ergot Derivatives		Mifepristone
Dihydroergotamine* (eg, *D.H.E. 45*)	Methylergonovine (eg, *Methergine*)	Mifepristone* (eg, *Korlym*)
Ergotamine* (*Ergomar*)		

Significance	Onset	Severity	Documentation
1	☐ Rapid	■ **Major**	☐ Established
	■ **Delayed**	☐ Moderate	☐ Probable
		☐ Minor	■ **Suspected**
			☐ Possible
			☐ Unlikely

Effects ERGOT DERIVATIVE plasma concentrations may be elevated, increasing the pharmacologic effects and risk of toxicity (eg, peripheral vasospasm, ischemia of the extremities).

Mechanism MIFEPRISTONE may inhibit ERGOT DERIVATIVE metabolism (CYP3A4).

Management Coadministration of DIHYDROERGOTAMINE or ERGOTAMINE with MIFEPRISTONE is contraindicated.[1]

Discussion

Because mifepristone inhibits CYP3A4, coadministration of mifepristone with a drug that is metabolized mainly or solely by CYP3A4 (eg, dihydroergotamine, ergotamine) is likely to increase plasma concentrations of the drug.[1] Therefore, the concurrent use of drugs with a narrow therapeutic index that are CYP3A4 substrates, such as dihydroergotamine and ergotamine, is contraindicated. The risk of ergotamine toxicity (eg, peripheral vasospasm, ischemia of the extremities) may be increased.

[1] *Korlym* [package insert]. Menlo Park, CA: Corcept Therapeutics Incorporated; February 2012.

* Asterisk indicates drugs cited in interaction reports. Based on pharmacologic and pharmacokinetic considerations, similar interactions may occur with other drugs that are listed.

Ergot Derivatives — *Nitrates*

Ergot Derivatives	Nitrates	
Dihydroergotamine* (eg, *D.H.E. 45*)	Amyl Nitrite (eg, *Amyl Nitrite Aspirols*)	Nitroglycerin* (eg, *Nitro-Bid*)
	Isosorbide Dinitrate* (eg, *Isordil*)	

Significance	Onset	Severity	Documentation
2	■ **Rapid**	□ Major	□ Established
	□ Delayed	■ **Moderate**	□ Probable
		□ Minor	■ **Suspected**
			□ Possible
			□ Unlikely

Effects The bioavailability of DIHYDROERGOTAMINE (oral form not available in US) may be increased, resulting in an increase in mean standing systolic BP. Functional antagonism between DIHYDROERGOTAMINE and NITROGLYCERIN may decrease the antianginal effects.

Mechanism NITROGLYCERIN, through increasing splanchnic blood flow, decreases the first-pass metabolism of DIHYDROERGOTAMINE, increasing its bioavailability. DIHYDROERGOTAMINE antagonizes coronary vasodilation.[1]

Management Increasing plasma concentrations of DIHYDROERGOTAMINE predisposes a patient to ergotism. DIHYDROERGOTAMINE dosages may need to be decreased. Monitor patients and counsel for signs of peripheral ischemia.

Discussion

The effects of oral nitroglycerin (1,200 mcg) on the bioavailability of oral dihydroergotamine were studied in 4 patients treated for autonomic insufficiency and postural hypotension.[2] Plasma dihydroergotamine levels and AUC increased with concomitant use when compared with dihydroergotamine alone; AUC increased 56% to 370%. Excretion was not altered. Standing systolic BP increased by a mean of 27% (most prominent 2 hr after dihydroergotamine dosing). IV dihydroergotamine antagonized coronary vasodilation.[1] Use caution with simultaneous use of dihydroergotamine and nitroglycerin in patients with angina pectoris.[3] In a subsequent study of the efficacy of nitroglycerin in dogs pretreated with dihydroergotamine, the antianginal effect of nitroglycerin was not affected by pretreatment with dihydroergotamine.[4] This is supported by findings that nitroglycerin and isosorbide dinitrate are effective antianginal agents in patients with ergot-induced ECG anomalies.[5]

1 Raberger G, et al. *Basic Res Cardiol.* 1976;71:645.
2 Bobik A, et al. *Clin Pharmacol Ther.* 1981;30:673.
3 Sievert H, et al. [in German]. *Dtsch Med Wochenschr.* 1986;111:1245.
4 Schneider W, et al. *Br J Pharmacol.* 1987;92:87.
5 Wendkos MH. *Am J Med Sci.* 1967;253:9.

* Asterisk indicates drugs cited in interaction reports. Based on pharmacologic and pharmacokinetic considerations, similar interactions may occur with other drugs that are listed.

Ergot Derivatives — *NNRT Inhibitors*

Dihydroergotamine* (eg, *D.H.E. 45*)	Ergotamine* (*Ergomar*)	Delavirdine* (*Rescriptor*)	Efavirenz* (*Sustiva*)

Significance	Onset	Severity	Documentation
1	□ Rapid ■ **Delayed**	■ **Major** □ Moderate □ Minor	□ Established □ Probable ■ **Suspected** □ Possible □ Unlikely

Effects The risk of ergot toxicity (peripheral vasospasm, ischemia of the extremities) may be increased.

Mechanism NON-NUCLEOSIDE REVERSE TRANSCRIPTASE (NNRT) INHIBITORS may interfere with the hepatic metabolism (CYP3A4) of the ERGOT DERIVATIVES.

Management Do not administer ERGOT DERIVATIVES concomitantly with NNRT INHIBITORS.

Discussion

Because of possible competition for metabolism, do not use ergot derivatives in patients receiving delavirdine or efavirenz.[1,2] Coadministration of delavirdine or efavirenz and an ergot preparation may lead to increased plasma concentrations of the ergot derivative and create the potential for serious adverse reactions (eg, ergotism).

The basis for this monograph is information on file with the manufacturers. Published clinical data are needed to further assess this interaction; however, because of the seriousness of this interaction, clinical evaluation in humans is not likely to be forthcoming.

[1] *Rescriptor* [package insert]. La Jolla, CA: Agouron Pharmaceuticals Inc.; April 1997.

[2] *Sustiva* [package insert]. Princeton, NJ: Bristol-Myers Squibb; September 1998.

* Asterisk indicates drugs cited in interaction reports.

Ergot Derivatives / *Protease Inhibitors*

Ergot Derivatives		Protease Inhibitors	
Dihydroergotamine* (eg, *D.H.E. 45*)	Methylergonovine* (eg, *Methergine*)	Amprenavir*	Lopinavir/Ritonavir* (*Kaletra*)
Ergonovine*		Atazanavir* (*Reyataz*)	Nelfinavir* (*Viracept*)
Ergotamine* (*Ergomar*)		Darunavir* (*Prezista*)	Ritonavir* (*Norvir*)
		Fosamprenavir* (*Lexiva*)	Saquinavir* (*Invirase*)
		Indinavir* (*Crixivan*)	

Significance	Onset	Severity	Documentation
1	☐ Rapid	■ **Major**	☐ Established
	■ **Delayed**	☐ Moderate	■ **Probable**
		☐ Minor	☐ Suspected
			☐ Possible
			☐ Unlikely

Effects The risk of ERGOT toxicity (peripheral vasospasm, ischemia of the extremities) may be increased.

Mechanism PROTEASE INHIBITORS may interfere with the hepatic metabolism (CYP3A4) of ERGOT DERIVATIVES.

Management Coadministration of PROTEASE INHIBITORS and ERGOT DERIVATIVES is contraindicated.[1-8]

Discussion

Ergot toxicity was reported in a 63-year-old man during coadministration of ergotamine and ritonavir.[9] The patient had been taking ergotamine tartrate 1 to 2 mg/day for 5 years when he was diagnosed with HIV and treated with ritonavir 600 mg every 12 hours. Ten days after starting treatment, he experienced subacute pain, paresthesia, skin paleness alternating with areas of cyanosis, and coldness in both arms. Ritonavir and ergotamine were stopped and his symptoms disappeared. A 40-year-old woman receiving nelfinavir developed ergotism (cyanosis and pain or edema of her extremities) on 2 occasions following self-administration of ergotamine for migraines.[10] Ergotism developed in 12 to 24 hours and resolved within 15 days. Additional cases of ergotism have been reported during coadministration of ergotamine and antiviral regimens, including indinavir,[11] ritonavir,[12,13] and ritonavir plus nelfinavir.[14] Death has been reported.[15] A 34-year-old woman infected with HIV receiving ritonavir 600 mg every 12 hours developed signs of severe vascular involvement and irreversible coma after receiving ergotamine 3 mg.[16]

[1] *Norvir* [package insert]. Abbott Park, IL: Abbott Laboratories; September 2001.
[2] *Fortovase* [package insert]. Nutley, NJ: Roche Pharmaceuticals; November 1997.
[3] *Agenerase* [package insert]. Research Triangle Park, NC: GlaxoSmithKline; April 1999.
[4] *Kaletra* [package insert]. Abbott Park, IL: Abbott Laboratories; September 2000.
[5] *Viracept* [package insert]. La Jolla, CA: Agouron Pharmaceuticals, Inc; December 2002.
[6] *Reyataz* [package insert]. Princeton, NJ: Bristol-Myers Squibb; June 2003.
[7] *Prezista* [package insert]. Raritan, NJ: Tibotec Therapeutics; June 2006.
[8] *Lexiva* [package insert]. Research Triangle Park, NC: GlaxoSmithKline; April 2010.
[9] Caballero-Granado FJ, et al. *Antimicrob Agents Chemother.* 1997;41(5):1207.
[10] Mortier E, et al. *Am J Med.* 2001;110(7):594.
[11] Rosenthal E, et al. *JAMA.* 1999;281(11):987.
[12] Liaudet L, et al. *BMJ.* 1999;318(7186):771.
[13] Vila A, et al. *Scand J Infect Dis.* 2001;33(10):788.
[14] Mitchell PB, et al. *Med J Aust.* 1999;171(9):502.
[15] Tribble MA, et al. *Headache.* 2002;42(7):694.
[16] Pardo Rey C, et al. *Clin Infect Dis.* 2003;37(5):e72.

* Asterisk indicates drugs cited in interaction reports.

Erlotinib — Proton Pump Inhibitors

Erlotinib	Proton Pump Inhibitors	
Erlotinib* (*Tarceva*)	Esomeprazole* (*Nexium*)	Pantoprazole* (eg, *Protonix*)
	Lansoprazole* (eg, *Prevacid*)	Rabeprazole* (*Aciphex*)
	Omeprazole* (eg, *Prilosec*)	

Significance	Onset	Severity	Documentation
2	□ Rapid ■ **Delayed**	□ Major ■ **Moderate** □ Minor	□ Established □ Probable ■ **Suspected** □ Possible □ Unlikely

Effects ERLOTINIB plasma concentrations may be reduced, decreasing the pharmacologic effects.

Mechanism Decreased solubility and absorption of ERLOTINIB.

Management If coadministration cannot be avoided, use the lowest effective dose of the PROTON PUMP INHIBITOR and closely monitor ERLOTINIB plasma concentrations and adjust the dose as needed. An alternative agent to suppress the pH of the upper GI tract may be needed.

Discussion

A 46-year-old woman with stage 4 non–small cell lung cancer was started on erlotinib 150 mg once daily as palliative therapy.[1] Subsequently, she reported a retrosternal burning sensation and was started on high-dose pantoprazole 8 mg/hr by continuous infusion. After 2 days, she was switched to oral pantoprazole 40 mg twice daily. During treatment with pantoprazole by continuous infusion, there was a drastic decrease in erlotinib concentrations to low and subtherapeutic levels. However, after changing to oral administration of omeprazole, erlotinib plasma concentrations returned to therapeutic values. Coadministration of erlotinib with omeprazole has been reported to decrease erlotinib AUC 46%. Because proton pump inhibitors affect the pH of the upper GI tract for an extended period, separating the administration times may not eliminate the interaction.[2] Avoid coadministration of erlotinib and proton pump inhibitors if possible.

1 Ter Heine R, et al. *Br J Clin Pharmacol.* 2010;70(6):908.

2 *Tarceva* [package insert]. Melville, NY: OSI Pharmaceuticals Inc; April 2010.

* Asterisk indicates drugs cited in interaction reports.

Erlotinib — *Rifamycins*

Erlotinib* (*Tarceva*)	Rifabutin* (*Mycobutin*) Rifampin* (eg, *Rifadin*)	Rifapentine* (*Priftin*)

Significance	Onset	Severity	Documentation
2	☐ Rapid ■ **Delayed**	☐ Major ■ **Moderate** ☐ Minor	☐ Established ☐ Probable ■ **Suspected** ☐ Possible ☐ Unlikely

Effects ERLOTINIB plasma concentrations may be reduced, decreasing the therapeutic effects.

Mechanism RIFAMYCINS may induce the metabolism (CYP3A4) of ERLOTINIB.

Management In patients receiving ERLOTINIB, consider alternative therapy with a drug that does not induce metabolism.[1] If alternative therapy is not available, consider increasing the dose of ERLOTINIB.

Discussion

In patients pretreated with rifampin, the AUC of erlotinib was reduced approximately 67%.[1] Consider treatment using an agent that does not induce erlotinib metabolism. If such treatment is not available, consider using a dose greater than erlotinib 150 mg.[1] It will be necessary to reduce the dose of erlotinib when rifampin therapy is discontinued.

Other CYP3A4 inducers, including carbamazepine (eg, *Tegretol*), phenobarbital (eg, *Luminal*), phenytoin (eg, *Dilantin*), and St. John's wort, may interact similarly.

[1] *Tarceva* [package insert]. Melville, NY: OSI Pharmaceuticals Inc; 2004.

* Asterisk indicates drugs cited in interaction reports.

Erythromycin — *Antacids*

Erythromycin	Antacids
Erythromycin Stearate*	Aluminum/Magnesium Hydroxide/Simethicone* (eg, *Mylanta*)

Significance	Onset	Severity	Documentation
5	■ **Rapid**	□ Major	□ Established
	□ Delayed	□ Moderate	□ Probable
		■ **Minor**	□ Suspected
			■ **Possible**
			□ Unlikely

Effects The pharmacologic effects of ERYTHROMYCIN may be increased.

Mechanism Unknown.

Management No special precautions appear to be necessary.

Discussion

Eight healthy adult volunteers participated in a randomized, crossover study evaluating the effect of antacid administration on the pharmacokinetics of erythromycin stearate.[1] All subjects received erythromycin 500 mg alone or with 30 mL of an antacid containing aluminum hydroxide 200 mg, magnesium hydroxide 200 mg and simethicone 20 mg per 5 mL. When they received both agents, the antacid was administered immediately after erythromycin. Individuals were crossed over to receive the alternate treatment after a 1-week washout period. Venous blood samples were obtained at various intervals for 12 hours following drug administration and the concentrations of erythromycin were determined. In addition, time to peak concentration, peak serum concentration, total area under the concentration-time curve and the elimination rate constant were determined for each phase of the investigation. Concurrent administration of erythromycin and antacid did not affect the time to peak concentration, peak serum concentration or total area under the concentration-time curve; however, there was a significant ($P < 0.02$) decrease in the mean elimination rate constant when erythromycin was given alone compared with erythromycin plus antacid (0.44 vs 0.2 hr^{-1}).

Because this was a single-dose investigation, additional studies are needed to determine the clinical significance of this finding in patients receiving a therapeutic course of erythromycin.

[1] Yamreudeewong W, et al. *Clin Pharm.* 1989;8:352.

* Asterisk indicates drugs cited in interaction reports.

Erythromycin — *Ethanol*

Erythromycin Ethylsuccinate* (eg, *E.E.S.*)	Ethanol*

Significance	Onset	Severity	Documentation
5	■ **Rapid**	□ Major	□ Established
	□ Delayed	□ Moderate	□ Probable
		■ **Minor**	□ Suspected
			□ Possible
			■ **Unlikely**

Effects The clinical effects of ERYTHROMYCIN ETHYLSUCCINATE may be decreased and delayed.

Mechanism ETHANOL may slow gastric emptying, delaying absorption of ERYTHROMYCIN ETHYLSUCCINATE.

Management It would be prudent to advise patients to avoid ingestion of ERYTHROMYCIN ETHYLSUCCINATE with ETHANOL.

Discussion

The effects of alcohol ingestion on the pharmacokinetics of erythromycin ethylsuccinate, 500 mg, were studied in nine healthy volunteers.[1] Compared with water, taking the antibiotic with alcohol decreased the area under the plasma concentration-time curve (AUC) of erythromycin ethylsuccinate by nearly 27% and decreased the peak serum concentration by 15%. In one subject, ingestion of the antibiotic with ethanol resulted in a 184% increase in the AUC of erythromycin.

[1] Morasso MI, et al. *Int J Clin Pharmacol Ther Toxicol.* 1990;28:426.

* Asterisk indicates drugs cited in interaction reports.

Estrogens — *Ascorbic Acid*

Ethinyl Estradiol* (*Estinyl*)	Ascorbic Acid* (eg, *Cevalin*)

Significance	Onset	Severity	Documentation
5	☐ Rapid	☐ Major	☐ Established
	■ **Delayed**	☐ Moderate	☐ Probable
		■ **Minor**	☐ Suspected
			■ **Possible**
			☐ Unlikely

Effects ASCORBIC ACID appears to increase plasma levels of ESTROGENS.

Mechanism Competitive inhibition of intestinal sulphation in the gut wall during absorption increases overall bioavailability of ESTROGENS.[2,4]

Management No clinically significant sequelae have been reported to date. Breakthrough bleeding has been reported in one patient. It was suggested that abrupt discontinuation of ASCORBIC ACID may prompt contraceptive failure. More definitive data are needed.

Discussion

Initially, Briggs[1] noted decreased leukocyte and platelet ascorbic acid levels in women taking oral contraceptives. A single dose trial in five women showed that 1 g ascorbic acid was associated with significantly higher plasma ethinyl estradiol concentrations.[2] Briggs subsequently compared 50 mg ascorbic acid with 1,000 mg in 2 groups of women to assess biological consequences. Over 2 months, patients took ascorbic acid daily; the second month was a crossover period. Significant differences in HDL, fibrinogen, Factor VII, Factor VIII, sex hormone binding globulin and ceruloplasmin were noted.[4] The clinical significance of these differences is unknown. Morris et al[3] describe breakthrough bleeding occurring in a patient on oral contraceptives who self-administered ascorbic acid 1 g for a cold. It was suggested that the breakthrough bleeding may have been a "withdrawal" effect because of decreasing estrogen levels when the ascorbic acid was discontinued. Plasma estrogen levels were not measured; however, the risk of contraceptive failure was a concern mentioned by the author.

1 Briggs MH, et al. *Nature.* 1972;238:277.
2 Back DJ. *Br Med J.* 1981;282:1516.
3 Morris JC, et al. *Br Med J.* 1981;283:503.
4 Briggs MH. *Br Med J.* 1981;283:1547.

* Asterisk indicates drugs cited in interaction reports.

Estrogens — *Barbiturates*

Estrogens		Barbiturates	
Conjugated Estrogens (eg, *Premarin*)	Estrone	Amobarbital (*Amytal*)	Pentobarbital
Esterified Estrogens (*Menest*)	Estropipate (eg, *Ogen*)	Butabarbital (eg, *Butisol*)	Phenobarbital* (eg, *Solfoton*)
Estradiol (eg, *Estrace*)	Ethinyl Estradiol*	Butalbital	Primidone (eg, *Mysoline*)
	Mestranol	Mephobarbital (*Mebaral*)	Secobarbital (*Seconal*)

Significance	Onset	Severity	Documentation
2	☐ Rapid ■ **Delayed**	☐ Major ■ **Moderate** ☐ Minor	☐ Established ☐ Probable ■ **Suspected** ☐ Possible ☐ Unlikely

Effects Contraceptive failure has been reported.[1-3] ORAL CONTRACEPTIVES (OCs) may worsen or stabilize epilepsy.[4-6]

Mechanism Induction of hepatic microsomal enzymes by BARBITURATES increases elimination of estrogenic substances, decreasing plasma concentration. OC-induced water retention may exacerbate seizures.[5,6]

Management Alternate methods of contraception are recommended[7]; ethinyl estradiol 80 mcg may give good cycle control.[8-10]

Discussion

The effect of OCs on seizure control are unconfirmed, with some patients worsening and some stabilizing. The major concern is the efficacy of OCs in preventing conception. Failure rates of OCs are higher in women taking antiepileptic agents with enzyme-inducing potential. In rats and humans, phenobarbital was shown to stimulate metabolism of estrogen compounds.[3,11] Also noted was a decreased rate of absorption as well as decreased AUC of estrogen by phenobarbital in rats.[12] Phenobarbital decreases plasma estrogen levels and increases sex hormone–binding globulins, thus decreasing unbound hormone.[3] Breakthrough bleeding and spotting are initial signs of contraceptive failure.[9,13] OC doses may be increased to estradiol 50 or 80 mcg, or alternative contraceptive measures may be considered. See also Contraceptives, Oral-Barbiturates.

[1] Janz D, et al. *Lancet.* 1974;1:1113.
[2] Coulam CB, et al. *Epilepsia.* 1979;20:519.
[3] Back DJ, et al. *Contraception.* 1980;22:495.
[4] Copeman H. *Med J Aust.* 1963;2:969.
[5] Anon. *Br Med J.* 1967;3:162.
[6] Espir M, et al. *Br Med J.* 1969;1:294.
[7] Laengner H, et al. *Lancet.* 1974;2:600.
[8] Anon. *Br Med J.* 1980;2:93.
[9] Back DJ, et al. *Drugs.* 1981;21:46.
[10] Mattson RH, et al. *JAMA.* 1986;256:238.
[11] Welch RM, et al. *J Pharmacol Exp Ther.* 1968;160:171.
[12] Dada OA, et al. *J Steroid Biochem.* 1983;19:821.
[13] Roberton YR, et al. *Curr Med Res Opin.* 1976;3:647.

* Asterisk indicates drugs cited in interaction reports. Based on pharmacologic and pharmacokinetic considerations, similar interactions may occur with other drugs that are listed.

Estrogens — *Bosentan*

Conjugated Estrogens (eg, *Premarin*)	Estropipate (eg, *Ogen*)	Bosentan* (*Tracleer*)
Esterified Estrogens	Ethinyl Estradiol*	
Estradiol (eg, *Estrace*)		

Significance	Onset	Severity	Documentation
1	☐ Rapid	■ **Major**	☐ Established
	■ **Delayed**	☐ Moderate	☐ Probable
		☐ Minor	■ **Suspected**
			☐ Possible
			☐ Unlikely

Effects BOSENTAN may impair the efficacy of ESTROGENS.

Mechanism Increased hepatic metabolism (CYP3A4) of ESTROGENS is suspected.

Management Inform women of the increased risk of ORAL CONTRACEPTIVE failure. Consider an alternative nonhormonal or additional method of contraception.

Discussion

The effect of bosentan on the pharmacokinetics of an oral contraceptive containing ethinyl estradiol 35 mcg plus norethindrone 1 mg was evaluated in 19 healthy women.[1] Using a randomized, crossover design, each woman received a single dose of the oral contraceptive alone and after 7 days of pretreatment with bosentan 125 mg twice daily. Compared with taking the oral contraceptive alone, bosentan administration reduced the AUC of norethindrone nearly 14% and ethinyl estradiol 31%, respectively. The maximum decrease in AUC of norethindrone and ethinyl estradiol in an individual subject was 56% and 66%, respectively. In the subject with the largest decrease in norethindrone AUC, ethinyl estradiol levels could not be measured. The C_{max} of the oral contraceptive components was not affected by bosentan.

[1] van Giersbergen PL, et al. *Int J Clin Pharmacol Ther.* 2006;44:113.

* Asterisk indicates drugs cited in interaction reports. Based on pharmacologic and pharmacokinetic considerations, similar interactions may occur with other drugs that are listed.

Estrogens — *Cimetidine*

Conjugated Estrogens (eg, *Premarin*)	Estrone	Cimetidine* (eg, *Tagamet*)
Esterified Estrogens (*Menest*)	Estropipate (*Ogen*)	
Estradiol* (eg, *Estrace*)	Ethinyl Estradiol	
	Mestranol	

Significance	Onset	Severity	Documentation
5	■ **Rapid**	□ Major	□ Established
	□ Delayed	□ Moderate	□ Probable
		■ **Minor**	□ Suspected
			■ **Possible**
			□ Unlikely

Effects CIMETIDINE elevates plasma ESTRADIOL concentrations in certain patients.

Mechanism Possible inhibition of oxidative metabolism of ESTROGENS by CIMETIDINE.

Management No special precautions appear necessary.

Discussion

The effects of cimetidine or ranitidine (eg, *Zantac*) treatment on estradiol biodisposition was studied in male patients.[1,2] Short-term parenteral administration of cimetidine as well as 2 weeks of oral cimetidine decreased the hepatic 2-hydroxylation of a test dose of estradiol.[2] The effect on hydroxylation also occurred to an equal degree with administration of cimetidine as either 400 or 800 mg twice daily.[1] Consequently, serum estradiol concentrations were elevated in both studies. In contrast, ranitidine did not affect estradiol biodisposition. Similar results were reported in women.[3] Estradiol hydroxylation was reduced in pre- and postmenopausal women when they received cimetidine 1,200 to 2,400 mg daily for 4 weeks. Serum estradiol levels increased from 30 to 60 pg/mL in postmenopausal women but did not change in premenopausal women. However, levels in postmenopausal women remained below those measured in the premenopausal group. The clinical importance of these effects is unknown.

[1] Galbraith RA, et al. *N Engl J Med.* 1989;321:269.
[2] Galbraith RA, et al. *Trans Assoc Am Physicians.* 1989;102:44.
[3] Michnovicz JJ, et al. *Metabolism.* 1991;40:170.

* Asterisk indicates drugs cited in interaction reports. Based on pharmacologic and pharmacokinetic considerations, similar interactions may occur with other drugs that are listed.

Estrogens | **Food**

Estradiol* (eg, *Estrace*)	Ethinyl Estradiol*	Grapefruit Juice*
Estrone*		

Significance	Onset	Severity	Documentation
5	■ **Rapid**	□ Major	□ Established
	□ Delayed	□ Moderate	□ Probable
		■ **Minor**	□ Suspected
			■ **Possible**
			□ Unlikely

Effects Serum ESTROGEN concentrations may be increased slightly.

Mechanism Possible inhibition of ESTROGEN metabolism (CYP-450 3A4).

Management Based on available data, no special precautions are needed.

Discussion

The effects of grapefruit juice on the bioavailability of a single oral dose of ethinyl estradiol 50 mcg were studied in 13 healthy women utilizing an open, randomized, crossover design.[1] When compared with herbal tea, grapefruit juice increased peak ethinyl estradiol concentrations 37% and the AUC 28%. In another open, randomized, crossover study in 8 ovariectomized women, grapefruit juice inhibited the metabolism of 17β-estradiol.[2] A single oral dose of micronized 17β-estradiol 2 mg was taken with and without grapefruit juice. Ingestion of grapefruit juice resulted in an increase in the AUC of combined estrogens (eg, 17β-estradiol and estrone). There was considerable interindividual variability.

[1] Weber A, et al. *Contraception.* 1996;53:41.

[2] Schubert W, et al. *Maturitas.* 1994;20:155.

* Asterisk indicates drugs cited in interaction reports.

Estrogens — *Hydantoins*

Conjugated Estrogens* (*Premarin*)	Estradiol (eg, *Estrace*)	Ethotoin (*Peganone*)	Phenytoin* (eg, *Dilantin*)
Esterified Estrogens (*Menest*)	Estropipate (eg, *Ogen*)	Fosphenytoin (*Cerebyx*)	

Significance	Onset	Severity	Documentation
2	☐ Rapid ■ **Delayed**	☐ Major ■ **Moderate** ☐ Minor	☐ Established ☐ Probable ■ **Suspected** ☐ Possible ☐ Unlikely

Effects Breakthrough bleeding, spotting, and pregnancy have resulted when these medications were used concurrently.[1-6] A loss of seizure control also has been suggested[7,8] but not confirmed.[9,10]

Mechanism Induction of hepatic microsomal enzymes, leading to increased metabolism of ESTROGEN compounds, has been suggested. Fluid retention may explain loss of seizure control. Protein binding of PHENYTOIN may be affected.[8,11,12]

Management Monitor patients for loss of seizure control. Increased doses of ESTRADIOL (ie, 50 or 80 mcg) may provide adequate cycle control[7,13]; however, consider alternate methods of contraception.

Discussion

Phenytoin enzyme induction is an accepted characteristic of this medication. Estrogenic substances are subject to enzyme induction; patients may have decreased estrogen plasma levels. Reviews of literature,[4,14,15] in addition to the cases cited previously, advocate caution in patients on concurrent therapy. Watch patients for breakthrough seizures. Bleeding, spotting, or amenorrhea are initial signals of contraceptive failure; estradiol 50 to 80 mcg may provide adequate control. However, advise patients of risks and counsel them to use alternative methods of contraception. See also Contraceptives, Hormonal-Hydantoins.

[1] Kenyon IE. *Br Med J.* 1972;1(5801):686.
[2] Janz D, et al. *Lancet.* 1974;1(7866):1113.
[3] Laengner H, et al. *Lancet.* 1974;2(7880):600.
[4] Coulam CB, et al. *Epilepsia.* 1979;20(5):519.
[5] Notelovitz M, et al. *N Engl J Med.* 1981;304(13):788.
[6] Haukkamaa M. *Contraception.* 1986;33(6):559.
[7] McArthur J. *Br Med J.* 1967;3:162.
[8] Kutt H, et al. *JAMA.* 1968;203(11):969.
[9] Copeman H. *Med J Aust.* 1963;2:969.
[10] Espir M, et al. *Br Med J.* 1969;1(5639):294.
[11] Hooper WD, et al. *Clin Pharmacol Ther.* 1973;15(3):276.
[12] DeLeacy EA, et al. *Br J Clin Pharmacol.* 1979;8:33.
[13] Mattson RH, et al. *JAMA.* 1986;256(2):238.
[14] Roberton YR, et al. *Curr Med Res Opin.* 1976;3(9):647.
[15] Anon. *Br Med J.* 1980;2:93.

* Asterisk indicates drugs cited in interaction reports. Based on pharmacologic and pharmacokinetic considerations, similar interactions may occur with other drugs that are listed.

Estrogens — *Modafinil*

Ethinyl Estradiol* (eg, *Femhrt*)	Modafinil* (*Provigil*)

Significance	Onset	Severity	Documentation
2	☐ Rapid	☐ Major	☐ Established
	■ **Delayed**	■ **Moderate**	☐ Probable
		☐ Minor	■ **Suspected**
			☐ Possible
			☐ Unlikely

Effects The efficacy of ESTROGENS may be impaired.

Mechanism Induction of GI (major) and hepatic (minor) metabolism (CYP3A4/5) of ETHINYL ESTRADIOL by MODAFINIL is suspected.

Management Inform women of the increased risk of ESTROGEN failure. An increased dose of ETHINYL ESTRADIOL may be needed for ESTROGEN replacement therapy.

Discussion

The effects of daily administration of modafinil on the pharmacokinetics of steady-state ethinyl estradiol were studied in 41 healthy women.[1] In a randomized, placebo-controlled, single-blind, single-period study, each subject was randomized to 1 of 2 treatment groups. The treatment spanned 2 consecutive 28-day menstrual cycles plus the first week of the third cycle (ie, 9 weeks). During this time, all subjects received a daily dose of an oral contraceptive containing ethinyl estradiol plus norgestimate. Starting on day 6, 7, or 8 of the second cycle, subjects received modafinil 200 mg/day for 7 days, followed by 400 mg/day for 21 days, taken with the subject's daily dose of the oral contraceptive. The protocol for the second group was the same as for the first, except subjects received matching placebo in place of modafinil for 28 days. Thirty-nine subjects completed the study. Modafinil administration decreased the mean AUC of ethinyl estradiol 18% compared with a 4% decrease with placebo, and decreased the mean peak plasma concentration 11% compared with 5% with placebo. See Contraceptives, Hormonal-Modafinil.

[1] Robertson P Jr, et al. *Clin Pharmacol Ther.* 2002;71(1):46.

* Asterisk indicates drugs cited in interaction reports.

Estrogens — *NNRT Inhibitors*

Estrogens	NNRT Inhibitors	
Ethinyl Estradiol*	Efavirenz (*Sustiva*)	Nevirapine* (*Viramune*)

Significance	Onset	Severity	Documentation
4	☐ Rapid	■ **Major**	☐ Established
	■ **Delayed**	☐ Moderate	☐ Probable
		☐ Minor	☐ Suspected
			■ **Possible**
			☐ Unlikely

Effects The efficacy of ESTROGENS may be reduced, increasing the incidence of menstrual abnormalities.

Mechanism Increased hepatic metabolism of ESTROGENS by NONNUCLEOSIDE REVERSE TRANSCRIPTASE (NNRT) INHIBITORS is suspected.

Management Inform women of the increased risk of ORAL CONTRACEPTIVE failure. Use an alternative nonhormonal or additional method of contraception. For indications other than contraception (eg, endometriosis), an adjustment of the ESTROGEN dose may be necessary.

Discussion

The effects of nevirapine on the pharmacokinetics of ethinyl estradiol 1 mg plus norethindrone 35 mcg (eg, *Ortho-Novum 1/35*) were evaluated in 10 HIV-1–infected women.[1] Each patient received nevirapine 200 mg once daily on days 2 to 15, followed by 200 mg twice daily on days 16 through 29. On days 0 and 30, single doses of ethinyl estradiol/norethindrone were administered. Coadministration of nevirapine with ethinyl estradiol/norethindrone reduced the median AUC of ethinyl estradiol 29%, decreased the terminal $t_{1/2}$ (from 15.7 to 11.6 hours), and reduced the mean residence time (from 16.1 to 11.7 hours). In addition, nevirapine decreased the AUC of norethindrone 18%. The steady-state pharmacokinetics of nevirapine were not altered by ethinyl estradiol/norethindrone administration.

[1] Mildvan D, et al. *J Acquir Immune Defic Syndr.* 2002;29(5):471.

* Asterisk indicates drugs cited in interaction reports. Based on pharmacologic and pharmacokinetic considerations, similar interactions may occur with other drugs that are listed.

Estrogens | **Rifamycins**

Conjugated Estrogens (*Premarin*)	Estrogenic Substance (eg, *Gynogen*)	Rifabutin (*Mycobutin*)	Rifapentine (*Priftin*)
Diethylstilbestrol (DES)	Estrone (eg, *Kestrone 5*)	Rifampin* (eg, *Rifadin*)	
Esterified Estrogens (eg, *Estratab*)	Estropipate (eg, *Ogen*)		
Estradiol* (eg, *Estrace*)	Ethinyl Estradiol* (*Estinyl*)		
Estriol			

Significance	Onset	Severity	Documentation
2	☐ Rapid	☐ Major	☐ Established
	■ **Delayed**	■ **Moderate**	☐ Probable
		☐ Minor	■ **Suspected**
			☐ Possible
			☐ Unlikely

Effects RIFAMYCINS may impair the effectiveness of ESTROGENS; menstrual disturbances have been noted.[1,2,4,9]

Mechanism RIFAMYCINS induce drug metabolizing enzymes of ESTROGENS in the liver[3,5-9]; metabolism is increased 4-fold in vitro[5] and in vivo.[7] AUC and half-life also are decreased.[8]

Management Consider alternate methods of contraception or raising the ESTROGEN dose.

Discussion

Pregnancy[1,6] and menstrual disturbances[1,2,4] have been reported with concomitant use of oral contraceptives or estrogens and rifampin. Spotting, intermenstrual bleeding, or amenorrhea were reported in 62 of 88 patients; 5 pregnancies also were reported.[1] Data indicate increased hepatic hydroxylation is responsible for the decreased half-life and AUC, and increased elimination.[3,5,7-9] While both rifampin and rifabutin affect the pharmacokinetics of ethinyl estradiol, the magnitude of the effects is greater with rifampin.[10,11] See also Contraceptives, Oral-Rifampin.

1 Nocke-Finck L, et al. *JAMA*. 1973;226:378.
2 Cohn HD. *JAMA*. 1974;228:828.
3 Bolt HM, et al. *Lancet*. 1974;1:1280.
4 Altschuler SL, et al. *Obstet Gynecol*. 1974;44:771.
5 Bolt HM, et al. *Eur J Clin Pharmacol*. 1975;8:301.
6 Skolnick JL, et al. *JAMA*. 1976;236:1382.
7 Bolt HM, et al. *Acta Endocrinol*. 1977;85:189.
8 Back DJ, et al. *Contraception*. 1980;21:135.
9 Joshi JV, et al. *Contraception*. 1980;21:617.
10 LeBel M, et al. *J Clin Pharmacol*. 1998;38:1042.
11 Barditch-Crovo P, et al. *Clin Pharmacol Ther*. 1999;65:428.

* Asterisk indicates drugs cited in interaction reports. Based on pharmacologic and pharmacokinetic considerations, similar interactions may occur with other drugs that are listed.

Estrogens — *Topiramate*

Estrogens		Topiramate
Chlorotrianisene (*Tace*)	Estrogenic Substance (eg, *Gynogen*)	Topiramate* (*Topamax*)
Conjugated Estrogens (*Premarin*)	Estrone (eg, *Aquest*)	
Esterified Estrogens (*Estratab, Menest*)	Estropipate (eg, *Ogen*)	
Estradiol (*Estrace*)	Ethinyl Estradiol* (*Estinyl*)	

Significance	Onset	Severity	Documentation
2	☐ Rapid	☐ Major	☐ Established
	■ **Delayed**	■ **Moderate**	☐ Probable
		☐ Minor	■ **Suspected**
			☐ Possible
			☐ Unlikely

Effects The efficacy of ESTROGENS may be decreased.

Mechanism TOPIRAMATE may increase the metabolism of ESTROGENS.

Management Inform women of the possible increased risk of ESTROGEN failure during concomitant administration of TOPIRAMATE. An alternate method of contraception or an increased ESTROGEN dose (greater than or equal to 35 mcg ETHINYL ESTRADIOL) should be considered.

Discussion

The effects of topiramate (doses less than or equal to 800 mg/day) on the pharmacokinetics of a combination oral contraceptive containing ethinyl estradiol 35 mcg and norethindrone 1 mg were studied in 12 women with epilepsy who were receiving stable doses (750 to 2,500 mg/day) of valproic acid (eg, *Depakene*).[1] After one cycle of the oral contraceptive, topiramate was administered during cycles 2 through 4. Topiramate administration reduced the ethinyl estradiol area under the plasma concentration-time curve (AUC) by 18% to 30% and plasma concentrations by 15% to 25%, while not affecting norethindrone pharmacokinetics. The effect on the AUC of ethinyl estradiol was dose-related. The effects of the ethinyl estradiol-norethindrone combination on topiramate pharmacokinetics were not studied.

[1] Rosenfeld WE, et al. *Epilepsia*. 1997;38:317.

* Asterisk indicates drugs cited in interaction reports. Based on pharmacologic and pharmacokinetic considerations, similar interactions may occur with other drugs that are listed.

Ethambutol — *Aluminum Salts*

Ethambutol	Aluminum Salts	
Ethambutol* (*Myambutol*)	Al Carbonate (*Basaljel*)	Dihydroxyaluminum Sodium Carbonate (*Rolaids*)
	Al Hydroxide* (eg, *Amphojel*)	Kaolin
	Al Magnesium Hydroxide* (eg, *Maalox*)	Magaldrate (eg, *Lowsium*)
	Attapulgite (eg, *Kaopectate*)	

Significance	Onset	Severity	Documentation
4	☐ Rapid	☐ Major	☐ Established
	■ **Delayed**	■ **Moderate**	☐ Probable
		☐ Minor	☐ Suspected
			■ **Possible**
			☐ Unlikely

Effects ALUMINUM SALTS delay and reduce the absorption of ETHAMBUTOL.

Mechanism Unknown.

Management Separate administration by several hours.

Discussion

This interaction was studied in 13 tuberculosis patients and 6 healthy controls receiving aluminum hydroxide.[1] Serum ethambutol levels were decreased in the first 4 hours after ethambutol administration. There are several limitations to the study. Changes in the area under the curve (AUC) were not mentioned; effects on gastric emptying were not noted; and the method used to assess gastric emptying was questionable. In another controlled, crossover study involving 14 healthy subjects, administration of ethambutol with 30 mL of aluminum-magnesium hydroxide reduced ethambutol peak plasma levels 29% and reduced the AUC 10% compared with fasting conditions.[2]

There is interindividual variation in the effect of aluminum salts on ethambutol absorption. Controlled studies are needed to assess this possible interaction.

[1] Mattila MJ, et al. *Br J Clin Pharmacol.* 1978;5:161.

[2] Peloquin CA, et al. *Antimicrob Agents Chemother.* 1999;43:568.

* Asterisk indicates drugs cited in interaction reports. Based on pharmacologic and pharmacokinetic considerations, similar interactions may occur with other drugs that are listed.

Ethanol — *Barbiturates*

Ethanol	Barbiturates	
Ethanol*	Amobarbital* (*Amytal*)	Phenobarbital*
	Butabarbital (eg, *Butisol*)	Primidone (eg, *Mysoline*)
	Butalbital	Secobarbital (*Seconal*)
	Mephobarbital (*Mebaral*)	Thiopental (*Pentothal*)
	Pentobarbital*	

Significance	Onset	Severity	Documentation
1	■ **Rapid**	■ **Major**	■ **Established**
	□ Delayed	□ Moderate	□ Probable
		□ Minor	□ Suspected
			□ Possible
			□ Unlikely

Effects Impaired hand-eye coordination,[9] additive CNS effects, and death[1] have been noted upon acute ingestion. Chronic ETHANOL ingestion may manifest as "drug tolerance."

Mechanism Acute ETHANOL ingestion inhibits hepatic microsomal enzymes, decreasing hepatic drug metabolism, thus decreasing clearance.[2,5] Chronic ETHANOL ingestion may increase clearance because of hepatic enzyme induction.[3]

Management Avoid concomitant use of BARBITURATES and ETHANOL. Tolerance is unpredictable since deaths have been reported.

Discussion

Small amounts of alcohol have been implicated in causing death in individuals also taking barbiturates or other sedatives.[1] While additive CNS effects may be involved, other data show the interaction to be complex. The half-lives of pentobarbital and ethanol increase with concomitant use.[2] The subjective and psychomotor effects of alcohol were potentiated by giving thiopental 4 hours earlier.[12] Studies on chronic alcohol ingestion indicate a decreased half-life of pentobarbital.[2,3] Conversely, phenobarbital decreases plasma alcohol concentrations in chronic alcoholics[7] and healthy volunteers.[4] While the mechanism is not fully understood, it appears that chronic alcoholics exhibit "tolerance" caused by a combination of enzyme induction and drug tolerance. With acute alcohol ingestion, inhibition at hepatic metabolic sites is believed to explain the increased CNS effects and deaths occurring at low plasma concentrations.[6,8,10,11]

[1] Gupta RC, et al. *Can Med Assoc J.* 1966;94:863.
[2] Rubin E, et al. *Am J Med.* 1970;49:801.
[3] Misra PS, et al. *Am J Med.* 1971;51:346.
[4] Mould GP, et al. *J Pharm Pharmacol.* 1972;24:894.
[5] Thomas BH, et al. *Biochem Pharmacol.* 1972;21:2605.
[6] Lieber CS. *Gastroenterology.* 1973;65:821.
[7] Mezey E, et al. *Gastroenterology.* 1974;66:248.
[8] Curry SH, et al. *J Pharm Pharmacol.* 1974;26:771.
[9] Saario I, et al. *Acta Pharmacol Toxicol.* 1976;38:382.
[10] Sellers EM, et al. *Clin Pharmacokinet.* 1978;3:440.
[11] Stead AH, et al. *Hum Toxicol.* 1983;2:5.
[12] Lichtor JL, et al. *Anesthesiology.* 1993;79:28.

* Asterisk indicates drugs cited in interaction reports. Based on pharmacologic and pharmacokinetic considerations, similar interactions may occur with other drugs that are listed.

Ethanol — *Benzodiazepines*

Ethanol	Benzodiazepines	
Ethanol*	Alprazolam* (*Xanax*)	Halazepam (*Paxipam*)
	Chlordiazepoxide* (eg, *Librium*)	Lorazepam* (eg, *Ativan*)
	Clonazepam (*Klonopin*)	Midazolam (*Versed*)
	Clorazepate (eg, *Tranxene*)	Oxazepam (eg, *Serax*)
	Diazepam* (eg, *Valium*)	Prazepam (*Centrax*)
	Estazolam (*ProSom*)	Quazepam (*Doral*)
	Flurazepam (eg, *Dalmane*)	Temazepam (eg, *Restoril*)
		Triazolam* (*Halcion*)

Significance	Onset	Severity	Documentation
2	■ **Rapid**	□ Major	■ **Established**
	□ Delayed	■ **Moderate**	□ Probable
		□ Minor	□ Suspected
			□ Possible
			□ Unlikely

Effects Increased CNS effects with acute ETHANOL ingestion. Tolerance may occur with chronic ETHANOL use.

Mechanism Possible additive or synergistic effect. Increased benzodiazepine absorption and decreased hepatic metabolism.[7,11,15,18,23]

Management Avoid concomitant use. Counsel patients about additive CNS effects and impairment of motor skills.

Discussion

This combination produces additive effects on psychomotor assessments, including driving skills.[3-6,9,12,16,17,19-22,24,25,27,28] Most studies involved healthy males in simulated environments and the results may not apply to the general population.[13] While effects with diazepam were consistent, those of chlordiazepoxide on alcohol were additive[12,22] or antagonistic.[1,2] Oral ethanol 4 hrs after IV midazolam did not further impair psychomotor performance or mood.[26] Pharmacokinetic changes were more prominent in alcoholics with impaired liver function.[7,8,18]

1 Goldberg L. *Psychosomatic Med.* 1966;28:570.
2 Dundee JW, et al. *Quart J Stud Alc.* 1971;32:960.
3 Linnoila M, et al. *Eur J Clin Pharmacol.* 1973;5:186.
4 Morland J, et al. *Acta Pharmacol Toxicol.* 1974;34:5.
5 Linnoila M, et al. *Clin Pharmacol Ther.* 1974;15:368.
6 Saario I, et al. *J Clin Pharmacol.* 1975;15:52.
7 Sellman R, et al. *Acta Pharmacol Toxicol.* 1975;36:25.
8 Sellman R, et al. *Acta Pharmacol Toxicol.* 1975;36:33.
9 Saario I. *Ann Clin Res.* 1976;8:117.
10 Thiessen JJ, et al. *J Clin Pharmacol.* 1976;16:345.
11 Hayes SL, et al. *N Engl J Med.* 1977;296:186.
12 MacLeod SM, et al. *Eur J Clin Pharmacol.* 1977;11:345.
13 Ascione FJ. *Drug Ther.* 1978;8:58.
14 Palva ES, et al. *Eur J Clin Pharmacol.* 1978;13:345.
15 Whiting B, et al. *Br J Clin Pharmacol.* 1979;7:95.
16 Divoll M, et al. *Psychopharmacology.* 1981;73:381.
17 Lehmann W, *Eur J Clin Pharmacol.* 1981;20:201.
18 Juhl RP, et al. *J Clin Pharmacol.* 1984;24:113.
19 Ochs HR, et al. *J Clin Psychopharmacol.* 1984;4:106.
20 Aranko K, et al. *Eur J Clin Pharmacol.* 1985;28:559.
21 Dorian P, et al. *Clin Pharmacol Ther.* 1985;37:558.
22 Okamoto M, et al. *Alcoholism: Clin Exper Res.* 1985;9:516.
23 Guthrie SK, et al. *Alcoholism: Clin Exper Res.* 1986;10:686.
24 Mamelak M, et al. *Sleep.* 1987;10(Suppl 1):79.
25 Linnoila M, et al. *Eur J Clin Pharmacol.* 1990;39:21.
26 Lichtor JL, et al. *Anesth Analg.* 1991;72:661.
27 Bond AJ, et al. *Eur J Clin Pharmacol.* 1992;42:495.
28 Allen D, et al. *Eur J Clin Pharmacol.* 1992;42:499.

* Asterisk indicates drugs cited in interaction reports. Based on pharmacologic and pharmacokinetic considerations, similar interactions may occur with other drugs that are listed.

Ethanol — *Bromocriptine*

Ethanol*	Bromocriptine* (*Parlodel*)

Significance	Onset	Severity	Documentation
4	☐ Rapid ■ **Delayed**	☐ Major ■ **Moderate** ☐ Minor	☐ Established ☐ Probable ☐ Suspected ■ **Possible** ☐ Unlikely

Effects Intolerance of BROMOCRIPTINE due to severity of side effects has been reported.

Mechanism ETHANOL is believed to enhance the sensitivity of dopamine receptors[3,4] to BROMOCRIPTINE.

Management Avoid ETHANOL in patients experiencing BROMOCRIPTINE side effects.

Discussion

In a study of the effects of bromocriptine in treating acromegaly, 5 of 73 patients experienced alcohol intolerance in addition to other side effects.[1] Patients were receiving 10 to 60 mg bromocriptine per day. A subsequent report described two cases of bromocriptine intolerance manifested by nausea and abdominal pain while receiving bromocriptine 5 mg/day.[2] Abstinence from alcohol decreased the side effects.

More definitive data are needed to assess the significance of this interaction.

[1] Wass JAH, et al. *Br Med J.* 1977;1:875.
[2] Ayres J. *N Engl J Med.* 1980;302:806.
[3] Borg V, et al. *Acta Psychiatr Scand.* 1982;65:101.
[4] Barbieri RL, et al. *Fertil Steril.* 1983;39:727.

* Asterisk indicates drugs cited in interaction reports.

Ethanol	***Cephalosporins***

Ethanol*	Cefamandole* (*Mandol*)	Ceforanide (*Precef*)
	Cefoperazone* (*Cefobid*)	Cefotetan* (*Cefotan*)
	Cefonicid (*Monocid*)	Moxalactam* (*Moxam*)

Significance	Onset	Severity	Documentation
2	■ **Rapid**	□ Major	□ Established
	□ Delayed	■ **Moderate**	■ **Probable**
		□ Minor	□ Suspected
			□ Possible
			□ Unlikely

Effects A disulfiram-like reaction manifested by flushing, tachycardia, bronchospasm, sweating, nausea and vomiting may occur when ETHANOL is ingested after a patient has taken a CEPHALOSPORIN with the methyltetrazolethiol moiety.

Mechanism Aldehyde dehydrogenase inhibition by methyltetrazolethiol moiety results in acetaldehyde accumulation. Occurrence and severity are unpredictable. Dose-response relationships and length of enzyme inhibition are unknown.

Management Warn patients of the reaction which may occur with concomitant ETHANOL ingestion. The reaction may occur immediately or after several days.

Discussion

Disulfiram reactions have been reported in patients and normal healthy volunteers who have ingested alcohol following administration of cefoperazone,[1,2,4] moxalactam,[3,7,8,10] cefamandole[5,6] and cefotetan.[13] These agents all contain the methyltetrazolethiol moiety which structurally resembles disulfiram. Cephalothin (eg, *Keflin*), cephradine (*Anspor, Velosef*), cefoxitin (*Mefoxin*), cefazolin (*Ancef, Kefzol*), cefotaxime (*Claforan*)[9] and ceftizoxime (*Cefizox*)[10] did not illustrate this reaction; they also do not possess the characteristic moiety. While cefonicid contains the moiety, data regarding the reaction are controversial.[12] Interestingly, reactions have been noted only when the antibiotic administration preceded alcohol consumption.[8,9] Based upon structural similarity, disulfiram-like reactions would be expected to occur with ceforanide, cefonicid, cefmetazole and cefmenoxime (latter two not available in the US); clinical data is lacking.[12]

1 Reeves DS, et al. *Lancet.* 1980;2:540.
2 Foster TS, et al. *Am J Hosp Pharm.* 1980;37:858.
3 Neu HC, et al. *Lancet.* 1980;1:1422.
4 McMahon FG. *JAMA.* 1980;243:2397.
5 Portier H, et al. *Lancet.* 1980;2:263.
6 Drummer S, et al. *N Engl J Med.* 1980;303:1417.
7 Brown KR, et al. *Ann Intern Med.* 1982;97:621.
8 Elenbaas RM, et al. *Clin Pharmacol Ther.* 1982;32:347.
9 Buening MK, et al. *Rev Infect Dis.* 1982;4(suppl):s555.
10 McMahon FG, et al. *J Antimicrob Chemother.* 1982;10 (suppl C):129.
11 Umeda S, et al. *Anesth Analg.* 1985;64:377.
12 Norrby SR. *Med Toxicol.* 1986;1:32. Review.
13 Kline SS, et al. *Antimicrob Agents Chemother.* 1987;31:1328.

* Asterisk indicates drugs cited in interaction reports. Based on pharmacologic and pharmacokinetic considerations, similar interactions may occur with other drugs that are listed.

Ethanol — *Chloral Hydrate*

Ethanol*	Chloral Hydrate* (eg, *Noctec*)

Significance	Onset	Severity	Documentation
2	■ **Rapid**	□ Major	■ **Established**
	□ Delayed	■ **Moderate**	□ Probable
		□ Minor	□ Suspected
			□ Possible
			□ Unlikely

Effects Concurrent ingestion of CHLORAL HYDRATE and ETHANOL synergistically increases CNS depression.[3-5] Disulfiram-like reactions, while rare, have been reported when alcohol is consumed after CHLORAL HYDRATE.[2,7,8]

Mechanism Metabolic competition in the alcohol dehydrogenase-mediated process is believed to explain the altered metabolism of CHLORAL HYDRATE.[2,3,9]

Management Due to the synergistic effects, discourage concomitant use. Patients at significant risks of disulfiram reactions should avoid concomitant use. Patients on this medication should be fully aware of the potential consequences of alcohol use.

Discussion

Enhanced CNS depression manifested by increased number of symptoms and increased severity of symptoms has been reported with concomitant use.[3-5] The mechanism for the synergism is believed to involve accelerated reduction of chloral hydrate to trichloroethanol through a coupled redox of chloral hydrate and ethanol catalyzed by aldehyde dehydrogenase.[6,7] Typically this reaction is associated with increased acetaldehyde levels; however, this has not been confirmed in these cases.

1 Asmussen E, et al. *Acta Pharmacol Toxicol.* 1948;4:311.
2 Anon. *JAMA.* 1958;167:273.
3 Kaplan HL, et al. *J Forensic Sci.* 1967;12:295.
4 Gessner PK, et al. *J Pharmacol Exp Ther.* 1967;156:602.
5 Gessner PK, et al. *J Pharmacol Exp Ther.* 1970;174:247.
6 Freeman J, et al. *Fed Proc.* 1970;29:275.
7 Sellers EM, et al. *Clin Pharmacol Ther.* 1972;13:37.
8 Sellers EM, et al. *Clin Pharmacol Ther.* 1972;13:50.
9 Wong LK, et al. *Biochem Pharmacol.* 1978;27:1019.

* Asterisk indicates drugs cited in interaction reports.

Ethanol ⨯ *Contraceptives, Hormonal*

Ethanol*
(Alcohol, Ethyl Alcohol)

Contraceptives, Oral*
(eg, *Ortho-Novum*)

Significance	Onset	Severity	Documentation
4	■ **Rapid**	□ Major	□ Established
	□ Delayed	■ **Moderate**	□ Probable
		□ Minor	□ Suspected
			■ **Possible**
			□ Unlikely

Effects ETHANOL serum concentrations and CNS effects may be increased.

Mechanism Possible enzyme inhibition.

Management Caution women that the effects of this interaction are unpredictable; increased CNS effects and impaired motor skills are possible.

Discussion

Reports of the influence of oral contraceptive use on the effects of alcohol ingestion are contradictory.[1,2] One study found a decrease in the elimination rate of alcohol.[1] During ingestion of a moderate amount of ethanol (0.52 g/kg), 20 women taking oral contraceptives were compared with 20 women who were not. Subjects taking oral contraceptives demonstrated decreases in the elimination and disappearance rates of ethanol. A second study involved 37 women who were light or moderate drinkers and had been taking oral contraceptives for at least 3 months.[2] Seventeen control subjects were not taking oral contraceptives. All women were studied between days 14 and 21 of their contraceptive/menstrual cycle. Plasma ethanol concentrations and tests of motor function were measured for 6 hours after ethanol 0.9 mg/kg was ingested over a 30-minute interval. The degree of impairment and mean recovery time were less in the oral contraceptive subjects than in the control group, suggesting that oral contraceptives may lead to ethanol tolerance.

[1] Jones MK, et al. *Alcohol Clin Exp Res.* 1984;8(1):24.

[2] Hobbes J, et al. *Clin Pharmacol Ther.* 1985;38(4):371.

* Asterisk indicates drugs cited in interaction reports.

Ethanol — *Disulfiram*

Ethanol* (Alcohol, Ethyl Alcohol)	Disulfiram* (eg, *Antabuse*)

Significance	Onset	Severity	Documentation
1	■ **Rapid**	■ **Major**	■ **Established**
	□ Delayed	□ Moderate	□ Probable
		□ Minor	□ Suspected
			□ Possible
			□ Unlikely

Effects Flushing and increased respiration, pulse rate, and cardiac output occur most commonly. Hypotension,[1] compensatory tachycardia,[1] and death also have been reported.[2-4]

Mechanism DISULFIRAM inhibits aldehyde dehydrogenase, the enzyme responsible for the oxidation of acetaldehyde to acetyl-CoA, causing accumulation of acetaldehyde.

Management Patients receiving DISULFIRAM should not be exposed to products or consume beverages containing ETHANOL. Make patients fully aware of the potential for this reaction.

Discussion

The characteristic "*Antabuse* reaction" was first noted to produce flushing of the face and general uneasiness.[5,6] Subsequently, this reaction, attributable to concomitant alcohol-disulfiram intake, was associated with the increased formation of acetaldehyde.[7] Acetaldehyde infused to attain levels of 0.32 to 0.7 mg/dL was accompanied by similar signs and symptoms.[8] Mild reactions have been associated with topical products containing alcohol.[9-12] However, in other instances, no effects have been noted from ear drops, nebulizers, or minimal sips of wine.[13] The reaction may be severe enough to cause polyneuritis,[14] esophageal rupture,[15] or death.[2-4] Delirium, without major autonomic symptoms, was reported in a 50-year-old woman during use of alcohol while taking disulfiram.[16] Reviews on the management of disulfiram-alcohol interactions state that the effects are often short-lived and without sequelae; however, severe reactions have occurred. Although the reaction usually lasts from 2 to 4 hours, the intensity and duration are directly related to the disulfiram dosage, the amount of alcohol ingested, and individual patient characteristics.[17-19]

[1] Roache JD, et al. *Drug Alcohol Depend.* 2011;119(1-2):37.
[2] Jones RO. *Can Med Assoc J.* 1949;60(6):609.
[3] van Ieperen L. *S Afr Med J.* 1984;66(5):165.
[4] Stransky G, et al. *J Anal Toxicol.* 1997;21(2):178.
[5] Hald J, et al. *Acta Pharmacol Toxicol.* 1948;4:285.
[6] Asmussen E, et al. *Acta Pharmacol Toxicol.* 1948;4:297.
[7] Hald J, et al. *Acta Pharmacol Toxicol.* 1948;4:305.
[8] Asmussen E, et al. *Acta Pharmacol Toxicol.* 1948;4:311.
[9] Mercurio F. *JAMA.* 1952;149:82.
[10] Stoll D, et al. *JAMA.* 1980;244(18):2045.
[11] Ellis CN, et al. *Arch Dermatol.* 1979;115(11):1367.
[12] Haddock NF, et al. *Arch Dermatol.* 1982;118(3):157.
[13] Rothstein E. *N Engl J Med.* 1970;283(17):936.
[14] Rothrock JF, et al. *Neurology.* 1984;34(3):357.
[15] Fernandez D. *N Engl J Med.* 1972;286(11):610.
[16] Park CW, et al. *Ann Pharmacother.* 2001;35(1):32.
[17] Elenbaas RM. *Am J Hosp Pharm.* 1977;34(8):827.
[18] Kitson TM. *J Stud Alcohol.* 1977;38(1):96.
[19] Kwentus J, et al. *J Stud Alcohol.* 1979;40(5):428.

* Asterisk indicates drugs cited in interaction reports.

Ethanol		**Furazolidone**
Ethanol*		Furazolidone*†

Significance	Onset	Severity	Documentation
2	■ **Rapid**	☐ Major	☐ Established
	☐ Delayed	■ **Moderate**	■ **Probable**
		☐ Minor	☐ Suspected
			☐ Possible
			☐ Unlikely

Effects A disulfiram-like reaction consisting of facial flushing, lightheadedness, weakness, lacrimation and conjunctivitis has been reported when ETHANOL was ingested after taking FURAZOLIDONE.[1]

Mechanism FURAZOLIDONE may inhibit the enzymes responsible for the conversion of acetaldehyde to acetate.

Management Caution patients to avoid alcohol ingestion.

Discussion

Calesnick[1] reported a disulfiram-like reaction in a patient who ingested beer after taking furazolidone. Kolodny also reported a similar reaction in a patient.[2] Dyspnea and wheezing accompanied flushing, all of which lasted one hour without significant sequelae. Kutnesov[4] reported similar reactions in 98 patients where the interaction was used as a deterrent to alcohol use. In reviewing the properties of furans, Chamberlain[3] reports that 43 cases are known, 14 of which were evoked in a laboratory setting. There has been no significant sequelae reported with this specific interaction; however, consider that acetaldehyde accumulation can be fatal. This reaction has not been reported to occur with nitrofurantoin (eg, *Macrodantin*).[5]

[1] Calesnick B. *Am J Med Sci.* 1958;236:736.
[2] Kolodny AL. *Md State Med J.* 1962;11:248.
[3] Chamberlain RE. *J Antimicrob Chemother.* 1976;2:325.
[4] Kuznetsov ON, et al. *Sov Med.* 1979;5:104.
[5] Rowles B, et al. *N Engl J Med.* 1982;306:113.

* Asterisk indicates drugs cited in interaction reports.
† Not available in the United States.

Ethanol — *Glutethimide*

Ethanol*	Glutethimide* (eg, *Doriden*)

Significance	Onset	Severity	Documentation
2	■ **Rapid**	□ Major	□ Established
	□ Delayed	■ **Moderate**	□ Probable
		□ Minor	■ **Suspected**
			□ Possible
			□ Unlikely

Effects Additive CNS depressant effects may occur when these agents are used together.

Mechanism Unsubstantiated; however, synergism with regard to CNS depressant effects is postulated.

Management Counsel patients to avoid concomitant use of alcohol. Use of this combination may impair reaction time and ability to drive or operate machinery.

Discussion

Additive CNS depression is suspect between combinations of drugs with CNS depressant activity. This was of particular concern with alcohol-glutethimide combinations since many patients exhibiting glutethimide intoxication also ingested alcohol.[1] To study this interaction Mould et al[2] reported 11% higher blood ethanol concentrations when glutethimide and alcohol were given versus alcohol alone. With concomitant use, a fall in urinary and plasma glutethimide levels was noted in the presence of alcohol. Psychomotor tests reflected changes in drug plasma concentration levels. Conversely, Saario et al[3] found no impairment in psychomotor performance from alcohol-glutethimide combinations.

Although conflicting, both studies reported results from single-dose ingestions. Data from studies using multiple dose combinations are warranted to fully substantiate the impact of this combination. Until these data are available, combination use should be avoided.

[1] Maher JF, et al. *Am J Med.* 1962;33:70.
[2] Mould GP, et al. *J Pharm Pharmacol.* 1972;24:894.
[3] Saario I, et al. *Acta Pharmacol Toxicol.* 1976;38:382.

* Asterisk indicates drugs cited in interaction reports.

Ethanol	***Histamine H_2 Antagonists***
Ethanol* (Alcohol, Ethyl Alcohol)	Cimetidine* (eg, *Tagamet*) Famotidine* (eg, *Pepcid*) Nizatidine (*Axid*) Ranitidine* (eg, *Zantac*)

Significance	Onset	Severity	Documentation
4	■ **Rapid**	☐ Major	☐ Established
	☐ Delayed	■ **Moderate**	☐ Probable
		☐ Minor	☐ Suspected
			■ **Possible**
			☐ Unlikely

Effects May increase peak plasma ETHANOL levels and AUC.

Mechanism HISTAMINE H_2 ANTAGONISTS may increase absorption and decrease gastric first-pass metabolism of ETHANOL by inhibiting gastric alcohol dehydrogenase activity.

Management Warn patients to avoid ETHANOL or use with caution.

Discussion

Data are conflicting. Increased peak ethanol levels and area under the concentration-time curve (AUC) were reported in 6 healthy males ingesting ethanol and cimetidine. Plasma levels were 10% higher in the treatment group vs the placebo group.[2] Intoxication was higher in the cimetidine-treated group. A 55-year-old male manifested disorientation and behavioral changes after consuming alcohol soon after stopping cimetidine.[3] In 20 healthy male volunteers, ranitidine and cimetidine, but not famotidine, decreased first-pass metabolism of ethanol, resulting in an increase in mean peak levels and AUC.[7] A study of ranitidine in 8 volunteers found increased gastric emptying and ethanol bioavailability.[18] Cimetidine, but not ranitidine or famotidine, slightly inhibited the metabolism of acetaldehyde.[5] In 24 male volunteers, famotidine increased ethanol AUC and peak serum level compared with placebo, but there was considerable intra-individual variation.[13] Other studies found that cimetidine, ranitidine, and famotidine do not alter the kinetics of ethanol[8,11,12,14,19] or blood alcohol levels after IV administration of ethanol.[6,7] Similarly, there were no changes in ethanol kinetics after low ethanol doses with cimetidine[20] or ranitidine[9,11] or high ethanol doses with ranitidine,[10,11,21] cimetidine,[10,21] or famotidine.[10,21] This interaction may occur only under specific conditions (eg, low-dose ethanol) and have minimal clinical importance.[13-17,19] Cimetidine may alleviate histamine-induced headaches from red wine,[4] and combined use of H_1 and H_2 antagonists may relieve alcohol-induced flushing.[1]

1 Tan OT, et al. *Lancet.* 1979;2:365.
2 Feely J, et al. *JAMA.* 1982;247:2819.
3 Harkness LL, et al. *J Clin Psychiatry.* 1983;44:75.
4 Glaser D, et al. *Ann Intern Med.* 1983;98:413.
5 Tanaka E, et al. *Br J Clin Pharmacol.* 1988;26:96.
6 Baldit C, et al. *Am J Gastroenterol.* 1988;83:700.
7 DiPadova C, et al. *JAMA.* 1992;267:83.
8 Jönsson KA, et al. *Eur J Clin Pharmacol.* 1992;42:209.
9 Fraser AG, et al. *Aliment Pharmacol Ther.* 1992;6:267.
10 Fraser AG, et al. *Aliment Pharmacol Ther.* 1992;6:693.
11 Kleine MW, et al. *Ann Pharmacother.* 1993;27:841.
12 Toon S, et al. *Clin Pharmacol Ther.* 1994;55:385.
13 Burnham DB, et al. *Aliment Pharmacol Ther.* 1994;8:55.
14 Mallat A, et al. *Br J Clin Pharmacol.* 1994;37:208.
15 Casini A, et al. *Ann Int Med.* 1994;120:90.
16 Marshall JM. *Ann Pharmacother.* 1994;28:55. Review.
17 Pipkin GA, et al. *Pharmacotherapy.* 1994;14:273. Review.
18 Amir I, et al. *Life Sci.* 1996;58:511.
19 Bye A, et al. *Br J Clin Pharmacol.* 1996;41:129.
20 Clemmensen JD, et al. *Scand J Gastroenterol.* 1997;32:217.
21 Czyzyk A, et al. *Arzneimittelfurschung.* 1997;47:746.

* Asterisk indicates drugs cited in interaction reports. Based on pharmacologic and pharmacokinetic considerations, similar interactions may occur with other drugs that are listed.

Ethanol — *Meprobamate*

Ethanol*	Meprobamate* (eg, *Equanil*)

Significance	Onset	Severity	Documentation
2	■ **Rapid**	□ Major	□ Established
	□ Delayed	■ **Moderate**	■ **Probable**
		□ Minor	□ Suspected
			□ Possible
			□ Unlikely

Effects Enhanced CNS depressant effects affecting coordination and judgment.

Mechanism Acute ETHANOL ingestion results in decreased clearance of drugs through inhibition of hepatic metabolic systems. With chronic ETHANOL ingestion, one may manifest tolerance presumably due to enhanced metabolic capacity.[3,4]

Management Warn patients of enhanced CNS depression when ETHANOL and MEPROBAMATE are combined. Effects may be pronounced impairing coordination, judgment and ability.

Discussion

Concern over the combined effects of meprobamate and alcohol prompted Zirkle et al[1] to study the effects of the combination on human ability, coordination and judgment. Using eight psychological tests, results confirmed impaired test performance when the drugs were combined versus taken separately. Synergy in CNS depressant effects for the combination has been noted and implicated in causing death.[2,5] A series of experiments attempted to predict the outcome of a mixture of drugs (alcohol and meprobamate) from the responses to individual components in normal subjects.[6-8] While inconsistent results were achieved, the model had some inherent problems. It was concluded that blood concentrations do not predict the outcome of combined drug use.

[1] Zirkle GA, et al. *JAMA*. 1960;173:1823.
[2] Felby S. *Acta Pharmacol Toxicol*. 1970;28:334.
[3] Rubin E, et al. *Am J Med*. 1970;49:801.
[4] Misra PS, et al. *Am J Med*. 1971;51:346.
[5] Anon. *JAMA*. 1972;219:508.
[6] Ashford JR, et al. *J Stud Alcohol*. 1975;Suppl 7:140.
[7] Cobby JM, et al. *J Stud Alcohol*. 1975;Suppl 7:162.
[8] Ashford JR, et al. *J Stud Alcohol*. 1975;Suppl 7:177.

* Asterisk indicates drugs cited in interaction reports.

Ethanol — *Metoclopramide*

Ethanol*	Metoclopramide* (eg, *Reglan*)

Significance	Onset	Severity	Documentation
4	■ **Rapid**	☐ Major	☐ Established
	☐ Delayed	■ **Moderate**	☐ Probable
		☐ Minor	☐ Suspected
			■ **Possible**
			☐ Unlikely

Effects METOCLOPRAMIDE increases the rate of absorption of ETHANOL.

Mechanism METOCLOPRAMIDE, by increasing gastric motility, decreases the time it takes ETHANOL to reach the small intestine from where it is rapidly absorbed.

Management Warn patients of altered absorption. Patients may feel the effects of alcohol, ie, sedation, with smaller amounts. Exercise caution when ETHANOL is taken with METOCLOPRAMIDE.

Discussion

Metoclopramide increased the rate of alcohol absorption in five normal healthy volunteers.[1] A significant increase in peak concentration was also noted. In a poorly reported second attempt to study this interaction, Gibbons et al reported elevated blood alcohol levels after metoclopramide ingestion.[2] In a further study of this interaction, Bateman et al reported an increased rate of absorption but no significant effect on peak plasma ethanol concentrations. Interestingly, significant sedation was noted when metoclopramide and alcohol were combined.[3]

[1] Finch JE, et al. *Br J Clin Pharmacol.* 1974;1:233.
[2] Gibbons DO, et al. *Clin Pharmacol Ther.* 1975;17:578.
[3] Bateman DN, et al. *Br J Clin Pharmacol.* 1978;6:401.

* Asterisk indicates drugs cited in interaction reports.

Ethanol — *Metronidazole*

Ethanol* (Alcohol, Ethyl Alcohol)	Metronidazole* (eg, *Flagyl*)

Significance	Onset	Severity	Documentation
2	■ **Rapid**	□ Major	□ Established
	□ Delayed	■ **Moderate**	□ Probable
		□ Minor	■ **Suspected**
			□ Possible
			□ Unlikely

Effects A disulfiram-like reaction (symptoms of flushing, palpitations, tachycardia, nausea, vomiting) may occur with concomitant ETHANOL and METRONIDAZOLE ingestion.

Mechanism It is postulated that METRONIDAZOLE inhibits aldehyde dehydrogenase, thus causing accumulation of acetaldehyde.

Management Warn patients of the potential interaction and advise them to avoid concomitant ETHANOL ingestion.

Discussion

A disulfiram-like reaction has been reported in patients who consume alcohol shortly after ingestion of metronidazole.[1-7] Vaginal suppositories also have been implicated in causing the reaction with alcohol ingestion.[8] In addition, alcohol contained in pharmaceuticals may cause a disulfiram-like reaction if administered concurrently with metronidazole.[9] A patient experienced multiple episodes of a disulfiram-like reaction during concomitant use of IV metronidazole and IV trimethoprim-sulfamethoxazole (TMP-SMZ), which is 10% ethanol.[9] Symptoms resolved when the IV TMP-SMZ was discontinued and did not recur during subsequent use of IV TMP SMZ in the absence of metronidazole. While the interaction is a concern, it is reported inconsistently, making the risk for most patients slight.[5] Careful review of published case reports questions the association between the disulfram-like reaction and concurrent use of ethanol and metronidazole.[10] In a double-blind study in 6 healthy volunteers, metronidazole 200 mg 3 times daily for 5 days did not affect acefaldehyde blood levels when ethanol (0.4g/kg) was ingested.[11] However, caution is still advised.

[1] Lehmann HE, et al. *Psychiatr Neurol.* 1966;152:395.
[2] Semer JM, et al. *Am J Psychiatry.* 1966;123:722.
[3] Lehmann HE, et al. *Curr Ther Res Clin Exp.* 1967;9:419.
[4] Gelder MG, et al. *Br J Psychiatry.* 1968;114:473.
[5] Penick SB, et al. *Am J Psychiatry.* 1969;125:1063.
[6] Tunguy-Desmarais GP. *S Afr Med J.* 1983;63:836.
[7] Alexander I. *Br J Clin Pract.* 1985;39:292.
[8] Plosker GL. *Clin Pharm.* 1987;6:189.
[9] Edwards DL, et al. *Clin Pharm.* 1986;5:999.
[10] Williams CS, et al. *Ann Pharmacother.* 2000;34:255.
[11] Visapää JP, et al. *Ann Pharmacother.* 2002;36:971.

* Asterisk indicates drugs cited in interaction reports.

Ethanol — *Phenothiazines*

Ethanol	Phenothiazines	
Ethanol* (Alcohol, Ethyl Alcohol)	Chlorpromazine* (eg, *Thorazine*)	Promethazine (eg, *Phenergan*)
	Fluphenazine* (eg, *Prolixin*)	Thioridazine*
	Perphenazine*	Trifluoperazine*
	Prochlorperazine (eg, *Compazine*)	

Significance	Onset	Severity	Documentation
2	■ **Rapid**	□ Major	□ Established
	□ Delayed	■ **Moderate**	■ **Probable**
		□ Minor	□ Suspected
			□ Possible
			□ Unlikely

Effects Enhanced CNS depression, most notably impairment of psychomotor skills, has been reported. Dystonic reactions may be precipitated by ALCOHOL.

Mechanism It is suspected that these agents act on different sites in the brain to produce CNS depression. Also, ALCOHOL may lower the threshold of resistance to neurotoxic side effects of the PHENOTHIAZINES, possibly through dopamine or calcium depletion.

Management Warn patients of enhanced CNS depression and the possibility of extrapyramidal side effects induced by concomitant ALCOHOL ingestion. Discourage concurrent use as psychomotor skills may be impaired.

Discussion

Combinations of phenothiazine drugs with alcohol have been reported to cause increased CNS depression.[1-8] Although several reports fail to distinguish between synergism vs addition, there is evidence to suggest that the 2 agents work on different sites in the brain, thus making the effects additive, not synergistic.[1,2,4] Subjective and objective assessment note the most marked effects on psychomotor skills[1,2,5,6,9] and behavioral changes.[3] Of concern are extrapyramidal reactions (dystonic reactions, acute akathisia) occurring in patients on phenothiazines after consuming alcohol. Symptoms abated with the use of antiparkinson agents. Discourage concomitant use of alcohol and phenothiazines.

1 Fazekas JF, et al. *Am J Med Sci.* 1955;230:128.
2 Zirkle GA, et al. *JAMA.* 1959;171:1496.
3 Sutherland VC, et al. *J Appl Physiol.* 1960;15:189.
4 Gebhart GF, et al. *Toxicol Appl Pharmacol.* 1969;15:405.
5 Milner G, et al. *Br J Psychiatry.* 1971;118:351.
6 Morselli PL, et al. *Arzneimittelforschung.* 1971;2:20.
7 Lutz EG. *JAMA.* 1976;236:2422.
8 Freed E. *Med J Aust.* 1981;2:44.
9 Saario I. *Ann Clin Res.* 1976;8:117.

* Asterisk indicates drugs cited in interaction reports. Based on pharmacologic and pharmacokinetic considerations, similar interactions may occur with other drugs that are listed.

Ethanol — *Procarbazine*

Ethanol*
(Alcohol, Ethyl Alcohol)

Procarbazine*
(*Matulane*)

Significance	Onset	Severity	Documentation
3	■ **Rapid**	□ Major	□ Established
	□ Delayed	□ Moderate	□ Probable
		■ **Minor**	■ **Suspected**
			□ Possible
			□ Unlikely

Effects Flushing of the face (red and hot) lasting a short while[1] has been reported in patients taking PROCARBAZINE and ETHANOL.[1-3]

Mechanism Unknown.

Management Advise patients receiving hydrazine compounds (PROCARBAZINE) of the occurrence of this effect with concomitant ingestion of ETHANOL. Discourage use of ETHANOL by these patients.

Discussion

While the true incidence of this interaction is unknown, flushing reactions have been reported by patients (5% to 23%) ingesting alcohol after receiving hydrazine compounds.[1-3]

[1] Mathe G, et al. *Lancet.* 1963;2:1077.
[2] Brule G, et al. *Cancer Chemother Rep.* 1965;44:31.
[3] Todd ID, et al. *Br Med J.* 1965;1:628.

* Asterisk indicates drugs cited in interaction reports.

Ethanol — *Tacrolimus*

Ethanol* (Alcohol, Ethyl Alcohol)	Tacrolimus* (*Protopic*)

Significance

3

Onset	Severity	Documentation
■ **Rapid**	□ Major	□ Established
□ Delayed	□ Moderate	□ Probable
	■ **Minor**	■ **Suspected**
		□ Possible
		□ Unlikely

Effects Risk of transient facial flushing may be increased.

Mechanism Unknown.

Management Warn patients applying topical TACROLIMUS of the increased risk of facial flushing with ALCOHOL ingestion. If flushing occurs following ALCOHOL ingestion, caution patients to avoid ALCOHOL as long as topical TACROLIMUS is being used.

Discussion

A 56-year-old woman being treated with tacrolimus 0.1% ointment for rosacea experienced facial flushing after drinking an alcoholic beverage.[1] She had been using tacrolimus ointment for 2 weeks. To determine if the reaction was clinically reproducible, the patient applied 0.1% tacrolimus ointment twice daily to her face. After 1 week of tacrolimus treatment, she ingested 50 mL of white wine. Twelve minutes later, she experienced facial erythema that faded after 45 minutes. One month after discontinuing tacrolimus, her alcohol tolerance was normal. Up to 7% of patients treated with topical tacrolimus experience alcohol intolerance. A similar interaction occurred in a 27-year-old woman using topical tacrolimus for vitiligo on the face, hands, and elbows.[2] After 1 month of using tacrolimus, the patient ingested 40 mL of wine. Within 5 minutes, she experienced facial flushing, periocular edema, intense itching, and skin irritation on the area of her face, but not other areas of her body, where tacrolimus was applied. The episode resolved within 30 minutes. A rechallenge with 10 mL of wine resulted in a less intense reaction that resolved within 10 minutes. Alcohol intolerance was reported in 3 infants receiving tacrolimus ointment for facial treatment of atopic dermatitis.[3] Facial erythema occurred in 2 of the children who received vitamin D in an alcoholic solution and 1 child who received an oral antihistamine solution containing 5% alcohol.

[1] Lübbe J, et al. *N Engl J Med.* 2004;351:2740.
[2] Morales-Molina JA, et al. *Ann Pharmacother.* 2005;39:772.
[3] Calza AM, et al. *Br J Dermatol.* 2005;152:565.

* Asterisk indicates drugs cited in interaction reports.

Ethanol	***Trimethoprim***
Ethanol* (Alcohol, Ethyl Alcohol)	Trimethoprim/Sulfamethoxazole* (eg, *Bactrim*)

Significance	Onset	Severity	Documentation
4	■ **Rapid** ☐ Delayed	☐ Major ■ **Moderate** ☐ Minor	☐ Established ☐ Probable ☐ Suspected ■ **Possible** ☐ Unlikely

Effects A disulfiram-like reaction including flushing, palpitations, tachycardia, nausea, and vomiting may occur.

Mechanism TRIMETHOPRIM/SULFAMETHOXAZOLE (TMP-SMZ) may inhibit acetaldehyde dehydrogenase, causing accumulation of acetaldehyde.

Management Advise patients to avoid concomitant ingestion of ETHANOL and TMP-SMZ.

Discussion

A disulfiram (*Antabuse*)-like reaction was reported in 2 patients who ingested ethyl alcohol while receiving TMP-SMZ.[1] Both patients were taking double-strength TMP-SMZ every 12 hours and experienced flushing, heart palpitations, dyspnea, headache, and nausea after two to three 12-ounce beers. Both patients then became drowsy and fell asleep. The next morning, symptoms were gone. In 1 patient, ingestion of 4 to 5 beers on the previous day while taking TMP-SMZ did not produce a reaction. In the second patient, symptoms occurred again the day after the first reaction when he ingested 6 ounces of beer. The reaction was similar to the previous day but resolved more quickly.

Intravenous TMP-SMZ contains 10% alcohol. This interaction does not appear to have been reported in patients receiving IV TMP-SMZ alone. However, metronidazole (eg, *Flagyl*), a drug that also interacts with ethanol to cause a disulfiram-like reaction, has been reported to interact with the alcohol contained in IV TMP-SMZ.[2]

[1] Heelon MW, et al. *Pharmacotherapy*. 1998;18:869.
[2] Edwards DL, et al. *Clin Pharm*. 1986;5:999.

* Asterisk indicates drugs cited in interaction reports.

Ethanol — *Verapamil*

Ethanol*	Verapamil* (eg, *Calan*)

Significance	Onset	Severity	Documentation
2	■ **Rapid**	□ Major	□ Established
	□ Delayed	■ **Moderate**	□ Probable
		□ Minor	■ **Suspected**
			□ Possible
			□ Unlikely

Effects Increased and prolonged CNS effects of ETHANOL affecting coordination and judgment.

Mechanism Unknown. Possibly inhibition of ETHANOL metabolism.

Management Caution patients to limit ETHANOL consumption while taking VERAPAMIL.

Discussion

The effects of verapamil on blood ethanol concentrations were investigated in a double-blind, placebo-controlled, randomized, crossover study.[1] During 2 phases, separated by a 2-week washout period, 10 healthy men received 80 mg verapamil or a placebo orally every 8 hours for 5 days as outpatients. On the sixth day, subjects were admitted to the hospital and continued to receive their outpatient treatment. Ethanol 0.8 g/kg was administered as a 20% oral solution. Mean peak ethanol concentrations were 17% higher (increased from 106 to 124 mg/dL) during verapamil administration and the area under the blood ethanol concentration-time curve (AUC) increased 30% (366 vs 475 mg•hr/dL). The percent increase in the blood ethanol AUC correlated significantly (P less than 0.05) with an increase in the area under the effect (ie, participant's subjective assessment of intoxication using a scale) versus time curve (from 10 to 14 cm/hr) and the duration of time ethanol concentrations remained above 100 mg/dL (0.2 to 1.3 hours; P less than 0.05). The time to peak ethanol concentration was not affected by verapamil.

[1] Bauer LA, et al. *Clin Pharmacol Ther.* 1992;52:6.

* Asterisk indicates drugs cited in interaction reports.

Etomidate — *Verapamil*

Etomidate* (*Amidate*)	Verapamil* (eg, *Calan*)

Significance	Onset	Severity	Documentation
4	■ **Rapid**	□ Major	□ Established
	□ Delayed	■ **Moderate**	□ Probable
		□ Minor	□ Suspected
			■ **Possible**
			□ Unlikely

Effects The anesthetic effect of ETOMIDATE may be increased with prolonged respiratory depression and apnea.

Mechanism Unknown.

Management Use this combination with caution. Monitor respiratory function and provide ventilatory support as required.

Discussion

Prolonged anesthesia and Cheyne-Stokes respiration was reported in 2 patients undergoing elective electrical cardioversion for supraventricular tachycardia. Both patients had received verapamil prior to etomidate induction.[1] One patient, a 71-year-old male with a long history of Wolff-Parkinson-White syndrome, was admitted to the hospital with a 3-hour episode of acute palpitations. Prior to admission, the patient had been maintained on chronic oral verapamil. Cardioversion was performed following an induction dose of etomidate 300 mcg/kg over 60 seconds. Following the procedure, the patient was unresponsive and apneic for 3 minutes, requiring ventilatory assistance. Cheyne-Stokes respiration was noted for an additional 15 minutes before consciousness was regained. The second patient, a 66-year-old man, was admitted to the hospital with a 6-hour history of acute palpitations. The patient had been receiving chronic oral disopyramide (eg, *Norpace*). IV administration of disopyramide 150 mg and verapamil 10 mg had no effect on the arrhythmia. An induction dose of 300 mcg/kg of IV etomidate was administered; however, because of a delay in the procedure, an additional dose of 120 mcg/kg was given after 10 minutes. Classic Cheyne-Stokes respiration was observed for 25 minutes and ventilatory support was required before the patient regained consciousness.

Additional studies are warranted to assess this possible interaction.

[1] Moore CA, et al. *Hosp Pharm.* 1989;24:24.

* Asterisk indicates drugs cited in interaction reports.

Etoposide — *Atovaquone*

Etoposide* (eg, *VePesid*)	Atovaquone* (*Mepron*)

Significance	Onset	Severity	Documentation
4	☐ Rapid ■ **Delayed**	☐ Major ■ **Moderate** ☐ Minor	☐ Established ☐ Probable ☐ Suspected ■ **Possible** ☐ Unlikely

Effects ETOPOSIDE plasma concentrations may be elevated, increasing the risk of toxicity.

Mechanism Unknown.

Management Closely monitor the patient for signs of ETOPOSIDE toxicity if these agents are used concurrently.

Discussion

The effect of atovaquone on the pharmacokinetics of etoposide was evaluated in 9 children with acute lymphoblastic leukemia or non-Hodgkin lymphoma.[1] Etoposide 300 mg/m^2 as a 2-hour IV infusion during weeks 46 and 54 was administered with cytarabine (eg, *Cytosar-U*). The week preceding etoposide administration, mercaptopurine (*Purinethol*) and methotrexate (eg, *Rheumatrex*) were administered. Patients were randomized to receive oral trimethoprim/sulfamethoxazole (eg, *Bactrim*) or atovaquone (45 mg/kg/day) in 2 divided doses during week 45, and in week 53 were crossed over to the alternate regimen. Compared with trimethoprim/sulfamethoxazole, atovaquone administration with etoposide increased the AUC of etoposide, etoposide catechol metabolite AUC, and the ratio of the catechol metabolite to etoposide AUC 8.6%, 28.4%, and 25.9%, respectively.

[1] van de Poll ME, et al. *Cancer Chemother Pharmacol.* 2001;47(6):467.

* Asterisk indicates drugs cited in interaction reports.

Etoposide — *Azole Antifungal Agents*

Etoposide	Azole Antifungal Agents	
Etoposide* (eg, *VePesid*)	Itraconazole (eg, *Sporanox*)	Posaconazole (*Noxafil*)
	Ketoconazole* (eg, *Nizoral*)	Voriconazole (*Vfend*)

Significance	Onset	Severity	Documentation
4	☐ Rapid	☐ Major	☐ Established
	■ **Delayed**	■ **Moderate**	☐ Probable
		☐ Minor	☐ Suspected
			■ **Possible**
			☐ Unlikely

Effects ETOPOSIDE serum concentrations may be elevated, increasing the risk of adverse reactions.

Mechanism Unknown.

Management Monitor complete blood cell count and adjust the ETOPOSIDE dose as needed.

Discussion

The effects of oral ketoconazole on the pharmacokinetics of oral etoposide were evaluated in 28 patients with solid tumors or lymphomas.[1] Three days prior to the treatment period, patients received etoposide 50 mg. During treatment, patients received ketoconazole 200 mg/day from day 1 to 22. Starting on day 2, escalating doses of etoposide (starting with 50 mg every other day and culminating with 50 mg alternating with 100 mg daily) were coadministered with ketoconazole. Ketoconazole increased the median AUC and reduced the clearance of etoposide 20% and 18%, respectively. Interpatient variability of AUC increased from 43% to 89%, and interpatient variability of clearance increased from 52% to 71%. Coadministration of ketoconazole and etoposide did not alter the toxicity of etoposide or improve the therapeutic index.

[1] Yong WP, et al. *Cancer Chemother Pharmacol.* 2007;60(6):811.

* Asterisk indicates drugs cited in interaction reports. Based on pharmacologic and pharmacokinetic considerations, similar interactions may occur with other drugs that are listed.

Etoposide		*Cyclosporine*
Etoposide* (eg, *VePesid*)		Cyclosporine* (eg, *Neoral*)

Significance	Onset	Severity	Documentation
2	□ Rapid	□ Major	■ **Established**
	■ **Delayed**	■ **Moderate**	□ Probable
		□ Minor	□ Suspected
			□ Possible
			□ Unlikely

Effects Serum ETOPOSIDE concentration may be elevated, resulting in increased toxicity.

Mechanism Decreased ETOPOSIDE renal clearance, possibly caused by inhibition of drug transport in the brush border of the proximal renal tubule. The decrease in nonrenal clearance is not as well understood, but may be caused by inhibition of ETOPOSIDE metabolism by CYCLOSPORINE.

Management Monitor complete blood cell count and adjust the dose of ETOPOSIDE as needed.

Discussion

The effects of high-dose continuous infusion of cyclosporine on the pharmacokinetics and pharmacodynamics of etoposide were studied in 16 patients with advanced cancer.[1] Compared with giving etoposide alone, coadministration of etoposide and cyclosporine resulted in a 59% increase in etoposide AUC, a 35% decrease in clearance, a 96% increase in mean residence time, a 73% increase in $t_{½}$ (from 6.6 to 11.4 hours), and a 12% increase in steady-state volume of distribution. Cyclosporine administration also demonstrated a concentration-dependent effect on etoposide pharmacokinetics. Cyclosporine concentration ranged from 297 to 5,073 ng/mL. Cyclosporine levels greater than 2,000 ng/mL produced a 33-fold greater percentage change in volume of distribution of etoposide, a 3.5-fold greater change in mean residence time, a 2.7-fold greater change in $t_{½}$, a 1.6-fold increase in AUC, and a 1.4-fold greater decrease in clearance compared with cyclosporine levels less than 2,000 ng/mL. The mean WBC nadir was lower during treatment with concentrations of cyclosporine greater than 2,000 ng/mL than with lower levels (WBC 1,600/mm^3 vs 900/mm^3). During coadministration of cyclosporine, renal and nonrenal clearance of etoposide decreased approximately 40% and 50%, respectively. These results have been confirmed in children[2] and adults.[3] Increases in etoposide AUC of approximately 100% were associated with increased toxicity.

[1] Lum BL, et al. *J Clin Oncol.* 1992;10(10):1635.
[2] Bisogno G, et al. *Br J Cancer.* 1998;77(12):2304.
[3] Lum BL, et al. *Cancer Chemother Pharmacol.* 2000;45(4):305.

* Asterisk indicates drugs cited in interaction reports.

Etoposide — *Food*

Etoposide* (eg, *Toposar*)	Grapefruit Juice*

Significance	Onset	Severity	Documentation
4	■ **Rapid**	□ Major	□ Established
	□ Delayed	■ **Moderate**	□ Probable
		□ Minor	□ Suspected
			■ **Possible**
			□ Unlikely

Effects ETOPOSIDE concentrations may be reduced, decreasing the pharmacologic effect.

Mechanism Unknown; however, possible alteration of intestinal P-glycoprotein–mediated transport.

Management Until more data are available, advise patients taking ETOPOSIDE to avoid concurrent ingestion of GRAPEFRUIT PRODUCTS and to take ETOPOSIDE with a liquid other than GRAPEFRUIT JUICE.

Discussion

In a randomized, crossover study, the effect of grapefruit juice on the systemic bioavailability of oral etoposide was investigated in 6 patients with a poor prognosis of relapsed small cell lung cancer.[1] Each patient was sequentially treated with etoposide 50 mg IV over 1 hour, 50 mg orally, or 50 mg orally 15 minutes after ingesting 100 mL of grapefruit juice. Compared with oral treatment without grapefruit juice, grapefruit juice ingestion decreased the etoposide AUC an average of 26.2%. The median absolute bioavailability was reduced nearly 21%. There was considerable interindividual variability of the AUC in all treatment groups.

Additional studies are needed to determine the mechanism of this interaction.

[1] Reif S, et al. *Eur J Clin Pharmacol.* 2002;58(7):491.

* Asterisk indicates drugs cited in interaction reports.

Etravirine — *Efavirenz*

Etravirine* (*Intelence*)		Efavirenz* (*Sustiva*)	
Significance	**Onset**	**Severity**	**Documentation**
4	□ Rapid ■ **Delayed**	□ Major ■ **Moderate** □ Minor	□ Established □ Probable □ Suspected ■ **Possible** □ Unlikely

Effects ETRAVIRINE plasma concentrations may be reduced, decreasing the pharmacologic effect.

Mechanism Increased ETRAVIRINE metabolism (CYP3A4) by EFAVIRENZ.

Management Avoid coadministration.

Discussion

The effects of efavirenz on the pharmacokinetics of etravirine were studied in 25 volunteers.[1] Using an open-label, randomized, prospective design, the pharmacokinetics of etravirine, given 400 mg once daily or 200 mg twice daily, were assessed before and after pretreatment with efavirenz 600 mg once daily for 14 days. Compared with administering etravirine alone, pretreatment with efavirenz decreased the etravirine C_{max}, C_{min}, and AUC approximately 22%, 33%, and 29%, respectively.

[1] Boffito M, et al. *J Acquir Immune Defic Syndr.* 2009;52(2):222.

* Asterisk indicates drugs cited in interaction reports.

Everolimus — *Azole Antifungal Agents*

Everolimus	Azole Antifungal Agents	
Everolimus* (eg, *Afinitor*)	Fluconazole (eg, *Diflucan*)	Ketoconazole* (eg, *Nizoral*)
	Itraconazole (eg, *Sporanox*)	Posaconazole (*Noxafil*)

Significance	Onset	Severity	Documentation
2	☐ Rapid ■ **Delayed**	☐ Major ■ **Moderate** ☐ Minor	☐ Established ☐ Probable ■ **Suspected** ☐ Possible ☐ Unlikely

Effects EVEROLIMUS plasma concentrations may be elevated, increasing the pharmacologic effects and adverse reactions.

Mechanism Inhibition of EVEROLIMUS metabolism (CYP3A4) by AZOLE ANTIFUNGAL AGENTS is suspected.

Management Avoid coadministration of EVEROLIMUS and an AZOLE ANTIFUNGAL AGENT. If coadministration cannot be avoided, use an antifungal agent with the least amount of CYP3A4 enzyme inhibition potential and adjust the EVEROLIMUS dose based on blood concentration monitoring.

Discussion

In a crossover study, the effects of ketoconazole on the pharmacokinetics of everolimus were evaluated in 12 healthy subjects.[1] Each subject received a single oral dose of everolimus 2 mg alone. On the fourth day of receiving ketoconazole 200 mg twice daily for 8 days, a single dose of everolimus 1 mg was administered. Compared with giving everolimus alone, coadministration of ketoconazole increased the C_{max} 3.9-fold, increased the AUC 15-fold, and prolonged the $t_{½}$ from 30 to 56 hours.

[1] Kovarik JM, et al. *J Clin Pharmacol.* 2005;45(5):514.

* Asterisk indicates drugs cited in interaction reports. Based on pharmacologic and pharmacokinetic considerations, similar interactions may occur with other drugs that are listed.

Everolimus — *Cyclosporine*

Everolimus* (eg, *Afinitor*)	Cyclosporine* (eg, *Neoral*)

Significance	Onset	Severity	Documentation
2	☐ Rapid ■ **Delayed**	☐ Major ■ **Moderate** ☐ Minor	☐ Established ☐ Probable ■ **Suspected** ☐ Possible ☐ Unlikely

Effects EVEROLIMUS blood concentrations may be elevated, increasing the pharmacologic effects and risk of adverse reactions.

Mechanism Inhibition of EVEROLIMUS metabolism (CYP3A4) and/or increased EVEROLIMUS bioavailability caused by inhibition of P-glycoprotein by CYCLOSPORINE is suspected.

Management Monitor the clinical response of the patient and EVEROLIMUS blood concentrations when CYCLOSPORINE is started or stopped. Adjust the EVEROLIMUS dose as needed.

Discussion

The effects of oral cyclosporine microemulsion formulation or suspension formulation on the pharmacokinetics of everolimus were evaluated in 24 healthy subjects.[1] Using an open-label, randomized, crossover design, each subject received a single oral dose of everolimus 2 mg alone and with cyclosporine 175 mg (microemulsion formulation) or cyclosporine 300 mg (suspension formulation). Simultaneous administration of everolimus with the cyclosporine microemulsion formulation increased the everolimus C_{max} and AUC 82% and 168%, respectively. Simultaneous administration of everolimus with the cyclosporine suspension formulation increased the everolimus AUC 74% but did not affect the C_{max}. Neither cyclosporine formulation affected the everolimus $t_{½}$.

[1] Kovarik JM, et al. *J Clin Pharmacol.* 2002;42(1):95.

* Asterisk indicates drugs cited in interaction reports.

Everolimus — *Macrolide & Related Antibiotics*

Everolimus	Macrolide & Related Antibiotics	
Everolimus* (eg, *Afinitor*)	Clarithromycin (eg, *Biaxin*)	Telithromycin (*Ketek*)
	Erythromycin* (eg, *Ery-Tab*)	

Significance	Onset	Severity	Documentation
2	□ Rapid	□ Major	□ Established
	■ **Delayed**	■ **Moderate**	□ Probable
		□ Minor	■ **Suspected**
			□ Possible
			□ Unlikely

Effects EVEROLIMUS plasma concentrations may be elevated, increasing the pharmacologic effects and adverse reactions.

Mechanism Inhibition of EVEROLIMUS metabolism (CYP3A4) by MACROLIDE and RELATED ANTIBIOTICS is suspected.

Management Avoid coadministration of EVEROLIMUS and MACROLIDE and RELATED ANTIBIOTICS. If coadministration cannot be avoided, use an alternative antibiotic with the least amount of CYP3A4 enzyme inhibition potential and adjust the EVEROLIMUS dose based on blood concentration monitoring.

Discussion

The effects of erythromycin on the pharmacokinetics of everolimus were evaluated in a crossover study in 16 healthy subjects.[1] Each subject received a single oral dose of everolimus 2 mg alone. On day 5 of receiving erythromycin 500 mg 3 times daily for 9 days, a single dose of everolimus 2 mg was administered. Compared with administering everolimus alone, coadministration of erythromycin increased the C_{max} 2-fold, increased the AUC 4.4-fold, and prolonged the $t_{1/2}$ from 32 to 44 hours.

[1] Kovarik JM, et al. *Eur J Clin Pharmacol.* 2005;61(1):35.

* Asterisk indicates drugs cited in interaction reports. Based on pharmacologic and pharmacokinetic considerations, similar interactions may occur with other drugs that are listed.

Everolimus — *Verapamil*

Everolimus* (eg, *Afinitor*)	Verapamil* (eg, *Calan*)

Significance	Onset	Severity	Documentation
2	☐ Rapid	☐ Major	☐ Established
	■ **Delayed**	■ **Moderate**	☐ Probable
		☐ Minor	■ **Suspected**
			☐ Possible
			☐ Unlikely

Effects EVEROLIMUS plasma concentrations may be elevated, increasing the pharmacologic effects and adverse reactions.

Mechanism Inhibition of CYP3A4 and P-glycoprotein by VERAPAMIL is suspected.

Management If coadministration of EVEROLIMUS and VERAPAMIL cannot be avoided, closely observe the clinical response of the patient when VERAPAMIL treatment is started or stopped. Adjust the EVEROLIMUS dose based on blood concentration monitoring and the VERAPAMIL dose based on blood pressure monitoring.

Discussion

The effects of verapamil on the pharmacokinetics of everolimus were studied in 16 healthy subjects.[1] In a crossover study, each subject received a single oral dose of everolimus 2 mg alone and on the second day of receiving verapamil 80 mg 3 times daily for 6 days. Compared with taking everolimus alone, coadministration of verapamil increased the everolimus C_{max} and AUC 2.3- and 3.5-fold, respectively. Verapamil predose concentrations doubled after a single dose of everolimus.

[1] Kovarik JM, et al. *Br J Clin Pharmacol.* 2005;60(4):434.

* Asterisk indicates drugs cited in interaction reports.

Exemestane — *Barbiturates*

Exemestane	Barbiturates	
Exemestane* (*Aromasin*)	Amobarbital (*Amytal*)	Pentobarbital
	Butabarbital (eg, *Butisol*)	Phenobarbital* (eg, *Solfoton*)
	Butalbital	Primidone (eg, *Mysoline*)
	Mephobarbital (*Mebaral*)	Secobarbital (*Seconal*)

Significance	Onset	Severity	Documentation
2	☐ Rapid	☐ Major	☐ Established
	■ **Delayed**	■ **Moderate**	☐ Probable
		☐ Minor	■ **Suspected**
			☐ Possible
			☐ Unlikely

Effects EXEMESTANE plasma concentrations may be reduced, decreasing the efficacy.

Mechanism Induction of EXEMESTANE metabolism (CYP3A4) by PHENOBARBITAL.

Management If PHENOBARBITAL is coadministered in patients receiving EXEMESTANE, the recommended dosage of EXEMESTANE is 50 mg once daily after a meal.[1] If PHENOBARBITAL is discontinued, reduce the EXEMESTANE dosage to 25 mg once daily with a meal.

Discussion

Because exemestane undergoes metabolism by CYP3A4, coadministration of phenobarbital is expected to decrease exemestane plasma concentrations.[1] Therefore, consider dosage adjustments in patients receiving exemestane when a strong CYP3A4 inducer (eg, phenobarbital) is started or stopped.

The basis for this monograph is information on file with the manufacturer. There are no clinical data with dose adjustments in patients receiving exemestane and phenobarbital. Studies are needed to determine the clinical importance of this interaction and if other barbiturates interact similarly.

[1] *Aromasin* [package insert]. New York, NY: Pfizer Inc; February 2007.

* Asterisk indicates drugs cited in interaction reports. Based on pharmacologic and pharmacokinetic considerations, similar interactions may occur with other drugs that are listed.

Exemestane — *Carbamazepine*

Exemestane* (*Aromasin*)	Carbamazepine* (eg, *Tegretol*)

Significance	Onset	Severity	Documentation
2	☐ Rapid ■ **Delayed**	☐ Major ■ **Moderate** ☐ Minor	☐ Established ☐ Probable ■ **Suspected** ☐ Possible ☐ Unlikely

Effects EXEMESTANE plasma concentrations may be reduced, decreasing the efficacy.

Mechanism Induction of EXEMESTANE metabolism (CYP3A4) by CARBAMAZEPINE.

Management If CARBAMAZEPINE is coadministered in patients receiving EXEMESTANE, the recommended dosage of EXEMESTANE is 50 mg once daily after a meal.[1] If CARBAMAZEPINE is discontinued, reduce the EXEMESTANE dosage to 25 mg once daily with a meal.

Discussion

Because exemestane undergoes metabolism by CYP3A4, coadministration of carbamazepine is expected to decrease exemestane plasma concentrations.[1] Therefore, consider dosage adjustments in patients receiving exemestane when a strong CYP3A4 inducer (eg, carbamazepine) is started or stopped.

The basis for this monograph is information on file with the manufacturer. There are no clinical data with dose adjustments in patients receiving exemestane and carbamazepine. Studies are needed to determine the clinical importance of this interaction.

[1] *Aromasin* [package insert]. New York, NY: Pfizer, Inc; February 2007.

* Asterisk indicates drugs cited in interaction reports.

Exemestane			***Hydantoins***
Exemestane* (*Aromasin*)		Fosphenytoin (*Cerebyx*)	Phenytoin* (eg, *Dilantin*)

Significance	Onset	Severity	Documentation
2	☐ Rapid ■ **Delayed**	☐ Major ■ **Moderate** ☐ Minor	☐ Established ☐ Probable ■ **Suspected** ☐ Possible ☐ Unlikely

Effects EXEMESTANE plasma concentrations may be reduced, decreasing the efficacy.

Mechanism Induction of EXEMESTANE metabolism (CYP3A4) by PHENYTOIN.

Management If PHENYTOIN is coadministered in patients receiving EXEMESTANE, the recommended dosage of EXEMESTANE is 50 mg once daily after a meal.[1] If PHENYTOIN is discontinued, reduce the EXEMESTANE dosage to 25 mg once daily with a meal.

Discussion

Because exemestane undergoes metabolism by CYP3A4, coadministration of phenytoin is expected to decrease exemestane plasma concentrations.[1] Therefore, consider dosage adjustments in patients receiving exemestane when a strong CYP3A4 inducer (eg, phenytoin) is started or stopped.

The basis for this monograph is information on file with the manufacturer. There are no clinical data with dose adjustments in patients receiving exemestane and phenytoin. Studies are needed to determine the clinical importance of this interaction.

[1] *Aromasin* [package insert]. New York, NY: Pfizer, Inc; February 2007.

* Asterisk indicates drugs cited in interaction reports. Based on pharmacologic and pharmacokinetic considerations, similar interactions may occur with other drugs that are listed.

Exemestane | **Rifamycins**

Exemestane* (*Aromasin*)	Rifabutin* (*Mycobutin*) Rifampin* (eg, *Rifadin*)	Rifapentine* (*Priftin*)

Significance	Onset	Severity	Documentation
2	☐ Rapid ■ **Delayed**	☐ Major ■ **Moderate** ☐ Minor	☐ Established ☐ Probable ■ **Suspected** ☐ Possible ☐ Unlikely

Effects EXEMESTANE plasma concentrations may be reduced, decreasing the efficacy.

Mechanism Induction of EXEMESTANE metabolism (CYP3A4) by RIFAMPIN.

Management If RIFAMPIN is coadministered in patients receiving EXEMESTANE, the recommended dosage of EXEMESTANE is 50 mg once daily after a meal.[1] If RIFAMPIN is discontinued, reduce the EXEMESTANE dosage to 25 mg once daily with a meal.

Discussion

The effects of rifampin on the pharmacokinetics of exemestane were studied in 10 healthy postmenopausal women.[1] Each subject was pretreated with rifampin 600 mg daily for 14 days followed by a single dose of exemestane 25 mg. Rifampin decreased the mean plasma exemestane C_{max} and AUC 41% and 54%, respectively. Therefore, consider dosage adjustments in patients receiving exemestane when a strong CYP3A4 inducer (eg, rifampin) is started or stopped.

The basis for this monograph is information on file with the manufacturer. Additional studies are needed to determine the clinical importance of this interaction and if other rifamycins interact similarly.

[1] *Aromasin* [package insert]. New York, NY: Pfizer, Inc; February 2007.

* Asterisk indicates drugs cited in interaction reports.

Exemestane | **St. John's Wort**

Exemestane*
(*Aromasin*)

St. John's Wort*

Significance	Onset	Severity	Documentation
2	☐ Rapid ■ **Delayed**	☐ Major ■ **Moderate** ☐ Minor	☐ Established ☐ Probable ■ **Suspected** ☐ Possible ☐ Unlikely

Effects EXEMESTANE plasma concentrations may be reduced, decreasing the efficacy.

Mechanism Induction of EXEMESTANE metabolism (CYP3A4) by ST. JOHN'S WORT.

Management Avoid concurrent use of ST. JOHN'S WORT in patients receiving EXEMESTANE. If ST. JOHN'S WORT cannot be avoided, the recommended dosage of EXEMESTANE is 50 mg once daily after a meal.[1] If ST. JOHN'S WORT is discontinued, reduce the EXEMESTANE dosage to 25 mg once daily with a meal.

Discussion

Because exemestane undergoes metabolism by CYP3A4, coadministration of St. John's wort is expected to decrease exemestane plasma concentrations.[1] Therefore, consider dosage adjustments in patients receiving exemestane when a strong CYP3A4 inducer (eg, St. John's wort) is started or stopped.

The basis for this monograph is information on file with the manufacturer. There are no clinical data with dose adjustments in patients receiving exemestane and St. John's wort. Studies are needed to determine the clinical importance of this interaction.

[1] *Aromasin* [package insert]. New York, NY: Pfizer, Inc; February 2007.

* Asterisk indicates drugs cited in interaction reports.

Ezetimibe — *Rifamycins*

Ezetimibe* (*Zetia*)	Rifampin* (eg, *Rifadin*)

Significance	Onset	Severity	Documentation
5	□ Rapid	□ Major	□ Established
	■ **Delayed**	□ Moderate	□ Probable
		■ **Minor**	□ Suspected
			■ **Possible**
			□ Unlikely

Effects Because enterosystemic recycling of EZETIMIBE is reduced, the cholesterol-lowering effect of EZETIMIBE may be decreased.

Mechanism Reduced enterosystemic recycling caused by inhibition of secretion of EZETIMIBE and its glucuronide metabolite by way of P-glycoprotein and multidrug resistance–associated protein 2.

Management Monitor patients receiving EZETIMIBE for a decrease in efficacy if RIFAMPIN is coadministered.

Discussion

The effects of rifampin on the disposition of ezetimibe were studied in 8 healthy subjects.[1] Using an open-label, randomized, crossover design, each subject received oral ezetimibe 20 mg alone and coadministered with rifampin 600 mg. Compared with administration of ezetimibe alone, rifampin administration increased the C_{max} of ezetimibe and its glucuronide metabolite more than 2-fold and decreased fecal excretion of ezetimibe. Also, the serum concentrations and AUC of the glucuronide metabolite were increased more than 2-fold. There was no change in systemic exposure to ezetimibe. The onset of the sterol-lowering effect of ezetimibe was shortened by coadministration of rifampin.

[1] Oswald S, et al. *Clin Pharmacol Ther.* 2006;80(5):477.

* Asterisk indicates drugs cited in interaction reports.

Famotidine — *Probenecid*

Famotidine*
(eg, *Pepcid*)

Probenecid*

Significance	Onset	Severity	Documentation
5	■ **Rapid**	□ Major	□ Established
	□ Delayed	□ Moderate	□ Probable
		■ **Minor**	□ Suspected
			■ **Possible**
			□ Unlikely

Effects The pharmacologic effects of FAMOTIDINE may be increased.

Mechanism PROBENECID appears to inhibit the renal tubular secretion of FAMOTIDINE.

Management Based on currently available data, no special precautions are needed.

Discussion

The effects of probenecid administration on the pharmacokinetics of famotidine were studied in 8 healthy men.[1] Each subject was evaluated on 2 separate occasions at 1-month intervals. Subjects received oral famotidine 20 mg alone or with probenecid 1,000 mg 2 hours before, 250 mg 1 hour before, and 250 mg simultaneously with famotidine (total probenecid dose, 1,500 mg orally). Coadministration of probenecid decreased the apparent volume of the central compartment of famotidine, increased the maximum serum concentration attained, and increased the famotidine AUC 81% for up to 10 hours. In addition, probenecid decreased the mean urinary excretion rate of unchanged famotidine, the mean renal clearance, the mean amount of unchanged famotidine excreted in the urine up to 24 hours, and the mean renal tubular secretion clearance of famotidine (from 196.2 to 22 mL/min).

Additional studies are needed to determine if this possible interaction is of clinical importance.

[1] Inotsume N, et al. *J Clin Pharmacol.* 1990;30(1):50.

* Asterisk indicates drugs cited in interaction reports.

Felbamate — **Gabapentin**

Felbamate* (*Felbatol*)	Gabapentin* (eg, *Neurontin*)

Significance	Onset	Severity	Documentation
4	☐ Rapid	☐ Major	☐ Established
	■ **Delayed**	■ **Moderate**	☐ Probable
		☐ Minor	☐ Suspected
			■ **Possible**
			☐ Unlikely

Effects FELBAMATE clearance may be decreased and the t½ prolonged, increasing the pharmacologic effects and adverse reactions of FELBAMATE.

Mechanism Competition for renal excretion sites is suspected.

Management Observe patients for changes in clinical response to FELBAMATE when GABAPENTIN is started or stopped. Adjust the dose of FELBAMATE as needed.

Discussion

Using a retrospective design, a pharmacokinetic interaction was identified during coadministration of felbamate and gabapentin.[1] In 40 observations of patients receiving felbamate monotherapy, the clearance and t½ of felbamate were 0.67 L/kg/day and 24 hours, respectively. Eleven patients were identified who were treated with felbamate and gabapentin concomitantly. In patients receiving both medications, the clearance of felbamate was 0.42 L/kg/day, and the t½ of felbamate was 35 hours. Thus, coadministration of gabapentin and felbamate resulted in a 37% reduction in felbamate clearance and a 46% prolongation in the t½. The effects of felbamate on gabapentin were not investigated.
This combination may be beneficial in treating patients with epilepsy.

[1] Hussein G, et al. *Neurology*. 1996;47(4):1106.

* Asterisk indicates drugs cited in interaction reports.

Felodipine — *Azole Antifungal Agents*

Felodipine	Azole Antifungal Agents	
Felodipine*	Itraconazole* (eg, *Sporanox*)	Posaconazole (*Noxafil*)
	Ketoconazole (eg, *Nizoral*)	Voriconazole (eg, *Vfend*)

Significance	Onset	Severity	Documentation
2	□ Rapid ■ **Delayed**	□ Major ■ **Moderate** □ Minor	□ Established □ Probable ■ **Suspected** □ Possible □ Unlikely

Effects Serum FELODIPINE concentrations may be increased. Peripheral edema has been reported.

Mechanism Possible inhibition of FELODIPINE metabolism (CYP3A4) by certain AZOLE ANTIFUNGAL AGENTS may occur.

Management Observe the clinical response of patients and monitor cardiovascular status when FELODIPINE and certain AZOLE ANTIFUNGAL AGENTS are coadministered. If an interaction is suspected, adjust the dose of FELODIPINE accordingly. Coadministration of FELODIPINE and ITRACONAZOLE is contraindicated.[1]

Discussion

A possible drug interaction has been reported in 2 hypertensive patients during coadministration of felodipine and itraconazole.[2] Both patients had been taking felodipine for 1 year without adverse reactions. Itraconazole treatment was initiated in 1 patient for tinea pedis. During the first week of treatment, the patient observed increased swelling of the lower extremities. When itraconazole treatment was discontinued, the edema subsided within 4 days. Swelling did not occur with felodipine alone. In the second patient, itraconazole was administered for onychomycosis. Within days, leg swelling occurred. Felodipine was discontinued, and itraconazole was given 7 days each month during the following 3 months without adverse reactions. When this patient was rechallenged with a single dose of felodipine on the last day of the itraconazole course, slight ankle swelling occurred and disappeared the following day. No swelling occurred on 2 rechallenges with felodipine alone. In addition, plasma felodipine concentrations were considerably higher when both drugs were coadministered compared with giving felodipine alone. In a study of 9 volunteers, itraconazole 200 mg/day for 4 days increased peak felodipine concentrations nearly 7-fold and the $t_{1/2}$ from 15 to 26 hours.[3] Bioavailability increased 6-fold. These changes were associated with an increase in heart rate and a decrease in BP. A similar interaction may occur with itraconazole and isradipine (eg, *DynaCirc*). See Nifedipine-Azole Antifungal Agents.

[1] *Sporanox* [package insert]. Raritan, NJ: Centocor Ortho Biotech Products; November 2011.
[2] Neuvonen PJ, et al. *J Am Acad Dermatol.* 1995;33(1):134.
[3] Jalava K, et al. *Clin Pharmacol Ther.* 1997;61(4):410.

* Asterisk indicates drugs cited in interaction reports. Based on pharmacologic and pharmacokinetic considerations, similar interactions may occur with other drugs that are listed.

Felodipine		***Barbiturates***	
Felodipine* (*Plendil*)		Amobarbital (eg, *Amytal*) Butabarbital (eg, *Butisol*) Butalbital Mephobarbital (*Mebaral*)	Pentobarbital Phenobarbital* Primidone (eg, *Mysoline*) Secobarbital (*Seconal*)

Significance	Onset	Severity	Documentation
2	☐ Rapid ■ **Delayed**	☐ Major ■ **Moderate** ☐ Minor	☐ Established ☐ Probable ■ **Suspected** ☐ Possible ☐ Unlikely

Effects The pharmacologic effects of FELODIPINE may be decreased.

Mechanism Unknown. However, the metabolism of FELODIPINE may be increased due to induction of mixed function oxidases by BARBITURATES, causing an increase in first-pass metabolism and decreased bioavailability.

Management Patients receiving long-term treatment with both drugs may require higher doses of FELODIPINE.

Discussion

The effect of long-term anticonvulsant therapy on the bioavailability of felodipine was studied in 10 epileptic patients.[1] Four patients were taking carbamazepine (eg, *Tegretol*), two were receiving phenytoin (eg, *Dilantin*), three were taking both drugs, and one patient was receiving phenobarbital. Twelve healthy volunteers, matched for age and sex with the treatment group, served as controls and were not receiving any regular medication. All 22 participants were given felodipine 5 mg twice daily for 4 days, and on the fifth day, they took 5 mg felodipine after breakfast. The mean peak plasma levels of felodipine on day 5 were greatly reduced in the epileptic patients compared with the controls (1.6 vs 8.9 nmol/L; $P < 0.01$). Felodipine was undetectable in the plasma of two patients. The area under the felodipine concentration-time curve was 2 nmol•hr/L in the patients compared with 30 nmol•hr/L in the controls ($P < 0.001$). The relative bioavailability of felodipine in the epileptic patients was 6.6% of that in the controls. The mean felodipine plasma half-life in the control group was 2.6 hours and could not be estimated in the epileptic patients. Carbamazepine, phenytoin and phenobarbital are potent inducers of the hepatic mixed function oxidase system. Because felodipine is extensively metabolized by these enzymes, enzyme induction is the most likely mechanism of this interaction.

Clinical trials are needed to determine the effect of each anticonvulsant.

[1] Capewell S, et al. *Lancet.* 1988;2:480.

* Asterisk indicates drugs cited in interaction reports. Based on pharmacologic and pharmacokinetic considerations, similar interactions may occur with other drugs that are listed.

Felodipine — *Carbamazepine*

Felodipine* (*Plendil*)	Carbamazepine* (eg, *Tegretol*)

Significance	Onset	Severity	Documentation
2	☐ Rapid	☐ Major	☐ Established
	■ **Delayed**	■ **Moderate**	☐ Probable
		☐ Minor	■ **Suspected**
			☐ Possible
			☐ Unlikely

Effects The pharmacologic effects of FELODIPINE may be decreased.

Mechanism Unknown. However, the metabolism of FELODIPINE may be increased due to induction of mixed function oxidases by CARBAMAZEPINE, causing an increase in first-pass metabolism and decreased bioavailability.

Management Patients receiving long-term treatment with CARBAMAZEPINE and FELODIPINE may require higher doses of FELODIPINE to achieve plasma levels equivalent to those of patients who are not receiving CARBAMAZEPINE concurrently.

Discussion

The effect of long-term anticonvulsant therapy on the bioavailability of felodipine was studied in 10 epileptic patients.[1] Four patients were taking carbamazepine, two were receiving phenytoin (eg, *Dilantin*), three were taking both drugs, and one patient was receiving phenobarbital. Twelve healthy volunteers, matched for age and sex with the treatment group, served as controls. None of the subjects in the control group were receiving any regular medication. All 22 participants were given felodipine 5 mg twice daily for 4 days, and on the fifth day, they took felodipine 5 mg after breakfast. The mean peak plasma levels of felodipine on day 5 were greatly reduced in the epileptic patients compared with the controls (1.6 vs 8.9 nmol/L; $P < 0.01$). Felodipine was undetectable in the plasma of two epileptic patients. The area under the felodipine concentration-time curve was 2 nmol•hr/L in the patients with epilepsy compared with 30 nmol•hr/L in the controls ($P < 0.001$). The relative bioavailability of felodipine in the epileptic patients was 6.6% of that in the controls. The mean felodipine plasma half-life in the control group was 2.6 hours and could not be estimated in the epileptic patients. Carbamazepine, phenytoin and phenobarbital are potent inducers of the hepatic mixed function oxidase system. Because felodipine is extensively metabolized by these enzymes, enzyme induction is the most likely mechanism of this interaction.

Clinical trials are needed to determine the effect of each anticonvulsant.

[1] Capewell S, et al. *Lancet.* 1988;2:480.

* Asterisk indicates drugs cited in interaction reports.

Felodipine — *Cimetidine*

Felodipine* (*Plendil*)	Cimetidine* (eg, *Tagamet*)

Significance	Onset	Severity	Documentation
4	☐ Rapid ■ **Delayed**	☐ Major ■ **Moderate** ☐ Minor	☐ Established ☐ Probable ☐ Suspected ■ **Possible** ☐ Unlikely

Effects Serum FELODIPINE levels may be increased, producing an increase in the pharmacologic and toxic effects of FELODIPINE.

Mechanism CIMETIDINE may inhibit the hepatic microsomal metabolism of FELODIPINE.

Management No special precautions appear to be necessary other than the usual monitoring of cardiovascular status.

Discussion

A preliminary report indicates that plasma levels of felodipine may be increased by cimetidine.[1] In a 2-way crossover study, 12 healthy men received cimetidine 1 g daily for 5 consecutive days. On the fifth day, each subject also received a single 10 mg dose of felodipine. During coadministration of the drugs, the area under the felodipine concentration-time curve increased from 53 to 83 nmol•hr/L ($P < 0.01$), and the maximum plasma felodipine concentration increased from 17 to 26.3 nmol/L ($P < 0.001$) compared with felodipine alone. Inhibition of felodipine metabolism by cimetidine may be involved.

Documentation for this possible interaction consists of an abstract. More substantive data are needed to evaluate the clinical importance of this reported interaction.

[1] Janzon K, et al. *Acta Pharmacol Toxicol.* 1986;59 (suppl V):98.258.

* Asterisk indicates drugs cited in interaction reports.

Felodipine | **Cyclosporine**

Felodipine*
(*Plendil*)

Cyclosporine*
(eg, *Neoral*)

Significance	Onset	Severity	Documentation
4	■ **Rapid**	□ Major	□ Established
	□ Delayed	■ **Moderate**	□ Probable
		□ Minor	□ Suspected
			■ **Possible**
			□ Unlikely

Effects The effects of FELODIPINE or CYCLOSPORINE may be increased.

Mechanism CYCLOSPORINE may inhibit the intestinal and hepatic metabolism (cytochrome P450 3A) of FELODIPINE.[1,2]

Management Because clinical data are not available, consider monitoring the response of the patient when coadministration of these agents is started, stopped, or changed in dosage. If an interaction is suspected, adjust therapy as needed.

Discussion

The pharmacokinetics of coadministered cyclosporine and felodipine were evaluated in 12 healthy men.[1] In addition, the effects of administration of these agents on 24-hour BP were studied. Using a double-blind, placebo-controlled, randomized, crossover design, each subject received a single dose of cyclosporine 5 mg/kg orally and extended release felodipine 10 mg together or separately with a placebo. Felodipine administration increased peak whole blood cyclosporine concentrations 16% but did not alter other cyclosporine pharmacokinetic parameters. In contrast, cyclosporine increased the area under the plasma concentration-time curve (AUC) of felodipine 58%, the peak plasma felodipine concentrations 151% and decreased the mean residence time 24% when compared with administration of felodipine plus placebo. The AUC of the dehydrofelodipine metabolite was increased 43%, and the peak concentrations of the metabolite were increased 84%. The mean 24-hour systolic and diastolic BPs were lower after felodipine plus placebo administration (121/68 mm Hg) or felodipine plus cyclosporine (122/68 mm Hg) compared with giving cyclosporine plus placebo (127/73 mm Hg). In a study of 22 renal transplant patients, cyclosporine levels were not affected by coadministration of felodipine 10 mg/day for 3 weeks.[3]

Evaluation of the clinical importance of this interaction in hypertensive patients is needed.

[1] Madsen JK, et al. *Eur J Clin Pharmacol.* 1996;50:203.
[2] Madsen JK, et al. *Eur J Clin Pharmacol.* 1997;52:161.
[3] Yildiz A, et al. *Nephron.* 1999;81:117.

* Asterisk indicates drugs cited in interaction reports.

Felodipine — *Erythromycin*

Felodipine* (*Plendil*)	Erythromycin* (eg, *Ery-Tab*)

Significance	Onset	Severity	Documentation
2	□ Rapid ■ **Delayed**	□ Major ■ **Moderate** □ Minor	□ Established □ Probable ■ **Suspected** □ Possible □ Unlikely

Effects The pharmacologic and adverse effects of FELODIPINE may be increased.

Mechanism The CYP-450 isoenzyme P-450 3A is known to metabolize other dihydropyridine calcium antagonists (eg, nifedipine) and is known to be inhibited by ERYTHROMYCIN. Thus, it is likely that the mechanism of this interaction is caused by inhibition of FELODIPINE metabolism by ERYTHROMYCIN.

Management Monitor the cardiovascular status of patients receiving FELODIPINE when treatment with ERYTHROMYCIN is initiated, altered, or discontinued. If an interaction is suspected, adjust the dose of FELODIPINE accordingly.

Discussion

Administration of erythromycin increased the effects of felodipine in a 43-year-old woman.[1] The patient had a family history of hypertension and was successfully treated for essential hypertension for 6 months with extended-release felodipine 10 mg/day. A 7-day course of enteric-coated erythromycin 250 mg twice daily was prescribed for the treatment of a respiratory tract infection. Within 3 days of treatment, she experienced increasing symptoms of palpitations, flushing, and ankle edema. The tachycardia kept the patient from performing her regular work. Upon physical examination, her BP was 110/70 mm Hg, and she had massive edema of her legs. Several days after completion of the antibiotic course, the patient's symptoms subsided. A trough serum felodipine level was 6 nmol/L at the end of coadministration with erythromycin compared with a level of less than 2 nmol/L measured 10 days after discontinuation of the antibiotic. In a randomized, crossover study involving 12 healthy men, extended-release felodipine 10 mg was administered with either water, grapefruit juice, or erythromycin 250 mg 4 times/day before and on the study day.[2] Compared with water, erythromycin increased the AUC of felodipine 52%, peak plasma felodipine concentrations 64%, and the felodipine $t_{1/2}$ 52%.

[1] Liedholm H, et al. *DICP*. 1991;25:1007.
[2] Bailey DG, et al. *Clin Pharmacol Ther*. 1996;60:25.

* Asterisk indicates drugs cited in interaction reports.

Felodipine — *Food*

Felodipine* (*Plendil*) | Grapefruit Juice*

Significance	Onset	Severity	Documentation
2	■ **Rapid**	□ Major	□ Established
	□ Delayed	■ **Moderate**	■ **Probable**
		□ Minor	□ Suspected
			□ Possible
			□ Unlikely

Effects Serum FELODIPINE concentrations may be elevated, producing an increase in pharmacologic and adverse effects.

Mechanism Inhibition of gut wall metabolism (CYP3A4) of FELODIPINE by furanocoumarins present in GRAPEFRUIT.[1-6]

Management Patients taking FELODIPINE should refrain from consuming GRAPEFRUIT JUICE.

Discussion

Coadministration of felodipine and grapefruit juice or unprocessed grapefruit has been associated with an increase in the bioavailability of felodipine,[1,2,6-9] as has coadministration with pure bergamottin.[10] The effects of concurrent felodipine 5 mg and ethanol 0.75 g/kg in grapefruit juice were studied in 10 patients with untreated, borderline hypertension, using a double-blind, placebo-controlled, crossover design.[7] Although felodipine plus ethanol enhanced the hemodynamic effects at 4 hours compared with felodipine alone, felodipine plasma concentrations in both treatment groups were greatly elevated over the findings of other published studies. One variation from other studies was that felodipine was given with grapefruit juice as opposed to water. Subsequently, in a crossover investigation, 6 men with borderline hypertension received felodipine 5 mg or nifedipine 10 mg (eg, *Procardia*) with water, grapefruit juice, or orange juice.[8] Compared with ingestion with water, the mean felodipine bioavailability with grapefruit juice was 284% higher. Felodipine taken with grapefruit juice had greater effects on diastolic pressure, heart rate, and vasodilation-associated side effects than when taken with water. In contrast, orange juice did not interact with felodipine. The bioavailability of nifedipine taken with grapefruit juice was 134% of the value compared with water. In 2 additional studies involving 18 healthy subjects, the effect of grapefruit juice on the actions of felodipine 5 mg was studied.[1,2] Compared with water, grapefruit juice produced an increase in the maximum serum level (127% to 310%) and the AUC (123% to 330%) of felodipine. Similar effects have been noted with extended-release felodipine administered with grapefruit juice.[3,5] In 9 healthy subjects, ingestion of grapefruit juice up to 24 hours before extended-release felodipine was shown to increase serum felodipine concentrations.[4]

1 Edgar B, et al. *Eur J Clin Pharmacol.* 1992;42:313.
2 Bailey DG, et al. *Clin Pharmacol Ther.* 1993;53:637.
3 Bailey DG, et al. *Br J Clin Pharmacol.* 1995;40:135.
4 Lundahl J, et al. *Eur J Clin Pharmacol.* 1995;49:61.
5 Bailey DG, et al. *Clin Pharmacol Ther.* 1996;60:25.
6 Bailey DG, et al. *Clin Pharmacol Ther.* 2000;68:468.
7 Bailey DG, et al. *Clin Invest Med.* 1989;12:357.
8 Bailey DG, et al. *Lancet.* 1991;337:268.
9 Dresser GK, et al. *Clin Pharmacol Ther.* 2000;68:28.
10 Goosen TC, et al. *Clin Pharmacol Ther.* 2004;76:607.

* Asterisk indicates drugs cited in interaction reports.

Felodipine — *Hydantoins*

Felodipine* (*Plendil*)	Ethotoin (*Peganone*)	Phenytoin* (eg, *Dilantin*)
	Fosphenytoin (*Cerebyx*)	

Significance	Onset	Severity	Documentation
2	☐ Rapid	☐ Major	☐ Established
	■ **Delayed**	■ **Moderate**	☐ Probable
		☐ Minor	■ **Suspected**
			☐ Possible
			☐ Unlikely

Effects The pharmacologic effects of FELODIPINE may be decreased.

Mechanism The metabolism of FELODIPINE may be increased because of induction of mixed-function oxidases by HYDANTOINS, causing an increase in first-pass metabolism and decreased bioavailability.

Management Patients receiving long-term treatment with HYDANTOINS and FELODIPINE may require higher doses of FELODIPINE to achieve plasma levels equivalent to those of patients who are not receiving HYDANTOINS concurrently.

Discussion

The effect of long-term anticonvulsant therapy on the bioavailability of felodipine was studied in 10 epileptic patients.[1] Four patients were taking carbamazepine (eg, *Tegretol*), 2 were receiving phenytoin, 3 were taking both drugs, and 1 patient was receiving phenobarbital. Twelve healthy volunteers, matched for age and sex with the treatment group, served as controls. None of the subjects in the control group were receiving any regular medication. All 22 participants were given felodipine 5 mg twice daily for 4 days; on day 5, they took felodipine 5 mg after breakfast. The mean peak plasma levels of felodipine on day 5 were greatly reduced in the epileptic patients compared with the controls (1.6 vs 8.9 nmol/L; $P < 0.01$). Felodipine was undetectable in the plasma of 2 epileptic patients. The felodipine AUC was 2 nmol•hr/L in the patients with epilepsy compared with 30 nmol•hr/L in the controls ($P < 0.001$). The relative bioavailability of felodipine in the epileptic patients was 6.6% of that in the controls. The mean felodipine plasma $t_{½}$ in the control group was 2.6 hours and could not be estimated in the epileptic patients. Carbamazepine, phenytoin, and phenobarbital are potent inducers of the hepatic mixed-function oxidase system. Because felodipine is extensively metabolized by these enzymes, enzyme induction is most likely the mechanism of this interaction.

Clinical trials are needed to determine the effect of each anticonvulsant.

[1] Capewell S, et al. *Lancet.* 1988;2:480.

* Asterisk indicates drugs cited in interaction reports. Based on pharmacologic and pharmacokinetic considerations, similar interactions may occur with other drugs that are listed.

Felodipine — *Oxcarbazepine*

Felodipine*
(*Plendil*)

Oxcarbazepine*
(*Trileptal*)

Significance	Onset	Severity	Documentation
4	☐ Rapid ■ **Delayed**	☐ Major ■ **Moderate** ☐ Minor	☐ Established ☐ Probable ☐ Suspected ■ **Possible** ☐ Unlikely

Effects The pharmacologic effects of FELODIPINE may be decreased.

Mechanism Unknown.

Management Closely monitor the patient's response to FELODIPINE when OXCARBAZEPINE is started, stopped, or changed in dosage. Adjust the dosage of FELODIPINE as needed.

Discussion

In an open-label investigation, the effect of single and repeated doses of oxcarbazepine on the pharmacokinetics of felodipine was studied in 8 healthy men.[1] Seven subjects completed the study. Felodipine 10 mg/day was administered to each subject for 13 consecutive days. On day 6, oxcarbazepine 600 mg was given in the morning, and, on days 7 to 13, each subject received oxcarbazepine 450 mg twice daily. Single-dose administration of oxcarbazepine did not affect the steady-state pharmacokinetics of felodipine or its pyridine metabolite. In contrast, multiple-dose oxcarbazepine administration decreased the felodipine AUC 28% and the peak concentration 34% (from 9.7 to 6.4 nmol/L). Despite the decrease, plasma felodipine concentrations remained within the recommended therapeutic range. The 28% reduction in felodipine AUC occurring with coadministration of oxcarbazepine is less than that which occurs with concomitant use of carbamazepine (94%; eg, *Tegretol*).[1] Therefore, if oxcarbazepine is substituted for carbamazepine in patients receiving felodipine, felodipine plasma concentrations may increase. See also Felodipine-Carbamazepine.

[1] Zaccara G, et al. *Ther Drug Monit.* 1993;15:39.

* Asterisk indicates drugs cited in interaction reports.

Felodipine — *Protease Inhibitors*

Felodipine	Protease Inhibitors	
Felodipine* (*Plendil*)	Amprenavir (*Agenerase*)	Lopinavir/Ritonavir (*Kaletra*)
	Atazanavir (*Reyataz*)	Nelfinavir* (*Viracept*)
	Fosamprenavir (*Lexiva*)	Ritonavir (*Norvir*)
	Indinavir (*Crixivan*)	Saquinavir (*Invirase*)

Significance	Onset	Severity	Documentation
4	☐ Rapid	☐ Major	☐ Established
	■ **Delayed**	■ **Moderate**	☐ Probable
		☐ Minor	☐ Suspected
			■ **Possible**
			☐ Unlikely

Effects FELODIPINE plasma concentrations may be elevated, increasing the pharmacologic and adverse effects.

Mechanism Inhibition of FELODIPINE metabolism (CYP3A4) by the PROTEASE INHIBITOR is suspected.

Management Observe the clinical response of the patient and monitor cardiovascular status when FELODIPINE and a PROTEASE INHIBITOR are given concurrently. If an interaction is suspected, consider adjusting the dosage of FELODIPINE or administering an alternative antihypertensive.

Discussion

A possible drug interaction between felodipine and nelfinavir was reported in a nurse.[1] Following an accidental needlestick from a patient known to be infected with HIV, the patient was treated with a regimen consisting of nelfinavir 2,000 mg/day, zidovudine (eg, *Retrovir*), and lamivudine (*Epivir*). She had been receiving metoprolol (eg, *Lopressor* 50 mg/day) plus felodipine 5 mg/day without any adverse reactions. Three days after starting the HIV treatment regimen, the patient developed bilateral leg edema, dizziness, fatigue, and orthostatic hypotension. The metoprolol and felodipine combination was stopped and, within 3 days, the leg edema and orthostatic hypotension subsided. A diuretic-based regimen was started for the patient's hypertension without recurrence of edema.

[1] Izzedine H, et al. *Clin Pharmacol Ther.* 2004;75:362.

* Asterisk indicates drugs cited in interaction reports. Based on pharmacologic and pharmacokinetic considerations, similar interactions may occur with other drugs that are listed.

Fenoprofen — *Barbiturates*

Fenoprofen	Barbiturates	
Fenoprofen* (eg, *Nalfon*)	Amobarbital (*Amytal*)	Pentobarbital
	Butabarbital (eg, *Butisol*)	Phenobarbital* (eg, *Solfoton*)
	Butalbital	Primidone (eg, *Mysoline*)
	Mephobarbital (*Mebaral*)	Secobarbital (*Seconal*)

Significance	Onset	Severity	Documentation
5	☐ Rapid ■ **Delayed**	☐ Major ☐ Moderate ■ **Minor**	☐ Established ☐ Probable ☐ Suspected ■ **Possible** ☐ Unlikely

Effects The pharmacologic effects of FENOPROFEN may be decreased.

Mechanism PHENOBARBITAL may increase the metabolism of FENOPROFEN by inducing hepatic enzymes.

Management Consider monitoring patients for decreased response to FENOPROFEN. Adjust the dose accordingly.

Discussion

The effect of 10 days of phenobarbital administration on the kinetics of IV fenoprofen was evaluated in 18 patients.[1] Three groups of 6 patients each received fenoprofen with either placebo, phenobarbital 15 mg every 6 hours, or phenobarbital 60 mg every 6 hours. A decreased AUC and increased elimination was found and attributed to increased metabolism. The clinical importance of this interaction is unclear.

[1] Helleberg L, et al. *Br J Clin Pharmacol.* 1974;1:371.

* Asterisk indicates drugs cited in interaction reports. Based on pharmacologic and pharmacokinetic considerations, similar interactions may occur with other drugs that are listed.

Fentanyl — *Mifepristone*

Fentanyl* (eg, *Sublimaze*)	Mifepristone* (eg, *Korlym*)

Significance	Onset	Severity	Documentation
1	☐ Rapid ■ **Delayed**	■ **Major** ☐ Moderate ☐ Minor	☐ Established ☐ Probable ■ **Suspected** ☐ Possible ☐ Unlikely

Effects FENTANYL plasma concentrations may be elevated, increasing the pharmacologic effects and risk of adverse reactions (eg, respiratory depression).

Mechanism MIFEPRISTONE may inhibit FENTANYL metabolism (CYP3A4).

Management Coadministration of FENTANYL with MIFEPRISTONE is contraindicated.[1]

Discussion

Because mifepristone inhibits CYP3A4, coadministration of mifepristone with a drug that is metabolized mainly or solely by CYP3A4 (eg, fentanyl) is likely to increase plasma concentrations of the drug.[1] Therefore, the concurrent use of drugs with a narrow therapeutic index that are CYP3A4 substrates, such as fentanyl, is contraindicated. The risk of fentanyl adverse reactions (eg, respiratory depression) may be increased.

[1] *Korlym* [package insert]. Menlo Park, CA: Corcept Therapeutics Incorporated; February 2012.

* Asterisk indicates drugs cited in interaction reports.

Fentanyl		**Rifamycins**	
Fentanyl* (eg, *Sublimaze*)		Rifabutin (*Mycobutin*) Rifampin* (eg, *Rifadin*)	Rifapentine (*Priftin*)

Significance	Onset	Severity	Documentation
2	■ **Rapid** □ Delayed	□ Major ■ **Moderate** □ Minor	□ Established □ Probable ■ **Suspected** □ Possible □ Unlikely

Effects FENTANYL plasma concentrations may be reduced, decreasing FENTANYL efficacy.

Mechanism Induction of FENTANYL metabolism (CYP3A4) by RIFAMYCINS is suspected.

Management Monitor the response of patients when a RIFAMYCIN is started or discontinued. Be prepared to adjust the FENTANYL dosage as needed.

Discussion

A possible interaction during coadministration of fentanyl and rifampin was reported in a 61-year-old man with recurrence of parotid gland adenocarcinoma.[1] The patient was switched to fentanyl 1.67 mg transdermal patches every 3 days after nausea and vomiting developed during oral morphine therapy. Fentanyl serum concentrations 48 and 72 hours after the first day of treatment were 0.9 and 0.77 ng/mL, respectively. The corresponding serum concentration to dose ratios were 0.54 and 0.46, respectively. Because of insufficient pain control, the fentanyl dosage was increased by 2.5 mg (25 mcg/h) every 3 days. Two days later, the patient developed severe pain. Fentanyl serum levels 48 and 72 hours after treatment were 0.53 ng/mL (serum concentration to dose ratio, 0.21) and 0.21 ng/mL (serum concentration to dose ratio, 0.08). The patient continued to complain of moderate pain with a dosage of fentanyl 7.5 mg (75 mcg/h) every 3 days and coadministration of loxoprofen.† A similar case of pain control failure with transdermal fentanyl (0.6 mg/day gradually increased to 2.5 mg/day) was reported in a 64-year-old man during coadministration of rifampin 450 mg/day.[2] When fentanyl 2.5 mg/day did not adequately control the pain, transdermal fentanyl was replaced with sustained-release morphine 180 mg/day.

[1] Takane H, et al. *Ann Pharmacother.* 2005;39(12):2139.

[2] Morii H, et al. *J Pain Symptom Manage.* 2007;33(1):5.

* Asterisk indicates drugs cited in interaction reports. Based on pharmacologic and pharmacokinetic considerations, similar interactions may occur with other drugs that are listed.
† Not available in the United States.

Fesoterodine | *Azole Antifungal Agents*

Fesoterodine* (*Toviaz*)	Fluconazole* (eg, *Diflucan*)	Ketoconazole* (eg, *Nizoral*)
	Itraconazole* (eg, *Sporanox*)	

Significance	Onset	Severity	Documentation
2	☐ Rapid	☐ Major	☐ Established
	■ **Delayed**	■ **Moderate**	☐ Probable
		☐ Minor	■ **Suspected**
			☐ Possible
			☐ Unlikely

Effects FESOTERODINE plasma concentrations may be elevated, increasing the pharmacologic effects and adverse reactions.

Mechanism Inhibition of metabolism (CYP3A4) of the active metabolite of FESOTERODINE by ITRACONAZOLE or KETOCONAZOLE.

Management The FESOTERODINE dose should not exceed 4 mg daily in patients receiving ITRACONAZOLE or KETOCONAZOLE.[1]

Discussion

The potential for an interaction between fesoterodine and ketoconazole was studied in 18 healthy men.[2] Six subjects were CYP2D6 poor metabolizers (PM) and 12 subjects were extensive metabolizers (EM). A single dose of fesoterodine 8 mg was administered alone and after pretreatment with ketoconazole 200 mg twice daily. Compared with fesoterodine alone, pretreatment with ketoconazole increased the C_{max} of the fesoterodine active metabolite, 5-hydroxymethyl tolterodine (5-HMT), from 3 to 6 ng/mL in EM subjects and from 6.4 to 13.4 ng/mL in PM subjects and the mean AUC approximately 132% and 146% in EM and PM subjects, respectively. Although fesoterodine is primarily metabolized by CYP2D6, 5-HMT is a CYP3A4 substrate.[2] Therefore, doses of fesoterodine greater than 4 mg daily are not recommended in patients taking strong CYP3A4 inhibitors, such as ketoconazole or itraconazole.[1,2] When fluconazole and fesoterodine were coadministered, there was a 27% increase in fesoterodine AUC, which was not considered to be clinically important.[3]

[1] *Toviaz* [package insert]. New York, NY: Pfizer; April 2008.

[2] Malhotra B, et al. *Eur J Clin Pharmacol.* 2009;65(6):551.

[3] Malhotra B, et al. *Br J Clin Pharmacol.* 2011;72(2):263.

* Asterisk indicates drugs cited in interaction reports.

Fesoterodine — *Macrolide & Related Antibiotics*

Fesoterodine	Macrolide & Related Antibiotics	
Fesoterodine* (*Toviaz*)	Clarithromycin* (eg, *Biaxin*)	Telithromycin (*Ketek*)
	Erythromycin* (eg, *Ery-Tab*)	

Significance	Onset	Severity	Documentation
2	☐ Rapid	☐ Major	☐ Established
	■ **Delayed**	■ **Moderate**	☐ Probable
		☐ Minor	■ **Suspected**
			☐ Possible
			☐ Unlikely

Effects FESOTERODINE plasma concentrations may be elevated, increasing the pharmacologic effects and adverse reactions.

Mechanism Inhibition of metabolism (CYP3A4) of the active metabolite of FESOTERODINE by MACROLIDE AND RELATED ANTIBIOTICS.

Management The FESOTERODINE dose should not exceed 4 mg daily in patients receiving CLARITHROMYCIN and possibly TELITHROMYCIN. In patients receiving ERYTHROMYCIN, assess the tolerability at FESOTERODINE 4 mg daily before increasing the dose to 8 mg daily.[1]

Discussion

Although fesoterodine is primarily metabolized by CYP2D6, the active metabolite of fesoterodine, 5-hydroxymethyl tolterodine (5-HMT), is a CYP3A4 substrate.[2] Therefore, doses of fesoterodine greater than 4 mg daily are not recommended in patients taking strong CYP3A4 inhibitors, such as clarithromycin.[1] The potential for an interaction between fesoterodine and strong CYP2D6 substrates (eg, clarithromycin, ketoconazole) was studied in 18 healthy men.[2] Six subjects were CYP2D6 poor metabolizers (PM) and 12 subjects were extensive metabolizers (EM). A single dose of fesoterodine 8 mg was administered alone and after pretreatment with ketoconazole 200 mg twice daily. Compared with fesoterodine alone, pretreatment with ketoconazole increased the C_{max} of 5-HMT from 3 to 6 ng/mL in EM subjects and from 6.4 to 13.4 ng/mL in PM subjects and the mean AUC approximately 132% and 146% in EM and PM subjects, respectively.

[1] *Toviaz* [package insert]. New York, NY: Pfizer Labs; April 2008.

[2] Malhotra B, et al. *Eur J Clin Pharmacol.* 2009;65(6):551.

* Asterisk indicates drugs cited in interaction reports. Based on pharmacologic and pharmacokinetic considerations, similar interactions may occur with other drugs that are listed.

Fesoterodine — *Rifamycins*

Fesoterodine	Rifamycins	
Fesoterodine* (*Toviaz*)	Rifabutin (*Mycobutin*)	Rifapentine (*Priftin*)
	Rifampin* (eg, *Rifadin*)	

Significance	Onset	Severity	Documentation
2	☐ Rapid	☐ Major	☐ Established
	■ **Delayed**	■ **Moderate**	☐ Probable
		☐ Minor	■ **Suspected**
			☐ Possible
			☐ Unlikely

Effects FESOTERODINE plasma concentrations may be reduced, decreasing the pharmacologic effects.

Mechanism Increased metabolism (CYP3A4) of the active metabolite of FESOTERODINE by RIFAMYCINS.

Management Concomitant use of FESOTERODINE with RIFAMYCINS is not recommended because the induction of CYP3A4 may lead to subtherapeutic plasma concentrations of the FESOTERODINE active metabolite, 5-hydroxymethyl tolterodine (5-HMT).[1]

Discussion

The effects of rifampin on the pharmacokinetics of fesoterodine were studied in 12 healthy men.[2] Four subjects were CYP2D6 poor metabolizers (PM) and 8 subjects were extensive metabolizers (EM). Using an open-label, sequential design, each subject received a single oral dose of fesoterodine 8 mg alone and after pretreatment with rifampin 600 mg twice daily for 7 days. Compared with administering fesoterodine alone, pretreatment with rifampin decreased the C_{max} of 5-HMT from 5.2 to 1.5 ng/mL in EM subjects and from 6.8 to 1.9 ng/mL in PM subjects and decreased the mean AUC (ie, exposure) approximately 77% and 78% in EM and PM subjects, respectively. Although fesoterodine is primarily metabolized by CYP2D6, 5-HMT is a CYP3A4 substrate. Therefore, administration of fesoterodine with strong CYP3A4 inducers may result in subtherapeutic 5-HMT plasma concentrations.[1]

[1] *Toviaz* [package insert]. New York, NY: Pfizer Labs; April 2008.

[2] Malhotra B, et al. *Eur J Clin Pharmacol.* 2009;65(6):551.

* Asterisk indicates drugs cited in interaction reports. Based on pharmacologic and pharmacokinetic considerations, similar interactions may occur with other drugs that are listed.

Fexofenadine — *Azole Antifungal Agents*

Fexofenadine* (eg, *Allegra*)	Itraconazole* (eg, *Sporanox*)

Significance	Onset	Severity	Documentation
3	■ **Rapid** □ Delayed	□ Major □ Moderate ■ **Minor**	□ Established □ Probable ■ **Suspected** □ Possible □ Unlikely

Effects FEXOFENADINE plasma concentrations may be elevated, increasing the pharmacologic (antihistaminic) effects and adverse reactions.

Mechanism The major mechanism appears to be ITRACONAZOLE inhibition of the P-gp transporter in the small intestine, which increases FEXOFENADINE absorption.

Management Observe patients for FEXOFENADINE adverse reactions.

Discussion

The effects of itraconazole on the pharmacokinetics and pharmacodynamics of fexofenadine were studied in 14 healthy men.[1] In a randomized, double-blind, crossover investigation, each subject received placebo or itraconazole 200 mg 1 hour before fexofenadine 180 mg. Compared with placebo, itraconazole increased the fexofenadine C_{max} and AUC more than 3-fold. In addition, itraconazole administration resulted in a higher suppression of the histamine-induced wheal-and-flare reaction compared with placebo. There were no changes in psychomotor performance. In a randomized, crossover study, 8 healthy subjects were pretreated with placebo or itraconazole 100 mg twice daily for 5 days; on day 5, each subject received a single dose of fexofenadine 120 mg.[2] Compared with placebo, itraconazole increased the fexofenadine C_{max} and AUC 2- and 3-fold, respectively. Fexofenadine renal clearance and elimination $t_{½}$ were not affected. In a double-blind, controlled study, itraconazole increased the AUC of S-fexofenadine and R-fexofenadine 4- and 3.1-fold, respectively.[3] The effect of itraconazole on fexofenadine kinetics appears to be independent of the itraconazole dose.[4]

1 Shon JH, et al. *Clin Pharmacol Ther.* 2005;78(2):191.
2 Shimizu M, et al. *Br J Clin Pharmacol.* 2006;61(5):538.
3 Tateishi T, et al. *Br J Clin Pharmacol.* 2008;65(5):693.
4 Uno T, et al. *Drug Metab Dispos.* 2006;34(11):1875.

* Asterisk indicates drugs cited in interaction reports.

Fexofenadine | **Food**

Fexofenadine* (eg, *Allegra*)	Apple Juice* Grapefruit Juice*	Orange Juice*

Significance	Onset	Severity	Documentation
3	■ **Rapid**	□ Major	□ Established
	□ Delayed	□ Moderate	□ Probable
		■ **Minor**	■ **Suspected**
			□ Possible
			□ Unlikely

Effects FEXOFENADINE plasma concentrations may be reduced, decreasing the clinical effect.

Mechanism Decreased absorption of FEXOFENADINE, resulting from inhibition of intestinal organic anion-transporting polypeptides by certain fruit juices, is suspected.

Management Patients may require a higher dose of FEXOFENADINE when taken with APPLE, GRAPEFRUIT, or ORANGE JUICE. Advise patients not to take FEXOFENADINE with these juices.

Discussion

The effects of normal-strength apple juice, normal- and 25% normal-strength grapefruit juice, and normal-strength orange juice on the pharmacokinetics of fexofenadine were studied in 10 healthy volunteers.[1] All subjects received fexofenadine 120 mg with 300 mL of water or apple, grapefruit, or orange juice, followed by 150 mL every 0.5 to 3 h (total volume, 1.2 L). Compared with water: 1) apple juice reduced the fexofenadine AUC 73%, C_{max} 72%, and urinary excretion 69%; 2) normal-strength grapefruit juice reduced the AUC 63%, C_{max} 62%, and urinary excretion 68%; 3) 25% normal-strength grapefruit juice decreased the AUC 23%, C_{max} 21%, and urinary excretion 21%; and 4) orange juice reduced the AUC 69%, C_{max} 67%, and urinary excretion 68%. The time to reach the C_{max} and the $t_{½}$ of fexofenadine were not affected by the juices. Individuals with the highest fexofenadine AUC with water experienced the greatest decrease with juice. The decrease in the AUC was greater with normal-strength grapefruit juice than with 25% normal-strength grapefruit juice. The effects of pretreatment with double-strength grapefruit juice (240 mL 3 times daily for 2 days) on the bioavailability of fexofenadine 60 mg was studied in 24 healthy adults.[2] Subjects received fexofenadine with 240 mL of grapefruit juice, followed by an additional 240 mL of grapefruit juice 2 hr later. Grapefruit juice decreased the rate and extent of fexofenadine absorption 30%, compared with taking fexofenadine without the juice. In a study of 12 subjects, fexofenadine 120 mg was administered with a 300 mL bolus or 1,200 mL over 3 hr of water or grapefruit juice.[3] Compared with 300 mL of water, 300 mL of juice decreased the AUC and C_{max} of fexofenadine 42% and 47%, respectively. Compared with 1,200 mL of water, 1,200 mL of grapefruit juice decreased the fexofenadine AUC and C_{max} 64% and 67%, respectively. Grapefruit juice or a solution of its bioflavonoid reduced the bioavailability of a single dose of fexofenadine.[4]

[1] Dresser GK, et al. *Clin Pharmacol Ther.* 2002;71(1):11.
[2] Banfield C, et al. *Clin Pharmacokinet.* 2002;41(4):311.
[3] Dresser GK, et al. *Clin Pharmacol Ther.* 2005;77(3):170.
[4] Bailey DG, et al. *Clin Pharmacol Ther.* 2007;81(4):495.

* Asterisk indicates drugs cited in interaction reports.

Fexofenadine — *Probenecid*

Fexofenadine* (eg, *Allegra*)	Probenecid*

Significance	Onset	Severity	Documentation
5	☐ Rapid ■ **Delayed**	☐ Major ☐ Moderate ■ **Minor**	☐ Established ☐ Probable ☐ Suspected ■ **Possible** ☐ Unlikely

Effects FEXOFENADINE AUC may be elevated by PROBENECID, increasing the risk of adverse reactions.

Mechanism PROBENECID may reduce the renal clearance of FEXOFENADINE.

Management Observe patients for FEXOFENADINE adverse reactions.

Discussion

The inhibitory effects of probenecid on fexofenadine transport were studied in 12 men.[1] In a randomized, crossover study, each subject received probenecid 1,000 mg twice daily for 6 days. At the beginning of the study and 1 hour after the last dose of probenecid, subjects received fexofenadine 120 mg. Probenecid administration increased fexofenadine AUC 1.5-fold and decreased renal clearance 27%. There was marked interindividual variation in fexofenadine pharmacokinetics. Similar results were reported in a study of 8 cystic fibrosis patients and 8 healthy volunteers.[2] Probenecid increased fexofenadine AUC and decreased the cumulative urinary excretion, total body clearance, and renal clearance of fexofenadine equally in cystic fibrosis patients and the healthy volunteers.

[1] Yasui-Furukori N, et al. *Clin Pharmacol Ther.* 2005;77(1):17.

[2] Liu S, et al. *J Clin Pharmacol.* 2008;48(8):957.

* Asterisk indicates drugs cited in interaction reports.

Fexofenadine — *Protease Inhibitors*

Fexofenadine* (eg, *Allegra*)	Indinavir (*Crixivan*)	Ritonavir* (*Norvir*)
	Lopinavir/Ritonavir* (*Kaletra*)	Saquinavir (*Invirase*)
	Nelfinavir (*Viracept*)	

Significance	Onset	Severity	Documentation
5	□ Rapid ■ **Delayed**	□ Major □ Moderate ■ **Minor**	□ Established □ Probable □ Suspected ■ **Possible** □ Unlikely

Effects FEXOFENADINE plasma concentrations may be elevated, increasing the risk of adverse reactions.

Mechanism Increased oral bioavailability of FEXOFENADINE caused by inhibition of hepatic P-glycoprotein.

Management Observe patients for FEXOFENADINE adverse reactions.

Discussion

The effects of single-dose and steady-state administration of lopinavir/ritonavir on the pharmacokinetics of fexofenadine were studied in 16 healthy volunteers.[1] Each subject received single-dose fexofenadine 120 mg alone, in combination with single-dose ritonavir 100 mg or lopinavir/ritonavir 400/100 mg, and in combination with steady-state lopinavir/ritonavir 400/100 mg twice daily for 11 days. Compared with giving fexofenadine alone, coadministration of single-dose ritonavir or lopinavir/ritonavir increased the fexofenadine AUC 2.2- and 4-fold, respectively. Steady-state lopinavir/ritonavir increased the fexofenadine AUC 2.9-fold. Thus, the effect of lopinavir/ritonavir on the AUC of fexofenadine was less with steady-state administration of lopinavir/ritonavir than with single-dose administration of lopinavir/ritonavir (ie, 4-fold vs 2.9-fold).

[1] van Heeswijk RP, et al. *J Clin Pharmacol.* 2006;46:758.

* Asterisk indicates drugs cited in interaction reports. Based on pharmacologic and pharmacokinetic considerations, similar interactions may occur with other drugs that are listed.

Fexofenadine — *Rifamycins*

Fexofenadine* (eg, *Allegra*)	Rifampin* (eg, *Rifadin*)

Significance	Onset	Severity	Documentation
3	☐ Rapid ■ **Delayed**	☐ Major ☐ Moderate ■ **Minor**	☐ Established ☐ Probable ■ **Suspected** ☐ Possible ☐ Unlikely

Effects The pharmacologic effect (ie, antihistaminic) of FEXOFENADINE may be decreased.

Mechanism RIFAMPIN-induced P-glycoprotein transporter expression in the small intestine, reducing the absorption of FEXOFENADINE, is suspected.

Management In patients receiving FEXOFENADINE, monitor for a decrease in antihistaminic effect if RIFAMPIN is coadministered.

Discussion

The effect of rifampin on the pharmacokinetics of fexofenadine was studied in 24 healthy volunteers.[1] Each subject received a dose of fexofenadine 60 mg alone and following treatment with rifampin 600 mg/day for 6 days. Compared with giving fexofenadine alone, pretreatment with rifampin increased the oral clearance of fexofenadine 87% to 169% and decreased the peak plasma concentration 32% to 51%. Rifampin did not affect the $t_{1/2}$ or renal clearance of fexofenadine. The effect of rifampin on fexofenadine pharmacokinetics was independent of age and sex.

[1] Hamman MA, et al. *Clin Pharmacol Ther.* 2001;69:114.

* Asterisk indicates drugs cited in interaction reports.

Fexofenadine — *St. John's Wort*

Fexofenadine* (eg, *Allegra*)	St. John's Wort*

Significance	Onset	Severity	Documentation
5	☐ Rapid	☐ Major	☐ Established
	■ **Delayed**	☐ Moderate	☐ Probable
		■ **Minor**	☐ Suspected
			■ **Possible**
			☐ Unlikely

Effects FEXOFENADINE plasma levels may be reduced, decreasing the pharmacologic effect. Increased FEXOFENADINE concentrations have been reported after a single dose of ST. JOHN'S WORT.

Mechanism ST. JOHN'S WORT may induce the enzymes responsible for the hepatic and intestinal metabolism (CYP3A4) of FEXOFENADINE, as well as the P-glycoprotein efflux transporter of FEXOFENADINE.

Management Advise patients that response to FEXOFENADINE may be altered by concurrent use of ST. JOHN'S WORT. If ST. JOHN'S WORT cannot be avoided, assess the patient's clinical response to FEXOFENADINE when ST. JOHN'S WORT is started or stopped. Adjust the dose of FEXOFENADINE as needed.

Discussion

Reports are conflicting. The effect of St. John's wort 900 mg/day for 12 days on the AUC of oral fexofenadine was assessed in 12 healthy subjects.[1] Compared with administration of fexofenadine alone, coadministration of St. John's wort decreased the AUC of fexofenadine 49%. In a study of 10 healthy volunteers, a single dose of St. John's wort 900 mg increased the peak plasma concentration of fexofenadine 60 mg 58%, compared with giving fexofenadine alone.[2] However, repetitive dosing of St. John's wort (300 mg 3 times/day for 14 days) did not affect single-dose fexofenadine plasma levels. The effects of St. John's wort on the pharmacokinetics of fexofenadine were studied in a 3-period, open-label investigation involving 12 healthy volunteers.[3] Each subject received a single oral dose of fexofenadine 60 mg before administration of St. John's wort, with a single dose of St. John's wort 900 mg, and after 2 weeks of receiving of St. John's wort 300 mg 3 times/day. The single dose of St. John's wort increased the peak plasma level of fexofenadine 45% and decreased the oral clearance 20%. Pretreatment of the subjects with St. John's wort for 2 weeks prior to administration of fexofenadine decreased the peak plasma level of fexofenadine 35% and increased the oral clearance 47%, essentially reversing the effects of single-dose administration of St. John's wort.

[1] Dresser GK, et al. *Clin Pharmacol Ther.* 2001;69(2):P23.
[2] Hamman MA, et al. *Clin Pharmacol Ther.* 2001;69(2):P53.
[3] Wang Z, et al. *Clin Pharmacol Ther.* 2002;71(6):414.

* Asterisk indicates drugs cited in interaction reports.

Fexofenadine — *Verapamil*

Fexofenadine* (eg, *Allegra*)	Verapamil* (eg, *Calan*)

Significance	Onset	Severity	Documentation
5	☐ Rapid ■ **Delayed**	☐ Major ☐ Moderate ■ **Minor**	☐ Established ☐ Probable ☐ Suspected ■ **Possible** ☐ Unlikely

Effects FEXOFENADINE plasma levels may be elevated by VERAPAMIL.

Mechanism VERAPAMIL inhibits P-glycoprotein transport of FEXOFENADINE.

Management No special precautions are needed.

Discussion

The inhibitory effects of verapamil on fexofenadine transport were studied in 12 men.[1] In a randomized, crossover study, each subject received verapamil 80 mg 3 times daily for 6 days. At the beginning of the study and 1 hour after the last dose of verapamil, subjects received fexofenadine 120 mg. Verapamil treatment increased the fexofenadine C_{max} 2.9-fold and the AUC 2.5-fold, compared with administration of fexofenadine alone. There was marked interindividual variation in fexofenadine pharmacokinetics. A similar study in 12 healthy subjects evaluated the effect of sustained-release verapamil 240 mg/day for 38 days on the disposition of fexofenadine.[2] The clearance of fexofenadine was reduced at day 1 and seemed maximal at day 10, but this effect was attenuated by day 38. The effect of verapamil on P-glycoprotein transport of fexofenadine was greater for S-fexofenadine compared with R-fexofenadine.[3]

[1] Yasui-Furukori N, et al. *Clin Pharmacol Ther.* 2005;77(1):17.
[2] Lemma GL, et al. *Clin Pharmacol Ther.* 2006;79(3):218.
[3] Sakugawa T, et al. *Br J Clin Pharmacol.* 2009;67(5):535.

* Asterisk indicates drugs cited in interaction reports.

Finasteride — *Terazosin*

Finasteride* (eg, *Proscar*)	Terazosin*

Significance	Onset	Severity	Documentation
5	☐ Rapid ■ **Delayed**	☐ Major ☐ Moderate ■ **Minor**	☐ Established ☐ Probable ☐ Suspected ■ **Possible** ☐ Unlikely

Effects The pharmacologic and adverse effects of FINASTERIDE may be increased.

Mechanism Unknown.

Management Based on available data, no special precautions are necessary. If an interaction is suspected, adjust the dose of FINASTERIDE as needed.

Discussion

The effects of doxazosin (eg, *Cardura*) or terazosin on the pharmacokinetics of finasteride were evaluated in 90 healthy male volunteers.[1] Each agent is indicated for the treatment of benign prostatic hyperplasia. In a randomized, placebo-controlled study, subjects were assigned to 1 of 6 treatment groups: doxazosin alone, doxazosin plus finasteride, terazosin alone, terazosin plus finasteride, placebo alone, or placebo plus finasteride. On day 1 of the study, subjects were started on doxazosin or terazosin 1 mg/day, and the doses were escalated to doxazosin 8 mg or terazosin 10 mg on days 31 through 45. Finasteride was administered in a single daily dose of 5 mg on days 36 through 45. The pharmacokinetic parameters of doxazosin and terazosin were not affected by coadministration of finasteride. The pharmacokinetics of finasteride were not affected by coadministration of doxazosin. However, terazosin administration significantly affected peak plasma concentrations and the AUC of finasteride ($P = 0.037$ and $P = 0.012$, respectively) on day 45 of the study (ie, after 10 days of coadministration of terazosin and finasteride) but not on day 40 (ie, after 5 days of coadministration). Compared with administering finasteride alone, coadministration of terazosin increased peak plasma concentrations of finasteride 16% (from 46.4 to 53.9 ng/mL) and the AUC 31%.

Although a statistically significant interaction between terazosin and finasteride has been demonstrated, additional studies are needed to determine if the interaction is clinically important.

[1] Vashi V, et al. *J Clin Pharmacol.* 1998;38(11):1072.

* Asterisk indicates drugs cited in interaction reports.

Fingolimod — *Beta-Blockers*

Fingolimod*
(*Gilenya*)

Acebutolol (eg, *Sectral*)
Atenolol* (eg, *Tenormin*)
Betaxolol (eg, *Kerlone*)
Bisoprolol (eg, *Zebeta*)
Carvedilol (eg, *Coreg*)
Esmolol (eg, *Brevibloc*)
Metoprolol (eg, *Lopressor*)
Nadolol (eg, *Corgard*)
Nebivolol (*Bystolic*)
Penbutolol (*Levatol*)
Pindolol
Propranolol (eg, *Inderal*)
Sotalol (eg, *Betapace*)
Timolol

Significance	Onset	Severity	Documentation
1	□ Rapid ■ **Delayed**	■ **Major** □ Moderate □ Minor	□ Established □ Probable ■ **Suspected** □ Possible □ Unlikely

Effects Increased bradycardia may occur.

Mechanism Bradycardic effect of both drugs may be additive.

Management Closely monitor patients during coadministration of FINGOLIMOD and BETA-BLOCKER therapy, especially during the start of concurrent treatment.

Discussion

The effects of combing a single dose of fingolimod with steady-state atenolol were evaluated in 25 healthy subjects.[1] Using a partially randomized, single-blind, crossover design, each subject received a single dose of fingolimod 5 mg (10 times the recommended dose) alone, atenolol 50 mg once daily for 5 days, or fingolimod 5 mg on day 5 of atenolol (50 mg) administration. The daytime mean heart rate was 15% lower when fingolimod and atenolol were administered concurrently compared with fingolimod alone. There was no clinically important change in mean arterial pressure when the drugs were coadministered compared with giving the drugs alone. The pharmacokinetics of fingolimod and atenolol were not altered during coadministration. Subjects with a stronger negative chronotropic response to fingolimod alone had minimal or no further reduction in heart rate when administered after pretreatment with atenolol.

[1] Kovarik JM, et al. *Eur J Clin Pharmacol.* 2008;64(5):457.

* Asterisk indicates drugs cited in interaction reports. Based on pharmacologic and pharmacokinetic considerations, similar interactions may occur with other drugs that are listed.

Fingolimod — *Ketoconazole*

Fingolimod* (*Gilenya*)	Ketoconazole* (eg, *Nizoral*)

Significance	Onset	Severity	Documentation
4	□ Rapid ■ **Delayed**	□ Major ■ **Moderate** □ Minor	□ Established □ Probable □ Suspected ■ **Possible** □ Unlikely

Effects FINGOLIMOD plasma concentrations may be elevated, increasing the pharmacologic effects and risk of adverse reactions (eg, bradycardia).

Mechanism Inhibition of FINGOLIMOD metabolism (CYP4F2) by KETOCONAZOLE is suspected.

Management Proactive FINGOLIMOD dose reduction is not needed; however, closely monitor patients for FINGOLIMOD adverse reactions if KETOCONAZOLE is given concurrently.

Discussion

In a 2-period, single-sequence, crossover study, the effects of ketoconazole on the pharmacokinetics of fingolimod were investigated in 22 healthy subjects.[1] Each subject received a single oral dose of fingolimod 5 mg (10 times the recommended dose) alone, and on day 4 of a 9-day course of ketoconazole 200 mg twice daily. Compared with receiving fingolimod alone, ketoconazole increased the fingolimod C_{max} and AUC 1.22- and 1.71-fold, respectively. The AUC of the active metabolite, fingolimod phosphate, increased 1.67-fold. Ketoconazole administration did not alter the T_{max} or $t_{½}$ of fingolimod. Fingolimod did not affect ketoconazole plasma concentrations.

[1] Kovarik JM, et al. *J Clin Pharmacol.* 2009;49(2):212.

* Asterisk indicates drugs cited in interaction reports.

Flecainide — *Amiodarone*

Flecainide*
(eg, *Tambocor*)

Amiodarone*
(eg, *Cordarone*)

Significance	Onset	Severity	Documentation
2	☐ Rapid ■ **Delayed**	☐ Major ■ **Moderate** ☐ Minor	☐ Established ☐ Probable ■ **Suspected** ☐ Possible ☐ Unlikely

Effects FLECAINIDE plasma levels may be increased.

Mechanism AMIODARONE may decrease the metabolism of FLECAINIDE.

Management Monitor patients closely when using this combination.[1] Adjusting FLECAINIDE dosage may be necessary. Decreasing FLECAINIDE dosage 33% to 50% has been advocated.[2]

Discussion

In 7 patients receiving flecainide, the flecainide doses were automatically decreased 33% to 50% when amiodarone was started.[2] Plasma flecainide levels increased in all patients. Few controls were implemented in this trial; however, data from 2 patients suggest the onset of the increased concentrations is early but may not fully manifest for 2 weeks. Seventy-eight patients with or without congestive heart failure were divided into groups receiving flecainide alone or in combination with amiodarone.[3] Amiodarone increased trough flecainide levels 25% in patients without heart failure and 90% when heart failure was present. In 9 patients, flecainide levels were compared before and after amiodarone administration. After a single loading dose of amiodarone compared with long-term administration for 4 to 12 weeks, flecainide levels increased 13% and 44%, respectively. In 12 healthy volunteers, amiodarone decreased flecainide clearance regardless of cytochrome P450 phenotype.[4] The ensuing increase in flecainide concentrations was probably responsible for the observed prolongation of the QRS interval during coadministration of amiodarone and flecainide compared with giving flecainide alone. A patient maintained on amiodarone therapy developed torsades de pointes shortly after addition of flecainide to her treatment.[5] Because neither drug alone has been reported to induce this effect, a subtle interaction may have produced the arrhythmia. However, administration of flecainide alone could not be ruled out as the cause. Additional studies to determine the clinical importance of this interaction are warranted.[6]

[1] Shea P, et al. *J Am Coll Cardiol.* 1986;7(5):1127.
[2] Rotmensch HH, et al. *Med Clin North Am.* 1988;72(2):321.
[3] Andrivet P, et al. *Intensive Care Med.* 1990;16(5):342.
[4] Leclercq JF, et al. *Cardiovasc Drugs Ther.* 1990;4(4):1161.
[5] Funck-Brentano C, et al. *Clin Pharmacol Ther.* 1994;55(3):256.
[6] Kantoch MJ. *Am J Cardiol.* 1995;75(12):862.

* Asterisk indicates drugs cited in interaction reports.

Flecainide — *Cimetidine*

Flecainide* (*Tambocor*)

Cimetidine* (*Tagamet*)

Significance	Onset	Severity	Documentation
4	☐ Rapid	☐ Major	☐ Established
	■ **Delayed**	■ **Moderate**	☐ Probable
		☐ Minor	☐ Suspected
			■ **Possible**
			☐ Unlikely

Effects CIMETIDINE is believed to increase area under the curve (AUC) and total renal excretion of FLECAINIDE.

Mechanism CIMETIDINE may either increase bioavailability or inhibit metabolism of FLECAINIDE.

Management Caution is warranted with concomitant use of CIMETIDINE and FLECAINIDE. Patients with compromised renal function may be at higher risk and require a tailoring of dosage.

Discussion

The pharmacokinetics of single doses of flecainide in the presence and absence of cimetidine were evaluated in 8 healthy males.[1] While no changes in half-life or renal clearance occurred, significant increases in AUC and total urinary excretion of flecainide were noted. The clinical significance of the interaction is unknown. Further research utilizing multiple dose techniques are warranted.

[1] Tjandra-Maga TB, et al. *Br J Clin Pharmacol.* 1986;22:108.

* Asterisk indicates drugs cited in interaction reports.

Flecainide — *Quinidine*

Flecainide* (*Tambocor*)	Quinidine*

Significance	Onset	Severity	Documentation
4	☐ Rapid	☐ Major	☐ Established
	■ **Delayed**	■ **Moderate**	☐ Probable
		☐ Minor	☐ Suspected
			■ **Possible**
			☐ Unlikely

Effects Plasma FLECAINIDE concentrations may be elevated, increasing the pharmacologic and toxic effects of FLECAINIDE.

Mechanism Unknown. Possibly due to inhibition of FLECAINIDE metabolism.

Management Monitor FLECAINIDE concentrations and adjust the dose accordingly.

Discussion

In a crossover study involving six healthy volunteers, concurrent administration of a subtherapeutic dose of oral quinidine and infusion of flecainide increased the half-life of flecainide.[1] One week apart, subjects received flecainide acetate 150 mg infused over 30 minutes either alone or after quinidine 50 mg was given orally the evening before the study day. During the study, all participants were under continuous electrocardiogram (ECG) monitoring. One subject was a poor metabolizer as assessed by hydroxylation phenotype using dextromethorphan. Sub-therapeutic doses of quinidine reduced the clearance and increased the half-life of flecainide, primarily by decreasing the non-renal clearance of flecainide by 26%. The subject with the lowest flecainide clearance was the poor metabolizer of dextromethorphan. The excretion of the metabolites of flecainide over 48 hours was reduced. Sub-therapeutic doses of quinidine did not alter the effects of flecainide on ECG intervals.

Controlled studies are needed to determine if this interaction is clinically important.

[1] Munafo A, et al. *Eur J Clin Pharmacol.* 1992;43:441.

* Asterisk indicates drugs cited in interaction reports.

Flecainide | **_Ritonavir_**

Flecainide*
(eg, *Tambocor*)

Ritonavir* (*Norvir*)

Significance	Onset	Severity	Documentation
1	☐ Rapid ■ **Delayed**	■ **Major** ☐ Moderate ☐ Minor	☐ Established ☐ Probable ■ **Suspected** ☐ Possible ☐ Unlikely

Effects Large increases in serum FLECAINIDE concentrations may occur, increasing the risk of FLECAINIDE toxicity.

Mechanism RITONAVIR may inhibit the metabolism (CYP2D6) of FLECAINIDE.

Management RITONAVIR is contraindicated in patients receiving FLECAINIDE.

Discussion

Flecainide slows cardiac conduction in most patients, producing dose-related increases in PR, QRS, and QT intervals. Ritonavir is expected to produce large increases in flecainide plasma concentrations, increasing the risk of toxicity.[1] Cardiovascular adverse reactions reported with flecainide include new or worsened arrhythmias, episodes of ventricular tachycardia or ventricular fibrillation that did not respond to resuscitation, new or worsened CHF, second- or third-degree atrioventricular block, sinus arrest, tachycardia, angina pectoris, bradycardia, hypertension, and hypotension. Flecainide therapy was associated with death in post-MI patients with asymptomatic premature ventricular contractions and nonsustained ventricular tachycardia.

The basis for this monograph is information on file with the manufacturer. Published clinical data are needed to further assess this interaction. However, because of the seriousness of the cardiac problems, clinical evaluation of this interaction in humans is not likely to be forthcoming.

[1] *Norvir* [package insert]. Abbott Park, IL: Abbott Laboratories; 1996.

* Asterisk indicates drugs cited in interaction reports.

Flecainide — *Serotonin Reuptake Inhibitors*

Flecainide*
(eg, *Tambocor*)

Duloxetine
(*Cymbalta*)
Fluoxetine
(eg, *Prozac*)

Paroxetine*
(eg, *Paxil*)

Significance	Onset	Severity	Documentation
4	☐ Rapid	☐ Major	☐ Established
	■ **Delayed**	■ **Moderate**	☐ Probable
		☐ Minor	☐ Suspected
			■ **Possible**
			☐ Unlikely

Effects FLECAINIDE plasma concentrations may be elevated, increasing the pharmacologic effects and risk of toxicity and prolonging the QT interval.

Mechanism Inhibition of FLECAINIDE metabolism (CYP2D6) by certain SRIs.

Management If coadministration cannot be avoided, close clinical and laboratory monitoring are warranted. Adjust the FLECAINIDE dose as needed. Citalopram (eg, *Celexa*) may be a safer SRI alternative.

Discussion

The effects of paroxetine on pharmacokinetic[1] and QTc[2] changes of flecainide were studied in healthy volunteers. Twenty-one subjects (7 extensive metabolizers, 7 intermediate metabolizers, and 7 poor metabolizers) received a single dose of flecainide 200 mg alone and after 7 days of pretreatment with paroxetine 20 mg daily.[1,2] Compared with giving flecainide alone, paroxetine pretreatment increased the mean residence time, AUC, and $t_{1/2}$ in the extensive and intermediate metabolizers.[1] Flecainide pharmacokinetics were not altered by paroxetine in the poor metabolizers. In addition, there was a greater prolongation in the QTc interval when flecainide was given after pretreatment with paroxetine, compared with administering flecainide alone.[2] The QTc prolongation was most pronounced in the extensive and intermediate metabolizers compared with the poor metabolizers. Delirium was reported in a 69-year-old woman on a stable dose of paroxetine 40 mg daily approximately 2 weeks after starting flecainide 100 mg twice daily.[3] Upon hospitalization, the flecainide dose was reduced to 50 mg twice daily and paroxetine was withheld. After 3 days, the patient's mental status improved.[1]

[1] Lim KS, et al. *Br J Clin Pharmacol.* 2008;66(5):660.
[2] Lim KS, et al. *Clin Ther.* 2010;32(4):659.
[3] Tsao YY, et al. *Ann Pharmacother.* 2009;43(7):1366.

* Asterisk indicates drugs cited in interaction reports. Based on pharmacologic and pharmacokinetic considerations, similar interactions may occur with other drugs that are listed.

Flecainide | *Urinary Acidifiers*

Flecainide* (eg, *Tambocor*)	Ammonium Chloride*	Sodium Acid Phosphate
	Potassium Acid Phosphate (eg, *K-Phos*)	

Significance	Onset	Severity	Documentation
5	☐ Rapid	☐ Major	☐ Established
	■ **Delayed**	☐ Moderate	☐ Probable
		■ **Minor**	☐ Suspected
			■ **Possible**
			☐ Unlikely

Effects Alterations in urinary excretion and plasma elimination of FLECAINIDE occur with changes in urinary pH.

Mechanism Ionization of FLECAINIDE and active tubular secretory mechanisms are believed to explain the pharmacokinetic changes.

Management Dosage alteration of FLECAINIDE caused by changes in urinary pH may be needed. Patients manifesting adverse reactions at low dosages of FLECAINIDE or unresponsive to high dosages of FLECAINIDE should receive urinary pH evaluation.

Discussion

Single dose studies in healthy volunteers note that acidic urine is associated with increased total urinary excretion, increased plasma elimination, and decreased AUC.[1,2] Flecainide t½ was 33 hours with an alkaline urine compared with 8.4 hours under acidic conditions.[3] While intersubject variation is high, intrasubject differences to changes in urinary pH are important. The overall clinical relevance of this effect is unknown; however, alteration in individual response should raise suspicion of the influence of urinary pH.

[1] Muhiddin KA, et al. *Br J Clin Pharmacol.* 1984;17(4):447.
[2] Johnston A, et al. *Br J Clin Pharmacol.* 1985;20(4):333.
[3] Nappi JM, et al. *Pharmacotherapy.* 1985;5(4):209.

* Asterisk indicates drugs cited in interaction reports. Based on pharmacologic and pharmacokinetic considerations, similar interactions may occur with other drugs that are listed.

Flecainide — *Urinary Alkalinizers*

Flecainide	Urinary Alkalinizers	
Flecainide* (*Tambocor*)	Potassium Citrate (*Urocit-K*)	Sodium Lactate
	Sodium Acetate	Tromethamine (eg, *Tham*)
	Sodium Bicarbonate*	
	Sodium Citrate (*Bicitra*)	

Significance	Onset	Severity	Documentation
5	☐ Rapid	☐ Major	☐ Established
	■ **Delayed**	☐ Moderate	☐ Probable
		■ **Minor**	☐ Suspected
			■ **Possible**
			☐ Unlikely

Effects The elimination half life and area under the concentration versus time curve (AUC) for flecainide are increased when the urine is alkalinized.

Mechanism FLECAINIDE urinary excretion decreases as the urine pH increases.

Management No alterations in FLECAINIDE therapy are needed unless the patient exhibits side effects or loss of arrhythmia control. Monitor patients as they begin or stop URINARY ALKALINIZERS for symptoms of alterations in serum FLECAINIDE concentrations.

Discussion

Muhiddin[1] studied six healthy adults after a single dose of flecainide. In a crossover design, their urine was acidified with ammonium chloride or alkalinized with sodium bicarbonate. In a later study, Johnston[2] studied eight healthy adults whose urine was alkalinized, acidified or untreated. Again a single dose of flecainide was given. Both studies noted few differences in the absorption parameters. However, as the urine pH increased, the elimination half-life and AUC of flecainide increased and urinary excretion decreased. Because the studies noted a high degree of intersubject variation in parameters, an individual response to the combination therapy would be difficult to predict.

[1] Muhiddin KA, et al. *Br J Clin Pharmacol.* 1984;17:447.

[2] Johnston A, et al. *Br J Clin Pharmacol.* 1985;20:333.

* Asterisk indicates drugs cited in interaction reports. Based on pharmacologic and pharmacokinetic considerations, similar interactions may occur with other drugs that are listed.

Fluconazole		***Cimetidine***
Fluconazole* (*Diflucan*)		Cimetidine* (*Tagamet*)

Significance	Onset	Severity	Documentation
4	■ **Rapid**	□ Major	□ Established
	□ Delayed	■ **Moderate**	□ Probable
		□ Minor	□ Suspected
			■ **Possible**
			□ Unlikely

Effects The plasma levels of FLUCONAZOLE may be reduced, which may decrease its antifungal activity.

Mechanism Unknown. Possible decreased absorption.

Management Based upon currently available data, no special precautions are necessary.

Discussion

Six healthy male volunteers received a single dose of fluconazole 100 mg.[1] After a 7-day washout period, each subject received a single 400 mg oral dose of cimetidine followed 2 hours later by 100 mg fluconazole. After coadministration of cimetidine and fluconazole, there was a 13% decrease in the area under the plasma concentration-time curve from 0 to 48 hours (from 54.1 to 47.1 mcg•hr/mL) and a 20% decrease in the maximum plasma concentration of fluconazole (from 2.5 to 2 mcg/mL). These changes were not considered to be clinically significant. See also Ketoconazole, Oral-Histamine H_2 Antagonists.

[1] Lazar JD, et al. *Reviews Infect Dis.* 1990;12 (Suppl 3):S327.

* Asterisk indicates drugs cited in interaction reports.

Fluorouracil — *Cimetidine*

Floxuridine (eg, *FUDR*)	Fluorouracil* (eg, *Adrucil*)	Cimetidine* (eg, *Tagamet*)

Significance	Onset	Severity	Documentation
4	☐ Rapid	☐ Major	☐ Established
	■ **Delayed**	■ **Moderate**	☐ Probable
		☐ Minor	☐ Suspected
			■ **Possible**
			☐ Unlikely

Effects The bioavailability of FLUOROURACIL may be increased by CIMETIDINE.

Mechanism Unknown.

Management Monitor patients for symptoms of FLUOROURACIL toxicity if the combination is used. Discontinue CIMETIDINE if necessary.

Discussion

The pharmacokinetic parameters of oral and IV fluorouracil were determined in 15 patients with carcinoma after pretreatment with a single cimetidine dose or cimetidine 100 mg/day for either 1 or 4 weeks.[1] Only after 4 weeks of pretreatment were significant alterations noted. The area under the fluorouracil concentration-time curve after oral and IV fluorouracil, and the maximum serum concentrations after oral administration were both increased after oral cimetidine dosing. No significant changes in elimination parameters were observed. Further study on the mechanisms of this possible interaction and the effect of other H_2 receptor antagonists is needed.

[1] Harvey VJ, et al. *Br J Clin Pharmacol.* 1984;18:421.

* Asterisk indicates drugs cited in interaction reports. Based on pharmacologic and pharmacokinetic considerations, similar interactions may occur with other drugs that are listed.

Fluoxetine	*Dextromethorphan*
Fluoxetine* (*Prozac*)	Dextromethorphan* (eg, *Benylin DM*)

Significance	Onset	Severity	Documentation
4	■ **Rapid** □ Delayed	□ Major ■ **Moderate** □ Minor	□ Established □ Probable □ Suspected ■ **Possible** □ Unlikely

Effects Hallucinations were reported during concurrent administration of FLUOXETINE and DEXTROMETHORPHAN.

Mechanism Unknown.

Management Consider recommending an alternative cough suppressant in patients receiving FLUOXETINE.

Discussion

Visual hallucinations were reported in a 32-year-old female patient during concurrent administration of fluoxetine and dextromethorphan.[1] The patient had a 20-year history of mood disorders. She was given fluoxetine 20 mg daily upon presentation with complaints of sadness, guilt, dissatisfaction, helplessness, hopelessness and insomnia. After 17 days of treatment, the patient took 2 teaspoonfuls of a cough syrup containing dextromethorphan for symptoms of a cold. The next morning she took fluoxetine and 2 teaspoonfuls of the cough syrup. Two hours later she experienced vivid hallucinations of bright colors and distortion of her surroundings. The hallucinations lasted 6 to 8 hours and were similar to those the patient had with LSD 12 years prior. The fluoxetine was discontinued without recurrence of the hallucinations.

[1] Achamallah NS. *Am J Psychiatry*. 1992;149:1406.

* Asterisk indicates drugs cited in interaction reports.

Fluvoxamine — *Food*

Fluvoxamine*
(eg, *Luvox*)

Grapefruit Juice*

Significance	Onset	Severity	Documentation
4	☐ Rapid	☐ Major	☐ Established
	■ **Delayed**	■ **Moderate**	☐ Probable
		☐ Minor	☐ Suspected
			■ **Possible**
			☐ Unlikely

Effects FLUVOXAMINE plasma concentrations may be elevated, increasing the pharmacologic and adverse effects.

Mechanism Inhibition of FLUVOXAMINE metabolism (intestinal CYP3A4) or altered p-glycoprotein-mediated transport by GRAPEFRUIT JUICE is suspected.

Management Caution patients receiving FLUVOXAMINE to avoid GRAPEFRUIT products and advise them to take FLUVOXAMINE with a liquid other than GRAPEFRUIT JUICE.

Discussion

In a randomized, crossover investigation, the effects of grapefruit juice on the pharmacokinetics of fluvoxamine were studied in 10 healthy men.[1] Each subject ingested 250 mL of regular strength grapefruit juice or water 3 times daily for 5 days. On day 6, they were given fluvoxamine (75 mg) with 250 mL of regular strength grapefruit juice or water. Grapefruit juice increased the mean peak concentration and AUC of fluvoxamine 1.3-fold and 1.6-fold, respectively. There were no changes in the $t_{½}$ or time to reach the peak plasma concentration of fluvoxamine.

[1] Hori H, et al. *J Clin Psychopharmacol.* 2003;23:422.

* Asterisk indicates drugs cited in interaction reports.

Folic Acid ✕ *Aminosalicylic Acid*

Folic Acid* (eg, *Folvite*) | Aminosalicylic Acid* (*PAS*)

Significance	Onset	Severity	Documentation
5	☐ Rapid	☐ Major	☐ Established
	■ **Delayed**	☐ Moderate	☐ Probable
		■ **Minor**	☐ Suspected
			■ **Possible**
			☐ Unlikely

Effects Decreased serum folate levels have been noted in patients taking aminosalicylic acid.

Mechanism Unknown. Aminosalicylic acid can cause diarrhea and steatorrhea. Low serum folate levels may be due to malabsorption.

Management Resolution of symptoms, including normalization of serum folate, occurred when aminosalicylic acid was stopped. It may be possible to administer exogenous folate, though no clinical data support this course.

Discussion

In three case reports,[1-3] patients taking 10 to 12 g aminosalicylic acid daily developed diarrhea after 1 to 6 months of therapy. A variety of abnormalities were noted including lower serum folate levels. These levels returned to normal after the aminosalicylic acid was stopped. No one administered folic acid. No specific effects were definitely attributable to folate deficiency, however 1 patient felt tired, 1 had macrocytosis, and 2 had vitamin B_{12} deficiency.

[1] Akhtar AJ, et al. *Tubercle.* 1968;49:328.
[2] Coltart DJ. *Br Med J.* 1969;1:825.
[3] Longstreth GF, et al. *Dig Dis.* 1972;17:731.

* Asterisk indicates drugs cited in interaction reports.

Folic Acid — *Sulfasalazine*

Folic Acid* (eg, *Folvite*)	Sulfasalazine* (eg, *Azulfidine*)

Significance	Onset	Severity	Documentation
3	☐ Rapid ■ **Delayed**	☐ Major ☐ Moderate ■ **Minor**	☐ Established ☐ Probable ■ **Suspected** ☐ Possible ☐ Unlikely

Effects Signs of FOLATE deficiency have been recorded including low serum folate, low red blood cell folate, megaloblastic anemia, macrocytosis and reticulocytosis. Specific symptoms related to the deficiency have not been recorded.

Mechanism Impairment of intestinal absorption of FOLATES and alteration in the hydrolysis or reduction of FOLATES.

Management Periodically monitor patients taking SULFASALAZINE. If FOLATE deficiency is noted, potential treatment measures include increasing dietary FOLATE, giving SULFASALAZINE between meals, and administering additional folic acid or folinic acid. Stopping the SULFASALAZINE usually results in return of values to normal, but this may not be viable or necessary if the other measures are attempted first.

Discussion

Folate deficiency has been associated with sulfasalazine therapy in patients with inflammatory bowel disease.[1,3,5-9] An antifolate effect in lymphocytes has been postulated as a possible mechanism for drug efficacy.[4] The clinical significance of this finding is still controversial as the incidence has ranged from 2.5% to 70% in the series of patients studied but few clinical symptoms directly related to the deficiency were described. Differences in patient populations and in defining deficiency may explain some variance. A variety of mechanisms for the folate deficiency have been postulated including impairment of GI absorption of folates,[5,10] inhibition of reduction and hydrolysis[2,5] and drug-induced hemolysis.[3,6] Also, patients may have complicating factors unrelated to sulfasalazine including the disease and nutritional deficiency.[6]

It is hard to obtain a true picture of the incidence and importance of this effect. Nonetheless, monitor patients taking sulfasalazine for inflammatory bowel disease periodically for folate deficiency and take appropriate measures if signs and symptoms develop.

1 Franklin JL, et al. *Gastroenterology*. 1973;64:517.
2 Selhub J, et al. *J Clin Invest*. 1978;61:221.
3 Elsborg L, et al. *Scand J Gastroenterol*. 1979;14:1019.
4 Baum CL, et al. *J Lab Clin Med*. 1981;97:779.
5 Halsted CH, et al. *N Engl J Med*. 1981;305:1513.
6 Swinson CM, et al. *Gut*. 1981;22:456.
7 Longstreth GF, et al. *Arch Intern Med*. 1983;143:902.
8 Goldberg J. *JAMA*. 1983;249:729.
9 Pironi L, et al. *Int J Clin Pharm Res*. 1988;8:143.
10 Darcy-Vrillon B, et al. *Am J Physiol*. 1988;255:G361.

* Asterisk indicates drugs cited in interaction reports.

Food — **Furazolidone**

Amine-Containing Foods*	Furazolidone*†

Significance	Onset	Severity	Documentation
1	■ **Rapid** □ Delayed	■ **Major** □ Moderate □ Minor	■ **Established** □ Probable □ Suspected □ Possible □ Unlikely

Effects Marked elevation of blood pressure, hypertensive crisis or hemorrhagic strokes may occur if AMINE-CONTAINING FOODS are consumed concurrently or after FURAZOLIDONE therapy.

Mechanism FURAZOLIDONE is an inhibitor of monoamine oxidase that metabolizes tyramine and other amines found in certain foods which, if unmetabolized or inadequately metabolized, can elevate blood pressure.

Management Monitor blood pressure closely. AMINE-CONTAINING FOODS should not be consumed for 2 to 4 weeks after FURAZOLIDONE is discontinued.

Discussion

The ability of furazolidone to increase the blood pressure response to tyramine has been demonstrated.[1,2] The risk of sudden and severe elevations of blood pressure if tyramine and amine-containing foods are consumed by patients receiving furazolidone therapy is great. Amines capable of elevating blood pressure including tyramine, are most prevalent in certain aged, overripe and fermented foods and drinks.[3,4] Broad beans, red wines (particularly chianti), yeast extract, some imported beers, chicken/beef liver, caviar, pickled herring, fermented sausage (eg, bologna, pepperoni, salami, summer sausage), overripe avocados and various cheeses (eg, boursault, brie, camembert, cheddar, emmenthaler, gruyere, mozzerella, parmesan, romano, roquefort, stilton) may produce marked elevations in blood pressure if consumed with or within 4 weeks after furazolidone therapy.

1 Pettinger WA, et al. *Clin Pharmacol Ther.* 1968;9:341.
2 Pettinger WA, et al. *Clin Pharmacol Ther.* 1968;9:442.
3 Maxwell MB. *Cancer Nurs.* 1980;1:451.
4 Anon. *Med Lett Drugs Ther.* 1980;22:58.

* Asterisk indicates drugs cited in interaction reports.
† Not available in the United States.

Food | **MAOIs**

Amine-Containing Foods*	Phenelzine* (*Nardil*)	Tranylcypromine* (*Parnate*)

Significance	Onset	Severity	Documentation
1	■ **Rapid** □ Delayed	■ **Major** □ Moderate □ Minor	■ **Established** □ Probable □ Suspected □ Possible □ Unlikely

Effects

Marked elevation of blood pressure, hypertensive crisis, or hemorrhagic strokes may occur if AMINE-CONTAINING FOODS are consumed concurrently with or after MAOI therapy.

Mechanism

The inhibition of monoamine oxidase impairs the normal metabolism of tyramine and other amines found in certain foods that may result in a marked elevation of blood pressure.

Management

Avoid FOODS HIGH IN AMINE CONTENT. Do not consume FOODS HIGH IN AMINE CONTENT for greater than or equal to 4 weeks after MAOI therapy is discontinued. Monitor blood pressure closely.

Discussion

Sudden and severe pressor responses to ingestion of foods high in amine content have occurred in patients taking MAOIs.[1-12] The incidence is high and health risks are great. The effects of MAOIs may persist for 2 to 4 weeks after the drug is discontinued.

Tyramine and other amines capable of elevating blood pressure are most prevalent in certain aged, overripe, and fermented foods and drinks. Broad beans, red wines (particularly Chianti), yeast extract, some imported beers (tap beers pose a greater risk than bottled beers[14]), chicken/beef liver, caviar, pickled herring, fermented sausage (eg, bologna, pepperoni, salami, summer sausage), overripe avocados, and various cheeses (eg, Boursault, Brie, Camembert, cheddar, Emmenthaler, Gruyere, mozzarella, Parmesan, Romano, Roquefort, Stilton) may produce marked elevations in blood pressure if taken with or a few weeks after MAOI therapy.[8,9,12] Fermented soybeans, bean curd, or soy sauce may also contain sufficient amounts of tyramine to cause a problem.[15] There is some concern that dietary supplements containing yeast and chocolates containing cocoa may also be a problem.[13]

[1] Blackwell B. *Lancet.* 1963;2:849.
[2] Foster AR, et al. *Lancet.* 1963;2:587.
[3] Horwitz D, et al. *JAMA.* 1964;188:1108.
[4] Nuessle WF, et al. *JAMA.* 1965;192:726.
[5] Hedberg DL, et al. *Am J Psychiatry.* 1966;122:933.
[6] Blackwell B, et al. *Br J Psychiatry.* 1967;113:349.
[7] Pettinger WA, et al. *Clin Pharmacol Ther.* 1968;9:341.
[8] Maxwell MB. *Cancer Nurs.* 1980;3:451.
[9] *Med Lett Drugs Ther.* 1980;22:58.
[10] Generali JA, et al. *DICP.* 1981;15:904.
[11] Davidson J, et al. *J Clin Psychiatry.* 1984;45:81.
[12] Walker JI, et al. *J Clin Psychiatry.* 1984;45:78.
[13] Sweet RA, et al. *J Clin Psychopharmacol.* 1991;11:331.
[14] Tailor SA, et al. *J Clin Psychopharmacol.* 1994;14:5.
[15] Wing YK, et al. *J Clin Psychopharmacol.* 1997;17:227.

* Asterisk indicates drugs cited in interaction reports.

Food — **Procarbazine**

Amine-Containing Foods*	Procarbazine* (*Matulane*)

Significance	Onset	Severity	Documentation
5	■ **Rapid**	□ Major	□ Established
	□ Delayed	□ Moderate	□ Probable
		■ **Minor**	□ Suspected
			■ **Possible**
			□ Unlikely

Effects A discomforting flush response, but no clinically significant elevation of blood pressure, has been reported when AMINE-CONTAINING FOODS are consumed by patients receiving PROCARBAZINE therapy.

Mechanism PROCARBAZINE inhibits monoamine oxidase (MAO) metabolizing enzymes. The concern that PROCARBAZINE, because of its weak effect on MAO, could inhibit metabolism of tyramine contained in certain foods and produce adverse elevations of blood pressure has not manifested itself clinically.

Management No contraindication between PROCARBAZINE and AMINE-CONTAINING FOODS exists. Dosage adjustments of PROCARBAZINE do not appear necessary. However, routine monitoring of blood pressure is encouraged.

Discussion

Although procarbazine is a weak inhibitor of monoamine oxidase (MAO), no significant adverse pressor effects have been reported.[2] Flushing has been reported in individuals taking procarbazine, but alcohol ingestion was also a factor[1,3,4]; a cause-effect relationship is not clear. Symptoms could be related to procarbazine-induced MAO inhibition, a disulfiram-like response to procarbazine, or coincidental factors.

Foods high in tyramine and other pressor amines are contained in certain aged, overripe and fermented foods and drinks. Foods with moderate-to-high amine content include broad beans, red wine (particularly Chianti), yeast extract, some imported beers, chicken/beef liver, caviar, pickled herring, fermented sausage (eg, bologna, pepperoni, salami, summer sausage), overripe avocados, and various cheeses (eg, Boursault, Brie, Camembert, cheddar, Emmenthaler, Gruyere, mozzarella, Parmesan, Romano, Roquefort, Stilton).[5-7] The need to restrict consumption of these foods and beverages while receiving procarbazine is not readily apparent.

[1] Mathe G, et al. *Lancet*. 1963;2:1077.
[2] DeVita VT, et al. *Proc Soc Exp Biol Med*. 1965;120:561.
[3] Brule G, et al. *Cancer Chemother Rep*. 1965;44:31.
[4] Todd ID. *BMJ*. 1965;1:628.
[5] Maxwell MB. *Cancer Nurs*. 1980;1:451.
[6] *Med Lett Drugs Ther*. 1980;22:58.
[7] Walker JI, et al. *J Clin Psychiatry*. 1984;45:78.

* Asterisk indicates drugs cited in interaction reports.

Fosamprenavir — *Rifamycins*

Fosamprenavir		Rifamycins	
Amprenavir*†		Rifabutin* (*Mycobutin*)	Rifapentine (*Priftin*)
Fosamprenavir* (*Lexiva*)		Rifampin* (eg, *Rifadin*)	

Significance	Onset	Severity	Documentation
2	☐ Rapid	☐ Major	☐ Established
	■ **Delayed**	■ **Moderate**	☐ Probable
		☐ Minor	■ **Suspected**
			☐ Possible
			☐ Unlikely

Effects RIFAMPIN may reduce AMPRENAVIR plasma levels, decreasing the pharmacologic effect. AMPRENAVIR may increase RIFABUTIN plasma levels, increasing the risk of adverse reactions.

Mechanism AMPRENAVIR may decrease RIFABUTIN metabolism (CYP3A4), while RIFAMPIN may increase AMPRENAVIR metabolism (CYP3A4).

Management Coadministration of FOSAMPRENAVIR and RIFAMPIN is contraindicated.[1] Carefully monitor the patient's response to FOSAMPRENAVIR, and observe the patient for adverse reactions during administration of RIFABUTIN or RIFAPENTINE. Be prepared to alter the dose of these agents as needed. Consider decreasing the dose of RIFABUTIN at least 50% when administering with FOSAMPRENAVIR.

Discussion

After oral administration, fosamprenavir is rapidly and almost completely hydrolyzed to amprenavir and inorganic phosphate in the gut epithelium during absorption.[1] The possibility of a pharmacokinetic interaction between amprenavir and rifabutin or rifampin was studied in 24 healthy men.[2] Using an open-label, parallel-group, 3-period design, all subjects received amprenavir 1,200 mg twice daily alone for 4 days, followed by either rifabutin 300 mg once daily (cohort 1) or rifampin 600 mg daily (cohort 2) alone for 14 days. Cohort 1 then received amprenavir plus rifabutin for 10 days, while cohort 2 received amprenavir plus rifampin for 4 days. Amprenavir increased the AUC of rifabutin and the 25-O-desacetylrifabutin metabolite 2.93- and 13.35-fold, respectively. Rifabutin did not affect the pharmacokinetics of amprenavir. Rifampin decreased the AUC of amprenavir 82%; however, amprenavir did not affect the pharmacokinetics of rifampin. Coadministration of amprenavir and rifabutin was poorly tolerated, and 5 subjects were withdrawn from the study because of adverse reactions (eg, diarrhea, fever, headache, myalgia, nausea, neutropenia). With respect to adverse reactions, amprenavir plus rifampin was well tolerated.

[1] *Lexiva* [package insert]. Research Triangle Park, NC: GlaxoSmithKline; April 2010.

[2] Polk RE, et al. *Antimicrob Agents Chemother.* 2001;45(2):502.

* Asterisk indicates drugs cited in interaction reports. Based on pharmacologic and pharmacokinetic considerations, similar interactions may occur with other drugs that are listed.
† Not available in the United States.

Foscarnet — *Cyclosporine*

Foscarnet* (*Foscavir*)	Cyclosporine* (eg, *Neoral*)

Significance	Onset	Severity	Documentation
1	☐ Rapid ■ **Delayed**	■ **Major** ☐ Moderate ☐ Minor	☐ Established ☐ Probable ■ **Suspected** ☐ Possible ☐ Unlikely

Effects The risk of renal failure may be increased.

Mechanism Possibly additive or synergistic nephrotoxicity.

Management Carefully monitor renal function. If nephrotoxicity occurs, it may be necessary to discontinue FOSCARNET treatment and manage the patient as needed.

Discussion

Reversible acute renal failure was reported in 2 patients during concurrent administration of foscarnet and cyclosporine.[1] One patient, a 21-year-old male who received a cadaveric renal transplant, was immunosuppressed with steroids and cyclosporine. After developing a cytomegalovirus (CMV) infection, foscarnet was administered at doses adjusted according to renal function. In addition, efforts were made to prevent the nephrotoxic effects of foscarnet by hydrating the patient with isotonic saline and by giving nifedipine (eg, *Procardia*). In spite of these precautions, the patient developed progressive, non-oliguric worsening of his renal function on the eighth day of foscarnet treatment. Foscarnet was discontinued, and, 9 days later, renal function was similar to that prior to foscarnet administration, and the CMV infection resolved. Cyclosporine blood concentrations were always within the therapeutic range. The second patient, a 38-year-old male who had received a liver transplant, was immunosuppressed with azathioprine (*Imuran*), cyclosporine, and steroids. Following the diagnosis of active chronic hepatitis due to hepatitis B, foscarnet therapy was started. Because renal function and serum bilirubin were normal, foscarnet was administered at usual doses. The patient was hydrated with isotonic saline before and after foscarnet administration. On the fifth day of foscarnet treatment, the patient developed acute renal failure. Cyclosporine blood concentrations were in the therapeutic range and the dose was not modified. Ten days after discontinuing foscarnet, renal function was normal. In neither patient did it appear that the renal failure was secondary to CMV nephritis or CMV-stimulated rejection.

[1] Morales JM, et al. *Nephrol Dial Transplant.* 1995;10:882.

* Asterisk indicates drugs cited in interaction reports.

Foscarnet — *Quinolones*

Foscarnet	Quinolones	
Foscarnet* (*Foscavir*)	Ciprofloxacin* (*Cipro*)	Norfloxacin (*Noroxin*)
	Enoxacin (*Penetrex*)	Ofloxacin (*Floxin*)
	Lomefloxacin (*Maxaquin*)	

Significance	Onset	Severity	Documentation
4	■ **Rapid**	□ Major	□ Established
	□ Delayed	■ **Moderate**	□ Probable
		□ Minor	□ Suspected
			■ **Possible**
			□ Unlikely

Effects The risk of seizures may be increased.

Mechanism Possible additive or synergistic epileptogenic activity.

Management Monitor patients for seizures during coadministration of FOSCARNET and CIPROFLOXACIN.

Discussion

Seizure occurrence during coadministration of foscarnet and ciprofloxacin was reported in 2male patients with AIDS, cytomegalovirus (CMV) retinitis and disseminated *Mycobacterium avium* complex (MAC) infection.[1] The first patient was admitted to the hospital for evaluation of headaches. Oral thrush and rash on the abdominal wall were found on physical examination, while neurologic examination detected headache. Treatment included foscarnet infusion over 2 hours, vancomycin (eg, *Vancocin*), rifampin (eg, *Rifadin*), clarithromycin (*Biaxin*), ciprofloxacin, fluconazole (*Diflucan*), morphine sulfate, cimetidine (eg, *Tagamet*), docusate sodium (eg, *Doxinate*), senna concentrate (eg, *Senokot*), calcium carbonate, magnesium oxide, and multiple vitamins. The patient's IV line infiltrated after he received approximately half of his first foscarnet dose. Nine hours after the foscarnet infusion, he experienced periods of confusion followed by tonic-clonic seizures that lasted approximately 1 minute. Later that day, he experienced similar seizure activity on completion of the foscarnet infusion. The patient experienced a third grand mal seizure approximately 45 minutes after the start of the second foscarnet dose. Foscarnet was stopped, and the patient was given phenytoin (eg, *Dilantin*). For approximately 18 hours after his last seizure, the patient was disoriented, lethargic and demonstrated periods of unresponsiveness to verbal commands. His mental status improved gradually over 36 hours after foscarnet therapy was stopped. The second patient had been on foscarnet for 10 days for CMV retinitis when ethambutol (*Myambutol*), pyrazinamide, rifampin, clofazimine (*Lamprene*) and ciprofloxacin were started for MAC infection. Within 36 hours of starting the multiple antimycobacterial drugs and within several minutes of initiating the foscarnet infusion, the patient experienced a seizure. Foscarnet was discontinued. Thirty minutes after his seizure abated, foscarnet was restarted and within 40 minutes, the patient experienced a grand mal seizure. The patient was rigid and displayed jerky movements of his extremities, bit his lips and was incontinent of bowel and bladder. The seizure subsided within 1 hour of stopping foscarnet.

[1] Fan-Harvard P, et al. *Ann Pharmacother.* 1994;28:869.

* Asterisk indicates drugs cited in interaction reports. Based on pharmacologic and pharmacokinetic considerations, similar interactions may occur with other drugs that are listed.

Gabapentin — *Beta-Blockers*

Gabapentin* (*Neurontin*)	Propranolol* (eg, *Inderal*)

Significance	Onset	Severity	Documentation
4	☐ Rapid	☐ Major	☐ Established
	■ **Delayed**	■ **Moderate**	☐ Probable
		☐ Minor	☐ Suspected
			■ **Possible**
			☐ Unlikely

Effects The risk of GABAPENTIN side effects (eg, movement disorders) may be increased.

Mechanism Unknown.

Management Closely monitor patients receiving GABAPENTIN for symptoms of movement disorders when PROPRANOLOL is started or increased in dose. If an interaction is suspected, adjust therapy as needed.

Discussion

Paroxysmal dystonic movements were reported in a 68-year-old man during coadministration of gabapentin and propranolol.[1] The patient had a 10-year history of essential tremor. Administration of propranolol 120 mg/day was mildly successful in relieving the patient's symptoms. Subsequently, propranolol was replaced by gabapentin 900 mg/day. The tremors worsened and 7 months later propranolol 80 mg/day was restarted. After 2 days of receiving both drugs, the patient developed paroxysmal dystonic movements in both hands. He experienced several episodes of dystonia daily, each lasting about 1 minute. Twenty days later, the propranolol dose was reduced to 40 mg/day and the dystonia immediately subsided. The patient was successfully maintained on gabapentin 900 mg/day and propranolol 40 mg/day.

[1] Palomeras E, et al. *Arch Neurol.* 2000;57;570.

* Asterisk indicates drugs cited in interaction reports.

Ganciclovir — *Zidovudine*

Ganciclovir* (eg, *Cytovene*)	Zidovudine* (*Retrovir*)

Significance	Onset	Severity	Documentation
1	☐ Rapid ■ **Delayed**	■ **Major** ☐ Moderate ☐ Minor	☐ Established ■ **Probable** ☐ Suspected ☐ Possible ☐ Unlikely

Effects Life-threatening hematologic toxicity may occur.

Mechanism Unknown.

Management Avoid coadministration of GANCICLOVIR and ZIDOVUDINE. Foscarnet (*Foscavir*) may be a suitable alternative to GANCICLOVIR in treating cytomegalovirus (CMV) infections in immunocompromised patients receiving ZIDOVUDINE.[1]

Discussion

The efficacy, safety, and pharmacokinetics of combined antiviral therapy with ganciclovir and zidovudine were studied in a prospective, phase 1, multicenter trial. Forty patients with AIDS and serious CMV disease participated in the investigation.[2] Prior to the start of the study, 13 patients had been receiving 600 to 1,200 mg/day of zidovudine, 18 patients had been on ganciclovir maintenance, and 10 patients had not received ganciclovir or zidovudine. During the trial, patients were treated with zidovudine 1,200 mg/day plus ganciclovir 5 mg/kg IV twice daily or zidovudine 600 mg/day plus ganciclovir 5 mg/kg IV twice daily for 2 weeks (induction), followed by zidovudine 600 mg/day plus ganciclovir 5 mg/kg IV daily 5 times weekly (maintenance). All 10 patients treated with zidovudine 1,200 mg/day plus ganciclovir developed severe hematologic toxicity. In the patients receiving the lower doses of zidovudine plus ganciclovir, 82% experienced hematologic toxicity, including anemia, neutropenia, and leukopenia. More than 80% of the patients receiving ganciclovir required dose reductions to 300 mg/day because of toxicity. The median time for toxicity to occur was 3 to 5 weeks, depending on the dose combination. There was no indication of improved efficacy resulting from combined use of these 2 antiviral agents. In fact, most patients remaining on the regimen for several months developed progressive CMV disease. Pharmacokinetic data indicate that the adverse hematologic effects resulted from combined toxicity rather than from a pharmacokinetic interaction. However, a pharmacokinetic study of 12 patients found that ganciclovir increased zidovudine plasma levels 61.6% and AUC 19.5%.[3] These increases may explain the higher rates of toxicities.

[1] Teich SA, et al. *Surv Ophthalmol.* 1992;37:19.
[2] Hochster H, et al. *Ann Intern Med.* 1990;113:111.
[3] Cimoch PJ, et al. *J Acquir Immune Defic Syndr Hum Retrovirol.* 1998;17:227.

* Asterisk indicates drugs cited in interaction reports.

Gefitinib — *Azole Antifungal Agents*

Gefitinib* (*Iressa*)	Fluconazole (eg, *Diflucan*)	Posaconazole (*Noxafil*)
	Itraconazole* (eg, *Sporanox*)	Voriconazole (*Vfend*)
	Ketoconazole (eg, *Nizoral*)	

Significance	Onset	Severity	Documentation
2	☐ Rapid	☐ Major	☐ Established
	■ **Delayed**	■ **Moderate**	☐ Probable
		☐ Minor	■ **Suspected**
			☐ Possible
			☐ Unlikely

Effects GEFITINIB plasma concentrations may be elevated, increasing the risk of adverse reactions.

Mechanism AZOLE ANTIFUNGAL AGENTS may inhibit the metabolism (CYP3A4) of GEFITINIB.

Management In patients receiving GEFITINIB, observe for an increase in adverse reactions if an AZOLE ANTIFUNGAL AGENT is added to the treatment regimen.

Discussion

The effects of itraconazole on the pharmacokinetics of gefitinib were investigated in 48 healthy subjects.[1] In an open-label, randomized, crossover study, each subject received a single dose of gefitinib 250 or 500 mg alone and after 4 days of itraconazole 200 mg/day. Although 3 subjects withdrew during the study, pharmacokinetic data for all subjects were included in the statistical analysis. Compared with administration of gefitinib alone, pretreatment with itraconazole increased the C_{max} of gefitinib 250 and 500 mg by 51% and 32%, respectively. The AUC for the 2 gefitinib doses increased 78% and 61%, respectively, while the $t_{½}$ increased 25% and 22%, respectively.

[1] Swaisland HC, et al. *Clin Pharmacokinet.* 2005;44(10):1067.

* Asterisk indicates drugs cited in interaction reports. Based on pharmacologic and pharmacokinetic considerations, similar interactions may occur with other drugs that are listed.

Gefitinib — **Hydantoins**

Gefitinib	Hydantoins	
Gefitinib* (*Iressa*)	Ethotoin (*Peganone*)	Phenytoin* (eg, *Dilantin*)
	Fosphenytoin (eg, *Cerebyx*)	

Significance	Onset	Severity	Documentation
2	☐ Rapid	☐ Major	☐ Established
	■ **Delayed**	■ **Moderate**	☐ Probable
		☐ Minor	■ **Suspected**
			☐ Possible
			☐ Unlikely

Effects GEFITINIB plasma concentrations may be reduced, decreasing the pharmacologic effects.

Mechanism Increased hepatic metabolism (CYP3A4) of GEFITINIB by HYDANTOINS.

Management Monitor the clinical response of the patient to GEFITINIB when the HYDANTOIN dose is started, stopped, or changed. Adjust the GEFITINIB dose as needed.

Discussion

The effect of phenytoin on the pharmacokinetics of gefitinib was studied in 18 healthy men.[1] Using an open-label, 2-phase, crossover design, each subject received oral gefitinib 250 mg alone and after 5 days of treatment with phenytoin 5 mg/kg daily. Compared with receiving gefitinib alone, pretreatment with phenytoin decreased the mean gefitinib C_{max}, T_{max}, and AUC by 26%, 12%, and 47%, respectively. The apparent gefitinib oral clearance increased 126%. Gefitinib was well tolerated when given alone or concurrently with phenytoin.

[1] Chhun S, et al. *Br J Clin Pharmacol.* 2009;68(2):226.

* Asterisk indicates drugs cited in interaction reports. Based on pharmacologic and pharmacokinetic considerations, similar interactions may occur with other drugs that are listed.

Gefitinib	*Rifamycins*	
Gefitinib* (*Iressa*)	Rifabutin (*Mycobutin*) Rifampin* (eg, *Rifadin*)	Rifapentine (*Priftin*)

Significance	Onset	Severity	Documentation
2	□ Rapid ■ **Delayed**	□ Major ■ **Moderate** □ Minor	□ Established □ Probable ■ **Suspected** □ Possible □ Unlikely

Effects GEFITINIB plasma concentrations may be reduced, decreasing efficacy.

Mechanism RIFAMYCINS may increase the metabolism (CYP3A4) of GEFITINIB.

Management Monitor the response to GEFITINIB when RIFAMYCIN therapy is started or stopped. Adjust the GEFITINIB dose as needed.

Discussion

The effects of rifampin on the pharmacokinetics of gefitinib were investigated in 18 healthy subjects.[1] In an open-label, randomized, crossover study, each subject received a single dose of gefitinib 500 mg alone and after 10 days of receiving rifampin 600 mg/day. Compared with receiving gefitinib alone, pretreatment with rifampin decreased the mean C_{max} and overall AUC of gefitinib 65% and 83%, respectively. The reduction in C_{max} occurred about 3 hours after the dose. In addition, the gefitinib $t_{½}$ was decreased 39%. Additional studies are needed to determine the effect of rifampin administration on the efficacy of gefitinib.

[1] Swaisland HC, et al. *Clin Pharmacokinet.* 2005;44(10):1067.

* Asterisk indicates drugs cited in interaction reports. Based on pharmacologic and pharmacokinetic considerations, similar interactions may occur with other drugs that are listed.

Gemcitabine — *Paclitaxel*

Gemcitabine* (*Gemzar*)	Paclitaxel* (eg, *Taxol*)

Significance	Onset	Severity	Documentation
4	□ Rapid ■ **Delayed**	□ Major ■ **Moderate** □ Minor	□ Established □ Probable □ Suspected ■ **Possible** □ Unlikely

Effects GEMCITABINE plasma concentrations may be elevated, increasing the pharmacologic and toxic effects.

Mechanism Unknown.

Management Carefully monitor the clinical response of the patient when PACLITAXEL is started or stopped. Assess the patient for GEMCITABINE toxicity during coadministration of PACLITAXEL.

Discussion

The effect of paclitaxel on the pharmacokinetics of gemcitabine, given at a fixed-dose rate, was assessed in 14 patients with advanced non-small-cell lung cancer.[1] Both drugs were administered intravenously. Patients received paclitaxel 110 mg/m^2 over 3 hr on days 1 and 8 prior to gemcitabine 800 mg/m^2 over 80 minutes on days 1 and 8 every 21 days. In order to determine the pharmacokinetics of gemcitabine in the absence of paclitaxel, paclitaxel was not administered on day 1 of cycle 1. Pharmacokinetic data were analyzed in 13 patients. The desired steady-state gemcitabine plasma concentration was achieved in 61% of the patients when gemcitabine was administered alone. When gemcitabine and paclitaxel were administered concurrently, 0 to 45% (depending on the treatment cycle) of the patients achieved the desired steady-state gemcitabine level. Paclitaxel decreased systemic clearance and volume of distribution of gemcitabine and increased the steady-state plasma concentration. There was greater interpatient variability in gemcitabine pharmacokinetics when the drug was given alone compared with coadministration of paclitaxel.

[1] Shord SS, et al. *Cancer Chemother Pharmacol.* 2003;51:328.

* Asterisk indicates drugs cited in interaction reports.

Gemfibrozil — *Colestipol*

Gemfibrozil* (eg, *Lopid*)	Colestipol* (eg, *Colestid*)

Significance	Onset	Severity	Documentation
5	☐ Rapid	☐ Major	☐ Established
	■ **Delayed**	☐ Moderate	☐ Probable
		■ **Minor**	☐ Suspected
			■ **Possible**
			☐ Unlikely

Effects Decreased pharmacologic effects of GEMFIBROZIL.

Mechanism Unknown. Possibly due to reduced GI absorption of GEMFIBROZIL.

Management Consider separating the administration times of these 2 drugs by at least 2 hours.

Discussion

In a randomized study, the effects of oral administration of colestipol 5 g on the oral bioavailability of gemfibrozil 600 mg were studied in 10 volunteers with hyperlipidemia (ie, fasting cholesterol concentration more than 240 mg/dL or triglyceride concentration more than 200 mg/dL).[1] Each subject received gemfibrozil alone, 2 hours before, 2 hours after, or with colestipol. When gemfibrozil was administered alone, 2 hours before, or 2 hours after colestipol, there was no significant difference in serum gemfibrozil concentration, peak concentration, T_{max}, serum elimination $t_{1/2}$, or AUC between the 3 treatment regimens. However, when gemfibrozil and colestipol were coadministered, there was a 33% decrease in the AUC for gemfibrozil compared with when the drug was given alone. The mean serum gemfibrozil concentrations were lower at the 0.5-, 1-, and 1.5-hour sampling times when gemfibrozil was administered with colestipol compared with the other 3 regimens.

[1] Forland SC, et al. *J Clin Pharmacol.* 1990;30(1):29.

* Asterisk indicates drugs cited in interaction reports.

Gemfibrozil — *Protease Inhibitors*

Gemfibrozil* (eg, *Lopid*)	Lopinavir/Ritonavir* (*Kaletra*)	Ritonavir* (*Norvir*)

Significance	Onset	Severity	Documentation
4	☐ Rapid ■ **Delayed**	☐ Major ■ **Moderate** ☐ Minor	☐ Established ☐ Probable ☐ Suspected ■ **Possible** ☐ Unlikely

Effects GEMFIBROZIL plasma concentrations may be reduced, decreasing the pharmacologic effects.

Mechanism Unknown; however, decreased GEMFIBROZIL absorption is suspected.

Management Monitor triglyceride concentrations when starting PROTEASE INHIBITORS. Adjust the GEMFIBROZIL dose as needed.

Discussion

In an open-label study, the effects of lopinavir/ritonavir on the pharmacokinetics of gemfibrozil were investigated in 15 healthy volunteers.[1] Each subject received a singe oral dose of gemfibrozil 600 mg before and after administration of lopinavir 400 mg/ritonavir 100 mg twice daily for 14 days. Compared with giving gemfibrozil alone, pretreatment with lopinavir/ritonavir decreased the gemfibrozil C_{max} and AUC approximately 32% and 40%, respectively. The gemfibrozil $t_{1/2}$ did not change.

[1] Busse KH, et al. *J Acquir Immune Defic Syndr.* 2009;52(2):235.

* Asterisk indicates drugs cited in interaction reports.

Glucagon — Beta-Blockers

Glucagon	Beta-Blockers	
Glucagon* (eg, *GlucaGen*)	Acebutolol (eg, *Sectral*)	Metoprolol* (eg, *Lopressor*)
	Atenolol (eg, *Tenormin*)	Nadolol (eg, *Corgard*)
	Betaxolol (eg, *Kerlone*)	Penbutolol (*Levatol*)
	Bisoprolol (eg, *Zebeta*)	Pindolol
	Carteolol (*Cartrol*)	Propranolol* (eg, *Inderal LA*)
	Esmolol (eg, *Brevibloc*)	Sotalol (eg, *Betapace*)
	Labetalol (eg, *Trandate*)	Timolol

Significance	Onset	Severity	Documentation
4	■ **Rapid**	□ Major	□ Established
	□ Delayed	■ **Moderate**	□ Probable
		□ Minor	□ Suspected
			■ **Possible**
			□ Unlikely

Effects The hyperglycemic effect of GLUCAGON administration may be blunted by BETA-BLOCKER therapy.

Mechanism Unknown.

Management Based on available clinical data, no special precautions are necessary. However, consider administering glucose instead of GLUCAGON for a hypoglycemic episode in a diabetic patient receiving a BETA-BLOCKER.

Discussion

Documentation for the interaction between glucagon and beta-blockers is indirect. In a study of healthy volunteers, propranolol blunted the normal hyperglycemic response to a glucagon dose.[1] Similarly, hemodialysis patients experienced blunted response to glucagon during propranolol or metoprolol administration.[2-4] The magnitude of the effect from metoprolol appears to be less than propranolol.[3] These findings imply that the hyperglycemic effect of glucagon needed for treatment of hypoglycemia may be decreased in diabetic patients receiving a beta-blocker. However, in a study of healthy volunteers who were hypoglycemic, either through starvation or insulin administration, intrinsic glucagon response was similar with or without propranolol administration, and no difference in glucose values was found.[5] This may indicate a difference in glucose homeostatic mechanisms during hypoglycemia. Consequently, it is not known if the effects of glucagon would be impaired by beta-blockers during hypoglycemia. In addition, glucagon has been used successfully to treat cardiovascular collapse during propranolol overdose, documenting that at least some of the effects of glucagon are independent of the adrenergic system.[6,7]

[1] Messerli FH, et al. *Int J Clin Pharmacol Biopharm.* 1976;14(3):189.
[2] Pun KK, et al. *Clin Nephrol.* 1984;21(4):235.
[3] Pun KK, et al. *Nephron.* 1985;39(3):175.
[4] Pun KK, et al. *Clin Nephrol.* 1986;26(5):222.
[5] Walter RM, et al. *J Clin Invest.* 1974;54(5):1214.
[6] Kosinski EJ, et al. *Arch Intern Med.* 1973;132(6):840.
[7] Smith RC, et al. *JAMA.* 1985;254(17):2412.

* Asterisk indicates drugs cited in interaction reports. Based on pharmacologic and pharmacokinetic considerations, similar interactions may occur with other drugs that are listed.

Glyburide — *Colesevelam*

Glyburide* (eg, *Diabeta*)	Colesevelam* (*Welchol*)

Significance	Onset	Severity	Documentation
2	☐ Rapid ■ **Delayed**	☐ Major ■ **Moderate** ☐ Minor	☐ Established ☐ Probable ■ **Suspected** ☐ Possible ☐ Unlikely

Effects The therapeutic efficacy of GLYBURIDE may be reduced.

Mechanism COLESEVELAM may bind with GLYBURIDE in the GI tract, decreasing GLYBURIDE absorption.

Management Administer GLYBURIDE at least 4 hours prior to COLESEVELAM.[1]

Discussion

Using an open-label, randomized design, the effects of colesevelam on the pharmacokinetics of glyburide were evaluated in healthy volunteers.[2] Eighteen subjects received glyburide 3 mg alone, simultaneously with colesevelam 3,750 mg, and 1 hour before colesevelam. Thirty-three subjects received glyburide alone and 4 hours before colesevelam. Simultaneous administration of colesevelam decreased the AUC and C_{max} of glyburide 32% and 47.2%, respectively. When glyburide was given 1 hour prior to colesevelam, the glyburide AUC and C_{max} were decreased 19.5% and 14.6%, respectively. When glyburide was administered 4 hours before colesevelam, no interaction was observed.

[1] *Welchol* [package insert]. Parsippany, NJ: Daiichi Sankyo Inc; February 2010.

[2] Brown KS, et al. *J Clin Pharmacol.* 2010;50(5):554.

* Asterisk indicates drugs cited in interaction reports.

Griseofulvin — *Barbiturates*

Griseofulvin	Barbiturates	
Griseofulvin* (eg, *Grifulvin V*)	Amobarbital (*Amytal*)	Phenobarbital* (eg, *Solfoton*)
	Butabarbital (eg, *Butisol*)	Primidone* (eg, *Mysoline*)
	Butalbital	Secobarbital (*Seconal*)
	Mephobarbital (*Mebaral*)	
	Pentobarbital	

Significance	Onset	Severity	Documentation
2	☐ Rapid	☐ Major	☐ Established
	■ **Delayed**	■ **Moderate**	☐ Probable
		☐ Minor	■ **Suspected**
			☐ Possible
			☐ Unlikely

Effects Serum levels of GRISEOFULVIN are decreased after pretreatment with PHENOBARBITAL.

Mechanism Decreased GRISEOFULVIN absorption and increased hepatic metabolism by PHENOBARBITAL have been suggested as potential mechanisms.

Management Separating drug administration times, giving the PHENOBARBITAL in divided doses, or increasing the GRISEOFULVIN dose may be helpful if therapeutic failures with GRISEOFULVIN occur. Also, consider stopping either drug or using alternative therapy.

Discussion

Studies in rats[1-4] and healthy humans[5-7] show pretreatment with phenobarbital or primidone[2] at a variety of doses and time courses will reduce the serum concentrations of griseofulvin. Although some studies[1-3] have described increased metabolism as a possible mechanism, one study[7] found that phenobarbital altered the concentration-time curve in 6 adults only after oral dosing of griseofulvin and not after IV dosing, suggesting altered absorption of griseofulvin was the cause. This was further supported by studies in rats using a variety of formulations and demonstration of physicochemical bonding of the 2 drugs in the laboratory.[4,8] Only 1 case of treatment failure with griseofulvin has been ascribed to the interaction.[6]

[1] Busfield D, et al. *Br J Pharmacol Chemother.* 1964;22:137.
[2] Kraml M, et al. *Proc Soc Exp Biol Med.* 1965;120(3):678.
[3] Lin C, et al. *Drug Metab Disp.* 1973;1(4):611.
[4] Jamali F, et al. *J Pharm Sci.* 1978;67(4):466.
[5] Busfield D, et al. *Lancet.* 1963;2:1042.
[6] Lorenc E. *Mo Med.* 1967;64(1):32.
[7] Riegelman S, et al. *JAMA.* 1970;213(3):426.
[8] Abougela AK, et al. *J Pharm Pharmacol.* 1976;28(suppl):44P.

* Asterisk indicates drugs cited in interaction reports. Based on pharmacologic and pharmacokinetic considerations, similar interactions may occur with other drugs that are listed.

Guanethidine — *CNS Stimulants*

Guanethidine*†	Amphetamine*	Mazindol (*Sanorex*)
	Benzphetamine (*Didrex*)	Methamphetamine* (eg, *Desoxyn*)
	Dextroamphetamine* (eg, *Dexedrine*)	Phendimetrazine (eg, *Bontril*)
	Diethylpropion	Phentermine (eg, *Ionamin*)
	Lisdexamfetamine (*Vyvanse*)	

Significance	Onset	Severity	Documentation
2	■ **Rapid**	□ Major	□ Established
	□ Delayed	■ **Moderate**	■ **Probable**
		□ Minor	□ Suspected
			□ Possible
			□ Unlikely

Effects CNS STIMULANTS can reverse the hypotensive effects of GUANETHIDINE.

Mechanism Unknown.

Management Monitor patients. If there is a loss of BP control, stop the CNS STIMULANT or switch to alternative hypotensive therapy. If the GUANETHIDINE dose is increased, hypotension may occur if the CNS STIMULANT is stopped.

Discussion

The antagonism of the hypotensive effects of guanethidine by amphetamines (eg, amphetamine, dextroamphetamine, methamphetamine) has been demonstrated in a variety of animal models[1-7] and in small, open-label studies in humans.[8,9] The exact mechanism remains controversial; however, animal studies suggest a variety of possible effects. Amphetamine may displace guanethidine from its receptor site, while not blocking the site from the effect of sympathetic impulses.[1,2,6,8] Others suggest the interaction is caused by a block of guanethidine uptake into nerve endings.[5,7,10,11] Amphetamine potentiates response to nerve stimulation by increasing norepinephrine release, therefore antagonizing guanethidine.[4,9] One report found the ability of amphetamine to inhibit compounds like guanethidine was inversely related to the compound's ability to deplete catecholamines.[6] Thus, the exact mechanism remains undetermined. Amphetamines appear to be the primary anorexiants studied. One brief report on the use of diethylpropion in obese, hypertensive patients showed no interaction.

[1] Day MD. *Br J Pharmacol Chemother.* 1962;18:421.
[2] Day MD, et al. *J Pharm Pharmacol.* 1962;14:541.
[3] Gokhale SD, et al. *Arch Int Pharmacodyn Ther.* 1966;160(2):321.
[4] Obianwu HO. *Acta Physiol Scand.* 1969;75(1):102.
[5] Gerkens JF, et al. *Br J Pharmacol.* 1969;35(3):563.
[6] Follenfant MJ, et al. *Br J Pharmacol.* 1970;38(4):792.
[7] Flegin OT, et al. *Br J Pharmacol.* 1970;39(1):253P.
[8] Gulati OD, et al. *Clin Pharmacol Ther.* 1966;7(4):510.
[9] Ober KF, et al. *Clin Pharmacol Ther.* 1973;14(2):190.
[10] Starke K. *Arch Int Pharmacodyn Ther.* 1972;195(2):309.
[11] Seedat YK, et al. *S Afr Med J.* 1974;48(14):569.

* Asterisk indicates drugs cited in interaction reports. Based on pharmacologic and pharmacokinetic considerations, similar interactions may occur with other drugs that are listed.
† Not available in the United States.

Guanethidine — *Haloperidol*

Guanethidine*†	Haloperidol* (eg, *Haldol*)

Significance	Onset	Severity	Documentation
4	□ Rapid	□ Major	□ Established
	■ **Delayed**	■ **Moderate**	□ Probable
		□ Minor	□ Suspected
			■ **Possible**
			□ Unlikely

Effects HALOPERIDOL antagonizes the hypotensive effect of GUANETHIDINE.

Mechanism May inhibit the amine uptake pump.

Management Avoid the combination if possible; discontinuing either drug should eliminate the interaction. The interaction may be minimized by increasing the GUANETHIDINE dose, but hypotension may occur if haloperidol is discontinued suddenly.

Discussion

Three hypertensive patients were stabilized on guanethidine (60, 90, and 150 mg) then given haloperidol (8, 6, and 9 mg).[1] A slight, but significant, increase in blood pressure was recorded. Further study on this interaction is needed.

[1] Janowsky DS, et al. *Am J Psychiatry.* 1973;130:808.

* Asterisk indicates drugs cited in interaction reports.
† Not available in the United States.

Guanethidine — *MAO Inhibitors*

Guanethidine	MAO Inhibitors	
Guanethidine*†	Isocarboxazid (*Marplan*)	Phenelzine (*Nardil*)
	Pargyline (*Eutonyl*)	Tranylcypromine (*Parnate*)

Significance	Onset	Severity	Documentation
4	■ **Rapid**	□ Major	□ Established
	□ Delayed	■ **Moderate**	□ Probable
		□ Minor	□ Suspected
			■ **Possible**
			□ Unlikely

Effects MONOAMINE OXIDASE INHIBITORS potentially inhibit the hypotensive effects of GUANETHIDINE.

Mechanism May inhibit amine uptake.

Management Monitor patients taking the combination and discontinue use of the monoamine oxidase inhibitor or switch to alternative hypotensive therapy if loss of blood pressure control occurs. Though it may be possible to increase the dose of GUANETHIDINE, little clinical data supports this and significant hypotension may be unmasked if the MONOAMINE OXIDASE INHIBITOR is suddenly discontinued.

Discussion

Various animal models have demonstrated that monoamine oxidase inhibitors can reverse, to varying degrees, the hypotensive effects of guanethidine.[1,4] Iverson[2] demonstrated that monoamine oxidase inhibitors can inhibit the uptake of norepinephrine into tissue. It has been postulated that this is how the drugs antagonize guanethidine. In a study of hypertensive patients[3] nialamide (not available in the US) partially reversed the hypotensive effects of guanethidine and restored the pressor response to cold.

[1] Day MD. *Br J Pharmacol.* 1962;18:421.
[2] Iverson LL. *J Pharm Pharmacol.* 1965;17:62.
[3] Gulati OD, et al. *Clin Pharmacol Ther.* 1966;7:510.
[4] Lee CH, et al. *Res Commun Chem Pathol Pharmacol.* 1980;30:3.

* Asterisk indicates drugs cited in interaction reports. Based on pharmacologic and pharmacokinetic considerations, similar interactions may occur with other drugs that are listed.
† Not available in the United States.

Guanethidine — *Maprotiline*

Guanethidine†	Maprotiline*

Significance	Onset	Severity	Documentation
5	□ Rapid ■ **Delayed**	□ Major ■ **Moderate** □ Minor	□ Established □ Probable □ Suspected □ Possible ■ **Unlikely**

Effects MAPROTILINE may reverse the hypotensive effects of GUANETHIDINE in certain patients.

Mechanism Unknown.

Management If hypertension occurs, may increase the dose of GUANETHIDINE or stop the MAPROTILINE. If the dose of guanethidine is increased, care must be taken to avoid suddenly discontinuing the maprotiline and thus unmasking the hypotensive effects of guanethidine.

Discussion

Two patients were given maprotiline after their blood pressure was stabilized on guanethidine.[2] Neither patient had a loss of blood pressure control, although one patient had a single value significantly above baseline. Later values were normal. In a related study in which bethanidine was used instead of guanethidine,[1] five of six patients maintained blood pressure. In one patient mean blood pressure increased 14% (lying) and 26% (standing).

A paucity of data does not support the interaction, however certain subsets of patients may be more susceptible. Further study is needed before maprotiline can be suggested as an alternative to other tricyclic antidepressants in patients taking guanethidine.

[1] Briant RH, et al. *Br J Clin Pharmacol.* 1974;1:113. [2] Smith AJ, et al. *J Int Med Res.* 1975;3(Suppl 2):55.

* Asterisk indicates drugs cited in interaction reports.
† Not available in the United States.

Guanethidine — Methylphenidate

Guanethidine	Methylphenidate
Guanethidine*†	Methylphenidate* (eg, *Ritalin*)

Significance	Onset	Severity	Documentation
4	■ **Rapid**	□ Major	□ Established
	□ Delayed	■ **Moderate**	□ Probable
		□ Minor	□ Suspected
			■ **Possible**
			□ Unlikely

Effects The hypotensive effects of GUANETHIDINE can be impaired by METHYLPHENIDATE. Arrhythmias were reported on one case.

Mechanism Unknown.

Management Little is known. Monitor blood pressure and heart rhythms if the combination is used. Stopping either drug, depending upon the clinical situation, should eliminate the effects that occur. Antiarrhythmics may be needed.

Discussion

Gulati[1] examined the effects of a variety of drugs, including methylphenidate, on the hypotensive effects of guanethidine. Guanethidine was given to hypertensive patients until their blood pressure had stabilized (approximately 2 weeks). The test drug was then given and the blood pressure and pressor response to cold measured at varying intervals. Sixteen patients were studied, but not every patient received every drug. It is unclear how many received methylphenidate, though every drug was given to at least 5 patients. At 6 hours methylphenidate partially restored the pressor response to cold and reversed the hypotensive effects of guanethidine.

In a single case,[2] a man who had been stabilized on guanethidine for several months developed hypotension and ventricular tachycardia 2 days after starting methylphenidate. Two hours after stopping both drugs and receiving propranolol (eg, *Inderal*) and procainamide (eg, *Procan*), his rhythm returned to normal.

[1] Gulati OD, et al. *Clin Pharmacol Ther.* 1966;7:510.

[2] Deshmankar BS, et al. *Can Med Assoc J.* 1967;97:1166.

* Asterisk indicates drugs cited in interaction reports.
† Not available in the United States.

Guanethidine — *Phenothiazines*

Guanethidine*†	Chlorpromazine* (eg, *Thorazine*)	Prochlorperazine* (eg, *Compazine*)
	Fluphenazine (eg, *Prolixin*)	Thioridazine
	Perphenazine	Trifluoperazine

Significance	Onset	Severity	Documentation
2	☐ Rapid	☐ Major	☐ Established
	■ **Delayed**	■ **Moderate**	■ **Probable**
		☐ Minor	☐ Suspected
			☐ Possible
			☐ Unlikely

Effects The hypotensive action of GUANETHIDINE is inhibited.

Mechanism Inhibition of the uptake of GUANETHIDINE into nerve endings where it exhibits its effects.

Management Switch to alternative antihypertensive therapy if GUANETHIDINE is no longer effective and continued antipsychotic therapy is necessary. Although it may be possible to raise the dose of GUANETHIDINE or lower the dose of PHENOTHIAZINES, this should be done cautiously and there is little clinical evidence to support this option.

Discussion

The antihypertensive effect of guanethidine has been reversed in animals[1-3] and humans[4,5] when phenothiazines, namely chlorpromazine, were added to the regimen. Blockade of amine uptake, and thus blockade of guanethidine uptake into its site of action at nerve endings, appears to be the mechanism.[2,6,7] The effect may be dose related[2,3]; in a single instance, 50 mg chlorpromazine[8] was used safely with guanethidine and 5 patients received a single dose of 25 mg prochlorperazine without experiencing loss of hypertensive control with guanethidine.[9] One antipsychotic agent, molindone, has been reported not to interact with guanethidine,[2,7] and this may represent an alternative.

1 Stone CA, et al. *J Pharmacol Exp Ther.* 1964;144:196.
2 Gilder DA, et al. *J Pharmacol Exp Ther.* 1976;198:255.
3 Rankin GO, et al. *Arch Int Pharmacodyn Ther.* 1982;260:130.
4 Fann WE, et al. *Lancet.* 1971;2:436.
5 Janowsky DS, et al. *Am J Psychiatry.* 1973;130:808.
6 Tuck D, et al. *Lancet.* 1971;2:492.
7 Simpson LL. *Am J Psychiatry.* 1979;136:1410.
8 Poe TE, et al. *Postgrad Med.* 1979;66:235.
9 Ober KE, et al. *Clin Pharmacol Ther.* 1973;14:190.

* Asterisk indicates drugs cited in interaction reports. Based on pharmacologic and pharmacokinetic considerations, similar interactions may occur with other drugs that are listed.

† Not available in the United States.

Guanethidine	***Sympathomimetics***	
Guanethidine*†	**Direct**	**Mixed**
	Dobutamine (*Dobutrex*)	Dopamine* (eg, *Intropin*)
	Epinephrine* (eg, *Adrenalin*)	Ephedrine*
	Norepinephrine* (eg, *Levophed*)	Mephentermine (*Wyamine*)
	Phenylephrine* (eg, *Neo-Synephrine*)	Metaraminol (*Aramine*)
		Pseudoephedrine (eg, *Sudafed*)

Significance	Onset	Severity	Documentation
2	■ **Rapid**	□ Major	□ Established
	□ Delayed	■ **Moderate**	□ Probable
		□ Minor	■ **Suspected**
			□ Possible
			□ Unlikely

Effects GUANETHIDINE potentiates effects of direct-acting SYMPATHOMIMETICS and inhibits effects of SYMPATHOMIMETICS that depend upon release of norepinephrine for activity. GUANETHIDINE hypotensive action may be reversed.

Mechanism GUANETHIDINE depletes norepinephrine stores; this may account for indirect SYMPATHOMIMETICS being less effective and receptors more sensitive to direct SYMPATHOMIMETICS.

Management Use alternative antihypertensive therapy. Be cautious when using this combination. Monitor BP.

Discussion

The effect of guanethidine on mydriasis caused by sympathomimetics has been studied. Mydriasis was intensified when sympathomimetics that act directly on alpha receptors (phenylephrine, epinephrine) were given,[1,2] but decreased when sympathomimetics that depend upon the release of norepinephrine for activity (ephedrine, dopamine) were administered.[2,3] In addition, norepinephrine's pressor action was intensified by guanethidine.[4,5] In 1 small study,[5] the combination increased the heart's sensitivity to norepinephrine-induced arrhythmias.

Ephedrine partially reversed hypotensive action of guanethidine after 2 hr but not at 6 hr[6]; similar effects were noted with bethanidine and phenylpropanolamine.[7] Thus, when guanethidine is used with a sympathomimetic, hypertension and arrhythmias can result because of decreased guanethidine effectiveness or increased sympathetic activity.

[1] Cooper B. *Med J Aust.* 1968;55:420.
[2] Sneddon JM, et al. *Arch Ophthalmol.* 1969;81:622.
[3] Spiers ASD, et al. *Br Med J.* 1969;4:333.
[4] Laurence DR, et al. *Br J Pharmacol.* 1963;21:403.
[5] Muelheims GH, et al. *Clin Pharmacol Ther.* 1965;6:757.
[6] Gulati OD, et al. *Clin Pharmacol Ther.* 1966;7:510.
[7] Misage JR, et al. *Br Med J.* 1970;4:347.

* Asterisk indicates drugs cited in interaction reports. Based on pharmacologic and pharmacokinetic considerations, similar interactions may occur with other drugs that are listed.
† Not available in the United States.

Guanethidine		*Thioxanthenes*
Guanethidine*†	Chlorprothixene (*Taractan*)	Thiothixene* (*Navane*)

Significance	Onset	Severity	Documentation
4	□ Rapid ■ **Delayed**	□ Major ■ **Moderate** □ Minor	□ Established □ Probable □ Suspected ■ **Possible** □ Unlikely

Effects The hypotensive action of GUANETHIDINE is antagonized.

Mechanism THIOXANTHENES may block neuronal uptake of GUANETHIDINE.

Management Monitor patients for loss of blood pressure control if the combination is used. Switch to alternative antihypertensive therapy if needed.

Discussion

Thiothixene caused a small but significant increase in blood pressure (126/87 vs 156/110 mm Hg) when used for a few days (specific time not stated) in one patient taking guanethidine.[1]

[1] Janowsky DS, et al. *Am J Psychiatry*. 1973;130:808.

* Asterisk indicates drugs cited in interaction reports. Based on pharmacologic and pharmacokinetic considerations, similar interactions may occur with other drugs that are listed.
† Not available in the United States.

Guanethidine — *Tricyclic Antidepressants*

Guanethidine	Tricyclic Antidepressants	
Guanethidine*†	Amitriptyline*	Imipramine* (eg, *Tofranil*)
	Amoxapine (*Asendin*)	Nortriptyline* (eg, *Pamelor*)
	Desipramine* (*Norpramin*, *Pertofrane*)	Protriptyline* (*Vivactil*)
	Doxepin* (eg, *Sinequan*)	Trimipramine (*Surmontil*)

Significance	Onset	Severity	Documentation
2	■ **Rapid**	□ Major	□ Established
	□ Delayed	■ **Moderate**	■ **Probable**
		□ Minor	□ Suspected
			□ Possible
			□ Unlikely

Effects The hypotensive action of GUANETHIDINE is inhibited.

Mechanism Inhibition of the uptake of GUANETHIDINE into the nerve terminal, its site of action.

Management Monitor blood pressure. Use alternative antihypertensive therapy to control blood pressure as needed.

Discussion

Animal studies have demonstrated tricyclic antidepressants can inhibit the effects of guanethidine[2,6] and case reports in man have demonstrated a loss of blood pressure control with combined guanethidine and tricyclic antidepressants.[1,4,5,7-9,11] Although the effects may begin within 24 hours,[4] the full effect may not be exhibited for days[7,8,11] and may continue after the antidepressant is stopped.[7,9] In the two studies where no interaction was seen, imipramine and amitriptyline were given as single doses and studied for only 12 and 8 hours respectively.[3,10] Thus, monitor a patient beginning the combination for several days to determine any necessary action. One group of researchers has demonstrated the interaction to be dose related for doxepin,[5,9] but this needs to be confirmed for other drugs.

[1] Leishman AWD, et al. *Lancet.* 1963;1:112.
[2] Stone CA, et al. *J Pharmacol Exp Ther.* 1964;144:196.
[3] Gulati OD, et al. *Clin Pharmacol Ther.* 1966;7:510.
[4] Mitchell JR, et al. *JAMA.* 1967;202:149.
[5] Oates JA, et al. *Psychosomatics.* 1969;10(suppl):12.
[6] Hanahoe THP, et al. *Arch Int Pharmacodyn.* 1969;182:349.
[7] Meyer JF, et al. *JAMA.* 1970;213:1487.
[8] Mitchell JR, et al. *J Clin Invest.* 1970;49:1596.
[9] Fann WE, et al. *Psychopharmacologia.* 1971;22:111.
[10] Ober KF, et al. *Clin Pharmacol Ther.* 1973;14:190.
[11] Poe TE, et al. *Postgrad Med.* 1979;66:235.

* Asterisk indicates drugs cited in interaction reports. Based on pharmacologic and pharmacokinetic considerations, similar interactions may occur with other drugs that are listed.
† Not available in the United States.

Guanfacine — *Barbiturates*

Guanfacine	Barbiturates	
Guanfacine* (eg, *Tenex*)	Amobarbital (*Amytal*)	Pentobarbital
	Butabarbital (eg, *Butisol*)	Phenobarbital* (eg, *Solfoton*)
	Butalbital	Primidone (eg, *Mysoline*)
	Mephobarbital (*Mebaral*)	Secobarbital (eg, *Seconal*)

Significance	Onset	Severity	Documentation
4	☐ Rapid	☐ Major	☐ Established
	■ **Delayed**	■ **Moderate**	☐ Probable
		☐ Minor	☐ Suspected
			■ **Possible**
			☐ Unlikely

Effects The antihypertensive effectiveness of GUANFACINE may be decreased.

Mechanism Increased GUANFACINE hepatic metabolism by BARBITURATES is suspected.

Management Monitor blood pressure when a BARBITURATE is started or discontinued in patients whose hypertension is controlled by GUANFACINE. Adjust the dose of GUANFACINE accordingly. When discontinuing GUANFACINE in patients receiving a concurrent BARBITURATE, taper the dosage of the antihypertensive agent.

Discussion

A single case of severe hypertension was observed following abrupt discontinuation of guanfacine in a 47-year-old woman with severe chronic renal insufficiency receiving concurrent phenobarbital. This withdrawal syndrome led to a kinetic study of guanfacine in the patient. During coadministration of both drugs, plasma concentration of guanfacine varied between 1.75 and 9.6 mcg/L, and the elimination $t_{½}$ was 5.1 hours. After discontinuation of phenobarbital, guanfacine concentrations ranged from 8.05 to 24.15 mcg/L, and the elimination $t_{½}$ was 20.5 hours.[1]

Additional documentation is needed to substantiate this possible interaction.

[1] Kiechel JR, et al. *Eur J Clin Pharmacol.* 1983;25(4):463.

* Asterisk indicates drugs cited in interaction reports. Based on pharmacologic and pharmacokinetic considerations, similar interactions may occur with other drugs that are listed.

Guanfacine	*Tricyclic Antidepressants*	
Guanfacine* (eg, *Tenex*)	Amitriptyline* Cyclobenzaprine (eg, *Flexeril*)	Imipramine* (eg, *Tofranil*)

Significance	Onset	Severity	Documentation
2	□ Rapid ■ **Delayed**	□ Major ■ **Moderate** □ Minor	□ Established □ Probable ■ **Suspected** □ Possible □ Unlikely

Effects The antihypertensive effect of GUANFACINE may be decreased.

Mechanism Inference by TRICYCLIC ANTIDEPRESSANTS is suspected with GUANFACINE uptake at the receptor site.

Management Monitor BP of patients receiving GUANFACINE when starting, stopping, or changing the dose of the TRICYCLIC ANTIDEPRESSANT. If an interaction is suspected, consider discontinuing the TRICYCLIC ANTIDEPRESSANT or using an antihypertensive agent with a different mechanism of action.

Discussion

Antagonism of the antihypertensive effects of guanfacine was reported in a 38-year-old woman on 2 separate occasions, following the coadministration of a tricyclic antidepressant.[1] The patient had a 2-year history of hypertension that was well controlled by guanfacine 2 mg at night. Amitriptyline 75 mg daily was prescribed for neuralgia accompanying a back injury. Prior to the administration of amitriptyline, her mean BP was 138/89 mm Hg. During the first week of concomitant amitriptyline administration, mean BP increased to 150/100 mm Hg. After 2 weeks, amitriptyline was discontinued because of drowsiness, and the patient's mean BP returned to previous levels (136/91 mm Hg) within 14 days. Similar changes in BP occurred 4 weeks later when imipramine 50 mg daily was prescribed. Two days after starting imipramine, her mean BP increased from 138/88 to 142/98 mm Hg. Six days later, imipramine was discontinued because of drowsiness, and her mean BP decreased to 137/90 mm Hg.

Cyclobenzaprine is structurally related to tricyclic antidepressants and may interact similarly.

[1] Buckley M, et al. *Lancet*. 1991;337(8750):1173.

* Asterisk indicates drugs cited in interaction reports. Based on pharmacologic and pharmacokinetic considerations, similar interactions may occur with other drugs that are listed.

Halofantrine | **Tetracyclines**

Halofantrine*†	Tetracycline* (eg, *Sumycin*)

Significance	Onset	Severity	Documentation
4	□ Rapid	□ Major	□ Established
	■ **Delayed**	■ **Moderate**	□ Probable
		□ Minor	□ Suspected
			■ **Possible**
			□ Unlikely

Effects Plasma concentrations of HALOFANTRINE and its active metabolite desbutylhalofantrine may be elevated, increasing the risk of toxicity.

Mechanism Unknown.

Management Carefully monitor patients for HALOFANTRINE adverse reactions if TETRACYCLINE is coadministered. If an interaction is suspected, adjust the dose as needed.

Discussion

The effects of tetracycline on the pharmacokinetics of halofantrine were studied in 8 healthy men.[1] In a crossover design, each subject received halofantrine 500 mg alone and with tetracycline 500 mg every 12 hours for 7 days. Compared with giving halofantrine alone, tetracycline increased halofantrine C_{max} 2.5-fold and AUC 2-fold, and prolonged the terminal $t_{½}$ from 91 to 157 hours. In addition, tetracycline administration increased the C_{max} and AUC of the major active halofantrine metabolite, desbutylhalofantrine, 2.5- and 1.8-fold, respectively.

[1] Bassi PU, et al. *Br J Clin Pharmacol.* 2004;58(1):52.

* Asterisk indicates drugs cited in interaction reports.
† Not available in the United States.

Haloperidol — *Anticholinergics*

Haloperidol*
(eg, *Haldol*)

Atropine
(eg, *Sal-Tropine*)
Belladonna
Benztropine*
(eg, *Cogentin*)
Biperiden
(*Akineton*)
Dicyclomine
(eg, *Bentyl*)
Glycopyrrolate
(eg, *Robinul*)
Hyoscyamine
(eg, *Anaspaz*)
Mepenzolate
(*Cantil*)
Methscopolamine
(eg, *Pamine*)
Orphenadrine
(eg, *Norflex*)
Oxybutynin
(eg, *Ditropan*)
Procyclidine*
(*Kemadrin*)
Propantheline
(eg, *Pro-Banthine*)
Scopolamine
(eg, *Scopace*)
Trihexyphenidyl*
(eg, *Trihexy*)

Significance	Onset	Severity	Documentation
2	□ Rapid	□ Major	□ Established
	■ **Delayed**	■ **Moderate**	□ Probable
		□ Minor	■ **Suspected**
			□ Possible
			□ Unlikely

Effects Effects are variable. Worsening of schizophrenic symptoms, decreased serum concentration of HALOPERIDOL, and development of tardive dyskinesia were reported when ANTICHOLINERGIC AGENTS were used with HALOPERIDOL.

Mechanism Unknown.

Management If coadministration of these agents cannot be avoided, closely monitor patients. Discontinue ANTICHOLINERGIC or tailor HALOPERIDOL if necessary.

Discussion

A series of articles[1-4] reported worsening of schizophrenia in patients taking haloperidol or chlorpromazine (eg, *Thorazine*) when benztropine or trihexyphenidyl was added to the drug regimen. The authors concluded that anticholinergic agents can worsen schizophrenia, whether given alone or with an antipsychotic agent,[5] and attributed the effect to central cholinergic pathways rather than pharmacokinetic interactions. Anticholinergics decreased the serum concentrations of various antipsychotic agents[6]; however, only 4 patients were taking haloperidol. Other studies have noted no change in serum levels[7,8] or therapeutic status[6,8,9] in patients taking anticholinergics. An animal study[10] indicated anticholinergic agents may promote tardive dyskinesia development.

[1] Singh MM, et al. *J Nerv Ment Dis.* 1973;157:50.
[2] Singh MM, et al. *Psychopharmacologia.* 1975;43:103.
[3] Singh MM, et al. *Psychopharmacologia.* 1975;43:115.
[4] Singh MM, et al. *J Nerv Ment Dis.* 1975;160:258.
[5] Singh MM, et al. *Neuropsychobiology.* 1979;5:74.
[6] Gautier J, et al. *Biol Psychiatry.* 1977;12:389.
[7] Linnoila M, et al. *Am J Psychiatry.* 1980;137:819.
[8] Altamura AC, et al. *Encephale.* 1986;12:31.
[9] Altamura AC, et al. *Acta Neurol.* 1986;8:19.
[10] Borison RL, et al. *Adv Biochem Psychopharmacol.* 1980;24:359.

* Asterisk indicates drugs cited in interaction reports. Based on pharmacologic and pharmacokinetic considerations, similar interactions may occur with other drugs that are listed.

Haloperidol — *Azole Antifungal Agents*

Haloperidol* (eg, *Haldol*)	Fluconazole (eg, *Diflucan*)	Ketoconazole (eg, *Nizoral*)
	Itraconazole* (eg, *Sporanox*)	

Significance	Onset	Severity	Documentation
2	☐ Rapid	☐ Major	☐ Established
	■ **Delayed**	■ **Moderate**	☐ Probable
		☐ Minor	■ **Suspected**
			☐ Possible
			☐ Unlikely

Effects HALOPERIDOL plasma concentrations may be elevated, increasing the risk of adverse reactions.

Mechanism Inhibition of HALOPERIDOL metabolism (CYP3A4) by AZOLE ANTIFUNGAL AGENTS is suspected.

Management Observe the clinical response to HALOPERIDOL when an AZOLE ANTIFUNGAL AGENT is started or stopped. Adjust the dose as needed. Plasma HALOPERIDOL levels may be helpful in managing patients.

Discussion

In an open-label study, the effects of itraconazole on the steady-state plasma concentrations of haloperidol and reduced haloperidol were investigated in 13 schizophrenic patients.[1] Eleven patients were given haloperidol 6 mg twice daily and 2 patients received 12 mg twice daily for 2 to 36 weeks. Each patient received itraconazole 200 mg/day for 7 days. Compared with haloperidol alone, coadministration of itraconazole resulted in an increase in the plasma levels of both haloperidol (from 13 to 16.9 ng/mL) and reduced haloperidol (from 4.9 to 6.1 ng/mL). One week after itraconazole was discontinued, plasma concentrations of haloperidol and reduced haloperidol were 13.5 and 4.9 ng/mL, respectively. During coadministration of itraconazole, neurologic adverse reactions were increased. In a crossover study, 15 healthy men were pretreated with itraconazole 200 mg or matching placebo twice daily for 10 days.[2] On day 7, subjects received a single oral dose of haloperidol 5 mg. Itraconazole increased haloperidol AUC 55% and adverse reaction scores compared with placebo.

[1] Yasui N, et al. *J Clin Psychopharmacol.* 1999;19:149. [2] Park JY, et al. *J Clin Psychopharmacol.* 2006;26:135.

* Asterisk indicates drugs cited in interaction reports. Based on pharmacologic and pharmacokinetic considerations, similar interactions may occur with other drugs that are listed.

Haloperidol — *Barbiturates*

Haloperidol	Barbiturates	
Haloperidol* (eg, *Haldol*)	Amobarbital (eg, *Amytal*)	Pentobarbital (eg, *Nembutal*)
	Butabarbital (eg, *Butisol*)	Phenobarbital*
	Butalbital	Primidone (eg, *Mysoline*)
	Mephobarbital (eg, *Mebaral*)	Secobarbital (eg, *Seconal*)

Significance	Onset	Severity	Documentation
4	☐ Rapid	☐ Major	☐ Established
	■ **Delayed**	■ **Moderate**	☐ Probable
		☐ Minor	☐ Suspected
			■ **Possible**
			☐ Unlikely

Effects PHENOBARBITAL may decrease serum concentrations of HALOPERIDOL. Haloperidol may have caused fatal hyperpyrexia in a single case when used for barbiturate withdrawal.

Mechanism PHENOBARBITAL may induce the metabolism of HALOPERIDOL.

Management Monitor for loss of control of psychiatric symptoms or side effects of HALOPERIDOL when PHENOBARBITAL is added to or deleted from the patient's regimen. Monitor body temperature, particularly when HALOPERIDOL is used for barbiturate withdrawal.

Discussion

Haloperidol and phenobarbital have been used together successfully for barbiturate withdrawal and schizophrenia.[1,5] In animals, haloperidol appears to have no effect on the serum concentrations[3] or the anticonvulsant activity of phenobarbital.[4] However, serum concentrations of haloperidol were lessened by concomitant administration of phenobarbital,[3,5] although the number of patients in these studies was limited and some patients were also receiving phenytoin.

One patient developed fatal hyperthermia after receiving haloperidol 50 mg IM for barbiturate withdrawal.[2] Though complicating factors were present, the haloperidol seemed to be the precipitating agent.

1 Snyder R. *Mil Med.* 1977;142:885.
2 Greenblatt DJ, et al. *J Clin Psychiatry.* 1978;39:673.
3 Linnoila M, et al. *Am J Psychiatry.* 1980;137:819.
4 Kleinrok Z, et al. *Epilepsia.* 1980;21:519.
5 Prakash R, et al. *J Clin Psychopharmacol.* 1984;4:362.

* Asterisk indicates drugs cited in interaction reports. Based on pharmacologic and pharmacokinetic considerations, similar interactions may occur with other drugs that are listed.

Haloperidol | **Carbamazepine**

Haloperidol* (eg, *Haldol*)	Carbamazepine* (eg, *Tegretol*)

Significance	Onset	Severity	Documentation
2	□ Rapid ■ **Delayed**	□ Major ■ **Moderate** □ Minor	□ Established □ Probable ■ **Suspected** □ Possible □ Unlikely

Effects The therapeutic effects of HALOPERIDOL may be decreased, while those of CARBAMAZEPINE may be increased.

Mechanism CARBAMAZEPINE may result in a dose-dependent increase in hepatic metabolism of HALOPERIDOL, while HALOPERIDOL may inhibit the metabolism of CARBAMAZEPINE.

Management If an interaction is suspected, consider adjusting the dose of therapy as indicated.

Discussion

Data conflict concerning the coadministration effect of carbamazepine and haloperidol.[1-11] Several reports have demonstrated carbamazepine to lower plasma haloperidol concentrations,[6-11] while 1 report found no effect.[1] In some patients, a marked decrease in the clinical efficacy of haloperidol was observed, including re-emergence of psychomotor agitation, obsessive-compulsive rituals, withdrawn behavior, auditory hallucinations, delusions, and inappropriate affect.[8,9] Other reports indicate that although carbamazepine may reduce haloperidol serum concentrations, patients may show no clinical change or may actually improve during coadministration of both drugs.[2,3,7,10] Administration of carbamazepine to patients receiving haloperidol has produced a 60% decrease in plasma haloperidol levels.[9] In some patients, haloperidol plasma levels may be undetectable.[9] In a study in 11 schizophrenic patients, haloperidol levels were 75%, 39%, and 15% of baseline with carbamazepine daily doses of 100, 300, and 600 mg, respectively, indicating a dose-dependent effect.[12] Two additional cases have been reported in which coadministration of carbamazepine and haloperidol to patients with rapid-cycling bipolar disorder has been associated with the occurrence of delirium.[4,5] In 1 patient, the drugs had been well tolerated when given alone.[5]

Serum carbamazepine concentrations were compared in 14 patients receiving carbamazepine and haloperidol and in 8 patients receiving carbamazepine alone.[11] Carbamazepine concentrations were 40% lower in patients receiving carbamazepine alone.

[1] Forsman A, et al. *Curr Ther Res Clin Exp.* 1977;21:245.
[2] Klein E, et al. *Arch Gen Psychiatry.* 1984;41:165.
[3] Ereshefsky L, et al. *J Clin Psychopharmacol.* 1984;4:138.
[4] Kanter GL, et al. *Am J Psychiatry.* 1984;141:1101.
[5] Yerevanian BI, et al. *Am J Psychiatry.* 1985;142:785.
[6] Kidron R, et al. *Biol Psychiatry.* 1985;20:219.
[7] Jann MW, et al. *J Clin Psychopharmacol.* 1985;5:106.
[8] Fast DK, et al. *Am J Psychiatry.* 1986;143:117.
[9] Arana GW, et al. *Am J Psychiatry.* 1986;143:650.
[10] Kahn EM, et al. *J Clin Psychopharmacol.* 1990;10:54.
[11] Iwahashi K, et al. *Clin Neuropharmacol.* 1995;18:233.
[12] Yasui-Furukori N, et al. *J Clin Psychopharmacol.* 2003;23:435.

* Asterisk indicates drugs cited in interaction reports.

Haloperidol | **Clozapine**

Haloperidol*
(eg, *Haldol*)

Clozapine*
(*Clozaril*)

Significance	Onset	Severity	Documentation
4	☐ Rapid	☐ Major	☐ Established
	■ **Delayed**	■ **Moderate**	☐ Probable
		☐ Minor	☐ Suspected
			■ **Possible**
			☐ Unlikely

Effects HALOPERIDOL plasma levels may be elevated, increasing the risk of side effects.

Mechanism Inhibition of HALOPERIDOL metabolism (CYP2D6) by CLOZAPINE is suspected.

Management Observe the clinical response of the patient to HALOPERIDOL when starting or stopping CLOZAPINE.

Discussion

A 40-year-old man treated with haloperidol experienced an elevated haloperidol plasma level during coadministration of clozapine.[1] The patient was started on clozapine (50 mg/day) for assaultive behaviors motivated by persecutory delusions. As a precaution, haloperidol 50 mg IM every 4 weeks was added to the patient's drug regimen, while clozapine was increased from 50 to 250 mg daily over a 12-day period. Two weeks after the first injection of haloperidol, while receiving clozapine 250 mg/day, the haloperidol plasma level was 166 ng/mL (therapeutic range, 5 to 12 ng/mL). Haloperidol was discontinued, and the patient was maintained on clozapine monotherapy. During a previous treatment, while the patient had been receiving a larger dose of haloperidol (150 mg IM every 2 weeks) and chlorpromazine (300 mg/day), his haloperidol plasma level was only 5.5 ng/mL.

[1] Allen SA. *J Clin Pharmacol.* 2000;40:1296.

* Asterisk indicates drugs cited in interaction reports.

Haloperidol — *Fluoxetine*

Haloperidol* (eg, *Haldol*)	Fluoxetine* (eg, *Prozac*)

Significance	Onset	Severity	Documentation
4	☐ Rapid ■ **Delayed**	☐ Major ■ **Moderate** ☐ Minor	☐ Established ☐ Probable ☐ Suspected ■ **Possible** ☐ Unlikely

Effects Coadministration of HALOPERIDOL and FLUOXETINE has been associated with severe extrapyramidal reactions.

Mechanism Unknown.

Management If extrapyramidal symptoms occur while a patient is receiving these drugs, consider discontinuing 1 or both agents.

Discussion

A 39-year-old woman developed intractable extrapyramidal symptoms while receiving haloperidol and fluoxetine for bipolar disorder.[1] The patient had been treated with haloperidol 2 to 5 mg/day for 2 years with and without benztropine (eg, *Cogentin*). At times, she experienced mild extrapyramidal symptoms that disappeared when the dose of haloperidol was decreased or the drug was discontinued. On this occasion, 5 days before stopping haloperidol, fluoxetine was started and the dose was increased over several days to 40 mg twice daily. After 2 weeks of fluoxetine therapy, the patient ingested 5 mg haloperidol on 2 consecutive mornings. She experienced severe tongue stiffness, parkinsonism, and akathisia. Haloperidol and fluoxetine were discontinued. The extrapyramidal symptoms slowly remitted over the following week. In a study of 8 psychotic patients receiving stable oral doses of haloperidol (mean, 14 mg/day), the addition of fluoxetine 20 mg/day for 7 to 10 days produced a 20% increase in mean haloperidol plasma levels. There was no change in extrapyramidal side effects.[2] Another patient developed catatonia, muteness, and stupor from coadministration of fluoxetine and haloperidol.[3] A study of 13 patients on stable doses of haloperidol demonstrated a 35% increase in haloperidol plasma levels after the addition of fluoxetine 20 mg/day.[4] One patient had an increase in extrapyramidal symptoms, while 6 had improvement in schizophrenic symptom scores. A similar study found limited value from fluoxetine augmentation of haloperidol therapy in schizophrenic patients.[5] There was a 28.5% increase in haloperidol plasma levels and 5 of 17 patients experienced aggravation of parkinsonian symptoms.

Additional studies are needed to document the importance of this possible interaction.

1 Tate JL. *Am J Psychiatry*. 1989;146:399.
2 Goff DC, et al. *Am J Psychiatry*. 1991;148:790.
3 Shad MU, et al. *J Clin Psychopharmacol*. 2001;21:119.
4 Avenoso A, et al. *Pharmacol Res*. 1997;35:335.
5 Shim JC, et al. *J Clin Psychopharmacol*. 2003;23:520.

* Asterisk indicates drugs cited in interaction reports.

Haloperidol — *Fluvoxamine*

Haloperidol* (eg, *Haldol*)	Fluvoxamine*

Significance	Onset	Severity	Documentation
4	☐ Rapid	☐ Major	☐ Established
	■ **Delayed**	■ **Moderate**	☐ Probable
		☐ Minor	☐ Suspected
			■ **Possible**
			☐ Unlikely

Effects Serum HALOPERIDOL concentrations may be elevated, increasing the pharmacologic and toxic effects.

Mechanism Inhibition of HALOPERIDOL metabolism by FLUVOXAMINE is suspected.

Management When starting therapy with HALOPERIDOL in patients receiving FLUVOXAMINE, consider giving a conservative dose of HALOPERIDOL and carefully titrating therapy. In patients stabilized on HALOPERIDOL, it may be necessary to alter the dose when starting or stopping FLUVOXAMINE. Serum HALOPERIDOL levels may be helpful in managing patients.

Discussion

Administration of fluvoxamine 150 to 300 mg/day to 4 patients with chronic schizophrenia maintained on haloperidol 15 to 60 mg/day plus benztropine (eg, *Cogentin*) 2 to 6 mg/day resulted in an increase in plasma haloperidol concentrations and impaired performance on tests of delayed recall memory and attentional function.[1] One patient became lethargic and experienced clinically significant exacerbation of preexisting confusion, poor concentration, and poor self-care while receiving fluvoxamine and haloperidol. In 2 patients, haloperidol serum concentrations did not plateau during the 6 weeks of fluvoxamine treatment and continued to decrease over 20 days after discontinuing fluvoxamine. In 3 patients who were receiving fluvoxamine 150 mg/day with haloperidol 2.5 to 15 mg/day, the average haloperidol plasma concentration increased 23%.[2] A study in 12 schizophrenic patients receiving haloperidol showed that fluvoxamine 25 to 150 mg/day increased haloperidol levels 39% to 60%.[3] The increases were not associated with increased adverse effects.

[1] Daniel DG, et al. *J Clin Psychopharmacol.* 1994;14:340.
[2] Vandel S, et al. *Pharmacol Res.* 1995;31:347.
[3] Yasui-Furukori N, et al. *Psychopharmacolgy.* 2004;171:223.

* Asterisk indicates drugs cited in interaction reports.

Haloperidol | *Hydantoins*

Haloperidol* (eg, *Haldol*)	Ethotoin (*Peganone*) Fosphenytoin (*Cerebyx*)	Phenytoin* (eg, *Dilantin*)

Significance	Onset	Severity	Documentation
5	☐ Rapid ■ **Delayed**	☐ Major ☐ Moderate ■ **Minor**	☐ Established ☐ Probable ☐ Suspected ■ **Possible** ☐ Unlikely

Effects HYDANTOINS may decrease the HALOPERIDOL serum concentration.

Mechanism Unknown. However, induction of HALOPERIDOL metabolism is suspected.

Management Monitor patients taking HALOPERIDOL for loss of control of psychiatric symptoms or for adverse reactions of HALOPERIDOL when a HYDANTOIN is added or discontinued, respectively.

Discussion

A single study[1] noted haloperidol serum concentrations were lower (19.4 vs 36.6 ng/mL after 42 days) in patients taking anticonvulsants compared with those not taking anticonvulsants. The study did not differentiate among patients taking phenobarbital (eg, *Solfoton*), phenytoin, or the combination.

An animal study suggests that haloperidol interferes with the anticonvulsant activity of phenytoin.[2] This has not been demonstrated clinically.

[1] Linnoila M, et al. *Am J Psychiatry*. 1980;137(7):819.

[2] Kleinrok Z, et al. *Epilepsia*. 1980;21(5):519.

* Asterisk indicates drugs cited in interaction reports. Based on pharmacologic and pharmacokinetic considerations, similar interactions may occur with other drugs that are listed.

Haloperidol — Lithium

Haloperidol* (eg, *Haldol*)	Lithium* (eg, *Lithobid*)

Significance	Onset	Severity	Documentation
1	☐ Rapid ■ **Delayed**	■ **Major** ☐ Moderate ☐ Minor	☐ Established ☐ Probable ■ **Suspected** ☐ Possible ☐ Unlikely

Effects Alterations in consciousness, encephalopathy, extrapyramidal effects, fever, leukocytosis, and increased serum enzymes.

Mechanism Unknown.

Management When this combination is used, monitor patients closely, particularly during the first 3 weeks of therapy. If an interaction is suspected, discontinue either drug. Institute supportive treatment for symptoms.

Discussion

Numerous retrospective and prospective studies have demonstrated that lithium and haloperidol can be used together safely with no increase in adverse reactions.[1-4] Nonetheless, several authors[5-14] have described patients taking the combination who developed, to varying degrees, weakness, lethargy, tremulousness, confusion, stupor, fever, severe extrapyramidal symptoms and dystonias, leukocytosis, elevated serum enzymes, and elevated blood urea nitrogen. Several patients were left with significant dyskinetic and parkinsonian sequelae.[5,8,10] Some have suggested that the syndrome was lithium toxicity; however, many patients had serum concentrations of lithium within the therapeutic range. Also, many features are similar to the neuroleptic malignant syndrome described for a variety of neuroleptic drugs (including haloperidol) both alone and in combination.[15] Therefore, haloperidol may be implicated. Electroencephalogram changes have been demonstrated in patients upon the addition of lithium to a haloperidol regimen, but not to other neuroleptics.[16] Clinical evidence and psychomotor testing suggest that the combination of haloperidol and lithium may produce brain damage.[17,18] Although another investigator found a direct correlation between neuroleptic dose and neurotoxicity, the maximum dose of haloperidol in affected patients ranges from 6 to 100 mg.[14]

1 Baastrup PC, et al. *JAMA*. 1976;236(23):2645.
2 Juhl RP, et al. *Dis Nerv Syst*. 1977;38(9):675.
3 Biederman J, et al. *Arch Gen Psychiatry*. 1979;36(3):327.
4 Goldney RD, et al. *Am J Psychiatry*. 1986;143(7):882.
5 Cohen WJ, et al. *JAMA*. 1974;230(9):1283.
6 Thornton WE, et al. *Can Psychiatry Assoc J*. 1975;20(4):281.
7 Loudon JB, et al. *Lancet*. 1976;2(7994):1088.
8 Spring G, et al. *Am J Psychiatry*. 1981;138(6):818.
9 Prakash R, et al. *Compr Psychiatry*. 1982;23(6):567.
10 Sandyk R, et al. *S Afr Med J*. 1983;64(22):875.
11 Keitner GI, et al. *J Clin Psychopharmacol*. 1984;4(2):104.
12 Jeffries J, et al. *Can J Psychiatry*. 1984;29(7):601
13 Addonizio G. *J Clin Psychopharmacol*. 1985;5(5):296.
14 Miller F, et al. *Hosp Community Psychiatry*. 1987;38(11):1219.
15 Gibb WR, et al. *Q J Med*. 1985;56(220):421.
16 Saran A, et al. *Neurophysiobiology*. 1989;20(3):152.
17 Thomas CJ. *Br J Psychiatry*. 1979;134:552.
18 Thomas C, et al. *Lancet*. 1982;1(8272):626.

* Asterisk indicates drugs cited in interaction reports.

Haloperidol — *Methyldopa*

Haloperidol*
(eg, *Haldol*)

Methyldopa*
(eg, *Aldomet*)

Significance	Onset	Severity	Documentation
4	□ Rapid	□ Major	□ Established
	■ **Delayed**	■ **Moderate**	□ Probable
		□ Minor	□ Suspected
			■ **Possible**
			□ Unlikely

Effects METHYLDOPA may potentiate the antipsychotic effects of HALOPERIDOL, or the combination may produce psychosis.

Mechanism Both drugs may additively reduce brain dopamine.

Management If psychological symptoms occur, discontinue either drug (depending upon the therapeutic situation) and substitute appropriate alternative therapy.

Discussion

An open study of 10 schizophrenic patients unresponsive to current therapy found that the combination of methyldopa 500 mg and haloperidol 10 mg improved the psychopathology of the patients within 2 weeks. No further improvement was noted at 4 weeks. All 10 patients exhibited extrapyramidal effects.[1] When haloperidol was given for situational anxiety to 2 patients taking methyldopa, both patients exhibited psychiatric symptoms (mental slowing and impairment, motor retardation, disorientation, and ideas of reference) that disappeared completely when haloperidol was stopped.[2] Similarly, a schizophrenic woman who had been manageable became irritable, aggressive, and assaultive when the combination was used.[3] She returned to her previous condition when hydrochlorothiazide (eg, *Esidrix*) was substituted for methyldopa.

Though the time course of the 3 case reports suggests a potential interaction, methyldopa alone may cause central effects. However, the first 2 patients had been taking methyldopa for 3 years and 18 months, respectively. The improvement of schizophrenic patients on the combination should be considered. The uncontrolled design of the study may have affected the results. Further study is needed to characterize this interaction.

[1] Chouinard G, et al. *Curr Ther Res.* 1973;15:473.
[2] Thornton WE. *N Engl J Med.* 1976;294:1222.
[3] Nadel I, et al. *Br J Psychiatry.* 1979;135:484.

* Asterisk indicates drugs cited in interaction reports.

Haloperidol — *Nefazodone*

Haloperidol* (eg, *Haldol*)	Nefazodone* (*Serzone*)

Significance	Onset	Severity	Documentation
4	□ Rapid ■ **Delayed**	□ Major ■ **Moderate** □ Minor	□ Established □ Probable □ Suspected ■ **Possible** □ Unlikely

Effects The pharmacologic and toxic effects of HALOPERIDOL may be increased.

Mechanism Unknown.

Management Observe patients for an increase in the response to HALOPERIDOL when NEFAZODONE is coadministered. If an interaction is suspected, it may be necessary to decrease the dose of HALOPERIDOL.

Discussion

Possible pharmacokinetic and pharmacodynamic drug interactions between haloperidol and nefazodone were investigated in a parallel-group, double-blind, placebo-controlled study involving 12 healthy male volunteers.[1] Each subject was randomly assigned to 1 of 2 treatment groups. Individuals in each group received either 5 mg of haloperidol or a placebo and either 200 mg of nefazodone or placebo. Compared with giving haloperidol alone, concurrent administration of haloperidol and nefazodone was associated with slight increases in the mean area under the plasma concentration-time curve (AUC; 36%), peak concentration (13%), and 12-hour concentration (37%) values for haloperidol. Only the increase in AUC was statistically significant ($P < 0.05$). Haloperidol did not affect the pharmacokinetics of nefazodone. Although the effects of haloperidol on several psychomotor performance tests were significantly altered, a consistent effect was not demonstrated.

Additional studies are needed to determine if a clinically important interaction occurs with concurrent administration of these agents.

[1] Barbhaiya RH, et al. *J Clin Psychopharmacol.* 1996;16:26.

* Asterisk indicates drugs cited in interaction reports.

Haloperidol — *NSAIDs*

Haloperidol* (eg, *Haldol*)	Indomethacin* (eg, *Indocin*)

Significance	Onset	Severity	Documentation
4	☐ Rapid ■ **Delayed**	☐ Major ■ **Moderate** ☐ Minor	☐ Established ☐ Probable ☐ Suspected ■ **Possible** ☐ Unlikely

Effects The incidence and severity of certain HALOPERIDOL side effects (eg, drowsiness, confusion) may be increased.

Mechanism Unknown.

Management Consider administering a neuroleptic other than HALOPERIDOL. If both drugs are administered concurrently, monitor patients for side effects.

Discussion

To determine whether haloperidol has synergistic action with indomethacin in reducing the pain of osteoarthritis, a placebo-controlled, double-blind crossover study was undertaken in 40 patients with osteoarthritis.[1] Patients were stabilized on indomethacin 25 mg 3 times daily, then allocated to receive indomethacin 25 mg 3 times daily plus either haloperidol 5 mg/day or a daily placebo at night for 28 days. After the recruitment of 20 patients, the study was discontinued on ethical grounds when 13 of 20 patients failed to complete the trial. Six patients receiving haloperidol experienced extreme drowsiness (a known side effect of haloperidol), 4 others complained of a variety of side effects that were also associated with haloperidol, and 1 patient experienced worsening of osteoarthritis. In addition to the 11 patients withdrawn from the haloperidol group, 2 patients were withdrawn from the placebo group for reasons unrelated to treatment. Although these side effects may have been caused by haloperidol alone, it is also possible that the adverse reactions were more intense than would be expected with haloperidol alone.

Additional documentation is needed to determine if the effects observed were caused by an interaction or to haloperidol alone, and if other NSAIDs would interact similarly.

[1] Bird HA, et al. *Lancet.* 1983;1:830.

* Asterisk indicates drugs cited in interaction reports.

Haloperidol — *Olanzapine*

Haloperidol* (eg, *Haldol*)	Olanzapine* (*Zyprexa*)

Significance	Onset	Severity	Documentation
4	☐ Rapid ■ **Delayed**	☐ Major ■ **Moderate** ☐ Minor	☐ Established ☐ Probable ☐ Suspected ■ **Possible** ☐ Unlikely

Effects Severe parkinsonism has been associated with concurrent use of these agents.

Mechanism Unknown.

Management Closely observe the patient for extrapyramidal side effects, including parkinsonism, during coadministration of HALOPERIDOL and OLANZAPINE. If an interaction is suspected, it may be necessary to discontinue one of the agents.

Discussion

A 67-year-old man with a long-standing history of bipolar disorder was admitted to the hospital after an episode of inappropriate and assaultive behavior.[1] Several weeks prior to admission, he had stopped taking his psychiatric medications, which included haloperidol 3 mg/day, benztropine (eg, *Cogentin*) 1 mg/day, and valproic acid (eg, *Depakene*). At the time of his hospitalization, he had mild symptoms of parkinsonism (mild cogwheeling rigidity, mildly festinating gait). Approximately 3 weeks after restarting his medication (including haloperidol 10 mg/day), the patient was stabilized and no longer assaultive. At this time, olanzapine 2.5 mg/day was initiated. On day 4, the olanzapine dose was increased to 5 mg/day, and the haloperidol dose was decreased to 8 mg/day. Two days later, the patient displayed symptoms of severe parkinsonism, with increased rigidity, mumbling speech, and an inability to walk. Three days after increasing the dose of benztropine to 1 mg 3 times daily and discontinuing haloperidol, the symptoms of parkinsonism resolved. Subsequently, benztropine was stopped, and the patient was maintained on olanzapine.

Additional data are needed to assess this possible interaction.

[1] Gomberg RF. *J Clin Psychopharmacol.* 1999;19:272.

* Asterisk indicates drugs cited in interaction reports.

Haloperidol		**Phenothiazines**	
Haloperidol* (eg, *Haldol*)		Chlorpromazine* (eg, *Thorazine*)	Promethazine* (eg, *Phenergan*)
		Fluphenazine (eg, *Prolixin*)	Thioridazine
		Perphenazine	

Significance	Onset	Severity	Documentation
4	■ **Rapid**	■ **Major**	□ Established
	□ Delayed	□ Moderate	□ Probable
		□ Minor	□ Suspected
			■ **Possible**
			□ Unlikely

Effects HALOPERIDOL plasma levels may be elevated, increasing the risk of side effects. The risk of life-threatening arrhythmias, including torsades de pointes, may be increased.

Mechanism Inhibition of HALOPERIDOL metabolism (CYP2D6) by certain PHENOTHIAZINES is suspected. Possible additive or synergistic prolongation of the QT interval.

Management Observe the clinical response of the patient to HALOPERIDOL when starting, stopping, or changing the dose of certain PHENOTHIAZINES.

Discussion

A 40-year-old man treated with haloperidol and chlorpromazine for assaultive behavior motivated by persecutory delusions, experienced an increase in haloperidol plasma levels when the chlorpromazine dose was gradually increased from 300 to 600 mg/day.[1] The effect of chlorpromazine on plasma concentrations of haloperidol and reduced haloperidol was studied in 43 schizophrenic men.[2] Chlorpromazine produced an average increase of 28.5% in haloperidol and 160.8% in reduced haloperidol plasma levels. However, there were wide interindividual variations in the effect of chlorpromazine on haloperidol. Administration of promethazine 150 mg/day for 1 week increased serum levels of both haloperidol 117% (from 12.7 to 27.6 mg/mL) and the reduced haloperidol metabolite.[3] There was no increase in haloperidol side effects.

Torsades de pointes and sudden death have been reported with phenothiazines[4] (particularly thioridazine[4-7] and mesoridazine[8]) and with haloperidol[4-7,9] (especially IV,[10-13] IM,[14] or high dosage[7]). The risk of cardiac arrhythmias, including torsades de pointes, may be increased when phenothiazines and haloperidol are coadministered.

1 Allen SA. *J Clin Pharmacol.* 2000;40:1296.
2 Suzuki Y, et al. *Ther Drug Monit.* 2001;23:363.
3 Suzuki A, et al. *Ther Drug Monit.* 2003;25:192.
4 Glassman AH, et al. *Am J Psychiatry.* 2001;158:1774.
5 Buckley NA, et al. *Drug Saf.* 2000;23:215.
6 Reilly JG, et al. *Lancet.* 2000;355:1048.
7 Liu BA, et al. *N Engl J Med.* 2004;351:1053.
8 Dallaire S, et al. *Can ADR Newsl.* 2001;11:1.
9 O'Brien JM, et al. *Ann Pharmacother.* 1999;33:1046.
10 Tisdale JE, et al. *J Clin Pharmacol.* 2001;41:1310.
11 Hatta K, et al. *J Clin Psychopharmacol.* 2001;21:257.
12 Douglas PH, et al. *Catheter Cardiovasc Interv.* 2000;50:352.
13 Perrault LP, et al. *Can J Anaesth.* 2000;47:251.
14 Harvey AT, et al. *J Clin Pharmacol.* 2004;44:1173.

* Asterisk indicates drugs cited in interaction reports. Based on pharmacologic and pharmacokinetic considerations, similar interactions may occur with other drugs that are listed.

Haloperidol — *Quinidine*

Haloperidol* (eg, *Haldol*)	Quinidine*

Significance	Onset	Severity	Documentation
4	☐ Rapid ■ **Delayed**	☐ Major ■ **Moderate** ☐ Minor	☐ Established ☐ Probable ☐ Suspected ■ **Possible** ☐ Unlikely

Effects Serum HALOPERIDOL concentrations may be elevated, increasing the pharmacologic and adverse effects.

Mechanism Unknown.

Management Carefully observe the clinical response of the patient during and soon after coadministration of HALOPERIDOL and QUINIDINE. Adjust the dose of HALOPERIDOL as indicated.

Discussion

The effect of oral quinidine bisulfate 250 mg on the pharmacokinetics of a single 5 mg oral dose of haloperidol or reduced haloperidol was studied in 12 healthy men.[1] The areas under the plasma concentration-time curve and the peak plasma concentrations of both haloperidol compounds were greater following coadministration of quinidine than when the compounds were taken alone. In addition, quinidine had no effect on the half-life of either compound.

Additional studies are needed to determine the clinical importance of this interaction in patients.

[1] Young D, et al. *Eur J Clin Pharmacol.* 1993;44:433.

* Asterisk indicates drugs cited in interaction reports.

Haloperidol — *Rifamycins*

Haloperidol* (eg, *Haldol*)	Rifabutin (*Mycobutin*)	Rifampin* (eg, *Rifadin*)

Significance	Onset	Severity	Documentation
2	☐ Rapid ■ **Delayed**	☐ Major ■ **Moderate** ☐ Minor	☐ Established ☐ Probable ■ **Suspected** ☐ Possible ☐ Unlikely

Effects RIFAMYCINS may decrease the plasma concentration and clinical effectiveness of HALOPERIDOL.

Mechanism Induction of HALOPERIDOL metabolism is suspected.

Management When adding or discontinuing RIFAMYCIN therapy in a patient receiving HALOPERIDOL, carefully monitor the clinical response of the patient. Adjust the HALOPERIDOL dose as indicated.

Discussion

The effects of rifampin on the plasma concentration and clinical response to haloperidol were assessed in 2 groups of patients with schizophrenia.[1] In group 1 (12 patients), trough haloperidol plasma concentrations decreased during coadministration of rifampin, and in group 2 (5 patients), haloperidol concentrations increased after rifampin was discontinued. The decreases in plasma haloperidol concentrations (approximately 63% of baseline at 3 days, 37% at 7 days, and 30% at 28 days) appeared to result in a reduction in the therapeutic effects of haloperidol. Six of 12 patients exhibited a 30% or more increase in their Brief Psychiatric Rating Scale score. After discontinuation of rifampin, there was a 3.3-fold increase in haloperidol plasma concentrations; however, there was no change in any clinical scale. Changes in plasma haloperidol concentrations seemed to level off 7 to 10 days after coadministration or at discontinuation of rifampin. In another report involving patients with schizophrenia receiving haloperidol with and without concurrent antituberculosis treatment, rifampin administration resulted in a decrease in haloperidol concentrations, which was associated with an increase in haloperidol clearance and a decrease in the $t_{½}$.[2]

[1] Kim YH, et al. *J Clin Psychopharmacol.* 1996;16(3):247.

[2] Takeda M, et al. *Clin Neuropharmacol.* 1986;9(4):386.

* Asterisk indicates drugs cited in interaction reports. Based on pharmacologic and pharmacokinetic considerations, similar interactions may occur with other drugs that are listed.

Haloperidol — *Tacrine*

Haloperidol* (eg, *Haldol*)	Tacrine* (*Cognex*)

Significance	Onset	Severity	Documentation
4	□ Rapid	□ Major	□ Established
	■ **Delayed**	■ **Moderate**	□ Probable
		□ Minor	□ Suspected
			■ **Possible**
			□ Unlikely

Effects Severe extrapyramidal symptoms may occur.

Mechanism Unknown.

Management Closely monitor the patient for extrapyramidal symptoms. If an interaction is suspected, it may be necessary to stop one or both drugs.

Discussion

In an 87-year-old man receiving haloperidol 5 mg/day for irrational behavior, severe parkinsonian symptoms developed 72 hours after adding tacrine 40 mg/day to his treatment regimen.[1] Symptoms included akinesia/bradykinesia, masked facies, shuffling gait, and lead-pipe rigidity. Both drugs were discontinued and his symptoms resolved within approximately 8 hours. Haloperidol alone was restarted without recurrence of the parkinsonian symptoms. In a 72-year-old woman receiving haloperidol 10 mg/day for severe progressive dementia, disabling parkinsonian symptoms occurred within 1 week of starting tacrine 40 mg/day.[2] Symptoms included severe akinesia, shuffling gait, masked facies, slurred speech, and pronounced rigidity and cogwheel signs. The haloperidol dose was tapered and then replaced with risperidone (eg, *Risperdal*). The parkinsonian symptoms resolved within a few days and did not recur even after the tacrine dose was increased.

[1] McSwain ML, et al. *J Clin Psychopharmacol.* 1995;15(4):284.

[2] Maany I. *Am J Psychiatry.* 1996;153(11):1504.

* Asterisk indicates drugs cited in interaction reports.

Halothane — *Rifampin*

Halothane*†	Rifampin* (eg, *Rifadin*)

Significance	Onset	Severity	Documentation
4	☐ Rapid	■ **Major**	☐ Established
	■ **Delayed**	☐ Moderate	☐ Probable
		☐ Minor	☐ Suspected
			■ **Possible**
			☐ Unlikely

Effects Hepatotoxicity and hepatic encephalopathy have been reported when RIFAMPIN and isoniazid were given after HALOTHANE anesthesia.

Mechanism Unknown. The combination of RIFAMPIN and HALOTHANE may enhance isoniazid hepatotoxicity.

Management Stop the antitubercular medication and treat the hepatotoxicity. Avoid giving RIFAMPIN-isoniazid shortly after HALOTHANE anesthesia.

Discussion

The combination of rifampin and isoniazid produced hepatotoxicity and hepatic encephalopathy in 4 patients when given after halothane anesthesia.[1-3] Symptoms noted were nausea, vomiting, weakness, shock, jaundice, altered consciousness, and coma; these appeared 3 to 9 days after surgery. One patient died[3]; however, the rifampin was discontinued in this patient on the day of surgery, and the isoniazid continued until symptoms developed 3 days later.

Two authors[2,3] believe the toxicity was due to the isoniazid and that the combination of rifampin and halothane accelerated the process. Similar effects were described in patients who received rifampin-isoniazid and other drugs (eg, phenobarbital, hydroxyzine, nitrous oxide) besides halothane.[2]

It is difficult to ascribe an interaction to halothane and rifampin alone. However, due to the potentially serious nature of the effect, use the drugs together with caution, and avoid the combination whenever possible if isoniazid is also used.

[1] Most JA, et al. *Am J Surg.* 1974;127(5):593.
[2] Pessayre D, et al. *Gastroenterology.* 1977;72(2):284.
[3] Bartelink AK, et al. *Tubercle.* 1983;64(2):125.

* Asterisk indicates drugs cited in interaction reports.
† Not available in the United States.

HCV Protease Inhibitors — *Barbiturates*

Boceprevir* (*Victrelis*)	Telaprevir* (*Incivek*)	Phenobarbital* (eg, *Luminal*)	
Significance	Onset	Severity	Documentation
1	☐ Rapid ■ **Delayed**	■ **Major** ☐ Moderate ☐ Minor	☐ Established ☐ Probable ■ **Suspected** ☐ Possible ☐ Unlikely

Effects HEPATITIS C VIRUS (HCV) PROTEASE INHIBITOR plasma concentrations may be reduced, leading to loss of virologic response. PHENOBARBITAL concentrations may be increased or decreased.

Mechanism HCV PROTEASE INHIBITOR metabolism (CYP3A4) may be increased by PHENOBARBITAL.

Management Coadministration of BOCEPREVIR and PHENOBARBITAL is contraindicated.[1] Coadminister TELAPREVIR and PHENOBARBITAL with caution; close clinical and laboratory monitoring of PHENOBARBITAL concentrations is recommended.[2] Dose titration is recommended to achieve the desired clinical response.

Discussion

Boceprevir and telaprevir are CYP3A4 and P-gp substrates. Concurrent use of strong CYP3A inducers, such as phenobarbital, may decrease boceprevir or telaprevir plasma concentrations, leading to a loss of virologic response.[1,2] Concomitant use of phenobarbital and boceprevir is contraindicated.[1] Coadministration of telaprevir with phenobarbital warrants close clinical and laboratory monitoring of phenobarbital concentrations and dose titration.[2]

The basis for this monograph is information on file with the manufacturer. Published clinical data are needed to further assess this interaction. Because of the seriousness of the interaction, clinical evaluation in humans is not likely to be forthcoming.

[1] *Victrelis* [package insert]. Whitehouse Station, NJ: Schering Corporation; May 2011.

[2] *Incivek* [package insert]. Cambridge, MA: Vertex Pharmaceuticals Incorporated; May 2011.

* Asterisk indicates drugs cited in interaction reports.

HCV Protease Inhibitors — Carbamazepine

Boceprevir* (*Victrelis*)	Telaprevir* (*Incivek*)	Carbamazepine* (eg, *Tegretol*)	
Significance	Onset	Severity	Documentation
1	☐ Rapid ■ **Delayed**	■ **Major** ☐ Moderate ☐ Minor	☐ Established ☐ Probable ■ **Suspected** ☐ Possible ☐ Unlikely

Effects HEPATITIS C VIRUS (HCV) PROTEASE INHIBITOR plasma concentrations may be reduced, leading to loss of virologic response. CARBAMAZEPINE concentrations may be elevated, increasing the risk of adverse reactions.

Mechanism HCV PROTEASE INHIBITOR metabolism (CYP3A4) may be increased by CARBAMAZEPINE while CARBAMAZEPINE metabolism (CYP3A4) may be inhibited.

Management Coadministration of BOCEPREVIR and CARBAMAZEPINE is contraindicated.[1] Coadminister TELAPREVIR and CARBAMAZEPINE with caution; close clinical and laboratory monitoring of CARBAMAZEPINE concentrations is recommended.[2] Dose titration is recommended to achieve the desired clinical response.

Discussion

Boceprevir and telaprevir are CYP3A4 and P-gp substrates. Concurrent use of strong CYP3A inducers, such as carbamazepine, may decrease boceprevir or telaprevir plasma concentrations, leading to a loss of virologic response.[1,2] Concomitant use of carbamazepine and boceprevir is contraindicated.[1] Coadministration of telaprevir with carbamazepine warrants close clinical and laboratory monitoring of carbamazepine concentrations and dose titration.[2]

The basis for this monograph is information on file with the manufacturer. Published clinical data are needed to further assess this interaction. Because of the seriousness of the interaction, clinical evaluation in humans is not likely to be forthcoming.

[1] *Victrelis* [package insert]. Whitehouse Station, NJ: Schering Corporation; May 2011.

[2] *Incivek* [package insert]. Cambridge, MA: Vertex Pharmaceuticals Incorporated; May 2011.

* Asterisk indicates drugs cited in interaction reports.

HCV Protease Inhibitors — *Hydantoins*

HCV Protease Inhibitors		Hydantoins	
Boceprevir* (*Victrelis*)	Telaprevir* (*Incivek*)	Ethotoin (*Peganone*) Fosphenytoin (eg, *Cerebyx*)	Phenytoin* (eg, *Dilantin*)

Significance	Onset	Severity	Documentation
1	☐ Rapid ■ **Delayed**	■ **Major** ☐ Moderate ☐ Minor	☐ Established ☐ Probable ■ **Suspected** ☐ Possible ☐ Unlikely

Effects HEPATITIS C VIRUS (HCV) PROTEASE INHIBITOR plasma concentrations may be reduced, leading to loss of virologic response. HYDANTOIN concentrations may be increased or decreased.

Mechanism HCV PROTEASE INHIBITOR metabolism (CYP3A4) may be increased by HYDANTOINS.

Management Coadministration of BOCEPREVIR and PHENYTOIN is contraindicated.[1] Coadminister TELAPREVIR and PHENYTOIN with caution; close clinical and laboratory monitoring of PHENYTOIN concentrations is recommended.[2] Dose titration is recommended to achieve the desired clinical response.

Discussion

Boceprevir and telaprevir are CYP3A4 and P-gp substrates. Concurrent use of strong CYP3A inducers, such as phenytoin, may decrease boceprevir or telaprevir plasma concentrations, leading to a loss of virologic response.[1,2] Concomitant use of phenytoin and boceprevir is contraindicated.[1] Coadministration of telaprevir with phenytoin warrants close clinical and laboratory monitoring of phenytoin concentrations and dose titration.[2]

The basis for this monograph is information on file with the manufacturer. Published clinical data are needed to further assess this interaction. Because of the seriousness of the interaction, clinical evaluation in humans is not likely to be forthcoming.

[1] *Victrelis* [package insert]. Whitehouse Station, NJ: Schering Corporation; May 2011.

[2] *Incivek* [package insert]. Cambridge, MA: Vertex Pharmaceuticals Incorporated; May 2011.

* Asterisk indicates drugs cited in interaction reports. Based on pharmacologic and pharmacokinetic considerations, similar interactions may occur with other drugs that are listed.

HCV Protease Inhibitors — *Rifamycins*

Boceprevir* (*Victrelis*)	Telaprevir* (*Incivek*)	Rifabutin* (*Mycobutin*) Rifampin* (eg, *Rifadin*)	Rifapentine (*Priftin*)

Significance	Onset	Severity	Documentation
1	☐ Rapid ■ **Delayed**	■ **Major** ☐ Moderate ☐ Minor	☐ Established ☐ Probable ■ **Suspected** ☐ Possible ☐ Unlikely

Effects HEPATITIS C VIRUS (HCV) PROTEASE INHIBITOR plasma concentrations may be reduced, leading to loss of virologic response. RIFAMYCIN plasma concentrations may be elevated, increasing the risk of adverse reactions.

Mechanism HCV PROTEASE INHIBITOR metabolism (CYP3A4) may be increased by RIFAMYCINS, while RIFAMYCIN metabolism (CYP3A4) may be decreased.

Management Coadministration of HCV PROTEASE INHIBITORS and RIFAMPIN is contraindicated. Coadministration of RIFABUTIN or RIFAPENTINE is not recommended.

Discussion

Boceprevir and telaprevir are CYP3A4 and P-gp substrates. Concurrent use of strong CYP3A inducers, such as rifampin, may decrease boceprevir or telaprevir plasma concentrations, leading to a loss of virologic response. Concomitant use of rifampin and boceprevir or telaprevir is contraindicated. Coadministration of boceprevir or telaprevir with rifabutin or rifapentine is not recommended.[1,2]

The basis for this monograph is information on file with the manufacturer. Published clinical data are needed to further assess this interaction. Because of the seriousness of the interaction, clinical evaluation in humans is not likely to be forthcoming.[1]

[1] *Victrelis* [package insert]. Whitehouse Station, NJ: Schering Corporation; May 2011.

[2] *Incivek* [package insert]. Cambridge, MA: Vertex Pharmaceuticals Incorporated; May 2011.

* Asterisk indicates drugs cited in interaction reports. Based on pharmacologic and pharmacokinetic considerations, similar interactions may occur with other drugs that are listed.

HCV Protease Inhibitors — *St. John's Wort*

Boceprevir* (*Victrelis*)	Telaprevir* (*Incivek*)	St. John's Wort*

Significance	Onset	Severity	Documentation
1	☐ Rapid ■ **Delayed**	■ **Major** ☐ Moderate ☐ Minor	☐ Established ☐ Probable ■ **Suspected** ☐ Possible ☐ Unlikely

Effects HEPATITIS C VIRUS (HCV) PROTEASE INHIBITOR plasma concentrations may be reduced, leading to loss of virologic response.

Mechanism HCV PROTEASE INHIBITOR metabolism (CYP3A4) may be increased by ST. JOHN'S WORT.

Management Coadministration of HCV PROTEASE INHIBITORS and ST. JOHN'S WORT is contraindicated.[1,2]

Discussion

Boceprevir and telaprevir are CYP3A4 and P-gp substrates. Concurrent use of CYP3A4 and/or P-gp inducers (eg, St. John's wort) may decrease boceprevir or telaprevir plasma concentrations, leading to a loss of virologic response. Concomitant use of St. John's wort and boceprevir or telaprevir is contraindicated.[1,2]

The basis for this monograph is information on file with the manufacturer. Published clinical data are needed to further assess this interaction. Because of the seriousness of the interaction, clinical evaluation in humans is not likely to be forthcoming.

[1] *Victrelis* [package insert]. Whitehouse Station, NJ: Schering Corporation; May 2011.

[2] *Incivek* [package insert]. Cambridge, MA: Vertex Pharmaceuticals Incorporated; May 2011.

* Asterisk indicates drugs cited in interaction reports.

Heparin — *Cephalosporins*

Heparin	Cefamandole*†	Cefoxitin*
	Cefazolin*	Ceftriaxone* (eg, *Rocephin*)
	Cefoperazone*†	
	Cefotetan	

Significance	Onset	Severity	Documentation
4	☐ Rapid	☐ Major	☐ Established
	■ **Delayed**	■ **Moderate**	☐ Probable
		☐ Minor	☐ Suspected
			■ **Possible**
			☐ Unlikely

Effects Increased risk of bleeding.

Mechanism Several CEPHALOSPORINS have caused coagulopathies. This might be additive with HEPARIN.

Management Monitor patients receiving the combination for bleeding and coagulopathies, and manage accordingly. Vitamin K has been used successfully to treat CEPHALOSPORIN-induced bleeding.

Discussion

Abnormalities in humoral and platelet-mediated coagulation tests[1-14] and clinically significant bleeding[1,2,4,5,7,9-14] have been reported with a variety of cephalosporins (cefazolin, cefoperazone, cefamandole, ceftriaxone, and cefoxitin). Several possible mechanisms have been suggested, including inhibition of adenosine diphosphate (ADP)–induced platelet aggregation, interference with vitamin K synthesis in the gut, and defective fibrinogen-fibrin polymerization. In only a few instances was heparin also used, and it did not appear to aggravate the situation.[4,7,9] Nonetheless, because heparin can also cause bleeding, monitor patients receiving the combination.

[1] Lerner PI, et al. *N Engl J Med.* 1974;290(23):1324.
[2] Khaleeli M, et al. *Blood.* 1976;48(5):791.
[3] Custer GM, et al. *Antimicrob Agents Chemother.* 1979;16(6):869.
[4] Reddy J, et al. *N Z Med J.* 1980;92(672):378.
[5] Rymer W, et al. *Drug Intell Clin Pharm.* 1980;14(11):780.
[6] Bang NU, et al. *Rev Infect Dis.* 1982;4(suppl):S546.
[7] Weitekamp MR, et al. *JAMA.* 1983;249(1):69.
[8] MacLennan FM, et al. *Lancet.* 1983;1(8335):1215.
[9] Haubenstock A, et al. *Lancet.* 1983;1(8335):1215.
[10] Fainstein V, et al. *J Infect Dis.* 1983;148(4):745.
[11] Joehl RJ, et al. *Arch Surg.* 1983;118(11):1259.
[12] Cristiano P. *Drug Intell Clin Pharm.* 1984;18(4):314.
[13] Meisel S. *Drug Intell Clin Pharm.* 1984;18(4):316.
[14] Parker SW, et al. *Lancet.* 1984;1(8384):1016.

* Asterisk indicates drugs cited in interaction reports. Based on pharmacologic and pharmacokinetic considerations, similar interactions may occur with other drugs that are listed.

† Not available in the United States.

Heparin ✕ **Nitroglycerin**

Heparin*	Nitroglycerin* (eg, *Nitrostat*)

Significance	Onset	Severity	Documentation
4	■ **Rapid**	☐ Major	☐ Established
	☐ Delayed	■ **Moderate**	☐ Probable
		☐ Minor	☐ Suspected
			■ **Possible**
			☐ Unlikely

Effects The pharmacologic effects of HEPARIN may be decreased.

Mechanism Unknown.

Management During coadministration of IV NITROGLYCERIN and HEPARIN, monitor the coagulation status of the patient and adjust the dose of HEPARIN accordingly.

Discussion

Data are conflicting. In a preliminary study, the presence of propylene glycol in IV nitroglycerin preparations was reported to interfere with the anticoagulant effect of heparin.[1] A subsequent, prospective investigation in 7 patients demonstrated that heparin resistance occurred whether or not the nitroglycerin preparation contained propylene glycol.[2] Increases in the infusion rate of nitroglycerin, in the presence of a constant infusion rate of heparin, were accompanied by a fall in the activated partial thromboplastin time (APTT). Conversely, when the nitroglycerin infusion rate was slowed, the APTT increased. Discontinuing nitroglycerin therapy during constant infusion of heparin resulted in a rebound overshoot with an increase in APTT to more than 3.5 times the control in 6 of 8 patients, including 2 patients receiving nitroglycerin without propylene glycol. A similar response occurred in a patient receiving 2 different preparations of IV nitroglycerin, one with and the other without propylene glycol.[3] In a group of 10 patients receiving heparin following coronary angioplasty, the APTT was not significantly different during the coadministration of nitroglycerin or 30 minutes after stopping the nitroglycerin infusion and continuing the same dose of heparin.[4] Similarly, in 8 volunteers, the APTT and thrombin time response to a single heparin 5,000 unit bolus was not affected by IV infusion of nitroglycerin.[5] In another study, there was no evidence of heparin resistance in 31 patients receiving concurrent nitroglycerin compared with 35 patients receiving heparin alone.[6] In 1 study, antithrombin III activity and APTT were lower in patients receiving nitroglycerin at high infusion rates of at least 350 mcg/min, suggesting a dose relationship.[7] A study of 22 patients found an inverse correlation between APTT ratio and nitroglycerin dose.[8] However, there was no difference in APTT ratio during coadministration and after stopping nitroglycerin.

Additional studies are needed to clarify the importance of this interaction.

1 Col J, et al. *Am Heart J.* 1985;110(1, pt 1):171.
2 Habbab MA, et al. *Arch Intern Med.* 1987;147(5):857.
3 Habbab MA, et al. *Ann Intern Med.* 1986;105(2):305.
4 Lepor NE, et al. *Clin Cardiol.* 1989;12(8):432.
5 Bode V, et al. *Arch Intern Med.* 1990;150(10):2117.
6 Koh KK, et al. *Am J Cardiol.* 1995;76(10):706.
7 Becker RC, et al. *Am Heart J.* 1990;119(6):1254.
8 Gonzalez ER, et al. *Ann Pharmacother.* 1992;26(12):1512.

* Asterisk indicates drugs cited in interaction reports.

Heparin ✕ NSAIDs

Heparin		NSAIDs	
Dalteparin (*Fragmin*)	Heparin*	Celecoxib (*Celebrex*)	Meclofenamate
Enoxaparin* (*Lovenox*)		Diclofenac (eg, *Cataflam*)	Mefenamic acid (eg, *Ponstel*)
		Etodolac	Meloxicam (eg, *Mobic*)
		Fenoprofen (eg, *Nalfon*)	Nabumetone
		Flurbiprofen (eg, *Ansaid*)	Naproxen (eg, *Naprosyn*)
		Ibuprofen (eg, *Motrin*)	Oxaprozin (eg, *Daypro*)
		Indomethacin* (eg, *Indocin*)	Piroxicam (eg, *Feldene*)
		Ketoprofen	Sulindac (eg, *Clinoril*)
		Ketorolac*	Tolmetin

Significance	Onset	Severity	Documentation
2	■ **Rapid**	□ Major	□ Established
	□ Delayed	■ **Moderate**	□ Probable
		□ Minor	■ **Suspected**
			□ Possible
			□ Unlikely

Effects Risk of hemorrhagic adverse reactions may be increased. Patent ductus arteriosus treatment failure has been reported with INDOMETHACIN.

Mechanism Inhibition of the clotting cascade and platelet hemostasis.

Management If HEPARIN and NSAID coadministration is required, conduct close clinical and laboratory monitoring.[1]

Discussion

An initial report indicates that there is an increased risk of bleeding with coadministration of low molecular weight heparin and modest doses of ketorolac, but the risk is slight.[2] In a randomized prospective study, 60 patients undergoing total hip replacement received enoxaparin 40 mg subcutaneously 12 hours preoperatively then every 24 hours for 10 days. In addition, each patient was given either ketorolac 30 mg IM on induction of anesthesia and once daily for 4 days postoperatively (34 patients) or an opioid analgesic plus acetaminophen (eg, *Tylenol*) (26 patients). There were no differences between the 2 groups of patients for intraoperative blood loss, postoperative drainage, transfusion requirements, bruising, wound oozing, and leg swelling. Major bleeding requiring 7 units of blood intraoperatively was reported in a patient taking oral NSAIDs who was given low molecular weight heparin prior to undergoing a spinal decompression operation.[3] Continuous exposure to heparin via central venous catheter was associated with patent ductus arteriosus treatment failure with indomethacin in very low birth weight infants.[4]

[1] *Lovenox* [package insert]. Greenville, NC: DSM pharmaceuticals, Inc; 2004.
[2] Weale AE, et al. *Ann R Coll Surg Engl.* 1995;77(1):35.
[3] Price AJ, et al. *Ann R Coll Surg Engl.* 1995;77(5):395.
[4] Ojala TH, et al. *Pediatr Crit Care Med.* 2007;8(3):258.

* Asterisk indicates drugs cited in interaction reports. Based on pharmacologic and pharmacokinetic considerations, similar interactions may occur with other drugs that are listed.

Heparin — *Penicillins*

Heparin	Penicillins	
Heparin*	Ampicillin* (eg, *Principen*)	Piperacillin*
	Nafcillin*	Ticarcillin* (*Ticar*)
	Oxacillin*	
	Penicillin G* (eg, *Pfizerpen*)	

Significance	Onset	Severity	Documentation
4	■ **Rapid**	□ Major	□ Established
	□ Delayed	■ **Moderate**	□ Probable
		□ Minor	□ Suspected
			■ **Possible**
			□ Unlikely

Effects Increased risk of bleeding.

Mechanism Parenteral PENICILLINS can produce alterations in platelet aggregation and coagulation tests. These effects might be additive with HEPARIN.

Management Monitor patients for coagulopathies and bleeding. Stop or decrease one of the drugs if necessary. Protamine sulfate may be useful for clinically important bleeding.

Discussion

A number of reports described abnormalities in coagulation tests, particularly increased bleeding times, decreased platelet aggregation, increased antithrombin III activity, and prolonged thrombin time,[1-7] in patients receiving parenteral penicillins. Overt bleeding occurred only when patients had another predisposing condition.[1,4,5,7,8] When concurrent heparin is used, additive or synergistic pharmacologic effects might predispose the patient to bleeding. However, little data support this postulation. Some of the patients were on dialysis and were probably receiving heparin,[4-6,8] but it was not clear whether heparin was involved in the bleeding. Surgical patients receiving ampicillin (route not stated) and cloxacillin† postoperatively were compared with patients not receiving the antibiotics.[7] All patients received heparin 5,000 units subcutaneously twice daily for 7 days. Increased bleeding time occurred in the patients receiving antibiotics. Whether this was due to the antibiotics alone or the combination was not determined. Thus, the clinical data do not clearly describe an interaction between heparin and parenteral penicillins. However, because of the known pharmacologic effects of both drugs, patients should be monitored when these drugs are used together.

[1] Brown CH 3rd, et al. *N Engl J Med.* 1974;291(6):265.
[2] Brown CH 3rd, et al. *Antimicrob Agents Chemother.* 1975;7(5):652.
[3] Brown CH 3rd, et al. *Blood.* 1976;47(6):949.
[4] Andrassy K, et al. *Lancet.* 1976;2(7994):1039.
[5] Andrassy K, et al. *Thromb Haemost.* 1976;36(1):115.
[6] Tabernero Romo JM, et al. *Clin Nephrol.* 1979;11(1):31.
[7] Wisloff F, et al. *Scand J Haematol.* 1983;31(2):97.
[8] Lurie A, et al. *S Afr Med J.* 1974;48(11):457.

* Asterisk indicates drugs cited in interaction reports.
† Not available in the United States.

Heparin | **Salicylates**

Heparin*	Aspirin* (eg, *Bayer*)

Significance	Onset	Severity	Documentation
1	■ **Rapid**	■ **Major**	□ Established
	□ Delayed	□ Moderate	■ **Probable**
		□ Minor	□ Suspected
			□ Possible
			□ Unlikely

Effects The risk of bleeding may be increased when ASPIRIN and HEPARIN are used together.

Mechanism ASPIRIN can inhibit platelet aggregation and has caused bleeding, which may be additive to HEPARIN anticoagulation.

Management Monitor coagulation parameters and signs of bleeding if the combination is used; treat symptomatically if bleeding occurs.

Discussion

Aspirin can impair platelet aggregation and prolong bleeding time.[1,2] Isolated case reports describe bleeding complications when aspirin and heparin were given concurrently[3,4]; although it was not always clear whether the combination was at fault. In a survey of 376 patients with GI bleeds, 1.2% of major bleeds were associated with use of heparin alone, 0.3% were associated with aspirin alone, and 0.7% were associated with heparin plus aspirin.[5] Thus, it did not appear that the combination was any worse than heparin alone. In a study involving patients with cerebral ischemia, no difference in bleeding rates occurred when short-term use of aspirin plus an anticoagulant (heparin or warfarin [eg, *Coumadin*]) was compared with use of an anticoagulant alone.[6] However, in a study of 2,656 patients taking heparin, aspirin use was associated with a 1.5 relative risk for a minor bleed and a 2.4 relative risk for a major bleed.[7] Use of enoxaparin with aspirin was associated with major bleeding events in 9 of 13 patients undergoing kidney or kidney/pancreas transplantation.[8] In a meta-analysis of 6 randomized studies involving patients with unstable angina, aspirin 75 to 325 mg/day plus IV heparin for 2 to 7 days produced a 33% reduction in risk of MI.[9] While the relative risk of major bleeding was 1.89 for the combination compared with aspirin alone, aspirin plus heparin was recommended because of the clinical benefit. In 41 patients on chronic aspirin therapy undergoing coronary endarterectomy, administration of heparin caused a temporary reversal of the antiplatelet effect of aspirin.[10] The effect persisted for up to 24 hr. See Anticoagulants-Salicylates.

[1] Weiss HJ, et al. *J Clin Invest.* 1968;47:2169.
[2] Zucker MB, et al. *J Lab Clin Med.* 1970;76:66.
[3] Niklasson PM, et al. *Scand J Infect Dis.* 1972;4:183.
[4] Yett HS, et al. *N Engl J Med.* 1978;298:1092.
[5] Jick H, et al. *Lancet.* 1978;2:87.
[6] Fagan SC, et al. *Ann Pharmacother.* 1994;28:441.
[7] Walker AM, et al. *JAMA.* 1980;244:1209.
[8] Shullo MA, et al. *Pharmacotherapy.* 2002;22:184.
[9] Oler A, et al. *JAMA.* 1996;276:811.
[10] Webster SE, et al. *J Vasc Surg.* 2004;40:463.

* Asterisk indicates drugs cited in interaction reports.

Heparin — Serotonin Reuptake Inhibitors

Heparin		Serotonin Reuptake Inhibitors	
Dalteparin (*Fragmin*)	Heparin	Citalopram (eg, *Celexa*)	Fluvoxamine
Enoxaparin (*Lovenox*)	Tinzaparin* (*Innohep*)	Escitalopram (*Lexapro*)	Paroxetine (eg, *Paxil*)
		Fluoxetine* (eg, *Prozac*)	Sertraline (*Zoloft*)

Significance	Onset	Severity	Documentation
4	□ Rapid	□ Major	□ Established
	■ **Delayed**	■ **Moderate**	□ Probable
		□ Minor	□ Suspected
			■ **Possible**
			□ Unlikely

Effects The risk of severe bleeding may be increased.

Mechanism Enhanced HEPARIN anticoagulant effects caused by SEROTONIN REUPTAKE INHIBITOR-induced impairment of platelet function.

Management Carefully monitor the coagulation status of the patient and observe the patient for bleeding. Adjust therapy as needed.

Discussion

Severe bleeding was reported in a 78-year-old woman during coadministration of fluoxetine and tinzaparin.[1] The patient had been taking fluoxetine for depression for more than 1 year when home treatment with subcutaneous injections of once daily tinzaparin was started for deep vein thrombosis. The patient had borderline renal function (plasma creatinine level 115 mcmol/L; Ccr less than 37 mL/min) but no history of abnormal bleeding. She was admitted to the emergency department because of abdominal pain 5 days after starting tinzaparin. At that time, her BP was 80/50 mm Hg, and her hemoglobin was 4.4 g/dL. She was given packed red blood cells, platelets, and fresh frozen plasma. Four liters of blood were evacuated from an intraperitoneal hematoma. All medications were discontinued. See also Anticoagulants-Serotonin Reuptake Inhibitors.

[1] de Maistre E, et al. *Am J Med.* 2002;113:530.

* Asterisk indicates drugs cited in interaction reports. Based on pharmacologic and pharmacokinetic considerations, similar interactions may occur with other drugs that are listed.

Heparin — *Streptokinase*

Heparin*	Streptokinase* (*Streptase*)

Significance	Onset	Severity	Documentation
4	■ **Rapid**	□ Major	□ Established
	□ Delayed	■ **Moderate**	□ Probable
		□ Minor	□ Suspected
			■ **Possible**
			□ Unlikely

Effects Relative resistance to HEPARIN anticoagulation may occur following administration of STREPTOKINASE as a systemic thrombolytic agent.

Mechanism Unknown.

Management Anticipate possible HEPARIN resistance with more frequent activated partial thromboplastin time (aPTT) guided dosage adjustments.

Discussion

In a retrospective study, 3 groups of patients were compared.[1] Fifty patients had received streptokinase for acute MI followed by heparin infusion. A second group consisted of 24 patients receiving heparin alone following MI. The last group of 11 patients received heparin alone for other indications. Results of the second and third group were combined. Compared with patients receiving both streptokinase and heparin, patients given heparin alone required a lower dose of heparin to achieve a therapeutic aPTT, and the time to reach it was shorter (3 vs 5 days). Despite the higher cumulative heparin dose employed in patients receiving streptokinase, the therapeutic aPTT was lower at 87 seconds (compared with 101 seconds), suggesting that partial resistance to heparin anticoagulation is induced by streptokinase. A nonstatistically significant trend toward warfarin (eg, *Coumadin*) resistance also was reported in the study. While careful and more aggressive heparin dose titration may be needed, the adverse clinical effects of the observed anticoagulation resistance after MI are speculative.

Additional prospective clinical trials are needed to confirm this possible interaction.

[1] Zahger D, et al. *Am J Cardiol.* 1990;66:28.

* Asterisk indicates drugs cited in interaction reports.

Histamine H_2 Antagonists — *Amiloride*

Histamine H_2 Antagonists	Amiloride
Cimetidine* (eg, *Tagamet*)	Amiloride* (*Midamor*)

Significance	Onset	Severity	Documentation
5	□ Rapid	□ Major	□ Established
	■ **Delayed**	□ Moderate	□ Probable
		■ **Minor**	□ Suspected
			■ **Possible**
			□ Unlikely

Effects AMILORIDE may decrease serum CIMETIDINE concentrations.

Mechanism Unknown.

Management Based on available information, no special precautions are necessary.

Discussion

Eight healthy volunteers received coadministration of amiloride 5 mg once daily and cimetidine 400 mg twice daily for 12 days.[1] The pharmacokinetics of both drugs during coadministration were studied and compared with baseline periods with either drug alone. When given with cimetidine, there was an apparent decrease in the oral bioavailability of amiloride, which was offset by a decrease in the fraction excreted unchanged by the kidney (reduction in renal clearance). In addition, the cimetidine AUC was decreased 14%. Plasma peak and trough drug concentrations also were decreased. Whether the pharmacologic actions of either drug were affected is unknown. Based on the change in AUC for cimetidine, the clinical effect should be minimal.

Additional studies are needed.

[1] Somogyi AA, et al. *Drug Metab Dispos.* 1989;17:190.

* Asterisk indicates drugs cited in interaction reports.

Histamine H_2 Antagonists — *Antacids*

Histamine H_2 Antagonists		Antacids	
Cimetidine* (eg, *Tagamet HB*)	Nizatidine* (eg, *Axid*)	Aluminum Hydroxide (eg, *Alternagel*)	Magnesium Hydroxide (eg, *Milk of Magnesia*)
Famotidine* (eg, *Pepcid*)	Ranitidine* (eg, *Zantac*)	Aluminum/Magnesium Hydroxide* (eg, *Mintox*)	

Significance	Onset	Severity	Documentation
5	□ Rapid	□ Major	□ Established
	■ **Delayed**	□ Moderate	□ Probable
		■ **Minor**	□ Suspected
			■ **Possible**
			□ Unlikely

Effects The bioavailability of H_2 ANTAGONISTS may be reduced.

Mechanism Reduced absorption of H_2 ANTAGONISTS by ANTACIDS is suspected.

Management Based on available data, no clinical intervention is needed. If an interaction is suspected, separate the oral administration of H_2 ANTAGONISTS and ANTACIDS by at least 2 hours.

Discussion

Single-dose studies involving patients and volunteers have produced conflicting results. Coadministration of high-potency antacids reduced the bioavailability of cimetidine 20% to 35%,[1-6] famotidine 19%, nizatidine 12%,[6] and ranitidine 20% to 40%,[6-8] compared with controls. It appears that antacids with lower acid-neutralizing capacity (eg, 48 to 80 mEq neutralizing capacity/dose) have little or no effect on H_2 antagonist bioavailability.[1,8-11] In a randomized, crossover study in 17 healthy volunteers, coadministration of an aluminum/magnesium hydroxide antacid and famotidine decreased famotidine bioavailability 10% to 15%.[12] The amount of this change is not expected to be clinically important. Separating the administration times of the antacid and H_2 antagonist by 1 to 2 hours appears to reduce or eliminate the reduction in H_2 antagonist bioavailability.[10,13]

The combination of H_2 antagonists with antacids is frequently used clinically. Although reduced bioavailability can occur when H_2 antagonists and antacids are coadministered, plasma concentrations of the H_2 antagonists usually exceed those considered to be therapeutic. In addition, clinical failures have not been reported with coadministration of H_2 antagonists and antacids.

1 Bodemar G, et al. *Gut.* 1978;19(10):A990.
2 Bodemar G, et al. *Lancet.* 1979;1(8113):444.
3 Gugler R, et al. *Eur J Clin Pharmacol.* 1981;20(3):225.
4 Steinberg WM, et al. *N Engl J Med.* 1982;307(7):400.
5 Russell WL, et al. *Dig Dis Sci.* 1984;29(5):385.
6 Bachmann KA, et al. *Scand J Gastroenterol Suppl.* 1994;206:14.
7 Mihaly GW, et al. *Br Med J (Clin Res Ed).* 1982;285(6347):998.
8 Albin H, et al. *Eur J Clin Pharmacol.* 1987;32(1):97.
9 Burland WL, et al. *Lancet.* 1976;2(7992):965.
10 Frislid K, et al. *Br Med J (Clin Res Ed).* 1983;286(6374):1358.
11 Donn KH, et al. *Pharmacotherapy.* 1984;4(2):89.
12 Lin JH, et al. *Br J Clin Pharmacol.* 1987;24(4):551.
13 Barzaghi N, et al. *Eur J Clin Pharmacol.* 1989;37(4):409.

* Asterisk indicates drugs cited in interaction reports. Based on pharmacologic and pharmacokinetic considerations, similar interactions may occur with other drugs that are listed.

HMG-CoA Reductase Inhibitors ✕ *Amiodarone*

HMG-CoA Reductase Inhibitors		Amiodarone
Atorvastatin (*Lipitor*)	Simvastatin* (eg, *Zocor*)	Amiodarone* (eg, *Cordarone*)
Lovastatin (eg, *Mevacor*)		

Significance	Onset	Severity	Documentation
1	□ Rapid ■ **Delayed**	■ **Major** □ Moderate □ Minor	□ Established □ Probable ■ **Suspected** □ Possible □ Unlikely

Effects Plasma concentrations of certain HMG-CoA REDUCTASE INHIBITORS may be elevated, increasing the risk of toxicity (eg, myositis, rhabdomyolysis).

Mechanism Inhibition of HMG-CoA REDUCTASE INHIBITOR metabolism (CYP2C9, CYP3A4) is suspected.

Management If coadministration of these agents cannot be avoided, use the lowest possible HMG-CoA REDUCTASE INHIBITOR dose. The dosage of LOVASTATIN[1] or SIMVASTATIN[2] should not exceed 40 or 20 mg/day, respectively, in patients taking AMIODARONE. Advise patients to immediately report any unexplained muscle pain, tenderness, or weakness. Pravastatin (eg, *Pravachol*) is not metabolized by CYP2C9 or CYP3A4 and may be a safer alternative.

Discussion

Several cases of rhabdomyolysis and azotemia, as well as increases in liver function tests have been reported when high-dose simvastatin 40 to 80 mg/day was given with amiodarone.[3-5] Severe myopathy developed in a 63-year-old man receiving simvastatin 40 mg/day 21 days after amiodarone 1,000 mg/day for 10 days and then 200 mg/day was added to his treatment regimen.[3] The patient developed diffuse muscle pain with generalized weakness, and his creatine kinase level was elevated, peaking at 40,392 units/L. Simvastatin and amiodarone were stopped. The creatine kinase normalized over the next 8 days, and the patient made an uneventful recovery. The pharmacokinetics of a single dose of simvastatin or pravastatin were studied in 12 healthy volunteers following 3 days of amiodarone 400 mg/day.[6] Amiodarone increased simvastatin lactone and simvastatin acid AUCs 73% and 78%, respectively. Pravastatin levels were not affected.

[1] *Mevacor* [package insert]. Whitehouse Station, NJ: Merck & Co Inc; 2007.
[2] *Zocor* [package insert]. Whitehouse Station, NJ: Merck & Co Inc; June 2008.
[3] Roten L, et al. *Ann Pharmacother.* 2004;38(6):978.
[4] Ricaurte B, et al. *Ann Pharmacother.* 2006;40(4):753.
[5] Wratchford P, et al. *Am J Health Syst Pharm.* 2003;60(7):698.
[6] Becquemont L, et al. *Clin Pharmacol Ther.* 2007;81(5):679.

* Asterisk indicates drugs cited in interaction reports. Based on pharmacologic and pharmacokinetic considerations, similar interactions may occur with other drugs that are listed.

HMG-CoA Reductase Inhibitors × Azole Antifungal Agents

HMG-CoA Reductase Inhibitors		Azole Antifungal Agents	
Atorvastatin* (*Lipitor*)	Pravastatin* (eg, *Pravachol*)	Fluconazole* (eg, *Diflucan*)	Posaconazole* (*Noxafil*)
Fluvastatin* (*Lescol*)	Simvastatin* (eg, *Zocor*)	Itraconazole* (eg, *Sporanox*)	Voriconazole (eg, *Vfend*)
Lovastatin* (eg, *Mevacor*)		Ketoconazole* (eg, *Nizoral*)	

Significance	Onset	Severity	Documentation
1	■ **Rapid** □ Delayed	■ **Major** □ Moderate □ Minor	□ Established ■ **Probable** □ Suspected □ Possible □ Unlikely

Effects Increased plasma levels and adverse reactions (eg, rhabdomyolysis) of HMG-CoA REDUCTASE INHIBITORS may occur.

Mechanism AZOLE ANTIFUNGAL AGENTS may inhibit the first-pass hepatic metabolism (CYP3A4; FLUCONAZOLE [CYP2C9]) of HMG-CoA REDUCTASE INHIBITORS.

Management ITRACONAZOLE is contraindicated with HMG-CoA REDUCTASE INHIBITORS metabolized by CYP3A4.[1] SIMVASTATIN is contraindicated with POSACONAZOLE.[2] If coadministration of other agents cannot be avoided, consider reducing the HMG-CoA REDUCTASE INHIBITOR dose and carefully monitor patient response. PRAVASTATIN levels are affected least and may be a preferable alternative.

Discussion

Rhabdomyolysis has been reported when simvastatin is taken with fluconazole,[3,4] itraconazole,[5] or ketoconazole.[6-8] Severe rhabdomyolysis was reported in a 63-year-old woman within 2 weeks of adding itraconazole to her treatment regimen, which included lovastatin and niacin (eg, *Niaspan*).[9] In an 84-year-old man receiving lovastatin, rhabdomyolysis occurred after starting high-dose ketoconazole (400 mg 3 times daily) for prostate cancer.[10] Fatal rhabdomyolysis was reported in a patient receiving fluconazole after the introduction of atorvastatin.[11] Itraconazole increased the average C_{max} of lovastatin acid (the active metabolite of lovastatin) 13-fold and AUC 20-fold in 12 healthy subjects.[12] One subject experienced a 10-fold increase in plasma creatine kinase within 24 hours of receiving lovastatin. Itraconazole increased the simvastatin AUC 19-fold in 10 healthy subjects. Pravastatin AUC increased less than 2-fold.[13] Itraconazole increased the AUC of atorvastatin and atorvastatin lactone between 2.5- and 4-fold.[14,15] Itraconazole had no effect on fluvastatin.[16] In 12 healthy volunteers, fluconazole increased the mean AUC of fluvastatin 81% and the mean C_{max} 44%, but had no effect on pravastatin.[17] Itraconazole produced clinically unimportant increases in the rosuvastatin C_{max} and AUC.[18]

1 *Sporanox* [package insert]. Titusville, NJ: Janssen Pharmaceutica, LP; January 2004.
2 *Noxafil* [package insert]. Kenilworth, NJ: Schering Corporation; September 2010.
3 Shaukat A, et al. *Ann Pharmacother.* 2003;37(7-8):1032.
4 Hazin R, et al. *J Natl Med Assoc.* 2008;100(4):444.
5 Horn M. *Arch Dermatol.* 1996;132(10):1254.
6 Gilad R, et al. *Clin Neuropharmacol.* 1999;22(5):295.
7 Itakura H, et al. *J Urol.* 2003;169(2):613.
8 Watkins JL, et al. *Ann Pharmacother.* 2011;45(2):e9.
9 Lees RS, et al. *N Engl J Med.* 1995;333(10):664.
10 Stein CA, et al. *Invest New Drugs.* 2007;25(3):277.
11 Kahri J, et al. *Eur J Clin Pharmacol.* 2005;60(12):905.
12 Neuvonen PJ, et al. *Clin Pharmacol Ther.* 1996;60(1):54.
13 Neuvonen PJ, et al. *Clin Pharmacol Ther.* 1998;63(3):332.
14 Kantola T, et al. *Clin Pharmacol Ther.* 1998;64(1):58.
15 Mazzu AL, et al. *Clin Pharmacol Ther.* 2000;68(4):391.
16 Kivistö KT, et al. *Br J Clin Pharmacol.* 1998;46(1):49.
17 Kantola T, et al. *Eur J Clin Pharmacol.* 2000;56(3):225.
18 Cooper KJ, et al. *Clin Pharmacol Ther.* 2003;73(4):322.

* Asterisk indicates drugs cited in interaction reports. Based on pharmacologic and pharmacokinetic considerations, similar interactions may occur with other drugs that are listed.

HMG-CoA Reductase Inhibitors — Baicalin

Rosuvastatin*
(*Crestor*)

Baicalin*†

Significance	Onset	Severity	Documentation
4	☐ Rapid	☐ Major	☐ Established
	■ **Delayed**	■ **Moderate**	☐ Probable
		☐ Minor	☐ Suspected
			■ **Possible**
			☐ Unlikely

Effects ROSUVASTATIN plasma concentrations may be reduced.

Mechanism Induction of ROSUVASTATIN hepatic uptake (OATP1B1) by BAICALIN.

Management Avoid BAICALIN administration in patients taking ROSUVASTATIN. Caution patients taking ROSUVASTATIN to consult their health care provider before taking herbal products.

Discussion

The effects of baicalin, a flavone glucuronide from the plant *Radix scutellariae*, on the pharmacokinetics of rosuvastatin were studied in 18 healthy men. The subjects were from different organic anion-transporting polypeptide 1B1 (OATP1B1) haplotype groups.[1] The study was a randomized, crossover design, in which subjects received placebo or baicalin 50 mg 3 times daily for 14 days. On day 15, a single oral dose of rosuvastatin 20 mg was administered. Compared with placebo, baicalin reduced the AUC of rosuvastatin. The decrease was in an OATP1B1 haplotype-dependent manner. The decreases in AUC in OATP1B1*1b/*1b, OATP1B1*1b/*15, and OATP1B1*15/*15 were 41.9%, 23.9%, and 1.76%, respectively.

[1] Fan L, et al. *Clin Pharmacol Ther.* 2008;83(3):471.

* Asterisk indicates drugs cited in interaction reports.
† Not available in the United States.

HMG-CoA Reductase Inhibitors — *Bile Acid Sequestrants*

HMG-CoA Reductase Inhibitors		Bile Acid Sequestrants	
Atorvastatin (*Lipitor*)	Pravastatin (eg, *Pravachol*)	Cholestyramine* (eg, *Questran*)	Colestipol (eg, *Colestid*)
Fluvastatin* (*Lescol*)	Simvastatin (eg, *Zocor*)		
Lovastatin (eg, *Mevacor*)			

Significance	Onset	Severity	Documentation
4	☐ Rapid	☐ Major	☐ Established
	■ **Delayed**	■ **Moderate**	☐ Probable
		☐ Minor	☐ Suspected
			■ **Possible**
			☐ Unlikely

Effects Pharmacologic effects of the HMG-CoA REDUCTASE INHIBITOR may be decreased.

Mechanism The HMG-CoA REDUCTASE INHIBITOR may adsorb to the BILE ACID SEQUESTRANT, reducing the GI absorption of the HMG-CoA REDUCTASE INHIBITOR.

Management Separate the administration times of the HMG-CoA REDUCTASE INHIBITOR and the BILE ACID SEQUESTRANT by as much as possible (at least 4 hr before the HMG-CoA REDUCTASE INHIBITOR), preferably giving the BILE ACID SEQUESTRANT before meals and the HMG-CoA REDUCTASE INHIBITOR in the evening.

Discussion

In a study of the effects of cholestyramine on the pharmacokinetics of fluvastatin, administration of fluvastatin 20 mg and cholestyramine 8 g at the same time decreased the AUC of fluvastatin 89% and C_{max} 96%.[1] When cholestyramine 8 g was ingested 4 hr prior to fluvastatin 20 mg, the AUC of fluvastatin was decreased 51%, and C_{max} was decreased 82%. However, the clinical efficacy of the combination was not affected when the administration times were separated by 4 hr. The effects of cholestyramine on the pharmacokinetics of cerivastatin† were studied in 12 healthy men.[2] Administration of both drugs at the same time decreased the bioavailability of cerivastatin 21% and C_{max} 41%. Administration of cholestyramine 1 hr prior to cerivastatin decreased the AUC of cerivastatin to a greater extent than separating the dosing times by 5 hr (16% vs 8% decrease, respectively). In both instances, pretreatment with cholestyramine decreased cerivastatin C_{max} 32%. In a study of 151 patients with hypercholesterolemia, fluvastatin 20 mg plus cholestyramine 4, 8, or 16 g daily demonstrated additive reducing effects on total cholesterol, LDL cholesterol, and apolipoprotein B.[3]

1 Smith HT, et al. *Am J Hypertens.* 1993;6(11, pt 2):375S.

2 Mück W, et al. *Int J Clin Pharmacol Ther.* 1997;35(6):250.

3 Hagen E, et al. *Eur J Clin Pharmacol.* 1994;46(5):445.

* Asterisk indicates drugs cited in interaction reports. Based on pharmacologic and pharmacokinetic considerations, similar interactions may occur with other drugs that are listed.

† Not available in the United States.

HMG-CoA Reductase Inhibitors — *Bosentan*

Atorvastatin (*Lipitor*)
Lovastatin (eg, *Mevacor*)
Simvastatin* (*Zocor*)

Bosentan* (*Tracleer*)

Significance	Onset	Severity	Documentation
4	☐ Rapid ■ **Delayed**	☐ Major ■ **Moderate** ☐ Minor	☐ Established ☐ Probable ☐ Suspected ■ **Possible** ☐ Unlikely

Effects Plasma concentrations of certain HMG-CoA REDUCTASE INHIBITORS may be reduced, decreasing the therapeutic effect.

Mechanism Induction of metabolism (CYP3A4) of certain HMG-CoA REDUCTASE INHIBITORS is suspected.

Management Monitor the clinical response of the patient and adjust therapy as needed.

Discussion

The effects of bosentan and simvastatin on the pharmacokinetics of each other were studied in 9 healthy men.[1] In a 3-period, randomized, crossover investigation, each subject received bosentan 125 mg twice daily alone for 5.5 days; simvastatin 40 mg once daily alone for 6 days; and bosentan 125 mg twice daily plus simvastatin 40 mg once daily for 5.5 and 6 days, respectively. Compared with administration of bosentan alone, coadministration of simvastatin did not affect the pharmacokinetics of bosentan or its metabolites. In contrast, coadministration of both agents reduced the AUC of simvastatin 34% and the AUC of the active β-hydroxyacid metabolite of simvastatin 46% compared with administration of simvastatin alone. Additional studies are needed to determine the clinical importance of this drug interaction.

[1] Dingemanse J, et al. *Clin Pharmacokinet.* 2003;42:293.

* Asterisk indicates drugs cited in interaction reports. Based on pharmacologic and pharmacokinetic considerations, similar interactions may occur with other drugs that are listed.

HMG-CoA Reductase Inhibitors — *Carbamazepine*

Atorvastatin (*Lipitor*)	Simvastatin* (*Zocor*)	Carbamazepine* (eg, *Tegretol*)
Lovastatin (eg, *Mevacor*)		

Significance	Onset	Severity	Documentation
2	☐ Rapid	☐ Major	☐ Established
	■ **Delayed**	■ **Moderate**	☐ Probable
		☐ Minor	■ **Suspected**
			☐ Possible
			☐ Unlikely

Effects Plasma concentrations of certain HMG-CoA REDUCTASE INHIBITORS may be reduced, decreasing the therapeutic effect (resulting in hypercholesterolemia).

Mechanism Increased metabolism (CYP3A4) of the HMG-CoA REDUCTASE INHIBITOR by CARBAMAZEPINE is suspected.

Management If coadministration of these agents cannot be avoided, closely monitor the clinical response of the patient. Pravastatin (*Pravachol*) and rosuvastatin (*Crestor*) are less likely to interact with CARBAMAZEPINE and may be suitable alternatives.

Discussion

The effects of carbamazepine on the pharmacokinetics of simvastatin were studied in 12 healthy men.[1] In a randomized, 2-phase crossover investigation, each subject received either no drug or 200 mg of carbamazepine once daily for 2 days followed by 300 mg twice daily for 12 days. On day 15, subjects received a single 80 mg dose of simvastatin. Compared with taking simvastatin alone, pretreatment with carbamazepine decreased the mean total AUC of simvastatin 75%, the C_{max} 68% (from 18.7 to 6 ng/mL), and shortened the $t_{½}$ from 5.9 to 3.7 hr. In addition, the AUC and C_{max} of the active metabolite of simvastatin, simvastatin acid, were decreased 82% and 68%, respectively.

[1] Ucar M, et al. *Eur J Clin Pharmacol.* 2004;59:879.

* Asterisk indicates drugs cited in interaction reports. Based on pharmacologic and pharmacokinetic considerations, similar interactions may occur with other drugs that are listed.

HMG-CoA Reductase Inhibitors — *Cilostazol*

Lovastatin* (eg, *Mevacor*)	Simvastatin (eg, *Zocor*)	Cilostazol* (eg, *Pletal*)

Significance	Onset	Severity	Documentation
4	□ Rapid	□ Major	□ Established
	■ **Delayed**	■ **Moderate**	□ Probable
		□ Minor	□ Suspected
			■ **Possible**
			□ Unlikely

Effects Plasma concentrations of certain HMG-CoA REDUCTASE INHIBITORS may be elevated by CILOSTAZOL, increasing the therapeutic and adverse reactions.

Mechanism CILOSTAZOL may inhibit the metabolism (CYP3A4) of certain HMG-CoA REDUCTASE INHIBITORS.

Management Monitor the patient's clinical response and adjust HMG-CoA REDUCTASE INHIBITOR therapy as needed.

Discussion

Using an open-label, multiple-dose design, the effect of cilostazol on the pharmacokinetics of lovastatin was assessed in 12 healthy volunteers.[1] Each subject received a single dose of lovastatin 80 mg on days 1, 7, and 9, as well as cilostazol 100 mg twice daily on days 2 to 8, followed by a dose of cilostazol 150 mg on day 9. Peak plasma concentrations of lovastatin, when given with cilostazol 100 or 150 mg, did not differ from those for lovastatin taken alone. The peak plasma concentration of the metabolite of lovastatin increased 68% and 120% when lovastatin was administered with cilostazol 100 or 150 mg, respectively. The AUC of lovastatin increased 1.6-fold with both doses of cilostazol, while the AUC of the metabolite of lovastatin increased 1.7- and 2-fold with the doses of cilostazol 100 and 150 mg, respectively. Peak plasma concentration and AUC of cilostazol decreased 14% and 15%, respectively, during coadministration of lovastatin.

Additional studies are needed to determine if this interaction is clinically important.

[1] Bramer SL, et al. *Clin Pharmacokinet.* 1999;37(suppl 2):69.

* Asterisk indicates drugs cited in interaction reports. Based on pharmacologic and pharmacokinetic considerations, similar interactions may occur with other drugs that are listed.

HMG-CoA Reductase Inhibitors — *Colchicine*

Atorvastatin* (*Lipitor*)	Pravastatin* (eg, *Pravachol*)	Colchicine*
Fluvastatin* (*Lescol*)	Rosuvastatin (*Crestor*)	
Lovastatin (eg, *Mevacor*)	Simvastatin* (eg, *Zocor*)	

Significance	Onset	Severity	Documentation
4	☐ Rapid	■ **Major**	☐ Established
	■ **Delayed**	☐ Moderate	☐ Probable
		☐ Minor	☐ Suspected
			■ **Possible**
			☐ Unlikely

Effects The risk of myopathy or rhabdomyolysis may be increased.

Mechanism Unknown.

Management If coadministration of these agents cannot be avoided, use with caution and closely monitor creatine kinase during concurrent use of these agents and after dose increases.

Discussion

Severe rhabdomyolysis was reported in a 45-year-old man receiving colchicine after atorvastatin therapy was started.[1] The patient had a history of nephrotic syndrome and amyloidosis. He had been receiving colchicine 1.5 mg daily for amyloidosis for 3 years without adverse reactions. Atorvastatin 10 mg daily was prescribed for hypercholesterolemia. Two weeks later, he experienced myalgia and decreased muscle strength. The patient was diagnosed with rhabdomyolysis. Laboratory tests found myoglobinuria, oliguric acute renal failure, and more than a 50-fold elevation in creatine kinase. His muscle strength improved when atorvastatin and colchicine were discontinued. Subsequently, he died after developing a nosocomial infection during his hospital stay. Acute myopathy has been reported in patients receiving long-term treatment with simvastatin[2,3] or pravastatin[4] after colchicine was added to their treatment regimen. Rhabdomyolysis occurred within 10 days of starting colchicine in a patient who had been receiving fluvastatin for 2 years.[5]

It should be noted that myopathy or rhabdomyolysis may occur with colchicine therapy alone.

[1] Tufan A, et al. *Ann Pharmacother.* 2006;40:1466.
[2] Hsu WC, et al. *Clin Neuropharmacol.* 2002;25:266.
[3] Baker SK, et al. *Muscle Nerve.* 2004;30:799.
[4] Alayli G, et al. *Ann Pharmacother.* 2005;39:1358.
[5] Atasoyu EM, et al. *Ann Pharmacother.* 2005;39:1368.

* Asterisk indicates drugs cited in interaction reports. Based on pharmacologic and pharmacokinetic considerations, similar interactions may occur with other drugs that are listed.

HMG-CoA Reductase Inhibitors — Cyclosporine

HMG-CoA Reductase Inhibitors		Cyclosporine
Atorvastatin* (eg, *Lipitor*)	Rosuvastatin* (*Crestor*)	Cyclosporine* (eg, *Neoral*)
Lovastatin* (eg, *Mevacor*)	Simvastatin* (eg, *Zocor*)	
Pravastatin* (eg, *Pravachol*)		

Significance	Onset	Severity	Documentation
1	□ Rapid	■ **Major**	□ Established
	■ **Delayed**	□ Moderate	■ **Probable**
		□ Minor	□ Suspected
			□ Possible
			□ Unlikely

Effects Increased levels and adverse reactions (eg, rhabdomyolysis) of HMG-CoA REDUCTASE INHIBITORS may occur.

Mechanism Decreased metabolism of certain HMG-CoA REDUCTASE INHIBITORS and increased bioavailability[1] are suspected.

Management If coadministration cannot be avoided, consider reducing the dose of the HMG-CoA REDUCTASE INHIBITOR; carefully monitor the response. Advise patients to report any unexplained muscle pain, tenderness, or weakness.

Discussion

Multiple case reports and retrospective analyses associated elevated stain levels and/or myolysis and rhabdomyolysis with coadministration of cyclosporine and lovastatin,[2-4] atorvastatin,[5,6] simvastatin,[7-11] rosuvastatin,[1] or pravastatin.[7] In some cases, rhabdomyolysis was accompanied by renal failure.[2-4,7,10,12] In most patients, symptoms improved over a few days, and creatine kinase returned to normal approximately 2 wk after stopping the HMG-CoA reductase inhibitor. Pravastatin levels were unchanged by cyclosporine in 23 patients, while 21 patients taking lovastatin had 40% to 50% increases in lovastatin levels after 28 days of cyclosporine therapy.[13] Increases in C_{max}[14] and AUC of simvastatin and pravastatin[14,15] were found in patients receiving cyclosporine. Lovastatin AUC was about 5 times higher in patients treated with cyclosporine compared with patients not receiving cyclosporine.[16] Atorvastatin AUC was increased 15-fold by cyclosporine.[17] Simvastatin was reported to increase the clearance of cyclosporine and its unbound fraction.[18] HMG-CoA reductase inhibitors do not alter cyclosporine dosage requirements.[13,19-22]

1 Simonson SG, et al. *Clin Pharmacol Ther.* 2004;76(2):167.
2 Norman DJ, et al. *N Engl J Med.* 1988;318(1):46.
3 Corpier CL, et al. *JAMA.* 1988;260(2):239.
4 Marais GE, et al. *Ann Intern Med.* 1990;112(3):228.
5 Maltz HC, et al. *Ann Pharmacother.* 1999;33(11):1176.
6 Hermann M, et al. *Clin Pharmacol Ther.* 2004;76(4):388.
7 Rodríguez JA, et al. *Transplant Proc.* 1999;31(6):2522.
8 Gruer PJ, et al. *Am J Cardiol.* 1999;84(7):811.
9 Cohen E, et al. *Transplantation.* 2000;70(1):119.
10 Weise WJ, et al. *Am J Med.* 2000;108(4):351.
11 Stirling CM, et al. *Nephrol Dial Transplant.* 2001;16(4):873.
12 East C, et al. *N Engl J Med.* 1988;318(1):47.
13 Kliem V, et al. *Transplant Proc.* 1996;28(6):3126.
14 Regazzi MB, et al. *Transplant Proc.* 1994;26(5):2644.
15 Park JW, et al. *Int J Clin Pharmacol Ther.* 2002;40(10):439.
16 Gullestad L, et al. *Transplant Proc.* 1999;31(5):2163.
17 Lemahieu WP, et al. *Am J Transplant.* 2005;5(9):2236.
18 Akhlaghi F, et al. *Br J Clin Pharmacol.* 1997;44(6):537.
19 Taylor PJ, et al. *Ann Pharmacother.* 2004;38(2):205.
20 Hermann M, et al. *Eur J Clin Pharmacol.* 2005;61(1):59.
21 Li PK, et al. *Int J Clin Pharmacol Ther.* 1995;33(4):246.
22 Holdaas H, et al. *Int J Clin Pharmacol Ther.* 2006;44(4):163.

* Asterisk indicates drugs cited in interaction reports.

HMG-CoA Reductase Inhibitors — *Delavirdine*

Atorvastatin* (eg, *Lipitor*)	Simvastatin* (eg, *Zocor*)	Delavirdine* (*Rescriptor*)
Lovastatin* (eg, *Mevacor*)		

Significance	Onset	Severity	Documentation
1	□ Rapid	■ **Major**	□ Established
	■ **Delayed**	□ Moderate	□ Probable
		□ Minor	■ **Suspected**
			□ Possible
			□ Unlikely

Effects Severe myopathy or rhabdomyolysis may occur because of increased HMG-CoA REDUCTASE INHIBITOR concentrations.

Mechanism Inhibition of HMG-CoA REDUCTASE INHIBITOR metabolism (CYP3A4) by DELAVIRDINE.

Management Concurrent use of LOVASTATIN or SIMVASTATIN with DELAVIRDINE is not recommended.[1] Use caution if DELAVIRDINE is administered with ATORVASTATIN or CERIVASTATIN† because the risk of myopathy, including rhabdomyolysis, may be increased. Use the lowest possible dose of ATORVASTATIN, CERIVASTATIN, or FLUVASTATIN.[1] Advise patients to report any unexplained muscle pain, tenderness, or weakness. Pravastatin is not metabolized by CYP3A4 and may be a safer alternative.[1]

Discussion

Acute tubular necrosis resulting from rhabdomyolysis was reported in a 63-year-old man during coadministration of atorvastatin and delavirdine.[2] The patient's hypercholesterolemia had been well controlled on atorvastatin 20 mg/day, which he had taken for 5 years. His HIV infection was controlled with indinavir (*Crixivan*), lamivudine (eg, *Epivir*), and stavudine (eg, *Zerit*). Two months before his hospitalization, delavirdine 400 mg every 8 hours was substituted for indinavir. One month later, the patient developed generalized malaise, leg and lower back pain, nausea, vomiting, and dark urine. He was diagnosed with acute renal failure due to rhabdomyolysis. All medications were withheld. His renal function improved 10 days later and was normal within 1 month. See HMG-CoA Reductase Inhibitors/NNRT Inhibitors.

[1] *Rescriptor* [package insert]. Research Triangle Park, NC: ViiV Healthcare; September 2010.

[2] Castro JG, et al. *Am J Med.* 2002;112(6):505.

* Asterisk indicates drugs cited in interaction reports.
† Not available in the United States.

HMG-CoA Reductase Inhibitors | **Diltiazem**

Atorvastatin* (*Lipitor*)	Simvastatin* (eg, *Zocor*)	Diltiazem* (eg, *Cardizem*)
Lovastatin* (eg, *Mevacor*)		

Significance	Onset	Severity	Documentation
1	☐ Rapid ■ **Delayed**	■ **Major** ☐ Moderate ☐ Minor	☐ Established ■ **Probable** ☐ Suspected ☐ Possible ☐ Unlikely

Effects Plasma concentrations of certain HMG-CoA REDUCTASE INHIBITORS may be elevated, increasing the risk of toxicity (eg, rhabdomyolysis, myositis).

Mechanism Possible inhibition of first-pass metabolism (CYP3A4) of the HMG-CoA REDUCTASE INHIBITOR.

Management If coadministration of these agents cannot be avoided, advise patients to report any unexplained muscle pain, tenderness, or weakness. Pravastatin (*Pravachol*) appears to be less likely to interact and may be a safer alternative.

Discussion

At least 6 cases of rhabdomyolysis have been reported in patients receiving diltiazem and statins concurrently (2 with atorvastatin[1,2] and 4 with simvastatin[2-4]). In some cases, preexisting renal dysfunction was present. Acute renal failure developed in 5 cases and required hemodialysis.[1-3] Two patients died from complications of acute renal failure, 1 died from unrelated causes, and 2 patients recovered. Diltiazem was started 1 or 3 weeks prior to development of rhabdomyolysis in 2 patients. In the other cases, there was a recent increase in the statin dose. The effects of diltiazem on the pharmacokinetics of lovastatin and pravastatin were studied in an open-label, 4-way crossover study in 10 subjects.[5] Each individual received a single dose of lovastatin or pravastatin with and without sustained-release diltiazem 120 mg twice daily during the 2 preceding weeks. Diltiazem did not affect the pharmacokinetics of pravastatin. In contrast, the AUC of lovastatin increased 257%, and the peak concentration increased 333%. However, IV administration of diltiazem did not affect lovastatin pharmacokinetics in 10 healthy volunteers.[6] In 10 healthy volunteers, diltiazem increased simvastatin AUC 387%, peak plasma levels 261%, and $t_{½}$ 129% compared with the control period. In a study of 30 patients, simvastatin 20 mg/day was given alone and with diltiazem 60 mg 3 times daily with no reports of creatine phosphokinase elevation or symptoms of rhabdomyolysis.[7] However, diltiazem did not enhance the lipid lowering effect of simvastatin. A 53-year-old man on a stable simvastatin regimen (40 mg/day) for 3 years developed hepatitis and rhabdomyolysis 3 months after starting diltiazem.[8] Steady-state concentrations of diltiazem were not affected by lovastatin, pravastatin,[5] or simvastatin.[4]

1 Lewin JJ III, et al. *Ann Pharmacother.* 2002;36(10):1546.
2 Gladding P, et al. *Ann Intern Med.* 2004;140(8):W31.
3 Peces R, et al. *Nephron.* 2001;89(1):117.
4 Mousa O, et al. *Clin Pharmacol Ther.* 2000;67(3):267.
5 Azie NE, et al. *Clin Pharmacol Ther.* 1998;64(4):369.
6 Masica AL, et al. *Br J Clin Pharmacol.* 2000;50(3):273.
7 You JH, et al. *J Clin Pharmacol.* 2010;50(10):1151.
8 Kanathur N, et al. *Tenn Med.* 2001;94(9):339.

* Asterisk indicates drugs cited in interaction reports.

HMG-CoA Reductase Inhibitors — *Fibers*

Atorvastatin (*Lipitor*)	Pravastatin (eg, *Pravachol*)	Oat Bran*
Fluvastatin (*Lescol*)	Simvastatin (eg, *Zocor*)	Pectin* (eg, *Kapectolin*)
Lovastatin* (eg, *Mevacor*)		

Significance	Onset	Severity	Documentation
4	☐ Rapid	☐ Major	☐ Established
	■ **Delayed**	■ **Moderate**	☐ Probable
		☐ Minor	☐ Suspected
			■ **Possible**
			☐ Unlikely

Effects Pharmacologic effects of HMG-CoA REDUCTASE INHIBITORS may be decreased.

Mechanism FIBERS, such as OAT BRAN and PECTIN, may decrease GI absorption of HMG-CoA REDUCTASE INHIBITORS.

Management If coadministration cannot be avoided, separate the administration times by as much as possible. Monitor the clinical response of the patient.

Discussion

Concurrent use of 50 to 100 g/day of oat bran and lovastatin 80 mg/day in patients with hypercholesterolemia resulted in increased LDL cholesterol compared with the use of lovastatin alone.[1] After stopping the oat bran, the LDL cholesterol decreased. Similarly, concomitant use of pectin 15 g/day and lovastatin 80 mg/day in patients with hypercholesterolemia resulted in increased LDL cholesterol compared with giving lovastatin alone.[1] After stopping the pectin, the LDL cholesterol decreased to previous levels.

Additional studies are needed to determine the clinical importance of this drug interaction and to determine whether HMG-CoA reductase inhibitors other than lovastatin are affected similarly.

[1] Richter WO, et al. *Lancet*. 1991;338(8768):706.

* Asterisk indicates drugs cited in interaction reports. Based on pharmacologic and pharmacokinetic considerations, similar interactions may occur with other drugs that are listed.

HMG-CoA Reductase Inhibitors — Fibric Acids

HMG-CoA Reductase Inhibitors		Fibric Acids	
Atorvastatin* (eg, *Lipitor*)	Rosuvastatin* (*Crestor*)	Fenofibrate* (eg, *Tricor*)	Gemfibrozil* (eg, *Lopid*)
Fluvastatin* (eg, *Lescol*)	Simvastatin* (eg, *Zocor*)		
Lovastatin* (eg, *Mevacor*)			
Pravastatin* (eg, *Pravachol*)			

Significance	Onset	Severity	Documentation
1	☐ Rapid ■ **Delayed**	■ **Major** ☐ Moderate ☐ Minor	☐ Established ■ **Probable** ☐ Suspected ☐ Possible ☐ Unlikely

Effects Severe myopathy or rhabdomyolysis may occur.

Mechanism Unknown.

Management If coadministration of these agents cannot be avoided, use with caution and closely monitor creatine kinase (CK).

Discussion

Myolysis and rhabdomyolysis, sometimes with renal failure, have been associated with the use of gemfibrozil and fluvastatin,[1] lovastatin,[2-4] atorvastatin,[5] or simvastatin,[6-8] as well as coadministration of fenofibrate and rosuvastatin.[9,10] Often, patients were taking multiple drugs. The FDA received 12 reports of cases of severe myopathy or rhabdomyolysis with serum CK levels greater than 10,000 units/L associated with concurrent lovastatin and gemfibrozil.[4] Four patients had myoglobinuria and 5 had acute renal failure. Symptoms resolved when both drugs were discontinued. The median CK level was 20 times higher (15,250 units/L) in patients receiving both drugs than in patients taking gemfibrozil alone and 30 times higher than in those receiving only lovastatin. In a case series of 80 patients, 3% developed myositis.[11] A retrospective evaluation of 70 patients receiving combined therapy for at least 6 months detected 5 cases of mild CK elevation and no myositis.[12] In a retrospective study of more than 250,000 patients, the incidence of rhabdomyolysis was 5.98 per 10,000 patient-years of therapy with fenofibrate or gemfibrozil plus atorvastatin, pravastatin, or simvastatin, compared with 2.82 or 0.44 per 10,000 patient-years with these fibrates or statins alone, respectively.[13] Using the database of a large US health insurer, there were more than 1.1 million patients who started HMG-CoA reductase inhibitor or fibric acid therapy.[14] The incidence of hospitalization due to rhabdomyolysis was increased approximately 3.3- and 12-fold for coadministration of fenofibrate or gemfibrozil, respectively, with an HMG-CoA reductase inhibitor compared with taking an HMG-CoA reductase inhibitor alone. In 12 patients receiving pravastatin with gemfibrozil, 1 developed asymptomatic elevation of CK levels.[15] Gemfibrozil increased the AUC of pravastatin,[16] atorvastatin,[17] simvastatin,[18] lovastatin,[19] and rosuvastatin.[20] In addition, increased C_{max} was reported with coadministration of gemfibrozil and pravastatin[19] or rosuvastatin.[20] Fenofibrate increased pravastatin AUC 28%.[21] The AUC and C_{max} of the N-desmethyl rosuvastatin metabolite decreased 48% and 39%, respectively. Fenofibrate does not appear to affect the pharmacokinetics of rosuvastatin,[22] although 1 case of severe rhabdomyolysis has been reported with the combination.[10] In an open-label, randomized study, fenofibrate did not affect the pharmacokinetics of atorvastatin.[23] In contrast, gemfibrozil increased the atorvastatin AUC 35%. A single dose of gemfibrozil did not affect plasma or biliary concentrations after single-dose administration of rosuvastatin.[24]

[1] Akoglu H, et al. *Ann Pharmacother.* 2007;41(1):143.
[2] East C, et al. *N Engl J Med.* 1988;318(1):47.
[3] Marais GE, et al. *Ann Intern Med.* 1990;112(3):228.
[4] Pierce LR, et al. *JAMA.* 1990;264(1):71.
[5] Duell PB, et al. *Am J Cardiol.* 1998;81(3):368.
[6] van Puijenbroek EP, et al. *J Intern Med.* 1996;240(6):403.
[7] Tal A, et al. *South Med J.* 1997;90(5):546.
[8] Federman DG, et al. *South Med J.* 2001;94(10):1023.
[9] Ireland JH, et al. *Ann Intern Med.* 2005;142(11):949.
[10] Dedhia V, et al. *J Assoc Physicians India.* 2007;55:152.
[11] Glueck CJ, et al. *Am J Cardiol.* 1992;70(1):1.
[12] Wirebaugh SR, et al. *Pharmacotherapy.* 1992;12(6):445.
[13] Graham DJ, et al. *JAMA.* 2004;292(21):2585.
[14] Amend KL, et al. *Ann Pharmacother.* 2011;45(10):1230.
[15] Pasternak RC, et al. *Ann Intern Med.* 1996;125(7):529.
[16] Kyrklund C, et al. *Clin Pharmacol Ther.* 2001;69(5):340.
[17] Backman JT, et al. *Clin Pharmacol Ther.* 2005;78(2):154.
[18] Backman JT, et al. *Clin Pharmacol Ther.* 2000;68(2):122.
[19] Kyrklund C, et al. *Clin Pharmacol Ther.* 2003;73(6):538.
[20] Schneck DW, et al. *Clin Pharmacol Ther.* 2004;75(5):455.
[21] Gustavson LE, et al. *J Clin Pharmacol.* 2005;45(8):947.
[22] Martin PD, et al. *Clin Ther.* 2003;25(2):459.
[23] Whitfield LR, et al. *J Clin Pharmacol.* 2011;51(3):378.
[24] Bergman E, et al. *J Clin Pharmacol.* 2010;50(9):1039.

*** Asterisk indicates drugs cited in interaction reports.**

HMG-CoA Reductase Inhibitors × *Food*

Atorvastatin* (eg, *Lipitor*)	Simvastatin* (eg, *Zocor*)	Grapefruit Juice*
Lovastatin* (eg, *Mevacor*)		

Significance	Onset	Severity	Documentation
4	■ **Rapid**	■ **Major**	□ Established
	□ Delayed	□ Moderate	□ Probable
		□ Minor	□ Suspected
			■ **Possible**
			□ Unlikely

Effects Increased serum levels and adverse reactions (eg, rhabdomyolysis) of certain HMG-CoA REDUCTASE INHIBITORS.

Mechanism Inhibition of first-pass metabolism (CYP3A4) of certain HMG-CoA REDUCTASE INHIBITORS in the small intestine.

Management Avoid coadministration of certain HMG-CoA REDUCTASE INHIBITORS with GRAPEFRUIT products. Take with liquids other than GRAPEFRUIT JUICE (GFJ). Fluvastatin (eg, *Lescol*) and pravastatin (eg, *Pravachol*) may be safer alternatives.

Discussion

The effect of 200 mL of double-strength GFJ 3 times daily for 2 days on lovastatin 80 mg was studied in 10 healthy volunteers.[1] On day 3, an additional 200 mL of GFJ or water was taken 30 and 90 min after lovastatin ingestion. GFJ increased the mean C_{max} of lovastatin 12-fold and its active metabolite, lovastatin acid, 4-fold. GFJ increased the AUC of lovastatin approximately 15-fold and lovastatin acid 5-fold. Lovastatin, lovastatin acid levels, and AUC increased in each subject. Regular-strength GFJ (8 oz) in the morning and lovastatin 40 mg in the evening increased the lovastatin AUC nearly 2-fold.[2] In 10 healthy volunteers, GFJ increased the mean C_{max} of simvastatin 9-fold and the mean AUC 16-fold.[3] The C_{max} and AUC of the active metabolite simvastatin acid increased about 7-fold. GFJ increased the mean AUC of active and total HMG-CoA reductase inhibitor 2.4- and 3.6-fold, respectively. Regular-strength GFJ increased simvastatin AUC and C_{max} 3.6- and 4.3-fold, respectively.[4] Rhabdomyolysis occurred in a woman who had tolerated simvastatin for 2 years.[5] Four days prior, she began eating 1 fresh grapefruit daily. The time course of this interaction was studied.[6] The simvastatin AUC increased 2.1- and 1.4-fold at 24 and 72 hours, respectively, after the ingestion of double-strength GFJ. Double-strength GFJ increased the atorvastatin AUC 2.5-fold.[7] The elimination $t_{½}$ increased from 7.8 to 13.3 hours. In a similar study, GFJ increased the atorvastatin AUC 1.4-fold and the AUC and C_{max} of the atorvastatin lactone metabolite 1.6- and 1.3-fold, respectively.[8] GFJ has little or no effect on pravastatin.[7,8] In a study in 8 healthy men, GFJ increased the mean AUC of atorvastatin acid 83%.[9] The effect of GFJ on the pharmacokinetics of atorvastatin was studied in hyperlipidemic patients.[10] Patients received atorvastatin with 300 mL of 100% GFJ daily for 90 days. Compared with baseline, GFJ increased atorvastatin serum concentrations 19% to 26%. Changes in lipid profiles were negligible and there were no adverse effects on liver function tests or creatine phosphokinase. Reduction of atorvastatin dose when moderate quantities of GFJ are ingested does not appear to be necessary.

[1] Kantola T, et al. *Clin Pharmacol Ther.* 1998;63(4):397.
[2] Rogers JD, et al. *Clin Pharmacol Ther.* 1999;66(4):358.
[3] Lilja JJ, et al. *Clin Pharmacol Ther.* 1998;64(5):477.
[4] Lilja JJ, et al. *Br J Clin Pharmacol.* 2004;58(1):56.
[5] Dreier JP, et al. *Neurology.* 2004;62(4):670.
[6] Lilja JJ, et al. *Clin Pharmacol Ther.* 2000;68(4):384.
[7] Lilja JJ, et al. *Clin Pharmacol Ther.* 1999;66(2):118.
[8] Fukazawa I, et al. *Br J Clin Pharmacol.* 2004;57(4):448.
[9] Ando H, et al. *Br J Clin Pharmacol.* 2005;60(5):494.
[10] Reddy P, et al. *Br J Clin Pharmacol.* 2011;72(3):434.

* Asterisk indicates drugs cited in interaction reports.

HMG-CoA Reductase Inhibitors — HCV Protease Inhibitors

HMG-CoA Reductase Inhibitors		HCV Protease Inhibitors	
Atorvastatin* (eg, *Lipitor*)	Pravastatin (eg, *Pravachol*)	Boceprevir* (*Victrelis*)	Telaprevir* (*Incivek*)
Fluvastatin (eg, *Lescol*)	Rosuvastatin (*Crestor*)		
Lovastatin* (eg, *Mevacor*)	Simvastatin* (eg, *Zocor*)		
Pitavastatin (*Livalo*)			

Significance	Onset	Severity	Documentation
1	□ Rapid ■ **Delayed**	■ **Major** □ Moderate □ Minor	□ Established □ Probable ■ **Suspected** □ Possible □ Unlikely

Effects HMG-CoA REDUCTASE INHIBITOR plasma concentrations may be elevated, increasing the pharmacologic effects and risk of myopathy and rhabdomyolysis.

Mechanism HMG-CoA REDUCTASE INHIBITOR metabolism (CYP3A) may be inhibited by HEPATITIS C VIRUS (HCV) PROTEASE INHIBITORS.

Management Coadministration of LOVASTATIN or SIMVASTATIN and HCV PROTEASE INHIBITORS is contraindicated.[1,2] In addition, coadministration of ATORVASTATIN and TELAPREVIR is contraindicated.[2] The maximum dose of ATORVASTATIN should not exceed 20 mg during concurrent use of BOCEPREVIR.[1] Use other HMG-CoA REDUCTASE INHIBITORS with caution and close clinical monitoring. FLUVASTATIN and PRAVASTATIN are not metabolized by CYP3A4 and may be less likely to interact.

Discussion

Boceprevir or telaprevir is contraindicated when coadministered with drugs that are highly dependent on CYP3A4 metabolism for clearance and for which elevated plasma concentrations are associated with serious and/or life-threatening adverse effects (eg, drugs with a narrow therapeutic index).[1,2] Pretreatment with telaprevir 750 mg every 8 hours for 7 days increased the C_{max} and AUC of a single oral dose of atorvastatin 20 mg approximately 11- and 8-fold, respectively, compared with atorvastatin alone.[2] Concomitant use of lovastatin and simvastatin is contraindicated in patients receiving boceprevir or telaprevir.[1,2] In addition, atorvastatin is contraindicated in patients receiving telaprevir.[2] Concurrent use of these agents may increase the risk of myopathy and rhabdomyolysis. In a study in 19 healthy volunteers receiving amlodipine 5 mg in combination with atorvastatin 20 mg, pretreatment with telaprevir 750 mg every 8 hours for 6 days increased the atorvastatin C_{max} and AUC 10.6- and 7.88-fold, respectively, compared with giving amlodipine/atorvastatin alone.[3]

1 *Victrelis* [package insert]. Whitehouse Station, NJ: Schering Corporation; May 2011.
2 *Incivek* [package insert]. Cambridge, MA: Vertex Pharmaceuticals Incorporated; May 2011.
3 Lee JE, et al. *Antimicrob Agents Chemother.* 2011;55(10):4569.

* Asterisk indicates drugs cited in interaction reports. Based on pharmacologic and pharmacokinetic considerations, similar interactions may occur with other drugs that are listed.

HMG-CoA Reductase Inhibitors — *Hydantoins*

HMG-CoA Reductase Inhibitors		Hydantoins
Atorvastatin* (eg, *Lipitor*)	Simvastatin* (eg, *Zocor*)	Fosphenytoin
Fluvastatin (eg, *Lescol*)		Phenytoin* (eg, *Dilantin*)

Significance	Onset	Severity	Documentation
4	☐ Rapid	☐ Major	☐ Established
	■ **Delayed**	■ **Moderate**	☐ Probable
		☐ Minor	☐ Suspected
			■ **Possible**
			☐ Unlikely

Effects Plasma concentrations of certain HMG-CoA REDUCTASE INHIBITORS may be decreased, producing a decrease in therapeutic effect (eg, hypercholesterolemia).

Mechanism Increased metabolism of the HMG-CoA REDUCTASE INHIBITORS is suspected.

Management Monitor the clinical response of the patient; if an interaction is suspected, it may be necessary to administer alternative therapy. Pravastatin (eg, *Pravachol*) is less likely to interact with PHENYTOIN and may be a suitable alternative.

Discussion

A possible interaction was reported in a 50-year-old woman with hypercholesterolemia and epilepsy during concurrent treatment with phenytoin and simvastatin or atorvastatin.[1] The patient was taking simvastatin 10 mg/day when her anticonvulsant therapy was changed from valproate sodium (eg, *Depacon*) to phenytoin 325 mg/day. Subsequently, the patient's total cholesterol increased from 9.4 to 16 mmol/L. Thereafter, successive changes in therapy included increasing the dosage of simvastatin to 40 mg/day, changing treatment to fluvastatin, then changing to atorvastatin (dosage increased stepwise to 80 mg/day). Throughout these changes, total cholesterol remained greater than 10 mmol/L. The dosage of phenytoin was decreased from 325 to 225 mg/day, then discontinued as the dosage of atorvastatin was increased from 40 to 80 mg/day. These changes were followed with a reduction in total cholesterol to 6.24 mmol/L. A 61-year-old man who had been taking phenytoin had an elevated lipid profile, despite taking 3 antiepileptic agents, including atorvastatin 80 mg daily.[2] After discontinuing phenytoin, his LDL decreased from 225 to 110 mg/dL. A 78-year-old woman stabilized on phenytoin and simvastatin experienced phenytoin toxicity, reduced simvastatin serum levels, and an increase in cholesterol after inadvertently doubling her phenytoin dose for a week.[3]

[1] Murphy MJ, et al. *Postgrad Med J.* 1999;75(884):359.
[2] Khandwala HM. *South Med J.* 2006;99(12):1385.
[3] Tan KM, et al. *Br J Clin Pharmacol.* 2008;65(1):147.

* Asterisk indicates drugs cited in interaction reports. Based on pharmacologic and pharmacokinetic considerations, similar interactions may occur with other drugs that are listed.

HMG-CoA Reductase Inhibitors — **_Imatinib_**

Atorvastatin (*Lipitor*)	Simvastatin* (eg, *Zocor*)	Imatinib* (*Gleevec*)
Lovastatin (eg, *Mevacor*)		

Significance	Onset	Severity	Documentation
2	□ Rapid ■ **Delayed**	□ Major ■ **Moderate** □ Minor	□ Established □ Probable ■ **Suspected** □ Possible □ Unlikely

Effects Plasma concentrations of certain HMG-CoA REDUCTASE INHIBITORS may be elevated, increasing the pharmacologic effects and risk of adverse reactions (eg, myopathy, rhabdomyolysis).

Mechanism Inhibition of HMG-CoA REDUCTASE INHIBITOR metabolism (CYP3A4) by IMATINIB is suspected.

Management Consider administering alternative therapy. Fluvastatin (*Lescol*), pravastatin (eg, *Pravachol*), and rosuvastatin (*Crestor*) are not metabolized by CYP3A4 and may be less likely to interact. Advise patients to report unexplained muscle pain, tenderness, or weakness.

Discussion

The effects of imatinib on the pharmacokinetics of simvastatin were studied in 20 patients with chronic myeloid leukemia.[1] In an open-label, nonrandomized study, each subject received simvastatin 40 mg on study day 1, imatinib 400 mg once daily on study days 2 to 7, and imatinib 400 mg plus simvastatin 40 mg on study day 8. Pretreatment with imatinib increased the simvastatin mean C_{max} and AUC 2- and 3.5-fold, respectively, compared with giving simvastatin alone. Total body clearance of simvastatin from the plasma was reduced 70%, and the mean $t_{½}$ was prolonged from 1.4 to 2.7 hours. Simvastatin administration did not affect imatinib pharmacokinetics.

[1] O'Brien SG, et al. *Br J Cancer.* 2003;89(10):1855.

* Asterisk indicates drugs cited in interaction reports. Based on pharmacologic and pharmacokinetic considerations, similar interactions may occur with other drugs that are listed.

HMG-CoA Reductase Inhibitors / *Isradipine*

HMG-CoA Reductase Inhibitors	Isradipine
Lovastatin* (eg, *Mevacor*)	Isradipine* (eg, *DynaCirc*)

Significance	Onset	Severity	Documentation
3	□ Rapid	□ Major	□ Established
	■ **Delayed**	□ Moderate	□ Probable
		■ **Minor**	■ **Suspected**
			□ Possible
			□ Unlikely

Effects Plasma concentrations of LOVASTATIN may be reduced, decreasing the pharmacologic effects. The change in LOVASTATIN levels appears to be greater in men than women.

Mechanism Unknown. Increased LOVASTATIN hepatic clearance secondary to increased hepatic blood flow is suspected.

Management Monitor the clinical response of the patient and adjust therapy as needed.

Discussion

Using a randomized, double-blind, crossover design, 6 healthy men and 6 healthy women volunteers received isradipine 5 mg twice daily, lovastatin 20 mg/day, or the combination of both drugs for 5 days.[1] In men, coadministration of isradipine reduced the lovastatin AUC 20% or 40%, depending on the assay method employed. In women, isradipine did not affect the AUC of lovastatin. There was a greater variance in lovastatin measurements in women than men. Half of the women had a decrease in the apparent clearance of lovastatin, while half had an increase. Lovastatin did not affect isradipine clearance in any subject.

[1] Zhou LX, et al. *J Pharmacol Exp Ther.* 1995;273(1):121.

* Asterisk indicates drugs cited in interaction reports.

HMG-CoA Reductase Inhibitors / *Macrolide & Related Antibiotics*

HMG-CoA Reductase Inhibitors		Macrolide & Related Antibiotics	
Atorvastatin* (eg, *Lipitor*)	Simvastatin* (eg, *Zocor*)	Clarithromycin* (eg, *Biaxin*)	Telithromycin* (*Ketek*)
Lovastatin* (eg, *Mevacor*)		Erythromycin* (eg, *Ery-Tab*)	

Significance	Onset	Severity	Documentation
1	☐ Rapid	■ **Major**	☐ Established
	■ **Delayed**	☐ Moderate	■ **Probable**
		☐ Minor	☐ Suspected
			☐ Possible
			☐ Unlikely

Effects Severe myopathy or rhabdomyolysis may occur because of increased HMG-CoA REDUCTASE INHIBITOR levels.

Mechanism Inhibition of metabolism (CYP3A4) is suspected.

Management If possible, administer alternative therapy. Fluvastatin (eg, *Lescol*), pravastatin (eg, *Pravachol*), and rosuvastatin (*Crestor*) are not metabolized by CYP3A4 and may be less likely to interact. Advise patients to report unexplained muscle pain, tenderness, or weakness.

Discussion

Multiple case reports have associated myopathy and rhabdomyolysis with coadministration of simvastatin and clarithromycin[1-3]; atorvastatin and clarithromycin[4]; and lovastatin with azithromycin, clarithromycin,[5] or erythromycin.[6-8] Case characteristics are as follows: 1) all patients had been on a stable, long-term HMG-CoA reductase inhibitor regimen with no evidence of myopathy or rhabdomyolysis; 2) myalgia and elevated creatine phosphokinase (CPK) developed 5 to 21 days after starting the macrolide; 3) increased lovastatin plasma levels were documented when measured[6,8]; 4) muscle biopsy was positive for myonecrosis secondary to toxin[1,8]; and 5) improvement was noted in symptoms and CPK following withdrawal of the HMG-CoA reductase inhibitor and IV hydration.[1,5,6] In 2 controlled studies, erythromycin had variable effects on the pharmacokinetics of simvastatin[9] and atorvastatin.[10] The C_{max} and AUC were increased 3.4- and 6.2-fold, respectively, for simvastatin and 38% and 33%, respectively, for atorvastatin. In 36 healthy subjects receiving atorvastatin 10 mg for 8 days and azithromycin 500 mg/day, clarithromycin 500 mg twice daily, or placebo on days 6 to 8, clarithromycin increased the AUC and C_{max} of atorvastatin 82% and 56%, respectively, compared with placebo.[11] The atorvastatin AUC increased between 2.6- and 2.7-fold in patients concurrently treated with clarithromycin whether or not patients expressed the CYP3A4 genotype.[12] There was no interaction when azithromycin was administered with atorvastatin. In 14 healthy volunteers, erythromycin slightly decreased rosuvastatin AUC and C_{max}.[13] In a pharmacokinetic study, simvastatin levels were elevated by telithromycin. A similar interaction may occur with atorvastatin or lovastatin.[14]

1 Lee AJ, et al. *Ann Pharmacother.* 2001;35(1):26.
2 Kahri AJ, et al. *Ann Pharmacother.* 2004;38(4):719.
3 Wagner J, et al. *J Neurol.* 2009;256(7):1182.
4 Sipe BE, et al. *Ann Pharmacother.* 2003;37(6):808.
5 Grunden JW, et al. *Ann Pharmacother.* 1997;31(7-8):859.
6 Ayanian JZ, et al. *Ann Intern Med.* 1988;109(8):682.
7 Corpier CL, et al. *JAMA.* 1988;260(2):239.
8 Spach DH, et al. *West J Med.* 1991;154(2):213.
9 Kantola T, et al. *Clin Pharmacol Ther.* 1998;64(2):177.
10 Siedlik PH, et al. *J Clin Pharmacol.* 1999;39(5):501.
11 Amsden GW, et al. *J Clin Pharmacol.* 2002;42(4):444.
12 Shin J, et al. *Pharmacotherapy.* 2011;31(10):942.
13 Cooper KJ, et al. *Eur J Clin Pharmacol.* 2003;59(1):51.
14 *Ketek* [package insert]. Kansas City, MO: Aventis Pharmaceuticals Inc; June 2004.

* Asterisk indicates drugs cited in interaction reports.

HMG-CoA Reductase Inhibitors — *Mifepristone*

Atorvastatin (eg, *Lipitor*)	Simvastatin* (eg, *Zocor*)	Mifepristone* (eg, *Korlym*)
Lovastatin* (eg, *Mevacor*)		

Significance	Onset	Severity	Documentation
1	☐ Rapid ■ **Delayed**	■ **Major** ☐ Moderate ☐ Minor	☐ Established ☐ Probable ■ **Suspected** ☐ Possible ☐ Unlikely

Effects Plasma concentrations of certain HMG-CoA REDUCTASE INHIBITORS may be elevated, increasing the pharmacologic effects and risk of adverse reactions (eg, myopathy, rhabdomyolysis).

Mechanism MIFEPRISTONE may inhibit the metabolism (CYP3A4) of certain HMG-CoA REDUCTASE INHIBITORS.

Management Coadministration of LOVASTATIN or SIMVASTATIN with MIFEPRISTONE is contraindicated.[1]

Discussion

Because mifepristone inhibits CYP3A4, coadministration of mifepristone with a drug that is metabolized mainly or solely by CYP3A4 (eg, lovastatin, simvastatin) is likely to increase plasma concentrations of the drug.[1] Concurrent use of mifepristone 1,200 mg daily for 10 days followed by a single dose of simvastatin 80 mg increased the simvastatin C_{max} and AUC by 7- and 10.4-fold, respectively, while increasing the simvastatin acid C_{max} and AUC by 18.2- and 15.7-fold, respectively. The risk of myopathy or rhabdomyolysis may be increased.

[1] *Korlym* [package insert]. Menlo Park, CA: Corcept Therapeutics Incorporated; February 2012.

* Asterisk indicates drugs cited in interaction reports. Based on pharmacologic and pharmacokinetic considerations, similar interactions may occur with other drugs that are listed.

HMG-CoA Reductase Inhibitors		***Nefazodone***
Atorvastatin (eg, *Lipitor*)	Simvastatin* (eg, *Zocor*)	Nefazodone*
Lovastatin (eg, *Mevacor*)		

Significance	Onset	Severity	Documentation
1	□ Rapid	■ **Major**	□ Established
	■ **Delayed**	□ Moderate	□ Probable
		□ Minor	■ **Suspected**
			□ Possible
			□ Unlikely

Effects With certain HMG-CoA REDUCTASE INHIBITORS, the risk of rhabdomyolysis and myositis may be increased.

Mechanism Possible NEFAZODONE inhibition of metabolism of HMG-CoA REDUCTASE INHIBITORS metabolized by CYP3A4.

Management If coadministration of these agents cannot be avoided, advise patients to report any unexplained muscle pain, tenderness, or weakness. Because CYP3A4 is not the principal isozyme responsible for fluvastatin (eg, *Lescol*) or pravastatin (eg, *Pravachol*) metabolism, these drugs may be less likely to interact and may be safer alternatives.

Discussion

Rhabdomyolysis has been reported in several patients receiving simvastatin with nefazodone[1-3] and in patients receiving simvastatin alone.[4] Myositis and rhabdomyolysis were reported in a 44-year-old man who had been asymptomatic while taking simvastatin 40 mg/day for 19 weeks.[1] One month after starting nefazodone 100 mg twice daily, the patient complained of tea-colored urine, which was thought to be a urinary tract infection. He was treated with amoxicillin/potassium clavulanate (eg, *Augmentin*). One month later, the patient still complained of tea-colored urine and severe myalgia in his thighs and calves. Following his physical examination and laboratory test results, rhabdomyolysis and myositis were diagnosed. Simvastatin and nefazodone were discontinued, and the patient was asymptomatic within 3 weeks. A 72-year-old man on a stable regimen that included simvastatin developed rhabdomyolysis 6 weeks after starting nefazodone.[2] Nefazodone was discontinued, and he was treated with hydration. The patient was continued on simvastatin and venlafaxine (eg, *Effexor*) without incident. A 79-year-old woman receiving nefazodone 150 mg twice daily without adverse reactions experienced rhabdomyolysis with elevated transaminase and creatine kinase levels 10 months after starting simvastatin 20 mg/day and 1 month after the dosage was increased to 40 mg/day.[5] Nefazodone and simvastatin were held, and transaminase and creatine kinase levels decreased over the next 3 days.

[1] Jacobson RH, et al. *JAMA*. 1997;277(4):296.
[2] Thompson M, et al. *Am J Psychiatry*. 2002;159(9):1607.
[3] Skrabal MZ, et al. *South Med J*. 2003;96(10):1034.
[4] Jody DN. *JAMA*. 1997;277(4):296.
[5] Karnik NS, et al. *Psychosomatics*. 2005;46(6):565.

* Asterisk indicates drugs cited in interaction reports. Based on pharmacologic and pharmacokinetic considerations, similar interactions may occur with other drugs that are listed.

HMG-CoA Reductase Inhibitors — *Niacin*

HMG-CoA Reductase Inhibitors		Niacin
Atorvastatin (eg, *Lipitor*)	Pravastatin (eg, *Pravachol*)	Niacin* (eg, *Niaspan*)
Ezetimibe/Simvastatin* (*Vytorin*)	Rosuvastatin (*Crestor*)	
Lovastatin* (eg, *Mevacor*)	Simvastatin (eg, *Zocor*)	

Significance	Onset	Severity	Documentation
4	☐ Rapid	☐ Major	☐ Established
	■ **Delayed**	■ **Moderate**	☐ Probable
		☐ Minor	☐ Suspected
			■ **Possible**
			☐ Unlikely

Effects Severe myopathy or rhabdomyolysis may occur with coadministration of these drugs.

Mechanism Unknown.

Management Advise patients receiving HMG-CoA REDUCTASE INHIBITORS and NIACIN to report any unexplained muscle pain, tenderness, or weakness.

Discussion

Myolysis and rhabdomyolysis (eg, muscle aches, tenderness, weakness) have been associated with coadministration of lovastatin and niacin.[1-3] Reports have involved case histories but no controlled studies. Patients were taking multiple medications, including cyclosporine (eg, *Neoral*) in 1 patient. In 1 case, the occurrence of rhabdomyolysis was accompanied by renal failure.[1] One patient, a 43-year-old man with familial hypercholesterolemia, had been taking lovastatin for nearly 2.5 years without evidence of myopathy.[2] Niacin therapy was started, and after the dosage was gradually increased to 2.5 g/day, the patient experienced mild back pain, darkened urine, and a creatine kinase (CK) level of 233,000 units/L. All drugs were discontinued, and the symptoms resolved over the next 2 weeks. A 77-year-old woman receiving lovastatin 40 mg/day developed muscle weakness, dark urine, and a CK level of 32,000 units/L when her niacin dosage was increased to 1 g/day.[3] Following discontinuation of both drugs, recovery was uneventful. Although a cause-and-effect relationship cannot be established in these patients, the temporal association between lovastatin administration and occurrence of the reaction has implicated niacin as a possible causative agent. In a study in 15 volunteers, coadministration of ER niacin 2,000 mg/day with ezetimibe 10 mg/simvastatin 20 mg increased the AUC of ezetimibe and simvastatin 26% and 35%, respectively.[4] These increases were not considered clinically important. See also Lovastatin-Cyclosporine.

[1] Norman DJ, et al. *N Engl J Med.* 1988;318(1):46.
[2] Reaven P, et al. *Ann Intern Med.* 1988;109(7):597.
[3] Cooke HM. *Hosp Pharm.* 1994;29:33.
[4] Kosoglou T, et al. *Eur J Clin Pharmacol.* 2011;67(5):483.

* Asterisk indicates drugs cited in interaction reports. Based on pharmacologic and pharmacokinetic considerations, similar interactions may occur with other drugs that are listed.

HMG-CoA Reductase Inhibitors — *NNRT Inhibitors*

HMG-CoA Reductase Inhibitors		NNRT Inhibitors	
Atorvastatin* (eg, *Lipitor*)	Pravastatin* (eg, *Pravachol*)	Efavirenz* (*Sustiva*)	Nevirapine (*Viramune*)
Lovastatin (eg, *Mevacor*)	Simvastatin* (eg, *Zocor*)		

Significance	Onset	Severity	Documentation
1	☐ Rapid ■ **Delayed**	■ **Major** ☐ Moderate ☐ Minor	☐ Established ☐ Probable ■ **Suspected** ☐ Possible ☐ Unlikely

Effects EFAVIRENZ and NEVIRAPINE may reduce HMG-CoA REDUCTASE INHIBITOR levels.

Mechanism EFAVIRENZ and NEVIRAPINE may induce CYP3A4 metabolism.

Management Monitor LDL levels after NNRT INHIBITORS are started or stopped.

Discussion

In a study in 42 patients, efavirenz 600 mg at bedtime reduced the AUC of atorvastatin, pravastatin, and simvastatin between 40% and 60%, decreasing the LDL-lowering effect.[1] In a retrospective study, 13 men infected with HIV who were receiving a stable efavirenz-based regimen and were started on simvastatin 20 mg/day were compared with 19 men not infected with HIV who were started on simvastatin 20 mg/day.[2] Simvastatin did not compromise viral or immunologic control in patients receiving the efavirenz-based regimen. However, there was a slight lessening of the LDL-lowering effect of simvastatin compared with giving simvastatin alone. See HMG-CoA Reductase Inhibitors/Delavirdine.

[1] Gerber JG, et al. *J Acquir Immune Defic Syndr.* 2005;39(3):307.

[2] Rahman AP, et al. *Pharmacotherapy.* 2008;28(7):913.

* Asterisk indicates drugs cited in interaction reports. Based on pharmacologic and pharmacokinetic considerations, similar interactions may occur with other drugs that are listed.

HMG-CoA Reductase Inhibitors — *Quinine*

HMG-CoA Reductase Inhibitors	Quinine
Atorvastatin* (*Lipitor*)	Quinine* (*Qualaquin*)

Significance	Onset	Severity	Documentation
4	■ **Rapid**	■ **Major**	□ Established
	□ Delayed	□ Moderate	□ Probable
		□ Minor	□ Suspected
			■ **Possible**
			□ Unlikely

Effects ATORVASTATIN plasma concentrations may be elevated, increasing the risk of severe myopathy or rhabdomyolysis.

Mechanism Inhibition of ATORVASTATIN first-pass metabolism (CYP3A4) by QUININE is suspected.

Management Until more information is available, consider avoiding this drug combination. Fluvastatin (*Lescol*) and pravastatin (eg, *Pravachol*) are not metabolized by CYP3A4 and may be less likely to interact. Advise patients to immediately report unexplained muscle pain, tenderness, or weakness.

Discussion

Rhabdomyolysis was reported in a 54-year-old woman after quinine was added to her drug regimen.[1] The patient had a history of dyslipidemia, hypertension, chronic back pain, and cholecystectomy. She was receiving atorvastatin 20 mg daily, amlodipine (eg, *Norvasc*), atenolol (eg, *Tenormin*), aspirin, and glucosamine. Upon developing nocturnal leg cramps, she took quinine 300 mg with atorvastatin. Within an hour, she developed nausea, vomiting, diarrhea, and abdominal pain. Soon, she experienced rigors, myalgia, dizziness, and peripheral paresthesia. She presented in the emergency department 2 hours after quinine ingestion. Following laboratory testing and repeat biochemistry evaluations, she was diagnosed with rhabdomyolysis, hemolytic-uremic syndrome, acute renal failure, acute hepatitis, and disseminated intravascular coagulation. She recovered with supportive treatment. The patient had a similar reaction 11 months prior after taking atorvastatin and a single dose of quinine 300 mg.

[1] Lim AK, et al. *Intern Med J.* 2006;36(7):465.

* Asterisk indicates drugs cited in interaction reports.

HMG-CoA Reductase Inhibitors — *Ranolazine*

Atorvastatin (*Lipitor*)	Simvastatin* (eg, *Zocor*)	Ranolazine* (*Ranexa*)
Lovastatin (eg, *Mevacor*)		

Significance	Onset	Severity	Documentation
1	☐ Rapid	■ **Major**	☐ Established
	■ **Delayed**	☐ Moderate	☐ Probable
		☐ Minor	■ **Suspected**
			☐ Possible
			☐ Unlikely

Effects Plasma concentrations of certain HMG-CoA REDUCTASE INHIBITORS may be elevated, increasing the risk of adverse reactions.

Mechanism Inhibition of certain HMG-CoA REDUCTASE INHIBITOR metabolism (CYP3A4) by RANOLAZINE.

Management In patients receiving RANOLAZINE, do not exceed a dose of SIMVASTATIN 20 mg daily.[1] Monitor patients for adverse reactions. Advise patients to immediately report any unexplained muscle pain, tenderness, or weakness. Pravastatin (eg, *Pravachol*) is not metabolized by CYP3A4 and may be a safer alternative.

Discussion

The effects of ranolazine on the pharmacokinetics of simvastatin were studied in 17 healthy subjects.[2] Using an open-label, multidose design, each subject received an initial dose of sustained-release ranolazine 1,750 mg followed by 1,000 mg twice daily for 7 days. During the last 4 days of ranolazine administration, simvastatin 80 mg daily was given. Compared with administration of simvastatin alone, coadministration of ranolazine sustained release increased the AUC and C_{max} of simvastatin, simvastatin acid, 2 simvastatin metabolites, and HMG-CoA reductase activity less than 2-fold. Simvastatin did not affect the pharmacokinetics of ranolazine. A 63-year-old man developed rhabdomyolysis shortly after ranolazine 500 mg daily was added to a stable simvastatin (80 mg daily) regimen.[3] Chronic renal failure may have contributed to the rhabdomyolysis.

[1] *Zocor* [package insert]. Whitehouse Station, NJ: Merck & Co Inc; October 2011.
[2] Jerling M, et al. *J Clin Pharmacol.* 2005;45(4):422.
[3] Hylton AC, et al. *Am J Health Syst Pharm.* 2010;67(21):1829.

* Asterisk indicates drugs cited in interaction reports. Based on pharmacologic and pharmacokinetic considerations, similar interactions may occur with other drugs that are listed.

HMG-CoA Reductase Inhibitors		***Rifamycins***	
Atorvastatin* (eg, *Lipitor*)	Pravastatin* (eg, *Pravachol*)	Rifabutin (*Mycobutin*)	Rifapentine (*Priftin*)
Fluvastatin (eg, *Lescol*)	Simvastatin* (eg, *Zocor*)	Rifampin* (eg, *Rifadin*)	
Lovastatin (eg, *Mevacor*)			

Significance	Onset	Severity	Documentation
2	□ Rapid	□ Major	□ Established
	■ **Delayed**	■ **Moderate**	□ Probable
		□ Minor	■ **Suspected**
			□ Possible
			□ Unlikely

Effects

HMG-CoA REDUCTASE INHIBITOR levels may be reduced, decreasing the pharmacologic effects. PRAVASTATIN levels may be increased in some patients.

Mechanism

RIFAMYCINS may induce first-pass metabolism (CYP3A4) and inhibit hepatic transported protein (OATP1B) of the HMG-CoA REDUCTASE INHIBITOR in the intestine and liver or may affect other intestinal transport mechanisms.

Management

Monitor the clinical response of patients. If an interaction is suspected, it may be necessary to administer alternative therapy or increase the dose of the HMG-CoA REDUCTASE INHIBITOR when a RIFAMYCIN is coadministered.

Discussion

In a randomized, crossover study, the effects of rifampin on the pharmacokinetics of simvastatin were investigated in 10 healthy volunteers.[1] Each subject was pretreated with rifampin 600 mg or placebo daily for 5 days. On day 6, a single oral dose of simvastatin 40 mg was administered. Compared with placebo, rifampin pretreatment reduced the AUCs of simvastatin and the active metabolite (simvastatin acid) 87% and 93%, respectively, as well as the C_{max} of both nearly 90% (eg, from 5.6 to 0.6 ng/mL for simvastatin). The elimination $t_{½}$ of simvastatin and simvastatin acid were not affected by rifampin pretreatment. In 10 volunteers, pravastatin pharmacokinetics were measured before and after 5 days of rifampin 600 mg/day.[2] Compared with placebo, rifampin reduced the AUC of pravastatin 69%; the $t_{½}$ did not change. While this change is relatively small, there was considerable individual variability in response. The reduction in AUC could be clinically important in some patients. In contrast, in a single-blind, placebo-controlled, crossover study, 12 healthy men received a single dose of rifampin or placebo after 9 days of pretreatment with pravastatin. Compared with placebo, rifampin increased the pravastatin AUC 182%, indicating that an interaction mechanism may be involved prior to enzyme induction.[3] The effect of rifampin 600 mg twice daily for 5 days on the kinetics of a single dose of atorvastatin 40 mg was evaluated in 10 healthy volunteers.[4] The AUCs of atorvastatin and atorvastatin lactone were 20% and 7%, respectively, of the values measured with placebo. The $t_{½}$ of atorvastatin was reduced from 10.3 to 2.7 hours. Administration of a single dose of rifampin to 11 healthy volunteers receiving atorvastatin 40 mg resulted in a nearly 7-fold increase in atorvastatin AUC.[5]

[1] Kyrklund C, et al. *Clin Pharmacol Ther.* 2000;68(6):592.
[2] Kyrklund C, et al. *Br J Clin Pharmacol.* 2004;57(2):181.
[3] Deng S, et al. *Clin Ther.* 2009;31(6):1256.
[4] Backman JT, et al. *Clin Pharmacol Ther.* 2005;78(2):154.
[5] Lau YY, et al. *Clin Pharmacol Ther.* 2007;81(2):194.

* Asterisk indicates drugs cited in interaction reports. Based on pharmacologic and pharmacokinetic considerations, similar interactions may occur with other drugs that are listed.

HMG-CoA Reductase Inhibitors	*Serotonin Reuptake Inhibitors*
Pravastatin* (eg, *Pravachol*)	Paroxetine* (eg, *Paxil*)

Significance	Onset	Severity	Documentation
4	☐ Rapid ■ **Delayed**	☐ Major ■ **Moderate** ☐ Minor	☐ Established ☐ Probable ☐ Suspected ■ **Possible** ☐ Unlikely

Effects Increased blood glucose concentrations may occur.

Mechanism Unknown.

Management Monitor blood glucose concentrations, especially in diabetic patients. If an interaction is suspected, it may be necessary to discontinue one of the agents and administer alternative therapy.

Discussion

A retrospective review of data mined from the FDA's Adverse Event Reports found an association between increased blood glucose concentrations and coadministration of pravastatin with paroxetine.[1] Mean random blood glucose concentrations were evaluated in 104 patients with diabetes and 136 without diabetes who received concurrent pravastatin and paroxetine. Blood glucose increased an average of 19 mg/dL (1 mmol/L) overall and 48 mg/dL (2.7 mmol/L) in individuals with diabetes. Neither drug administered alone was associated with a change in blood glucose concentrations.

[1] Tatonetti NP, et al. *Clin Pharmacol Ther*. 2011;90(1):133.

* Asterisk indicates drugs cited in interaction reports.

HMG-CoA Reductase Inhibitors — Sildenafil

Atorvastatin (*Lipitor*)	Simvastatin* (eg, *Zocor*)	Sildenafil* (eg, *Viagra*)
Lovastatin (eg, *Mevacor*)		

Significance	Onset	Severity	Documentation
4	☐ Rapid	☐ Major	☐ Established
	■ **Delayed**	■ **Moderate**	☐ Probable
		☐ Minor	☐ Suspected
			■ **Possible**
			☐ Unlikely

Effects The risk of rhabdomyolysis and myositis may be increased.

Mechanism Inhibition of metabolism (CYP3A4) of certain HMG-CoA REDUCTASE INHIBITORS is suspected.

Management Advise patients to report any unexplained muscle pain, tenderness, or weakness.

Discussion

A possible case of rhabdomyolysis was reported in a 76-year-old man during concomitant use of simvastatin and sildenafil.[1] The patient had a history of hypertension and hypercholesterolemia and was receiving simvastatin 10 mg/day for at least 3 years and atenolol (eg, *Tenormin*). He complained of erectile dysfunction and was prescribed sildenafil 50 mg to be taken 2 hours prior to sexual activity. His previous physical examination was normal. Twelve days later, he presented to the clinic with a 3-day history of severe muscle aches that occurred 8 to 10 hours after the use of sildenafil and resolved over the next 3 days. At the time of his physical examination, he was asymptomatic and had no muscle tenderness. His laboratory results showed a mild elevation in creatine phosphokinase and serum urea nitrogen and an increase in creatinine and potassium levels. Simvastatin was immediately discontinued.

[1] Gutierrez CA. *Am Fam Physician.* 2001;63(4):636.

* Asterisk indicates drugs cited in interaction reports. Based on pharmacologic and pharmacokinetic considerations, similar interactions may occur with other drugs that are listed.

HMG-CoA Reductase Inhibitors		*St. John's Wort*	
Atorvastatin* (*Lipitor*)	Simvastatin* (eg, *Zocor*)	St. John's Wort*	
Lovastatin (eg, *Mevacor*)			

Significance	Onset	Severity	Documentation
2	☐ Rapid	☐ Major	☐ Established
	■ **Delayed**	■ **Moderate**	☐ Probable
		☐ Minor	■ **Suspected**
			☐ Possible
			☐ Unlikely

Effects Plasma levels of certain HMG-CoA REDUCTASE INHIBITORS may be reduced, decreasing the cholesterol-lowering effect of the HMG-CoA REDUCTASE INHIBITOR.

Mechanism Induction by ST. JOHN'S WORT of first-pass metabolism (CYP3A4) of certain HMG-CoA REDUCTASE INHIBITORS in the small intestine and liver is suspected.

Management Although the clinical importance of this interaction has not been studied, advise patients taking certain HMG-CoA REDUCTASE INHIBITORS to avoid use of ST. JOHN'S WORT. Because pravastatin (eg, *Pravachol*) is not metabolized by CYP3A4, it is less likely to interact with ST. JOHN'S WORT and may be a suitable alternative.

Discussion

The effects of St. John's wort on the pharmacokinetics of simvastatin and pravastatin were studied in 16 healthy men.[1] Using a double-blind, crossover, placebo-controlled design, each subject received St. John's wort (standardized to hypericin 0.3%) or a matching placebo 3 times daily for 14 days. In addition to St. John's wort, the 14th day, 8 subjects received a single oral dose of pravastatin 20 mg, and 8 subjects received a single oral dose of simvastatin 10 mg. Compared with placebo, administration of St. John's wort decreased the AUC of the active metabolite of simvastatin, simvastatin hydroxy acid, 62%. St. John's wort did not affect pravastatin plasma concentrations. Administration of St. John's wort to 16 patients on stable doses of atorvastatin increased total and LDL cholesterol 7% and 11%, respectively, compared with baseline.[2]

The ingredients of most herbal products are not standardized. It is unclear whether herbal products contain ingredients other than those listed on the label or purported to be present that could interact with HMG-CoA reductase inhibitors. See also Rosuvastatin-St. John's Wort.

[1] Sugimoto K, et al. *Clin Pharmacol Ther.* 2001;70(6):518.

[2] Andrén L, et al. *Eur J Clin Pharmacol.* 2007;63(10):913.

* Asterisk indicates drugs cited in interaction reports. Based on pharmacologic and pharmacokinetic considerations, similar interactions may occur with other drugs that are listed.

HMG-CoA Reductase Inhibitors — Tacrolimus

Atorvastatin (*Lipitor*)	Simvastatin* (eg, *Zocor*)	Tacrolimus* (eg, *Prograf*)
Lovastatin (eg, *Mevacor*)		

Significance	Onset	Severity	Documentation
4	☐ Rapid	■ **Major**	☐ Established
	■ **Delayed**	☐ Moderate	☐ Probable
		☐ Minor	☐ Suspected
			■ **Possible**
			☐ Unlikely

Effects Plasma concentrations of certain HMG-CoA REDUCTASE INHIBITORS may be elevated, increasing the risk of toxicity (eg, myositis, rhabdomyolysis).

Mechanism Possible inhibition of HMG-CoA REDUCTASE INHIBITOR metabolism (CYP3A4) by TACROLIMUS.

Management If coadministration cannot be avoided, advise patients to report any unexplained muscle pain, tenderness, or weakness. Fluvastatin (*Lescol*) or pravastatin (eg, *Pravachol*), which are not metabolized by CYP3A4, may be less likely to interact and may be safer alternatives.

Discussion

A 51-year-old woman receiving tacrolimus 1 to 2 mg daily was admitted to the hospital with severe muscle pain approximately 6 weeks after her simvastatin dosage was increased from 10 to 20 mg/day and 5 weeks after fusidic acid† 500 mg 3 times daily was started.[1] The serum creatine kinase concentration was 24,000 units/mL. Simvastatin and fusidic acid were stopped immediately, and treatment with saline and mannitol was started. Simvastatin was replaced with fluvastatin 40 mg/day without incident. Rhabdomyolysis has not been reported previously with coadministration of simvastatin and tacrolimus. Because rhabdomyolysis has been reported in patients treated concurrently with simvastatin and fusidic acid, the latter drug cannot be ruled out as a cause or risk factor in the development of rhabdomyolysis in this patient. See HMG-CoA Reductase Inhibitors-Cyclosporine.

[1] Kotanko P, et al. *Nephron.* 2002;90(2):234.

* Asterisk indicates drugs cited in interaction reports. Based on pharmacologic and pharmacokinetic considerations, similar interactions may occur with other drugs that are listed.
† Not available in the United States.

HMG-CoA Reductase Inhibitors — *Verapamil*

Atorvastatin* (*Lipitor*)	Simvastatin* (eg, *Zocor*)	Verapamil* (eg, *Calan*)
Lovastatin* (eg, *Mevacor*)		

Significance	Onset	Severity	Documentation
2	☐ Rapid	☐ Major	☐ Established
	■ **Delayed**	■ **Moderate**	■ **Probable**
		☐ Minor	☐ Suspected
			☐ Possible
			☐ Unlikely

Effects Certain HMG-CoA REDUCTASE INHIBITOR plasma levels may be elevated, increasing the risk of toxicity (eg, myositis, rhabdomyolysis). VERAPAMIL levels may be elevated, increasing the pharmacologic effects and risk of toxicity.

Mechanism Possible inhibition of first-pass metabolism (CYP3A4) of the HMG-CoA REDUCTASE INHIBITOR. ATORVASTATIN and LOVASTATIN may inhibit VERAPAMIL absorption (via P-glycoprotein inhibition) and/or metabolism (CYP3A4).

Management If coadministration of these agents cannot be avoided, administer a conservative dose of the HMG-CoA REDUCTASE INHIBITOR and advise patients to report any unexplained muscle pain, tenderness, or weakness. Monitor the clinical response and for adverse reactions to VERAPAMIL. Adjust the dose as needed. Because CYP3A4 is not the principal isozyme responsible for the metabolism of fluvastatin (*Lescol*), rosuvastatin (*Crestor*), and pravastatin (eg, *Pravachol*), these drugs may be less likely to interact and may be safer alternatives.

Discussion

In a randomized, double-blind, crossover study, the effects of verapamil on the pharmacokinetics of simvastatin were studied in 12 healthy volunteers.[1] Each subject received verapamil 240 mg/day or placebo. On the second day, oral simvastatin 40 mg was administered. Verapamil increased the mean C_{max} of simvastatin 2.6-fold and the AUC 4.6-fold. The AUC of simvastatin increased in each subject. In addition, verapamil increased the peak concentrations of the active simvastatin acid metabolite 3.4-fold and the AUC 2.8-fold. In an analysis of the data from 27 healthy subjects, extended-release verapamil increased simvastatin C_{max} and AUC 5- and 4-fold, respectively.[2] There were no changes in the C_{max} and AUC of pravastatin. In a study of 12 healthy men, atorvastatin 40 mg coadministered with verapamil 60 mg resulted in a 42.8% increase in the verapamil AUC compared with administering verapamil alone.[3] Fourteen healthy men received verapamil 60 mg orally with and without lovastatin 20 mg.[4] Compared with receiving verapamil alone, coadministration of lovastatin increased verapamil AUC and C_{max} 62.8% and 32.1%, respectively.

[1] Kantola T, et al. *Clin Pharmacol Ther.* 1998;64(2):177.
[2] Jacobson TA. *Am J Cardiol.* 2004;94(9):1140.
[3] Choi DH, et al. *Eur J Clin Pharmacol.* 2008;64(5):445.
[4] Choi DH, et al. *Eur J Clin Pharmacol.* 2010;66(3):285.

* Asterisk indicates drugs cited in interaction reports.

Hydantoins | **Acyclovir**

Hydantoins	Acyclovir
Phenytoin* (eg, *Dilantin*)	Acyclovir* (eg, *Zovirax*)

Significance	Onset	Severity	Documentation
4	☐ Rapid	☐ Major	☐ Established
	■ **Delayed**	■ **Moderate**	☐ Probable
		☐ Minor	☐ Suspected
			■ **Possible**
			☐ Unlikely

Effects Serum PHENYTOIN concentrations may be decreased, resulting in a decrease in activity.

Mechanism Unknown.

Management Consider monitoring patients for a change in PHENYTOIN activity if ACYCLOVIR is started or stopped. Adjust the dose of PHENYTOIN as indicated.

Discussion

Decreased antiepileptic activity occurred in a 7-year-old boy with severe symptomatic partial epilepsy receiving phenytoin, valproic acid, and nitrazepam† several days after starting treatment with acyclovir.[1] Prior to receiving acyclovir, the patient's clinical status had been stable for the preceding 2 years while he was receiving phenytoin and valproic acid 1,000 mg twice daily. Plasma phenytoin concentrations were 18 and 19 mcg/mL, while his trough and peak valproic acid concentrations were 35 and 70 mcg/mL, respectively. The boy's pediatrician prescribed acyclovir 1 g/day for throat and mouth lesions suspected to be caused by a virus. Ten days prior to starting acyclovir treatment, phenytoin and valproic acid plasma concentrations were 17 and 32 mcg/mL, respectively. Seizure frequency was fewer than 1 per month. Four days after the start of acyclovir treatment, the patient was admitted to the hospital for previously scheduled verification of his antiepileptic regimen. At this time, his trough and peak phenytoin concentrations were 5 and 7.1 mcg/mL, while valproic acid concentrations were 22 and 50 mcg/mL. Acyclovir treatment was discontinued 2 days after hospitalization. Six days later, phenytoin and valproic acid concentrations were still low, and the next day the patient had 25 serial partial seizures. The phenytoin dose was increased, and plasma concentrations increased to values of 23 to 24 mcg/mL after 10 days. Valproic acid concentrations returned to initial values without dose modification. Seizure frequency was 2 to 3 per week. The phenytoin dose was reduced, and plasma trough and peak concentrations decreased to 14 and 15 mcg/mL, respectively. The patient's clinical, electroecephalogram (EEG), and antiepileptic drug status remained stable over the next 10 months.

[1] Parmeggiani A, et al. *Ther Drug Monit.* 1995;17(3):312.

* Asterisk indicates drugs cited in interaction reports.
† Not available in the United States.

Hydantoins — *Allopurinol*

Ethotoin (*Peganone*)	Mephenytoin†	Allopurinol* (eg, *Zyloprim*)
Fosphenytoin (*Cerebyx*)	Phenytoin* (eg, *Dilantin*)	

Significance	Onset	Severity	Documentation
4	□ Rapid	□ Major	□ Established
	■ **Delayed**	■ **Moderate**	□ Probable
		□ Minor	□ Suspected
			■ **Possible**
			□ Unlikely

Effects Serum HYDANTOIN concentrations may be increased, resulting in toxicity.

Mechanism HYDANTOIN metabolism may be inhibited.

Management Monitor patients taking HYDANTOINS if ALLOPURINOL is started or stopped. Tailor the dose of the HYDANTOIN as needed.

Discussion

In a single case of a boy with Lesch-Nyhan syndrome, the maximum clearance rate of phenytoin was decreased when allopurinol was given.[1] Serum concentrations of phenytoin increased, although the only side effect noted was somnolence. This patient was taking other anticonvulsants (the doses remained constant), and some of the serum phenytoin concentrations were not measured at steady state.

Controlled studies are needed to verify and determine the importance of this possible interaction.

[1] Yokochi K, et al. *Ther Drug Monit.* 1982;4:353.

* Asterisk indicates drugs cited in interaction reports. Based on pharmacologic and pharmacokinetic considerations, similar interactions may occur with other drugs that are listed.

† Not available in the United States.

Hydantoins — *Amiodarone*

Ethotoin (*Peganone*)	Mephenytoin†	Amiodarone* (*Cordarone*)
Fosphenytoin (*Cerebyx*)	Phenytoin* (eg, *Dilantin*)	

Significance	Onset	Severity	Documentation
2	☐ Rapid	☐ Major	☐ Established
	■ **Delayed**	■ **Moderate**	■ **Probable**
		☐ Minor	☐ Suspected
			☐ Possible
			☐ Unlikely

Effects Increased serum HYDANTOIN concentrations with symptoms of toxicity. HYDANTOINS may decrease AMIODARONE serum levels.

Mechanism Probably decreased metabolism of HYDANTOINS and increased metabolism of AMIODARONE.

Management Monitor drug concentrations and observe the patient for toxicity or loss of therapeutic effect when this combination is used. Be prepared to adjust the dose of either agent. Because effects may be delayed for several weeks, long-term monitoring is necessary.

Discussion

Serum phenytoin concentrations increased by as much as 2-fold with toxicity (eg, ataxia, nystagmus, lethargy, vertigo, confusion) when amiodarone was started in patients previously stabilized on phenytoin.[2-4,8] Amiodarone can inhibit hepatic metabolism and increase the half-life of phenytoin by 30% to 150% and decrease the clearance by 25% to 61%.[5,6] A single-dose study in seven healthy volunteers demonstrated that amiodarone decreased phenytoin clearance from 1.57 to 1.17 L/hr with changes in the protein binding;[5] with chronic amiodarone and phenytoin dosing, clearance decreased from 1.29 to 0.93 L/hr.[6] Both phenytoin and amiodarone are highly protein bound, and phenytoin can increase amiodarone binding.[1]

Conversely, coadministration of oral phenytoin 2 to 4 mg/kg/day for 2 weeks to five healthy volunteers receiving oral amiodarone 200 mg/day for 4 weeks resulted in a 49% reduction in observed vs predicted amiodarone serum levels.[7] The clinical importance of this interaction needs to be determined.

1 Lalloz MRA, et al. *J Pharm Pharmacol.* 1984;36:366.
2 Gore JM, et al. *Am J Cardiol.* 1984;54:1145.
3 McGovern B, et al. *Ann Intern Med.* 1984;101:650.
4 Shackleford EJ, et al. *DICP.* 1987;21:921.
5 Nolan PE Jr, et al. *Clin Pharmacol Ther.* 1989;46:43.
6 Nolan PE Jr, et al. *Am J Cardiol.* 1990;65:1252.
7 Nolan PE Jr, et al. *J Clin Pharmacol.* 1990;30:1112.
8 Ahmad S. *J Am Geriatr Soc.* 1995;12:1449.

* Asterisk indicates drugs cited in interaction reports. Based on pharmacologic and pharmacokinetic considerations, similar interactions may occur with other drugs that are listed.
† Not available in the United States.

Hydantoins			***Antacids***
Ethotoin (*Peganone*)	Phenytoin* (eg, *Dilantin*)	Aluminum Hydroxide* (eg, *Amphojel*)	Calcium Carbonate* (eg, *Tums*)
		Aluminum/ Magnesium Hydroxide* (eg, *Maalox*)	Magnesium Hydroxide* (eg, *Dulcolax*)

Significance	Onset	Severity	Documentation
5	□ Rapid ■ **Delayed**	□ Major □ Moderate ■ **Minor**	□ Established □ Probable □ Suspected ■ **Possible** □ Unlikely

Effects Both the AUC and serum concentration of PHENYTOIN are reduced by ANTACIDS. Loss of seizure control may result.

Mechanism Decreased rate and extent of absorption of PHENYTOIN.

Management Separate the dose of PHENYTOIN and ANTACID by several hours if possible. Monitor seizure activity and PHENYTOIN serum concentrations.

Discussion

Evidence of the interaction is conflicting. Although 2 patients had poor seizure control after antacids were started, no interaction was seen in 2 studies of 8 healthy volunteers.[1,2] A third study of 12 patients taking long-term phenytoin found no effect of calcium carbonate and a very slight but statistically significant decrease in serum phenytoin concentration (from 40.4 to 35.4 mcmol/L) after magnesium trisilicate-aluminum hydroxide.[3] A decrease in the AUC of phenytoin after aluminum-magnesium hydroxide and after calcium carbonate but not after aluminum hydroxide-magnesium trisilicate was seen in 8 volunteers, although there were considerable differences in interindividual response to the antacid.[4,5] Both the rate and extent of absorption were decreased; a similar finding was noted in another study in 6 healthy subjects.[6] Phenytoin bioavailability is highly variable and can be affected by many factors, including product formulation, diet, and individual variation.[7] In many of these studies, the number of subjects was small, the dosage form and dose of phenytoin varied, the dose and administration of antacid varied, and the phenytoin was not at steady state. All of these factors could affect the bioavailability of phenytoin.[7,8] Therefore, it will be difficult to predict whether an individual would be affected by the interaction.

[1] O'Brien LS, et al. *Br J Clin Pharmacol.* 1978;6(2):176.
[2] Chapron DJ, et al. *Arch Neurol.* 1979;36(7):436.
[3] Kulshrestha VK, et al. *Br J Clin Pharmacol.* 1978;6(2):177.
[4] Garnett WR, et al. *Arch Neurol.* 1980;37(7):467.
[5] Carter BL, et al. *Ther Drug Monit.* 1981;3(4):333.
[6] McElnay JC, et al. *Br J Clin Pharmacol.* 1982;13(4):501.
[7] Cacek AT. *Ther Drug Monit.* 1986;8(2):166.
[8] D'Arcy PF, et al. *Drug Intell Clin Pharm.* 1987;21(7-8):607.

* Asterisk indicates drugs cited in interaction reports. Based on pharmacologic and pharmacokinetic considerations, similar interactions may occur with other drugs that are listed.

Hydantoins — *Anticoagulants*

Hydantoins		Anticoagulants
Ethotoin (*Peganone*)	Phenytoin* (eg, *Dilantin*)	Dicumarol*†
Fosphenytoin (*Cerebyx*)		Warfarin* (eg, *Coumadin*)

Significance	Onset	Severity	Documentation
2	□ Rapid	□ Major	□ Established
	■ **Delayed**	■ **Moderate**	■ **Probable**
		□ Minor	□ Suspected
			□ Possible
			□ Unlikely

Effects Increased HYDANTOIN serum concentrations with possible toxicity. Increased PT and an increased risk of bleeding.

Mechanism Several mechanisms may be involved.

Management Monitor patients for signs or symptoms of altered response to HYDANTOINS or ANTICOAGULANTS while receiving the combination or when starting or stopping either drug.

Discussion

Increases in serum phenytoin concentration and $t_{½}$ have been seen with dicumarol,[1,2] warfarin,[3] and phenprocoumon,[†,2] while one brief report[4] described symptoms of phenytoin toxicity when warfarin was added to the drug regimen. However, the latter report did not measure serum concentrations, and another[2] found that warfarin and phenindione[†] had no effect on phenytoin. Further information is needed on the effect of anticoagulants on phenytoin.

Phenytoin increased PT when it was added to the regimen of patients taking warfarin, resulting in severe bleeding.[3,5-7] However, a delayed effect of decreased PT was seen in one patient in one study[7] and another[8] noted decreased dicumarol concentrations after long-term phenytoin administration. Subsequent study did not demonstrate any effects when phenytoin was given with phenprocoumon.[9] The mechanism for an interaction is not clear. Phenytoin may initially displace warfarin from protein binding sites followed by enzyme induction increasing metabolism[7]; however, phenytoin had no effect on dicumarol binding.[8] The S- and R-isomer ratio may be changed, altering the amount of the more active S-isomer.[3]

[1] Hansen JM, et al. *Lancet.* 1966;2(7457):265.
[2] Skovsted L, et al. *Acta Med Scand.* 1976;199(6):513.
[3] Taylor JW, et al. *Drug Intell Clin Pharm.* 1980;14:669.
[4] Rothermich NO. *Lancet.* 1966;2:640.
[5] Nappi JM. *Ann Intern Med.* 1979;90(5):852.
[6] Levine M, et al. *Clin Pharm.* 1984;3(2):200.
[7] Panegyres PK, et al. *Postgrad Med J.* 1991;67(783):98.
[8] Hansen JM, et al. *Acta Med Scand.* 1971;189(1-2):15.
[9] Chrishe HW, et al. *Eur J Clin Invest.* 1974;4:331.

* Asterisk indicates drugs cited in interaction reports. Based on pharmacologic and pharmacokinetic considerations, similar interactions may occur with other drugs that are listed.
† Not available in the United States.

Hydantoins | **Antineoplastic Agents**

Fosphenytoin (*Cerebyx*)	Phenytoin* (eg, *Dilantin*)	Bleomycin* (eg, *Blenoxane*)	Cisplatin*
		Carboplatin*	Methotrexate* (eg, *Trexall*)
		Carmustine* (eg, *BiCNU*)	Vinblastine* (eg, *Velban*)

Significance	Onset	Severity	Documentation
2	☐ Rapid	☐ Major	☐ Established
	■ **Delayed**	■ **Moderate**	☐ Probable
		☐ Minor	■ **Suspected**
			☐ Possible
			☐ Unlikely

Effects Serum concentrations of PHENYTOIN may be decreased, resulting in a loss of therapeutic effect.

Mechanism Decreased absorption or increased metabolism of PHENYTOIN.

Management Monitor PHENYTOIN serum levels and adjust the PHENYTOIN dosage appropriately. IV PHENYTOIN may be useful.

Discussion

Decreased phenytoin concentrations shortly after beginning a course of chemotherapy have been observed in several patients.[1] Seizures were precipitated in some patients,[2,3,5-7] and another patient had toxic concentrations of phenytoin between chemotherapy courses when the phenytoin dose was not decreased following completion of chemotherapy.[1] The mechanism is not clear and may be partially related to the different combinations of drugs. The absorption of phenytoin decreased significantly to 22% in one study.[3] However, another investigation noted reduced serum concentrations with IV dosing,[4] and pharmacokinetic studies indicated an increase in the metabolism of phenytoin. Another study noted both effects in a series of treatments in one patient.[5] Three cases of acute phenytoin toxicity associated with uracil plus tegafur† reinforces the need to monitor phenytoin levels closely.[8]

Additional studies evaluating the effects of individual drugs are needed.

[1] Fincham RW, et al. *Ther Drug Monit.* 1979;1(2):277.
[2] Bollini P, et al. *Epilepsia.* 1983;24(1):75.
[3] Sylvester RK, et al. *Ther Drug Monit.* 1984;6(3):302.
[4] Jarosinski PF, et al. *J Pediatr.* 1988;112(6):996.
[5] Neef C, et al. *Clin Pharmacol Ther.* 1988;43(4):372.
[6] Grossman SA, et al. *Am J Med.* 1989;87(5):505.
[7] Dofferhoff AS, et al. *Am J Med.* 1990;89(2):247.
[8] Wakisaka S, et al. *Fukuoka Igaku Zasshi.* 1990;81(4):192.

* Asterisk indicates drugs cited in interaction reports. Based on pharmacologic and pharmacokinetic considerations, similar interactions may occur with other drugs that are listed.

† Not available in the United States.

Hydantoins			*Barbiturates*
Ethotoin (*Peganone*) Fosphenytoin (*Cerebyx*)	Phenytoin* (eg, *Dilantin*)	Amobarbital (*Amytal*) Butabarbital (eg, *Butisol*) Butalbital Mephobarbital (*Mebaral*)	Pentobarbital Phenobarbital* (eg, *Solfoton*) Secobarbital (*Seconal*)

Significance	Onset	Severity	Documentation
5	☐ Rapid ■ **Delayed**	☐ Major ☐ Moderate ■ **Minor**	☐ Established ☐ Probable ☐ Suspected ■ **Possible** ☐ Unlikely

Effects Addition of HYDANTOINS may increase BARBITURATE serum concentrations. The effect of BARBITURATES on HYDANTOINS is unpredictable.

Mechanism Alterations in metabolism.

Management Monitor serum concentrations of both drugs, seizure activity, and clinical symptoms, particularly when initiating or discontinuing either drug.

Discussion

The effect of adding phenobarbital to phenytoin therapy appears unpredictable. Although serum concentrations and $t_{½}$ of phenytoin usually decreased with concurrent phenobarbital,[1-5] other studies have demonstrated increased levels[3,6,7] or no change.[3,5,8,9] Great interindividual variations were noted, and some investigations did not take into account the dose-related pharmacokinetics of phenytoin. A well-controlled study demonstrated that phenobarbital had no effect on the pharmacokinetics of phenytoin[9]; however, only 6 patients were studied. In many instances changes were small, and only 1 investigation reported clinical toxicity from phenytoin.[5] The effect of phenytoin on phenobarbital has not been studied as thoroughly. Generally, serum phenobarbital concentrations increased after phenytoin was given[5,10,11] or the dose was increased,[12] but one trial reported a decrease in concentration.[4] Dose, time course, and individual characteristics may affect the final serum concentrations and drug effects. Therefore, predicting the end results from the combination is difficult. Individual monitoring is needed, particularly when starting or stopping either drug. In one study,[13] phenytoin and phenytoin metabolites caused false-positive results for phenobarbital in urine when using the Abbott TDx analyzer.

1 Buchanan RA, et al. *Pediatrics.* 1969;43(1):114.
2 Kristensen M, et al. *Acta Med Scand.* 1969;185(4):347.
3 Kutt H, et al. *Neurology.* 1969;19(6):611.
4 Sotaniemi E, et al. *Ann Clin Res.* 1970;2(3):223.
5 Morselli PL, et al. *Ann NY Acad Sci.* 1971;179:88.
6 Kokenge R, et al. *Neurology.* 1965;15:823.
7 Muller FO, et al. *S Afr Med J.* 1977;52(9):356.
8 Booker HE, et al. *Neurology.* 1971;21(4):383.
9 Browne TR, et al. *Neurology.* 1988;38(7):639.
10 Lambie DG, et al. *Lancet.* 1976;2(7982):386.
11 Nishihara K, et al. *Folia Psychiatr Neurol Jpn.* 1979;33(3):315.
12 Kuranari M, et al. *Ann Pharmacother.* 1995;29(1):83.
13 Siff KS, et al. *Clin Chem.* 1988;34(6):1359.

* Asterisk indicates drugs cited in interaction reports. Based on pharmacologic and pharmacokinetic considerations, similar interactions may occur with other drugs that are listed.

Hydantoins — *Benzodiazepines*

Hydantoins		Benzodiazepines	
Ethotoin (*Peganone*)	Mephenytoin†	Alprazolam (eg, *Xanax*)	Lorazepam (eg, *Ativan*)
Fosphenytoin (*Cerebyx*)	Phenytoin* (eg, *Dilantin*)	Chlordiazepoxide* (eg, *Librium*)	Midazolam* (eg, *Versed*)
		Clorazepate (eg, *Tranxene*)	Oxazepam* (eg, *Serax*)
		Diazepam* (eg, *Valium*)	Quazepam (*Doral*)
		Estazolam (eg, *ProSom*)	Temazepam (eg, *Restoril*)
		Flurazepam (eg, *Dalmane*)	Triazolam (eg, *Halcion*)

Significance	Onset	Severity	Documentation
2	☐ Rapid	☐ Major	☐ Established
	■ **Delayed**	■ **Moderate**	☐ Probable
		☐ Minor	■ **Suspected**
			☐ Possible
			☐ Unlikely

Effects Serum HYDANTOIN concentrations may be increased, resulting in toxicity, but data conflict. PHENYTOIN may increase OXAZEPAM and MIDAZOLAM clearance.

Mechanism Possibly alteration of HYDANTOIN and BENZODIAZEPINE metabolism.

Management Monitor serum HYDANTOIN levels and effects when BENZODIAZEPINES are started or stopped. In some situations, a larger BENZODIAZEPINE dose may be needed.

Discussion

Serum phenytoin concentrations increased with concurrent chlordiazepoxide or diazepam,[1-6] and symptoms of phenytoin toxicity were observed in some cases.[2,4-6] In 2 patients, the apparent 50% saturation concentration and maximum reaction velocity of phenytoin were decreased with diazepam vs phenytoin alone.[5] However, some reports do not describe an interaction, and others[7,8] have found lower than expected phenytoin concentrations. In 1 report, phenytoin increased the clearance and shortened the $t_{½}$ of oxazepam.[9] In a study of 6 epileptic patients and 7 control subjects receiving carbamazepine or phenytoin and oral midazolam, the $t_{½}$, the AUC, and the peak concentration of midazolam were decreased 94%, 92%, and 42%, respectively, compared with the control subjects.[10] The sedative effects were greatly reduced in epileptic patients receiving either phenytoin or carbamazepine. Controlled studies are needed.

1 Kutt H, et al. *JAMA*. 1968;203:167.
2 Vajda FJE, et al. *Br Med J*. 1971;1:346.
3 Kariks J, et al. *Med J Aust*. 1971;2:368.
4 Shuttleworth E, et al. *JAMA*. 1974;230:1170.
5 Rogers HJ, et al. *J Neurol Neurosurg Psychiatry*. 1977;40:890.
6 Murphy A, et al. *Ann Pharmacother*. 2003;37:659.
7 Houghton GW, et al. *Br J Clin Pharmacol*. 1974;1:344P.
8 Siris JH, et al. *N Y State J Med*. 1974;74:1554.
9 Scott AK, et al. *Br J Clin Pharmacol*. 1983;16:441.
10 Backman JT, et al. *Epilepsia*. 1996;37:253.

* Asterisk indicates drugs cited in interaction reports. Based on pharmacologic and pharmacokinetic considerations, similar interactions may occur with other drugs that are listed.
† Not available in the United States.

Hydantoins — *Carbamazepine*

Ethotoin (*Peganone*)	Mephenytoin†	Carbamazepine* (eg, *Tegretol*)
Fosphenytoin (*Cerebyx*)	Phenytoin* (eg, *Dilantin*)	

Significance	Onset	Severity	Documentation
2	☐ Rapid	☐ Major	☐ Established
	■ **Delayed**	■ **Moderate**	☐ Probable
		☐ Minor	■ **Suspected**
			☐ Possible
			☐ Unlikely

Effects PHENYTOIN decreases serum carbamazepine levels. The effect of CARBAMAZEPINE on PHENYTOIN is variable.

Mechanism Probable alteration in metabolism, including increased metabolism of CARBAMAZEPINE resulting from enzyme induction. CARBAMAZEPINE may reduce the bioavailability of PHENYTOIN.

Management Monitor serum concentrations of both drugs, particularly when starting or stopping 1 drug. Alter dose as needed to maintain therapeutic effects and avoid toxicity.

Discussion

Phenytoin (PH) can reduce carbamazepine (CBZ) serum concentrations, probably as a result of enzyme induction.[1-8] The effect of CBZ on PH is more variable. Increased,[6,9,10] decreased,[11-13] and no change in serum PH levels[2,10] have been reported. There is no clear explanation for the varied results. Although enzyme induction by CBZ can explain the low PH levels, there is also evidence that CBZ may reduce PH bioavailability.[13] One study found as CBZ increased PH levels, these higher PH concentrations subsequently induced CBZ metabolism, resulting in lower than expected CBZ concentrations.[6,10] One study reported PH toxicity from higher concentrations.[10] Increased seizure activity has not been seen.[4]

Phenytoin has reversed CBZ-induced water retention.[4,14]

1 Christiansen J, et al. *Acta Neurol Scand.* 1973;49:543.
2 Cereghino JJ, et al. *Clin Pharmacol Ther.* 1975;18:733.
3 Lander CM, et al. *Proc Aust Assoc Neurol.* 1977;14:184.
4 Perucca E, et al. *J Neurol Neurosurg Psychiatry.* 1980;43:540.
5 McKauge L, et al. *Ther Drug Monit.* 1981;3:63.
6 Zielinski JJ, et al. *Ther Drug Monit.* 1987;9:21.
7 Morris JC, et al. *Neurology.* 1987;37:1111.
8 Ramsay RE, et al. *Ther Drug Monit.* 1990;12:235.
9 Gratz ES, et al. *Neurology.* 1982;32:A223.
10 Zielinski JJ, et al. *Ther Drug Monit.* 1985;7:51.
11 Hansen JM, et al. *Clin Pharmacol Ther.* 1971;12:539.
12 Windorfer A, et al. *Neuropaediatrie.* 1977;8:29.
13 Lai ML, et al. *Eur J Clin Pharmacol.* 1992;43:201.
14 Sordillo P, et al. *Arch Intern Med.* 1978;138:299.

* Asterisk indicates drugs cited in interaction reports. Based on pharmacologic and pharmacokinetic considerations, similar interactions may occur with other drugs that are listed.
† Not available in the United States.

Hydantoins — *Chloral Hydrate*

Hydantoins		Chloral Hydrate
Ethotoin (*Peganone*)	Phenytoin* (eg, *Dilantin*)	Chloral Hydrate* (eg, *Somnote*)
Fosphenytoin (*Cerebyx*)		

Significance	Onset	Severity	Documentation
4	☐ Rapid	☐ Major	☐ Established
	■ **Delayed**	■ **Moderate**	☐ Probable
		☐ Minor	☐ Suspected
			■ **Possible**
			☐ Unlikely

Effects The elimination of PHENYTOIN is increased, perhaps reducing therapeutic action.

Mechanism Enhanced microsomal enzyme activity, increasing the metabolism of PHENYTOIN.

Management Monitor PHENYTOIN actions and serum concentrations if CHLORAL HYDRATE is started or stopped; tailor the PHENYTOIN dose as needed.

Discussion

A single, small study in healthy volunteers found administration of chloral hydrate and phenazone for 13 days decreased the $t_{1/2}$ of a single dose of phenytoin from 20 to 14 hours, while clearance increased from 2 to 4 hours.[1] Antipyrine $t_{1/2}$ was also decreased. Additional studies are needed.

[1] Riddell JG, et al. *Br J Clin Pharmacol.* 1980;9(1):118P.

* Asterisk indicates drugs cited in interaction reports. Based on pharmacologic and pharmacokinetic considerations, similar interactions may occur with other drugs that are listed.

Hydantoins — *Chloramphenicol*

Hydantoins		Chloramphenicol
Ethotoin (*Peganone*)	Phenytoin* (eg, *Dilantin*)	Chloramphenicol* (eg, *Chloromycetin*)
Fosphenytoin* (*Cerebyx*)		

Significance	Onset	Severity	Documentation
2	☐ Rapid	☐ Major	☐ Established
	■ **Delayed**	■ **Moderate**	☐ Probable
		☐ Minor	■ **Suspected**
			☐ Possible
			☐ Unlikely

Effects Increased serum PHENYTOIN concentrations with potential toxicity. CHLORAMPHENICOL concentrations also may change.

Mechanism Alteration in PHENYTOIN metabolism.

Management If CHLORAMPHENICOL must be used in a patient taking PHENYTOIN, closely monitor serum concentrations of both drugs and adjust the dose as needed.

Discussion

Concurrent chloramphenicol increased serum phenytoin concentrations in several patients, often with symptoms of phenytoin toxicity.[1-8] A retrospective study discovered patients taking phenytoin and chloramphenicol had a greater incidence of phenytoin toxicity than patients taking phenytoin and tetracycline or taking chloramphenicol.[9] Although no specific studies have been done, it is likely chloramphenicol interferes with the phenytoin metabolism.[4,9-11]

Two studies have examined the effect of phenytoin on chloramphenicol with conflicting results.[10,12] In 1 patient, chloramphenicol peak and trough concentrations were decreased by phenytoin.[12] In the other study, all 11 patients receiving phenytoin and chloramphenicol had potentially toxic peak chloramphenicol serum concentrations compared with 9 of 17 patients receiving chloramphenicol alone.[10] Phenytoin may have complex effects on chloramphenicol by inducing hepatic microsomal enzymes and competing for binding in hepatocytes.

[1] Christensen LK, et al. *Lancet.* 1969;2(7635):1397.
[2] Ballek RE, et al. *Lancet.* 1973;1(7795):150.
[3] Houghton GW, et al. *Int J Clin Pharmacol Biopharm.* 1975;12(1-2):210.
[4] Rose JQ, et al. *JAMA.* 1977;237(24):2630.
[5] Koup JR, et al. *Clin Pharmacol Ther.* 1978;24(5):571.
[6] Vincent FM, et al. *Ann Neurol.* 1978;3(5):469.
[7] Greenlaw CW. *Drug Intell Clin Pharm.* 1979;13:609.
[8] Saltiel M, et al. *Drug Intell Clin Pharm.* 1980;14:221.
[9] Harper JM, et al. *Drug Intell Clin Pharm.* 1979;13:425.
[10] Krasinski K, et al. *Pediatr Infect Dis.* 1982;1(4):232.
[11] Ogutu BR, et al. *Br J Clin Pharmacol.* 2002;54(6):635.
[12] Powell DA, et al. *J Pediatr.* 1981;98(6):1001.

* Asterisk indicates drugs cited in interaction reports. Based on pharmacologic and pharmacokinetic considerations, similar interactions may occur with other drugs that are listed.

Hydantoins		***Chlorpheniramine***
Fosphenytoin (*Cerebyx*)	Phenytoin* (eg, *Dilantin*)	Chlorpheniramine* (eg, *Chlor-Trimeton*)

Significance	Onset	Severity	Documentation
4	☐ Rapid ■ **Delayed**	☐ Major ■ **Moderate** ☐ Minor	☐ Established ☐ Probable ☐ Suspected ■ **Possible** ☐ Unlikely

Effects Serum PHENYTOIN levels may be increased, resulting in an increase in the pharmacologic and toxic effects.

Mechanism Inhibition of hepatic metabolism of PHENYTOIN by CHLORPHENIRAMINE is suspected.

Management Consider monitoring serum PHENYTOIN levels and observing patients for PHENYTOIN toxicity or a decrease in PHENYTOIN activity if CHLORPHENIRAMINE is started or stopped. Adjust the PHENYTOIN dosage as needed.

Discussion

A 17-year-old girl with a history of generalized tonic-clonic and psychomotor seizures developed drowsiness, ataxia, diplopia, tinnitus, and occipital headaches with vomiting while receiving phenytoin 100 mg 3 times daily, chlorpheniramine 4 mg 3 times daily, and phenobarbital 30 mg 2 times daily.[1] Chlorpheniramine was stopped and both anticonvulsants were continued. Plasma levels of phenytoin were in the toxic range while the patient received all 3 drugs. Phenytoin levels decreased to within the therapeutic range after chlorpheniramine was discontinued, and the dosage of phenytoin was lowered to 50 mg 3 times daily. Neurologic signs and symptoms resolved with the fall in plasma phenytoin levels. A 28-year-old woman with a 10-year history of epilepsy was being maintained with several anticonvulsants, including phenytoin 250 mg/day.[2] The patient developed symptoms of phenytoin toxicity following the addition of chlorpheniramine 12 to 16 mg/day to her treatment regimen. Symptoms resolved after the antihistamine was discontinued.

Controlled studies are needed to confirm this drug interaction and to assess the clinical consequences.

[1] Pugh RN, et al. *Br J Clin Pharmacol.* 1975;2(2):173.

[2] Ahmad S, et al. *J Neurol Neurosurg Psychiatry.* 1975;38(3):225.

* Asterisk indicates drugs cited in interaction reports. Based on pharmacologic and pharmacokinetic considerations, similar interactions may occur with other drugs that are listed.

Hydantoins — Cimetidine

Ethotoin (*Peganone*)	Phenytoin* (eg, *Dilantin*)	Cimetidine* (eg, *Tagamet*)
Fosphenytoin (*Cerebyx*)		

Significance	Onset	Severity	Documentation
2	☐ Rapid	☐ Major	■ **Established**
	■ **Delayed**	■ **Moderate**	☐ Probable
		☐ Minor	☐ Suspected
			☐ Possible
			☐ Unlikely

Effects Serum HYDANTOIN levels may be elevated, increasing the pharmacologic effects.

Mechanism Inhibition of hepatic metabolism by CIMETIDINE.

Management Monitor serum HYDANTOIN levels and observe the patient's response when starting or stopping CIMETIDINE. Adjust the HYDANTOIN dosage as needed.

Discussion

In studies and case reports involving epileptic patients receiving treatment with phenytoin, coadministration of cimetidine consistently produced an increase in serum phenytoin levels[1-6] and symptoms of phenytoin toxicity were observed in some patients.[1,3-5] Similar findings, with levels increased by as much as 140%,[7] were observed during retrospective chart review of inpatients receiving cimetidine and phenytoin concomitantly,[8] in nonepileptic patients given phenytoin for neurological or cardiovascular indications,[9] and in healthy volunteers receiving cimetidine (400 to 2,400 mg/day) and phenytoin (250 or 500 mg as single doses).[7,10,11] There is evidence that the increase in serum phenytoin level is dose-dependent.[7] One study of 9 stable phenytoin-treated patients did not find an interaction with cimetidine 200 mg twice daily for 2 weeks.[12]

Increased incidence of agranulocytosis during coadministration of cimetidine and phenytoin has been postulated; however, additional documentation is needed.[13,14] Ranitidine (eg, *Zantac*) and famotidine (eg, *Pepcid*) do not appear to interact with phenytoin,[3,15] although in 1 case, following phenytoin discontinuation, ranitidine delayed the decrease in phenytoin concentration.[16] Controlled studies are needed to clarify this interaction.

1 Hetzel DJ, et al. *Br Med J.* 1981;282(6275):1512.
2 Algozzine GJ, et al. *Ann Intern Med.* 1981;95(2):244.
3 Watts RW, et al. *Br J Clin Pharmacol.* 1983;15(4):499.
4 Salem RB, et al. *Epilepsia.* 1983;24(3):284.
5 Phillips P, et al. *Med J Aust.* 1984;141(9):602.
6 Levine M, et al. *Neurology.* 1985;35(4):562.
7 Bartle WR, et al. *Clin Pharmacol Ther.* 1983;33(5):649.
8 Griffin JW, et al. *Am J Med.* 1984;77(5B):85.
9 Neuvonen PJ, et al. *Eur J Clin Pharmacol.* 1981;21(3):215.
10 Frigo GM, et al. *Eur J Clin Pharmacol.* 1983;25(1):135.
11 Iteogu MO, et al. *Clin Pharm.* 1983;2(4):302.
12 Rafi JA, et al. *Ann Pharmacother.* 1999;33(7-8):769.
13 Al-Kawas FH, et al. *Ann Intern Med.* 1979;90(6):992.
14 Sazie E, et al. *Ann Intern Med.* 1980;93(1):151.
15 Sambol NC, et al. *Br J Clin Pharmacol.* 1989;27(1):83.
16 Tse CS, et al. *Ann Pharmacother.* 1993;27(12):1448.

* Asterisk indicates drugs cited in interaction reports. Based on pharmacologic and pharmacokinetic considerations, similar interactions may occur with other drugs that are listed.
† Not available in the United States.

Hydantoins | **Colesevelam**

Ethotoin (*Peganone*)	Phenytoin* (eg, *Dilantin*)	Colesevelam* (*Welchol*)

Significance	Onset	Severity	Documentation
2	□ Rapid ■ **Delayed**	□ Major ■ **Moderate** □ Minor	□ Established □ Probable ■ **Suspected** □ Possible □ Unlikely

Effects The therapeutic efficacy of HYDANTOINS may be reduced.

Mechanism COLESEVELAM may bind with HYDANTOINS in the GI tract, decreasing HYDANTOIN absorption.

Management Administer HYDANTOINS at least 4 hours prior to COLESEVELAM.[1] Monitor PHENYTOIN concentrations and the clinical response. Adjust the PHENYTOIN dose as needed.

Discussion

Increased seizure activity or decreased phenytoin concentrations have been reported in patients receiving colesevelam during postmarketing experience. Because these reports are voluntary and from a population of uncertain size, it is not possible to reliably estimate the frequency or establish a causal relationship to drug exposure.[1]

[1] *Welchol* [package insert]. Parsippany, NJ: Daiichi Sakyo Inc; February 2010.

* Asterisk indicates drugs cited in interaction reports. Based on pharmacologic and pharmacokinetic considerations, similar interactions may occur with other drugs that are listed.

Hydantoins — *Diazoxide*

Fosphenytoin (*Cerebyx*)	Phenytoin* (eg, *Dilantin*)	Diazoxide* (*Proglycem*)

Significance	Onset	Severity	Documentation
2	□ Rapid ■ **Delayed**	□ Major ■ **Moderate** □ Minor	□ Established □ Probable ■ **Suspected** □ Possible □ Unlikely

Effects PHENYTOIN serum levels may be decreased, resulting in a possible decrease in the anticonvulsant actions of PHENYTOIN.

Mechanism Increased PHENYTOIN metabolism is suspected.

Management Monitor PHENYTOIN serum levels and observe patients for a decrease in PHENYTOIN activity or an increase in toxicity if DIAZOXIDE is added to or discontinued from the treatment regimen. Tailor the PHENYTOIN dosage as needed.

Discussion

Two children being treated for hypoglycemia and convulsions with diazoxide and phenytoin experienced subtherapeutic serum phenytoin levels and inadequate seizure control despite large dosages of phenytoin 17 and 29 mg/kg/day, respectively.[1] Following discontinuation of diazoxide, therapeutic phenytoin serum levels were achieved with dosages of 6.6 and 10 mg/kg/day, respectively. When diazoxide administration was stopped following subtotal pancreatectomy in 1 patient, phenytoin toxicity occurred with doses of phenytoin that had previously failed to produce therapeutic serum concentrations. Under controlled conditions, serum phenytoin levels decreased to undetectable levels after reinstituting diazoxide administration. A similar case was reported in a boy 5 and ½ years of age treated with diazoxide (10 mg/kg/day for 4.5 years) for hypoglycemia and with phenytoin 5 mg/kg/day for convulsions.[2] In addition, the patient experienced symptomatic hypoglycemia when phenytoin was coadministered with diazoxide, which reversed when phenytoin was discontinued.

Additional studies are warranted.

[1] Roe TF, et al. *J Pediatr.* 1975;87(3):480.

[2] Petro DJ, et al. *J Pediatr.* 1976;89(2):331.

* Asterisk indicates drugs cited in interaction reports. Based on pharmacologic and pharmacokinetic considerations, similar interactions may occur with other drugs that are listed.

Hydantoins — *Disulfiram*

Ethotoin (*Peganone*)	Phenytoin* (eg, *Dilantin*)	Disulfiram* (*Antabuse*)
Fosphenytoin (*Cerebyx*)		

Significance	Onset	Severity	Documentation
2	■ **Rapid**	□ Major	■ **Established**
	□ Delayed	■ **Moderate**	□ Probable
		□ Minor	□ Suspected
			□ Possible
			□ Unlikely

Effects Serum HYDANTOIN levels may be increased, resulting in an increase in the pharmacologic and toxic effects of HYDANTOINS.

Mechanism DISULFIRAM inhibits the hepatic microsomal enzyme metabolism of HYDANTOINS. In addition, DISULFIRAM may interfere with the rate of elimination of HYDANTOINS by noncompetitive mechanisms.

Management Monitor serum HYDANTOIN levels and observe patients for HYDANTOIN toxicity or a decrease in HYDANTOIN activity if DISULFIRAM is added to or discontinued from the treatment regimen. Adjust the HYDANTOIN dosage as needed.

Discussion

Several studies and case histories have demonstrated that disulfiram coadministration significantly increases serum phenytoin levels, which may result in phenytoin toxicity.[1-7] In a study of 4 epileptic patients receiving long-term treatment with phenytoin, coadministration of disulfiram produced a 100% to 500% increase in serum phenytoin levels.[2] The rise was rapid, occurring within 4 hours of the first dose of disulfiram. Phenytoin levels increased throughout the 9-day course of therapy and continued to rise for several days after disulfiram was discontinued. In another investigation, a 73% increase in the $t_{1/2}$ and a 34% decrease in the metabolic clearance rate of phenytoin were observed in 5 volunteers following the coadministration of disulfiram.[4]

1 Kiorboe E. *Epilepsia.* 1966;7(3):246.
2 Olesen OV. *Acta Pharmacol Toxicol.* 1966;24(4):317.
3 Olesen OV. *Arch Neurol.* 1967;16(6):642.
4 Svendsen TL, et al. *Eur J Clin Pharmacol.* 1976;9(5-6):439.
5 Taylor JW, et al. *Am J Hosp Pharm.* 1981;38(1):93.
6 Brown CG, et al. *Ann Emerg Med.* 1983;12(5):310.
7 Taylor JW, et al. *Drug Intell Clin Pharm.* 1984;18:499.

* Asterisk indicates drugs cited in interaction reports. Based on pharmacologic and pharmacokinetic considerations, similar interactions may occur with other drugs that are listed.

Hydantoins			***Erlotinib***
Ethotoin (*Peganone*) Fosphenytoin (*Cerebyx*)	Phenytoin* (eg, *Dilantin*)	Erlotinib* (*Tarceva*)	

Significance	Onset	Severity	Documentation
2	□ Rapid ■ **Delayed**	□ Major ■ **Moderate** □ Minor	□ Established □ Probable ■ **Suspected** □ Possible □ Unlikely

Effects

HYDANTOIN concentrations may be elevated, increasing the pharmacologic effects and adverse reactions. Plasma levels of ERLOTINIB may be reduced, decreasing the efficacy.

Mechanism

The mechanism for the increase in HYDANTOIN levels is unknown; however, HYDANTOINS increase the metabolism (CYP3A4) of ERLOTINIB.

Management

Use of alternative treatment that lacks CYP3A4-inducing activity is recommended.[1] If alternative therapy is not available, consider increasing the ERLOTINIB starting dose at 2-wk intervals. If the dose of ERLOTINIB is adjusted upward, reduce to the indicated starting dose immediately after stopping the HYDANTOIN. In addition, monitor HYDANTOIN concentrations and observe the clinical response of patients when starting, stopping, or changing the ERLOTINIB dose. Adjust the HYDANTOIN dose as needed.

Discussion

Elevated phenytoin levels were reported in a 52-year-old woman receiving phenytoin 100 mg twice daily after starting therapy with erlotinib 150 mg daily.[2] Phenytoin was prescribed after the patient, who was being treated for cancer, developed headache and focal seizures in her right hand. Her cancer progressed and erlotinib was added to her treatment regimen. Two weeks later, her phenytoin concentration increased from 5 to 6 mg/dL to 19.81 mg/dL. The phenytoin dosage was reduced to 100 or 200 mg daily on alternate days. Over the next 2 weeks, the phenytoin serum concentration increased to 25.3 mg/dL. She developed dysarthria, poor balance, and ataxia. Phenytoin was withheld for 3 days and the serum level decreased to 16 mg/dL. The phenytoin dosage was reduced to 100 mg/day and, after 3 weeks, her phenytoin level was 13.48 mg/dL.

Because erlotinib is metabolized by CYP3A4, inducers of this isozyme are expected to decrease erlotinib plasma concentrations.[1] This is supported by a 67% to 80% decrease in the erlotinib AUC when coadministered with rifampin (eg, *Rifadin*), a drug that induces the CYP3A4 isozyme.[1]

[1] *Tarceva* [package insert]. Melville, NY: OSI Pharmaceuticals; March 2007.

[2] Grenader T, et al. *Lung Cancer*. 2007;57(3):404.

* Asterisk indicates drugs cited in interaction reports. Based on pharmacologic and pharmacokinetic considerations, similar interactions may occur with other drugs that are listed.

Hydantoins — *Felbamate*

Ethotoin (*Peganone*)	Phenytoin* (eg, *Dilantin*)	Felbamate* (*Felbatol*)
Fosphenytoin (eg, *Cerebyx*)		

Significance	Onset	Severity	Documentation
2	☐ Rapid	☐ Major	☐ Established
	■ **Delayed**	■ **Moderate**	■ **Probable**
		☐ Minor	☐ Suspected
			☐ Possible
			☐ Unlikely

Effects Serum HYDANTOIN concentrations may be increased, possibly resulting in an increase in the pharmacologic and toxic effects of HYDANTOINS. PHENYTOIN also may decrease FELBAMATE concentrations.

Mechanism Inhibition of HYDANTOIN metabolism by FELBAMATE is suspected. In addition, PHENYTOIN may increase the metabolism of FELBAMATE.

Management During any change in drug therapy, monitor HYDANTOIN and FELBAMATE concentrations and observe for changes in seizure control. In addition, observe for HYDANTOIN toxicity if FELBAMATE is added to the treatment schedule. When adding FELBAMATE to PHENYTOIN therapy, consider reducing the PHENYTOIN dose approximately 20%.

Discussion

In patients with epilepsy stabilized on phenytoin and carbamazepine, the addition of felbamate to the therapeutic regimen caused an increase in serum phenytoin concentrations and a decrease in plasma carbamazepine levels.[1-3] While receiving felbamate therapy, patients usually required a 10% to 30% reduction in phenytoin dosage. When the dose of felbamate is tapered, serum phenytoin concentrations may decrease, and it may be necessary to increase the dose of phenytoin to maintain adequate seizure control.[1] There is wide interindividual variation in the pharmacokinetic effects of this interaction.

Phenytoin also increases felbamate clearance, decreasing serum concentrations of felbamate.[4]

[1] Fuerst RH, et al. *Epilepsia.* 1988;29(4):488.
[2] Graves NM, et al. *Epilepsia.* 1989;30(2):225.
[3] Sachdeo R, et al. *Epilepsia.* 1999;40(8):1122.
[4] Wagner ML, et al. *Epilepsia.* 1991;32(3):398.

* Asterisk indicates drugs cited in interaction reports. Based on pharmacologic and pharmacokinetic considerations, similar interactions may occur with other drugs that are listed.

Hydantoins | **Fluconazole**

Ethotoin (*Peganone*) Fosphenytoin	Phenytoin* (eg, *Dilantin*)	Fluconazole* (eg, *Diflucan*)

Significance	Onset	Severity	Documentation
2	☐ Rapid ■ **Delayed**	☐ Major ■ **Moderate** ☐ Minor	☐ Established ■ **Probable** ☐ Suspected ☐ Possible ☐ Unlikely

Effects HYDANTOIN serum concentrations may be increased, producing an increase in the pharmacologic and toxic effects of HYDANTOINS.

Mechanism FLUCONAZOLE may inhibit the hepatic metabolism of HYDANTOINS.

Management Monitor HYDANTOIN serum concentrations and observe for HYDANTOIN toxicity or a decrease in HYDANTOIN activity if FLUCONAZOLE is started or stopped. Adjust the HYDANTOIN dosage as needed.

Discussion

In a placebo-controlled study, the effects of fluconazole 200 mg/day on the AUC of a single dose of phenytoin 250 mg IV were studied in 19 healthy volunteers.[1] Coadministration of fluconazole and phenytoin produced a mean increase of 75% in phenytoin AUC. In a similar study of 20 healthy volunteers, coadministration of fluconazole 200 mg/day and phenytoin 200 mg orally for 2 days followed by a single dose of 250 mg IV produced a mean increase of 75% in AUC and an increase of 128% in the minimum plasma phenytoin level.[2] In a placebo-controlled study, 9 healthy volunteers received fluconazole 400 mg/day, ketoconazole (eg, *Nizoral*) 400 mg/day, or placebo for 6 days.[3] A single oral dose of phenytoin 250 mg was given on day 5. At 48 hours, phenytoin serum levels during fluconazole administration were 132% higher than with placebo, and there was a 33% increase in the phenytoin AUC. By contrast, ketoconazole did not produce a change in phenytoin pharmacokinetics. Four patients developed increased phenytoin serum levels and symptoms of phenytoin toxicity following the addition of fluconazole to their treatment regimens.[4-6] A 59-year-old woman, who was a CYP2C9 fast metabolizer, developed phenytoin toxicity after starting fluconazole therapy.[7] See also Hydantoins-Voriconazole and Itraconazole-Hydantoins.

[1] Lazar JD, et al. *Rev Infect Dis.* 1990;12(suppl 3):S327.
[2] Blum RA, et al. *Clin Pharmacol Ther.* 1991;49(4):420.
[3] Touchette MA, et al. *Br J Clin Pharmacol.* 1992;34(1):75.
[4] Mitchell AS, et al. *BMJ.* 1989;298(6683):1315.
[5] Howitt KM, et al. *Med J Aust.* 1989;151(10):603.
[6] Cadle RM, et al. *Ann Pharmacother.* 1994;28(2):191.
[7] Helldén A, et al. *Eur J Clin Pharmacol.* 2010;66(8):791.

* Asterisk indicates drugs cited in interaction reports. Based on pharmacologic and pharmacokinetic considerations, similar interactions may occur with other drugs that are listed.

Hydantoins — *Fluoxetine*

Hydantoins		Fluoxetine
Ethotoin (*Peganone*)	Phenytoin* (eg, *Dilantin*)	Fluoxetine* (eg, *Prozac*)
Fosphenytoin (*Cerebyx*)		

Significance	Onset	Severity	Documentation
2	☐ Rapid	☐ Major	☐ Established
	■ **Delayed**	■ **Moderate**	☐ Probable
		☐ Minor	■ **Suspected**
			☐ Possible
			☐ Unlikely

Effects Serum HYDANTOIN concentrations may be elevated, producing an increase in the pharmacologic and toxic effects.

Mechanism Inhibition of HYDANTOIN metabolism by FLUOXETINE.

Management Monitor HYDANTOIN levels and observe patients for toxicity or a loss of activity if FLUOXETINE is started or stopped. Adjust the HYDANTOIN dose as needed.

Discussion

Phenytoin toxicity has been described in 2 patients following the addition of fluoxetine to their treatment schedule.[1] The first patient, an 84-year-old woman, was treated with phenytoin 300 mg/day (plasma concentration, 15 mcg/mL) following removal of a chronic subdural hematoma. Two months later, she developed a depressive syndrome. Fluoxetine 20 mg/day was started, and the dose was increased to 40 mg/day after 10 days. Five days after starting treatment with fluoxetine, she developed signs and symptoms of phenytoin toxicity. The serum phenytoin concentration was 35 mcg/mL. The doses of both drugs were reduced gradually, and the patient's signs and symptoms became normal within 4 weeks. Symptoms of phenytoin toxicity did not recur when fluoxetine was reinstated at the original dose. In the second patient, a 57-year-old woman, phenytoin 400 mg/day (serum concentration, 11.5 mcg/mL) was administered for generalized secondary partial epilepsy developing after an embolic cerebral infarction. One year later, the patient became depressed, and fluoxetine 20 mg/day was prescribed. Ten days later, she experienced signs and symptoms of phenytoin toxicity. Her phenytoin serum concentration was 47 mcg/mL. Within 3 weeks of discontinuing fluoxetine, the signs and symptoms of phenytoin toxicity completely resolved. Four weeks after stopping fluoxetine, the plasma phenytoin concentration was 20 mcg/mL. Numerous other cases of a clinically important interaction between phenytoin and fluoxetine have been reported to the FDA.[2,3] Several of these patients required hospitalization. Loss of therapeutic efficacy associated with decreased phenytoin levels were reported after discontinuation of fluoxetine.[4]

[1] Jalil P. *J Neurol Neurosurg Psychiatry.* 1992;55:412.
[2] *FDA Med Bull.* 1994;24:3.
[3] Shader RI, et al. *J Clin Psychopharmacol.* 1994;14:375.
[4] Shad MU, et al. *J Clin Psychopharmacol.* 1999;19:471.

* Asterisk indicates drugs cited in interaction reports. Based on pharmacologic and pharmacokinetic considerations, similar interactions may occur with other drugs that are listed.

Hydantoins — *Fluvoxamine*

Hydantoins		Fluvoxamine
Ethotoin (*Peganone*)	Phenytoin* (eg, *Dilantin*)	Fluvoxamine*
Fosphenytoin (*Cerebyx*)		

Significance	Onset	Severity	Documentation
2	□ Rapid	□ Major	□ Established
	■ **Delayed**	■ **Moderate**	□ Probable
		□ Minor	■ **Suspected**
			□ Possible
			□ Unlikely

Effects HYDANTOIN serum concentrations may be elevated, increasing the pharmacologic and toxic effects.

Mechanism Inhibition of HYDANTOIN metabolism (CYP2C9 and CYP2C19) is suspected.

Management Monitor HYDANTOIN serum concentrations and observe patients for toxicity or a decrease in anticonvulsant activity if FLUVOXAMINE is started or stopped. Adjust the HYDANTOIN dose as needed.

Discussion

A 45-year-old woman with a history of generalized tonic-clonic seizures was receiving phenytoin 300 mg/day.[1] Her phenytoin serum concentration was 16.6 mcg/mL. She was started on fluvoxamine 50 mg/day for depression, and ataxia was observed 4 weeks later. Phenytoin serum concentration was 49.1 mcg/mL at that time. The dose of phenytoin was gradually reduced to 200 mg/day while fluvoxamine was withdrawn. There was a progressive recovery from the symptoms of phenytoin toxicity. The phenytoin serum concentration was 24.7 mcg/mL 2 weeks after fluvoxamine withdrawal. See also Hydantoins-Fluoxetine and Hydantoins-Sertraline.

[1] Mamiya K, et al. *Ther Drug Monit.* 2001;23:75.

* Asterisk indicates drugs cited in interaction reports. Based on pharmacologic and pharmacokinetic considerations, similar interactions may occur with other drugs that are listed.

Hydantoins — *Folic Acid*

Hydantoins		Folic Acid
Ethotoin (*Peganone*)	Mephenytoin†	Folic Acid* (eg, *Folvite*)
Fosphenytoin (*Cerebyx*)	Phenytoin* (eg, *Dilantin*)	

Significance	Onset	Severity	Documentation
2	☐ Rapid	☐ Major	☐ Established
	■ **Delayed**	■ **Moderate**	☐ Probable
		☐ Minor	■ **Suspected**
			☐ Possible
			☐ Unlikely

Effects Serum HYDANTOIN concentrations may be decreased, resulting in a possible decrease of pharmacologic effects.

Mechanism Unknown. However, an alteration of a metabolic process is suspected.

Management Monitor serum HYDANTOIN concentrations and observe for decreased HYDANTOIN activity or increased toxicity if FOLIC ACID is started or stopped. Adjust the HYDANTOIN dosage as needed.

Discussion

Low folate concentrations were observed in 27% to 91% of patients receiving long-term phenytoin therapy; however, megaloblastic anemia occurred in fewer than 1% of the patients.[1-3] The effects of folic acid on the pharmacokinetics of phenytoin are conflicting. Although the majority of reports indicate folic acid decreases serum phenytoin levels in certain patients,[3-13] resulting in an increased incidence of seizures,[1,3,5,8,13] no controlled studies have demonstrated any change in seizure frequency in patients treated with folic acid compared with placebo.[6,9] In 1 study, patients showed a decrease in seizure frequency.[14] In another study, folic acid 1 or 5 mg did not change serum phenytoin concentrations with long-term phenytoin administration.[15] In most reports, the folic acid dose administered ranged from 5 mg/wk to 30 mg/day and was associated with a 7.5% to 56% decrease in serum phenytoin levels.[1,4,6-13,16] In a patient who had been seizure-free for 3 yr, decreased phenytoin levels occurred after starting folic acid.[17]

The conflicting data are expected because only certain patients appear to be affected by this interaction, and controlled studies would need to be long term.[2,18]

[1] MacCosbe PE, et al. *Clin Pharm.* 1983;2:362.
[2] Rivey MP, et al. *Drug Intell Clin Pharm.* 1984;18:292.
[3] Seligmann H, et al. *Clin Neuropharmacol.* 1999;22:268.
[4] Kutt H, et al. *Neurology.* 1966;16:594.
[5] Reynolds EH, et al. *Lancet.* 1967;1:1086.
[6] Jensen ON, et al. *Arch Neurol.* 1970;22:181.
[7] Olesen OV, et al. *Acta Pharmacol Toxicol.* 1970;28:265.
[8] Baylis EM, et al. *Lancet.* 1971;1:62.
[9] Mattson RH, et al. *Arch Neurol.* 1973;29:78.
[10] Furlanut M, et al. *Clin Pharmacol Ther.* 1978;24:294.
[11] Inoue F. *Clin Pharm.* 1982;1:372.
[12] Berg MJ, et al. *Ther Drug Monit.* 1983;5:389.
[13] Berg MJ, et al. *Ther Drug Monit.* 1983;5:395.
[14] Gibberd FB, et al. *Eur J Clin Pharmacol.* 1981;19:57.
[15] Berg MJ, et al. *Epilepsia.* 1992;33:712.
[16] Lewis DP, et al. *Ann Pharmacother.* 1995;29:726.
[17] Steinweg DL, et al. *Neurolgy.* 2005;64:1982.
[18] Yuen GJ, et al. *Clin Pharm.* 1984;3:116.

* Asterisk indicates drugs cited in interaction reports. Based on pharmacologic and pharmacokinetic considerations, similar interactions may occur with other drugs that are listed.
† Not available in the United States.

Hydantoins — *Gabapentin*

Fosphenytoin (*Cerebyx*)	Phenytoin* (eg, *Dilantin*)	Gabapentin* (*Neurontin*)

Significance	Onset	Severity	Documentation
4	□ Rapid ■ **Delayed**	□ Major ■ **Moderate** □ Minor	□ Established □ Probable □ Suspected ■ **Possible** □ Unlikely

Effects Serum PHENYTOIN concentrations may be elevated, increasing the risk of toxicity.

Mechanism Unknown.

Management Monitor serum PHENYTOIN concentrations and observe the clinical response of the patient. Adjust the dose of PHENYTOIN as indicated.

Discussion

Increased serum phenytoin concentrations have been reported in a 31-year-old male patient following the addition of gabapentin to his antiepileptic regimen.[2] The patient had a 21-year-history of epilepsy with complex partial and secondarily generalized seizures. For 2 years, the patient had been receiving phenytoin 300 mg/day, carbamazepine (eg, *Tegretol*) 1400 mg/day, and clobazam (eg, *Mogadon*; not available in the US) 20 mg/day. The phenytoin serum concentration was 42 mcmol/L (therapeutic range, 40 to 80 mcmol/L = 10 to 20 mcg/mL). Without changing the dose of these 3 drugs, gabapentin was started at 300 mg/day, and the dose was increased to 600 mg/day after 1 week. The patient reported dizziness and imbalance, and gabapentin was discontinued halfway through the second week. However, symptoms continued, and the patient experienced dysarthria, horizontal jerk nystagmus, and ataxia. The serum phenytoin concentration 1.5 weeks after stopping gabapentin was 177 mcmol/L. Phenytoin therapy was stopped for 1.5 weeks, and the serum concentration decreased to 68 mcmol/L. Upon rechallenge with phenytoin and gabapentin, the serum phenytoin concentration was 136 mcmol/L after 1 week of concurrent therapy. When gabapentin was discontinued, the phenytoin concentration decreased. A 25% increase in the serum phenytoin concentration was noted in one trial in which patients received gabapentin 900 mg/day; however, no change in serum phenytoin concentrations were found with daily doses of 300 or 600 mg of gabapentin.[1]

Additional investigations are needed to confirm this potential interaction.

[1] Crawford P, et al. *J Neurol Neurosurg Psychiatry.* 1987;50:682.

[2] Tyndel F. *Lancet.* 1994;343:1363.

* Asterisk indicates drugs cited in interaction reports. Based on pharmacologic and pharmacokinetic considerations, similar interactions may occur with other drugs that are listed.

Hydantoins — *Gamma Globulin*

Hydantoins		Gamma Globulin
Ethotoin (*Peganone*)	Mephenytoin†	Gamma Globulin* (eg, *Sandoglobulin*)
Fosphenytoin (*Cerebyx*)	Phenytoin* (eg, *Dilantin*)	

Significance	Onset	Severity	Documentation
4	☐ Rapid	■ **Major**	☐ Established
	■ **Delayed**	☐ Moderate	☐ Probable
		☐ Minor	☐ Suspected
			■ **Possible**
			☐ Unlikely

Effects The risk of HYDANTOIN-induced hypersensitivity myocarditis may be increased.

Mechanism Unknown.

Management Monitor hematologic findings (eg, leucocyte counts, especially eosinophils) and cardiac function (blood pressure, ECG abnormalities) if these agents are coadministered.

Discussion

Fatal hypersensitivity myocarditis occurred in a 43-year-old male patient during concurrent administration of phenytoin and gamma globulin.[2] He had been receiving phenytoin for 8 years and had infrequently taken acetaminophen (eg, *Tylenol*) and nizatidine (*Axid*). The patient was admitted to the hospital with symptoms of progressive pain, numbness and paresis on the legs for 5 days. He was diagnosed with Guillain-Barré syndrome and intravenous gamma globulin 0.4 g/kg daily was started. On the second day after the last administration of gamma globulin, the patient complained of abdominal pain, aching shoulders and backache. Subsequently, he developed hypotension and died. Autopsy confirmed Guillain-Barré syndrome and found hypersensitivity myocarditis.

A cause-and-effect relationship between the reaction and the coadministration of phenytoin and gamma globulin was not established. Cardiac arrhythmia may result from autonomic failure in Guillain-Barré syndrome; however, the autopsy findings suggested cardiac failure due to acute hypersensitivity myocarditis. Hypersensitivity myocarditis has been reported with phenytoin therapy as well as with numerous other drugs.[1] Because patients often receive more than one drug, establishing a causative association is difficult.[2] Additional documentation is needed to confirm this possible drug interaction.

[1] Fenoglio JJ, et al. *Hum Pathol.* 1981;12:900.
[2] Koehler PJ, et al. *J Neurol.* 1996;243:366.

* Asterisk indicates drugs cited in interaction reports. Based on pharmacologic and pharmacokinetic considerations, similar interactions may occur with other drugs that are listed.
† Not available in the United States.

Hydantoins — *Ibuprofen*

Fosphenytoin (*Cerebyx*)	Phenytoin* (eg, *Dilantin*)	Ibuprofen* (eg, *Motrin*)

Significance	Onset	Severity	Documentation
4	☐ Rapid ■ **Delayed**	☐ Major ■ **Moderate** ☐ Minor	☐ Established ☐ Probable ☐ Suspected ■ **Possible** ☐ Unlikely

Effects Serum PHENYTOIN concentrations may be increased, resulting in an increase in the pharmacologic and toxic effects of PHENYTOIN.

Mechanism Unknown. However, IBUPROFEN is suspected to inhibit the hepatic metabolism of PHENYTOIN.

Management Consider monitoring serum PHENYTOIN concentrations and observe the patient for PHENYTOIN toxicity or a decrease in PHENYTOIN activity if IBUPROFEN is added to or discontinued from the treatment regimen. Tailor the PHENYTOIN dosage as needed.

Discussion

The effect of ibuprofen administration 1600 mg/day for 7 days on the pharmacokinetics of a single oral dose of phenytoin 300 mg was studied in 10 healthy male volunteers.[2] Although ibuprofen increased the free fraction of phenytoin from a mean value of 6.9% to 7.8%, the half-life, clearance, and volume of distribution of phenytoin were not affected by ibuprofen administration. However, a 38-year-old woman taking phenytoin 300 mg/day for 5 years for grand mal epilepsy developed phenytoin toxicity and elevated serum concentrations 1 week after starting treatment with ibuprofen 1600 mg/day for degenerative rheumatic disease.[1] Phenytoin was stopped for 3 days, and ibuprofen was discontinued completely. Serum phenytoin concentrations returned to the therapeutic range within 10 days. The patient had been experiencing ataxia and nystagmus, which disappeared 3 weeks later, and truncal and head tremor, which resolved in an additional 2 weeks.

Additional studies are needed to determine if there is a clinically important interaction between these drugs.

[1] Sandyk R. *S Afr Med J.* 1982;62:592.

[2] Bachmann KA, et al. *Br J Clin Pharmacol.* 1986;21:165.

* Asterisk indicates drugs cited in interaction reports. Based on pharmacologic and pharmacokinetic considerations, similar interactions may occur with other drugs that are listed.

Hydantoins — *Influenza Virus Vaccine*

Fosphenytoin (*Cerebyx*)	Phenytoin* (eg, *Dilantin*)	Influenza Virus Vaccine* (eg, *Fluzone*)

Significance	Onset	Severity	Documentation
5	☐ Rapid ■ **Delayed**	☐ Major ☐ Moderate ■ **Minor**	☐ Established ☐ Probable ☐ Suspected ■ **Possible** ☐ Unlikely

Effects Alterations in both total and free serum PHENYTOIN concentrations have been reported following INFLUENZA VIRUS VACCINE.

Mechanism Unknown.

Management Based on current documentation, no clinical interventions appear to be needed.

Discussion

Influenza virus vaccine has been reported to increase, decrease, or have no effect on total serum phenytoin concentrations.[1-4] In each study, patients received chronic treatment with phenytoin for seizure disorders and were administered influenza virus vaccine 0.5 mL. In 1 study, 7 epileptic patients experienced a significant reduction in total serum phenytoin concentration following influenza vaccination; however, these changes were not considered clinically significant.[1] In another investigation, no change in phenytoin concentration was observed in 15 epileptic patients on day 7 or 14 after vaccination; however, a temporary increase of 46% to 170% was measured in 4 patients.[2] In 2 of these patients, the increase was attributed to influenza virus vaccine administration. In another study, patients demonstrated an increase in the mean total serum phenytoin concentration from 9.5 to 15.16 mcg/mL on day 7 after receiving the influenza vaccine.[3] These values returned to baseline by day 14. In a report involving 8 patients, a transient increase in total serum phenytoin concentration was measured on day 2 following influenza virus vaccine, but there was a gradual, prolonged reduction in free phenytoin concentration beginning after vaccination that became lower than prevaccination values by day 14.[4] No changes in seizure frequency occurred.

Because of the small number of patients in each of these studies, no conclusion can be reached. Additional research is needed to determine the effect of influenza virus vaccine on phenytoin treatment.

[1] Sawchuk RJ, et al. *Ther Drug Monit.* 1979;1(2):285.
[2] Levine M, et al. *Clin Pharm.* 1984;3(5):505.
[3] Jann MW, et al. *Clin Pharm.* 1986;5(10):817.
[4] Smith CD, et al. *Clin Pharm.* 1988;7(11):828.

* Asterisk indicates drugs cited in interaction reports. Based on pharmacologic and pharmacokinetic considerations, similar interactions may occur with other drugs that are listed.

Hydantoins — *Isoniazid*

Ethotoin (*Peganone*)	Phenytoin* (eg, *Dilantin*)	Isoniazid* (eg, *Nydrazid*)
Fosphenytoin (*Cerebyx*)		

Significance	Onset	Severity	Documentation
2	□ Rapid	□ Major	■ **Established**
	■ **Delayed**	■ **Moderate**	□ Probable
		□ Minor	□ Suspected
			□ Possible
			□ Unlikely

Effects HYDANTOIN serum concentrations may be increased, producing an increase in the pharmacologic and toxic effects of HYDANTOINS. In common therapeutic doses, phenytoin toxicity appears to be most notable in patients who are slow acetylators of ISONIAZID.

Mechanism ISONIAZID inhibits the hepatic microsomal enzyme metabolism of HYDANTOINS.

Management Monitor HYDANTOIN serum concentrations and observe patients for HYDANTOIN toxicity or a decrease in HYDANTOIN activity if ISONIAZID is added to or discontinued from the treatment regimen. Adjust the HYDANTOIN dosage as needed.

Discussion

This interaction is well established, with documentation provided from clinical studies and case reports.[1-8] The incidence of patients experiencing CNS toxicity while receiving phenytoin and isoniazid concomitantly ranges from 11% to 27%,[1,3-5] compared with 3% of patients administered phenytoin alone.[1,5] Patients who have received phenytoin 300 mg daily for years without adverse reactions have developed symptoms of toxicity after the start of isoniazid treatment.[2] Isoniazid produces a reversible inhibition of phenytoin metabolism. Phenytoin toxicity development during coadministration of isoniazid appears to occur predominantly in patients who are slow acetylators of isoniazid.[3,4]

[1] Murray FJ. *Am Rev Respir Dis.* 1962;86:729.
[2] Kutt H, et al. *Neurology.* 1966;16(6):594.
[3] Brennan RW, et al. *Neurology.* 1970;20(7):687.
[4] Kutt H, et al. *Am Rev Respir Dis.* 1970;101(3):377.
[5] Miller RR, et al. *Chest.* 1979;75(3):356.
[6] Sandyk R. *S Afr Med J.* 1982;61(11):382.
[7] Witmer DR, et al. *Drug Intell Clin Pharm.* 1984;18(6):483.
[8] Thulasimnay M, et al. *Tubercle.* 1984;65(3):229.

* Asterisk indicates drugs cited in interaction reports. Based on pharmacologic and pharmacokinetic considerations, similar interactions may occur with other drugs that are listed.

Hydantoins — *Loxapine*

Fosphenytoin (*Cerebyx*)	Phenytoin* (eg, *Dilantin*)	Loxapine* (eg, *Loxitane*)

Significance	Onset	Severity	Documentation
4	☐ Rapid ■ **Delayed**	☐ Major ■ **Moderate** ☐ Minor	☐ Established ☐ Probable ☐ Suspected ■ **Possible** ☐ Unlikely

Effects Serum PHENYTOIN levels may be decreased, resulting in a decrease in the pharmacologic effects of PHENYTOIN.

Mechanism LOXAPINE is suspected to increase PHENYTOIN metabolism.

Management Consider monitoring serum PHENYTOIN levels and observing patients for a decrease in PHENYTOIN activity or an increase in toxicity if LOXAPINE is added to or discontinued from the treatment regimen. Tailor the PHENYTOIN dosage as needed.

Discussion

Loxapine was reported to decrease serum phenytoin levels in a 23-year-old man with mental retardation receiving the drug for frequent, aggressive outbursts.[1] Initial treatment with phenytoin 400 mg daily alone produced serum levels of 10 mcg/mL. Because the aggressive outbursts persisted, loxapine 20 mg daily was added to his treatment regimen. After approximately 3 months of concurrent treatment, the serum phenytoin level was discovered on routine screening to be 6.9 mcg/mL. The dose of phenytoin was increased to 460 mg daily, and the dose of loxapine was increased to 40 mg daily. Serum phenytoin levels approximately 1 month later were 7.5 mcg/mL. A drug interaction was suspected and loxapine was discontinued. Ten days later, with no change in phenytoin dosage, serum phenytoin levels increased to 16.5 mcg/mL.

Additional studies to confirm this potential interaction and to evaluate the clinical significance are warranted.

[1] Ryan GM, et al. *Drug Intell Clin Pharm.* 1977;11:428.

* Asterisk indicates drugs cited in interaction reports. Based on pharmacologic and pharmacokinetic considerations, similar interactions may occur with other drugs that are listed.

Hydantoins			*Methylphenidate*
Fosphenytoin (*Cerebyx*)	Phenytoin* (eg, *Dilantin*)	Methylphenidate* (eg, *Ritalin*)	

Significance	Onset	Severity	Documentation
4	□ Rapid ■ **Delayed**	□ Major ■ **Moderate** □ Minor	□ Established □ Probable □ Suspected ■ **Possible** □ Unlikely

Effects Serum PHENYTOIN levels may be increased, resulting in an increase in the pharmacologic and toxic effects of PHENYTOIN.

Mechanism Unknown.

Management Consider monitoring serum PHENYTOIN levels and observing patients for PHENYTOIN toxicity or a decrease in PHENYTOIN activity if METHYLPHENIDATE is added to or discontinued from the treatment regimen. Tailor the PHENYTOIN dosage as needed.

Discussion

A 5-year-old boy with epilepsy was being treated with phenytoin and primidone (eg, *Mysoline*).[1] Methylphenidate 10 mg twice daily was added to his drug regimen to treat hyperkinetic behavior. Within 1 week after increasing the dosage of methylphenidate to 20 mg twice daily, ataxia was noted; the dosage was reduced to 10 mg in the morning and 20 mg at night, and the ataxia subsided. Phenytoin levels increased into the toxic range during coadministration with methylphenidate and did not return to baseline values until 6 weeks after methylphenidate treatment was discontinued. A 10-year-old boy experienced a phenytoin plasma level of 56 mcg/mL 1 month after the start of methylphenidate therapy.[2] The boy had headaches, nausea, and dizziness. Subsequently, he developed seizures, and both drugs were discontinued. However, in this case report, the possibility of an accidental overdose could not be ruled out. In 2 other hyperkinetic children, serum levels of phenytoin were not elevated by the coadministration of methylphenidate. In 2 subsequent studies, methylphenidate administration did not significantly alter plasma phenytoin levels.[3,4]

Because of the small number of patients involved in these reports, additional studies are needed to assess the potential interaction between phenytoin and methylphenidate.

[1] Garrettson LK, et al. *JAMA*. 1969;207(11):2053.
[2] Ghofrani M. *Develop Med Child Neurol*. 1988;30(2):267.
[3] Mirkin BL, et al. *Neurology*. 1971;21(11):1123.
[4] Kupferberg HJ, et al. *Clin Pharmacol Ther*. 1972;13(2):201.

* Asterisk indicates drugs cited in interaction reports. Based on pharmacologic and pharmacokinetic considerations, similar interactions may occur with other drugs that are listed.

Hydantoins | **Metronidazole**

Ethotoin (*Peganone*)	Phenytoin* (eg, *Dilantin*)	Metronidazole* (eg, *Flagyl*)
Fosphenytoin (*Cerebyx*)		

Significance	Onset	Severity	Documentation
4	□ Rapid	□ Major	□ Established
	■ **Delayed**	■ **Moderate**	□ Probable
		□ Minor	□ Suspected
			■ **Possible**
			□ Unlikely

Effects The pharmacologic effects of HYDANTOINS may be increased.

Mechanism Hepatic metabolism of HYDANTOINS may be inhibited by METRONIDAZOLE.

Management No special precautions appear necessary. Monitor HYDANTOIN plasma levels and adjust the dose accordingly.

Discussion

The effect of metronidazole on the clearance of phenytoin was studied in healthy volunteers.[1] Subjects received a single dose of phenytoin 300 mg IV on 2 occasions. One trial served as the control. Metronidazole 250 mg orally 3 times daily was administered beginning 4 days prior to and continuing through the duration of the study. Metronidazole increased the volume of distribution of phenytoin (0.42 to 0.49 L/kg; $P < 0.025$), prolonged the elimination $t_{1/2}$ of phenytoin (16.4 to 23.4 hours; $P < 0.02$), and reduced the total clearance of phenytoin 15% (from 0.33 to 0.28 mL/min/kg; $P < 0.005$). Because of the narrow therapeutic index of phenytoin, this effect could be clinically significant.

Additional studies are needed to assess the clinical importance of this possible interaction.

[1] Blyden GT, et al. *J Clin Pharmacol.* 1988;28(3):240.

* Asterisk indicates drugs cited in interaction reports. Based on pharmacologic and pharmacokinetic considerations, similar interactions may occur with other drugs that are listed.

Hydantoins ╳ **Miconazole**

Ethotoin (*Peganone*)	Phenytoin* (eg, *Dilantin*)	Miconazole*
Fosphenytoin (*Cerebyx*)		

Significance	Onset	Severity	Documentation
4	□ Rapid	□ Major	□ Established
	■ **Delayed**	■ **Moderate**	□ Probable
		□ Minor	□ Suspected
			■ **Possible**
			□ Unlikely

Effects Serum HYDANTOIN levels may be increased, resulting in increased pharmacologic and toxic effects of HYDANTOINS.

Mechanism MICONAZOLE is suspected to inhibit the hepatic metabolism of HYDANTOINS.

Management Consider monitoring serum HYDANTOIN levels and observing patients for HYDANTOIN toxicity or a decrease in HYDANTOIN activity if MICONAZOLE is added to or discontinued from the treatment regimen. Tailor the HYDANTOIN dosage as needed.

Discussion

Increased phenytoin plasma levels were reported in a 51-year-old man during the coadministration of phenytoin with miconazole and flucytosine (*Ancobon*).[1] The patient had been receiving phenytoin 300 mg/day for 20 years for epilepsy. Following the diagnosis of severe hemoptysis associated with pulmonary aspergillosis, miconazole 500 mg every 8 hours and oral flucytosine 2 g every 6 hours were added to his treatment regimen. Three days later, the patient developed nystagmus, which was attributed to miconazole, and the dosage of the antifungal agent was decreased to 400 mg every 8 hours; however, the symptoms persisted. One week later, the patient's plasma phenytoin level was 43 mcg/mL. Phenytoin was discontinued for 12 days, and miconazole and flucytosine were stopped for 4 days. During this time, the patient's symptoms subsided, and the phenytoin plasma levels decreased to 9.8 mcg/mL. Phenytoin therapy was reinstituted at 100 mg/day, and 20 days later, the plasma level was 23 mcg/mL. Miconazole and flucytosine therapy was discontinued again, and after 10 days, plasma phenytoin concentrations decreased to 14.3 mcg/mL.

It is not possible to determine whether flucytosine contributed to this possible interaction; however, miconazole is suspected to be the most likely cause because it is a potent inhibitor of hepatic microsomal enzymes.

[1] Rolan PE, et al. *Br Med J.* 1983;287(6407):1760.

* Asterisk indicates drugs cited in interaction reports. Based on pharmacologic and pharmacokinetic considerations, similar interactions may occur with other drugs that are listed.

Hydantoins — *Nifedipine*

Hydantoins	Nifedipine
Phenytoin* (eg, *Dilantin*)	Nifedipine* (eg, *Procardia*)

Significance	Onset	Severity	Documentation
4	□ Rapid	□ Major	□ Established
	■ **Delayed**	■ **Moderate**	□ Probable
		□ Minor	□ Suspected
			■ **Possible**
			□ Unlikely

Effects Plasma PHENYTOIN concentrations may be elevated, increasing the risk of toxicity.

Mechanism Unknown.

Management Observe the patient for PHENYTOIN toxicity and monitor PHENYTOIN concentrations when starting or stopping NIFEDIPINE. Adjust the PHENYTOIN dose as needed.

Discussion

A 57-year-old man with grand mal epilepsy was well controlled for 10 years with phenytoin 300 mg/day.[1] Four weeks after nifedipine was added to the patient's drug regimen for control of angina, he exhibited symptoms of CNS toxicity (eg, nystagmus, ataxia, dysarthria, slurred speech), and a presumptive diagnosis of phenytoin toxicity was made. The phenytoin plasma concentration was 30.4 mcg/mL. Nifedipine was discontinued. Over the next 2 weeks, the patient's symptoms improved, and the phenytoin plasma concentration was measured at 10.5 mcg/mL. Two weeks later, the patient's symptoms had completely resolved.

[1] Ahmad S. *J Am Coll Cardiol.* 1984;3:1582.

* Asterisk indicates drugs cited in interaction reports.

Hydantoins — *Nitrofurantoin*

Fosphenytoin (*Cerebyx*)	Phenytoin* (eg, *Dilantin*)	Nitrofurantoin* (eg, *Furadantin*)

Significance	Onset	Severity	Documentation
4	□ Rapid ■ **Delayed**	□ Major ■ **Moderate** □ Minor	□ Established □ Probable □ Suspected ■ **Possible** □ Unlikely

Effects Serum PHENYTOIN levels may be decreased, resulting in a possible decrease in the pharmacologic effects of PHENYTOIN.

Mechanism Unknown.

Management Consider monitoring serum PHENYTOIN levels and observing patients for a decrease in PHENYTOIN activity or an increase in toxicity if NITROFURANTOIN is added to or discontinued from the treatment regimen. Tailor the PHENYTOIN dosage as needed.

Discussion

Following surgery for a brain tumor, left-sided seizures developed in a 51-year-old man.[1] The seizures were controlled by phenytoin 300 mg/day. Upon diagnosis of a urinary tract infection, the patient was started on nitrofurantoin 200 mg/day. The next day, the patient experienced a left-sided motor seizure, and the dose of phenytoin was increased to 350 mg/day. Eight days later, the patient had another focal seizure, and the dose of phenytoin was increased to 400 mg/day. When nitrofurantoin was discontinued 6 days later, phenytoin levels increased, necessitating a decrease in the phenytoin dose to 300 mg/day.

[1] Heipertz R, et al. *J Neurol.* 1978;218(4):297.

* Asterisk indicates drugs cited in interaction reports. Based on pharmacologic and pharmacokinetic considerations, similar interactions may occur with other drugs that are listed.

Hydantoins | **Omeprazole**

Hydantoins		Omeprazole
Ethotoin (*Peganone*)	Phenytoin* (eg, *Dilantin*)	Omeprazole* (eg, *Prilosec*)
Fosphenytoin (*Cerebyx*)		

Significance	Onset	Severity	Documentation
4	□ Rapid	□ Major	□ Established
	■ **Delayed**	■ **Moderate**	□ Probable
		□ Minor	□ Suspected
			■ **Possible**
			□ Unlikely

Effects Serum HYDANTOIN levels may be increased, resulting in an increase in the pharmacologic and toxic effects.

Mechanism OMEPRAZOLE appears to inhibit the oxidative hepatic metabolism of HYDANTOINS.

Management Consider monitoring serum HYDANTOIN levels and observing patients for HYDANTOIN toxicity or a decrease in HYDANTOIN activity if OMEPRAZOLE is added or discontinued. Tailor the HYDANTOIN dosage as needed.

Discussion

In 8 healthy subjects, omeprazole increased serum phenytoin levels, prolonged the elimination $t_{½}$, and decreased the total systemic clearance of phenytoin.[1] Each subject received omeprazole 40 mg orally for 8 days before breakfast. On the seventh day, a single dose of phenytoin 250 mg was infused over 30 minutes. Omeprazole caused a small but consistent increase in the serum phenytoin level in each subject. Compared with administration of phenytoin alone, coadministration of omeprazole produced a 15% decrease (from 25.1 to 21.4 mL/kg•hr) in phenytoin plasma clearance and an average increase of 27% (from 20.7 to 26.3 hr) in the elimination $t_{½}$ of phenytoin. In another investigation, the effects of omeprazole on the kinetics of oral phenytoin were studied in a double-blind crossover trial involving 10 healthy men.[2] In random order, each subject received either omeprazole 40 mg orally or a matching placebo every morning for 9 days. After an overnight fast, a single oral dose of phenytoin 300 mg was taken on the seventh day of omeprazole or placebo administration. The phenytoin AUC was increased 25% (from 121 to 151 mcg•hr/mL) by concurrent omeprazole therapy. However, in 1 subject, the AUC decreased, while in another, the change was minimal. C_{max}, time to C_{max}, and apparent elimination $t_{½}$ of phenytoin were not significantly affected.

Conversely, in 8 epileptic patients maintained on phenytoin, omeprazole 20 mg/day for 3 weeks did not affect phenytoin plasma levels.[3] These results may reflect the lower omeprazole dose as compared with the previous 2 studies.

[1] Gugler R, et al. *Gastroenterology.* 1985;89(6):1235.
[2] Prichard PJ, et al. *Br J Clin Pharmacol.* 1987;24(4):543.
[3] Andersson T, et al. *Ther Drug Monit.* 1990;12(4):329.

* Asterisk indicates drugs cited in interaction reports. Based on pharmacologic and pharmacokinetic considerations, similar interactions may occur with other drugs that are listed.

Hydantoins | **Paroxetine**

Phenytoin* (eg, *Dilantin*) | Paroxetine* (eg, *Paxil*)

Significance	Onset	Severity	Documentation
4	☐ Rapid ■ **Delayed**	☐ Major ■ **Moderate** ☐ Minor	☐ Established ☐ Probable ☐ Suspected ■ **Possible** ☐ Unlikely

Effects Serum PHENYTOIN concentrations may be decreased by concurrent administration of PAROXETINE, decreasing the pharmacologic effects of PHENYTOIN.

Mechanism Unknown.

Management If an interaction is suspected, it may be necessary to adjust the dose of PHENYTOIN when starting, stopping, or changing the dose of PAROXETINE. Observe the clinical response of the patient. Serum PHENYTOIN concentrations may be useful in adjusting the dose.

Discussion

In vitro studies have not found paroxetine to alter the plasma protein binding of phenytoin or vice versa.[1] The effects of oral administration of phenytoin 300 mg daily for 14 days on the pharmacokinetics of a single oral dose of paroxetine 30 mg were studied in 7 subjects.[1] Phenytoin administration produced a 27% decrease in the AUC of paroxetine and a 28% decrease in the $t_{1/2}$. The effects of oral administration of paroxetine 30 mg daily for 14 days on the pharmacokinetics of a single oral dose of phenytoin 300 mg were studied in 12 subjects.[1] Paroxetine administration produced a 12% decrease in the mean AUC of phenytoin. In contrast, paroxetine did not alter phenytoin concentrations in 6 epileptic patients receiving each drug for many days.[2] Phenytoin may have caused lower paroxetine concentrations than if paroxetine had been administered alone. However, this was not specifically studied.

[1] Kaye CM, et al. *Acta Psychiatr Scand.* 1989;80(1):60. [2] Andersen BB, et al. *Epilepsy Res.* 1991;10(2-3):201.

* Asterisk indicates drugs cited in interaction reports.

Hydantoins | **Phenacemide**

Ethotoin (*Peganone*) Fosphenytoin	Phenytoin* (eg, *Dilantin*)	Phenacemide*†

Significance	Onset	Severity	Documentation
2	☐ Rapid ■ **Delayed**	☐ Major ■ **Moderate** ☐ Minor	☐ Established ☐ Probable ■ **Suspected** ☐ Possible ☐ Unlikely

Effects Serum HYDANTOIN levels may be increased, producing increased pharmacologic and toxic effects of HYDANTOINS.

Mechanism PHENACEMIDE may inhibit the hepatic microsomal enzyme metabolism of HYDANTOINS.

Management Monitor serum HYDANTOIN levels and observe the patient for HYDANTOIN toxicity or a decrease in HYDANTOIN activity if PHENACEMIDE is added to or discontinued from the treatment regimen. Tailor the HYDANTOIN dosage as needed.

Discussion

Increased serum phenytoin levels[1-3] and $t_{1/2}$[1,2] have been measured during coadministration of ethylphenacemide.[†] A phenytoin serum level in the toxic range was estimated in 1 patient when ethylphenacemide was coadministered.[3]

This interaction has not been reported with concomitant therapy with phenytoin and phenacemide, but is expected to occur.

[1] Huisman JW, et al. *Epilepsia.* 1970;11(2):207.
[2] Houghton GW, et al. *Int J Clin Pharmacol Biopharm.* 1975;12(1-2):210.
[3] Ahmad S, et al. *J Neurol Neurosurg Psychiatry.* 1975;38(3):225.

* Asterisk indicates drugs cited in interaction reports. Based on pharmacologic and pharmacokinetic considerations, similar interactions may occur with other drugs that are listed.
† Not available in the United States.

Hydantoins / *Phenothiazines*

Hydantoins	Phenothiazines	
Fosphenytoin	Chlorpromazine*	Prochlorperazine*
Phenytoin* (eg, *Dilantin*)	Fluphenazine	Thioridazine*
	Perphenazine	Trifluoperazine

Significance	Onset	Severity	Documentation
4	☐ Rapid	☐ Major	☐ Established
	■ **Delayed**	■ **Moderate**	☐ Probable
		☐ Minor	☐ Suspected
			■ **Possible**
			☐ Unlikely

Effects Possible increase in the pharmacologic effects of PHENYTOIN and a decrease in those of certain PHENOTHIAZINES.

Mechanism Unknown.

Management Monitor plasma PHENYTOIN levels and observe the patient for signs of PHENYTOIN toxicity. Tailor the dose as needed.

Discussion

Although thioridazine has no consistent effect on phenytoin levels,[1] in a study involving epileptic patients receiving phenytoin, a 44% and 33% decrease in serum phenytoin levels occurred following initiation of treatment with or increasing the dose of, respectively, chlorpromazine, mesoridazine, or thioridazine.[2] Decreasing or discontinuing the phenothiazines produced a 55% and 71% increase, respectively, in the serum phenytoin level. There was a clear trend toward toxic phenytoin serum levels when the dose of the phenothiazine was reduced or discontinued. However, 2 patients receiving phenytoin 300 mg/day experienced elevated serum phenytoin levels and toxicity during coadministration of thioridazine.[3] Both drugs were discontinued. After restarting phenytoin, therapeutic levels of the drug were maintained at phenytoin 300 mg/day. In a study of 5 epileptic patients, the addition of chlorpromazine increased the serum phenytoin level 59% in 1 patient.[4] This occurred after 1 month of therapy. In a study in which epileptic patients received multiple drug therapy, serum phenytoin levels were higher in those also treated with chlorpromazine compared with patients receiving similar regimens without the phenothiazine.[5] In 2 patients, the therapeutic effectiveness of thioridazine decreased following the addition of phenytoin to the treatment regimen.[6]

[1] Gay PE, et al. *Neurology*. 1983;33(12):1631.
[2] Haidukewych D, et al. *Ther Drug Monit*. 1985;7(4):401.
[3] Vincent FM. *Ann Intern Med*. 1980;93(1):56.
[4] Houghton GW, et al. *Int J Clin Pharmacol Biopharm*. 1975;12(1-2):210.
[5] Bielmann P, et al. *Int J Clin Pharmacol Biopharm*. 1978;16(6):268.
[6] Marcoux AW. *Hosp Pharm*. 1986;21:889.

* Asterisk indicates drugs cited in interaction reports. Based on pharmacologic and pharmacokinetic considerations, similar interactions may occur with other drugs that are listed.

Hydantoins | *Piperine*

Phenytoin* (eg, *Dilantin*)	Piperine*

Significance	Onset	Severity	Documentation
4	☐ Rapid	☐ Major	☐ Established
	■ **Delayed**	■ **Moderate**	☐ Probable
		☐ Minor	☐ Suspected
			■ **Possible**
			☐ Unlikely

Effects PHENYTOIN concentrations may be elevated, increasing the pharmacologic effects and risk of adverse reactions.

Mechanism Unknown.

Management Caution patient receiving PHENYTOIN to consult their health care provider before using herbal products or receiving other complementary/alternative therapies (eg, Ayurvedic medicine).

Discussion

Piperine is a major alkaloidal component of black pepper and long pepper. The effects of a single dose of piperine on the steady-state pharmacokinetics of phenytoin were studied in 2 groups of 10 adult epileptic patients.[1] One group of patients was receiving phenytoin 150 mg twice daily and the second group was receiving phenytoin 200 mg twice daily for at least 2 months when a single dose of piperine 20 mg was administered. Patients received the piperine dose with their morning dose of phenytoin. In patients who had been receiving phenytoin 150 mg twice daily, piperine slightly increased the phenytoin C_{max} and AUC (approximately 10% and 9%, respectively) compared with administering phenytoin alone. When piperine was given to patients receiving phenytoin 200 mg twice daily, the C_{max} and AUC increased approximately 22% and 17%, respectively. The elimination rate of phenytoin was not affected in either group. Because phenytoin has a narrow therapeutic index, additional studies are needed to determine the clinical importance of multiple-dose and long-term administration of piperine on phenytoin therapy.

[1] Pattanaik S, et al. *Phytother Res.* 2006;20(8):683.

* Asterisk indicates drugs cited in interaction reports.

Hydantoins | **Propoxyphene**

Phenytoin* (eg, *Dilantin*) | Propoxyphene* (eg, *Darvon*)

Significance	Onset	Severity	Documentation
5	☐ Rapid ■ **Delayed**	☐ Major ☐ Moderate ■ **Minor**	☐ Established ☐ Probable ☐ Suspected ☐ Possible ■ **Unlikely**

Effects Serum PHENYTOIN levels may be increased, resulting in an increase in the pharmacologic effects of PHENYTOIN. However, a clinically important interaction would not be expected with therapeutic doses of PROPOXYPHENE.

Mechanism Unknown.

Management Based upon currently available documentation, no clinical interventions appear necessary.

Discussion

In a study involving 6 patients receiving phenytoin 300 to 500 mg/day concurrently with propoxyphene 65 mg 3 times a day, slight increases in phenytoin serum levels and the AUC were observed after 1 week.[1] Additional treatment with both drugs produced a further increase in phenytoin levels. Serum phenytoin levels in the toxic range have been reported in one epileptic patient who periodically took large doses of propoxyphene (up to 600 mg/day).[2]

Additional studies are needed to determine the clinical significance of this reported interaction.

[1] Hansen BS, et al. *Acta Neurol Scand.* 1980;61:357.

[2] Kutt H. *Ann N Y Acad Sci.* 1971;179:705.

* Asterisk indicates drugs cited in interaction reports.

Hydantoins — *Pyridoxine*

Fosphenytoin (*Cerebyx*)	Phenytoin* (eg, *Dilantin*)	Pyridoxine* (Vitamin B_6)

Significance	Onset	Severity	Documentation
4	☐ Rapid	☐ Major	☐ Established
	■ **Delayed**	■ **Moderate**	☐ Probable
		☐ Minor	☐ Suspected
			■ **Possible**
			☐ Unlikely

Effects Serum PHENYTOIN concentrations may be decreased, resulting in a possible decrease in the pharmacologic effects of PHENYTOIN.

Mechanism Unknown.

Management Consider monitoring serum PHENYTOIN concentrations and observing the patient for a decrease in PHENYTOIN activity or an increase in toxicity if PYRIDOXINE is started or stopped. Tailor the PHENYTOIN dosage as needed.

Discussion

Decreased phenytoin serum concentrations were observed in patients during coadministration of pyridoxine 80 to 400 mg/day for 12 days to 4 weeks.[1] However, phenytoin serum levels did not decrease in all patients receiving pyridoxine.

Additional documentation is needed to assess the clinical importance of this possible interaction.

[1] Hansson O, et al. *Lancet.* 1976;1:256.

* Asterisk indicates drugs cited in interaction reports. Based on pharmacologic and pharmacokinetic considerations, similar interactions may occur with other drugs that are listed.

Hydantoins		*Pyrimidine Analogs*	
Ethotoin (*Peganone*)	Phenytoin* (eg, *Dilantin*)	Capecitabine* (*Xeloda*)	Fluorouracil* (eg, *Adrucil*)
Fosphenytoin			

Significance	Onset	Severity	Documentation
2	□ Rapid	□ Major	□ Established
	■ **Delayed**	■ **Moderate**	□ Probable
		□ Minor	■ **Suspected**
			□ Possible
			□ Unlikely

Effects Plasma HYDANTOIN concentrations may be elevated, increasing the pharmacologic and toxic effects.

Mechanism Inhibition of HYDANTOIN metabolism (CYP2C9) by PYRIMIDINE ANALOGS is suspected.

Management In patients receiving phenytoin, closely monitor HYDANTOIN plasma levels and observe the clinical response when starting or stopping PYRIMIDINE ANALOGS.

Discussion

Several case reports document increased phenytoin levels in a patient receiving 5-fluorouracil.[1-3] A 66-year-old man with a history of chronic schizophrenia, epilepsy, and arthritis had been receiving phenytoin 300 mg/day.[1] His medication regimen, including phenytoin, had remained stable for more than 4 years. The most recent phenytoin plasma concentration was 10.6 mcg/mL. The patient was started on IV fluorouracil 750 mg and leucovorin calcium as adjuvant chemotherapy for colon cancer. Eleven weeks after starting fluorouracil, the patient experienced unsteadiness and had fallen on several occasions. Chemotherapy was withheld, and his plasma phenytoin level was measured as 36 mcg/mL. The dose of phenytoin was reduced to 200 mg/day and later to 160 mg/day. The plasma phenytoin level decreased to 13 mcg/mL; however, the patient's gait remained slow and ataxic. Chemotherapy was resumed, and the patient remained on 160 mg/day of phenytoin. When chemotherapy was completed and discontinued, the phenytoin level was less than 1 mcg/mL. After the dose of phenytoin was increased to 300 mg/day, the plasma phenytoin level increased to 11 mcg/mL. A similar case was reported in a 50-year-old woman who experienced marked ataxia and blurred vision during coadministration of fluorouracil and phenytoin.[2] At least 4 other cases were reported in phenytoin-treated patients given 5-fluorouracil or capecitabine.[3,4] The symptoms were associated with elevated phenytoin levels.

[1] Gilbar PJ, et al. *Ann Pharmacother.* 2001;35(11):1367.
[2] Rosemergy I, et al. *N Z Med J.* 2002;115(1159):U124.
[3] Brickell K, et al. *Br J Cancer.* 2003;89(4):615.
[4] Privitera M, et al. *Anticancer Drugs.* 2011;22(10):1027.

* Asterisk indicates drugs cited in interaction reports. Based on pharmacologic and pharmacokinetic considerations, similar interactions may occur with other drugs that are listed.

Hydantoins ✕ **Quinolones**

Hydantoins	Quinolones
Fosphenytoin Phenytoin* (eg, *Dilantin*)	Ciprofloxacin* (eg, *Cipro*)

Significance	Onset	Severity	Documentation
4	☐ Rapid ■ **Delayed**	☐ Major ■ **Moderate** ☐ Minor	☐ Established ☐ Probable ☐ Suspected ■ **Possible** ☐ Unlikely

Effects Serum PHENYTOIN concentrations may be reduced, producing a decrease in the therapeutic effects.

Mechanism Unknown.

Management Monitor serum PHENYTOIN levels and observe patients for a loss of drug activity if CIPROFLOXACIN is added to their treatment schedule. Adjust the dose of PHENYTOIN as needed.

Discussion

Several cases of marked reduction in phenytoin levels and ensuing seizure activity were reported during coadministration of ciprofloxacin and phenytoin.[1-5] A 78-year-old man was hospitalized for fever and weakness caused by left lobe abscess secondary to aspiration pneumonia. Upon admission, the patient was receiving phenytoin 300 mg/day for a medical history of seizures. After a course of therapy with ceftriaxone (eg, *Rocephin*) failed, ciprofloxacin 400 mg IV every 12 hours was initiated. The patient's serum phenytoin level decreased from 14.7 mcg/mL on day 6 to 6.3 mcg/mL on day 8, and breakthrough seizures occurred. Following the seizures, the dose of phenytoin was increased to 400 mg/day. On day 9, the serum phenytoin level was 4.8 mcg/mL. When the dose of phenytoin was increased to 500 mg/day, no seizures occurred (serum phenytoin concentration, 8 to 11 mcg/mL). On day 20, ciprofloxacin was discontinued and phenytoin treatment was maintained at 500 mg/day. Phenytoin concentrations increased to 13.7 mcg/mL. A 61-year-old man receiving phenytoin 100 mg 3 times daily had a stable phenytoin level (12.6 mcg/mL).[2] Oral ciprofloxacin 750 mg twice daily was given for aspiration pneumonia. Two days later, phenytoin levels decreased to 2.5 mcg/mL, and the patient seized. His phenytoin dosage was gradually titrated to 200 mg 3 times daily. Ciprofloxacin was stopped, and the dose of phenytoin was continued upon discharge. The patient then became toxic and presented to the emergency room with a phenytoin level of 42.8 mcg/mL. Four healthy volunteers received phenytoin 200 mg/day for 14 days.[6] On day 10, ciprofloxacin 500 mg twice daily for 4 days was started. While the results of the study are limited by the small sample size, neither the AUC nor the peak phenytoin concentration were affected. However, 1 patient had a marked reduction in AUC.

1 Dillard ML, et al. *Ann Pharmacother.* 1992;26(2):263.
2 Pollak PT, et al. *Ann Pharmacother.* 1997;31(1):61.
3 Brouwers PJ, et al. *Ann Pharmacother.* 1997;31(4):498.
4 McLeod R, et al. *Ann Pharmacother.* 1998;32(10):1110.
5 Otero MJ, et al. *Ann Pharmacother.* 1999;33(2):251.
6 Job ML, et al. *Ther Drug Monit.* 1994;16(4):427.

* Asterisk indicates drugs cited in interaction reports. Based on pharmacologic and pharmacokinetic considerations, similar interactions may occur with other drugs that are listed.

Hydantoins — *Ranitidine*

Hydantoins		Ranitidine
Ethotoin (*Peganone*)	Phenytoin* (eg, *Dilantin*)	Ranitidine* (eg, *Zantac*)
Fosphenytoin (*Cerebyx*)		

Significance	Onset	Severity	Documentation
4	☐ Rapid	☐ Major	☐ Established
	■ **Delayed**	■ **Moderate**	☐ Probable
		☐ Minor	☐ Suspected
			■ **Possible**
			☐ Unlikely

Effects HYDANTOIN serum concentrations may be increased, producing an increase in the pharmacologic and toxic effects of HYDANTOINS.

Mechanism Possible inhibition of hepatic metabolism of HYDANTOINS.

Management Consider observing patients for changes in clinical response and monitoring HYDANTOIN serum concentrations when RANITIDINE is started or stopped. Adjust the dose of the HYDANTOIN as indicated.

Discussion

Elevated phenytoin serum concentrations following coadministration of ranitidine were reported in a 77-year-old man.[1] The patient had a 1-year history of severe stroke and slight right-side paralysis. Phenytoin 100 mg 3 times daily was administered for a new-onset seizure occurring 4 weeks prior to his hospital admission. The patient was discharged with a stated dosage of phenytoin 300 mg oral suspension 3 times daily. Five days after discharge, he was placed on ranitidine 150 mg twice daily. When the patient returned to the hospital because of abdominal pain, the phenytoin plasma concentration was 43 mcg/mL (therapeutic range, 10 to 20 mcg/mL). Phenytoin therapy was discontinued, but 6 days later, the concentration was 26 mcg/mL. An interaction with ranitidine was suspected, and the H_2 antagonist was discontinued. Subsequently, phenytoin plasma concentrations decreased.

Baseline phenytoin plasma concentrations were not given for this case report. In addition, the effects of phenytoin dose-dependent elimination were not ruled out. It is possible that phenytoin metabolism had approached saturation, producing increased phenytoin serum concentrations. Controlled studies are needed to confirm this possible drug interaction.

[1] Tse CS, et al. *Ann Intern Med.* 1994;120(10):892.

* Asterisk indicates drugs cited in interaction reports. Based on pharmacologic and pharmacokinetic considerations, similar interactions may occur with other drugs that are listed.

Hydantoins		*Rifamycins*	
Ethotoin (*Peganone*) Fosphenytoin (*Cerebyx*)	Phenytoin* (eg, *Dilantin*)	Rifabutin (*Mycobutin*)	Rifampin* (eg, *Rifadin*)

Significance	Onset	Severity	Documentation
2	☐ Rapid ■ **Delayed**	☐ Major ■ **Moderate** ☐ Minor	☐ Established ☐ Probable ■ **Suspected** ☐ Possible ☐ Unlikely

Effects HYDANTOIN serum levels may be decreased, resulting in a possible decrease in pharmacologic effects of HYDANTOINS.

Mechanism RIFAMPIN increases the hepatic microsomal enzyme metabolism of HYDANTOINS.

Management Monitor HYDANTOIN serum levels and observe patients for a decrease in HYDANTOIN activity or an increase in toxicity if RIFAMPIN is added to or discontinued from the treatment regimen. Tailor the HYDANTOIN dosage as needed.

Discussion

The effect of rifampin 450 mg/day on the clearance of phenytoin was studied in 6 patients with arteriosclerotic disorders and 14 patients with pulmonary tuberculosis receiving isoniazid (eg, *Nydrazid*) and ethambutol (eg, *Myambutol*) in addition to rifampin 450 mg/day.[1] Following 10 to 14 days of treatment with rifampin as the only interacting drug, phenytoin clearance increased from a mean value of 46.7 to 97.8 mL/min (109%), while the $t_{½}$ decreased from 784 to 369 minutes (53%). In patients with tuberculosis receiving rifampin, ethambutol, and isoniazid, clearance increased from 47.1 to 81.3 mL/min (73%) and the $t_{½}$ decreased from 755 to 401 minutes (47%). The volume of distribution was unchanged in both groups. In addition, no difference was measured between fast and slow acetylators of phenytoin. In an 82-year-old man with generalized seizures being treated with rifampin 600 mg/day and ethambutol 1,200 mg/day for pulmonary tuberculosis, it was necessary to decrease the dose of phenytoin from 375 to 325 mg/day after discontinuing the antitubercular treatment.[2] Prior to reducing the dose of phenytoin, serum levels had increased from 13 to 22 mg/L.

[1] Kay L, et al. *Br J Clin Pharmacol.* 1985;20(4):323.

[2] Abajo FJ. *BMJ.* 1988;297(6655):1048.

* Asterisk indicates drugs cited in interaction reports. Based on pharmacologic and pharmacokinetic considerations, similar interactions may occur with other drugs that are listed.

Hydantoins | **Salicylates**

Hydantoins		Salicylates	
Ethotoin (*Peganone*)	Mephenytoin†	Aspirin* (eg, *Bayer*)	Salsalate (eg, *Disalcid*)
Fosphenytoin (*Cerebyx*)	Phenytoin* (eg, *Dilantin*)	Bismuth Subsalicylate (eg, *Pepto-Bismol*)	Sodium Salicylate
		Choline Salicylate (*Arthropan*)	Sodium Thiosalicylate (eg, *Rexolate*)
		Magnesium Salicylate (eg, *Doan's*)	

Significance	Onset	Severity	Documentation
5	☐ Rapid	☐ Major	☐ Established
	■ **Delayed**	☐ Moderate	☐ Probable
		■ **Minor**	☐ Suspected
			☐ Possible
			■ **Unlikely**

Effects

The pharmacologic and toxic effects of HYDANTOINS may be increased by coadministration of high doses of SALICYLATES.

Mechanism

SALICYLATES compete with HYDANTOINS for attachment to plasma proteins.

Management

Based upon currently available documentation, no clinical interventions appear required. If symptoms of HYDANTOIN toxicity manifest, tailor the dose as needed.

Discussion

In vitro studies demonstrate competition between phenytoin and salicylates for protein binding sites.[1,2] This finding has been substantiated by single-dose phenytoin studies; however, no change in the free levels of phenytoin was demonstrated.[3,4] In a study involving 10 healthy subjects, the effects of increasing salicylate doses on protein binding of phenytoin at therapeutic steady-state levels were investigated.[5] The highest dose of salicylate, 975 mg every 4 hours, produced a statistically significant decrease in serum phenytoin levels and a rise in salivary concentration. The magnitude of this change was small (16%) and would not be expected to be clinically significant. No significant changes in serum or salivary levels of phenytoin were found with low or intermediate doses of salicylate, 325 mg and 650 mg every 4 hours for 48 hours, respectively. Administration of aspirin 600 mg 4 times daily to six epileptic patients maintained on phenytoin resulted in a statistically significant decrease in total serum phenytoin levels; however, saliva and free phenytoin levels were not reduced.[6] Neither loss of seizure control nor toxicity was observed. A 34-year-old patient receiving concurrent phenytoin 350 mg and aspirin 975 mg at bedtime demonstrated elevated serum phenytoin levels and mild nystagmus and serum folate deficiency.[7]

[1] Lunde PKM, et al. *Clin Pharmacol Ther.* 1970;11:846.
[2] Odar-Cederlof I, et al. *Clin Pharmacol Ther.* 1976;20:36.
[3] Paxton JW. *Clin Pharmacol Ther.* 1980;27:170.
[4] Fraser DG, et al. *Clin Pharmacol Ther.* 1980;27:165.
[5] Leonard RF, et al. *Clin Pharmacol Ther.* 1981;29:56.
[6] Olanow CW, et al. *Neurology.* 1981;31:341.
[7] Inoue F, et al. *Neurology.* 1983;33:115.

* Asterisk indicates drugs cited in interaction reports. Based on pharmacologic and pharmacokinetic considerations, similar interactions may occur with other drugs that are listed.
† Not available in the United States.

Hydantoins — **Sertraline**

Ethotoin (*Peganone*)	Mephenytoin†	Sertraline* (*Zoloft*)
Fosphenytoin (*Cerebyx*)	Phenytoin* (eg, *Dilantin*)	

Significance	Onset	Severity	Documentation
2	☐ Rapid	☐ Major	☐ Established
	■ **Delayed**	■ **Moderate**	☐ Probable
		☐ Minor	■ **Suspected**
			☐ Possible
			☐ Unlikely

Effects Serum hydantoin concentrations may be elevated, producing an increase in the pharmacologic and toxic effects.

Mechanism Possible inhibition of metabolism of HYDANTOINS by SERTRALINE.

Management Monitor serum hydantoin concentrations and observe the clinical response of the patient when SERTRALINE therapy is started, stopped or changed in dosage. Adjust the HYDANTOIN dose accordingly.

Discussion

Increased serum phenytoin concentrations occurred in 2 patients being treated for a seizure disorder upon adding sertraline to their drug treatment regimens.[1] Each patient was receiving multiple drug therapy for other conditions. Sertraline was added to their drug regimens for the treatment of depression. One patient, a 78-year-old male, was receiving phenytoin 300 mg/day when sertraline, 25 mg at night, was started. Within 1 week, the serum phenytoin concentration increased from 6.7 mcg/mL to 14.6 mcg/mL (values for this patient were corrected for hypoalbuminemia). Upon increasing the sertraline dose stepwise to 75 mg/day, the phenytoin concentration increased to 36.8 mcg/mL. Phenytoin treatment was withheld, but the serum concentration continued to increase to 47.7 mcg/mL. Subsequently, the serum phenytoin concentration decreased to 21 mcg/mL, and phenytoin was restarted at 200 mg/day, while the daily dose of sertraline was increased to 100 mg. The patient was discharged on these doses of phenytoin (non-steady-state serum concentration, 11.5 mcg/mL) and sertraline. At no time did the patient report experiencing signs or symptoms of phenytoin toxicity. The second patient, an 85-year-old male, was receiving phenytoin 260 mg/day (serum concentration, 15.6 mcg/mL) when sertraline 25 mg every other day was initiated. One week later, his phenytoin concentration was 20 mcg/mL. The phenytoin dose was decreased to 200 mg/day, while the sertraline dose was increased to 25 mg/day. Upon experiencing increasing agitation, sertraline was discontinued. No further agitation was reported. The patient's steady-state phenytoin concentration, while continuing on 200 mg phenytoin daily, was 10.5 mcg/mL. See also Hydantoins-Fluoxetine and Hydantoins-Paroxetine.

[1] Haselberger MB, et al. *J Clin Psychopharmacol.* 1997;17:107.

* Asterisk indicates drugs cited in interaction reports. Based on pharmacologic and pharmacokinetic considerations, similar interactions may occur with other drugs that are listed.
† Not available in the United States.

Hydantoins		*Succinimides*	
Ethotoin (*Peganone*) Fosphenytoin (*Cerebyx*)	Mephenytoin† Phenytoin* (eg, *Dilantin*)	Ethosuximide* (*Zarontin*) Methsuximide* (*Celontin*)	Phensuximide (*Milontin*)

Significance	Onset	Severity	Documentation
4	☐ Rapid ■ **Delayed**	☐ Major ■ **Moderate** ☐ Minor	☐ Established ☐ Probable ☐ Suspected ■ **Possible** ☐ Unlikely

Effects Serum hydantoin levels may be increased, resulting in increased pharmacologic and toxic effects of HYDANTOINS.

Mechanism Unknown. However, SUCCINIMIDES are suspected to inhibit the hepatic metabolism of HYDANTOINS.

Management Consider monitoring serum hydantoin levels and observing the patient for HYDANTOIN toxicity or a decrease in HYDANTOIN activity if SUCCINIMIDES are added to or discontinued from the treatment regimen. Tailor the HYDANTOIN dosage as needed.

Discussion

In an uncontrolled study involving hospitalized epileptic patients, mean serum phenytoin levels increased by 78% upon the addition of methsuximide to the treatment regimen.[3] In another report of 12 seizure patients, 10 patients experienced a mean increase of 43.4% in plasma phenytoin concentration during concurrent administration of methsuximide, while in two patients, serum phenytoin concentration decreased.[5] Two cases of elevated serum phenytoin levels with signs of toxicity have been reported during coadministration of ethosuximide.[1,2] In both patients, plasma phenytoin concentrations decreased when the dose of phenytoin was reduced. However, in one study of epileptic patients, coadministration of ethosuximide and phenytoin did not affect plasma phenytoin levels.[4]

Well-controlled studies are needed to determine the clinical significance of this possible interaction.

[1] Frantzen E, et al. *Acta Neurol Scand.* 1967;43:440.
[2] Dawson GW, et al. *Ann Neurol.* 1978;4:583.
[3] Rambeck B. *Epilepsia.* 1979;20:147.
[4] Smith GA, et al. *Clin Pharmacokinet.* 1979;4:38.
[5] Browne TR, et al. *Neurology.* 1983;33:414.

* Asterisk indicates drugs cited in interaction reports. Based on pharmacologic and pharmacokinetic considerations, similar interactions may occur with other drugs that are listed.
† Not available in the United States.

Hydantoins — *Sucralfate*

Phenytoin* (eg, *Dilantin*)	Sucralfate* (*Carafate*)

Significance	Onset	Severity	Documentation
2	□ Rapid ■ **Delayed**	□ Major ■ **Moderate** □ Minor	□ Established □ Probable ■ **Suspected** □ Possible □ Unlikely

Effects The anticonvulsant action of PHENYTOIN may be reduced.

Mechanism Absorption of orally administered PHENYTOIN may be reduced by coadministration with SUCRALFATE.

Management Consider monitoring the patient for a change in PHENYTOIN activity if SUCRALFATE is added to or discontinued from the treatment regimen. Tailor the dose of PHENYTOIN as needed.

Discussion

Two studies in healthy volunteers have demonstrated a significant ($P < 0.005$) decrease in phenytoin absorption as measured by the area under the concentration-time curve (AUC).[1,2] In a double-blind, placebo-controlled investigation of 8 subjects, 1 g of sucralfate reduced the absorption of phenytoin 300 mg 20%.[1] In a study involving 9 subjects, sucralfate administration decreased the AUC measured from 0 to 48 hours and 0 to 120 hours 9.5% and 7.7%, respectively.[2] However, in 2 subjects the AUC was increased.

Multiple-dose studies are needed to determine whether the extent of absorption is decreased. Although small decreases in phenytoin absorption have been observed, this change may be significant in certain patients stabilized on phenytoin.

[1] Smart HL, et al. *Br J Clin Pharmacol.* 1985;20:238.
[2] Hall TG, et al. *Drug Intell Clin Pharm.* 1986;20:607.

* Asterisk indicates drugs cited in interaction reports.

Hydantoins — *Sulfonamides*

Ethotoin (*Peganone*) Fosphenytoin	Phenytoin* (eg, *Dilantin*)	Sulfadiazine*	Sulfamethizole*†

Significance	Onset	Severity	Documentation
2	☐ Rapid ■ **Delayed**	☐ Major ■ **Moderate** ☐ Minor	☐ Established ■ **Probable** ☐ Suspected ☐ Possible ☐ Unlikely

Effects Serum HYDANTOIN levels may be increased, resulting in an increase in the pharmacologic and toxic effects of HYDANTOINS.

Mechanism SULFONAMIDES inhibit the hepatic microsomal enzyme metabolism of HYDANTOINS.

Management Monitor serum HYDANTOIN levels and observe the patient for HYDANTOIN toxicity or a decrease in HYDANTOIN activity if SULFONAMIDES are added to or discontinued from the treatment regimen. Tailor the HYDANTOIN dosage as needed.

Discussion

The effect of sulfamethizole on the metabolism of a single dose of phenytoin was studied in 8 patients.[1] Phenytoin $t_{1/2}$ increased from 11.8 to 19.6 hours (66%), and the mean metabolic clearance rate decreased from 43.7 to 28.1 mL/min (36%) during concurrent administration of sulfamethizole. In 4 patients on long-term phenytoin treatment, 1 week of sulfamethizole treatment produced an increase in serum phenytoin levels in 3 of 4 patients.

In a single-dose investigation, the effects of sulfaphenazole,† sulfadiazine, sulfamethizole, and trimethoprim/sulfamethoxazole (eg, *Bactrim*) on phenytoin $t_{1/2}$ and metabolic clearance rate were studied.[2] The phenytoin $t_{1/2}$ was increased 237%, 80%, 66%, and 39%, respectively, while metabolic clearance was decreased 67%, 45%, 36%, and 27%, respectively, by each agent. Sulfamethoxazole alone increased the phenytoin $t_{1/2}$ 15%, but did not significantly alter metabolic clearance. In an additional 17 epileptic patients, sulfonamide coadministration increased steady-state serum phenytoin levels by as much as 50%. A study of 796 patients hospitalized for phenytoin toxicity found an association with use of trimethoprim/sulfamethoxazole within 30 days prior to hospitalization (odds ratio, 2.11; 95% confidence interval, 1.24 to 3.6) compared with matched controls who did not receive trimethoprim/sulfamethoxazole.[3] See also Hydantoins-Trimethoprim.

1 Lumholtz B, et al. *Clin Pharmacol Ther.* 1975;17:(6)731.
2 Hansen JM, et al. *Acta Med Scand Suppl.* 1979;624:106.
3 Antoniou T, et al. *Br J Clin Pharmacol.* 2011;71(4):544.

* Asterisk indicates drugs cited in interaction reports. Based on pharmacologic and pharmacokinetic considerations, similar interactions may occur with other drugs that are listed.
† Not available in the United States.

Hydantoins		**Ticlopidine**
Ethotoin (*Peganone*)	Phenytoin* (eg, *Dilantin*)	Ticlopidine*
Fosphenytoin		

Significance	Onset	Severity	Documentation
2	□ Rapid	□ Major	□ Established
	■ **Delayed**	■ **Moderate**	■ **Probable**
		□ Minor	□ Suspected
			□ Possible
			□ Unlikely

Effects Plasma HYDANTOIN concentrations may be increased, resulting in an increase in adverse effects. HYDANTOIN levels may increase slowly over a 1-month period.

Mechanism Inhibition of HYDANTOIN hepatic metabolism.

Management Monitor HYDANTOIN levels and observe the patient's clinical response when the dose of TICLOPIDINE is started, stopped, or changed. Adjust the PHENYTOIN dose as needed.

Discussion

Several patients, well controlled on stable doses of phenytoin, experienced increases in plasma phenytoin levels and CNS toxicity when ticlopidine was added to their treatment regimens.[1-4] One patient, a 65-year-old man with a history of seizures, was receiving phenytoin 250 mg/day (plasma levels, 19 mg/L) and clobazam† when ticlopidine 250 mg/day was started.[1] One week later, the patient experienced vertigo, ataxia, and somnolence. The phenytoin level had increased to 34 mg/L. After reducing the dose of phenytoin to 200 mg/day, the level decreased to 18 to 19 mg/L. To determine if a drug interaction was involved, ticlopidine was stopped for 1 month, after which the phenytoin plasma level decreased to 8 mg/L. During this time, the patient experienced complex partial seizures. When ticlopidine was restarted, phenytoin levels increased to 19 mg/L within 1 month. The patient was later maintained seizure-free, without toxicity, on a treatment regimen of phenytoin 200 mg/day, clobazam, and ticlopidine 250 mg/day. A 63-year-old man, stabilized with phenytoin 400 mg/day, complained of dizziness, ataxia, and drowsiness within 3 weeks of starting ticlopidine, 250 mg twice daily.[2] His phenytoin plasma level had increased during treatment with both drugs from 19.9 to 35 mg/L and continued to rise over the next 3 days to 41 mg/L. After stopping ticlopidine and decreasing the phenytoin dosage to 300 mg/day, the patient's symptoms improved over a 2-week period. Subsequently, the patient had several complex partial seizures and complete amnesia for long periods of time. His phenytoin level was 9.1 mg/L. Ticlopidine 250 mg twice daily for 2 weeks inhibited the clearance of phenytoin in 6 patients on stable phenytoin doses (levels 6 to 12 mcg/mL).[5]

[1] Riva R, et al. *Neurology.* 1996;46(4):1172.
[2] Privitera M, et al. *Arch Neurol.* 1996;53(11):1191.
[3] Donahue SR, et al. *Clin Pharmacol Ther.* 1997;62(5):572.
[4] Klaassen SL. *Ann Pharmacother.* 1998;32(12):1295.
[5] Donahue S, et al. *Clin Pharmacol Ther.* 1999;66(6):563.

* Asterisk indicates drugs cited in interaction reports. Based on pharmacologic and pharmacokinetic considerations, similar interactions may occur with other drugs that are listed.
† Not available in the United States.

Hydantoins — *Trazodone*

Fosphenytoin (*Cerebyx*)	Phenytoin* (eg, *Dilantin*)	Trazodone*

Significance	Onset	Severity	Documentation
4	☐ Rapid ■ **Delayed**	☐ Major ■ **Moderate** ☐ Minor	☐ Established ☐ Probable ☐ Suspected ■ **Possible** ☐ Unlikely

Effects The pharmacologic effects of PHENYTOIN may be increased by TRAZODONE. Limited evidence suggests that elevated PHENYTOIN plasma levels resulting in toxicity could occur.

Mechanism Unknown.

Management If an interaction is suspected, consider lowering the dose of PHENYTOIN during coadministration of TRAZODONE. Measure PHENYTOIN levels and adjust the dose accordingly.

Discussion

A case of phenytoin toxicity associated with coadministration of trazodone has been reported in a 33-year-old man with paranoid schizophrenia and generalized seizures.[1] The plasma phenytoin level was 17.8 mcg/mL prior to the implementation of trazodone therapy. Trazodone was started at a dosage of 200 mg daily and increased to 500 mg daily. During this period, the phenytoin dosage remained at 300 mg daily. While receiving both drugs, the patient reported increasing weakness and dizziness. At this time, his phenytoin level was 46 mcg/mL. Upon reducing the phenytoin dosage to 200 mg daily and decreasing the trazodone dosage to 400 mg daily, serum phenytoin levels returned to within the normal therapeutic range and the patient's weakness and dizziness subsided.

A causal relationship was not established in this case. Lack of adequate patient data makes it difficult to draw any conclusions. Additional documentation is needed.

[1] Dorn JM. *J Clin Psychiatry*. 1986;47(2):89.

* Asterisk indicates drugs cited in interaction reports. Based on pharmacologic and pharmacokinetic considerations, similar interactions may occur with other drugs that are listed.

Hydantoins — *Tricyclic Antidepressants*

Fosphenytoin (*Cerebyx*)	Phenytoin* (eg, *Dilantin*)	Imipramine* (eg, *Tofranil*)

Significance	Onset	Severity	Documentation
4	☐ Rapid	☐ Major	☐ Established
	■ **Delayed**	■ **Moderate**	☐ Probable
		☐ Minor	☐ Suspected
			■ **Possible**
			☐ Unlikely

Effects Serum PHENYTOIN levels may be increased, resulting in an increase in the pharmacologic and toxic effects of PHENYTOIN.

Mechanism Unknown.

Management Monitor serum PHENYTOIN levels and observe patients for PHENYTOIN toxicity or a decrease in PHENYTOIN activity if IMIPRAMINE is added to or discontinued from the treatment regimen. Tailor the PHENYTOIN dosage as needed.

Discussion

An increase in serum phenytoin levels was observed in 2 epileptic patients during concomitant treatment with imipramine 75 mg daily.[1] In both patients, phenytoin levels increased during concurrent imipramine administration and returned to their original values when the antidepressant was discontinued. In one case, although the upper limit of the therapeutic range (10 to 20 mcg/mL) was not exceeded, the patient developed mild symptoms of phenytoin toxicity, including drowsiness, incoordination, and behavioral changes, which reversed upon discontinuation of imipramine therapy. In a previous study of 5 patients, nortriptyline (eg, *Aventyl*) produced a slight, but not statistically significant, increase in serum phenytoin levels.[2] In 3 patients receiving amitriptyline and phenytoin concurrently, no significant change in phenytoin elimination was measured.[3]

Additional studies are needed to assess the clinical significance of this possible interaction.

[1] Pond SM, et al. *Clin Pharmacol Ther.* 1975;18(2):191.

[2] Houghton GW, et al. *Int J Clin Pharmacol Biopharm.* 1975;12(1-2):210.

[3] Perucca E, et al. *Br J Clin Pharmacol.* 1977;4(4):485.

* Asterisk indicates drugs cited in interaction reports. Based on pharmacologic and pharmacokinetic considerations, similar interactions may occur with other drugs that are listed.

Hydantoins — *Trimethoprim*

Ethotoin (*Peganone*)	Phenytoin* (eg, *Dilantin*)	Trimethoprim* (eg, *Primsol*)
Fosphenytoin		

Significance	Onset	Severity	Documentation
2	□ Rapid	□ Major	□ Established
	■ **Delayed**	■ **Moderate**	■ **Probable**
		□ Minor	□ Suspected
			□ Possible
			□ Unlikely

Effects Serum HYDANTOIN concentrations may be increased, producing an increase in the pharmacologic and toxic effects of HYDANTOINS.

Mechanism TRIMETHOPRIM inhibits the hepatic metabolism of HYDANTOINS.

Management Monitor serum HYDANTOIN concentrations and observe patients for HYDANTOIN toxicity or a decrease in HYDANTOIN activity if TRIMETHOPRIM is added to or discontinued from the treatment regimen. Tailor the HYDANTOIN dosage as needed.

Discussion

In 8 subjects, the administration of trimethoprim plus sulfamethoxazole (eg, *Bactrim*) for 1 week increased the $t_{1/2}$ of a single dose of phenytoin 39% and decreased the metabolic clearance 27%.[1] Pretreatment of 7 subjects with trimethoprim 320 mg/day alone prolonged the $t_{1/2}$ of phenytoin 51% and reduced the metabolic clearance rate 30%; pretreatment of 9 patients with sulfamethoxazole 1.6 g/day alone increased the $t_{1/2}$ of phenytoin 15% but did not alter its metabolic clearance rate significantly. In a 4-year-old patient also receiving sulfamethoxazole plus trimethoprim, phenytoin toxicity was noted.[2] Prior to taking the anti-infective combination, the patient's serum phenytoin concentration was 62 mcmol/L (therapeutic range, 53 to 70 mcmol/L). Forty-eight hours after addition of sulfamethoxazole plus trimethoprim to the patient's drug regimen, the serum phenytoin concentration was 79 mcmol/L. Sulfamethoxazole plus trimethoprim was discontinued, and in 48 hours the serum phenytoin concentration decreased to 59 mcmol/L. A study of 796 patients hospitalized for phenytoin toxicity found an association with use of trimethoprim/sulfamethoxazole within 30 days prior to hospitalization (odds ratio, 2.11; 95% confidence interval, 1.24 to 3.6) compared with matched controls who did not receive trimethoprim/sulfamethoxazole.[3]

[1] Hansen JM, et al. *Acta Med Scand Suppl.* 1979;624:106.
[2] Gillman MA, et al. *Ann Intern Med.* 1985;102(4):559.
[3] Antoniou T, et al. *Br J Clin Pharmacol.* 2011;71(4):544.

* Asterisk indicates drugs cited in interaction reports. Based on pharmacologic and pharmacokinetic considerations, similar interactions may occur with other drugs that are listed.

Hydantoins — *Valproic Acid*

Ethotoin (*Peganone*) Fosphenytoin	Phenytoin* (eg, *Dilantin*)	Divalproex Sodium (eg, *Depakote*)	Valproic Acid* (eg, *Depakene*)

Significance	Onset	Severity	Documentation
2	□ Rapid ■ **Delayed**	□ Major ■ **Moderate** □ Minor	□ Established ■ **Probable** □ Suspected □ Possible □ Unlikely

Effects HYDANTOIN effects may be enhanced, while those of VALPROIC ACID may be decreased. HYDANTOIN toxicity may occur at therapeutic total plasma concentrations.

Mechanism VALPROIC ACID displaces HYDANTOIN from plasma protein[1-13] and may inhibit HYDANTOIN metabolism.[4,5,8] HYDANTOIN increases VALPROIC ACID metabolism.

Management Monitor the free fraction of HYDANTOIN and serum VALPROIC ACID levels. Interpret total HYDANTOIN plasma levels, considering the increase in the free fraction of the drug. Observe patients for HYDANTOIN toxicity or loss of therapeutic effects. Tailor the dose of either drug as needed.

Discussion

Valproic acid may decrease total phenytoin levels,[1,2,5-7,9,14,15] increase total phenytoin levels,[1,15,16] increase the free fraction of phenytoin,[2-7,9-13,17] and have no effect on phenytoin levels.[1,7-9,15,18] The concentration of unbound phenytoin is not altered.[2,6,7] Phenytoin toxicity has occurred with total phenytoin levels in the therapeutic range.[8,12] Nine of 11 epileptic patients on stable doses of phenytoin and valproic acid experienced increased phenytoin levels (increases of 21% to 72%) when valproic acid tablets were replaced with the same dose of a slow-release formulation.[19] Two patients experienced toxicity. Decreased phenytoin levels also were reported.[2,7,14] Phenytoin has decreased valproic acid serum levels.[10,15,18,20] Diurnal variations in protein displacement of phenytoin by valproic acid complicate this interaction.[9,13]

[1] Wilder BJ, et al. *Neurology.* 1978;28(9, pt 1):892.
[2] Mattson RH, et al. *Ann Neurol.* 1978;3(1):20.
[3] Dahlqvist R, et al. *Br J Clin Pharmacol.* 1979;8(6):547.
[4] Bruni J, et al. *Neurology.* 1980;30(11):1233.
[5] Perucca E, et al. *Clin Pharmacol Ther.* 1980;28(6):779.
[6] Monks A, et al. *Clin Pharmacol Ther.* 1980;27(1):89.
[7] Tsanaclis LM, et al. *Br J Clin Pharmacol.* 1984;18(1):17.
[8] Palm R, et al. *Br J Clin Pharmacol.* 1984;17(5):597.
[9] Riva R, et al. *Neurology.* 1985;35(4):510.
[10] Bourgeois BF. *Am J Med.* 1988;84(1A):29.
[11] Haidukewych D, et al. *Ther Drug Monit.* 1989;11(2):134.
[12] Johnson GJ, et al. *Br J Clin Pharmacol.* 1989;27(6):843.
[13] May T, et al. *Ther Drug Monit.* 1990;12(2):124.
[14] Bruni J, et al. *Neurology.* 1979;29(6):904.
[15] Henriksen O, et al. *Acta Neurol Scand.* 1982;65(5):504.
[16] Windorfer A Jr, et al. *Acta Paediatr Scand.* 1975;64(5):771.
[17] Mamiya K, et al. *Clin Neuropharmacol.* 2002;25(4):230.
[18] Reunanen MI, et al. *Curr Ther Res.* 1980;28(13):456.
[19] Suzuki Y, et al. *Eur J Clin Pharmacol.* 1995;48(1):61.
[20] de Wolff FA, et al. *Neuropediatrics.* 1982;13(1):10.

* Asterisk indicates drugs cited in interaction reports. Based on pharmacologic and pharmacokinetic considerations, similar interactions may occur with other drugs that are listed.

Hydantoins — *Voriconazole*

Ethotoin (*Peganone*)	Phenytoin* (eg, *Dilantin*)	Voriconazole* (eg, *Vfend*)
Fosphenytoin		

Significance	Onset	Severity	Documentation
1	□ Rapid	■ **Major**	□ Established
	■ **Delayed**	□ Moderate	□ Probable
		□ Minor	■ **Suspected**
			□ Possible
			□ Unlikely

Effects HYDANTOIN plasma levels may be elevated, increasing the risk of toxicity, while VORICONAZOLE plasma levels may be reduced, decreasing the efficacy.

Mechanism VORICONAZOLE inhibits the metabolism of HYDANTOINS, while HYDANTOINS induce the metabolism of VORICONAZOLE.

Management Monitor HYDANTOIN levels and adjust the dose as needed. In addition, it may be necessary to increase the dose of VORICONAZOLE during coadministration with a HYDANTOIN.

Discussion

The effects of voriconazole and phenytoin on the pharmacokinetics of one another were studied in healthy men.[1] In 1 study, subjects received voriconazole 200 and 400 mg twice daily with placebo or phenytoin 300 mg/day. Compared with placebo, phenytoin decreased the C_{max} and AUC of voriconazole approximately 50% and 70%, respectively. Increasing the dosage of voriconazole from 200 to 400 mg twice daily compensated for the interaction. In the second study, subjects received phenytoin 300 mg in the morning (days 2 to 17) with placebo or voriconazole 400 mg twice daily on days 8 to 17. Compared with placebo, voriconazole increased the C_{max} and AUC of phenytoin approximately 70% and 80%, respectively. Four patients did not achieve adequate voriconazole levels, despite doubling the dose when phenytoin was coadministered.[2,3] However, voriconazole dose adjustment and IV administration may compensate for this interaction.[4] See also Hydantoins-Fluconazole and Itraconazole-Hydantoins.

[1] Purkins L, et al. *Br J Clin Pharmacol.* 2003;56(suppl 1):37.
[2] Gerzenshtein L, et al. *Ann Pharmacother.* 2005;39(7-8):1342.
[3] Alffenaar JW, et al. *Br J Clin Pharmacol.* 2009;68(3):462.
[4] Spriet I, et al. *Br J Clin Pharmacol.* 2010;69(6):701.

* Asterisk indicates drugs cited in interaction reports. Based on pharmacologic and pharmacokinetic considerations, similar interactions may occur with other drugs that are listed.

Hydralazine — *Enteral Nutrition*

Hydralazine*	Enteral Nutrition* (eg, *Ensure*)

Significance	Onset	Severity	Documentation
4	☐ Rapid	☐ Major	☐ Established
	■ **Delayed**	■ **Moderate**	☐ Probable
		☐ Minor	☐ Suspected
			■ **Possible**
			☐ Unlikely

Effects Depending on the rate of nutrient administration, HYDRALAZINE plasma concentrations may be altered.

Mechanism Absorption and/or disposition kinetics of HYDRALAZINE appear to be altered by food and ENTERAL NUTRITION.

Management In patients receiving HYDRALAZINE and ENTERAL NUTRITION concurrently, carefully monitor the response and adjust the HYDRALAZINE dose as needed.

Discussion

The effects of food or enteral nutrition on hydralazine bioavailability were studied in 8 healthy subjects.[1] Each subject received hydralazine 50 mg as an oral solution during fasting, with a standard breakfast, with a bolus of enteral nutrients, and with slow infusion of enteral nutrients administered via nasogastric tube. The AUC and C_{max} were highest under fasting and slow infusion conditions compared with administration with the standard breakfast or enteral bolus. The rate of nutrient administration appeared to have a greater effect on hydralazine pharmacokinetics than the physical form of the nutrient. Because oral hydralazine is usually given with food, it is noteworthy that compared with the standard breakfast, hydralazine AUC and C_{max} were 2.6- and 7.5-fold higher, respectively, when administered with slow infusion enteral nutrition.

[1] Semple HA, et al. *Ther Drug Monit.* 1991;13(4):304.

* Asterisk indicates drugs cited in interaction reports.

Hydralazine ✕ *Indomethacin*

Hydralazine*	Indomethacin* (eg, *Indocin*)

Significance	Onset	Severity	Documentation
5	☐ Rapid	☐ Major	☐ Established
	■ **Delayed**	☐ Moderate	☐ Probable
		■ **Minor**	☐ Suspected
			■ **Possible**
			☐ Unlikely

Effects The pharmacologic effects of HYDRALAZINE may be decreased.

Mechanism Unknown.

Management No special precautions appear necessary. If an interaction is suspected, consider increasing the dose of HYDRALAZINE during coadministration with INDOMETHACIN.

Discussion

In a double-blind, crossover, randomized trial involving 11 healthy subjects, indomethacin decreased but did not abolish the vasodilator effect of hydralazine.[1] All subjects received oral indomethacin (four 50 mg doses) or placebo at 6-hour intervals, followed by 2 IV doses of hydralazine 0.15 mg/kg administered 30 minutes apart. During placebo administration, the initial dose of hydralazine was followed by a prompt decrease in mean arterial pressure. Following pretreatment with indomethacin, the first dose of hydralazine did not decrease arterial BP. There was a lowering of BP after the second dose of hydralazine; however, the change in BP was less than that observed during the placebo phases.

Additional studies in hypertensive patients receiving hydralazine are needed to determine the clinical importance of this possible interaction.

[1] Cinquegrani MP, et al. *Clin Pharmacol Ther.* 1986;39(5):564.

* Asterisk indicates drugs cited in interaction reports.

Imatinib — *Azole Antifungal Agents*

Imatinib* (*Gleevec*)	Fluconazole (eg, *Diflucan*) Itraconazole (eg, *Sporanox*) Ketoconazole* (eg, *Nizoral*)	Posaconazole (*Noxafil*) Voriconazole* (eg, *Vfend*)

Significance	Onset	Severity	Documentation
4	■ **Rapid** □ Delayed	□ Major ■ **Moderate** □ Minor	□ Established □ Probable □ Suspected ■ **Possible** □ Unlikely

Effects IMATINIB plasma concentrations may be elevated, increasing the pharmacologic and toxic effects.

Mechanism Inhibition of IMATINIB metabolism (CYP3A4) by AZOLE ANTIFUNGAL AGENTS is suspected.

Management Closely monitor patients and adjust therapy as needed.

Discussion

The effects of ketoconazole on the pharmacokinetics of imatinib were studied in 14 healthy subjects.[1] Using a randomized, crossover design, each subject received a single oral dose of imatinib 200 mg alone and with a single oral dose of ketoconazole 400 mg. Compared with giving imatinib alone, coadministration with ketoconazole increased the imatinib C_{max} 26% and the 24-hour AUC 40%. The apparent clearance of imatinib decreased approximately 29%. The C_{max} and 24-hour AUC of the imatinib metabolite CGP74588 decreased approximately 23% and 13%, respectively. There was no change in the $t_{1/2}$ of imatinib. Coadministration of imatinib and ketoconazole increased the exposure to imatinib 40% compared with giving imatinib alone. A severe pustular eruption and elevated imatinib plasma levels were reported in a 42-year-old man during coadministration of imatinib and voriconazole.[2]

[1] Dutreix C, et al. *Cancer Chemother Pharmacol.* 2004;54(4):290.

[2] Gambillara E, et al. *Dermatology.* 2005;211(4):363.

* Asterisk indicates drugs cited in interaction reports. Based on pharmacologic and pharmacokinetic considerations, similar interactions may occur with other drugs that are listed.

Imatinib — *Rifamycins*

Imatinib* (*Gleevec*)	Rifabutin (*Mycobutin*)	Rifapentine (*Priftin*)
	Rifampin* (eg, *Rifadin*)	

Significance	Onset	Severity	Documentation
2	□ Rapid	□ Major	□ Established
	■ **Delayed**	■ **Moderate**	□ Probable
		□ Minor	■ **Suspected**
			□ Possible
			□ Unlikely

Effects IMATINIB plasma concentrations may be reduced, decreasing the therapeutic effect.

Mechanism Increased metabolism (CYP3A4) of IMATINIB by RIFAMYCINS.

Management In patients receiving IMATINIB, closely monitor the clinical response when RIFAMYCIN therapy is started or stopped. Consider alternative agents for RIFAMYCIN therapy.

Discussion

The effects of rifampin on the pharmacokinetics of imatinib were investigated in 14 healthy subjects.[1] Each subject received a single oral dose of imatinib 400 mg alone and after 7 days of pretreatment with rifampin 600 mg once daily. Compared with administration of imatinib alone, coadministration with rifampin decreased the mean imatinib C_{max} 54% and decreased the AUC during the first 24 hr 68%, while the clearance was increased 385%. The mean C_{max} and 24-hr AUC of the main imatinib metabolite, CGP74588, increased 89% and 24%, respectively. There were large variations in the pharmacokinetics of imatinib; however, the interaction occurred in all subjects.

[1] Bolton AE, et al. *Cancer Chemother Pharmacol.* 2004;53:102.

* Asterisk indicates drugs cited in interaction reports. Based on pharmacologic and pharmacokinetic considerations, similar interactions may occur with other drugs that are listed.

Imatinib | **St. John's Wort**

Imatinib* (*Gleevec*)	St. John's Wort*

Significance	Onset	Severity	Documentation
4	□ Rapid	□ Major	□ Established
	■ **Delayed**	■ **Moderate**	□ Probable
		□ Minor	□ Suspected
			■ **Possible**
			□ Unlikely

Effects Plasma concentrations of IMATINIB may be reduced, decreasing the clinical effect.

Mechanism ST. JOHN'S WORT increases the metabolism (CYP3A4) of IMATINIB.

Management Advise patients taking IMATINIB to avoid ST. JOHN'S WORT. Caution patients not to use herbal products and IMATINIB without consulting their health care provider.

Discussion

The effects of St. John's wort on the pharmacokinetics of imatinib were studied in 12 healthy subjects.[1] Each subject received an oral dose of imatinib 400 mg on days 1 and 15, and St. John's wort 300 mg 3 times daily on days 3 to 17. Compared with receiving imatinib alone, coadministration of St. John's wort increased the clearance of imatinib 43% (from 12.5 to 17.9 L/hr) and decreased the AUC 30%, the $t_{½}$ 30% (from 12.8 to 9 hr), and the C_{max} 18% (from 2.2 to 1.8 mcg/mL). In an open-label, crossover study, 10 healthy volunteers received a single dose of imatinib 400 mg before and after 2 weeks of treatment with St. John's wort 300 mg 3 times daily.[2] Compared with taking imatinib alone, pretreatment with St. John's wort reduced the imatinib AUC 32%, the C_{max} 29% (from 1.8 to 1.28 mcg/mL), and the $t_{½}$ 21% (from 13.5 to 10.7 hr).

[1] Frye RF, et al. *Clin Pharmacol Ther.* 2004;76:323.
[2] Smith P. *Pharmacotherapy.* 2004;24:1508.

* Asterisk indicates drugs cited in interaction reports.

Indinavir — *Delavirdine*

Indinavir* (*Crixivan*)	Delavirdine* (*Rescriptor*)

Significance	Onset	Severity	Documentation
2	□ Rapid ■ **Delayed**	□ Major ■ **Moderate** □ Minor	□ Established ■ **Probable** □ Suspected □ Possible □ Unlikely

Effects INDINAVIR plasma concentrations may be elevated, increasing the pharmacologic and adverse effects.

Mechanism Possibly decreased metabolism (CYP3A4) and postabsorptive clearance of INDINAVIR.

Management Closely monitor patients and adjust therapy as needed.

Discussion

The effect of delavirdine on the pharmacokinetics of indinavir was evaluated in 14 healthy men.[1] Using an open-label design, each subject received a single 800 mg dose of indinavir on day 1, a 400 mg dose on day 9, and a 600 mg dose on day 10. All subjects received delavirdine 400 mg 3 times daily on days 2 through 10. Single doses of indinavir did not affect the pharmacokinetics of delavirdine. Compared with giving indinavir alone, coadministration of indinavir and delavirdine increased the 8-hr postdose plasma concentrations of the 400 and 600 mg doses of indinavir 143% and 414%, respectively. In 12 of the 14 subjects receiving the 400 mg dose and in all 14 subjects receiving the 600 mg dose of indinavir with delavirdine, plasma indinavir concentrations were greater than the corresponding values determined after giving 800 mg of indinavir alone.

Additional studies are needed to determine if the pharmacokinetic effects of this interaction can be beneficial in reducing the frequency of indinavir dosing.

[1] Ferry JJ, et al. *J Acquir Immune Defic Syndr Hum Retrovirol.* 1998;18:252.

* Asterisk indicates drugs cited in interaction reports.

Indinavir — *Didanosine*

Indinavir* (*Crixivan*)	Didanosine* (eg, *Videx*)

Significance	Onset	Severity	Documentation
2	■ **Rapid** ☐ Delayed	☐ Major ■ **Moderate** ☐ Minor	☐ Established ☐ Probable ■ **Suspected** ☐ Possible ☐ Unlikely

Effects The therapeutic effects of INDINAVIR may be decreased by the buffered formulation of DIDANOSINE.

Mechanism The buffers in DIDANOSINE may decrease the absorption of INDINAVIR.

Management Administer INDINAVIR and buffered formulation of DIDANOSINE at least 1 hr apart on an empty stomach. Enteric-coated DIDANOSINE is unlikely to interact.

Discussion

Gastric acid degrades didanosine; therefore, buffers are present in didanosine to increase pH. Administer didanosine and indinavir at least 1 hr apart on an empty stomach because a normal stomach pH may be necessary for optimal indinavir absorption.[1] The effects of enteric-coated didanosine on the pharmacokinetics of indinavir plus ritonavir were studied in 8 volunteers.[2] Using a crossover design, subjects received the combination of indinavir/ritonavir with breakfast and with enteric-coated didanosine with breakfast and 2 hours after breakfast. Enteric-coated didanosine did not affect the pharmacokinetics of indinavir or ritonavir. In another study, neither buffered nor enteric-coated didanosine affected the pharmacokinetics of amprenavir.[3] Amprenavir may be considered as an alternative protease inhibitor.

[1] *Crixivan* [package insert]. White House Station, NJ: Merck & Co., Inc.; 1996.

[2] la Porte C, et al. *J Clin Pharmacol.* 2005;45:211.

[3] Shelton MJ, et al. *Pharmacotherapy.* 2003;23:835.

* Asterisk indicates drugs cited in interaction reports.

Indinavir — *Food*

Indinavir* (*Crixivan*)	Grapefruit Juice*

Significance	Onset	Severity	Documentation
3	■ **Rapid**	□ Major	□ Established
	□ Delayed	□ Moderate	□ Probable
		■ **Minor**	■ **Suspected**
			□ Possible
			□ Unlikely

Effects Taking INDINAVIR with GRAPEFRUIT JUICE may delay the time to reach INDINAVIR peak plasma concentrations.

Mechanism Ingestion of INDINAVIR with GRAPEFRUIT JUICE may delay INDINAVIR absorption because of an increase in gastric pH.

Management Based on available data, a single dose of INDINAVIR can be taken safely with a GRAPEFRUIT product. However, until more data are available, it would be prudent for patients taking INDINAVIR to avoid chronic ingestion of GRAPEFRUIT products.

Discussion

The effects of double-strength grapefruit juice on the systemic bioavailability of indinavir and gastric pH were studied in 14 HIV-infected subjects.[1] Using a randomized, crossover, open-label design, each subject received an oral dose of indinavir 800 mg with 180 mL of double-strength grapefruit juice or water. Compared with water, grapefruit juice increased the median gastric pH by nearly 2 units (from 1.5 to 3.3) and slightly delayed the absorption of indinavir. The time to reach indinavir peak plasma levels was delayed from 1.12 to 1.56 hr. There were no statistically significant differences in indinavir C_{max} or AUC when indinavir was taken with grapefruit juice compared with water. The manufacturer of indinavir states that administration of a single oral dose of indinavir 400 mg with 240 mL of grapefruit juice decreased the AUC of indinavir 26%; however, no dosage modification was recommended.[2] The effects of single-strength grapefruit juice on the pharmacokinetics of indinavir 800 mg every 8 hr for 4 doses were investigated in an open-label crossover study involving 13 healthy volunteers.[3] Compared with water, grapefruit juice did not alter the pharmacokinetics of indinavir.

Additional studies are needed to determine the effect of chronic ingestion of grapefruit juice on the pharmacokinetics of indinavir. Because grapefruit juice inhibits the CYP3A4 isozyme and indinavir is a substrate for CYP3A4, investigation of the effect of grapefruit juice on indinavir metabolism is warranted.

[1] Shelton MJ, et al. *J Clin Pharmacol.* 2001;41:435.
[2] *Crixivan* [package insert]. White House Station, NJ: Merck & Co., Inc.; 2001.
[3] Penzak SR, et al. *J Clin Pharmacol.* 2002;42:1165.

* Asterisk indicates drugs cited in interaction reports.

Indinavir — *Rifamycins*

Indinavir* (*Crixivan*)	Rifabutin* (*Mycobutin*) Rifampin* (eg, *Rifadin*)	Rifapentine* (*Priftin*)

Significance	Onset	Severity	Documentation
2	□ Rapid	□ Major	□ Established
	■ **Delayed**	■ **Moderate**	■ **Probable**
		□ Minor	□ Suspected
			□ Possible
			□ Unlikely

Effects RIFAMYCINS may decrease INDINAVIR serum concentrations. In addition, INDINAVIR may elevate serum RIFABUTIN and RIFAMPIN concentrations, increasing the risk of toxicity.

Mechanism INDINAVIR may decrease RIFAMYCIN metabolism (CYP3A4), while RIFAMYCINS may increase the metabolism of INDINAVIR by inducing the enzyme.

Management It is recommended that the dose of RIFABUTIN be reduced to half the standard dose when administered with INDINAVIR.[1] Concurrent use of RIFAMPIN and INDINAVIR is not recommended. Use RIFAPENTINE with extreme caution, if at all, in patients also taking INDINAVIR.[2]

Discussion

Administration of indinavir 800 mg every 8 hours with rifabutin 300 mg once daily for 10 days resulted in a 32% decrease in the AUC of indinavir and a 204% increase in the rifabutin AUC.[1] In a study of 6 HIV-infected patients, rifampin 300 mg daily for 4 days reduced the indinavir mean blood level 87%.[3] Because rifampin is a potent inducer of CYP3A4, rifampin administration could produce marked decreases in serum indinavir concentrations.[1] In a study of 11 HIV-infected patients, indinavir 800 mg 3 times daily increased the AUC of rifampin 73%.[4] Likewise, in 2 studies of indinavir plus rifabutin administered to healthy volunteers, there was a decrease in the AUC of indinavir while the AUC and C_{max} of rifabutin increased 2.73- and 2.34-fold, respectively.[5] See also Ritonavir-Rifamycins.

[1] *Crixivan* [package insert]. White House Station, NJ: Merck & Co, Inc.; 1996.
[2] *Priftin* [package insert]. Bridgewater, NJ: Aventis Pharmaceuticals; 1998.
[3] Justesen US, et al. *Clin Infect Dis.* 2004;38(3):426.
[4] Jaruratanasirikul S, et al. *J Pharm Pharmacol.* 2001; 53(3):409.
[5] Kraft WK, et al. *J Clin Pharmacol.* 2004;44(3):305.

* Asterisk indicates drugs cited in interaction reports.

Indinavir — *Ritonavir*

Indinavir* (*Crixivan*)	Ritonavir* (*Norvir*)

Significance	Onset	Severity	Documentation
2	☐ Rapid ■ **Delayed**	☐ Major ■ **Moderate** ☐ Minor	☐ Established ■ **Probable** ☐ Suspected ☐ Possible ☐ Unlikely

Effects INDINAVIR plasma concentrations may be elevated, increasing the pharmacologic effects and adverse reactions.

Mechanism Possibly decreased metabolism (CYP3A4) and postabsorptive clearance of INDINAVIR.

Management Closely monitor patients and adjust therapy as needed.

Discussion

The effect of ritonavir on the pharmacokinetics of indinavir 800 mg every 8 hr for 3 doses or 400 or 600 mg single doses was studied in 39 healthy adult volunteers.[1] At steady state, ritonavir 200, 300, or 400 mg every 12 hr increased indinavir plasma concentrations 21% to 110% and the AUC 185% to 475% compared with administration of indinavir alone. For a constant dose of indinavir, increasing the dose of ritonavir produced similar AUCs, peak concentrations, and 12-hr concentrations of indinavir. For a constant dose of ritonavir, increasing the dose of indinavir produced proportional increases in AUC, less than proportional increases in peak concentration, and slightly more than proportional increases in the 12-hr concentration of indinavir. Intersubject variability in the AUC and trough concentrations of indinavir was reduced by ritonavir administration. In a study in HIV infected Thai patients, coadministration of indinavir 800 mg every 12 hr and ritonavir 100 mg every 12 hr increased the median indinavir AUC 135% compared with patients taking indinavir 800 mg every 8 hr alone.[2] Pharmacokinetic analysis of patients receiving indinavir and ritonavir found that ritonavir decreased the clearance of indinavir 64.6%.[3] In 19 HIV-infected children, adequate indinavir concentrations were achieved with reduced dosages of indinavir 220 to 300 mg/m^2 when boosted with either 100 mg or full-dose ritonavir.[4] This interaction is suspected to have caused hyperbilirubinemia and jaundice in a 27-year-old woman.[5]

[1] Hsu A, et al. *Antimicrob Agents Chemother.* 1998;42(11):2784.

[2] Burger D, et al. *J Antimicrob Chemother.* 2003;51(5):1231.

[3] Kappelhoff BS, et al. *Br J Clin Pharmacol.* 2005;60(3):276.

[4] Plipat N, et al. *Pediatr Infect Dis J.* 2007;26(1):86.

[5] Rayner CR, et al. *Ann Pharmacother.* 2001;35(11):1391.

* Asterisk indicates drugs cited in interaction reports.

Indomethacin — *Antacids*

Indomethacin* (eg, *Indocin*)	Aluminum Hydroxide/Magnesium Hydroxide* (eg, *Maalox*)

Significance	Onset	Severity	Documentation
5	☐ Rapid	☐ Major	☐ Established
	■ **Delayed**	☐ Moderate	☐ Probable
		■ **Minor**	☐ Suspected
			■ **Possible**
			☐ Unlikely

Effects The therapeutic actions of INDOMETHACIN may be reduced.

Mechanism It is suspected that INDOMETHACIN'S GI absorption may be reduced by ANTACIDS.

Management Based upon currently available documentation, no clinical interventions appear required.

Discussion

While aluminum-magnesium-containing antacids have been reported to delay the rate of indomethacin absorption[1,2] and increase[1] and decrease its bioavailability,[2,3] sodium bicarbonate has been documented to enhance the rate of the GI absorption of indomethacin.[2]

Additional studies are needed to assess the clinical importance of this possible interaction and determine how other antacids may affect the absorption of indomethacin.

[1] Emori HW, et al. *Ann Rheum Dis.* 1976;35:333.
[2] Garnham JC, et al. *Postgrad Med J.* 1977;53:126.
[3] Galeazzi RL. *Eur J Clin Pharmacol.* 1977;12:65.

* Asterisk indicates drugs cited in interaction reports.

Indomethacin — *Diflunisal*

Indomethacin* (eg, *Indocin*)	Diflunisal*

Significance	Onset	Severity	Documentation
4	☐ Rapid	☐ Major	☐ Established
	■ **Delayed**	■ **Moderate**	☐ Probable
		☐ Minor	☐ Suspected
			■ **Possible**
			☐ Unlikely

Effects Plasma levels of INDOMETHACIN may be increased, producing an increase in the incidence and severity of adverse reactions.

Mechanism Unknown. However, DIFLUNISAL is suspected of inhibiting the metabolism of INDOMETHACIN.

Management Consider observing the patient for an increase in INDOMETHACIN toxicity if DIFLUNISAL is added to the treatment regimen.

Discussion

In an open, randomized trial involving 2 parallel groups of 8 volunteers, a pharmacokinetic interaction was demonstrated during coadministration of diflunisal 500 mg twice daily and indomethacin 50 mg twice daily.[1] Patients received 7 days of indomethacin or diflunisal, followed by 7 days of coadministration of both drugs, then 7 days of indomethacin administration alone. The steady-state plasma concentration and AUC of indomethacin were increased 2- to 3-fold during coadministration of diflunisal, while both total clearance and volume of distribution were decreased. The urinary recovery of unchanged and total indomethacin over 1 dosage interval was also decreased. In addition, the number of CNS and GI adverse reactions during the periods when indomethacin was administered alone were 20 and 15, compared with an incidence of 24 and 113 when combined dosing of indomethacin and diflunisal was preceded by 7 days of administration of indomethacin or diflunisal, respectively. The highest plasma levels of indomethacin were measured in the latter group of subjects. Subjective adverse reactions (eg, sleepiness, headache, light-headedness, dizziness) were more intense and of a longer duration during combined treatment with both drugs compared with administration of indomethacin alone.

[1] Van Hecken A, et al. *Eur J Clin Pharmacol.* 1989;36(5):507.

* Asterisk indicates drugs cited in interaction reports.

Influenza Virus Vaccine, Intranasal — *Aspirin*

Influenza Virus Vaccine, Intranasal* (eg, *Influenza [H1N1] virus vaccine*)	Aspirin* (eg, *Norwich Extra-Strength*)

Significance	Onset	Severity	Documentation
1	■ **Rapid**	■ **Major**	□ Established
	□ Delayed	□ Moderate	□ Probable
		□ Minor	■ **Suspected**
			□ Possible
			□ Unlikely

Effects Risk of Reye syndrome may be increased.

Mechanism Unknown.

Management INTRANASAL FLU VACCINE is contraindicated in children and adolescents on aspirin therapy.

Discussion

Because of the association of Reye syndrome with aspirin and wild-type influenza infection, intranasal influenza virus vaccines are contraindicated in children and adolescents (2 to 17 years of age) on aspirin therapy.[1]

The basis for this monograph is information on file with the manufacturer. Because of the seriousness of the possible reaction, clinical evaluation of this interaction in children and adolescents is not likely to be forthcoming.

[1] *Influenza Virus Vaccine, Intranasal* [package insert]. Gaithersburg, MD: MedImmune LLC; September 2009.

* Asterisk indicates drugs cited in interaction reports.

Influenza Virus Vaccine, Live — *Oseltamivir*

Influenza Virus Vaccine, Live* (eg, *FluMist*)	Oseltamivir* (*Tamiflu*)

Significance	Onset	Severity	Documentation
2	■ **Rapid**	□ Major	□ Established
	□ Delayed	■ **Moderate**	□ Probable
		□ Minor	■ **Suspected**
			□ Possible
			□ Unlikely

Effects The clinical effect of live attenuated INFLUENZA VIRUS VACCINE may be decreased by OSELTAMIVIR.

Mechanism Inhibition of LIVE VACCINE VIRUS replication by OSELTAMIVIR is suspected.

Management Do not give live attenuated INFLUENZA VIRUS VACCINE within 14 days before or 48 hours after OSELTAMIVIR administration, unless medically indicated.[1]

Discussion

The concomitant use of oseltamivir and intranasal live attenuated influenza virus vaccine has not been studied. However, because of the potential for oseltamivir to inhibit replication of live vaccine virus, do not administer live attenuated influenza vaccine within 14 days before or 48 hours after oseltamivir administration, unless medically indicated.[1] Trivalent inactivated influenza vaccine can be administered at any time relative to oseltamivir administration.

The basis for this monograph is information on file with the manufacturer.

[1] *Tamiflu* [package insert]. Foster City, CA: Gilead Sciences Inc; February 2010.

* Asterisk indicates drugs cited in interaction reports.

Influenza Virus Vaccine, Live / *Zanamivir*

Influenza Virus Vaccine Live* (eg, *FluMist*)	Zanamivir* (*Relenza*)

Significance	Onset	Severity	Documentation
2	■ **Rapid**	□ Major	□ Established
	□ Delayed	■ **Moderate**	□ Probable
		□ Minor	■ **Suspected**
			□ Possible
			□ Unlikely

Effects The clinical effect of live attenuated INFLUENZA VIRUS VACCINE may be decreased by ZANAMIVIR.

Mechanism Inhibition of LIVE VACCINE VIRUS replication by ZANAMIVIR is suspected.

Management Live attenuated INFLUENZA VIRUS VACCINE should not be given within 14 days before or 48 hours after ZANAMIVIR administration, unless medically indicated.[1]

Discussion

The concomitant use of zanamivir and intranasal live attenuated influenza virus vaccine has not been studied. However, because of the potential for zanamivir to inhibit replication of live vaccine virus, live attenuated influenza vaccine should not be administered within 14 days before or 48 hours after zanamivir administration, unless medically indicated.[1] Trivalent inactivated influenza vaccine can be administered at any time relative to zanamivir administration.

The basis for this monograph is information on file with the manufacturer.

[1] *Relenza* [package insert]. Research Triangle Park, NC: Glaxo SmithKline; October 2008.

* Asterisk indicates drugs cited in interaction reports.

Insulin — *Beta-Blockers (Cardiosel.)*

Insulin	Beta-Blockers (Cardiosel.)	
Insulin*	Acebutolol* (eg, *Sectral*)	Esmolol (eg, *Brevibloc*)
	Atenolol* (eg, *Tenormin*)	Metoprolol* (eg, *Lopressor*)
	Betaxolol (eg, *Kerlone*)	

Significance	Onset	Severity	Documentation
5	■ **Rapid**	□ Major	□ Established
	□ Delayed	□ Moderate	□ Probable
		■ **Minor**	□ Suspected
			■ **Possible**
			□ Unlikely

Effects May see an increase in the hypoglycemic effect of INSULIN.

Mechanism Unknown. However, inhibition of hepatic glycogenolysis by BETA-BLOCKERS is suspected to be a contributing factor.

Management Based upon currently available documentation, no clinical interventions appear to be required.

Discussion

Data from studies evaluating the effect of metoprolol on insulin-induced hypoglycemia are conflicting. While one trial has found that metoprolol potentiates the hypoglycemic action of insulin[1] and delays glucose recovery,[1-5] others have not shown metoprolol to intensify the hypoglycemic effect of insulin[4,6,7] or impair glucose recovery.[6-8] Acebutolol has been reported to increase insulin-induced hypoglycemia, but not to affect glucose recovery[1,9] or to have no effect on either phase.[10] Atenolol has not differed from placebo in its actions on the metabolic responses to acute hypoglycemia,[9,11] but has decreased glucose uptake and reduced insulin sensitivity.[5] The cardioselective beta-blockers decreased the tachycardia and/or palpitations associated with insulin-induced hypoglycemia, indicating effective beta blockade[1-11]; however, symptoms of hypoglycemia were not masked.[3,7,8]

Based on the majority of studies, administration of a cardioselective beta-blocking agent to insulin-dependent diabetics requiring a beta-blocker is preferable to using a nonselective agent. See also Insulin/Beta-Blockers, Nonselective.

1 Newman RJ. *Br Med J.* 1976;2(6033):447.
2 Davidson NMcD, et al. *Scot Med J.* 1976;22:69.
3 Viberti GC, et al. *Metabolism.* 1980;29(9):866.
4 Popp DA, et al. *Diabetes Care.* 1984;7(3):243.
5 Pollare T, et al. *BMJ.* 1989:298(6681):1152.
6 Lager I, et al. *Lancet.* 1979;1(8114):458.
7 Viberti GC, et al. *Metabolism.* 1980;29(9):873.
8 Ostman J, et al. *Acta Med Scand.* 1982;211(5):381.
9 Deacon SP, et al. *Br Med J.* 1977;2(6097):1255.
10 Grimaldi A, et al. *Curr Ther Res.* 1984;36:361.
11 Deacon SP, et al. *Br Med J.* 1976;2(6030):272.

* Asterisk indicates drugs cited in interaction reports. Based on pharmacologic and pharmacokinetic considerations, similar interactions may occur with other drugs that are listed.

Insulin ✕ Beta-Blockers (Nonsel.)

Insulin	Beta-Blockers (Nonsel.)	
Insulin*	Carteolol (*Cartrol*)	Pindolol* (eg, *Visken*)
	Nadolol (eg, *Corgard*)	Propranolol* (eg, *Inderal*)
	Penbutolol (*Levatol*)	Timolol* (eg, *Blocadren*)

Significance	Onset	Severity	Documentation
2	■ **Rapid**	□ Major	■ **Established**
	□ Delayed	■ **Moderate**	□ Probable
		□ Minor	□ Suspected
			□ Possible
			□ Unlikely

Effects Prolonged hypoglycemia with masking of hypoglycemic symptoms (ie, tachycardia).

Mechanism BETA-BLOCKERS blunt sympathetic mediated responses to hypoglycemia.

Management If BETA-BLOCKERS cannot be avoided, use with caution in diabetic patients. BETA-BLOCKERS with selectivity or intrinsic sympathomimetic activity are preferable. Monitor patients closely for signs of hypoglycemia (eg, diaphoresis) that are not affected by beta blockade. Patients who continue to experience hypoglycemia should have their insulin dosages reduced if the BETA-BLOCKER cannot be discontinued.

Discussion

Hypoglycemia with use of nonselective beta-adrenergic blockers in diabetics is well documented.[1-3,9,11,12,14] Possible mechanisms mediating the enhanced hypoglycemic response include masking of signs and symptoms, potentiation of the effect of insulin and sulfonylureas, and prolongation of the recovery time to normal glucose levels.[8] Diabetic patients have deficient glucagon secretory responses to hypoglycemia; therefore, enhanced epinephrine secretion is critical in the correction of hypoglycemia in this patient population.[7] Both nonselective and selective beta-blockers will blunt the tachycardic response to hypoglycemia, but agents with selectivity or intrinsic sympathomimetic activity may not prolong the recovery time to normal blood glucose in mild or moderate hypoglycemia.[4-6,10,12] Systemic absorption of ophthalmic timolol may alter the hypoglycemic response to insulin.[13]

[1] Abramson EA, et al. *Lancet.* 1966;2:1386.
[2] Kotler MN, et al. *Lancet.* 1966;2:1389.
[3] Lloyd-Mostyn RH, et al. *Lancet.* 1975;1:1213.
[4] Newman RJ. *BMJ.* 1976;2:447.
[5] Deacon SP, et al. *BMJ.* 1977;2:1255.
[6] Lager I, et al. *Lancet.* 1979;1:458.
[7] Cryer PE. *Diabetes.* 1981;30:261.
[8] Ostman J. *Acta Med Scand Suppl.* 1983;672:69.
[9] Kleinbaum J, et al. *Diabetes Care.* 1984;7:155.
[10] Popp DA, et al. *Diabetes Care.* 1984;7:243.
[11] Mann SJ, et al. *Arch Intern Med.* 1984;144:2427.
[12] Grimaldi A, et al. *Curr Ther Res.* 1984;36:361.
[13] Munroe WP, et al. *DICP.* 1985;19:85.
[14] Shorr RI, et al. *JAMA.* 1997;278:40.

* Asterisk indicates drugs cited in interaction reports. Based on pharmacologic and pharmacokinetic considerations, similar interactions may occur with other drugs that are listed.

Insulin — Clofibrate

Insulin	Clofibrate
Insulin*	Clofibrate* (*Atromid-S*)

Significance	Onset	Severity	Documentation
3	☐ Rapid	☐ Major	☐ Established
	■ **Delayed**	☐ Moderate	☐ Probable
		■ **Minor**	■ **Suspected**
			☐ Possible
			☐ Unlikely

Effects Enhanced hypoglycemic response to INSULIN.

Mechanism Unknown (see Discussion).

Management Monitor patient for signs and symptoms of hypoglycemia. If appropriate, reduce the dose of INSULIN accordingly and monitor blood glucose levels.

Discussion

Clofibrate 2 g/day produces statistically significant reductions in fasting plasma glucose, ketone bodies, free fatty acids, triglycerides, and cholesterol with no change in free insulin or glucagon levels.[1-6] Patients with adult onset diabetes mellitus appear to have the greatest reduction in blood glucose levels while most juvenile onset diabetics exhibit no hypoglycemic response to concomitant therapy.[1-5] Glucose tolerance tests are improved with clofibrate therapy in a large percentage of nondiabetic patients with hypertriglyceridemia and in previously untreated diabetics with or without lipid abnormalities. In adult onset diabetics, the mild fall in blood glucose may be preceded by a fall in triglycerides or free fatty acids. However, a reduction in insulin resistance and an increase in insulin receptor affinity also occurs in some patients.[3,4,6]

During the first week of therapy, closely monitor patients receiving these agents concurrently for signs and symptoms of hypoglycemia. If blood glucose levels fall significantly, reduce insulin dosages accordingly.

[1] Miller RD. *J Atheroscler Res.* 1963;3:694.
[2] Danowski TS, et al. *Clin Pharmacol Ther.* 1965;6:716.
[3] Ferrari C, et al. *Metabolism.* 1977;26:129.
[4] Schade DS, et al. *Metabolism.* 1978;27:461.
[5] Twomey C, et al. *Ir J Med Sci.* 1979;148:31.
[6] Murakami K, et al. *Br J Clin Pharmacol.* 1984;17:89.

* Asterisk indicates drugs cited in interaction reports.

Insulin | **Diltiazem**

Insulin* | Diltiazem* (*Cardizem*)

Significance	Onset	Severity	Documentation
4	■ **Rapid**	□ Major	□ Established
	□ Delayed	■ **Moderate**	□ Probable
		□ Minor	□ Suspected
			■ **Possible**
			□ Unlikely

Effects The hypoglycemic effect of INSULIN may be decreased.

Mechanism Unknown.

Management No special precautions appear necessary. If an interaction is suspected, consider increasing the dose of INSULIN. Blood glucose determinations may provide useful information.

Discussion

Insulin resistance was observed in a 39-year-old female with a 29-year history of insulin-dependent diabetes mellitus.[1] While receiving diltiazem, 90 mg every 6 hours, the patient's insulin requirements increased significantly. Due to the presence of intractable hyperglycemia, diltiazem was discontinued.

A causal relationship was not established in this case. Additional documentation is needed to determine the clinical significance of this possible interaction.

[1] Pershadsingh HA, et al. *JAMA*. 1987;257:930.

* Asterisk indicates drugs cited in interaction reports.

Insulin — *Ethanol*

Insulin*

Ethanol*

Significance	Onset	Severity	Documentation
1	■ **Rapid**	■ **Major**	□ Established
	□ Delayed	□ Moderate	■ **Probable**
		□ Minor	□ Suspected
			□ Possible
			□ Unlikely

Effects The serum glucose-lowering action of INSULIN may be potentiated.

Mechanism Enhanced release of INSULIN following a glucose load and inhibition of gluconeogenesis.

Management If ETHANOL is to be ingested, it should be done in moderation, taken with a meal, and the patient should be monitored closely for hypoglycemia.

Discussion

The effect of ethanol on glucose homeostasis is quite complex and varies depending upon the circumstances.[1-15] In the fasting state, ethanol administration does not alter basal insulin secretion, but may induce hypoglycemia and enhance the hypoglycemic response to exogenous insulin by inhibition of gluconeogenesis. Acute ethanol administration may improve glucose tolerance by enhancing the insulin response to a glucose load. However, ethanol does not appear to directly enhance peripheral glucose utilization.

Discourage the insulin-treated patient with diabetes mellitus from ingesting ethanol in the fasting state. If ethanol is to be ingested, it should be done in moderation, along with the usual meal, and the caloric value included in the diet. Closer monitoring of blood glucose concentrations during ethanol ingestion may be the best approach for early identification and subsequent treatment of hypoglycemia.

[1] Field JB, et al. *J Clin Invest.* 1963;42:497.
[2] Freinkel N, et al. *J Clin Invest.* 1963;42:1112.
[3] Arky RA, et al. *JAMA.* 1968;206:575.
[4] Metz R, et al. *Diabetes.* 1969;18:517.
[5] Friedenberg R, et al. *Diabetes.* 1971;20:397.
[6] Bagdade JD, et al. *Diabetes.* 1972;21:65.
[7] Siegal AM, et al. *Diabetes.* 1972;21:157.
[8] Turner RC, et al. *Metabolism.* 1973;22:111.
[9] Kalkhoff RK, et al. *Diabetes.* 1973;22:372.
[10] Kuhl C, et al. *Diabetes.* 1974;23:821.
[11] McMonagle J, et al. *Metabolism.* 1975;24:625.
[12] Nikkila EA, et al. *Diabetes.* 1975;24:933.
[13] Priem HA, et al. *Metabolism.* 1976;25:397.
[14] Joffe BI, et al. *Br Med J.* 1977;2:678.
[15] Kolaczynski JW, et al. *J Clin Endocrinol Metab.* 1988;67:384.

* Asterisk indicates drugs cited in interaction reports.

Insulin — *Fenfluramine*

Insulin*	Fenfluramine*†

Significance	Onset	Severity	Documentation
2	□ Rapid ■ **Delayed**	□ Major ■ **Moderate** □ Minor	■ **Established** □ Probable □ Suspected □ Possible □ Unlikely

Effects FENFLURAMINE potentiates the hypoglycemic effect of INSULIN.

Mechanism Potentiation of INSULIN'S action at the receptor site with enhanced glucose uptake and decreased glucose production.

Management In insulin-treated patients with diabetes mellitus, closely monitor blood glucose concentrations and tailor the INSULIN regimen as needed to avoid hypoglycemia.

Discussion

Fenfluramine is an anorectic agent that may potentiate the hypoglycemic effect of insulin in patients with diabetes mellitus.[1-8] In a group of 21 patients with Type II diabetes mellitus, single oral doses of fenfluramine significantly reduced post-prandial hyperglycemia, while minimally affecting fasting blood glucose concentrations.[1] However, when administered daily for 4 weeks to patients with Type II diabetes mellitus who were inadequately controlled with diet and glyburide, oral fenfluramine significantly reduced fasting blood glucose concentrations. Similarly, a 7-week course of fenfluramine significantly improved both fasting and post-prandial blood glucose concentrations when compared to placebo in patients with diabetes.[7] Glucose control in normal individuals is not significantly affected by fenfluramine.

The hypoglycemic action of fenfluramine occurs due to potentiation of insulin activity at the receptor site with increased peripheral glucose uptake or decreased hepatic glucose production, independent of changes in insulin secretion or body weight. Monitor blood glucose concentrations closely in patients with diabetes mellitus when fenfluramine is started and make adjustments in the insulin regimen as needed to avoid hypoglycemia.

1 Turtle JR, et al. *Diabetes*. 1973;22:858.
2 Harrison LC, et al. *Postgrad Med J*. 1975;51(Suppl 1):110.
3 Pasquine TA, et al. *Proc Soc Exp Biol Med*. 1981;166:241.
4 Salmela PI, et al. *Diabetes Care*. 1981;4:535.
5 Barseghian G, et al. *Eur J Pharmacol*. 1983;96:53.
6 Verdy M, et al. *Int J Obes*. 1983;7:289.
7 Pestell RG, et al. *Diabetes Care*. 1989;12:252.
8 Storlien LH, et al. *Diabetes*. 1989;38:499.

* Asterisk indicates drugs cited in interaction reports.
†Not available in the United States.

Insulin — *MAOIs*

Insulin*

Isocarboxazid* (*Marplan*)
Pargyline* (*Eutonyl*)
Phenelzine* (*Nardil*)
Tranylcypromine* (*Parnate*)

Significance	Onset	Severity	Documentation
2	☐ Rapid	☐ Major	■ **Established**
	■ **Delayed**	■ **Moderate**	☐ Probable
		☐ Minor	☐ Suspected
			☐ Possible
			☐ Unlikely

Effects Coadministration of MAOIs may potentiate the hypoglycemic response to INSULIN and delay recovery from hypoglycemia.

Mechanism Stimulation of INSULIN secretion and inhibition of gluconeogenesis.

Management Blood glucose concentrations should be monitored closely and adjustments in INSULIN dosage should be made as necessary.

Discussion

MAOIs enhance the hypoglycemic response to insulin by stimulation of endogenous insulin secretion and inhibition of gluconeogenesis.[1-12] The hypoglycemic potency of individual MAOIs is variable and independent of their ability to inhibit monoamine oxidase. The onset of effect is delayed, often requiring several weeks to fully manifest. In patients with diabetes mellitus, the hypoglycemic effect has persisted for several weeks after discontinuation of the agent. In insulin treated patients with diabetes mellitus, blood glucose concentrations should be monitored closely after institution of the MAOIs and adjustments in the patient's insulin regimen should be made as needed to avoid hypoglycemia.

[1] Weiss J, et al. *Ann NY Acad Sci.* 1959;80:854.
[2] Cooper AJ, et al. *Lancet.* 1964;1:1133.
[3] Wickstrom L, et al. *Lancet.* 1964;2:995.
[4] Barrett AM, et al. *J Pharm Pharmacol.* 1965;17:19.
[5] Cooper AJ, et al. *Lancet.* 1966;1:407.
[6] Cooper AJ, et al. *Diabetes.* 1967;16:272.
[7] Bressler R, et al. *Diabetes.* 1968;17:617.
[8] Adnitt PI. *Diabetes.* 1968;17:628.
[9] Potter WZ, et al. *Diabetes.* 1969;18:538.
[10] Aleyassine H, et al. *Am J Physiol.* 1972;222:565.
[11] Aleyassine H, et al. *Endocrinology.* 1975;96:702.
[12] Feldman JM, et al. *Diabetologia.* 1975;11:487.

* Asterisk indicates drugs cited in interaction reports.

Insulin		**Salicylates**	
Insulin*		Aspirin* (eg, *Bayer*)	Salsalate (eg, *Disalcid*)
		Bismuth Subsalicylate (*Pepto-Bismol*)	Sodium Salicylate* (eg, *Uracel 5*)
		Choline Salicylate (*Arthropan*)	Sodium Thiosalicylate (eg, *Tusal*)
		Magnesium Salicylate (eg, *Doan's*)	

Significance	Onset	Severity	Documentation
2	□ Rapid	□ Major	□ Established
	■ **Delayed**	■ **Moderate**	■ **Probable**
		□ Minor	□ Suspected
			□ Possible
			□ Unlikely

Effects The serum glucose-lowering action of INSULIN may be potentiated.

Mechanism Basal INSULIN concentrations are increased, and the acute INSULIN response to a glucose load is enhanced.

Management Monitor blood glucose concentrations and tailor the INSULIN regimen as needed.

Discussion

Salicylates (ie, sodium salicylate and aspirin) significantly increase basal insulin secretion, the acute insulin response to a glucose load, and secondary insulin release in both normal subjects and patients with Type II diabetes mellitus.[1-17] These effects have been associated with lower glucose concentrations in patients with diabetes, while glucose tolerance is generally unchanged in normal individuals. In many cases, the chronic administration of salicylates allowed downward dosage adjustments or discontinuation of insulin therapy. The hypoglycemic effect appears to be greater at higher glucose concentrations. In insulin-treated patients who are receiving high doses of salicylates, blood glucose concentrations should be monitored closely to evaluate the hypoglycemic response.

1 Hecht A, et al. *Metabolism.* 1959;8:418.
2 Reid J, et al. *Br Med J.* 1959;1:897.
3 Gilgore SG, et al. *Metabolism.* 1961;10:419.
4 Anderson WF, et al. *Gerontol Clin.* 1963;5:234.
5 Kaye R, et al. *Am J Dis Child.* 1966;112:52.
6 Field JB, et al. *Lancet.* 1967;1:1191.
7 Robertson RP, et al. *J Clin Invest.* 1977;60:747.
8 Robertson RP, et al. *Trans Assoc Am Phys.* 1977;90:353.
9 Giugliano D, et al. *Diabetologia.* 1978;14:359.
10 Chen M, et al. *Diabetes.* 1978;27:750.
11 Micossi P, et al. *Diabetes.* 1978;27:1196.
12 Robertson RP, et al. *Adv Exp Med Biol.* 1979;119:227.
13 McRae JR, et al. *Adv Prost Thrombox Res.* 1980;8:1287.
14 Metz SA, et al. *Adv Prost Thrombox Res.* 1980;8:1291.
15 Prince RL, et al. *Metabolism.* 1981;30:293.
16 Baron SH. *Diabetes Care.* 1982;5:64. Review.
17 Philipps AF, et al. *Am J Obstet Gynecol.* 1984;148:481.

* Asterisk indicates drugs cited in interaction reports. Based on pharmacologic and pharmacokinetic considerations, similar interactions may occur with other drugs that are listed.

Insulin — *Tetracyclines*

Insulin	Tetracyclines	
Insulin*	Demeclocycline (*Declomycin*)	Oxytetracycline* (eg, *Terramycin*)
	Doxycycline* (eg, *Vibramycin*)	Tetracycline (eg, *Achromycin V*)
	Minocycline (*Minocin*)	

Significance	Onset	Severity	Documentation
4	□ Rapid	□ Major	□ Established
	■ **Delayed**	■ **Moderate**	□ Probable
		□ Minor	□ Suspected
			■ **Possible**
			□ Unlikely

Effects The ability of INSULIN to produce hypoglycemia may be potentiated.

Mechanism Increased extra-pancreatic response to INSULIN.

Management In patients with diabetes mellitus, blood glucose concentrations should be monitored closely; tailor the INSULIN regimen as needed to avoid hypoglycemia.

Discussion

The tetracyclines may reduce blood glucose concentrations both in the fasting state and in response to a glucose load.[1-8] This effect has occurred despite a lowering of circulating insulin concentrations and an increase in granulation of the beta cells of the pancreas in those obese animals with underlying beta cell dysfunction. This effect appears to occur only in response to exogenous insulin administration and does not appear to influence glucose control in the individual with normal glucose tolerance. While controlled clinical trials are still needed, monitor blood glucose concentrations closely and tailor the insulin regimen as needed to avoid hypoglycemia.

[1] Miller JB. *Br Med J.* 1966;2:1007.
[2] Hiatt N, et al. *Diabetes.* 1970;19:307.
[3] New Zealand Committee on Adverse Drug Reactions. *NZ Dent J.* 1975;71:28.
[4] Phillips PJ, et al. *Ann Intern Med.* 1977;86:111.
[5] El-Denshary ESM, et al. *Diabete Metab.* 1977;3:3.
[6] Begin-Heick N, et al. *Diabetes.* 1979;28:65.
[7] Dalpe-Scott M, et al. *Diabetes.* 1982;31:53.
[8] Dalpe-Scott M, et al. *Diabetes.* 1983;32:932.

* Asterisk indicates drugs cited in interaction reports. Based on pharmacologic and pharmacokinetic considerations, similar interactions may occur with other drugs that are listed.

Interferon Alfa — *Corticosteroids*

Interferon Alfa	Corticosteroids	
Interferon Alfa* (eg, *Intron A*)	Betamethasone (*Celestone*)	Hydrocortisone (eg, *Cortef*)
	Corticotropin (eg, *ACTH*)	Methylprednisolone (eg, *Medrol*)
	Cortisone	Prednisolone (eg, *Prelone*)
	Cosyntropin (*Cortrosyn*)	Prednisone* (eg, *Sterapred*)
	Dexamethasone (eg, *Decadron*)	Triamcinolone (eg, *Kenalog*)
	Fludrocortisone (eg, *Florinef*)	

Significance	Onset	Severity	Documentation
5	☐ Rapid	☐ Major	☐ Established
	■ **Delayed**	☐ Moderate	☐ Probable
		■ **Minor**	☐ Suspected
			■ **Possible**
			☐ Unlikely

Effects Possible inhibition of antiviral activity of INTERFERON ALFA by CORTICOSTEROIDS.

Mechanism Unknown.

Management Based on available clinical data, no special precautions are needed.

Discussion

In a study of 20 healthy volunteers, a single dose of 18 million units of interferon alfa was administered alone or concurrently with prednisone 40 mg/day for 6 days, starting the day before interferon administration.[1] Antiviral activity was measured by harvesting peripheral monocytes and measuring the activity of the enzyme 2′-5′-oligoadenylate synthetase and the resistance to vesicular stomatitis virus infection in vitro. Prednisone decreased the former but did not alter experimental viral infection. In addition, prednisone did not diminish the adverse reactions caused by interferon. These data suggest the potential for a prednisone-induced decrease in antiviral effectiveness to interferon, which is consistent with the immunosuppressive action of corticosteroids.

Additional studies are needed to determine the clinical importance of this interaction.

[1] Witter FR, et al. *Clin Pharmacol Ther.* 1988;44(2):239.

* Asterisk indicates drugs cited in interaction reports. Based on pharmacologic and pharmacokinetic considerations, similar interactions may occur with other drugs that are listed.

Interleukins — *Corticosteroids*

Interleukins	Corticosteroids	
Aldesleukin* (Interleukin [IL]-2; *Proleukin*)	Betamethasone (*Celestone*)	Hydrocortisone (eg, *Cortef*)
	Budesonide (eg, *Entocort EC*)	Methylprednisolone (eg, *Medrol*)
	Corticotropin (ACTH)	Prednisolone (eg, *Prelone*)
	Cortisone	Prednisone (eg, *Sterapred*)
	Cosyntropin (*Cortrosyn*)	Triamcinolone (eg, *Kenolog*)
	Dexamethasone* (eg, *Decadron*)	
	Fludrocortisone (eg, *Florinef*)	

Significance	Onset	Severity	Documentation
2	☐ Rapid	☐ Major	☐ Established
	■ **Delayed**	■ **Moderate**	☐ Probable
		☐ Minor	■ **Suspected**
			☐ Possible
			☐ Unlikely

Effects Therapeutic effects of ALDESLEUKIN may be decreased.

Mechanism Unknown.

Management Avoid coadministration of ALDESLEUKIN and CORTICOSTEROIDS.[1]

Discussion

Coadministration of aldesleukin and dexamethasone may reduce the toxic and therapeutic effects of aldesleukin.[2-5] In 19 patients with advanced carcinoma receiving aldesleukin plus dexamethasone, the maximum tolerated dose of aldesleukin was approximately 3-fold higher and organ dysfunction and hypotension were markedly reduced, compared with patients in a National Cancer Institute protocol who were treated with aldesleukin alone.[2] However, only 1 patient treated with aldesleukin plus dexamethasone showed partial tumor regression, and 2 patients demonstrated minimal tumor regression. In a study in 33 patients with advanced cancer, patients receiving dexamethasone tolerated larger doses of aldesleukin and experienced less toxicity, compared with patients not receiving dexamethasone.[5] However, 9 of 27 patients receiving aldesleukin and lymphokine-activated killer cells showed cancer regression, while none of the 6 patients receiving the same regimen plus dexamethasone demonstrated cancer regression.

1 *Proleukin* [package insert]. Emeryville, CA: Chiron Corporation; September 2000.
2 Mier JW, et al. *Blood.* 1990;76(10):1933.
3 Shiloni E, et al. *Blood.* 1991;78(5):1389.
4 Mier JW. *Blood.* 1991;78(5):1390.
5 Vetto JT, et al. *J Clin Oncol.* 1987;5(3):496.

* Asterisk indicates drugs cited in interaction reports. Based on pharmacologic and pharmacokinetic considerations, similar interactions may occur with other drugs that are listed.

Irinotecan — *Hydantoins*

Irinotecan* (eg, *Camptosar*)	Ethotoin (*Peganone*)	Phenytoin* (eg, *Dilantin*)
	Fosphenytoin	

Significance	Onset	Severity	Documentation
4	☐ Rapid	■ **Major**	☐ Established
	■ **Delayed**	☐ Moderate	☐ Probable
		☐ Minor	☐ Suspected
			■ **Possible**
			☐ Unlikely

Effects Antitumor activity of IRINOTECAN may be reduced.

Mechanism HYDANTOINS may increase the metabolism (CYP3A4) of IRINOTECAN.

Management It may be necessary to adjust the dose of IRINOTECAN when HYDANTOINS are started or stopped.

Discussion

The effects of phenytoin on the pharmacokinetics of irinotecan and its metabolites were evaluated in a 15-year-old boy with recurrent metastatic pinealoblastoma.[1] During the patient's therapy, he received varying doses of irinotecan. However, the pharmacokinetics of irinotecan were evaluated during 2 cycles in which the patient received 50 mg/m^2 doses of irinotecan (ie, cycle 1 without phenytoin and cycle 6 with phenytoin). Coadministration of phenytoin decreased the AUC of irinotecan 63% and increased the clearance by 168%. In addition, the AUC of the active metabolite of irinotecan, SN-38, was decreased 60%. The AUC of the inactive metabolite of irinotecan was increased 16%.

[1] Murry DJ, et al. *J Pediatr Hematol Oncol.* 2002;24(2):130.

* Asterisk indicates drugs cited in interaction reports. Based on pharmacologic and pharmacokinetic considerations, similar interactions may occur with other drugs that are listed.

Irinotecan — *Methimazole*

Irinotecan* (eg, *Camptosar*)	Methimazole* (eg, *Tapazole*)

Significance	Onset	Severity	Documentation
4	☐ Rapid ■ **Delayed**	☐ Major ■ **Moderate** ☐ Minor	☐ Established ☐ Probable ☐ Suspected ■ **Possible** ☐ Unlikely

Effects Plasma and GI concentrations of the active IRINOTECAN metabolite (SN-38) may be elevated, increasing the risk of toxicity (eg, diarrhea).

Mechanism Unknown. However, induction of uridine diphosphate glucuronosyltransferase 1A by METHIMAZOLE is suspected to be partly involved.

Management Coadminister with caution. Closely monitor patients for IRINOTECAN toxicity.

Discussion

The pharmacokinetics and pharmacodynamics of irinotecan were followed in a 53-year-old man receiving irinotecan for colorectal cancer and methimazole for Graves disease.[1] Although the irinotecan AUC was not affected by methimazole cotreatment, plasma concentrations of the active irinotecan metabolite SN-38 and inactive irinotecan metabolites SN-38-glucuronide were increased 14% and 67%, respectively, compared with irinotecan monotherapy. The risk of intestinal toxicity may be increased when SN-38-glucuronide is excreted in the gut and converted to SN-38 by deglucuronidation by intestinal bacteria.

[1] van der Bol JM, et al. *Cancer Chemother Pharmacol.* 2011;67(1):231.

* Asterisk indicates drugs cited in interaction reports.

Irinotecan		**Milk Thistle**	
Irinotecan* (eg, *Camptosar*)		Milk Thistle*	
Significance	**Onset**	**Severity**	**Documentation**
5	□ Rapid ■ **Delayed**	□ Major □ Moderate ■ **Minor**	□ Established □ Probable □ Suspected □ Possible ■ **Unlikely**

Effects Short-term and more prolonged ingestion of MILK THISTLE have no pronounced effect on IRINOTECAN pharmacokinetics.

Mechanism Plasma concentrations of the principal component of MILK THISTLE (silybin) are too low to affect CYP3A4.

Management Based on available data, no special precautions are needed.

Discussion

The effect of short-term (4 days) and more prolonged (12 days) administration of milk thistle (principal component, silymarin) on the pharmacokinetics of irinotecan was studied in 6 cancer patients.[1] During the study, patients were treated with irinotecan 125 mg/m^2 as a 90-minute infusion once weekly for 4 consecutive weeks. Four days before the second dose of irinotecan, patients began taking milk thistle seed extract (80% silymarin) 200 mg 3 times daily for 14 days. Administration of milk thistle for 4 days or 12 days had no pronounced effect on irinotecan pharmacokinetics. The only effect of milk thistle administration was a slight decrease in the AUC ratio of the irinotecan metabolite (7-ethyl-10-hydroxycamptothecin) to irinotecan, which decreased from 2.58% on day 1 to 2.17% on day 15. This change is not expected to be clinically important.

[1] van Erp NP, et al. *Clin Cancer Res.* 2005;11(21):7800.

* Asterisk indicates drugs cited in interaction reports.

Irinotecan — *Protease Inhibitors*

Irinotecan* (*Camptosar*)	Lopinavir/Ritonavir* (*Kaletra*)

Significance	Onset	Severity	Documentation
2	□ Rapid ■ **Delayed**	□ Major ■ **Moderate** □ Minor	□ Established □ Probable ■ **Suspected** □ Possible □ Unlikely

Effects Plasma concentrations of the active IRINOTECAN metabolite (SN-38) may be elevated, increasing the risk of toxicity (eg, neutropenia, diarrhea).

Mechanism LOPINAVIR/RITONAVIR may inhibit IRINOTECAN metabolism (CYP3A4), inhibit transporter-mediated excretion of IRINOTECAN in the urine and bile, and inhibit conversion of the active metabolite of IRINOTECAN (SN-38) to the inactive glucuronide metabolite (SN-38G) by the UDP-glucuronyl transferase 1A1 isoform.

Management Closely monitor patients for IRINOTECAN toxicity.

Discussion

Irinotecan is a prodrug that is converted in the liver to a potent topoisomerase inhibitor (SN-38).[1] Inactivation of SN-38 occurs by conversion to the glucuronide (SN-38G). In a prospective, open-label, randomized investigation, the effects of lopinavir/ritonavir on the pharmacokinetics of irinotecan were studied in 7 HIV-infected patients with Kaposi sarcoma.[1] Coadministration of irinotecan with lopinavir/ritonavir reduced the clearance of irinotecan 47%, reduced the AUC of an inactive irinotecan metabolite (APC) 81%, and inhibited the formation of SN-38G. These effects resulted in an increase in irinotecan availability for conversion to SN-38 and reduced inactivation to SN-38G, leading to a 204% increase in the SN-38 AUC.

[1] Corona G, et al. *Clin Pharmacol Ther*. 2008;83(4):601.

* Asterisk indicates drugs cited in interaction reports.

Irinotecan — *St. John's Wort*

Irinotecan* (eg, *Camptosar*)	St. John's Wort*

Significance	Onset	Severity	Documentation
2	□ Rapid	□ Major	□ Established
	■ **Delayed**	■ **Moderate**	□ Probable
		□ Minor	■ **Suspected**
			□ Possible
			□ Unlikely

Effects Reduced plasma levels of the active metabolite (SN-38) of IRINOTECAN, resulting in decreased efficacy.

Mechanism The precise mechanism is unknown; however, the metabolism (CYP3A4) of IRINOTECAN appears to be altered by ST. JOHN'S WORT.

Management Patients receiving IRINOTECAN should not take ST. JOHN'S WORT.

Discussion

The effect of St. John's wort on the metabolism of irinotecan was studied in 5 cancer patients.[1] Using an open-label, randomized, crossover design, irinotecan (350 mg/m^2 as a 90-minute continuous IV infusion) was administered once every 3 weeks. Fourteen days before the start of the first or second irinotecan administration, patients started taking St. John's wort 300 mg 3 times daily with each meal for 18 days. The nadir leukocyte and neutrophil counts decreased 56% and 63%, respectively, during administration of irinotecan alone, compared with 8.6% and 4.3%, respectively, during concurrent ingestion of St. John's wort. Compared with irinotecan alone, the AUC of the irinotecan active metabolite SN-38 decreased 42% during coadministration of St. John's wort.

[1] Mathijssen RH, et al. *J Natl Cancer Inst.* 2002;94(16):1247.

* Asterisk indicates drugs cited in interaction reports.

Iron Salts — *ACE Inhibitors*

Iron Salts		ACE Inhibitors	
Ferrous Sulfate* (eg, *Feosol*)	Iron Dextran (eg, *InFeD*)	Benazepril (eg, *Lotensin*)	Moexipril (eg, *Univasc*)
		Captopril* (eg, *Capoten*)	Perindopril (*Aceon*)
		Enalapril* (eg, *Vasotec*)	Quinapril (eg, *Accupril*)
		Fosinopril (eg, *Monopril*)	Ramipril (*Altace*)
		Lisinopril (eg, *Zestril*)	Trandolapril (*Mavik*)

Significance	Onset	Severity	Documentation
4	■ **Rapid**	□ Major	□ Established
	□ Delayed	■ **Moderate**	□ Probable
		□ Minor	□ Suspected
			■ **Possible**
			□ Unlikely

Effects Adverse systemic reactions to IV IRON administration, including fever, arthralgia, and hypotension, may occur. Oral FERROUS SULFATE may reduce CAPTOPRIL blood levels.

Mechanism ACE INHIBITORS may decrease the catabolism of kinins, which may augment IV IRON systemic effects. FERROUS SULFATE may promote the formation of an inactive CAPTOPRIL disulfide dimer.

Management Because of the seriousness of this reaction, consider using an alternative to one of these agents. Oral CAPTOPRIL and FERROUS SULFATE should not be taken at the same time; separate administration times by at least 2 hours.

Discussion

Three patients developed severe systemic reactions, including diffuse erythema, hypotension, nausea, vomiting, diarrhea, abdominal cramps, and fever, during coadministration of enalapril (5 mg/day in 1 patient and 20 mg/day in 2 patients) and IV ferrigluconate†.[1] All patients recovered from the reaction 20 minutes after stopping the iron injection and administering IV hydrocortisone (eg, *Solu-Cortef*) 200 mg. In 1 of the patients, subsequent treatment with ferrigluconate or enalapril alone did not result in an adverse systemic reaction. In 15 other patients who received IV ferrigluconate without being given enalapril, adverse reactions did not occur.

Seven healthy volunteers received oral captopril 25 mg with oral ferrous sulfate 300 mg or placebo.[2] Ferrous sulfate decreased the AUC of unconjugated captopril 37%. However, there was no difference in systolic or diastolic BP.

[1] Rolla G, et al. *J Allergy Clin Immunol.* 1994;93:1074.
[2] Schaefer JP, et al. *Br J Clin Pharmacol.* 1998;46:377.

* Asterisk indicates drugs cited in interaction reports. Based on pharmacologic and pharmacokinetic considerations, similar interactions may occur with other drugs that are listed.
† Not available in the United States.

Iron Salts — **Antacids**

Iron Salts		Antacids
Ferrous Fumarate* (eg, *Femiron*)	Ferrous Sulfate* (eg, *Mol-Iron*)	Antacids* (eg, *Maalox*)
Ferrous Gluconate* (eg, *Fergon*)	Iron Polysaccharide (eg, *Hytinic*)	

Significance	Onset	Severity	Documentation
3	□ Rapid	□ Major	□ Established
	■ **Delayed**	□ Moderate	□ Probable
		■ **Minor**	■ **Suspected**
			□ Possible
			□ Unlikely

Effects GI absorption of IRON may be reduced by ANTACIDS.

Mechanism Reduction in IRON solubility because of an increase in gastric pH or formation of an insoluble salt.

Management In order to avoid a possible interaction, separate administration times whenever possible.

Discussion

Simultaneous administration of antacids may reduce the oral absorption of iron as a result of a reduction in the solubility of iron because of an increase in gastric pH or the formation of an insoluble salt.[1-6] In vitro studies reveal that the solubility of iron may be lower at a higher pH (pH greater than 4.5 to 5) and decrease as interaction time increases.[3-5] The solubility of the fumarate, gluconate, and carbonate salts may be affected by pH to a greater extent than the sulfate salt.[4] Although a comparison of the different antacid preparations is difficult because of the variability in acid-neutralizing capacity, iron solubility may be reduced to a greater extent with calcium carbonate and sodium bicarbonate than with magnesium and aluminum hydroxide.[3] In vivo, coadministration of magnesium trisilicate reduced mean oral iron absorption from 30.5% to 11.7%.[1] Similarly, iron absorption was reduced from a mean of 47.2% to 12.3% in 5 patients receiving concurrent aluminum hydroxide.[2] In healthy, iron-replete subjects, single doses of calcium carbonate and calcium acetate decreased iron absorption from ferrous sulfate.[7] Sevelamer (*Renagel*) did not affect iron absorption.

In order to avoid a possible interaction, it is reasonable to separate administration times of antacids and iron preparations, whenever possible. However, the clinical significance of this interaction on a patient's erythropoietic response to iron has not been well evaluated.

[1] Hall GJ, et al. *Med J Aust.* 1969;2:95.
[2] Rastogi SP, et al. *Kidney Int.* 1975;8:417.
[3] Ekenved G, et al. *Scand J Haematol Suppl.* 1976;28:65.
[4] Coste JF, et al. *Curr Ther Res.* 1977;22:205.
[5] Corby DG, et al. *J Toxicol Clin Toxicol.* 1985-86;23:489.
[6] O'Neil-Cutting MA, et al. *JAMA.* 1986;255:1468.
[7] Pruchnicki MC, et al. *J Clin Pharmacol.* 2002;42:1171.

* Asterisk indicates drugs cited in interaction reports. Based on pharmacologic and pharmacokinetic considerations, similar interactions may occur with other drugs that are listed.

Iron Salts — *Chloramphenicol*

Iron Salts		Chloramphenicol
Ferrous Fumarate (eg, *Femiron*)	Iron Dextran* (eg, *Imferon*)	Chloramphenicol* (*Chloromycetin*)
Ferrous Gluconate (eg, *Fergon*)	Iron Polysaccharide (eg, *Hytinic*)	
Ferrous Sulfate (eg, *Mol-Iron*)		

Significance	Onset	Severity	Documentation
2	☐ Rapid	☐ Major	☐ Established
	■ **Delayed**	■ **Moderate**	☐ Probable
		☐ Minor	■ **Suspected**
			☐ Possible
			☐ Unlikely

Effects Serum IRON levels may be increased by CHLORAMPHENICOL.

Mechanism Decreased IRON clearance and erythropoiesis due to direct bone marrow toxicity from CHLORAMPHENICOL.

Management If bone marrow suppression occurs, choose an alternative antimicrobial agent, if possible. If CHLORAMPHENICOL must be continued, monitor iron stores and appropriately alter the IRON regimen.

Discussion

As a result of a dose-dependent, direct toxic effect on the bone marrow, chloramphenicol may inhibit heme synthesis, reduce iron clearance, and possibly increase serum and intramitochondrial iron.[1-5] In patients with bone marrow suppression, serum iron levels usually begin to rise within 5 to 7 days of the start of chloramphenicol therapy and begin to fall within 3 to 4 days after drug withdrawal. If bone marrow suppression occurs, select an alternative antimicrobial agent, if possible, in order to avoid the development of a severe anemia. If chloramphenicol must be continued in a patient who has developed bone marrow suppression, monitor iron stores and adjust the iron regimen as necessary to avoid iron overload.

[1] Rubin D, et al. *J Clin Invest.* 1958;37:1286.
[2] Saidi P, et al. *J Lab Clin Med.* 1961;57:247.
[3] Jiji RM, et al. *Arch Intern Med.* 1963;111:70.
[4] Scott JL, et al. *N Engl J Med.* 1965;272:1137.
[5] Haile CA. *South Med J.* 1977;70:479

* Asterisk indicates drugs cited in interaction reports. Based on pharmacologic and pharmacokinetic considerations, similar interactions may occur with other drugs that are listed.

Iron Salts — *Histamine H_2 Antagonists*

Ferrous Fumarate (eg, *Hemocyte*)	Ferrous Sulfate* (eg, *Feosol*)	Cimetidine* (eg, *Tagamet*)	Nizatidine (eg, *Axid*)
Ferrous Gluconate (eg, *Fergon*)	Iron Polysaccharide (eg, *ProFe*)	Famotidine (eg, *Pepcid*)	Ranitidine (eg, *Zantac*)

Significance	Onset	Severity	Documentation
5	☐ Rapid ■ **Delayed**	☐ Major ☐ Moderate ■ **Minor**	☐ Established ☐ Probable ☐ Suspected ■ **Possible** ☐ Unlikely

Effects The oral absorption of IRON may be impaired by HISTAMINE H_2 ANTAGONISTS.

Mechanism Reduction in IRON solubility because of an increased gastric pH.

Management Administer IRON preparation at least 1 hour prior to the HISTAMINE H_2 ANTAGONIST. If an interaction is still suspected, reduce the dose of the HISTAMINE H_2 ANTAGONIST or administer supplemental IRON parenterally.

Discussion

The oral absorption of iron has been reduced when coadministered with antacid preparations because of the increase in pH or ion complexation with reduced solubility.[1-3] In 1 study, absorption of dietary nonheme iron following a single oral dose of cimetidine 300 mg was reduced by 28% compared with baseline.[4] Absorption was decreased by 42% when the cimetidine dose was increased to 600 mg and decreased by 65% when an additional 300 mg was administered 1 hour postprandially. However, another investigation noted stable serum iron concentrations associated with rising hemoglobin in 64 patients receiving long-term treatment with cimetidine 400 to 800 mg daily.[5] In 1 study, persistent anemia and iron depletion occurred in a patient receiving concomitant oral cimetidine (1 g/day) and ferrous sulfate for 2 months, with subsequent improvement 30 days after reducing the cimetidine dose to 400 mg/day. Ferrous sulfate did not affect the absorption or the plasma levels of cimetidine or famotidine.[6]

Evidence is insufficient to suggest that a clinically important decrease in the erythropoietic response to oral iron salts would occur in patients also being treated with a histamine H_2 antagonist.[7,8]

1 Hall GJ, et al. *Med J Aust.* 1969;2(2):95.
2 Ekenved G, et al. *Scand J Haematol Suppl.* 1976;28:65.
3 Coste J, et al. *Curr Ther Res.* 1977;22:205.
4 Esposito R. *Lancet.* 1977;2(8048):1132.
5 Rosner F. *Lancet.* 1978;1:95.
6 Partlow ES, et al. *Clin Pharmacol Ther.* 1996;59(4):389.
7 Skikne BS, et al. *Gastroenterology.* 1981;81(6):1068.
8 Walan A, et al. *Scand J Gastroenterol Suppl.* 1985;111:24.

* Asterisk indicates drugs cited in interaction reports. Based on pharmacologic and pharmacokinetic considerations, similar interactions may occur with other drugs that are listed.

Iron Salts — *Proton Pump Inhibitors*

Ferrous Fumarate (eg, *Hemocyte*)	Ferrous Sulfate* (eg, *Feosol*)	Esomeprazole (*Nexium*)	Pantoprazole (eg, *Protonix*)
Ferrous Gluconate (eg, *Fergon*)	Iron Polysaccharide (eg, *Nu-Iron*)	Lansoprazole (eg, *Prevacid*)	Rabeprazole (*Aciphex*)
		Omeprazole* (eg, *Prilosec*)	

Significance	Onset	Severity	Documentation
4	□ Rapid ■ **Delayed**	■ **Major** □ Moderate □ Minor	□ Established □ Probable □ Suspected ■ **Possible** □ Unlikely

Effects Oral absorption of IRON may be impaired by PROTON PUMP INHIBITORS.

Mechanism PROTON PUMP INHIBITOR–induced achlorhydria may impair the absorption of orally administered IRON SALTS.

Management If PROTON PUMP INHIBITOR therapy cannot be discontinued, parenteral administration of the IRON SALT may be a suitable alternative.

Discussion

Iron-deficiency anemia was reported in 2 patients who failed to respond to oral iron replacement therapy.[1] The anemia was the result of GI bleeding. Both patients had been receiving long-term omeprazole therapy. Failure of the patients to respond to oral iron replacement therapy was attributed to malabsorption of the iron as a result of omeprazole-induced achlorhydria. After discontinuing omeprazole, both patients responded appropriately to continued oral iron replacement.

[1] Sharma VR, et al. *South Med J.* 2004;97(9):887.

* Asterisk indicates drugs cited in interaction reports. Based on pharmacologic and pharmacokinetic considerations, similar interactions may occur with other drugs that are listed.

Iron Salts | **_Zinc Salts_**

Iron Salts		Zinc Salts	
Ferrous Fumarate (eg, *Hemocyte*)	Ferrous Sulfate* (eg, *Feosol*)	Zinc Gluconate	Zinc Sulfate*
Ferrous Gluconate (eg, *Fergon*)	Iron Polysaccharide (eg, *ProFe*)		

Significance	Onset	Severity	Documentation
3	☐ Rapid ■ **Delayed**	☐ Major ☐ Moderate ■ **Minor**	☐ Established ☐ Probable ■ **Suspected** ☐ Possible ☐ Unlikely

Effects Bioavailability of IRON may be decreased.

Mechanism Unknown.

Management Separate the administration times of IRON and ZINC by as much as possible.

Discussion

The effects of 2 zinc sulfate doses on the bioavailability of radiotracer-labeled iron sulfate were studied in 14 healthy women.[1] An aqueous solution of elemental iron as ferrous sulfate was ingested alone and with an aqueous solution of zinc sulfate 0.59 mg (molar ratio zinc:iron was 1:1). After 14 days, each subject ingested a second solution with ferrous sulfate 10 mg alone and with zinc 11.71 mg (molar ratio zinc:iron was 1:1). Compared with ingesting ferrous sulfate alone, the lower doses of zinc and ferrous sulfate did not affect the bioavailability of iron. However, at the higher dose, zinc reduced iron bioavailability by 56%. Consider this potential interaction when iron and zinc supplements are taken concurrently.

[1] Olivares M, et al. *Nutrition*. 2007;23(4):292.

* Asterisk indicates drugs cited in interaction reports. Based on pharmacologic and pharmacokinetic considerations, similar interactions may occur with other drugs that are listed.

Isoniazid — *Aluminum Salts*

Isoniazid*	Aluminum Hydroxide* (eg, *Alternagel*)	Attapulgite (eg, *Diarrest*)

Significance	Onset	Severity	Documentation
5	■ **Rapid**	□ Major	□ Established
	□ Delayed	□ Moderate	□ Probable
		■ **Minor**	□ Suspected
			■ **Possible**
			□ Unlikely

Effects Serum concentrations of ISONIAZID may be decreased because of a reduction in oral absorption by ALUMINUM SALTS.

Mechanism Unknown; possibly due to a delay in gastric emptying, complexation with ALUMINUM, or a reduction in solubility.

Management To avoid a possible interaction, ISONIAZID may be administered 1 to 2 hours before any ALUMINUM-containing compounds.

Discussion

Preliminary evidence suggests that coadministration of isoniazid and aluminum-containing antacids may decrease isoniazid serum concentrations achieved after an oral dose.[1,2] Although not fully elucidated, delayed gastric emptying, complexation with aluminum, or a reduction in solubility are possible mechanisms for impaired isoniazid absorption. In a crossover study of 10 patients receiving isoniazid 300 mg orally, coadministration with aluminum hydroxide decreased the 1-hour and peak concentrations of isoniazid. In contrast, however, 1 patient had higher serum isoniazid concentrations following aluminum hydroxide administration.[1]

Although the clinical importance of such an interaction has not been determined, separation of isoniazid and aluminum administration times by a minimum of 1 to 2 hours may be a reasonable approach to avoid any possible interaction.

[1] Hava M, et al. *Eur J Pharmacol.* 1973;22(2):156.
[2] Hurwitz A, et al. *Am Rev Respir Dis.* 1974;109(1):41.

* Asterisk indicates drugs cited in interaction reports. Based on pharmacologic and pharmacokinetic considerations, similar interactions may occur with other drugs that are listed.

Isoniazid		***Aminosalicylic Acid***

Isoniazid* (eg, *Nydrazid*) | Aminosalicylic Acid* (PAS)

Significance	Onset	Severity	Documentation
5	☐ Rapid ■ **Delayed**	☐ Major ☐ Moderate ■ **Minor**	☐ Established ☐ Probable ☐ Suspected ☐ Possible ■ **Unlikely**

Effects The elimination half-life and serum concentrations of ISONIAZID may be increased by AMINOSALICYCLIC ACID.

Mechanism Possible competitive inhibition of N-acetylation of ISONIAZID.

Management Special precautions are not deemed necessary.

Discussion

Para-aminosalicylic acid may competitively inhibit N-acetylation of isoniazid and, thereby, increase isoniazid serum concentrations and elimination half-life.[1-9] Some authors found this effect to be greater in patients who were rapid acetylators and to increase as the dose of para-aminosalicylic acid was increased.[3,8] In vitro, one study found para-aminosalicylic acid to significantly increase the antimycobacterial activity of isoniazid only at low isoniazid concentrations.[9] This interaction appears to lack any clinical significance and, therefore, special precautions for concurrent administration of these two agents are not deemed necessary.

[1] Lauener H, et al. *Am Rev Resp Dis.* 1959;80:26.
[2] Peters JH. *Am Rev Resp Dis.* 1960;82:153.
[3] Kreukniet J, et al. *Scand J Resp Dis.* 1967;47:236.
[4] Tiitinen H, et al. *Arzneimittelforschung.* 1968;18:623.
[5] Tiitinen H. *Scand J Resp Dis.* 1969;50:281.
[6] Lehmann J. *Scand J Resp Dis.* 1969;50:169.
[7] Boman G, et al. *Acta Pharmacol Toxicol.* 1970;28(suppl):15.
[8] Hanngren A, et al. *Scand J Resp Dis.* 1970;51:61.
[9] Mattila MJ, et al. *Arzneimittelforschung.* 1972;22:1769.

* Asterisk indicates drugs cited in interaction reports.

Isoniazid — *Beta-Adrenergic Blockers*

Isoniazid* (eg, *Nydrazid*)	Propranolol* (eg, *Inderal*)

Significance	Onset	Severity	Documentation
5	■ **Rapid** □ Delayed	□ Major □ Moderate ■ **Minor**	□ Established □ Probable □ Suspected □ Possible ■ **Unlikely**

Effects The pharmacologic effects of ISONIAZID may be increased.

Mechanism Unknown.

Management No special precautions appear necessary.

Discussion

The effect of propranolol on isoniazid elimination was investigated in six healthy males.[1] Subjects were studied after an overnight fast on two occasions, one week apart. During a control period, isoniazid kinetics were determined following an IV injection of 600 mg of the drug. On the second occasion, in addition to the isoniazid dose, 40 mg propranolol was administered orally every 8 hours starting 3 days prior to and during the 8-hour investigation. Isoniazid clearance with propranolol pretreatment was approximately 3 L/hour (21%) lower than during the control period ($P < 0.01$).

[1] Santoso B. *Int J Clin Pharmacol Ther Toxicol.* 1985;23:134.

* Asterisk indicates drugs cited in interaction reports.

Isoniazid — *Corticosteroids*

Isoniazid	Corticosteroids	
Isoniazid* (eg, *Nydrazid*)	Betamethasone (eg, *Celestone*)	Methylprednisolone (eg, *Medrol*)
	Cortisone (eg, *Cortone*)	Paramethasone (*Haldrone*)
	Desoxycorticosterone	Prednisolone* (eg, *Prelone*)
	Dexamethasone (eg, *Decadron*)	Prednisone (eg, *Deltasone*)
	Fludrocortisone (*Florinef*)	Triamcinolone (eg, *Kenalog*)
	Hydrocortisone (eg, *Cortef*)	

Significance	Onset	Severity	Documentation
5	☐ Rapid	☐ Major	☐ Established
	■ **Delayed**	☐ Moderate	☐ Probable
		■ **Minor**	☐ Suspected
			■ **Possible**
			☐ Unlikely

Effects Serum concentrations of ISONIAZID may be decreased by CORTICOSTEROIDS.

Mechanism Possible increase in hepatic acetylation or renal clearance of ISONIAZID.

Management Special precautions are not deemed necessary.

Discussion

Limited data available suggest that single doses of prednisolone may decrease serum isoniazid concentrations by increasing the acetylation rate in slow acetylators and increasing the renal clearance in both slow and rapid acetylators.[1] In addition, one clinical trial suggests that isoniazid may inhibit endogenous cortisol oxidation.[2] The clinical significance of either interaction has not been determined, and so special precautions are not currently deemed necessary.

[1] Raghupati Sarma G, et al. *Antimicrob Agents Chemother.* 1980;18:661.

[2] Brodie MJ, et al. *Clin Pharmacol Ther.* 1981;30:363.

* Asterisk indicates drugs cited in interaction reports. Based on pharmacologic and pharmacokinetic considerations, similar interactions may occur with other drugs that are listed.

Isoniazid			*Meperidine*
Isoniazid* (eg, *Nydrazid*)		Meperidine* (eg, *Demerol*)	
Significance	Onset	Severity	Documentation
4	■ **Rapid** □ Delayed	□ Major ■ **Moderate** □ Minor	□ Established □ Probable □ Suspected ■ **Possible** □ Unlikely

Effects Hypotensive episode or CNS depression may occur when these agents are given together.

Mechanism Unclear, but may be related to inhibition of monoamine oxidase by ISONIAZID.

Management Use this combination with caution. Monitor blood pressure frequently when beginning therapy. If hypotension occurs, supportive therapy may be required.

Discussion

One case report found that a 75 mg IM dose of meperidine given 1 hour after the first dose of isoniazid (30 mg/day) produced an interaction resulting in lethargy and hypotension within 20 minutes.[2] The patient recovered spontaneously, and therapy was changed to morphine sulfate with no recurrence of symptoms. Isoniazid has been shown to inhibit monoamine oxidase,[1] and the drug interaction between meperidine and monoamine oxidase inhibitors has been shown to produce a similar pharmacologic effect.

[1] Vitek V, et al. *Biochem Pharmacol*. 1965;14:1417.

[2] Gannon R, et al. *Ann Intern Med*. 1983;99:415.

* Asterisk indicates drugs cited in interaction reports.

Isoniazid — *Rifampin*

Isoniazid* (eg, *Nydrazid*)	Rifampin* (eg, *Rifadin*)

Significance	Onset	Severity	Documentation
1	☐ Rapid ■ **Delayed**	■ **Major** ☐ Moderate ☐ Minor	☐ Established ■ **Probable** ☐ Suspected ☐ Possible ☐ Unlikely

Effects Hepatotoxicity may occur at a rate higher than with either agent alone.

Mechanism Possibly an alteration in the metabolism of isoniazid caused by RIFAMPIN.

Management If alterations in liver function tests occur, consider discontinuation of one or both of these agents. Although discontinuation of therapy is usually sufficient, close monitoring is necessary due to the severity of the reaction.

Discussion

In patients receiving both isoniazid and rifampin, an increased incidence of hepatotoxicity has been observed.[4,8] This reaction may be associated with an alteration in isoniazid metabolic pathways by rifampin. Rifampin appears to induce a secondary pathway of isoniazid metabolism,[7,10] while having little net effect on the primary pathway.[1,5,6,9,10] The secondary pathway produces hydrazine and isonicotinic acid directly from isoniazid.[7,10] Hydrazine is a proven hepatotoxin, mutagen and carcinogen in animals.[7,10] Hepatotoxicity has occurred more often in slow vs fast acetylators of isoniazid.[10] Hydrazine levels have been shown to be higher in slow acetylators.[7,10] Thus, it is possible that hydrazine contributes to the hepatotoxicity seen in this interaction. Pharmacokinetic parameters of isoniazid are relatively stable in the presence of rifampin.[1-3,6,10]

The frequency of hepatotoxicity with this combination in adults implies that the effects are additive rather than synergistic.[11] Children appear to be more susceptible to the interaction than adults.[11]

1 Venho VMK, et al. *Ann Clin Res.* 1971;3:277.
2 Acocella G, et al. *Gut.* 1972;13:47.
3 Boman G, et al. *Eur J Clin Pharmacol.* 1974;7:217.
4 Pessayre D, et al. *Gastroenterology.* 1977;72:284.
5 Llorens J, et al. *Chemotherapy.* 1978;24:97.
6 Raghupati Sarma G, et al. *Antimicrob Agents Chemother.* 1980;18:661.
7 Beever IW, et al. *Br J Clin Pharmacol.* 1982;13:599p.
8 O'Brien RJ, et al. *Pediatrics.* 1983;72:491.
9 Timbrell JA, et al. *Human Toxicol.* 1985;4:279.
10 Raghupati Sarma G, et al. *Am Rev Resp Dis.* 1986;133:1072.
11 Steele MA, et al. *Chest.* 1991;99:465. Review.

* Asterisk indicates drugs cited in interaction reports.

Isoniazid — *Valproic Acid*

Isoniazid* (eg, *Nydrazid*)	Divalproex Sodium (*Depakote*)	Valproic Acid* (eg, *Depakene*)

Significance	Onset	Severity	Documentation
5	□ Rapid	□ Major	□ Established
	■ **Delayed**	■ **Moderate**	□ Probable
		□ Minor	□ Suspected
			□ Possible
			■ **Unlikely**

Effects The toxic effects of both drugs may be increased. Elevated valproic acid levels were reported in one patient.

Mechanism ISONIAZID may inhibit valproic acid metabolism.

Management If an interaction is suspected, measure valproic acid levels and liver function tests. If toxicity, increased serum valproic acid levels, or evidence of liver dysfunction occur, consider an alternative anticonvulsant.

Discussion

A 13-year-old girl with a history of epilepsy since the age of 9 months was treated with valproic acid for 10 years and was seizure-free for several years.[1] Upon developing tuberculosis, she was treated with isoniazid. During concurrent administration of isoniazid and valproic acid, loss of seizure control, elevated liver enzymes and CNS side effects, including drowsiness and vomiting, were observed. The altered liver enzymes and CNS side effects occurred only when the drugs were administered concomitantly, and not when either drug was given alone. A 5-year-old girl receiving valproic acid 600 mg/day experienced increased serum valproic acid levels (to 139 mcg/mL) with associated trauma and lethargy when isoniazid 200 mg daily was added to her treatment regimen.[2] Her valproic acid dose was reduced. After completion of isoniazid therapy, valproic acid levels decreased with ensuing seizures and the dose of the anticonvulsant was titrated to 600 mg daily. The patient was a slow isoniazid acetylator.

A causal relationship was not established in these cases. Controlled clinical studies are needed.

[1] Dockweiler U. *Lancet.* 1987;2:152.

[2] Jonville AP, et al. *Eur J Clin Pharmacol.* 1991;40:197.

* Asterisk indicates drugs cited in interaction reports. Based on pharmacologic and pharmacokinetic considerations, similar interactions may occur with other drugs that are listed.

Itraconazole — *Hydantoins*

Itraconazole* (eg, *Sporanox*)	Ethotoin (*Peganone*)	Phenytoin* (eg, *Dilantin*)
	Fosphenytoin	

Significance	Onset	Severity	Documentation
2	☐ Rapid	☐ Major	☐ Established
	■ **Delayed**	■ **Moderate**	☐ Probable
		☐ Minor	■ **Suspected**
			☐ Possible
			☐ Unlikely

Effects The pharmacologic effects of ITRACONAZOLE may be decreased, while those of HYDANTOINS may be increased.

Mechanism Increased metabolism of ITRACONAZOLE is suspected, while HYDANTOIN metabolism may be inhibited.

Management Until more clinical data are available, avoid concomitant use of ITRACONAZOLE and HYDANTOINS, if possible.

Discussion

The pharmacokinetics of single doses of itraconazole and phenytoin when given alone and after long-term administration of the other drug were studied in 32 healthy men.[1] The subjects were randomized into 2 groups. Volunteers in group 1 were given a single oral dose of itraconazole 200 mg alone and after 15 days of oral phenytoin 300 mg/day. The participants in group 2 received a single oral dose of phenytoin 300 mg alone and after 15 days of oral itraconazole 200 mg/day. Twenty-eight subjects completed the study. Phenytoin decreased the AUC of itraconazole 93% and the $t_{½}$ 83% (from 22.3 to 3.8 hours). In addition, itraconazole C_{max} decreased 83% (from 215 to 37 ng/mL). The AUC of one of the metabolites of itraconazole (hydroxyitraconazole) decreased 95%, and the $t_{½}$ decreased 74% (from 11.3 to 2.9 hours). Itraconazole increased the AUC of phenytoin 10%, while no changes occurred in other pharmacokinetic parameters. See also Hydantoins-Fluconazole and Hydantoins-Miconazole.

[1] Ducharme MP, et al. *Clin Pharmacol Ther.* 1995;58(6):617.

* Asterisk indicates drugs cited in interaction reports. Based on pharmacologic and pharmacokinetic considerations, similar interactions may occur with other drugs that are listed.

Ixabepilone — *Azole Antifungal Agents*

Ixabepilone	Azole Antifungal Agents	
Ixabepilone* (*Ixempra*)	Itraconazole* (eg, *Sporanox*)	Posaconazole* (*Noxafil*)
	Ketoconazole* (eg, *Nizoral*)	Voriconazole* (eg, *Vfend*)

Significance	Onset	Severity	Documentation
2	☐ Rapid	☐ Major	☐ Established
	■ **Delayed**	■ **Moderate**	☐ Probable
		☐ Minor	■ **Suspected**
			☐ Possible
			☐ Unlikely

Effects IXABEPILONE plasma concentrations may be elevated, increasing the risk of IXABEPILONE toxicity.

Mechanism AZOLE ANTIFUNGAL AGENTS inhibit the metabolism (CYP3A4) of IXABEPILONE.

Management Avoid coadministration of IXABEPILONE and AZOLE ANTIFUNGAL AGENTS. If these agents must be used concurrently, consider reducing the IXABEPILONE dosage to 20 mg/m^2 every 3 weeks.[1] If the AZOLE ANTIFUNGAL AGENT is discontinued, allow a washout period of approximately 1 week before adjusting the dose of IXABEPILONE up to the indicated dose.

Discussion

CYP3A4 is the major isozyme responsible for the metabolism of ixabepilone. Coadministration of strong inhibitors of CYP3A4 (eg, ketoconazole) is expected to increase ixabepilone plasma concentrations. Coadministration of ixabepilone and ketoconazole increased ixabepilone AUC 79% compared with administration of ixabepilone alone.[1] Therefore, if alternative treatment cannot be given, consider adjusting the ixabepilone dosage in patients receiving a strong CYP3A4 inhibitor (eg, ketoconazole) concurrently. Closely monitor patients for acute toxicities (eg, frequent monitoring of peripheral blood cell counts between ixabepilone cycles). The effects of ketoconazole on the pharmacokinetics and pharmacodynamics of ixabepilone were studied in 27 patients who had advanced malignancies.[2] Coadministration of ketoconazole and ixabepilone increased the ixabepilone AUC 79% compared with giving ixabepilone alone. When administered with ketoconazole, the maximum tolerated ixabepilone dose was 25 mg/m^2 compared with the recommended dose of 40 mg/m^2 when ixabepilone is given alone.

[1] *Ixempra* [package insert]. Princeton, NJ: Bristol-Myers Squibb; October 2007.

[2] Goel S, et al. *Clin Cancer Res*. 2008;14(9):2701.

* Asterisk indicates drugs cited in interaction reports.

Ixabepilone ✕ **Capecitabine**

Ixabepilone* (*Ixempra*)	Capecitabine* (*Xeloda*)

Significance	Onset	Severity	Documentation
1	☐ Rapid ■ **Delayed**	■ **Major** ☐ Moderate ☐ Minor	☐ Established ☐ Probable ■ **Suspected** ☐ Possible ☐ Unlikely

Effects The risk of neurotoxicity and neutropenia-related death may be increased in patients with hepatic function impairment.

Mechanism Unknown. Possible additive toxicity including neutropenia. IXABEPILONE exposure is increased in patients with elevated AST or bilirubin.

Management Coadministration of IXABEPILONE and CAPECITABINE is contraindicated in patients with AST or ALT greater than 2.5 times the upper limit of normal (ULN) or bilirubin greater than 1 times the ULN.

Discussion

Coadministration of ixabepilone and capecitabine is indicated for the treatment of patients with metastatic or locally advanced breast cancer resistant to anthracycline and taxane treatment, or whose cancer is taxane resistant and for whom additional anthracycline treatment is contraindicated. However, coadministration of ixabepilone and capecitabine is contraindicated in patients with AST or ALT greater than 2.5 times the ULN or bilirubin greater than 1 times the ULN because of an increased risk of toxicity and neutropenia-related death. In patients receiving combined treatment with ixabepilone and capecitabine, neutropenia-related death was reported to be 29% (5 of 17) in patients with AST or ALT greater than 2.5 times the ULN or bilirubin greater than 1 times the ULN, compared with 0.4% of 240 patients receiving ixabepilone monotherapy.[1]

The basis for this monograph is information on file with the manufacturer. Because of the seriousness of the adverse reactions, clinical evaluation of this interaction in humans is not likely to be forthcoming.

[1] *Ixempra* [package insert]. Princeton, NJ: Bristol-Myers Squibb; October 2009.

* Asterisk indicates drugs cited in interaction reports.

Ixabepilone — *Macrolide & Related Antibiotics*

Ixabepilone* (*Ixempra*)	Clarithromycin* (eg, *Biaxin*)	Telithromycin* (*Ketek*)

Significance	Onset	Severity	Documentation
2	☐ Rapid ■ **Delayed**	☐ Major ■ **Moderate** ☐ Minor	☐ Established ☐ Probable ■ **Suspected** ☐ Possible ☐ Unlikely

Effects IXABEPILONE plasma concentrations may be elevated, increasing the risk of IXABEPILONE toxicity.

Mechanism MACROLIDE AND RELATED ANTIBIOTICS inhibit the metabolism (CYP3A4) of IXABEPILONE.

Management Avoid coadministration of IXABEPILONE and MACROLIDE AND RELATED ANTIBIOTICS. If these agents must be used concurrently, consider reducing the dosage of XABEPILONE to 20 mg/m^2 every 3 weeks.[1] If the MACROLIDE OR RELATED ANTIBIOTIC is discontinued, allow a washout period of approximately 1 week before upwardly adjusting the IXABEPILONE dose to the indicated dose.

Discussion

CYP-450 3A4 is the major isozyme responsible for the metabolism of ixabepilone.[1] Coadministration of strong inhibitors of CYP3A4 (eg, clarithromycin) is expected to increase ixabepilone plasma concentrations. Therefore, if alternative treatment cannot be given, consider adjusting the ixabepilone dosage in patients concurrently receiving a strong CYP3A4 inhibitor (eg, clarithromycin). Closely monitor patients for acute toxicities (eg, frequent monitoring of peripheral blood cell counts between ixabepilone cycles).

The basis for this monograph is information on file with the manufacturer.[1] Studies are needed to determine the clinical importance of this interaction and the effect of other macrolide and related antibiotics on ixabepilone metabolism.

[1] *Ixempra* [package insert]. Princeton, NJ: Bristol-Myers Squibb; October 2007.

* Asterisk indicates drugs cited in interaction reports.

Ixabepilone | **Nefazodone**

Ixabepilone*
(*Ixempra*)

Nefazodone*

Significance	Onset	Severity	Documentation
2	☐ Rapid ■ **Delayed**	☐ Major ■ **Moderate** ☐ Minor	☐ Established ☐ Probable ■ **Suspected** ☐ Possible ☐ Unlikely

Effects IXABEPILONE plasma concentrations may be elevated, increasing the risk of IXABEPILONE toxicity.

Mechanism NEFAZODONE inhibits the metabolism (CYP3A4) of IXABEPILONE.

Management Avoid coadministration of IXABEPILONE and NEFAZODONE. If these agents must be used concurrently, consider reducing the dosage of IXABEPILONE to 20 mg/m^2 every 3 weeks.[1] If NEFAZODONE is discontinued, allow a washout period of approximately 1 week before upwardly adjusting the IXABEPILONE dose to the indicated dose.

Discussion

CYP-450 3A4 is the major isozyme responsible for the metabolism of ixabepilone.[1] Coadministration of strong inhibitors of CYP3A4 (eg, nefazodone) is expected to increase ixabepilone plasma concentrations. Therefore, if alternative treatment cannot be given, consider reducing the ixabepilone dosage in patients concurrently receiving a strong CYP3A4 inhibitor (eg, nefazodone). Closely monitor patients for acute toxicities (eg, frequent monitoring of peripheral blood cell counts between ixabepilone cycles).

The basis for this monograph is information on file with the manufacturer.[1] Studies are needed to determine the clinical importance of this interaction.

[1] *Ixempra* [package insert]. Princeton, NJ: Bristol-Myers Squibb; October 2007.

* Asterisk indicates drugs cited in interaction reports.

Ixabepilone — *NNRT Inhibitors*

Ixabepilone* (*Ixempra*)	Delavirdine* (*Rescriptor*)

Significance	Onset	Severity	Documentation
2	☐ Rapid	☐ Major	☐ Established
	■ **Delayed**	■ **Moderate**	☐ Probable
		☐ Minor	■ **Suspected**
			☐ Possible
			☐ Unlikely

Effects IXABEPILONE plasma concentrations may be elevated, increasing the risk of IXABEPILONE toxicity.

Mechanism DELAVIRDINE inhibits the metabolism (CYP3A4) of IXABEPILONE.

Management Avoid coadministration of IXABEPILONE and DELAVIRDINE. If these agents must be used concurrently, consider reducing the dosage of IXABEPILONE to 20 mg/m^2 every 3 weeks.[1] If DELAVIRDINE is discontinued, allow a washout period of approximately 1 week before upwardly adjusting the IXABEPILONE dose to the indicated dose.

Discussion

CYP-450 3A4 is the major isozyme responsible for the metabolism of ixabepilone.[1] Coadministration of strong inhibitors of CYP3A4 (eg, delavirdine) is expected to increase ixabepilone plasma concentrations. Therefore, if alternative treatment cannot be given, consider adjusting the ixabepilone dosage in patients concurrently receiving a strong CYP3A4 inhibitor (eg, delavirdine). Closely monitor patients for acute toxicities (eg, frequent monitoring of peripheral blood cell counts between ixabepilone cycles).

The basis for this monograph is information on file with the manufacturer.[1] Studies are needed to determine the clinical importance of this interaction and the effect of other NNRT inhibitors on ixabepilone metabolism.

[1] *Ixempra* [package insert]. Princeton, NJ: Bristol-Myers Squibb; October 2007.

* Asterisk indicates drugs cited in interaction reports.

Ixabepilone — *Protease Inhibitors*

Ixabepilone	Protease Inhibitors	
Ixabepilone* (*Ixempra*)	Amprenavir*†	Ritonavir* (*Norvir*)
	Atazanavir* (*Reyataz*)	Saquinavir* (*Invirase*)
	Indinavir* (*Crixivan*)	
	Nelfinavir* (*Viracept*)	

Significance	Onset	Severity	Documentation
2	□ Rapid	□ Major	□ Established
	■ **Delayed**	■ **Moderate**	□ Probable
		□ Minor	■ **Suspected**
			□ Possible
			□ Unlikely

Effects IXABEPILONE plasma concentrations may be elevated, increasing the risk of IXABEPILONE toxicity.

Mechanism PROTEASE INHIBITORS inhibit the metabolism (CYP3A4) of IXABEPILONE.

Management Avoid coadministration of IXABEPILONE and PROTEASE INHIBITORS. If these agents must be used concurrently, consider reducing the dosage of IXABEPILONE to 20 mg/m^2 every 3 weeks.[1] If the PROTEASE INHIBITOR is discontinued, allow a washout period of approximately 1 week before upwardly adjusting the IXABEPILONE dose to the indicated dose.

Discussion

CYP-450 3A4 is the major isozyme responsible for the metabolism of ixabepilone.[1] Coadministration of strong inhibitors of CYP3A4 (eg, indinavir) is expected to increase ixabepilone plasma concentrations. Therefore, if alternative treatment cannot be given, consider adjusting the ixabepilone dosage in patients concurrently receiving a strong CYP3A4 inhibitor (eg, indinavir). Closely monitor patients for acute toxicities (eg, frequent monitoring of peripheral blood cell counts between ixabepilone cycles).

The basis for this monograph is information on file with the manufacturer.[1] Studies are needed to determine the clinical importance of this interaction and the effect of other protease inhibitors on ixabepilone metabolism.

[1] *Ixempra* [package insert]. Princeton, NJ: Bristol-Myers Squibb; October 2007.

* Asterisk indicates drugs cited in interaction reports.
† Not available in the United States.

Ketamine — *Halothane*

Ketamine* (eg, *Ketalar*)	Halothane*

Significance	Onset	Severity	Documentation
2	■ **Rapid**	□ Major	■ **Established**
	□ Delayed	■ **Moderate**	□ Probable
		□ Minor	□ Suspected
			□ Possible
			□ Unlikely

Effects Hypotension and decreased cardiac output may occur following the addition of KETAMINE to patients receiving HALOTHANE.

Mechanism Unknown.

Management Use this combination with caution. Monitor blood pressure frequently. If an interaction occurs, supportive therapy (including the use of atropine) may be necessary.

Discussion

Studies have shown that administration of ketamine (2 mg/kg or 75 mg/m^2) to patients anesthetized with halothane (0.3% to 1.5%) can produce dramatic decreases in blood pressure,[1-3] cardiac output, and stroke volume.[3] Heart rate was noted to decrease slightly in one study,[2] but not in the others.[1,3] Effects were seen within 2 to 3 minutes and were still present up to 30 minutes after coadministration.[1,3]

[1] Stanley TH. *Anesthesiology*. 1973;39(6):648.
[2] Johnston RR, et al. *Anesth Analg*. 1974;53(4):496.
[3] Bidwai AV, et al. *Anesth Analg*. 1975;54(5):588.

* Asterisk indicates drugs cited in interaction reports.

Ketamine — *Thyroid Hormones*

Ketamine		Thyroid Hormones	
Ketamine* (eg, *Ketalar*)		Levothyroxine* (eg, *Synthroid*)	Liotrix (*Thyrolar*)
		Liothyronine (eg, *Cytomel*)	Thyroid (eg, *Armour Thyroid*)

Significance	Onset	Severity	Documentation
5	■ **Rapid**	□ Major	□ Established
	□ Delayed	■ **Moderate**	□ Probable
		□ Minor	□ Suspected
			□ Possible
			■ **Unlikely**

Effects Hypertension and tachycardia may be seen during coadministration of KETAMINE and THYROID HORMONES.

Mechanism Unknown.

Management If an interaction is suspected, treat patients symptomatically.

Discussion

One paper reported 2 cases of patients on levothyroxine who developed severe hypertension (240/140 and 210/130 mm Hg) and tachycardia (190 and 150 bpm) following the administration of ketamine 125 to 150 mg for elective surgery.[1] Both patients had normal baseline blood pressures and heart rates. Their supraventricular tachycardias were successfully treated with propranolol 1 mg by slow IV push. Later in their procedures, additional doses of ketamine 25 to 50 mg were given and did not produce alterations in blood pressure or heart rate.

It is unclear whether these reactions could have been caused by ketamine alone.

[1] Kaplan JA, et al. *Anesthesiology*. 1971;35:229.

* Asterisk indicates drugs cited in interaction reports. Based on pharmacologic and pharmacokinetic considerations, similar interactions may occur with other drugs that are listed.

Ketoconazole — *Antacids*

Ketoconazole	Antacids	
Ketoconazole* (eg, *Nizoral*)	Aluminum Hydroxide (eg, *Amphojel*)	Magnesium Hydroxide (eg, *Milk of Magnesia*)
	Aluminum/ Magnesium Hydroxide	Sodium Bicarbonate*

Significance	Onset	Severity	Documentation
2	☐ Rapid ■ **Delayed**	☐ Major ■ **Moderate** ☐ Minor	☐ Established ☐ Probable ■ **Suspected** ☐ Possible ☐ Unlikely

Effects The therapeutic effects of KETOCONAZOLE may be reduced.

Mechanism Possibly decreased bioavailability of KETOCONAZOLE. This appears to be related to a reduced tablet dissolution in the presence of higher gastric pH.

Management Consider giving ANTACIDS at least 2 hours after KETOCONAZOLE, although efficacy has not been established.

Discussion

A single case report found ketoconazole 200 mg/day to be ineffective in treating cryptococcal suppurative arthritis in a patient with systemic lupus erythematosus and severe renal impairment. Concomitant therapy included sodium bicarbonate, aluminum oxide, and cimetidine (eg, *Tagamet*), with dosages adjusted for renal failure. After discontinuing cimetidine and altering administration time of sodium bicarbonate and aluminum oxide to 2 hours after the ketoconazole dose, the patient responded.[1] The administration of a single dose of an aluminum-magnesium antacid to 4 patients produced a 41% decrease in AUC compared with control patients. This was not statistically significant, possibly because of the small sample size.[2] In vitro, ketoconazole dissolution was directly related to pH. At pH 2 or 3, dissolution was more than 85% after 5 minutes, but at pH 6 only 10% was dissolved after 60 minutes.[3] In a study involving 12 healthy volunteers, achlorhydria was simulated by administering cimetidine 300 mg and sodium bicarbonate 2 g prior to ketoconazole 200 mg.[4] This combination produced a marked reduction in peak ketoconazole concentration from 4.37 to 0.32 mcg/mL and a decrease in the AUC from 15.25 to 1.29 mcg•hr/mL. While the effects of both drugs cannot be separated, this study demonstrated that decreased gastric acidity impairs ketoconazole absorption. By contrast, fluconazole (eg, *Diflucan*), a related antifungal agent, was unaffected by coadministration with an aluminum-magnesium antacid.[5] See also Ketoconazole-Histamine H_2 Antagonists.

[1] Van Der Meer JW, et al. *J Antimicrob Chemother.* 1980;6:552.
[2] Brass C, et al. *Antimicrob Agents Chemother.* 1982;21:151. (erratum *Antimicrob Agents Chemother.* 1982;21:692).
[3] Carlson JA, et al. *Am J Hosp Pharm.* 1983;40:1334.
[4] Lelawongs P, et al. *Clin Pharm.* 1988;7:228.
[5] Thorpe JE, et al. *Antimicrob Agents Chemother.* 1990;34:2032.

* Asterisk indicates drugs cited in interaction reports. Based on pharmacologic and pharmacokinetic considerations, similar interactions may occur with other drugs that are listed.

Ketoconazole — *Isoniazid*

Ketoconazole* (eg, *Nizoral*)	Isoniazid* (eg, *Nydrazid*)

Significance	Onset	Severity	Documentation
4	☐ Rapid	☐ Major	☐ Established
	■ **Delayed**	■ **Moderate**	☐ Probable
		☐ Minor	☐ Suspected
			■ **Possible**
			☐ Unlikely

Effects The therapeutic benefit of KETOCONAZOLE may be attenuated.

Mechanism Unknown. (See discussion.)

Management Avoid concomitant use if possible. Monitoring of KETOCONAZOLE serum levels or antifungal activity may be necessary.

Discussion

Concomitant use of isoniazid and ketoconazole decreased the ketoconazole serum concentration and AUC approximately 80% and resulted in antifungal treatment failure. This was seen regardless of whether the drugs were given together or 12 hr apart.[1] Two other cases have been reported in which isoniazid had a similar effect on ketoconazole.[2,3] In both of these cases, the patient was also taking rifampin (eg, *Rifadin*). The ketoconazole AUC decreased 78% with the addition of isoniazid.[2] Ketoconazole, isoniazid, and rifampin were not detected in 1 patient taking the 3 agents concomitantly.[3] The mechanism of this interaction is unknown, but is probably not related to GI absorption because there was no change in ketoconazole concentrations when the administration times were altered.

[1] Engelhard D, et al. *N Engl J Med.* 1984;311:1681.

[2] Brass C, et al. *Antimicrob Agents Chemother.* 1982;21:151. (erratum *Antimicrob Agents Chemother.* 1982;21:692.)

[3] Abadie-Kemmerly S, et al. *Ann Intern Med.* 1988;109:844. (erratum *Ann Intern Med.* 1989;111:96.)

* Asterisk indicates drugs cited in interaction reports.

Ketoconazole — *Sucralfate*

Ketoconazole*
(eg, *Nizoral*)

Sucralfate*
(eg, *Carafate*)

Significance	Onset	Severity	Documentation
4	■ **Rapid** □ Delayed	□ Major ■ **Moderate** □ Minor	□ Established □ Probable □ Suspected ■ **Possible** □ Unlikely

Effects The therapeutic effects of KETOCONAZOLE may be reduced.

Mechanism Unknown. Likely caused by a decrease in KETOCONAZOLE bioavailability.

Management When the clinical situation permits, administer KETOCONAZOLE at least 2 hr before SUCRALFATE.

Discussion

In a randomized, crossover investigation, coadministration of ketoconazole and sucralfate produced a 20% decrease in the bioavailability of ketoconazole.[1] Subjects received a single oral dose of ketoconazole 400 mg (control group) or sucralfate 1 g orally 4 times/day for 2 days prior to the administration of ketoconazole 400 mg, then 1 g sucralfate (extemporaneously compounded as a suspension) 5 min before the 400 mg dose of ketoconazole. A decrease in the peak serum ketoconazole concentration (from a mean of 8.2 to 5.39 mcg/mL) occurred in 5 subjects during coadministration of sucralfate compared with the control treatment and a slight increase was observed in 1. Five subjects showed an increase in the time to reach peak ketoconazole concentration (mean increase 1.75 to 3.42 hr) while 1 subject had no change. A decrease in the AUC was measured in 5 subjects during sucralfate administration compared with the control group (mean decrease from 37.05 to 29.17 mg•hr/L) while 1 subject exhibited an increase. Compared with the control group, there was a 20% decrease in bioavailability for ketoconazole during coadministration with sucralfate.

[1] Piscitelli SC, et al. *Antimicrob Agents Chemother.* 1991;35:1765.

* Asterisk indicates drugs cited in interaction reports.

Ketorolac — *Probenecid*

Ketorolac*
(eg, *Toradol*)

Probenecid*

Significance	Onset	Severity	Documentation
1	☐ Rapid ■ **Delayed**	■ **Major** ☐ Moderate ☐ Minor	☐ Established ☐ Probable ■ **Suspected** ☐ Possible ☐ Unlikely

Effects Serum KETOROLAC concentrations may be elevated, increasing the toxicity (eg, renal, GI, hematologic).

Mechanism PROBENECID may decrease the clearance of KETOROLAC.

Management Coadministration is contraindicated.

Discussion

The coadministration of ketorolac and probenecid is contraindicated.[1] Coadministration of ketorolac and probenecid resulted in a decrease in ketorolac clearance, an increase in plasma ketorolac concentrations, and a 2-fold increase in the terminal $t_{½}$ (from 6.6 to 15.1 hr). The total AUC increased 3-fold (from 5.4 to 17.8 mcg•hr/mL). The basis for the contraindication appears to be the possible increase in serum ketorolac concentrations. Ketorolac is a potent nonsteroidal anti-inflammatory analgesic and increasing serum concentrations of the drug may increase the risk of developing serious adverse reactions, including renal and GI effects and the risk of bleeding. Probenecid has been found to increase serum concentrations and the toxicity of other NSAIDs; however, the clinical importance of these interactions does not appear to be as important as with ketorolac because of their relative NSAID effect. See also NSAIDs-Probenecid.

The basis for this monograph is information on file with the manufacturer. Published clinical data are needed to further assess this interaction.

[1] Manufacturer's information. Ketorolac (*Toradol*). Roche Laboratories, Inc. December 1994.

* Asterisk indicates drugs cited in interaction reports.

Ketorolac — *Salicylates*

Ketorolac* (eg, *Toradol*)	Aspirin* (eg, *Bayer*)

Significance	Onset	Severity	Documentation
1	☐ Rapid ■ **Delayed**	■ **Major** ☐ Moderate ☐ Minor	☐ Established ☐ Probable ■ **Suspected** ☐ Possible ☐ Unlikely

Effects Increased risk of serious KETOROLAC-related side effects.

Mechanism SALICYLATES may displace KETOROLAC from protein binding sites. Possible synergistic side effects.

Management KETOROLAC is contraindicated in patients receiving ASPIRIN.

Discussion

In vitro investigations indicated that at therapeutic concentrations of salicylates (300 mcg/mL) there is a 2-fold increase in unbound plasma ketorolac concentrations (from 99.2% to 97.5%).[1] Ketorolac is also contraindicated in patients receiving other NSAIDs.[1]

The basis for this monograph is information on file with the manufacturer. Although ketorolac is an NSAID, it is being considered separately from other NSAIDs because it is contraindicated in patients receiving aspirin. See also NSAIDs-Salicylates.

[1] Product information. Ketorolac (*Toradol*). Roche Laboratories. July 1995.

* Asterisk indicates drugs cited in interaction reports.

Labetalol — *Cimetidine*

Labetalol* (eg, *Normodyne*)	Cimetidine* (*Tagamet*)

Significance	Onset	Severity	Documentation
4	■ **Rapid**	□ Major	□ Established
	□ Delayed	■ **Moderate**	□ Probable
		□ Minor	□ Suspected
			■ **Possible**
			□ Unlikely

Effects Increased hypotensive effect of LABETALOL.

Mechanism Increased bioavailability.

Management Monitor patient for hypotension and reduce the dose of LABETALOL accordingly.

Discussion

The effects of labetalol 200 mg orally with cimetidine 400 mg every 6 hours were evaluated in 6 patients.[1,2] There was no significant change in the half-life or clearance of labetalol, but the bioavailability was increased 56% and the AUC 66%. Most patients exhibited a slight hypotensive response, but the change in blood pressure did not reach statistical significance. Interestingly, the patient with the greatest increase in plasma labetalol levels exhibited the greatest reduction in blood pressure. A case report involving a 64-year-old patient receiving both labetalol and cimetidine suggested an interaction between the two agents that resulted in prolonged and excessive hypotension after surgery.[3]

Monitor patients for excessive hypotension when these two agents are given concurrently. If an interaction is suspected, reduce the dose of labetalol accordingly.

[1] Daneshmend TK, et al. *Lancet.* 1981;1:565.
[2] Daneshmend TK, et al. *Br J Clin Pharmacol.* 1984;18:393.
[3] Durant PAC, et al. *Br J Anaesth.* 1984;56:917.

* Asterisk indicates drugs cited in interaction reports.

Labetalol — *Glutethimide*

Labetalol* (eg, *Normodyne*)	Glutethimide* (eg, *Doriden*)

Significance	Onset	Severity	Documentation
5	■ **Rapid**	□ Major	□ Established
	□ Delayed	□ Moderate	□ Probable
		■ **Minor**	□ Suspected
			■ **Possible**
			□ Unlikely

Effects Reduction of hypotensive action of LABETALOL.

Mechanism Microsomal enzyme induction.

Management Consider increasing the dose of LABETALOL during coadministration of GLUTETHIMIDE. Monitor the patient's blood pressure response and adjust the dose accordingly.

Discussion

Glutethimide 500 mg was administered at bedtime to five healthy volunteers for 28 days prior to receiving labetalol 200 mg orally.[1] The bioavailability of labetalol was decreased by 43%, but there were no statistically significant changes in heart rate or blood pressure. The proposed mechanism for the interaction was induction of microsomal enzymes by glutethimide. Glutethimide has no effect on labetalol given intravenously.

The significance of this interaction is poorly defined, and the possibility of it occurring is not strong. If an interaction is suspected, monitor the patient closely for changes in blood pressure before increasing the labetalol dose accordingly.

[1] Daneshmend TK, et al. *Br J Clin Pharmacol.* 1984;18:393.

* Asterisk indicates drugs cited in interaction reports.

Labetalol — *Inhalation Anesthetics*

Labetalol	Inhalation Anesthetics	
Labetalol* (eg, *Normodyne*)	Desflurane (*Suprane*)	Isoflurane* (eg, *Forane*)
	Enflurane* (*Ethrane*)	Sevoflurane (*Ultane*)
	Halothane* (eg, *Fluothane*)	

Significance	Onset	Severity	Documentation
2	■ **Rapid**	□ Major	□ Established
	□ Delayed	■ **Moderate**	■ **Probable**
		□ Minor	□ Suspected
			□ Possible
			□ Unlikely

Effects Excessive hypotension.

Mechanism Additive myocardial depressant effects.

Management Use LABETALOL and HALOTHANE together with caution and monitor blood pressure closely. To minimize hypotensive effects, the concentration of HALOTHANE should not exceed 3%.

Discussion

Halothane in concentrations of 0.8% to 1.2% reduces arterial blood pressure by decreasing cardiac output (20% to 50%) and by blunting the baroreceptor response to hypotension. Labetalol, a combined alpha and beta blocker, produces synergistic myocardial depressant effects when given with halothane resulting in a significant reduction in cardiac output and blood pressure.[1,2] The degree and duration of the interaction is dose dependent and may be controlled by adjusting the concentration of halothane. Scott et al, found that patients receiving a single 25 mg dose of IV labetalol did not exhibit excessive hypotensive reactions until the halothane concentration reached 3%.[2] Patients receiving oral labetalol prior to surgery are also at risk for hypotension and should be monitored closely throughout the surgical procedure.[3] The interaction has also been documented with enflurane and isoflurane and appears to be ideal for inducing deliberate hypotension in some types of surgery.[4]

Patients receiving both labetalol and halothane should be monitored closely for excessive hypotension, and the concentration of halothane should be reduced accordingly if necessary.

1 Scott DB, et al. *Br J Clin Pharmacol.* 1976;3(suppl):817.
2 Scott DB, et al. *Anaesthesia.* 1978;33:145.
3 Hunter JM. *Anaesthesia.* 1979;34:257.
4 Toivonen J, et al. *Acta Anaesthesiol Scand.* 1989;33:283.

* Asterisk indicates drugs cited in interaction reports. Based on pharmacologic and pharmacokinetic considerations, similar interactions may occur with other drugs that are listed.

Lamivudine — *Trimethoprim*

Lamivudine	Trimethoprim	
Lamivudine* (*Epivir*)	Trimethoprim (eg, *Proloprim*)	Trimethoprim/Sulfamethoxazole* (eg, *Bactrim*)

Significance	Onset	Severity	Documentation
5	■ **Rapid**	□ Major	□ Established
	□ Delayed	□ Moderate	□ Probable
		■ **Minor**	□ Suspected
			□ Possible
			■ **Unlikely**

Effects Plasma lamivudine concentrations may be increased.

Mechanism TRIMETHOPRIM appears to inhibit the renal secretion of LAMIVUDINE.

Management Based upon available data, no special precautions are necessary.

Discussion

The effects of trimethoprim-sulfamethoxazole (TMP-SMX) on the pharmacokinetics of lamivudine, and vice versa, were studied in 14 asymptomatic subjects with human immunodeficiency virus (HIV).[1] In a randomized, two-way, crossover study, each subject received an oral dose of 300 mg of lamivudine alone or oral trimethoprim-sulfamethoxazole (160/800 mg) daily for 4 days, followed by a dose simultaneously with 300 mg of lamivudine on the fifth day. Compared with giving lamivudine alone, concomitant administration of TMP-SMX increased the area under the plasma concentration-time curve of lamivudine by 43%, decreased the oral clearance by 30% and decreased the renal clearance by 35%. Administration of a single dose of lamivudine with the fifth dose of TMP-SMX did not alter the pharmacokinetics of TMP-SMX. There were no differences in side effects between the treatment groups.

[1] Moore KHP, et al. *Clin Pharmacol Ther.* 1996;59:550.

* Asterisk indicates drugs cited in interaction reports. Based on pharmacologic and pharmacokinetic considerations, similar interactions may occur with other drugs that are listed.

Lamotrigine | **Acetaminophen**

Lamotrigine* (*Lamictal*)	Acetaminophen* (eg, *Tylenol*)

Significance	Onset	Severity	Documentation
4	☐ Rapid ■ **Delayed**	☐ Major ■ **Moderate** ☐ Minor	☐ Established ☐ Probable ☐ Suspected ■ **Possible** ☐ Unlikely

Effects Serum lamotrigine concentrations may be reduced, producing a decrease in therapeutic effects.

Mechanism Unknown.

Management A clinically important interaction is unlikely to occur with a single dose or several doses of ACETAMINOPHEN. With chronic administration of ACETAMINOPHEN, if an interaction is suspected, it may be necessary to adjust the dose of LAMOTRIGINE. Observe the clinical response of the patient, and adjust the LAMOTRIGINE dose as indicated.

Discussion

Utilizing a double-blind, randomized, crossover, placebo controlled design, the effects of multiple oral doses of acetaminophen, 2700 mg daily, on a single oral dose of lamotrigine (150 mg) were studied in eight healthy volunteers.[1] Acetaminophen administration decreased the area under the plasma concentration-time curve of lamotrigine from 229 to 191.2 mcg•hr/mL (17%) and the half-life from 35.7 to 30.2 hr (15%). These decreases were statistically significant (p = 0.01). In addition, the percentage of the β-glucuronidase hydrolyzable conjugate of lamotrigine recovered in the urine was significantly higher (72.5%) compared with acetaminophen administration (65.9%, p = 0.05).

Controlled clinical studies are needed to determine if the magnitude of the effects of acetaminophen on lamotrigine serum concentrations are sufficient enough to produce a clinically important drug interaction.

[1] Depot M. et al. *Clin Pharmacol Ther.* 1990;48:346.

* Asterisk indicates drugs cited in interaction reports.

Lamotrigine — *Carbamazepine*

Lamotrigine* (eg, *Lamictal*) | Carbamazepine* (eg, *Tegretol*)

Significance	Onset	Severity	Documentation
2	☐ Rapid ■ **Delayed**	☐ Major ■ **Moderate** ☐ Minor	☐ Established ■ **Probable** ☐ Suspected ☐ Possible ☐ Unlikely

Effects Serum LAMOTRIGINE levels and efficacy may be reduced. Serum levels of the active epoxide metabolite of CARBAMAZEPINE (CBZ) may be elevated, increasing CBZ toxicity.

Mechanism LAMOTRIGINE metabolism may be increased. LAMOTRIGINE may increase CBZ toxicity.

Management It may be necessary to adjust the dose of LAMOTRIGINE when the dose of CBZ is started, stopped, or changed. Observe clinical response and adjust the LAMOTRIGINE dose as needed. When adding LAMOTRIGINE to regimens including CBZ, monitor for CBZ toxicity and reduce the dose if noted.

Discussion

A dose-dependent decrease in lamotrigine $t_{1/2}$ (1.7 hours per CBZ 100 mg) was reported in the range of CBZ 800 to 1,600 mg/day.[1] The manufacturer of lamotrigine reports that CBZ may decrease steady-state lamotrigine serum levels 40%.[2] A similar drug interaction may occur with other enzyme-inducing antiepileptic agents, including phenobarbital, phenytoin (eg, *Dilantin*), and primidone (eg, *Mysoline*).[2] Two studies have demonstrated a decrease in lamotrigine $t_{1/2}$ in children taking enzyme-inducers, including CBZ.[3,4] A potential interaction between lamotrigine and CBZ, as well as the epoxide metabolite of carbamazepine (CBZ-E), was reported in 9 patients.[5] Lamotrigine 100 to 300 mg/day administration was associated with a variable increase or decrease in serum CBZ levels (a mean rise of 16%) and a 45% increase in trough steady-state plasma CBZ-E level. The CBZ to CBZ-E ratio increased 19%. Four patients displayed symptoms of CBZ toxicity (eg, dizziness, nausea, diplopia) that resolved when the CBZ dose was decreased. In 2 patients, CBZ-E levels increased when the dose of lamotrigine was increased. In 9 of 47 patients on stable CBZ regimens, CNS toxicity developed after starting lamotrigine.[6] No change in serum levels of CBZ or CBZ-E was noted. Other investigators have not found lamotrigine to alter the disposition of CBZ-E.[7,8]

1 Jawad S, et al. *Epilepsy Res.* 1987;1(3):194.
2 *Lamictal* [package insert]. Research Park Triangle, NC: GlaxoSmithKline; December 1994.
3 Vauzelle-Kervroedan F, et al. *Br J Clin Pharmacol.* 1996;41(4):325.
4 Eriksson AS, et al. *Epilepsia.* 1996;37(8):769.
5 Warner T, et al. *Epilepsy Res.* 1992;11(2):147.
6 Besag FM, et al. *Epilepsia.* 1998;39(2):183.
7 Pisani F, et al. *Epilepsy Res.* 1994;19(3):245.
8 Malminiemi K, et al. *Int J Clin Pharmacol Ther.* 2000;38(11):540.

* Asterisk indicates drugs cited in interaction reports.

Lamotrigine — *Contraceptives, Hormonal*

Lamotrigine* (eg, *Lamictal*)	Contraceptives, Oral* (eg, *Desogen*)

Significance	Onset	Severity	Documentation
2	☐ Rapid ■ **Delayed**	☐ Major ■ **Moderate** ☐ Minor	☐ Established ■ **Probable** ☐ Suspected ☐ Possible ☐ Unlikely

Effects LAMOTRIGINE plasma concentrations may be reduced, decreasing the therapeutic effect.

Mechanism Increased LAMOTRIGINE metabolism (glucuronidation) by HORMONAL CONTRACEPTIVE use is suspected.

Management Observe the clinical response and adjust the LAMOTRIGINE dose as needed when HORMONAL CONTRACEPTIVES are started or stopped.

Discussion

Lamotrigine plasma concentrations in 7 women decreased during coadministration of oral contraceptives consisting of ethinyl estradiol plus desogestrel, ethinyl estradiol plus norethindrone, and norethindrone alone.[1] Two women were taking lamotrigine when oral contraceptives were started. In both individuals, lamotrigine plasma levels decreased and seizures occurred 1 to 2 months after starting oral contraceptives. Two women were taking lamotrigine when oral contraceptives were discontinued. In 1 woman, lamotrigine plasma levels increased 1 week after discontinuing oral contraceptive use. Three weeks later, she developed symptoms of lamotrigine toxicity (eg, dizziness, double vision, nausea), necessitating a decrease in the lamotrigine dosage. One woman discontinued oral contraceptive use to become pregnant. Several months after a successful pregnancy, to achieve lamotrigine plasma levels similar to those attained while she was taking the oral contraceptive, it was necessary to reduce the lamotrigine dose. Three women were taking lamotrigine when oral contraceptives were started and discontinued. Seizure control deteriorated after oral contraceptives were started, and lamotrigine plasma levels decreased. After discontinuing the oral contraceptives, lamotrigine plasma levels increased and one of the patients developed symptoms of lamotrigine toxicity. In 22 women taking lamotrigine (dosage range, 25 to 700 mg/day) plus an oral contraceptive, lamotrigine levels decreased 54% compared with lamotrigine alone.[2] In women taking lamotrigine and oral contraceptives concurrently, lamotrigine clearance was increased from 49 L per 24 hr to 126 L per 24 hr compared with women receiving lamotrigine alone.[3] Lamotrigine levels were decreased in a study of 45 women using combination estrogen-progestin contraceptives, but not in women using progestin only.[4] In 8 women taking lamotrigine and oral contraceptives, which involved a hormonal contraceptive–free week every 4 weeks, lamotrigine plasma levels increased 27% by the end of the hormone-free week.[5] Similarly, in a double-blind study, when women on chronic lamotrigine therapy stopped their oral contraceptive use for 1 month, lamotrigine levels increased 84%.[6] See Lamotrigine-Progestins.

[1] Sabers A, et al. *Epilepsy Res.* 2001;47(1-2):151.
[2] Sabers A, et al. *Neurology.* 2003:61(4):570.
[3] Wegner I, et al. *Neurology.* 2009;73(17):1388.
[4] Reimers A, et al. *Epilepsia.* 2005;46(9):1414.
[5] Contin M, et al. *Epilepsia.* 2006;47(9):1573.
[6] Christensen J, et al. *Epilepsia.* 2007;48(3)484.

* Asterisk indicates drugs cited in interaction reports.

Lamotrigine — *Orlistat*

Lamotrigine* (eg, *Lamictal*)	Orlistat* (eg, *Xenical*)

Significance	Onset	Severity	Documentation
4	□ Rapid ■ **Delayed**	□ Major ■ **Moderate** □ Minor	□ Established □ Probable □ Suspected ■ **Possible** □ Unlikely

Effects LAMOTRIGINE plasma concentrations may be reduced, decreasing the therapeutic effects.

Mechanism LAMOTRIGINE absorption may be decreased by ORLISTAT.

Management If this combination cannot be avoided, observe the clinical response of the patient and adjust the LAMOTRIGINE dose as needed when ORLISTAT is started or stopped.

Discussion

An 18-year-old woman with epilepsy presented with increased seizure frequency.[1] Her antiepileptic medication consisted of lamotrigine 200 mg daily. After starting orlistat 120 mg 3 times daily for obesity, her seizure frequency increased from 1 per month to more than 1 per week. She was admitted to the hospital for further evaluation. On admission, her lamotrigine plasma concentration was 8 mmol/L (normal, 0 to 15 mmol/L).

[1] Bigham S, et al. *Epilepsia.* 2006;47(12):2207.

* Asterisk indicates drugs cited in interaction reports.

Lamotrigine — *Oxcarbazepine*

Lamotrigine* (eg, *Lamictal*)	Oxcarbazepine* (eg, *Trileptal*)

Significance	Onset	Severity	Documentation
4	☐ Rapid ■ **Delayed**	☐ Major ■ **Moderate** ☐ Minor	☐ Established ☐ Probable ☐ Suspected ■ **Possible** ☐ Unlikely

Effects LAMOTRIGINE serum concentrations may be reduced, decreasing the therapeutic effects.

Mechanism OXCARBAZEPINE may induce the metabolism of LAMOTRIGINE.

Management It may be necessary to adjust the dose of LAMOTRIGINE when the dose of OXCARBAZEPINE is started, stopped, or changed. Observe the clinical response of patients, and adjust the dose of LAMOTRIGINE as needed.

Discussion

Data are conflicting. In a retrospective evaluation, the influence of oxcarbazepine on lamotrigine serum concentrations was investigated.[1] The effect of oxcarbazepine on lamotrigine levels was compared with the effect of carbamazepine on lamotrigine serum levels in epileptic patients with and without valproic acid (eg, *Depakene*) coadministration. Oxcarbazepine administration reduced serum concentrations of lamotrigine 29% compared with a 54% reduction by carbamazepine. Administration of valproic acid increased lamotrigine serum concentrations approximately 211%; however, the increase was smaller when oxcarbazepine (111%) or carbamazepine (21%) also was administered. In patients receiving lamotrigine, if oxcarbazepine is substituted for carbamazepine, lamotrigine plasma concentrations may increase. In another study, lamotrigine increased concentrations of the active 10-mono-hydroxy metabolite of oxcarbazepine.[2] A study in healthy volunteers receiving lamotrigine or oxcarbazepine alone and in combination found no differences in the pharmacokinetics of lamotrigine or oxcarbazepine when used in combination, compared with monotherapy.[3] Additional studies are needed to determine if these changes in concentration are clinically important. See also Lamotrigine-Carbamazepine.

[1] May TW, et al. *Ther Drug Monit.* 1999;21(2):175.
[2] Guénault N, et al. *Eur J Clin Pharmacol.* 2003;59(10):781.
[3] Theis JG, et al. *Neuropsychopharmacology.* 2005;30(12):2269.

* Asterisk indicates drugs cited in interaction reports.

Lamotrigine — *Progestins*

Lamotrigine* (eg, *Lamictal*)	Norethindrone* (eg, *Aygestin*)

Significance	Onset	Severity	Documentation
4	□ Rapid ■ **Delayed**	□ Major ■ **Moderate** □ Minor	□ Established □ Probable □ Suspected ■ **Possible** □ Unlikely

Effects LAMOTRIGINE plasma concentrations may be reduced, decreasing the therapeutic effect.

Mechanism Increased LAMOTRIGINE metabolism (glucuronidation) by PROGESTIN use is suspected.

Management It may be necessary to adjust the dose of LAMOTRIGINE when NORETHINDRONE is started or stopped. Observe the clinical response of patients, and adjust the dose of LAMOTRIGINE as needed.

Discussion

A 28-year-old woman with complex partial seizures discontinued norethindrone 0.35 mg in order to become pregnant.[1] Before stopping norethindrone, she was seizure-free while receiving lamotrigine 300 mg/day. Her lamotrigine plasma levels were stable with values of 13 to 14 mcmol/L during the last 6 months before discontinuing the oral contraceptive. Seven months after a successful pregnancy, her lamotrigine dose was 300 mg/day, and the plasma concentration was 10 mcmol/L higher (ie, 23 mcmol/L) than before pregnancy. The dose of lamotrigine was decreased to 200 mg/day, and the plasma level was 16 mcmol/L 3 weeks after restarting the norethindrone. See Lamotrigine-Contraceptives, Hormonal.

[1] Sabers A, et al. *Epilepsy Res.* 2001;47(1-2):151.

* Asterisk indicates drugs cited in interaction reports.

Lamotrigine — *Protease Inhibitors*

Lamotrigine* (eg, *Lamictal*)	Lopinavir/Ritonavir* (*Kaletra*)	Ritonavir (*Norvir*)

Significance	Onset	Severity	Documentation
4	☐ Rapid	☐ Major	☐ Established
	■ **Delayed**	■ **Moderate**	☐ Probable
		☐ Minor	☐ Suspected
			■ **Possible**
			☐ Unlikely

Effects LAMOTRIGINE plasma concentrations may be reduced, decreasing the efficacy.

Mechanism Induction of LAMOTRIGINE glucuronidation by RITONAVIR is suspected.

Management It may be necessary to adjust the dose of LAMOTRIGINE when LOPINAVIR/RITONAVIR is started or stopped. Closely monitor the clinical response and adjust the LAMOTRIGINE dose as needed.

Discussion

The effect of lopinavir/ritonavir on the pharmacokinetics of lamotrigine was studied in healthy subjects.[1] Lamotrigine 50 mg daily was administered on days 1 and 2, then increased to 100 mg twice daily on days 3 through 23. Lopinavir 400 mg/ritonavir 100 mg twice daily was added on day 11. Depending on the decrease in lamotrigine trough levels between days 10 and 20, the dose of lamotrigine was adjusted. Compared with giving lamotrigine alone, the mean decrease in lamotrigine trough level between days 10 and 20 was 55.4%. In addition, the lamotrigine $t_{1/2}$ was shortened, exposure was decreased, and clearance was increased. Based on this decrease, the dosage of lamotrigine was increased to 200 mg twice daily in all subjects and administered with lopinavir/ritonavir to day 31. After adjusting the dosage of lamotrigine to 200 mg twice daily, the AUC on day 31 was bioequivalent to day 10. Lamotrigine did not appear to affect the pharmacokinetics of lopinavir/ritonavir. In an open-label study involving 17 healthy men, atazanavir/ritonavir decreased the AUC of single-dose lamotrigine 32%; however, atazanavir administration alone had no effect on lamotrigine pharmacokinetics.[2]

[1] van der Lee MJ, et al. *Clin Pharmacol Ther.* 2006;80(2):159.

[2] Burger DM, et al. *Clin Pharmacol Ther.* 2008;84(6):698.

* Asterisk indicates drugs cited in interaction reports. Based on pharmacologic and pharmacokinetic considerations, similar interactions may occur with other drugs that are listed.

Lamotrigine — *Rifamycins*

Lamotrigine	Rifamycins	
Lamotrigine* (eg, *Lamictal*)	Rifabutin (*Mycobutin*)	Rifapentine (*Priftin*)
	Rifampin* (eg, *Rifadin*)	

Significance	Onset	Severity	Documentation
2	☐ Rapid	☐ Major	☐ Established
	■ **Delayed**	■ **Moderate**	☐ Probable
		☐ Minor	■ **Suspected**
			☐ Possible
			☐ Unlikely

Effects LAMOTRIGINE plasma levels may be reduced, decreasing the pharmacologic effects.

Mechanism Induction of hepatic enzymes responsible for the glucuronidation of LAMOTRIGINE is suspected.

Management It may be necessary to adjust the dose of LAMOTRIGINE when starting, stopping, or changing the dose of the RIFAMYCIN. Observe the clinical response of the patient and adjust the dose of LAMOTRIGINE as needed.

Discussion

The effects of rifampin and cimetidine (eg, *Tagamet*) on the pharmacokinetics and pharmacodynamics of lamotrigine were studied in 10 healthy male volunteers.[1] Using a randomized, placebo-controlled, open-label, crossover design, each subject received a single lamotrigine 25 mg dose after 5 days of pretreatment with cimetidine 400 mg twice daily, rifampin 600 mg daily, or placebo. Compared with placebo, cimetidine did not affect the pharmacokinetics or pharmacodynamics of lamotrigine. In contrast, rifampin increased the clearance over bioavailability (CL/F) of lamotrigine by 97% (from 2.6 to 5.13 L/h) and the amount of lamotrigine excreted in the urine as the glucuronide metabolite by 36% (from 8.9 to 12.12 mg), while decreasing the mean total AUC by 44%, the half-life by 41% (from 23.8 to 14.1 hours), and the mean residence time by 17%. No differences were found in the renal clearance, C_{max} of lamotrigine, T_{max}, or electroencephalographic parameters of lamotrigine during the trial periods.

[1] Ebert U, et al. *Eur J Clin Pharmacol.* 2000;56(4):299.

* Asterisk indicates drugs cited in interaction reports. Based on pharmacologic and pharmacokinetic considerations, similar interactions may occur with other drugs that are listed.

Lamotrigine — *Sertraline*

Lamotrigine* (eg, *Lamictal*)	Sertraline* (eg, *Zoloft*)

Significance	Onset	Severity	Documentation
4	☐ Rapid ■ **Delayed**	☐ Major ■ **Moderate** ☐ Minor	☐ Established ☐ Probable ☐ Suspected ■ **Possible** ☐ Unlikely

Effects LAMOTRIGINE plasma concentrations may be elevated, increasing the risk of toxicity.

Mechanism Unknown.

Management In patients receiving LAMOTRIGINE, monitor the clinical response of the patient when the SERTRALINE dose is started, stopped, or changed. Adjust the LAMOTRIGINE dose as needed.

Discussion

Increased lamotrigine concentrations were reported in 2 patients after sertraline was added to their treatment regimen.[1] One patient, a 39-year-old woman, had been maintained on lamotrigine 200 mg daily. After starting sertraline 25 mg daily, the patient complained of cognitive impairment and confusion. The lamotrigine blood concentration increased from 2.5 to 5.1 mcg/mL 6 weeks after starting sertraline. Subsequently, the sertraline dose was increased to 50 mg daily and the lamotrigine dose was decreased to 100 mg daily. Within 3 weeks the impaired cognition and confusion cleared. The lamotrigine concentration remained stable at 3.1 mcg/mL. The second patient, a 17-year-old girl, had been maintained on lamotrigine 450 mg daily when sertraline 75 mg daily was started. Six weeks after increasing her lamotrigine dose to 600 mg daily, she complained of decreased cognition, fatigue, and sedation. The lamotrigine blood concentration was 19.3 mcg/mL. The sertraline dose was decreased to 50 mg daily and the lamotrigine dose was increased to 800 mg daily. Although the lamotrigine dose was increased, the blood concentration decreased to 9.8 mcg/mL.

[1] Kaufman KR, et al. *Seizure.* 1998;7(2):163.

* Asterisk indicates drugs cited in interaction reports.

Lamotrigine — *Succinimides*

Lamotrigine	Succinimides	
Lamotrigine* (eg, *Lamictal*)	Ethosuximide (eg, *Zarontin*)	Phensuximide (*Milontin*)
	Methsuximide* (*Celontin*)	

Significance	Onset	Severity	Documentation
2	□ Rapid	□ Major	□ Established
	■ **Delayed**	■ **Moderate**	□ Probable
		□ Minor	■ **Suspected**
			□ Possible
			□ Unlikely

Effects LAMOTRIGINE serum concentrations may be reduced, decreasing the therapeutic effects.

Mechanism SUCCINIMIDES may induce the metabolism of LAMOTRIGINE.

Management It may be necessary to adjust the dose of LAMOTRIGINE when starting, stopping, or changing the dose of SUCCINIMIDE therapy. Observe the clinical response of the patient and adjust the dose of LAMOTRIGINE as needed.

Discussion

In a retrospective evaluation, the influence of methsuximide on lamotrigine serum concentrations was investigated.[1] The effect of methsuximide on lamotrigine levels was compared with and without concurrent valproic acid (eg, *Depakene*) administration. Methsuximide administration reduced serum concentrations of lamotrigine 70% compared with lamotrigine monotherapy. Administration of valproic acid increased lamotrigine serum concentrations approximately 211%; however, the increase was smaller (8%) when methsuximide was administered concurrently. The effect of methsuximide on lamotrigine plasma concentrations was studied in 16 patients (age range, 9 to 19 years) with epilepsy.[2] During concomitant methsuximide administration, mean lamotrigine plasma levels decreased 53% (from 13.4 to 6.3 mg/L) and increased when methsuximide was discontinued. Several patients experienced a deterioration in seizure control when methsuximide was started and an improvement when it was stopped. Comedication with other antiepileptic agents (eg, valproic acid) was being received by 14 of the 16 patients.

[1] May TW, et al. *Ther Drug Monit.* 1999;21(2):175.
[2] Besag FMC, et al. *Epilepsia.* 2000;41(5):624.

* Asterisk indicates drugs cited in interaction reports. Based on pharmacologic and pharmacokinetic considerations, similar interactions may occur with other drugs that are listed.

Lamotrigine		**Valproic Acid**
Lamotrigine* (eg, *Lamictal*)	Divalproex Sodium* (eg, *Depakote*) Valproate Sodium* (eg, *Depacon*)	Valproic Acid* (eg, *Depakene*)

Significance	Onset	Severity	Documentation
2	□ Rapid ■ **Delayed**	□ Major ■ **Moderate** □ Minor	□ Established ■ **Probable** □ Suspected □ Possible □ Unlikely

Effects Serum VALPROIC ACID concentrations may be decreased, while LAMOTRIGINE levels and toxicity may be increased.

Mechanism Possible inhibition of LAMOTRIGINE metabolism.

Management Patients receiving combined antiepileptic therapy require careful monitoring when another agent is started, stopped, or changed in dosage.

Discussion

Data indicate that lamotrigine decreases serum valproic acid levels 25%.[1,2] In a double-blind, placebo-controlled investigation, lamotrigine did not alter the plasma valproic acid level.[3] In 6 healthy men, valproic acid reduced the total clearance of lamotrigine 21% and increased elimination t½ from 37.4 to 48.3 hr, compared with giving lamotrigine alone.[4] In a study of 16 epileptic patients, valproic acid doubled the elimination t½ of lamotrigine.[5] Similar results have been reported in other studies,[2,6] including one involving young children.[6] Maximal inhibition of lamotrigine occurs with valproic acid levels of approximately 20 mcg/mL, which correspond to approximately 250 mg/day.[7] The interaction may improve antiepileptic efficacy[8,9]; however, disabling tremor,[10] neurotoxicity,[11] vomiting,[12] and Stevens-Johnson syndrome[2] caused by lamotrigine toxicity have been reported.

Patients receiving enzyme-inducing antiepileptics (eg, carbamazepine [eg, *Tegretol*], phenytoin [eg, *Dilantin*], phenobarbital [eg, *Luminal*], primidone [eg, *Mysoline*]) demonstrated a mean lamotrigine plasma elimination t½ of 14 hr compared with 30 hr in patients taking sodium valproate plus an enzyme-inducing antiepileptic agent.[13] The latter value is similar to lamotrigine t½ during monotherapy,[14] indicating that valproic acid may counteract the enzyme inducer.[13,15] If valproic acid is discontinued in a patient receiving lamotrigine and an enzyme-inducing antiepileptic, serum lamotrigine levels may decrease.[15]

1 *Lamictal* [package insert]. Philadelphia, PA: GlaxoSmithKline; December 1994.
2 Anderson GD, et al. *Clin Pharmacol Ther.* 1996;60(2):145.
3 Binnie CD, et al. *Epilepsy Res.* 1989;4(3):222.
4 Yuen AW, et al. *Br J Clin Pharmacol.* 1992;33(5):511.
5 Binnie CD, et al. *Epilepsia.* 1986;27(3):248.
6 Vauzelle-Kervroëdan F, et al. *Br J Clin Pharmacol.* 1996;41(4):325.
7 Gidal BE, et al. *Epilepsy Res.* 2003;57(2-3):85.
8 Pisani F, et al. *Lancet.* 1993;341(8854):1224.
9 Morris RG, et al. *Ther Drug Monit.* 2000;22(6):656.
10 Reutens DC, et al. *Lancet.* 1993;342(8864):185.
11 Burneo JG, et al. *Neurology.* 2003;60(12):1991.
12 Greiner C, et al. *Pharmacopsychiatry.* 2007;40(6):287.
13 Jawad S, et al. *Epilepsy Res.* 1987;1(3):194.
14 Cohen AF, et al. *Clin Pharmacol Ther.* 1987;42(5):535.
15 Brodie MJ. *Lancet.* 1992;339(8806):1397.

* Asterisk indicates drugs cited in interaction reports.

Lapatinib — *Azole Antifungal Agents*

Lapatinib* (*Tykerb*)	Itraconazole* (eg, *Sporanox*)	Posaconazole (*Noxafil*)
	Ketoconazole* (eg, *Nizoral*)	Voriconazole* (eg, *Vfend*)

Significance	Onset	Severity	Documentation
2	☐ Rapid	☐ Major	☐ Established
	■ **Delayed**	■ **Moderate**	☐ Probable
		☐ Minor	■ **Suspected**
			☐ Possible
			☐ Unlikely

Effects LAPATINIB plasma concentrations may be elevated, increasing the risk of LAPATINIB toxicity.

Mechanism Inhibition of LAPATINIB metabolism (CYP3A4) by AZOLE ANTIFUNGAL AGENTS.

Management Avoid coadministration of LAPATINIB and AZOLE ANTIFUNGAL AGENTS. If these agents must be used concurrently, a dosage reduction of LAPATINIB to 500 mg daily is recommended.[1] One week after the AZOLE ANTIFUNGAL AGENT is discontinued, adjust the dose of LAPATINIB upward to the indicated dosage.

Discussion

Because lapatinib undergoes extensive metabolism by CYP3A4, coadministration of strong inhibitors of CYP3A4 (eg, ketoconazole) is expected to alter lapatinib plasma concentrations.[1] In healthy subjects receiving ketoconazole 200 mg twice daily for 7 days, the lapatinib AUC was increased and the $t_{½}$ was prolonged 3.6- and 1.7-fold, respectively, compared with controls.[2] Therefore, consider dosage adjustments for patients receiving lapatinib and a strong CYP3A4 inhibitor concurrently.

Studies are needed to determine the clinical importance of this interaction and the effect of other azole antifungal agents on lapatinib metabolism.

[1] *Tykerb* [package insert]. Research Triangle Park, NC: GlaxoSmithKline; August 2007.

[2] Smith DA, et al. *Br J Clin Pharmacol.* 2009;67(4):421.

* Asterisk indicates drugs cited in interaction reports. Based on pharmacologic and pharmacokinetic considerations, similar interactions may occur with other drugs that are listed.

Lapatinib — *Barbiturates*

Lapatinib* (*Tykerb*)	Phenobarbital* (eg, *Solfoton*)	Primidone (eg, *Mysoline*)

Significance	Onset	Severity	Documentation
2	☐ Rapid ■ **Delayed**	☐ Major ■ **Moderate** ☐ Minor	☐ Established ☐ Probable ■ **Suspected** ☐ Possible ☐ Unlikely

Effects LAPATINIB plasma concentrations may be reduced, decreasing the efficacy.

Mechanism Induction of LAPATINIB metabolism (CYP3A4) by PHENOBARBITAL.

Management Avoid coadministration of LAPATINIB and PHENOBARBITAL. If these agents must be used concurrently, gradually titrate the dosage of LAPATINIB from 1,250 to 4,500 mg/day based on tolerability. If PHENOBARBITAL is discontinued, reduce LAPATINIB to the indicated dose.

Discussion

Because lapatinib undergoes extensive metabolism by CYP3A4, coadministration of a strong inducer of CYP3A4 (eg, phenobarbital) is expected to decrease lapatinib plasma concentrations.[1] Therefore, consider dosage adjustments in patients receiving lapatinib when a strong CYP3A4 inducer is started or stopped.

The basis for this monograph is information on file with the manufacturer. There are no clinical data with dose adjustments in patients receiving lapatinib and phenobarbital. Studies are needed to determine the clinical importance of this interaction and the effect of other barbiturates on lapatinib metabolism.

[1] *Tykerb* [package insert]. Research Triangle Park, NC: GlaxoSmithKline; August 20, 2007.

* Asterisk indicates drugs cited in interaction reports. Based on pharmacologic and pharmacokinetic considerations, similar interactions may occur with other drugs that are listed.

Lapatinib — *Carbamazepine*

Lapatinib* (*Tykerb*)	Carbamazepine* (eg, *Tegretol*)

Significance	Onset	Severity	Documentation
2	☐ Rapid ■ **Delayed**	☐ Major ■ **Moderate** ☐ Minor	☐ Established ☐ Probable ■ **Suspected** ☐ Possible ☐ Unlikely

Effects LAPATINIB plasma concentrations may be reduced, decreasing the efficacy.

Mechanism Induction of LAPATINIB metabolism (CYP3A4) by CARBAMAZEPINE.

Management Avoid coadministration of LAPATINIB and CARBAMAZEPINE. If these agents must be used concurrently, titrate the dosage of LAPATINIB gradually from 1,250 to 4,500 mg/day based on tolerability.[1] If CARBAMAZEPINE is discontinued, reduce the LAPATINIB dose to the indicated dosage.

Discussion

Because lapatinib undergoes extensive metabolism by CYP3A4, coadministration of a strong inducer of CYP3A4 (eg, carbamazepine) is expected to decrease lapatinib plasma concentrations.[1] In healthy subjects receiving carbamazepine 100 mg twice daily for 3 days and 200 mg twice daily for 17 days, the lapatinib AUC was decreased approximately 72%.[2] Therefore, consider dosage adjustments in patients receiving lapatinib when carbamazepine is started or stopped.

1 *Tykerb* [package insert]. Research Triangle Park, NC: GlaxoSmithKline; August 20, 2007.

2 Smith DA, et al. *Br J Clin Pharmacol.* 2009;67(4):421.

* Asterisk indicates drugs cited in interaction reports.

Lapatinib		**Corticosteroids**
Lapatinib* (*Tykerb*)		Dexamethasone* (eg, *Decadron*)

Significance	Onset	Severity	Documentation
2	□ Rapid ■ **Delayed**	□ Major ■ **Moderate** □ Minor	□ Established □ Probable ■ **Suspected** □ Possible □ Unlikely

Effects LAPATINIB plasma concentrations may be reduced, decreasing the efficacy.

Mechanism Induction of LAPATINIB metabolism (CYP3A4) by DEXAMETHASONE.

Management Avoid coadministration of LAPATINIB and DEXAMETHASONE. If these agents must be used concurrently, gradually titrate the dose of LAPATINIB from 1,250 to 4,500 mg/day based on tolerability. If DEXAMETHASONE is discontinued, reduce LAPATINIB to the indicated dose.

Discussion

Because lapatinib undergoes extensive metabolism by CYP3A4, coadministration of a strong inducer of CYP3A4 (eg, dexamethasone) is expected to decrease lapatinib plasma concentrations.[1] Therefore, consider dosage adjustments in patients receiving lapatinib when a strong CYP3A4 inducer is started or stopped.

The basis for this monograph is information on file with the manufacturer. There are no clinical data with dose adjustments in patients receiving lapatinib and dexamethasone. Studies are needed to determine the clinical importance of this interaction and the effect of other corticosteroids on lapatinib metabolism.

[1] *Tykerb* [package insert]. Research Triangle Park, NC: GlaxoSmithKline; August 20, 2007.

* Asterisk indicates drugs cited in interaction reports.

Lapatinib — *Food*

Lapatinib* (*Tykerb*)	Grapefruit Juice*

Significance	Onset	Severity	Documentation
2	□ Rapid ■ **Delayed**	□ Major ■ **Moderate** □ Minor	□ Established □ Probable ■ **Suspected** □ Possible □ Unlikely

Effects LAPATINIB plasma concentrations may be elevated, increasing the risk of LAPATINIB toxicity.

Mechanism Inhibition of LAPATINIB metabolism (CYP3A4) in the small intestine by GRAPEFRUIT.

Management Avoid coadministration of LAPATINIB and GRAPEFRUIT. Administer LAPATINIB with a liquid other than GRAPEFRUIT JUICE.

Discussion

Because lapatinib undergoes extensive metabolism by CYP3A4, ingestion of lapatinib and grapefruit juice, an inhibitor of CYP3A4, is expected to increase lapatinib plasma concentrations.[1] Therefore, patients taking lapatinib should avoid grapefruit.[1]

The basis for this monograph is information on file with the manufacturer. There are no clinical data with dose adjustments in patients receiving lapatinib and grapefruit. Studies are needed to determine the clinical importance of this interaction.

[1] *Tykerb* [package insert]. Research Triangle Park, NC: GlaxoSmithKline; August 20, 2007.

* Asterisk indicates drugs cited in interaction reports.

Lapatinib			*Hydantoins*
Lapatinib* (*Tykerb*)		Fosphenytoin (*Cerebyx*)	Phenytoin* (eg, *Dilantin*)

Significance	Onset	Severity	Documentation
2	☐ Rapid	☐ Major	☐ Established
	■ **Delayed**	■ **Moderate**	☐ Probable
		☐ Minor	■ **Suspected**
			☐ Possible
			☐ Unlikely

Effects LAPATINIB plasma concentrations may be reduced, decreasing the efficacy.

Mechanism Induction of LAPATINIB metabolism (CYP3A4) by HYDANTOINS.

Management Avoid coadministration of LAPATINIB and HYDANTOINS. If these agents must be used concurrently, gradually titrate the dose of LAPATINIB from 1,250 up to 4,500 mg/day based on tolerability. If the HYDANTOIN is discontinued, reduce LAPATINIB to the indicated dose.

Discussion

Because lapatinib undergoes extensive metabolism by CYP3A4, coadministration of a strong inducer of CYP3A4 (eg, phenytoin) is expected to decrease lapatinib plasma concentrations.[1] Therefore, consider adjusting the dosage in patients receiving lapatinib when a strong CYP3A4 inducer is started or stopped.

The basis for this monograph is information on file with the manufacturer. There are no clinical data with dose adjustments in patients receiving lapatinib and a hydantoin. Studies are needed to determine the clinical importance of this interaction and the effect of other hydantoins on lapatinib metabolism.

[1] *Tykerb* [package insert]. Research Triangle Park, NC: GlaxoSmithKline; August 20, 2007.

* Asterisk indicates drugs cited in interaction reports. Based on pharmacologic and pharmacokinetic considerations, similar interactions may occur with other drugs that are listed.

Lapatinib — *Macrolide & Related Antibiotics*

Lapatinib* (*Tykerb*)	Clarithromycin* (eg, *Biaxin*)	Telithromycin* (*Ketek*)

Significance	Onset	Severity	Documentation
2	☐ Rapid ■ **Delayed**	☐ Major ■ **Moderate** ☐ Minor	☐ Established ☐ Probable ■ **Suspected** ☐ Possible ☐ Unlikely

Effects LAPATINIB plasma concentrations may be elevated, increasing the risk of LAPATINIB toxicity.

Mechanism Inhibition of LAPATINIB metabolism (CYP3A4) by MACROLIDE AND RELATED ANTIBIOTICS.

Management Avoid coadministration of LAPATINIB and MACROLIDE AND RELATED ANTIBIOTICS. If these agents must be used concurrently, a dosage reduction of LAPATINIB to 500 mg daily is recommended. One week after the MACROLIDE AND RELATED ANTIBIOTIC is discontinued, adjust the dose of LAPATINIB upward to the indicated dosage.

Discussion

Because lapatinib undergoes extensive metabolism by CYP3A4, coadministration of strong inhibitors of CYP3A4 (eg, clarithromycin) is expected to alter lapatinib plasma concentrations.[1] Therefore, consider dosage adjustments for patients receiving lapatinib and a strong CYP3A4 inhibitor concurrently.

The basis for this monograph is information on file with the manufacturer. There are no clinical data with dose adjustments in patients receiving lapatinib and a strong CYP3A4 inhibitor. Studies are needed to determine the clinical importance of this interaction and the effect of other macrolide and related antibiotics on lapatinib metabolism.

[1] *Tykerb* [package insert]. Research Triangle Park, NC: GlaxoSmithKline; August 20, 2007.

* Asterisk indicates drugs cited in interaction reports.

Lapatinib / *Nefazodone*

Lapatinib*
(*Tykerb*)

Nefazodone*

Significance	Onset	Severity	Documentation
2	☐ Rapid	☐ Major	☐ Established
	■ **Delayed**	■ **Moderate**	☐ Probable
		☐ Minor	■ **Suspected**
			☐ Possible
			☐ Unlikely

Effects LAPATINIB plasma concentrations may be elevated, increasing the risk of LAPATINIB toxicity.

Mechanism Inhibition of LAPATINIB metabolism (CYP3A4) by NEFAZODONE.

Management Avoid coadministration of LAPATINIB and NEFAZODONE. If these agents must be used concurrently, a dosage reduction of LAPATINIB to 500 mg daily is recommended. One week after NEFAZODONE is discontinued, adjust the dose of LAPATINIB upward to the indicated dosage.

Discussion

Because lapatinib undergoes extensive metabolism by CYP3A4, coadministration of strong inhibitors of CYP3A4 (eg, nefazodone) is expected to alter lapatinib plasma concentrations.[1] Therefore, consider dosage adjustments for patients receiving lapatinib and a strong CYP3A4 inhibitor concurrently.

The basis for this monograph is information on file with the manufacturer. There are no clinical data with dose adjustments in patients receiving lapatinib and a strong CYP3A4 inhibitor. Studies are needed to determine the clinical importance of this interaction.

[1] *Tykerb* [package insert]. Research Triangle Park, NC: GlaxoSmithKline; August 20, 2007.

* Asterisk indicates drugs cited in interaction reports.

Lapatinib — *Protease Inhibitors*

Lapatinib	Protease Inhibitors	
Lapatinib* (*Tykerb*)	Atazanavir* (*Reyataz*)	Ritonavir* (*Norvir*)
	Indinavir* (*Crixivan*)	Saquinavir* (*Invirase*)
	Nelfinavir* (*Viracept*)	

Significance	Onset	Severity	Documentation
2	□ Rapid	□ Major	□ Established
	■ **Delayed**	■ **Moderate**	□ Probable
		□ Minor	■ **Suspected**
			□ Possible
			□ Unlikely

Effects LAPATINIB plasma concentrations may be elevated, increasing the risk of LAPATINIB toxicity.

Mechanism Inhibition of LAPATINIB metabolism (CYP3A4) by PROTEASE INHIBITORS.

Management Avoid coadministration of LAPATINIB and PROTEASE INHIBITORS. If these agents must be used concurrently, a dosage reduction of LAPATINIB to 500 mg daily is recommended. One week after the PROTEASE INHIBITOR is discontinued, adjust the dose of LAPATINIB upward to the indicated dosage.

Discussion

Because lapatinib undergoes extensive metabolism by CYP3A4, coadministration of strong inhibitors of CYP3A4 (eg, indinavir) is expected to alter lapatinib plasma concentrations.[1] Therefore, consider dosage adjustments for patients receiving lapatinib and a strong CYP3A4 inhibitor concurrently.

The basis for this monograph is information on file with the manufacturer. There are no clinical data with dose adjustments in patients receiving lapatinib and a strong CYP3A4 inhibitor. Studies are needed to determine the clinical importance of this interaction and the effect of other protease inhibitors on lapatinib metabolism.

[1] *Tykerb* [package insert]. Research Triangle Park, NC: GlaxoSmithKline; August 20, 2007.

* Asterisk indicates drugs cited in interaction reports.

Lapatinib | **Rifamycins**

Lapatinib* (*Tykerb*)		Rifabutin* (*Mycobutin*) Rifampin* (eg, *Rifadin*)	Rifapentine* (*Priftin*)

Significance	Onset	Severity	Documentation
2	□ Rapid	□ Major	□ Established
	■ **Delayed**	■ **Moderate**	□ Probable
		□ Minor	■ **Suspected**
			□ Possible
			□ Unlikely

Effects LAPATINIB plasma concentrations may be reduced, decreasing the efficacy.

Mechanism Induction of LAPATINIB metabolism (CYP3A4) by RIFAMYCINS.

Management Avoid coadministration of LAPATINIB and RIFAMYCINS. If these agents must be used concurrently, gradually titrate the dose of LAPATINIB from 1,250 to 4,500 mg/day based on tolerability. If RIFAMYCIN is discontinued, reduce LAPATINIB to the indicated dose.

Discussion

Because lapatinib undergoes extensive metabolism by CYP3A4, coadministration of a strong inducer of CYP3A4 (eg, rifampin) is expected to decrease lapatinib plasma concentrations.[1] Therefore, consider dosage adjustments in patients receiving lapatinib when a strong CYP3A4 inducer is started or stopped.

The basis for this monograph is information on file with the manufacturer. There are no clinical data with dose adjustments in patients receiving lapatinib and a strong CYP3A4 inducer. Studies are needed to determine the clinical importance of this interaction.

[1] *Tykerb* [package insert]. Research Triangle Park, NC: GlaxoSmithKline; August 20, 2007.

* Asterisk indicates drugs cited in interaction reports.

Lapatinib — *St. John's Wort*

Lapatinib* (*Tykerb*)	St. John's Wort*

Significance	Onset	Severity	Documentation
2	☐ Rapid	☐ Major	☐ Established
	■ **Delayed**	■ **Moderate**	☐ Probable
		☐ Minor	■ **Suspected**
			☐ Possible
			☐ Unlikely

Effects LAPATINIB plasma concentrations may be reduced, decreasing the efficacy.

Mechanism Induction of LAPATINIB metabolism (CYP3A4) by ST. JOHN'S WORT.

Management Avoid coadministration of LAPATINIB and ST. JOHN'S WORT. Caution patients taking LAPATINIB to inform their health care provider before taking ST. JOHN'S WORT.

Discussion

Because lapatinib undergoes extensive metabolism by CYP3A4, coadministration of a strong inducer of CYP3A4 (eg, St. John's wort) is expected to decrease lapatinib plasma concentrations.[1] Therefore, advise patients taking lapatinib to avoid St. John's wort.

The basis for this monograph is information on file with the manufacturer. There are no clinical data with dose adjustments in patients receiving lapatinib and St. John's wort. Studies are needed to determine the clinical importance of this interaction.

[1] *Tykerb* [package insert]. Research Triangle Park, NC: GlaxoSmithKline; August 20, 2007.

* Asterisk indicates drugs cited in interaction reports.

Leflunomide | **Methotrexate**

Leflunomide*
(eg, *Arava*)

Methotrexate*
(eg, *Rheumatrex*)

Significance	Onset	Severity	Documentation
1	☐ Rapid	■ **Major**	☐ Established
	■ **Delayed**	☐ Moderate	☐ Probable
		☐ Minor	■ **Suspected**
			☐ Possible
			☐ Unlikely

Effects Risk of serious adverse reactions, including hepatotoxicity and hematologic toxicity (eg, agranulocytosis, pancytopenia, thrombocytopenia), may be increased.

Mechanism Additive or synergistic effects.

Management If coadministration of LEFLUNOMIDE and METHOTREXATE cannot be avoided, monitor ALT, AST, serum albumin, platelets, WBC, and hemoglobin or hematocrit monthly.

Discussion

No pharmacokinetic interaction was found in 30 patients receiving leflunomide (100 mg daily for 2 days followed by 10 to 20 mg daily) and methotrexate (10 to 25 mg/week) with folate.[1] However, the risk of hepatotoxicity was increased. In addition to hepatotoxicity, hematologic toxicity (eg, pancytopenia) has been reported with coadministration of leflunomide and methotrexate.[2,3] In a report of 18 cases of pancytopenia associated with leflunomide, 13 of which were accessed through the Adverse Drug Reaction Advisory Committee in Australia, 14 patients were receiving concurrent methotrexate therapy.[2] In general, the pancytopenia was severe, requiring hospitalization, withdrawal of immunosuppressive therapy, intensive support therapy, and treatment of neutropenic sepsis. Four of 5 patients who died were receiving leflunomide and methotrexate concomitantly. The mean time of onset of pancytopenia in patients receiving concurrent leflunomide and methotrexate was 4 months, with a range of 23 days to 4 years.

[1] *Arava* [package insert]. Kansas City, MO: Aventis Pharmaceuticals Inc; October 2005.

[2] Chan J, et al. *Ann Pharmacother.* 2004;38(7-8):1206.

[3] Hill RL, et al. *Ann Pharmacother.* 2003;37(1):149.

* Asterisk indicates drugs cited in interaction reports.

Levetiracetam — *Valproic Acid*

Levetiracetam* (*Keppra*)	Divalproex Sodium (*Depakote*)	Valproic Acid (eg, *Depakene*)
	Valproate Sodium* (eg, *Depacon*)	

Significance	Onset	Severity	Documentation
4	□ Rapid	□ Major	□ Established
	■ **Delayed**	■ **Moderate**	□ Probable
		□ Minor	□ Suspected
			■ **Possible**
			□ Unlikely

Effects The risk of occurrence of acute psychiatric symptoms, including agitation, anxiety, and/or sleeplessness, may be increased.

Mechanism Unknown; however, a pharmacodynamic interaction is suspected.

Management Closely monitor patients during coadministration of LEVETIRACETAM and VALPROIC ACID for psychiatric disturbances. Be prepared to adjust therapy as needed.

Discussion

Psychiatric disturbances were reported in a 48-year-old woman with a history of complex partial seizures during treatment with levetiracetam and valproate sodium.[1] The patient was admitted to the hospital after experiencing complex partial seizures during the preceding 5 months. At admission, she was receiving valproate sodium 500 mg twice daily. Levetiracetam 500 mg twice daily was added to the valproate sodium therapy, and the patient was discharged from the hospital 3 days later. Several days later, seizure activity resumed, and the dosage of levetiracetam was increased to 1,500 mg/day. On this regimen, no epileptic symptoms occurred; however, 13 days later she experienced agitation, anxiety, and sleeplessness. Valproate sodium was replaced with carbamazepine (titrated to 400 mg twice daily). Complete remission of the psychiatric symptoms occurred over the next 5 days. During the 6-month follow-up period, neuropsychological evaluation and blood chemical tests were normal. In 23 children with partial-onset seizures receiving valproic acid, coadministration of levetiracetam did not alter valproic acid plasma levels.[2]

[1] Siniscalchi A, et al. *Ann Pharmacother.* 2007;41(3):527.

[2] Otoul C, et al. *Epilepsia.* 2007;48(11):2111.

* Asterisk indicates drugs cited in interaction reports. Based on pharmacologic and pharmacokinetic considerations, similar interactions may occur with other drugs that are listed.

Levodopa — *Antacids*

Levodopa	Antacids	
Levodopa* (*Larodopa*)	Aluminum Hydroxide* (eg, *Amphojel*)	Magnesium Hydroxide (eg, *Dulcolax*)
	Aluminum Hydroxide/ Magnesium Hydroxide* (eg, *Maalox*)	

Significance	Onset	Severity	Documentation
4	☐ Rapid	☐ Major	☐ Established
	■ **Delayed**	■ **Moderate**	☐ Probable
		☐ Minor	☐ Suspected
			■ **Possible**
			☐ Unlikely

Effects Effectiveness of LEVODOPA may be increased.

Mechanism ANTACIDS decrease gastric emptying times, allowing for more rapid and complete intestinal LEVODOPA absorption.

Management No clinical interventions appear necessary.

Discussion

Only 1 case report has demonstrated this interaction clinically.[1] In this case, a parkinsonian patient did not improve on levodopa 5 g/day until 30 mL of an antacid was given prior to each levodopa dose. He was subsequently stabilized on the antacid and levodopa 3 g/day.

Small open-label studies of the effect of an antacid (usually a magnesium hydroxide and aluminum hydroxide combination) on levodopa absorption have found a decrease in gastric emptying time,[1,2] an increase in time to peak for levodopa,[1-3] and an increase in total levodopa AUC.[2] However, another study found that only certain subjects had an increase in peak levodopa concentrations following antacid administration.[4] In addition, there have been reports[4] and small studies[5] that did not show any clinical benefit from the addition of an antacid to levodopa therapy. Therefore, it appears that only certain subjects may benefit from this interaction.

1 Rivera-Calimlim L, et al. *Br Med J.* 1970;4(5727):93.
2 Rivera-Calimlim L, et al. *Eur J Clin Invest.* 1971;1(5):313.
3 Pocelinko R, et al. *Clin Pharmacol Ther.* 1972;13:149.
4 Leon AS, et al. *J Clin Pharmacol New Drugs.* 1972;12(7):263.
5 Lau E, et al. *Clin Neuropharmacol.* 1986;9(5):477.

* Asterisk indicates drugs cited in interaction reports. Based on pharmacologic and pharmacokinetic considerations, similar interactions may occur with other drugs that are listed.

Levodopa — *Anticholinergics*

Levodopa	Anticholinergics	
Levodopa* (eg, *Larodopa*)	Anisotropine (*Valpin 50*)	Methixene
	Atropine	Methscopolamine (*Pamine*)
	Belladonna	Orphenadrine (*Disipal*)
	Benztropine (*Cogentin*)	Oxybutynin (*Ditropan*)
	Biperiden (*Akineton*)	Oxyphencyclimine (*Daricon*)
	Clidinium (*Quarzan*)	Oxyphenonium (*Atrenyl*)
	Dicyclomine (eg, *Bentyl*)	Procyclidine (*Kemadrin*)
	Ethopropazine (*Parsidol*)	Propantheline (eg, *Pro-Banthine*)
	Glycopyrrolate (eg, *Robinul*)	Scopolamine (eg, *Triptone*)
	Hexocyclium (eg, *Tral*)	Thiphenamil
	Hyoscyamine (eg, *Anaspaz*)	Tridihexethyl (*Pathilon*)
	Isopropamide (*Darbid*)	Trihexyphenidyl* (eg, *Artane*)
	Mepenzolate (*Cantil*)	
	Methantheline (*Banthine*)	

Significance	Onset	Severity	Documentation
5	☐ Rapid	☐ Major	☐ Established
	■ **Delayed**	☐ Moderate	☐ Probable
		■ **Minor**	☐ Suspected
			■ **Possible**
			☐ Unlikely

Effects The therapeutic utility of LEVODOPA may be reduced.

Mechanism Probably ANTICHOLINERGIC-associated decreased gastric motility resulting in increased gastric deactivation of LEVODOPA and decreased intestinal absorption.

Management The dose of LEVODOPA can be increased or the dose of ANTICHOLINERGIC may be decreased.

Discussion

A case report of a Parkinsonian patient on homatropine (not available in the US) found that his response to levodopa was slow and required a much higher dose to achieve efficacy.[2] It was postulated that a homatropine-associated decrease in gastric motility resulted in increased gastric metabolism and decreased intestinal absorption of levodopa. Similar effects were seen in three of six healthy volunteers and four of six Parkinson patients who experienced a delayed time to peak and reduced peak concentrations of levodopa following pretreatment with trihexyphenidyl.[3] Other reports refute these findings. Hughes et al[1] found no increase in levodopa effects when anticholinergics were removed from the therapy, and Bergmann et al[4] found that pretreatment of Parkinson patients with anticholinergics (mostly trihexyphenidyl) was not associated with any significant difference in levodopa blood levels. Thus, the clinical importance of this interaction may only be important in patients with abnormal gastric motility.

[1] Hughes RC, et al. *Br Med J.* 1971;2:487.
[2] Fermaglich J, et al. *Dis Nerv Syst.* 1972;33:624.
[3] Algeri S, et al. *Eur J Pharmacol.* 1976;35:293.
[4] Bergmann S, et al. *Br J Clin Pharmacol.* 1974;1:417.

* Asterisk indicates drugs cited in interaction reports. Based on pharmacologic and pharmacokinetic considerations, similar interactions may occur with other drugs that are listed.

Levodopa — *Benzodiazepines*

Levodopa	Benzodiazepines	
Levodopa* (eg, *Larodopa*)	Alprazolam (*Xanax*)	Halazepam (*Paxipam*)
	Chlordiazepoxide* (eg, *Librium*)	Lorazepam (eg, *Ativan*)
	Clonazepam (*Klonopin*)	Oxazepam (eg, *Serax*)
	Clorazepate (eg, *Tranxene*)	Prazepam (*Centrax*)
	Diazepam* (eg, *Valium*)	Temazepam (eg, *Restoril*)
	Flurazepam (eg, *Dalmane*)	Triazolam (*Halcion*)

Significance	Onset	Severity	Documentation
5	■ **Rapid**	□ Major	□ Established
	□ Delayed	□ Moderate	□ Probable
		■ **Minor**	□ Suspected
			■ **Possible**
			□ Unlikely

Effects LEVODOPA'S therapeutic value may be attenuated.

Mechanism Unknown.

Management No clinical interventions appear required. Consider discontinuing the BENZODIAZEPINE if a problem arises.

Discussion

Several studies and case reports have noted that the addition of diazepam[1,4] or chlordiazepoxide[3,5] to a Parkinson patient stabilized on levodopa can cause rapid deterioration (less than 24 hours) of Parkinsonian control. Some patients have returned to a nearly pre-levodopa level of control. Another report told of inadequate improvement on initial levodopa treatment until the patient's chlordiazepoxide was discontinued.[2]

Patients returned to their previous baseline within a few days or weeks following discontinuation of the benzodiazepine.[1,3,5]

[1] Hunter KR, et al. *Lancet.* 1970;2:1283.
[2] Schwarz GA, et al. *Med Clin N Am.* 1970;54:773.
[3] Mackie L. *BMJ.* 1971;1:651.
[4] Wodak J, et al. *Med J Aust.* 1972;2:1277.
[5] Yosselson-Superstine S, et al. *Ann Intern Med.* 1982;96:259.

* Asterisk indicates drugs cited in interaction reports. Based on pharmacologic and pharmacokinetic considerations, similar interactions may occur with other drugs that are listed.

Levodopa — *Clonidine*

Levodopa*	Clonidine* (eg, *Catapres*)

Significance	Onset	Severity	Documentation
4	☐ Rapid ■ **Delayed**	☐ Major ■ **Moderate** ☐ Minor	☐ Established ☐ Probable ☐ Suspected ■ **Possible** ☐ Unlikely

Effects The effectiveness of LEVODOPA may be reduced.

Mechanism Unknown.

Management Data do not indicate that clinical interventions are necessary.

Discussion

A double-blind, crossover study was conducted in 6 parkinsonian patients, 2 patients stabilized on levodopa/carbidopa (eg, *Sinemet*) and 4 patients stabilized on piribedil†. This group found that clonidine (mean dose, 0.7 mg) increased overall parkinsonian signs by 31%. Measures of rigidity and akinesia were significantly different from the placebo period.[1] Another study found no difference in levodopa-stabilized patients with the addition of clonidine.[2] These results were unexpected because a beneficial effect from clonidine plus levodopa was anticipated.

[1] Shoulson I, et al. *Neuropharmacology.* 1976;15(1):25. [2] Tarsy D, et al. *Arch Neurol.* 1975;32(2):134.

* Asterisk indicates drugs cited in interaction reports.
† Not available in the United States.

Levodopa | *Enteral Nutrition*

Levodopa*	Enteral Nutrition, High Protein*

Significance	Onset	Severity	Documentation
4	□ Rapid ■ **Delayed**	□ Major ■ **Moderate** □ Minor	□ Established □ Probable □ Suspected ■ **Possible** □ Unlikely

Effects ENTERAL NUTRITION with protein supplementation may decrease LEVODOPA efficacy. A neuroleptic malignant-like syndrome resulting from acute lowering of dopaminergic activity has been reported.

Mechanism Because of the protein content, ENTERAL NUTRITION with protein supplementation may decrease intestinal LEVODOPA absorption.

Management If there is a decrease in control of Parkinson disease symptoms, it may be necessary to alter protein administration to minimize the decrease in control.

Discussion

Decreased control of Parkinson disease symptoms in a patient receiving levodopa was reported after enteral nutrition was started.[1] The patient, a 77-year-old man with Parkinson disease, was admitted to the intensive care unit for an intracerebral hemorrhage. Continuous enteral nutrition support with 1.4 g/kg of protein was provided via an oral gastric tube. The patient's medications, consisting of immediate-release carbidopa 25 mg/levodopa 100 mg (1.5 tablets 4 times daily), pramipexole (eg, *Mirapex*), and entacapone (*Comtan*), were continued during hospitalization. The patient developed severe rigidity, and the amount of protein in the enteral feeding was decreased to 0.9 g/kg/day. The administration of the enteral nutrition was changed from continuous to bolus feeding (every 4 hours), with levodopa administered between boluses. On this regimen, parkinsonian symptoms improved markedly. A 63-year-old man was receiving levodopa/carbidopa and enteral nutrition that provided 0.88 g/kg/day of protein.[2] Within 24 hours of being changed to an enteral nutrition formula that provided 1.8 g/kg/day of protein, he developed a neuroleptic malignant-like syndrome with mental status changes, fever, rigidity, increased WBC, and acute renal function impairment. The patient began to improve after being switched to a low-protein formula.

[1] Cooper MK, et al. *Ann Pharmacother.* 2008;42(3):439. [2] Bonnici A, et al. *Ann Pharmacother.* 2010;44(9):1504.

* Asterisk indicates drugs cited in interaction reports.

Levodopa — *Furazolidone*

Levodopa* (*Larodopa*)	Furazolidone*†

Significance	Onset	Severity	Documentation
4	■ **Rapid** □ Delayed	■ **Major** □ Moderate □ Minor	□ Established □ Probable □ Suspected ■ **Possible** □ Unlikely

Effects Both the efficacy and adverse reactions, specifically hypertensive crisis, of LEVODOPA may be increased. This may be seen for several weeks after stopping FURAZOLIDONE therapy.

Mechanism Speculative. Chronic use of FURAZOLIDONE can result in inhibition of monoamine oxidase. LEVODOPA-produced dopamine may increase efficacy and adverse reactions centrally and precipitate a hypertensive crisis peripherally.

Management If possible, do not coadminister these drugs. If hypertensive crisis occurs, phentolamine (eg, *Regitine*) may be useful.

Discussion

No clinical examples of this interaction were found. However, furazolidone has been shown to be a potent inhibitor of monoamine oxidase with chronic therapy (5 or more days),[1] and levodopa has been shown to produce hypertension episodes in subjects receiving other monoamine oxidase inhibitors.[2] Carbidopa (*Sinemet*) in high doses (300 to 400 mg) may partially prevent this hypertensive episode, but response is highly variable.[2] Because of the potential seriousness of the interaction, this combination should be avoided. See also Levodopa-MAOIs.

[1] Pettinger WA, et al. *Clin Pharmacol Ther.* 1968;9(4):442.

[2] Teychenne PF, et al. *Clin Pharmacol Ther.* 1975;18(3):273.

* Asterisk indicates drugs cited in interaction reports.
† Not available in the United States.

Levodopa — *Hydantoins*

Levodopa	Hydantoins	
Levodopa* (*Larodopa*)	Ethotoin (*Peganone*)	Phenytoin* (eg, *Dilantin*)
	Fosphenytoin (*Cerebyx*)	

Significance	Onset	Severity	Documentation
2	□ Rapid	□ Major	□ Established
	■ **Delayed**	■ **Moderate**	□ Probable
		□ Minor	■ **Suspected**
			□ Possible
			□ Unlikely

Effects LEVODOPA efficacy may be reduced.

Mechanism Unknown.

Management Use this combination with caution. If an interaction is suspected, consider changing the HYDANTOIN therapy.

Discussion

The clinical effects of phenytoin on 7 patients taking levodopa for Parkinson disease (5 cases) or chronic manganese poisoning (2 cases) were evaluated.[1] A few days after the addition of phenytoin 300 to 500 mg, the subjects with Parkinson disease experienced a return of rigidity and hypokinesia, but tremor re-emergence was not noted. The chronic manganese-poisoning patients also returned to nearly prelevodopa-like conditions. Following discontinuation of the phenytoin, patients returned to baseline within 2 weeks. Avoid this combination if alternative therapies are available.

[1] Mendez JS, et al. *Arch Neurol.* 1975;32(1):44.

* Asterisk indicates drugs cited in interaction reports. Based on pharmacologic and pharmacokinetic considerations, similar interactions may occur with other drugs that are listed.

Levodopa — *Iron Salts*

Levodopa*	Ferrous Fumarate	Ferrous Sulfate*
(*Larodopa*)	(eg, *Hemocyte*)	(eg, *Feosol*)
	Ferrous Gluconate	Iron Polysaccharide
	(eg, *Fergon*)	(eg, *Niferex*)

Significance	Onset	Severity	Documentation
2	☐ Rapid	☐ Major	☐ Established
	■ **Delayed**	■ **Moderate**	■ **Probable**
		☐ Minor	☐ Suspected
			☐ Possible
			☐ Unlikely

Effects The pharmacologic effect of LEVODOPA may be decreased.

Mechanism LEVODOPA appears to form chelates with IRON SALTS, decreasing LEVODOPA absorption and serum levels.

Management Separate the administration times by as much as possible. Observe the patient's clinical response and increase the dose of LEVODOPA accordingly.

Discussion

The effects of ferrous sulfate on the bioavailability of levodopa and levodopa plus carbidopa (*Lodosyn*) have been studied.[1] In one investigation, 8 healthy subjects were randomized to take levodopa 250 mg with or without ferrous sulfate 325 mg.[1] Seven days later, the alternative treatment was taken. During administration of ferrous sulfate, serum levodopa levels were reduced 55%, and the AUC was decreased 51%. There was wide individual variability. However, subjects with high peak levodopa levels and a large AUC with levodopa alone demonstrated the greatest reduction in serum concentrations when ferrous sulfate was ingested. The second study involved 9 patients with idiopathic Parkinson disease.[2] All patients had taken levodopa plus carbidopa at dosages between 100 mg/10 mg 2 times daily and 100 mg/25 mg 8 times daily for more than 2 years. Patients were also receiving various other antiparkinsonian medications and were clinically stable. In this randomized, double-blind, crossover design, patients received either placebo or ferrous sulfate 325 mg administered with levodopa plus carbidopa (100 mg/25 mg). The alternative therapy was administered 24 hours later. Ferrous sulfate produced a 47% decrease in peak plasma levodopa levels and a 30% reduction in the AUC. Peak serum carbidopa concentrations were reduced 77%, and the AUC was decreased 82% when ingested with ferrous sulfate. In some patients, carbidopa levels were reduced below the limits of assay detection. In addition to decreases in levodopa and carbidopa levels, there was a loss of clinical efficacy with concurrent ferrous sulfate ingestion. Patients in whom ferrous sulfate produced the largest reduction in the levodopa AUC demonstrated the greatest decrease in levodopa/carbidopa efficacy.

[1] Campbell NR, et al. *Clin Pharmacol Ther.* 1989;45(3):220.

[2] Campbell NR, et al. *Br J Clin Pharmacol.* 1990;30(4):599.

* Asterisk indicates drugs cited in interaction reports. Based on pharmacologic and pharmacokinetic considerations, similar interactions may occur with other drugs that are listed.

Levodopa | **Kava**

Levodopa* (*Larodopa*)	Kava*

Significance	Onset	Severity	Documentation
4	☐ Rapid	☐ Major	☐ Established
	■ **Delayed**	■ **Moderate**	☐ Probable
		☐ Minor	☐ Suspected
			■ **Possible**
			☐ Unlikely

Effects KAVA may decrease LEVODOPA efficacy.

Mechanism Antagonism of dopamine is suspected.

Management Until more data are available, patients taking LEVODOPA should avoid KAVA.

Discussion

A 76-year-old woman with Parkinson disease who was receiving levodopa 500 mg/day experienced increasing problems with motor fluctuations and dyskinesia.[1] Her general practitioner had prescribed kava extract 150 mg twice daily for inner tension. Within 10 days of starting kava, she noted a dramatic increase in the duration and number of daily "off" periods. Within 2 days of discontinuing kava, the patient returned to her normal baseline pattern.

[1] Schelosky L, et al. *J Neurol Neurosurg Psychiatry*. 1995;58(5):639.

* Asterisk indicates drugs cited in interaction reports.

Levodopa — *MAOIs*

Levodopa*
(*Larodopa*)

Isocarboxazid (*Marplan*)	Rasagiline (*Azilect*)
Linezolid (*Zyvox*)	Selegiline (eg, *Eldepryl*)
Phenelzine* (*Nardil*)	Tranylcypromine* (eg, *Parnate*)

Significance	Onset	Severity	Documentation
1	■ **Rapid**	■ **Major**	■ **Established**
	□ Delayed	□ Moderate	□ Probable
		□ Minor	□ Suspected
			□ Possible
			□ Unlikely

Effects Hypertensive reactions occur if LEVODOPA is administered to patients receiving MAOIs.

Mechanism Inhibited peripheral metabolism of LEVODOPA-derived dopamine with increased levels at dopamine receptors.

Management Do not coadminister. The monoamine oxidase (MAO)–type B inhibitor SELEGILINE is not associated with a hypertensive reaction and is used therapeutically in combination with LEVODOPA and dopa decarboxylase inhibitors.

Discussion

Coadministration of levodopa and MAOIs has caused hypertensive reactions.[1,2] These effects appear within 1 hour[2] and seem to be dose related. Patients may experience flushing, light-headedness, and palpitations.[2] Cardiac arrhythmias are theoretically possible.[3] One patient receiving phenelzine 15 mg 3 times daily received levodopa 50 mg with a systolic blood pressure response of up to 180 mm Hg. The effect was terminated with phentolamine.[4] This interaction was studied in a patient with idiopathic orthostatic hypotension. However, the patient was sensitive to small changes in the levodopa dose and experienced a hypertensive episode with retinal hemorrhages during titration.[5]

Dopamine alone produces substantial and sustained hypertensive effects in patients taking MAOIs.[6] Levodopa administered to patients taking MAOIs substantially increased urinary dopamine levels and reduced Parkinson disease control.[7] In addition, carbidopa (*Lodosyn*) administration seems to eliminate or blunt the hypertensive response.[8] Selegiline is a selective monoamine type B inhibitor. It has been used with levodopa and a peripheral dopa decarboxylase inhibitor for Parkinson disease.[9] Selegiline does not appear to increase levodopa plasma concentrations.[10]

1 Schildkraut JJ, et al. *Ann NY Acad Sci.* 1963;107:1005.
2 Friend DG, et al. *Clin Pharmacol Ther.* 1965;6:362.
3 Goldberg LI, et al. *Clin Pharmacol Ther.* 1971;12(2):376.
4 Hunter KR, et al. *Br Med J.* 1970;3(5719):388.
5 Sharpe J, et al. *Can Med Assoc J.* 1972;107(4):296.
6 Horwitz D, et al. *J Lab Clin Med.* 1960;56:747.
7 Kott E, et al. *N Engl J Med.* 1971;284(7):395.
8 Teychenne PF, et al. *Clin Pharmacol Ther.* 1975;18(3):273.
9 Birkmayer W, et al. *Lancet.* 1977;1(8009):439.
10 Roberts J, et al. *Br J Clin Pharmacol.* 1995;40(4):404.

* Asterisk indicates drugs cited in interaction reports. Based on pharmacologic and pharmacokinetic considerations, similar interactions may occur with other drugs that are listed.

Levodopa ✕ *Methionine*

Levodopa* (*Larodopa*)	Methionine* (eg, *Uracid*)

Significance	Onset	Severity	Documentation
4	☐ Rapid ■ **Delayed**	☐ Major ■ **Moderate** ☐ Minor	☐ Established ☐ Probable ☐ Suspected ■ **Possible** ☐ Unlikely

Effects The clinical utility of LEVODOPA may be decreased.

Mechanism Unknown.

Management No clinical interventions appear to be needed. Consider stopping METHIONINE or increasing the dose of LEVODOPA if conditions warrant action.

Discussion

One small, randomized, double-blind, placebo-controlled trial in 14 patients found that methionine 4.5 g/day supplementation caused a deterioration in the clinical signs of Parkinson disease (eg, bradykinesia, psychiatric symptoms, rigidity, tremor). All patients were on a low-methionine diet (0.5 g/day) and remained on their stabilized doses of levodopa throughout the 8-day study. Differences were significant by day 6 of methionine supplementation.[1]

[1] Pearce LA, et al. *Neurology.* 1974;24(1):46.

* Asterisk indicates drugs cited in interaction reports.

Levodopa — *Metoclopramide*

Levodopa*
(*Larodopa*)

Metoclopramide*
(eg, *Reglan*)

Significance	Onset	Severity	Documentation
4	☐ Rapid ■ **Delayed**	☐ Major ■ **Moderate** ☐ Minor	☐ Established ☐ Probable ☐ Suspected ■ **Possible** ☐ Unlikely

Effects The effects of METOCLOPRAMIDE on gastric emptying and lower esophageal pressure are decreased by LEVODOPA. METOCLOPRAMIDE may increase the bioavailability of LEVODOPA.

Mechanism LEVODOPA and METOCLOPRAMIDE have opposite effects on dopamine receptors.

Management METOCLOPRAMIDE may not be effective in patients receiving LEVODOPA. Because of its dopamine-antagonizing effects, METOCLOPRAMIDE is relatively contraindicated in patients with Parkinson disease.

Discussion

In 12 healthy volunteers and 1 patient with Parkinson disease, the use of metoclopramide doubled levodopa bioavailability.[1] Increased gastric emptying may rapidly deliver drugs to the small intestine, causing saturation of first-pass metabolism. While this effect may be of potential use in enhancing levodopa delivery to patients, metoclopramide may also adversely affect disease control. This is possibly due to antagonism of CNS dopamine receptors. There is one case report of a hypertensive crisis with the combination of metoclopramide and carbidopa/levodopa (eg, *Sinemet*) in a 60-year-old woman.[2] There is no clear explanation for this reaction other than increased bioavailability yielding high dopamine levels. However, the patient was on a low carbidopa/levodopa dose of 5/50 mg 3 times daily for one day when the reaction occurred.

In single-dose studies using healthy subjects, levodopa inhibited the increase in lower esophageal pressure normally seen with metoclopramide therapy.[3] Likewise, metoclopramide restored delayed gastric emptying induced by levodopa to normal.[4] Both observations document a dopamine receptor mechanism for metoclopramide in the GI tract. They also indicate a pharmacologic antagonism between the 2 drugs. While this antagonism is, in theory, clinically relevant, metoclopramide is contraindicated in patients taking levodopa. Metoclopramide may worsen Parkinson disease through a CNS inhibition of dopamine receptors.

[1] Mearrick PT, et al. *Aust NZ J Med.* 1974;4(2):144.
[2] Rampton DS. *Br Med J.* 1977;2(6087):607.
[3] Baumann HW, et al. *Dig Dis Sci.* 1979;24(4):289.
[4] Berkowitz DM, et al. *Clin Pharmacol Ther.* 1980;27(3):414.

* Asterisk indicates drugs cited in interaction reports.

Levodopa — *Papaverine*

Levodopa* (eg, *Larodopa*)	Ethaverine (eg, *Ethaquin*)	Papaverine* (eg, *Pavabid*)

Significance	Onset	Severity	Documentation
4	☐ Rapid	☐ Major	☐ Established
	■ **Delayed**	■ **Moderate**	☐ Probable
		☐ Minor	☐ Suspected
			■ **Possible**
			☐ Unlikely

Effects Loss of Parkinson's disease control following the introduction of PAPAVERINE.

Mechanism Unknown.

Management Although the interaction is poorly documented, avoidance of PAPAVERINE in LEVODOPA-treated patients is reasonable.

Discussion

One study reported experience in five patients being treated with levodopa.[1] They lost control of Parkinson's disease after papaverine therapy. For example, a 71-year-old woman had gradual recurrence of Parkinson's disease over 4 weeks when given papaverine 100 mg daily. When papaverine was discontinued, the patient improved. Similarly, another study alluded to several cases and described two female Parkinson's patients who had a reversal of the levodopa effect.[3] It was noted that patients recovered 5 to 6 days after stopping papaverine. Further support that papaverine may affect dopaminergic neurons is offered by another study that reported three patients with tardive dyskinesia who had some improvement in their movement disorder with papaverine 300 to 600 mg/day.[2] On the contrary, in a controlled trial in nine patients receiving papaverine 150 mg every day, no effect on Parkinson's disease was detected.[4]

While the documentation for the interaction between levodopa and papaverine is sparse, the dubious benefit of papaverine as a cerebral vasodilator indicates that avoidance of the combination is rational.

1 Duvoisin RC. *JAMA*. 1975;231:845.
2 Gardos G, et al. *N Engl J Med*. 1975;292:1355.
3 Posner DM. *JAMA*. 1975;233:768.
4 Montastruc JL, et al. *Ann Neurol*. 1987;22:558.

* Asterisk indicates drugs cited in interaction reports. Based on pharmacologic and pharmacokinetic considerations, similar interactions may occur with other drugs that are listed.

Levodopa — *Penicillamine*

Levodopa* (eg, *Larodopa*)	Penicillamine* (eg, *Cuprimine*)

Significance	Onset	Severity	Documentation
4	☐ Rapid	☐ Major	☐ Established
	■ **Delayed**	■ **Moderate**	☐ Probable
		☐ Minor	☐ Suspected
			■ **Possible**
			☐ Unlikely

Effects Serum levodopa concentrations may be elevated, increasing the pharmacologic and toxic effects of LEVODOPA.

Mechanism Unknown.

Management Observe the clinical response of the patient to LEVODOPA when starting or stopping PENICILLAMINE. If an interaction is suspected, adjust the dose of LEVODOPA as indicated.

Discussion

A 42-year-old male patient with a 5-year history of levodopa therapy for Parkinson's disease was admitted to the hospital for readjustment of his drug regimen.[1] High doses of levodopa plus a dopa-decarboxylase inhibitor reduced parkinsonian symptoms but induced dyskinesia, whereas concurrent administration of levodopa and bromocriptine (eg, *Prolactin*) did not increase efficacy. Treatment with D-penicillamine 600 mg daily was instituted because of relatively low levels of serum copper and ceruloplasmin. Penicillamine improved parkinsonian symptoms by increasing serum levodopa concentrations; however, symptoms of dyskinesia were also increased.

[1] Mizuta E, et al. *Clin Neuropharmacol.* 1993;16:448.

* Asterisk indicates drugs cited in interaction reports.

Levodopa — *Phenothiazines*

Levodopa	Phenothiazines	
Levodopa* (eg, *Larodopa*)	Acetophenazine (*Tindal*)	Promazine (eg, *Sparine*)
	Chlorpromazine* (eg, *Thorazine*)	Promethazine (eg, *Phenergan*)
	Ethopropazine (*Parsidol*)	Propiomazine (*Largon*)
	Fluphenazine (eg, *Prolixin*)	Thiethylperazine (*Torecan*)
	Methdilazine (*Tacaryl*)	Thioridazine
	Methotrimeprazine (*Levoprome*)	Trifluoperazine
	Perphenazine	Triflupromazine (*Vesprin*)
	Prochlorperazine (eg, *Compazine*)	Trimeprazine (*Temaril*)

Significance	Onset	Severity	Documentation
4	☐ Rapid	☐ Major	☐ Established
	■ **Delayed**	■ **Moderate**	☐ Probable
		☐ Minor	☐ Suspected
			■ **Possible**
			☐ Unlikely

Effects Stimulation of growth hormone secretion by LEVODOPA may be inhibited by PHENOTHIAZINES. The antiparkinsonian effects of LEVODOPA may also be inhibited.

Mechanism PHENOTHIAZINES may inhibit dopamine receptors in the central nervous system.

Management In patients with parkinsonism, monitor for loss of therapeutic effect if a PHENOTHIAZINE is started. If an interaction is suspected, consider stopping the PHENOTHIAZINE.

Discussion

The effects of oral chlorpromazine on levodopa-induced stimulation of growth hormone was studied in six adult men.[1] All subjects had responded to oral administration of 1 g levodopa (mean growth hormone response 34 ng/mL). When chlorpromazine preceded levodopa administration the mean peak growth hormone response decreased to 4.6 ng/mL.

Additional studies are needed to determine whether phenothiazine administration would alter the response of patients receiving levodopa with and without carbidopa (*Lodosyn*) for parkinsonism. Since phenothiazine can cause extrapyramidal effects, avoid use in patients with parkinsonism. Levodopa does not appear to be effective in treating phenothiazine-induced pseudo-parkinsonism. See also Levodopa-Anticholinergics.

[1] Mims RB, et al. *J Clin Endocrinol Metab.* 1975;40:256.

* Asterisk indicates drugs cited in interaction reports. Based on pharmacologic and pharmacokinetic considerations, similar interactions may occur with other drugs that are listed.

Levodopa		*Pyridoxine*
Levodopa* (eg, *Larodopa*)		Pyridoxine*

Significance	Onset	Severity	Documentation
2	■ **Rapid**	□ Major	■ **Established**
	□ Delayed	■ **Moderate**	□ Probable
		□ Minor	□ Suspected
			□ Possible
			□ Unlikely

Effects PYRIDOXINE reduces the effectiveness of LEVODOPA in Parkinson's disease.

Mechanism PYRIDOXINE increases the peripheral metabolism of LEVODOPA. Consequently, lower levels are available for penetration into the central nervous system.

Management This interaction is of importance in patients treated with LEVODOPA alone. Avoid giving PYRIDOXINE. In patients taking levodopa/carbidopa (eg, *Sinemet*) combinations, the effect of PYRIDOXINE is minimal to negligible.

Discussion

An interaction between pyridoxine and levodopa is supported by several studies. Leon et al[3] studied four patients given pyridoxine 50 mg/day. Three of the four patients had clinical deterioration of their Parkinson's disease associated with 65.9% lower dopa plasma levels. Pyridoxine not only reverses the beneficial effects of levodopa but the side effects as well. In one patient, involuntary muscle spasms quickly reversed with parenteral pyridoxine.[1] While it has been theorized that levodopa may promote pyridoxine deficiency, no such cases were detected in a large series.[7] Conversely, it seems unnecessary to promote a pyridoxine-deficient diet in patients taking levodopa as the interaction has only been seen with large pyridoxine doses. Pyridoxine interferes with levodopa-induced increases in growth hormone[9] as used in some diagnostic tests. When the combination of levodopa and carbidopa *(Sinemet)* is used, the interaction is negligible or beneficial.[2] Klawans studied seven patients and found no effect of pyridoxine.[4] In another study, carbidopa (*Lodosyn*) reduced daily levodopa requirements by 30%. The addition of pyridoxine 600 mg/day to levodopa/carbidopa did not improve Parkinson's disease control, but two patients required higher carbidopa doses.[5] Using mice, higher dopamine levels were achieved with pyridoxine/carbidopa/levodopa although these levels were not very different from levodopa/carbidopa.[6] In 15 patients taking levodopa/carbidopa, administration of pyridoxine very slightly reduced the area under the dopa concentration vs time curve (AUC) while it markedly increased the excretion of urinary dopa.[8] These observations support the lack of adverse effect of pyridoxine in carbidopa/levodopa-treated patients.

[1] Jameson HD. *JAMA*. 1970;211:1700.
[2] Yahr MD, et al. *JAMA*. 1971; 216:2141.
[3] Leon AS, et al. *JAMA*. 1971;218:1924.
[4] Klawans HL, et al. *J Neurol Neurosurg Psychiatry*. 1971;34:682.
[5] Papavasiliou PS, et al. *N Engl J Med*. 1972;285:8.
[6] Mars H, et al. *JAMA*. 1972;219:1764.
[7] Yahr MD, et al. *JAMA*. 1972;220:861.
[8] Mars H. *Arch Neurol*. 1974;30:444.
[9] Mims RB, et al. *J Clin Endocrinol Metab*. 1975;40:256.

* Asterisk indicates drugs cited in interaction reports.

Levodopa — *Tacrine*

Levodopa* (eg, *Larodopa*)	Tacrine* (*Cognex*)

Significance	Onset	Severity	Documentation
4	☐ Rapid ■ **Delayed**	☐ Major ■ **Moderate** ☐ Minor	☐ Established ☐ Probable ☐ Suspected ■ **Possible** ☐ Unlikely

Effects The effects of LEVODOPA in patients with parkinsonism may be inhibited.

Mechanism Possible worsening of cholinergic activity in patients with parkinsonism due to central cholinesterase inhibitor activity of TACRINE.

Management Patients with parkinsonism should be carefully monitored if TACRINE is administered. Adjust the dose of the antiparkinson agent or TACRINE as indicated.

Discussion

A 67-year-old female patient with Alzheimer's disease and mild parkinsonism was treated with tacrine.[1] The patient had a 2 to 3 year history of progressive decline in memory and poor recent memory recall. The patient was started on 10 mg tacrine 4 times daily; after 6 weeks, the dose was increased to 20 mg 4 times daily. Two weeks later, the patient presented in the emergency department with severe tremor, nocturnal restlessness, stiffness of the limbs and stumbling gait. Tacrine was continued and carbidopa-levodopa (eg, *Sinemet*) was started. A dose of 12.5/50 mg carbidopa/levodopa, 3 to 4 times daily, produced prompt improvement in the tremor, gait instability and limb rigidity. Four weeks later, the dose of tacrine was increased to 30 mg 4 times daily; 2 days later, the patient developed marked tremor and became depressed and despondent. The next day, the dose of tacrine was decreased to 20 mg 4 times daily and carbidopa/levodopa was continued at 12.5/50 mg 4 times daily. There were no further adverse symptoms. One month later, physical examination revealed no action tremor, extreme slowness in movement and only mild intermittent rest tremor.

Although not a drug interaction, it remains to be determined whether tacrine could unmask mild or latent Parkinson's disease.

[1] Ott BR, et al. *Clin Neuropharmacol.* 1992;15:322.

* Asterisk indicates drugs cited in interaction reports.

Levodopa — *Tricyclic Antidepressants*

Levodopa	Tricyclic Antidepressants	
Levodopa* (eg, *Larodopa*)	Amitriptyline*	Nortriptyline (eg, *Aventyl*)
	Amoxapine	Protriptyline (eg, *Vivactil*)
	Desipramine (eg, *Norpramin*)	Trimipramine (*Surmontil*)
	Doxepin (eg, *Sinequan*)	
	Imipramine (eg, *Tofranil*)	

Significance	Onset	Severity	Documentation
4	■ **Rapid**	□ Major	□ Established
	□ Delayed	■ **Moderate**	□ Probable
		□ Minor	□ Suspected
			■ **Possible**
			□ Unlikely

Effects TRICYCLIC ANTIDEPRESSANTS (TCAs) delay the absorption of LEVODOPA and may decrease its bioavailability. Hypertensive episodes have also been reported.

Mechanism Unknown.

Management No special precautions appear necessary.

Discussion

Imipramine decreased the urinary excretion of levodopa, dopamine, and their metabolites in 4 healthy volunteers.[1] The mechanism appears to be reduced oral absorption caused by delayed gastric emptying.[2] Apparently the more gradual absorption of levodopa results in more peripheral metabolism and ultimately less drug at the site of action, as suggested in a rat study.[3] This implies reduced levodopa efficacy in Parkinson disease. However, large clinical studies are needed to document this potential interaction.

In 2 case reports, hypertensive episodes have been attributed to the combination of TCAs and levodopa. A 60-year-old woman with hypertension taking low-dose (20 mg/day) amitriptyline received levodopa/carbidopa (eg, *Sinemet*) and metoclopramide (eg, *Reglan*). Beginning in 24 hr, BP reached 270/140 mm Hg. The reaction resolved upon discontinuation of all medications.[4] In the other report, an 82-year-old woman on levodopa/carbidopa received imipramine (25 mg 3 times daily). Her BP rose to 210/110 mm Hg during the second day of combined therapy. This rapidly resolved after discontinuation of imipramine. The patient had a similar episode with amitriptyline 25 mg 3 times daily.[5] Antidepressants are occasionally used in Parkinson disease patients; no adverse effects or decreased control have been noted.[6] Hypertensive episodes, if related to the combination, must occur infrequently.

1 Messiha FS, et al. *Biochem Pharmacol.* 1974;23:1503.
2 Morgan JP, et al. *Neurology.* 1975;25:1029.
3 Morgan JP, et al. *J Pharmacol Exp Ther.* 1975;192:451.
4 Rampton DS. *Br Med J.* 1977;2:607.
5 Edwards M. *Practitioner.* 1982;226:1447.
6 Andersen J, et al. *Acta Neurol Scand.* 1980;62:210.

* Asterisk indicates drugs cited in interaction reports. Based on pharmacologic and pharmacokinetic considerations, similar interactions may occur with other drugs that are listed.

Levomethadyl — *Azole Antifungal Agents*

Levomethadyl* (*ORLAAM*)	Itraconazole* (*Sporanox*)

Significance	Onset	Severity	Documentation
1	□ Rapid ■ **Delayed**	■ **Major** □ Moderate □ Minor	□ Established □ Probable ■ **Suspected** □ Possible □ Unlikely

Effects LEVOMETHADYL plasma concentrations may be elevated, increasing the risk of life-threatening cardiac arrhythmias, including torsades de pointes.

Mechanism ITRACONAZOLE may inhibit the hepatic metabolism (CYP3A4) of LEVOMETHADYL.

Management Coadministration of LEVOMETHADYL and ITRACONAZOLE is contraindicated.

Discussion

Levomethadyl may prolong the QT interval and is metabolized by CYP3A4.[1] Thus, coadministration of itraconazole and levomethadyl may result in increased plasma concentrations of levomethadyl, which could lead to potentially serious and life-threatening cardiac arrhythmias.[1]

The basis for this monograph is information on file with the manufacturer. Published clinical data are needed to further assess this interaction. Because of the seriousness of the cardiac events, clinical evaluation of this interaction in humans is not likely to be forthcoming.

[1] *Sporanox* [package insert]. Titusville, NJ: Janssen Pharmaceutica, LP; January 2004.

* Asterisk indicates drugs cited in interaction reports.

Lidocaine ✕ *Amiodarone*

Lidocaine* (eg, *Xylocaine*)	Amiodarone (eg, *Cordarone*)

Significance	Onset	Severity	Documentation
4	■ **Rapid**	□ Major	□ Established
	□ Delayed	■ **Moderate**	□ Probable
		□ Minor	□ Suspected
			■ **Possible**
			□ Unlikely

Effects Serum LIDOCAINE concentrations may be increased, possibly producing LIDOCAINE toxicity. The effect may be seen with local anesthetic doses.

Mechanism AMIODARONE or 1 of its metabolites may inhibit LIDOCAINE metabolism (CYP3A4).

Management Monitor cardiac function and observe patients for symptoms of LIDOCAINE toxicity when AMIODARONE is added to the treatment regimen. Monitoring serum LIDOCAINE levels may be useful in managing the patient.

Discussion

A 71-year-old man taking digoxin (eg, *Lanoxin*), enalapril (*Vasotec*), amitriptyline, and temazepam (eg, *Restoril*) was hospitalized with a history of sustained monomorphic ventricular tachycardia (VT) and atrial fibrilation.[1] Sustained VT was induced, but procainamide (eg, *Procanbid*) failed to control it and was stopped. Lidocaine IV was administered as a 75 mg bolus followed by a 2 mg/min infusion. Amiodarone 600 mg twice daily was started the next day. Twelve hours later, the serum lidocaine level was 5.4 mg/L (therapeutic, 1.5 to 5.5 mg/L). Two days later, the patient experienced a seizure. The lidocaine level was 12.6 mg/L, and the drug was stopped. Within 13 hr, the lidocaine level was 2 mg/L. A 64-year-old man taking amiodarone 600 mg/day underwent permanent pacemaker implantation under local anesthesia with 15 mL of 2% lidocaine.[2] The patient developed sinus bradycardia and sinoatrial arrest 25 minutes after receiving local anesthesia. He responded to CPR and administration of atropine and isoproterenol (eg, *Isuprel*). In 10 patients, no change in lidocaine pharmacokinetics was noted when 1 mg/kg lidocaine was given before and after at least 4 weeks of therapy with amiodarone 200 to 400 mg/day following variable loading doses.[3] The pharmacokinetics of a single 1 mg/kg IV lidocaine dose were studied in 6 patients after a 6-day amiodarone loading dose and after 19 to 21 days of therapy.[4] A small decrease in lidocaine clearance and an increase in the AUC were noted.

Additional studies with lidocaine infusions are needed to clarify this interaction.

[1] Keidar S, et al. *Am Heart J.* 1982;104:1384.
[2] Siegmund JB, et al. *J Cardiovasc Pharmacol.* 1993;21:513.
[3] Nattel S, et al. *Am J Cardiol.* 1994;73:92.
[4] Ha HR, et al. *J Cardiovasc Pharmacol.* 1996;28:533.

* Asterisk indicates drugs cited in interaction reports. Based on pharmacologic and pharmacokinetic considerations, similar interactions may occur with other drugs that are listed.

Lidocaine — *Beta-Blockers*

Lidocaine		Beta-Blockers	
Lidocaine* (eg, *Xylocaine*)		Atenolol* (eg, *Tenormin*)	Pindolol* (eg, *Visken*)
		Metoprolol* (eg, *Lopressor*)	Propranolol* (eg, *Inderal*)
		Nadolol* (eg, *Corgard*)	

Significance	Onset	Severity	Documentation
2	■ **Rapid**	□ Major	■ **Established**
	□ Delayed	■ **Moderate**	□ Probable
		□ Minor	□ Suspected
			□ Possible
			□ Unlikely

Effects BETA-BLOCKERS cause higher LIDOCAINE levels. LIDOCAINE toxicity may manifest.

Mechanism Reduced hepatic LIDOCAINE metabolism and possibly a minor component of diminished hepatic blood flow.

Management Slower rate of bolus LIDOCAINE infusions may prevent high peak levels and toxicity. During continuous infusions, monitor LIDOCAINE levels and tailor doses as needed; interaction most significant for PROPRANOLOL.

Discussion

In multiple controlled studies, the clearance of lidocaine has been reduced by pretreatment with propranolol.[1-5] One study reported a reduction in single-dose lidocaine clearance of 40% after propranolol 80 mg was given orally for 3 days. During the continuous lidocaine infusion study, steady-state levels rose from 3.02 to 3.9 mcg/mL in 7 volunteers.[1] Lidocaine toxicity has also been reported,[6] possibly caused by a reduction in hepatic blood flow from beta-blockade. Because lidocaine is a high-extraction ratio drug, its clearance is dependent upon liver blood flow.[1,7] In a study of other beta-blockers, it was unclear if they equally modified hepatic blood flow.[8] In any event, propranolol reduced liver blood flow 11%.[5] This would not explain the consistently larger reduction in clearance. Because propranolol inhibits hepatic metabolic enzymes[9] and the oral bioavailability is increased 100%[5] (largely independent of liver blood flow), a more likely explanation is reduced hepatic lidocaine metabolism.[7] Neither pindolol[2] nor atenolol[10] have affected lidocaine pharmacokinetics. Nadolol increased lidocaine levels similar to propranolol.[4] Metoprolol did not affect lidocaine clearance following a single lidocaine dose.[10,11] Conversely, lidocaine's clearance was reduced from 0.88 to 0.61 L/hr•kg by 1 pretreatment day of metoprolol 200 mg. This effect was less than the decrease induced by propranolol (0.47 L/hr•kg).[3]

1. Ochs HR, et al. *N Engl J Med.* 1980;303:373.
2. Svendsen TL, et al. *Br J Clin Pharmacol.* 1982;13 (suppl 2):223S.
3. Conrad KA, et al. *Clin Pharmacol Ther.* 1983;33:133.
4. Schneck DW, et al. *Clin Pharmacol Ther.* 1984;36:584.
5. Bax ND, et al. *Br J Clin Pharmacol.* 1985;19:597.
6. Graham CF, et al. *N Engl J Med.* 1981;304:1301.
7. Lewis RV, et al. *Med Toxicol.* 1986;1:343.
8. Parker G, et al. *J Clin Pharmacol.* 1984;24:493.
9. Bax ND, et al. *Drugs.* 1983;25 (suppl 2):121.
10. Miners JO, et al. *Br J Clin Pharmacol.* 1984;18:853.
11. Jordo L, et al. *Int J Clin Pharmacol Ther Toxicol.* 1984;22:312.

* Asterisk indicates drugs cited in interaction reports.

Lidocaine — *Fluvoxamine*

Lidocaine* (eg, *Xylocaine*)	Fluvoxamine*

Significance	Onset	Severity	Documentation
4	□ Rapid ■ **Delayed**	□ Major ■ **Moderate** □ Minor	□ Established □ Probable □ Suspected ■ **Possible** □ Unlikely

Effects LIDOCAINE plasma concentrations may be elevated during IV infusion, increasing the risk of toxicity.

Mechanism Inhibition of LIDOCAINE metabolism (CYP1A2) by FLUVOXAMINE may occur.

Management Monitor cardiac function and observe the patient for symptoms of LIDOCAINE toxicity when starting FLUVOXAMINE. Monitoring LIDOCAINE concentrations may be useful in managing the patient.

Discussion

The effect of erythromycin (eg, *Ery-Tab*) and fluvoxamine on the pharmacokinetics of IV lidocaine was studied in 9 healthy volunteers.[1] In a double-blind, randomized, 3-way crossover investigation, each subject ingested fluvoxamine 100 mg and placebo, fluvoxamine 100 mg and erythromycin 1,500 mg, or their respective placebo for 5 days. On day 6, lidocaine 1.5 mg/kg was administered IV over 60 minutes. Giving fluvoxamine alone decreased lidocaine clearance 41% and prolonged the elimination $t_{½}$ 35% (from 2.6 to 3.5 hours). After administration of fluvoxamine plus erythromycin, lidocaine clearance was 21% less than during fluvoxamine alone and 53% less than during placebo administration. The $t_{½}$ of lidocaine was longer (4.3 hours) during coadministration with erythromycin plus fluvoxamine than during placebo (2.6 hours) or fluvoxamine (3.5 hours). Fluvoxamine alone or in combination with erythromycin did not affect the lidocaine steady-state volume of distribution. Fluvoxamine alone and in combination with erythromycin decreased the C_{max} and AUC of 1 of the major lidocaine metabolites (monoethylglycinexylidide). The ratio of the AUC of the metabolite to the AUC of lidocaine was decreased, and the $t_{½}$ of the metabolite was prolonged. The decrease in the AUC of the lidocaine metabolite was greater with fluvoxamine alone, compared with the decrease during coadministration of fluvoxamine and erythromycin.

[1] Olkkola KT, et al. *Anesth Analg.* 2005;100:1352.

* Asterisk indicates drugs cited in interaction reports.

Lidocaine | *Histamine H_2 Antagonists*

Lidocaine* (eg, *Xylocaine*)	Cimetidine* (eg, *Tagamet*)

Significance	Onset	Severity	Documentation
2	■ **Rapid**	□ Major	■ **Established**
	□ Delayed	■ **Moderate**	□ Probable
		□ Minor	□ Suspected
			□ Possible
			□ Unlikely

Effects Decreased LIDOCAINE clearance with possible toxicity.

Mechanism Possibly inhibition of lidocaine hepatic metabolism and decreased hepatic blood flow.[11]

Management Monitor the patient for signs of lidocaine toxicity and measure lidocaine plasma levels. Tailor the lidocaine dose as needed. Use an alternative H_2 antagonist such as ranitidine (eg, *Zantac*) or famotidine (eg, *Pepcid*) if possible.

Discussion

An interaction between cimetidine and lidocaine is demonstrated by several well-designed studies. However, the effect on lidocaine pharmacokinetics has varied. Apparently the method of lidocaine or cimetidine administration affects the interaction. In an initial report, 6 subjects were given a single IV lidocaine bolus infusion before and after pretreatment with oral cimetidine 1,200 mg in 4 divided doses. There was a 50% increase in peak lidocaine concentration associated with a reduction in clearance and a small reduction in volume of distribution and fraction unbound.[1] In a similar single–dose experiment using healthy volunteers, the bioavailability of oral lidocaine also increased.[2] The clearance has been reported as reduced 20%[2,3] to 30%.[4] With the combination, toxicity consisting of paresthesias and lightheadedness has been associated with higher lidocaine plasma levels.[1] In 2 studies of patients receiving lidocaine infusions, cimetidine 300 mg every 6 hours produced a 75% increase in steady-state lidocaine levels; toxicity was reported in 2 patients.[5] Conversely, an uncontrolled study using cimetidine infusions did not detect a consistent increase in lidocaine levels.[6] The lidocaine AUC and elimination $t_{½}$ were prolonged with oral but not IV cimetidine.[7] Famotidine[8] and ranitidine, either alone[9,10] or when compared with cimetidine,[11,12] have produced negligible effects upon lidocaine pharmacokinetics or toxicity. It appears that famotidine, ranitidine, and perhaps other H_2 antagonists, are safer for use.

1 Feely J, et al. *Ann Intern Med.* 1982;96:592.
2 Wing LM, et al. *Clin Pharmacol Ther.* 1984;35:695.
3 Abernethy DR, et al. *Clin Pharmacol Ther.* 1985;38:342.
4 Bauer LA, et al. *Am Heart J.* 1984;108:413.
5 Knapp AB, et al. *Ann Intern Med.* 1983;98:174.
6 Patterson JH, et al. *J Clin Pharmacol.* 1985;25:607.
7 Powell JR, et al. *Clin Pharm.* 1986;5:993.
8 Kishikawa K, et al. *Anaesthesia.* 1990;45:719.
9 Feely J, et al. *Br J Clin Pharmacol.* 1983;15:378.
10 Robson RA, et al. *Br J Clin Pharmacol.* 1985;20:170.
11 Jackson JE, et al. *Clin Pharmacol Ther.* 1983;33:255.
12 Jackson JE, et al. *Clin Pharmacol Ther.* 1985;37:544.

* Asterisk indicates drugs cited in interaction reports.

Lidocaine ✕ *Macrolide & Related Antibiotics*

Lidocaine	Macrolide & Related Antibiotics	
Lidocaine* (eg, *Xylocaine*)	Clarithromycin (eg, *Biaxin*)	Telithromycin (*Ketek*)
	Erythromycin* (eg, *Ery-Tab*)	

Significance	Onset	Severity	Documentation
4	☐ Rapid	☐ Major	☐ Established
	■ **Delayed**	■ **Moderate**	☐ Probable
		☐ Minor	☐ Suspected
			■ **Possible**
			☐ Unlikely

Effects LIDOCAINE plasma concentrations may be elevated during IV infusion, increasing the risk of toxicity.

Mechanism Inhibition of LIDOCAINE metabolism (CYP3A4) by MACROLIDE and RELATED ANTIBIOTICS may occur.

Management Monitor cardiac function and observe patients for symptoms of LIDOCAINE toxicity when starting a MACROLIDE or RELATED ANTIBIOTIC. Monitoring LIDOCAINE concentrations may be useful in managing patients.

Discussion

The effect of erythromycin and fluvoxamine on the pharmacokinetics of IV lidocaine was studied in 9 healthy volunteers.[1] In a double-blind, randomized, 3-way crossover investigation, each subject ingested fluvoxamine 100 mg and placebo, fluvoxamine 100 mg and erythromycin 1,500 mg, or their respective placebo for 5 days. On the sixth day, lidocaine 1.5 mg/kg was administered IV over 60 minutes. Giving fluvoxamine alone decreased lidocaine clearance 41% and prolonged the elimination $t_{1/2}$ 35% (from 2.6 to 3.5 hours). After administration of fluvoxamine plus erythromycin, lidocaine clearance was 21% less than during fluvoxamine alone and 53% less than during placebo administration. The $t_{1/2}$ of lidocaine was longer (4.3 hours) during coadministration with erythromycin plus fluvoxamine than during placebo (2.6 hours) or fluvoxamine (3.5 hours). Fluvoxamine alone or in combination with erythromycin did not affect the lidocaine steady-state volume of distribution. Fluvoxamine alone and in combination with erythromycin decreased the C_{max} and AUC of 1 of the major lidocaine metabolites (monoethylglycinexylidide). The ratio of AUC of the metabolite to the AUC of lidocaine was decreased and the $t_{1/2}$ of the metabolite was prolonged. The decrease in the AUC of the lidocaine metabolite was greater with fluvoxamine alone, compared with the decrease during coadministration of fluvoxamine and erythromycin.

[1] Olkkola KT, et al. *Anesth Analg.* 2005;100:1352.

* Asterisk indicates drugs cited in interaction reports. Based on pharmacologic and pharmacokinetic considerations, similar interactions may occur with other drugs that are listed.

Lidocaine — *Mexiletine*

Lidocaine* (eg, *Xylocaine*)	Mexiletine* (*Mexitil*)

Significance	Onset	Severity	Documentation
4	■ **Rapid**	□ Major	□ Established
	□ Delayed	■ **Moderate**	□ Probable
		□ Minor	□ Suspected
			■ **Possible**
			□ Unlikely

Effects MEXILETINE may cause increased serum lidocaine concentrations, producing LIDOCAINE toxicity, or additive pharmacologic effects may be producing neurotoxicity.

Mechanism Unknown.

Management Consider measuring plasma lidocaine concentrations and observing the patient for symptoms of LIDOCAINE toxicity during coadministration of MEXILETINE.

Discussion

A 54-year-old woman was being considered for heart transplantation.[1] In addition to mexiletine 300 mg every 12 hours, she was receiving captopril (eg, *Capoten*), potassium chloride, ranitidine (eg, *Zantac*), and digoxin (eg, *Lanoxin*). As part of her work-up for transplantation, she was scheduled for right heart catheterization. On the day of catheterization, the patient experienced esophageal burning with belching and was given an antacid and 5 mL oral viscous lidocaine 2% (100 mg). She was given a second dose of lidocaine 25 mL (500 mg) 1 hr after the initial dose. Within minutes, the patient reported double vision. Her pulse was 106 beats/min and blood pressure 90/70 mm Hg. She then experienced blurred vision, slow and garbled speech, muscle fasciculations, nystagmus, and reported a "thick" tongue. Her serum lidocaine level was found to be 26.9 mcmol/L (therapeutic range, 6.4 to 21.3 mcmol/L). The reaction experienced by this patient may have resulted from administration of excessive lidocaine and not a drug interaction. In the presence of inflamed esophageal tissue, lidocaine absorption could be increased. The second patient was hospitalized for episodic sustained ventricular tachycardia.[2] While receiving mexiletine 300 mg 3 times daily and procainamide (eg, *Pronestyl*), a lidocaine 2 mg/min infusion following an 80 mg bolus was started. Ten hours later the patient experienced diffuse polymyoclonus that resolved when lidocaine was stopped. An 80-year-old man receiving mexiletine experienced toxic lidocaine concentrations with severe adverse effects (eg, involuntary motion and systemic muscular stiffness) during concurrent IV lidocaine infusion.[3]

[1] Geraets DR, et al. *Ann Pharmacother.* 1992;26:1380.
[2] Christie JM, et al. *Anesth Analg.* 1993;77:1291.
[3] Maeda Y, et al. *Clin Pharmacol Ther.* 2002;71:389.

* Asterisk indicates drugs cited in interaction reports.

Lidocaine ✕ *Procainamide*

Lidocaine* (eg, *Xylocaine*)	Procainamide* (eg, *Pronestyl*)

Significance	Onset	Severity	Documentation
4	■ **Rapid** □ Delayed	□ Major ■ **Moderate** □ Minor	□ Established □ Probable □ Suspected ■ **Possible** □ Unlikely

Effects Additive cardiodepressant action. Potential for conduction abnormalities.

Mechanism The independent cardiotoxicity of each drug may be additive.

Management Use the combination of LIDOCAINE and PROCAINAMIDE with caution, particularly if both are given IV to patients with preexisting conduction abnormalities or postmyocardial infarct. Although combined use may be reasonable in selected situations, electrocardiographic monitoring is recommended.

Discussion

The IV administration of procainamide prolonged conduction through the His-Purkinje fibers in 15 of 16 patients. Additionally, there was a BP drop of about 10 mm Hg.[1] The adverse reactions of procainamide are dose and serum-level related, with cardiac conduction disturbances commonly observed at levels of 12 mcg/mL or higher.[2] Likewise, lidocaine given by bolus IV injections can also cause various degrees of heart block in patients with preexisting conduction abnormalities.[3] It is possible for the combination of these 2 drugs to have additive negative effects on the heart. In a single study, procainamide did not alter lidocaine infusion levels.[4] However, a pharmacodynamic interaction was demonstrated in animal experiments.[5] Dogs with experimentally induced MI experienced negative effects from the combination. There was an additive reduction in cardiac output, ventricular contractility, and mean aortic pressure as compared with either drug alone. Published adverse reactions of the combination are limited to a single case of restlessness and visual hallucinations.[6] However, lidocaine alone can cause these reactions when given by rapid, repeated IV boluses.[7] It is unknown if the combination of drugs was actually responsible for the reaction. No reports of adverse cardiac reactions are available. Nonetheless, because the conduction abnormalities are possible with either drug, it is likely that an additive adverse reaction may not be recognized as such and, therefore, may be underreported.

1 Josephson ME, et al. *Am J Cardiol.* 1974;33:596.
2 Koch-Weser J, et al. *JAMA.* 1971;215:1454.
3 Gupta PK, et al. *Am J Cardiol.* 1974;33:487.
4 Karlsson E, et al. *Eur J Clin Pharmacol.* 1974;7:455.
5 Cote P, et al. *Am J Cardiol.* 1973;32:937.
6 Ilyas M, et al. *Lancet.* 1969;2:1368.
7 Gianelly R, et al. *N Engl J Med.* 1967;277:1215.

* Asterisk indicates drugs cited in interaction reports.

Lidocaine — *Propafenone*

Lidocaine* (eg, *Xylocaine*)	Propafenone* (eg, *Rythmol*)

Significance	Onset	Severity	Documentation
5	■ **Rapid**	□ Major	□ Established
	□ Delayed	□ Moderate	□ Probable
		■ **Minor**	□ Suspected
			■ **Possible**
			□ Unlikely

Effects Increased CNS adverse reactions of LIDOCAINE and PROPAFENONE.

Mechanism Unknown. Inhibition of LIDOCAINE metabolism or additive CNS adverse reactions may be contributing factors.

Management Consider observing patients for increased CNS adverse reactions during coadministration of PROPAFENONE and LIDOCAINE.

Discussion

In a randomized, single-blind, 2-way, crossover study involving 11 extensive metabolizers and 1 poor metabolizer, oral propafenone produced a slight, but probably clinically unimportant, decrease in the steady-state volume of distribution (V_{SS}) of continuously infused lidocaine.[1] Patients were randomly assigned to receive placebo or propafenone 225 mg orally every 8 hours for 6 days. On the morning of day 5, each participant was given a loading dose of lidocaine 1.5 mg/kg over 10 minutes, followed by a continuous infusion of 2 mg/kg/hr for 22 hours. In the 11 extensive metabolizers, propafenone caused a small (7%), but statistically significant ($P \leq 0.05$), increase in the lidocaine AUC and systemic clearance compared with placebo. In the individual who was a poor metabolizer, lidocaine clearance and V_{SS} increased 21% and 59%, respectively. The V_{SS} of lidocaine was not altered by propafenone in extensive metabolizers. Compared with placebo, propafenone prolonged the PR and QRS intervals 10% and 15%, respectively. Two subjects experiencing mild CNS reactions to propafenone (eg, dysguesia, light-headedness, paresthesia) before lidocaine administration experienced more serious CNS reactions during concurrent infusion of lidocaine.

[1] Ujhelyi MR, et al. *Clin Pharmacol Ther.* 1993;53:38.

* Asterisk indicates drugs cited in interaction reports.

Lidocaine | **Quinolones**

Lidocaine* (eg, *Xylocaine*)	Ciprofloxacin* (eg, *Cipro*)	Norfloxacin (*Noroxin*)

Significance	Onset	Severity	Documentation
4	□ Rapid ■ **Delayed**	□ Major ■ **Moderate** □ Minor	□ Established □ Probable □ Suspected ■ **Possible** □ Unlikely

Effects LIDOCAINE plasma levels may be elevated, increasing the risk of toxicity.

Mechanism CIPROFLOXACIN may inhibit the metabolism (CYP1A2) of LIDOCAINE.

Management Monitor cardiac function and observe patients for symptoms of LIDOCAINE toxicity when CIPROFLOXACIN is added to the treatment regimen.

Discussion

The effects of ciprofloxacin on the pharmacokinetics of lidocaine were studied in a randomized, double-blind, crossover investigation.[1] Nine healthy volunteers received oral ciprofloxacin 500 mg or placebo twice daily for 2.5 days. On day 3, a single IV dose of lidocaine 1.5 mg/kg was given over 60 minutes. Compared with placebo, ciprofloxacin increased the mean C_{max} and AUC of lidocaine by 12% and 26%, respectively. The mean plasma clearance of lidocaine was decreased by 22%. In addition, ciprofloxacin decreased the AUC of the monoethylglycinexylidide and 3-hydroxylidocaine metabolites of lidocaine by 21% and 14%, respectively.

[1] Isohanni MH, et al. *Eur J Anaesthesiol.* 2005;22(10):795.

* Asterisk indicates drugs cited in interaction reports. Based on pharmacologic and pharmacokinetic considerations, similar interactions may occur with other drugs that are listed.

Lincosamides — *Aluminum Salts*

Lincosamides		Aluminum Salts	
Clindamycin* (eg, *Cleocin*)	Lincomycin* (*Lincocin*)	Aluminum Carbonate Aluminum Hydroxide (eg, *Alternagel*) Aluminum Phosphate	Attapulgite (eg, *Diarrest*) Kaolin* Magaldrate

Significance	Onset	Severity	Documentation
2	☐ Rapid ■ **Delayed**	☐ Major ■ **Moderate** ☐ Minor	☐ Established ☐ Probable ■ **Suspected** ☐ Possible ☐ Unlikely

Effects GI absorption is decreased for LINCOMYCIN and delayed for CLINDAMYCIN when they are administered with KAOLIN-PECTIN antidiarrheals.

Mechanism KAOLIN-PECTIN adsorption of LINCOMYCIN and CLINDAMYCIN occurs.

Management Administer KAOLIN-PECTIN suspension 2 hours before LINCOMYCIN or CLINDAMYCIN.

Discussion

When lincomycin and kaolin-pectin suspension were administered orally at the same time to 8 volunteers, only 9% of the lincomycin was absorbed.[1] Coadministration of clindamycin and kaolin-pectin suspension in 16 volunteers resulted in a 61% decrease in the peak serum clindamycin concentration.[2] Time to peak serum clindamycin concentration also was delayed from 1 to approximately 2.5 hours. However, the total amount of clindamycin absorbed was not altered.

[1] Wagner JG. *Can J Pharm Sci.* 1966;1:55.

[2] Albert KS, et al. *J Pharm Sci.* 1978;67(11):1579.

* Asterisk indicates drugs cited in interaction reports. Based on pharmacologic and pharmacokinetic considerations, similar interactions may occur with other drugs that are listed.

Linezolid	*Macrolide Antibiotics*	
Linezolid* (*Zyvox*)	Clarithromycin* (eg, *Biaxin*)	Erythromycin (eg, *Ery-Tab*)

Significance	Onset	Severity	Documentation
4	☐ Rapid ■ **Delayed**	☐ Major ■ **Moderate** ☐ Minor	☐ Established ☐ Probable ☐ Suspected ■ **Possible** ☐ Unlikely

Effects LINEZOLID serum concentrations may be elevated, increasing the pharmacologic effects and risk of adverse reactions.

Mechanism P-glycoprotein inhibition by MACROLIDE ANTIBIOTICS may increase LINEZOLID intestinal absorption.

Management Increased therapeutic drug monitoring is warranted when LINEZOLID and a MACROLIDE ANTIBIOTIC are coadministered. Be prepared to alter the LINEZOLID dose when the MACROLIDE ANTIBIOTIC is started or stopped.

Discussion

Increased linezolid serum concentrations were reported in a 42-year-old man with smear-positive pulmonary tuberculosis after clarithromycin was started.[1] The patient had been receiving linezolid 300 mg twice daily when clarithromycin 1,000 mg daily was initiated. There was approximately a 272% increase in the linezolid AUC after starting clarithromycin. In addition, the time to the C_{max} was delayed. The linezolid dose was decreased to 150 mg twice daily, and after 6 months, sputum cultures and smear microscopy were negative.

[1] Bolhuis MS, et al. *Antimicrob Agents Chemother*. 2010;54(12):5418.

* Asterisk indicates drugs cited in interaction reports. Based on pharmacologic and pharmacokinetic considerations, similar interactions may occur with other drugs that are listed.

Linezolid — *MAOIs*

Linezolid* (eg, *Zyvox*)	Isocarboxazid* (*Marplan*)	Selegiline* (eg, *Eldepryl*)
	Phenelzine* (eg, *Nardil*)	Tranylcypromine* (eg, *Parnate*)
	Rasagiline* (*Azilect*)	

Significance	Onset	Severity	Documentation
2	■ **Rapid**	□ Major	□ Established
	□ Delayed	■ **Moderate**	□ Probable
		□ Minor	■ **Suspected**
			□ Possible
			□ Unlikely

Effects The risk of adverse reactions may be increased.

Mechanism Unknown.

Management LINEZOLID is contraindicated in patients taking MAOIs or within 2 weeks of taking these agents.[1]

Discussion

Linezolid is a reversible, nonselective MAOI. Do not administer linezolid to patients taking agents that inhibit MAO A or B (eg, isocarboxazid, phenelzine) or within 2 weeks of taking these agents.[1]

The basis for this monograph is information on file with the manufacturer. Published clinical data are needed to further assess this interaction.

[1] *Zyvox* [package insert]. New York, NY: Pharmacia & Upjohn Company; December 2009.

* Asterisk indicates drugs cited in interaction reports.

Linezolid — *Rifamycins*

Linezolid* (*Zyvox*)	Rifampin* (eg, *Rifadin*)

Significance	Onset	Severity	Documentation
4	■ **Rapid**	□ Major	□ Established
	□ Delayed	■ **Moderate**	□ Probable
		□ Minor	□ Suspected
			■ **Possible**
			□ Unlikely

Effects LINEZOLID serum concentrations may be reduced, decreasing the pharmacologic effects.

Mechanism Increased metabolism (CYP3A4) and/or intestinal excretion of LINEZOLID caused by induction of P-gp by RIFAMPIN is suspected.

Management In patients receiving LINEZOLID, monitor the clinical response when RIFAMPIN is started or stopped. Be prepared to adjust therapy as needed.

Discussion

A possible interaction between linezolid and rifampin was reported in a study involving 8 healthy men.[1] Each subject received linezolid 600 mg IV. The next day, they received simultaneous IV doses of linezolid 600 mg and rifampin 600 mg. Compared with linezolid serum concentrations obtained the previous day, linezolid concentrations were reduced 10%, 20%, and 35% when measured 6, 9, and 12 hours, respectively, after coadministration of linezolid and rifampin. In an open-label, multidose, crossover study in 16 healthy subjects, coadministration of linezolid and rifampin reduced linezolid AUC and C_{max} 32% and 21%, respectively.[2] Decreased linezolid levels were reported in a 31-year-old woman receiving IV linezolid and rifampin for methicillin-resistant *Staphylococcus aureus*.[3] Linezolid levels increased after rifampin was discontinued.

1 Egle H, et al. *Clin Pharmacol Ther.* 2005;77(5):451.
2 Gandelman K, et al. *J Clin Pharmacol.* 2011;51(2):229.
3 Gebhart BC, et al. *Pharmacotherapy.* 2007;27(3):476.

* Asterisk indicates drugs cited in interaction reports.

Lithium | **ACE Inhibitors**

Lithium	ACE Inhibitors	
Lithium* (eg, *Lithobid*)	Benazepril (eg, *Lotensin*)	Moexipril (eg, *Univasc*)
	Captopril	Perindopril (eg, *Aceon*)
	Enalapril* (eg, *Vasotec*)	Quinapril (eg, *Accupril*)
	Fosinopril (eg, *Monopril*)	Ramipril (eg, *Altace*)
	Lisinopril* (eg, *Zestril*)	Trandolapril (eg, *Mavik*)

Significance	Onset	Severity	Documentation
2	☐ Rapid	☐ Major	☐ Established
	■ **Delayed**	■ **Moderate**	☐ Probable
		☐ Minor	■ **Suspected**
			☐ Possible
			☐ Unlikely

Effects Elevated serum LITHIUM levels with neurotoxicity may occur.

Mechanism Unknown. Dehydration appears to increase the effects.

Management Monitor serum LITHIUM levels and observe patients for signs of LITHIUM toxicity. Consider an alternative antihypertensive agent.

Discussion

Elevated serum lithium levels occurred in patients receiving lithium and an ACE inhibitor.[1-5] Lithium levels increased nearly 4-fold in a patient after enalapril was added.[1] This was accompanied by symptoms of lithium toxicity. When both drugs were discontinued, symptoms reversed and serum lithium levels decreased. A 49-year-old woman developed elevated lithium levels and lithium toxicity 3 weeks after the substitution of lisinopril for clonidine.[3] The patient had diarrhea prior to the incident. All medications were stopped and she was treated. She recovered within 3 days. Another patient was well maintained for more than 6 months with sodium restriction and hydrochlorothiazide (eg, *Microzide*), enalapril, and lithium.[2] Following volume loss associated with diarrhea, lithium levels increased 5-fold. A woman receiving lithium carbonate, theophylline, loxapine (eg, *Loxitane*), and benztropine (eg, *Cogentin*) developed acute lithium toxicity several months after lisinopril was started.[4] All medications were discontinued, and over the next 48 hours, lithium levels decreased; however, neurotoxicity persisted for several days. Nine healthy volunteers received lithium carbonate 450 mg alone every 12 hours for 10 days, followed by lithium carbonate plus enalapril 10 mg daily for 10 days, then lithium carbonate alone for an additional 6 days; no change in serum lithium concentrations occurred.[6] In a retrospective study of 20 patients, administration of an ACE inhibitor resulted in a 26% reduction in clearance and a 35% increase in lithium levels.[7] Patients 50 years and older had a larger decrease in lithium clearance than those younger than 50 years.

[1] Douste-Blazy P, et al. *Lancet.* 1986;1(8485):1448.
[2] Navis GJ, et al. *Am J Med.* 1989;86(5):621.
[3] Baldwin CM, et al. *DICP.* 1990;24(10):946.
[4] Griffin JH, et al. *DICP.* 1991;25(1):101.
[5] Correa FJ, et al. *Am J Med.* 1992;93(1):108.
[6] DasGupta K, et al. *J Clin Psychiatry.* 1992;53(11):398.
[7] Finley PR, et al. *J Clin Psychopharmacol.* 1996;16(1):68.

* Asterisk indicates drugs cited in interaction reports. Based on pharmacologic and pharmacokinetic considerations, similar interactions may occur with other drugs that are listed.

Lithium — *Angiotensin II Receptor Antagonists*

Lithium	Angiotensin II Receptor Antagonists	
Lithium* (eg, *Lithobid*)	Candesartan* (*Atacand*)	Losartan* (eg, *Cozaar*)
	Eprosartan (*Teveten*)	Telmisartan (*Micardis*)
	Irbesartan (*Avapro*)	Valsartan* (*Diovan*)

Significance	Onset	Severity	Documentation
2	☐ Rapid	☐ Major	☐ Established
	■ **Delayed**	■ **Moderate**	☐ Probable
		☐ Minor	■ **Suspected**
			☐ Possible
			☐ Unlikely

Effects Plasma LITHIUM concentrations may be elevated, resulting in an increase in the pharmacologic and toxic effects of LITHIUM (eg, ataxia, confusion, delirium).

Mechanism ANGIOTENSIN II RECEPTOR ANTAGONISTS may decrease LITHIUM renal excretion by enhancing its reabsorption.

Management Monitor patients for possible LITHIUM toxicity and adjust the LITHIUM dose as needed.

Discussion

Lithium toxicity occurred in a 77-year-old woman following addition of losartan to her drug regimen.[1] Her plasma lithium level had been stable for many years, with a level of 0.63 mmol/L 1 to 2 months prior to starting losartan. Because of persistent high BP, losartan 50 mg/day was administered. Five weeks later, the patient was hospitalized with a 10 day history of lithium toxicity symptoms. Her plasma lithium level was 2 mmol/L. When lithium and losartan were discontinued, her symptoms disappeared. Two days after stopping both drugs, the plasma lithium level was 0.55 mmol/L. Lithium was reinstated with coadministration of nicardipine (eg, *Cardene*) 100 mg/day. Lithium toxicity did not recur. Elevated lithium plasma levels and toxicity were reported in a 51-year-old woman after valsartan was added to her treatment regimen.[2] She had been taking lithium 750 mg at bedtime for 6 years when valsartan 80 mg/day was started. Within 11 days of starting valsartan, her lithium plasma level increased 75% to 1.4 mmol/L and she exhibited symptoms of lithium toxicity. Valsartan was discontinued and diltiazem was started. Within 5 days, her lithium levels decreased and her symptoms resolved. Lithium toxicity (eg, agitation, ataxia, disorientation, increased confusion) and elevated lithium levels were reported in a 58-year-old woman stabilized on lithium therapy approximately 7 weeks after starting candesartan.[3] Both drugs were stopped, and the patient was treated. Lithium treatment was restarted without incidence.

[1] Blanche P, et al. *Eur J Clin Pharmacol.* 1997;52(6):501.
[2] Leung M, et al. *J Clin Psychopharmacol.* 2000;20(3):392.
[3] Zwanzger P, et al. *J Clin Psychiatry.* 2001;62(3):208.

* Asterisk indicates drugs cited in interaction reports. Based on pharmacologic and pharmacokinetic considerations, similar interactions may occur with other drugs that are listed.

Lithium — **Anorexiants**

Lithium* (eg, *Eskalith*)	Mazindol* (eg, *Sanorex*)

Significance	Onset	Severity	Documentation
5	□ Rapid ■ **Delayed**	□ Major ■ **Moderate** □ Minor	□ Established □ Probable □ Suspected □ Possible ■ **Unlikely**

Effects MAZINDOL may raise LITHIUM levels and caused LITHIUM-poisoning in one case.

Mechanism Unknown.

Management No clinical interventions appear necessary. Regular counseling about maintaining a constant dietary sodium intake is needed regardless of the method for weight reduction.

Discussion

In the only published case report, a patient developed lithium toxicity 3 days after beginning 2 mg/day mazindol for weight reduction. A lithium level of 3.2 mEq/L was measured 6 days later.[2] It is possible that alterations in diet could have changed daily sodium intake. During sodium depletion lithium toxicity can occur. Lithium toxicity has also been suspected in a patient on a weight reduction diet without appetite suppressant drugs.[1] Further clinical experience is needed to confirm an interaction between lithium and anorexiants.

[1] Furlong FW. *Can Psychiatr Assoc J.* 1973;18:75. [2] Hendy MS, et al. *BMJ.* 1980;280:684.

* Asterisk indicates drugs cited in interaction reports.

Lithium — *Benzodiazepines*

Lithium* (eg, *Eskalith*)	Diazepam* (eg, *Valium*)

Significance	Onset	Severity	Documentation
4	☐ Rapid	☐ Major	☐ Established
	■ **Delayed**	■ **Moderate**	☐ Probable
		☐ Minor	☐ Suspected
			■ **Possible**
			☐ Unlikely

Effects Hypothermia has been reported to occur during coadministration of LITHIUM and DIAZEPAM.

Mechanism Unknown.

Management No clinical interventions appear to be required.

Discussion

In a 38-year-old mentally retarded woman, diazepam 20 to 30 mg/day together with lithium carbonate induced several episodes of hypothermia.[1] During a controlled investigation of the same patient, three separate instances of severe hypothermia were documented with an onset between 4 hours to 17 days. Temperatures as low as 32° C produced coma. The mechanism is unknown, but hypothyroidism was excluded. This single case study suggests an interaction due to positive rechallenges and the fact that neither drug alone produced hypothermia.

In one case, long-term administration of alprazolam and lithium did not produce adverse effects.[2] In a study of ten volunteers, alprazolam 1 mg twice daily produced slightly increased steady-state lithium levels, which were not clinically significant.[3] Alprazolam pharmacokinetics were unchanged.

[1] Naylor GJ, et al. *BMJ.* 1977;2:22.
[2] Cerra D, et al. *Am J Psychiatry.* 1986;143:552.
[3] Evans RL, et al. *J Clin Psychopharmacol.* 1990:10:355.

* Asterisk indicates drugs cited in interaction reports.

Lithium | **Caffeine**

Lithium*
(eg, *Lithobid*)

Caffeine*
(eg, *NoDoz*)

Significance	Onset	Severity	Documentation
4	☐ Rapid	☐ Major	☐ Established
	■ **Delayed**	■ **Moderate**	☐ Probable
		☐ Minor	☐ Suspected
			■ **Possible**
			☐ Unlikely

Effects CAFFEINE may reduce serum LITHIUM concentrations.

Mechanism CAFFEINE may enhance renal elimination of LITHIUM.

Management Caution patients who ingest large amounts of CAFFEINE (at least 4 cups of coffee daily) to inform their health care providers before eliminating CAFFEINE. Monitoring of serum LITHIUM concentrations and adjustments in their LITHIUM dosage may be necessary.

Discussion

Two patients on stable lithium dosages for bipolar disorder developed mild to moderate lithium tremor and were advised to discontinue caffeine ingestion (coffee).[1] In both patients, the intensity of the tremor increased. In 1 patient receiving lithium 1,500 mg who stopped ingesting 17 cups of coffee per day, the serum lithium concentration increased almost 50%. A 20% reduction in the lithium dosage was required to decrease the lithium level and intensity of the tremor. The second patient, who was taking lithium 450 mg, also required a lithium dosage reduction, but serum lithium concentrations were not monitored. The effect of caffeine withdrawal on serum lithium concentrations was evaluated in 11 lithium-treated patients who consumed 4 to 8 cups of coffee daily.[2] Patients were maintained on lithium 600 to 1,200 mg/day. Lithium serum concentrations increased 24% when caffeine was eliminated from the patients' diets and returned to baseline when coffee was reinstated. However, increases in serum lithium levels occurred in only 8 of the 11 patients. Caffeine present in daily consumption of large quantities of a cola beverage has been reported to decrease lithium plasma concentrations.[3]

[1] Jefferson JW. *J Clin Psychiatry*. 1988;49(2):72.
[2] Mester R, et al. *Biol Psychiatry*. 1995;37(5):348.
[3] Kralovec K, et al. *J Clin Psychopharmacol*. 2011;31(4):543.

* Asterisk indicates drugs cited in interaction reports.

Lithium — *Calcitonin*

Lithium* (eg, *Lithobid*)	Calcitonin-Human (*Cibacalcin*)	Calcitonin-Salmon* (eg, *Fortical*)

Significance	Onset	Severity	Documentation
4	☐ Rapid ■ **Delayed**	☐ Major ■ **Moderate** ☐ Minor	☐ Established ☐ Probable ☐ Suspected ■ **Possible** ☐ Unlikely

Effects LITHIUM serum levels may be reduced, decreasing the therapeutic effect.

Mechanism Unknown. Decreased LITHIUM intestinal absorption or increased renal excretion is suspected.

Management Observe the clinical response of the patient and monitor LITHIUM serum concentrations. Adjust the LITHIUM dose as needed.

Discussion

The effects of calcitonin-salmon treatment on lithium pharmacokinetics were studied in 4 manic-depressive women stabilized on lithium 300 mg twice daily for at least 10 years.[1] Each patient was being followed for osteoporosis and received 100 units of calcitonin-salmon by subcutaneous injection for 3 consecutive days. Compared with baseline lithium serum levels, lithium concentrations were reduced in all patients during calcitonin administration. The average decrease in lithium serum concentrations after calcitonin injection was 30% of the baseline value. Minimum lithium serum levels fell below the lower limit of the therapeutic range (ie, 0.6 to 1.2 mmol/L) for at least 1 measurement in each patient. Urinary lithium clearance was assessed in 2 patients and was increased in both patients.

[1] Passiu G, et al. *Int J Clin Pharmacol Res*. 1998;18(4):179.

* Asterisk indicates drugs cited in interaction reports. Based on pharmacologic and pharmacokinetic considerations, similar interactions may occur with other drugs that are listed.

Lithium — *Carbamazepine*

Lithium* (eg, *Eskalith*)	Carbamazepine* (eg, *Tegretol*)

Significance	Onset	Severity	Documentation
2	□ Rapid	□ Major	□ Established
	■ **Delayed**	■ **Moderate**	□ Probable
		□ Minor	■ **Suspected**
			□ Possible
			□ Unlikely

Effects Some patients may develop adverse CNS effects, consisting of lethargy, muscular weakness, ataxia, tremor, and hyperreflexia, despite therapeutic levels of both drugs.

Mechanism Unknown.

Management Monitor patients for signs of neurotoxicity. If these develop, 1 of the 2 drugs may need to be discontinued.

Discussion

Following the initial description of the efficacy of carbamazepine in treating bipolar depression,[2] there have been several reports of the combined use of lithium and carbamazepine. Combination therapy is claimed to have a synergistic effect in controlling manic episodes as well as rapid-cycling bipolar affective disorder[11] and is generally well tolerated.[3,5,6,8,10] However, other information suggests that the combination may be associated with neurotoxicity. In a study of patients with lithium-induced diabetes insipidus, about 50% of patients experienced CNS side effects.[1] In a controlled investigation of a single patient, CNS toxicity developed 3 days after starting both lithium and carbamazepine.[4] The patient experienced ataxia, tremors, and muscle hyperreflexia despite therapeutic carbamazepine and lithium levels. Neither drug alone caused these effects, but neurotoxicity recurred with a rechallenge with the combination. In other reports, similar neurotoxic signs and symptoms have been observed between 3 and 14 days after initiating combined therapy.[7,9,13] In most cases, neurotoxicity resolved after stopping all medications; however, 1 case of irreversible tardive dystonia has been reported after 7 years of combined lithium and carbamazepine therapy.[12] It appears that some patients can tolerate the combined use of carbamazepine and lithium whereas others cannot. Because of the potential therapeutic benefit, combined therapy may be justified. Further experience is needed to characterize the patients who may be at risk for this potential interaction.

1 Ghose K. *Br Med J.* 1980;280:1122.
2 Ballenger JC, et al. *Am J Psychiatry.* 1980;137:782.
3 Lipinski JF, et al. *Am J Psychiatry.* 1982;139:948.
4 Chaudhry RP, et al. *J Clin Psychiatry.* 1983;44:30.
5 Keisling R. *Arch Gen Psychiatry.* 1983;40:223.
6 Moss GR, et al. *Arch Gen Psychiatry.* 1983;40:588.
7 Andrus PF, et al. *J Clin Psychiatry.* 1984;45:525.
8 Post RM, et al. *Arch Gen Psychiatry.* 1984;41:210.
9 Shukla S, et al. *Am J Psychiatry.* 1984;141:1604.
10 Klein EM. *Isr J Psychiatry Relat Sci.* 1987;24:295.
11 Laird LK, et al. *Pharmacotherapy.* 1987;7:130.
12 Lazarus A. *J Clin Psychopharmacol.* 1994;14:146.
13 Marcoux A. *Ann Pharmacother.* 1996;30:547.

* Asterisk indicates drugs cited in interaction reports.

Lithium	***Carbonic Anhydrase Inh.***
Lithium* (eg, *Eskalith*)	Acetazolamide* (eg, *Diamox*) Dichlorphenamide (*Daranide*) Methazolamide (eg, *Neptazane*)

Significance	Onset	Severity	Documentation
5	☐ Rapid ■ **Delayed**	☐ Major ☐ Moderate ■ **Minor**	☐ Established ☐ Probable ☐ Suspected ■ **Possible** ☐ Unlikely

Effects Possibly reduced serum LITHIUM levels resulting in a decrease in therapeutic response.

Mechanism Increased renal LITHIUM clearance is suspected.

Management No special precautions appear necessary.

Discussion

The administration of a single acetazolamide dose (500 to 750 mg) to 6 volunteers caused a 31% increase in the lithium excretion fraction. Urine sodium and potassium excretion also increased, indicating that a diuretic effect was attained with this acetazolamide dose.[1] Lithium levels could potentially decrease because of the increased renal clearance. It is not known if this effect would be sustained with repeated acetazolamide dosing, because the diuretic effect of acetazolamide may dissipate after a few doses. Nonetheless, acetazolamide has been used with apparent success in the management of lithium intoxication in combination with sodium bicarbonate and mannitol.[2] While the patient had minimal toxicity despite a high lithium level, it is not known if any of the drugs used were protective. However, the lithium level data indicated increased elimination. See also Lithium-Urinary Alkalinizers.

[1] Thomsen K, et al. *Am J Physiol.* 1968;215:823.

[2] Horowitz LC, et al. *N Engl J Med.* 1970;281:1369.

* Asterisk indicates drugs cited in interaction reports. Based on pharmacologic and pharmacokinetic considerations, similar interactions may occur with other drugs that are listed.

Lithium — *Clozapine*

Lithium*	Clozapine*
(eg, *Eskalith*)	(eg, *Clozaril*)

Significance	Onset	Severity	Documentation
4	☐ Rapid	☐ Major	☐ Established
	■ **Delayed**	■ **Moderate**	☐ Probable
		☐ Minor	☐ Suspected
			■ **Possible**
			☐ Unlikely

Effects Diabetic ketoacidosis may occur.

Mechanism Unknown.

Management Based on available data, no special precautions are warranted.

Discussion

Diabetic ketoacidosis has been reported in two patients receiving lithium after the addition of clozapine to their drug regimen.[1,2] Signs or symptoms of lithium toxicity were not reported in either patient. Diabetic ketoacidosis occurred within 6 weeks of starting clozapine, and insulin-dependent diabetes was still present 2 years after clozapine was discontinued in one patient. Neither patient had a history of hyperglycemia; however, one patient had a family history of diabetes.

Controlled studies are needed to determine if this is a drug-drug interaction or an idiosyncratic adverse reaction.

[1] Koval MS, et al. *Am J Psychiatry.* 1994;151:1520. [2] Peterson GA, et al. *Am J Psychiatry.* 1996;153:737.

* Asterisk indicates drugs cited in interaction reports.

Lithium — *Diltiazem*

Lithium* (eg, *Lithobid*)	Diltiazem* (eg, *Cardizem*)

Significance	Onset	Severity	Documentation
4	☐ Rapid ■ **Delayed**	☐ Major ■ **Moderate** ☐ Minor	☐ Established ☐ Probable ☐ Suspected ■ **Possible** ☐ Unlikely

Effects Neurotoxicity and psychotic symptoms have been reported.

Mechanism Unknown.

Management Monitor patients for signs of neurotoxicity during coadministration of these drugs.

Discussion

Two patients developed neurotoxic or psychotic symptoms during coadministration of diltiazem and lithium.[1,2] In both cases, symptoms resolved when both drugs were discontinued and did not recur when lithium was restarted. Although it was not possible to definitely attribute these symptoms to a drug interaction, the temporal association between the occurrence of the reactions and the coadministration of the drugs is suggestive of an interaction. The diagnosis of an interaction is confounded in one patient because the reaction could have been caused by thiothixene-induced extrapyramidal effects rather than an interaction between lithium and diltiazem.[3] In addition, the patient was receiving several other medications that may have interacted with lithium. With increasing age, neurotoxicity has been reported to occur more frequently, even in patients with serum lithium levels less than 0.42 mEq/L.[4]

Additional studies are needed to assess the clinical importance of this possible interaction. See also Lithium-Verapamil.

[1] Valdiserri EV. *J Clin Psychiatry.* 1985;46(12):540.
[2] Binder EF, et al. *Arch Intern Med.* 1991;151(2):373.
[3] Flicker MR, et al. *J Clin Psychiatry.* 1988;49(8):325.
[4] Price WA, et al. *J Clin Psychiatry.* 1987;48(3):124.

* Asterisk indicates drugs cited in interaction reports.

Lithium | **Fluvoxamine**

Lithium* (eg, *Lithobid*)	Fluvoxamine*

Significance	Onset	Severity	Documentation
4	□ Rapid ■ **Delayed**	□ Major ■ **Moderate** □ Minor	□ Established □ Probable □ Suspected ■ **Possible** □ Unlikely

Effects Coadministration of LITHIUM and FLUVOXAMINE may produce severe somnolence.

Mechanism Increased 5-hydroxytryptamine concentrations in the brain is suspected.

Management Caution patients of the possible sedative effect and observe closely during initial treatment. If this interaction occurs, it may be necessary to stop one of the drugs.

Discussion

Irresistible somnolence was reported in a 39-year-old woman with a history of bipolar affective swings during coadministration of slow-release lithium 400 mg daily and fluvoxamine.[1] All medication was stopped, and the next day she was fully conscious and became mildly elated. Lithium 800 mg at night was restarted 10 days later, and satisfactory serum concentrations were achieved. There were no reported adverse reactions with treatment with either drug alone.

Additional controlled investigations are needed to determine whether this is an idiosyncratic reaction or a drug interaction.

[1] Evans M, et al. *Br J Psychiatry*. 1990;156:286.

* Asterisk indicates drugs cited in interaction reports.

Lithium — *Hydantoins*

Lithium* (eg, *Eskalith*)	Phenytoin* (eg, *Dilantin*)

Significance	Onset	Severity	Documentation
5	□ Rapid	□ Major	□ Established
	■ **Delayed**	■ **Moderate**	□ Probable
		□ Minor	□ Suspected
			□ Possible
			■ **Unlikely**

Effects LITHIUM toxicity may occur despite therapeutic lithium levels.

Mechanism Unknown.

Management No clinical interventions appear required. If LITHIUM toxicity is suspected, consider decreasing the LITHIUM dose.

Discussion

At least three cases of a possible lithium-phenytoin interaction have occurred.[1-3] In one case, a 26-year-old man taking phenytoin and phenobarbital was treated with lithium carbonate 1200 mg/day. Lithium levels decreased from initially therapeutic values, requiring an increase in lithium dose to 2400 mg/day. With this increase, lithium toxicity developed despite levels in the therapeutic range. Lithium was discontinued, and 1 week later, the patient developed shaking and hypereflexia and became comatose.[1] Toxicity was most severe 7 days after stopping lithium. In the second report, a patient was being treated with phenytoin 300 mg/day. Lithium carbonate 1200 mg/day was added, achieving a level of 0.6 mEq/L. After 2 years the patient experienced lithium toxicity consisting of polyuria and tremor despite a normal lithium level. These effects disappeared after stopping phenytoin and starting carbamazepine (eg, *Tegretol*).[2] In the third case, a patient on phenytoin was begun on lithium carbonate 1200 mg/day. Three days later he had a level of 2 mEq/L and signs and symptoms consistent with lithium intoxication. Whether phenytoin contributed at all to the high level or toxicity in this patient is unknown.

Current data do not correlate lithium toxicity to phenytoin coadministration. Controlled investigations are needed to establish an interaction.

[1] Speirs J, et al. *Br Med J.* 1978;1:815.
[2] MacCallum WAG. *Br Med J.* 1980;280:610.
[3] Salem RB, et al. *Drug Intell Clin Pharm.* 1980;14:622.

* Asterisk indicates drugs cited in interaction reports.

Lithium | **Iodide Salts**

Lithium	Iodide Salts	
Lithium* (eg, *Eskalith*)	Calcium Iodide	Iodine
	Hydrogen Iodide (*Hydriodic Acid*)	Potassium Iodide* (eg, *SSKI*)
	Iodide	Sodium Iodide
	Iodinated Glycerol (eg, *Organidin*)	

Significance	Onset	Severity	Documentation
2	☐ Rapid	☐ Major	☐ Established
	■ **Delayed**	■ **Moderate**	☐ Probable
		☐ Minor	■ **Suspected**
			☐ Possible
			☐ Unlikely

Effects LITHIUM with IODIDES may act synergistically to more readily produce hypothyroidism.

Mechanism Unknown.

Management Generally avoid IODIDES in patients taking LITHIUM. If hypothyroidism or goiter develop, thyroid hormone will decrease symptoms and reverse goiter.

Discussion

Lithium causes changes in the function of the thyroid gland, resulting in goiter with or without hypothyroidism. Furthermore, it appears that these changes are caused by interference with normal iodine use in the thyroid gland. Of 330 patients in one series, 12 developed goiters between 5 and 24 months after beginning lithium therapy. Despite the goiters, these patients were euthyroid. Goiters were reduced in size by administration of dessicated thyroid.[1] In other cases, however, hypothyroidism has ensued.[2,3,8] In lithium-induced hypothyroidism, concomitantly administered iodides may contribute to the development of hypothyroidism.[4,5] Typically, hypothyroidism manifests as increased weight gain, lethargy, myxedema and laboratory test changes supporting the hypothyroid state.[3,6] In one case, heart failure was observed.[7] Hypothyroidism can be managed by the administration of thyroid hormones. Shopsin described two cases in whom the synergism between lithium and iodine was studied.[6] Both patients had developed hypothyroidism from lithium therapy. In one patient, lithium was stopped with resolution of symptoms and correction of abnormally low thyroxine levels over 12 weeks. The patient was then given 30 drops/day of saturated solution of potassium iodide (*SSKI*). After a few weeks, symptoms and laboratory evidence of hypothyroidism recurred. In the second case, addition of *SSKI* to lithium caused a further increase in serum TSH levels, a decrease in thyroxine and triiodothyronine to hypothyroid levels as well as clinical evidence of hypothyroidism. Confirmation of these observations was made in a clinical study using ten patients compared to five control subjects.[8]

1 Schou M, et al. *Br Med J.* 1968;3:710.
2 Shopsin B, et al. *Compr Psychiatry.* 1969;10:215.
3 Luby ED, et al. *JAMA.* 1971;218:1298.
4 Wiener JD. *JAMA.* 1972;220:587.
5 Jorgensen JV, et al. *JAMA.* 1973;223:192.
6 Shopsin B, et al. *Am J Med.* 1973;55:695.
7 Swedberg K, et al. *Acta Med Scand.* 1974;196:279.
8 Spaulding SW, et al. *Acta Endocrinol.* 1977;84:290.

* Asterisk indicates drugs cited in interaction reports. Based on pharmacologic and pharmacokinetic considerations, similar interactions may occur with other drugs that are listed.

Lithium	***Loop Diuretics***	
Lithium* (eg, *Eskalith*)	Bumetanide* (eg, *Bumex*)	Furosemide* (eg, *Lasix*)
	Ethacrynic Acid* (*Edecrin*)	Torsemide (eg, *Demadex*)

Significance	Onset	Severity	Documentation
2	☐ Rapid ■ **Delayed**	☐ Major ■ **Moderate** ☐ Minor	☐ Established ☐ Probable ■ **Suspected** ☐ Possible ☐ Unlikely

Effects Increased plasma LITHIUM concentrations with an increased risk of toxicity may occur.

Mechanism Unknown.

Management Observe the patient for LITHIUM toxicity; monitor plasma LITHIUM level and adjust LITHIUM doses as needed.

Discussion

In a single-dose study, the effects of furosemide 40 to 80 mg, ethacrynic acid 50 to 100 mg, and several nonloop diuretics were investigated. Neither furosemide nor ethacrynic acid affected the renal elimination of a single lithium carbonate 600 mg dose.[1] Lithium toxicity has been described following the administration of furosemide. However, the evaluation of these reports is confounded by other factors. In 1 case, the patient received furosemide plus sodium restriction, which led to dehydration and a lithium level of 3.05 mEq/L.[2] In another case, the lithium level was normal, but the patient developed lithium neurotoxicity that persisted even after the discontinuation of furosemide.[3] In the third case report, IV furosemide resulted in a deep coma over a few hours and a lithium level of 2.3 mEq/L.[4] The atypical nature of the toxicity in this patient (including deep coma, ileus, and muscular rigidity) plus his coexisting diseases do not clearly relate furosemide to the ensuing events. A patient's serum lithium level increased 45% to 100% with bumetanide therapy[5]; however, no toxicity resulted. In another case report, the lithium level during bumetanide administration rose from 0.7 to 2.3 mEq/L and was associated with symptoms of lithium toxicity.[6] Sodium restriction may have caused the patient to be sensitive to the changes. In the only study investigating the effect of long-term furosemide therapy on lithium levels, no difference was detected during combination therapy vs lithium alone.[7] In addition, lithium clearance appears to be reliably affected by IV furosemide.[8] However, a case-control study evaluating hospital admissions for lithium toxicity in patients older than 65 years of age found an association with coadministration of loop diuretics.[9] See also Lithium-Thiazide Diuretics.

[1] Thomsen K, et al. *Am J Physiol.* 1968;215:823.
[2] Hurtig HI, et al. *N Engl J Med.* 1974;290:748.
[3] Thornton WE, et al. *Can Psychiatr Assoc J.* 1975;20:281.
[4] Oh TE. *Anaesth Intens Care.* 1977;5:60.
[5] Kerry RJ, et al. *Br Med J.* 1980;281:371.
[6] Huang LG. *J Clin Psychopharmacol.* 1990;10:228.
[7] Jefferson JW, et al. *JAMA.* 1979;241:1134.
[8] Atherton JC, et al. *Clin Sci.* 1987;73:645.
[9] Juurlink DN, et al. *J Am Geriatr Soc.* 2004;52:794

* Asterisk indicates drugs cited in interaction reports. Based on pharmacologic and pharmacokinetic considerations, similar interactions may occur with other drugs that are listed.

Lithium | **Methyldopa**

Lithium*
(eg, *Eskalith*)

Methyldopa*
(eg, *Aldomet*)

Significance	Onset	Severity	Documentation
4	☐ Rapid ■ **Delayed**	☐ Major ■ **Moderate** ☐ Minor	☐ Established ☐ Probable ☐ Suspected ■ **Possible** ☐ Unlikely

Effects Symptoms of LITHIUM toxicity (eg, drowsiness, ataxia, diarrhea, blurred vision, weakness), with or without increased LITHIUM serum concentrations, have been reported with concurrent METHYLDOPA therapy.

Mechanism Unknown.

Management Monitor the patient for LITHIUM toxicity. If toxicity develops, temporarily discontinue LITHIUM until resolution. Consider an alternative antihypertensive medication.

Discussion

Numerous case reports describe a potential interaction between lithium and methyldopa. However, there are no controlled investigations. In a 45-year-old woman, methyldopa 1 g/day caused symptoms consistent with lithium toxicity despite a lithium serum level within the therapeutic range.[1] Another case similarly described lithium toxicity with a normal lithium level after lithium was given for 2 days to a patient taking methyldopa.[5] In two other reports, lithium toxicity developed after methyldopa therapy was begun and was associated with moderately increased lithium levels (1.5 and 1.87 mEq/L, respectively).[2,6] In an attempt to further elucidate this interaction, one investigator self-administered the combination and described symptoms of lithium toxicity with a lithium level of 0.8 mEq/L.[3] This was verified by another group of investigators who also self-administered the combination.[4]

Controlled studies are needed to further characterize this interaction and its mechanism.

1 Byrd GJ. *JAMA*. 1975;233:320.
2 O'Regan JB. *Can Med Assoc J*. 1976;115:385.
3 Byrd GJ. *Clin Toxicol*. 1977;11:1.
4 Walker N, et al. *DICP*. 1980;14:638.
5 Osanloo E, et al. *Ann Intern Med*. 1980;92:433.
6 Yassa R. *Can Med Assoc J*. 1986;134:141.

* Asterisk indicates drugs cited in interaction reports.

Lithium — *Metronidazole*

Lithium* (eg, *Lithobid*)	Metronidazole* (eg, *Flagyl*)

Significance	Onset	Severity	Documentation
4	☐ Rapid	☐ Major	☐ Established
	■ **Delayed**	■ **Moderate**	☐ Probable
		☐ Minor	☐ Suspected
			■ **Possible**
			☐ Unlikely

Effects Increased risk of LITHIUM toxicity.

Mechanism Unknown.

Management If an interaction is suspected, it may be necessary to decrease the dose of LITHIUM or discontinue one of the agents.

Discussion

Possible lithium nephrotoxicity was reported in 2 women during coadministration of metronidazole.[1] Both patients had been stabilized on lithium therapy when a 1-week course of metronidazole was prescribed for vaginitis. One patient developed increased serum creatinine levels and plasma lithium concentrations 12 to 17 days after starting metronidazole. One month later, both levels were still elevated and the patient complained of polyuria and nocturia. The dose of lithium was decreased from 1,500 to 900 mg/day, and there was a decrease in her serum lithium concentrations as well as in her symptoms of polyuria and nocturia; however, serum creatinine remained elevated at 2 mg/dL 5 months after metronidazole was discontinued. In the second patient, serum creatinine levels increased, as did her serum sodium, although there was no change in plasma lithium concentrations. After she became confused, lithium was discontinued and serum creatinine levels returned to normal, while the hypernatremia persisted.

[1] Teicher MH, et al. *JAMA*. 1987;257(24):3365.

* Asterisk indicates drugs cited in interaction reports.

Lithium | **NSAIDs**

Lithium*
(eg, *Lithobid*)

Celecoxib*
(*Celebrex*)
Diclofenac*
(eg, *Voltaren*)
Etodolac
Fenoprofen
(eg, *Nalfon*)
Flurbiprofen
Ibuprofen* (eg, *Motrin*)
Indomethacin*
(eg, *Indocin*)
Ketoprofen
Ketorolac* (eg, *Toradol*)
Meclofenamate
Meclofenamic Acid
(eg, *Ponstel*)
Meloxicam* (eg, *Mobic*)
Nabumetone
Naproxen* (eg, *Naprosyn*)
Oxaprozin
(eg, *Daypro*)
Piroxicam* (eg, *Feldene*)
Rofecoxib*†
Sulindac* (eg, *Clinoril*)
Tolmetin

Significance	Onset	Severity	Documentation
2	☐ Rapid	☐ Major	■ **Established**
	■ **Delayed**	■ **Moderate**	☐ Probable
		☐ Minor	☐ Suspected
			☐ Possible
			☐ Unlikely

Effects Increased pharmacologic and toxic effects of LITHIUM.

Mechanism NSAID interference with renal prostaglandin production may reduce renal elimination of LITHIUM.

Management When an NSAID is started or stopped, monitor LITHIUM levels every 4 to 5 days until stable and observe patients for clinical changes. Adjust LITHIUM dosage as needed.

Discussion

The addition of ibuprofen 1,200 to 1,800 mg/day,[1-4] indomethacin 150 mg/day,[5-9] naproxen 750 mg/day,[10] piroxicam 20 mg/day,[11-14] diclofenac 75 to 150 mg/day,[15,16] sulindac 300 mg/day,[17] meloxicam 15 mg/day,[18] rofecoxib,[19,20] celecoxib,[21] or ketorolac 30 mg/day[22,23] to stable lithium dosage regimens may reduce lithium clearance and elevate lithium levels. These effects develop over 5 to 10 days, resulting in 16% to 150% increases in lithium levels, and may produce lithium toxicity.[1,2,10-14,24] Lithium serum levels usually return to pretreatment values within 7 days of discontinuing the NSAID. Clinically important interactions between NSAIDs and lithium rarely occur.[4,23,25] In healthy men, naproxen sodium taken in the OTC dose (220 mg every 8 h) for 5 days did not increase serum lithium levels.[26] Sulindac had no effect on, or somewhat decreased, lithium levels.[10,27,28] Lithium AUC increased 21% when administered with meloxicam.[18]

1 Kristoff CA, et al. *Clin Pharm.* 1986;5(1):51.
2 Ragheb M. *J Clin Psychiatry.* 1987;48(4):161.
3 Bailey CE, et al. *South Med J.* 1989;82(9):1197.
4 Khan IH. *BMJ.* 1991;302(6791):1537.
5 Frölich JC, et al. *Br Med J.* 1979;1(6171):1115.
6 Ragheb M, et al. *J Clin Psychiatry.* 1980;41(11):397.
7 Reimann IW, et al. *Arch Gen Psychiatry.* 1983;40(3):283.
8 Herschberg SN, et al. *Am Fam Physician.* 1983;28(2):155.
9 Reimann IW, et al. *Eur J Clin Pharmacol.* 1985;29(4):435.
10 Ragheb M, et al. *J Clin Psychopharmacol.* 1986;6(3):150.
11 Kerry RJ, et al. *Lancet.* 1983;1(8321):418.
12 Walbridge DG, et al. *Br J Psychiatry.* 1985;147:206.
13 Nadarajah J, et al. *Ann Rheum Dis.* 1985;44(7):502.
14 Harrison TM, et al. *Br J Psychiatry.* 1986;149:124.
15 Reimann IW, et al. *Clin Pharmacol Ther.* 1981;30(3):348.
16 Monji A, et al. *Clin Neuropharmacol.* 2002;25(5):241.
17 Jones MT, et al. *J Clin Psychiatry.* 2000;61(7):527.
18 Türck D, et al. *Br J Clin Pharmacol.* 2000;50(3):197.
19 Sajbel TA, et al. *Pharmacotherapy.* 2001;21:380.
20 Lundmark J, et al. *Br J Clin Pharmacol.* 2002;53(4):403.
21 Slørdal L, et al. *Br J Clin Pharmacol.* 2003;55(4):413.
22 Langlois R, et al. *CMAJ.* 1994;150(9):1455.
23 Cold JA, et al. *J Clin Psychopharmacol.* 1998;18(1):33.
24 Ragheb M. *J Clin Psychopharmacol.* 1990;10(5):350.
25 Stein G, et al. *Psychol Med.* 1988;18(3):535.
26 Levin GM, et al. *J Clin Psychopharmacol.* 1998;18(3):237.
27 Furnell MM, et al. *Drug Intell Clin Pharm.* 1985;19(5):374.
28 Miller LG, et al. *J Fam Pract.* 1989;28(5):592.

* Asterisk indicates drugs cited in interaction reports. Based on pharmacologic and pharmacokinetic considerations, similar interactions may occur with other drugs that are listed.
† Not available in the United States.

Lithium — Serotonin Reuptake Inhibitors

Lithium	Serotonin Reuptake Inhibitors	
Lithium* (eg, *Lithobid*)	Citalopram (eg, *Celexa*)	Milnacipran (*Savella*)
	Escitalopram (*Lexapro*)	Paroxetine (eg, *Paxil*)
	Fluoxetine (eg, *Prozac*)	Sertraline (eg, *Zoloft*)
	Fluvoxamine (eg, *Luvox*)	Venlafaxine* (eg, *Effexor*)

Significance	Onset	Severity	Documentation
2	☐ Rapid	☐ Major	☐ Established
	■ **Delayed**	■ **Moderate**	☐ Probable
		☐ Minor	■ **Suspected**
			☐ Possible
			☐ Unlikely

Effects Elevated LITHIUM levels and neurotoxicity may occur. Serotonin syndrome (eg, agitation, altered consciousness, ataxia, myoclonus, overactive reflexes, shivering) may occur.

Mechanism Unknown.

Management Closely monitor patients. Serotonin syndrome requires immediate medical attention, including withdrawal of the serotonergic agent and supportive care. Administration of an antiserotonergic agent (eg, cyproheptadine) may be helpful.

Discussion

A 44-year-old woman on long-term lithium treatment developed stiffness in her legs and arms, dizziness, dysarthria, an ataxic gait, and an elevated lithium serum level (1.7 mEq/L) a few days after adding fluoxetine to her treatment regimen.[1] Approximately 1 week after discontinuing fluoxetine and reducing the lithium dose, neurologic symptoms disappeared and serum lithium levels fell to 0.9 mEq/L. Elevation in lithium levels without toxicity was reported in 2 patients.[2] In a study of 10 healthy volunteers, there was no effect on the single-dose pharmacokinetics of lithium by either a single dose of fluoxetine 60 mg or 7 days of pretreatment with fluoxetine 20 mg 3 times daily.[3] In another study, 110 patients receiving fluoxetine and lithium were compared with 110 cohort controls receiving fluoxetine alone for 7 weeks prior to starting lithium.[4] Although not statistically significant, there was an increased rate of minor adverse reactions during coadministration of fluoxetine and lithium. A 71-year-old woman developed confusion, moderate tremor, hyporeflexia, and myoclonus while receiving venlafaxine 150 mg and lithium 600 mg daily.[5] She was diagnosed with serotonin syndrome, and both drugs were stopped. All signs of serotonin syndrome subsided 3 days later. Venlafaxine was reintroduced and slowly titrated to 225 mg daily without recurrence of serotonin syndrome symptoms.

[1] Salama AA, et al. *Am J Psychiatry.* 1989;146(2):278.
[2] Hadley A, et al. *Am J Psychiatry.* 1989;146(12):1637.
[3] Breuel HP, et al. *Int J Clin Pharmacol Ther.* 1995;33(7):415.
[4] Bauer M, et al. *J Clin Psychopharmacol.* 1996;16(2):130.
[5] Adan-Manes J, et al. *J Clin Pharm Ther.* 2006;31(4):397.

* Asterisk indicates drugs cited in interaction reports. Based on pharmacologic and pharmacokinetic considerations, similar interactions may occur with other drugs that are listed.

Lithium — Tetracyclines

Lithium* (eg, *Lithobid*)	Doxycycline* (eg, *Vibramycin*)	Tetracycline* (eg, *Sumycin*)

Significance	Onset	Severity	Documentation
4	☐ Rapid ■ **Delayed**	☐ Major ■ **Moderate** ☐ Minor	☐ Established ☐ Probable ☐ Suspected ■ **Possible** ☐ Unlikely

Effects Increased LITHIUM plasma levels with lithium poisoning.

Mechanism Unknown.

Management No clinical interventions appear necessary. If an interaction is suspected, monitor LITHIUM plasma levels.

Discussion

In a single case report, a 30-year-old woman maintained on sustained-release lithium carbonate 1,600 mg was given tetracycline 250 mg 3 times daily after an initial 500 mg dose. Two days later, she presented with an elevated lithium plasma level and signs and symptoms consistent with lithium poisoning (drowsiness, slurred speech, thirst, tremor). Her lithium levels increased from a previously stable baseline level of 0.81 mmol/L to a maximum of 2.75 mmol/L. Upon discontinuation of tetracycline and lithium, her lithium plasma level decreased and lithium toxicity resolved.[1] The conclusions of this report have been questioned.[2] To study this potential interaction, a crossover controlled investigation was conducted using 13 volunteers.[3] A lithium dosage of 900 mg/day produced an average lithium level of 0.51 mmol/L. Tetracycline 1 g/day did not affect lithium levels nor did it cause any changes in lithium adverse reactions. A 68-year-old bipolar depressive man on a stable dosage of lithium 1,500 mg/day (level, 0.8 to 1.1 mEq/L) was given doxycycline 100 mg twice daily for bronchitis.[4] He experienced symptoms of lithium toxicity immediately after starting the antibiotic, and they increased further over the next week. A lithium level of 1.8 mEq/L was measured just before the antibiotic was stopped, and the lithium dosage was reduced to 1,200 mg/day. Over the next 3 days, symptoms resolved and lithium levels returned to the therapeutic range.

[1] McGennis AJ. *Br Med J.* 1978;1(6121):1183.
[2] Malt U. *Br Med J.* 1978;2(6135):502.
[3] Fankhauser MP, et al. *Clin Pharm.* 1988;7(4):314.
[4] Miller SC. *J Clin Psychopharmacol.* 1997;17(1):54.

* Asterisk indicates drugs cited in interaction reports.

Lithium | **Theophyllines**

Lithium	Theophyllines	
Lithium* (eg, *Eskalith*)	Aminophylline* (eg, *Somophyllin*)	Oxtriphylline (eg, *Choledyl*)
	Dyphylline (eg, *Lufyllin*)	Theophylline* (eg, *Bronkodyl*)

Significance	Onset	Severity	Documentation
4	☐ Rapid	☐ Major	☐ Established
	■ **Delayed**	■ **Moderate**	☐ Probable
		☐ Minor	☐ Suspected
			■ **Possible**
			☐ Unlikely

Effects THEOPHYLLINE administration reduces plasma LITHIUM levels. When measured 11 hours after the dose, lithium levels decreased by 21%.

Mechanism THEOPHYLLINE enhances the renal elimination of LITHIUM.

Management It is difficult to predict if the relatively small decrease in LITHIUM levels would cause clinical deterioration of the patient's manic-depressive condition. If deterioration is suspected, measure lithium levels and tailor doses as needed.

Discussion

In a study using 6 healthy volunteers, the administration of oral aminophylline in a single 1 g dose caused a 58% increase in the lithium excretion fraction (lithium clearance/creatinine clearance).[1] Aminophylline exerted a diuretic effect since the renal excretion of sodium and potassium also significantly increased. In a more detailed pharmacokinetic investigation, lithium carbonate was administered on a daily basis to 10 healthy subjects. After one week, theophylline was given in doses titrated to a therapeutic level over 1 week. At the end of the theophylline period, a lithium pharmacokinetic analysis was performed. During theophylline administration, lithium levels were significantly lower than in the control period. For example, at 11 hours lithium levels were an average of 21% lower (decreased from 0.78 to 0.62 mmol/L). The lithium half-life was similarly affected; however, the volume of distribution did not change. There was some evidence that the magnitude of the change was related to the serum theophylline level.[3,4] While it appears that some reduction in lithium levels may occur, no instance of loss of therapeutic control due to the interaction has been published. In fact, in one report, safe use of this combination was possible with careful lithium dose titration.[2]

[1] Thomsen K, et al. *Am J Physiol.* 1968;215:823.
[2] Sierles FS, et al. *Am J Psychiatry.* 1982;139:117.
[3] Perry PJ, et al. *Acta Psychiatr Scand.* 1984;69:528.
[4] Cook BL, et al. *J Clin Psychiatry.* 1985;46:278.

* Asterisk indicates drugs cited in interaction reports. Based on pharmacologic and pharmacokinetic considerations, similar interactions may occur with other drugs that are listed.

Lithium	**Thiazide Diuretics**	
Lithium* (eg, *Eskalith*)	Bendroflumethiazide* (*Naturetin*)	Indapamide (*Lozol*)
	Benzthiazide (eg, *Aquatag*)	Methyclothiazide* (eg, *Enduron*)
	Chlorothiazide* (eg, *Diuril*)	Metolazone (eg, *Zaroxolyn*)
	Chlorthalidone* (eg, *Hygroton*)	Polythiazide (*Renese*)
	Hydrochlorothiazide* (eg, *HydroDiuril*)	Quinethazone (*Hydromox*)
	Hydroflumethiazide* (eg, *Saluron*)	Trichlormethiazide (eg, *Naqua*)

Significance	Onset	Severity	Documentation
2	☐ Rapid ■ **Delayed**	☐ Major ■ **Moderate** ☐ Minor	■ **Established** ☐ Probable ☐ Suspected ☐ Possible ☐ Unlikely

Effects THIAZIDE DIURETICS increase serum lithium levels. LITHIUM toxicity has occurred.

Mechanism Decreased renal LITHIUM clearance.

Management Monitor plasma lithium levels and observe the patient for symptoms of toxicity. Adjust the dose accordingly.

Discussion

Long-term use of thiazides can decrease lithium clearance and has resulted in toxicity.[1-15] A patient stabilized on lithium 300 mg twice daily developed ataxia, tremor and muscle twitching after taking an unspecified amount of chlorthalidone. Her lithium level was 3.7 mEq/L.[10] In another case, lithium toxicity (3.9 mEq/L) resembled mania and was treated by hemodialysis.[13] It appears that the reduction in lithium clearance is dependent upon the thiazide dose.[6] Despite the interaction between lithium and thiazides, they have been used together for therapeutic reasons.[2,4,5,9,12] Of 13 patients treated with thiazides and lithium, seven developed some degree of lithium toxicity. However, lithium levels were also stabilized with improved manic-depressive control and a reduction in nephrogenic diabetes insipidus.[5] Lithium and thiazides can be administered safely, provided close lithium level monitoring is instituted.[7] See also Lithium-Loop Diuretics.

1 Thomsen K, et al. *Am J Physiol.* 1968;215:823.
2 Levy ST, et al. *Am J Psychiatry.* 1973;130:1014.
3 Petersen V, et al. *Br Med J.* 1974;3:143.
4 MacNeil S, et al. *Lancet.* 1975;1:1295.
5 Himmelhoch JM, et al. *Am J Psychiatry.* 1977;134:149.
6 Himmelhoch JM, et al. *Clin Pharmacol Ther.* 1977;22:225.
7 Solomon K. *South Med J.* 1978;71:1098.
8 Jefferson JW, et al. *JAMA.* 1979;241:1134.
9 Maletzky BM. *J Clin Psychiatry.* 1979;40:317.
10 Solomon JG. *Psychosomatics.* 1980;21:425.
11 Mehta BR, et al. *Postgrad Med J.* 1980;56:783.
12 Constandis DD, et al. *Am J Surg.* 1981;141:741.
13 Nurnberger JI. *J Nerv Ment Dis.* 1985;173:316.
14 Dorevitch A, et al. *Am J Psychiatry.* 1986;143:257.
15 Hanna ME, et al. *J Clin Psychopharmacol.* 1990;10:379.

* Asterisk indicates drugs cited in interaction reports. Based on pharmacologic and pharmacokinetic considerations, similar interactions may occur with other drugs that are listed.

Lithium — *Topiramate*

Lithium* (eg, *Eskalith*)	Topiramate* (*Topamax*)

Significance	Onset	Severity	Documentation
4	☐ Rapid ■ **Delayed**	☐ Major ■ **Moderate** ☐ Minor	☐ Established ☐ Probable ☐ Suspected ■ **Possible** ☐ Unlikely

Effects LITHIUM serum concentrations may be elevated, increasing the risk of toxicity.

Mechanism Competition for renal excretion between LITHIUM and TOPIRAMATE is suspected.

Management In patients receiving LITHIUM, closely monitor LITHIUM serum levels when starting, stopping, or changing the TOPIRAMATE dose. Observe the patient for LITHIUM toxicity when starting or changing the TOPIRAMATE dose. Adjust the LITHIUM dose as needed.

Discussion

At least 2 cases of elevated lithium serum concentrations and symptoms of toxicity have been reported during coadministration of topiramate and lithium.[1,2] One patient, a 26-year-old woman with type I bipolar disorder, was well maintained on lithium 900 to 1,200 mg/day.[1] She experienced increased lithium serum levels (from 0.82 to 1.24 mmol/L) and symptoms of toxicity after topiramate 75 mg/day was added to her treatment regimen. Her serum lithium levels increased to 1.97 mmol/L despite decreasing the lithium dose to 750 mg/day. Lithium was discontinued, and levels returned to the therapeutic range within 4 days. During this time, the patient experienced symptoms of lithium toxicity (ie, worsening concentration, confusion, lethargy), which disappeared when lithium serum levels returned to the therapeutic range. Lithium was restarted and therapeutic concentrations (0.67 mmol/L) were achieved at 450 mg/day. The second patient, a 42-year-old woman with type II bipolar disorder, was on a stable regimen of lithium 1,500 mg and topiramate 500 mg daily. Lithium levels increased (from 0.5 to 1.4 mEq/L) and she experienced neurotoxicity when the dose of topiramate was increased from 500 to 800 mg/day.[2] Upon stopping lithium and continuing topiramate, symptoms disappeared over the next 4 days. Two months later, lithium was restarted and, while receiving lithium 1,200 mg/day and topiramate 500 mg/day, the lithium trough serum level was 0.5 mEq/L.

[1] Abraham G, et al. *J Clin Psychopharmacol.* 2004;24:565.

[2] Pinninti NR, et al. *J Clin Psychopharmacol.* 2002;22:340.

* Asterisk indicates drugs cited in interaction reports.

Lithium | **Urea**

Lithium*
(eg, *Eskalith*)

Urea*
(*Ureaphil*)

Significance	Onset	Severity	Documentation
4	□ Rapid ■ **Delayed**	□ Major ■ **Moderate** □ Minor	□ Established □ Probable □ Suspected ■ **Possible** □ Unlikely

Effects The therapeutic effectiveness of LITHIUM may be reduced by UREA.

Mechanism UREA may enhance the renal elimination of LITHIUM.

Management No special precautions appear necessary.

Discussion

In a single study using six healthy volunteers, lithium excretion was increased by urea. The volunteers received between 60 and 83 g of urea over 5 hours. Their urinary lithium clearance was measured over 7 hours. The fractional clearance of lithium, defined as the lithium clearance over the creatinine clearance, was increased around 36% by urea.[1] It is unknown whether patients receiving lithium would actually experience a sustained change in their lithium levels from urea administration. Furthermore, it is unlikely that patients would receive such high urea doses for prolonged periods of time. As a reference point, maximum recommended urea doses in controlling increased intracranial or intraocular pressure are 120 g/24 hours.

[1] Thomsen K, et al. *Am J Physiol.* 1968;215:823.

* Asterisk indicates drugs cited in interaction reports.

Lithium — *Urinary Alkalinizers*

Lithium	Urinary Alkalinizers	
Lithium* (eg, *Eskalith*)	Potassium Citrate (eg, *Urocit-K*)	Sodium Citrate
	Sodium Acetate	Sodium Lactate
	Sodium Bicarbonate*	Tromethamine (eg, *Tham*)

Significance	Onset	Severity	Documentation
2	☐ Rapid	☐ Major	☐ Established
	■ **Delayed**	■ **Moderate**	☐ Probable
		☐ Minor	■ **Suspected**
			☐ Possible
			☐ Unlikely

Effects Alkalinization of the urine reduces LITHIUM plasma levels and could possibly decrease LITHIUM's effectiveness.

Mechanism Enhanced renal lithium clearance.

Management Avoid the administration of regular or large doses of URINARY ALKALINIZERS to patients receiving LITHIUM. Sodium bicarbonate is a component of some *otc* antacids. Patients should read labels carefully.

Discussion

In a study using six healthy volunteers, Thomsen et al, administered sodium bicarbonate in a dose of approximately 5 g hourly for 5 hours (total of 245 mEq) which caused a 27% increase in the lithium excretion fraction (lithium/creatinine clearance).[1] The urinary pH was alkalinized to a pH between 7 and 8. It was postulated that the increase in lithium elimination occurs due to the need to eliminate cations as excess base is removed from the body in the urine. In agreement with these observations, two brief reports described patients who had low lithium plasma levels during consumption of over-the-counter products containing sodium bicarbonate.[2,4] While in no case was a lack of therapeutic efficacy reported, it is possible that reduction in lithium levels via this interaction could result in resurgence of manic symptoms.

In a single case report, urinary alkalinization was used therapeutically in the management of lithium poisoning. During forced alkaline diuresis (achieved with IV sodium bicarbonate or other bases), lithium levels dropped from 4 to 0.7 mEq/L over 48 hours.[3] It was suggested that forced alkiline diuresis may be an alternative to hemodialysis in treating lithium intoxication.

[1] Thomsen K, et al. *Am J Physiol.* 1968;215:823.
[2] Arthur RK. *Med J Aust.* 1975;2:918.
[3] Forrest JAH. *Postgrad Med J.* 1975;51:189.
[4] McSwiggan C. *Med J Aust.* 1978;1:38.

* Asterisk indicates drugs cited in interaction reports. Based on pharmacologic and pharmacokinetic considerations, similar interactions may occur with other drugs that are listed.

Lithium | **Verapamil**

Lithium* (eg, *Eskalith*)	Verapamil* (eg, *Calan*)

Significance	Onset	Severity	Documentation
4	☐ Rapid	☐ Major	☐ Established
	■ **Delayed**	■ **Moderate**	☐ Probable
		☐ Minor	☐ Suspected
			■ **Possible**
			☐ Unlikely

Effects Both a reduction in lithium levels causing decreased antimanic control and lithium toxicity have been reported.

Mechanism Unknown.

Management Use this combination cautiously. Closely monitor the patient for signs of neurotoxicity. Lithium plasma levels may not be predictive of such toxicity.

Discussion

In one case report, verapamil 160 mg/day was added as an antimanic agent to the drug regimen of a 32-year-old woman without adverse effects. This patient improved and was able to discontinue lithium therapy.[1] In two other cases, the addition of verapamil 320 mg/day for cardiovascular indications resulted in a decrease in lithium levels.[2] In one patient, manic symptoms recurred and were controlled with an increase in lithium dose. In the second patient, the lithium excretion fraction (lithium clearance/creatinine clearance) had increased from 0.14 to 0.2. However, two other reports describe lithium toxicity that developed after approximately 1 week of verapamil administration despite lithium levels within the therapeutic range.[3,4] In one of these cases the reaction was confirmed upon rechallenge.[3] Choreoathetosis developed in a 66-year-old patient 4 days after adding verapamil 360 mg daily to a stable lithium regimen.[7] The involuntary movements disappeared 4 days after discontinuing verapamil. Two cases of bradycardia have been associated with the use of this combination.[6] In a long-term crossover comparison of lithium with verapamil, patients showed additive effects during the brief period when lithium levels were still present and verapamil was started.[5]

[1] Gitlin MJ, et al. *J Clin Psychopharmacol.* 1984;4:341.
[2] Weinrauch LA, et al. *Am Heart J.* 1984;108:1378.
[3] Price WA, et al. *J Clin Pharmacol.* 1986;26:717.
[4] Price WA, et al. *J Am Geriatr Soc.* 1987;35:177.
[5] Giannini AJ, et al. *J Clin Pharmacol.* 1987;27:980.
[6] Dubovsky SL, et al. *J Clin Psychiatry.* 1987;48:371.
[7] Helmuth D, et al. *J Clin Psychopharmacol.* 1989;9:454.

* Asterisk indicates drugs cited in interaction reports.

Loop Diuretics | **ACE Inhibitors**

Loop Diuretics		ACE Inhibitors	
Bumetanide* (*Bumex*)	Furosemide* (eg, *Lasix*)	Benazepril (*Lotensin*)	Lisinopril (eg, *Zestril*)
Ethacrynic Acid (*Edecrin*)	Torsemide (*Demadex*)	Captopril* (*Capoten*)	Quinapril (*Accupril*)
		Enalapril (*Vasotec*)	Ramipril (*Altace*)
		Fosinopril (*Monopril*)	

Significance	Onset	Severity	Documentation
3	☐ Rapid ■ **Delayed**	☐ Major ☐ Moderate ■ **Minor**	☐ Established ☐ Probable ■ **Suspected** ☐ Possible ☐ Unlikely

Effects The effects of LOOP DIURETICS may be decreased.

Mechanism Possibly inhibition of angiotensin II production by the ACE INHIBITOR.

Management Fluid status and body weight of the patient should be carefully monitored in patients receiving a LOOP DIURETIC when treatment with an ACE INHIBITOR is started.

Discussion

In a double-blind investigation, the effects of captopril on the diuretic and sodium excreting actions of furosemide were studied in 25 male patients with stable chronic heart failure.[1] Three weeks prior to admission, each patient was placed on a stabilized sodium diet (approximately 120 mmol/day). Patients were randomized, in a double-blind design, into two groups. Group 1 received placebo at 9 am, 2 pm and 10 pm on day 1 and at 9 am on day 2, while group 2 received a first dose of placebo and matching captopril tablets for the remaining three doses. At 1 pm on both days, each patient received his usual dose of oral furosemide. In the placebo group, furosemide produced a 214% increase in urine flow on the first day and a 280% increase on day 2. In the captopril group, pre-treatment with captopril attenuated the effect of furosemide. The increase in urinary flow was 225% on day 1 (furosemide plus placebo) and 128% on day 2 (furosemide plus captopril). In the placebo group, furosemide produced an 870% increase in sodium excretion on day 1 and 1172% increase on day 2. In the captopril group, captopril did not alter baseline sodium excretion but attenuated the effect of furosemide on sodium excretion. The increase in sodium excretion was 623% on day 1 (furosemide plus placebo) and 242% on day 2 (furosemide plus captopril). While placebo administration did not alter baseline creatinine clearance, pretreatment with captopril abolished the increase in creatinine clearance obtained with furosemide. Captopril also blunted the increase in urinary albumin excretion after furosemide.

[1] McLay JS, et al. *Am Heart J.* 1993;126:879.

* Asterisk indicates drugs cited in interaction reports. Based on pharmacologic and pharmacokinetic considerations, similar interactions may occur with other drugs that are listed.

Loop Diuretics | **Acetaminophen**

Bumetanide (*Bumex*)	Furosemide* (eg, *Lasix*)	Acetaminophen* (eg, *Tylenol*)
Ethacrynic Acid (*Edecrin*)	Torsemide (*Demadex*)	

Significance	Onset	Severity	Documentation
5	□ Rapid	□ Major	□ Established
	■ **Delayed**	□ Moderate	□ Probable
		■ **Minor**	□ Suspected
			□ Possible
			■ **Unlikely**

Effects The effects of the LOOP DIURETIC may be decreased.

Mechanism ACETAMINOPHEN may decrease renal prostaglandin excretion and decrease plasma renin activity.

Management Based on currently available clinical data, no special precautions are needed.

Discussion

The effects of acetaminophen on the pharmacological actions of furosemide were studied in 10 healthy female volunteers.[1] Following 2 days of administration of placebo or acetaminophen (1 g 4 times daily), a single 20 mg IV dose of furosemide was given. After furosemide administration, the rate of prostaglandin E_2 excretion increased from 18.5 to 46.6 ng/hr, in the first 30 minutes. However, with acetaminophen pretreatment, the increase in prostaglandin E_2 excretion was blunted, increasing from 7.6 to 23.2 ng/hr. The decrease in prostaglandin E_2 excretion was due to a lower baseline excretion of prostaglandin E_2. A similar effect was seen with 6-keto prostaglandin $F_{1\alpha}$. After pre-treatment with acetaminophen, the mean basal excretion rate of 6-keto prostaglandin $F_{1\alpha}$ was less with acetaminophen than with placebo (38.7 vs 61.7 ng/hr). In the 6 hours after furosemide administration, the mean excretion rate of 6-keto prostaglandin $F_{1\alpha}$ was significantly lower ($P < 0.05$) with acetaminophen pre-treatment than with placebo (183 vs 306 ng/hr). Furosemide-induced increase in plasma renin activity was also significantly ($P < 0.01$) reduced by acetaminophen (4.3 vs 2.7 ng/mL•hr). However, acetaminophen pre-treatment had little effect on the diuretic or sodium excretion action of furosemide.

[1] Martin U, et al. *Br J Clin Pharmacol.* 1994;37:464.

* Asterisk indicates drugs cited in interaction reports. Based on pharmacologic and pharmacokinetic considerations, similar interactions may occur with other drugs that are listed.

Loop Diuretics — *Barbiturates*

Loop Diuretics	Barbiturates	
Furosemide* (eg, *Lasix*)	Phenobarbital*	Primidone (eg, *Mysoline*)

Significance	Onset	Severity	Documentation
5	□ Rapid	□ Major	□ Established
	■ **Delayed**	□ Moderate	□ Probable
		■ **Minor**	□ Suspected
			□ Possible
			■ **Unlikely**

Effects Controversial. See discussion.

Mechanism Unknown.

Management No clinical interventions appear required.

Discussion

In a study of epileptic patients receiving both phenytoin (eg, *Dilantin*) and phenobarbital, there was a delay and a reduction in the diuretic effect to a single oral furosemide test dose. Additionally, the effect to an intravenous furosemide dose was similarly reduced by about 50% as judged from a reduction in the amount of urine output during the study.[1] However, it was not possible to tell whether these effects were those of phenytoin, phenobarbital, or the combination. In a subsequent study using 5 normal volunteers, 15 days of phenobarbital 100 mg at bedtime did not affect the area under the plasma concentration curve or the metabolic clearance of furosemide. Urine output was not influenced by phenobarbital. Only a small and insignificant decrease in total furosemide body clearance occurred which, if anything, is in the opposite direction of that expected from the previous study.[2] Lastly, no case reports of a clinical adverse effect from this interaction were located in the medical literature.

In summary, it is unlikely that an interaction between phenobarbital and furosemide is either clinically significant or real.

[1] Ahmad S. *BMJ.* 1974;3:657.

[2] Lambert C, et al. *Clin Pharmacol Ther.* 1983;34:170.

* Asterisk indicates drugs cited in interaction reports. Based on pharmacologic and pharmacokinetic considerations, similar interactions may occur with other drugs that are listed.

Loop Diuretics | *Cholestyramine*

Furosemide* (eg, *Lasix*)	Cholestyramine* (eg, *Questran*)

Significance	Onset	Severity	Documentation
2	■ **Rapid**	□ Major	□ Established
	□ Delayed	■ **Moderate**	□ Probable
		□ Minor	■ **Suspected**
			□ Possible
			□ Unlikely

Effects Absorption of FUROSEMIDE is decreased by CHOLESTYRAMINE. A decrease in pharmacologic effects may be expected.

Mechanism CHOLESTYRAMINE (an anion exchange resin) binds FUROSEMIDE.

Management Separate CHOLESTYRAMINE and FUROSEMIDE administration by as much time as possible (at least 2 hours).

Discussion

In a controlled study involving 6 healthy adults, cholestyramine 8 g was administered 5 minutes after furosemide 40 mg.[1] When cholestyramine was ingested after furosemide, there was a 95% decrease in the total urinary excretion of furosemide and a 94% decrease in the furosemide AUC compared with taking furosemide alone. This resulted in a decreased diuretic effect. Sodium excretion was not measured.

Additional studies are needed to clarify the clinical importance of this interaction.

[1] Neuvonen PJ, et al. *Br J Clin Pharmacol.* 1988;25:229.

* Asterisk indicates drugs cited in interaction reports.

Loop Diuretics — *Cisplatin*

Loop Diuretics		Cisplatin
Bumetanide* (eg, *Bumex*)	Furosemide* (eg, *Lasix*)	Cisplatin*
Ethacrynic Acid* (*Edecrin*)	Torsemide (eg, *Demadex*)	

Significance	Onset	Severity	Documentation
2	■ **Rapid**	□ Major	□ Established
	□ Delayed	■ **Moderate**	□ Probable
		□ Minor	■ **Suspected**
			□ Possible
			□ Unlikely

Effects Additive ototoxicity.

Mechanism Unknown.

Management Avoid this combination if possible. If it becomes necessary to use LOOP DIURETICS in CISPLATIN-treated patients, perform hearing tests to detect early hearing loss. Such hearing loss would be the dose-limiting toxicity of the diuretic.

Discussion

The additive ototoxic effects of loop diuretics and cisplatin are suggested by their independent ototoxicity. Human experimentation on this subject would be unethical; therefore, animal models have been studied. In 62 guinea pigs, cisplatin 7 mg/kg or ethacrynic acid 50 mg/kg produced reversible ototoxicity as measured using cochlear microphonics and the Preyer reflex threshold. In contrast, the combination of the 2 drugs caused permanent damage to hearing function.[1] Similar observations were also made using guinea pigs treated with combinations of cisplatin and bumetanide, furosemide, ethacrynic acid, or piretanide. An anatomical defect consisting of loss of cochlear hair cells was documented in support of these observations.[2] From these animal experiments it may be concluded that the combination of cisplatin and a loop diuretic has the potential to cause significant ototoxicity far beyond that expected from either agent alone. Therefore, cautious use of the combination is advisable despite the fact that no human case reports document this interaction.

[1] Komune S, et al. *Arch Otolaryngol.* 1981;107:594.

[2] Brummett RE. *Scand Audiol Suppl.* 1981;14 suppl:215.

* Asterisk indicates drugs cited in interaction reports. Based on pharmacologic and pharmacokinetic considerations, similar interactions may occur with other drugs that are listed.

Loop Diuretics — *Clofibrate*

Furosemide* (eg, *Lasix*)	Clofibrate* (eg, *Atromid-S*)

Significance	Onset	Severity	Documentation
5	☐ Rapid	☐ Major	☐ Established
	■ **Delayed**	■ **Moderate**	☐ Probable
		☐ Minor	☐ Suspected
			☐ Possible
			■ **Unlikely**

Effects Exaggerated diuretic response to LOOP DIURETICS.

Mechanism An increase in the free (active) fraction of LOOP DIURETICS as a result of their displacement from protein binding sites by CLOFIBRATE has been proposed but not established.

Management Observe for exaggerated diuresis from a LOOP DIURETIC during concurrent clofibrate use. If an excessive diuretic response occurs, consider lowering the dose of one or both drugs, or discontinue CLOFIBRATE.

Discussion

Muscle pain and cramping, often associated with elevated serum transaminase and creatine phosphokinase (CPK) concentrations, were recorded after initiation of clofibrate therapy in five of six patients maintained on furosemide for nephrotic syndrome.[2] In three of these patients, an increased response to furosemide was observed as evidenced by excessive diuresis, polydipsia and weight loss. Symptoms resolved with lower doses or discontinuation of clofibrate. The excessive diuresis was attributed to displacement of furosemide from its protein binding sites and the muscle pain and cramping to consequent fluid and electrolyte depletion. However, this reversible muscle pain syndrome was also reported in a series of five patients treated with clofibrate for hyperlipoproteinemia in whom there was no mention of furosemide use or of excessive diuresis.[1]

[1] Langer T, et al. *N Engl J Med.* 1968;279:856. [2] Bridgman JF, et al. *Lancet.* 1972;2:506.

* Asterisk indicates drugs cited in interaction reports.

Loop Diuretics | *Colestipol*

Furosemide* (eg, *Laxix*)	Colestipol* (*Colestid*)

Significance	Onset	Severity	Documentation
2	■ **Rapid** ☐ Delayed	☐ Major ■ **Moderate** ☐ Minor	☐ Established ☐ Probable ■ **Suspected** ☐ Possible ☐ Unlikely

Effects Absorption of FUROSEMIDE is decreased by COLESTIPOL. A decrease in pharmacologic effects may be expected.

Mechanism COLESTIPOL (an anion exchange resin) binds FUROSEMIDE.

Management COLESTIPOL should be taken as long as possible (at least 2 hours) after FUROSEMIDE.

Discussion

In a controlled study involving six healthy adults, 10 g of colestipol was administered 5 minutes after 40 mg of furosemide.[1] When colestipol was ingested after furosemide, there was an 80% decrease in the total urinary excretion of furosemide and a 79% decrease in the area under the furosemide plasma concentration-time curve compared with taking furosemide alone. This resulted in a decreased diuretic effect. Sodium excretion was not measured.

Additional studies are needed to clarify the clinical importance of this interaction.

[1] Neuvonen PJ, et al. *Br J Clin Pharmacol.* 1988;25:229.

* Asterisk indicates drugs cited in interaction reports.

Loop Diuretics — *Ginseng*

Bumetanide (eg, *Bumex*)	Furosemide* (eg, *Lasix*)	Ginseng*
Ethacrynic Acid (eg, *Edecrin*)	Torsemide (*Demadex*)	

Significance	Onset	Severity	Documentation
4	☐ Rapid	☐ Major	☐ Established
	■ **Delayed**	■ **Moderate**	☐ Probable
		☐ Minor	☐ Suspected
			■ **Possible**
			☐ Unlikely

Effects The diuretic effect of the LOOP DIURETIC may be reduced.

Mechanism Nephrotoxicity involving the loop of Henle has been proposed.

Management Caution patients receiving a LOOP DIURETIC to consult their health care provider before using nonprescription or herbal products. If GINSENG cannot be avoided, the patient's response to LOOP DIURETIC treatment should be carefully assessed when GINSENG is started or stopped. Adjust the dose as needed.

Discussion

A 63-year-old man with membranous glomerulonephritis, receiving furosemide and cyclosporine (eg, *Neoral*), was hospitalized for edema and hypertension approximately 10 days after he started taking daily nutritional products, which included 10 to 12 tablets daily of ginseng (containing germanium; *Uncle Hsu's Korean ginseng*).[1] While in the hospital, the patient did not receive any nutritional products and responded to IV furosemide 240 mg every 8 hours. He was discharged on 80 mg twice daily of furosemide. Following discharge, the patient again started taking nutritional supplements. Over the next 2 weeks, in spite of an increase in the dose of furosemide to 240 mg twice daily, his weight increased 27 lbs and he developed worsening edema and hypertension. Upon readmission to the hospital, the nutritional supplements were withheld, and IV furosemide 240 mg every 8 hours was restarted. Over the next 48 hours, the patient responded to the diuretic, and his weight and blood pressure decreased. Although a causal relationship was not established between ginseng ingestion and refractoriness to furosemide, the temporal association suggests that ginseng may have induced resistance to the diuretic.

The ingredients of many herbal products are not standardized. It is unclear if herbal products contain ingredients other than those listed on the label or purported to be present that could interact with diuretic therapy.

[1] Becker BN, et al. *JAMA*. 1996;276:606.

* Asterisk indicates drugs cited in interaction reports. Based on pharmacologic and pharmacokinetic considerations, similar interactions may occur with other drugs that are listed.

Loop Diuretics — *Hydantoins*

Loop Diuretics	Hydantoins
Furosemide* (eg, *Lasix*)	Phenytoin* (eg, *Dilantin*)

Significance	Onset	Severity	Documentation
3	☐ Rapid	☐ Major	☐ Established
	■ **Delayed**	☐ Moderate	☐ Probable
		■ **Minor**	■ **Suspected**
			☐ Possible
			☐ Unlikely

Effects PHENYTOIN may reduce the diuretic effects of FUROSEMIDE.

Mechanism Reduced oral absorption of FUROSEMIDE. Additional mechanisms may exist.

Management Increased FUROSEMIDE doses may be needed in patients receiving PHENYTOIN. Monitor diuretic response.

Discussion

In one study, 17 patients were receiving phenytoin with phenobarbital and, in a few cases, other anticonvulsants.[1] When compared to a group of healthy individuals, the diuretic response to oral or IV furosemide was reduced as measured by urinary output. The reduction in the diuretic response was 68%, 51% and 50% for 20 mg oral, 40 mg oral or 20 mg IV doses, respectively. In addition, the diuretic response to oral furosemide was delayed in those patients receiving anticonvulsants.[1] While the study clearly documented an effect, it was not possible to tell which anticonvulsant was causing it. Furthermore, since the patients received furosemide test doses, it is unknown if the therapeutic effect would be modified in actual patients requiring furosemide.

In another report, five volunteers were studied before and after 1 week of phenytoin 300 mg daily. Phenytoin reduced the absorption of a 20 mg furosemide dose; the absolute bioavailability was 81% before and 39% after phenytoin. In parallel with these absorption changes, the maximal furosemide concentration was reduced from 2.24 to 1.22 mcg/mL. Since there was no change in the clearance of furosemide, the reduction in serum concentration was attributable to decreased absorption alone.[2] However, this would not explain the reduction in diuretic response after an IV furosemide dose, as observed in the previous study. Clearly the mechanism and clinical significance of this interaction requires further study.

[1] Ahmad S. *BMJ.* 1974;3:657.

[2] Fine A, et al. *BMJ.* 1977;2:1061.

* Asterisk indicates drugs cited in interaction reports.

Loop Diuretics — *NSAIDs*

Loop Diuretics		NSAIDs	
Bumetanide* (eg, *Bumex*)	Furosemide* (eg, *Lasix*)	Ibuprofen* (eg, *Motrin*)	Sulindac* (eg, *Clinoril*)
Ethacrynic Acid (*Edecrin*)	Torsemide (*Demadex*)	Indomethacin* (eg, *Indocin*)	

Significance	Onset	Severity	Documentation
3	■ **Rapid**	□ Major	□ Established
	□ Delayed	□ Moderate	■ **Probable**
		■ **Minor**	□ Suspected
			□ Possible
			□ Unlikely

Effects Effects of the LOOP DIURETICS may be decreased.

Mechanism Possible inhibitions of prostaglandins responsible for maintaining renal hemodynamics.[3,6,21]

Management May need a higher dose of the LOOP DIURETIC. Consider other anti-inflammatory agents if diuresis is inadequate.

Discussion

Indomethacin can increase BP and decrease sodium excretion in healthy and hypertensive patients.[2,3,6] In hypertensive patients receiving unspecified diuretics, ibuprofen was associated with increased BP when compared with placebo.[17] In combination with furosemide or bumetanide, indomethacin has been associated with decreased sodium excretion and urine volume.[1,4,5,7-15] Sulindac has been reported to affect bumetanide similarly.[18] In healthy volunteers pretreated with ibuprofen 600 mg twice/day there was no interference with furosemide.[16] However, ibuprofen inhibited furosemide diuresis in volunteers on sodium-restricted diets.[20] Salt depletion exaggerating indomethacin inhibition of furosemide diuresis has also been reported.[19] Changes in the pharmacokinetics of furosemide were not responsible for the observed effects.[4,7] Case reports describe worsening heart failure, fluid overload, and diuretic refractoriness to furosemide and bumetanide.[12-14] A case report noted marked improvement in diuresis when indomethacin was changed to flurbiprofen (eg, *Ansaid*).[12] Deterioration of CHF following ibuprofen 1200 mg/day occurred in a previously well-controlled patient. Response to furosemide was blunted until ibuprofen was discontinued.[13] However, a randomized, double-blind, crossover study of 19 patients showed that meloxicam (*Mobic*) did not alter the pharmacokinetics or pharmacodynamics of furosemide.[21]

1 Patak RV, et al. *Prostaglandins*. 1975;10:649.
2 Donker AJ, et al. *Nephron*. 1976;17:288.
3 Frolich JC, et al. *Circ Res*. 1976;39:447.
4 Smith DE, et al. *J Pharmacokinet Biopharm*. 1979;7:265.
5 Brater DC. *J Pharmacol Exp Ther*. 1979;210:386.
6 Brater DC. *Clin Pharmacol Ther*. 1979;25:322.
7 Chennavasin P, et al. *J Pharmacol Exp Ther*. 1980;215:77.
8 Brater DC, et al. *Clin Pharmacol Ther*. 1980;27:421.
9 Pedrinelli R, et al. *Clin Pharmacol Ther*. 1980;28:722.
10 Brater C, et al. *J Clin Pharmacol*. 1981;21:647.
11 Kaufman J, et al. *J Clin Pharmacol*. 1981;21:663.
12 Allan SG, et al. *BMJ*. 1981;283:1611.
13 Laiwah AC, et al. *BMJ*. 1981;283:714.
14 Poe TE, et al. *J Fam Pract*. 1983;16:610.
15 Ahmad S. *Am J Cardiol*. 1984;54:246.
16 Riley LJ Jr, et al. *Nephron*. 1985;41:283.
17 Radack KL, et al. *Ann Intern Med*. 1987;107:628.
18 Skinner MH, et al. *Clin Pharmacol Ther*. 1987;42:542.
19 Herchuelz A, et al. *J Pharmacol Exp Ther*. 1989;248:1175.
20 Passmore AP, et al. *Br J Clin Pharmacol*. 1990;29:311.
21 Müller FO, et al. *Br J Clin Pharmacol*. 1997;44:393.

* Asterisk indicates drugs cited in interaction reports. Based on pharmacologic and pharmacokinetic considerations, similar interactions may occur with other drugs that are listed.

Loop Diuretics — *Orlistat*

Loop Diuretics	Orlistat
Furosemide* (eg, *Lasix*)	Orlistat* (*Xenical*)

Significance	Onset	Severity	Documentation
5	☐ Rapid ■ **Delayed**	☐ Major ☐ Moderate ■ **Minor**	☐ Established ☐ Probable ☐ Suspected ■ **Possible** ☐ Unlikely

Effects The $t_{½}$ of FUROSEMIDE may be prolonged, effecting diuresis.

Mechanism Unknown.

Management Based on available data, no special precautions are necessary with short-term therapy. However, until more information is available, it may be prudent to monitor the patient for electrolyte abnormalities if therapy is long-term.

Discussion

In an open-label, crossover investigation, the effects of orlistat on the pharmacokinetics of furosemide were studied in 6 healthy men.[1] Each subject received 50 mg of orlistat 3 times/day mid-meal for 8 days. Furosemide (40 mg) was administered in single doses twice, once before and once at the end of orlistat treatment. Compared with giving furosemide alone, administration after orlistat pretreatment prolonged the $t_{½}$ of furosemide 21% (from 1.4 to 1.7 hr).

[1] Weber C, et al. *Eur J Clin Pharmacol.* 1996;51:87.

* Asterisk indicates drugs cited in interaction reports.

Loop Diuretics — *Probenecid*

Loop Diuretics		Probenecid
Bumetanide* (eg, *Bumex*)	Furosemide* (eg, *Lasix*)	Probenecid*
Ethacrynic Acid* (*Edecrin*)	Torsemide (eg, *Demadex*)	

Significance	Onset	Severity	Documentation
5	■ **Rapid** □ Delayed	□ Major □ Moderate ■ **Minor**	□ Established □ Probable □ Suspected □ Possible ■ **Unlikely**

Effects The actions of LOOP DIURETICS may be reduced.

Mechanism PROBENECID may decrease distribution of LOOP DIURETICS to sites of action within the renal tubular lumen.

Management No clinical interventions appear required.

Discussion

Although probenecid appears to decrease the clearance of furosemide, the net effects on diuresis are not altered. Increased plasma concentrations result in an increased net diuresis over longer time intervals.[1-4] Diuretic response is related more closely to urinary excretion than to plasma concentrations.[5] The effects of probenecid on bumetanide are unclear. Two reports suggest decreased early responses[6,7]; yet others were unable to detect any influences on sodium or water excretion.[8-10]

Ethacrynic acid clearance was inhibited by probenecid in animals.[11] No human studies are available.

1 Honari J, et al. *Clin Pharmacol Ther.* 1977;22:395.
2 Homeida M, et al. *Clin Pharmacol Ther.* 1977;22:402.
3 Brater DC. *Clin Pharmacol Ther.* 1978;24:548.
4 Chennavasin P, et al. *Kidney Int.* 1979;16:187.
5 Odlind B, et al. *Clin Pharmacol Ther.* 1980;27:784.
6 Lant AF. *Postgrad Med J.* 1975;51(suppl 6):35.
7 Velasquez MT, et al. *J Clin Pharmacol.* 1981;21:657.
8 Brater DC, et al. *Clin Pharmacol Ther.* 1980;27:246.
9 Brater DC, et al. *J Clin Pharmacol.* 1981;21:311.
10 Brater DC, et al. *J Clin Pharmacol.* 1981;21:647.
11 Beyer KH, et al. *J Pharmacol Exp Ther.* 1965;147:1.

* Asterisk indicates drugs cited in interaction reports. Based on pharmacologic and pharmacokinetic considerations, similar interactions may occur with other drugs that are listed.

Loop Diuretics — *Salicylates*

Loop Diuretics		Salicylates	
Bumetanide (eg, *Bumex*)	Furosemide* (eg, *Lasix*)	Aspirin* (eg, *Bayer*)	Salsalate (eg, *Amigesic*)
Ethacrynic Acid (*Edecrin*)	Torsemide (eg, *Demadex*)	Bismuth Subsalicylate (eg, *Pepto-Bismol*)	Sodium Salicylate
		Choline Salicylate	Sodium Thiosalicylate
		Magnesium Salicylate (eg, *Doan's*)	

Significance	Onset	Severity	Documentation
5	☐ Rapid	☐ Major	☐ Established
	■ **Delayed**	☐ Moderate	☐ Probable
		■ **Minor**	☐ Suspected
			■ **Possible**
			☐ Unlikely

Effects The diuretic response to LOOP DIURETICS may be impaired in patients with cirrhosis and ascites.

Mechanism Unknown.

Management No clinical interventions are generally required. For patients with cirrhosis and ascites requiring LOOP DIURETICS, use SALICYLATES with caution.

Discussion

In 6 patients with cirrhosis and ascites, preadministration of IV lysine acetylsalicylate decreased urine volume and sodium excretion following furosemide 40 mg IV. The patients served as their own control.[1] Other studies in healthy volunteers have failed to demonstrate antagonism of furosemide-induced diuresis with low or high doses of aspirin[2-4] or with the fluorinated salicylate derivative diflunisal (eg, *Dolobid*).[5]

Further study is needed in patients with CHF, renal dysfunction, and cirrhosis to evaluate the importance of salicylate derivatives on the response to loop diuretics.

[1] Planas R, et al. *Gastroenterology*. 1983;84:247.
[2] Berg KJ. *Eur J Clin Pharmacol*. 1977;11:117.
[3] Bartoli E, et al. *J Clin Pharmacol*. 1980;20:452.
[4] Wilson TW, et al. *J Clin Pharmacol*. 1986;26:100.
[5] Tobert JA, et al. *Clin Pharmacol Ther*. 1980;27:289.

* Asterisk indicates drugs cited in interaction reports. Based on pharmacologic and pharmacokinetic considerations, similar interactions may occur with other drugs that are listed.

Loop Diuretics — *Thiazide Diuretics*

Loop Diuretics		Thiazide Diuretics	
Bumetanide*	Torsemide* (eg, *Demadex*)	Bendroflumethiazide*†	Indapamide
Ethacrynic Acid (*Edecrin*)		Chlorothiazide (eg, *Diuril*)	Methyclothiazide (eg, *Enduron*)
Furosemide* (eg, *Lasix*)		Chlorthalidone (eg, *Hygroton*)	Metolazone* (eg, *Zaroxolyn*)
		Hydrochlorothiazide* (eg, *HydroDIURIL*)	

Significance	Onset	Severity	Documentation
2	■ **Rapid**	□ Major	□ Established
	□ Delayed	■ **Moderate**	■ **Probable**
		□ Minor	□ Suspected
			□ Possible
			□ Unlikely

Effects Both groups have synergistic effects that may result in profound diuresis and serious electrolyte abnormalities.

Mechanism The two classes of agents exhibit their diuretic action at different sites in the renal tubules.

Management Carefully titrate with small or intermittent doses. Monitor patients for dehydration and electrolyte abnormalities during combined therapy.

Discussion

Coadministration of a loop diuretic and a thiazide diuretic leads to greater sodium, potassium, and chloride excretion and diuresis than with either agent alone. This response has been observed in bumetanide-treated patients with CHF who received bendroflumethiazide,[1] patients with refractory edema on maximal furosemide doses who received metolazone,[2] and patients with azotemia unresponsive to large doses of furosemide who also received hydrochlorothiazide.[3] When loop and thiazide diuretics have been administered for therapeutic benefit,[2,3] some patients have experienced rapid diuresis with deterioration in renal function and severe hypokalemia requiring massive potassium supplementation. A patient receiving concurrent metolazone and furosemide experienced a decrease in serum potassium from 3.7 to 2.9 mEq/L, even with the administration of potassium supplements 200 mEq/day.[3] The addition of hydrochlorothiazide to high-dose furosemide (greater than 250 mg/day) was effective in patients with severe CHF, even in those with renal function impairment.[4] However, it was necessary to aggressively manage hypokalemia. Sodium excretion was increased by coadministration of hydrochlorothiazide and torsemide, compared with giving either diuretic alone.[5] In this single-dose study, torsemide had a potassium- and magnesium-sparing effect.

One study failed to demonstrate an interaction between metolazone and furosemide in healthy volunteers,[6] while a second study did not find an interaction between hydrochlorothiazide and furosemide in patients with nephrotic syndrome.[7]

1 Sigurd B, et al. *Am Heart J.* 1975;89(2):163.
2 Epstein M, et al. *Curr Ther Res Clin Exp.* 1977;21:656.
3 Wollam GL, et al. *Am J Med.* 1982;72(6):929.
4 Dormans TP, et al. *Eur Heart J.* 1996;17(12):1867.
5 Knauf H, et al. *Eur J Clin Pharmacol.* 2009;65(5):465.
6 Marone C, et al. *Eur J Clin Invest.* 1985;15(5):253.
7 Nakahama H, et al. *Nephron.* 1988;49(3):223.

* Asterisk indicates drugs cited in interaction reports. Based on pharmacologic and pharmacokinetic considerations, similar interactions may occur with other drugs that are listed.
† Not available in the United States.

Loperamide — *Azole Antifungal Agents*

Loperamide	Azole Antifungal Agents	
Loperamide* (eg, *Imodium A-D*)	Itraconazole* (eg, *Sporanox*)	Voriconazole (*Vfend*)
	Ketoconazole (eg, *Nizoral*)	

Significance	Onset	Severity	Documentation
4	☐ Rapid	☐ Major	☐ Established
	■ **Delayed**	■ **Moderate**	☐ Probable
		☐ Minor	☐ Suspected
			■ **Possible**
			☐ Unlikely

Effects LOPERAMIDE plasma concentrations may be elevated, increasing the risk of adverse reactions.

Mechanism Inhibition of LOPERAMIDE metabolism (CYP3A4), as well as inhibition of gut wall P-glycoprotein.

Management In patients receiving LOPERAMIDE, monitor for an increase in CNS opioid effects (eg, respiratory depression) if an AZOLE ANTIFUNGAL AGENT and/or gemfibrozil (eg, *Lopid*) are coadministered.

Discussion

The effects of itraconazole, gemfibrozil, and their combination on loperamide were studied in 12 healthy volunteers.[1] Using a randomized, crossover, 4–phase design, each subject received itraconazole 100 mg (first dose 200 mg), gemfibrozil 600 mg, both itraconazole and gemfibrozil, or placebo, 2 times/day for 5 days. On day 3, subjects took a single dose of loperamide 4 mg. Compared with placebo, itraconazole increased the loperamide C_{max} 2.9-fold, the AUC 3.8-fold, and prolonged the $t_{½}$ from 11.9 to 18.7 hours. The combination of itraconazole and gemfibrozil increased the loperamide C_{max} 4.2-fold, the AUC 12.6-fold, and prolonged the $t_{½}$ from 11.9 to 36.9 hours. The plasma AUC ratio of the metabolite N-desmethylloperamide to loperamide was reduced 65% and 88% by itraconazole and itraconazole combined with gemfibrozil, respectively. No differences occurred in the Digit Symbol Substitution Test or subjective drowsiness between phases.

[1] Niemi M, et al. *Eur J Clin Pharmacol.* 2006;62(6):463.

* Asterisk indicates drugs cited in interaction reports. Based on pharmacologic and pharmacokinetic considerations, similar interactions may occur with other drugs that are listed.

Loperamide — *Cholestyramine*

Loperamide* (eg, *Imodium A-D*)	Cholestyramine* (eg, *Questran*)

Significance	Onset	Severity	Documentation
5	☐ Rapid ■ **Delayed**	☐ Major ☐ Moderate ■ **Minor**	☐ Established ☐ Probable ☐ Suspected ☐ Possible ■ **Unlikely**

Effects The actions of LOPERAMIDE may be reduced.

Mechanism Unknown.

Management No clinical interventions appear required.

Discussion

One group of clinicians reported a situation of extreme intestinal fluid loss in a 55-year-old man following colon resection and an ileostomy. Treatment with cholestyramine 2 g every 4 hours and loperamide 2 mg every 6 hours was initiated. Cholestyramine was then discontinued, and loperamide was continued alone. Intestinal fluid losses were less with loperamide alone than with the combination. In vitro evidence suggests that cholestyramine can bind loperamide and may decrease its absorption.[1]

Further evaluation is needed before an interaction can be confirmed.

[1] Ti TY, et al. *Can Med Assoc J.* 1978;119:607.

* Asterisk indicates drugs cited in interaction reports.

Loperamide ✕ **Fibric Acids**

Loperamide* (eg, *Imodium A-D*)	Gemfibrozil* (eg, *Lopid*)

Significance	Onset	Severity	Documentation
4	☐ Rapid	☐ Major	☐ Established
	■ **Delayed**	■ **Moderate**	☐ Probable
		☐ Minor	☐ Suspected
			■ **Possible**
			☐ Unlikely

Effects LOPERAMIDE plasma concentrations may be elevated, increasing the risk of adverse reactions.

Mechanism Inhibition of LOPERAMIDE metabolism (CYP2C8) as well as inhibition of gut wall P-glycoprotein.

Management In patients receiving LOPERAMIDE, monitor for an increase in CNS opioid effects (eg, respiratory depression) if GEMFIBROZIL and/or itraconazole (eg, *Sporanox*) are coadministered.

Discussion

The effects of gemfibrozil, itraconazole, and their combination on loperamide were studied in 12 healthy volunteers.[1] Using a randomized, crossover, 4-phase design, each subject received gemfibrozil 600 mg, itraconazole 100 mg (first dose 200 mg), both gemfibrozil and itraconazole, or placebo, 2 times/day for 5 days. On day 3, subjects took a single dose of loperamide 4 mg. Compared with placebo, gemfibrozil increased the loperamide C_{max} 1.6-fold, the AUC 2.2-fold, and prolonged the $t_{1/2}$ from 11.9 to 16.7 hours. The combination of gemfibrozil and itraconazole increased the loperamide C_{max} 4.2-fold, the AUC 12.6-fold, and prolonged the $t_{1/2}$ from 11.9 to 36.9 hours. The plasma AUC ratio of the metabolite N-desmethylloperamide to loperamide was reduced 46% and 88% by gemfibrozil and gemfibrozil combined with itraconazole, respectively. No differences occurred in the Digit Symbol Substitution Test or subjective drowsiness between phases.

[1] Niemi M, et al. *Eur J Clin Pharmacol.* 2006;62:463.

* Asterisk indicates drugs cited in interaction reports.

Loperamide — *Quinidine*

Loperamide (eg, *Imodium*)	Quinidine*

Significance	Onset	Severity	Documentation
4	■ **Rapid**	□ Major	□ Established
	□ Delayed	■ **Moderate**	□ Probable
		□ Minor	□ Suspected
			■ **Possible**
			□ Unlikely

Effects LOPERAMIDE plasma concentrations and the risk of respiratory depression may be increased.

Mechanism Inhibition of P-glycoprotein transport may increase LOPERAMIDE penetration into the CNS and also increase LOPERAMIDE absorption from the GI tract.

Management In patients receiving LOPERAMIDE, monitor for an increase in CNS opioid effects (eg, respiratory depression) if QUINIDINE is coadministered.

Discussion

The effect of quinidine on loperamide CNS penetration was studied in 8 healthy men.[1] Each subject received loperamide 16 mg with quinidine 600 mg or placebo. When given with placebo, loperamide produced no respiratory depression; however, when administered with quinidine, respiratory depression occurred. In addition, quinidine administration increased the loperamide AUC 2.5-fold. Impaired ventilatory response to CO_2 occurred after quinidine administration but not placebo, indicating that the respiratory depression was independent of changes in loperamide plasma concentration.

[1] Sadeque AJ, et al. *Clin Pharmacol Ther.* 2000;68:231.

* Asterisk indicates drugs cited in interaction reports.

Loperamide | **Ritonavir**

Loperamide*
(eg, *Imodium*)

Ritonavir*
(*Norvir*)

Significance	Onset	Severity	Documentation
3	☐ Rapid	☐ Major	☐ Established
	■ **Delayed**	☐ Moderate	☐ Probable
		■ **Minor**	■ **Suspected**
			☐ Possible
			☐ Unlikely

Effects LOPERAMIDE plasma concentrations may be increased.

Mechanism RITONAVIR may inhibit LOPERAMIDE metabolism (CYP3A4).

Management Based on available data, no special precautions appear to be needed. In patients receiving RITONAVIR, it may be possible to reduce the dose of LOPERAMIDE without reducing the efficacy.

Discussion

The effects of ritonavir on the pharmacokinetics and pharmacodynamics of loperamide were studied in 12 healthy volunteers.[1] In a randomized, double-blind, crossover study, each subject received a single dose of loperamide 16 mg with ritonavir 600 mg or placebo. Compared with placebo, coadministration of loperamide with ritonavir increased the C_{max} of loperamide 17%, increased the time to reach the peak level 56%, increased the AUC 223%, decreased the oral clearance 70%, and increased the amount of loperamide excreted in the urine 181%. Ritonavir administration delayed the formation of the major metabolite of loperamide, desmethylloperamide. Ritonavir did not affect the pharmacodynamics of loperamide as measured by pupil diameter, pain threshold, pain tolerance, and transcutaneous Po_2 and Pco_2. Lack of penetration through the blood-brain barrier appears to have prevented untoward effects from the increased loperamide plasma levels.

[1] Tayrouz Y, et al. *Clin Pharmacol Ther*. 2001;70:405.

* Asterisk indicates drugs cited in interaction reports.

Lopinavir/Ritonavir | **Echinacea**

Lopinavir/Ritonavir* (*Kaletra*)	Echinacea*

Significance	Onset	Severity	Documentation
5	☐ Rapid	☐ Major	☐ Established
	■ **Delayed**	☐ Moderate	☐ Probable
		■ **Minor**	☐ Suspected
			■ **Possible**
			☐ Unlikely

Effects Preliminary data indicate there is no interaction between ECHINACEA and LOPINAVIR/RITONAVIR.

Mechanism Although ECHINACEA induces CYP3A activity, it is possible that the pharmacokinetics of LOPINAVIR may not be altered because of the presence of RITONAVIR, a potent CYP3A inhibitor.

Management Based on available data, no special precautions are necessary when ECHINACEA is used by patients treated with the LOPINAVIR/RITONAVIR combination.

Discussion

In a study involving 13 healthy volunteers, each subject received lopinavir 400 mg/ritonavir 100 mg twice daily for 29.5 days.[1] Starting on day 16, subjects received *Echinacea purpurea* 500 mg 3 times daily for 28 days, 14 days in combination with lopinavir/ritonavir and 14 days with echinacea alone. Neither lopinavir nor ritonavir pharmacokinetics were affected by concurrent use of echinacea. Although echinacea induced CYP3A activity, it is possible that echinacea does not alter lopinavir pharmacokinetics because of the presence of ritonavir, a potent CYP3A inhibitor.

[1] Penzak SR, et al. *Pharmacotherapy*. 2010;30(8):797.

* Asterisk indicates drugs cited in interaction reports.

Loratadine — *Azole Antifungal Agents*

Loratadine	Azole Antifungal Agents	
Loratadine* (eg, *Claritin*)	Fluconazole (eg, *Diflucan*)	Posaconazole (*Noxafil*)
	Itraconazole (eg, *Sporanox*)	Voriconazole (eg, *Vfend*)
	Ketoconazole* (eg, *Nizoral*)	

Significance	Onset	Severity	Documentation
4	☐ Rapid	☐ Major	☐ Established
	■ **Delayed**	■ **Moderate**	☐ Probable
		☐ Minor	☐ Suspected
			■ **Possible**
			☐ Unlikely

Effects LORATADINE plasma concentrations may be elevated, increasing the risk of adverse reactions.

Mechanism AZOLE ANTIFUNGAL AGENTS inhibit the metabolism (CYP3A4) of LORATADINE.

Management Observe patients receiving LORATADINE for an increase in adverse reactions during coadministration of an AZOLE ANTIFUNGAL AGENT.

Discussion

In a randomized study, the effects of ketoconazole on the pharmacokinetics and pharmacodynamics of loratadine were investigated in 62 healthy men.[1] Each subject received loratadine 10 mg daily or placebo alone, followed by 8 days of either ketoconazole 450 mg daily plus loratadine or ketoconazole 400 mg daily plus placebo. Compared with giving loratadine alone, coadministration of ketoconazole increased the AUC of loratadine and its active metabolite, desloratadine, 4.5- and 1.9-fold, respectively. Ketoconazole increased the mean QTc interval; however, coadministration of ketoconazole and loratadine resulted in a nonsignificant mean increase in the QTc compared with ketoconazole plus placebo.

[1] Chaikin P, et al. *Br J Clin Pharmacol.* 2005;59(3):346.

* Asterisk indicates drugs cited in interaction reports. Based on pharmacologic and pharmacokinetic considerations, similar interactions may occur with other drugs that are listed.

Loratadine — *Nefazodone*

Loratadine*
(eg, *Claritin*)

Nefazodone*

Significance	Onset	Severity	Documentation
4	□ Rapid ■ **Delayed**	■ **Major** □ Moderate □ Minor	□ Established □ Probable □ Suspected ■ **Possible** □ Unlikely

Effects LORATADINE plasma levels may be elevated, producing a modest prolongation in the QTc interval.

Mechanism Unknown.

Management Until more data are available, consider use of alternative therapy. Cetirizine (*Zyrtec*) and fexofenadine (*Allegra*) do not appear to affect the QTc interval and may be safer alternatives to LORATADINE.

Discussion

The effect of coadministration of nefazodone and loratadine on electrocardiographic QTc prolongation was studied in healthy men and women.[1] Using a randomized, double-blind, parallel group design, subjects received loratadine 20 mg/day plus placebo, loratadine 20 mg/day plus nefazodone 300 mg every 12 hours, or placebo plus nefazodone 300 mg every 12 hours. Compared with placebo, administration of nefazodone with loratadine increased the dose interval AUC of loratadine and its metabolite 39% and 12%, respectively. The mean QTc interval was unchanged by administration of either loratadine or nefazodone alone. However, coadministration of loratadine and nefazodone prolonged the QTc interval. The prolongation was positively correlated with the loratadine plasma concentration. Several points have been made regarding the data presented and question the use of these data to determine the importance of the QTc changes.[2] In addition, it is not known if the clinically recommended dose of loratadine 10 mg/day would have the same effect.

[1] Abernethy DR, et al. *Clin Pharmacol Ther.* 2001;69:96.

[2] Barbey JT. *Clin Pharmacol Ther.* 2002;71:403.

* Asterisk indicates drugs cited in interaction reports.

Losartan | **Azole Antifungal Agents**

Losartan* (*Cozaar*)	Fluconazole* (eg, *Diflucan*)

Significance	Onset	Severity	Documentation
3	☐ Rapid	☐ Major	☐ Established
	■ **Delayed**	☐ Moderate	☐ Probable
		■ **Minor**	■ **Suspected**
			☐ Possible
			☐ Unlikely

Effects The antihypertensive and adverse effects of LOSARTAN may be increased.

Mechanism Possibly inhibition of metabolism (CYP2C9) of LOSARTAN by FLUCONAZOLE.

Management Closely monitor blood pressure response to LOSARTAN when FLUCONAZOLE is started, stopped, or changed in dosage.

Discussion

The effects of administration of fluconazole at steady state on the steady-state pharmacokinetics of eprosartan (*Teveten*), losartan, and the active metabolite of losartan (E 3174) were evaluated in 32 healthy men.[1] Each subject was randomly assigned to receive oral eprosartan 300 mg every 12 hours or oral losartan 100 mg/day for 20 days. In addition, each subject received oral fluconazole 200 mg once daily on days 11 through 20 in an open-labeled, parallel group study. Fluconazole administration did not affect the pharmacokinetics of eprosartan. However, coadministration of fluconazole and losartan increased the AUC and peak plasma concentration of losartan 69% and 31%, respectively, compared with taking losartan alone. The AUC and peak plasma concentrations of the active metabolite of losartan (E 3174) decreased 41% and 54%, respectively, following coadministration of fluconazole and losartan.

[1] Kazierad DJ, et al. *Clin Pharmacol Ther*. 1997;62:417.

* Asterisk indicates drugs cited in interaction reports.

Losartan | **Berberine**

Losartan*
(eg, *Cozaar*)

Berberine*

Significance	Onset	Severity	Documentation
4	☐ Rapid ■ **Delayed**	☐ Major ■ **Moderate** ☐ Minor	☐ Established ☐ Probable ☐ Suspected ■ **Possible** ☐ Unlikely

Effects The hypotensive effect of LOSARTAN may be decreased.

Mechanism Inhibition of LOSARTAN metabolism (CYP2C9) to its active metabolite (E-3174) by BERBERINE is suspected.

Management Instruct patients taking LOSARTAN to avoid BERBERINE.

Discussion

The effects of berberine (a plant alkaloid found in herbs such as goldenseal) on the pharmacokinetics of losartan were evaluated in 17 healthy men.[1] Using a randomized, crossover design, each subject received either placebo or berberine 300 mg 3 times daily for 14 days. Losartan 30 mg was administered before and at the end of the 14 days. Compared with placebo, berberine ingestion increased the ratio of losartan to E-3174 by 2-fold.

[1] Guo Y, et al. *Eur J Clin Pharmacol.* 2012;68(2):213.

* Asterisk indicates drugs cited in interaction reports.

Losartan | **Food**

Losartan*
(eg, *Cozaar*)

Grapefruit Juice*

Significance	Onset	Severity	Documentation
5	□ Rapid	□ Major	□ Established
	■ **Delayed**	□ Moderate	□ Probable
		■ **Minor**	□ Suspected
			□ Possible
			■ **Unlikely**

Effects The rate and magnitude of LOSARTAN metabolism to its major active metabolite may be decreased, possibly reducing the therapeutic effects.

Mechanism Simultaneous inhibition of CYP3A4 metabolism and activation of P-gp efflux.

Management Based on available data, a clinically important interaction is unlikely. However, caution patients to take LOSARTAN with a liquid other than GRAPEFRUIT JUICE.

Discussion

The effect of grapefruit juice on the pharmacokinetics of losartan and its major active metabolite E-3174 was studied in 9 healthy volunteers.[1] In a randomized, crossover study, each subject received losartan 50 mg with 200 mL of 100% natural grapefruit juice or water. The time lapse for the appearance of losartan in the plasma was increased by administration with grapefruit juice compared with water (0.6 vs 1.3 hours). The mean residence time and $t_{½}$ of the E-3174 metabolite were longer when losartan was taken with grapefruit juice. Administration of losartan with grapefruit juice increased the ratio of the losartan AUC to its metabolite 41%, indicating the magnitude of metabolic conversion.

Additional studies are needed to determine the effect of chronic ingestion of grapefruit juice on the pharmacokinetics of losartan.

[1] Zaidenstein R, et al. *Ther Drug Monit.* 2001;23(4):369.

* Asterisk indicates drugs cited in interaction reports.

Losartan — *Hydantoins*

Losartan* (eg, *Cozaar*)		Fosphenytoin (*Cerebyx*)	Phenytoin* (eg, *Dilantin*)

Significance	Onset	Severity	Documentation
4	☐ Rapid ■ **Delayed**	☐ Major ■ **Moderate** ☐ Minor	☐ Established ☐ Probable ☐ Suspected ■ **Possible** ☐ Unlikely

Effects The antihypertensive effects of LOSARTAN may be decreased because of decreased exposure to the active carboxylic acid metabolite (E3174).

Mechanism Inhibition of LOSARTAN metabolism (CYP2C9) to its active carboxylic acid metabolite (E-3174) by PHENYTOIN.

Management Monitor BP response to LOSARTAN when starting, stopping, or changing the PHENYTOIN dose.

Discussion

The potential for a 2-way pharmacokinetic interaction between losartan and phenytoin was evaluated in 16 healthy volunteers.[1] Using a 3-period crossover design, each subject received phenytoin 4 mg/kg/day (max, 400 mg/day) alone, losartan 50 mg twice daily alone, and phenytoin plus losartan for 9 days. Compared with taking losartan alone, coadministration of phenytoin increased the losartan mean AUC 29% and reduced the AUC of the active carboxylic acid metabolite of losartan, E-3174, by 63%. This effect was seen in the CYP2C9 wild-type genotype. Compared with taking phenytoin alone, losartan had no effect on the pharmacokinetics of phenytoin.

[1] Fischer TL, et al. *Clin Pharmacol Ther.* 2002;72(3):238.

* Asterisk indicates drugs cited in interaction reports. Based on pharmacologic and pharmacokinetic considerations, similar interactions may occur with other drugs that are listed.

Losartan — *Indomethacin*

Losartan* (eg, *Cozaar*)	Indomethacin* (eg, *Indocin*)

Significance	Onset	Severity	Documentation
2	☐ Rapid	☐ Major	☐ Established
	■ **Delayed**	■ **Moderate**	☐ Probable
		☐ Minor	■ **Suspected**
			☐ Possible
			☐ Unlikely

Effects The hypotensive effect of LOSARTAN may be reduced.

Mechanism Unknown.

Management Monitor BP and consider discontinuing INDOMETHACIN or using an alternative antihypertensive agent if an interaction is suspected.

Discussion

The effect of coadministration of indomethacin on the antihypertensive effect of captopril and losartan was evaluated in 216 men and women with essential hypertension.[1] In a multicenter, randomized, double-blind, parallel study, subjects received 6 weeks of treatment with either captopril (started at 25 mg twice daily for 1 week, then increased to 50 mg twice daily for 5 weeks) or losartan (50 mg daily). This was followed by 1 week of concurrent treatment with indomethacin 75 mg daily. After 6 weeks of therapy, captopril and losartan reduced the mean 24-hour systolic (captopril, −8.6 mm Hg; losartan, −7.9 mm Hg) and diastolic (captopril, −5.6 mm Hg; losartan, −5.3 mm Hg) BPs. Coadministration of indomethacin with both antihypertensive agents resulted in an increase in mean 24-hour systolic (captopril, 4.6 mm Hg; losartan, 3.8 mm Hg) and diastolic (captopril, 2.7 mm Hg; losartan, 2.2 mm Hg) BPs from values measured at week 6. During indomethacin therapy, 67% of the captopril-treated patients and 68.5% of the losartan-treated patients had an increase in ambulatory diastolic BP. Indomethacin attenuated the nighttime diastolic BP in patients receiving captopril but did not affect losartan-treated patients. See also ACE Inhibitors-Indomethacin.

[1] Conlin PR, et al. *Hypertension*. 2000;36(3):461.

* Asterisk indicates drugs cited in interaction reports.

Losartan | **Milk Thistle**

Losartan*
(*Cozaar*)

Milk Thistle*

Significance	Onset	Severity	Documentation
4	☐ Rapid	☐ Major	☐ Established
	■ **Delayed**	■ **Moderate**	☐ Probable
		☐ Minor	☐ Suspected
			■ **Possible**
			☐ Unlikely

Effects The hypotensive effect of LOSARTAN may be decreased.

Mechanism Inhibition of LOSARTAN metabolism (CYP2C9 and CYP3A4) to its active metabolite (E3174) by MILK THISTLE is suspected.

Management If coadministration cannot be avoided, closely monitor BP response. If an interaction is suspected, discontinue MILK THISTLE.

Discussion

The effects of silymarin, a purified extract from the milk thistle plant, on the pharmacokinetics of losartan and its active metabolite, E3174, were studied in 12 healthy men.[1] In addition, the relationship of CYP genotypes to the magnitude of the effects was assessed. Using a 2-phase, randomized, crossover design, each subject received losartan 50 mg alone and after 14 days of receiving placebo or silymarin 140 mg 3 times daily. Compared with placebo, pretreatment with silymarin increased the losartan AUC approximately 108% in subjects with the CYP2C9*1/*1 genotype but not in individuals with the CYP2C9*1/*3 genotype. The AUC of the E3174 metabolite decreased with silymarin pretreatment in both the CYP2C9*1/*1 and CYP2C9*1/*3 genotypes approximately 17% and 13%, respectively. The metabolic ratio of losartan decreased approximately 55% after silymarin pretreatment in subjects with the CYP2C9*1/*1 genotype, but not in individuals with the CYP2C9*1/*3 genotype. Thus, silymarin inhibits the metabolism of losartan to E3174, and the magnitude of the interaction differs based on the CYP2C9 genotype.

[1] Han Y, et al. *Eur J Clin Pharmacol.* 2009;65(6):585.

* Asterisk indicates drugs cited in interaction reports.

Losartan — *Rifamycins*

Losartan		Rifamycins	
Losartan* (eg, *Cozaar*)		Rifabutin (*Mycobutin*)	Rifapentine (*Priftin*)
		Rifampin* (eg, *Rifadin*)	

Significance	Onset	Severity	Documentation
4	☐ Rapid	☐ Major	☐ Established
	■ **Delayed**	■ **Moderate**	☐ Probable
		☐ Minor	☐ Suspected
			■ **Possible**
			☐ Unlikely

Effects LOSARTAN plasma concentrations may be reduced, decreasing the antihypertensive effects.

Mechanism RIFAMYCINS may increase the metabolism of LOSARTAN.

Management Observe the clinical response of patients when a RIFAMYCIN is started or stopped. Adjust therapy as needed.

Discussion

The effects of rifampin on the pharmacokinetics of losartan and the active metabolite of losartan (E-3174) were studied in 10 healthy volunteers.[1] In a prospective, open-label, nonrandomized investigation, each subject received losartan 50 mg/day alone (baseline) or with rifampin 300 mg twice daily for 7 days. On day 8 of each phase, another dose of losartan was administered, and blood samples were collected at various time intervals between 0.5 and 32 hours. Rifampin decreased the AUC of losartan 35% and increased the oral clearance 60%, while the AUC of the E-3174 metabolite was decreased 40%. The $t_{1/2}$ values of losartan and E-3174 were decreased approximately 50%.

[1] Williamson KM, et al. *Clin Pharmacol Ther*. 1998;63(3):316.

* Asterisk indicates drugs cited in interaction reports. Based on pharmacologic and pharmacokinetic considerations, similar interactions may occur with other drugs that are listed.

Lovastatin — *Danazol*

Lovastatin* (eg, *Mevacor*)	Danazol* (*Danazol*)

Significance	Onset	Severity	Documentation
4	☐ Rapid ■ **Delayed**	■ **Major** ☐ Moderate ☐ Minor	☐ Established ☐ Probable ☐ Suspected ■ **Possible** ☐ Unlikely

Effects Severe myopathy or rhabdomyolysis may occur with coadministration of these drugs.

Mechanism Unknown.

Management When possible, consider avoiding this drug combination and administering alternative therapy. Advise patients receiving LOVASTATIN to report any unexplained muscle pain, tenderness, or weakness.

Discussion

Myoglobulinuria and rhabdomyolysis were reported in a 72-year-old man receiving a drug regimen consisting of aspirin (eg, *Bayer*), dipyridamole (eg, *Persantine*), lovastatin, danazol, prednisone (eg, *Sterapred*), and doxycycline (eg, *Vibramycin*).[1] The symptoms resolved, and laboratory results returned to normal within 2 weeks of stopping lovastatin, danazol, and aspirin. Additional data are needed to determine if this reaction was the result of a drug interaction or caused by lovastatin alone.

[1] Dallaire M, et al. *CMAJ*. 1994;150(12):1991.

* Asterisk indicates drugs cited in interaction reports.

Lovastatin — *Protease Inhibitors*

Lovastatin	Protease Inhibitors	
Lovastatin* (eg, *Mevacor*)	Atazanavir* (*Reyataz*)	Lopinavir/Ritonavir (*Kaletra*)
	Darunavir* (*Prezista*)	Nelfinavir* (*Viracept*)
	Fosamprenavir* (*Lexiva*)	Ritonavir* (*Norvir*)
	Indinavir (*Crixivan*)	Saquinavir (*Invirase*)

Significance	Onset	Severity	Documentation
1	□ Rapid	■ **Major**	□ Established
	■ **Delayed**	□ Moderate	□ Probable
		□ Minor	■ **Suspected**
			□ Possible
			□ Unlikely

Effects LOVASTATIN plasma levels may be elevated, increasing the risk of adverse reactions (eg, rhabdomyolysis).

Mechanism PROTEASE INHIBITORS may inhibit the metabolism (CYP3A4) of LOVASTATIN.

Management LOVASTATIN is contraindicated in patients receiving DARUNAVIR,[1] FOSAMPRENAVIR,[2] or NELFINAVIR.[3] In addition, do not coadminister LOVASTATIN with RITONAVIR[4] or ATAZANAVIR.[5]

Discussion

Atazanavir, nelfinavir, and ritonavir inhibit CYP3A4.[3-5] Coadministration of atazanavir, nelfinavir, or ritonavir with drugs that are metabolized by CYP3A4 (eg, lovastatin) may result in increased plasma concentrations of the other drug (eg, lovastatin), increasing and prolonging the therapeutic effects and adverse reactions.[3,4] See Atorvastatin-Protease Inhibitors, Pravastatin-Ritonavir, and Simvastatin-Protease Inhibitors.

The basis for this monograph is information on file with the manufacturers. Because of the seriousness of the adverse reactions, clinical evaluation of this interaction in humans is not likely to be forthcoming.

1 *Prezista* [package insert]. Raritan, NJ: Tibotec Therapeutics; October 2008.
2 *Lexiva* [package insert]. Research Triangle Park, NC: GlaxoSmithKline; April 2010.
3 *Viracept* [package insert]. La Jolla, CA: Agouron Pharmaceuticals Inc; 2002.
4 *Norvir* [package insert]. Abbott Park, IL: Abbott Laboratories; 2001.
5 *Reyataz* [package insert]. Princeton, NJ: Bristol-Myers Squibb Co; 2003.

* Asterisk indicates drugs cited in interaction reports. Based on pharmacologic and pharmacokinetic considerations, similar interactions may occur with other drugs that are listed.

Macrolide Antibiotics — *Atovaquone*

Azithromycin* (eg, *Zithromax*)	Atovaquone* (*Mepron*)

Significance	Onset	Severity	Documentation
5	☐ Rapid	☐ Major	☐ Established
	■ **Delayed**	■ **Moderate**	☐ Probable
		☐ Minor	☐ Suspected
			☐ Possible
			■ **Unlikely**

Effects AZITHROMYCIN serum concentrations may be reduced, decreasing the pharmacologic effects.

Mechanism Unknown.

Management Based on available data, no special precautions appear necessary. Closely monitor the patient's response and adjust therapy as needed.

Discussion

The effects of atovaquone on the pharmacokinetics of azithromycin were studied in 10 children (4 to 13 years of age) with HIV infection.[1] In a randomized, crossover study with each phase lasting 10 days, subjects received azithromycin 5 mg/kg/day alone or simultaneously with atovaquone 30 mg/kg/day prior to the phase in which both drugs were given 12 hours apart. Although there was no statistically significant difference in mean azithromycin pharmacokinetic parameters in the 3 phases, steady-state values of azithromycin AUC were lower in all patients (in whom the data were sufficient to analyze) who were receiving the simultaneous regimen compared with patients who received azithromycin alone. Similarly, the azithromycin C_{max} was lower in 6 of 7 patients receiving the simultaneous regimen.

A larger study is needed to determine if the effect of atovaquone on azithromycin pharmacokinetics and efficacy is statistically significant and clinically important.

[1] Ngo LY, et al. *Antimicrob Agents Chemother.* 1999;43(6):1516.

* Asterisk indicates drugs cited in interaction reports.

Macrolide & Related Antibiotics — *Diltiazem*

Macrolide & Related Antibiotics		Diltiazem
Clarithromycin (eg, *Biaxin*)	Telithromycin (*Ketek*)	Diltiazem* (eg, *Cardizem*)
Erythromycin* (eg, *Ery-Tab*)		

Significance	Onset	Severity	Documentation
1	☐ Rapid	■ **Major**	☐ Established
	■ **Delayed**	☐ Moderate	☐ Probable
		☐ Minor	■ **Suspected**
			☐ Possible
			☐ Unlikely

Effects Elevated plasma concentrations of MACROLIDE and RELATED ANTIBIOTICS, increasing the risk of cardiotoxicity. DILTIAZEM concentrations may be elevated, increasing the risk of hypotension.

Mechanism Inhibition of CYP3A4 metabolism by both MACROLIDE and RELATED ANTIBIOTIC and DILTIAZEM is suspected.

Management Until more data are available, avoid coadministration of MACROLIDE and RELATED ANTIBIOTICS and DILTIAZEM, if possible.

Discussion

A Medicaid cohort including more than 1.2 million person-years of follow-up and 1,476 cases of confirmed sudden death from cardiac causes was analyzed.[1] There was no increase in risk of sudden death among former users of erythromycin or among patients who were currently taking amoxicillin. Also, there was no increase in risk of sudden death among patients who were currently taking amoxicillin and CYP3A inhibitors or patients who were currently taking amoxicillin or erythromycin and had previously taken CYP3A inhibitors. However, the rate of sudden death from cardiac causes was 5 times higher among patients who took CYP3A inhibitors and erythromycin concurrently compared with patients who took neither CYP3A inhibitors nor erythromycin or amoxicillin. One death occurred in a patient taking concurrent erythromycin and diltiazem and 2 deaths occurred in patients receiving erythromycin and verapamil (eg, *Calan*). There were no sudden deaths from cardiac causes in patients receiving erythromycin and other calcium channel blockers that do not appreciably inhibit CYP3A (eg, nifedipine [eg, *Procardia*]). A population-based study of 7,100 elderly patients hospitalized due to hypotension found an association between coadministration of calcium channel blockers and erythromycin or clarithromycin, but not azithromycin.[2] Forty percent of the patients were receiving diltiazem. See Verapamil-Macrolide & Related Antibiotics.

[1] Ray WA, et al. *N Engl J Med.* 2004;351(11):1089.

[2] Wright AJ, et al. *CMAJ.* 2011;183(3):303.

* Asterisk indicates drugs cited in interaction reports. Based on pharmacologic and pharmacokinetic considerations, similar interactions may occur with other drugs that are listed.

Macrolide Antibiotics — *Food*

Clarithromycin* (eg, *Biaxin*)	Erythromycin* (eg, *Ery-Tab*)	Food*	Grapefruit Juice*

Significance	Onset	Severity	Documentation
1	☐ Rapid ■ **Delayed**	■ **Major** ☐ Moderate ☐ Minor	☐ Established ☐ Probable ■ **Suspected** ☐ Possible ☐ Unlikely

Effects Reduced antimicrobial effectiveness of ERYTHROMYCIN stearate and certain ERYTHROMYCIN base formulations. GRAPEFRUIT may elevate MACROLIDE ANTIBIOTIC levels, increasing the risk of side effects.

Mechanism FOOD may decrease GI absorption of nonenteric-coated ERYTHROMYCIN base tablets and stearate. GRAPEFRUIT may inhibit the metabolism (CYP3A4) in the small intestine.

Management Administer ERYTHROMYCIN stearate and nonenteric-coated ERYTHROMYCIN base tablets at least 2 hr before or after a meal. Administer MACROLIDE ANTIBIOTICS with a liquid other than GRAPEFRUIT JUICE.

Discussion

In 6 healthy volunteers, grapefruit juice increased the mean C_{max} of erythromycin 52% and AUC 49%, compared with water.[1] Grapefruit juice may increase the time to reach clarithromycin C_{max}.[2] Grapefruit juice does not appear to affect telithromycin (*Ketek*) kinetics.[3]

Erythromycin base – Enteric-coated tablet may be taken without regard to meals.[4] However, administer capsules containing enteric-coated pellets (eg, *Eryc*), tablets containing polymer-coated particles (*PCE Dispertab*), and film-coated tablets at least 2 hr before or after a meal to achieve optimal blood levels. Erythromycin was 28% bioavailable following administration of the polymer-coated particles formulation with a high-fat meal.[5]

Erythromycin stearate – Serum levels may be reduced when administered with food.[6] Optimum levels are obtained when administered at least 1 hr before or 2 hr after meals. High blood levels were achieved when administered immediately before a meal.[7]

Erythromycin estolate and ethylsuccinate – Comparable serum levels may be achieved in the fasting and nonfasting states. Food may enhance the absorption of erythromycin estolate[8] and ethylsuccinate.[9] Because erythromycin estolate, ethylsuccinate, and the enteric-coated tablet base formulations may be given without regard to meals, give these preparations with food to reduce the occasional occurrence of GI side effects.

Clarithromycin – Food may enhance absorption of clarithromycin.[10]

1 Kanazawa S, et al. *Eur J Clin Pharmacol.* 2001;56:799.
2 Cheng KL, et al. *Antimicrob Agents Chemother.* 1998;42:927.
3 Shi J, et al. *Pharmacotherapy.* 2005;25:42.
4 Welling PG. *J Pharmacokinet Biopharm.* 1977;5:291.
5 Randinitis EJ, et al. *J Clin Pharmacol.* 1989;29:79.
6 Welling PG, et al. *J Pharm Sci.* 1978;67:764.
7 Malmborg AS. *J Antimicrob Chemother.* 1979;5:591.
8 Welling PG, et al. *J Pharm Sci.* 1979;68:150.
9 Coyne TC, et al. *J Clin Pharmacol.* 1978;18:194.
10 Chu S, et al. *J Clin Pharmacol.* 1992;32:32.

* Asterisk indicates drugs cited in interaction reports.

Macrolide Antibiotics | **Histamine H_2 Antagonists**

Macrolide Antibiotics	Histamine H_2 Antagonists
Clarithromycin* (eg, *Biaxin*)	Cimetidine* (eg, *Tagamet*)

Significance	Onset	Severity	Documentation
4	☐ Rapid	☐ Major	☐ Established
	■ **Delayed**	■ **Moderate**	☐ Probable
		☐ Minor	☐ Suspected
			■ **Possible**
			☐ Unlikely

Effects The antimicrobial effects of CLARITHROMYCIN may be decreased.

Mechanism Unknown.

Management Closely monitor the response to CLARITHROMYCIN therapy. Adjust therapy as needed.

Discussion

In an open-label, randomized, crossover study, the effects of oral cimetidine on the pharmacokinetics of clarithromycin were investigated in 12 healthy subjects.[1] Each subject received a single dose of clarithromycin 500 mg alone and with cimetidine 800 mg dosed to steady state. Cimetidine administration resulted in prolonged clarithromycin absorption. This was evidenced by a 46% decrease in the peak plasma concentrations of clarithromycin and a 43% decrease in the peak plasma concentrations of an active metabolite, 14-OH-clarithromycin (OHC). There was a 68% increase in the time to reach OHC peak concentrations. In addition, the $t_{½}$ of clarithromycin and OHC increased 75% and 82%, respectively. No changes were seen in the oral clearance or AUC of clarithromycin or OHC.

[1] Amsden GW, et al. *Antimicrob Agents Chemother*. 1998;42:1578.

* Asterisk indicates drugs cited in interaction reports.

Macrolide & Related Antibiotics — *Quinolones*

Azithromycin (eg, *Zithromax*)	Erythromycin* (eg, *Ery-Tab*)	Gatifloxacin* (*Zymar*)	Moxifloxacin* (*Avelox*)
Clarithromycin (eg, *Biaxin*)	Telithromycin (*Ketek*)	Levofloxacin* (*Levaquin*)	Sparfloxacin*†

Significance	Onset	Severity	Documentation
1	□ Rapid ■ **Delayed**	■ **Major** □ Moderate □ Minor	□ Established □ Probable ■ **Suspected** □ Possible □ Unlikely

Effects The risk of life-threatening cardiac arrhythmias, including torsades de pointes, may be increased.

Mechanism Unknown.

Management SPARFLOXACIN is contraindicated in patients receiving drugs that prolong the QTc interval (eg, ERYTHROMYCIN).[1] Avoid LEVOFLOXACIN and use GATIFLOXACIN and MOXIFLOXACIN with caution in patients receiving MACROLIDE AND RELATED ANTIBIOTICS.

Discussion

Because torsades de pointes has been reported in patients receiving sparfloxacin with amiodarone (eg, *Cordarone*) or disopyramide (eg, *Norpace*), sparfloxacin is contraindicated in patients receiving these antiarrhythmic agents, other QTc-prolonging drugs (eg, erythromycin), or drugs known to cause torsades de pointes.[1,2] Pharmacokinetic studies between gatifloxacin or moxifloxacin and other drugs that prolong the QT interval have not been performed; therefore, use gatifloxacin and moxifloxacin with caution when erythromycin is coadministered.[3,4] Levofloxacin has been associated with prolongation of the QT interval and infrequent cases of cardiac arrhythmias. The risk may be reduced by avoiding coadministration with drugs that prolong the QT interval.[5]

The basis for this monograph is information on file with the manufacturers. Because of the seriousness of the cardiac problems, clinical evaluation of this interaction in humans is not likely to be forthcoming. Additional data are needed to determine the magnitude of the effect of other quinolone antibiotics on the QT interval.

1 Thomas M, et al. *Br J Clin Pharmacol.* 1996;41(2):77.
2 *Zagam* [package insert]. Research Triangle Park, NC: Bertek Pharmaceuticals, Inc; November 1996.
3 *Avelox* [package insert]. West Haven, CT: Bayer Pharmaceuticals Corp; November 2000.
4 *Tequin* [package insert]. Princeton, NJ: Bristol-Myers Squibb Company; March 2004.
5 *Levoquin* [package insert]. Raritan, NJ: Ortho-McNeil Pharmaceuticals, Inc; February 2004.

* Asterisk indicates drugs cited in interaction reports. Based on pharmacologic and pharmacokinetic considerations, similar interactions may occur with other drugs that are listed.
†Not available in the US.

Macrolide & Related Antibiotics		Rifamycins	
Clarithromycin* (eg, *Biaxin*)	Telithromycin* (*Ketek*)	Rifabutin* (*Mycobutin*)	Rifapentine (*Priftin*)
Erythromycin (eg, *Ery-Tab*)		Rifampin (eg, *Rifadin*)	

Significance	Onset	Severity	Documentation
2	☐ Rapid	☐ Major	☐ Established
	■ **Delayed**	■ **Moderate**	■ **Probable**
		☐ Minor	☐ Suspected
			☐ Possible
			☐ Unlikely

Effects Decreased antimicrobial effects of MACROLIDE AND RELATED ANTIBIOTICS. Increased frequency of GI and RIFAMYCIN adverse reactions.

Mechanism Inhibition of RIFAMYCIN metabolism. Increased MACROLIDE AND RELATED ANTIBIOTIC metabolism.

Management If these agents are used concurrently, monitor for increased RIFAMYCIN adverse reactions and a decrease in the response to the MACROLIDE OR RELATED ANTIBIOTIC. Avoid coadministration of TELITHROMYCIN and a RIFAMYCIN.[1] Azithromycin (eg, *Zithromax*) does not undergo metabolism and may be a safer alternative.[2]

Discussion

In a study of clarithromycin and rifabutin in 34 HIV-infected volunteers, a bidirectional drug interaction was found.[3] When rifabutin was added to the clarithromycin regimen, the clarithromycin AUC decreased 44% and the AUC of the 14-hydroxy metabolite of clarithromycin increased 57%. The decrease in clarithromycin AUC was significant between days 15 and 42 ($P < 0.004$) but not between days 14 and 15. In 1 subject, clarithromycin AUC increased 49%. When clarithromycin was started in subjects receiving rifabutin, the rifabutin AUC increased 99%, and the AUC of the rifabutin metabolite (25-0-desacetyl-rifabutin) increased 375%. Most of the changes occurred between days 14 and 15. In 1 subject, the AUC of rifabutin decreased 39%. Nearly 66% of the subjects reported nausea, vomiting, or diarrhea during coadministration of these drugs. A study comparing the effects of azithromycin or clarithromycin on rifabutin pharmacokinetics was terminated because of a high incidence of neutropenia, possibly caused by the drug combination.[4] Clarithromycin increased rifabutin and rifabutin metabolite levels 400% and 3,700%, respectively. Azithromycin caused a slight decrease in rifabutin levels. There was no pharmacokinetic interaction between azithromycin and rifabutin[5]; however, the combination was poorly tolerated because of GI symptoms and neutropenia.

[1] *Ketek* [package insert]. Kansas City, MO: Aventis Pharmaceuticals, Inc; June 2004.
[2] von Rosensteil NA, et al. *Drug Saf.* 1995;13(2):105.
[3] Hafner R, et al. *Antimicrob Agents Chemother.* 1998;42(3):631.
[4] Apseloff G, et al. *J Clin Pharmacol.* 1998;38(9):830.
[5] Hafner R, et al. *Antimicrob Agents Chemother.* 2001;45(5):1572.

* Asterisk indicates drugs cited in interaction reports. Based on pharmacologic and pharmacokinetic considerations, similar interactions may occur with other drugs that are listed.

Magnesium Sulfate — *Nifedipine*

Magnesium Sulfate*	Nifedipine* (eg, *Procardia*)

Significance	Onset	Severity	Documentation
4	■ **Rapid**	■ **Major**	□ Established
	□ Delayed	□ Moderate	□ Probable
		□ Minor	□ Suspected
			■ **Possible**
			□ Unlikely

Effects Neuromuscular blockade and hypotension have occurred with coadministration of NIFEDIPINE and MAGNESIUM SULFATE.

Mechanism Unknown.

Management Consider closely monitoring the clinical response of the patient and providing supportive treatment as needed.

Discussion

Neuromuscular blockade occurred in a 22-year-old pregnant woman during coadministration of nifedipine and magnesium sulfate.[1] The patient was admitted to the hospital at 32 weeks' gestation with regular uterine contractions of 45 seconds' duration and 50% effacement of the cervix. Nifedipine 60 mg orally was initiated over the next 3 hours, which resulted in a marked decrease in the duration and frequency of contractions; the patient was subsequently maintained on nifedipine 20 mg every 8 hours. When contractions recurred 12 hours later, the patient was started on IV magnesium sulfate. After administration of magnesium sulfate 500 mg, she developed jerky movements of the extremities, complained of difficulty in swallowing, had paradoxical respirations, and was unable to lift her head. Magnesium was discontinued, and the muscle weakness reversed over the next 25 minutes. In another report, 2 women with preeclampsia treated with oral methyldopa 2 g and IV magnesium sulfate 20 g/day developed profound hypotension 45 minutes after the addition of oral nifedipine 10 mg to their treatment regimen.[2] BP returned to previous levels within 30 minutes (75 minutes after nifedipine administration).

[1] Snyder SW, et al. *Am J Obstet Gynecol.* 1989;161(1):35.

[2] Waisman GD, et al. *Am J Obstet Gynecol.* 1988;159(2):308.

* Asterisk indicates drugs cited in interaction reports.

MAOIs — *Cyclobenzaprine*

Isocarboxazid* (*Marplan*)	Rasagiline* (*Azilect*)	Cyclobenzaprine* (eg, *Flexeril*)
Linezolid* (*Zyvox*)	Selegiline (eg, *Eldepryl*)	
Phenelzine* (*Nardil*)	Tranylcypromine* (eg, *Parnate*)	

Significance	Onset	Severity	Documentation
1	■ **Rapid** □ Delayed	■ **Major** □ Moderate □ Minor	□ Established □ Probable ■ **Suspected** □ Possible □ Unlikely

Effects The risk of hypertensive crises, convulsions, and death may be increased.

Mechanism Unknown.

Management Coadministration of MAOIs and CYCLOBENZAPRINE is contraindicated.[1] Do not administer CYCLOBENZAPRINE with or within 14 days of discontinuing an MAOI.

Discussion

Hyperpyretic crisis, seizures, and death have occurred in patients receiving cyclobenzaprine concurrently with an MAOI.[1] In addition, severe CNS toxicity associated with hyperpyrexia and death have been reported with coadministration of TCAs and selective or nonselective MAOIs.[2] Cyclobenzaprine is structurally related to TCAs. Coadministration of cyclobenzaprine with an MAOI or within 14 days after their discontinuation is contraindicated.[1]

The basis for this monograph is information on file with the manufacturer. Published clinical data are needed to further assess this interaction. Because of the seriousness of the interaction, clinical evaluation in humans is not likely to be forthcoming. See also Tricyclic Antidepressants-MAOIs.

[1] *Flexeril* [package insert]. West Point, PA: Merck & Co Inc; February 2003.

[2] *Azilect* [package insert]. Kfar Saba, Israel: Teva Pharmaceuticals Industries Ltd; May 2006.

* Asterisk indicates drugs cited in interaction reports. Based on pharmacologic and pharmacokinetic considerations, similar interactions may occur with other drugs that are listed.

MAOIs | **Ginseng**

Isocarboxazid (*Marplan*)	Tranylcypromine (eg, *Parnate*)	Ginseng*
Phenelzine* (eg, *Nardil*)		

Significance	Onset	Severity	Documentation
4	□ Rapid	□ Major	□ Established
	■ **Delayed**	■ **Moderate**	□ Probable
		□ Minor	□ Suspected
			■ **Possible**
			□ Unlikely

Effects Manic-like symptoms, headache, and tremulousness have been reported.

Mechanism Unknown.

Management Advise patients to avoid concomitant use of MAOIs and GINSENG when possible.

Discussion

A 64-year-old woman experienced headache, insomnia, and tremulousness on 2 occasions while taking phenelzine and ginseng.[1] She did not experience these symptoms while taking phenelzine or ginseng alone. Manic-like symptoms occurred in a 42-year-old woman in association with concomitant use of phenelzine, ginseng, and bee pollen.[2] Other medications the patient was taking included triazolam (eg, *Halcion*) and lorazepam (eg, *Ativan*).

The ingredients of many herbal products are not standardized. It is unclear if herbal products contain ingredients other than those listed on the label or purported to be present that could interact with MAOIs.

[1] Shader RI, et al. *J Clin Psychopharmacol.* 1985;5(2):65.

[2] Jones BD, et al. *J Clin Psychopharmacol.* 1987;7(3):201.

* Asterisk indicates drugs cited in interaction reports. Based on pharmacologic and pharmacokinetic considerations, similar interactions may occur with other drugs that are listed.

MAOIs — *Tapentadol*

MAOIs		Tapentadol
Isocarboxazid* (*Marplan*)	Rasagiline* (*Azilect*)	Tapentadol* (*Nucynta*)
Linezolid* (*Zyvox*)	Selegiline* (eg, *Eldepryl*)	
Phenelzine* (eg, *Nardil*)	Tranylcypromine* (eg, *Parnate*)	

Significance	Onset	Severity	Documentation
1	■ **Rapid**	■ **Major**	□ Established
	□ Delayed	□ Moderate	□ Probable
		□ Minor	■ **Suspected**
			□ Possible
			□ Unlikely

Effects The risk of adverse cardiovascular events may be increased.

Mechanism Pharmacologic effects of both agents may be additive.

Management Concomitant use or use within 14 days of each other is contraindicated.[1]

Discussion

Tapentadol is contraindicated in patients receiving MAOIs or who have taken an MAOI within the last 14 days.[1] Coadministration may result in potential additive effects on norepinephrine concentrations, which may result in adverse cardiovascular events.

[1] *Nucynta* [package insert]. Titusville, NJ: Janssen Pharmaceuticals Inc; August 2011.

* Asterisk indicates drugs cited in interaction reports.

MAOIs | **Tetrabenazine**

Isocarboxazid* (*Marplan*)	Rasagiline* (*Azilect*)	Tetrabenazine* (*Xenazine*)
Linezolid* (*Zyvox*)	Selegiline* (eg, *Eldepryl*)	
Phenelzine* (*Nardil*)	Tranylcypromine* (eg, *Parnate*)	

Significance	Onset	Severity	Documentation
2	■ **Rapid**	□ Major	□ Established
	□ Delayed	■ **Moderate**	□ Probable
		□ Minor	■ **Suspected**
			□ Possible
			□ Unlikely

Effects Risk of hypertension and CNS adverse reactions (eg, confusion, disorientation, excitability, restlessness) may be increased.

Mechanism Unknown; however, TETRABENAZINE reversibly inhibits vesicular monoamine transporter type 2 (VMAT2), resulting in decreased uptake of monoamine into synaptic vesicles and depletion of monoamine stores.

Management Coadministration of TETRABENAZINE and MAOIs is contraindicated.

Discussion

Tetrabenazine reversibly inhibits VMAT2, resulting in decreased uptake of monoamine into synaptic vesicles and depletion of monoamine stores.[1] Tetrabenazine administration may reversibly deplete monoamine (eg, dopamine, histamine, norepinephrine, serotonin) from nerve terminals.

[1] *Xenazine* [package insert]. Washington, DC: Prestwick Pharmaceuticals; May 2008.

* Asterisk indicates drugs cited in interaction reports.

MAOIs — *L-Tryptophan*

MAOIs		L-Tryptophan
Isocarboxazid (*Marplan*)	Rasagiline* (*Azilect*)	L-Tryptophan*†
Linezolid* (*Zyvox*)	Selegiline* (eg, *Eldepryl*)	
Phenelzine* (*Nardil*)	Tranylcypromine* (eg, *Parnate*)	

Significance	Onset	Severity	Documentation
1	■ **Rapid** □ Delayed	■ **Major** □ Moderate □ Minor	□ Established □ Probable ■ **Suspected** □ Possible □ Unlikely

Effects Serotonin syndrome, including CNS irritability, motor weakness, shivering, myoclonus, and altered consciousness, may occur.

Mechanism The serotonergic effects of these agents may be additive.

Management Avoid coadministration of an MAOI and L-TRYPTOPHAN.

Discussion

Serotonin syndrome symptoms have been reported in patients receiving an MAOI and L-tryptophan concomitantly.[1-5] A 42-year-old woman experienced delirium, including bizarre and inappropriate behavior, shortly after taking phenelzine 45 mg/day and L-tryptophan 2,040 mg.[5] Both drugs were discontinued, and she was fully alert and oriented within 8 hours. An acute behavioral and neurologic syndrome was reported in a 21-year-old man taking phenelzine 90 mg/day immediately after taking L-tryptophan 6 g.[1] His abnormal status resolved within 24 hours of withholding therapy. Delirium was reported in 8 patients during coadministration of tranylcypromine 40 to 130 mg/day and L-tryptophan 1 to 6 g/day.[3] Delirium resolved within 12 hours to 4 days of stopping both medications. Death from toxic encephalopathy with multisystem failures caused by neuroleptic syndrome occurred in a 45-year-old woman taking tranylcypromine, L-tryptophan 500 mg, and fluoxetine (eg, *Prozac*).[6] In a 63-year-old man taking lithium (eg, *Lithobid*), tranylcypromine, and L-tryptophan 2 g, self-limiting twice-daily episodes of hyperventilation, diaphoresis, shivering, hyperthermia, increased tone, and hyperreflexia occurred over a period of 2 weeks.[4] The episodes stopped and did not recur after L-tryptophan was discontinued. Three patients receiving phenelzine 60 to 105 mg/day developed a transient syndrome of myoclonus, hyperreflexia, quivering jaw, chattering teeth, and diaphoresis shortly after L-tryptophan 2 g was added.[2] Two cases of hypomania were reported after the addition of L-tryptophan to phenelzine or tranylcypromine.[7] See Serotonin Reuptake Inhibitors-L-Tryptophan.

[1] Thomas JM, et al. *Am J Psychiatry*. 1984;141(2):281.
[2] Levy AB, et al. *Can J Psychiatry*. 1985;30(6):434.
[3] Pope HG, et al. *Am J Psychiatry*. 1985;142(4):491.
[4] Price WA, et al. *J Clin Pharmacol*. 1986;26(1):77.
[5] Alvine G, et al. *J Clin Psychiatry*. 1990;51(7):311.
[6] Kline SS, et al. *Clin Pharm*. 1989;8(7):510.
[7] Goff DC. *Am J Psychiatry*. 1985;142(12):1487.
[8] *FDA Drug Bull*. 1990;20(1):2.

* Asterisk indicates drugs cited in interaction reports. Based on pharmacologic and pharmacokinetic considerations, similar interactions may occur with other drugs that are listed.

† The FDA requested a nationwide recall of all nonprescription supplements that contain L-tryptophan as a sole major component because of a possible link with eosinophilia myalgia.[8]

Maprotiline / *Beta-Blockers*

Maprotiline*	Propranolol* (eg, *Inderal*)

Significance	Onset	Severity	Documentation
4	☐ Rapid	☐ Major	☐ Established
	■ **Delayed**	■ **Moderate**	☐ Probable
		☐ Minor	☐ Suspected
			■ **Possible**
			☐ Unlikely

Effects Adverse reactions to MAPROTILINE may be enhanced.

Mechanism Unknown.

Management Consider reducing the MAPROTILINE dosage.

Discussion

A 40-year-old man experienced sedation, dry mouth, blurred vision, tremor, and poor balance 30 days after beginning propranolol 120 mg/day. The trough maprotiline serum concentration had increased from 311 ng/mL (prior to propranolol) to 530 ng/mL. Plasma levels returned to 380 ng/mL 3 weeks after propranolol was discontinued.[1] Another suspected interaction was reported in a 43-year-old man who developed terrifying visual hallucinations less than 2 weeks after adding maprotiline 200 mg/day to propranolol 120 mg/day.[2] Symptoms resolved when maprotiline was discontinued.

The fundamentals of this interaction remain elusive. More data incorporating information about other available beta-blockers are necessary.

[1] Tollefson G, et al. *Am J Psychiatry*. 1984;141(1):148.

[2] Saiz-Ruiz J, et al. *J Clin Psychopharmacol*. 1988;8(1):77.

* Asterisk indicates drugs cited in interaction reports.

Maprotiline — *Risperidone*

Maprotiline*	Risperidone* (*Risperdal*)

Significance	Onset	Severity	Documentation
4	□ Rapid ■ **Delayed**	□ Major ■ **Moderate** □ Minor	□ Established □ Probable □ Suspected ■ **Possible** □ Unlikely

Effects MAPROTILINE plasma concentrations may be elevated, increasing the risk of adverse reactions.

Mechanism Inhibition of MAPROTILINE metabolism (CYP2D6) by RISPERIDONE is suspected.

Management In patients receiving MAPROTILINE, observe the clinical response when RISPERIDONE is started or stopped. Adjust therapy as needed.

Discussion

Increased maprotiline plasma concentrations during coadministration of risperidone were reported in 3 patients.[1] Two patients were receiving maprotiline 150 mg/day and 1 was receiving 175 mg/day for severe depressive episodes when risperidone was started. One patient received risperidone 1 mg/day, while the dose of risperidone was titrated over 5 days to 5 mg/day in another patient, and titrated to 12 mg/day within 1 week in the remaining patient. Coadministration of maprotiline and risperidone resulted in a 40% to 60% increase in maprotiline plasma levels. After starting risperidone therapy, maprotiline plasma levels increased over a 10-day period in 1 patient and reached steady state in the 2 other patients after 6 and 7 weeks, respectively. One patient gradually developed anticholinergic adverse reactions that decreased in severity when the doses of maprotiline and risperidone were decreased.

[1] Normann C, et al. *J Clin Psychopharmacol.* 2002;22(1):92.

* Asterisk indicates drugs cited in interaction reports.

Maraviroc — *St. John's Wort*

Maraviroc* (*Selzentry*)	St. John's Wort*

Significance	Onset	Severity	Documentation
2	☐ Rapid	☐ Major	☐ Established
	■ **Delayed**	■ **Moderate**	☐ Probable
		☐ Minor	■ **Suspected**
			☐ Possible
			☐ Unlikely

Effects MARAVIROC plasma concentrations may be reduced, resulting in a loss of virologic response and possible resistance.

Mechanism Increased hepatic metabolism (CYP3A4) of MARAVIROC by ST. JOHN'S WORT.

Management Do not coadminister MARAVIROC and ST. JOHN'S WORT. Caution patients taking MARAVIROC to consult their health care provider before using nonprescription or herbal products.

Discussion

In vitro studies indicate that CYP3A4 is the major enzyme responsible for maraviroc metabolism.[1] Maraviroc is a substrate of CYP3A and P-glycoprotein and its pharmacokinetics are likely to be affected by inhibitors and inducers (eg, St. John's wort) of these enzymes. Coadministration of maraviroc and St. John's wort (*Hypericum perforatum*) or products containing St. John's wort is not recommended. Coadministration of maraviroc and St. John's wort is expected to result in a loss of virologic response and possible maraviroc resistance.[1]

The basis for this monograph is information on file with the manufacturer. Studies are needed to determine the clinical importance of this interaction.

[1] *Selzentry* [package insert]. New York, NY: Pfizer, Inc; August 2007.

* Asterisk indicates drugs cited in interaction reports.

Mebendazole — *Carbamazepine*

Mebendazole* (*Vermox*)	Carbamazepine* (eg, *Tegretol*)

Significance	Onset	Severity	Documentation
4	☐ Rapid	☐ Major	☐ Established
	■ **Delayed**	■ **Moderate**	☐ Probable
		☐ Minor	☐ Suspected
			■ **Possible**
			☐ Unlikely

Effects Pharmacologic effects of MEBENDAZOLE may be decreased.

Mechanism Unknown.

Management No special precautions appear necessary. If an interaction is suspected, consider increasing the dose of MEBENDAZOLE during coadministration of CARBAMAZEPINE. Measure MEBENDAZOLE plasma levels and adjust the dose accordingly.

Discussion

In patients treated for inoperable infections due to *Echinococcus multilocularis* or *granulosus*, plasma mebendazole levels were analyzed retrospectively together with patient data, including age, sex, weight, type of hydatid disease, dose and duration of mebendazole therapy and concurrent medications.[1] The lowest median plasma levels occurred in patients who were receiving carbamazepine and mebendazole concomitantly for echinococcal infections of the central nervous system. When carbamazepine was discontinued and treatment was changed to valproic acid (*Depakene*), plasma mebendazole levels increased in each instance.

[1] Luder PJ, et al. *Eur J Clin Pharmacol.* 1986;31:443.

* Asterisk indicates drugs cited in interaction reports.

Mebendazole — *Hydantoins*

Mebendazole* (*Vermox*)	Phenytoin* (eg, *Dilantin*)

Significance	Onset	Severity	Documentation
4	☐ Rapid	☐ Major	☐ Established
	■ **Delayed**	■ **Moderate**	☐ Probable
		☐ Minor	☐ Suspected
			■ **Possible**
			☐ Unlikely

Effects Pharmacologic effects of MEBENDAZOLE may be decreased.

Mechanism Unknown.

Management No special precautions appear necessary. If an interaction is suspected, consider increasing the dose of MEBENDAZOLE during coadministration with HYDANTOINS. Measure MEBENDAZOLE plasma levels and adjust the dose accordingly.

Discussion

In patients treated for inoperable infections due to *Echinococcus multilocularis* or *granulosus*, plasma mebendazole levels were analyzed retrospectively together with patient data, including age, sex, weight, type of hydatid disease, dose and duration of mebendazole therapy and concurrent medications.[1] The lowest median plasma levels occurred in patients who were receiving phenytoin and mebendazole concomitantly for echinococcal infections of the central nervous system. When phenytoin was discontinued and treatment was changed to valproic acid (eg, *Depakene*), plasma mebendazole levels increased in each instance.

[1] Luder PJ, et al. *Eur J Clin Pharmacol.* 1986;31:443.

* Asterisk indicates drugs cited in interaction reports.

Mecamylamine — *Urinary Alkalinizers*

Mecamylamine	Urinary Alkalinizers	
Mecamylamine* (*Inversine*)	Potassium Citrate (*Urocit-K*)	Sodium Lactate
	Sodium Acetate	Tromethamine (*Tham*)
	Sodium Bicarbonate	
	Sodium Citrate (*Citra pH*)	

Significance	Onset	Severity	Documentation
4	□ Rapid	□ Major	□ Established
	■ **Delayed**	■ **Moderate**	□ Probable
		□ Minor	□ Suspected
			■ **Possible**
			□ Unlikely

Effects The blood pressure lowering action of MECAMYLAMINE may be amplified or prolonged in the presence of alkaline urine.

Mechanism Renal excretion of MECAMYLAMINE decreases as urinary pH increases as a result of urinary alkalinization. In addition to the more prolonged course of action that could be expected, the consequent accumulation of MECAMYLAMINE could produce a more intense hypotensive effect.

Management Closely observe the patient for clinical signs of hypotension, and monitor blood pressure during the combined use of MECAMYLAMINE and agents that can produce alkaline urine. The dose of MECAMYLAMINE may need to be lowered.

Discussion

In a study involving an unknown number of hypertensive patients,[1] the effect of urinary pH on the excretion of mecamylamine was demonstrated. When urinary pH was 6.5 or less, approximately 50% of the drug was recovered 12 hours after administration in 1 patient and after 24 hours in the other. When urinary pH was at least 7.5, less than 10% of the drug was recovered during the same time periods. Thus, use of mecamylamine in patients who sustain alkaline urinary pHs could produce unexpectedly prolonged and intense hypotensive effects.

[1] Allanby KD, et al. *BMJ.* 1957;4:1219.

* Asterisk indicates drugs cited in interaction reports. Based on pharmacologic and pharmacokinetic considerations, similar interactions may occur with other drugs that are listed.

Mefenamic Acid — *Magnesium Salts*

Mefenamic Acid	Magnesium Salts	
Mefenamic Acid* (*Ponstel*)	Magnesium Carbonate (eg, *Marblen*)	Magnesium Oxide (eg, *Mag-Ox 400*)
	Magnesium Citrate	Magnesium Sulfate (*Epsom Salt*)
	Magnesium Gluconate (eg, *Almora*)	Magnesium Trisilicate
	Magnesium Hydroxide* (eg, *Milk of Magnesia*)	

Significance	Onset	Severity	Documentation
5	■ **Rapid**	□ Major	□ Established
	□ Delayed	□ Moderate	□ Probable
		■ **Minor**	□ Suspected
			■ **Possible**
			□ Unlikely

Effects May see an increase in the rate of onset of activity of MEFENAMIC ACID.

Mechanism Increased rate of absorption of MEFENAMIC ACID.

Management Based on currently available information, no special precautions are necessary.

Discussion

Using a randomized, crossover design, the effects of magnesium hydroxide 85, 425, or 1700 mg or water on the absorption of mefenamic acid 500 mg were studied in healthy volunteers.[1] Magnesium hydroxide increased the rate of absorption and the peak plasma concentration of mefenamic acid, while the peak time, the half-life of absorption, and the mean residence time were shortened. Only the 1700 mg dose of magnesium hydroxide increased the area under the concentration-time curve. This effect of magnesium hydroxide was prevented by aluminum hydroxide.

[1] Neuvonen PJ, et al. *Eur J Clin Pharmacol.* 1988;35:495.

* Asterisk indicates drugs cited in interaction reports. Based on pharmacologic and pharmacokinetic considerations, similar interactions may occur with other drugs that are listed.

Mefloquine — *Azole Antifungal Agents*

Mefloquine	Azole Antifungal Agents	
Mefloquine*	Itraconazole (eg, *Sporanox*)	Posaconazole (*Noxafil*)
	Ketoconazole* (eg, *Nizoral*)	Voriconazole (*Vfend*)

Significance	Onset	Severity	Documentation
4	□ Rapid	□ Major	□ Established
	■ **Delayed**	■ **Moderate**	□ Probable
		□ Minor	□ Suspected
			■ **Possible**
			□ Unlikely

Effects MEFLOQUINE plasma concentrations may be elevated, increasing the pharmacologic effects and risk of adverse reactions.

Mechanism Inhibition of MEFLOQUINE metabolism (CYP3A4) by AZOLE ANTIFUNGAL AGENTS.

Management Avoid coadministration. KETOCONAZOLE should not be administered within 15 weeks of the last MEFLOQUINE dose due to the risk of potentially fatal QT interval prolongation.[1]

Discussion

The effect of ketoconazole on mefloquine plasma concentrations was studied in 8 healthy men.[2] Using an open-label, randomized, 2-phase, crossover design, each subject received a single oral dose of mefloquine 500 mg alone or with ketoconazole 400 mg daily for 10 days. Coadministration of mefloquine with ketoconazole increased the mefloquine AUC and C_{max} 79% and 64%, respectively, and prolonged the $t_{½}$ 39% (from approximately 323 to 448 hours) compared with mefloquine alone.

[1] *Lariam* [package insert]. Nutley, NJ: Roche Laboratories Inc; August 2009.

[2] Ridtitid W, et al. *J Clin Pharm Ther.* 2005;30(3):285.

* Asterisk indicates drugs cited in interaction reports. Based on pharmacologic and pharmacokinetic considerations, similar interactions may occur with other drugs that are listed.

Mefloquine — *Halofantrine*

Mefloquine* | Halofantrine*

Significance	Onset	Severity	Documentation
1	■ **Rapid**	■ **Major**	☐ Established
	☐ Delayed	☐ Moderate	☐ Probable
		☐ Minor	■ **Suspected**
			☐ Possible
			☐ Unlikely

Effects The risk of life-threatening cardiac arrhythmias may be increased.

Mechanism Possible additive prolongation of the QT interval.

Management Do not give HALOFANTRINE simultaneously with, or subsequent to, MEFLOQUINE.

Discussion

Halofantrine prolongs the QT interval at recommended therapeutic doses.[1] Serious ventricular arrhythmias, sometimes associated with sudden death, have been reported.[1] Data on the use of halofantrine subsequent to mefloquine suggest a potentially fatal prolongation of the QT interval of the ECG.[2] Therefore, halofantrine is not recommended for use in combination with, or subsequent to, mefloquine.[1,2]

The basis for this monograph is information on file with the manufacturers. Because of the seriousness of the cardiac problems, clinical evaluation of this interaction in humans is not likely to be forthcoming.

[1] *Halfan* [package insert]. Parsippany, NJ: SmithKline Beecham; August 1997.

[2] *Lariam* [package insert]. Nutley, NJ: Roche Laboratories; August 1994.

* Asterisk indicates drugs cited in interaction reports.

Mefloquine | **Metoclopramide**

Mefloquine*

Metoclopramide* (eg, *Reglan*)

Significance	Onset	Severity	Documentation
4	■ **Rapid** □ Delayed	□ Major ■ **Moderate** □ Minor	□ Established □ Probable □ Suspected ■ **Possible** □ Unlikely

Effects Serum MEFLOQUINE concentrations may be elevated, possibly increasing toxicity (cardiovascular, GI, CNS).

Mechanism Possible increased gastric emptying could increase the rate of MEFLOQUINE absorption in the small intestine.

Management Consider observing patients for increased MEFLOQUINE toxicity if METOCLOPRAMIDE is administered. If an interaction is suspected, decrease the dose of MEFLOQUINE.

Discussion

The effects of oral administration of metoclopramide 10 mg on the single-dose pharmacokinetics of oral mefloquine 750 mg were studied in 7 healthy men.[1] In the presence of metoclopramide, the apparent absorption $t_{1/2}$ of mefloquine decreased 25%, C_{max} increased 31%, and AUC in the first 24 hours increased 37%. However, there were no changes in the total AUC or the elimination $t_{1/2}$. Thus, metoclopramide increased the rate of mefloquine absorption but did not change the amount of absorption. There was no evidence of increased mefloquine toxicity.

[1] Na Bangchang K, et al. *Br J Clin Pharmacol.* 1991;32(5):640.

* Asterisk indicates drugs cited in interaction reports.

Meglitinides		***Cyclosporine***
Nateglinide (*Starlix*)	Repaglinide* (*Prandin*)	Cyclosporine* (eg, *Neoral*)

Significance	Onset	Severity	Documentation
2	☐ Rapid ■ **Delayed**	☐ Major ■ **Moderate** ☐ Minor	☐ Established ☐ Probable ■ **Suspected** ☐ Possible ☐ Unlikely

Effects MEGLITINIDE plasma concentrations and pharmacologic effects may be increased.

Mechanism CYCLOSPORINE may inhibit MEGLITINIDE metabolism (CYP3A4) and organic anion transporting polypeptide 1B1-mediated hepatic uptake.

Management In patients receiving MEGLITINIDES, carefully monitor blood glucose levels when starting or stopping CYCLOSPORINE. Be prepared to adjust the MEGLITINIDE dose as needed.

Discussion

The effects of cyclosporine on the pharmacokinetics and pharmacodynamics of repaglinide were studied in 12 healthy men.[1] Using a randomized, crossover design, each subject ingested cyclosporine 100 mg or placebo every 12 hours for 2 doses. One hour after the second dose, each subject received repaglinide 0.25 mg. Compared with placebo, cyclosporine increased the mean repaglinide plasma concentration 175% and the total AUC 244%. The amounts of unchanged repaglinide and its M2 and M4 metabolites excreted in the urine increased 2.7-, 7.5-, and 5-fold, respectively. In addition, cyclosporine decreased the ratio of M1 to repaglinide 62%. Cyclosporine did not affect the elimination $t_{1/2}$ or renal clearance of repaglinide or the amount of M1 excreted in the urine. The greatest increase in the blood glucose-lowering effect of repaglinide occurred in the subject with the greatest pharmacokinetic interaction. In vitro, cyclosporine inhibited formation of M1 and M2 but not M4.

[1] Kajosaari LI, et al. *Clin Pharmacol Ther.* 2005;78:388.

* Asterisk indicates drugs cited in interaction reports. Based on pharmacologic and pharmacokinetic considerations, similar interactions may occur with other drugs that are listed.

Meglitinides — **Food**

Nateglinide (*Starlix*)	Repaglinide* (*Prandin*)	Grapefruit Juice*

Significance	Onset	Severity	Documentation
4	■ **Rapid** □ Delayed	□ Major ■ **Moderate** □ Minor	□ Established □ Probable □ Suspected ■ **Possible** □ Unlikely

Effects Bioavailability of the MEGLITINIDE may be increased slightly.

Mechanism Metabolism (CYP3A4) of the MEGLITINIDE in the gut may be inhibited.

Management Until more data are available, advise patients to avoid coadministration of a MEGLITINIDE with GRAPEFRUIT JUICE. Caution patients to take the MEGLITINIDE with a liquid other than GRAPEFRUIT juice.

Discussion

The effect of grapefruit juice on the pharmacokinetics of repaglinide given at 2 different doses was studied in 36 healthy men.[1] Using a randomized, crossover design, each subject ingested 300 mL of water or grapefruit juice 2 hours before administration of a single dose of repaglinide 0.25 mg or 2 mg. Grapefruit juice caused a statistically significant ($P = 0.005$) increase in the mean AUC (19%), compared with water. There was no difference in blood glucose concentrations with or without grapefruit juice. The effect of grapefruit juice on the repaglinide AUC was greater at the low dose of repaglinide (ie, 0.25 mg) than at the therapeutic dose (ie, 2 mg).

Studies in patients with type 2 diabetes are needed to determine the clinical importance of this interaction.

[1] Bidstrup TB, et al. *Br J Clin Pharmacol.* 2005;61:49.

* Asterisk indicates drugs cited in interaction reports. Based on pharmacologic and pharmacokinetic considerations, similar interactions may occur with other drugs that are listed.

Meglitinides — Rifamycins

Nateglinide* (*Starlix*)	Repaglinide* (*Prandin*)	Rifabutin (*Mycobutin*) Rifampin* (eg, *Rifadin*)	Rifapentine (*Priftin*)

Significance	Onset	Severity	Documentation
2	□ Rapid ■ **Delayed**	□ Major ■ **Moderate** □ Minor	□ Established □ Probable ■ **Suspected** □ Possible □ Unlikely

Effects MEGLITINIDE plasma concentrations and pharmacologic effects may be decreased.

Mechanism RIFAMYCINS may increase metabolism (CYP3A4) of the MEGLITINIDE during the first-pass and elimination phases.

Management In patients receiving a MEGLITINIDE, closely monitor blood glucose levels when starting or stopping RIFAMYCIN therapy. Adjust the MEGLITINIDE dose as needed.

Discussion

The effects of rifampin on the pharmacokinetics and pharmacodynamics of repaglinide were studied in 9 healthy volunteers.[1] Using a randomized, 2-phase, crossover design, each subject was pretreated for 5 days with rifampin 600 mg or a matched placebo. On day 6, a single oral dose of repaglinide 0.5 mg was given. Compared with placebo, rifampin decreased the AUC of repaglinide 57% and C_{max} 41% (from 9.6 to 5.6 ng/mL) and shortened the $t_{½}$ 27% (from 1.5 to 1.1 hr). The range of the decrease in AUC and C_{max} was from 30% to 78% and 15% to 73%, respectively. In addition, rifampin reduced the blood glucose decremental AUC (0 to 3 hr) 76% and the maximum decrease in blood glucose concentration 38% (from 1.6 to 1 mmol/L). The decrease in repaglinide plasma levels resulted in an increase in blood glucose concentrations. However, smaller changes were reported in another study.[2] The AUC and C_{max} of repaglinide were reduced 31% and 26%, respectively. The effect of rifampin on the pharmacokinetics of nateglinide was studied in 10 volunteers.[3] The AUC of nateglinide was reduced 24% and the $t_{½}$ from 1.6 to 1.3 hr. No change in blood glucose levels was detected.

[1] Niemi M, et al. *Clin Pharmacol Ther.* 2000;68:495.
[2] Hatorp V, et al. *J Clin Pharmacol.* 2003;43:649.
[3] Niemi M, et al. *Br J Clin Pharmacol.* 2003;56:427.

* Asterisk indicates drugs cited in interaction reports. Based on pharmacologic and pharmacokinetic considerations, similar interactions may occur with other drugs that are listed.

Melatonin — **Caffeine**

Melatonin*	Caffeine*

Significance	Onset	Severity	Documentation
5	■ **Rapid** □ Delayed	□ Major □ Moderate ■ **Minor**	□ Established □ Probable □ Suspected ■ **Possible** □ Unlikely

Effects MELATONIN plasma concentrations may be elevated, increasing the effects (eg, drowsiness).

Mechanism Inhibition of MELATONIN first-pass metabolism (CYP1A2) by CAFFEINE is suspected.

Management Based on available data, no special precautions are necessary. Advise patients that drowsiness occurring with MELATONIN may be increased.

Discussion

The effect of caffeine on the pharmacokinetics of melatonin was investigated in 12 healthy subjects (6 smokers and 6 nonsmokers).[1] Each subject was given melatonin 6 mg alone and with 200 mg of caffeine 1 hr before and 1 and 3 hr after melatonin ingestion. Compared with taking melatonin alone, caffeine increased the C_{max} and AUC of melatonin 137% and 120%, respectively. The effect was more pronounced in nonsmokers compared with smokers.

[1] Härtter S, et al. *Br J Clin Pharmacol.* 2003;56:679.

* Asterisk indicates drugs cited in interaction reports.

Melatonin | **Fluvoxamine**

Melatonin* | Fluvoxamine*

Significance	Onset	Severity	Documentation
5	■ **Rapid**	□ Major	□ Established
	□ Delayed	□ Moderate	□ Probable
		■ **Minor**	□ Suspected
			■ **Possible**
			□ Unlikely

Effects Plasma concentrations of MELATONIN may be elevated, increasing the effects.

Mechanism FLUVOXAMINE inhibits the hepatic metabolism (CYP1A2) of MELATONIN.[1,2]

Management Based on available data, no special precautions are needed.

Discussion

Because fluvoxamine is known to elevate endogenous melatonin plasma concentrations, the effect of fluvoxamine on the pharmacokinetics of oral melatonin ingestion was studied in 5 healthy men.[3] One subject was a CYP2D6 poor metabolizer. On day 1 of the study, each subject received a single oral dose of melatonin 5 mg. One week later, all subjects ingested a single oral dose of fluvoxamine 50 mg at 7 AM and a single oral dose of melatonin 5 mg at 10 AM. Coadministration of fluvoxamine resulted in a 23-fold increase in the AUC and a 12-fold increase (from 2.18 to 25.1 ng/mL) in the peak plasma concentration of melatonin. The effect of fluvoxamine on melatonin pharmacokinetics was more pronounced and of longer duration in the CYP2D6 poor metabolizer. All subjects reported remarkable drowsiness after melatonin intake. The drowsiness was more pronounced with fluvoxamine coadministration. The effect of fluvoxamine on melatonin secretion could not be excluded.

[1] Härtter S, et al. *J Clin Psychopharmacol.* 2001;21:167.

[2] Facciolà G, et al. *Eur J Clin Pharmacol.* 2001;56:881.

[3] Härtter S, et al. *Clin Pharmacol Ther.* 2000;67:1.

* Asterisk indicates drugs cited in interaction reports.

Melphalan — *Interferon Alfa*

Melphalan* (*Alkeran*)	Interferon alfa-2a* (*Roferon A*)	Interferon alfa-2b* (*Intron A*)

Significance	Onset	Severity	Documentation
5	■ **Rapid** □ Delayed	□ Major □ Moderate ■ **Minor**	□ Established □ Probable □ Suspected ■ **Possible** □ Unlikely

Effects Serum MELPHALAN concentrations may be decreased.

Mechanism Possibly increased elimination of MELPHALAN because of INTERFERON ALFA-induced fever.

Management Based on available clinical data, no special precautions are needed.

Discussion

The pharmacokinetics of a single dose of melphalan 0.25 mg/kg administered alone or with interferon alfa 7 million units/m^2 given IM 5 hr prior to melphalan were studied in 10 patients with multiple myeloma.[1] The AUC, normalized to the dose and weight of the patient, was decreased by interferon (from an average of 1.66 to 1.44 mcg•hr/mL). This resulted from an apparent increase in the clearance as evidenced by a shorter $t_{½}$ in all patients. In addition, the AUC was correlated to body temperature, raising the possibility that the interaction is mediated through fever induced by interferon alfa administration. There was large interpatient variability in the AUC. In some cases, the variability was greater than the difference between pre- and post-interferon values. It is possible that the increase in body temperature may increase the alkylating action of melphalan, countering the possible reduction in activity from the decrease in the AUC. There are no clinical correlates for this interaction.

Additional studies are needed to confirm this possible interaction.

[1] Ehrsson H, et al. *Clin Pharmacol Ther.* 1990;47:86.

* Asterisk indicates drugs cited in interaction reports.

Meperidine — *Barbiturates*

Meperidine	Barbiturates	
Meperidine* (eg, *Demerol*)	Amobarbital (eg, *Amytal*)	Pentobarbital (eg, *Nembutal*)
	Aprobarbital (*Alurate*)	Phenobarbital*
	Butabarbital (eg, *Butisol*)	Primidone (eg, *Mysoline*)
	Butalbital	Secobarbital (eg, *Seconal*)
	Mephobarbital (*Mebaral*)	Talbutal (*Lotusate*)
	Metharbital (*Gemonil*)	

Significance	Onset	Severity	Documentation
5	■ **Rapid**	□ Major	□ Established
	□ Delayed	□ Moderate	□ Probable
		■ **Minor**	□ Suspected
			■ **Possible**
			□ Unlikely

Effects CNS depressant side effects of MEPERIDINE may be prolonged.

Mechanism The CNS depression of the combination appears to be additive.

Management Consider smaller doses of MEPERIDINE should an interaction be suspected.

Discussion

Stambaugh et al reported enhanced and prolonged sedation in a 31-year-old female receiving post-operative meperidine and phenobarbital for seizure prophylaxis. Additional evaluation revealed that phenobarbital stimulated the formation of normeperidine (a major meperidine metabolite).[1] Although the normeperidine production could account for these symptoms, it is usually regarded as a CNS stimulant, twice as potent as meperidine as a convulsive agent.[3]

In an investigation of 12 healthy subjects, 30 mg of phenobarbital 3 times daily for 14 days was associated with an increased clearance rate of meperidine and increased cumulative excretion of normeperidine.[2] Phenobarbital abused by a methadone maintenance patient was also associated with decreased methadone plasma levels and the onset of opiate withdrawal symptoms.[4]

Whether increased metabolism of meperidine is associated with clinically relevant symptoms is unclear. Consider dosage adjustment of meperidine if excessive sedation occurs.

[1] Stambaugh JE, et al. *Lancet.* 1977;1:398.
[2] Stambaugh JE, et al. *J Clin Pharmacol.* 1978;18:482.
[3] Mather LE, et al. *Clin Pharmacokinet.* 1978;3:352.
[4] Liu S-J, et al. *Am J Psychiatry.* 1984;141:1287.

* Asterisk indicates drugs cited in interaction reports. Based on pharmacologic and pharmacokinetic considerations, similar interactions may occur with other drugs that are listed.

Meperidine — *Furazolidone*

Meperidine* (eg, *Demerol*)	Furazolidone*†

Significance	Onset	Severity	Documentation
4	■ **Rapid**	■ **Major**	□ Established
	□ Delayed	□ Moderate	□ Probable
		□ Minor	□ Suspected
			■ **Possible**
			□ Unlikely

Effects Effects are difficult to characterize, but may include agitation, seizures, diaphoresis, fever, and progress to coma and apnea.

Mechanism Unknown.

Management Avoid this drug combination.

Discussion

Although case reports of an interaction are lacking, the serious nature of meperidine/ monoamine oxidase inhibitor toxicity warrants caution when coadministering these agents.[1] See Meperidine-Monoamine Oxidase Inhibitors.

Furazolidone possesses significant monoamine oxidase inhibitor activity[2] and the possibility of a similar interaction should dictate caution in administering meperidine. Should a strong analgesic be required within 2 weeks of discontinuing furazolidone, morphine is considered the drug of choice.[3]

[1] Goldberg LI. *JAMA*. 1964;190:456.
[2] Pettinger WA, et al. *Clin Pharmacol Ther*. 1968;9:442.
[3] Brown B, et al. *Br J Psychiatry*. 1987;151:210. Review.

* Asterisk indicates drugs cited in interaction reports.
† Not available in the United States.

Meperidine | **Hydantoins**

Meperidine* (eg, *Demerol*)	Ethotoin (*Peganone*)	Phenytoin* (eg, *Dilantin*)
	Fosphenytoin (*Cerebyx*)	

Significance	Onset	Severity	Documentation
5	□ Rapid	□ Major	□ Established
	■ **Delayed**	□ Moderate	□ Probable
		■ **Minor**	□ Suspected
			■ **Possible**
			□ Unlikely

Effects The therapeutic actions of MEPERIDINE may be reduced, while adverse reactions might be enhanced.

Mechanism PHENYTOIN appears to increase the metabolism of MEPERIDINE to normeperidine.

Management If unexpected adverse reactions appear, consider using an alternate analgesic.

Discussion

Phenytoin 300 mg/day administered for 10 days to 4 healthy young men increased meperidine clearance 25% and decreased the elimination $t_{1/2}$ of IV meperidine 33%. Phenytoin also increased the serum concentrations of normeperidine, a metabolite that has been associated with agitation, lethargy, and seizures.[1] Methadone metabolism increased, and withdrawal symptoms occurred in 5 men who enrolled in a methadone maintenance program and received phenytoin 300 mg/day for 6 days.[2]

More data are needed to determine the clinical importance of this possible interaction.

[1] Pond SM, et al. *Clin Pharmacol Ther.* 1981;30(5):680. [2] Tong TG, et al. *Ann Intern Med.* 1981;94(3):349.

* Asterisk indicates drugs cited in interaction reports. Based on pharmacologic and pharmacokinetic considerations, similar interactions may occur with other drugs that are listed.

Meperidine | **MAOIs**

Meperidine* (eg, *Demerol*)	Isocarboxazid (*Marplan*)	Rasagiline (*Azilect*)
	Linezolid* (*Zyvox*)	Selegiline* (eg, *Eldepryl*)
	Phenelzine* (*Nardil*)	Tranylcypromine* (eg, *Parnate*)

Significance	Onset	Severity	Documentation
1	■ **Rapid**	■ **Major**	□ Established
	□ Delayed	□ Moderate	■ **Probable**
		□ Minor	□ Suspected
			□ Possible
			□ Unlikely

Effects Coadministration may result in agitation, diaphoresis, fever, and seizures, which may progress to coma, apnea, and death. These reactions may occur several weeks following withdrawal of the MAOI.

Mechanism Unknown.

Management Coadministration of these agents is contraindicated.

Discussion

Because of the severity of this drug interaction, although unpredictable,[1] avoid meperidine administration in patients receiving MAOIs. Numerous case reports with various nonselective MAOIs, which included fatalities,[2] have established the importance of this interaction.[3-9] Symptoms were reversed in some instances with corticosteroids or chlorpromazine.[4,5] Although morphine (eg, *MS Contin*) may have caused a similar reaction in 1 case report,[10] it is considered the narcotic analgesic of choice in patients with a history of MAOI therapy.[11,12] A life-threatening reaction was reported in a patient receiving selegiline after meperidine was added to the treatment regimen.[13] Serotonin syndrome was reported in a 27-year-old man shortly after he started linezolid and meperidine.[14]

Administer other narcotic analgesics with caution. Information concerning the potential of this interaction with similar agents is limited.

[1] Evans-Prosser CD. *Br J Anaesth.* 1968;40(4):279.
[2] Goldberg LI. *JAMA.* 1964;190:456.
[3] Mitchell RS. *Ann Intern Med.* 1955;42(2):417.
[4] Papp C, et al. *Br Med J.* 1958;2(5103):1070.
[5] Shee JC. *Br Med J.* 1960;2(5197):507.
[6] Palmer H. *Br Med J.* 1960;2(5203):944.
[7] Denton PH, et al. *Br Med J.* 1962;2(5321):1752.
[8] Vigran IM. *JAMA.* 1964;187:953.
[9] Jounela AJ, et al. *N Engl J Med.* 1973;288(26):1411.
[10] Barry BJ. *Anaesth Intensive Care.* 1979;7(2):194.
[11] Browne B, et al. *Br J Psychiatry.* 1987;151:210.
[12] Rossiter A, et al. *Hosp Formul.* 1993;28:692.
[13] Zornberg GL, et al. *Lancet.* 1991;337(8735):246.
[14] Das PK, et al. *Clin Infect Dis.* 2008;46(2):264.

* Asterisk indicates drugs cited in interaction reports. Based on pharmacologic and pharmacokinetic considerations, similar interactions may occur with other drugs that are listed.

Meperidine — *Phenothiazines*

Meperidine* (eg, *Demerol*)	Chlorpromazine* (eg, *Thorazine*)

Significance	Onset	Severity	Documentation
2	■ **Rapid**	□ Major	□ Established
	□ Delayed	■ **Moderate**	■ **Probable**
		□ Minor	□ Suspected
			□ Possible
			□ Unlikely

Effects Excessive sedation and hypotension may occur with concurrent administration of PHENOTHIAZINES and MEPERIDINE.

Mechanism Additive CNS depressant and cardiovascular effects.

Management The benefit-to-risk ratio does not support administering this particular combination.

Discussion

Although uncontrolled observations have supported concurrent administration of these agents to minimize narcotic dosage and control nausea and vomiting,[1-3] serious additive adverse effects may outweigh the benefits.[5] In 1 study, respiratory depression was more severe and extended when meperidine plus chlorpromazine were administered concomitantly than with meperidine alone.[4] In a study of 10 healthy subjects, meperidine and chlorpromazine compared with meperidine and placebo resulted in increased lethargy and hypotension.[6] Lethargy appeared to correlate with increased excretion of normeperidine and normeperidinic acid. The importance of this finding is unclear because these metabolites are not known to cause CNS depression.

Because both meperidine and phenothiazines are known to cause CNS depression and orthostatic hypotension, additive effects appear to account for the adverse experiences described.

[1] Sadove MS, et al. *JAMA*. 1954;155:626.
[2] Jackson GL, et al. *Ann Intern Med*. 1956;45:640.
[3] Dundee JW. *Br J Anaesth*. 1957;29:28.
[4] Lambertsen CJ, et al. *J Pharmacol Exp Ther*. 1961;131:381.
[5] Hoffman JC, et al. *Anesthesiology*. 1970;32:325.
[6] Stambaugh JE, et al. *J Clin Pharmacol*. 1981;21:140.

* Asterisk indicates drugs cited in interaction reports.

Meperidine | ***Ritonavir***

Meperidine*
(eg, *Demerol*)

Ritonavir*
(eg, *Norvir*)

Significance	Onset	Severity	Documentation
2	☐ Rapid ■ **Delayed**	☐ Major ■ **Moderate** ☐ Minor	☐ Established ☐ Probable ■ **Suspected** ☐ Possible ☐ Unlikely

Effects Reduced MEPERIDINE and increased normeperidine serum levels may occur, possibly decreasing efficacy but increasing neurologic toxicity.

Mechanism RITONAVIR may enhance the metabolism of MEPERIDINE.

Management RITONAVIR is contraindicated in patients receiving MEPERIDINE.

Discussion

The manufacturer of ritonavir cautions that ritonavir is expected to produce large increases in meperidine plasma concentrations, increasing the risk of toxicity.[1] Toxic effects of meperidine include increased and decreased CNS side effects, seizures, and cardiac arrhythmias. A study of 8 healthy subjects found the opposite results.[2] Each subject received a single 50 mg oral meperidine dose before and after 10 days of ritonavir administration. Peak meperidine serum levels and area under the plasma concentration-time curve (AUC) decreased 56% and 67%, respectively. By contrast, normeperidine AUC increased 47%. These results suggest that ritonavir increases the metabolic conversion of meperidine to normeperidine.

The basis for this monograph is information on file with the manufacturer. Published clinical data are needed to further assess this interaction.

[1] Product Information. Ritonavir (*Norvir*). Abbott Laboratories. February 1996.

[2] Piscitelli SC, et al. *Pharmacotherapy*. 2000;20:549.

* Asterisk indicates drugs cited in interaction reports.

Mepivacaine — *Beta-Blockers*

Mepivacaine* (eg, *Carbocaine*)	Propranolol* (eg, *Inderal*)

Significance	Onset	Severity	Documentation
5	■ **Rapid**	□ Major	□ Established
	□ Delayed	□ Moderate	□ Probable
		■ **Minor**	□ Suspected
			■ **Possible**
			□ Unlikely

Effects MEPIVACAINE plasma concentrations may be elevated, increasing the pharmacologic and toxic effects.

Mechanism Inhibition of MEPIVACAINE metabolism (CYP1A2) by PROPRANOLOL and reduced hepatic blood flow are suspected.

Management In patients receiving PROPRANOLOL, administer MEPIVACAINE with caution and closely monitor the patient during the procedure and for 45 minutes following the MEPIVACAINE injection. Adjust the MEPIVACAINE dose as needed.

Discussion

The effect of propranolol on mepivacaine serum concentrations was studied in 10 patients undergoing dental scaling and root planing of maxillary molars.[1] Each subject was pretreated with oral propranolol 30 mg or placebo 2 hours prior to receiving a single dose of mepivacaine 51 mg for posterior superior alveolar nerve block. Compared with placebo, pretreatment with propranolol increased mepivacaine C_{max} from 1.214 to 2.249 mcg/mL. No signs of mepivacaine toxicity were noted. Mepivacaine pharmacodynamics were not affected. See Lidocaine-Beta-Blockers.

[1] Popescu SM, et al. *Oral Surg Oral Med Oral Pathol Oral Radiol Endod.* 2008;105(4):e19.

* Asterisk indicates drugs cited in interaction reports.

Metformin / *Acarbose*

Metformin	Acarbose
Metformin* (*Glucophage*)	Acarbose* (*Precose*)

Significance	Onset	Severity	Documentation
5	■ **Rapid**	□ Major	□ Established
	□ Delayed	□ Moderate	□ Probable
		■ **Minor**	□ Suspected
			■ **Possible**
			□ Unlikely

Effects The onset of the effects of METFORMIN may be delayed following the initial dose.

Mechanism ACARBOSE may delay the intestinal absorption of METFORMIN.

Management Based on available data, no special precautions are needed.

Discussion

The influence of acarbose (100 mg) on the bioavailability of metformin (1 g) was investigated in a randomized, placebo-controlled, double-blind, crossover study in 6 healthy male volunteers.[1] Acarbose administration reduced both the peak serum concentration of metformin and the area under the concentration-time curve (0 to 9 hours) 35% ($p < 0.05$). The 24-hour urinary excretion of metformin was not affected by acarbose administration. Thus, acarbose reduced the acute bioavailability of metformin, possibly by delaying intestinal absorption. The effect was most pronounced during the first 3 hours following coadministration of acarbose and metformin.

[1] Scheen AJ, et al. *Eur J Clin Invest.* 1994;24(suppl 3):50.

* Asterisk indicates drugs cited in interaction reports.

Metformin × *Anticholinergics*

Metformin	Anticholinergics	
Metformin* (*Glucophage*)	Atropine (eg, *Sal-Tropine*)	Methscopolamine (eg, *Pamine*)
	Belladonna	Orphenadrine (eg, *Norflex*)
	Benztropine (*Cogentin*)	Oxybutynin (*Ditropan*)
	Biperiden (*Akineton*)	Procyclidine (*Kemadrin*)
	Dicyclomine (eg, *Bentyl*)	Propantheline*
	Glycopyrrolate (eg, *Robinul*)	Scopolamine (eg, *Scopace*)
	Hyoscyamine (eg, *Anaspaz*)	Trihexyphenidyl (eg, *Artane*)
	Mepenzolate (*Cantil*)	

Significance	Onset	Severity	Documentation
5	■ **Rapid**	□ Major	□ Established
	□ Delayed	□ Moderate	□ Probable
		■ **Minor**	□ Suspected
			■ **Possible**
			□ Unlikely

Effects METFORMIN plasma levels may be elevated, increasing the pharmacologic and adverse effects.

Mechanism ANTICHOLINERGICS may slow GI motility, increasing absorption of METFORMIN from the small intestine.

Management In patients receiving METFORMIN, observe the clinical response when starting or stopping ANTICHOLINERGICS. Be prepared to adjust the dose of METFORMIN.

Discussion

The effects of altered gastric emptying and GI motility, induced by metoclopramide (eg, *Reglan*) and propantheline, on the absorption of metformin were studied in 11 healthy volunteers.[1] In an open-label, 3-treatment, 3-period crossover investigation, each subject received metformin 550 mg alone, 5 minutes after a 10 mg IV dose of metoclopramide, and 30 minutes after a 30 mg oral dose of propantheline. Giving metoclopramide before metformin did not affect the disposition of metformin. However, pretreatment with propantheline increased the area under the plasma concentration-time curve of metformin 19% and increased the amount of metformin excreted unchanged in the urine 26%. Propantheline slowed gastric emptying and extended the mean time to empty 50% of radiolabeled metformin from the stomach. No serious side effects were reported in any of the treatment groups.

[1] Marathe PH, et al. *Br J Clin Pharmacol.* 2000;50:325.

* Asterisk indicates drugs cited in interaction reports. Based on pharmacologic and pharmacokinetic considerations, similar interactions may occur with other drugs that are listed.

Metformin — *Cimetidine*

Metformin* (eg, *Glucophage*)	Cimetidine* (eg, *Tagamet*)

Significance	Onset	Severity	Documentation
4	■ **Rapid**	□ Major	□ Established
	□ Delayed	■ **Moderate**	□ Probable
		□ Minor	□ Suspected
			■ **Possible**
			□ Unlikely

Effects Serum concentrations of METFORMIN may be elevated, increasing the pharmacologic effects.

Mechanism CIMETIDINE reduces the renal clearance of METFORMIN by inhibiting renal tubular secretion.

Management Carefully monitor patients. It may be necessary to decrease or increase the dose of METFORMIN when CIMETIDINE therapy is started or stopped.

Discussion

The effect of cimetidine on the pharmacokinetics of metformin was studied in 7 healthy subjects.[1] Each subject received metformin 250 mg once daily for 10 days and cimetidine 400 mg twice daily between days 6 and 10. Cimetidine increased peak serum concentrations of metformin 81% ($P < 0.008$) and the AUC 50% ($P < 0.008$). There was no difference in the time required to reach peak metformin serum concentrations. Cimetidine reduced the average renal clearance of metformin 27%, with the effect being time-dependent and significant up to 6 hours after cimetidine administration. The effects of the increased metformin concentrations were noted in the biochemical consequences to metformin (eg, increased lactate/pyruvate ratio). Metformin had negligible effects on the pharmacokinetics of cimetidine.

[1] Somogyi A, et al. *Br J Clin Pharmacol.* 1987;23:545.

* Asterisk indicates drugs cited in interaction reports.

Metformin — *Guar Gum*

Metformin* (eg, *Glucophage*)	Guar Gum*

Significance	Onset	Severity	Documentation
5	■ **Rapid** □ Delayed	□ Major □ Moderate ■ **Minor**	□ Established □ Probable □ Suspected ■ **Possible** □ Unlikely

Effects The hypoglycemic effects of METFORMIN may be decreased.

Mechanism GUAR GUM decreases the absorption of METFORMIN.

Management Based upon available data, no special precautions are needed. In patients receiving large doses of GUAR GUM, monitor the clinical response and adjust the dose as needed.

Discussion

Guar gum is a dietary fiber used as a thickening agent in food and medicinals.[1] Although not labeled for these uses, in large doses (eg, 10 to 15 g/day), guar gum has been shown to decrease serum total cholesterol, LDL levels, and postprandial glucose and insulin levels. The effects of guar gum on metformin 1,700 mg were studied in 6 healthy subjects.[2] When compared with a meal consisting of carbohydrate 35 g, mean serum metformin concentrations were decreased between 1.5 and 5 hours after ingesting guar gum 10 g. The metformin AUC decreased 39%. Guar gum decreased the absorption rate of metformin over the first 6 hours after coadministration.

[1] DerMarderosian A, ed. Guar Gum. In: *The Review of Natural Products*. St. Louis, MO: Facts and Comparisons; 1993.

[2] Gin H, et al. *Horm Metab Res*. 1989;21:81.

* Asterisk indicates drugs cited in interaction reports.

Metformin | **Iodinated Contrast Materials, Parenteral**

Metformin*
(eg, *Glucophage*)

Iodinated Contrast Materials, Parenteral* (eg, Iothalamate "*Cysto-Conray*")

Significance	Onset	Severity	Documentation
1	■ **Rapid**	■ **Major**	□ Established
	□ Delayed	□ Moderate	□ Probable
		□ Minor	■ **Suspected**
			□ Possible
			□ Unlikely

Effects Increased risk of METFORMIN-induced lactic acidosis.

Mechanism IODINATED CONTRAST MATERIAL–induced renal failure can interfere with the renal elimination of METFORMIN.

Management Coadministration of parenteral IODINATED CONTRAST MATERIALS and METFORMIN is contraindicated. Temporarily stop METFORMIN therapy.

Discussion

Although not a drug interaction, metformin administration is contraindicated in patients who are going to receive parenteral iodinated contrast materials.[1] These materials can lead to acute renal failure, particularly in diabetic patients, and have been associated with lactic acidosis in patients receiving metformin. These reactions were attributed to accumulation of high blood concentrations of metformin resulting from impairment of the renal clearance of metformin during acute renal failure.[2] Metformin does not undergo hepatic metabolism or biliary excretion and is excreted unchanged in the urine. Isolated case reports have been documented.[2] One study found that nearly 4% of patients with diabetes mellitus and normal renal function developed contrast material–associated neuropathy.[3] In addition, about 8% of patients with diabetes mellitus who were receiving metformin and whose baseline serum creatinine levels were below 1.5 mg/dL had an increased risk of lactic acidosis, requiring the withholding of metformin beyond 48 hours after IV contrast material administration. If a radiologic study involving the use of iodinated contrast materials (eg, IV urogram, IV cholangiography, angiography, scans with contrast materials) is planned, withhold metformin therapy at the time of, prior to, and for 48 hours after the procedure. Metformin administration may be reinstated only after renal function has been reevaluated and found to be normal.[1]

[1] *Glucophage* [package insert]. Princeton, NJ: Bristol-Myers Squibb Company; March 2004.
[2] Dachman AH. *Radiology*. 1995;197(2):545.
[3] Parra D, et al. *Pharmacotherapy*. 2004;24(8):987.

* Asterisk indicates drugs cited in interaction reports.

Methadone — *Barbiturates*

Methadone	Barbiturates	
Methadone* (eg, *Dolophine*)	Amobarbital	Phenobarbital* (eg, *Luminal*)
	Butabarbital (eg, *Butisol*)	Primidone (eg, *Mysoline*)
	Butalbital (eg, *Florinal*)	Secobarbital (*Seconal*)
	Pentobarbital* (*Nembutal*)	

Significance	Onset	Severity	Documentation
2	☐ Rapid	☐ Major	☐ Established
	■ **Delayed**	■ **Moderate**	☐ Probable
		☐ Minor	■ **Suspected**
			☐ Possible
			☐ Unlikely

Effects The actions of METHADONE may be reduced. Patients receiving long-term METHADONE treatment may experience opiate withdrawal symptoms.

Mechanism Unknown. Possibly caused by increased hepatic metabolism of METHADONE by BARBITURATES.

Management A higher dose of METHADONE may be required during coadministration of BARBITURATES.

Discussion

In 1 case, a 28-year-old former heroin addict maintained on methadone 95 mg/day experienced opiate withdrawal symptoms and later admitted to the abuse of phenobarbital for the previous month.[1] Symptoms seemed to correlate with lower mean trough plasma methadone concentrations and mean peak plasma methadone concentrations. Six weeks after discontinuing the barbiturate abuse, methadone plasma concentrations had increased to their original level. The patient reported feeling good. In a study of 43 heroin addicts in a methadone maintenance program, 5 patients also admitted to the abuse of barbiturates.[2] The patients' methadone levels were less than 100 ng/mL. Although they had no signs of withdrawal, they performed poorly in the program. Four of the patients were subsequently detoxified from barbiturates or ceased abuse on their own. All patients had increased serum methadone concentrations. One patient exhibited methadone toxicity.

[1] Liu SJ, et al. *Am J Psychiatry*. 1984;141(10):1287.

[2] Bell J, et al. *Clin Pharmacol Ther*. 1988;43(6):623.

* Asterisk indicates drugs cited in interaction reports. Based on pharmacologic and pharmacokinetic considerations, similar interactions may occur with other drugs that are listed.

Methadone — *Carbamazepine*

Methadone* (eg, *Dolophine*)	Carbamazepine* (eg, *Tegretol*)

Significance	Onset	Severity	Documentation
5	☐ Rapid ■ **Delayed**	☐ Major ☐ Moderate ■ **Minor**	☐ Established ☐ Probable ☐ Suspected ■ **Possible** ☐ Unlikely

Effects The pharmacologic effects of METHADONE may be decreased. Patients receiving METHADONE in maintenance programs for narcotic abuse may experience withdrawal symptoms.

Mechanism Increased hepatic metabolism of METHADONE is suspected.

Management A higher METHADONE dose may be required in patients receiving CARBAMAZEPINE concurrently.

Discussion

Trough plasma methadone levels were measured in 43 heroin-addicted patients complaining of withdrawal symptoms.[1] Low methadone serum levels were documented in 10 patients who were taking an enzyme-inducing drug. Four patients were taking phenobarbital, 5 patients were receiving phenytoin (eg, *Dilantin*), and 1 patient was taking carbamazepine. (See also Methadone-Barbiturates and Methadone-Hydantoins.)

Controlled clinical studies are needed to determine the importance of this possible interaction.

[1] Bell J, et al. *Clin Pharmacol Ther.* 1988;43(6):623.

* Asterisk indicates drugs cited in interaction reports.

Methadone — Fluvoxamine

Methadone* (eg, *Dolophine*)	Fluvoxamine* (eg, *Luvox*)

Significance	Onset	Severity	Documentation
2	☐ Rapid	☐ Major	☐ Established
	■ **Delayed**	■ **Moderate**	☐ Probable
		☐ Minor	■ **Suspected**
			☐ Possible
			☐ Unlikely

Effects Increased serum METHADONE concentrations with possible toxicity.

Mechanism FLUVOXAMINE may inhibit the hepatic metabolism of METHADONE.

Management Start and stop FLUVOXAMINE therapy with caution in patients receiving METHADONE maintenance treatment.

Discussion

In 5 patients with affective disorders who were receiving methadone maintenance treatment for opiate addiction, addition of fluvoxamine 50 to 250 mg/day produced a 20% to 100% increase in methadone plasma concentration-to-dose ratios.[1] Symptoms of opioid intoxication occurred in 1 patient during coadministration of both drugs, while withdrawal symptoms were experienced by another patient within 5 days of stopping fluvoxamine. This report indicates that it may take 2 to 3 weeks for the interaction to be detectable. Respiratory depression developed in a 28-year-old woman receiving methadone 70 mg/day after 3 weeks of fluvoxamine 100 mg/day.[2] It was necessary to decrease the methadone dose to 50 mg/day. A 38-year-old woman experienced heroin withdrawal symptoms despite a high methadone dose (ie, 200 mg/day).[3] Methadone levels were low or undetectable. Fluvoxamine therapy was added to increase methadone levels. Her withdrawal symptoms disappeared within 1 week and her methadone levels increased, causing the patient to be oversedated.

[1] Bertschy G, et al. *Ther Drug Monit.* 1994;16(1):42.
[2] Alderman CP, et al. *Aust N Z J Psychiatry.* 1999;33(1):99.
[3] DeMaria PA, et al. *J Addict Dis.* 1999;18(4):5.

* Asterisk indicates drugs cited in interaction reports.

Methadone — *Food*

Methadone*
(eg, *Dolophine*)

Grapefruit Juice*

Significance	Onset	Severity	Documentation
4	☐ Rapid	☐ Major	☐ Established
	■ **Delayed**	■ **Moderate**	☐ Probable
		☐ Minor	☐ Suspected
			■ **Possible**
			☐ Unlikely

Effects METHADONE serum concentrations may be elevated, increasing the pharmacologic effects and adverse reactions.

Mechanism GRAPEFRUIT JUICE may inhibit METHADONE metabolism (CYP3A4) in the small intestine.

Management Until more clinical data are available, avoid coadministration of METHADONE with GRAPEFRUIT products. Advise patients to take METHADONE with a liquid other than GRAPEFRUIT JUICE.

Discussion

The effects of grapefruit juice ingestion on the steady-state pharmacokinetics of methadone were studied in 8 patients undergoing maintenance treatment.[1] For 5 days, subjects ingested 200 mL of water approximately 30 minutes before methadone intake and again 30 minutes later with methadone. After a 2-week washout period, the same subjects ingested regular-strength grapefruit juice 120 mL approximately 30 minutes before taking methadone and again 30 minutes later with methadone. Compared with water, administration of methadone with grapefruit juice increased the mean AUC of methadone 17%. There were similar increases in peak concentrations and decreases in apparent clearance of methadone. There was a considerable range in effect among the patients. Time to peak levels, terminal $t_{1/2}$, and apparent volume of distribution were not affected. No symptoms of overmedication were reported by patients or observed by investigators. In another study, grapefruit juice decreased the methadone metabolite/methadone AUC ratio after oral administration of methadone, but had no effect on methadone plasma levels.[2]

[1] Benmebarek M, et al. *Clin Pharmacol Ther.* 2004;76(1):55.

[2] Kharasch ED, et al. *Clin Pharmacol Ther.* 2004;76(3):250.

* Asterisk indicates drugs cited in interaction reports.

Methadone — *Hydantoins*

Methadone* (eg, *Dolophine*)	Ethotoin (*Peganone*) Fosphenytoin	Phenytoin* (eg, *Dilantin*)

Significance	Onset	Severity	Documentation
2	☐ Rapid ■ **Delayed**	☐ Major ■ **Moderate** ☐ Minor	☐ Established ☐ Probable ■ **Suspected** ☐ Possible ☐ Unlikely

Effects The actions of METHADONE may be reduced. Patients receiving long-term METHADONE treatment may experience withdrawal symptoms.

Mechanism HYDANTOINS appear to increase the metabolic clearance of METHADONE.

Management A higher dose of METHADONE may be required during coadministration of HYDANTOINS.

Discussion

A case report described the onset of narcotic withdrawal symptoms in a 46-year-old former heroin addict treated with phenytoin for traumatic neuropathy.[1] Symptoms improved with the same dose of methadone 3 to 4 days following phenytoin discontinuation. In a methadone treatment program, serum methadone concentrations were low in 4 patients also taking phenytoin.[2] Three of these patients had recently started phenytoin and were experiencing signs of opiate withdrawal. A controlled study evaluated 5 men in a methadone maintenance program. Phenytoin 300 mg/day was administered for 4 days.[3] Opiate withdrawal symptoms occurred by day 3 or 4 in all subjects. These withdrawal symptoms were associated with decreases of more than 50% in trough methadone concentrations and AUC during phenytoin therapy.

[1] Finelli PF. *N Engl J Med.* 1976;294(4):227.
[2] Bell J, et al. *Clin Pharmacol Ther.* 1988;43(6):623.
[3] Tong TG, et al. *Ann Intern Med.* 1981;94(3):349.

* Asterisk indicates drugs cited in interaction reports. Based on pharmacologic and pharmacokinetic considerations, similar interactions may occur with other drugs that are listed.

Methadone — *MAOIs*

Methadone* (eg, *Dolophine*)	Rasagiline* (*Azilect*)	Selegiline* (eg, *Emsam*)

Significance	Onset	Severity	Documentation
1	☐ Rapid ■ **Delayed**	■ **Major** ☐ Moderate ☐ Minor	☐ Established ☐ Probable ■ **Suspected** ☐ Possible ☐ Unlikely

Effects The risk of life-threatening adverse reactions, including serotonin syndrome, may be increased.

Mechanism Unknown.

Management Coadministration of METHADONE and RASAGILINE or SELEGILINE is contraindicated.[1,2] After stopping treatment with METHADONE, allow at least 7 days to elapse before starting therapy with SELEGILINE.[2] At least 14 days should elapse between discontinuing RASAGILINE and starting treatment with METHADONE.[1]

Discussion

Severe adverse reactions may occur when methadone and rasagiline or selegiline are given concurrently.[1,2] Serious and sometimes fatal CNS toxicity, including serotonin syndrome, has been reported with coadministration of selegiline with certain other drugs, including narcotic analgesics.[2] Serotonin syndrome is characterized by agitation, altered consciousness, ataxia, myoclonus, overactive reflexes, and shivering. Because of the risk of life-threatening adverse reactions, selegiline or rasagiline should not be used in combination with methadone.[1,2]

[1] *Azilect* [package insert]. North Wales, PA: Teva Pharmaceuticals; December 2009.

[2] *Emsam* [package insert]. Tampa, FL: Somerset Pharmaceuticals; June 2007.

* Asterisk indicates drugs cited in interaction reports.

Methadone	**Narcotic Agonists-Antagonists**	
Methadone* (eg, *Dolophine*)	Buprenorphine (eg, *Buprenex*) Butorphanol	Nalbuphine*

Significance	Onset	Severity	Documentation
2	■ **Rapid** □ Delayed	□ Major ■ **Moderate** □ Minor	□ Established □ Probable ■ **Suspected** □ Possible □ Unlikely

Effects NARCOTIC AGONISTS-ANTAGONISTS may decrease or potentiate the pharmacologic effects of METHADONE.

Mechanism NARCOTIC AGONISTS-ANTAGONISTS potentiate or block the effect of METHADONE by competitively binding with opiate receptors.

Management Closely monitor patients receiving METHADONE for withdrawal symptoms or an increase in METHADONE action (eg, increased adverse reactions) when starting or stopping a NARCOTIC AGONIST-ANTAGONIST. Adjust the METHADONE dosage as needed.

Discussion

In patients receiving short-term methadone administration, the effect of nalbuphine is expected to be additive or agonistic with methadone, possibly warranting a dose reduction in either or both drugs. In contrast, in patients receiving long-term methadone therapy (eg, methadone maintenance), the effect of nalbuphine is expected to be antagonistic, precipitating withdrawal symptoms.[1] The subjective, physiologic, and behavioral effects of nalbuphine were studied in 5 methadone-dependent men.[2] Each subject was stabilized on methadone 30 mg/day for at least 14 days. Escalating doses of IM nalbuphine (0.75, 1.5, 3, and 6 mg) were administered to each subject. The ascending dose series was stopped whenever a subject's reaction was so intense that he threatened to discontinue participation in the study or the investigator judged it unethical to administer higher doses. In methadone-dependent subjects, nalbuphine increased systolic and diastolic BP, decreased skin temperature, and increased pupil diameter. Nalbuphine administration did not result in any effect on psychomotor or cognitive performance measurements. Nalbuphine increased the observer-rated Adjective Rating Scale for Withdrawal and total Himmelsbach Item Scale scores, which measured opioid abstinence signs and symptoms. There was no evidence that nalbuphine produced any opioid agonist-like effects in the methadone-dependent subjects.

[1] *Nubain* [package insert]. Chadds Ford, PA: Endo Pharmaceuticals; January 2005.

[2] Preston KL, et al. *J Pharmacol Exp Ther.* 1989;248(3):929.

* Asterisk indicates drugs cited in interaction reports. Based on pharmacologic and pharmacokinetic considerations, similar interactions may occur with other drugs that are listed.

Methadone | **NNRT Inhibitors**

Methadone* (eg, *Dolophine*) | Efavirenz* (*Sustiva*) | Nevirapine* (eg, *Viramune*)

Significance	Onset	Severity	Documentation
2	☐ Rapid ■ **Delayed**	☐ Major ■ **Moderate** ☐ Minor	☐ Established ■ **Probable** ☐ Suspected ☐ Possible ☐ Unlikely

Effects METHADONE action may be reduced, resulting in opiate withdrawal symptoms.

Mechanism Increased METHADONE hepatic metabolism (CYP2B6 and CYP3A4).[1]

Management Anticipate an increase in the METHADONE dose when starting treatment with an NNRT INHIBITOR. Monitor patients for opiate withdrawal symptoms during cotherapy. Monitor for signs of METHADONE overdose if the NNRT INHIBITOR is discontinued. Adjust the METHADONE dose as needed.

Discussion

Opiate withdrawal symptoms have been reported in patients receiving methadone after starting treatment with efavirenz or nevirapine.[2-8] In 1 patient, withdrawal symptoms persisted despite an increase in the methadone dose.[2] It was necessary to discontinue efavirenz or nevirapine for the symptoms to resolve. Opiate withdrawal symptoms have occurred as soon as 2 days[2] and as long as 28 days[6] after starting nevirapine or efavirenz.[2-7] In the cases presented, it was necessary to increase the methadone dose 13% to 133% to control or resolve withdrawal symptoms.[3-7,9-11]Coadministration of methadone and efavirenz or nevirapine has resulted in a decrease of approximately 50% in the AUC[1,6,8-10] and peak concentration[6] of methadone. The degree of induction of methadone metabolism by nevirapine is similar with administration of nevirapine 200 mg once daily, compared with 400 mg once daily.[10]

1 Kharasch ED, et al. *Clin Pharmacol Ther.* 2012;91(4):673.
2 Pinzani V, et al. *Ann Pharmacother.* 2000;34(3):405.
3 Altice FL, et al. *AIDS.* 1999;13(8):957.
4 Otero MJ, et al. *AIDS.* 1999;13(8):1004.
5 Marzolini C, et al. *AIDS.* 2000;14(9):1291.
6 Boffito M, et al. *AIDS Res Hum Retroviruses.* 2002;18(5):341.
7 Clarke SM, et al. *Br J Clin Pharmacol.* 2001;51(3):213.
8 Clarke SM, et al. *Clin Infect Dis.* 2001;33(9):1595.
9 Stocker H, et al. *Antimicrob Agents Chemother.* 2004;48(11):4148.
10 Arroyo E, et al. *Eur J Clin Pharmacol.* 2007;63(7):669.
11 Tossonian HK, et al. *J Acquir Immune Defic Syndr.* 2007;45(3):324.

* Asterisk indicates drugs cited in interaction reports.

Methadone — *Peginterferon Alfa-2b*

Methadone* (eg, *Dolophine*)	Peginterferon Alfa-2b* (eg, *Peg-Intron*)

Significance	Onset	Severity	Documentation
5	☐ Rapid ■ **Delayed**	☐ Major ☐ Moderate ■ **Minor**	☐ Established ☐ Probable ☐ Suspected ■ **Possible** ☐ Unlikely

Effects METHADONE plasma concentrations may be increased slightly.

Mechanism Inhibition of METHADONE metabolism by PEGINTERFERON ALFA-2B is suspected.

Management Based on available data, no special precautions are necessary.

Discussion

The effects of peginterferon alfa-2b on the pharmacokinetics of methadone were evaluated in 19 adults with hepatitis C virus infection who were enrolled in a methadone maintenance program.[1] In an open-label investigation, each subject received oral methadone 40 mg/day and subcutaneous peginterferon alfa-2b 1.5 mcg/kg/wk. Before the first dose and after the fourth dose (day 23) of peginterferon alfa-2b, methadone serial blood samples were collected. Following administration of peginterferon alfa-2b, exposure to methadone was increased approximately 15%. The magnitude of the increase in methadone exposure is not expected to be clinically important.

[1] Gupta SK, et al. *J Clin Pharmacol.* 2007;47(5):604.

* Asterisk indicates drugs cited in interaction reports.

Methadone — *Protease Inhibitors*

Methadone	Protease Inhibitors	
Methadone* (eg, *Dolophine*)	Darunavir* (*Prezista*)	Nelfinavir* (*Viracept*)
	Lopinavir/Ritonavir* (*Kaletra*)	Ritonavir* (*Norvir*)

Significance	Onset	Severity	Documentation
2	☐ Rapid	☐ Major	☐ Established
	■ **Delayed**	■ **Moderate**	☐ Probable
		☐ Minor	■ **Suspected**
			☐ Possible
			☐ Unlikely

Effects The pharmacologic effects of METHADONE may be decreased. Patients receiving METHADONE maintenance treatment may experience opiate withdrawal symptoms.

Mechanism Increased hepatic metabolism and renal clearance of METHADONE.

Management Closely observe patients receiving METHADONE for withdrawal symptoms when starting certain PROTEASE INHIBITORS. Increase the METHADONE dose as needed. If the PROTEASE INHIBITOR is stopped, METHADONE levels may increase, necessitating a decrease in the METHADONE dose.

Discussion

The safety of methadone 50 to 120 mg/day maintenance treatment was assessed in 10 patients seropositive for HIV and receiving protease inhibitors.[1] Adding nelfinavir in 2 patients and ritonavir in 1 patient decreased the steady-state levels of methadone 40% to 50%. When indinavir (*Crixivan*) was started in 6 patients and saquinavir (*Invirase*) in 1 patient, methadone levels were unchanged. A 51-year-old man with HIV receiving methadone maintenance therapy experienced methadone withdrawal after ritonavir, saquinavir, and stavudine (eg, *Zerit*) were added to his treatment regimen.[2] It is likely that ritonavir precipitated opiate withdrawal. A controlled study of 12 HIV-negative volunteers evaluated the effect of ritonavir on the pharmacokinetics of R- or S-methadone given orally or IV.[3] Ritonavir increased the renal clearance and hepatic methadone N-demethylation 40% to 50% and 50% to 80%, respectively, despite more than a 70% inhibition of intestinal and hepatic CYP3A by ritonavir.[3,4] Adding lopinavir/ritonavir to a stable methadone regimen resulted in an average reduction of 36% in the methadone AUC in 8 patients.[5] In 4 other studies of patients on methadone maintenance treatment, atazanavir,[6] fosamprenavir/ritonavir,[7] nelfinavir,[8] and darunavir/ritonavir[9] administration decreased plasma levels of the active and inactive methadone enantiomers. However, no patient showed signs of methadone withdrawal or required methadone dose adjustments.[5,7,9-11] Similarly, no withdrawal occurred in 18 patients receiving methadone maintenance after the addition of lopinavir/ritonavir.[10] In a 53-year-old woman infected with HIV, discontinuation of lopinavir/ritonavir was associated with an increase in methadone level, prolongation of the QT interval, and development of torsades de pointes.[12] Other risk factors contributing to the development of torsades were present. Patients starting atazanavir (*Reyataz*) with or without ritonavir or lopinavir/ritonavir required no adjustment in methadone dosage.[13] In 12 patients on stable methadone treatment studied before and after 14 days of saquinavir 1,600 mg/day plus ritonavir 100 mg/day, the pharmacokinetics of the R- and S-enantiomers of methadone were unchanged.[11] Similarly, no changes were seen in methadone levels in healthy volunteers receiving indinavir[14] or ritonavir plus indinavir.[15]

1 Beauverie P, et al. *AIDS*. 1998;12(18):2510.
2 Geletko SM, et al. *Pharmacotherapy*. 2000;20(1):93.
3 Kharasch ED, et al. *Clin Pharmacol Ther*. 2008;84(4):497.
4 Kharasch ED, et al. *Clin Pharmacol Ther*. 2008;84(4):506.
5 Clarke S, et al. *Clin Infect Dis*. 2002;34(8):1143.
6 Hsyu PH, et al. *Biopharm Drug Dispos*. 2006;27(2):61.
7 Cao YJ, et al. *Pharmacotherapy*. 2008;28(7):863.
8 Friedland G, et al. *AIDS*. 2005;19(15):1635.
9 Sekar VS, et al. *J Clin Pharmacol*. 2011;51(2):271.
10 Stevens RC, et al. *J Acquir Immune Defic Syndr*. 2003;33(5):650.
11 Shelton MJ, et al. *J Clin Pharmacol*. 2004;44(3):293.
12 Lüthi B, et al. *Eur J Clin Microbiol Infect Dis*. 2007;26(5):367.
13 Tossonian HK, et al. *J Aquir Immune Defic Syndr*. 2007;45(3):324.
14 Kharasch ED, et al. *Anesthesiology*. 2012;116(2):432.
15 Kharasch ED, et al. *Anesthesiology*. 2009;110(3):660.

* Asterisk indicates drugs cited in interaction reports.

Methadone — *Quetiapine*

Methadone* (eg, *Dolophine*) | Quetiapine* (*Seroquel*)

Significance	Onset	Severity	Documentation
4	☐ Rapid	☐ Major	☐ Established
	■ **Delayed**	■ **Moderate**	☐ Probable
		☐ Minor	☐ Suspected
			■ **Possible**
			☐ Unlikely

Effects METHADONE plasma levels may be elevated, increasing the pharmacologic effects and adverse reactions.

Mechanism Inhibition of METHADONE metabolism (CYP2D6) by QUETIAPINE is suspected.

Management In patients receiving METHADONE, monitor the clinical status when starting or stopping QUETIAPINE. Be prepared to adjust the METHADONE dose as needed.

Discussion

The effects of quetiapine on steady-state plasma concentrations of methadone were evaluated in 14 patients on methadone maintenance treatment.[1] Patients were receiving methadone for at least 1 month, with an unchanged dose for at least 7 days, prior to the start of quetiapine (mean dose, 138 mg/day). Quetiapine administration resulted in mean increases in (R)-methadone (the active methadone isomer) concentration/dose ratios of 7%, 21%, and 30% in CYP2D6 poor metabolizers, heterozygous extensive metabolizers (EMs), and homozygous EMs, respectively. No signs of overmedication with the increased methadone plasma levels were reported by the staff or patients.

[1] Uehlinger C, et al. *J Clin Psychopharmacol.* 2007;27(3):273.

* Asterisk indicates drugs cited in interaction reports.

Methadone — *Quinolones*

Methadone	Quinolones	
Methadone* (eg, *Dolophine*)	Ciprofloxacin* (eg, *Cipro*)	Moxifloxacin* (*Avelox*)
	Gatifloxacin* (*Zymar*)	Norfloxacin (*Noroxin*)
	Levofloxacin* (eg, *Levaquin*)	

Significance	Onset	Severity	Documentation
1	□ Rapid	■ **Major**	□ Established
	■ **Delayed**	□ Moderate	□ Probable
		□ Minor	■ **Suspected**
			□ Possible
			□ Unlikely

Effects METHADONE plasma levels may be elevated by CIPROFLOXACIN and NORFLOXACIN, increasing pharmacologic effects and adverse reactions. Coadministration of METHADONE and GATIFLOXACIN, LEVOFLOXACIN, or MOXIFLOXACIN may increase the risk of life-threatening cardiac arrhythmias, including torsades de pointes.

Mechanism Inhibition of METHADONE metabolism (CYP1A2 and 3A4). Possible additive prolongation of the QT interval with METHADONE and certain QUINOLONES. In addition, METHADONE inhibits cardiac potassium channels.

Management Carefully monitor the clinical response to METHADONE when certain QUINOLONES are started or stopped. Consider alternative therapy with a QUINOLONE antibiotic that does not prolong the QT interval. If coadministration cannot be avoided, closely monitor CV status, including QT interval prolongation, especially in patients with a history of cardiac conduction abnormalities, increased risk of cardiac dysrhythmia, or risk of hypokalemia or hypomagnesemia.

Discussion

A 42-year-old woman was treated successfully for pain with oral methadone 140 mg/day for longer than 6 yr.[1] Two days after starting ciprofloxacin 750 mg twice daily, the patient became sedated and confused, and her hospital stay was extended. Trimethoprim/sulfamethoxazole (eg, *Bactrim*) was substituted for ciprofloxacin, and the patient's symptoms reversed within 48 hr. On 3 other occasions while receiving methadone, the patient became sedated when ciprofloxacin was administered for urinary tract infections. Following the first administration, the patient's sedation reversed after stopping ciprofloxacin. During the last administration, sedation was accompanied by respiratory depression, which reversed with administration of naloxone (eg, *Narcan*). Use extreme caution when giving methadone with drugs known to prolong the QT interval.[2] See Appendix: Drug-Induced Prolongation of the QT Interval and Torsades de Pointes.

[1] Herrlin K, et al. *Lancet.* 2000;356(9247):2069.

[2] *Dolophine* [package insert]. Columbus, OH: Roxane Laboratories, Inc; October 2006.

* Asterisk indicates drugs cited in interaction reports. Based on pharmacologic and pharmacokinetic considerations, similar interactions may occur with other drugs that are listed.

Methadone	*Rifamycins*
Methadone* (eg, *Dolophine*)	Rifampin* (eg, *Rifadin*)

Significance	Onset	Severity	Documentation
2	□ Rapid	□ Major	■ **Established**
	■ **Delayed**	■ **Moderate**	□ Probable
		□ Minor	□ Suspected
			□ Possible
			□ Unlikely

Effects The actions of METHADONE may be reduced. Patients receiving chronic METHADONE treatment may experience withdrawal symptoms.

Mechanism RIFAMPIN primarily appears to stimulate the hepatic and intestinal metabolism of METHADONE.

Management A higher dose of METHADONE may be required during coadministration of RIFAMPIN.

Discussion

A 70% incidence of opiate withdrawal symptoms occurred in a population of 30 patients receiving methadone maintenance when rifampin therapy was initiated for tuberculosis.[1] No withdrawal symptoms occurred in 26 patients treated with an antitubercular regimen not including rifampin. Further evaluation of 6 patients identified a 33% to 68% decrease in methadone plasma levels during rifampin treatment. In 4 of 6 patients, urinary excretion of pyrrolidine, a major methadone metabolite, was increased 150%. A case report of a 24-year-old female addict associated opiate withdrawal symptoms with the administration of an antitubercular regimen containing rifampin 5 days earlier.[2] In a similar case, a 40-year-old woman suffered opioid withdrawal symptoms associated with decreased methadone concentrations.[3] The effects of rifampin on the pharmacokinetics of single-dose oral and IV methadone were studied in 12 healthy volunteers.[4] Rifampin decreased methadone plasma levels and oral bioavailability. The AUC of orally administered methadone decreased 77%.

[1] Kreek MJ, et al. *N Engl J Med.* 1976;294:1104.
[2] Bending MR, et al. *Lancet.* 1977;1:1211.
[3] Raistrick D, et al. *BMJ.* 1996;313:925.
[4] Kharasch ED, et al. *Clin Pharmacol Ther.* 2004;76:250.

* Asterisk indicates drugs cited in interaction reports.

Methadone — *Somatostatin*

Methadone*
(eg, *Dolophine*)

Somatostatin*†

Significance	Onset	Severity	Documentation
4	■ **Rapid** □ Delayed	□ Major ■ **Moderate** □ Minor	□ Established □ Probable □ Suspected ■ **Possible** □ Unlikely

Effects The analgesic effect of METHADONE may be reduced.

Mechanism Unknown.

Management If a decrease or loss in analgesia occurs, consider discontinuing SOMATOSTATIN.

Discussion

A 20-year-old woman with left leg pain caused by chondrosarcoma was in good pain control while receiving oral methadone 4 mg 3 times/day.[1] Her pain increased after starting subcutaneous somatostatin 3 mg over 8 hr as part of an antineoplastic regimen. The dose of methadone was increased to 10 mg 3 times/day, which the patient reported to be completely ineffective. Methadone was changed to subcutaneous morphine 30 mg every 4 hr without success. When somatostatin was switched to IV administration over a 24-hr period, the patient's pain increased during the night and day despite continuous subcutaneous administration of morphine 300 mg/day plus an additional 4 to 5 bolus doses of 20 mg as needed. No improvement in pain control occurred, even with spinal administration of morphine. After discontinuing somatostatin, pain intensity was reduced more than 50% with spinal administration of morphine 20 mg/day. Myosis and sedation occurred for the first time. See also Morphine-Somatostatin.

[1] Ripamonti C, et al. *Ann Oncol.* 1998;9:921.

* Asterisk indicates drugs cited in interaction reports.
†Not available in the US.

Methadone — *St. John's Wort*

Methadone* (eg, *Dolophine*)		St. John's Wort*

Significance	Onset	Severity	Documentation
4	☐ Rapid	☐ Major	☐ Established
	■ **Delayed**	■ **Moderate**	☐ Probable
		☐ Minor	☐ Suspected
			■ **Possible**
			☐ Unlikely

Effects The pharmacologic effects of METHADONE may be reduced, resulting in opiate withdrawal symptoms.

Mechanism Increased hepatic metabolism (CYP3A4) or altered P-glycoprotein-mediated transport of METHADONE by ST. JOHN'S WORT is suspected.

Management Caution patients receiving METHADONE to consult their health care provider before using nonprescription or herbal products. The use of ST. JOHN'S WORT should be avoided in patients receiving METHADONE. If ST. JOHN'S WORT cannot be avoided, observe the patient for opiate withdrawal symptoms. Monitor for signs of METHADONE overdose if ST. JOHN'S WORT is discontinued. Adjust the METHADONE dose as needed.

Discussion

Methadone steady-state trough plasma concentrations were measured in 4 addict patients before and after starting St. John's wort 900 mg/day.[1] In these patients, a median treatment period of 31 days with St. John's wort resulted in a median decrease in the methadone plasma concentration of 47% compared with the original concentrations. Two patients reported symptoms consistent with methadone withdrawal and asked for an increase and/or a splitting of their daily methadone dose.

[1] Eich-Höchli D, et al. *Pharmacopsychiatry*. 2003;36:35.

* Asterisk indicates drugs cited in interaction reports.

Methadone — *Urinary Acidifiers*

Methadone	Urinary Acidifiers	
Methadone* (eg, *Dolophine*)	Ammonium Chloride*	Sodium Acid Phosphate
	Potassium Acid Phosphate (*K-Phos Original*)	

Significance	Onset	Severity	Documentation
3	□ Rapid	□ Major	□ Established
	■ **Delayed**	□ Moderate	□ Probable
		■ **Minor**	■ **Suspected**
			□ Possible
			□ Unlikely

Effects URINARY ACIDIFIERS increase the renal clearance of METHADONE.

Mechanism Clearance is increased because of increased ionization.

Management URINARY ACIDIFIERS can be used to increase the total body clearance of METHADONE in overdose situations.

Discussion

Several studies have shown that patients with a high clearance rate of methadone also have a low urine pH.[1-3] One study of 5 healthy volunteers found that the administration of 20 g of ammonium chloride and sodium carbonate over 3 days each resulted in a mean methadone elimination half-life of 19.5 hours following ammonium chloride, compared with 42.1 hours following sodium carbonate.[4]

[1] Inturrisi CE, et al. *Clin Pharmacol Ther.* 1972;13:633.
[2] Inturrisi CE, et al. *Clin Pharmacol Ther.* 1972;13:923.
[3] Bellward GD, et al. *Clin Pharmacol Ther.* 1977;22:92.
[4] Nilsson M-I, et al. *Eur J Clin Pharmacol.* 1982;22:337.

* Asterisk indicates drugs cited in interaction reports. Based on pharmacologic and pharmacokinetic considerations, similar interactions may occur with other drugs that are listed.

Methenamine — *Urinary Alkalinizers*

Methenamine	Urinary Alkalinizers	
Methenamine* (eg, *Mandelamine*)	Potassium Citrate* (eg, *Urocit-K*)	Sodium Citrate*
	Sodium Acetate*	Sodium Lactate*
	Sodium Bicarbonate*	Tromethamine* (eg, *Tham*)

Significance	Onset	Severity	Documentation
5	☐ Rapid	☐ Major	☐ Established
	■ **Delayed**	☐ Moderate	☐ Probable
		■ **Minor**	☐ Suspected
			■ **Possible**
			☐ Unlikely

Effects ALKALINIZING agents may interfere with the antibacterial activity of the METHENAMINE compounds.

Mechanism METHENAMINE activity is a function of formaldehyde generation in the urine, occurring in an acid milieu. ALKALINIZATION would theoretically counteract a favorable environment.

Management When possible, avoid agents that tend to alkalinize urine. Monitoring urinary pH may assist. Alternatively, use other effective urinary antimicrobials.

Discussion

Once methenamine is excreted from the kidneys, it is hydrolyzed to formaldehyde and ammonia in an acidic environment. It is this form that has antibacterial action. Antimicrobial potency is related to urinary pH; it is doubtful that sufficient formaldehyde is generated above a urine pH of 6.5. Numerous in vitro and in vivo studies appear to bear this out; however, controversy exists on the clinical significance of wide fluctuations of urinary pH.[1-7] There is a paucity of good clinical data.

Despite this lack of supportable evidence, it is prudent to avoid agents known to alkalinize urine when methenamine therapy is in progress. If therapeutic efficacy is in doubt, use an alternative antimicrobial.

[1] Zangwill DP, et al. *Arch Intern Med.* 1962;110:801.
[2] Gandelman AL, et al. *J Urol.* 1967;97:533.
[3] Miller H, et al. *Invest Urol.* 1970;8:21.
[4] Musher DM, et al. *Antimicrob Agents Chemother.* 1974;6:708.
[5] Musher DM, et al. *Invest Urol.* 1976;13:380.
[6] Pearman JW, et al. *Invest Urol.* 1978;16:91.
[7] Kevorkian CG, et al. *Mayo Clin Proc.* 1984;59:523.

* Asterisk indicates drugs cited in interaction reports.

Methotrexate | *Acitretin*

Methotrexate*	Acitretin*
(eg, *Rheumatrex*)	(*Soriatane*)

Significance	Onset	Severity	Documentation
1	□ Rapid	■ **Major**	□ Established
	■ **Delayed**	□ Moderate	□ Probable
		□ Minor	■ **Suspected**
			□ Possible
			□ Unlikely

Effects The risk of hepatitis may be increased.

Mechanism Unknown; however, increased METHOTREXATE plasma concentrations may be involved.

Management Coadministration of METHOTREXATE and ACITRETIN is contraindicated.

Discussion

Acitretin is a metabolite of the retinoid etretinate.[1] Because an increased risk of hepatitis has been reported with coadministration of methotrexate and etretinate, concomitant use of methotrexate and acitretin is contraindicated.[1]

The basis for this monograph is information on file with the manufacturer. Published clinical data are needed to further assess this interaction. However, because of the seriousness of the reaction, clinical evaluation in humans is not likely to be forthcoming.

[1] *Soriatane* [package insert]. Florence, KY: Roche Pharmaceuticals, Inc.; 2003.

* Asterisk indicates drugs cited in interaction reports.

Methotrexate — *Aminoglycosides*

Methotrexate	Aminoglycosides	
Methotrexate* (eg, *Rheumatrex*)	Kanamycin* (eg, *Kantrex*)	Paromomycin* (*Humatin*)
	Neomycin* (eg, *Neo-frandin*)	

Significance	Onset	Severity	Documentation
4	□ Rapid	□ Major	□ Established
	■ **Delayed**	■ **Moderate**	□ Probable
		□ Minor	□ Suspected
			■ **Possible**
			□ Unlikely

Effects The antitumorigenic actions of METHOTREXATE may be decreased.

Mechanism METHOTREXATE'S GI absorption appears to be reduced.

Management Consider parenteral use of METHOTREXATE if oral AMINOGLYCOSIDES are being coadministered.

Discussion

Methotrexate absorption is dose-dependent. At doses less than 30 mg/m^2, absorption is rapid and complete but is unpredictable above this level. Metabolism by intestinal bacteria may inactivate up to 30% of an oral dose. One would anticipate that sterilization of the bowel with nonabsorbable antibiotics, such as the aminoglycosides, would increase methotrexate absorption.[1] However, controlled evaluations have demonstrated an opposite effect. Neomycin 500 mg every 6 hr for 3 days decreased methotrexate's 24-hr AUC 50%.[1] A combination of paromomycin 800 mg, polymyxin B 100 mg, vancomycin 500 mg, and nystatin 800,000 units 4 times/day for 6 weeks decreased methotrexate absorption 44% in patients receiving intensive chemotherapy for bronchogenic carcinoma.[2]

When oral nonabsorbable aminoglycoside antibiotics are utilized, consider coadministration of IV methotrexate.

[1] Shen DD, et al. *Clin Pharmacokinet.* 1978;3:1.

[2] Cohen MH, et al. *Cancer.* 1976;38:1556.

* Asterisk indicates drugs cited in interaction reports.

Methotrexate — *Aminoquinolines*

Methotrexate* (eg, *Rheumatrex*)	Chloroquine* (*Aralen*)	Hydroxychloroquine (eg, *Plaquenil*)

Significance	Onset	Severity	Documentation
5	☐ Rapid	☐ Major	☐ Established
	■ **Delayed**	☐ Moderate	☐ Probable
		■ **Minor**	☐ Suspected
			■ **Possible**
			☐ Unlikely

Effects The antirheumatic effect of METHOTREXATE may be decreased.

Mechanism Unknown; however, CHLOROQUINE may reduce the bioavailability of METHOTREXATE.

Management Monitor the clinical response of the patient. If an interaction is suspected, it may be necessary to increase the dose of METHOTREXATE.

Discussion

The effects of a single dose of chloroquine on the pharmacokinetics of low-dose methotrexate were evaluated in 11 patients with rheumatoid arthritis.[1] After an overnight fast, patients received the regular weekly oral dose of methotrexate 15 mg alone, and 1 week later, each patient received 15 mg of methotrexate plus chloroquine 250 mg. In 9 of the 11 patients, chloroquine reduced the AUC of methotrexate. The median value of the AUC was decreased 28%; ($P = 0.03$). In 8 of the 11 patients, chloroquine reduced peak serum methotrexate concentrations. The median decrease in methotrexate levels was from 606 to 488 nanomole/L (19%). This change did not reach statistical significance ($P = 0.06$).

[1] Seideman P, et al. *Arthritis Rheum.* 1994;37:830.

* Asterisk indicates drugs cited in interaction reports. Based on pharmacologic and pharmacokinetic considerations, similar interactions may occur with other drugs that are listed.

Methotrexate — *Amiodarone*

Methotrexate* (eg, *Rheumatrex*)	Amiodarone* (eg, *Cordarone*)

Significance	Onset	Severity	Documentation
4	☐ Rapid	■ **Major**	☐ Established
	■ **Delayed**	☐ Moderate	☐ Probable
		☐ Minor	☐ Suspected
			■ **Possible**
			☐ Unlikely

Effects METHOTREXATE toxicity may be increased.

Mechanism Unknown.

Management Consider monitoring patients receiving METHOTREXATE for signs of toxicity if treatment with AMIODARONE is initiated.

Discussion

A 79-year-old woman maintained on methotrexate for 2 years developed ulcerated skin lesions following the addition of amiodarone to her therapy.[1] The patient was taking methotrexate 17.5 mg/week for severe psoriasis. She was hospitalized for worsening psoriasis and episodes of prolonged palpitations accompanied by dizziness and breathlessness. Other therapy the patient had been receiving when she was admitted to the hospital included furosemide (eg, *Lasix*), amiloride (*Midamor*), isosorbide mononitrate (eg, *Ismo*), digoxin (eg, *Lanoxin*), and dothiepin (not available in the United States). The patient was started on amiodarone for uncontrolled atrial fibrillation. Amiodarone therapy consisted of a loading dose of 200 mg 3 times/day for 1 week, 200 mg twice a day for an additional week, and then a maintenance dose of 200 mg/day. After 2 weeks, many of her psoriatic plaques became tender, red, and eroded together. Methotrexate was discontinued and the lesions healed.

[1] Reynolds NJ, et al. *BMJ.* 1989;299:980.

* Asterisk indicates drugs cited in interaction reports.

Methotrexate — *Caffeine*

Methotrexate* (eg, *Rheumatrex*)	Caffeine*

Significance	Onset	Severity	Documentation
4	☐ Rapid ■ **Delayed**	☐ Major ■ **Moderate** ☐ Minor	☐ Established ☐ Probable ☐ Suspected ■ **Possible** ☐ Unlikely

Effects The antirheumatic effect of METHOTREXATE may be reduced.

Mechanism Unknown; however, because CAFFEINE is an adenosine receptor antagonist, it may interfere with the effects of METHOTREXATE.

Management Monitor the clinical response of the patient. If an interaction is suspected and the patient's CAFFEINE intake is high, it may be necessary to reduce CAFFEINE ingestion.

Discussion

In an open-label, nonrandomized, observational investigation, the effects of low (less than 120 mg/day), medium (120 to 180 mg/day), and high (greater than 180 mg/day) caffeine intake (approximately 66 mg/cup of instant or 135 mg/cup of brewed coffee) on the efficacy of methotrexate were studied in 39 patients with rheumatoid arthritis.[1] Rheumatoid arthritis disease activity was evaluated before starting methotrexate therapy and at monthly intervals for 3 months. Patients in the high caffeine intake group experienced less improvement in morning stiffness and joint pain than patients in the low caffeine intake group. The response of patients in the medium caffeine intake group did not differ statistically from the low or high caffeine intake groups.

[1] Nesher G, et al. *Arthritis Rheum.* 2003;48:571.

* Asterisk indicates drugs cited in interaction reports.

Methotrexate — *Cyclosporine*

Methotrexate*
(eg, *Rheumatrex*)

Cyclosporine*
(eg, *Neoral*)

Significance	Onset	Severity	Documentation
2	☐ Rapid	☐ Major	☐ Established
	■ **Delayed**	■ **Moderate**	☐ Probable
		☐ Minor	■ **Suspected**
			☐ Possible
			☐ Unlikely

Effects METHOTREXATE plasma levels may be elevated, increasing the pharmacologic and adverse effects.

Mechanism Blocking of the oxidation of METHOTREXATE to its relatively inactive metabolite by CYCLOSPORINE is suspected.

Management In patients receiving METHOTREXATE, monitor the clinical response when CYCLOSPORINE is started or stopped. Adjust the METHOTREXATE dose as needed.

Discussion

The effects of oral administration of cyclosporine and methotrexate on the pharmacokinetics of each drug were evaluated in 30 patients with rheumatoid arthritis.[1] On day 1 of the study, methotrexate was discontinued in patients who had been receiving stable weekly doses of methotrexate (7.5 to 22.5 mg/week). Cyclosporine (1.5 mg/kg every 12 hr) was started on day 8. On day 23, methotrexate was restarted. During each phase, drug and drug metabolite concentrations in the blood and urine were measured. Coadministration of cyclosporine and methotrexate increased the mean peak plasma level of methotrexate 26% and the mean AUC 18%, and decreased the AUC of the 7-hydroxymethotrexate (7-OH-MTX) metabolite 80% compared with giving methotrexate alone. The urinary excretion of the 7-OH-MTX metabolite was reduced 87% in 13 patients who received a 10-mg dose of methotrexate. Methotrexate did not affect the pharmacokinetics of cyclosporine or its metabolites.

[1] Fox RI, et al. *Rheumatology*. 2003;42:989.

* Asterisk indicates drugs cited in interaction reports.

Methotrexate — *Dantrolene*

Methotrexate* (eg, *Rheumatrex*)	Dantrolene* (eg, *Dantrium*)

Significance	Onset	Severity	Documentation
4	■ **Rapid**	■ **Major**	□ Established
	□ Delayed	□ Moderate	□ Probable
		□ Minor	□ Suspected
			■ **Possible**
			□ Unlikely

Effects METHOTREXATE plasma concentrations may be elevated, increasing the risk of toxicity.[1]

Mechanism Altered METHOTREXATE protein binding is suspected.

Management Use with caution, monitoring for signs of METHOTREXATE toxicity. Consider longer leucovorin rescue when giving high-dose METHOTREXATE.

Discussion

A 16-year-old girl receiving high-dose methotrexate for nonmetastatic femoral osteosarcoma and dantrolene for pain displayed high plasma methotrexate concentrations (418 mcmol/L) after the first course of methotrexate 18 g.[1] Intensification of urine alkalinization and increased leucovorin rescue (100 mg/m^2 every 3 hours) were administered immediately and dantrolene was discontinued. A bacterial enzyme that allows hydrolysis of methotrexate to a nontoxic metabolite was administered as soon as it was available (first dose at 54 hours and a second dose at 78 hours). The threshold value, determining the end of methotrexate rescue, was reached 13 days after the start of the methotrexate infusion. Signs of methotrexate toxicity that were present included cytolytic hepatitis without hepatic failure, renal failure with tubulointerstitial nephropathy, and succession of grade 1 thrombocytopenia and grade 4 mucositis. The patient experienced a seizure on day 9 as a result of elevated BP. Methotrexate treatment was resumed at a lower dose (10 g) 3 weeks later and was well tolerated, with a standard decrease in plasma concentrations. An interaction with dantrolene was considered to be the probable cause of the methotrexate toxicity.

[1] André N, et al. *Ann Pharmacother*. 2006;40(9):1695.

* Asterisk indicates drugs cited in interaction reports.

Methotrexate — *Folic Acid*

Methotrexate* (eg, *Rheumatrex*)	Folic Acid* (eg, *Folvite*)

Significance	Onset	Severity	Documentation
4	☐ Rapid	☐ Major	☐ Established
	■ **Delayed**	■ **Moderate**	☐ Probable
		☐ Minor	☐ Suspected
			■ **Possible**
			☐ Unlikely

Effects The antipsoriatic effect of METHOTREXATE may be reduced.

Mechanism Unknown.

Management If an interaction is suspected, consider tailoring the METHOTREXATE dose based on therapeutic response.

Discussion

The effect of oral folic acid on low-dose oral methotrexate during the remission-induction phase of psoriasis treatment was studied in 20 patients with moderate to severe plaque psoriasis.[1] In an open-label, crossover study, patients were treated with methotrexate alone or with methotrexate plus folic acid 20 mg/week for 16 weeks. There was a marked difference in the efficacy of remission-induction therapy in favor of methotrexate monotherapy compared with coadministration of folic acid, irrespective of pretreatment folate levels. The percent improvement of skin impairment using the psoriasis area and severity index was nearly 2-fold greater in patients receiving methotrexate monotherapy compared with methotrexate plus folic acid.

[1] Chládek J, et al. *Eur J Clin Pharmacol.* 2008;64(4):347.

* Asterisk indicates drugs cited in interaction reports.

Methotrexate — *Food*

Methotrexate* (eg, *Rheumatrex*)	Cola Beverages*

Significance	Onset	Severity	Documentation
4	■ **Rapid**	□ Major	□ Established
	□ Delayed	■ **Moderate**	□ Probable
		□ Minor	□ Suspected
			■ **Possible**
			□ Unlikely

Effects Elevated METHOTREXATE serum concentrations, possibly increasing the risk of METHOTREXATE toxicity (eg, renal failure).

Mechanism Possible decrease in pH-dependent renal clearance of METHOTREXATE.

Management Patients taking METHOTREXATE should avoid COLA BEVERAGES 24 hours before and during METHOTREXATE administration and until METHOTREXATE is completely eliminated.

Discussion

Delayed methotrexate elimination in a 56-year-old man was attributed to drinking a cola beverage.[1] Recurrent urinary acidity occurred in the patient despite administration of large amounts of sodium bicarbonate. Acute renal failure was diagnosed 24 hours after methotrexate infusion. Urinary pH was observed to decrease from 8.5 to 6.5 after the patient had consumed 330 mL of a cola beverage. He was asked to stop drinking cola on the third day after methotrexate infusion and the urinary pH was maintained at 8 or greater. Renal function returned to normal 56 days after methotrexate administration.

[1] Santucci R, et al. *Br J Clin Pharmacol.* 2010;70(5):762.

* Asterisk indicates drugs cited in interaction reports.

Methotrexate ⨯ *Haloperidol*

Methotrexate* (eg, *Rheumatrex*)	Haloperidol* (eg, *Haldol*)

Significance	Onset	Severity	Documentation
4	☐ Rapid ■ **Delayed**	☐ Major ■ **Moderate** ☐ Minor	☐ Established ☐ Probable ☐ Suspected ■ **Possible** ☐ Unlikely

Effects The risk of METHOTREXATE-induced dermatologic conditions (eg, photosensitivity dermatitis) may be increased.

Mechanism Unknown.

Management Monitor patients receiving METHOTREXATE for possible photosensitivity recall phenomenon when HALOPERIDOL is started. During coadministration of both agents, advise patients to avoid exposure to sunlight and to use sunscreen or wear protective clothing when outdoors.

Discussion

Pellagra-like photosensitivity dermatitis was reported in a 41-year-old man whose psoriasis was well controlled on methotrexate when haloperidol was added to his treatment regimen.[1] The patient had been taking oral methotrexate 15 mg/week for 10 months. Haloperidol treatment, 1.5 mg twice weekly, was started for a psychotic illness. Two weeks after initiating haloperidol, the patient experienced a sudden onset of redness and swelling of his face and hands together with redness and watering of his eyes. Physical examination revealed edema, erythema, scaling, and erosions over his face and anterior aspect of the neck and dorsi of both hands that was demarcated to photo-exposed areas. Results of a skin biopsy from the dorsum of the hand were consistent with subacute dermatitis. Pellagra-like photosensitivity was considered. Haloperidol was stopped, emollients were administered, and a multivitamin (with niacin 100 mg and riboflavin 10 mg) was given 3 times a day. Within 5 days, dermatologic, oral, and eye symptoms resolved. Administration of the next weekly dose of methotrexate resulted in a severe relapse of the dermatitis within 24 hours, despite the patient being indoors and on the multivitamin preparation. Methotrexate and the multivitamin supplement were stopped, and within 1 week, the dermatitis resolved. Two weeks later, the patient was restarted on methotrexate without relapse of the dermatitis.

[1] Thami GP, et al. *Postgrad Med J.* 2002;78:116.

* Asterisk indicates drugs cited in interaction reports.

Methotrexate — *NSAIDs*

Methotrexate	NSAIDs	
Methotrexate* (eg, *Rheumatrex*)	Diclofenac* (eg, *Voltaren*)	Meclofenamate
	Etodolac (eg, *Lodine*)	Mefenamic Acid (*Ponstel*)
	Fenoprofen (eg, *Nalfon*)	Nabumetone (eg, *Relafen*)
	Flurbiprofen* (eg, *Ansaid*)	Naproxen* (eg, *Naprosyn*)
	Ibuprofen* (eg, *Motrin*)	Oxaprozin (eg, *Daypro*)
	Indomethacin* (eg, *Indocin*)	Piroxicam (eg, *Feldene*)
	Ketoprofen* (eg, *Oruvail*)	Sulindac (eg, *Clinoril*)
	Ketorolac (eg, *Toradol*)	Tolmetin* (eg, *Tolectin*)

Significance	Onset	Severity	Documentation
1	☐ Rapid	■ **Major**	☐ Established
	■ **Delayed**	☐ Moderate	☐ Probable
		☐ Minor	■ **Suspected**
			☐ Possible
			☐ Unlikely

Effects Increased METHOTREXATE (MTX) toxicity, which is less likely to occur with weekly low-dose MTX regimens for rheumatoid arthritis (RA) and other inflammatory diseases.[1]

Mechanism Reduced renal clearance is suspected.

Management Consider longer leucovorin rescue when giving NSAIDs and MTX at antineoplastic doses. Monitor for renal impairment that could predispose to MTX toxicity, for signs of MTX toxicity,[2,3] and MTX levels if indicated.

Discussion

NSAIDs have been associated with severe toxic reactions or reduced MTX clearance.[4-8] Ketoprofen was implicated in 4 cases of high-dose MTX toxicity. Renal function was adequate prior to therapy, but 3 patients developed renal impairment and severe toxicity, and subsequently died. Two patients showed marked impairment of MTX clearance.[9] A study of 7 children given oral MTX and NSAIDs for RA demonstrated a prolonged MTX $t_{1/2}$.[10] There was wide variation in the effect of NSAIDs on MTX clearance. A woman with RA taking MTX developed hematemesis, diarrhea with melena, nausea, and weakness approximately 1 week after starting flurbiprofen.[8] In a double-blind study in RA patients, naproxen and ibuprofen reduced the systemic clearance of MTX 22% and 40%, respectively.[11] Ketoprofen, celecoxib,[12] rofecoxib,[13] flurbiprofen, and piroxicam did not alter MTX clearance when given to adult RA patients receiving stable weekly doses of MTX.[14] This interaction occurs rarely but can have severe consequences.

1 Franck H, et al. *Clin Rheumatol.* 1996;15:266.
2 Small RE, et al. *Am Pharm.* 1994;NS34:3.
3 Kremer JM, et al. *J Rheumatol.* 1995;22:2072.
4 Maiche AG. *Lancet.* 1986;1:1390.
5 Singh RR, et al. *Lancet.* 1986;1:1390.
6 Stockley IH. *Drug Intell Clin Pharm.* 1987;21:546.
7 Kraus A, et al. *J Rheumatol.* 1991;18:1274.
8 Frenia ML, et al. *Ann Pharmacother.* 1992;26:234.
9 Thyss A, et al. *Lancet.* 1986;1:256.
10 Dupuis LL, et al. *J Rheumatol.* 1990;17:1469.
11 Tracy TS, et al. *Eur J Clin Pharmacol.* 1992;42:121.
12 Karim A, et al. *J Rheumatol.* 1999;26:2539.
13 Schwartz JI, et al. *J Clin Pharmacol.* 2001;41:1120.
14 Tracy TS, et al. *Br J Clin Pharmacol.* 1994;37:453.

* Asterisk indicates drugs cited in interaction reports. Based on pharmacologic and pharmacokinetic considerations, similar interactions may occur with other drugs that are listed.

Methotrexate — *Omeprazole*

Methotrexate* (eg, *Rheumatrex*)	Omeprazole* (eg, *Prilosec*)

Significance	Onset	Severity	Documentation
4	■ **Rapid** □ Delayed	■ **Major** □ Moderate □ Minor	□ Established □ Probable □ Suspected ■ **Possible** □ Unlikely

Effects Increased serum METHOTREXATE concentrations, possibly increasing the risk of METHOTREXATE toxicity.

Mechanism Possible decrease in the renal clearance of METHOTREXATE.

Management If possible, consider stopping OMEPRAZOLE treatment several days prior to giving METHOTREXATE. Consider administering an H_2 antagonist (eg, ranitidine [eg, *Zantac*]) instead of OMEPRAZOLE.

Discussion

A 41-year-old man with osteosarcoma and a history of Hodgkin disease exhibited elevated plasma methotrexate concentrations during coadministration of omeprazole.[1] The patient was receiving bleomycin, cyclophosphamide, and dactinomycin (eg, *Cosmegen*). He then received high-dose methotrexate 12 g/m^2 with leucovorin rescue. At this time, he was taking a number of medications, including omeprazole. During the first cycle of therapy, the patient's plasma methotrexate concentrations remained elevated for several days. His renal function was healthy. He was aggressively hydrated, his urine alkalinized, and leucovorin administered for 8 days. None of the medications the patient was taking were known to inhibit methotrexate elimination. However, omeprazole treatment was stopped. After discontinuing omeprazole, the patient's serum methotrexate concentration decreased rapidly and displayed normal kinetics for 3 consecutive cycles. An 11-year-old boy received 5 chemotherapy cycles involving high-dose methotrexate.[2] During the first cycle, he also received omeprazole 20 mg twice daily. Methotrexate $t_{1/2}$ was 65% longer during this cycle compared with the next 4 cycles, which did not include omeprazole.

[1] Reid T, et al. *Cancer Chemother Pharmacol.* 1993;33(1):82.

[2] Beorlegui B, et al. *Ann Pharmacother.* 2000;34(9):1024.

* Asterisk indicates drugs cited in interaction reports.

Methotrexate — *Pantoprazole*

Methotrexate* (eg, *Rheumatrex*)	Pantoprazole* (eg, *Protonix*)

Significance	Onset	Severity	Documentation
4	□ Rapid	■ **Major**	□ Established
	■ **Delayed**	□ Moderate	□ Probable
		□ Minor	□ Suspected
			■ **Possible**
			□ Unlikely

Effects The risk of METHOTREXATE adverse effects (eg, myalgia) may be increased.

Mechanism Interference with the renal elimination of the 7-hydroxymethotrexate metabolite by PANTOPRAZOLE is suspected.

Management Observe patients receiving METHOTREXATE for an increase in adverse effects during coadministration of PANTOPRAZOLE.

Discussion

A 59-year-old man experienced severe myalgia and bone pain when methotrexate and pantoprazole were coadministered.[1] The patient was receiving methotrexate 15 mg IM once weekly for T-cell lymphoma, which had relapsed while receiving interferon alfa-2a (*Roferon-A*). Treatment with oral pantoprazole 20 mg/day was started for a Barrett esophagus. He was also receiving atenolol (eg, *Tenormin*) for hypertension. After the first injection of methotrexate, the patient experienced severe generalized myalgia and bone pain, which led to partial immobility beginning 3 to 4 h after the injection and lasting for several days. The symptoms occurred over the following 4 methotrexate cycles, and a drug interaction was suspected. Ranitidine (eg, *Zantac*) was substituted for pantoprazole and the symptoms subsided dramatically and then disappeared. When the patient was rechallenged with pantoprazole, the symptoms recurred but did not reappear when pantoprazole was not administered. Pantoprazole did not affect the concentration-time curve of methotrexate; however, the AUC and $t_{1/2}$ of the 7-hydroxymethotrexate metabolite were increased 71% and 123%, respectively, when methotrexate and pantoprazole were coadministered compared with giving methotrexate alone. A 53-year-old woman receiving high-dose methotrexate IV (3,000 mg/m^2) and pantoprazole 20 mg/day experienced high (20.5 mcmol/L at 36 hours) and prolonged methotrexate concentrations, leading to acute renal failure.[2]

[1] Tröger U, et al. *BMJ.* 2002;324(7352):1497.

[2] Ranchon F, et al. *Chemotherapy.* 2011;57(3):225.

* Asterisk indicates drugs cited in interaction reports.

Methotrexate — *Penicillins*

Methotrexate	Penicillins	
Methotrexate* (eg, *Rheumatrex*)	Amoxicillin* (eg, *Amoxil*)	Penicillin G (eg, *Pfizerpen*)
	Ampicillin (eg, *Principen*)	Penicillin V (eg, *Veetids*)
	Carbenicillin (*Geocillin*)	Piperacillin*
	Dicloxacillin	Ticarcillin (*Ticar*)
	Oxacillin*	

Significance	Onset	Severity	Documentation
1	□ Rapid	■ **Major**	□ Established
	■ **Delayed**	□ Moderate	■ **Probable**
		□ Minor	□ Suspected
			□ Possible
			□ Unlikely

Effects Serum METHOTREXATE (MTX) concentrations may be elevated, increasing the risk of toxicity.

Mechanism Competitive inhibition of renal tubular secretion of MTX.

Management Monitor patients for MTX toxicity and measure MTX concentrations twice a week for at least the first 2 weeks. The dose and duration of leucovorin rescue may need to be increased. If a broad-spectrum parenteral antibiotic is needed, ceftazidime (eg, *Fortaz*) may be less likely to interact.

Discussion

A 16-yr-old patient receiving 10 cycles of MTX treatment experienced a decrease in plasma clearance, an increase in mean residence time, an increase in the t½ of MTX, and evidence of toxicity (renal failure, myelosuppression) during cycle 10, compared with cycles 1 through 9.[1] The only difference between cycle 10 and the previous cycles was the coadministration of amoxicillin. There are other reports of a possible MTX-penicillin interaction.[2-5] The t½ of MTX was more than doubled in a 15-yr-old patient during administration of mezlocillin and MTX.[2] In another report, neutropenia occurred during low-dose MTX therapy and various penicillins.[3] A patient developed leukopenia, thrombocytopenia, increased liver function tests, mucositis, and skin ulcers during coadministration of MTX, penicillin, and furosemide (eg, *Lasix*).[4] An 8-year-old patient experienced reduced MTX clearance without evidence of toxicity during piperacillin coadministration, compared with ceftazidime administration or when MTX was given alone.[5] Elevated MTX levels occurred in a 50-yr-old woman while receiving piperacillin/tazobactam (*Zosyn*).[6] MTX concentrations decreased only after the antibiotic was discontinued. An 18-yr-old man experienced marked elevations of MTX plasma levels and toxicity during coadministration of oxacillin.[7] A previous course of MTX, without oxacillin, was tolerated without incident.

[1] Nierenberg DW, et al. *Arch Dermatol.* 1983;119(6):449.
[2] Mayall B, et al. *Med J Aust.* 1991;155(7):480.
[3] Dean R, et al. *Am J Pediatr Hematol Oncol.* 1992;14(1):88.
[4] Ronchera CL, et al. *Ther Drug Monit.* 1993;15(5):375.
[5] Yamamoto K, et al. *Ann Pharmacother.* 1997;31(10):1261.
[6] Zarychanski R, et al. *J Antimicrob Chemother.* 2006;58(1):228.
[7] Titier K, et al. *Ther Drug Monit.* 2002;24(4):570.

* Asterisk indicates drugs cited in interaction reports. Based on pharmacologic and pharmacokinetic considerations, similar interactions may occur with other drugs that are listed.

Methotrexate — *Probenecid*

Methotrexate* (eg, *Rheumatrex*)	Probenecid*

Significance	Onset	Severity	Documentation
1	■ **Rapid**	■ **Major**	□ Established
	□ Delayed	□ Moderate	■ **Probable**
		□ Minor	□ Suspected
			□ Possible
			□ Unlikely

Effects METHOTREXATE plasma levels, therapeutic effects, and toxicity may be enhanced.

Mechanism PROBENECID appears to impair renal excretion of METHOTREXATE.

Management Decreased METHOTREXATE dosage and prolonged leucovorin (eg, *Wellcovorin*) rescue may be required to avoid undue toxicity risk when PROBENECID is administered concomitantly. Monitor METHOTREXATE serum concentrations; adjust the dose accordingly.

Discussion

Investigations in animals and humans have consistently demonstrated impaired clearance of methotrexate by probenecid.[1-7] A 67-year-old woman with rheumatoid arthritis developed pancytopenia from low-dose oral methotrexate 7.5 mg/week after the addition of probenecid 1 g/day.[8] Methotrexate is cleared renally by glomerular filtration and tubular secretion.[1] Probenecid, which blocks the renal secretion of many organic acids, also appears to block methotrexate. Methotrexate plasma levels are increased 3- to 4-fold with coadministration of probenecid.

Animal studies indicate that biliary excretion may also be impaired by probenecid.[2,3] Whether this contributes to the decreased methotrexate clearance in humans remains to be clarified.

[1] Bourke RS, et al. *Cancer Res.* 1975;35:110.
[2] Kates RE, et al. *Biochem Pharmacol.* 1976;25:1485.
[3] Kates RE, et al. *J Pharm Sci.* 1976;65:1348.
[4] Aherne GW, et al. *BMJ.* 1978;1:1097.
[5] Israili ZH, et al. *Am Assoc Cancer Res.* 1978;19:194.
[6] Howell SB, et al. *Clin Pharmacol Ther.* 1979;26:641.
[7] Lilly MB, et al. *Cancer Chemother Pharmacol.* 1985;15:220.
[8] Basin KS, et al. *J Rheumatol.* 1991;18:609.

* Asterisk indicates drugs cited in interaction reports.

Methotrexate — *Procarbazine*

Methotrexate* (eg, *Rheumatrex*)	Procarbazine* (*Matulane*)

Significance	Onset	Severity	Documentation
4	□ Rapid	■ **Major**	□ Established
	■ **Delayed**	□ Moderate	□ Probable
		□ Minor	□ Suspected
			■ **Possible**
			□ Unlikely

Effects The nephrotoxicity of METHOTREXATE may be increased.

Mechanism Unknown.

Management Consider allowing an interval of at least 72 hours between the administration of the final dose of PROCARBAZINE and the initiation of a high-dose METHOTREXATE infusion.

Discussion

Three cases of renal impairment occurred following the combined administration of high-dose methotrexate 2 g/m^2 IV over 6 hours on days 15, 22, and 29 and procarbazine 100 mg/m^2/day for 14 days.[1] Procarbazine was administered on days 1 through 14, and the first dose of methotrexate was infused within 48 hours following the completion of procarbazine therapy. All patients had normal renal function, and no patient had a history of kidney disease. Standard high-dose methotrexate administration precautions were followed, including prehydration and posthydration, alkalinization of the urine, and adequate leucovorin (eg, *Wellcovorin*) rescue. Deterioration in renal function was observed 24 to 48 hours after methotrexate administration. With the onset of renal impairment, the second dose of methotrexate was delayed in 2 patients, and chemotherapy was discontinued in the third. In all patients, 3 months after the study, serum creatinine remained within normal limits.

Impaired renal function can occur with the administration of high-dose methotrexate alone; however, the temporal association between administration of methotrexate and procarbazine, as well as the observed changes in renal function, suggest that the reaction may be caused by an interaction between the drugs. Additional clinical data are needed.

[1] Price P, et al. *Cancer Chemother Pharmacol.* 1988;21:265.

* Asterisk indicates drugs cited in interaction reports.

Methotrexate — *Salicylates*

Methotrexate	Salicylates	
Methotrexate* (eg, *Rheumatrex*)	Aspirin* (eg, *Bayer*)	Salsalate (eg, *Salsitab*)
	Bismuth Subsalicylate (eg, *Pepto-Bismol*)	Sodium Salicylate*
	Choline Magnesium Salicylate* (eg, *Tricosal*)	Sodium Thiosalicylate (eg, *Thiocyl*)
	Magnesium Salicylate (eg, *Doan's*)	

Significance	Onset	Severity	Documentation
1	■ **Rapid**	■ **Major**	□ Established
	□ Delayed	□ Moderate	□ Probable
		□ Minor	■ **Suspected**
			□ Possible
			□ Unlikely

Effects Increased toxic effects of METHOTREXATE may occur.

Mechanism SALICYLATES may decrease METHOTREXATE renal clearance and plasma protein binding.

Management Decreased doses of METHOTREXATE or prolonged regimens of leucovorin rescue may be indicated when SALICYLATES are coadministered. Consider monitoring METHOTREXATE plasma levels to guide dosage adjustment.

Discussion

Salicylates in vitro can decrease methotrexate plasma protein binding 20% to 60%.[1,2] Infusions of salicylate appear to reduce the clearance of methotrexate up to 35% in patients with malignancy.[3] In 9 patients with rheumatoid arthritis, choline magnesium salicylate increased the unbound fraction of methotrexate and reduced systemic clearance of methotrexate 24%.[4] Increased methotrexate toxicity (eg, pancytopenia, epidermal necrolysis, GI toxicity) associated with salicylates has been reported in patients with psoriasis or malignancy.[5,6] Animal studies in mice have noted decreased survival and greater bone marrow suppression when salicylates were combined with methotrexate.

Although human data are retrospective and anecdotal, the severity of this possible adverse interaction warrants close patient monitoring.

1 Dixon RL, et al. *Fed Proc.* 1965;24:454.
2 Taylor JR, et al. *Arch Dermatol.* 1977;113(5):588.
3 Liegler DG, et al. *Clin Pharmacol Ther.* 1969;10(6):849.
4 Tracy TS, et al. *Eur J Clin Pharmacol.* 1992;42(2):121.
5 Baker H. *Br J Dermatol.* 1970;82(1):65.
6 Mandel MA. *Plast Reconstr Surg.* 1976;57(6):733.

* Asterisk indicates drugs cited in interaction reports. Based on pharmacologic and pharmacokinetic considerations, similar interactions may occur with other drugs that are listed.

Methotrexate — *Sulfonamides*

Methotrexate	Sulfonamides	
Methotrexate* (eg, *Rheumatrex*)	Sulfadiazine	Trimethoprim-Sulfamethoxazole* (eg, *Bactrim*)
	Sulfamethoxazole*†	
	Sulfasalazine (eg, *Azulfidine*)	
	Sulfisoxazole* (*Gantrisin Pediatric*)	

Significance	Onset	Severity	Documentation
1	□ Rapid	■ **Major**	□ Established
	■ **Delayed**	□ Moderate	□ Probable
		□ Minor	■ **Suspected**
			□ Possible
			□ Unlikely

Effects SULFONAMIDES may increase the risk of METHOTREXATE (MTX)-induced bone marrow suppression. MTX may predispose patients to TRIMETHOPRIM-SULFAMETHOXAZOLE (TMP-SMZ)–induced megaloblastic anemia.

Mechanism SULFONAMIDES displace MTX from protein-binding sites and decrease renal clearance of MTX.[1-3] MTX may induce folate deficiency, which develops into acute megaloblastic anemia upon administration of TMP-SMZ.

Management If SULFONAMIDES cannot be avoided, closely monitor patients for signs of hematologic toxicity.

Discussion

Hematologic toxicity (eg, bone marrow hypoplasia, megaloblastic pancytopenia, pancytopenia) has occurred in patients receiving MTX and TMP-SMZ or TMP alone (eg, *Proloprim*).[4-9] A 74-year-old woman taking MTX 10 mg/wk for 2 years for rheumatoid arthritis developed severe pancytopenia and died of infectious complications after receiving TMP-SMZ.[10] Sulfamethizole† may displace a highly protein-bound cytotoxic 7-hydroxy metabolite of MTX.[11] In 9 children with leukemia, coadministration of MTX with TMP-SMZ produced an increase in the unbound fraction of MTX (from 38% to 52%) and a slower free MTX renal clearance (from 12.1 to 5.6 mL/kg/min). Whether these pharmacokinetic effects are responsible for the toxicities is unknown. Two case reports describe the onset of acute megaloblastic anemia in patients receiving MTX shortly after TMP-SMZ therapy was started.[12,13] See also Methotrexate-Trimethoprim.

[1] Liegler DG, et al. *Clin Pharmacol Ther.* 1969;10(6):849.
[2] Nierenberg DW. *J Pharmacol Exp Ther.* 1983;226(1):1.
[3] Dixon RL, et al. *Fed Proc.* 1965;24:454.
[4] Thomas MH, et al. *J Rheumatol.* 1986;13(2):440.
[5] Maricic M, et al. *Arthritis Rheum.* 1986;29(1):133.
[6] Frain JB. *J Rheumatol.* 1987;14(1):176.
[7] Ng HW, et al. *Br Med J (Clin Res Ed).* 1987;295(6601):752.
[8] Govert JA, et al. *Ann Intern Med.* 1992;117(10):877.
[9] Ferrazzini G, et al. *J Pediatr.* 1990;117(5):823.
[10] Groenendal H, et al. *Clin Exp Dermatol.* 1990;15(5):358.
[11] Slørdal L, et al. *Lancet.* 1988;1(8585):591.
[12] Kobrinsky NL, et al. *Ann Intern Med.* 1981;94(6):780.
[13] Dan M, et al. *Isr J Med Sci.* 1984;20(3):262.

* Asterisk indicates drugs cited in interaction reports. Based on pharmacologic and pharmacokinetic considerations, similar interactions may occur with other drugs that are listed.

† Not available in the United States.

Methotrexate — *Tetracyclines*

Methotrexate* (eg, *Rheumatrex*)	Doxycycline* (eg, *Vibramycin*)	Tetracycline* (eg, *Sumycin*)

Significance	Onset	Severity	Documentation
4	☐ Rapid	■ **Major**	☐ Established
	■ **Delayed**	☐ Moderate	☐ Probable
		☐ Minor	☐ Suspected
			■ **Possible**
			☐ Unlikely

Effects METHOTREXATE concentrations may be elevated, increasing the risk of toxicity (eg, bone marrow suppression).

Mechanism Unknown.

Management If DOXYCYCLINE cannot be avoided in patients receiving high-dose METHOTREXATE, closely monitor METHOTREXATE plasma concentrations and patients for signs and symptoms of toxicity.

Discussion

A possible drug interaction between high-dose methotrexate 12 g/m^2 and doxycycline was reported in a 17-year-old girl (body surface area, 1.52 m^2) with high-degree osteosarcoma in her left femur.[2] The patient was admitted to the hospital for her eleventh postoperative cycle of high-dose methotrexate. During a previous hospitalization, the distal third of her femur was amputated. One day prior to the current admission, the patient developed a palpebral abscess in her left eye. On admission, she had a slight fever and was treated with tobramycin 0.3% ophthalmic solution (eg, *Tobrex*), hydrocortisone plus chloramphenicol ointment (eg, *Ophthocort*), and oral doxycycline 100 mg every 12 hours. Her laboratory data showed grade 2 hematologic toxicity. Because of the absence of fever and mild hematologic recovery, the patient received methotrexate 18 g as a 12-hour IV infusion. The patient developed facial erythema, malaise, and vomiting in the first 24 hours after chemotherapy. These did not occur following the first 10 postoperative cycles of high-dose methotrexate. An interaction with doxycycline was suspected, and the antibiotic was discontinued while topical therapy was continued. The first blood count, performed on day 6 after methotrexate infusion, showed grade 3 hematologic toxicity. Leucovorin calcium (eg, *Wellcovorin*) rescue was continued until all signs and symptoms of toxicity disappeared. The patient's hospital stay was prolonged to 11 days, compared with 7.7 days during the first 10 postoperative high-dose methotrexate cycles. In addition, the methotrexate plasma concentrations and half-life were prolonged. A 39-year-old man with psoriasis who was well-maintained on methotrexate treatment for 18 weeks suddenly developed cytotoxicity after the addition of tetracycline to his treatment regimen.[1] Methotrexate was withdrawn. When tetracycline therapy was completed and methotrexate resumed, the patient had no further complications.

[1] Turck M. *Hosp Pract.* 1984;19:175.

[2] Tortajada-Ituren JJ, et al. *Ann Pharmacother.* 1999;33:804.

* Asterisk indicates drugs cited in interaction reports.

Methotrexate			***Trimethoprim***
Methotrexate* (eg, *Rheumatrex*)		Trimethoprim* (eg, *Proloprim*)	Trimethoprim-Sulfamethoxazole (eg, *Septra*)

Significance	Onset	Severity	Documentation
1	□ Rapid ■ **Delayed**	■ **Major** □ Moderate □ Minor	□ Established □ Probable ■ **Suspected** □ Possible □ Unlikely

Effects TRIMETHOPRIM may increase the risk of METHOTREXATE-induced bone marrow suppression and megaloblastic anemia.

Mechanism METHOTREXATE and TRIMETHOPRIM are folate antagonists and may have a synergistic effect on folate metabolism.

Management If this drug combination cannot be avoided, closely monitor the patient for signs of hematologic toxicity. Leucovorin calcium (eg, *Wellcovorin*) may be necessary to treat megaloblastic anemia and neutropenia resulting from folic acid deficiency.

Discussion

Necrotic skin ulceration and pancytopenia were reported in an 80-year-old woman during concurrent administration of methotrexate 25 mg by injection and trimethoprim.[1] The patient had a 24-year history of psoriasis. Five days before the sixth injection of methotrexate, the patient was started on trimethoprim 200 mg twice daily for a UTI. Other factors may have predisposed this patient to methotrexate toxicity. For example, in addition to undetected deterioration in renal function, she was receiving naproxen (eg, *Naprosyn*), which may reduce methotrexate clearance and increase the risk of methotrexate toxicity (see also Methotrexate-NSAIDs). In another report, an 81-year-old woman on low-dose methotrexate 7.5 mg/week for approximately 12 months was given trimethoprim 200 mg/day for a UTI.[2] Within 1 week, she became profoundly neutropenic and died of infectious complications. See also Methotrexate-Sulfonamides.

[1] Ng HW, et al. *BMJ.* 1987;295:752.

[2] Steuer A, et al. *Br J Rheumatol.* 1998;37:105.

* Asterisk indicates drugs cited in interaction reports.

Methotrexate — *Urinary Alkalinizers*

Methotrexate	Urinary Alkalinizers	
Methotrexate* (eg, *Rheumatrex*)	Potassium Acetate	Sodium Citrate (*Citra pH*)
	Potassium Citrate (*Urocit-K*)	Sodium Lactate
	Sodium Acetate	Tromethamine (*Tham*)
	Sodium Bicarbonate* (eg, *Neut*)	

Significance	Onset	Severity	Documentation
5	■ **Rapid**	□ Major	□ Established
	□ Delayed	□ Moderate	□ Probable
		■ **Minor**	□ Suspected
			■ **Possible**
			□ Unlikely

Effects The pharmacologic actions of METHOTREXATE may be reduced.

Mechanism Urinary alkalinization increases the renal excretion of METHOTREXATE.

Management No clinical interventions appear required.

Discussion

Methotrexate toxicity is correlated with high plasma concentrations persisting beyond 48 to 72 hours.[1] Methods to prevent toxicity have included adequate hydration, leucovorin (eg, *Wellcovorin*) rescue, and urinary alkalinization.[2] Alkalinization of the urine to a pH of at least 8 increases renal clearance and decreases methotrexate plasma levels.[3]

[1] Stoller RG, et al. *N Engl J Med.* 1977;297:630.
[2] Nirenberg A, et al. *Cancer Treat Rep.* 1977;61:779.
[3] Sand TE, et al. *Eur J Clin Pharmacol.* 1981;19:453.

* Asterisk indicates drugs cited in interaction reports. Based on pharmacologic and pharmacokinetic considerations, similar interactions may occur with other drugs that are listed.

Methotrexate		***Vancomycin***
Methotrexate* (eg, *Rheumatrex*)		Vancomycin* (eg, *Vancocin*)

Significance	Onset	Severity	Documentation
4	□ Rapid	■ **Major**	□ Established
	■ **Delayed**	□ Moderate	□ Probable
		□ Minor	□ Suspected
			■ **Possible**
			□ Unlikely

Effects METHOTREXATE serum concentrations may be elevated and clearance may be delayed, increasing the risk of toxicity (eg, myelosuppression).

Mechanism Delayed excretion of METHOTREXATE caused by subclinical nephrotoxicity induced by VANCOMYCIN is suspected.

Management When VANCOMYCIN is administered prior to METHOTREXATE (eg, up to 10 days prior), assess glomerular filtration rate and adjust the METHOTREXATE dose as needed.

Discussion

Two patients, a 29-year-old man and a 29-year-old woman, experienced a possible drug interaction when methotrexate was administered following recent exposure to vancomycin.[1] Both patients were being treated for femoral osteosarcoma with alternating chemotherapy, which consisted of high-dose methotrexate (12 g/m^2 IV), cisplatin (eg, *Platinol-AQ*), doxorubicin (eg, *Adriamycin RDF*), and ifosfamide (eg, *Ifex*). In both patients, during initial treatment cycles, methotrexate serum concentrations decreased to safe levels of 0.2 mcmol/L within 72 hr. However, when vancomycin (1 g twice daily) was given 8 to 10 days prior to methotrexate administration, methotrexate serum concentrations were elevated and clearance was markedly prolonged, requiring 170 to 231 hr to decline to below 0.2 mcmol/L. Although there were no signs of overt renal impairment at the time of methotrexate administration, subclinical renal impairment was documented by impaired glomerular filtration. Subsequently, when methotrexate was given without recent exposure to vancomycin, methotrexate was cleared within 72 hr.

Additional documentation is needed to confirm this possible drug interaction and to clarify the mechanism.

[1] Blum R, et al. *Ann Oncol.* 2002;13:327.

* Asterisk indicates drugs cited in interaction reports.

Methoxyflurane | **_Aminoglycosides, Parent._**

Methoxyflurane	Aminoglycosides, Parent.	
Methoxyflurane* (*Penthrane*)	Amikacin (*Amikin*)	Netilmicin (*Netromycin*)
	Gentamicin* (eg, *Garamycin*)	Streptomycin
	Kanamycin* (eg, *Kantrex*)	Tobramycin (*Nebcin*)
	Neomycin (*Mycifradin*)	

Significance	Onset	Severity	Documentation
4	■ **Rapid**	■ **Major**	□ Established
	□ Delayed	□ Moderate	□ Probable
		□ Minor	□ Suspected
			■ **Possible**
			□ Unlikely

Effects Enhanced renal toxicity may occur.

Mechanism Additive or perhaps even synergistic renal toxicity appears probable.

Management Avoid coadministration if possible; seek alternative agents. If coadministration is necessary, monitor renal function closely and tailor AMINOGYCOSIDE dosage as needed.

Discussion

Methoxyflurane[1,3,5] and aminoglycoside antibiotics[7] have both been documented to cause significant nephrotoxicity. Because their individual mechanisms appear to be different, additive or synergistic nephrotoxicity is possible. Kanamycin[2] and gentamicin[2,4-6] have been specifically implicated in interacting adversely with methoxyflurane in both man[2,5,6] and animals.[4] However, there appears to be very few real cases reported and no controlled studies. The importance of this interaction lies primarily in the known pharmacology of the individual agents.

[1] Mazze RI, et al. *JAMA*. 1971;216:278.
[2] Cousins MJ, et al. *Lancet*. 1972;1:751.
[3] Hollenberg NK, et al. *N Engl J Med*. 1972;286:877.
[4] Barr GA, et al. *Br J Anaesth*. 1973;45:306.
[5] Mazze RI, et al. *Br J Anaesth*. 1973;45:394.
[6] Churchill D, et al. *Am J Med*. 1974;56:575.
[7] Kucers A, et al. *The Use of Antibiotics*.. 4th ed. Phil: JB Lippincott, 1987.

* Asterisk indicates drugs cited in interaction reports. Based on pharmacologic and pharmacokinetic considerations, similar interactions may occur with other drugs that are listed.

Methoxyflurane — *Barbiturates*

Methoxyflurane	Barbiturates	
Methoxyflurane* (*Penthrane*)	Amobarbital (eg, *Amytal*)	Pentobarbital* (eg, *Nembutal*)
	Aprobarbital (*Alurate*)	Phenobarbital*
	Butabarbital (eg, *Butisol*)	Primidone (eg, *Mysoline*)
	Butalbital	Secobarbital* (eg, *Seconal*)
	Mephobarbital (*Mebaral*)	Talbutal (*Lotusate*)
	Metharbital (*Gemonil*)	

Significance	Onset	Severity	Documentation
2	■ **Rapid**	□ Major	□ Established
	□ Delayed	■ **Moderate**	□ Probable
		□ Minor	■ **Suspected**
			□ Possible
			□ Unlikely

Effects Enhanced renal toxicity may occur.

Mechanism BARBITURATES appear to stimulate degradation of METHOXYFLURANE, perhaps to nephrotoxic metabolites.

Management If possible, do not administer METHOXYFLURANE in the presence of enzyme inducers such as BARBITURATES. Because enzyme induction dissipates slowly, be wary of the combination for several weeks following withdrawal of BARBITURATES. Monitor renal function closely.

Discussion

Methoxyflurane's nephrotoxic potential is well documented[2,3] as is the barbiturate property of stimulating liver microsomal enzymes to increase metabolism of drugs so degraded. Several studies, all in rats, have demonstrated that the barbiturates induce the metabolism of methoxyflurane to the nephrotoxic metabolites, fluorinated compounds and oxalate.[1,4-7] At least 2 cases of human renal toxicity have been published.[2,8]

This interaction is well documented in the laboratory but human data is lacking. However, the weight of evidence warrants caution when using these agents together and avoidance of coadministration when possible.

[1] Son SL, et al. *Br J Anaesth.* 1972;44:1224.
[2] Cousins MJ, et al. *JAMA.* 1973;225:1611.
[3] Churchill D, et al. *Am J Med.* 1974;56:575
[4] Mazze RI, et al. *J Pharmacol Exp Ther.* 1974;190:523.
[5] Cousins MJ, et al. *J Pharmacol Exp Ther.* 1974;190:530.
[6] Cook TL, et al. *Anesth Analg.* 1975;54:829.
[7] Brodeur J, et al. *Toxicol Appl Pharmacol.* 1976;37:349.
[8] Churchill D, et al. *Can Med Assoc J.* 1976;114:326.

* Asterisk indicates drugs cited in interaction reports. Based on pharmacologic and pharmacokinetic considerations, similar interactions may occur with other drugs that are listed.

Methoxyflurane — *Tetracyclines*

Methoxyflurane	Tetracyclines	
Methoxyflurane* (*Penthrane*)	Demeclocycline (*Declomycin*)	Minocycline (*Minocin*)
	Doxycycline (eg, *Vibramycin*)	Oxytetracycline* (eg, *Terramycin*)
	Methacycline (*Rondomycin*)	Tetracycline* (eg, *Achromycin V*)

Significance	Onset	Severity	Documentation
1	■ **Rapid**	■ **Major**	□ Established
	□ Delayed	□ Moderate	□ Probable
		□ Minor	■ **Suspected**
			□ Possible
			□ Unlikely

Effects Enhanced renal toxicity may occur.

Mechanism Speculative, but includes TETRACYCLINE-induced METHOXYFLURANE biotransformation and impairment of renal excretion of toxic metabolites.

Management Do not coadminister; if possible, seek alternative agents.

Discussion

Methoxyflurane[3,5,9] and tetracyclines[12] are both documented to cause nephrotoxicity. Numerous case reports exist implicating the combination of methoxyflurane and tetracylines to be additive or synergistic in causing renal dysfunction; deaths have also been reported.[1,2,4,6-11] Animal experiments also suggest some additive activity.[10] However, controlled trials are absent and some speculate that much of the nephrotoxicity is attributable to prolonged methoxyflurane administration.[8,11]

More data and preferably controlled studies are needed to clarify whether or not a real interaction exists.

[1] Kuzucu EY. *JAMA*. 1970;211:1162.
[2] Albers DD, et al. *J Urol*. 1971;106:348.
[3] Mazze RI, et al. *JAMA*. 1971;216:278.
[4] Proctor EA, et al. *Br Med J*. 1971;4:661.
[5] Hollenberg NK, et al. *N Engl J Med*. 1972;286:877.
[6] Cousins MJ, et al. *Lancet*. 1972;1:752.
[7] Stoelting RK, et al. *Anesth Analg*. 1973;52:431.
[8] Cousins MJ, et al. *JAMA*. 1973;225:1611.
[9] Churchill D, et al. *Am J Med*. 1974;56:575.
[10] Rosenberg PH, et al. *Acta Pharmacol Toxicol*. 1974;34:46.
[11] Dryden GE. *Anesth Analg*. 1974;53:383.
[12] Kucers A, et al. *The Use of Antibiotics*.. 4th ed. Phil:JB Lippincott, 1987.

* Asterisk indicates drugs cited in interaction reports. Based on pharmacologic and pharmacokinetic considerations, similar interactions may occur with other drugs that are listed.

Methyldopa | **Barbiturates**

Methyldopa* (eg, *Aldomet*)	Phenobarbital*	Primidone (eg, *Mysoline*)

Significance	Onset	Severity	Documentation
5	☐ Rapid ■ **Delayed**	☐ Major ☐ Moderate ■ **Minor**	☐ Established ☐ Probable ☐ Suspected ☐ Possible ■ **Unlikely**

Effects The actions of METHYLDOPA may be reduced.

Mechanism Unknown.

Management No clinical interventions appear required.

Discussion

Kaldor et al evaluated the effect of phenobarbital on serum catecholamines as an indirect measure of methyldopa. The results implied that phenobarbital may increase the metabolic clearance of methyldopa.[1] However, subsequent reports utilizing direct plasma measurements of methyldopa and alpha methyldopa-O-sulfate, found no evidence of an effect by phenobarbital.[2,3]

This interaction appears unlikely.

[1] Kaldor A, et al. *Br Med J.* 1971;3:518.
[2] Kristensen M, et al. *Br Med J.* 1973;1:49.
[3] Kristensen M, et al. *Clin Pharmacol Ther.* 1973;14:139.

* Asterisk indicates drugs cited in interaction reports. Based on pharmacologic and pharmacokinetic considerations, similar interactions may occur with other drugs that are listed.

Methyldopa — *Beta-Blockers (Nonsel.)*

Methyldopa	Beta-Blockers (Nonsel.)	
Methyldopa*	Carteolol (*Cartrol*)	Pindolol (eg, *Visken*)
	Nadolol (eg, *Corgard*)	Propranolol* (eg, *Inderal*)
	Oxprenolol*†	Timolol (eg, *Blocadren*)
	Penbutolol (*Levatol*)	

Significance	Onset	Severity	Documentation
4	■ **Rapid**	□ Major	□ Established
	□ Delayed	■ **Moderate**	□ Probable
		□ Minor	□ Suspected
			■ **Possible**
			□ Unlikely

Effects Hypertensive crisis.

Mechanism Alpha-adrenergic–mediated vasoconstriction effects of the METHYLDOPA metabolite alpha-methyldopa norepinephrine are unopposed because of beta-blockade.

Management Closely monitor for acute BP increases during combined METHYLDOPA and BETA-BLOCKER use. If acute increases in BP occur, treat with alpha-adrenergic blocking agents such as phentolamine.

Discussion

A rapid and fatal increase in BP occurred in a severely hypertensive patient maintained on methyldopa shortly after injection of propranolol.[1] The incremental increase in BP was reversed by phentolamine. A serious increase in BP occurred in another severely hypertensive patient maintained on oxprenolol[†] and methyldopa after ingestion of phenylpropanolamine[†] for relief of cold symptoms.[2] BP returned to baseline after phenylpropanolamine was discontinued.

The risk of serious increases in BP when methyldopa is combined with beta-adrenergic blockers is not clear. They have been used together effectively in the treatment of hypertension[3] and methyldopa alone has been associated with paradoxical increases in BP.[4] The risk may be limited to severely hypertensive patients or those exposed to excessive endogenous or exogenous sympathetic agonists.[1,3,5]

1 Nies AS, et al. *Clin Pharmacol Ther.* 1973;14(5):823.
2 McLaren EH. *Br Med J.* 1976;2(6030):283.
3 Petrie JC, et al. *Br Med J.* 1976;2(6028):137.
4 Zehnle CG. *Am J Hosp Pharm.* 1981;38(11):1774.
5 Swan B. *JAMA.* 1975;232:1281.

* Asterisk indicates drugs cited in interaction reports. Based on pharmacologic and pharmacokinetic considerations, similar interactions may occur with other drugs that are listed.
†Not available in the US.

Methyldopa — *Levodopa*

Methyldopa*	Levodopa* (*Larodopa*)

Significance	Onset	Severity	Documentation
5	■ **Rapid**	□ Major	□ Established
	□ Delayed	□ Moderate	□ Probable
		■ **Minor**	□ Suspected
			■ **Possible**
			□ Unlikely

Effects BP-lowering effects of METHYLDOPA may be potentiated by LEVODOPA. Central effects of LEVODOPA in Parkinson disease may be potentiated by METHYLDOPA.

Mechanism The mechanism for the BP-lowering effects of METHYLDOPA and LEVODOPA are unknown. Potentiation of LEVODOPA's central effects may result from METHYLDOPA inhibition of peripheral dopa-decarboxylase, making more LEVODOPA available to cross the blood-brain barrier.

Management Observe for hypotension or signs of LEVODOPA toxicity. If either occurs, consider decreasing the dose of METHYLDOPA or LEVODOPA, or use an alternative antihypertensive agent.

Discussion

Attempts have been made to potentiate the action of levodopa in the treatment of Parkinson disease by combining it with methyldopa.[1-5] The use of this combination in the treatment of Parkinson disease has produced variable clinical success with some patients improving, some remaining the same, and others worsening.[1,2,4,5] In one study that assessed the hemodynamic consequences of combining methyldopa and levodopa in Parkinson patients,[3] standing BP was lower when the 2 drugs were used together than when either was used alone, but no symptoms were reported. The effect of methyldopa and levodopa on BP overall has been inconsistent.[1-5]

During combined use of methyldopa and levodopa, monitor BP and watch for signs of levodopa toxicity. This combination may permit or require reduction of the levodopa dosage.

[1] Fermaglich J, et al. *Neurology.* 1971;21:408.
[2] Sweet RD, et al. *Clin Pharmacol Ther.* 1972;13(1):23.
[3] Gibberd FB, et al. *Br Med J.* 1973;2(5858):90.
[4] Fermaglich J, et al. *Lancet.* 1973;1(7814):1261.
[5] Mones RJ. *NY State J Med.* 1974;74(1):47.

* Asterisk indicates drugs cited in interaction reports.

Methyldopa — *MAOIs*

Methyldopa	MAOIs	
Methyldopa*	Isocarboxazid (*Marplan*)	Tranylcypromine (eg, *Parnate*)
	Pargyline*	
	Phenelzine (*Nardil*)	

Significance	Onset	Severity	Documentation
2	☐ Rapid	☐ Major	☐ Established
	■ **Delayed**	■ **Moderate**	☐ Probable
		☐ Minor	■ **Suspected**
			☐ Possible
			☐ Unlikely

Effects Loss of BP control or signs of central stimulation (eg, excitation, hallucinations).

Mechanism Metabolites of METHYLDOPA stimulate release of endogenous catecholamines that are usually metabolized by MAOIs, thereby leading to excessive sympathetic stimulation.

Management Coadministration is contraindicated.[1]

Discussion

Hallucinations were reported in a 55-year-old patient maintained on the MAOI pargyline after the addition of methyldopa.[2] The hallucinations resolved upon discontinuation of both drugs and did not recur when pargyline was reinstituted. Animal studies have suggested that metabolites of methyldopa release endogenous catecholamines that are subject to metabolism by MAOIs.[3,4]

[1] *Methyldopa* [package insert]. Sellersville, PA: Teva Pharmaceuticals; December 2008.
[2] Paykel ES. *Br Med J.* 1966;1(5490):803.
[3] Van Rossum J. *Lancet.* 1963;1(7287):950.
[4] Van Rossum J, et al. *J Pharm Pharmacol.* 1963;15:493.

* Asterisk indicates drugs cited in interaction reports.

Methyldopa — *Phenothiazines*

Methyldopa*	Trifluoperazine*

Significance	Onset	Severity	Documentation
5	☐ Rapid	☐ Major	☐ Established
	■ **Delayed**	■ **Moderate**	☐ Probable
		☐ Minor	☐ Suspected
			☐ Possible
			■ **Unlikely**

Effects Serious elevations in BP.

Mechanism Unknown.

Management Closely observe BP when METHYLDOPA and a PHENOTHIAZINE are used concurrently. If BP increases, discontinue either or both of the agents.

Discussion

Serious elevations in BP were recorded after initiating methyldopa therapy in a patient maintained on trifluoperazine. BP returned to previous levels after discontinuation of trifluoperazine.[1] However, a case of worsening hypertension associated with methyldopa in a patient not maintained on a phenothiazine has also been reported. In addition, an animal study failed to demonstrate an interaction between methyldopa and chlorpromazine that resulted in hemodynamic manifestations.[2,3]

[1] Westervelt FB Jr, et al. *JAMA*. 1974;227(5):557.
[2] Levine RJ, et al. *N Engl J Med*. 1966;275(17):946.
[3] Rankin GO, et al. *Arch Int Pharmacodyn Ther*. 1982;260(1):130.

* Asterisk indicates drugs cited in interaction reports.

Methyldopa — *Tricyclic Antidepressants*

Methyldopa	Tricyclic Antidepressants	
Methyldopa* (eg, *Aldomet*)	Amitriptyline*	Imipramine (eg, *Tofranil*)
	Amoxapine (eg, *Asendin*)	Nortriptyline (eg, *Pamelor*)
	Clomipramine (eg, *Anafranil*)	Protriptyline (eg, *Vivactil*)
	Desipramine (eg, *Norpramin*)	Trimipramine (*Surmontil*)
	Doxepin (eg, *Sinequan*)	

Significance	Onset	Severity	Documentation
5	□ Rapid	□ Major	□ Established
	■ **Delayed**	■ **Moderate**	□ Probable
		□ Minor	□ Suspected
			□ Possible
			■ **Unlikely**

Effects TRICYCLIC ANTIDEPRESSANT reversal or attenuation of the hypotensive effects of METHYLDOPA.

Mechanism TRICYCLIC ANTIDEPRESSANT interference with the central actions of METHYLDOPA has been proposed.

Management Monitor blood pressure after initiation of a TRICYCLIC ANTIDEPRESSANT in patients maintained on METHYLDOPA.

Discussion

Loss of blood pressure control was reported after initiation of amitriptyline in a hypertensive patient maintained on methyldopa.[1] Subsequent animal studies provided evidence that tricyclic antidepressants could modestly attenuate the hypotensive effects of methyldopa.[3,4] However, in clinical investigations involving both hypertensive and normotensive subjects, the hypotensive effects of methyldopa were not affected by concurrent use of a tricyclic antidepressant.[2,5] Therefore, tricyclic antidepressants are not contraindicated in hypertensive patients maintained on methyldopa, but monitor blood pressure during combined use.

[1] White AG. *Lancet*. 1965;2:441.
[2] Mitchell JR, et al. *J Clin Invest*. 1970;49:1596.
[3] Kale AK, et al. *Eur J Pharmacol*. 1970;9:120.
[4] van Zwieten PA, et al. *Arch Int Pharmacodyn*. 1975;214:12.
[5] Reid JL, et al. *Eur J Clin Pharmacol*. 1979;16:75.

* Asterisk indicates drugs cited in interaction reports.

Methylphenidate — *Carbamazepine*

Methylphenidate* (eg, *Ritalin*)	Carbamazepine* (eg, *Tegretol*)

Significance	Onset	Severity	Documentation
4	☐ Rapid	☐ Major	☐ Established
	■ **Delayed**	■ **Moderate**	☐ Probable
		☐ Minor	☐ Suspected
			■ **Possible**
			☐ Unlikely

Effects METHYLPHENIDATE blood concentrations may be reduced, leading to a decrease in pharmacologic effects.

Mechanism Unknown.

Management In patients receiving METHYLPHENIDATE, carefully monitor the clinical response when starting, stopping, or changing the dose of CARBAMAZEPINE.

Discussion

Methylphenidate blood concentrations decreased in a 13-year-old girl with attention deficit hyperactivity disorder (ADHD) after starting therapy with carbamazepine.[2] The patient was receiving methylphenidate 20 mg 3 times daily and risperidone (*Risperdal*) 2 mg at bedtime. Risperidone was discontinued because the patient complained of weight gain. She was later started on carbamazepine 200 mg at bedtime because of modest effect on weight gain. At this time, the peak morning concentration of methylphenidate and ritalinic acid was 5.3 ng/mL (therapeutic 5 to 20 ng/mL). The patient's ADHD symptoms worsened as the carbamazepine dose was increased to 200 mg twice daily and 400 mg at bedtime. Approximately 6 weeks later, her methylphenidate and ritalinic acid strict 2-hour peak blood level decreased to 4.2 ng/mL. One month later, the carbamazepine dose was increased to 300 mg twice daily and 400 mg at bedtime. The methylphenidate and ritalinic acid blood concentration decreased to 2.4 ng/mL, even though the methylphenidate dose was increased to 35 mg 3 times daily because her ADHD symptoms worsened. Two months later, her dose of methylphenidate was increased to 60 mg 3 times daily and carbamazepine was increased to 1200 mg/day to achieve the benefits from methylphenidate therapy she had before starting carbamazepine. A 7-year-old boy with severe mental retardation and ADHD failed to respond to methylphenidate 20 mg every 4 hours.[1] His dose of thiothixene (eg, *Navane*) was increased from 6 to 10 mg/day to enhance the effects of methylphenidate and to reduce aggressiveness. In addition, he was receiving carbamazepine for grand mal epilepsy. Neither thiothixene nor methylphenidate or their metabolites could be measured in the blood. Despite increases in the dose of methylphenidate to 30 mg every 4 hours and thiothixene to 20 mg/day, no clinical evidence of either drug could be found.

[1] Behar D, et al. *J Am Acad Child Adolesc Psychiatry.* 1998;37:1128.

[2] Schaller JL, et al. *J Am Acad Child Adolesc Psychiatry.* 1999;38:112.

* Asterisk indicates drugs cited in interaction reports.

Methylphenidate — *Ethanol*

Methylphenidate*
(eg, *Ritalin*)

Ethanol*
(Alcohol, Ethyl Alcohol)

Significance	Onset	Severity	Documentation
4	☐ Rapid ■ **Delayed**	☐ Major ■ **Moderate** ☐ Minor	☐ Established ☐ Probable ☐ Suspected ■ **Possible** ☐ Unlikely

Effects METHYLPHENIDATE plasma concentrations may be elevated, increasing the risk of adverse reactions, including abuse liability.

Mechanism Inhibition of METHYLPHENIDATE hydrolysis by ALCOHOL is suspected.

Management Patients taking METHYLPHENIDATE should abstain from ALCOHOL use. When treating adult attention deficit hyperactivity disorder in patients with comorbid ALCOHOL abuse, consider an alternative treatment to METHYLPHENIDATE. Atomoxetine (*Strattera*) may be a safer alternative.

Discussion

In an open-label, randomized, crossover study, the effects of alcohol ingestion on the pharmacokinetics and pharmacodynamics of methylphenidate were investigated in 20 men and women.[1] Each individual received immediate-release methylphenidate 0.3 mg/kg 30 minutes before or after ingestion of orange juice and soda containing alcohol 0.6 g/kg. In addition, each subject received methylphenidate 0.3 mg/kg, followed 30 minutes later by orange juice and soda containing no alcohol. Compared with taking methylphenidate without alcohol, ingestion of alcohol 30 minutes before or after methylphenidate increased the methylphenidate C_{max} and AUC approximately 40% and 25%, respectively. In general, women reported greater subjective stimulant effects to methylphenidate than men, in spite of lower mean methylphenidate C_{max} and AUC values.

[1] Patrick KS, et al. *Clin Pharmacol Ther*. 2007;81(3):346.

* Asterisk indicates drugs cited in interaction reports.

Methylphenidate — *MAOIs*

Methylphenidate		MAOIs	
Dexmethylphenidate* (eg, *Focalin*)	Methylphenidate* (eg, *Ritalin*)	Isocarboxazid* (*Marplan*)	Rasagiline* (*Azilect*)
		Linezolid* (*Zyvox*)	Selegiline* (eg, *Eldepryl*)
		Phenelzine* (*Nardil*)	Tranylcypromine* (eg, *Parnate*)

Significance	Onset	Severity	Documentation
1	□ Rapid	■ **Major**	□ Established
	■ **Delayed**	□ Moderate	□ Probable
		□ Minor	■ **Suspected**
			□ Possible
			□ Unlikely

Effects Hypertensive crisis.

Mechanism Unknown.

Management Monitor BP during combined MAOI and METHYLPHENIDATE use. DEXMETHYLPHENIDATE is contraindicated in patients receiving MAOI therapy and also within a minimum of 14 days after discontinuation of an MAOI.[1]

Discussion

Dexmethylphenidate, the d-threo-enantiomer of racemic (ie, d- and l-threo-enantiomers) methylphenidate, is the more pharmacologically active enantiomer.[1] The manufacturer of dexmethylphenidate states that hypertensive crises may result with coadministration of an MAOI. A single case report with a questionable cause-effect relationship is the only documentation of this interaction. A patient receiving tranylcypromine presented to an emergency room in hypertensive crisis 15 days after methylphenidate was added to the patient's therapy.[2] No other information was provided to rule out other causes, such as dietary consideration. See also CNS Stimulants-MAOIs.

[1] *Focalin* [package insert]. East Hanover, NJ: Novartis Pharmaceutical Corp; November 2001.

[2] Sherman M, et al. *Am J Psychiatry*. 1964;120:1019.

* Asterisk indicates drugs cited in interaction reports.

Methylphenidate — *St. John's Wort*

Methylphenidate* (eg, *Ritalin*)	St. John's Wort*

Significance	Onset	Severity	Documentation
4	☐ Rapid ■ **Delayed**	☐ Major ■ **Moderate** ☐ Minor	☐ Established ☐ Probable ☐ Suspected ■ **Possible** ☐ Unlikely

Effects Efficacy of METHYLPHENIDATE may be reduced.

Mechanism Unknown.

Management Avoid concurrent use of METHYLPHENIDATE and ST. JOHN'S WORT.

Discussion

A 22-year-old man, showing improvement in attention deficit hyperactivity disorder symptomatology while on a stable regimen of methylphenidate 20 mg daily, experienced diminished methylphenidate efficacy after he self-medicated with St. John's wort 600 mg daily for 4 months.[1] He became more inattentive. His condition improved 3 weeks after discontinuing St. John's wort.

[1] Niederhofer H. *Med Hypotheses*. 2007;68(5):1189.

* Asterisk indicates drugs cited in interaction reports.

Metrizamide — Phenothiazines

Metrizamide	Phenothiazines	
Metrizamide* (*Amipaque*)	Acetophenazine (*Tindal*)	Promazine (eg, *Sparine*)
	Chlorpromazine* (eg, *Thorazine*)	Promethazine (eg, *Phenergan*)
	Ethopropazine (*Parsidol*)	Propiomazine (*Largon*)
	Fluphenazine (eg, *Prolixin*)	Thiethylperazine (*Torecan*)
	Methdilazine (*Tacaryl*)	Thioridazine
	Methotrimeprazine (*Levoprome*)	Trifluoperazine
	Perphenazine	Triflupromazine (*Vesprin*)
	Prochlorperazine (eg, *Compazine*)	Trimeprazine (*Temaril*)

Significance	Onset	Severity	Documentation
2	■ **Rapid**	□ Major	□ Established
	□ Delayed	■ **Moderate**	□ Probable
		□ Minor	■ **Suspected**
			□ Possible
			□ Unlikely

Effects The possibility of seizure may be increased during subarachnoid injection of METRIZAMIDE in patients maintained on a PHENOTHIAZINE.

Mechanism A lowering of the seizure threshold by the combined use of METRIZAMIDE and a PHENOTHIAZINE has been proposed.

Management Discontinue PHENOTHIAZINE therapy at least 48 hours in advance of METRIZAMIDE use. In the event that seizures occur, treat with phenobarbital.

Discussion

Clinical seizure activity in one patient and epileptogenic EEG patterns in another were reported among a large series of patients who had undergone myelography with metrizamide.[1,2] The 2 patients with seizure activity were distinguished from the other patients by their maintenance phenothiazine therapy. Subsequent animal studies provided further evidence that a greater likelihood of seizures may exist when metrizamide is used in patients maintained on a phenothiazine.[3,5] In addition, animal data suggested that phenothiazines should be discontinued 48 hours in advance of metrizamide use and in the event of seizure, phenobarbital may be the antiseizure drug of choice.[3] However, in a series of 100 patients admitted for myelography with metrizamide, no seizure activity was observed and no attempts were made to discontinue phenothiazine therapy in advance.[4]

[1] Hindmarsh T, et al. *Acta Radiol Diag*. 1975;16:129.
[2] Hindmarsh T. *Acta Radiol Diag*. 1975;16:209.
[3] Gonsette RE, et al. *Neuroradiology*. 1977;14:27.
[4] Hauge O, et al. *AJR*. 1982;139:357.
[5] Maly P, et al. *Neuroradiology*. 1984;26:235.

* Asterisk indicates drugs cited in interaction reports. Based on pharmacologic and pharmacokinetic considerations, similar interactions may occur with other drugs that are listed.

Metronidazole — *Barbiturates*

Metronidazole	Barbiturates	
Metronidazole* (eg, *Flagyl*)	Amobarbital (eg, *Amytal*)	Pentobarbital (eg, *Nembutal*)
	Aprobarbital (*Alurate*)	Phenobarbital*
	Butabarbital (eg, *Butisol*)	Primidone (eg, *Mysoline*)
	Butalbital	Secobarbital (eg, *Seconal*)
	Mephobarbital (*Mebaral*)	Talbutal (*Lotusate*)
	Metharbital (*Gemonil*)	

Significance	Onset	Severity	Documentation
2	☐ Rapid	☐ Major	☐ Established
	■ **Delayed**	■ **Moderate**	☐ Probable
		☐ Minor	■ **Suspected**
			☐ Possible
			☐ Unlikely

Effects Therapeutic failure of METRONIDAZOLE.

Mechanism BARBITURATE induction of METRONIDAZOLE metabolism resulting in more rapid elimination and lower serum concentrations.

Management Observe for METRONIDAZOLE treatment failure in patients receiving a BARBITURATE concurrently, and if necessary, increase the METRONIDAZOLE dose accordingly. Alternatively, use higher initial METRONIDAZOLE doses in patients also receiving a BARBITURATE.

Discussion

Barbiturate induction of metronidazole metabolism has been demonstrated to varying degrees in patients,[1-3,5] animals,[4] and in vitro.[6] Treatment failures have been reported when conventional doses of metronidazole have been used in patients maintained on phenobarbital.[1,2] Investigations into these metronidazole failures revealed unexpectedly short elimination half-lives (3.5 hours) and higher metabolite to metronidazole ratios (0.5-1.9). Clinical success has been achieved with higher metronidazole doses.

[1] Mead PB, et al. *N Engl J Med.* 1982;306:1490.
[2] Gupte S. *N Engl J Med.* 1983;308:529.
[3] Loft S, et al. *Eur J Clin Pharmacol.* 1987;32:35.
[4] Mannisto PT, et al. *Pharmacol Toxicol.* 1987;60:24.
[5] Eradiri O, et al. *Biopharm Drug Dispos.* 1988;9:219.
[6] Loft S, et al. *Biochem Pharmacol.* 1989;38:1125.

* Asterisk indicates drugs cited in interaction reports. Based on pharmacologic and pharmacokinetic considerations, similar interactions may occur with other drugs that are listed.

Metronidazole — *Cimetidine*

Metronidazole* (eg, *Flagyl*)	Cimetidine* (*Tagamet*)

Significance	Onset	Severity	Documentation
5	☐ Rapid	☐ Major	☐ Established
	■ **Delayed**	☐ Moderate	☐ Probable
		■ **Minor**	☐ Suspected
			■ **Possible**
			☐ Unlikely

Effects Decreased METRONIDAZOLE clearance and increased serum concentrations.

Mechanism CIMETIDINE inhibition of METRONIDAZOLE hepatic metabolism has been proposed, but not established.

Management Observe for METRONIDAZOLE toxicity during concurrent CIMETIDINE use. If METRONIDAZOLE toxicity occurs, consider discontinuing or lowering the dose of METRONIDAZOLE.

Discussion

The results of studies investigating the interaction of metronidazole and cimetidine have been equivocal. In 1 study involving 6 healthy volunteer subjects,[1] metronidazole clearance decreased by 29% from control after 6 days of cimetidine 800 mg/day. However, subsequent studies involving small numbers of volunteers or patients with Crohn Disease did not confirm the alterations in metronidazole pharmacokinetics during concurrent cimetidine use.[2-4] In none of the studies were there any reports of metronidazole toxicity during concurrent cimetidine use.

[1] Gugler R, et al. *N Engl J Med.* 1983;309:1518.
[2] Loft S, et al. *Eur J Clin Pharmacol.* 1987;32:35.
[3] Loft S, et al. *Eur J Clin Pharmacol.* 1988;35:65.
[4] Eradiri O, et al. *Biopharm Drug Dispos.* 1988;9:219.

* Asterisk indicates drugs cited in interaction reports.

Metyrapone — *Cyproheptadine*

Metyrapone* (*Metopirone*)	Cyproheptadine* (*Periactin*)

Significance	Onset	Severity	Documentation
2	■ **Rapid** ☐ Delayed	☐ Major ■ **Moderate** ☐ Minor	☐ Established ■ **Probable** ☐ Suspected ☐ Possible ☐ Unlikely

Effects Subnormal pituitary-adrenal responses to METYRAPONE.

Mechanism A reduction in the ACTH secretion expected after METYRAPONE administration by CYPROHEPTADINE.

Management Discontinue CYPROHEPTADINE use before or avoid its use during assessment of pituitary-adrenal axis function assessment with METYRAPONE.

Discussion

The expected pituitary-adrenal response to metyrapone was diminished during concurrent cyproheptadine administration in patients with Carcinoid Syndrome and in volunteer subjects. This interaction appears to be caused by a subnormal ACTH release in response to metyrapone by cyproheptadine and may involve cyproheptadine antiserotonin actions.[1,2] Cyproheptadine should be avoided or discontinued before metyrapone is used for pituitary-adrenal axis assessment.

[1] Plonk J, et al. *Metabolism.* 1975;24:1035.

[2] Plonk J, et al. *J Clin Endocrinol Metab.* 1976;42:291.

* Asterisk indicates drugs cited in interaction reports.

Metyrapone | **Hydantoins**

Metyrapone		Hydantoins	
Metyrapone* (*Metopirone*)		Ethotoin (*Peganone*)	Phenytoin* (eg, *Dilantin*)
		Fosphenytoin (*Cerebyx*)	

Significance	Onset	Severity	Documentation
2	□ Rapid	□ Major	■ **Established**
	■ **Delayed**	■ **Moderate**	□ Probable
		□ Minor	□ Suspected
			□ Possible
			□ Unlikely

Effects Subnormal pituitary-adrenal responses to oral METYRAPONE.

Mechanism HYDANTOIN induction of METYRAPONE first-pass hepatic extraction, resulting in insufficient amounts available to inhibit 11 beta-hydroxylase.

Management Consider using oral METYRAPONE doses up to twice the usual dose when assessing pituitary-adrenal axis function in patients maintained on HYDANTOINS. Discontinue HYDANTOINS when possible.

Discussion

Administration of oral metyrapone to patients maintained on phenytoin resulted in subnormal increases in plasma 11-deoxycortisol and adrenocorticotropic hormone concentrations as well as urinary excretion of 17-hydroxycorticosteroids.[1-3] An animal study provided evidence that phenytoin induces first-pass hepatic extraction of metyrapone, substantially reducing bioavailability.[4] Thus, less metyrapone is available to inhibit 11 beta-hydroxylase, leading to subnormal responses. Doubling the oral dose of IV administration of metyrapone restored the expected response in one study.[3]

[1] Krieger DT, *J Clin Endocrinol Metab.* 1962;22:490.
[2] Werk EE Jr, et al. *J Clin Endocrinol Metab.* 1967;27(9):1358.
[3] Meikle AW, et al. *J Clin Endocrinol Metab.* 1969;29(12):1553.
[4] Jubiz W, et al. *Endocrinology.* 1970;86(2):328.

* Asterisk indicates drugs cited in interaction reports. Based on pharmacologic and pharmacokinetic considerations, similar interactions may occur with other drugs that are listed.

Mexiletine — *Fluvoxamine*

Mexiletine* (eg, *Mexitil*)	Fluvoxamine* (eg, *Luvox*)

Significance	Onset	Severity	Documentation
4	☐ Rapid ■ **Delayed**	☐ Major ■ **Moderate** ☐ Minor	☐ Established ☐ Probable ☐ Suspected ■ **Possible** ☐ Unlikely

Effects MEXILETINE serum levels may be elevated, increasing the therapeutic effects and adverse reactions.

Mechanism Inhibition of MEXILETINE metabolism by FLUVOXAMINE is suspected.

Management Carefully monitor mexiletine serum concentrations and observe the clinical response of the patient to MEXILETINE when starting or stopping FLUVOXAMINE. If an interaction is suspected, adjust the MEXILETINE dose as needed.

Discussion

The effect of fluvoxamine on the pharmacokinetics of mexiletine was studied in 6 healthy Japanese men.[1] In a 2-phase, randomized, crossover study, each subject received 200 mg of mexiletine alone or following 50 mg twice daily of fluvoxamine for 7 days. Compared with giving mexiletine alone, coadministration of fluvoxamine resulted in a 55% increase in the mexiletine AUC and a 16% increase (from 0.536 to 0.623 mcg/mL) in peak serum concentration. Pretreatment with fluvoxamine produced a 38% decrease in the oral clearance of mexiletine.

[1] Kusumoto M, et al. *Clin Pharmacol Ther.* 2001;69(3):104.

* Asterisk indicates drugs cited in interaction reports.

Mexiletine — *Hydantoins*

Mexiletine* (eg, *Mexitil*)	Ethotoin (*Peganone*) Fosphenytoin (*Cerebyx*)	Phenytoin* (eg, *Dilantin*)

Significance	Onset	Severity	Documentation
2	☐ Rapid ■ **Delayed**	☐ Major ■ **Moderate** ☐ Minor	☐ Established ☐ Probable ■ **Suspected** ☐ Possible ☐ Unlikely

Effects Increased MEXILETINE clearance during coadministration of HYDANTOINS leading to lower steady-state plasma MEXILETINE concentrations and possibly loss of effectiveness.

Mechanism HYDANTOIN induction of MEXILETINE hepatic metabolism.

Management Monitor plasma MEXILETINE concentrations and observe for loss of MEXILETINE effectiveness during coadministration of HYDANTOINS. Increase MEXILETINE dose according to plasma concentration changes and clinical requirements.

Discussion

Low plasma mexiletine concentrations in 3 patients maintained on phenytoin led to a pharmacokinetic analysis involving 6 healthy volunteers.[1] After 1 week of phenytoin ingestion, the mexiletine AUC and plasma elimination $t_{1/2}$ decreased approximately 50%. Peak plasma mexiletine concentrations were not affected. Although steady-state plasma mexiletine concentrations could be expected to decrease during concomitant hydantoin therapy, loss of efficacy as a result of this interaction has not been reported. Lidocaine metabolism also may be affected by antiepileptic drugs.[2]

[1] Begg EJ, et al. *Br J Clin Pharmacol.* 1982;14(2):219.

[2] Perucca E, et al. *Br J Clin Pharmacol.* 1979;8(1):21.

* Asterisk indicates drugs cited in interaction reports. Based on pharmacologic and pharmacokinetic considerations, similar interactions may occur with other drugs that are listed.

Mexiletine — *Propafenone*

Mexiletine* (*Mexitil*)	Propafenone* (eg, *Rythmol*)

Significance	Onset	Severity	Documentation
2	☐ Rapid	☐ Major	☐ Established
	■ **Delayed**	■ **Moderate**	☐ Probable
		☐ Minor	■ **Suspected**
			☐ Possible
			☐ Unlikely

Effects MEXILETINE plasma concentrations may be elevated in extensive metabolizers, increasing the risk of side effects.

Mechanism PROPAFENONE may inhibit the metabolism (CYP2D6) of MEXILETINE.

Management Monitor plasma levels of MEXILETINE and observe the clinical response when PROPAFENONE is started or stopped. If both agents are started at the same time, slowly titrate the dose of each agent.

Discussion

The potential pharmacokinetic and electrophysiological interactions between mexiletine and propafenone were studied in 15 healthy men.[1] The investigation was conducted on 12 consecutive days. Each subject, 8 extensive metabolizers and 7 poor metabolizers of cytochrome P450 2D6, received oral doses of mexiletine 100 mg every 12 hr (from day 1 to 8) and propafenone 150 mg every 12 hr (from day 5 to 12). Mean plasma concentrations of both R-(-)- and S-(+)-mexiletine enantiomers were higher in poor metabolizers than in extensive metabolizers. Propafenone administration did not alter the plasma levels of R-(-)- and S-(+)-mexiletine in poor metabolizers; however, propafenone increased plasma levels of both enantiomers in the extensive metabolizers. When mexiletine was administered alone, the oral and nonrenal clearances of R-(-)- and S-(+)-mexiletine were 1.6- and 1.5-fold greater in extensive metabolizers than in poor metabolizers. Propafenone administration decreased the clearance of R-(-)- and S-(+)-mexiletine to values similar to those of the poor metabolizers and did not affect the clearance of mexiletine in poor metabolizers. The renal clearance of R-(-)- and S-(+)-mexiletine was not affected in extensive or poor metabolizers by propafenone administration. Coadministration of propafenone inhibited the formation of the 3 major metabolites of mexiletine, hydroxymethylmexiletine, p-hydroxymexiletine, and m-hydroxymexiletine, in extensive metabolizers 71%, 67%, and 73%, respectively. Administration of mexiletine did not alter the pharmacokinetics of propafenone. Coadministration of mexiletine and propafenone did not affect electrocardiographic measurements.

[1] Labbé L, et al. *Clin Pharmacol Ther.* 2000;68:44.

* Asterisk indicates drugs cited in interaction reports.

Mexiletine — *Quinolones*

Mexiletine*		Ciprofloxacin* (eg, *Cipro*)	Norfloxacin (*Noroxin*)
(*Mexitil*)		Lomefloxacin (*Maxaquin*)	Ofloxacin (eg, *Floxin*)

Significance	Onset	Severity	Documentation
4	☐ Rapid ■ **Delayed**	☐ Major ■ **Moderate** ☐ Minor	☐ Established ☐ Probable ☐ Suspected ■ **Possible** ☐ Unlikely

Effects Plasma MEXILETINE concentrations may be elevated, possibly producing an increase in therapeutic effects and side effects.

Mechanism QUINOLONE antibiotics may inhibit the hepatic metabolism (cytochrome P4501A2) of MEXILETINE.

Management Observe the clinical response of the patient to MEXILETINE when starting or stopping QUINOLONE antibiotics. If an interaction is suspected, adjust the dose of MEXILETINE as indicated.

Discussion

The effects of ciprofloxacin on the clearance of mexiletine were studied in healthy subjects (10 smokers, 9 nonsmokers).[1] The oral and metabolic clearance of mexiletine was greater in smokers than in nonsmokers. The administration of ciprofloxacin 750 mg twice daily for 5 days, starting 3 days prior to the administration of mexiletine, decreased oral and metabolic clearance of mexiletine in smokers and nonsmokers without changing renal mexiletine clearance. These results indicate that ciprofloxacin inhibits the hepatic metabolism of mexiletine.

[1] Labbé L, et al. *Ther Drug Monit.* 2004;26:492.

* Asterisk indicates drugs cited in interaction reports. Based on pharmacologic and pharmacokinetic considerations, similar interactions may occur with other drugs that are listed.

Mexiletine — *Rifampin*

Mexiletine*
(*Mexitil*)

Rifampin*
(eg, *Rifadin*)

Significance	Onset	Severity	Documentation
4	☐ Rapid	☐ Major	☐ Established
	■ **Delayed**	■ **Moderate**	☐ Probable
		☐ Minor	☐ Suspected
			■ **Possible**
			☐ Unlikely

Effects Increased MEXILETINE clearance leading to lower steady-state plasma concentrations and possibly loss of effectiveness.

Mechanism RIFAMPIN induction of MEXILETINE hepatic metabolism.

Management Monitor plasma MEXILETINE concentrations and observe for loss of MEXILETINE effectiveness during concurrent use of RIFAMPIN. Increase MEXILETINE dose according to plasma concentration changes and clinical requirements.

Discussion

In a study involving 8 healthy volunteers, total mexiletine clearance decreased after 10 days of rifampin ingestion.[1] The decrease in total clearance was explained by a decrease in nonrenal clearance. Peak plasma mexiletine concentrations and rate of absorption were not affected, but mexiletine plasma elimination half-life decreased from 8.5 to 5 hours. Although steady-state plasma mexiletine concentrations could be expected to decrease during concomitant rifampin therapy, loss of mexiletine efficacy as a result of this interaction has not been reported.

[1] Pentikainen PJ, et al. *Eur J Clin Pharmacol.* 1982;23:261.

* Asterisk indicates drugs cited in interaction reports.

Mexiletine | *Urinary Acidifiers*

Mexiletine	Urinary Acidifiers	
Mexiletine* (*Mexitil*)	Ammonium Chloride* Potassium Acid Phosphate (*K-Phos Original*)	Sodium Acid Phosphate

Significance	Onset	Severity	Documentation
4	■ **Rapid** □ Delayed	□ Major ■ **Moderate** □ Minor	□ Established □ Probable □ Suspected ■ **Possible** □ Unlikely

Effects Loss of MEXILETINE effectiveness might occur.

Mechanism Renal MEXILETINE clearance is increased as urine pH decreases, which can result in lower steady-state plasma concentrations.

Management Observe for loss of MEXILETINE effectiveness or decreases in plasma concentrations if drugs or foods that can lower urinary pH are used concurrently. Should MEXILETINE failure occur, discontinue the specific drug or diet or tailor MEXILETINE doses as needed.

Discussion

Renal clearance of mexiletine is related to urinary pH.[1-6] More than 50% of a mexiletine dose can be excreted in acidic urine, whereas renal excretion of mexiletine is virtually nil in alkaline urine.[1-6] The increased renal clearance of mexiletine in acidic urine; however, has variable effects on total clearance. Shorter plasma mexiletine elimination half-lives have been reported by some investigators,[1-4] but others have shown that the effects on total clearance are subject to interpatient variability.[6] The degree to which the increase in mexiletine renal clearance affects total clearance and steady-state plasma concentrations appears to be dependent on corresponding increases in nonrenal clearance and changes in volume of distribution.[6]

No clinical mexiletine failures, as a consequence of concurrent use of urinary acidifiers, have been reported.

1 Kiddie MA, et al. *Br J Clin Pharmacol.* 1974;1:229.
2 Prescott LF, et al. *Postgrad Med J.* 1977;53(suppl 1):50.
3 Kaye CM, et al. *Postgrad Med J.* 1977;53(suppl 1):56.
4 Beckett AH, et al. *Postgrad Med J.* 1977;53(suppl 1):60.
5 Johnston A, et al. *Br J Clin Pharmacol.* 1979;8:349.
6 Mitchell BG, et al. *Br J Clin Pharmacol.* 1983;16:281.

* Asterisk indicates drugs cited in interaction reports. Based on pharmacologic and pharmacokinetic considerations, similar interactions may occur with other drugs that are listed.

Mirtazapine — *Hydantoins*

Mirtazapine	Hydantoins	
Mirtazapine* (*Remeron*)	Ethotoin (*Peganone*)	Phenytoin* (eg, *Dilantin*)
	Fosphenytoin (*Cerebyx*)	

Significance	Onset	Severity	Documentation
2	☐ Rapid ■ **Delayed**	☐ Major ■ **Moderate** ☐ Minor	☐ Established ☐ Probable ■ **Suspected** ☐ Possible ☐ Unlikely

Effects MIRTAZAPINE plasma concentrations may be reduced, decreasing the pharmacologic effects.

Mechanism Induction of MIRTAZAPINE metabolism (CYP3A3/4) by HYDANTOINS is suspected.

Management In patients receiving MIRTAZAPINE, closely monitor the clinical response when starting, stopping, or changing the HYDANTOIN dose. Adjust MIRTAZAPINE therapy as needed.

Discussion

The effects of mirtazapine and phenytoin on the steady-state pharmacokinetics of each other were studied in an open-label, randomized, parallel-groups, multiple-dose investigation.[1] Nine subjects completed treatment consisting of phenytoin 200 mg/day for 17 days plus mirtazapine (15 mg/day for 2 days [days 11 and 12] and 30 mg/day for 5 days [days 13 to 17]). Eight subjects completed treatment consisting of mirtazapine 15 mg/day for 2 days followed by 30 mg/day for 15 days plus phenytoin 200 mg/day from day 8 to 17. Mirtazapine did not affect the steady-state pharmacokinetics of phenytoin as measured by the AUC and peak concentration. However, the addition of phenytoin to an existing daily regimen of mirtazapine resulted in a 47% decrease in the AUC of mirtazapine and a mean decrease in the peak concentration from 69.7 to 46.9 ng/mL.

[1] Spaans E, et al. *Eur J Clin Pharmacol.* 2002;58:423.

* Asterisk indicates drugs cited in interaction reports. Based on pharmacologic and pharmacokinetic considerations, similar interactions may occur with other drugs that are listed.

Mirtazapine | **Serotonin Reuptake Inhibitors**

Mirtazapine* (eg, *Remeron*)	Fluoxetine* (eg, *Prozac*)	Fluvoxamine*

Significance	Onset	Severity	Documentation
4	□ Rapid ■ **Delayed**	□ Major ■ **Moderate** □ Minor	□ Established □ Probable □ Suspected ■ **Possible** □ Unlikely

Effects MIRTAZAPINE plasma concentrations may be elevated, increasing the pharmacologic and adverse reactions.

Mechanism Inhibition of MIRTAZAPINE metabolism by FLUVOXAMINE is suspected.

Management In patients receiving MIRTAZAPINE, observe the clinical response when FLUVOXAMINE is started or stopped. Be prepared to adjust the MIRTAZAPINE dose as needed. Monitoring serum MIRTAZAPINE levels may be useful in managing patients.

Discussion

A 3- to 4-fold increase in mirtazapine serum levels was reported in 2 patients after fluvoxamine was added to their treatment regimens.[1] The first patient, a 17-year-old boy with major depression, was taking mirtazapine 15 mg/day for 2 months. Nine days after increasing the mirtazapine dose to 30 mg/day, the plasma concentration was 20 ng/mL. Nine days later, to augment the effect of mirtazapine, fluvoxamine 100 mg/day was started. One week later, the mirtazapine level was 60 ng/mL. The patient reported feeling anxious, and the dose of mirtazapine was reduced to 15 mg/day. The second patient, a 43-year-old woman, was started on mirtazapine 15 mg/day for major depression. One week after starting mirtazapine, the plasma level was 10 ng/mL. At this time, fluvoxamine 50 mg/day was started, and, 3 days later, the plasma mirtazapine concentration was 20 ng/mL. Two weeks later, the level had increased to 40 ng/mL. No adverse reactions were noted. In another report, agitation, restlessness, tremors, twitching, and "feeling like she could crawl out of her skin" were reported in a 26-year-old woman on a stable fluvoxamine 200 mg/day regimen 4 days after mirtazapine 30 mg/day was added to her therapy.[2] Symptoms consistent with restless leg syndrome were reported in 3 of 5 patients receiving fluoxetine 20 mg/day and mirtazapine 15 mg/day concurrently.[3] However, mirtazapine plasma levels were not measured in this or previous case reports.

[1] Anttila AK, et al. *Ann Pharmacother.* 2001;35(10):1221.
[2] Demers JC, et al. *Ann Pharmacother.* 2001;35(10):1217.
[3] Prospero-Garcia KA, et al. *J Clin Psychiatry.* 2006;67(11):1820.

* Asterisk indicates drugs cited in interaction reports.

Mitotane — **Spironolactone**

Mitotane*
(*Lysodren*)

Spironolactone*
(eg, *Aldactone*)

Significance	Onset	Severity	Documentation
4	☐ Rapid	■ **Major**	☐ Established
	■ **Delayed**	☐ Moderate	☐ Probable
		☐ Minor	☐ Suspected
			■ **Possible**
			☐ Unlikely

Effects Adrenolytic effects of MITOTANE may be blocked by SPIRONOLACTONE.

Mechanism Unknown.

Management Observe for diminished or absent clinical and biochemical signs of MITOTANE efficacy during SPIRONOLACTONE coadministration. Consider discontinuation of SPIRONOLACTONE if expected effects of MITOTANE are not achieved.

Discussion

Mitotane was added to spironolactone for the treatment of Cushing syndrome in a 65-year-old woman. After 5 months of therapy with both agents, no evidence of mitotane activity had been observed. Spironolactone was discontinued and symptoms consistent with mitotane activity (eg, severe nausea, profuse diarrhea) appeared within 24 to 48 hours.[1] In another report, antagonism of mitotane activity was not observed during 5 days of concurrent use with spironolactone.[2]

Although evidence in support of this interaction is lacking, the consequences as a result of this interaction could be grave; mitotane is the only agent known to prolong survival in inoperable adrenocortical carcinoma.[2] Therefore, if concurrent spironolactone is required, confirm clinical and biochemical efficacy of mitotane, otherwise discontinue spironolactone.

[1] Wortsman J, et al. *JAMA*. 1977;238(23):2527.

[2] May CA, et al. *Drug Intell Clin Pharm*. 1986;20(1):24.

* Asterisk indicates drugs cited in interaction reports.

Modafinil | **MAOIs**

Modafinil* (*Provigil*)	Isocarboxazid (*Marplan*)	Tranylcypromine* (eg, *Parnate*)
	Phenelzine (*Nardil*)	

Significance	Onset	Severity	Documentation
4	☐ Rapid	■ **Major**	☐ Established
	■ **Delayed**	☐ Moderate	☐ Probable
		☐ Minor	☐ Suspected
			■ **Possible**
			☐ Unlikely

Effects Risk of MODAFINIL adverse reactions may be increased.

Mechanism Unknown.

Management Observe the clinical response of patients. If an interaction is suspected, be prepared to adjust therapy as needed.

Discussion

Acute chorea, confusion, and hyperthermia occurred in a 34-year-old woman during coadministration of modafinil and tranylcypromine.[1] The patient was on a stable dose of tranylcypromine (80 mg daily) for refractory depression. Three days after starting modafinil 200 mg daily to improve wakefulness, the patient experienced restlessness, tics, inappropriate verbal responses, severe choreiform movements in all limbs, lip smacking, and rhythmic rapid tongue protrusions. Her neck was in opisthotonos with rhythmic bilateral rotations. Her temperature increased to 38°C (100.4°F), remained elevated for 24 hours, then normalized. Both drugs were discontinued and symptoms resolved within 2 days.

[1] Vytopil M, et al. *Am J Psychiatry*. 2007;164(4):684.

* Asterisk indicates drugs cited in interaction reports. Based on pharmacologic and pharmacokinetic considerations, similar interactions may occur with other drugs that are listed.

Montelukast — *Barbiturates*

Montelukast	Barbiturates
Montelukast* (*Singulair*)	Phenobarbital* (eg, *Luminal*)

Significance	Onset	Severity	Documentation
4	☐ Rapid	☐ Major	☐ Established
	■ **Delayed**	■ **Moderate**	☐ Probable
		☐ Minor	☐ Suspected
			■ **Possible**
			☐ Unlikely

Effects MONTELUKAST plasma concentrations may be reduced, decreasing the pharmacologic effect.

Mechanism PHENOBARBITAL may increase the hepatic metabolism of MONTELUKAST.

Management In patients receiving MONTELUKAST, monitor the clinical response when starting or stopping PHENOBARBITAL. Adjust the dose of MONTELUKAST as needed.

Discussion

The effect of phenobarbital on the pharmacokinetics of montelukast was evaluated in a placebo-controlled, parallel study involving 14 healthy subjects.[1] A single oral dose of montelukast 10 mg was given alone and after administration of phenobarbital 100 mg daily for 14 days. Compared with placebo, phenobarbital administration decreased the AUC of montelukast 38% and the C_{max} 20%.

Additional studies are needed to determine the clinical importance of this interaction and the magnitude of the effect of other barbiturates on the pharmacokinetics of montelukast.

[1] Holland S, et al. *Clin Pharmacol Ther.* 1998;63:231.

* Asterisk indicates drugs cited in interaction reports.

Montelukast — *Gemfibrozil*

Montelukast* (*Singulair*)	Gemfibrozil* (eg, *Lopid*)

Significance	Onset	Severity	Documentation
4	☐ Rapid	☐ Major	☐ Established
	■ **Delayed**	■ **Moderate**	☐ Probable
		☐ Minor	☐ Suspected
			■ **Possible**
			☐ Unlikely

Effects MONTELUKAST plasma concentrations may be elevated, increasing the pharmacologic effects and risk of adverse reactions.

Mechanism Inhibition of MONTELUKAST metabolism (CYP2C8) by GEMFIBROZIL.

Management Monitor the clinical response when GEMFIBROZIL is started or stopped. Adjust the MONTELUKAST dose as needed.

Discussion

The effects of gemfibrozil on the pharmacokinetics of montelukast were studied in 10 healthy subjects.[1] In a randomized, crossover study, each subject received a single dose of montelukast 10 mg alone and after pretreatment with gemfibrozil 600 mg or placebo twice daily for 3 days. Compared with placebo, pretreatment with gemfibrozil increased the montelukast AUC and C_{max} 4.5- and 1.5-fold, respectively, and prolonged the montelukast elimination $t_{1/2}$ by 3-fold. Increased AUC, C_{max}, and $t_{1/2}$ occurred in all subjects.

[1] Karonen T, et al. *Clin Pharmacol Ther*. 2010;88(2):223.

* Asterisk indicates drugs cited in interaction reports.

Moricizine — *Cimetidine*

Moricizine	Cimetidine
Moricizine*†	Cimetidine* (eg, *Tagamet*)

Significance	Onset	Severity	Documentation
2	□ Rapid	□ Major	□ Established
	■ **Delayed**	■ **Moderate**	□ Probable
		□ Minor	■ **Suspected**
			□ Possible
			□ Unlikely

Effects The pharmacologic and toxic effects of MORICIZINE may be increased.

Mechanism CIMETIDINE may inhibit the enzymes responsible for the hepatic metabolism of MORICIZINE.

Management Consider monitoring the ECG when starting, stopping, or changing the dose of CIMETIDINE.

Discussion

The effects of cimetidine on the pharmacokinetics and pharmacodynamics of moricizine were investigated in 8 healthy men.[1] The study was performed in 2 phases separated by 1 week. During the first phase of the investigation, a single oral dose of moricizine 500 mg was taken after an overnight fast. In the second phase of the study after a 1-week washout period, subjects received cimetidine 300 mg orally every 6 hours for 1 week. On the following day, while cimetidine was continued, subjects received a single dose of moricizine 500 mg. Moricizine had no effect on the pharmacokinetics of cimetidine. However, cimetidine increased the plasma concentrations of moricizine, producing a 39% increase in the AUC of moricizine and a 50% decrease in the clearance of moricizine. The moricizine terminal elimination $t_{½}$ increased from 3.4 to 4.6 hours. Although moricizine prolonged the PR and QRS intervals, no further detectable prolongation of these intervals was observed when cimetidine and moricizine were coadministered.

Additional studies are needed to further evaluate the clinical importance of the pharmacokinetic interaction.

[1] Biollaz J, et al. *Clin Pharmacol Ther.* 1985;37(6):665.

* Asterisk indicates drugs cited in interaction reports.
† Not available in United States.

Morphine — *Lidocaine*

Morphine* (eg, *Astramorph*)	Lidocaine* (eg, *Xylocaine*)

Significance	Onset	Severity	Documentation
4	■ **Rapid**	□ Major	□ Established
	□ Delayed	■ **Moderate**	□ Probable
		□ Minor	□ Suspected
			■ **Possible**
			□ Unlikely

Effects Respiratory depression and loss of consciousness may occur.

Mechanism Synergistic effect between these agents, possibly because of reduced intracellular calcium levels in opioid-sensitive CNS sites.

Management Carefully observe patients for increased narcosis and be prepared to administer naloxone if needed.

Discussion

A case of possible potentiation of narcosis was reported after systemic administration of lidocaine to a 74-year-old man receiving morphine and fentanyl (eg, *Sublimaze*).[1] The patient, scheduled for elective coronary artery bypass grafting, received intrathecal fentanyl 100 mcg and morphine 0.5 mg, IV etomidate (eg, *Amidate*), midazolam, and succinylcholine (eg, *Anectine*) for anesthetic induction. Sevoflurane (eg, *Ultane*), propofol (eg, *Diprivan*), and cisatracurium (*Nimbex*) were administered for anesthetic maintenance. When the patient was alert and stable, he was transferred to the surgical intensive care unit. Four hours after the last dose of opioid was given, the patient had an episode of ventricular tachycardia and IV lidocaine was administered. Over the next 5 minutes, the patient's ventilatory rate slowed and he lost consciousness. Within 1 to 2 minutes of administering naloxone 0.2 mg, the patient was able to breathe on his own and he was mentally alert.

Additional studies are needed to assess this possible drug interaction.

[1] Jensen E, et al. *Anesth Analg.* 1999;89(3):758.

* Asterisk indicates drugs cited in interaction reports.

Morphine — *Remifentanil*

Morphine* (eg, *Roxanol*)	Remifentanil* (*Ultiva*)

Significance	Onset	Severity	Documentation
2	■ **Rapid**	□ Major	□ Established
	□ Delayed	■ **Moderate**	□ Probable
		□ Minor	■ **Suspected**
			□ Possible
			□ Unlikely

Effects The analgesic effect of MORPHINE may be decreased.

Mechanism Unknown; however, acute opioid tolerance and postanesthetic hyperalgesia have been proposed as a possible cause.

Management Observe the patient's clinical response to MORPHINE analgesia following surgery utilizing REMIFENTANIL. Be prepared to titrate MORPHINE dose to higher levels than expected.

Discussion

The effect of remifentanil on acute opioid tolerance was evaluated in 49 adult patients undergoing abdominal surgery.[1] Patients were randomly assigned to receive desflurane (*Suprane*) kept constant at 0.5 minimum alveolar concentrations and a remifentanil infusion titrated to autonomic responses (remifentanil group) or a constant infusion of remifentanil and desflurane titrated to autonomic responses (desflurane group). All patients received a 0.15 mg/kg bolus of morphine 40 minutes before the end of surgery. Subsequent morphine administration was initially titrated by postanesthesia care nurses until patients could utilize a PCA device to control their pain. Patients and nurses were blinded to group assignment. The rate of remifentanil infusion was greater in the remifentanil group than in the desflurane group. In addition, compared with the desflurane group, postoperative pain scores were greater in the remifentanil group, patients required morphine earlier, and needed 84% more morphine (59 vs 32 mg) in the first 24 postoperative hours.

[1] Guignard B, et al. *Anesthesiology*. 2000;93:409.

* Asterisk indicates drugs cited in interaction reports.

Morphine — *Rifamycins*

Morphine	Rifamycins	
Morphine* (eg, *Roxanol*)	Rifabutin (*Mycobutin*)	Rifapentine (*Priftin*)
	Rifampin* (eg, *Rifadin*)	

Significance	Onset	Severity	Documentation
2	☐ Rapid	☐ Major	☐ Established
	■ **Delayed**	■ **Moderate**	☐ Probable
		☐ Minor	■ **Suspected**
			☐ Possible
			☐ Unlikely

Effects The analgesic effects of MORPHINE may be decreased.

Mechanism Unknown.

Management Observe the patient's clinical response to MORPHINE analgesia. It may be necessary to administer an alternative analgesic.

Discussion

The influence of rifampin on the analgesic effects and pharmacokinetics of morphine was studied in 10 healthy male subjects.[1] Using a randomized, double-blind, placebo-controlled, double-crossover design, each subject received rifampin 600 mg/day on days 5 through 18 of the study. In addition, on days 1, 4, 15, and 18, each subject received morphine 10 mg or placebo. The effects of morphine on pain were assessed using the cold pressor test. Compared with placebo, the pain threshold was increased during morphine administration. In contrast, no analgesia from morphine was noted when rifampin was given concomitantly. Although there was considerable interindividual variability, overall rifampin administration resulted in a 27% reduction in the area under the plasma concentration-time curve (AUC) of morphine and a 45% reduction in peak plasma concentration. In addition, the AUCs of the morphine metabolites (morphine-6-glucuronide [active] and morphine-3-glucuronide [no analgesic activity]) were reduced.

[1] Fromm MF, et al. *Pain.* 1997;72:261.

* Asterisk indicates drugs cited in interaction reports. Based on pharmacologic and pharmacokinetic considerations, similar interactions may occur with other drugs that are listed.

Morphine | **Somatostatin**

Morphine*
(eg, *MS Contin*)

Somatostatin*†

Significance	Onset	Severity	Documentation
4	■ **Rapid**	□ Major	□ Established
	□ Delayed	■ **Moderate**	□ Probable
		□ Minor	□ Suspected
			■ **Possible**
			□ Unlikely

Effects The analgesic effect of MORPHINE may be reduced.

Mechanism Unknown.

Management If a decrease or loss in analgesia occurs, consider discontinuing SOMATOSTATIN.

Discussion

A 20-year-old woman with left leg pain caused by chondrosarcoma had good pain control while receiving oral methadone 4 mg 3 times daily.[1] Her pain increased after starting subcutaneous somatostatin 3 mg over 8 hours as part of an antineoplastic regimen. The dosage of methadone was increased to 10 mg 3 times daily, which the patient reported to be completely ineffective. Methadone was changed to subcutaneous morphine 30 mg every 4 hours without success. When somatostatin was switched to IV administration over a 24-hour period, the patient's pain increased during the night and day, despite continuous subcutaneous administration of morphine 300 mg/day plus an additional 4 to 5 bolus doses of 20 mg as needed. No improvement in pain control occurred, even with spinal administration of morphine. After discontinuing somatostatin, pain intensity was reduced more than 50% with spinal administration of morphine 20 mg/day. Myosis and sedation occurred for the first time. Loss of pain control with morphine despite increases in the dose was described in 2 additional patients with severe cancer pain after somatostatin was added to their treatment regimens.

[1] Ripamonti C, et al. *Ann Oncol.* 1998;9(8):921.

* Asterisk indicates drugs cited in interaction reports.
† Available under orphan drug status.

Mycophenolate — *Amoxicillin/Clavulanate*

Mycophenolate Mofetil* (eg, *CellCept*)	Mycophenolate Sodium (*Myfortic*)	Amoxicillin/Clavulanate* (eg, *Augmentin*)
Mycophenolate Mofetil Hydrochloride (*CellCept*)		

Significance	Onset	Severity	Documentation
2	□ Rapid	□ Major	□ Established
	■ **Delayed**	■ **Moderate**	□ Probable
		□ Minor	■ **Suspected**
			□ Possible
			□ Unlikely

Effects MYCOPHENOLIC ACID plasma concentrations may be reduced, decreasing the pharmacologic effects.

Mechanism Decreased MYCOPHENOLIC ACID enterohepatic recirculation due to the effects of AMOXICILLIN/CLAVULANATE on intestinal flora is suspected.

Management Closely monitor MYCOPHENOLIC ACID concentrations and the response to therapy when starting or stopping AMOXICILLIN/CLAVULANATE. Adjust the MYCOPHENOLATE dose as needed.

Discussion

A 37-year-old man was receiving mycophenolate mofetil 2,000 mg/day as part of his treatment regimen following a renal transplant.[1] Subsequently, he received amoxicillin/clavulanate for a lower respiratory tract infection. One week later, the mycophenolic acid AUC decreased by 39%. A 14-year-old boy was receiving mycophenolate mofetil 2,000 mg as part of his treatment regimen following his second renal transplant.[1] Upon developing a urinary tract infection, he received amoxicillin/clavulanate. The mycophenolate acid AUC was not determined at that time. However, measurements of the mycophenolic acid AUC during amoxicillin/clavulanate administration and 5 days after discontinuation of the antibiotic showed a 91% increase in mycophenolic acid AUC following discontinuation of amoxicillin/clavulanate. In a multivariate analysis of factors affecting 12-hour trough concentrations of total mycophenolic acid in renal transplant patients, treatment with amoxicillin/clavulanate was associated with a reduction in mycophenolic acid concentrations.[2] The extent and time course of mycophenolic acid predose concentration reduction during amoxicillin/clavulanate administration was studied in renal transplant patients.[3] Amoxicillin/clavulanate administration resulted in a decrease in the 12-hour predose mycophenolic acid level to 46% of baseline within 3 days of starting the antibiotic. Mycophenolic acid levels spontaneously recovered to 79% of baseline after 14 days of amoxicillin/clavulanate coadministration. Mycophenolic acid concentrations normalized within 3 days of stopping the antibiotic.

[1] Ratna P, et al. *Transplantation.* 2011;91(6):e36.
[2] Borrows R, et al. *Ther Drug Monit.* 2005;27(4):442.
[3] Borrows R, et al. *Ther Drug Monit.* 2007;29(1):122.

* Asterisk indicates drugs cited in interaction reports. Based on pharmacologic and pharmacokinetic considerations, similar interactions may occur with other drugs that are listed.

Mycophenolate — *Cyclosporine*

Mycophenolate		Cyclosporine
Mycophenolate Mofetil* (eg, *CellCept*)	Mycophenolate Sodium (*Myfortic*)	Cyclosporine* (eg, *Neoral*)
Mycophenolate Mofetil Hydrochloride (*CellCept*)		

Significance	Onset	Severity	Documentation
2	☐ Rapid	☐ Major	☐ Established
	■ **Delayed**	■ **Moderate**	■ **Probable**
		☐ Minor	☐ Suspected
			☐ Possible
			☐ Unlikely

Effects CYCLOSPORINE may decrease MYCOPHENOLIC ACID trough levels.

Mechanism CYCLOSPORINE reduces MYCOPHENOLIC ACID enterohepatic recirculation.

Management In patients receiving MYCOPHENOLATE, monitor MYCOPHENOLIC ACID concentrations and the response to therapy when CYCLOSPORINE is started or stopped.

Discussion

In a longitudinal study, the effect of discontinuing cyclosporine on mycophenolic acid trough levels was assessed in 52 renal transplant patients.[1] For 6 months after renal transplantation, each patient was treated with mycophenolate mofetil 1 g twice daily, prednisone 0.1 mg/kg/day, and cyclosporine (target trough levels, 125 to 175 ng/mL). Six months after transplantation, 19 patients were randomized to continue treatment with the triple-drug regimen, cyclosporine was discontinued in 19 patients, and prednisone was stopped in 14 patients. Three months later (at month 9), mycophenolic acid levels were lower in patients receiving concomitant cyclosporine than in patients receiving only mycophenolate mofetil and prednisone. After discontinuing cyclosporine, median mycophenolic acid trough levels increased 69% (from 1.87 to 3.16 mg/L). Mycophenolic acid trough levels in patients receiving the triple-drug regimen or mycophenolate mofetil and cyclosporine did not change, compared with patients receiving mycophenolate mofetil and prednisone. In 8 patients, changing from cyclosporine therapy to tacrolimus increased the mycophenolic acid AUC 46%.[2] In other studies, a similar increase in mycophenolic acid levels occurred after cyclosporine discontinuation.[3,4] The effect declined after 6 months. The mycophenolic acid AUC was lower when mycophenolate mofetil was coadministered with cyclosporine compared with sirolimus (*Rapamune*).[5-8] Animal data[9] and studies in renal transplant patients[6,7,10] suggest the mechanism for this interaction is a reduction in mycophenolic acid enterohepatic recirculation.

1 Gregoor PJ, et al. *Transplantation.* 1999;68(10):1603.
2 Park JM, et al. *Ther Drug Monit.* 2008;30(5):591.
3 Shipkova M, et al. *Ther Drug Monit.* 2001;23(6):717.
4 Kuypers DR, et al. *Clin Pharmacokinet.* 2009;48(5):329.
5 Büchler M, et al. *Clin Pharmacol Ther.* 2005;78(1):34.
6 Cattaneo D, et al. *Am J Transplant.* 2005;5(12):2937.
7 Picard N, et al. *Br J Clin Pharmacol.* 2006;62(4):477.
8 Pescovitz MD, et al. *Br J Clin Pharmacol.* 2007;64(6):758.
9 van Gelder T, et al. *Ther Drug Monit.* 2001;23(2):119.
10 Yau WP, et al. *J Clin Pharmacol.* 2009;49(6):684.

* Asterisk indicates drugs cited in interaction reports. Based on pharmacologic and pharmacokinetic considerations, similar interactions may occur with other drugs that are listed.

Mycophenolate | **Iron Salts**

Mycophenolate		Iron Salts	
Mycophenolate Mofetil* (*CellCept*)	Mycophenolate Sodium (*Myfortic*)	Ferrous Fumarate (eg, *Hemocyte*)	Ferrous Sulfate* (eg, *Feosol*)
Mycophenolate Mofetil Hydrochloride (*CellCept*)		Ferrous Gluconate (eg, *Fergon*)	Iron Polysaccharide* (eg, *Niferex*)

Significance	Onset	Severity	Documentation
4	■ **Rapid**	□ Major	□ Established
	□ Delayed	■ **Moderate**	□ Probable
		□ Minor	□ Suspected
			■ **Possible**
			□ Unlikely

Effects Simultaneous administration may decrease MYCOPHENOLIC ACID plasma levels and the clinical effect of MYCOPHENOLATE.

Mechanism Absorption of MYCOPHENOLATE may be decreased, possibly by the formation of a drug-iron complex in the GI tract.

Management Monitor MYCOPHENOLIC ACID levels and adjust the dose as needed. Because MYCOPHENOLATE is rapidly absorbed, separate the administration by as much time as possible.

Discussion

Data are conflicting. In a randomized, crossover investigation, the effect of iron on the absorption of mycophenolate mofetil was studied in 7 healthy volunteers.[1] Each subject received 4 capsules of mycophenolate mofetil 250 mg alone and concomitantly with 2 tablets of sustained-release iron, each containing ferrous sulfate 525 mg (elemental iron ion 105 mg). When mycophenolate mofetil was taken with iron, the mean AUC for mycophenolate mofetil decreased 91%, and the mean peak plasma concentration decreased 94% (from 20.1 to 1.3 mcg/mL). However, 3 other studies found no effect of oral iron on mycophenolate bioavailability.[2-4] Single-[2] and multiple-dose[3,4] administration of ferrous sulfate[2-4] or iron polysaccharide complex[2] given 4 hours after mycophenolate mofetil did not reduce systemic exposure to mycophenolic acid, as measured by the AUC, compared with mycophenolate mofetil alone.

[1] Morii M, et al. *Clin Pharmacol Ther.* 2000;68(6):613.
[2] Gelone DK, et al. *Pharmacotherapy.* 2007;27(9):1272.
[3] Mudge DW, et al. *Transplantation.* 2004;77(2):206.
[4] Lorenz M, et al. *Am J Kidney Dis.* 2004;43(6):1098.

* Asterisk indicates drugs cited in interaction reports. Based on pharmacologic and pharmacokinetic considerations, similar interactions may occur with other drugs that are listed.

Mycophenolate — *Metronidazole*

Mycophenolate		Metronidazole
Mycophenolate Mofetil* (*CellCept*)	Mycophenolate Sodium (*Myfortic*)	Metronidazole* (eg, *Flagyl*)
Mycophenolate Mofetil Hydrochloride (*CellCept*)		

Significance	Onset	Severity	Documentation
5	□ Rapid	□ Major	□ Established
	■ **Delayed**	□ Moderate	□ Probable
		■ **Minor**	□ Suspected
			■ **Possible**
			□ Unlikely

Effects METRONIDAZOLE may decrease MYCOPHENOLIC ACID concentrations.

Mechanism Reduction in enterohepatic recirculation of MYCOPHENOLIC ACID and mycophenolic acid glucuronide by METRONIDAZOLE is suspected.

Management In patients receiving MYCOPHENOLATE, monitor the response to therapy when starting or stopping METRONIDAZOLE.

Discussion

The effects of administration of metronidazole plus norfloxacin (*Noroxin*) on the pharmacokinetics of mycophenolate mofetil were studied in 11 healthy subjects.[1] Each subject received a single dose of mycophenolate mofetil 1 g alone and on day 4 of administration of norfloxacin 400 mg twice daily, metronidazole 500 mg 3 times daily, and the combination of norfloxacin plus metronidazole. Nine subjects completed all 4 treatment periods. Compared with administration of mycophenolate mofetil alone, the AUC of mycophenolic acid was reduced 10%, 19%, and 33% when administered with norfloxacin, metronidazole, or norfloxacin plus metronidazole, respectively. During the corresponding periods, the AUC of the metabolite mycophenolic acid glucuronide was reduced 10%, 27%, and 41%, respectively. Thus, the effect of the combination of norfloxacin and metronidazole on the AUC of mycophenolic acid and mycophenolic acid glucuronide appears to be additive.

[1] Naderer OJ, et al. *J Clin Pharmacol.* 2005;45(2):219.

* Asterisk indicates drugs cited in interaction reports. Based on pharmacologic and pharmacokinetic considerations, similar interactions may occur with other drugs that are listed.

Mycophenolate — *Proton Pump Inhibitors*

Mycophenolate		Proton Pump Inhibitors	
Mycophenolate Mofetil* (eg, *CellCept*)	Mycophenolate Sodium (*Myfortic*)	Dexlansoprazole (*Dexilant*)	Omeprazole* (eg, *Prilosec*)
Mycophenolate Mofetil Hydrochloride (*CellCept*)		Esomeprazole (eg, *Nexium*)	Pantoprazole* (eg, *Protonix*)
		Lansoprazole* (eg, *Prevacid*)	Rabeprazole (*Aciphex*)

Significance	Onset	Severity	Documentation
2	□ Rapid ■ **Delayed**	□ Major ■ **Moderate** □ Minor	□ Established ■ **Probable** □ Suspected □ Possible □ Unlikely

Effects MYCOPHENOLIC ACID concentrations may be reduced, decreasing the efficacy.

Mechanism Impaired MYCOPHENOLATE MOFETIL absorption due to incomplete dissolution in the stomach at increased pH.[1]

Management If PROTON PUMP INHIBITORS must be used, monitor MYCOPHENOLIC ACID concentrations and adjust the dose as needed.

Discussion

In a retrospective investigation, the effects of lansoprazole and rabeprazole on mycophenolic acid pharmacokinetics were studied in 61 patients 1 year after renal transplantation.[2] Thirty-nine patients were receiving mycophenolate mofetil 0.5 to 2 g/day, lansoprazole 30 mg once daily (n = 22), or rabeprazole 10 mg once daily (n = 17). The control group (n = 22) discontinued lansoprazole or rabeprazole 6 months after transplantation but continued taking mycophenolate mofetil. Lansoprazole decreased the mean C_{max} and AUC of mycophenolic acid 30% and 25%, respectively, and delayed the T_{max} compared with the control group. The mycophenolic acid AUC was lower in individuals with the CYP2C19 *1/*2 + *1/*3 genotype than in those with the CYP2C19 *1/*1 genotype. Lansoprazole did not reduce mycophenolic acid enterohepatic recirculation. Rabeprazole did not affect the pharmacokinetics of mycophenolic acid. The mycophenolic acid dose-adjusted AUC was lower (41.7 mg/L) in heart transplant recipients when mycophenolate mofetil and pantoprazole were coadministered compared with patients receiving mycophenolate mofetil alone (59.5 mg/L).[3] In addition, heart transplant rejection episodes were higher in patients receiving mycophenolate mofetil plus pantoprazole compared with mycophenolate mofetil alone (33.3% compared with 8.3%, respectively). In healthy subjects, mycophenolic acid C_{max} and AUC decreased 57% and 27%, respectively, when mycophenolate mofetil was coadministered with pantoprazole compared with giving mycophenolate mofetil alone.[4] In contrast, pantoprazole did not affect the pharmacokinetics of enteric-coated mycophenolate sodium. Similarly, omeprazole decreased mycophenolic acid C_{max} and AUC following administration of mycophenolate mofetil but did not affect the pharmacokinetics of enteric-coated mycophenolate sodium.[1] In a pharmacokinetic study in 22 heart transplant patients, pantoprazole decreased mycophenolic acid trough concentrations, C_{max}, and AUC (24%, 41%, and 25%, respectively) compared with giving mycophenolate alone.[5] Similarly, pantoprazole lowered the mycophenolic acid AUC 37% in patients with autoimmune disease.[6] In recent recipients of kidney transplants, there was no overall difference in mycophenolic acid AUC at day 5 whether patients were taking a proton pump inhibitor (most frequently omeprazole or pantoprazole) concurrently or receiving mycophenolate mofetil alone.[7] However, the 2- and 12-hour mycophenolic acid concentrations were lower in patients receiving a proton pump inhibitor.

[1] Kees MG, et al. *J Clin Pharmacol.* 2012;52(8):1265.
[2] Miura M, et al. *Ther Drug Monit.* 2008;30(1):46.
[3] Kofler S, et al. *J Heart Lung Transplant.* 2009;28(6):605.
[4] Rupprecht K, et al. *J Clin Pharmacol.* 2009;49(10):1196.
[5] Kofler S, et al. *Am J Transplant.* 2009;9(7):1650.
[6] Schaier M, et al. *Rheumatology (Oxford).* 2010;49(11):2061.
[7] Kiberd BA, et al. *Ther Drug Monit.* 2011;33(1):120.

* Asterisk indicates drugs cited in interaction reports. Based on pharmacologic and pharmacokinetic considerations, similar interactions may occur with other drugs that are listed.

Mycophenolate — *Quinolones*

Mycophenolate Mofetil* (*CellCept*)	Mycophenolate Sodium (*Myfortic*)	Ciprofloxacin* (eg, *Cipro*)	Norfloxacin* (*Noroxin*)
Mycophenolate Mofetil Hydrochloride (*CellCept*)			

Significance	Onset	Severity	Documentation
2	□ Rapid	□ Major	□ Established
	■ **Delayed**	■ **Moderate**	□ Probable
		□ Minor	■ **Suspected**
			□ Possible
			□ Unlikely

Effects NORFLOXACIN may decrease MYCOPHENOLIC ACID concentrations.

Mechanism Reduction in enterohepatic recirculation of MYCOPHENOLIC ACID and MYCOPHENOLIC ACID glucuronide by NORFLOXACIN is suspected.

Management In patients receiving MYCOPHENOLATE, monitor the response to therapy when NORFLOXACIN is started or stopped.

Discussion

The effects of metronidazole (eg, *Flagyl*) administration plus norfloxacin on the pharmacokinetics of mycophenolate mofetil were studied in 11 healthy subjects.[1] Each subject received a single dose of mycophenolate mofetil 1 g alone and on day 4 of administration of norfloxacin 400 mg twice daily, metronidazole 500 mg 3 times daily, and the combination of norfloxacin plus metronidazole. Nine subjects completed all 4 treatment periods. Compared with administration of mycophenolate mofetil alone, the AUC of mycophenolic acid was reduced 10%, 19%, and 33% when administered with norfloxacin, metronidazole, or norfloxacin plus metronidazole, respectively. During the corresponding periods, the AUC of the metabolite mycophenolic acid glucuronide was reduced 10%, 27%, and 41%, respectively. Thus, the effect of the combination of norfloxacin and metronidazole on the AUC of mycophenolic acid and mycophenolic acid glucuronide appears to be additive. A 17-year-old woman received IV mycophenolate 1,800 mg daily following a bone marrow transplant.[2] Eight days later, the mycophenolic acid AUC had decreased approximately 65%. A drug interaction with IV ciprofloxacin was suspected.

[1] Naderer OJ, et al. *J Clin Pharmacol.* 2005;45(2):219.

[2] Goutelle S, et al. *Pharmacotherapy.* 2011;31(1):36e.

* Asterisk indicates drugs cited in interaction reports. Based on pharmacologic and pharmacokinetic considerations, similar interactions may occur with other drugs that are listed.

Mycophenolate — *Rifamycins*

Mycophenolate		Rifamycins	
Mycophenolate Mofetil (*CellCept*)	Mycophenolate Sodium (*Myfortic*)	Rifabutin (*Mycobutin*)	Rifapentine (*Priftin*)
Mycophenolate Mofetil Hydrochloride* (*CellCept*)		Rifampin* (eg, *Rifadin*)	

Significance	Onset	Severity	Documentation
2	☐ Rapid	☐ Major	☐ Established
	■ **Delayed**	■ **Moderate**	☐ Probable
		☐ Minor	■ **Suspected**
			☐ Possible
			☐ Unlikely

Effects RIFAMYCINS may reduce MYCOPHENOLIC ACID plasma concentrations, decreasing efficacy.

Mechanism Multiple mechanisms are suspected, including simultaneous induction of renal, hepatic, and GI uridine diphosphate-glucuronosyltransferases and organic anion transporters with subsequent inhibition of enterohepatic MYCOPHENOLIC ACID recirculation.

Management In patients receiving RIFAMYCINS and MYCOPHENOLATE, closely monitor MYCOPHENOLIC ACID concentrations and adjust the MYCOPHENOLATE dose as needed when RIFAMYCIN therapy is started or stopped.

Discussion

A drug interaction between rifampin and mycophenolate mofetil was reported in a 51-year-old man.[1] In addition to other medications he was receiving (eg, tacrolimus [*Prograf*]), the patient was started on rifampin 600 mg daily 13 days after receiving his transplant. While attempting to control the interaction between tacrolimus and rifampin, the dose requirements for mycophenolate mofetil increased from 2 to 6 g daily without achieving the mycophenolic acid target trough plasma level of 2.5 mcg/mL. The highest mycophenolic acid level measured with mycophenolic mofetil 2 g daily was 0.84 mg/L on postoperative day 44. Increasing the mycophenolate mofetil dose to 6 g daily resulted in a maximum mycophenolic acid trough plasma concentration of 3.16 mg/L on postoperative day 81. Rifampin therapy resulted in more than a 2-fold decrease in dose-corrected exposure to mycophenolic acid. After rifampin was discontinued, the effects of rifampin were reversed over a 2-week period. There was a 221% increase in the mycophenolic acid dose-corrected AUC and a 69% decrease in total body clearance after rifampin was discontinued. Eight renal transplant patients receiving mycophenolate mofetil were given rifampin 600 mg daily for 8 days.[2] Rifampin administration decreased the mean AUC and trough levels of mycophenolic acid 17.5% and 48.8%, respectively. No adverse reactions were reported.

[1] Kuypers DR, et al. *Clin Pharmacol Ther.* 2005;78(1):81.

[2] Naesens M, et al. *Clin Pharmacol Ther.* 2006;80(5):509.

* Asterisk indicates drugs cited in interaction reports. Based on pharmacologic and pharmacokinetic considerations, similar interactions may occur with other drugs that are listed.

Mycophenolate — *Sirolimus*

Mycophenolate		Sirolimus
Mycophenolate Mofetil* (eg, *CellCept*)	Mycophenolate Sodium (*Myfortic*)	Sirolimus* (*Rapamune*)
Mycophenolate Mofetil Hydrochloride (*CellCept*)		

Significance	Onset	Severity	Documentation
2	□ Rapid	□ Major	□ Established
	■ **Delayed**	■ **Moderate**	□ Probable
		□ Minor	■ **Suspected**
			□ Possible
			□ Unlikely

Effects MYCOPHENOLIC ACID trough plasma concentrations may be elevated, increasing the risk of adverse reactions.

Mechanism Unknown.

Management Perform therapeutic drug monitoring of MYCOPHENOLIC ACID during coadministration of SIROLIMUS. Adjust the dose of MYCOPHENOLATE as needed.

Discussion

The effects of cyclosporine (eg, *Neoral*) and sirolimus on the pharmacokinetics of mycophenolic acid were studied in cadaveric kidney transplant patients.[1] Thirteen patients received sirolimus 15 mg on day 1 and 10 mg on days 2 and 3, followed by a dosage adjustment to achieve trough blood concentrations between 10 and 20 ng/mL. Seventeen patients were started on day 1 at a dosage of cyclosporine 8 mg/kg/day, followed by a dosage adjustment to obtain cyclosporine trough blood concentrations between 200 and 300 ng/mL during month 1 and between 150 and 250 ng/mL during months 2 and 3 after transplantation. All patients received induction therapy with antithymocyte globulin (*Thymoglobulin*), prednisolone (eg, *Prelone*), and mycophenolate mofetil, which was started at 2 g/day and decreased only with the occurrence of adverse reactions. The AUCs for mycophenolic acid during coadministration of sirolimus at 2 weeks, 1 month, and 2 months were increased 88%, 50%, and 49%, respectively, compared with the same time points during coadministration of cyclosporine. The WBC was lower in the group receiving cotreatment with sirolimus at months 1 and 2 compared with cyclosporine. Exposure to mycophenolate, as measured by the AUC:dose ratio, was 50% higher in kidney transplant patients during coadministration of sirolimus compared with cyclosporine coadministration.[2] The drug with which mycophenolate was interacting was not determined. See Mycophenolate-Cyclosporine and Mycophenolate-Tacrolimus.

[1] Büchler M, et al. *Clin Pharmacol Ther.* 2005;78(1):34. [2] Picard N, et al. *Br J Clin Pharmacol.* 2006;62(4):477.

* Asterisk indicates drugs cited in interaction reports. Based on pharmacologic and pharmacokinetic considerations, similar interactions may occur with other drugs that are listed.

Mycophenolate — *Tacrolimus*

Mycophenolate		Tacrolimus
Mycophenolate Mofetil* (eg, *CellCept*)	Mycophenolate Sodium (*Myfortic*)	Tacrolimus* (eg, *Prograf*)
Mycophenolate Mofetil Hydrochloride (*CellCept*)		

Significance	Onset	Severity	Documentation
4	☐ Rapid	☐ Major	☐ Established
	■ **Delayed**	■ **Moderate**	☐ Probable
		☐ Minor	☐ Suspected
			■ **Possible**
			☐ Unlikely

Effects MYCOPHENOLIC ACID trough plasma concentrations may be elevated, increasing the risk of adverse reactions.

Mechanism Unknown.

Management Monitor MYCOPHENOLIC ACID plasma levels and adjust the dose of MYCOPHENOLATE as needed.

Discussion

A possible pharmacokinetic interaction between mycophenolate mofetil and tacrolimus was evaluated in 15 consecutive renal transplant patients receiving mycophenolate plus methylprednisolone with cyclosporine (eg, *Neoral*) (10 patients) or tacrolimus (5 patients).[1] Compared with cyclosporine coadministration, tacrolimus increased the mean mycophenolate trough plasma level 82%, despite a 12% lower dose of mycophenolate. The pharmacokinetic profiles of 13 pediatric renal transplant patients who received mycophenolate alone were compared with 15 children receiving mycophenolate in combination with cyclosporine and 14 children receiving mycophenolate with tacrolimus.[2] Compared with the patients receiving cyclosporine, the dose of mycophenolate was 48% lower in the patients receiving concomitant tacrolimus. Mycophenolate mofetil does not appear to alter the pharmacokinetics of tacrolimus.[3] A study of 71 renal transplant patients did not find an interaction between mycophenolate and tacrolimus.[4] However, increased tacrolimus levels were reported in an 8-year-old boy during coadministration of mycophenolate.[5] The pharmacokinetics of mycophenolic acid were studied in 23 kidney transplant patients receiving tacrolimus or sirolimus.[6] The mycophenolic acid AUC was more than 2-fold higher when mycophenolate mofetil was given with tacrolimus compared with coadministration with sirolimus.

[1] Hübner GI, et al. *Ther Drug Monit.* 1999;21(5):536.
[2] Filler G, et al. *Pediatr Nephrol.* 2000;14(2):100.
[3] Pirsch J, et al. *J Clin Pharmacol.* 2000;40(5):527.
[4] Kagaya H, et al. *J Clin Pharm Ther.* 2008;33(2):193.
[5] Frühwirth M, et al. *Pediatr Transplant.* 2001;5(2):132.
[6] Braun F, et al. *Clin Pharmacol Ther.* 2009;86(4):411.

* Asterisk indicates drugs cited in interaction reports. Based on pharmacologic and pharmacokinetic considerations, similar interactions may occur with other drugs that are listed.

Mycophenolate — *Thiazolidinediones*

Mycophenolate Mofetil* (eg, *CellCept*) Mycophenolate Mofetil Hydrochloride (*CellCept Intravenous*)	Mycophenolate Sodium (*Myfortic*)	Rosiglitazone* (*Avandia*)

Significance	Onset	Severity	Documentation
4	☐ Rapid ■ **Delayed**	☐ Major ■ **Moderate** ☐ Minor	☐ Established ☐ Probable ☐ Suspected ■ **Possible** ☐ Unlikely

Effects MYCOPHENOLIC ACID concentrations may be elevated, increasing the pharmacologic effects and risk of adverse reactions.

Mechanism Decreased MYCOPHENOLATE metabolism by ROSIGLITAZONE is suspected.

Management Measure MYCOPHENOLIC ACID concentrations and the response of the patient when ROSIGLITAZONE is started or stopped. Adjust the MYCOPHENOLATE dose as needed.

Discussion

Severe anemia was reported in a 47-year-old man during coadministration of mycophenolate mofetil 500 mg twice daily and rosiglitazone 4 mg daily.[1] The patient was taking maintenance immunosuppressive treatment, which included mycophenolate mofetil, following a cadaveric renal allograft. Subsequently, he was entered into a pilot study evaluating the metabolic and renal effects of rosiglitazone in proteinuric renal transplant recipients. After starting rosiglitazone, he experienced a progressive decline in RBC count. Three months after the start of rosiglitazone, the mycophenolic acid AUC was 2-fold higher than baseline measurements. Rosiglitazone was discontinued and a progressive increase in RBC count and reduction of mycophenolic acid AUC occurred.

[1] Cattaneo D, et al. *Transplantation.* 2008;85(6):921.

* Asterisk indicates drugs cited in interaction reports. Based on pharmacologic and pharmacokinetic considerations, similar interactions may occur with other drugs that are listed.

Nalidixic Acid — *Melphalan*

Nalidixic Acid* (*NegGram*)	Melphalan* (*Alkeran*)

Significance	Onset	Severity	Documentation
1	☐ Rapid	■ **Major**	☐ Established
	■ **Delayed**	☐ Moderate	☐ Probable
		☐ Minor	■ **Suspected**
			☐ Possible
			☐ Unlikely

Effects Increased risk of GI toxicity, including hemorrhagic ulcerative colitis or intestinal necrosis.

Mechanism Unknown.

Management Coadministration of NALIDIXIC ACID and MELPHALAN is contraindicated.

Discussion

Coadministration of nalidixic acid and melphalan is contraindicated because of increased risk of serious GI toxicity, including hemorrhagic ulcerative colitis or intestinal necrosis.[1] Serious GI toxicity has been associated with concomitant use of nalidixic acid and melphalan.

The basis for this monograph is information on file with the manufacturer.[1] Published clinical data are needed to further assess this interaction. However, because of the seriousness of the GI toxicity that may occur, clinical evaluation of this interaction in humans is not likely to be forthcoming.

[1] *NegGram* [package insert]. Philadelphia, PA: GlaxoSmithKline; March 5, 2007.

* Asterisk indicates drugs cited in interaction reports.

Nateglinide — *Fluconazole*

Nateglinide* (*Starlix*)	Fluconazole* (eg, *Diflucan*)

Significance	Onset	Severity	Documentation
4	□ Rapid ■ **Delayed**	□ Major ■ **Moderate** □ Minor	□ Established □ Probable □ Suspected ■ **Possible** □ Unlikely

Effects FLUCONAZOLE administration may increase and prolong the blood glucose-lowering effects of NATEGLINIDE.

Mechanism Inhibition of NATEGLINIDE (CYP2C9 and, to a lesser degree, CYP3A4) metabolism by FLUCONAZOLE is suspected.

Management In patients receiving NATEGLINIDE, carefully monitor blood glucose levels when starting or stopping FLUCONAZOLE therapy. Adjust the NATEGLINIDE dose as needed.

Discussion

The effects of fluconazole on the pharmacokinetics and pharmacodynamics of nateglinide were studied in 10 healthy volunteers.[1] In a 2-phase, randomized, double-blind, crossover investigation, each subject received fluconazole 200 mg (400 mg on day 1) or placebo once daily for 4 days. On day 4, they received a single dose of nateglinide 30 mg. Fluconazole administration increased the AUC 48% and prolonged the $t_{1/2}$ from 1.6 to 1.9 hours, compared with placebo. The nateglinide peak plasma concentration was unchanged, indicating that the interaction mainly occurs during the elimination phase. Fluconazole decreased the peak plasma levels of the M7 metabolite of nateglinide 34% and prolonged the $t_{1/2}$ from 2.2 to 3.5 hours. See Repaglinide-Azole Antifungal Agents.

[1] Niemi M, et al. *Clin Pharmacol Ther.* 2003;74(1):25.

* Asterisk indicates drugs cited in interaction reports.

Nateglinide — *Sulfinpyrazone*

Nateglinide* (*Starlix*)	Sulfinpyrazone* (eg, *Anturane*)

Significance	Onset	Severity	Documentation
4	☐ Rapid	☐ Major	☐ Established
	■ **Delayed**	■ **Moderate**	☐ Probable
		☐ Minor	☐ Suspected
			■ **Possible**
			☐ Unlikely

Effects NATEGLINIDE plasma concentrations may be elevated, increasing the pharmacologic and adverse effects.

Mechanism Inhibition of NATEGLINIDE metabolism (CYP2C9) by SULFINPYRAZONE is suspected.

Management In patients receiving NATEGLINIDE, carefully monitor blood glucose levels when starting or stopping SULFINPYRAZONE. Adjust the dose of NATEGLINIDE as needed.

Discussion

The effects of sulfinpyrazone on the pharmacokinetics of nateglinide were evaluated in 16 healthy subjects.[1] In a randomized, open-label, crossover study, each subject received a single oral dose of nateglinide 120 mg alone and after 7 days of administration of sulfinpyrazone 200 mg twice daily. Compared with taking nateglinide alone, sulfinpyrazone administration increased the nateglinide AUC approximately 28%. Sulfinpyrazone administration did not affect the C_{max}, time to reach the C_{max}, or the $t_{1/2}$ of nateglinide. Both treatments were safe and well tolerated.

Because of the moderate effect of sulfinpyrazone on nateglinide pharmacokinetics in this investigation, additional studies are needed to determine the clinical importance of this possible interaction.

[1] Sabia H, et al. *Eur J Clin Pharmacol.* 2004;60(6):407.

* Asterisk indicates drugs cited in interaction reports.

Nefazodone — *Selective Serotonin Reuptake Inhibitors*

Nefazodone*	Fluoxetine* (eg, *Prozac*)	Paroxetine* (eg, *Paxil*)

Significance	Onset	Severity	Documentation
4	■ **Rapid**	■ **Major**	□ Established
	□ Delayed	□ Moderate	□ Probable
		□ Minor	□ Suspected
			■ **Possible**
			□ Unlikely

Effects Serotonin syndrome, including irritability, increased muscle tone, shivering, myoclonus, and altered consciousness, may occur.

Mechanism Possibly an additive or synergistic effect of combining 2 SSRIs.

Management If combined administration of 2 SSRIs is necessary, start with a low dose of NEFAZODONE or an SSRI and carefully monitor. In addition, if changing SSRIs, consider the residual effects of agents with a long t½ and allow a sufficient washout period.

Discussion

A 51-year-old woman with bipolar affective disorder was diaphoretic with dilated pupils, dry mouth, uncoordinated body tremors, flailing arms, and twitching when she was brought to the emergency room.[1] The patient had been taking nefazodone for approximately 6 months. The dose was tapered over a 2-week period and stopped 2 days prior to her hospital admission. One day before admission, she took paroxetine and valproic acid (eg, *Depakene*). The patient's condition responded to treatment with IV diazepam (eg, *Valium*) and benztropine (eg, *Cogentin*). A rechallenge with paroxetine 7 days after nefazodone was discontinued did not produce any adverse reactions. Serotonin syndrome symptoms (eg, ataxia, confusion, myoclonus, visual hallucinations) occurred in a 50-year-old man who incorrectly continued taking fluoxetine 40 mg/day while being switched to nefazodone 100 mg twice daily.[2] Symptoms developed 6 days after combined use and disappeared 4 days after stopping both drugs.

A similar reaction may occur with the combined use of other SSRIs (eg, citalopram [eg, *Celexa*], duloxetine [*Cymbalta*], fluvoxamine [eg, *Luvox CR*], sertraline [*Zoloft*], venlafaxine [*Effexor*]).

[1] John L, et al. *Ann Emerg Med.* 1997;29(2):287.

[2] Smith DL, et al. *J Clin Psychiatry.* 2000;61(2):146.

* Asterisk indicates drugs cited in interaction reports.

Nelfinavir — *Rifamycins*

Nelfinavir	Rifamycins	
Nelfinavir* (*Viracept*)	Rifabutin* (*Mycobutin*)	Rifapentine (*Priftin*)
	Rifampin* (eg, *Rifadin*)	

Significance	Onset	Severity	Documentation
2	☐ Rapid	☐ Major	☐ Established
	■ **Delayed**	■ **Moderate**	■ **Probable**
		☐ Minor	☐ Suspected
			☐ Possible
			☐ Unlikely

Effects RIFAMYCINS may decrease NELFINAVIR serum concentrations, decreasing the pharmacologic effects.

Mechanism Possible increase in metabolism (CYP3A4) of NELFINAVIR induced by RIFAMYCINS.

Management RIFAMPIN and NELFINAVIR should not be administered together.[1] It is recommended that the dose of RIFABUTIN be reduced to one-half the usual dose when coadministered with NELFINAVIR.[1] Contact the CDC for current guidelines regarding management of drug therapy in patients who are diagnosed as having tuberculosis but are already receiving a protease inhibitor for HIV infection or are being considered for protease inhibitor therapy. (CDC web page: http://www.cdc.gov; National Institutes of Health AIDS treatment guideline: 1-800-448-0440)

Discussion

In a randomized, 2-way, crossover study, the effect of rifampin on the pharmacokinetics of nelfinavir was evaluated in 12 healthy volunteers.[2] Each subject received nelfinavir 750 mg alone every 8 hours for 16 doses, and with rifampin 600 mg daily for 7 doses. Rifampin administration increased the oral clearance of nelfinavir 467% (37.4 to 212 L/hr). Seven patients with HIV-related tuberculosis were given rifabutin twice weekly plus isoniazid for at least 2 weeks when an antiretroviral regimen containing nelfinavir was started.[3] A pharmacokinetic analysis after a median of 21 days found no change in nelfinavir or its M8 metabolite. On average, the AUC of rifabutin was elevated 22%.

[1] *Viracept* [package insert]. New York, NY: Pfizer; March 1997.
[2] Yuen GJ, et al. *Clin Pharmacol Ther.* 1997;61:147.
[3] Benator DA, et al. *Pharmacotherapy.* 2007;27(6):793.

* Asterisk indicates drugs cited in interaction reports. Based on pharmacologic and pharmacokinetic considerations, similar interactions may occur with other drugs that are listed.

Niacin — *Salicylates*

Niacin* (Nicotinic Acid; eg, *Niaspan*)	Aspirin* (eg, *Bayer*)

Significance	Onset	Severity	Documentation
5	■ **Rapid**	□ Major	□ Established
	□ Delayed	□ Moderate	□ Probable
		■ **Minor**	□ Suspected
			□ Possible
			■ **Unlikely**

Effects Elevated NICOTINIC ACID plasma levels during coadministration of ASPIRIN.

Mechanism Unknown.

Management Based on available information, no special precautions are needed.

Discussion

A study in 6 healthy volunteers described elevations in plasma nicotinic acid concentration following coadministration of aspirin 1,000 mg orally and the IV infusion of varying doses of nicotinic acid.[1] Coincident with the increase in nicotinic acid levels was a marked reduction in the concentration of a nicotinic acid metabolite, nicotinuric acid, indicating that metabolism might have been inhibited by aspirin. In theory, this could result in increased nicotinic acid adverse reactions, particularly flushing. However, it has also been demonstrated that the administered dose of aspirin decreases flushing in individuals taking large doses of nicotinic acid.[2] Therefore, it is unlikely that this pharmacokinetic interaction produces deleterious effects. Further study is needed to determine if the antilipidemic effect of nicotinic acid is potentiated.

[1] Ding RW, et al. *Clin Pharmacol Ther.* 1989;46(6):642. [2] Wilkin JK, et al. *Clin Pharmacol Ther.* 1982;31(4):478.

* Asterisk indicates drugs cited in interaction reports.

Nicardipine — *Food*

Nicardipine* (eg, *Cardene*)	Grapefruit Juice*

Significance	Onset	Severity	Documentation
2	■ **Rapid**	□ Major	□ Established
	□ Delayed	■ **Moderate**	□ Probable
		□ Minor	■ **Suspected**
			□ Possible
			□ Unlikely

Effects NICARDIPINE plasma concentrations may be elevated, increasing the pharmacologic effects and adverse reactions.

Mechanism Inhibition of gut wall metabolism (CYP3A4) of NICARDIPINE by GRAPEFRUIT JUICE is suspected.

Management Avoid coadministration of NICARDIPINE with GRAPEFRUIT products. Caution patients to take NICARDIPINE with a liquid other than GRAPEFRUIT JUICE.

Discussion

The effect of grapefruit juice on the pharmacokinetics of nicardipine was studied in an open-label, crossover investigation.[1] On different occasions, 6 healthy volunteers received racemic nicardipine 40 mg orally or 2 mg IV. On each occasion, subjects ingested 300 mL of water or concentrated grapefruit juice 30 minutes prior to nicardipine administration. When nicardipine was administered orally, compared with water, grapefruit juice increased the AUC of (+)- and (-)-nicardipine 43% and 84%, respectively, and decreased the clearance 26% and 42%, respectively. One and 2 hours after oral administration of nicardipine, the heart rate increased following the consumption of grapefruit juice compared with water. Grapefruit juice did not alter the pharmacokinetics of IV-administered racemic nicardipine. The $t_{1/2}$ values for oral and IV nicardipine did not differ between the water and grapefruit phases.

[1] Uno T, et al. *Eur J Clin Pharmacol.* 2000;56(9-10):643.

* Asterisk indicates drugs cited in interaction reports.

Nicotine — *Food*

Nicotine* (eg, *Commit*)	Grapefruit Juice*

Significance	Onset	Severity	Documentation
5	☐ Rapid ■ **Delayed**	☐ Major ☐ Moderate ■ **Minor**	☐ Established ☐ Probable ☐ Suspected ■ **Possible** ☐ Unlikely

Effects The clinical consequences of this interaction are expected to be minimal.

Mechanism Inhibition of metabolism (CYP2A6) and increased renal clearance of NICOTINE by GRAPEFRUIT JUICE.

Management Based on available data, no special precautions are necessary.

Discussion

The effects of grapefruit juice on the pharmacokinetics of nicotine were studied in 10 healthy nonsmokers.[1] Each subject received oral nicotine 2 mg, as deuterium-labeled nicotine, with 250 mL of full-strength grapefruit juice, half-strength grapefruit juice, or water. The metabolic conversion of nicotine to cotinine was inhibited approximately 15% and 2.5% when ingested with full-strength and half-strength grapefruit juice, respectively, compared with ingestion with water. The time to C_{max} of cotinine was delayed approximately 47% and 8%, respectively, and the C_{max} was decreased approximately 18% and 4.5%, respectively, compared with ingestion with water. Because the inhibition of hepatic metabolism of nicotine is offset by the increase in renal clearance of nicotine, the net effect on oral nicotine clearance appears to be negligible. This interaction is not expected to be clinically important.

[1] Hukkanen J, et al. *Clin Pharmacol Ther.* 2006;80(5):522.

* Asterisk indicates drugs cited in interaction reports.

Nifedipine		*Azole Antifungal Agents*	
Nifedipine* (eg, *Procardia*)		Itraconazole* (eg, *Sporanox*)	Posaconazole (*Noxafil*)
		Ketoconazole (eg, *Nizoral*)	Voriconazole* (*Vfend*)

Significance	Onset	Severity	Documentation
2	☐ Rapid	☐ Major	☐ Established
	■ **Delayed**	■ **Moderate**	☐ Probable
		☐ Minor	■ **Suspected**
			☐ Possible
			☐ Unlikely

Effects Serum NIFEDIPINE concentrations may be increased. Peripheral edema and hypotension have been reported.

Mechanism Possible inhibition of NIFEDIPINE metabolism (CYP3A4) by certain AZOLE ANTIFUNGAL AGENTS.

Management Observe the clinical response of patients and monitor CV status when NIFEDIPINE and certain AZOLE ANTIFUNGAL AGENTS are coadministered. If an interaction is suspected, adjust the NIFEDIPINE dose accordingly.

Discussion

Pitting edema of the lower extremities was reported in a 74-year-old woman following the addition of itraconazole to her long-term drug regimen that included nifedipine, methylprednisolone (eg, *Medrol*), propranolol (eg, *Inderal*), and sulindac (eg, *Clinoril*).[1] However, the possibility of a drug interaction was not considered. In this report, a second patient who was not taking nifedipine experienced a similar toxic response while receiving itraconazole. Subsequently, a second case of edema during coadministration of nifedipine and itraconazole was reported, and the possibility of an interaction was taken into account.[2] A 68-year-old woman who had been taking nifedipine, atenolol (eg, *Tenormin*), medroxyprogesterone (eg, *Provera*), conjugated estrogens (eg, *Premarin*), and vitamins for 2 to 3 years was started on itraconazole 200 mg twice daily for 1 week every month for 3 courses to treat pedal onychomycosis. During the first 2 courses of itraconazole therapy, the patient developed ankle edema 2 to 3 days after starting itraconazole, which resolved 2 to 3 days after the antifungal agent was stopped. The patient did not develop ankle edema during the third course of itraconazole treatment, at which time serum concentrations of nifedipine, itraconazole, and the active metabolite of itraconazole (hydroxyitraconazole) were measured. Trough serum concentrations of nifedipine were increased 4-fold when itraconazole was administered. In addition, the median BP during nifedipine administration was 147/83 mm Hg, compared with 128/72 mm Hg when itraconazole was given concomitantly. In a 48-year-old man receiving nifedipine 40 mg daily, BP decreased from 130 to 146/70 to 88 mm Hg to 76/48 mm Hg within 1 day of receiving IV voriconazole.[3] See also Felodipine-Azole Antifungal Agents.

[1] Rosen T. *Arch Dermatol.* 1994;130(2):260.
[2] Tailor SA, et al. *Arch Dermatol.* 1996;132(3):350.
[3] Kato J, et al. *Eur J Clin Pharmacol.* 2009;65(3):323.

* Asterisk indicates drugs cited in interaction reports. Based on pharmacologic and pharmacokinetic considerations, similar interactions may occur with other drugs that are listed.

Nifedipine — *Barbiturates*

Nifedipine	Barbiturates	
Nifedipine* (eg, *Procardia*)	Amobarbital (*Amytal*)	Phenobarbital* (eg, *Solfoton*)
	Butabarbital (eg, *Butisol*)	Primidone* (eg, *Mysoline*)
	Mephobarbital (*Mebaral*)	Secobarbital (*Seconal*)
	Pentobarbital*	

Significance	Onset	Severity	Documentation
2	☐ Rapid	☐ Major	☐ Established
	■ **Delayed**	■ **Moderate**	☐ Probable
		☐ Minor	■ **Suspected**
			☐ Possible
			☐ Unlikely

Effects Decreased serum NIFEDIPINE concentrations, possibly reducing efficacy.

Mechanism Enhanced metabolic clearance caused by enzyme induction.

Management Titrate dose according to response. A larger dose of NIFEDIPINE may be needed.

Discussion

The effect of pretreatment with phenobarbital 100 mg daily for 8 days on the pharmacokinetics of a single dose of nifedipine 20 mg was studied in 15 healthy volunteers.[1] Compared with baseline values, total clearance increased from 1,088 to 2,981 mL/min, and the AUC decreased from 343 to 135 ng•hr/mL. Consequently, plasma nifedipine concentrations were markedly reduced.

Clinical trials are needed to determine the therapeutic implications of this interaction.

[1] Schellens JH, et al. *J Pharmacol Exp Ther.* 1989;249(2):638.

* Asterisk indicates drugs cited in interaction reports. Based on pharmacologic and pharmacokinetic considerations, similar interactions may occur with other drugs that are listed.

Nifedipine — *Cisapride*

Nifedipine* (eg, *Procardia*)	Cisapride* (*Propulsid*)

Significance	Onset	Severity	Documentation
2	■ **Rapid**	□ Major	□ Established
	□ Delayed	■ **Moderate**	□ Probable
		□ Minor	■ **Suspected**
			□ Possible
			□ Unlikely

Effects Serum NIFEDIPINE concentrations may be elevated, increasing the therapeutic and adverse effects.

Mechanism Possible increased rate of NIFEDIPINE absorption, resulting from enhanced GI motility.

Management Monitor the patient for altered effects of NIFEDIPINE when starting or stopping CISAPRIDE therapy. Adjust the dose of NIFEDIPINE as needed.

Discussion

The effects of cisapride administration on nifedipine serum concentrations and pharmacologic activity were evaluated in 20 inpatients with mild-to-moderate essential hypertension.[1] Each patient received 20 mg of sustained release nifedipine alone and after 2.5 mg of cisapride. When cisapride and nifedipine were administered concurrently, the serum nifedipine concentration at 1 hour after administration was similar to when nifedipine was given alone. However, compared with nifedipine monotherapy, cisapride administration increased nifedipine serum concentrations at 2, 3 and 4 hours after administration by 93%, 107% and 60%, respectively. Cisapride administration decreased the mean blood pressure at 3 hours after administration of nifedipine by 22.5% compared with 12.6% when patients received nifedipine alone.

The effects of cisapride on steady-state concentrations of sustained release nifedipine need to be determined. In addition, because both cisapride and nifedipine are metabolized by the CYP 3A4 isozyme, the effects on hepatic and gut wall metabolism need to be studied.

[1] Satoh C, et al. *Intern Med.* 1996;35:941.

* Asterisk indicates drugs cited in interaction reports.

Nifedipine **_Cyclosporine_**

Nifedipine* (eg, *Procardia*)	Cyclosporine* (eg, *Neoral*)

Significance	Onset	Severity	Documentation
4	☐ Rapid	☐ Major	☐ Established
	■ **Delayed**	■ **Moderate**	☐ Probable
		☐ Minor	☐ Suspected
			■ **Possible**
			☐ Unlikely

Effects The pharmacologic and toxic effects of NIFEDIPINE may be increased.

Mechanism Unknown, possibly inhibition of the metabolism of NIFEDIPINE.

Management Consider observing patients receiving NIFEDIPINE for changes in clinical response and for side effects during concurrent treatment with CYCLOSPORINE. Adjust the dose of NIFEDIPINE as needed.

Discussion

The occurrence of an unpleasant burning sensation in 1 patient and a rash in a second patient during coadministration of nifedipine and cyclosporine prompted a study for a possible interaction between these 2 drugs.[1] In 8 psoriatic patients, the mean percentage recovery of the principle metabolite of nifedipine was 51% to 75% after taking a single dose of nifedipine alone compared with 34% to 58% while taking cyclosporine 3 to 4 mg/kg daily. The decrease in recovery of the nifedipine metabolite was attributed to the inhibition of nifedipine metabolism by cyclosporine.

Controlled studies are needed to determine the clinical importance of this possible interaction.

[1] McFadden JP, et al. *BMJ.* 1989;299:1224.

* Asterisk indicates drugs cited in interaction reports.

Nifedipine — *Diltiazem*

Nifedipine* (eg, *Procardia*)	Diltiazem* (eg, *Cardizem*)

Significance	Onset	Severity	Documentation
3	■ **Rapid**	□ Major	□ Established
	□ Delayed	□ Moderate	□ Probable
		■ **Minor**	■ **Suspected**
			□ Possible
			□ Unlikely

Effects DILTIAZEM increases plasma NIFEDIPINE concentrations and NIFEDIPINE increases plasma DILTIAZEM concentrations. The pharmacologic and toxic effects of NIFEDIPINE or DILTIAZEM may be increased.

Mechanism Possibly caused by reduced hepatic clearance.

Management Observe patients for increased side effects of NIFEDIPINE or DILTIAZEM and adjust the doses as needed.

Discussion

Based on treadmill exercise tolerance, combined use of nifedipine and diltiazem in 11 patients with classic angina produced greater antianginal efficacy than nifedipine alone.[1] Trough nifedipine concentrations increased from 34.8 to 106.4 ng/mL. Diltiazem concentrations were unchanged. Subsequently, 2 pharmacokinetic studies conducted in healthy volunteers were reported.[2,3] In 1 study, administration of diltiazem 60 mg 3 times daily to patients receiving nifedipine 20 mg produced a mean increase of 140% in the AUC of nifedipine.[3] The second study compared the effects of placebo or diltiazem 30 or 90 mg 3 times daily on nifedipine.[2] A dose-dependent increase in the AUC was observed. The nifedipine $t_{1/2}$ was prolonged from 2.54 hr with placebo to 3.4 and 3.47 hr with coadministration of diltiazem 30 or 90 mg, respectively. Likewise, the C_{max} of diltiazem was increased by nifedipine.[4] A report involving the combined use of diltiazem and nifedipine in 9 patients with variant angina suggests that the incidence of adverse effects is greater when both drugs are given together than with either agent alone.[5] All patients taking the combination developed side effects. A case of paralytic ileus has been reported.[6]

The effects of diltiazem on other dihydropyridine calcium channel blockers (eg, amlodipine [eg, *Norvasc*], nicardipine [eg, *Cardene*]) are unknown.

[1] Toyosaki N, et al. *Circulation*. 1988;77:1370.
[2] Tateishi T, et al. *J Clin Pharmacol*. 1989;29:994.
[3] Ohashi K, et al. *J Cardiovasc Pharmacol*. 1990;15:96.
[4] Tateishi T, et al. *J Clin Pharmacol*. 1993;33:738.
[5] Prida XE, et al. *J Am Coll Cardiol*. 1987;9:412.
[6] Harada T, et al. *Cardiology*. 2002;97:113.

* Asterisk indicates drugs cited in interaction reports.

Nifedipine — *Food*

Nifedipine* (eg, *Procardia*)	Food*	Grapefruit Juice*

Significance	Onset	Severity	Documentation
2	■ **Rapid**	□ Major	□ Established
	□ Delayed	■ **Moderate**	□ Probable
		□ Minor	■ **Suspected**
			□ Possible
			□ Unlikely

Effects FOOD is not likely to change the actions of NIFEDIPINE. However, GRAPEFRUIT JUICE may increase the bioavailability and activity of NIFEDIPINE.

Mechanism FOOD may slow the rate but not the extent of absorption of NIFEDIPINE. GRAPEFRUIT JUICE appears to inhibit first-pass metabolism (CYP3A4) of NIFEDIPINE.

Management NIFEDIPINE may be given without regard to meals. Avoid coadministration of NIFEDIPINE with GRAPEFRUIT products. Caution patients to take NIFEDIPINE with liquids other than GRAPEFRUIT JUICE.

Discussion

The effects of fasting, a low-fat (high-carbohydrate) meal, and a high-fat meal on the bioavailability of nifedipine 10 mg capsules were evaluated in 15 healthy subjects.[1] Food reduced the C_{max} and prolonged the time to peak concentration of nifedipine but did not alter the AUC. The AUC of nifedipine increased 134% when the 10 mg capsule was taken with grapefruit juice.[2] In 1 patient, enhanced hypotensive effects occurred.[3] In 8 healthy subjects, the C_{max} and AUC increased 40% and 15%, respectively, when a nifedipine 20 mg tablet was taken with grapefruit juice compared with ingestion with water.[4] Studies of the extended-release tablet formulation of nifedipine (eg, *Procardia XL*) indicate that food slightly alters the early rate of absorption but does not change the extent of drug availability.[5] Administration of this product after a meal resulted in a higher peak level (28%) and a shorter time to maximum plasma drug concentration as compared with the fasting state. However, the peak level still was much lower than that obtained with the use of the capsule (immediate-release) formulation. There was no evidence of dose dumping. In a study of a sustained-release formulation of nifedipine that is not available in the US, food increased the peak concentration and AUC.[6] However, in a study of another sustained-release product (also not available in the US), food did not affect the bioavailability of nifedipine.[7] These observations demonstrate the importance of evaluating the potential for interaction with food with each formulation of the drug.

[1] Reitberg DP, et al. *Clin Pharmacol Ther.* 1987;42:72.
[2] Bailey DG, et al. *Lancet.* 1991;337:268.
[3] Pisarik P. *Arch Fam Med.* 1996;5:413.
[4] Azuma J, et al. *Curr Ther Res.* 1998;59:619.
[5] Chung M, et al. *Am J Med.* 1987;83(6B):10.
[6] Ueno K, et al. *DICP.* 1989;23:662.
[7] Ueno K, et al. *DICP.* 1991;25:317.

* Asterisk indicates drugs cited in interaction reports.

Nifedipine — *Histamine H_2 Antagonists*

Nifedipine*
(eg, *Procardia*)

Cimetidine*
(eg, *Tagamet*)

Significance	Onset	Severity	Documentation
2	☐ Rapid ■ **Delayed**	☐ Major ■ **Moderate** ☐ Minor	☐ Established ☐ Probable ■ **Suspected** ☐ Possible ☐ Unlikely

Effects The effects of NIFEDIPINE may be increased.

Mechanism Undetermined, but the hepatic metabolism of NIFEDIPINE may be decreased.

Management Monitor patients for altered effects of NIFEDIPINE when initiating, discontinuing, or altering the dose of CIMETIDINE. Adjust the dose of NIFEDIPINE accordingly.

Discussion

Cimetidine increases the AUC and peak plasma levels of nifedipine.[1-5] Six healthy volunteers given nifedipine 40 mg/day exhibited an 80% increase in peak plasma level and AUC and a nearly 40% decrease in plasma clearance of nifedipine during coadministration of cimetidine 1 g/day.[2] Twelve healthy volunteers received cimetidine 800 mg/day for 5 days with nifedipine as a single 20 mg dose on day 5 or as a 10 mg dose 3 times daily for 5 days. This resulted in an 80% increase in the AUC of nifedipine compared with placebo.[3] However, only the multiple-dose study demonstrated an increase in peak plasma concentrations. Cimetidine increased the hypotensive actions of nifedipine in 7 patients with hypertension. In a controlled study of 11 healthy volunteers, cimetidine 1.2 g/day increased the AUC of nifedipine 80% and 65% during single and multiple dosing of nifedipine, respectively.[4] In addition to increased nifedipine blood levels, heart rate was increased during cimetidine administration.

Data from studies with ranitidine (eg, *Zantac*) have shown either a small increase in nifedipine plasma levels and AUC[1,2] or no changes.[3-5]

1 Kirch W, et al. *Dtsch Med Wochenschr.* 1983;108(46):1757.
2 Kirch W, et al. *Clin Pharmacol Ther.* 1985;37:204.
3 Smith SR, et al. *Br J Clin Pharmacol.* 1987;23(3):311.
4 Schwartz JB, et al. *Clin Pharmacol Ther.* 1988;43(6):673.
5 Khan A, et al. *Br J Clin Pharmacol.* 1991;32(4):519.

* Asterisk indicates drugs cited in interaction reports.

Nifedipine — **Macrolide & Related Antibiotics**

Nifedipine	Macrolide & Related Antibiotics	
Nifedipine* (eg, *Procardia*)	Clarithromycin* (eg, *Biaxin*)	Telithromycin (*Ketek*)
	Erythromycin* (eg, *Ery-Tab*)	

Significance	Onset	Severity	Documentation
1	☐ Rapid	■ **Major**	☐ Established
	■ **Delayed**	☐ Moderate	☐ Probable
		☐ Minor	■ **Suspected**
			☐ Possible
			☐ Unlikely

Effects NIFEDIPINE plasma concentrations may be elevated, increasing the pharmacologic effects and risk of adverse reactions (eg, severe hypotension).

Mechanism Inhibition of NIFEDIPINE metabolism (CYP3A4) by MACROLIDE AND RELATED ANTIBIOTICS.

Management Closely monitor for increased NIFEDIPINE pharmacologic response and for signs of toxicity. In patients already receiving NIFEDIPINE, azithromycin may be less likely to interact.

Discussion

A 77-year-old man with uncontrollable hypertension who was taking sustained-release nifedipine 60 mg twice daily as part of his antihypertensive regimen developed shock, heart block, and multiorgan failure 2 days after clarithromycin (500 mg every 12 hours) was started.[1] Upon admission to the hospital the patient showed reduced consciousness, hypotension (BP 80/40 mm Hg), bradycardia (40 bpm), tachypnea with cyanosis, cold limbs, and absent peripheral pulses. On admission, his antihypertensive medications were stopped and clarithromycin was continued. His acidosis and hyperkalemia were treated and norepinephrine was started to control his BP. Once his clinical status and BP were adequately controlled, the patient was discharged on nifedipine 60 mg daily, furosemide (eg, *Lasix*), and clarithromycin. In a population-based, case-crossover study involving patients 66 years and older, coadministration of clarithromycin or erythromycin and a calcium channel blocker (including nifedipine) increased the risk of hypotension.[2]

[1] Gerónimo-Pardo M, et al. *Ann Pharmacother.* 2005;39(3):538.

[2] Wright AJ, et al. *CMAJ.* 2011;183(3):303.

* Asterisk indicates drugs cited in interaction reports. Based on pharmacologic and pharmacokinetic considerations, similar interactions may occur with other drugs that are listed.

Nifedipine — *Melatonin*

Nifedipine* (eg, *Procardia*)	Melatonin*

Significance	Onset	Severity	Documentation
2	☐ Rapid	☐ Major	☐ Established
	■ **Delayed**	■ **Moderate**	☐ Probable
		☐ Minor	■ **Suspected**
			☐ Possible
			☐ Unlikely

Effects MELATONIN may interfere with the antihypertensive effect of NIFEDIPINE.

Mechanism Unknown.

Management Caution patients to consult their health care provider regarding the use of OTC or herbal products. If MELATONIN cannot be avoided, carefully assess the patient's response to NIFEDIPINE treatment when MELATONIN is started or stopped. Adjust the dose as needed.

Discussion

The effect of evening ingestion of melatonin on the antihypertensive action of nifedipine GI therapeutic system (GITS) was evaluated in 47 patients with mild to moderate essential hypertension.[1] Using a double-blind, randomized, placebo-controlled, crossover design, each subject took nifedipine 30 or 60 mg once daily at 8:30 AM for at least 3 months. Subjects were randomized to receive placebo or an immediate-release formulation of melatonin 5 mg at 10:30 PM for 4 weeks. Compared with placebo, in patients taking nifedipine, melatonin ingestion produced an increase in BP throughout the day (ie, 24-hour period; 6.5 mm Hg increase in systolic BP; 4.9 mm Hg increase in diastolic BP). The increase in systolic BP with melatonin was highest during the afternoon and first part of the night. The increase in the diastolic BP was greatest in the morning. In addition, melatonin ingestion resulted in a 3.9 bpm increase in heart rate throughout the 24-hour period, being highest in the morning. Patients taking melatonin reported drowsiness in the morning and weakness more often than patients taking placebo.

The ingredients of many herbal products are not standardized. It is unclear if herbal products contain ingredients other than those listed on the label or purported to be present that could interact with nifedipine therapy.

[1] Lusardi P, et al. *Br J Clin Pharmacol.* 2000;49(5):423.

* Asterisk indicates drugs cited in interaction reports.

Nifedipine — *Omeprazole*

Nifedipine* (eg, *Procardia*)	Omeprazole* (*Prilosec*)

Significance	Onset	Severity	Documentation
5	□ Rapid ■ **Delayed**	□ Major □ Moderate ■ **Minor**	□ Established □ Probable □ Suspected □ Possible ■ **Unlikely**

Effects Serum NIFEDIPINE concentrations may be increased. The relatively small increase is not likely to result in a clinically important interaction.

Mechanism Unknown.

Management Based on currently available data, no special precautions are needed.

Discussion

The effects of therapeutic doses of oral omeprazole on the pharmacokinetics of oral nifedipine as well as the effects on heart rate and BP were studied in 10 healthy subjects.[1] The pharmacokinetics of a single oral dose of nifedipine 10 mg were investigated following administration of placebo, a single oral dose of omeprazole 20 mg (enteric-coated granules in capsules), and after the last dose of 8 days of treatment with omeprazole 20 mg once daily. There were no significant changes in any of the pharmacokinetic parameters of nifedipine following single-dose administration of omeprazole. However, short-term administration of omeprazole significantly ($P = 0.006$) increased nifedipine's AUC. When taken 30 minutes after the eighth dose of omeprazole, the AUC of nifedipine was 26% greater compared with placebo treatment and 20% larger compared with single-dose omeprazole treatment. All other pharmacokinetic parameters, including $t_{½}$, AUC of the metabolite of nifedipine (dehydronifedipine), and the 8 -hr urinary recovery of the metabolite were not different between treatment periods. In addition, the BP and heart rate of the subjects were not different between treatments.

Compared to the large therapeutic index of nifedipine and the wide range of intra- and inter-individual variability caused by other factors, the relatively small increase in AUC is not likely to result in a clinically important interaction between nifedipine and omeprazole.

[1] Soons PA, et al. *Eur J Clin Pharmacol.* 1992;42:319.

* Asterisk indicates drugs cited in interaction reports.

Nifedipine — *Orlistat*

Nifedipine* (eg, *Procardia*)	Orlistat* (*Xenical*)

Significance	Onset	Severity	Documentation
5	☐ Rapid ■ **Delayed**	☐ Major ☐ Moderate ■ **Minor**	☐ Established ☐ Probable ☐ Suspected ■ **Possible** ☐ Unlikely

Effects The time to reach peak plasma concentration for NIFEDIPINE may be increased.

Mechanism Unknown.

Management Based on available date, no special precautions are necessary. Be prepared to make appropriate changes in dosage if an interaction is suspected.

Discussion

In an open-label, crossover investigation, the effects of orlistat on the pharmacokinetics of nifedipine were studied in 8 healthy men.[1] Each subject received 50 mg of orlistat 3 times/day mid-meal for 7 days. Nifedipine (20 mg slow-release tablet) was administered in single doses twice, once before and once at the end of orlistat treatment. Compared with giving nifedipine alone, administration after orlistat pretreatment increased the time to reach the peak concentration of nifedipine 62% (from 1.3 to 2.3 hr).

[1] Weber C, et al. *Eur J Clin Pharmacol.* 1996;51:87.

* Asterisk indicates drugs cited in interaction reports.

Nifedipine — *Penicillins*

Nifedipine* (eg, *Procardia*)	Nafcillin*

Significance	Onset	Severity	Documentation
3	☐ Rapid	☐ Major	☐ Established
	■ **Delayed**	☐ Moderate	☐ Probable
		■ **Minor**	■ **Suspected**
			☐ Possible
			☐ Unlikely

Effects NIFEDIPINE plasma concentrations may be reduced, decreasing the therapeutic effect.

Mechanism Induction of NIFEDIPINE metabolism (CYP3A4) by NAFCILLIN is suspected.

Management In patients receiving NIFEDIPINE, closely observe the clinical response when starting or stopping NAFCILLIN. If an interaction is suspected, adjust the dose of NIFEDIPINE as needed.

Discussion

Using a randomized, placebo-controlled, crossover design, the effects of nafcillin on the pharmacokinetics of nifedipine were investigated in 9 healthy subjects.[1] Individuals received pretreatment with nafcillin 500 mg or placebo 4 times/day for 5 days. On the study day after an overnight fast, each subject received an oral dose of nifedipine 10 mg. Compared with taking nifedipine alone, pretreatment with nafcillin decreased the average $t_{1/2}$ of nifedipine 62% (from 2.9 to 1.1 hours) and the AUC 63%, while the total plasma clearance was increased 145% (from 56.5 to 138.5 L/hr).

[1] Lang CC, et al. *Br J Clin Pharmacol.* 2003;55(6):588.

* Asterisk indicates drugs cited in interaction reports.

Nifedipine — *Protease Inhibitors*

Nifedipine	Protease Inhibitors	
Nifedipine* (eg, *Procardia*)	Atazanavir (*Reyataz*)	Nelfinavir* (*Viracept*)
	Darunavir (*Prezista*)	Ritonavir* (*Norvir*)
	Fosamprenavir (*Lexiva*)	Saquinavir (*Invirase*)
	Indinavir* (*Crixivan*)	Tipranavir (*Aptivus*)
	Lopinavir/Ritonavir* (*Kaletra*)	

Significance	Onset	Severity	Documentation
2	☐ Rapid ■ **Delayed**	☐ Major ■ **Moderate** ☐ Minor	☐ Established ☐ Probable ■ **Suspected** ☐ Possible ☐ Unlikely

Effects NIFEDIPINE plasma levels may be elevated, increasing the risk of adverse reactions (eg, severe hypotension, renal failure).

Mechanism Inhibition of NIFEDIPINE metabolism (CYP3A4) by RITONAVIR is suspected.

Management If coadministration of these agents cannot be avoided, closely monitor for adverse reactions. Be prepared to reduce the NIFEDIPINE dose if needed.

Discussion

Hypotension and renal failure were reported in a 47-year-old HIV-infected man on 3 occasions during coadministration of nifedipine 30 mg every 12 hours and lopinavir/ritonavir.[1] In the latter 2 instances, the patient was receiving nifedipine and, within 2 days of reinstating lopinavir/ritonavir, severe hypotension (eg, 90/50 mm Hg), edema, malaise, and renal failure developed. In each occasion, the patient's condition improved when nifedipine and lopinavir/ritonavir were discontinued. A 51-year-old HIV-infected man with hypertension, whose drug regimen included nifedipine 60 mg daily, experienced dizziness, fatigue, and hypotension, as well as complete heart block after starting antiretroviral therapy that included nelfinavir.[2] The ECG abnormalities reversed within 24 hours of stopping antiretroviral therapy; however, orthostatic symptoms occurred when nelfinavir was restarted. His antiretroviral regimen was changed. Subsequently, when indinavir and ritonavir were administered, orthostatic symptoms occurred again. His orthostatic changes were managed with a 50% reduction in the nifedipine dose.

[1] Baeza MT, et al. *AIDS*. 2007;21(1):119.

[2] Rossi DR, et al. *Pharmacotherapy*. 2002;22(10):1312.

* Asterisk indicates drugs cited in interaction reports. Based on pharmacologic and pharmacokinetic considerations, similar interactions may occur with other drugs that are listed.

Nifedipine — *Rifamycins*

Nifedipine* (eg, *Procardia*)	Rifabutin (*Mycobutin*) Rifampin* (eg, *Rifadin*)	Rifapentine (*Priftin*)

Significance	Onset	Severity	Documentation
2	☐ Rapid ■ **Delayed**	☐ Major ■ **Moderate** ☐ Minor	☐ Established ■ **Probable** ☐ Suspected ☐ Possible ☐ Unlikely

Effects The therapeutic effects of NIFEDIPINE may be reduced.

Mechanism Possibly caused by increased gut wall metabolism (CYP3A4) of NIFEDIPINE induced by RIFAMYCINS.

Management Monitor BP and for angina symptoms. Adjust the NIFEDIPINE dose accordingly or consider an alternative antihypertensive medication.

Discussion

Rifampin has been reported to interfere with the clinical effects of long-acting nifedipine.[1] A 72-year-old woman with essential hypertension had been well controlled with long-acting nifedipine 40 mg twice daily. Following a positive skin test and histological features suggestive of tuberculosis, the patient was started on a regimen of rifampin 450 mg daily, isoniazid (eg, *Nydrazid*), and ethambutol (*Myambutol*). During concurrent antituberculosis treatment, the patient's BP gradually increased, reaching approximately 200/110 mm Hg after 2 weeks. Rifampin was presumed to be attenuating the effect of nifedipine and was discontinued. The other antitubercular agents were continued. In addition, the alpha-blocker bunazosin† was administered. The BP gradually decreased. Elevation in BP recurred when rifampin was restarted. Plasma nifedipine levels and AUC were measured during concomitant rifampin loading and administration of long-acting nifedipine 20 mg twice daily. Compared with administering nifedipine alone, peak plasma nifedipine levels decreased from 66.6 to 28.4 ng/mL, and the AUC decreased 61% during coadministration of rifampin. In a study of 6 healthy volunteers, administration of rifampin caused a decrease in the $t_{1/2}$ of nifedipine from 2.3 to 1.7 hours.[2] However, the reduction in nifedipine levels was more pronounced when nifedipine was given orally as compared with IV. This demonstrates a larger extraction of nifedipine in the gut wall.

A similar interaction may be expected with nicardipine (eg, *Cardene*) and rifampin. See also Verapamil-Rifampin.

[1] Tada Y, et al. *Am J Med Sci.* 1992;303(1):25.

[2] Holtbecker N, et al. *Drug Metab Dispos.* 1996;24(10):1121.

* Asterisk indicates drugs cited in interaction reports. Based on pharmacologic and pharmacokinetic considerations, similar interactions may occur with other drugs that are listed.

† Not available in the US.

Nifedipine — *Serotonin Reuptake Inhibitors*

Nifedipine* (eg, *Procardia*)	Fluoxetine* (eg, *Prozac*)	Nefazodone

Significance	Onset	Severity	Documentation
4	☐ Rapid ■ **Delayed**	☐ Major ■ **Moderate** ☐ Minor	☐ Established ☐ Probable ☐ Suspected ■ **Possible** ☐ Unlikely

Effects Pharmacologic effects and adverse reactions of NIFEDIPINE may be increased.

Mechanism Certain SRIs may inhibit the metabolism (CYP3A4) of NIFEDIPINE.

Management In patients receiving NIFEDIPINE, closely observe the clinical response when an SRI is started or stopped.

Discussion

A 76-year-old woman with a history of diabetic peripheral neuropathy, hypertension, hiatal hernia, and mitral valve prolapse was maintained on sustained-release nifedipine 60 mg/day and trazodone.[1] After she was diagnosed with depression, fluoxetine 20 mg every other day was started, and trazodone was discontinued. Three days later, treatment with lorazepam (eg, *Ativan*) and acetaminophen plus oxycodone (eg, *OxyContin*) was started. One week after starting fluoxetine, the patient complained of flushing and excessive warmth without night sweats. The dose of nifedipine was reduced to 30 mg/day, and the patient's complaints diminished over the following 2 to 3 weeks.

Additional studies are needed to determine the clinical importance of this possible interaction.

[1] Sternbach H. *J Clin Psychopharmacol.* 1991;11(6):390.

* Asterisk indicates drugs cited in interaction reports. Based on pharmacologic and pharmacokinetic considerations, similar interactions may occur with other drugs that are listed.

Nilotinib		*Azole Antifungal Agents*	
Nilotinib* (*Tasigna*)		Itraconazole* (eg, *Sporanox*)	Posaconazole (*Noxafil*)
		Ketoconazole* (eg, *Nizoral*)	Voriconazole* (eg, *Vfend*)

Significance	Onset	Severity	Documentation
1	□ Rapid ■ **Delayed**	■ **Major** □ Moderate □ Minor	□ Established □ Probable ■ **Suspected** □ Possible □ Unlikely

Effects NILOTINIB plasma concentrations may be elevated, increasing the risk of adverse reactions, including life-threatening cardiac arrhythmias (eg, torsades de pointes).

Mechanism Inhibition of NILOTINIB metabolism (CYP3A4) by AZOLE ANTIFUNGAL AGENTS is suspected.

Management Avoid concurrent use of NILOTINIB and AZOLE ANTIFUNGAL AGENTS.[1] If coadministration cannot be avoided, closely monitor for adverse reactions, including QT prolongation. NILOTINIB dosage adjustments may be needed when an AZOLE ANTIFUNGAL AGENT is started or stopped.

Discussion

In healthy subjects, administration of ketoconazole 400 mg once daily for 6 days increased the nilotinib AUC approximately 3-fold. Nilotinib has been associated with concentration-dependent QT prolongation. Administration of strong CYP3A4 inhibitors, such as ketoconazole, may increase nilotinib plasma concentrations and should be avoided. If a strong CYP3A4 inhibitor is discontinued, allow a washout period before the nilotinib dose is adjusted upward to the indicated dose.[1] In an open-label study, the effects of ketoconazole on the pharmacokinetics of nilotinib were evaluated in 25 healthy subjects.[2] Each subject received a single oral dose of nilotinib 200 mg alone and after 4 days of receiving ketoconazole 400 mg once daily. Compared with receiving nilotinib alone, pretreatment with ketoconazole increased the nilotinib C_{max} and AUC 1.8- and 3-fold, respectively. In addition, the mean $t_{1/2}$ of nilotinib was prolonged from 15.2 to 32.7 hours.

[1] *Tasigna* [package insert]. East Hanover, NJ: Novartis Pharmaceuticals Corporation; October 2007.

[2] Tanaka C, et al. *J Clin Pharmacol.* 2011;51(1):75.

* Asterisk indicates drugs cited in interaction reports. Based on pharmacologic and pharmacokinetic considerations, similar interactions may occur with other drugs that are listed.

Nilotinib — *Food*

Nilotinib* (*Tasigna*)	Grapefruit Juice*

Significance	Onset	Severity	Documentation
1	☐ Rapid ■ **Delayed**	■ **Major** ☐ Moderate ☐ Minor	☐ Established ☐ Probable ■ **Suspected** ☐ Possible ☐ Unlikely

Effects NILOTINIB plasma concentrations may be elevated, increasing the risk of adverse reactions, including life-threatening cardiac arrhythmias (eg, torsades de pointes).

Mechanism Inhibition of intestinal first-pass metabolism (CYP3A4) of NILOTINIB by GRAPEFRUIT products is suspected.

Management Avoid taking NILOTINIB with GRAPEFRUIT products.[1] Advise patients to take NILOTINIB with a liquid other than GRAPEFRUIT JUICE.

Discussion

Data from coadministration of nilotinib with ketoconazole indicate that CYP3A4 inhibitors increase nilotinib plasma concentrations.[1] Nilotinib has been associated with concentration-dependent QT prolongation. Grapefruit products may also increase nilotinib plasma concentrations and should be avoided.[1,2] There are no clinical data with dose adjustments in patients receiving nilotinib and grapefruit products, including grapefruit juice. The effects of grapefruit juice on the pharmacokinetics of nilotinib were studied in 21 healthy men.[2] Using an open-label, randomized, crossover design, each subject received a single dose of nilotinib 400 mg with 240 mL of double-strength grapefruit juice or 240 mL of water. Compared with water, grapefruit juice increased the nilotinib C_{max} and AUC 60% and 29%, respectively, but did not affect the T_{max} or elimination $t_{½}$.

[1] *Tasigna* [package insert]. East Hanover, NJ: Novartis Pharmaceuticals Corporation; October 2007.

[2] Yin OQ, et al. *J Clin Pharmacol.* 2010;50(2):188.

* Asterisk indicates drugs cited in interaction reports.

Nilotinib | **Macrolide & Related Antibiotics**

Nilotinib*	Azithromycin*	Erythromycin
(*Tasigna*)	(eg, *Zithromax*)	(eg, *Ery-Tab*)
	Clarithromycin*	Telithromycin*
	(eg, *Biaxin*)	(*Ketek*)

Significance	Onset	Severity	Documentation
1	☐ Rapid	■ **Major**	☐ Established
	■ **Delayed**	☐ Moderate	☐ Probable
		☐ Minor	■ **Suspected**
			☐ Possible
			☐ Unlikely

Effects NILOTINIB plasma concentrations may be elevated, increasing the risk of adverse reactions, including life-threatening cardiac arrhythmias (eg, torsades de pointes).

Mechanism Inhibition of NILOTINIB metabolism (CYP3A4) by MACROLIDE and RELATED ANTIBIOTICS is suspected.

Management Avoid concurrent use of NILOTINIB and MACROLIDE and RELATED ANTIBIOTICS.[1] If coadministration cannot be avoided, closely monitor for adverse reactions, including QT prolongation. NILOTINIB dosage adjustments may be needed when a MACROLIDE or RELATED ANTIBIOTIC is started or stopped.

Discussion

Data from coadministration of nilotinib with ketoconazole indicate that CYP3A4 inhibitors increase nilotinib plasma concentrations. Nilotinib has been associated with concentration-dependent QT prolongation.[1] Administration of strong CYP3A4 inhibitors, such as clarithromycin, may increase nilotinib plasma concentrations; avoid coadministration. If a strong CYP3A4 inhibitor is discontinued, allow a washout period before the nilotinib dose is adjusted upward to the indicated dose.[1] There are no clinical data with dose adjustments in patients receiving nilotinib and strong CYP3A4 inhibitors.

The basis for this interaction is information on file with the manufacturer. Published clinical data are needed to further assess this interaction. Because of the seriousness of the cardiac problem, clinical evaluation of this interaction in humans is not likely to be forthcoming.

[1] *Tasigna* [package insert]. East Hanover, NJ: Novartis Pharmaceuticals Corporation; October 2007.

* Asterisk indicates drugs cited in interaction reports. Based on pharmacologic and pharmacokinetic considerations, similar interactions may occur with other drugs that are listed.

Nilotinib | **Nefazodone**

Nilotinib*
(*Tasigna*)

Nefazodone*

Significance	Onset	Severity	Documentation
1	☐ Rapid ■ **Delayed**	■ **Major** ☐ Moderate ☐ Minor	☐ Established ☐ Probable ■ **Suspected** ☐ Possible ☐ Unlikely

Effects NILOTINIB plasma concentrations may be elevated, increasing the risk of adverse reactions, including life-threatening cardiac arrhythmias (eg, torsades de pointes).

Mechanism Inhibition of NILOTINIB metabolism (CYP3A4) by NEFAZODONE is suspected.

Management Avoid concurrent use of NILOTINIB and NEFAZODONE.[1] If coadministration cannot be avoided, closely monitor for adverse reactions, including QT prolongation. NILOTINIB dosage adjustments may be needed when NEFAZODONE is started or stopped.

Discussion

Data from coadministration of nilotinib with ketoconazole indicate that CYP3A4 inhibitors increase nilotinib plasma concentrations.[1] Nilotinib has been associated with concentration-dependent QT prolongation.[1] Administration of strong CYP3A4 inhibitors, such as nefazodone, may increase nilotinib plasma concentrations; avoid coadministration. If a strong CYP3A4 inhibitor is discontinued, allow a washout period before the nilotinib dose is adjusted upward to the indicated dose.[1] There are no clinical data with dose adjustments in patients receiving nilotinib and strong CYP3A4 inhibitors.

The basis for this interaction is information on file with the manufacturer. Published clinical data are needed to further assess this interaction. Because of the seriousness of the cardiac problem, clinical evaluation of this interaction in humans is not likely to be forthcoming.

[1] *Tasigna* [package insert]. East Hanover, NJ: Novartis Pharmaceuticals Corporation; October 2007.

* Asterisk indicates drugs cited in interaction reports.

Nilotinib — *Protease Inhibitors*

Nilotinib	Protease Inhibitors	
Nilotinib* (*Tasigna*)	Atazanavir* (*Reyataz*)	Nelfinavir* (*Viracept*)
	Fosamprenavir (*Lexiva*)	Ritonavir* (*Norvir*)
	Indinavir* (*Crixivan*)	Saquinavir* (*Invirase*)
	Lopinavir/Ritonavir (*Kaletra*)	

Significance	Onset	Severity	Documentation
1	☐ Rapid	■ **Major**	☐ Established
	■ **Delayed**	☐ Moderate	☐ Probable
		☐ Minor	■ **Suspected**
			☐ Possible
			☐ Unlikely

Effects NILOTINIB plasma concentrations may be elevated, increasing the risk of adverse reactions, including life-threatening cardiac arrhythmias (eg, torsades de pointes).

Mechanism Inhibition of NILOTINIB metabolism (CYP3A4) by PROTEASE INHIBITORS is suspected.

Management Avoid concurrent use of NILOTINIB and PROTEASE INHIBITORS.[1] If coadministration cannot be avoided, closely monitor for adverse reactions, including QT prolongation. NILOTINIB dosage adjustments may be needed when a PROTEASE INHIBITOR is started or stopped.

Discussion

Data from coadministration of nilotinib with ketoconazole indicate that CYP3A4 inhibitors increase nilotinib plasma concentrations.[1] Nilotinib has been associated with concentration-dependent QT prolongation. Administration of strong CYP3A4 inhibitors, such as ritonavir, may increase nilotinib plasma concentrations and should be avoided. If a strong CYP3A4 inhibitor is discontinued, allow a washout period before the nilotinib dose is adjusted upward to the indicated dose. There are no clinical data with dose adjustments in patients receiving nilotinib and strong CYP3A4 inhibitors.

The basis for this interaction is information on file with the manufacturer. Published clinical data are needed to further assess this interaction. Because of the seriousness of the cardiac problem, clinical evaluation of this interaction in humans is not likely to be forthcoming.

[1] *Tasigna* [package insert]. East Hanover, NJ: Novartis Pharmaceuticals Corporation; October 2007.

* Asterisk indicates drugs cited in interaction reports. Based on pharmacologic and pharmacokinetic considerations, similar interactions may occur with other drugs that are listed.

Nilotinib — *Proton Pump Inhibitors*

Nilotinib	Proton Pump Inhibitors	
Nilotinib* (*Tasigna*)	Esomeprazole* (*Nexium*)	Pantoprazole (eg, *Protonix*)
	Lansoprazole (eg, *Prevacid*)	Rabeprazole (*Aciphex*)
	Omeprazole (eg, *Prilosec*)	

Significance	Onset	Severity	Documentation
2	■ **Rapid** □ Delayed	□ Major ■ **Moderate** □ Minor	□ Established □ Probable ■ **Suspected** □ Possible □ Unlikely

Effects NILOTINIB plasma concentrations may be reduced, decreasing the pharmacologic effects.

Mechanism NILOTINIB pH-dependent solubility may be reduced, decreasing NILOTINIB GI absorption.

Management Coadminister with caution. Separating the administration times is not likely to circumvent the interaction. However, administration of an antacid or histamine H_2 blocker several hours before or after NILOTINIB may be considered as an alternative to the PROTON PUMP INHIBITOR.

Discussion

Because nilotinib solubility decreases at a higher pH, drugs such as proton pump inhibitors that elevate gastric pH by inhibiting gastric acid secretion may decrease the solubility of nilotinib and reduce its bioavailability.[1] In an open-label, 2-period, sequential study, the effect of esomeprazole on the pharmacokinetics of nilotinib was evaluated in 15 subjects.[2] Each subject received a single dose of nilotinib 400 mg on days 1 and 13 and esomeprazole 40 mg once daily on days 8 through 13. Compared with giving nilotinib alone, administration of nilotinib with steady-state esomeprazole decreased the nilotinib C_{max} and AUC 27% and 34%, respectively. Nilotinib T_{max} was prolonged from 4 to 6 hours. Increasing the dose of nilotinib is not likely to make up for the decrease in drug exposure.[1] In addition, because proton pump inhibitors affect the pH of the upper GI tract for an extended period, separating the doses may not circumvent the interaction.[1]

[1] *Tasigna* [package insert]. East Hanover, NJ: Novartis Pharmaceuticals Corporation; June 2010.

[2] Yin OQ, et al. *J Clin Pharmacol*. 2010;50(8):960.

* Asterisk indicates drugs cited in interaction reports. Based on pharmacologic and pharmacokinetic considerations, similar interactions may occur with other drugs that are listed.

Nilotinib — Rifamycins

Nilotinib	Rifamycins	
Nilotinib* (*Tasigna*)	Rifabutin (*Mycobutin*)	Rifapentine (*Priftin*)
	Rifampin* (eg, *Rifadin*)	

Significance	Onset	Severity	Documentation
2	□ Rapid	□ Major	□ Established
	■ **Delayed**	■ **Moderate**	□ Probable
		□ Minor	■ **Suspected**
			□ Possible
			□ Unlikely

Effects NILOTINIB plasma concentrations may be reduced, decreasing the pharmacologic effects.

Mechanism RIFAMYCINS may increase the metabolism (CYP3A4) of NILOTINIB.

Management If concurrent use cannot be avoided, monitor the clinical response and adjust the NILOTINIB dose as needed.

Discussion

In an open-label study, the effects of rifampin on the pharmacokinetics of nilotinib were evaluated in 15 healthy subjects.[1] Each subject received a single oral dose of nilotinib 200 mg alone and after 9 days of receiving rifampin 600 mg once daily. Compared with receiving nilotinib alone, pretreatment with rifampin decreased the nilotinib C_{max} and AUC 64% and 80%, respectively. In addition, the mean $t_{1/2}$ of nilotinib was shortened from 18.8 to 14.6 hours and the apparent oral clearance increased from 45.2 to 215.9 L/hr (approximately 4.8-fold). The median T_{max} of nilotinib increased from 3 to 4 hours.

[1] Tanaka C, et al. *J Clin Pharmacol.* 2011;51(1):75.

* Asterisk indicates drugs cited in interaction reports. Based on pharmacologic and pharmacokinetic considerations, similar interactions may occur with other drugs that are listed.

Nilotinib — **St. John's Wort**

Nilotinib*
(*Tasigna*)

St. John's Wort*

Significance	Onset	Severity	Documentation
2	☐ Rapid ■ **Delayed**	☐ Major ■ **Moderate** ☐ Minor	☐ Established ☐ Probable ■ **Suspected** ☐ Possible ☐ Unlikely

Effects NILOTINIB plasma concentrations may be reduced, decreasing the efficacy.

Mechanism Induction of NILOTINIB metabolism (CYP3A4) by ST. JOHN'S WORT.

Management Avoid concurrent use of NILOTINIB and ST. JOHN'S WORT.[1] If coadministration cannot be avoided, carefully titrate the dose of NILOTINIB upward. If ST. JOHN'S WORT is discontinued, reduce the NILOTINIB dose to the indicated dose.

Discussion

Data from coadministration of nilotinib with rifampin indicate that CYP3A4 inducers decrease systemic exposure (AUC) to nilotinib. St. John's wort, a CYP3A4 inducer, may also decrease system exposure to nilotinib.[1] Therefore, caution patients taking nilotinib to avoid taking St. John's wort.

The basis for this monograph is information on file with the manufacturer. Published clinical data are needed to assess the clinical importance of this interaction.

[1] *Tasigna* [package insert]. East Hanover, NJ: Novartis Pharmaceuticals Corporation; October 2007.

* Asterisk indicates drugs cited in interaction reports.

Nimodipine — **Food**

Nimodipine*
(eg, *Nimotop*)

Grapefruit Juice*

Significance	Onset	Severity	Documentation
2	☐ Rapid ■ **Delayed**	☐ Major ■ **Moderate** ☐ Minor	☐ Established ☐ Probable ■ **Suspected** ☐ Possible ☐ Unlikely

Effects NIMODIPINE plasma concentrations may be elevated, increasing the pharmacologic effects and adverse reactions.

Mechanism GRAPEFRUIT JUICE may inhibit the first-pass metabolism (CYP3A4) of NIMODIPINE.

Management Caution patients receiving NIMODIPINE to avoid GRAPEFRUIT products, and advise patients to take NIMODIPINE with a liquid other than GRAPEFRUIT JUICE.

Discussion

The effects of grapefruit juice ingestion on the pharmacokinetics of nimodipine and its metabolites were studied in a randomized, crossover investigation.[1] Eight healthy men received a single dose of nimodipine 30 mg with 250 mL of water or grapefruit juice. Compared with water, grapefruit juice ingestion increased the AUC and C_{max} of nimodipine 51% and 24%, respectively. The ratios of the nimodipine metabolite AUC to nimodipine AUC were decreased slightly by grapefruit juice ingestion. In addition, there was a more pronounced hemodynamic effect (eg, increased heart rate) when nimodipine was taken with grapefruit juice.

[1] Fuhr U, et al. *Int J Clin Pharmacol Ther*. 1998;36(3):126.

* Asterisk indicates drugs cited in interaction reports.

Nisoldipine | **Azole Antifungal Agents**

Nisoldipine	Azole Antifungal Agents	
Nisoldipine* (eg, *Sular*)	Fluconazole (eg, *Diflucan*)	Posaconazole (*Noxafil*)
	Itraconazole* (eg, *Sporanox*)	Voriconazole (eg, *Vfend*)
	Ketoconazole* (eg, *Nizoral*)	

Significance	Onset	Severity	Documentation
2	☐ Rapid ■ **Delayed**	☐ Major ■ **Moderate** ☐ Minor	☐ Established ☐ Probable ■ **Suspected** ☐ Possible ☐ Unlikely

Effects Serum NISOLDIPINE concentrations may be elevated, increasing the pharmacologic effects and adverse reactions.

Mechanism Possible inhibition of NISOLDIPINE metabolism (CYP3A4) by the AZOLE ANTIFUNGAL AGENT. FLUCONAZOLE, especially 200 mg/day or more, may inhibit CYP3A4.[1]

Management If this drug combination cannot be avoided, observe the clinical response of patients and monitor cardiovascular status when NISOLDIPINE and an AZOLE ANTIFUNGAL AGENT are coadministered. If an interaction is suspected, adjust the dose of NISOLDIPINE accordingly. Coadministration of NISOLDIPINE and ITRACONAZOLE is contraindicated.[2]

Discussion

The effect of ketoconazole on the pharmacokinetics of nisoldipine was studied in 7 healthy volunteers.[3] Using a nonblind, randomized, crossover design, subjects received a single dose of nisoldipine 5 mg immediate release alone or on day 5 of pretreatment with ketoconazole 200 mg/day. Compared with administration of nisoldipine alone, coadministration with ketoconazole increased the mean AUC of nisoldipine 25-fold and C_{max} 11-fold (from 1.06 to 12.1 mcg/L). Coadministration of nisoldipine and ketoconazole increased the AUC of the 2-hydroxyisobutyl-metabolite M9 of nisoldipine 25-fold and C_{max} 7-fold (from 1.87 to 12.8 mcg/L).

A similar effect would be expected with coadministration of the nisoldipine extended-release formulation; however, because first-pass metabolism would be reduced, the magnitude of the interaction may be smaller. See also Felodipine-Azole Antifungal Agents and Nifedipine-Azole Antifungal Agents.

[1] Goa KL, et al. *Drugs.* 1995;50(4):658.
[2] *Sporanox* [package insert]. Raritan, NJ: Centocor Ortho Biotech; April 2011.
[3] Heinig R, et al. *Eur J Clin Pharmacol.* 1999;55(1):57.

* Asterisk indicates drugs cited in interaction reports. Based on pharmacologic and pharmacokinetic considerations, similar interactions may occur with other drugs that are listed.

Nisoldipine | **Food**

Nisoldipine* (eg, *Sular*)

Grapefruit Juice*

Significance	Onset	Severity	Documentation
2	■ **Rapid**	□ Major	□ Established
	□ Delayed	■ **Moderate**	■ **Probable**
		□ Minor	□ Suspected
			□ Possible
			□ Unlikely

Effects Serum NISOLDIPINE concentrations may be elevated, producing an increase in pharmacologic effects and adverse reactions.

Mechanism Possibly caused by inhibition of first-pass NISOLDIPINE metabolism (CYP3A4). This effect may last up to 3 days after stopping daily GRAPEFRUIT JUICE ingestion.[1]

Management Avoid coadministration of NISOLDIPINE with GRAPEFRUIT products. Caution patients to take NISOLDIPINE with liquids other than GRAPEFRUIT JUICE.

Discussion

The pharmacokinetics of nisoldipine 20 mg extended-release tablets (coat-core) were studied in 12 healthy men.[2] Each subject was administered nisoldipine with 250 mL of water, 250 mL of grapefruit juice, or encapsulated naringin powder (naringin is the major flavonoid present in grapefruit juice). Compared with water, grapefruit juice increased the nisoldipine C_{max} 4-fold and the AUC 2-fold, and decreased the T_{max} 58%. The encapsulated naringin powder did not affect nisoldipine pharmacokinetics. Similar pharmacologic changes were reported in 2 additional studies involving 16 healthy subjects.[1,3]

This drug interaction may occur with other dihydropyridine calcium channel blockers (eg, nifedipine [eg, *Procardia*]); however, the magnitude of the interactions may vary. See also Felodipine-Food and Nifedipine-Food.

[1] Takanaga H, et al. *Clin Pharmacol Ther.* 2000;67(3);201.

[2] Bailey DG, et al. *Clin Pharmacol Ther.* 1993;54(6):589.

[3] Azuma J, et al. *Curr Ther Res Clin Exp.* 1998;59(9);619.

* Asterisk indicates drugs cited in interaction reports.

Nisoldipine — *Hydantoins*

Nisoldipine	Hydantoins	
Nisoldipine* (*Sular*)	Ethotoin (*Peganone*)	Mephenytoin†
	Fosphenytoin	Phenytoin* (eg, *Dilantin*)

Significance	Onset	Severity	Documentation
2	☐ Rapid	☐ Major	☐ Established
	■ **Delayed**	■ **Moderate**	☐ Probable
		☐ Minor	■ **Suspected**
			☐ Possible
			☐ Unlikely

Effects The pharmacologic effects of NISOLDIPINE may be decreased.

Mechanism HYDANTOINS may increase the first-pass metabolism of NISOLDIPINE, decreasing its bioavailability.

Management Monitor the cardiovascular status of patients receiving NISOLDIPINE when HYDANTOIN therapy is started, stopped, or adjusted in dose. Patients receiving long-term treatment with HYDANTOINS may require larger doses of NISOLDIPINE than patients who are not receiving HYDANTOINS.

Discussion

The effects of phenytoin on the pharmacokinetics of nisoldipine were evaluated by comparing 2 matched groups of subjects.[1] One group consisted of 12 patients with epilepsy who had been receiving long-term therapy with phenytoin 200 to 450 mg/day and had stable plasma phenytoin concentrations over the previous 3 months. The second group included 12 drug-free healthy subjects (control group). Because it was anticipated that phenytoin might reduce nisoldipine plasma concentrations, leading to assay problems, the dose of nisoldipine administered to patients with epilepsy was twice as large as the dose administered to the control subjects (a single 40 mg dose vs a 20 mg dose, respectively). Before analysis, nisoldipine C_{max} and AUCs were normalized for a 20 mg dose in the patients with epilepsy. Although the dose of nisoldipine was twice as large in the patients with epilepsy, extremely low plasma nisoldipine concentrations, with undetectable concentrations at most sampling times, occurred in a substantial proportion of the patients. The mean dose-normalized C_{max} of nisoldipine was 0.19 mcg/L in the patients with epilepsy compared with 1.06 mcg/L in the control subjects. In addition, the dose-normalized mean AUCs were approximately 10-fold lower in the patients with epilepsy than in the control group. Both groups demonstrated interindividual variability, which was greater in the patients with epilepsy. See also Felodipine-Hydantoins and Verapamil-Hydantoins.

[1] Michelucci R, et al. *Epilepsia.* 1996;37(11):1107.

* Asterisk indicates drugs cited in interaction reports. Based on pharmacologic and pharmacokinetic considerations, similar interactions may occur with other drugs that are listed.
† Not available in the United States.

Nitrates | **Avanafil**

Nitrates		Avanafil
Amyl nitrite*	Nitroglycerin* (eg, *Nitrostat*)	Avanafil* (*Stendra*)
Isosorbide dinitrate* (eg, *Isordil*)		
Isosorbide mononitrate* (eg, *ISMO*)		

Significance	Onset	Severity	Documentation
1	■ **Rapid**	■ **Major**	□ Established
	□ Delayed	□ Moderate	□ Probable
		□ Minor	■ **Suspected**
			□ Possible
			□ Unlikely

Effects Severe hypotension may occur.

Mechanism AVANAFIL potentiates the hypotensive effects of NITRATES.

Management Coadministration of AVANAFIL with NITRATES (regularly or intermittently) is contraindicated.[1] If a patient has taken AVANAFIL, and nitrate administration is medically necessary due to a life-threatening situation, allow at least 12 hours to elapse after the last dose of AVANAFIL before considering NITRATE administration. In such situations, administer NITRATES only under close medical supervision and provide appropriate hemodynamic monitoring.

Discussion

Administration of avanafil with any form of organic nitrates, either regularly or intermittently, is contraindicated. Avanafil has been shown to potentiate the hypotensive effects of nitrates. The degree of interaction between nitroglycerin and avanafil was assessed in a double-blind, randomized, crossover study in healthy men.[1] Each subject received avanafil 200 mg and placebo in random order. Subjects received a single dose of sublingual nitroglycerin 0.4 mg following their dose of trial drug. Overall, 15% of subjects treated with placebo and 28% of subjects treated with avanafil had clinically important decreases in standing blood pressure (ie, decreases greater than or equal to 30 mm Hg).

The basis for this monograph is information on file with the manufacturer. Published clinical data are needed to further assess this interaction.

[1] *Stendra* [package insert]. Mountain View, CA: Vivus Inc; April 2012.

* Asterisk indicates drugs cited in interaction reports.

Nitrates / *Salicylates*

Nitroglycerin* (eg, *NitroMist*)	Aspirin* (eg, *Bayer*)

Significance	Onset	Severity	Documentation
5	■ **Rapid**	☐ Major	☐ Established
	☐ Delayed	☐ Moderate	☐ Probable
		■ **Minor**	☐ Suspected
			■ **Possible**
			☐ Unlikely

Effects Analgesic doses of ASPIRIN may increase serum concentrations and enhance the actions of NITROGLYCERIN.

Mechanism Alteration of prostaglandin concentrations by ASPIRIN may play a role.

Management If exaggerated responses to NITROGLYCERIN occur (eg, headache, syncope), consider discontinuing ASPIRIN or tailoring the dose of NITROGLYCERIN.

Discussion

The possible interaction between aspirin and nitroglycerin in 7 healthy volunteers was investigated.[1,2] The effects of nitroglycerin 0.8 mg sublingual spray were assessed by the decrease in diastolic arterial pressure, increase in heart rate, and decrease in M-mode echocardiographic end-diastolic and end-systolic diameters of the left ventricle. Measurements were performed before, during, and 30 minutes after nitroglycerin. Each of the following trials was repeated 3 times in each volunteer in random order: nitroglycerin without aspirin pretreatment and nitroglycerin 1 hour after aspirin 1 g. Aspirin 1 g increased the effects of nitroglycerin on diastolic BP and left ventricular end-diastolic and end-systolic diameters. Aspirin 1 g increased mean nitroglycerin plasma levels (54%) and heart rate. Some animal data indicate indomethacin (eg, *Indocin*) may modify nitroglycerin's effects via prostaglandin inhibition.[3] Platelet aggregation time is additively prolonged by aspirin and IV nitroglycerin.[4] This may be a therapeutic benefit in patients with acute MI.[3]

Clinical studies are needed to determine if other forms of nitroglycerin, other salicylates, or other NSAIDs interact in a similar manner.

[1] Rey E, et al. *Eur J Clin Pharmacol.* 1983;25(6):779.
[2] Weber S, et al. *J Cardiovasc Pharmacol.* 1983;5(5):874.
[3] Morcillio E, et al. *Am J Cardiol.* 1980;45(1):53.
[4] Karlberg KE, et al. *Am J Cardiol.* 1993;71(4):361.

* Asterisk indicates drugs cited in interaction reports.

Nitrates — Sildenafil

Amyl Nitrite
Isosorbide Dinitrate (eg, *Isordil*)
Isosorbide Mononitrate* (eg, *ISMO*)
Nitroglycerin* (eg, *Nitrostat*)

Sildenafil* (eg, *Viagra*)

Significance	Onset	Severity	Documentation
1	■ **Rapid**	■ **Major**	□ Established
	□ Delayed	□ Moderate	□ Probable
		□ Minor	■ **Suspected**
			□ Possible
			□ Unlikely

Effects Severe hypotension may occur.

Mechanism SILDENAFIL potentiates the hypotensive effects of NITRATES and enhances the effect of nitric oxide and nitric acid donor drugs by inhibiting phosphodiesterase type 5, which is responsible for degradation of cyclic guanosine monophosphate (cGMP) in the corpus cavernosum. Increased cGMP produces smooth muscle relaxation in the corpus cavernosum, which allows inflow of blood.

Management Concomitant use of any form of organic NITRATES and SILDENAFIL is contraindicated. Carefully screen patients for NITRATE use before prescribing or dispensing SILDENAFIL. In emergency situations, determine if patients with chest pain have taken SILDENAFIL during the previous 24 hr before administering a NITRATE.

Discussion

Sildenafil potentiates the hypotensive effects of nitrates and is therefore contraindicated in patients using any form of an organic nitrate, including nitroglycerin (NTG).[1] Deaths have occurred in several patients taking sildenafil. It has not been determined if the drug was responsible for the deaths or if the deaths occurred coincidentally. In patients with stable angina, the effects of sildenafil on BP were investigated in 2 double-blind, placebo-controlled, randomized, crossover studies involving isosorbide mononitrate (ISMN) and NTG.[2] In 16 men receiving sildenafil or placebo after 7 days of ISMN 20 mg twice daily, sildenafil caused a 27 mm Hg reduction in systolic BP compared with placebo. Fifteen men received NTG 0.5 mg sublingually 1 hr after sildenafil or placebo. Compared with placebo, sildenafil caused a 10 mm Hg greater reduction in systolic and a 9 mm Hg greater reduction in diastolic BP. Dizziness, sweating, postural hypotension, and headache occurred more frequently with sildenafil. In a placebo-controlled study, the safety of an NTG IV infusion was evaluated in 34 men with coronary artery disease.[3] Each patient received a single dose of sildenafil 100 mg. The NTG infusion was gradually titrated to limit the drop in BP or increase in heart rate. The median NTG dose tolerated for patients receiving sildenafil was 80 mcg/min, compared with 160 mcg/min for placebo. In healthy men, compared with administration of sublingual nitroglycerin and placebo, coadministration of sildenafil and sublingual nitroglycerin resulted in a decrease in BP for up to 1 hr after sildenafil administration; whereas, in patients with angina, the decrease in BP persisted for up to 8 hr.[4]

[1] *Viagra* [package insert]. New York, NY: Pfizer Labs; 1998.
[2] Webb DJ, et al. *J Am Coll Cardiol.* 2000;36(1):25.
[3] Parker JD, et al. *Crit Care Med.* 2007;35(8):1863.
[4] Oliver JJ, et al. *Br J Clin Pharmacol.* 2009;67(4):403.

* Asterisk indicates drugs cited in interaction reports. Based on pharmacologic and pharmacokinetic considerations, similar interactions may occur with other drugs that are listed.

Nitrates — *Tadalafil*

Amyl Nitrite Isosorbide Dinitrate (eg, *Isordil*) Isosorbide Mononitrate (eg, *ISMO*)	Nitroglycerin* (eg, *Nitrostat*)	Tadalafil* (eg, *Cialis*)

Significance	Onset	Severity	Documentation
1	■ **Rapid** ☐ Delayed	■ **Major** ☐ Moderate ☐ Minor	☐ Established ☐ Probable ■ **Suspected** ☐ Possible ☐ Unlikely

Effects Severe hypotension may occur.

Mechanism TADALAFIL potentiates the hypotensive effects of NITRATES.

Management Concomitant use of TADALAFIL and NITRATES (regularly or intermittently) or nitric oxide donors is contraindicated.[1] Carefully screen patients for NITRATE use before prescribing or dispensing TADALAFIL.

Discussion

The time course of the interaction between tadalafil and sublingual nitroglycerin was evaluated in 150 men.[1] Using a randomized, placebo-controlled, double-blind, 2-period, crossover design, each subject received placebo or tadalafil to steady state (20 mg daily for 7 days). Sublingual nitroglycerin (0.4 mg) was administered at 2, 4, 8, 24, 48, 72, and 96 hours after tadalafil or placebo. Nitroglycerin administration at 4, 8, and 24 hours resulted in a standing systolic BP less than 85 mm Hg in more tadalafil-treated subjects compared with placebo, with no difference in response to nitroglycerin at 48, 72, and 96 hours. A similar response occurred for standing diastolic BP (less than 45 mm Hg), decrease in systolic BP (more than 30 mm Hg), and decrease in diastolic BP (more than 20 mm Hg). In addition, nitroglycerin induced greater mean maximal decreases in standing systolic BP at 8 and 24 hours after taking tadalafil compared with placebo, while no difference occurred with nitroglycerin at 48, 72, or 96 hours. Compensatory heart rate responses, resulting from nitroglycerin-induced decreases in BP, were similar after tadalafil or placebo administration.[2]

[1] *Cialis* [package insert]. Indianapolis, IN: Eli Lilly and Company; January 2008.

[2] Kloner RA, et al. *J Am Coll Cardiol.* 2003;42(10):1855.

* Asterisk indicates drugs cited in interaction reports. Based on pharmacologic and pharmacokinetic considerations, similar interactions may occur with other drugs that are listed.

Nitrates — *Vardenafil*

Nitrates		Vardenafil
Amyl Nitrite Isosorbide Dinitrate (eg, *Isordil*) Isosorbide Mononitrate (eg, *ISMO*)	Nitroglycerin* (eg, *Nitroglyn*)	Vardenafil* (*Levitra*)

Significance	Onset	Severity	Documentation
1	■ **Rapid** □ Delayed	■ **Major** □ Moderate □ Minor	□ Established □ Probable ■ **Suspected** □ Possible □ Unlikely

Effects Severe hypotension may occur.

Mechanism VARDENAFIL potentiates the hypotensive effects of NITRATES.

Management Concomitant use of VARDENAFIL and NITRATES (regularly or intermittently) or nitric oxide donors is contraindicated. Carefully screen patients for NITRATE use before prescribing or dispensing VARDENAFIL.

Discussion

The BP and heart rate response to 0.4 mg nitroglycerin (NTG) sublingually was evaluated in 18 healthy subjects following pretreatment with vardenafil 20 mg at various times prior to NTG administration.[1] Vardenafil produced an additional time-related decrease in BP and increase in heart rate in association with NTG administration. The BP-lowering effects of NTG were observed when vardenafil was administered 1 or 4 hr before NTG; increases in heart rate were observed when vardenafil was given 1,4, or 8 hr before NTG. These effects were not observed when vardenafil was taken 24 hr before NTG.

The basis for this monograph is information on file with the manufacturer. Published clinical data are needed to further assess this interaction.

[1] *Levitra* [package insert]. West Haven, CT: Bayer Pharmaceuticals Corporation; 2003.

* Asterisk indicates drugs cited in interaction reports. Based on pharmacologic and pharmacokinetic considerations, similar interactions may occur with other drugs that are listed.

Nitrofurantoin — *Anticholinergics*

Nitrofurantoin*
(eg, *Macrodantin*)

Anisotropine
Atropine*
Belladonna
Benztropine (eg, *Cogentin*)
Biperiden (*Akineton*)
Clidinium (*Quarzan*)
Dicyclomine (eg, *Bentyl*)
Glycopyrrolate (eg, *Robinul*)
Hyoscyamine (eg, *Anaspaz*)
Mepenzolate (*Cantil*)
Methantheline (*Banthine*)
Methscopolamine (*Pamine*)
Orphenadrine (eg, *Norflex*)
Oxybutynin (eg, *Ditropan*)
Procyclidine (*Kemadrin*)
Propantheline* (eg, *Pro-Banthine*)
Scopolamine
Tridihexethyl (*Pathilon*)
Trihexyphenidyl (eg, *Trihexy-5*)

Significance	Onset	Severity	Documentation
5	☐ Rapid	☐ Major	☐ Established
	■ **Delayed**	☐ Moderate	☐ Probable
		■ **Minor**	☐ Suspected
			☐ Possible
			■ **Unlikely**

Effects ANTICHOLINERGICS may increase plasma concentration of NITROFURANTOIN, possibly increasing adverse effects.

Mechanism Delayed gastric emptying by ANTICHOLINERGICS may increase NITROFURANTOIN bioavailability.[1]

Management Based on available data, no clinical intervention is needed.

Discussion

Six healthy subjects were administered a single oral dose of nitrofurantoin 100 mg with 100 mL of water.[1] In crossover design, 3 subjects received propantheline 30 mg 45 minutes prior to nitrofurantoin administration while the other 3 subjects received only nitrofurantoin. One week later, the trial was reversed. All subjects fasted overnight and for 4 hr after drug administration. A statistically significant increase in nitrofurantoin excretion occurred when propantheline was coadministered, compared with the control condition. No statistical significance was observed for differences in urinary volume or urinary pH between the 2 conditions. Thus, it appears that a delay in gastric emptying may increase the bioavailability of nitrofurantoin. In 10 healthy volunteers, atropine 0.5 mg given SC 30 minutes before nitrofurantoin alone retarded the absorption of the antibiotic, while excretion of nitrofurantoin was delayed to 4 to 8 hr.[2]

[1] Jaffe JM. *J Pharm Sci.* 1975;64:1729.

[2] Mannisto P. *Int J Clin Pharmacol Biopharm.* 1978;16:223.

* Asterisk indicates drugs cited in interaction reports. Based on pharmacologic and pharmacokinetic considerations, similar interactions may occur with other drugs that are listed.

Nitrofurantoin		**Magnesium Salts**
Nitrofurantoin* (eg, *Macrodantin*)	Magaldrate (eg, *Riopan*) Magnesium Carbonate* (eg, *Marblen*) Magnesium Citrate Magnesium Gluconate (eg, *Magonate*)	Magnesium Hydroxide* (eg, *Milk of Magnesia*) Magnesium Oxide* (eg, *Mag-Ox*) Magnesium Trisilicate*

Significance	Onset	Severity	Documentation
3	□ Rapid ■ **Delayed**	□ Major □ Moderate ■ **Minor**	□ Established □ Probable ■ **Suspected** □ Possible □ Unlikely

Effects The anti-infective capabilities of NITROFURANTOIN may be reduced.

Mechanism Adsorption onto MAGNESIUM SALTS may occur, reducing NITROFURANTOIN bioavailability.

Management Avoid this combination when possible. If impossible, separate administration times as much as possible, or use an aluminum-based antacid.

Discussion

One study demonstrated that nitrofurantoin adsorbed in vitro onto magnesium trisilicate (99.3%), while 26% to 53% was absorbed onto bismuth oxycarbonate, talc, kaolin, and magnesium oxide. Aluminum hydroxide and calcium carbonate showed minor adsorptive properties.[3] This study also found that coadministration of nitrofurantoin with magnesium trisilicate to healthy subjects reduced both the rate and extent of its excretion, probably reflecting a decrease in rate and extent of absorption. Ten healthy volunteers were given nitrofurantoin 100 mg with 50 mL of a magnesium-aluminum antacid.[2] The bioavailability of nitrofurantoin was decreased ≈ 25%. The clinical importance of this effect remains to be determined.[4]

An earlier report stated that an interaction between nitrofurantoin and antacids had been widely reported in reviews without the support of controlled clinical studies.[1] This report's data from volunteers demonstrated that aluminum hydroxide gel given concomitantly with nitrofurantoin did not alter the absorption rate of nitrofurantoin, the concentration of nitrofurantoin in the urine, or the urinary pH between treatments with nitrofurantoin alone and nitrofurantoin plus the antacid.

1 Jaffe JM, et al. *DICP.* 1976;10:419.
2 Mannisto P. *Int J Clin Pharmacol Biopharm.* 1978;16:223.
3 Naggar VF, et al. *Clin Pharmacol Ther.* 1979;25:857.
4 D'Arcy PF, et al. *DICP.* 1987;21:607.

* Asterisk indicates drugs cited in interaction reports. Based on pharmacologic and pharmacokinetic considerations, similar interactions may occur with other drugs that are listed.

NNRT Inhibitors / *Histamine H_2 Antagonists*

NNRT Inhibitors	Histamine H_2 Antagonists
Etravirine* (*Intelence*)	Ranitidine* (eg, *Zantac*)

Significance	Onset	Severity	Documentation
5	☐ Rapid ■ **Delayed**	☐ Major ☐ Moderate ■ **Minor**	☐ Established ☐ Probable ☐ Suspected ■ **Possible** ☐ Unlikely

Effects ETRAVIRINE plasma concentrations may be reduced slightly.

Mechanism Unknown.

Management Based on available information, no special precautions are necessary.

Discussion

The effect of steady-state ranitidine on the pharmacokinetics of etravirine was evaluated in 16 healthy volunteers.[1] Using an open-label, randomized, one-way, crossover design, each subject received ranitidine 150 mg twice daily for 11 days. A single dose of etravirine 100 mg was administered before starting ranitidine and on day 8 of ranitidine administration. Compared with administering etravirine alone, pretreatment with ranitidine decreased the etravirine AUC 16%, which is not expected to be clinically important. There was no change in the etravirine C_{max}.

[1] Schöller-Gyüre M, et al. *Br J Clin Pharmacol.* 2008;66(4):508.

* Asterisk indicates drugs cited in interaction reports.

NNRT Inhibitors — **Hydantoins**

NNRT Inhibitors		Hydantoins	
Delavirdine (*Rescriptor*)	Etravirine (*Intelence*)	Ethotoin (*Peganone*)	Phenytoin* (eg, *Dilantin*)
Efavirenz* (*Sustiva*)	Nevirapine (*Viramune*)	Fosphenytoin (eg, *Cerebyx*)	

Significance	Onset	Severity	Documentation
4	☐ Rapid ■ **Delayed**	☐ Major ■ **Moderate** ☐ Minor	☐ Established ☐ Probable ☐ Suspected ■ **Possible** ☐ Unlikely

Effects NNRT INHIBITOR plasma concentrations may be reduced, decreasing the efficacy. Plasma HYDANTOIN levels may be elevated, increasing the risk of toxicity.

Mechanism HYDANTOINS may increase the hepatic metabolism (CYP3A4 and/or CYP2B6) of NNRT INHIBITORS. Inhibition of HYDANTOIN metabolism (CYP2C9 and/or CYP2C19) by NNRT INHIBITORS is suspected.

Management Closely monitor NNRT INHIBITOR and HYDANTOIN levels when these agents are coadministered to avoid potential treatment failure and toxicity, respectively. Adjust the dosages as needed.

Discussion

Lower than expected levels of efavirenz (0.34 mcg/mL) and elevated phenytoin levels occurred in a 39-year-old man with advanced HIV infection, cytomegalovirus retinitis, and probable toxoplasmic encephalitis.[1] Because of concern that the reduced efavirenz levels were caused by an interaction with phenytoin, the phenytoin dosage was rapidly tapered, alternative anticonvulsant therapy was initiated (for tonic-clonic seizures), and the efavirenz dosage was increased from 600 to 800 mg/day. Approximately 18 days after phenytoin was discontinued, efavirenz concentrations increased to 2.5 mcg/mL, and the dosage was reduced to 600 mg/day. During coadministration of efavirenz and phenytoin, phenytoin plasma concentrations increased from 11.5 to 23.5 mg/L, despite a stable dosage of phenytoin 300 mg twice daily. A 35-year-old man was receiving efavirenz 800 mg daily as part of his antiretroviral therapy when phenytoin 400 mg twice daily was added to his treatment regimen for a seizure disorder.[2] Two weeks later, efavirenz levels were undetectable. Phenytoin was discontinued, and the efavirenz dosage was increased to 600 mg twice daily, which resulted in therapeutic efavirenz levels.

[1] Robertson SM, et al. *Clin Infect Dis*. 2005;41(2):e15. [2] Spak CW, et al. *AIDS*. 2008;22(1):164.

* Asterisk indicates drugs cited in interaction reports. Based on pharmacologic and pharmacokinetic considerations, similar interactions may occur with other drugs that are listed.

NNRT Inhibitors	***Proton Pump Inhibitors***
Etravirine* (*Intelence*)	Omeprazole* (eg, *Prilosec*)

Significance	Onset	Severity	Documentation
5	☐ Rapid ■ **Delayed**	☐ Major ☐ Moderate ■ **Minor**	☐ Established ☐ Probable ☐ Suspected ■ **Possible** ☐ Unlikely

Effects ETRAVIRINE plasma concentrations may be increased.

Mechanism Unknown.

Management Based on available information, no special precautions are necessary. If an interaction is suspected, consider adjusting the ETRAVIRINE dose.

Discussion

The effect of steady-state omeprazole on the pharmacokinetics of etravirine was evaluated in 17 healthy volunteers.[1] Using an open-label, randomized, one-way, crossover design, each subject received omeprazole 40 mg daily for 11 days. A single dose of etravirine 100 mg was administered before starting omeprazole and on day 8 of omeprazole administration. Compared with administering etravirine alone, pretreatment with omeprazole increased the etravirine AUC 41%. There was no change in the etravirine C_{max}. Because of the safety profile of etravirine, the increase in etravirine exposure is not expected to be clinically important.

[1] Schöller-Gyüre M, et al. *Br J Clin Pharmacol.* 2008;66(4):508.

* Asterisk indicates drugs cited in interaction reports.

NNRT Inhibitors — Rifamycins

NNRT Inhibitors		Rifamycins	
Efavirenz* (*Sustiva*)	Nevirapine* (eg, *Viramune*)	Rifabutin* (*Mycobutin*)	Rifapentine* (*Priftin*)
Etravirine* (*Intelence*)		Rifampin* (eg, *Rifadin*)	

Significance	Onset	Severity	Documentation
2	☐ Rapid	☐ Major	☐ Established
	■ **Delayed**	■ **Moderate**	■ **Probable**
		☐ Minor	☐ Suspected
			☐ Possible
			☐ Unlikely

Effects NNRT INHIBITOR plasma concentrations and RIFAMYCIN levels may be reduced, decreasing the efficacy of both drugs.

Mechanism RIFAMYCINS may increase the hepatic metabolism of the NNRT INHIBITOR.

Management Monitor NNRT INHIBITOR plasma levels and adjust the dose as needed. An empiric increase in RIFABUTIN dosage to 450 to 600 mg/day is recommended during coadministration of EFAVIRENZ. Do not use ETRAVIRINE with RIFAMPIN or RIFAPENTINE. RIFABUTIN may be administered with ETRAVIRINE in certain instances.[1]

Discussion

The effects of nevirapine and rifampin oral administration on the pharmacokinetics of each other were evaluated in 9 patients infected with HIV admitted to the hospital with tuberculosis.[2] Four patients were receiving nevirapine 200 mg twice daily and concurrent nucleoside analogs. The remaining 5 patients had not received antiviral treatment that included nevirapine or protease inhibitors. Antituberculosis treatment was started and consisted of rifampin 600 mg daily, isoniazid (eg, *Nydrazid*), pyrazinamide, and ethambutol (eg, *Myambutol*). Rifampin administration decreased nevirapine AUC 31% and C_{max} from 5.6 to 4.5 mcg/mL, compared with nevirapine pharmacokinetics prior to rifampin administration. Nevirapine did not alter the pharmacokinetics of rifampin. Studies showed a 17.7% to 39% decrease in nevirapine trough levels with coadministration of rifampin.[3,4] However, virological response was unaltered in 1 study.[3] In another report, rifampin reduced nevirapine AUC 46%.[5] The effects of rifampin on the pharmacokinetics of nevirapine were studied in 16 patients infected with HIV.[6] Nevirapine AUC was 40% lower during coadministration of rifampin compared with after discontinuation of rifampin. Subtherapeutic levels of nevirapine occurred in 6 patients, with therapeutic failure occurring in 1 patient. Increasing the nevirapine dosage from 200 to 300 mg twice daily overcame the interaction. Subtherapeutic rifabutin plasma levels were measured in a patient receiving efavirenz despite administration of megadoses of rifabutin (1,350 mg daily).[7] Rifabutin levels increased when efavirenz was stopped and nevirapine was started. In another study, increasing the rifabutin dosage from 300 to 600 mg twice weekly was sufficient to maintain therapeutic rifabutin levels in most patients receiving efavirenz.[8] Use of a rifampin-based regimen resulted in subtherapeutic efavirenz concentrations in 2 patients with tuberculosis.[9] In contrast, 58 patients, coinfected with HIV and tuberculosis, were randomized to receive efavirenz during or after completion of their rifampin-containing regimen.[10] Efavirenz clearance was reduced 29.5%. In healthy volunteers, coadministration of efavirenz with rifampin decreased the efavirenz AUC 18%.[11] However, the variability in response between subjects suggested that the interaction may be clinically relevant in some individuals. See Delavirdine-Rifamycins, Rilpivirine-Rifamycins.

[1] *Intelence* [package insert]. Raritan, NJ: Tibotec Therapeutics; January 2008.
[2] Ribera E, et al. *J Acquir Immune Defic Syndr.* 2001;28(5):450.
[3] Manosuthi W, et al. *Clin Infect Dis.* 2006;43(2):253.
[4] Elsherbiny D, et al. *Eur J Clin Pharmacol.* 2009;65(1):71.
[5] Ramachandran G, et al. *J Acquir Immune Defic Syndr.* 2006;42(1):36.
[6] Cohen K, et al. *J Antimicrob Chemother.* 2008;61(2):389.
[7] Edelstein HE, et al. *AIDS.* 2004;18(12):1748.
[8] Weiner M, et al. *Clin Infect Dis.* 2005;41(9):1343.
[9] Cabrera SE, et al. *AIDS.* 2008;22(18):2549.
[10] Gengiah TN, et al. *Eur J Clin Pharmacol.* 2012;68(5):689.
[11] Kwara A, et al. *Antimicrob Agents Chemother.* 2011;55(7):3527.

* Asterisk indicates drugs cited in interaction reports.

NNRT Inhibitors — *St. John's Wort*

Delavirdine (*Rescriptor*)	Nevirapine* (*Viramune*)	St. John's Wort*
Efavirenz (*Sustiva*)		

Significance	Onset	Severity	Documentation
4	☐ Rapid	☐ Major	☐ Established
	■ **Delayed**	■ **Moderate**	☐ Probable
		☐ Minor	☐ Suspected
			■ **Possible**
			☐ Unlikely

Effects NNRT INHIBITOR plasma concentrations may be reduced, decreasing the clinical efficacy.

Mechanism ST. JOHN'S WORT may increase the hepatic metabolism of the NNRT INHIBITOR.

Management Caution patients receiving NNRT INHIBITORS to consult their health care provider before using nonprescription or herbal products. If ST. JOHN'S WORT cannot be avoided, carefully assess the response to NNRT INHIBITOR treatment when ST. JOHN'S WORT is started or stopped. Adjust the dose as needed.

Discussion

Five patients treated with nevirapine for more than 1 year had been taking St. John's wort concurrently for several months.[1] Each patient had at least 1 nevirapine plasma level measurement with and without coadministration of St. John's wort. Because some measurements of nevirapine were consistently lower on certain occasions, a nonlinear, mixed-effect modeling analysis was performed to determine if the lower concentrations were caused by St. John's wort ingestion. It was calculated that St. John's wort increased the oral clearance of nevirapine 35%, resulting in decreased exposure to nevirapine.

[1] de Maat MM, et al. *AIDS*. 2001;15:420.

* Asterisk indicates drugs cited in interaction reports. Based on pharmacologic and pharmacokinetic considerations, similar interactions may occur with other drugs that are listed.

NNRT Inhibitors | **Thiazolidinediones**

Nevirapine* (*Viramune*) | Rosiglitazone* (*Avandia*)

Significance	Onset	Severity	Documentation
4	□ Rapid	□ Major	□ Established
	■ **Delayed**	■ **Moderate**	□ Probable
		□ Minor	□ Suspected
			■ **Possible**
			□ Unlikely

Effects NEVIRAPINE plasma concentrations may be reduced, decreasing the efficacy.

Mechanism Unknown.

Management Carefully monitor NEVIRAPINE plasma levels and observe the clinical response of patients when ROSIGLITAZONE is started or stopped. Be prepared to adjust the NEVIRAPINE dose as needed.

Discussion

The effects of rosiglitazone on the bioavailability of nevirapine, efavirenz (*Sustiva*), and ritonavir-boosted lopinavir (*Kaletra*) treatment were studied before and at 28 days of rosiglitazone therapy in 18 HIV-infected patients.[1] In addition to the study drugs, all patients received appropriate antiretroviral co-medication. All subjects received rosiglitazone 4 mg/day, 10 subjects received efavirenz 600 mg/day, 4 received nevirapine 200 mg twice daily, and 4 received lopinavir/ritonavir 400 per 100 mg twice daily. Rosiglitazone did not affect the pharmacokinetics of efavirenz or lopinavir. However, rosiglitazone therapy decreased the C_{max} of nevirapine. In addition, the minimum plasma concentration of nevirapine was less than 3,400 ng/mL in 2 patients on day 1 and in all 4 patients on day 28.

Because of the small sample size, larger trials are needed to confirm this possible interaction and to assess the clinical importance.

[1] Oette M, et al. *J Antimicrob Chemother*. 2005;56:416.

* Asterisk indicates drugs cited in interaction reports.

Nondepol. Muscle Relaxants — Aminoglycosides

Nondepol. Muscle Relaxants		Aminoglycosides	
Atracurium*	Rocuronium* (eg, *Zemuron*)	Amikacin	Netilmicin*†
Cisatracurium (*Nimbex*)	Tubocurarine*†	Gentamicin*	Streptomycin*
Gallamine*†	Vecuronium	Kanamycin*	Tobramycin* (eg, *Tobrex*)
Pancuronium*		Neomycin* (eg, *Neo-Fradin*)	

Significance	Onset	Severity	Documentation
1	■ **Rapid**	■ **Major**	□ Established
	□ Delayed	□ Moderate	■ **Probable**
		□ Minor	□ Suspected
			□ Possible
			□ Unlikely

Effects The actions of NONDEPOLARIZING MUSCLE RELAXANTS may be enhanced (eg, protracted respiratory depression).

Mechanism Possible pharmacologic synergism.

Management Administer this combination only when necessary, then tailor dosage of the NONDEPOLARIZING MUSCLE RELAXANT, based on neuromuscular response. Provide ventilatory support as indicated.

Discussion

It is well documented through animal experiments that aminoglycoside antibiotics have neuromuscular-blocking capabilities and that combination with a nondepolarizing muscle relaxant results in synergistic blocking action.[1-5] Aminoglycosides appear to produce both a presynaptic inhibition of acetylcholine release and a postsynaptic reduction of sensitivity of the postjunctional membrane to acetylcholine. Severe apnea (sometimes fatal) and respiratory paralysis in a child have occurred when agents of these 2 classes were administered together.[6-15]

1 Timmerman JC, et al. *Toxicology.* 1959;1(3):299.
2 Barnett A, et al. *Arch Int Pharmacodyn Ther.* 1969;181(1):109.
3 Singh YN, et al. *Br J Anaesth.* 1978;50(2):109.
4 Burkett L, et al. *Anesth Analg.* 1979;58(2):107.
5 Chapple DJ, et al. *Br J Anaesth.* 1983;55(suppl 1):17S.
6 Bodley PO, et al. *Anaesthesia.* 1962;17(4):438.
7 Emery ER. *Anaesthesia.* 1963;18(1):57.
8 Pinkerton HH, et al. *Scott Med J.* 1964;9:256.
9 Viljoen JF. *S Afr Med J.* 1966;40(39):963.
10 Warner WA, et al. *JAMA.* 1971;215(7):1153.
11 Levä nen J, et al. *Ann Clin Res.* 1975;7(1):47.
12 Geha DG, et al. *Anesth Analg.* 1976;55(3):343.
13 Waterman PM, et al. *Anesth Analg.* 1977;56(4):587.
14 Sinha SK, et al. *Arch Dis Child.* 1984;59(1):73.
15 Hasfurther DL, et al. *Can J Anaesth.* 1996;43(6):617

* Asterisk indicates drugs cited in interaction reports. Based on pharmacologic and pharmacokinetic considerations, similar interactions may occur with other drugs that are listed.
† Not available in the United States.

Nondepol. Muscle Relaxants — Benzodiazepines

Nondepol. Muscle Relaxants		Benzodiazepines	
Atracurium*	Rocuronium (eg, *Zemuron*)	Alprazolam (eg, *Xanax*)	Lorazepam* (eg, *Ativan*)
Cisatracurium (eg, *Nimbex*)	Tubocurarine*†	Chlordiazepoxide (eg, *Librium*)	Oxazepam*
Pancuronium*	Vecuronium*	Clonazepam (eg, *Klonopin*)	Quazepam (*Doral*)
		Clorazepate (eg, *Tranxene*)	Temazepam (eg, *Restoril*)
		Diazepam* (eg, *Valium*)	Triazolam (eg, *Halcion*)
		Flurazepam	

Significance	Onset	Severity	Documentation
4	■ **Rapid**	□ Major	□ Established
	□ Delayed	■ **Moderate**	□ Probable
		□ Minor	□ Suspected
			■ **Possible**
			□ Unlikely

Effects BENZODIAZEPINES may potentiate, counteract, or have no effect on the actions of NONDEPOLARIZING MUSCLE RELAXANTS.

Mechanism Undetermined.

Management Major problems have not been reported. Monitor patients for respiratory distress.

Discussion

The effects of benzodiazepines on muscle contraction are ascribed mainly to an action on spinal and supraspinal mechanisms; however, peripheral effects on neuromuscular transmission or muscle itself has been suggested in skeletal, smooth, and heart muscle. The interactions of benzodiazepines with nondepolarizing muscle relaxants are unclear.[1] Some investigations indicated that diazepam increased the duration of action of gallamine† and tubocurarine.[2-4] However, other studies could not substantiate the findings[5,6] with diazepam, lorazepam, or oxazepam and various neuromuscular blockers.[1,5-13] Reversal of blockade has been noted.[14] These highly variable results may be due to differing study protocols, animal species, and individual pharmacology of benzodiazepines.[1,13,15]

1 Driessen JJ, et al. *Br J Anaesth.* 1984;56(10):1131.
2 Stovner J, et al. *Acta Anaesthesiol Scand Suppl.* 1965;24:223.
3 Feldman SA, et al. *Br Med J.* 1970;1(5697):691.
4 Feldman SA, et al. *Br Med J.* 1970;2(5705):336.
5 Webb SN, et al. *Br Med J.* 1971;3(5775):640.
6 Dretchen K, et al. *Anesthesiology.* 1971;34(5):463.
7 Stovner J, et al. *Lancet.* 1965;2(7425):1298.
8 Hunter AR. *Br J Anaesth.* 1967;39(8):632.
9 Bradshaw EG, et al. *Br J Anaesth.* 1979;51(10):955.
10 Asbury AJ, et al. *Br J Anaesth.* 1981;53(8):859.
11 Chapple DJ, et al. *Br J Anaesth.* 1983;55(suppl 1):17S.
12 Wali FA. *Acta Anaesthesiol Scand.* 1985;29(8):785.
13 Driessen JJ, et al. *Acta Anaesthesiol Scand.* 1986;30(8):642.
14 Sharma KK, et al. *J Pharm Pharmacol.* 1978;30(1):64.
15 Driessen JJ, et al. *J Pharm Pharmacol.* 1984;36(4):244.

* Asterisk indicates drugs cited in interaction reports. Based on pharmacologic and pharmacokinetic considerations, similar interactions may occur with other drugs that are listed.

† Not available in the United States.

Nondepol. Muscle Relaxants — Beta-Blockers

Nondepol. Muscle Relaxants		Beta-Blockers	
Atracurium*	Tubocurarine*†	Esmolol* (eg, *Brevibloc*)	Propranolol* (eg, *Inderal LA*)
Rocuronium* (eg, *Zemuron*)		Pindolol*	

Significance	Onset	Severity	Documentation
4	■ **Rapid**	☐ Major	☐ Established
	☐ Delayed	■ **Moderate**	☐ Probable
		☐ Minor	☐ Suspected
			■ **Possible**
			☐ Unlikely

Effects BETA-BLOCKERS may potentiate, counteract, delay, or have no effect on the actions of NONDEPOLARIZING MUSCLE RELAXANTS.

Mechanism Undetermined; possibly relates to a local anesthetic effect at the postsynaptic membrane.

Management Monitor patients for respiratory distress and response to the muscle relaxant. Provide life support if necessary.

Discussion

Propranolol 120 mg/day was used in 2 patients who were thyrotoxic and administered tubocurarine during surgery; propranolol appeared to prolong the duration of tubocurarine.[1] Animal studies have shown a similar effect.[2,3] Beta-blockers have also been reported to aggravate or unmask myasthenia gravis or induce the myasthenic syndrome.[4] However, studies in humans and animals have indicated that beta-blockers have shortened the recovery time from tubocurarine and gallamine[†5-7]; pindolol had little effect.[7] Esmolol increased the onset of action of rocuronium from 93 to 118 seconds.[8] Propranolol and atracurium have been noted not to interact in cats.[9]

Propranolol blocks the acetylcholine binding site at the postsynaptic membrane in a manner similar to local anesthetics, independent of their catecholamine interaction.[4,10]

1 Rozen MS, et al. *Med J Aust.* 1972;1(10):467.
2 Usubiaga JE. *Anesthesiology.* 1968;29(3):484.
3 Harrah MD, et al. *Anesthesiology.* 1970;33(4):406.
4 Ostergaard D, et al. *Med Toxicol Adverse Drug Exp.* 1989;4(5):351.
5 Wislicki L, et al. *Br J Anaesth.* 1967;39(12):939.
6 Varma YS, et al. *Indian J Med Res.* 1972;60(2):266.
7 Varma YS, et al. *Indian J Med Res.* 1973;61(9):1382.
8 Szmuk P, et al. *Anesth Analg.* 2000;90(5):1217.
9 Chapple DJ, et al. *Br J Anaesth.* 1983;55(suppl 1):17S.
10 Herishanu Y, et al. *Ann Intern Med.* 1975;83(6):834

* Asterisk indicates drugs cited in interaction reports.
† Not available in the United States.

Nondepol. Muscle Relaxants — Carbamazepine

Atracurium*	Rocuronium* (eg, *Zemuron*)	Carbamazepine* (eg, *Tegretol*)
Cisatracurium* (*Nimbex*)	Vecuronium*	
Pancuronium*		

Significance	Onset	Severity	Documentation
2	■ **Rapid**	□ Major	□ Established
	□ Delayed	■ **Moderate**	■ **Probable**
		□ Minor	□ Suspected
			□ Possible
			□ Unlikely

Effects NONDEPOLARIZING MUSCLE RELAXANTS may have a shorter than expected duration or be less effective when the patient also is receiving CARBAMAZEPINE (CBZ).

Mechanism Unknown.

Management Monitor patients for reduced muscle relaxant effectiveness and increase the dose of the NONDEPOLARIZING MUSCLE RELAXANT accordingly.

Discussion

In 18 adult patients undergoing craniotomy or cerebrovascular surgery, 9 received CBZ for at least 1 month prior to surgery and 9 received no CBZ.[1] Patients receiving CBZ recovered approximately 65% faster from pancuronium blockade than did controls. There was an inverse correlation between CBZ daily dose and times to recovery; there was no correlation with plasma CBZ levels. Recovery from atracurium was approximately 42% faster in 14 epileptic patients receiving CBZ than in 21 nonepileptic patients receiving only atracurium.[2] Similarly, 18 patients receiving CBZ plus phenytoin (eg, *Dilantin*) or valproic acid (eg, *Depakene*) recovered from atracurium 70% faster than control patients. Similar findings were reported for rocuronium in 11 patients pretreated with CBZ compared with 11 control patients.[3] For vecuronium, the interaction is partly explained by pharmacokinetic changes.[4,5] In 10 patients receiving CBZ, vecuronium clearance increased 137% when compared with the control group. Vecuronium clearance increased 208% in 10 children receiving CBZ compared with 10 control children.[5] Alternatively, pancuronium and CBZ may compete for sites at the neuromuscular junction.[1,6] Patients on long-term anticonvulsant therapy (CAT), including 10 patients taking CBZ, required higher cisatracurium infusion rates and exhibited more rapid recovery of muscle function than patients not receiving CAT.[7] Cisatracurium clearance was 26% greater in patients receiving concurrent CAT.

[1] Roth S, et al. *Anesthesiology.* 1987;66(5):691.
[2] Tempelhoff R, et al. *Anesth Analg.* 1990;71(6):665.
[3] Spacek A, et al. *Anesthesiology.* 1999;90(1):109.
[4] Alloul K, et al. *Anesthesiology.* 1996;84(2):330.
[5] Soriano SG, et al. *Br J Anaesth.* 2001;86(2):223.
[6] Ostergaard D, et al. *Med Toxicol Adverse Drug Exp.* 1989;4(5):351.
[7] Richard A, et al. *Anesth Analg.* 2005;100(2):538.

* Asterisk indicates drugs cited in interaction reports.

Nondepol. Muscle Relaxants — *Corticosteroids*

Atracurium Cisatracurium (*Nimbex*) Pancuronium*	Rocuronium* (eg, *Zemuron*) Tubocurarine*† Vecuronium*	Betamethasone* (*Celestone*) Corticotropin* (*Acthar HP*) Cortisone Cosyntropin (eg, *Cortrosyn*) Dexamethasone (eg, *Baycadron*) Fludrocortisone	Hydrocortisone* (eg, *Cortef*) Methylprednisolone (eg, *Medrol*) Prednisolone* (eg, *Prelone*) Prednisone* (eg, *Millipred*) Triamcinolone (eg, *Kenalog*)

Significance	Onset	Severity	Documentation
4	■ **Rapid** ☐ Delayed	☐ Major ■ **Moderate** ☐ Minor	☐ Established ☐ Probable ☐ Suspected ■ **Possible** ☐ Unlikely

Effects CORTICOSTEROIDS may decrease the actions of NONDEPOLARIZING MUSCLE RELAXANTS.

Mechanism Unknown; however, CORTICOSTEROIDS may decrease the sensitivity of the end plate.

Management Patients may require higher doses of NONDEPOLARIZING MUSCLE RELAXANTS.

Discussion

Antagonism of pancuronium-induced blockade occurred in 2 patients on long-term corticosteroid therapy.[1,2] In 2 patients with myasthenia, corticotropin antagonized the effects of tubocurarine,[3] but prednisone appeared to have no effect.[4] The short-term effect of corticosteroids in cats appears to be a potentiation of pancuronium-induced blockade.[5,6] Resistance to vecuronium has occurred in 2 neurosurgical patients receiving preoperative betamethasone therapy. A subsequent retrospective evaluation of 50 cases revealed a higher vecuronium dosage requirement (134 mcg/kg/h) in patients pretreated with betamethasone compared with patients who were not pretreated (76 mcg/kg/h).[7] In patients with inflammatory bowel disease, prednisolone increased the onset and reduced the duration of rocuronium neuromuscular blockade.[8]

[1] Laflin MJ. *Anesthesiology.* 1977;47(5):471.
[2] Meyers EF. *Anesthesiology.* 1977;46(2):148.
[3] Griggs RC, et al. *Trans Am Neurol Assoc.* 1968;93:216.
[4] Lake CL. *Anesth Analg.* 1978;57(1):132.
[5] Durant NN, et al. *Anesthesiology.* 1982;57(suppl 3A):A266.
[6] Ostergaard D, et al. *Med Toxicol Adverse Drug Exp.* 1989;4(5):351.
[7] Parr SM, et al. *Anaesth Intensive Care.* 1991;19(1):103.
[8] Soltész S, et al. *Acta Anaesthesiol Scand.* 2009;53(4):443.

* Asterisk indicates drugs cited in interaction reports. Based on pharmacologic and pharmacokinetic considerations, similar interactions may occur with other drugs that are listed.
† Not available in the United States.

Nondepol. Muscle Relaxants — Cyclosporine

Nondepol. Muscle Relaxants		Cyclosporine
Atracurium Cisatracurium (*Nimbex*) Pancuronium*	Rocuronium (eg, *Zemuron*) Vecuronium*	Cyclosporine* (eg, *Neoral*)

Significance	Onset	Severity	Documentation
2	■ **Rapid** □ Delayed	□ Major ■ **Moderate** □ Minor	□ Established □ Probable ■ **Suspected** □ Possible □ Unlikely

Effects Prolonged neuromuscular blockade.

Mechanism Unknown.

Management Monitor for neuromuscular blockade and respiratory depression. Provide ventilatory support if needed.

Discussion

Coadministration of cyclosporine and the nondepolarizing muscle relaxants pancuronium and vecuronium may produce prolonged neuromuscular blockade.[1-3] A 15-year-old girl with a 5-year history of acute lymphocytic leukemia was anesthetized with fentanyl (eg, *Sublimaze*), thiopental (*Pentothal*), and vecuronium 0.1 mg/kg for endoscopy and bone marrow aspiration.[4] Immunosuppressive therapy consisted of IV cyclosporine 20 mg twice daily. Anesthesia was maintained with nitrous oxide, oxygen, and isoflurane (eg, *Forane*). Despite attempts to reverse neuromuscular blockade with edrophonium (*Enlon*), atropine, and neostigmine (eg, *Prostigmin*), neuromuscular function did not return for more than 3 hours after vecuronium administration. In a second report, a 54-year-old woman was scheduled to have a right posterior clipping of a communicating artery aneurysm.[1] Two years earlier, the patient had received a renal allograft. Immunosuppression was maintained with azathioprine (eg, *Imuran*), cyclosporine 300 mg/day, and prednisone (eg, *Sterapred*) daily. The patient also was receiving nifedipine (eg, *Procardia*) and furosemide (eg, *Lasix*) for chronic hypertension. Anesthesia induction consisted of fentanyl, thiopental, and pancuronium 5.5 mg, and was maintained with nitrous oxide and isoflurane. After surgery, residual neuromuscular blockade was reversed with atropine and neostigmine. In the recovery room, edrophonium was administered for signs of residual paralysis. Over the next 5 minutes, the patient's paralysis improved, and she was extubated. However, increasing respiratory distress was noted, necessitating reintubation. The patient was successfully extubated 4 hours later. A study of 4 patients demonstrated potentiation of vecuronium effects with a cyclosporine infusion.[3]

[1] Crosby E, et al. *Can J Anaesth.* 1988;35(3, pt 1):300.
[2] Sharpe MD, et al. *Can J Anaesth.* 1992;39(5, pt 2):A126.
[3] Ganjoo P, et al. *Can J Anaesth.* 1994;41(10):1017.
[4] Wood GG. *Can J Anaesth.* 1989;36(3, pt 1):358.

* Asterisk indicates drugs cited in interaction reports. Based on pharmacologic and pharmacokinetic considerations, similar interactions may occur with other drugs that are listed.

Nondepol. Muscle Relaxants — *Hydantoins*

Atracurium*	Rocuronium* (eg, *Zemuron*)	Fosphenytoin (eg, *Cerebyx*)	Phenytoin* (eg, *Dilantin*)
Cisatracurium* (*Nimbex*)	Vecuronium*		
Pancuronium*			

Significance	Onset	Severity	Documentation
2	■ **Rapid**	□ Major	■ **Established**
	□ Delayed	■ **Moderate**	□ Probable
		□ Minor	□ Suspected
			□ Possible
			□ Unlikely

Effects NONDEPOLARIZING MUSCLE RELAXANTS may have a shorter than expected duration or be less effective.

Mechanism PHENYTOIN may increase NONDEPOLARIZING MUSCLE RELAXANT metabolism and has prejunctional effects similar to NONDEPOLARIZING MUSCLE RELAXANTS.

Management NONDEPOLARIZING MUSCLE RELAXANT dosage may need to be increased. Monitor for reduced effectiveness.

Discussion

Phenytoin has been reported to potentiate[1,2] and antagonize the effects of nondepolarizing muscle relaxants (eg, pancuronium).[3-8] Vecuronium clearance was increased 168% and the $t_{1/2}$ was decreased 49% in 10 children receiving phenytoin compared with 10 control patients.[9] Similarly, vecuronium clearance was increased 138% in patients taking phenytoin compared with patients not on long-term phenytoin therapy.[10] A study of 5 patients on long-term phenytoin therapy reported greater cisatracurium infusion requirements and faster spontaneous reversal of muscle paralysis compared with patients not receiving long-term phenytoin therapy.[11] Rocuronium clearance was increased and a higher dose was needed in 10 patients undergoing craniotomy while receiving phenytoin compared with 11 patients not receiving phenytoin.[12] The effects of phenytoin on atracurium are conflicting.[6,13]

1 Norris FH Jr, et al. *Neurology.* 1964;14:869.
2 Gandhi IC, et al. *Arzneimittelforschung.* 1976;26(2):258.
3 Messick JM, et al. *Anesth Analg.* 1982;61(2):203.
4 Chen J, et al. *Anesthesiology.* 1983;59(3):A288.
5 Ornstein E, et al. *Anesthesiology.* 1985;63(3):294.
6 Ornstein E, et al. *Anesthesiology.* 1985;63:A331.
7 Ornstein E, et al. *Anesth Analg.* 1986;65(suppl 2):S116.
8 Liberman BA, et al. *Int J Clin Pharmacol Ther Toxicol.* 1988;26(8):371.
9 Soriano SG, et al. *Br J Anaesth.* 2001;86(2):223.
10 Wright PM, et al. *Anesthesiology.* 2004;100(3):626.
11 Richard A, et al. *Anesth Analg.* 2005;100(2):538.
12 Fernández-Candil J, et al. *Eur J Clin Pharmacol.* 2008;64(8):795.
13 Tempelhoff R, et al. *Anesth Analg.* 1990;71(6):665.

* Asterisk indicates drugs cited in interaction reports. Based on pharmacologic and pharmacokinetic considerations, similar interactions may occur with other drugs that are listed.

Nondepol. Muscle Relaxants ✕ Inhalation Anesthetics

Atracurium*	Rocuronium (eg, *Zemuron*)	Enflurane* (eg, *Ethrane*)	Methoxyflurane*†
Cisatracurium (*Nimbex*)	Tubocurarine*†	Halothane*†	Nitrous Oxide*†
Pancuronium*	Vecuronium*	Isoflurane* (eg, *Forane*)	

Significance	Onset	Severity	Documentation
1	■ **Rapid**	■ **Major**	■ **Established**
	□ Delayed	□ Moderate	□ Probable
		□ Minor	□ Suspected
			□ Possible
			□ Unlikely

Effects INHALATION ANESTHETICS potentiate the actions of the NONDEPOLARIZING MUSCLE RELAXANTS.

Mechanism Potentiation of pharmacologic actions.

Management Monitor respiratory function and adjust the dose of both agents. Provide ventilatory support.

Discussion

Inhalational anesthetics enhance nondepolarizing neuromuscular blockade in a dose-dependent and, with atracurium, time-dependent manner.[1-14]

The potency and the duration of action of neuromuscular relaxants are increased, although prolonged recovery has not been documented. The maintenance dose of the neuromuscular blocking agent may need to be reduced 25% to 30%. Longer-acting nondepolarizing relaxants, such as pancuronium and d-tubocurarine, are more affected than the intermediate-acting drugs atracurium and vecuronium.[6-9,12,13]

Enflurane, methoxyflurane, and isoflurane are more effective than halothane in potentiating neuromuscular blocking agents. However, halothane is more potent than cyclopropane. Nitrous oxide has been demonstrated to increase the neuromuscular blocking effect of pancuronium and d-tubocurarine.

[1] Miller RD, et al. *Anesthesiology.* 1971;35(1):38.
[2] Miller RD, et al. *Anesthesiology.* 1971;35(5):509.
[3] Miller RD, et al. *Anesthesiology.* 1972;37(6):573.
[4] Fogdall RP, et al. *Anesthesiology.* 1975;42(2):173.
[5] Vitez TS. *Anesth Analg.* 1978;57(1):116.
[6] Duncalf D, et al. *Anesthesiology.* 1981;55:A203.
[7] Ramsey FM, et al. *Anesthesiology.* 1982;57:A255.
[8] Rupp SM, et al. *Br J Anaesth.* 1983;55(suppl 1):67S.
[9] Rupp SM, et al. *Anesthesiology.* 1984;60(2):102.
[10] Bennett MJ, et al. *Anesthesiology.* 1985;62(6):759.
[11] Brandom BW, et al. *Anesth Analg.* 1985;64(5):471.
[12] Ostergaard D, et al. *Med Toxicol Adverse Drug Exp.* 1989;4(5):351.
[13] Swen J, et al. *Anesth Analg.* 1989;69(6):752.
[14] Withington DE, et al. *Anesth Analg.* 1991;72(4):469.

* Asterisk indicates drugs cited in interaction reports. Based on pharmacologic and pharmacokinetic considerations, similar interactions may occur with other drugs that are listed.

† Not available in the United States.

Nondepol. Muscle Relaxants — *Ketamine*

Nondepol. Muscle Relaxants		Ketamine
Atracurium*	Rocuronium (*Zemuron*)	Ketamine* (eg, *Ketalar*)
Cisatracurium (*Nimbex*)	Tubocurarine*†	
Pancuronium*		

Significance	Onset	Severity	Documentation
2	■ **Rapid**	□ Major	□ Established
	□ Delayed	■ **Moderate**	■ **Probable**
		□ Minor	□ Suspected
			□ Possible
			□ Unlikely

Effects KETAMINE may enhance the actions of the NONDEPOLARIZING MUSCLE RELAXANTS, possibly contributing to profound and severe respiratory depression.

Mechanism An increase in acetylcholine release and a decrease in postsynaptic membrane sensitivity is suspected.

Management If coadministration is necessary, use with caution and proper dosage tailoring; monitor for respiratory distress. Provide life support if needed.

Discussion

Laboratory data and human experience document a potentiation of ketamine on the actions of tubocurarine and atracurium.[1-6] Laboratory data (positive) and clinical experience (negative) conflict as to an interaction between ketamine and pancuronium.[2] In 20 patients receiving ketamine 2 mg/kg followed by an infusion of 2 mg/kg/h and IV atracurium 0.5 mg/kg, the average time to 25% recovery from atracurium was prolonged by 8 minutes as compared with a control group not receiving ketamine.[5]

1 Cronnelly R, et al. *Eur J Pharmacol.* 1973;22(1):17.
2 Johnston RR, et al. *Anesth Analg.* 1974;53(4):496.
3 Kraunak P, et al. *Br J Anaesth.* 1977;49(8):765.
4 Amaki Y, et al. *Anesth Analg.* 1978;57(2):238.
5 Toft P, et al. *Br J Anaesth.* 1989;62(3):319.
6 Ostergaard D, et al. *Med Toxicol Adverse Drug Exp.* 1989;4(5):351.

* Asterisk indicates drugs cited in interaction reports. Based on pharmacologic and pharmacokinetic considerations, similar interactions may occur with other drugs that are listed.
† Not available in the United States.

Nondepol. Muscle Relaxants / *Lincosamides*

Nondepol. Muscle Relaxants		Lincosamides	
Atracurium	Rocuronium (*Zemuron*)	Clindamycin* (eg, *Cleocin*)	Lincomycin* (*Lincocin*)
Cisatracurium (*Nimbex*)	Tubocurarine*†		
Pancuronium*	Vecuronium		

Significance	Onset	Severity	Documentation
2	■ **Rapid**	□ Major	□ Established
	□ Delayed	■ **Moderate**	□ Probable
		□ Minor	■ **Suspected**
			□ Possible
			□ Unlikely

Effects LINCOSAMIDES may enhance the actions of the NONDEPOLARIZING MUSCLE RELAXANTS, possibly contributing to profound and severe respiratory depression.

Mechanism Apparent potentiation or additive pharmacologic actions.

Management Avoid the combination if possible. If concurrent use is considered necessary, monitor for respiratory distress; provide life support if needed. Anticholinesterases or calcium has benefited in some cases.

Discussion

Clindamycin and lincomycin appear to augment the effects of nondepolarizing muscle relaxants; although controversy exists, they have neuromuscular blocking action of their own.[1-7] Laboratory data[2-5] and human experience[6-8] document the interaction. The mechanism of action is complex. Acetylcholine release is inhibited (prejunctional effect), the ion channel conductance is impaired (postjunctional effect), and muscle contractility is depressed. Anticholinesterases have been successful and unsuccessful in reversing pancuronium-induced neuromuscular blockade.[1,6]

There is a case report of an interaction between succinylcholine (eg, *Anectine*) and these antibiotics.[9] See also Succinylcholine-Lincosamides.

1 Fogdall RP, et al. *Anesthesiology.* 1974;41(4):407.
2 Samuelson RJ, et al. *Anesth Analg.* 1975;54(1):103.
3 Wright JM, et al. *Can J Physiol Pharmacol.* 1976;54(6):937.
4 Becker LD, et al. *Anesthesiology.* 1976;45(1):84.
5 Rubbo JT, et al. *Anesth Analg.* 1977;56(3):329.
6 Booij LH, et al. *Anesth Analg.* 1978;57(3):316.
7 Ostergaard D, et al. *Med Toxicol Adverse Drug Exp.* 1989:4(5):351.
8 Sloan PA, et al. *Anesth Analg.* 2002;94(1):123.
9 Avery D, et al. *Dis Nerv Syst.* 1977;38(6):473.

* Asterisk indicates drugs cited in interaction reports. Based on pharmacologic and pharmacokinetic considerations, similar interactions may occur with other drugs that are listed.

† Not available in the United States.

Nondepol. Muscle Relaxants — Lithium

Cisatracurium (*Nimbex*)	Pancuronium*	Lithium* (eg, *Lithobid*)
Gallamine*†	Tubocurarine*†	

Significance	Onset	Severity	Documentation
4	■ **Rapid**	□ Major	□ Established
	□ Delayed	■ **Moderate**	□ Probable
		□ Minor	□ Suspected
			■ **Possible**
			□ Unlikely

Effects LITHIUM may cause prolonged recovery time from NONDEPOLARIZING MUSCLE RELAXANTS, possibly resulting in profound and severe respiratory depression.

Mechanism Unknown. However, LITHIUM may affect acetylcholine activity at the nerve terminal.

Management Be aware of coadministration; tailor dosage of NONDEPOLARIZING MUSCLE RELAXANTS dosage and provide life support if needed.

Discussion

A woman had received lithium carbonate 1,200 mg/day for 3 days prior to undergoing surgery, in which pancuronium 0.06 mg/kg was administered.[1] The patient required more than 3 times the normal time for 80% recovery. Laboratory experiments have demonstrated a synergistic combination of lithium and pancuronium or tubocurarine.[2-4] However, data is also conflicting.[2,5-7] One study in dogs indicates that gallamine may be less likely to interact.[4] A suggested mechanism of action is that lithium reduces the synthesis and release of acetylcholine at the nerve terminal.

[1] Borden H, et al. *Can Anaesth Soc J.* 1974;21(1):79.
[2] Reimherr FW, et al. *Am J Psychiatry.* 1977;134(2):205.
[3] Basuray BN, et al. *Eur J Pharmacol.* 1977;45(1):79.
[4] Hill GE, et al. *Anesthesiology.* 1977;46(2):122.
[5] Martin BA, et al. *Am J Psychiatry.* 1982;139(10):1326.
[6] Waud BE, et al. *Anesth Analg.* 1982;61(5):399.
[7] Ostergaard D, et al. *Med Toxicol Adverse Drug Exp.* 1989;4(5):351.

* Asterisk indicates drugs cited in interaction reports. Based on pharmacologic and pharmacokinetic considerations, similar interactions may occur with other drugs that are listed.
† Not available in the United States.

Nondepol. Muscle Relaxants × Loop Diuretics

Nondepol. Muscle Relaxants		Loop Diuretics	
Atracurium	Rocuronium (eg, *Zemuron*)	Bumetanide	Torsemide (eg, *Demadex*)
Cisatracurium (*Nimbex*)	Tubocurarine*†	Ethacrynic Acid (*Edecrin*)	
Pancuronium*	Vecuronium	Furosemide* (eg, *Lasix*)	

Significance	Onset	Severity	Documentation
4	■ **Rapid** □ Delayed	□ Major ■ **Moderate** □ Minor	□ Established □ Probable □ Suspected ■ **Possible** □ Unlikely

Effects LOOP DIURETICS may potentiate or antagonize the actions of NONDEPOLARIZING MUSCLE RELAXANTS, possibly depending on dosage.

Mechanism Complicated (see discussion).

Management Monitor the patient for neuromuscular blockade and respiratory depression. Provide life support when necessary.

Discussion

Three men were given tubocurarine during surgery. They developed increased neuromuscular blockade when given furosemide and mannitol (eg, *Osmitrol*).[1] Laboratory experiments have indicated that the interaction may be dose dependent or biphasic; high doses (1 to 4 mg/kg) antagonize tubocurarine neuromuscular blockade, whereas low doses (0.1 to 10 mcg/kg) enhance the blockade.[2-4]

These effects may relate to diuretic-induced hypokalemia, increasing sensitivity to the nondepolarizing neuromuscular relaxants.[4-6] In addition, the biphasic nature of the interaction may be explained by diuretic enzyme inhibition, protein kinase inhibition at low doses and phosphodiesterase inhibition at high diuretic doses.[4]

1 Miller RD, et al. *Anesthesiology*. 1976;45(4):442.
2 Azar I, et al. *Anesth Analg*. 1980;59(1):55.
3 Scappaticci KA, et al. *Anesthesiology*. 1982;57(5):381.
4 Ostergaard D, et al. *Med Toxicol Adverse Drug Exp*. 1989;4(5):351.
5 Hunter AR. *Br Med J*. 1956;2(4998):919.
6 Taylor GJ. *Anaesthesia*. 1963;18(1):9.

* Asterisk indicates drugs cited in interaction reports. Based on pharmacologic and pharmacokinetic considerations, similar interactions may occur with other drugs that are listed.

† Not available in the United States.

Atracurium Cisatracurium (eg, *Nimbex*) Pancuronium*	Rocuronium* (eg, *Zemuron*) Vecuronium*	Magnesium Sulfate*

Significance	Onset	Severity	Documentation
2	■ **Rapid** □ Delayed	□ Major ■ **Moderate** □ Minor	□ Established □ Probable ■ **Suspected** □ Possible □ Unlikely

Effects MAGNESIUM SULFATE may potentiate the actions of NONDEPOLARIZING MUSCLE RELAXANTS, possibly resulting in profound and severe respiratory depression.

Mechanism Probable potentiation of pharmacologic actions.

Management Coadminister these agents carefully; tailor the NONDEPOLARIZING MUSCLE RELAXANT dosage as needed and monitor for respiratory distress. Provide life support if necessary.

Discussion

Magnesium sulfate, widely used for preeclamptic hyperreflexia, also has actions at the neuromuscular junction site to decrease the release of acetylcholine and reduce the postjunctional membrane sensitivity; it also decreases the excitability of the muscle fiber membrane.[1] Magnesium sulfate–induced potentiation of nondepolarizing muscle relaxants, resulting in respiratory depression, has been demonstrated in the laboratory and via case reports, primarily in obstetric patients.[1-6] In cats, the plasma concentration of magnesium is linearly and inversely related to the dose requirements of pancuronium.[4] Using a double-blind, randomized, placebo-controlled design, the effects of magnesium sulfate IV on the neuromuscular-blocking requirements of rocuronium were studied in 61 children with cerebral palsy undergoing orthopedic surgery.[7] The rocuronium requirements were less and pain scores were lower during the entire postoperative period in the group concurrently receiving magnesium sulfate compared with placebo. Magnesium sulfate has decreased muscle fasciculations associated with succinylcholine (eg, *Anectine*).[8]

1 Ostergaard D, et al. *Med Toxicol Adverse Drug Exp.* 1989;4(5):351.
2 Giesecke AH Jr, et al. *Anesth Analg.* 1968;47(6):689.
3 Ghoneim MM, et al. *Anesthesiology.* 1970;32(1):23.
4 Lee C, et al. *Anesthesiology.* 1982;57:A392.
5 Sinatra RS, et al. *Anesth Analg.* 1985;64(12):1220.
6 Sloan PA, et al. *Anesth Analg.* 2002;94(1):123.
7 Na HS, et al. *Br J Anaesth.* 2010;104(3):344.
8 Aldrete JA, et al. *Can Anaesth Soc J.* 1970;17(5):477.

* Asterisk indicates drugs cited in interaction reports. Based on pharmacologic and pharmacokinetic considerations, similar interactions may occur with other drugs that are listed.

Nondepol. Muscle Relaxants ✕ *Nitrates*

Gallamine Triethiodide*† Pancuronium | Nitroglycerin* (eg, *Nitrostat*)

Significance	Onset	Severity	Documentation
4	■ **Rapid**	□ Major	□ Established
	□ Delayed	■ **Moderate**	□ Probable
		□ Minor	□ Suspected
			■ **Possible**
			□ Unlikely

Effects NITROGLYCERIN may potentiate the actions of PANCURONIUM, possibly resulting in profound and severe respiratory depression.

Mechanism Undetermined.

Management Monitor patients for respiratory distress. Provide life support if needed.

Discussion

Based on clinical observation of prolonged pancuronium-induced blockade in the presence of IV nitroglycerin, experiments were conducted in cats.[1,2] In 2 separate investigations, pancuronium was the only nondepolarizing muscle relaxant to have its action prolonged. This action appeared to be at least partially dose-dependent, and it was necessary for the nitroglycerin to be present before pancuronium was administered.

Gallamine, tubocurarine, and succinylcholine (eg, *Anectine*) all were unaltered by preadministration of IV nitroglycerin.[1,2] The block was reversible with neostigmine (eg, *Prostigmin*).

[1] Glisson SN, et al. *Anesthesiology.* 1979;51(1):47. [2] Glisson SN, et al. *Anesth Analg.* 1980;59(2):117.

* Asterisk indicates drugs cited in interaction reports. Based on pharmacologic and pharmacokinetic considerations, similar interactions may occur with other drugs that are listed.

† Not available in the United States.

Nondepol. Muscle Relaxants — *Piperacillin*

Atracurium	Pancuronium	Piperacillin*
Cisatracurium (*Nimbex*)	Vecuronium*	

Significance	Onset	Severity	Documentation
5	■ **Rapid**	■ **Major**	□ Established
	□ Delayed	□ Moderate	□ Probable
		□ Minor	□ Suspected
			□ Possible
			■ **Unlikely**

Effects PIPERACILLIN may potentiate NONDEPOLARIZING MUSCLE RELAXANTS, producing protracted respiratory depression.

Mechanism Unknown.

Management Consider monitoring postoperative neuromuscular and respiratory function in patients receiving NONDEPOLARIZING MUSCLE RELAXANTS and PIPERACILLIN concurrently.

Discussion

A case of recurrent paralysis occurred following administration of piperacillin to a 29-year-old man who had undergone neuromuscular blockade with vecuronium.[1] The patient was admitted for an exploratory laparotomy for abdominal stab wounds. The patient received vecuronium 4 mg (an additional 2 mg dose was administered 35 minutes later to facilitate abdominal closure). In the recovery room, the patient received an infusion of piperacillin 3 g. Thirty minutes after the start of the piperacillin infusion, the patient's heart rate was 40 bpm, he was blinking his eyes, having difficulty breathing, and could not lift his extremities or head. The patient did not respond to naloxone 0.2 mg. The patient's lungs were manually ventilated. He demonstrated a strong sustained tetanus to 50 hertz stimulation of the ulnar nerve 5 minutes after receiving atropine 0.8 mg and neostigmine 2.5 mg. He was discharged to the ward 2.5 hours after admission. In a study, 27 patients undergoing major surgeries received vecuronium 0.08 mg/kg for muscle relaxation and antibiotic prophylaxis with piperacillin or cefoxitin (mofoxin[†] [control group]).[2] Five patients distributed between the 2 antibiotics experienced slight prolongation of the time to recovery of baseline twitch. The duration of prolongation was not considered clinically important. Neuromuscular blockade was not prolonged.

Additional studies are needed to confirm this possible interaction.

[1] Mackie K, et al. *Anesthesiology*. 1990;72(3):561.
[2] Condon RE, et al. *Am Surg*. 1995;61(5):403.

* Asterisk indicates drugs cited in interaction reports. Based on pharmacologic and pharmacokinetic considerations, similar interactions may occur with other drugs that are listed.
† Not available in the United States.

Nondepol. Muscle Relaxants		**Polypeptide Antibiotics**	
Atracurium*	Tubocurarine*†	Bacitracin* (eg, *Baciim*)	Polymyxin B*
Cisatracurium (*Nimbex*)	Vecuronium*	Capreomycin (*Capastat*)	Vancomycin* (eg, *Vancocin*)
Pancuronium*		Colistimethate* (eg, *Coly-Mycin M*)	

Significance	Onset	Severity	Documentation
2	■ **Rapid** □ Delayed	□ Major ■ **Moderate** □ Minor	□ Established ■ **Probable** □ Suspected □ Possible □ Unlikely

Effects Neuromuscular blockade may be enhanced.

Mechanism POLYPEPTIDE ANTIBIOTICS may affect presynaptic and postsynaptic myoneural function and act synergistically with NONDEPOLARIZING MUSCLE RELAXANTS.

Management Avoid this combination if possible. When necessary, monitor the neuromuscular function closely, titrate the dose of NONDEPOLARIZING MUSCLE RELAXANTS, and be prepared to provide mechanical respiratory support as needed.

Discussion

Evidence of additive neuromuscular blockade between nondepolarizing muscle relaxants and polypeptide antibiotic combinations have generally been accepted clinically. Various antibiotics, including colistimethate, polymyxin B, bacitracin, and vancomycin, have been demonstrated in numerous laboratory animals and in clinical reports to potentiate the neuromuscular blockade activity of nondepolarizing muscle relaxants such as pancuronium, d-tubocurarine, atracurium, and vecuronium.[1-10] Prolongation of neuromuscular blockade for 21 hours has been reported.[5] In a patient receiving vecuronium, IV infusion of vancomycin enhanced vercuronium-induced muscle relaxation and temporarily reversed recovery in response to edrophonium administration.[10]

[1] Timmerman JC, et al. *Toxicology.* 1959;1(3):299.
[2] Zauder HL, et al. *Can Anaesth Soc J.* 1966;13(6):607.
[3] Lindesmith LA, et al. *Ann Intern Med.* 1968;68(2):318.
[4] Gebbie D. *Anesth Analg.* 1971;50(1):109.
[5] Fogdall RP, et al. *Anesthesiology.* 1974;40(1):84.
[6] Van Nyhuis LS, et al. *Anesth Analg.* 1976;55(2):224.
[7] Burkett L, et al. *Anesth Analg.* 1979;58(2):107.
[8] Chapple DJ, et al. *Br J Anaesth.* 1983;55(suppl 1):17S.
[9] Kronenfeld MA, et al. *Anesthesiology.* 1986;65(1):93.
[10] Huang KC, et al. *Anesth Analg.* 1990;71(2):194.

* Asterisk indicates drugs cited in interaction reports. Based on pharmacologic and pharmacokinetic considerations, similar interactions may occur with other drugs that are listed.

† Not available in the United States.

Nondepol. Muscle Relaxants — *Quinine Derivatives*

Atracurium	Rocuronium (eg, *Zemuron*)	Quinidine*
Cisatracurium (*Nimbex*)	Vecuronium	Quinine* (*Qualaquin*)
Pancuronium*		

Significance	Onset	Severity	Documentation
2	■ **Rapid**	□ Major	□ Established
	□ Delayed	■ **Moderate**	□ Probable
		□ Minor	■ **Suspected**
			□ Possible
			□ Unlikely

Effects NONDEPOLARIZING MUSCLE RELAXANT effects may be enhanced by QUININE and QUININE DERIVATIVES.

Mechanism Probably additive or synergistic pharmacologic effects.

Management Close monitoring of neuromuscular function is necessary; titrate the dose of NONDEPOLARIZING MUSCLE RELAXANTS and provide mechanical respiratory support when needed.

Discussion

The interaction between quinidine and neuromuscular blocking agents was studied in laboratory animals and described in case reports.[1-4] One study reported a 47-year-old patient with malaria receiving quinine 1,800 mg daily who developed recurarization after reversal from anesthesia and administration of pancuronium 6 mg.[5] A similar case was reported involving quinidine, a d-stereoisomer of quinine.[3] The neuromuscular blockade secondary to d tubocurarine and succinylcholine (eg, *Anectine*) after quinidine was almost doubled in intensity and duration.[4]

Additional studies are needed to clarify the clinical relevance of this potentially life-threatening interaction. See also Succinylcholine-Quinine Derivatives.

[1] Grogono AW. *Lancet.* 1963;2(7316):1039.
[2] Schmidt JL, et al. *JAMA.* 1963;183:669.
[3] Way WI, et al. *JAMA.* 1967;200(2):153.
[4] Miller RD, et al. *Anesthesiology.* 1967;28(6):1036.
[5] Sher MH, et al. *Anaesth Intensive Care.* 1983;11(3):241.

* Asterisk indicates drugs cited in interaction reports. Based on pharmacologic and pharmacokinetic considerations, similar interactions may occur with other drugs that are listed.

Nondepol. Muscle Relaxants — *Ranitidine*

Nondepol. Muscle Relaxants		Ranitidine
Atracurium*	Rocuronium (eg, *Zemuron*)	Ranitidine* (eg, *Zantac*)
Cisatracurium (*Nimbex*)	Tubocurarine*†	
Pancuronium*	Vecuronium	

Significance	Onset	Severity	Documentation
4	■ **Rapid**	□ Major	□ Established
	□ Delayed	■ **Moderate**	□ Probable
		□ Minor	□ Suspected
			■ **Possible**
			□ Unlikely

Effects RANITIDINE may induce profound resistance to the neuromuscular blocking effects of NONDEPOLARIZING MUSCLE RELAXANTS.

Mechanism Unknown.

Management If difficulty is experienced, the dosage of the NONDEPOLARIZING MUSCLE RELAXANT may need to be titrated upwards. If unsuccessful, attempt neuromuscular blockade with another NONDEPOLARIZING MUSCLE RELAXANT.

Discussion

In a case report, a 30-year-old woman pretreated with oral ranitidine 300 mg daily for 3 weeks underwent vagotomy and gastrojejunostomy. Difficulty was experienced in producing muscle paralysis following adequate doses of 3 consecutive nondepolarizing muscle relaxants tubocurarine, pancuronium, and atracurium.[1] Because there were no other adequate explanations for the resistance to neuromuscular blockade in this patient, a drug interaction was speculated as the cause.

More studies are needed to clarify the clinical relevance of this possible drug interaction.

[1] Katende RS, et al. *Mt Sinai J Med.* 1987;54(4):330.

* Asterisk indicates drugs cited in interaction reports. Based on pharmacologic and pharmacokinetic considerations, similar interactions may occur with other drugs that are listed.

† Not available in the United States.

Nondepol. Muscle Relaxants ✕ **Theophyllines**

Nondepol. Muscle Relaxants		Theophyllines	
Atracurium	Rocuronium (eg, *Zemuron*)	Aminophylline*	Theophylline* (eg, *Theo-24*)
Cisatracurium (*Nimbex*)	Tubocurarine*†	Dyphylline (eg, *Lufyllin*)	
Pancuronium*	Vecuronium		

Significance	Onset	Severity	Documentation
2	■ **Rapid**	□ Major	□ Established
	□ Delayed	■ **Moderate**	□ Probable
		□ Minor	■ **Suspected**
			□ Possible
			□ Unlikely

Effects A dose-dependent reversal of neuromuscular blockade induced by NONDEPOLARIZING MUSCLE RELAXANTS may occur.

Mechanism Antagonistic activity is speculated.

Management Higher dosage of the NONDEPOLARIZING MUSCLE RELAXANT may be necessary when used in combination with THEOPHYLLINE.

Discussion

In an in vitro study, theophylline demonstrated a dose-dependent reversal effect on tubocurarine-induced neuromuscular blockade.[1] Two case reports speculated that aminophylline was the cause of resistance in pancuronium-induced neuromuscular blockade.[2,3] A third patient, a 48-year-old male, had responded to pancuronium. However, following aminophylline therapy, the patient could not be paralyzed.[4] He did respond to a normal dose of vecuronium. In another study, a 61-year-old male stabilized on aminophylline developed sudden supraventricular tachycardia following pancuronium administration; however, firm evidence supporting this potential interaction has not been established.[5]

More clinical data are needed to clarify the significance of this interaction.

[1] Dretchen KL, et al. *Anesthesiology.* 1976;45(6):604.
[2] Doll DC, et al. *Anesth Analg.* 1979;58(2):139.
[3] Azar I, et al. *Can Anaesth Soc J.* 1982;29(3):280.
[4] Daller JA, et al. *Crit Care Med.* 1991;19(7):983.
[5] Belani KG, et al. *Anesth Analg.* 1982;61(5):473.

* Asterisk indicates drugs cited in interaction reports. Based on pharmacologic and pharmacokinetic considerations, similar interactions may occur with other drugs that are listed.
† Not available in the United States.

Nondepol. Muscle Relaxants — Thiazide Diuretics

Nondepol. Muscle Relaxants		Thiazide Diuretics	
Atracurium	Rocuronium (eg, *Zemuron*)	Chlorothiazide* (eg, *Diuril*)	Indapamide
Cisatracurium (*Nimbex*)	Vecuronium	Chlorthalidone (eg, *Thalitone*)	Methyclothiazide
Pancuronium*		Hydrochlorothiazide (eg, *Microzide*)	Metolazone (eg, *Zaroxolyn*)

Significance	Onset	Severity	Documentation
4	■ **Rapid** □ Delayed	□ Major ■ **Moderate** □ Minor	□ Established □ Probable □ Suspected ■ **Possible** □ Unlikely

Effects NONDEPOLARIZING MUSCLE RELAXANT effects may be enhanced. Respiratory depression may be prolonged.

Mechanism DIURETICS may induce hypokalemia, which increases resistance to depolarization by hyperpolarizing the end plate membrane, thereby enhancing the myoneural blockade.

Management If hypokalemia cannot be corrected, a lower dosage of NONDEPOLARIZING MUSCLE RELAXANTS may be needed.

Discussion

Laboratory animal data and clinical case reports have suggested that hypokalemia may enhance the myoneural blockade of d-tubocurarine and gallamine.[1-7] In a study involving cat anterior tibialis-peroneal nerve preparation, the infusion rate of pancuronium required to maintain a 90% depression of twitch tension was reduced by 43.5% after hypokalemia was induced by long-term administration of chlorothiazide. A 45.9% reduction of neostigmine dosage was needed to achieve a 50% antagonism of pancuronium-induced depression of twitch tension.[7]

More data are needed for confirmation of this interaction, but avoidance of hypokalemia in patients receiving nondepolarizing muscle relaxant appears justified.

1 Hunter AR. *Br Med J.* 1956;2(4998):919.
2 Scott WE, et al. *Br Med J.* 1956;2(5002):1174.
3 Gray TC, et al. *Br Med J.* 1956;2(5005):1365.
4 Taylor GJ. *Anaesthesia.* 1963;18(1):9.
5 Gessa GL, et al. *Arch Int Pharmacodyn Ther.* 1963;144:258.
6 Sphire RD. *Anesth Analg.* 1964;43:690.
7 Miller RD, et al. *Br J Anaesth.* 1978;50(6):541.

* Asterisk indicates drugs cited in interaction reports. Based on pharmacologic and pharmacokinetic considerations, similar interactions may occur with other drugs that are listed.

Nondepol. Muscle Relaxants — *Thiopurines*

Nondepol. Muscle Relaxants		Thiopurines	
Atracurium	Rocuronium (eg, *Zemuron*)	Azathioprine* (eg, *Imuran*)	Mercaptopurine (eg, *Purinethol*)
Cisatracurium (*Nimbex*)	Tubocurarine*†		
Gallamine Triethiodide*†	Vecuronium		
Pancuronium*			

Significance	Onset	Severity	Documentation
2	■ **Rapid**	□ Major	□ Established
	□ Delayed	■ **Moderate**	□ Probable
		□ Minor	■ **Suspected**
			□ Possible
			□ Unlikely

Effects The pharmacological actions of the NONDEPOLARIZING MUSCLE RELAXANTS may be decreased or reversed.

Mechanism Possibly caused by inhibition of phosphodiesterase in the motor nerve terminal, thereby exerting its anticurare action.

Management Close monitoring of respiratory function is critical. NONDEPOLARIZING MUSCLE RELAXANT dosage increase may be necessary with combination therapy.

Discussion

Laboratory animal data and case reports revealed that neuromuscular blockade induced by d-tubocurarine, pancuronium, or gallamine may be reversed by azathioprine.[1,2] In a study of 15 patients pretreated with IV azathioprine, a 2- to 4-fold increase in d-tubocurarine was needed to achieve curare action.[2] Hypokalemia, secondary to nausea and vomiting and subsequent to azathioprine, was suggested as a possible cause of anticurare action.[2] In another study utilizing anesthetized cats, azathioprine did not significantly alter the neuromuscular blocking action of atracurium.[3]

More data are needed to clarify the clinical relevance of this interaction.

[1] Vetten KB. *S Afr Med J.* 1973;47(18):767.
[2] Dretchen KL, et al. *Anesthesiology.* 1976;45(6):604.
[3] Chapple DJ, et al. *Br J Anaesth.* 1983;55(suppl 1):17S.

* Asterisk indicates drugs cited in interaction reports. Based on pharmacologic and pharmacokinetic considerations, similar interactions may occur with other drugs that are listed.
† Not available in the United States.

Nondepol. Muscle Relaxants — Trimethaphan

Atracurium	Tubocurarine*†	Trimethaphan*†
Pancuronium	Vecuronium	

Significance	Onset	Severity	Documentation
2	■ **Rapid**	□ Major	□ Established
	□ Delayed	■ **Moderate**	□ Probable
		□ Minor	■ **Suspected**
			□ Possible
			□ Unlikely

Effects Prolonged apnea may occur with combination therapy.

Mechanism Probably due to curare-like effect of TRIMETHAPHAN augmenting the neuromuscular blockade of the NONDEPOLARIZING MUSCLE RELAXANT.

Management Avoid this combination if possible. If necessary, provide mechanical respiratory support and adjust the dose of the NONDEPOLARIZING MUSCLE RELAXANT.

Discussion

Experimental animal and human data suggest that trimethaphan can prolong myoneural blockade achieved by tubocurarine, hexamethonium,† and alcuronium.†[1-3] Respiratory arrest was reported after large doses of trimethaphan were administered to control hypertension.[4] A direct effect of trimethaphan on the respiratory center has been postulated.

Although clinical documentation for this interaction is limited, data are sufficient to warrant using alternative antihypertensive medication when administering nondepolarizing muscle relaxants.

[1] Deacock AR, et al. *Br J Anaesth.* 1958;30(5):217.
[2] Wilson SL, et al. *Anesth Analg.* 1976;55(3):353.
[3] Nakamura K, et al. *Anaesthesia.* 1980;35(12):1202.
[4] Dale RC, et al. *Arch Intern Med.* 1976;136(7):816.

* Asterisk indicates drugs cited in interaction reports. Based on pharmacologic and pharmacokinetic considerations, similar interactions may occur with other drugs that are listed.
† Not available in the United States.

Nondepol. Muscle Relaxants — *Verapamil*

Atracurium	Rocuronium (eg, *Zemuron*)	Verapamil* (eg, *Calan*)
Cisatracurium (*Nimbex*)	Tubocurarine*†	
Pancuronium*	Vecuronium*	

Significance	Onset	Severity	Documentation
2	■ **Rapid**	□ Major	□ Established
	□ Delayed	■ **Moderate**	□ Probable
		□ Minor	■ **Suspected**
			□ Possible
			□ Unlikely

Effects NONDEPOLARIZING MUSCLE RELAXANT effects may be enhanced. Respiratory depression may be prolonged.

Mechanism Probably involves blockade of calcium channels in skeletal muscle at the postsynaptic muscle membrane site.

Management Avoid combination therapy if possible. Adjust the NONDEPOLARIZING MUSCLE RELAXANT dosage and monitor respiratory function; provide mechanical ventilatory support.

Discussion

Experimental animal data suggest the presence of minimal neuromuscular blockade with verapamil alone and through interaction with nondepolarizing muscle relaxants.[1-11] Case reports also substantiate an interaction between verapamil and nondepolarizing muscle relaxants.[8,12,13] A 61-year-old man maintained on verapamil 240 mg/day for hypertension received pancuronium for abdominal surgery. Prolonged skeletal muscle paralysis occurred despite repeated attempts to reverse the effects with neostigmine (eg, *Prostigmin*).[12] In another case, a marked degree of residual neuromuscular blockade was exhibited following pancuronium and tubocurarine in a 55-year-old man maintained on verapamil 120 mg/day. Reversal of neuromuscular blockade was achieved with edrophonium (*Enlon*) but not neostigmine.[11] An interaction between nifedipine (eg, *Procardia*) and nondepolarizing muscle relaxants also occurred in a study using anesthetized cats.[9]

1 Kraynack BJ, et al. *Anesthesiology*. 1982;57:A265.
2 Bikhazi GB, et al. *Anesthesiology*. 1982;57:A268.
3 Lawson NW, et al. *Anesth Analg*. 1983;62(1):50.
4 Carpenter RL, et al. *Anesthesiology*. 1983;59:A272.
5 Kraynack BJ, et al. *Can Anaesth Soc J*. 1983;30(3, pt 1):242.
6 Kraynack BJ, et al. *Anesth Analg*. 1983;62(9):827.
7 Durant NN, et al. *Anesthesiology*. 1984;60(4):298.
8 van Poorten JF, et al. *Anesth Analg*. 1984;63(2):155.
9 Anderson KA, et al. *Br J Anaesth*. 1985;57(8):775.
10 Bikhazi GB, et al. *Anesth Analg*. 1985;64(5):505.
11 Wali FA. *Acta Anaesthesiol Scand*. 1987;31(1):15.
12 Jones RM, et al. *Anesth Analg*. 1985;64(10):1021.
13 Carlos R, et al. *Clin Ther*. 1986;9(1):22.

* Asterisk indicates drugs cited in interaction reports. Based on pharmacologic and pharmacokinetic considerations, similar interactions may occur with other drugs that are listed.
† Not available in the United States.

NSAIDs — Azole Antifungal Agents

NSAIDs		Azole Antifungal Agents	
Celecoxib (*Celebrex*)	Meclofenamate	Fluconazole* (eg, *Diflucan*)	Voriconazole* (*Vfend*)
Diclofenac* (eg, *Cataflam*)	Mefenamic acid (*Ponstel*)	Itraconazole* (eg, *Sporanox*)	
Etodolac	Meloxicam (eg, *Mobic*)		
Fenoprofen (eg, *Nalfon*)	Nabumetone		
Flurbiprofen* (eg, *Ansaid*)	Naproxen (eg, *Naprosyn*)		
Ibuprofen* (eg, *Motrin*)	Oxaprozin (eg, *Daypro*)		
Indomethacin (eg, *Indocin*)	Piroxicam (eg, *Feldene*)		
Ketoprofen	Sulindac (eg, *Clinoril*)		
Ketorolac	Tolmetin		

Significance	Onset	Severity	Documentation
2	☐ Rapid ■ **Delayed**	☐ Major ■ **Moderate** ☐ Minor	☐ Established ☐ Probable ■ **Suspected** ☐ Possible ☐ Unlikely

Effects NSAID plasma concentrations may be elevated, increasing the pharmacologic and adverse reactions. ITRACONAZOLE may lower NSAID plasma levels, reducing the efficacy.

Mechanism Inhibition of NSAID metabolism (CYP2C9) by FLUCONAZOLE and VORICONAZOLE is suspected.

Management Observe the clinical response of the patient and adjust the NSAID dose as needed.

Discussion

The effects of fluconazole on the pharmacokinetics of flurbiprofen were evaluated in 14 healthy subjects.[1] In a randomized, crossover study, each subject received a single dose of flurbiprofen 100 mg after 2 doses of fluconazole 200 mg or placebo. Compared with placebo, fluconazole increased the flurbiprofen AUC 81%, reduced flurbiprofen clearance to approximately 55% of placebo, and prolonged the $t_{1/2}$ from 3.3 to 5.3 hours. The effects of fluconazole or voriconazole on the pharmacokinetics of S-(+)- and R-(-)-ibuprofen were studied in 12 healthy men.[2] Using a crossover design, each subject received a single oral dose of racemic ibuprofen 400 mg alone and after pretreatment with fluconazole (400 mg on day 1 and 200 mg on day 2) or voriconazole (400 mg twice daily on day 1 and 200 mg on day 2). The pharmacokinetics of R-(-)-ibuprofen were affected to a minor degree. However, fluconazole and voriconazole increased exposure to S-(+)-ibuprofen 1.8- and 2-fold, respectively. The effects of voriconazole on the pharmacokinetics of diclofenac were studied in 10 healthy men.[3] Voriconazole increased the diclofenac AUC and C_{max} 78% and 114%, respectively. The $t_{1/2}$ remained unchanged. Voriconazole increased the AUC and $t_{1/2}$ of meloxicam 47% and 51%, respectively.[4] In contrast, when subjects received itraconazole, there was a 37% decrease in meloxicam AUC and a loss of effect as measured by thromboxane B_2 formation.

[1] Greenblatt DJ, et al. *Clin Pharmacol Ther.* 2006;79(1):125.

[2] Hynninen VV, et al. *Antimicrob Agents Chemother.* 2006;50(6):1967.

[3] Hynninen VV, et al. *Fundam Clin Pharmacol.* 2007;21(6):651.

[4] Hynninen VV, et al. *Antimicrob Agent Chemother.* 2009;53(2):587.

* Asterisk indicates drugs cited in interaction reports. Based on pharmacologic and pharmacokinetic considerations, similar interactions may occur with other drugs that are listed.

NSAIDs		***Bile Acid Sequestrants***	
Diclofenac* (eg, *Cataflam*)	Sulindac* (eg, *Clinoril*)	Cholestyramine* (eg, *Questran*)	Colestipol* (eg, *Colestid*)
Piroxicam* (eg, *Feldene*)			

Significance	Onset	Severity	Documentation
3	□ Rapid	□ Major	□ Established
	■ **Delayed**	□ Moderate	■ **Probable**
		■ **Minor**	□ Suspected
			□ Possible
			□ Unlikely

Effects The pharmacologic effects of the NSAID may be decreased.

Mechanism Plasma clearance of PIROXICAM is increased, and GI absorption of the NSAID is decreased.

Management If an interaction is suspected, consider increasing the dose of the NSAID during administration of CHOLESTYRAMINE.

Discussion

The effects of oral cholestyramine on the pharmacokinetics of oral piroxicam were studied in 8 healthy volunteers.[1] On 2 occasions, single oral doses of piroxicam 20 mg were given followed by either cholestyramine 4 g 3 times daily or placebo for 10 days. The first dose of cholestyramine was given 3.5 hours after piroxicam. Compared with placebo, cholestyramine enhanced piroxicam elimination as demonstrated by an increase in oral clearance and a corresponding decrease in $t_{½}$ (28.1 vs 46.8 hours). In a pharmacokinetic study, cholestyramine was given in multiple doses for 5 days beginning 24 hours after a single dose of piroxicam 20 mg.[2] Compared with a control period, the $t_{½}$ of piroxicam decreased from 53.1 to 29.6 hours in 8 young adults and from 52.3 to 27.3 hours in 7 elderly subjects, indicating that a mechanism besides interference with the absorption of piroxicam may be involved. The effect of cholestyramine 8 g or colestipol 10 g on the absorption of a single dose of diclofenac 100 mg was studied in 6 healthy volunteers.[3] Compared with water, cholestyramine and colestipol reduced the AUC of diclofenac 62% and 33%, respectively, and the peak plasma level 75% and 58%, respectively. No adverse reactions occurred with diclofenac or cholestyramine. In a single-dose study, cholestyramine decreased plasma levels of sulindac and its active metabolite.[4] Staggering the administration times of cholestyramine and sulindac by 3 hours did not prevent the interaction. This may be caused by enterohepatic recirculation of sulindac. Similar, but quantitatively different, effects were observed when the NSAIDs meloxicam (eg, *Mobic*) and tenoxicam† were administered IV to patients receiving oral cholestyramine, indicating that these NSAIDs undergo enterohepatic recirculation.[1,5]

[1] Guentert TW, et al. *Eur J Clin Pharmacol.* 1988;34(3):283.
[2] Ferry DG, et al. *Eur J Clin Pharmacol.* 1990;39(6):599.
[3] al-Balla SR, et al. *Int J Clin Pharmacol Ther.* 1994;32(8):441.
[4] Malloy MJ, et al. *Int J Clin Pharmacol Ther.* 1994;32(6):286.
[5] Busch U, et al. *Eur J Clin Pharmacol.* 1995;48(3-4):269.

* Asterisk indicates drugs cited in interaction reports.
† Not available in the US.

NSAIDs | **Bisphosphonates**

NSAIDs		Bisphosphonates	
Diclofenac (eg, *Cataflam*)	Meloxicam (eg, *Mobic*)	Alendronate* (eg, *Fosamax*)	Pamidronate (eg, *Aredia*)
Etodolac	Nabumetone	Etidronate (eg, *Didronel*)	Risedronate (*Actonel*)
Fenoprofen (eg, *Nalfon*)	Naproxen* (eg, *Naprosyn*)	Ibandronate (*Boniva*)	Tiludronate (*Skelid*)
Flurbiprofen	Oxaprozin (eg, *Daypro*)		
Ibuprofen (eg, *Motrin*)	Piroxicam (eg, *Feldene*)		
Indomethacin (eg, *Indocin*)	Sulindac (eg, *Clinoril*)		
Ketoprofen	Tolmetin		
Ketorolac			
Meclofenamate			
Mefenamic Acid (*Ponstel*)			

Significance	Onset	Severity	Documentation
4	☐ Rapid	☐ Major	☐ Established
	■ **Delayed**	■ **Moderate**	☐ Probable
		☐ Minor	☐ Suspected
			■ **Possible**
			☐ Unlikely

Effects The risk of gastric ulceration may be increased.

Mechanism NSAIDs and BISPHOSPHONATES may be synergistic with respect to causing gastric ulcers.

Management Use caution when coadministering these agents. Carefully monitor patients for possible GI adverse reactions, especially gastric ulceration.

Discussion

The risk of occurrence of gastric ulcer during coadministration of alendronate and naproxen was studied in 26 healthy volunteers.[1] The investigation was an endoscopist-blind, randomized, crossover trial in which each subject received either alendronate 10 mg/day or naproxen 500 mg twice daily for 10 days or coadministration of alendronate 10 mg/day and naproxen 500 mg twice daily for 10 days. During the 10 days, gastric ulcers developed in 2 subjects receiving alendronate alone, in 3 subjects receiving naproxen alone, and in 10 subjects receiving both drugs concurrently. Other adverse reactions also occurred more frequently with coadministration of alendronate and naproxen than with either drug alone. A retrospective, case-control study found no evidence of an increased risk of upper GI bleeding in patients taking an NSAID and bisphosphonate concurrently compared with an NSAID alone.[2]

[1] Graham DY, et al. *Arthritis Rheum.* 1999;42(suppl):S291.

[2] Etminan M, et al. *Aliment Pharmacol Ther.* 2009;29(11):1188.

* Asterisk indicates drugs cited in interaction reports. Based on pharmacologic and pharmacokinetic considerations, similar interactions may occur with other drugs that are listed.

NSAIDs — *Gemfibrozil*

Ibuprofen* (eg, *Motrin*)	Gemfibrozil* (eg, *Lopid*)

Significance	Onset	Severity	Documentation
4	☐ Rapid	☐ Major	☐ Established
	■ **Delayed**	■ **Moderate**	☐ Probable
		☐ Minor	☐ Suspected
			■ **Possible**
			☐ Unlikely

Effects IBUPROFEN plasma levels may be elevated, increasing the pharmacologic effects and adverse reactions.

Mechanism Inhibition of IBUPROFEN metabolism (CYP2C8) by GEMFIBROZIL is suspected.

Management Observe patients for an increase in IBUPROFEN adverse reactions and adjust the dose as needed.

Discussion

The effect of gemfibrozil on the pharmacokinetics of ibuprofen was studied in 10 healthy volunteers.[1] In a randomized, 2-phase, crossover study, each subject received gemfibrozil 600 mg or placebo twice daily for 3 days. On day 3, racemic ibuprofen 400 mg was administered. Compared with placebo, gemfibrozil increased the AUC of R-ibuprofen 34% and increased the elimination t½ of R- and S-ibuprofen 54% and 34%, respectively.

Additional studies are needed to determine the clinical importance of this interaction.

[1] Tornio A, et al. *Eur J Clin Pharmacol.* 2007;63(5):463.

* Asterisk indicates drugs cited in interaction reports.

NSAIDs | ***Hibiscus sabdariffa***

Diclofenac* (eg, *Cataflam*)	Hibiscus sabdariffa*

Significance	Onset	Severity	Documentation
4	□ Rapid	□ Major	□ Established
	■ **Delayed**	■ **Moderate**	□ Probable
		□ Minor	□ Suspected
			■ **Possible**
			□ Unlikely

Effects DICLOFENAC urinary excretion may be decreased.

Mechanism Unknown.

Management Until more data are available, patients taking DICLOFENAC should avoid routine use of beverages made from flowers of *HIBISCUS SABDARIFFA*.

Discussion

The effects of a beverage of water extract of *H. sabdariffa* on renal excretion of diclofenac were studied in 12 healthy volunteers.[1] Using a 2-way, randomized, crossover design, each subject ingested 300 mL of *H. sabdariffa* water extract daily for 2 days (equivalent to anthocyanins 8.18 mg), prepared from the dried calyx. On day 3, the beverage was ingested with diclofenac 25 mg. As a control, diclofenac was ingested with water. Compared with ingestion of diclofenac with water, the *H. sabdariffa* water extract decreased the urinary excretion of diclofenac approximately 38%. There were wide interindividual variations in the amount of diclofenac excreted.

[1] Fakeye TO, et al. *Phytother Res.* 2007;21(1):96.

* Asterisk indicates drugs cited in interaction reports.

NSAIDs		***Histamine H_2 Antagonists***	
Diclofenac* (eg, *Cataflam*)	Meclofenamate	Cimetidine* (eg, *Tagamet*)	Nizatidine (eg, *Axid*)
Etodolac	Mefenamic Acid (eg, *Ponstel*)	Famotidine* (eg, *Pepcid*)	Ranitidine* (eg, *Zantac*)
Fenoprofen (eg, *Nalfon*)	Nabumetone		
Flurbiprofen* (eg, *Ansaid*)	Naproxen* (eg, *Naprosyn*)		
Ibuprofen* (eg, *Motrin*)	Oxaprozin (eg, *Daypro*)		
Indomethacin* (eg, *Indocin*)	Piroxicam* (eg, *Feldene*)		
Ketoprofen	Sulindac* (eg, *Clinoril*)		
Ketorolac	Tolmetin		

Significance	Onset	Severity	Documentation
5	☐ Rapid ■ **Delayed**	☐ Major ☐ Moderate ■ **Minor**	☐ Established ☐ Probable ☐ Suspected ☐ Possible ■ **Unlikely**

Effects The therapeutic actions of NSAIDs may be altered.

Mechanism Unknown.

Management No clinical interventions appear necessary.

Discussion

In 10 rheumatoid arthritis patients, chronic cimetidine use decreased the mean steady-state plasma indomethacin levels 18%,[1] although another study found a small increase.[3] Urinary excretion of total indomethacin decreased 26%. No clinical changes were found. Studies of cimetidine and NSAIDs (eg, flurbiprofen, ibuprofen, naproxen, piroxicam, sulindac) also failed to show a clinically important interaction.[2-7] However, cimetidine increased peak serum ibuprofen and sulindac levels 14% and 57%, respectively; the effect on clearance was less.[2,5] The $t_{1/2}$ of naproxen was reduced approximately 50% by cimetidine, famotidine, and ranitidine.[8,9] Cimetidine increased the piroxicam AUC 16% but did not alter the elimination kinetics.[5] Cimetidine, but not ranitidine, caused small (less than 15%) increases in the flurbiprofen AUC.[7] Ranitidine does not appear to affect ibuprofen kinetics.[5,10] Indomethacin and sulindac increased the bioavailability of cimetidine and ranitidine.[2] In 14 volunteers, famotidine increased peak serum diclofenac levels 21% and decreased time to reach the peak 27%.[11] These results may indicate early dissolution of diclofenac because of gastric pH changes.

1 Howes CA, et al. *Eur J Clin Pharmacol.* 1983;24(1):99.
2 Delhotal-Landes B, et al. *Clin Pharmacol Ther.* 1988;44(4):442.
3 Holford NH, et al. *Clin Pharmacol Ther.* 1981;29:251.
4 Conrad KA, et al. *Br J Clin Pharmacol.* 1984;18(4):624.
5 Ochs HR, et al. *Clin Pharmacol Ther.* 1985;38(6):648.
6 Mailhot C, et al. *Pharmacotherapy.* 1986;6(3):112.
7 Small RE, et al. *J Clin Pharmacol.* 1990;30(7):660.
8 Vree TB, et al. *Br J Clin Pharmacol.* 1993;35(5):467.
9 Vree TB, et al. *Int J Clin Pharmacol Ther Toxicol.* 1993;31(12):597.
10 Small RE, et al. *Clin Pharm.* 1991;10(11):870.
11 Suryakumar J, et al. *Drug Invest.* 1992:4:66.

* Asterisk indicates drugs cited in interaction reports. Based on pharmacologic and pharmacokinetic considerations, similar interactions may occur with other drugs that are listed.

NSAIDs — Probenecid

NSAIDs		Probenecid
Diclofenac (eg, *Cataflam*)	Mefenamic Acid (eg, *Ponstel*)	Probenecid*
Etodolac	Nabumetone	
Fenoprofen (eg, *Nalfon*)	Naproxen* (eg, *Naprosyn*)	
Flurbiprofen (eg, *Ocufen*)	Oxaprozin (eg, *Daypro*)	
Ibuprofen (eg, *Motrin*)	Piroxicam (eg, *Feldene*)	
Indomethacin* (eg, *Indocin*)	Sulindac (eg, *Clinoril*)	
Ketoprofen*	Tolmetin	
Meclofenamate		

Significance	Onset	Severity	Documentation
2	☐ Rapid	☐ Major	☐ Established
	■ **Delayed**	■ **Moderate**	☐ Probable
		☐ Minor	■ **Suspected**
			☐ Possible
			☐ Unlikely

Effects Toxicity of NSAIDs may be enhanced.

Mechanism Plasma clearance of NSAIDs is reduced via renal and biliary pathways.

Management No immediate intervention appears necessary. If toxicity occurs, tailor the dose of PROBENECID accordingly.

Discussion

The influence of probenecid on the clearance of indomethacin,[1-5] ketoprofen,[6,7] and naproxen[8] was investigated. In a study of 9 healthy subjects, probenecid doubled peak concentrations of indomethacin.[2] In another study of 17 patients with arthritis, the AUC of indomethacin 75 mg/day increased 63.7% when probenecid 1 g/day was added; decreased biliary clearance of indomethacin was speculated.[4] These kinetic changes are considered therapeutic and desirable because plasma concentration swings are minimized,[7] and a decrease in joint inflammation can be achieved.[3,4] However, an increase in the incidence of adverse reactions (eg, confusion, epigastric pain, headache, nausea, tinnitus) and an increase in serum urea nitrogen was reported in a 60-year-old patient with hyperuricemia with stable, mild renal function impairment.[5] Kinetic interference with the elimination of ketoprofen 67% and 74% on the unbound moiety was reported in a crossover study involving 6 healthy subjects.[7] In another study of 6 healthy volunteers, probenecid 2 g/day decreased the renal tubular secretion, $t_{1/2}$, and metabolism of a single oral dose of naproxen 500 mg.[8] Plasma $t_{1/2}$ was prolonged from 14 to 37 hours, steady-state plasma levels were increased 50%, and naproxen conjugate excretion in the urine was reduced 66% after combination therapy.

1 Skeith MD, et al. *Clin Pharmacol Ther.* 1968;9(1):89.
2 Emori W, et al. *Clin Pharmacol Ther.* 1973;14:134.
3 Brooks PM, et al. *Br J Clin Pharmacol.* 1974;1(4):287.
4 Baber N, et al. *Clin Pharmacol Ther.* 1978;24(3):298.
5 Sinclair H, et al. *Br J Rheumatol.* 1986;25(3):316.
6 Wollheim FA, et al. *Eur J Clin Pharmacol.* 1981;20(6):423.
7 Upton RA, et al. *Clin Pharmacol Ther.* 1982;31(6):705.
8 Runkel R, et al. *Clin Pharmacol Ther.* 1978;24(6):706.

* Asterisk indicates drugs cited in interaction reports. Based on pharmacologic and pharmacokinetic considerations, similar interactions may occur with other drugs that are listed.

NSAIDs ✕ **Salicylates**

NSAIDs		Salicylates
Celecoxib (*Celebrex*)	Mefenamic Acid (*Ponstel*)	Aspirin* (eg, *Bayer*)
Diclofenac (eg, *Cataflam*)	Meloxicam (eg, *Mobic*)	
Etodolac	Nabumetone	
Fenoprofen* (eg, *Nalfon*)	Naproxen* (eg, *Naprosyn*)	
Flurbiprofen* (eg, *Ocufen*)	Oxaprozin (eg, *Daypro*)	
Ibuprofen* (eg, *Motrin*)	Piroxicam (eg, *Feldene*)	
Indomethacin* (eg, *Indocin*)	Sulindac (eg, *Clinoril*)	
Ketoprofen	Tolmetin*	
Meclofenamate*		

Significance	Onset	Severity	Documentation
1	☐ Rapid ■ **Delayed**	■ **Major** ☐ Moderate ☐ Minor	☐ Established ☐ Probable ■ **Suspected** ☐ Possible ☐ Unlikely

Effects Cardioprotective effect of low-dose ASPIRIN may be reduced. These agents also are gastric irritants.

Mechanism Competitive inhibition of the acetylation site of cyclooxygenase in the platelet is suspected.

Management Consider using analgesics that do not interfere with antiplatelet effect (eg, acetaminophen). In patients receiving IBUPROFEN and ASPIRIN, administer IBUPROFEN at least 8 hours before or 30 minutes after immediate-release ASPIRIN. Administer an NSAID at least 1 hour after taking enteric-coated ASPIRIN for cardioprotective action.

Discussion

Ibuprofen 400 mg may interfere with the cardioprotective effect of immediate-release, low-dose aspirin (81 mg)[1,2]; however, occasional use of ibuprofen is not likely to have the same result.[1] At least 15 studies have found an increase in mortality risk related to coadministration of ibuprofen and aspirin. Additional studies are needed to determine the effect of: 1) ibuprofen doses less than 400 mg on the antiplatelet effect of aspirin; 2) enteric-coated aspirin with ibuprofen; 3) daily enteric-coated, single- and low-dose aspirin with multiple daily doses of ibuprofen; and 4) other NSAIDs on the cardioprotective effect of aspirin. One study found no increased risk of MI in patients receiving aspirin and ibuprofen compared with aspirin alone.[3] In a study of 10 healthy volunteers, administration of aspirin 325 mg 2 hours after taking ibuprofen 400 mg resulted in antiplatelet effects that were the same as those that occurred with ibuprofen alone. Also, in 18 patients taking aspirin for stroke prevention, coadministration of ibuprofen or naproxen antagonized the antiplatelet effect of aspirin.[4] However, the antiplatelet effect of aspirin 100 mg/day was not affected after 4 days of coadministration of acetaminophen (eg, *Tylenol*), diclofenac, or naproxen.[5] In a study in healthy subjects, ibuprofen administration reduced the inhibitory effect of aspirin on thromboxane production in platelets, while there was no interference when aspirin was coadministered with diclofenac.[6] A 7-year-old boy with Kawasaki disease experienced myocardial ischemia resulting from a medium-sized coronary artery aneurysm occluded with thrombi during regression.[7] The event was attributed to ibuprofen blocking aspirin-induced platelet inhibition. See also Ketorolac-Salicylates.

1 *The Green Sheet.* 2006;6(9, pt 2). http://www.greensheet.com/gsonline_pdfs/060902.pdf. Published September 25, 2006. Accessed April 24, 2012.

2 Food and Drug Administration. Ibuprofen and aspirin taken together. Food and Drug Administration website. http://www.fda.gov/Safety/MedWatch/SafetyInformation/SafetyAlertsforHumanMedicalProducts/ucm150611.htm. Published September 8, 2006. Accessed April 24, 2012.

3 Patel TN, et al. *Arch Intern Med.* 2004;164(8):852.

4 Gengo FM, et al. *J Clin Pharmacol.* 2008;48(1):117.

5 Galliard-Grigioni KS, et al. *Eur J Pharmacol.* 2009;609(1-3):96.

6 Schuijt MP, et al. *Br J Pharmacol.* 2009;157(6):931.

7 Sohn S, et al. *Pediatr Cardiol.* 2008;29(1):153.

* Asterisk indicates drugs cited in interaction reports. Based on pharmacologic and pharmacokinetic considerations, similar interactions may occur with other drugs that are listed.

NSAIDs | **Selective Serotonin Reuptake Inhibitors**

Diclofenac (eg, *Cataflam*)
Etodolac
Fenoprofen (eg, *Nalfon*)
Flurbiprofen (eg, *Ansaid*)
Ibuprofen (eg, *Motrin*)
Indomethacin (eg, *Indocin*)
Ketoprofen
Ketorolac
Meclofenamate
Mefenamic Acid (eg, *Ponstel*)
Meloxicam (eg, *Mobic*)
Nabumetone
Naproxen (eg, *Naprosyn*)
Oxaprozin (eg, *Daypro*)
Piroxicam (eg, *Feldene*)
Sulindac (eg, *Clinoril*)
Tolmetin

Citalopram* (eg, *Celexa*)
Duloxetine (*Cymbalta*)
Escitalopram (*Lexapro*)
Fluoxetine* (eg, *Prozac*)
Fluvoxamine* (eg, *Luvox*)
Paroxetine* (eg, *Paxil*)
Sertraline* (eg, *Zoloft*)

Significance	Onset	Severity	Documentation
2	☐ Rapid	☐ Major	☐ Established
	■ **Delayed**	■ **Moderate**	■ **Probable**
		☐ Minor	☐ Suspected
			☐ Possible
			☐ Unlikely

Effects The risk of upper GI bleeding may be increased.

Mechanism Unknown.

Management If coadministration of these agents cannot be avoided, consider shortening NSAID treatment duration, decreasing the NSAID dose, or replacing NSAIDs with acetaminophen (eg, *Tylenol*) or the SSRI with a TCA. If GI adverse reactions occur, consider interventional therapy (eg, proton pump inhibitor) or discontinuing the SSRI or NSAID and giving alternative therapy.

Discussion

The relationship between TCA or SSRI usage, with or without NSAIDs, and risk of GI adverse reactions was investigated in a population-based cohort study.[1] Data on drug usage in 180,000 patients from 16 Dutch pharmacies were analyzed. There were 1,960 patients with no prescription for TCAs, SSRIs, NSAIDs, or peptic ulcer drugs 6 months prior to the study. The outcome measurement for SSRI adverse reactions was the number of first prescriptions for peptic ulcer drugs prescribed 2 days after starting antidepressant usage, with or without NSAIDs, until 10 days after the last dose. SSRI and NSAID coadministration increased the risk of GI adverse reactions 10-fold compared with taking SSRIs alone. The study did not report individual NSAIDs or SSRIs with respect to relative risk of GI adverse reactions. Further studies are needed to determine if certain NSAIDs or SSRIs have a lower risk of causing GI adverse reactions when coadministered. It has not been determined if coadministration of an SSRI and a cyclooxygenase-2 selective NSAID (eg, celecoxib [*Celebrex*]) increases the risk of GI adverse reactions compared with giving either agent alone. Two studies found that SSRIs increased risk of upper GI bleeding. Coadministration of NSAIDs and SSRIs increased the risk of GI hemorrhage (nearly 4-fold in one study).[2,3] A meta-analysis of 4 observational studies reported that SSRIs increase the odds ratio for occurrence of upper GI bleeding to 2.36 and that coadministration of an SSRI and NSAID increase the odds ratio to 6.33.[4]

[1] de Jong JC, et al. *Br J Clin Pharmacol.* 2003;55(6):591.
[2] de Abajo FJ, et al. *BMJ.* 1999;319(7217):1106.
[3] Dalton SO, et al. *Arch Intern Med.* 2003;163(1):59.
[4] Loke YK, et al. *Aliment Pharmacol Ther.* 2008;27(1):31.

* Asterisk indicates drugs cited in interaction reports. Based on pharmacologic and pharmacokinetic considerations, similar interactions may occur with other drugs that are listed.

NSAIDs | **St. John's Wort**

Ibuprofen*
(eg, *Motrin*)

St. John's wort*

Significance	Onset	Severity	Documentation
5	☐ Rapid	☐ Major	☐ Established
	■ **Delayed**	☐ Moderate	☐ Probable
		■ **Minor**	☐ Suspected
			■ **Possible**
			☐ Unlikely

Effects Mean residence time of IBUPROFEN may be reduced.

Mechanism Unknown.

Management Based on available data, no special precautions are necessary.

Discussion

The effects of St. John's wort on the pharmacokinetics of ibuprofen were studied in 8 healthy men.[1] Each subject received a single oral dose of ibuprofen 400 mg alone and after 21 days of administration of St. John's wort 300 mg 3 times daily (standardized with hypericin 0.3%). Compared with administration of ibuprofen alone, pretreatment with St. John's wort for 21 days did not affect the C_{max} or AUC of either the S(+)- or R(−)-ibuprofen enantiomers. However, the mean residence time of the S(+)-ibuprofen enantiomer was reduced. No dose adjustment in ibuprofen appears to be warranted when coadministered with St. John's wort.

[1] Bell EC, et al. *Ann Pharmacother.* 2007;41(2):229.

* Asterisk indicates drugs cited in interaction reports.

NSAIDs — **Sucralfate**

Diclofenac* (eg, *Cataflam*)	Sucralfate* (eg, *Carafate*)

Significance	Onset	Severity	Documentation
3	☐ Rapid ■ **Delayed**	☐ Major ☐ Moderate ■ **Minor**	☐ Established ☐ Probable ■ **Suspected** ☐ Possible ☐ Unlikely

Effects The pharmacologic effects of DICLOFENAC may be decreased.

Mechanism The absorption of DICLOFENAC may be decreased; however, the precise mechanism is not known.

Management Monitor the clinical response of the patient and adjust the dose of DICLOFENAC as needed. SUCRALFATE does not appear to alter the bioavailability of ketoprofen (eg, *Orudis*) or naproxen (eg, *Naprosyn*).

Discussion

The effects of sucralfate on the pharmacokinetics of diclofenac were studied in 18 healthy men.[1] Using an open, randomized, 2-period crossover design, each subject received diclofenac 105 mg as a suspension either alone or after 5 days of pretreatment with sucralfate 2 g twice daily. Pretreatment with sucralfate decreased the AUC of diclofenac 20% and the peak plasma concentration of diclofenac 38% (from 1,135 to 701 ng/mL). Although the peak concentration was decreased, there was no delay in absorption.

In an open-labeled study involving healthy volunteers, sucralfate did not alter the pharmacokinetics of ketoprofen or naproxen.[2]

[1] Pedrazzoli JJ, et al. *Br J Clin Pharmacol.* 1997;43:104. [2] Caille G, et al. *Am J Med.* 1989;86(6A):38.

* Asterisk indicates drugs cited in interaction reports.

Olanzapine — *Carbamazepine*

Olanzapine* (*Zyprexa*)	Carbamazepine* (eg, *Tegretol*)

Significance	Onset	Severity	Documentation
3	☐ Rapid ■ **Delayed**	☐ Major ☐ Moderate ■ **Minor**	☐ Established ☐ Probable ■ **Suspected** ☐ Possible ☐ Unlikely

Effects OLANZAPINE plasma concentrations may be reduced, decreasing the pharmacologic effects.

Mechanism Induction of hepatic microsomal enzymes (CYP1A2) by CARBAMAZEPINE is suspected.

Management Observe the clinical response of the patient. If an interaction is suspected, adjust the dose of OLANZAPINE as needed.

Discussion

The effect of carbamazepine on the pharmacokinetics of olanzapine was assessed in 11 healthy men.[1] A single dose of olanzapine 10 mg was administered alone and again after 14 days of treatment with carbamazepine 200 mg twice daily. Compared with administration of olanzapine alone, coadministration of carbamazepine resulted in a 25% decrease in the peak plasma concentration of olanzapine, a 34% decrease in the AUC, a 20% decrease in the elimination $t_{1/2}$, and an 18% increase in the volume of distribution. Because of the wide therapeutic index of olanzapine, the magnitude of these pharmacokinetic changes was not expected to be clinically important. Free and glucuronidated olanzapine concentrations were measured in 15 patients taking olanzapine alone and 16 patients taking concurrent carbamazepine.[2] The concentration to dose ratio of free olanzapine was 38% lower in patients taking olanzapine plus carbamazepine whereas glucuronidated olanzapine was higher, suggesting carbamazepine had induced olanzapine metabolism. Decreased olanzapine plasma concentrations during coadministration of carbamazepine 600 mg/day and olanzapine 15 mg/day were reported in a 23-year-old paranoid schizophrenic patient.[3] Prior to discontinuing carbamazepine, the olanzapine plasma level was 21 ng/mL. Over the week following discontinuation of carbamazepine, the olanzapine level increased 114% (to 45 ng/mL). Six weeks later, the dose of olanzapine was reduced to 10 mg/day with a corresponding decrease in the plasma level.

Additional studies are needed to determine the clinical importance of this interaction.

[1] Lucas RA, et al. *Eur J Clin Pharmacol.* 1998;54:639.
[2] Linnet K, et al. *Ther Drug Monit.* 2002;24:512.
[3] Licht RW, et al. *J Clin Psychopharmacol.* 2000;20:110.

* Asterisk indicates drugs cited in interaction reports.

Olanzapine — *Fluoxetine*

Olanzapine* (eg, *Zyprexa*)	Fluoxetine* (eg, *Prozac*)

Significance	Onset	Severity	Documentation
3	☐ Rapid ■ **Delayed**	☐ Major ☐ Moderate ■ **Minor**	☐ Established ☐ Probable ■ **Suspected** ☐ Possible ☐ Unlikely

Effects OLANZAPINE plasma concentrations may be slightly elevated.

Mechanism Inhibition of OLANZAPINE metabolism (CYP2D6) by FLUOXETINE is suspected.

Management Based on available data, no special precautions are necessary. If an interaction is suspected, adjust the dose of OLANZAPINE as needed.

Discussion

The effects of single and repeat administration of fluoxetine on the pharmacokinetics of single dose olanzapine were studied in 15 healthy subjects.[1] Using an open-label, single-sequence crossover design of 3 treatment periods, each subject received 1) a single 5 mg olanzapine dose, 2) a single 60 mg fluoxetine dose followed 1 hr later by a single 5 mg olanzapine dose, and 3) fluoxetine 60 mg/day for 8 days followed by a 5 mg olanzapine dose 1 hr after the last fluoxetine dose. Compared with administering olanzapine alone, single-dose administration of fluoxetine increased the peak concentration and the olanzapine AUC 18%. After multiple dosing of fluoxetine, olanzapine peak concentrations were increased 15%. Neither dosing regimen affected the $t_{1/2}$ nor time to reach olanzapine peak concentrations. No serious or unexpected adverse events occurred. See Olanzapine/Fluvoxamine.

[1] Gossen D, et al. *AAPS PharmSci.* 2002;4:E11.

* Asterisk indicates drugs cited in interaction reports.

Olanzapine		*Fluvoxamine*
Olanzapine* (*Zyprexa*)		Fluvoxamine*

Significance	Onset	Severity	Documentation
4	□ Rapid ■ **Delayed**	□ Major ■ **Moderate** □ Minor	□ Established □ Probable □ Suspected ■ **Possible** □ Unlikely

Effects OLANZAPINE plasma concentrations may be elevated, increasing the pharmacologic and adverse effects.

Mechanism Inhibition of OLANZAPINE metabolism (CYP1A2) by FLUVOXAMINE is suspected.

Management Observe the clinical response to OLANZAPINE when starting, stopping, or changing the dose of FLUVOXAMINE. Adjust the OLANZAPINE dose as needed. Monitoring OLANZAPINE plasma levels may be useful in managing patients.

Discussion

Elevated olanzapine plasma levels and side effects were reported in a 21-year-old woman during coadministration of fluvoxamine 150 mg/day and olanzapine 15 mg/day.[1] The patient had mydriasis, a slight tremor of both hands, and rigid movement. The olanzapine plasma level was 120 mcg/L. The dose of olanzapine was reduced to 10 mg/day, which resulted in a plasma level of 93 mcg/L. The dose of olanzapine was further reduced to 5 mg/day, resulting in a plasma level of 38 mcg/L. Over the next 2 weeks, the tremor and rigidity resolved, but the mydriasis persisted. Fluvoxamine was discontinued, and paroxetine (eg, *Paxil*) 20 mg/day was started, resulting in an olanzapine plasma level of 22 mcg/L. Utilizing data from a therapeutic drug monitoring service, the effect of fluvoxamine on the ratio of olanzapine plasma concentration to daily dose (C/D) was assessed.[2] Patients received olanzapine alone, olanzapine plus fluvoxamine, or olanzapine plus sertraline (*Zoloft*). Patients coadministered olanzapine and fluvoxamine had a mean C/D ratio that was 2.3-fold higher than patients receiving olanzapine alone. The ratio was increased as much as 4.2-fold in some individuals. In contrast, there was no difference in the C/D ratio of olanzapine given alone compared with coadministration with sertraline. In a prospective study of 8 olanzapine-treated schizophrenic patients, olanzapine levels increased between 12% to 112% after 8 weeks of fluvoxamine 100 mg/day.[3] There was no increase in adverse reactions, and some patients appeared to improve clinically. A study of 12 volunteers taking fluvoxamine 100 mg/day found nearly a 76% increase in olanzapine AUC.[4] The $t_{1/2}$ of olanzapine increased from 32.2 to 46.1 hours. Similar results were found in a study of 12 schizophrenic patients.[5]

[1] de Jong J, et al. *Psychopharmacology.* 2001;155:219.
[2] Weigmann H, et al. *Ther Drug Monit.* 2001;23:410.
[3] Hiemke C, et al. *J Clin Psychopharmacol.* 2002;22:502.
[4] Wang CY, et al. *J Clin Pharmacol.* 2004;44:785.
[5] Chiu CC, et al. *J Clin Pharmacol.* 2004;44:1385.

* Asterisk indicates drugs cited in interaction reports.

Olanzapine — *Probenecid*

Olanzapine* (*Zyprexa*)	Probenecid*

Significance	Onset	Severity	Documentation
4	☐ Rapid	☐ Major	☐ Established
	■ **Delayed**	■ **Moderate**	☐ Probable
		☐ Minor	☐ Suspected
			■ **Possible**
			☐ Unlikely

Effects OLANZAPINE plasma levels may be elevated, increasing the pharmacologic and adverse effects.

Mechanism PROBENECID appears to inhibit the metabolism (glucuronidation) of OLANZAPINE.

Management Closely monitor the clinical response of patients to OLANZAPINE when starting, stopping, or changing the dose of PROBENECID. Be prepared to adjust the OLANZAPINE dose as needed.

Discussion

In a single-dose, randomized, double-blind, crossover study, the effects of probenecid on the disposition of olanzapine were analyzed in 14 healthy subjects.[1] Each subject received olanzapine 5 mg alone and with probenecid. Probenecid 500 mg twice daily was given 1 day before the antipsychotic agent and for 2 days thereafter. Compared with administration of olanzapine alone, probenecid administration increased the olanzapine mean AUC 26%, mean peak plasma concentration 19%, and mean rate of absorption 57%. The clinical importance of this interaction cannot be determined from these data. Long-term studies are needed to assess this drug interaction.

[1] Markowitz JS, et al. *Clin Pharmacol Ther.* 2002;71:30.

* Asterisk indicates drugs cited in interaction reports.

Olanzapine — *Protease Inhibitors*

Olanzapine* (*Zyprexa*)	Lopinavir/Ritonavir* (*Kaletra*)	Ritonavir* (*Norvir*)

Significance	Onset	Severity	Documentation
2	□ Rapid	□ Major	□ Established
	■ **Delayed**	■ **Moderate**	□ Probable
		□ Minor	■ **Suspected**
			□ Possible
			□ Unlikely

Effects OLANZAPINE plasma concentrations may be reduced, decreasing the therapeutic effects.

Mechanism Increased metabolism (CYP1A2) or glucuronide conjugation of OLANZAPINE by RITONAVIR is suspected.

Management Observe the clinical response of the patient to OLANZAPINE when RITONAVIR is started or stopped. Adjust the dose of OLANZAPINE as needed.

Discussion

In an open-label investigation, the effect of ritonavir on the pharmacokinetics of olanzapine was evaluated in 14 healthy volunteers.[1] Each subject received a single dose of olanzapine 10 mg alone and after pretreatment with ritonavir 300 mg twice daily for 3 days, 400 mg twice daily for 4 days, and 500 mg twice daily for 4 days. Compared with taking olanzapine alone, pretreatment with ritonavir reduced the AUC of olanzapine 53%, the $t_{½}$ 50% (from 32 to 16 hours), and the C_{max} 40% (from 15 to 9 ng/mL). The oral clearance of olanzapine increased 115%.

[1] Penzak SR, et al. *J Clin Psychopharmacol.* 2002;22(4):366.

* Asterisk indicates drugs cited in interaction reports.

Olanzapine — *Quinolones*

Olanzapine* (*Zyprexa*)	Ciprofloxacin* (eg, *Cipro*)	Norfloxacin (*Noroxin*)

Significance	Onset	Severity	Documentation
4	□ Rapid ■ **Delayed**	□ Major ■ **Moderate** □ Minor	□ Established □ Probable □ Suspected ■ **Possible** □ Unlikely

Effects OLANZAPINE plasma concentrations may be elevated, increasing the risk of adverse reactions (eg, sedation, orthostatic hypotension).

Mechanism Certain QUINOLONE antibiotics may inhibit the metabolism (CYP1A2) of OLANZAPINE.

Management Observe the clinical response of the patient and adjust the dose of OLANZAPINE as needed.

Discussion

Increased olanzapine plasma levels were reported in a 54-year-old woman during coadministration of ciprofloxacin.[1] The patient had a history of major depressive disorder with psychotic features. She was hospitalized because of suicidal ideation. At admission, she was receiving olanzapine 10 mg in the evening, in addition to nefazodone, atenolol (eg, *Tenormin*), levothyroxine (eg, *Synthroid*), and phenytoin (eg, *Dilantin*). After admission, nefazodone was tapered and discontinued over a 3-day period. Ciprofloxacin 250 mg twice daily was started for a suspected urinary tract infection. During coadministration of olanzapine and ciprofloxacin, plasma olanzapine levels were more than 2-fold higher than when the patient received olanzapine alone (32.6 vs 14.6 ng/mL). The patient did not appear to experience any adverse reactions relating to the increased olanzapine plasma levels.

Additional studies are needed to determine the clinical importance of this interaction.

[1] Markowitz JS, et al. *J Clin Psychopharmacol.* 1999;19(3):289.

* Asterisk indicates drugs cited in interaction reports. Based on pharmacologic and pharmacokinetic considerations, similar interactions may occur with other drugs that are listed.

Olanzapine — *Valproic Acid Derivatives*

Olanzapine* (*Zyprexa*)	Divalproex Sodium* (eg, *Depakote*)	Valproic Acid* (eg, *Depakene*)

Significance	Onset	Severity	Documentation
4	☐ Rapid ■ **Delayed**	☐ Major ■ **Moderate** ☐ Minor	☐ Established ☐ Probable ☐ Suspected ■ **Possible** ☐ Unlikely

Effects The incidence of hepatic enzyme elevations may be increased, increasing the risk of hepatic adverse reactions. OLANZAPINE levels may be decreased.

Mechanism Unknown.

Management In patients receiving OLANZAPINE, DIVALPROEX, or a combination of the 2 drugs, monitor AST and ALT levels every 3 to 4 months during the first year. If there are no elevations in AST or ALT after 1 year, consider decreasing the frequency of monitoring to every 6 months.

Discussion

In a retrospective, uncontrolled study, the effect of divalproex, olanzapine, and a combination of the 2 drugs on hepatic enzyme elevations was evaluated in 52 children 4 to 18 years of age.[1] Patients were included in the study if they had serum levels of ALT, AST, or lactate dehydrogenase (LDH) measured during divalproex or olanzapine treatment. Compared with administration of divalproex or olanzapine alone, mean and peak hepatic enzyme levels were higher with coadministration of these agents. At least 1 peak enzyme elevation above the normal range occurred in all 12 patients receiving divalproex and olanzapine concomitantly. At least 1 peak enzyme level was elevated in 59% of the 17 patients receiving olanzapine alone and 26% of the 23 patients receiving divalproex alone. In 42% of the combined therapy group, at least 1 enzyme level remained elevated above normal during the observed course of treatment. In addition, coadministration of divalproex and olanzapine was associated with higher peak enzyme levels than monotherapy with either drug. In most instances, the peak and mean enzyme levels were less than 3 times the upper limit of the normal range. Treatment was discontinued in 2 patients receiving concurrent divalproex and olanzapine because of development of pancreatitis in 1 patient and steatohepatitis in the other. Preliminary information from an uncontrolled case series of 4 patients suggests that olanzapine plasma levels decrease between 32% and 79% after the addition of valproic acid.[2] Valproate was administered to 18 patients receiving stable olanzapine doses.[3] Olanzapine blood levels decreased from a baseline of 32.9 ng/mL to 27.4 and 26.9 ng/mL at 2 and 4 weeks, respectively.

[1] Gonzalez-Heydrich J, et al. *J Am Acad Child Adolesc Psychiatry*. 2003;42(10):1227.
[2] Bergemann N, et al. *J Clin Psychopharmacol*. 2006;26(4):432.
[3] Spina E, at al. *Ther Drug Monit*. 2009;31(6):758.

* Asterisk indicates drugs cited in interaction reports.

Ondansetron — *Rifamycins*

Ondansetron* (eg, *Zofran*)	Rifabutin (*Mycobutin*)	Rifapentine (*Priftin*)
	Rifampin* (eg, *Rifadin*)	

Significance	Onset	Severity	Documentation
2	☐ Rapid	☐ Major	☐ Established
	■ **Delayed**	■ **Moderate**	☐ Probable
		☐ Minor	■ **Suspected**
			☐ Possible
			☐ Unlikely

Effects Plasma concentrations of ONDANSETRON may be reduced, decreasing its antiemetic effect.

Mechanism Induction of hepatic metabolism (CYP3A4) of ONDANSETRON by RIFAMYCINS is suspected.

Management If a drug interaction is suspected, consider use of an alternative antiemetic.

Discussion

The effect of rifampin on the pharmacokinetics of ondansetron was studied in 10 healthy volunteers.[1] Using a randomized, crossover, placebo-controlled design, each subject received rifampin 600 mg or placebo once daily for 5 days. On day 6 (13 hours after the last dose of rifampin), ondansetron 8 mg was administered orally or IV. Compared with placebo, pretreatment with rifampin decreased the mean AUC of oral ondansetron 65%, the mean peak concentration 49% (from 27.2 to 13.8 ng/mL), and the mean elimination $t_{½}$ 38% (from 4.5 to 2.8 hours). Pretreatment with rifampin decreased the mean bioavailability of oral ondansetron from 60% to 40%. Pretreatment with rifampin increased the clearance of IV ondansetron 83% and reduced the mean $t_{½}$ 46% (from 5.2 to 2.8 hours) and the AUC 48%.

[1] Villikka K, et al. *Clin Pharmacol Ther.* 1999;65(4):377.

* Asterisk indicates drugs cited in interaction reports. Based on pharmacologic and pharmacokinetic considerations, similar interactions may occur with other drugs that are listed.

Opioid Analgesics — *Azole Antifungal Agents*

Opioid Analgesics		Azole Antifungal Agents	
Alfentanil* (eg, *Alfenta*)	Methadone* (eg, *Dolophine*)	Fluconazole* (eg, *Diflucan*)	Miconazole* (eg, *Oravig*)
Buprenorphine (eg, *Buprenex*)	Oxycodone* (eg, *OxyContin*)	Itraconazole* (eg, *Sporanox*)	Posaconazole (*Noxafil*)
Fentanyl* (eg, *Fentora*)	Sufentanil (eg, *Sufenta*)	Ketoconazole* (eg, *Nizoral*)	Voriconazole* (eg, *Vfend*)

Significance	Onset	Severity	Documentation
1	■ **Rapid** ☐ Delayed	■ **Major** ☐ Moderate ☐ Minor	☐ Established ■ **Probable** ☐ Suspected ☐ Possible ☐ Unlikely

Effects The pharmacologic effects and adverse reactions of certain OPIOID ANALGESICS may be increased.

Mechanism Possible inhibition of certain OPIOID ANALGESIC metabolism (CYP3A4) by AZOLE ANTIFUNGAL AGENTS.

Management Use caution when administering certain OPIOID ANALGESICS to patients receiving AZOLE ANTIFUNGAL AGENTS. Monitor for prolonged or recurrent respiratory depression. It may be necessary to administer a lower dose of the OPIOID ANALGESIC. Coadministration of METHADONE with ITRACONAZOLE is contraindicated.[1]

Discussion

The effects of oral and IV fluconazole on alfentanil were studied in 9 healthy volunteers.[2] Using a randomized, double-blind, placebo-controlled design, each subject received a single oral dose of fluconazole 400 mg and IV saline infusion, an oral placebo and an IV infusion of fluconazole 400 mg, or an oral placebo and an IV saline infusion. Alfentanil 20 mcg/kg IV infused over 2 minutes was administered 60 minutes after the oral dose of fluconazole or placebo. IV and oral fluconazole decreased the clearance of alfentanil 58% and 55%, respectively, while prolonging the elimination $t_{½}$ 80% (from 1.5 to 2.7 h) and 67% (from 1.5 to 2.5 h), respectively. In addition, IV and oral fluconazole increased the alfentanil AUC 107% and 97%, respectively. Although no serious adverse reactions occurred in any of the subjects, oral and IV fluconazole increased alfentanil-induced respiratory depression by decreasing the respiratory rate 10% to 15%. In a 46-year-old man, 8 days after the transdermal fentanyl dosage was increased to 150 mcg/h, fluconazole 50 mg/day was started for oral candidiasis.[3] He died 3 days later. The cause of death was attributed to fatal respiratory depression resulting from elevated fentanyl levels caused by an interaction with fluconazole. In healthy subjects, oral voriconazole decreased the mean plasma clearance of IV alfentanil 85%, increased the AUC 6-fold, and prolonged the elimination $t_{½}$ from 1.5 to 6.6 h.[4] Similarly, oral voriconazole or fluconazole given to 12 healthy subjects decreased the mean plasma clearance of IV fentanyl 23% and 16%, respectively, while increasing the AUC 1.4- and 1.3-fold, respectively.[5] The $t_{½}$ was not changed. Twelve healthy volunteers received a single oral dose of oxycodone after pretreatment with voriconazole or placebo for 4 days.[6] Compared with placebo, voriconazole increased the oxycodone C_{max} and AUC 1.7- and 3.6-fold, respectively. The oxycodone $t_{½}$ increased from 3.5 to 7.1 h. Ketoconazole increased the AUC of orally administered oxycodone 2.4-fold[7] and increased the pharmacodynamic effects.[7,8] Itraconazole increased the AUC of orally administered oxycodone 1.4-fold,[9] while simultaneous inhibition of CYP3A4 (by itraconazole) and CYP2D6 (by paroxetine) metabolism increased the AUC of oxycodone 2.9-fold.[10] Miconazole oral gel 3 times daily increased the oxycodone AUC 1.6-fold but caused minimal changes in the pharmacodynamic response.[11] In a study in 23 men on individualized methadone therapy, compared with placebo, voriconazole increased the C_{max} and AUC of the active enantiomer (R)-methadone approximately 31% and 47%, respectively, and increased the (S)-methadone enantiomer C_{max} and AUC approximately 65% and 103%, respectively.[12] Patients showed no signs of opioid withdrawal or methadone toxicity. Methadone did not affect voriconazole pharmacokinetics. A 26-year-old woman receiving long-term methadone therapy was started on voriconazole for suspected aspergillosis.[13] Four days later, she presented with ventricular bigeminy associated with high plasma concentrations of methadone and voriconazole. Omeprazole may have contributed to the interaction.

[1] *Sporanox* [package insert]. Raritan, NJ: Centacor Ortho Biotech Products LP; November 2011.
[2] Palkama VJ, et al. *Anesth Analg.* 1998;87(1):190.
[3] Hallberg P, et al. *Eur J Clin Pharmacol.* 2006;62(6):491.
[4] Saari TI, et al. *Clin Pharmacol Ther.* 2006;80(5):502.
[5] Saari TI, et al. *Eur J Clin Pharmacol.* 2008;64(1):25.
[6] Hagelberg NM, et al. *Eur J Clin Pharmacol.* 2009;65(3):263.
[7] Kummer O, et al. *Eur J Clin Pharmacol.* 2011;67(1):63.
[8] Samer CF, et al. *Br J Pharmacol.* 2010;160(4):919.
[9] Saari TI, et al. *Eur J Clin Pharmacol.* 2010;66(4):387.
[10] Grönlund J, et al. *Br J Clin Pharmacol.* 2010;70(1):78.
[11] Grönlund J, et al. *Antimicrob Agents Chemother.* 2011;55(3):1063.
[12] Liu P, et al. *Antimicrob Agents Chemother.* 2007;51(1):110.
[13] Scholler J, et al. *Int J Clin Pharm.* 2011;33(6):905.

* Asterisk indicates drugs cited in interaction reports. Based on pharmacologic and pharmacokinetic considerations, similar interactions may occur with other drugs that are listed.

Opioid Analgesics | **Benzodiazepines**

Opioid Analgesics		Benzodiazepines	
Buprenorphine* (eg, *Buprenex*)	Methadone* (eg, *Dolophine*)	Alprazolam* (eg, *Xanax*)	Lorazepam (eg, *Ativan*)
		Chlordiazepoxide*	Midazolam
		Clonazepam (eg, *Klonopin*)	Oxazepam*
		Clorazepate (eg, *Tranxene*)	Quazepam (*Doral*)
		Diazepam* (eg, *Valium*)	Temazepam (eg, *Restoril*)
		Estazolam	Triazolam (eg, *Halcion*)
		Flurazepam	

Significance	Onset	Severity	Documentation
1	■ **Rapid**	■ **Major**	□ Established
	□ Delayed	□ Moderate	□ Probable
		□ Minor	■ **Suspected**
			□ Possible
			□ Unlikely

Effects Increased risk of sedation and life-threatening respiratory depression, especially with overdosage.

Mechanism Synergistic effects of OPIOIDS and BENZODIAZEPINES.

Management Use with caution in patients in METHADONE maintenance programs (eg, supervised ingestion) or patients receiving OPIOIDS for pain management. Subjective and performance responses may be altered. Caution patients against driving or operating machinery while taking these agents.

Discussion

In a double-blind study, subjective drug effects (eg, drug-liking, sedation) and performance responses (eg, reaction time, digit symbol substitution task) were affected by diazepam in patients receiving methadone[1-3] or buprenorphine.[1,3] The effects were dose- and time-related, reaching a maximum of approximately 1 to 2 hours after coadministration of these agents.[1] Information is available regarding illicit use of methadone with benzodiazepines.[4] In a review of 101 deaths in which methadone was detected in the blood, methadone was the sole intoxicant in 15 cases; benzodiazepines were the most frequently detected cointoxicants in 60 cases and were the only cointoxicants in 30 cases. Compared with methadone intoxication alone, cointoxication with benzodiazepines increased methadone plasma levels more than 2-fold. Coadministration of methadone and benzodiazepines was identified as a contributing[5] or major risk factor for premature mortality.[6]

[1] Lintzeris N, et al. *J Clin Psycopharmacol.* 2006;26(3):274.
[2] Preston KL, et al. *Clin Pharmacol Ther.* 1984;36(4):534.
[3] Lintzeris N, et al. *Drug Alcohol Depend.* 2007;91(2-3):187.
[4] Mikolaenko I, et al. *Am J Forensic Med Pathol.* 2002;23(3):299.
[5] Caplehorn JR, et al. *Aust N Z J Public Health.* 2002;26(4):358.
[6] Ernst E, et al. *Aust N Z J Public Health.* 2002;26(4):364.

* Asterisk indicates drugs cited in interaction reports. Based on pharmacologic and pharmacokinetic considerations, similar interactions may occur with other drugs that are listed.

Opioid Analgesics — *Diltiazem*

Alfentanil (eg, *Alfenta*)	Sufentanil (eg, *Sufenta*)	Diltiazem* (eg, *Cardizem*)
Fentanyl* (eg, *Sublimaze*)		

Significance	Onset	Severity	Documentation
1	☐ Rapid ■ **Delayed**	■ **Major** ☐ Moderate ☐ Minor	☐ Established ☐ Probable ■ **Suspected** ☐ Possible ☐ Unlikely

Effects OPIOID ANALGESIC plasma concentrations may be elevated, increasing the pharmacologic effects and risk of toxicity (eg, severe respiratory depression).

Mechanism Inhibition of OPIOID ANALGESIC metabolism (CYP3A4) by DILTIAZEM.

Management Closely monitor the clinical response of patients. Monitor patients for signs of opioid toxicity over an extended period of time and increase the OPIOID ANALGESIC dosage conservatively when necessary.[1]

Discussion

An 85-year-old man receiving fentanyl 25 mcg/h experienced hypoactive delirium, somnolence, and pinpoint pupils 3 days after diltiazem was started for supraventricular tachycardia.[2] The fentanyl dose had not been changed over the preceding 2 weeks. The patient became more alert within hours of discontinuing the fentanyl drip.

[1] *Abstral* [package insert]. Bedminster, NJ: ProStrakan Inc; January 2011.

[2] Levin TT, et al. *Gen Hosp Psychiatry.* 2010;32(6):648.e9.

* Asterisk indicates drugs cited in interaction reports. Based on pharmacologic and pharmacokinetic considerations, similar interactions may occur with other drugs that are listed.

Opioid Analgesics — *Histamine H_2 Antagonists*

Opioid Analgesics		Histamine H_2 Antagonists
Alfentanil (eg, *Alfenta*)	Morphine* (eg, *Oramorph*)	Cimetidine* (eg, *Tagamet*)
Buprenorphine (eg, *Buprenex*)	Nalbuphine	
Butorphanol	Opium* (eg, *Paregoric*)	
Codeine	Oxycodone (eg, *OxyContin*)	
Fentanyl (eg, *Sublimaze*)	Oxymorphone (eg, *Opana*)	
Hydromorphone (eg, *Dilaudid*)	Pentazocine (*Talwin*)	
Levorphanol	Sufentanil (eg, *Sufenta*)	
Meperidine* (eg, *Demerol*)		
Methadone* (eg, *Dolophine*)		

Significance

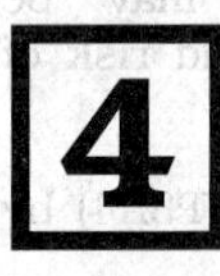

Onset	Severity	Documentation
■ **Rapid**	■ **Major**	□ Established
□ Delayed	□ Moderate	□ Probable
	□ Minor	□ Suspected
		■ **Possible**
		□ Unlikely

Effects The actions of OPIOID ANALGESICS may be enhanced, resulting in toxicity.

Mechanism Decreased OPIOID ANALGESIC metabolism is suspected.

Management If CNS depression manifests, withdraw the drugs. If needed, give a narcotic antagonist (eg, naloxone [eg, *Narcan*]).

Discussion

Potentially fatal respiratory depression occurred in patients receiving cimetidine with morphine or opium and methadone.[1-3] In a randomized, crossover study, 8 healthy volunteers were subjectively more sedated when given cimetidine 600 mg with morphine 10 mg IM.[4] In addition, cimetidine premedication caused more profound respiratory depression, delayed recovery, and produced a slight increase in morphine serum levels. However, these effects were judged to be clinically insignificant in healthy subjects. Cimetidine did not affect morphine kinetics in healthy volunteers.[5,6] In 8 volunteers, 7 days of cimetidine 1,200 mg/day reduced meperidine clearance 22%.[7] Normeperidine levels also were lower. Ranitidine (eg, *Zantac*) does not appear to change meperidine kinetics.[8] Clinical importance has not been determined. Cimetidine's effects on other narcotic analgesics are not known. This combination may attenuate cardiovascular responses to narcotic-induced histamine release.[9]

1 Fine A, et al. *Can Med Assoc J.* 1981;124(11):1434.
2 Lam AM. *Can Med Assoc J.* 1981;125(8):820.
3 Sorkin EM, et al. *Drug Intell Clin Pharm.* 1983;17(1):60.
4 Lam AM, et al. *Can Anaesth Soc J.* 1984;31(1):36.
5 Mojaverian P, et al. *Br J Clin Pharmacol.* 1982;14(6):809.
6 Reilly PE, et al. *Biochem Pharmacol.* 1984;33(7):1151.
7 Guay DR, et al. *Br J Clin Pharmacol.* 1984;18(6):907.
8 Guay DR, et al. *Br J Clin Pharmacol.* 1985;20(1):55.
9 Philbin DM, et al. *Anesthesiology.* 1981;55(3):292.

* Asterisk indicates drugs cited in interaction reports. Based on pharmacologic and pharmacokinetic considerations, similar interactions may occur with other drugs that are listed.

Opioid Analgesics — *Macrolide & Related Antibiotics*

Opioid Analgesics		Macrolide & Related Antibiotics	
Buprenorphine (eg, *Buprenex*)	Oxycodone* (eg, *OxyContin*)	Clarithromycin* (eg, *Biaxin*)	Telithromycin (*Ketek*)
Codeine	Sufentanil (eg, *Sufenta*)	Erythromycin (eg, *Ery-Tab*)	
Fentanyl* (eg, *Duragesic*)			
Methadone (eg, *Dolophine*)			

Significance	Onset	Severity	Documentation
1	☐ Rapid	■ **Major**	☐ Established
	■ **Delayed**	☐ Moderate	☐ Probable
		☐ Minor	■ **Suspected**
			☐ Possible
			☐ Unlikely

Effects OPIOID ANALGESIC plasma concentrations may be elevated, increasing the pharmacologic effects and toxicity.

Mechanism Inhibition of OPIOID ANALGESIC metabolism (CYP3A4) by MACROLIDE AND RELATED ANTIBIOTICS.

Management Use caution when administering OPIOID ANALGESICS to patients receiving MACROLIDE AND RELATED ANTIBIOTICS. Monitor for symptoms of opioid toxicity (eg, excessive drowsiness, respiratory depression). It may be necessary to administer a lower OPIOID ANALGESIC dose.

Discussion

An 81-year-old man with chronic obstructive pulmonary disease was receiving transdermal fentanyl 200 mcg/h with the patch changed every 48 hours.[1] Within 36 hours after receiving the first dose of clarithromycin 500 mg twice daily for *Helicobacter pylori*, the patient was unresponsive to verbal or tactile stimuli. He had pinpoint pupils, hypoventilation, profound hypoxemia, and a respiratory rate of 2 breaths per minute. Following administration of naloxone 0.4 mg IV, he promptly regained consciousness, and his respiratory rate increased to 30 breaths per minute with associated tachycardia, agitation, and respiratory distress. The fentanyl patch was discontinued, and his withdrawal symptoms were managed with subcutaneous morphine. The following day, he was alert and conversive, with normal respiration and oxygen saturation. Transdermal fentanyl 100 mcg/h was resumed and well tolerated. The effects of telithromycin on the pharmacokinetics of oxycodone were studied in 11 healthy subjects.[2] In a randomized, crossover study, each subject was pretreated with oral telithromycin 800 mg daily or placebo for 4 days. On day 3, subjects received oxycodone 10 mg. Compared with placebo, telithromycin increased the oxycodone AUC 80% and decreased the noroxycodone metabolite 46%. The pharmacodynamic effects of oxycodone were modestly increased. Ten young and 10 elderly healthy subjects received clarithromycin 500 mg or placebo twice daily for 5 days.[3] A single dose of oxycodone 100 mg was administered on day 4. Compared with placebo, clarithromycin increased oxycodone AUC 2- and 2.3-fold in young and elderly subjects, respectively. However, there was no change in the pharmacodynamic effects of oxycodone.

[1] Horton R, et al. *J Pain Symptom Manage.* 2009;37(6):e2.
[2] Grönlund J, et al. *J Clin Pharmacol.* 2010;50(1):101.
[3] Liukas A, et al. *J Clin Psychopharmacol.* 2011;31(3):302.

* Asterisk indicates drugs cited in interaction reports. Based on pharmacologic and pharmacokinetic considerations, similar interactions may occur with other drugs that are listed.

Opioid Analgesics — *Protease Inhibitors*

Opioid Analgesics		Protease Inhibitors	
Alfentanil (eg, *Alfenta*)	Oxycodone* (eg, *Oxycontin*)	Atazanavir* (*Reyataz*)	Nelfinavir (*Viracept*)
Buprenorphine* (eg, *Buprenex*)	Sufentanil (eg, *Sufenta*)	Darunavir (*Prezista*)	Ritonavir* (*Norvir*)
Fentanyl* (eg, *Fentora*)		Fosamprenavir (*Lexiva*)	Saquinavir* (*Invirase*)
		Indinavir (*Crixivan*)	Tipranavir (*Aptivus*)
		Lopinavir/Ritonavir* (*Kaletra*)	

Significance	Onset	Severity	Documentation
1	☐ Rapid	■ **Major**	☐ Established
	■ **Delayed**	☐ Moderate	☐ Probable
		☐ Minor	■ **Suspected**
			☐ Possible
			☐ Unlikely

Effects OPIOID ANALGESIC plasma concentrations may be increased and the t½ prolonged, increasing the risk of adverse reactions (eg, respiratory depression).

Mechanism Possible inhibition of OPIOID ANALGESIC metabolism (CYP3A4) in the gut wall and liver.

Management In patients receiving PROTEASE INHIBITORS, closely monitor respiratory function during OPIOID ANALGESIC administration and for a longer period than usual after stopping the OPIOID ANALGESIC. If the OPIOID ANALGESIC is administered continuously, it may be necessary to reduce the OPIOID ANALGESIC dose.

Discussion

The effect of ritonavir on fentanyl pharmacokinetics was assessed in 11 healthy volunteers.[1] Each subject received ritonavir or placebo for 3 days. Three doses of oral ritonavir 200 mg were given on day 1, and 3 doses of ritonavir 300 mg were administered on day 2. On the morning of day 3, the last dose of ritonavir 300 mg or placebo was given. On day 2, approximately 2 hours after the afternoon dose of ritonavir or placebo, fentanyl 5 mcg/kg was injected IV over 2 min. The mean fentanyl plasma level 18 hours after injection in the ritonavir phase was at the same level as at 4 hours during the placebo phase. Compared with placebo, ritonavir decreased the fentanyl plasma clearance 67%, increased the elimination t½ from 9.4 to 20.1 hours, and increased the AUC 174%. In 6 subjects, secondary fentanyl C_{max} occurred 5 and 9 hours after fentanyl administration. Eight of 11 subjects reported nausea. Increased buprenorphine adverse reactions have been reported in at least 3 patients during coadministration of atazanavir plus ritonavir.[2] Adverse reactions improved when the buprenorphine dose was reduced. In 10 HIV-positive opioid-dependent volunteers, administration of ritonavir increased the buprenorphine AUC 57%.[3] In contrast, in 12 healthy subjects, administration of lopinavir/ritonavir did not affect the buprenorphine AUC.[4] In a randomized, crossover study in 12 healthy volunteers, coadministration of oxycodone with ritonavir or lopinavir/ritonavir increased the oxycodone AUC 3- and 2.6-fold, respectively, compared with placebo.[5] In addition, the mean elimination t½ of oxycodone was increased.

1 Olkkola KT, et al. *Anesthesiology*. 1999;91(3):681.
2 Bruce RD, et al. *AIDS*. 2006;20(5):783.
3 McCance-Katz EF, et al. *Clin Infect Dis*. 2006;43(suppl 4):S235.
4 Bruce RD, et al. *J Acquir Immune Defic Syndr*. 2010;54(5):511.
5 Nieminen TH, et al. *Eur J Clin Pharmacol*. 2010;66(10):977.

* Asterisk indicates drugs cited in interaction reports. Based on pharmacologic and pharmacokinetic considerations, similar interactions may occur with other drugs that are listed.

Oseltamivir — *Probenecid*

Oseltamivir* (*Tamiflu*)	Probenecid*

Significance	Onset	Severity	Documentation
4	□ Rapid	□ Major	□ Established
	■ **Delayed**	■ **Moderate**	□ Probable
		□ Minor	□ Suspected
			■ **Possible**
			□ Unlikely

Effects OSELTAMIVIR plasma concentrations may be elevated, increasing the pharmacologic effects and risk of adverse reactions.

Mechanism PROBENECID may decrease renal tubular secretion of OSELTAMIVIR.

Management Coadminister with caution. Monitor patients for OSELTAMIVIR adverse reactions.

Discussion

In a randomized, open-label, crossover study, the effects of probenecid on oseltamivir pharmacokinetics were evaluated in 21 healthy individuals.[1] Coadministration of probenecid 200 mg daily for 2 days decreased the renal elimination of oseltamivir 61%, resulting in a 154% increase in the oseltamivir AUC. Compared with administration of oseltamivir alone, the rate of adverse reactions was approximately twice as high when oseltamivir was coadministered with probenecid (18% compared with 35%). Coadministration of oseltamivir and probenecid was associated with a case of thrombocytopenia in a 68-year-old woman.[2] However, thrombocytopenia has been reported with administration of oseltamivir or probenecid alone.

[1] Wattanagoon Y, et al. *Antimicrob Agents Chemother.* 2009;53(3):945.

[2] Raisch DW, et al. *Pharmacotherapy.* 2009;29(8):988.

* Asterisk indicates drugs cited in interaction reports.

Oxycodone | **Food**

Oxycodone* (eg, *OxyContin*)	Grapefruit Juice*

Significance	Onset	Severity	Documentation
4	□ Rapid	□ Major	□ Established
	■ **Delayed**	■ **Moderate**	□ Probable
		□ Minor	□ Suspected
			■ **Possible**
			□ Unlikely

Effects OXYCODONE plasma concentrations may be elevated, increasing the pharmacologic effects and risk of adverse reactions.

Mechanism GRAPEFRUIT JUICE inhibits OXYCODONE first-pass metabolism (CYP3A4) in the small intestine.

Management Until more information is available, avoid administration of OXYCODONE with GRAPEFRUIT PRODUCTS and advise patients to take OXYCODONE with a liquid other than GRAPEFRUIT JUICE.

Discussion

The effects of grapefruit juice on the pharmacokinetics of oxycodone were studied in 12 healthy volunteers.[1] Using a randomized, cross-over design, each subject ingested 200 mL of grapefruit juice or water 3 times a day for 5 days. On day 4, an oral dose of oxycodone 10 mg was administered. Compared with water, grapefruit juice increased the mean oxycodone AUC 1.7-fold, the C_{max} 1.5-fold, and prolonged the $t_{1/2}$ by 1.2-fold. Formation of the oxycodone metabolites noroxycodone and noroxymorphone were decreased, while formation of oxymorphone was increased. The analgesic effect was not affected.

[1] Nieminen TH, et al. *Basic Clin Pharmacol Toxicol.* 2010;107(4):782.

* Asterisk indicates drugs cited in interaction reports.

Oxycodone — *Rifamycins*

Oxycodone	Rifamycins	
Oxycodone* (eg, *OxyContin*)	Rifabutin (*Mycobutin*)	Rifapentine (*Priftin*)
	Rifampin* (eg, *Rifadin*)	

Significance	Onset	Severity	Documentation
2	☐ Rapid	☐ Major	☐ Established
	■ **Delayed**	■ **Moderate**	☐ Probable
		☐ Minor	■ **Suspected**
			☐ Possible
			☐ Unlikely

Effects OXYCODONE plasma concentrations may be reduced, decreasing the pharmacologic effects (eg, pain management). Oral bioavailability of OXYCODONE is decreased.

Mechanism Increased OXYCODONE metabolism (CYP3A4) by RIFAMYCINS. Oral bioavailability of OXYCODONE is decreased.

Management Observe the clinical response of the patient. Adjust the OXYCODONE dose as needed.

Discussion

The effects of rifampin on the pharmacologic effects and metabolism of oxycodone were studied in 12 volunteers.[1] Each subject received IV oxycodone 0.1 mg/kg or oral oxycodone 15 mg after 5 doses of placebo or rifampin 600 mg daily. Compared with placebo, rifampin decreased the AUC of IV and oral oxycodone 53% and 86%, respectively. Oral bioavailability of oxycodone decreased from 69% to 21%. The ratios of plasma metabolite-to-parent drug for noroxycodone and noroxymorphone were greatly increased by rifampin. The pharmacologic effects of oxycodone, as measured by self-reported drowsiness, drug effect, deterioration of performance, and cold pain sensitivity, were decreased. In addition, rifampin reduced the miotic effect of IV oxycodone and oxycodone-associated heterotropia after oral oxycodone.

[1] Nieminen TH, et al. *Anesthesiology*. 2009;110(6):1371.

* Asterisk indicates drugs cited in interaction reports. Based on pharmacologic and pharmacokinetic considerations, similar interactions may occur with other drugs that are listed.

Oxycodone | **St. John's Wort**

Oxycodone* (eg, *OxyContin*)	St. John's Wort*

Significance	Onset	Severity	Documentation
4	☐ Rapid	☐ Major	☐ Established
	■ **Delayed**	■ **Moderate**	☐ Probable
		☐ Minor	☐ Suspected
			■ **Possible**
			☐ Unlikely

Effects OXYCODONE plasma concentrations may be reduced.

Mechanism Increased metabolism of OXYCODONE (CYP3A4) by ST. JOHN'S WORT.

Management If coadministration cannot be avoided, it may be necessary to increase the OXYCODONE dose when coadministering with ST. JOHN'S WORT and to reduce the dose when discontinuing ST. JOHN'S WORT. Advise patients taking OXYCODONE to inform their health care provider before taking nonprescription or herbal products.

Discussion

The effects of St. John's wort on the pharmacokinetics of oxycodone were studied in 12 healthy subjects.[1] Using a placebo-controlled, randomized, cross-over design, each subject received St. John's wort 300 mg 3 times daily or placebo for 15 days. On day 14, oxycodone 15 mg was administered. Compared with placebo, St. John's wort decreased oxycodone C_{max} and AUC 29% and 50%, respectively. St. John's wort shortened the oxycodone $t_{1/2}$ from 3.8 to 3 hours. In addition, St. John's wort decreased the subjective drug effects of oxycodone.

[1] Nieminen TH, et al. *Eur J Pain.* 2010;14(8):854.

* Asterisk indicates drugs cited in interaction reports.

Paclitaxel — *Amifostine*

Paclitaxel* (eg, *Abraxane*)	Amifostine* (eg, *Ethyol*)

Significance	Onset	Severity	Documentation
4	☐ Rapid ■ **Delayed**	☐ Major ■ **Moderate** ☐ Minor	☐ Established ☐ Probable ☐ Suspected ■ **Possible** ☐ Unlikely

Effects PACLITAXEL plasma concentrations may be reduced, decreasing the pharmacologic effects and adverse reactions.

Mechanism Unknown.

Management In patients receiving PACLITAXEL, closely monitor the response when starting or stopping AMIFOSTINE. Adjust therapy as needed.

Discussion

The effects of amifostine (500 mg IV over 15 minutes just prior to paclitaxel administration) on the pharmacokinetics of low-dose paclitaxel (80 mg/m^2 given as a 1-hour infusion) were studied in patients with nonresectable or metastatic non–small cell lung cancer.[1] Compared with treatment cycles in which paclitaxel was administered alone, paclitaxel C_{max} was decreased approximately 20%, and residence time in the plasma was prolonged during treatment cycles with coadministration of paclitaxel and amifostine.

Additional studies are needed to determine the effects of amifostine on paclitaxel safety and efficacy.

[1] Juan O, et al. *Chemotherapy*. 2005;51(4):200.

* Asterisk indicates drugs cited in interaction reports.

Paclitaxel — *Clindamycin*

Paclitaxel* (eg, *Abraxane*)	Clindamycin* (eg, *Cleocin*)

Significance	Onset	Severity	Documentation
4	☐ Rapid	☐ Major	☐ Established
	■ **Delayed**	■ **Moderate**	☐ Probable
		☐ Minor	☐ Suspected
			■ **Possible**
			☐ Unlikely

Effects PACLITAXEL cell uptake may be increased, increasing the pharmacologic and toxic effects.

Mechanism Unknown. Possibly displacement of PACLITAXEL from alpha-1 acid glycoprotein.

Management Observe patients for signs of PACLITAXEL toxicity. Be prepared to adjust the PACLITAXEL dose as needed.

Discussion

The effects of clindamycin on the pharmacokinetics of paclitaxel were evaluated in 16 women with advanced ovarian cancer.[1] Patients received paclitaxel 175 mg/m^2 by 3-hour infusion alone and with clindamycin 600 and 1,200 mg. The sequence of the 3 treatment regimens was randomly assigned. Paclitaxel C_{max} and AUC were higher when the drug was given alone than when it was administered with clindamycin 1,200 mg. When given with clindamycin 600 mg, paclitaxel C_{max} and AUC did not show a statistically significant difference between paclitaxel alone and with clindamycin 1,200 mg. There were no differences in incidence or grade of toxicity between the treatment groups.

Additional studies are needed to determine the clinical importance of this possible interaction.

[1] Fruscio R, et al. *Cancer Chemother Pharmacol.* 2006;58(3):319.

* Asterisk indicates drugs cited in interaction reports.

Pancuronium — *Thiotepa*

Pancuronium* (*eg, Pavulon*)	Thiotepa* (*Thioplex*)

Significance	Onset	Severity	Documentation
4	■ **Rapid**	□ Major	□ Established
	□ Delayed	■ **Moderate**	□ Probable
		□ Minor	□ Suspected
			■ **Possible**
			□ Unlikely

Effects The neuromuscular blocking effects of PANCURONIUM may be increased. Prolonged apnea may occur.

Mechanism Unknown.

Management No special therapeutic managements appear necessary. Close monitoring of neuromuscular function may be needed.

Discussion

Laboratory animal data suggested that thiotepa (triethylenethiophosphoramide) did not possess significant myoneural blockade when administered alone.[1,3] However, in an isolated case report, a 58-year-old myasthenic woman maintained with pyridostigmine (eg, *Mestinon*) 480 mg daily developed prolonged muscular paralysis and respiratory depression when pancuronium and thiotepa were administered intraperitoneally for laparotomy, despite repeated doses of neostigmine (eg, *Prostigmin*).[2]

No other reports of similar neuromuscular blockade interaction have been reported with other nondepolarizing muscle relaxants. Additional studies are needed to better establish this interaction.

[1] Kurek EJ, et al. *Can Fed Biol Sci.* 1976;19:103.
[2] Bennett EJ, et al. *Anesthesiology.* 1977;46:220.
[3] Rylett BJ, et al. *Can J Physiol Pharmacol.* 1977;55:769.

* Asterisk indicates drugs cited in interaction reports.

Paroxetine — *Barbiturates*

Paroxetine	Barbiturates	
Paroxetine* (*Paxil*)	Amobarbital (*Amytal*)	Pentobarbital (eg, *Nembutal*)
	Aprobarbital (*Alurate*)	Phenobarbital*
	Butabarbital (eg, *Butisol*)	Primidone (eg, *Mysoline*)
	Butalbital	Secobarbital (eg, *Seconal*)
	Mephobarbital (*Mebaral*)	

Significance	Onset	Severity	Documentation
5	☐ Rapid	☐ Major	☐ Established
	■ **Delayed**	☐ Moderate	☐ Probable
		■ **Minor**	☐ Suspected
			■ **Possible**
			☐ Unlikely

Effects Serum PAROXETINE concentrations may be decreased, reducing the clinical effect.

Mechanism Possibly, BARBITURATES increase the hepatic metabolism of PAROXETINE.

Management If an interaction is suspected, it may be necessary to adjust the dose of PAROXETINE when starting, stopping, or changing the dose of the BARBITURATE.

Discussion

The effects of multiple dose administration of phenobarbital on the pharmacokinetics of a single oral 30 mg dose of paroxetine were studied in ten healthy subjects.[1] Based on the group mean values for the area under the plasma concentration-time curve (AUC), half-life and maximum concentrations (C_{max}) achieved for paroxetine, there were no statistically significant differences between administration of paroxetine alone or with phenobarbital. However, on a patient by patient basis, individual differences in AUC, C_{max} and half-life were observed. The AUC of paroxetine was decreased in six subjects after treatment with phenobarbital. In a study involving 12 healthy volunteers, administration of either paroxetine or amobarbital alone caused subjects to feel less alert, attentive, energetic or well-coordinated.[2] However, concurrent administration of paroxetine and amobarbital failed to affect these subjective CNS assessments more than those of giving either drug alone.

Controlled trials are needed to determine if the combined effects of administering paroxetine and barbiturates are greater than giving either agent alone.

[1] Greb WH, et al. *Acta Psychiatr Scand.* 1989;80 (suppl 350):95.

[2] Cooper SM, et al. *Acta Psychiatr Scand.* 1989;80 (suppl 350):53.

* Asterisk indicates drugs cited in interaction reports. Based on pharmacologic and pharmacokinetic considerations, similar interactions may occur with other drugs that are listed.

Paroxetine — *Protease Inhibitors*

Paroxetine* (eg, *Paxil*)	Fosamprenavir* (*Lexiva*)	Ritonavir* (*Norvir*)

Significance	Onset	Severity	Documentation
4	☐ Rapid ■ **Delayed**	☐ Major ■ **Moderate** ☐ Minor	☐ Established ☐ Probable ☐ Suspected ■ **Possible** ☐ Unlikely

Effects PAROXETINE plasma concentrations may be reduced, decreasing the efficacy.

Mechanism Unknown; however, displacement of PAROXETINE from protein binding sites is suspected to be partially involved.

Management Closely observe the clinical response of patients and titrate the PAROXETINE dosage as needed when starting or stopping FOSAMPRENAVIR and/or RITONAVIR.

Discussion

The effects of a 2-way pharmacokinetic drug interaction between fosamprenavir (a prodrug of amprenavir) plus ritonavir administration on paroxetine were evaluated in 23 healthy subjects.[1] In an open-label study, 13 subjects received paroxetine 20 mg daily alone for 10 days. Following a 16-day washout period, they received paroxetine 20 mg daily, fosamprenavir 700 mg twice daily, and ritonavir 100 mg twice daily for 10 days. A second group of 13 patients received the regimens in reverse order. Three subjects did not complete the study. Paroxetine did not affect the pharmacokinetics of amprenavir or ritonavir. However, compared with paroxetine alone, administration of fosamprenavir and ritonavir with paroxetine decreased paroxetine plasma exposure 55% and increased the free fraction of paroxetine (unbound paroxetine divided by the total unbound and bound paroxetine concentrations) 30%. No serious adverse reactions were reported.

[1] van der Lee MJ, et al. *Antimicrob Agents Chemother*. 2007;51(11):4098.

* Asterisk indicates drugs cited in interaction reports.

Pazopanib		**Azole Antifungal Agents**	
Pazopanib* (*Votrient*)		Itraconazole (eg, *Sporanox*)	Ketoconazole* (eg, *Nizoral*)

Significance	Onset	Severity	Documentation
2	☐ Rapid ■ **Delayed**	☐ Major ■ **Moderate** ☐ Minor	☐ Established ☐ Probable ■ **Suspected** ☐ Possible ☐ Unlikely

Effects PAZOPANIB plasma concentrations may be elevated, increasing the pharmacologic effects and risk of adverse reactions.

Mechanism Inhibition of PAZOPANIB metabolism (CYP3A4) by AZOLE ANTIFUNGAL AGENTS.

Management If coadministration cannot be avoided, limit the PAZOPANIB dosage to 400 mg once daily.[1] Monitor the patient and reduce the PAZOPANIB dosage further if adverse reactions occur.

Discussion

Coadministration of pazopanib and strong CYP3A4 inhibitors (eg, ketoconazole) may increase pazopanib plasma concentrations; avoid coadministration. If coadministration of a strong CYP3A4 inhibitor is warranted, reduce the dosage of pazopanib to 400 mg once daily.[1] Additional dosage reductions may be necessary if adverse reactions occur during therapy. The recommended dosage reduction is predicted to adjust the pazopanib AUC to the range observed without coadministration of a strong CYP3A4 inhibitor. However, there are no clinical data with this dosage adjustment in patients receiving strong CYP3A4 inhibitors.

The basis for this monograph is information on file with the manufacturer. Published clinical data are needed to further assess this interaction.

[1] *Votrient* [package insert]. Research Triangle Park, NC: GlaxoSmithKline; October 2009.

* Asterisk indicates drugs cited in interaction reports. Based on pharmacologic and pharmacokinetic considerations, similar interactions may occur with other drugs that are listed.

Pazopanib — *Food*

Pazopanib* (*Votrient*)	Grapefruit Juice*

Significance	Onset	Severity	Documentation
2	☐ Rapid	☐ Major	☐ Established
	■ **Delayed**	■ **Moderate**	☐ Probable
		☐ Minor	■ **Suspected**
			☐ Possible
			☐ Unlikely

Effects PAZOPANIB plasma concentrations may be elevated, increasing the pharmacologic effects and risk of adverse reactions.

Mechanism Inhibition of PAZOPANIB metabolism (CYP3A4) by GRAPEFRUIT JUICE.

Management GRAPEFRUIT JUICE should be avoided in patients taking PAZOPANIB.[1] Administer PAZOPANIB with a liquid other than GRAPEFRUIT JUICE.

Discussion

Coadministration of pazopanib and grapefruit juice may increase pazopanib plasma concentrations and should be avoided.[1] However, there are no clinical data for patients taking pazopanib and ingesting grapefruit juice.

The basis for this monograph is information on file with the manufacturer. Published clinical data are needed to further assess this interaction.

[1] *Votrient* [package insert]. Research Triangle Park, NC: GlaxoSmithKline; October 2009.

* Asterisk indicates drugs cited in interaction reports.

Pazopanib | **Macrolide & Related Antibiotics**

Pazopanib* (*Votrient*)	Clarithromycin* (eg, *Biaxin*)	Telithromycin (*Ketek*)

Significance	Onset	Severity	Documentation
2	□ Rapid ■ **Delayed**	□ Major ■ **Moderate** □ Minor	□ Established □ Probable ■ **Suspected** □ Possible □ Unlikely

Effects PAZOPANIB plasma concentrations may be elevated, increasing the pharmacologic effects and risk of adverse reactions.

Mechanism Inhibition of PAZOPANIB metabolism (CYP3A4) by MACROLIDE AND RELATED ANTIBIOTICS.

Management If coadministration cannot be avoided, limit the dosage to PAZOPANIB 400 mg once daily.[1] Monitor the patient and reduce the PAZOPANIB dosage further if adverse reactions occur.

Discussion

Coadministration of pazopanib and strong CYP3A4 inhibitors (eg, clarithromycin) may increase pazopanib plasma concentrations and should be avoided. If coadministration of a strong CYP3A4 inhibitor is warranted, the dose of pazopanib should be reduced to 400 mg once daily.[1] Additional dose reductions may be necessary if adverse reactions occur during therapy. The recommended dose reduction is predicted to adjust the pazopanib AUC to the range observed without coadministration of a strong CYP3A4 inhibitor. However, there are no clinical data with this dosage adjustment in patients receiving strong CYP3A4 inhibitors.

The basis for this monograph is information on file with the manufacturer. Published clinical data are needed to further assess this interaction.

[1] *Votrient* [package insert]. Research Triangle Park, NC: GlaxoSmithKline; October 2009.

* Asterisk indicates drugs cited in interaction reports. Based on pharmacologic and pharmacokinetic considerations, similar interactions may occur with other drugs that are listed.

Pazopanib — *Protease Inhibitors*

Pazopanib* (*Votrient*)	Indinavir (*Crixivan*)	Ritonavir* (*Norvir*)
	Nelfinavir (*Viracept*)	Saquinavir (*Invirase*)

Significance	Onset	Severity	Documentation
2	☐ Rapid ■ **Delayed**	☐ Major ■ **Moderate** ☐ Minor	☐ Established ☐ Probable ■ **Suspected** ☐ Possible ☐ Unlikely

Effects PAZOPANIB plasma concentrations may be elevated, increasing the pharmacologic effects and risk of adverse reactions.

Mechanism Inhibition of PAZOPANIB metabolism (CYP3A4) by PROTEASE INHIBITORS.

Management If coadministration cannot be avoided, limit the PAZOPANIB dosage to 400 mg once daily.[1] Monitor the patient and reduce the PAZOPANIB dosage further if adverse reactions occur.

Discussion

Coadministration of pazopanib and strong CYP3A4 inhibitors (eg, ritonavir) may increase pazopanib plasma concentrations; avoid coadministration. If coadministration of a strong CYP3A4 inhibitor is warranted, reduce the dosage of pazopanib to 400 mg once daily.[1] Additional dosage reductions may be necessary if adverse reactions occur during therapy. The recommended dosage reduction is predicted to adjust the pazopanib AUC to the range observed without coadministration of a strong CYP3A4 inhibitor. However, there are no clinical data with this dosage adjustment in patients receiving strong CYP3A4 inhibitors.

The basis for this monograph is information on file with the manufacturer. Published clinical data are needed to further assess this interaction.

[1] *Votrient* [package insert]. Research Triangle Park, NC: GlaxoSmithKline; October 2009.

* Asterisk indicates drugs cited in interaction reports. Based on pharmacologic and pharmacokinetic considerations, similar interactions may occur with other drugs that are listed.

Pazopanib | **Rifamycins**

Pazopanib* (*Votrient*)	Rifampin* (eg, *Rifadin*)

Significance	Onset	Severity	Documentation
2	☐ Rapid ■ **Delayed**	☐ Major ■ **Moderate** ☐ Minor	☐ Established ☐ Probable ■ **Suspected** ☐ Possible ☐ Unlikely

Effects PAZOPANIB plasma concentrations may be reduced, decreasing the pharmacologic effects.

Mechanism RIFAMYCINS may increase PAZOPANIB metabolism (CYP3A4).

Management Avoid coadministration of PAZOPANIB and strong CYP3A4 inducers (eg, RIFAMPIN).[1]

Discussion

Coadministration of pazopanib and strong CYP3A4 inducers (eg, rifampin) may decrease pazopanib plasma concentrations and should be avoided.[1] Do not administer pazopanib to long-term users of strong CYP3A4 inducers (eg, rifampin).

The basis for this monograph is information on file with the manufacturer. Published clinical data are needed to further assess this interaction.

[1] *Votrient* [package insert]. Research Triangle Park, NC: GlaxoSmithKline; October 2009.

* Asterisk indicates drugs cited in interaction reports.

Penicillamine — *Aluminum Salts*

Penicillamine	Aluminum Salts	
Penicillamine* (eg, *Cuprimine*)	Aluminum Carbonate (*Basaljel*)	Kaolin
	Aluminum Hydroxide* (eg, *Amphojel*)	Magaldrate (eg, *Riopan*)
	Attapulgite (eg, *Kaopectate* tabs)	Sucralfate (*Carafate*)

Significance	Onset	Severity	Documentation
2	□ Rapid	□ Major	□ Established
	■ **Delayed**	■ **Moderate**	■ **Probable**
		□ Minor	□ Suspected
			□ Possible
			□ Unlikely

Effects PENICILLAMINE's effectiveness may be lessened or negated.

Mechanism Probably by formation of a physical or chemical complex with ALUMINUM, thereby decreasing GI absorption of PENICILLAMINE.

Management Separating dose administration times may prevent problems. If necessary, tailor the dose of PENICILLAMINE accordingly during coadministration therapy with ALUMINUM SALTS.

Discussion

In six healthy males, the kinetic profile of penicillamine was investigated after a single 500 mg dose of penicillamine: After an overnight fast; after a standard breakfast; after 300 mg ferrous sulfate (eg, *Mol-Iron*); and after 30 mL of aluminum and magnesium hydroxide and simethicone (*Maalox Plus*).[1] This was done in a randomized, crossover design. The mean peak plasma concentrations of total penicillamine were markedly decreased to 52%, 35% and 66% as compared with the fasting period. In another study, four healthy subjects each received penicillamine 500 mg under three different treatment plans, A) after an overnight fast, B) fasting but immediately following 30 mL of aluminum and magnesium hydroxide and simethicone (*Aludrox*), C) fasting but immediately following 7.06 g of sodium bicarbonate. The time to achieve maximum concentration was shorter for both A and B groups with B significantly smaller than other treatment plans.[2]

It is suggested that chelation is the predominant cause of reduced penicillamine absorption when given with antacids containing polyvalent metal ions.

[1] Osman MA, et al. *Clin Pharmacol Ther.* 1983;33:465. [2] Ifan A, et al. *Biopharm Drug Disp.* 1986;7:401.

* Asterisk indicates drugs cited in interaction reports. Based on pharmacologic and pharmacokinetic considerations, similar interactions may occur with other drugs that are listed.

Penicillamine — *Chloroquine*

Penicillamine* (eg, *Cuprimine*)	Chloroquine* (*Aralen*)

Significance	Onset	Severity	Documentation
4	☐ Rapid	☐ Major	☐ Established
	■ **Delayed**	■ **Moderate**	☐ Probable
		☐ Minor	☐ Suspected
			■ **Possible**
			☐ Unlikely

Effects The pharmacologic and toxic effects of PENICILLAMINE may be increased.

Mechanism Unknown.

Management Based on currently available data, no special precautions appear necessary.

Discussion

The pharmacokinetic effects of coadministration of penicillamine with chloroquine were studied in six patients with rheumatoid arthritis.[1] Patients received penicillamine 250 mg daily for at least 3 months. Coadministration of a single dose of chloroquine phosphate 250 mg significantly increased the area under the penicillamine plasma concentration-time curve from a mean of 1.54 hr•mcg/mL to 2.34 hr•mcg/mL ($P < 0.01$).

Additional studies are needed to determine the mechanism and clinical significance of this potential interaction.

[1] Seideman P, et al. *J Rheumatol.* 1989;16:473.

* Asterisk indicates drugs cited in interaction reports.

Penicillamine — *Food*

Penicillamine* (eg, *Cuprimine*)	Food*

Significance	Onset	Severity	Documentation
2	☐ Rapid	☐ Major	☐ Established
	■ **Delayed**	■ **Moderate**	☐ Probable
		☐ Minor	■ **Suspected**
			☐ Possible
			☐ Unlikely

Effects The therapeutic effectiveness of PENICILLAMINE may be decreased by food.

Mechanism Decreased GI absorption of PENICILLAMINE possibly due to formation of complexes with certain dietary components and increased inactivation of the drug in the GI tract.

Management Administer PENICILLAMINE on an empty stomach, at least one hour before meals or two hours after meals, and at least one hour apart from any other drug, food or milk.

Discussion

Investigation have shown that plasma levels of penicillamine are reduced when the drug is taken after meals.[1,2] In a randomized crossover study of six healthy volunteers, the absorption of a single 500 mg dose of penicillamine was studied after an overnight fast and after a standard breakfast.[3] Compared to the fasting control period, the mean cumulative relative fraction of penicillamine absorbed was 52% after food.

By administering penicillamine at least 1 hour before or 2 hours after food, it should be possible to avoid significant reductions in absorption of the drug.

[1] Bergstrom RF, et al. *Clin Pharmacol Ther.* 1981;30:404.

[2] Schuna A, et al. *J Rheumatol.* 1983;10:95.

[3] Osman MA, et al. *Clin Pharmacol Ther.* 1983;33:465.

* Asterisk indicates drugs cited in interaction reports.

Penicillamine — *Indomethacin*

Penicillamine* (eg, *Cuprimine*)	Indomethacin* (*Indocin*)

Significance	Onset	Severity	Documentation
4	□ Rapid	□ Major	□ Established
	■ **Delayed**	■ **Moderate**	□ Probable
		□ Minor	□ Suspected
			■ **Possible**
			□ Unlikely

Effects The pharmacologic and toxic effects of PENICILLAMINE may be increased.

Mechanism Unknown.

Management Based on currently available data, no special precautions appear necessary.

Discussion

The pharmacokinetic effects of coadministration of penicillamine with indomethacin were studied in six patients with rheumatiod arthritis.[1] Patients received penicillamine 250 mg daily for at least 3 months. Coadministration of a single dose of 50 mg indomethacin significantly increased the area under the concentration-time curve from a mean of 1.54 hr•mcg/mL to 2.09 hr•mcg/mL ($P < 0.05$).

Additional studies are needed to determine the mechanism and clinical significance of this potential interaction.

[1] Seidman P, et al. *J Rheumatol.* 1989;16:473.

* Asterisk indicates drugs cited in interaction reports.

Penicillamine — *Iron Salts*

Penicillamine	Iron Salts	
Penicillamine* (eg, *Cuprimine*)	Ferrous Fumarate* (eg, *Femiron*)	Ferrous Sulfate* (eg, *Mol-Iron*)
	Ferrous Gluconate (eg, *Fergon*)	Iron Polysaccharide (eg, *Hytinic*)

Significance	Onset	Severity	Documentation
2	☐ Rapid ■ **Delayed**	☐ Major ■ **Moderate** ☐ Minor	☐ Established ■ **Probable** ☐ Suspected ☐ Possible ☐ Unlikely

Effects PENICILLAMINE's effectiveness may be lessened.

Mechanism Marked reduction in GI absorption of PENICILLAMINE with IRON SALTS may be due to chelation.

Management Take PENICILLAMINE on an empty stomach, between meals with water, or unaccompanied by IRON preparations.

Discussion

Plasma levels of penicillamine are inhibited by ferrous salts when coadministered.[1-4] In a controlled study of 5 healthy subjects, a single oral dose of 250 mg/day panicillamine and 90 mg of ferrous sulfate was administered.[1] The mean 24-hour urinary copper extraction (μg) was 16 after iron, 163.5 after penicillamine and 45.4 after both were given together in the same dose. In a randomized, crossover study of six healthy men, plasma levels of penicillamine were reduced to 35% of those from the fasting dose after ferrous sulfate.[3] One study also reported a decrease in intestinal resorption of penicillamine, thereby resulting in a 70% reduction of peak penicillamine plasma levels and 48-hour urinary excretion, after a single 1 g oral dose of penicillamine and 600 mg ferrous fumarate.[4]

The clinical significance of this interaction is apparent in patients with Wilson's disease but remain undetermined in the patient with rheumatiod arthritis.

[1] Lyle WH. *Lancet.* 1976;2:420.
[2] Lyle WH, et al. *Proc Roy Soc Med.* 1977;70 (suppl 3):48.
[3] Osman MA, et al. *Clin Pharmacol Ther.* 1983;33:465.
[4] Muijsers AO, et al. *Arthritis Rheum.* 1984;27:1362.

* Asterisk indicates drugs cited in interaction reports. Based on pharmacologic and pharmacokinetic considerations, similar interactions may occur with other drugs that are listed.

Penicillamine — *Magnesium Salts*

Penicillamine	Magnesium Salts	
Penicillamine* (eg, *Cuprimine*)	Magaldrate (eg, *Riopan*)	Mg Hydroxide* (*Milk of Magnesia*)
	Mg Carbonate (eg, *Marblen*)	Mg Oxide (eg, *Mag-Ox*)
	Mg Citrate (eg, *Citroma*)	Mg Sulfate (*Epsom Salts*)
	Mg Gluconate	Mg Trisilicate

Significance	Onset	Severity	Documentation
3	☐ Rapid	☐ Major	☐ Established
	■ **Delayed**	☐ Moderate	☐ Probable
		■ **Minor**	■ **Suspected**
			☐ Possible
			☐ Unlikely

Effects Pharmacologic actions of PENICILLAMINE may be attenuated.

Mechanism Poor GI absorption of PENICILLAMINE may be a result of chelation or adsorption with MAGNESIUM ions.

Management Take PENICILLAMINE on an empty stomach or between meals with water and unaccompanied by MAGNESIUM SALTS.

Discussion

Plasma levels of penicillamine, urinary recovery of total penicillamine (reduced and oxidized) and urinary excretion of copper were examined in a randomized crossover study of six healthy subjects.[1] Single oral doses of 500 mg penicillamine were administered after A) an overnight fast, B) a standard breakfast, C) 300 mg ferrous sulfate, or D) 30 mL antacid (*Maalox Plus*, contains aluminum hydroxide, magnesium hydroxide and simethicone). Penicillamine levels were reduced to 52%, 35% and 66% of those from the fasting dose, after food, ferrous salts and antacid, respectively. Urinary excretion of copper correlated closely with plasma levels of reduced penicillamine and urinary excretion of total penicillamine ranging from 0.58 mg for treatment A and 0.36 for treatment D. No differentiation was attempted between the aluminum or magnesium component of the antacid as the cause of this interaction. In another in vitro study, a small binding of penicillamine to colloidal aluminum hydroxide-magnesium hydroxide antacid was reported.[2] The degree of adsorption of penicillamine to antacid was low and clinically insignificant.

Data conflict. The clinical significance of this interaction has yet to be defined.

[1] Osman MA, et al. *Clin Pharmacol Ther.* 1983;33:465. [2] Allgayer H, et al. *Arznelm-Forsch.* 1983;33:417.

* Asterisk indicates drugs cited in interaction reports. Based on pharmacologic and pharmacokinetic considerations, similar interactions may occur with other drugs that are listed.

Penicillamine — *Probenecid*

Penicillamine* (eg, *Cuprimine*)	Probenecid*

Significance	Onset	Severity	Documentation
4	☐ Rapid	☐ Major	☐ Established
	■ **Delayed**	■ **Moderate**	☐ Probable
		☐ Minor	☐ Suspected
			■ **Possible**
			☐ Unlikely

Effects — Pharmacologic effects of PENICILLAMINE may be attenuated by PROBENECID.

Mechanism — Possibly due to a reduced PENICILLAMINE metabolite excretion through the urine.

Management — For patients with cystinuria, avoid coadministration of PENICILLAMINE and PROBENECID; the use of alternative hypouricemic agents may be therapeutically advantageous.

Discussion

In a single dose study of two cystinuric patients, each received 500 mg penicillamine and probenecid 1 g simultaneously after an overnight fast.[1] Substantial increases in cystine excretion were observed in both patients; decreased excretion of cysteine-penicillamine mixed disulfide (CSSC) and penicillamine-penicillamine disulfide (PSSP) metabolites was observed. Probenecid also decreased the urinary excretion of both penicillamine metabolites in one of five patients with rheumatoid arthritis.

Although data is limited, it appears that coadministration of probenecid is contraindicated in hyperuricemic cystinuric patients. What this means for patients with rheumatoid arthritis or Wilson's disease has yet to be established.

[1] Yu T-F, et al. *J Rheumatol.* 1984;11:467.

* Asterisk indicates drugs cited in interaction reports.

Penicillins — Allopurinol

Penicillins	Allopurinol
Ampicillin* (eg, *Omnipen*)	Allopurinol* (eg, *Zyloprim*)

Significance	Onset	Severity	Documentation
2	□ Rapid	□ Major	□ Established
	■ **Delayed**	■ **Moderate**	□ Probable
		□ Minor	■ **Suspected**
			□ Possible
			□ Unlikely

Effects The rate of AMPICILLIN-induced skin rash appears much higher when coadministered with ALLOPURINOL than with either drug by itself.

Mechanism ALLUPURINOL may potentiate AMPICILLIN rashes through an unknown mechanism.

Management Be alert for allergic-type rashes. If a skin rash appears, consider lowering the dose of ALLOPURINOL or alternative drug therapy.

Discussion

Epidemiologic studies suggest that allopurinol may enhance the allergenicity of ampicillin.[1,4] The incidence of skin rash in patients receiving combination therapy is approximately 13.9% to 22.4% as compared with ampicillin 5.9% to 7.5% or allopurinol 2.1% administered alone. However, it is not clear whether the potentiation is secondary to hyperuricemia or allopurinol when data on uric acid levels were lacking. A significantly increased occurrence of penicillin allergy was also confirmed in hyperuricemic patients without symptoms. A higher but not statistically significant increase was found in reaction to other antibiotics in the same group of patients.[2] In another report, two cases of toxic epidermal necrolysis have been reported when ampicillin was coadministered with allopurinol.[3]

[1] Boston Collaborative Drug Surveillance Program. *N Engl J Med.* 1972;286:505.
[2] Fessel WJ, et al. *Arch Intern Med.* 1973;132:44.
[3] Ellman MH, et al. *Arch Dermatol.* 1975;111:986.
[4] Jick H, et al. *J Clin Pharmacol.* 1981;21:456.

* Asterisk indicates drugs cited in interaction reports.

Penicillins × *Amiloride*

Amoxicillin* (eg, *Amoxil*)	Amiloride* (*Midamor*)

Significance	Onset	Severity	Documentation
3	□ Rapid ■ **Delayed**	□ Major □ Moderate ■ **Minor**	□ Established □ Probable ■ **Suspected** □ Possible □ Unlikely

Effects The therapeutic activity of AMOXICILLIN may be reduced.

Mechanism AMILORIDE may reduce the absorption of AMOXICILLIN, possibly by interfering with the sodium-hydrogen exchanger.

Management Observe the clinical response of the patient. If a decrease in antibiotic efficacy is suspected, a larger dose of AMOXICILLIN may be needed.

Discussion

The effects of amiloride on the absorption of amoxicillin were studied in eight healthy male volunteers.[1] Each subject received oral administration of 1 g amoxicillin suspension 2 hours after receiving a single oral dose of amiloride with water or water alone. The same procedure was followed with 1 g of amoxicillin IV. Amiloride did not affect the disposition of IV amoxicillin. However, the bioavailability of oral amoxicillin was decreased from 74% to 54% by administration of oral amiloride, the peak serum concentration of amoxicillin was decreased by 25%, and the time to reach peak serum concentration was delayed by 60%.

[1] Westphal JF, et al. *Clin Pharmacol Ther.* 1995;57:257.

* Asterisk indicates drugs cited in interaction reports.

Penicillins		***Aminoglycosides***
Penicillin V* (eg, *Beepen VK*)		Neomycin* (eg, *Mycifradin*)

Significance	Onset	Severity	Documentation
5	□ Rapid ■ **Delayed**	□ Major □ Moderate ■ **Minor**	□ Established □ Probable □ Suspected ■ **Possible** □ Unlikely

Effects The therapeutic activity of oral PENICILLIN may be reduced.

Mechanism GI absorption of oral PENICILLIN may be impaired by NEOMYCIN.

Management Avoid combination therapy if possible. When necessary, tailor the dose of PENICILLIN as needed.

Discussion

The effect of orally administered neomycin 12 g/day on the GI absorption of a single dose 400,000 units penicillin V was studied in five healthy subjects for a 7-day period.[1] A significant reduction of 55% penicillin serum concentration and a decrease of 58% in 24-hour urinary recovery were reported. Reports of a similar interaction between other oral penicillins and aminoglycosides are lacking. The clinical relevance of this interaction remains to be determined.

[1] Cheng SH, et al. *N Engl J Med.* 1962;267:1296.

* Asterisk indicates drugs cited in interaction reports.

Penicillins — *Chloramphenicol*

Penicillins		Chloramphenicol
Amoxicillin (eg, *Amoxil*)	Oxacillin	Chloramphenicol (eg, *Chloromycetin*)
Ampicillin* (eg, *Principen*)	Penicillin G* (eg, *Pfizerpen*)	
Carbenicillin (*Geocillin*)	Penicillin V (eg, *Veetids*)	
Dicloxacillin	Piperacillin (*Pipracil*)	
Nafcillin	Ticarcillin (*Ticar*)	

Significance	Onset	Severity	Documentation
4	□ Rapid	□ Major	□ Established
	■ **Delayed**	■ **Moderate**	□ Probable
		□ Minor	□ Suspected
			■ **Possible**
			□ Unlikely

Effects Synergistic effects may develop in the treatment of certain microorganisms, but antagonism has also been reported in animal studies.

Mechanism Obscure and not fully established.

Management No clinical interventions appear to be required.

Discussion

Early animal studies and laboratory data showed antagonistic effects between penicillin and chloramphenico.[1-2] In a large-scale clinical study of 268 patients (2 months to over 60 years of age) with acute bacterial meningitis, a higher mortality rate (11.4%), was reported in the ampicillin plus chloramphenicol group compared with 4.1% when administered ampicillin alone.[3] Separate studies investigated bacterial meningitis or severe pneumonia in children receiving either chloramphenicol IM injection alone or chloramphenicol plus penicillin IV injection.[4,5] Sequential analysis showed no difference in mortality between the 2 treatment plans. Conversely, combination synergisms have been reported.[6,7] Simultaneous administration of high-dose penicillin was also reported to increase the serum level of nonglucuronidated chloramphenicol in children of various age groups.[8,9]

Clinical data, though limited, have convinced many clinicians to initiate combination therapy of ampicillin and chloramphenicol in view of the increasing resistance to ampicillin among *Haemophilus influenzae*.[10] The advent of potent, broad-spectrum cephalosporins has been advocated as an alternative to ampicillin and chloramphenicol combination therapy in meningitis.

1 Jawetz E, et al. *Arch Intern Med.* 1951;87:349.
2 Wallace JF, et al. *J Lab Clin Med.* 1967;70:408.
3 Wehrle PF, et al. *Ann N Y Acad Sci.* 1967;145:488.
4 Shann F, et al. *Lancet.* 1985;2:681.
5 Shann F, et al. *Lancet.* 1985;2:684.
6 Gjessing HC, et al. *Br J Vener Dis.* 1967;43:133.
7 De Ritis F, et al. *Br Med J.* 1972;4:17.
8 Windorfer A. *Z Kinderheilkd.* 1972;112:79.
9 Windorfer A, et al. *Eur J Pediatr.* 1977;124:129.
10 Whitby M, et al. *Drugs.* 1986;31:266.

* Asterisk indicates drugs cited in interaction reports. Based on pharmacologic and pharmacokinetic considerations, similar interactions may occur with other drugs that are listed.

Penicillins | **Erythromycin**

Penicillins		Erythromycin
Amoxicillin (eg, *Amoxil*)	Oxacillin	Erythromycin* (eg, *Ery-Tab*)
Ampicillin* (eg, *Principen*)	Penicillin G* (eg, *Pfizerpen*)	
Carbenicillin (*Geocillin*)	Penicillin V* (eg, *Veetids*)	
Cloxacillin	Piperacillin (*Pipracil*)	
Dicloxacillin	Ticarcillin (*Ticar*)	
Nafcillin		

Significance	Onset	Severity	Documentation
5	□ Rapid	□ Major	□ Established
	■ **Delayed**	□ Moderate	□ Probable
		■ **Minor**	□ Suspected
			■ **Possible**
			□ Unlikely

Effects Therapeutic effects of a PENICILLIN and ERYTHROMYCIN coadministration are unpredictable.

Mechanism Unknown.

Management No clinical interventions appear required.

Discussion

In vitro tests and clinical studies have demonstrated both antagonism and synergism with combined use of penicillin and erythromycin.[1-10] In a study involving 315 cases of uncomplicated scarlatina, patients were treated with penicillin V, erythromycin, or a combination of the two.[1] Based on the duration of fever and of positive cultures, the combination therapy showed inferior effects as compared with the other groups. Other in vitro studies also reported the antagonistic effects of erythromycin combination with ampicillin against various pathogenic organisms of the respiratory tract[9] and with penicillin or ampicillin against *Listeria monocytogenes*.[10] In contrast, synergistic effects have been demonstrated by erythromycin and ampicillin against in vitro *Nocardia asteroides* and in pulmonary nocardiosis.[6,7] Similar synergism between erythromycin and penicillin G against *Staphylococcus aureus* also has been reported.[2,3,8]

Data conflict. Based on available data, synergistic effects of combined penicillins and erythromycin therapy are more convincing when bactericidal effects are desirable.

[1] Strom J. *Antibiot Chemother.* 1961;11:694.
[2] Herrel WE, et al. *Antibiot Chemother.* 1961;11:727.
[3] Oswald EJ, et al. *Antimicrob Agents Chemother.* 1961;904.
[4] Manten A, et al. *Chemioterapia.* 1964;8:21.
[5] Kabins SA. *JAMA.* 1972;219:206.
[6] Bach MC, et al. *JAMA.* 1973;224:1378.
[7] Finland M, et al. *Antimicrob Agents Chemother.* 1974;5:344.
[8] Allen NE, et al. *Antimicrob Agents Chemother.* 1978;13:849.
[9] Cohn JR, et al. *Antimicrob Agents Chemother.* 1980;18:872.
[10] Penn RL, et al. *Antimicrob Agents Chemother.* 1982;22:289.

* Asterisk indicates drugs cited in interaction reports. Based on pharmacologic and pharmacokinetic considerations, similar interactions may occur with other drugs that are listed.

Penicillins — *Food*

Penicillins		Food
Ampicillin* (eg, *Omnipen*)	Nafcillin* (eg, *Unipen*)	Food*
Carbenicillin Indanyl Sodium* (*Geocillin*)	Oxacillin* (eg, *Prostaphlin*)	
Cloxacillin* (eg, *Tegopen*)	Penicillin G*	
Dicloxacillin* (eg, *Dynapen*)		

Significance	Onset	Severity	Documentation
2	□ Rapid	□ Major	□ Established
	■ **Delayed**	■ **Moderate**	□ Probable
		□ Minor	■ **Suspected**
			□ Possible
			□ Unlikely

Effects Antimicrobial effectiveness of the interacting PENICILLINS may be reduced by food.

Mechanism Food may delay or reduce the GI absorption of the interacting PENICILLINS.

Management Administer the interacting PENICILLINS at least 1 hour before or 2 hours after meals.

Discussion

The influence of food on the GI absorption of the penicillin derivatives has been the subject of a number of studies. Although the results of some studies are conflicting, the available information is sufficient to establish guidelines for the administration of oral penicillin.

Penicillin G is highly susceptible to the action of gastric acid and is more rapidly inactivated when given with food. Ampicillin administration with food has resulted in a significant decrease in the absorption and peak serum concentrations.[5,6] Oxacillin absorption was delayed or reduced when given immediately after a meal.[3] The absorption of cloxacillin, dicloxacillin and nafcillin also appears to be delayed by food. Little information is available regarding the influence of food on the absorption of carbenicillin indanyl sodium. In the absence of data, give this agent on an empty stomach. A potential exists for food to delay and reduce the absorption of each of the penicillin derivatives discussed. To achieve optimal absorption, give these agents at least 1 hour before or 2 hours after meals. Food may reduce and delay peak penicillin V serum levels.[1,2] However, blood levels of penicillin V are only slightly higher when the drug is given on an empty stomach, and it can be given with meals without a loss of efficacy. Peak serum levels of amoxicillin (eg, *Amoxil*) have been reported to be the same when the drug is given in both fasting and nonfasting states.[4] Food also has been reported to reduce the absorption of this antibiotic.[6] Amoxicillin is well absorbed and may be given without regard to meals.

[1] McCarthy CG, et al. *NEJM.* 1960;263:315.
[2] Cronk GA, et al. *Am J Med Sci.* 1960;240:219.
[3] Klein JO, et al. *Am J Med Sci.* 1963;245:399.
[4] Neu HC. *J Infect Dis.* 1974;129:S123.
[5] Neuvonen PJ, et al. *J Int Med Res.* 1977;5:71.
[6] Welling PG, et al. *J Pharm Sci.* 1977;66:549.

* Asterisk indicates drugs cited in interaction reports.

Penicillins | **Khat**

Amoxicillin* (eg, *Amoxil*) | Ampicillin* (eg, *Omnipen*) | Khat*

Significance	Onset	Severity	Documentation
4	☐ Rapid	☐ Major	☐ Established
	■ **Delayed**	■ **Moderate**	☐ Probable
		☐ Minor	☐ Suspected
			■ **Possible**
			☐ Unlikely

Effects Antimicrobial effectiveness of the interacting PENICILLIN may be reduced.

Mechanism Possible delayed or reduced GI absorption of the interacting PENICILLIN.

Management Administration of the interacting PENICILLIN 2 hours after khat chewing does not appear to affect the bioavailability of the antibiotic.

Discussion

Using a crossover design, the effects of khat chewing on the bioavailability of ampicillin and amoxicillin were studied in eight healthy adult male Yemeni volunteers.[1] The percentage of the dose of unchanged ampicillin excreted in the urine, the peak excretion and the time to reach the peak were reduced by khat chewing, except when the antibiotic was administered 2 hours after chewing khat. The decrease in ampicillin bioavailability was greatest when the antibiotic was administered midway through the 4-hour khat chewing session.

Compared with taking amoxicillin alone under fasting conditions, the percentage of the dose of unchanged amoxicillin excreted in the urine and the peak excretion were reduced when amoxicillin was taken midway through the 4-hour khat chewing session. This monograph is presented to illustrate potential unexpected interactions that may occur between medication administration and use or abuse of natural products. The ingredients of khat are not standardized; therefore, it is unclear if the product contains ingredients other than khat that could affect the absorption of interacting penicillins.

[1] Attef OA, et al. *J Antimicrob Chemother.* 1997;39:523.

* Asterisk indicates drugs cited in interaction reports.

Penicillins — *Tetracyclines*

Penicillins		Tetracyclines	
Amoxicillin (eg, *Amoxi*)	Penicillin G* (*Pfizerpen*)	Demeclocycline (eg, *Declomycin*)	Minocycline (eg, *Minocin*)
Ampicillin (eg, *Principen*)	Penicillin V	Doxycycline (eg, *Vibramycin*)	Tetracycline* (eg, *Sumycin*)
Dicloxacillin	Piperacillin		
Nafcillin	Ticarcillin		
Oxacillin			

Significance	Onset	Severity	Documentation
2	☐ Rapid ■ **Delayed**	☐ Major ■ **Moderate** ☐ Minor	☐ Established ☐ Probable ■ **Suspected** ☐ Possible ☐ Unlikely

Effects Pharmacologic and therapeutic action of PENICILLINS could be reduced.

Mechanism The bacteriostatic action of TETRACYCLINES may withhold part of the microorganisms from the bactericidal activity of PENICILLINS.

Management Consider avoiding this combination if at all possible.

Discussion

In vitro data and clinical studies suggest that the bacteriostatic actions of tetracycline derivatives may impair the bactericidal effects of penicillins.[1-5] In a study of 43 patients with pneumococcal meningitis, the fatality rate was lower among those receiving penicillin alone (30%) than those receiving penicillin plus chlortetracycline† (79%).[2] In another study of 315 patients with uncomplicated scarlatina, the combination of penicillin and chlortetracycline exhibited no improvement compared with chlortetracycline alone based on the occurrence of sinusitis and otitis.[4] Researchers studied 36 adults with pneumococcal meningitis; the mortality rate for those patients treated with penicillin plus a tetracycline derivative was 85% (6 of 7 patients) compared with 33% and 59% mortality rates from patients treated with aqueous procaine penicillin or erythromycin, respectively.[4] Conversely, in a controlled study involving 50 patients with pneumococcal pneumonia, patient response of the group treated with penicillin and chlortetracycline was similar to patient response of a control group treated with penicillin alone.[6]

[1] Gunnison JB, et al. *Proc Soc Exp Biol Med.* 1950;75(2):549.
[2] Lepper MH, et al. *AMA Arch Intern Med.* 1951;88(4):489.
[3] Strom J. *Antibiot Med Clin Ther.* 1955;1(1):6.
[4] Olsson RA, et al. *AMA Ann Intern Med.* 1961;55:545.
[5] Jawetz E. *West J Med.* 1975;123(2):87.
[6] Ahern JJ, et al. *AMA Arch Intern Med.* 1953;91(2):197.

* Asterisk indicates drugs cited in interaction reports. Based on pharmacologic and pharmacokinetic considerations, similar interactions may occur with other drugs that are listed.

† Not available in the United States.

Pentoxifylline | **_Cimetidine_**

Pentoxifylline* (eg, *Trental*)	Cimetidine* (eg, *Tagamet*)

Significance	Onset	Severity	Documentation
3	☐ Rapid	☐ Major	☐ Established
	■ **Delayed**	☐ Moderate	☐ Probable
		■ **Minor**	■ **Suspected**
			☐ Possible
			☐ Unlikely

Effects The pharmacologic effects of PENTOXIFYLLINE may be increased.

Mechanism Inhibition of hepatic microsomal enzymes by CIMETIDINE may result in decreased PENTOXIFYLLINE metabolism.

Management No special precautions are necessary. If an interaction is suspected, adjust the dose of PENTOXIFYLLINE accordingly or select a histamine H_2 antagonist that does not affect metabolism.

Discussion

A randomized, crossover investigation was conducted in 10 healthy men to determine if cimetidine alters pentoxifylline metabolism.[1] The study consisted of 2 phases separated by 3 weeks: 1) each subject was randomly assigned to receive pentoxifylline 400 mg every 8 hours alone or with cimetidine 300 mg 4 times daily for 6 days; 2) each patient was subsequently crossed over to receive the alternative therapy in an identical fashion to the first phase. During cimetidine and pentoxifylline coadministration, the apparent oral clearance of pentoxifylline was reduced by 21.5%, and the average steady-state plasma concentrations were increased by 27.4%. Both of these changes were statistically significant ($P < 0.02$ and $P < 0.05$, respectively). In addition, cimetidine significantly ($P < 0.05$) increased the pentoxifylline AUC at steady-state by 26.2%. While there was considerable intersubject variability, pentoxifylline plasma levels approximately doubled in 2 patients while 1 subject experienced a slight decrease. The AUC of 2 metabolites of pentoxifylline increased significantly ($P < 0.02$ and $P < 0.05$), and 1 decreased slightly.

Additional studies are needed to determine the clinical importance of this interaction. Famotidine (eg, *Pepcid*) and nizatidine (eg, *Axid*) is not expected to affect the metabolism of pentoxifylline.

[1] Mauro VF, et al. *J Clin Pharmacol.* 1988;28(7):649.

* Asterisk indicates drugs cited in interaction reports.

Phenformin — *Beta-Blockers*

Phenformin	Beta-Blockers	
Phenformin*†	Acebutolol (eg, *Sectral*)	Nadolol (eg, *Corgard*)
	Atenolol (eg, *Tenormin*)	Penbutolol (*Levatol*)
	Betaxolol (*Kerlone*)	Pindolol (eg, *Visken*)
	Carteolol (*Cartrol*)	Propranolol* (eg, *Inderal*)
	Esmolol (eg, *Brevibloc*)	Timolol (eg, *Blocadren*)
	Metoprolol (eg, *Lopressor*)	

Significance	Onset	Severity	Documentation
4	□ Rapid	□ Major	□ Established
	■ **Delayed**	■ **Moderate**	□ Probable
		□ Minor	□ Suspected
			■ **Possible**
			□ Unlikely

Effects The therapeutic effects of PHENFORMIN may be enhanced and hypoglycemic symptoms may be masked by BETA-BLOCKERS.

Mechanism Unknown.

Management Monitor blood glucose and adjust the PHENFORMIN dose as needed.

Discussion

Laboratory data and case reports suggest the interference of propranolol with insulin.[1-7] Based on pharmacologic activity of phenformin, a similar interaction is anticipated. Beta-adrenergic receptor blockade by propranolol can obscure the reactive symptoms of hypoglycemia and may dampen plasma glucose rebound.[1,3] Hypoglycemia has not been shown to be associated with the use of atenolol.[7]

1 Abramson EA, et al. *Lancet.* 1966;2(7478):1386.
2 Kotler MN, et al. *Lancet.* 1966;2(7478):1389.
3 Abramson EA, et al. *Diabetes.* 1968;17(3):141.
4 McMurtry RJ. *Ann Intern Med.* 1974;80(5):669.
5 Molnar GW, et al. *Clin Pharmacol Ther.* 1974;15(5):490.
6 Lloyd-Mostyn RH, et al. *Lancet.* 1975;1(7918):1213.
7 Deacon SP, et al. *Br Med J.* 1976;2(6030):272.

* Asterisk indicates drugs cited in interaction reports. Based on pharmacologic and pharmacokinetic considerations, similar interactions may occur with other drugs that are listed.
†Not available in the US.

Phenformin — *Ethanol*

Phenformin*†	Ethanol* (Alcohol, Ethyl Alcohol)

Significance	Onset	Severity	Documentation
2	☐ Rapid	☐ Major	☐ Established
	■ **Delayed**	■ **Moderate**	■ **Probable**
		☐ Minor	☐ Suspected
			☐ Possible
			☐ Unlikely

Effects Pharmacologic effects of PHENFORMIN may be increased by ETHANOL. The rate of occurrence of hyperlacticacidemia may be enhanced.

Mechanism Possibly caused by impaired gluconeogenesis, increased lactate production, and decreased lactate utilization.

Management Avoid excessive ETHANOL ingestion in PHENFORMIN-treated patients.

Discussion

Experimental and clinical hypoglycemias have been reported in healthy patients and in patients with abnormal carbohydrate metabolism after acute ethanol ingestion.[1-7] Increased incidence of lactic acidosis has also been demonstrated by ethanol-phenformin synergism,[8,9] but the exact mechanism of this interaction has not been elucidated. Based on similar pharmacologic considerations, hypoglycemia is expected with concomitant use of phenformin and ethanol.

1 Field JB, et al. *J Clin Invest.* 1963;42:497.
2 Freinkel N, et al. *J Clin Invest.* 1963;42(7):1112.
3 Davidson MB, et al. *N Engl J Med.* 1966;275(16):886.
4 Arky RA, et al. *JAMA.* 1968;206(3):575.
5 Johnson HK, et al. *Am J Med.* 1968;45(1):98.
6 Shirriffs GG, et al. *Br Med J.* 1970;3(5721):506.
7 Isaacs P. *Br Med J.* 1970;3(5725):773.
8 Lacher J, et al. *Clin Pharmacol Ther.* 1966;7(4):477.
9 Kreisberg RA, et al. *J Clin Endocrinol Metab.* 1972;34(1):29.

* Asterisk indicates drugs cited in interaction reports.
†Not available in the US.

Phenmetrazine — *Barbiturates*

Phenmetrazine	Barbiturates
Phenmetrazine*†	Amobarbital* (eg, *Amytal*)

Significance	Onset	Severity	Documentation
4	☐ Rapid	☐ Major	☐ Established
	■ **Delayed**	■ **Moderate**	☐ Probable
		☐ Minor	☐ Suspected
			■ **Possible**
			☐ Unlikely

Effects Decreased anorexic effect of PHENMETRAZINE.

Mechanism Reduced CNS stimulation.

Management If an interaction is suspected, monitor the patient for loss of anorexiant effect; discontinue the BARBITURATE if necessary.

Discussion

Thirty-nine patients receiving either phenmetrazine 25 mg 3 times daily or phenmetrazine 25 mg 3 times daily with amobarbital 30 mg 3 times daily were studied over a 2-month period.[1] Eighty-two percent of the patients on phenmetrazine alone lost weight compared with 64% of patients on the combination of phenmetrazine and amobarbital. In addition, 7 patients gained weight on the combination. It was concluded that amobarbital reduced the CNS stimulation necessary for full anorexiant action.

[1] Hadler AJ. *Curr Ther Res Clin Exp.* 1969;11(12):750.

* Asterisk indicates drugs cited in interaction reports.
†Not available in the US.

Phenothiazines — *Aluminum Salts*

Phenothiazines		Aluminum Salts	
Chlorpromazine* (eg, *Thorazine*)	Promethazine (eg, *Phenergan*)	Aluminum Carbonate (*Basaljel*)	Kaolin*†
Fluphenazine* (eg, *Prolixin*)	Thiethylperazine (*Torecan*)	Aluminum Hydroxide* (eg, *AlternaGEL*)	Magaldrate (eg, *Riopan*)
Methotrimeprazine (*Levoprome*)	Thioridazine*	Attapulgite* (eg, *Kaopectate*)	
Perphenazine	Triflupromazine* (*Vesprin*)		
Prochlorperazine* (eg, *Compazine*)			

Significance	Onset	Severity	Documentation
5	□ Rapid	□ Major	□ Established
	■ **Delayed**	□ Moderate	□ Probable
		■ **Minor**	□ Suspected
			■ **Possible**
			□ Unlikely

Effects Pharmacologic and therapeutic action of PHENOTHIAZINES could be reduced.

Mechanism The formation of insoluble physical or chemical complexes may impair GI absorption of PHENOTHIAZINES.

Management Space the administration of ANTACIDS at least 1 hour before or 2 hours after CHLORPROMAZINE ingestion. An ionic antacid (ie, calcium carbonate) may be an alternative.

Discussion

The adsorption interaction of activated attapulgite alone or plus pectin on the bioavailability of promazine (not available in the US) has been reported in in vivo and in vitro studies.[1,2] In 10 patients, an aluminum-magnesium hydroxide antacid (*Aludrox*), acting as a physical absorbent coadministered with chlorpromazine, decreased the urinary chlorpromazine efficacy.[2,3] In another study of 6 psychiatric patients, plasma chlorpromazine levels were reduced following the use of a gel-type antacid (*Gelusil*) compared with chlorpromazine given alone.[4] Deterioration of therapeutic efficacy, described as relapsed psychosis, has been reported in a patient treated with chlorpromazine and liquid antacid, simultaneously.[5] In contrast, research showed that there was no alteration of chlorpromazine blood levels when 16 patients were given a magnesium-aluminum hydroxide antacid.[6] More controlled studies are needed to clarify the exact role of antacids on the bioavailability and clinical efficacy of phenothiazines.

1 Sorby DL. *J Pharm Sci.* 1965;54:677.
2 Sorby DL, et al. *J Pharm Sci.* 1966;55:504.
3 Forrest FM, et al. *Biol Psychiatry.* 1970;2:53.
4 Fann WE, et al. *J Clin Pharmacol.* 1973;13:388.
5 Fann WE, et al. *Clin Pharmacol Ther.* 1973;14:135.
6 Pinell OC, et al. *Clin Pharmacol Ther.* 1978;23:125.

* Asterisk indicates drugs cited in interaction reports. Based on pharmacologic and pharmacokinetic considerations, similar interactions may occur with other drugs that are listed.
†Not available in the US.

Phenothiazines	*Antiarrhythmic Agents*	
Thioridazine*	Amiodarone* (eg, *Cordarone*)	Procainamide* (eg, *Procanbid*)
	Bretylium*	Quinidine*
	Disopyramide* (eg, *Norpace*)	Sotalol* (eg, *Betapace*)

Significance	Onset	Severity	Documentation
1	☐ Rapid	■ **Major**	☐ Established
	■ **Delayed**	☐ Moderate	☐ Probable
		☐ Minor	■ **Suspected**
			☐ Possible
			☐ Unlikely

Effects The risk of life-threatening cardiac arrhythmias, including torsades de pointes, may be increased.

Mechanism Possibly synergistic or additive prolongation of the corrected QT (QTc) interval.

Management THIORIDAZINE is contraindicated in patients receiving certain ANTIARRHYTHMIC AGENTS.

Discussion

Sudden, unexplained deaths have been reported in patients receiving drugs that prolong the QTc interval. Do not use thioridazine with other agents that prolong the QTc interval. Thioridazine causes dose-related prolongation of the QTc interval, and other drugs that prolong the QTc interval (eg, amiodarone, sotalol)[1] have been associated with fatal arrhythmias.[2] In addition to other drugs that prolong the QTc interval, certain factors may increase the risk of occurrence of torsades de pointes and sudden death in association with thioridazine, including bradycardia, hypokalemia, drugs that reduce the clearance of thioridazine, and congenital prolongation of the QTc interval.

The basis for this monograph is information on file with the manufacturer. Because of the seriousness of the cardiac problems, clinical evaluation of this interaction in humans is not likely to be forthcoming.

[1] Thomas M, et al. *Br J Clin Pharmacol.* 1996;41:77.

[2] Product information. Thioridazine (*Mellaril*). Novartis Pharmaceutical Corporation. 2000.

* Asterisk indicates drugs cited in interaction reports.

Phenothiazines — *Anticholinergics*

Phenothiazines		Anticholinergics	
Chlorpromazine* (eg, *Thorazine*)	Promethazine (eg, *Phenergan*)	Atropine (*Sal-Tropine*)	Orphenadrine* (eg, *Orphengesic*)
Fluphenazine (eg, *Prolixin*)	Thiethylperazine (*Torecan*)	Belladonna	Oxybutynin (eg, *Ditropan*)
Methotrimeprazine (*Levoprome*)	Thioridazine*	Benztropine* (eg, *Cogentin*)	Procyclidine* (*Kemadrin*)
Perphenazine*	Trifluoperazine	Biperiden (*Akineton*)	Propantheline (eg, *Pro-Banthine*)
Prochlorperazine (eg, *Compazine*)		Clidinium (*Quarzan*)	Scopolamine (eg, *Scopace*)
		Dicyclomine (eg, *Bentyl*)	Trihexyphenidyl* (eg, *Artane*)
		Hyoscyamine (eg, *Anaspaz*)	
		Mepenzolate (*Cantil*)	

Significance	Onset	Severity	Documentation
2	☐ Rapid	☐ Major	☐ Established
	■ **Delayed**	■ **Moderate**	☐ Probable
		☐ Minor	■ **Suspected**
			☐ Possible
			☐ Unlikely

Effects Therapeutic effects of PHENOTHIAZINES may be decreased by centrally-acting ANTICHOLINERGICS.

Mechanism ANTICHOLINERGICS probably antagonize PHENOTHIAZINES by direct CNS pathways involving cholinergic mechanisms. Acceleration of PHENOTHIAZINE gut metabolism has also been postulated.

Management Individualize the dose of PHENOTHIAZINES as needed.

Discussion

Data conflict. An increase in anticholinergic side effects including adynamic ileus, hyperpyrexia, and neurological deficits is reported experientially and clinically.[1,3,4,6,8] Hypoglycemic coma developed in a 53-year-old woman treated with chlorpromazine and orphenadrine.[2] The hypoglycemia rapidly responded to glucose and stopped when combination therapy was discontinued. In addition to the beneficial effect of alleviating extrapyramidal symptoms of neuroleptics, the therapeutic effects of anticholinergic agents used to treat Parkinson's disease may be antagonized as reflected in deterioration of social behavior and cognitive functions.[9] A decrease in the plasma level of oral phenothiazines was reported.[5,7,10,11,12] Higher chlorpromazine levels have occurred with trihexyphenidyl.[13]

1 Gershon S, et al. *Clin Pharmacol Ther.* 1965;6:749.
2 Buckle RM, et al. *Br Med J.* 1967;4:599.
3 Warnes H, et al. *Can Med Assoc J.* 1967;96:1112.
4 Zelman S, et al. *Am J Psychiatry.* 1970;126:1787.
5 Rivera-Calimlim L, et al. *Clin Pharmacol Ther.* 1973;14:978.
6 Giordano J, et al. *South Med J.* 1975;68:351.
7 Rivera-Calimlim L, et al. *Am J Psychiatry.* 1976;133:646.
8 Mann SC, et al. *Am J Psychiatry.* 1978;135:1097.
9 Singh MM, et al. *Neuropsychobiology.* 1979;5:74.
10 Hansen LB, et al. *Br J Clin Pharmacol.* 1979;7:75.
11 Simpson GM, et al. *Arch Gen Psychiatry.* 1980;37:205.
12 Linnoila M, et al. *Am J Psychiatry.* 1980;137:819.
13 Rockland L, et al. *Can J Psychiatry.* 1990;35:604.

* Asterisk indicates drugs cited in interaction reports. Based on pharmacologic and pharmacokinetic considerations, similar interactions may occur with other drugs that are listed.

Phenothiazines — *Ascorbic Acid*

Phenothiazines	Ascorbic Acid
Fluphenazine* (eg, *Prolixin*)	Ascorbic Acid* (eg, *Cevalin*)

Significance	Onset	Severity	Documentation
5	☐ Rapid	☐ Major	☐ Established
	■ **Delayed**	☐ Moderate	☐ Probable
		■ **Minor**	☐ Suspected
			■ **Possible**
			☐ Unlikely

Effects Pharmacologic and therapeutic action of FLUPHENAZINE could be reduced.

Mechanism Unknown.

Management No clinical interventions appear necessary. Tailor the dose of FLUPHENAZINE as needed.

Discussion

In an isolated case report, a 23-year-old man was treated with oral fluphenazine 15 mg for control of his mania. He was also receiving ascorbic acid (vitamin C) 1 g for ascorbic acid deficiency.[1] His fluphenazine steady-state levels declined steadily from 0.93 to 0.705 ng/mL over 14 days and his clinical response worsened with an increase in irritability and provocative behavior that necessitated discontinuation of ascorbic acid therapy and additional psychotropic medication.

More data is needed to establish the clinical significance of this interaction.

[1] Dysken MW, et al. *JAMA*. 1979;241:2008.

* Asterisk indicates drugs cited in interaction reports.

Phenothiazines — *Barbiturates*

Phenothiazines		Barbiturates	
Acetophenazine	Promazine (eg, *Sparine*)	Amobarbital (eg, *Amytal*)	Pentobarbital (eg, *Nembutal*)
Chlorpromazine* (eg, *Thorazine*)	Promethazine (eg, *Phenergan*)	Aprobarbital (*Alurate*)	Phenobarbital*
Fluphenazine (eg, *Prolixin*)	Thioridazine*	Butabarbital (eg, *Butisol*)	Primidone (eg, *Mysoline*)
Perphenazine	Trifluoperazine	Butalbital	Secobarbital (eg, *Seconal*)
Prochlorperazine (eg, *Compazine*)	Triflupromazine (*Vesprin*)	Mephobarbital (*Mebaral*)	

Significance	Onset	Severity	Documentation
5	□ Rapid	□ Major	□ Established
	■ **Delayed**	□ Moderate	□ Probable
		■ **Minor**	□ Suspected
			■ **Possible**
			□ Unlikely

Effects Pharmacologic effects of PHENOTHIAZINES may be reduced. Plasma levels of BARBITURATES may also be decreased by PHENOTHIAZINES.

Mechanism Possibly due to stimulation of hepatic microsomal enzymes by BARBITURATES.

Management If an interaction is suspected, tailor the dose of PHENOTHIAZINES as needed.

Discussion

Concomitant use of phenobarbital 150 mg/day for 3 weeks resulted in a significant reduction of chlorpromazine plasma levels in 12 psychiatric patients.[5] No overall deterioration of clinical effectiveness was reported, although a reduction of blood pressure and pulse rate were observed in patients treated with combination therapy. This kinetic change was supported by other studies demonstrating reduced serum levels and enhanced renal elimination of chlorpromazine during phenobarbital coadministration.[1-3] Similar plasma level reductions have been reported using mesoridazine,[7] but the influence of phenobarbital on thioridazine has not been clearly defined.[6] One study also reported a substantial reduction of phenobarbital plasma level by 25% when administered with thioridazine 100 to 200 mg/day compared with phenobarbital given alone.[8] Conversely, another study reported that thioridazine did not interfere with phenobarbital plasma levels when given concomitantly with phenytoin (eg, *Dilantin*).[4]

Although data are limited, the influence of barbiturates on the reduction of other phenothiazine blood levels is a distinct possibility.

[1] Dundee JW, et al. *Anesth Analg.* 1958;37:12.
[2] Forrest FM, et al. *Biol Psychiatry.* 1970;2:53.
[3] Curry SH, et al. *Arch Gen Psychiatry.* 1970;22:209.
[4] Siris JH, et al. *NY State J Med.* 1974;9:1554.
[5] Loga S, et al. *Br J Clin Pharmacol.* 1975;2:197.
[6] Ellenor GL, et al. *Res Commun Chem Pathol Pharmacol.* 1978;21:185.
[7] Linnoila M, et al. *Am J Psychiatry.* 1980;137:819.
[8] Gay PE, et al. *Neurology.* 1983;33:1631.

* Asterisk indicates drugs cited in interaction reports. Based on pharmacologic and pharmacokinetic considerations, similar interactions may occur with other drugs that are listed.

Phenothiazines — *Cimetidine*

Chlorpromazine* (eg, *Thorazine*)		Cimetidine* (eg, *Tagamet*)	
Significance	Onset	Severity	Documentation
5	☐ Rapid	☐ Major	☐ Established
	■ **Delayed**	☐ Moderate	☐ Probable
		■ **Minor**	☐ Suspected
			■ **Possible**
			☐ Unlikely

Effects The therapeutic action of CHLORPROMAZINE could be decreased.

Mechanism Reduced GI absorption of CHLORPROMAZINE caused by CIMETIDINE; however, reduced metabolism of CHLORPROMAZINE confounds the assessment.

Management No clinical interventions appear necessary. Tailor the dose of CHLORPROMAZINE as needed.

Discussion

Researchers studied a series of eight patients receiving cimetidine 1 g/day for 7 days and chlorpromazine 75 to 450 mg/day for 3 months to 14 years.[1] Evidence from the urinary excretion data suggested inhibition of chlorpromazine metabolism by cimetidine, but a 36% reduction of steady plasma levels of chlorpromazine during coadministration with cimetidine was suggestive of a decreased absorption mechanism overriding the metabolic change.

No clinical response in correlation with a reduced plasma level of chlorpromazine was reported. Further studies are needed to establish the clinical significance of this interaction.

[1] Howes CA, et al. *Eur J Clin Pharmacol.* 1983;24:99.

* Asterisk indicates drugs cited in interaction reports.

Phenothiazines — *Clonidine*

Chlorpromazine (eg, *Thorazine*)	Fluphenazine* (eg, *Prolixin*)	Clonidine* (eg, *Catapres*)

Significance	Onset	Severity	Documentation
4	■ **Rapid**	☐ Major	☐ Established
	☐ Delayed	■ **Moderate**	☐ Probable
		☐ Minor	☐ Suspected
			■ **Possible**
			☐ Unlikely

Effects The antihypertensive effects of CLONIDINE may be increased and the antipsychotic effects of FLUPHENAZINE may be decreased.

Mechanism Alpha-adrenergic blocking effect of FLUPHENAZINE may potentiate the hypotensive effects of CLONIDINE. The dopamine-blocking activity of FLUPHENAZINE may leave the alpha-adrenergic simulation effect of CLONIDINE unopposed.

Management No special precautions appear necessary.

Discussion

A case of acute organic brain syndrome was reported in a 33-year-old patient treated concomitantly with clonidine 0.2 mg/day and fluphenazine 50 mg IM biweekly.[1] He exhibited signs of delirium, agitation, short-term memory loss and confusion which abated within 72 hours when clonidine was discontinued. His mental status deteriorated again rapidly when rechallenged with clonidine. In another case, a 51-year-old patient treated with clonidine 0.1 mg for hypertension and chlorpromazine 100 mg orally for anxiety developed dizziness and a significant systolic blood pressure reduction from 160 to 76 mmHg in 70 minutes.[2] The hypotensive episode was not associated with bradycardia or tachycardia and responded to fluid replacement.

More data are needed to define the clinical relevance of this interaction.

[1] Allen RM, et al. *J Clin Psychiatry*. 1979;40:236.
[2] Fruncillo RJ, et al. *Am J Psychiatry*. 1985;142:274.

* Asterisk indicates drugs cited in interaction reports.

Phenothiazines — *Contraceptives, Hormonal*

Chlorpromazine* (eg, *Thorazine*)	Contraceptives, Oral* (eg, *Ovral-28*)

Significance	Onset	Severity	Documentation
4	□ Rapid ■ **Delayed**	□ Major ■ **Moderate** □ Minor	□ Established □ Probable □ Suspected ■ **Possible** □ Unlikely

Effects CHLORPROMAZINE plasma concentrations may be elevated, increasing the risk of side effects.

Mechanism Unknown.

Management Monitor patients receiving CHLORPROMAZINE for side effects if ORAL CONTRACEPTIVES are coadministered.

Discussion

A possible drug interaction was reported in a 21-year-old woman receiving chlorpromazine (100 mg 3 times/day) after she took an oral contraceptive containing ethinyl estradiol 50 mcg plus norgestrel 0.5 mg.[1] The patient was a subject in a population pharmacokinetic study of chlorpromazine. Chlorpromazine was well tolerated during the first week of the study; however, on day 12, she presented with severe tremor and dyskinesias. It was discovered that she had taken an oral contraceptive 8 days after starting the study. When the oral contraceptive was taken concurrently, chlorpromazine plasma concentrations were approximately 6-fold higher than levels measured during the first week of the study (134 vs 839 ng/mL).

[1] Chetty M, et al. *Ther Drug Monit.* 2001;23:556.

* Asterisk indicates drugs cited in interaction reports.

Phenothiazines — *Disulfiram*

Perphenazine*	Disulfiram* (*Antabuse*)

Significance	Onset	Severity	Documentation
5	☐ Rapid	☐ Major	☐ Established
	■ **Delayed**	☐ Moderate	☐ Probable
		■ **Minor**	☐ Suspected
			■ **Possible**
			☐ Unlikely

Effects The therapeutic action of PERPHENAZINE could be reduced.

Mechanism Unknown.

Management No special precautions appear to be necessary. Consider switching to a parenteral form of PERPHENAZINE.

Discussion

In a 26-year-old psychotic patient previously stabilized with oral perphenazine 16 mg/day,[1] plasma perphenazine concentrations became subtherapeutic and the sulfoxide metabolite concentration was markedly increased when disulfiram was coadministered, despite no change in the perphenazine dosage regimen. Subsequent clinical improvement was achieved when perphenazine enanthate IM was administered.

More data are required to better define this possible interaction.

[1] Hansen LB, et al. *Lancet.* 1982;2(8313):1472.

* Asterisk indicates drugs cited in interaction reports.

Phenothiazines — *Duloxetine*

Phenothiazines	Duloxetine
Thioridazine*	Duloxetine* (*Cymbalta*)

Significance	Onset	Severity	Documentation
1	☐ Rapid ■ **Delayed**	■ **Major** ☐ Moderate ☐ Minor	☐ Established ☐ Probable ■ **Suspected** ☐ Possible ☐ Unlikely

Effects THIORIDAZINE plasma concentrations may be elevated, increasing the risk of life-threatening ventricular arrhythmias and sudden death.

Mechanism Inhibition of THIORIDAZINE metabolism (CYP2D6) by DULOXETINE.

Management Do not coadminister THIORIDAZINE with DULOXETINE.[1]

Discussion

Duloxetine is a moderate inhibitor of CYP2D6.[1] Therefore, coadministration of duloxetine with other drugs that are metabolized by CYP2D6 and have a narrow therapeutic index (eg, thioridazine) should be approached with caution or avoided. Thioridazine can prolong the QT interval and, because of the risk of serious ventricular arrhythmias and sudden death associated with increased plasma levels of thioridazine, duloxetine and thioridazine should not be given concomitantly.[1]

The basis for this monograph is information on file with the manufacturer. Because of the seriousness of the cardiac problems, clinical evaluation of this interaction in humans is not likely to be forthcoming.

[1] *Cymbalta* [package insert]. Indianapolis, IN: Eli Lilly and Company; 2004.

* Asterisk indicates drugs cited in interaction reports.

Phenothiazines — *Fluoxetine*

Chlorpromazine* (eg, *Thorazine*)	Thioridazine*	Fluoxetine* (eg, *Prozac*)

Significance	Onset	Severity	Documentation
1	□ Rapid	■ **Major**	□ Established
	■ **Delayed**	□ Moderate	□ Probable
		□ Minor	■ **Suspected**
			□ Possible
			□ Unlikely

Effects PHENOTHIAZINE plasma concentrations may be elevated, increasing the risk of life-threatening cardiac arrhythmias, including torsades de pointes.

Mechanism FLUOXETINE may inhibit the metabolism (CYP2D6) of PHENOTHIAZINES.

Management THIORIDAZINE is contraindicated in patients receiving FLUOXETINE.[1] Closely monitor ECG when coadministering FLUOXETINE and a PHENOTHIAZINE.

Discussion

Sudden, unexplained deaths have been reported in patients receiving drugs that prolong the QTc interval. Because thioridazine causes dose-related prolongation of the QTc interval, drugs such as fluoxetine that inhibit the metabolism of thioridazine may produce increased levels of thioridazine, augmenting thioridazine-induced QTc interval prolongation and increasing the risk of potentially fatal cardiac arrhythmias, such as torsades de pointes.[1] Do not use thioridazine with other drugs that inhibit CYP-450 2D6 (CYP2D6) or with agents that may interfere with thioridazine clearance. In addition to agents that reduce the clearance of thioridazine, certain factors may increase the risk of the occurrence of life-threatening arrhythmias in association with thioridazine, including bradycardia, hypokalemia, concomitant use of drugs that prolong the QTc interval, and congenital prolongation of the QTc interval. A 35-year-old woman, diagnosed with paranoid schizophrenia, was taking chlorpromazine 200 mg/day for 3 years.[2] Upon hospitalization for depression, she was started on fluoxetine. When she complained of hearing increasing voices, she was given chlorpromazine 50 mg orally. Shortly thereafter, she became dizzy, collapsed, and lost consciousness for several seconds. An ECG documented prolongation of the QTc interval from 402 to 524 msec. Both medications were stopped, and the prolongation resolved.

[1] *Mellaril* [package insert]. East Hanover, NJ: Novartis Pharmaceutical Corporation; 2000.

[2] Adetunji B, et al. *J Clin Psychopharmacol.* 2006;26:438.

* Asterisk indicates drugs cited in interaction reports.

Phenothiazines — *Fluvoxamine*

Thioridazine*	Fluvoxamine*

Significance	Onset	Severity	Documentation
1	☐ Rapid ■ **Delayed**	■ **Major** ☐ Moderate ☐ Minor	☐ Established ☐ Probable ■ **Suspected** ☐ Possible ☐ Unlikely

Effects Plasma THIORIDAZINE concentrations may be elevated, increasing the pharmacologic and adverse effects, including life-threatening cardiac arrhythmias.

Mechanism Inhibition of THIORIDAZINE metabolism is suspected.

Management THIORIDAZINE is contraindicated in patients receiving FLUVOXAMINE.[1]

Discussion

The effect of fluvoxamine on the pharmacokinetics of thioridazine was studied in 10 male schizophrenic inpatients.[2] All patients were receiving chronic treatment with a mean dose of thioridazine 88 mg/day (range, 20 to 200 mg/day) at bedtime. Fluvoxamine 25 mg twice daily was added to each patient's thioridazine regimen for 1 week. Plasma concentrations of thioridazine and 2 active metabolites (ie, mesoridazine and sulforidazine) were measured during treatment with thioridazine alone, after 1 week of concurrent fluvoxamine, and 2 weeks after fluvoxamine was discontinued. Coadministration of thioridazine and fluvoxamine increased thioridazine plasma concentrations 3-fold (from 0.4 to 1.21 mcmol/L), mesoridazine concentrations 3-fold (from 0.65 to 2 mcmol/L), and sulforidazine concentrations 2.7-fold (from 0.21 to 0.56 mcmol/L). In 3 patients, plasma concentrations of thioridazine and its metabolites were still elevated 2 weeks after fluvoxamine discontinuation. See Phenothiazines-Fluoxetine and Phenothiazines-Paroxetine.

[1] *Mellaril* [package insert]. East Hanover, NJ: Novartis Pharmaceutical Corporation; 2000.

[2] Carrillo JA, et al. *J Clin Psychopharmacol.* 1999;19:494.

* Asterisk indicates drugs cited in interaction reports.

Phenothiazines — **Hydroxyzine**

Chlorpromazine* (eg, *Thorazine*)	Promethazine (eg, *Phenergan*)	Hydroxyzine* (eg, *Vistaril*)
Fluphenazine	Thioridazine*	
Perphenazine	Trifluoperazine*	
Prochlorperazine (eg, *Compazine*)		

Significance	Onset	Severity	Documentation
5	☐ Rapid	☐ Major	☐ Established
	■ **Delayed**	☐ Moderate	☐ Probable
		■ **Minor**	☐ Suspected
			■ **Possible**
			☐ Unlikely

Effects The pharmacologic and therapeutic actions of the PHENOTHIAZINES could be reduced.

Mechanism Unknown.

Management No special precautions appear necessary. If an interaction is suspected, consider increasing the dose of PHENOTHIAZINES.

Discussion

In a double-blind, controlled study, researchers reported that the combined use of oral hydroxyzine 100 mg and usual doses of phenothiazines (eg, chlorpromazine, thioridazine, trifluoperazine) produced a reduction of antipsychotic effects in 19 psychotic patients, as assessed by the independently administered Hostility and Direction of Hostility Questionnaire.[1]

Additional studies are needed to establish this interaction.

[1] Ross EK, et al. *Dis Nerv Syst.* 1970;31:412.

* Asterisk indicates drugs cited in interaction reports. Based on pharmacologic and pharmacokinetic considerations, similar interactions may occur with other drugs that are listed.

Phenothiazines — *Lithium*

Chlorpromazine* (eg, *Thorazine*)	Promethazine (eg, *Phenergan*)	Lithium* (eg, *Eskalith*)
Fluphenazine*	Thioridazine*	
Perphenazine*	Trifluoperazine	
Prochlorperazine (eg, *Compazine*)		

Significance	Onset	Severity	Documentation
4	☐ Rapid	☐ Major	☐ Established
	■ **Delayed**	■ **Moderate**	☐ Probable
		☐ Minor	☐ Suspected
			■ **Possible**
			☐ Unlikely

Effects LITHIUM with PHENOTHIAZINE may induce disorientation, unconsciousness, and extrapyramidal symptoms.

Mechanism Unknown.

Management If an interaction is suspected, consider discontinuation or a reduction in the dose of 1 or both agents.

Discussion

In a survey of reports, 39 patients developed neurotoxicity while receiving lithium and a neuroleptic.[1] The most frequent symptoms were confusion, disorientation, and unconsciousness (81.5%); extrapyramidal symptoms (73.7%); cerebellar signs (26.3%); fever (18.4%); and pyramidal symptoms (15.8%). Serum lithium levels were less than 1.5 mEq/L in 91.2% of the cases. Slow-wave electroencephalogram changes were common (90%). Symptoms reversed following discontinuation of 1 or both agents in 89.5% of patients. Similar symptoms have been described in a number of other cases.[2-9] In some, therapy was reinitiated with no recurrence of symptoms.[4-6] Lithium reduced mean peak serum chlorpromazine concentrations 40.3% and AUC 26.6%.[10,11] Another study found elevated lithium concentrations and ratios in patients on phenothiazines.[12]

[1] Prakash R, et al. *Compr Psychiatry.* 1982;23:567.
[2] Charney DS, et al. *Br J Psychiatry.* 1979;135:418.
[3] Spring GK. *J Clin Psychiatry.* 1979;40:135.
[4] Singh SV. *Lancet.* 1982;2:278.
[5] Addonizio G. *J Clin Psychopharmacol.* 1985;5:296.
[6] Bailine SH, et al. *Biol Psychiatry.* 1986;21:834.
[7] Yassa R. *J Clin Psychiatry.* 1986;47:90.
[8] Sachdev PS. *Am J Psychiatry.* 1986;143:942.
[9] McGennis AJ. *Br J Psychiatry.* 1983;142:99.
[10] Rivera-Calimlim L, et al. *Am J Psychiatry.* 1976;133:646.
[11] Rivera-Calimlim L, et al. *Clin Pharmacol Ther.* 1978;23:451.
[12] Levy DL, et al. *Arch Gen Psychiatry.* 1985;42:335.

* Asterisk indicates drugs cited in interaction reports. Based on pharmacologic and pharmacokinetic considerations, similar interactions may occur with other drugs that are listed.

Phenothiazines — *Midodrine*

Promethazine* (eg, *Phenergan*)	Midodrine* (eg, *ProAmatine*)

Significance	Onset	Severity	Documentation
4	■ **Rapid**	□ Major	□ Established
	□ Delayed	■ **Moderate**	□ Probable
		□ Minor	□ Suspected
			■ **Possible**
			□ Unlikely

Effects The risk of akathisia may be increased, which may be potentially hazardous when patients are driving or performing other tasks.

Mechanism Unknown.

Management If these agents are prescribed concurrently, caution patients of the possible risk of akathisia and advise caution while driving or performing other potentially dangerous tasks until tolerance is determined.

Discussion

The effect of promethazine on the positive effects of midodrine on orthostatic hypotension was evaluated in 9 healthy subjects.[1] One subject withdrew prior to testing. Using a randomized design, each subject received midodrine 10 mg or matching placebo, followed 60 minutes later by promethazine 25 mg IV infused over 12 minutes or placebo. An unexpected degree of akathisia was observed during the study. None of the participants receiving either of the placebos or midodrine alone experienced akathisia. Akathisia occurred in 6 subjects receiving midodrine and promethazine concurrently. Akathisia occurred in 4 of these 6 participants while receiving promethazine alone. However, the akathisia was more severe than occurred with promethazine alone.

[1] Platts SH, et al. *JAMA*. 2006;295:2000.

* Asterisk indicates drugs cited in interaction reports.

Phenothiazines — *Paroxetine*

Phenothiazines		Paroxetine
Chlorpromazine (eg, *Thorazine*)	Promethazine (eg, *Phenergan*)	Paroxetine* (*Paxil*)
Fluphenazine (eg, *Prolixin*)	Thiethylperazine (*Torecan*)	
Methotrimeprazine (*Levoprome*)	Thioridazine*	
Perphenazine*	Trifluoperazine	
Prochlorperazine (eg, *Compazine*)		

Significance	Onset	Severity	Documentation
2	☐ Rapid	☐ Major	☐ Established
	■ **Delayed**	■ **Moderate**	■ **Probable**
		☐ Minor	☐ Suspected
			☐ Possible
			☐ Unlikely

Effects PHENOTHIAZINE plasma levels may be elevated, increasing the pharmacologic and adverse effects, including the risk of life-threatening cardiac arrhythmias with THIORIDAZINE.

Mechanism Decreased metabolism (CYP2D6) of the PHENOTHIAZINE.

Management THIORIDAZINE is contraindicated in patients receiving PAROXETINE.[2] It may be necessary to decrease the usual starting dose of other PHENOTHIAZINES in patients who are at steady-state concentrations of PAROXETINE. In patients receiving a PHENOTHIAZINE, carefully observe the clinical response when starting, stopping, or changing the dose of PAROXETINE. Adjust the PHENOTHIAZINE dose as needed.

Discussion

The effects of paroxetine pretreatment on the pharmacokinetics and CNS action of perphenazine were investigated in 8 healthy subjects who were extensive metabolizers for cytochrome P450 2D6 (CYP2D6).[1] Each subject received a single oral dose of perphenazine 0.11 mg/kg or placebo on 2 occasions. Subjects received paroxetine 20 mg/day for 10 days. At the completion of paroxetine administration, perphenazine and placebo administration were repeated. Paroxetine administration resulted in a 2- to 21-fold decrease in CYP2D6 activity. Following pretreatment with paroxetine, perphenazine peak plasma levels increased 2- to 13-fold (mean increase, approximately 6-fold), with a similar increase in the AUC of perphenazine (mean increase, approximately 7-fold). The increases in plasma perphenazine levels were associated with an increase in CNS side effects, including excessive sedation, extrapyramidal effects, and impaired psychomotor performance and memory. See Phenothiazines-Fluoxetine and Phenothiazines-Fluvoxamine.

[1] Ozdemir V, et al. *Clin Pharmacol Ther.* 1997;62:334.

[2] Product Information. Thioridazine (*Mellaril*). Novartis Pharmaceutical Corporation. 2000.

* Asterisk indicates drugs cited in interaction reports. Based on pharmacologic and pharmacokinetic considerations, similar interactions may occur with other drugs that are listed.

Phenothiazines — *Pimozide*

Phenothiazines	Pimozide
Thioridazine*	Pimozide* (*Orap*)

Significance	Onset	Severity	Documentation
1	☐ Rapid	■ **Major**	☐ Established
	■ **Delayed**	☐ Moderate	☐ Probable
		☐ Minor	■ **Suspected**
			☐ Possible
			☐ Unlikely

Effects The risk of life-threatening cardiac arrhythmias, including torsades de pointes, may be increased.

Mechanism Possibly synergistic or additive prolongation of the corrected QT (QTc) interval.

Management THIORIDAZINE is contraindicated in patients receiving PIMOZIDE.

Discussion

Sudden, unexplained deaths have been reported in patients receiving drugs that prolong the QTc interval. Do not use thioridazine with other agents that prolong the QTc interval. Thioridazine causes dose-related prolongation of the QTc interval and other drugs that prolong the QTc interval (eg, pimozide)[1] have been associated with fatal arrhythmias.[2] In addition to other agents that prolong the QTc interval, certain factors may increase the risk of occurrence of torsades de pointes and sudden death in association with thioridazine, including bradycardia, hypokalemia, drugs that reduce the clearance of thioridazine, and congenital prolongation of the QTc interval.

The basis for this monograph is information on file with the manufacturer. Because of the seriousness of the cardiac problems, clinical evaluation of this interaction in humans is not likely to be forthcoming.

[1] Thomas M, et al. *Br J Clin Pharmacol.* 1996;41:77.

[2] Product information. Thioridazine (*Mellaril*). Novartis Pharmaceutical Corporation. 2000.

* Asterisk indicates drugs cited in interaction reports.

Phenothiazines — *Piperazine*

Chlorpromazine*	Piperazine*†

Significance	Onset	Severity	Documentation
5	■ **Rapid**	■ **Major**	□ Established
	□ Delayed	□ Moderate	□ Probable
		□ Minor	□ Suspected
			□ Possible
			■ **Unlikely**

Effects There is an unlikely possibility that PIPERAZINE may predispose a patient to PHENOTHIAZINE-induced convulsions.

Mechanism Unknown.

Management A patient who is receiving a PHENOTHIAZINE and requires PIPERAZINE may need to be closely monitored after receiving the drug.

Discussion

After discovering a case of a child on chlorpromazine who developed convulsions several days after treatment with piperazine for pinworms, the combination was tested in 9 goats and 6 dogs.[1] Chlorpromazine 4.5 to 10 mg/kg produced signs of ataraxia when infused IV. When piperazine 220 mg/kg was added, severe clonic convulsions and respiratory arrest occurred in all of the animals. The usual veterinary dose of chlorpromazine was noted to be 1.1 to 2.2 mg/kg.

In a subsequent report, chlorpromazine 10 mg/kg or less was administered IV with and without piperazine citrate 200 mg/kg.[2] No animals exhibited adverse effects. The report also noted personal communication with one of the authors who said that the previous results were unable to be repeated.

[1] Boulos BM, et al. *N Engl J Med.* 1969;280(22):1245.

[2] Armbrecht BH. *N Engl J Med.* 1970;282(26):1490.

* Asterisk indicates drugs cited in interaction reports.
† Not available in the United States.

Phenothiazines | **Quinolones**

Chlorpromazine*	Thioridazine*	Levofloxacin* (eg, *Levaquin*)	Moxifloxacin* (eg, *Avelox*)

Significance	Onset	Severity	Documentation
1	☐ Rapid ■ **Delayed**	■ **Major** ☐ Moderate ☐ Minor	☐ Established ☐ Probable ■ **Suspected** ☐ Possible ☐ Unlikely

Effects The risk of life-threatening cardiac arrhythmias, including torsades de pointes, may be increased.

Mechanism Unknown.

Management Avoid LEVOFLOXACIN administration,[1] and use MOXIFLOXACIN[2] with caution in patients receiving drugs that prolong the QTc interval (eg, certain PHENOTHIAZINES).[3] Other QUINOLONE antibiotics that do not prolong the QTc interval or are not metabolized by the CYP3A4 isozyme may be suitable alternatives.

Discussion

Because torsades de pointes has been reported in patients receiving sparfloxacin[†] with amiodarone (eg, *Cordarone*) or disopyramide (eg, *Norpace*), sparfloxacin is contraindicated in patients receiving these antiarrhythmic agents or other QTc-prolonging drugs (eg, phenothiazines) or drugs known to cause torsades de pointes.[1-3] Moxifloxacin has prolonged the QT interval in some patients.[2] Because studies between moxifloxacin and drugs that prolong the QTc interval have not been performed, use moxifloxacin with caution when drugs that prolong the QT interval (eg, certain phenothiazines) are coadministered.[2] Levofloxacin has been associated with prolongation of the QT interval and infrequent cases of cardiac arrhythmias.[1]

[1] *Levaquin* [package insert]. Raritan, NJ: Ortho-McNeil Pharmaceuticals Inc; February 2004.

[2] *Avelox* [package insert]. West Haven, CT: Bayer Health Care; April 2004.

[3] Thomas M, et al. *Br J Clin Pharmacol.* 1996;41(2):77.

* Asterisk indicates drugs cited in interaction reports.

† Not available in the United States.

Phenothiazines — *Venlafaxine*

Trifluoperazine*	Venlafaxine* (*Effexor*)

Significance	Onset	Severity	Documentation
4	■ **Rapid**	■ **Major**	□ Established
	□ Delayed	□ Moderate	□ Probable
		□ Minor	□ Suspected
			■ **Possible**
			□ Unlikely

Effects Neuroleptic malignant syndrome, including pyrexia, muscular rigidity, tremor, and labile BP, may occur.

Mechanism Unknown. VENLAFAXINE may augment TRIFLUOPERAZINE dopamine-receptor inhibition.

Management If administration of this combination cannot be avoided, start with low doses of VENLAFAXINE or PHENOTHIAZINE and carefully monitor the patient.

Discussion

A 44-year-old man who had been taking trifluoperazine 1 mg 3 times daily for 10 yr for anxiety developed symptoms consistent with neuroleptic malignant syndrome 12 hr after the first dose of venlafaxine 75 mg, which was prescribed for depressive symptoms.[1] The patient presented with profound anxiety and malaise, profuse sweating, tremor, and rigidity. His BP fluctuated between 130/80 and 165/100 mm Hg, with a pulse of 163 bpm, temperature 38.3°C, and respiration of 25 breaths/min. His creatine phosphokinase and neutrophils were elevated. All psychotropic medication was discontinued. He was given a single dose of dantrolene (*Dantrium*) 70 mg and bromocriptine (eg, *Parlodel*) 15 mg twice daily for 48 hr. The patient's vital signs returned to normal within 24 hr of admission, and he completely recovered. Trifluoperazine was restarted without incident.

[1] Nimmagadda SR, et al. *Lancet.* 2000;355:289.

* Asterisk indicates drugs cited in interaction reports.

Phenytoin | **Protease Inhibitors**

Phenytoin* (eg, *Dilantin*)	Lopinavir/Ritonavir* (*Kaletra*)

Significance	Onset	Severity	Documentation
4	☐ Rapid ■ **Delayed**	☐ Major ■ **Moderate** ☐ Minor	☐ Established ☐ Probable ☐ Suspected ■ **Possible** ☐ Unlikely

Effects In a 2-way interaction, LOPINAVIR/RITONAVIR and PHENYTOIN plasma concentrations may be reduced, decreasing the therapeutic effects.

Mechanism PHENYTOIN may induce LOPINAVIR/RITONAVIR metabolism (CYP3A4), while LOPINAVIR/RITONAVIR may induce PHENYTOIN metabolism (CYP2C9).

Management Closely monitor PHENYTOIN concentrations when LOPINAVIR/RITONAVIR is coadministered. Adjustments in the dosage or alterations in the PHENYTOIN or LOPINAVIR/RITONAVIR regimens may be necessary.

Discussion

The effects of phenytoin and lopinavir/ritonavir on the pharmacokinetics of each other were studied in an open-label, randomized investigation.[1] In 1 arm of the study, lopinavir/ritonavir 400 mg/100 mg twice daily was administered to 12 healthy subjects for 22 days. Phenytoin 300 mg daily was given concurrently on days 11 through 22. In the second arm of the study, 12 healthy subjects received phenytoin 300 mg daily for 23 days. Eight subjects completed the study. Lopinavir/ritonavir 400 mg/100 mg twice daily was administered concomitantly on days 12 through 23. Plasma samples were collected on days 11 and 22. Following addition of phenytoin to the lopinavir/ritonavir regimen, lopinavir AUC decreased 30% and the plasma concentration decreased 41%. Following addition of lopinavir/ritonavir to phenytoin administration, the phenytoin AUC and plasma concentration decreased 23% and 25%, respectively.

[1] Lim ML, et al. *J Acquir Immune Defic Syndr.* 2004;36:1034.

* Asterisk indicates drugs cited in interaction reports.

Phosphodiesterase Type 5 Inhibitors — Azole Antifungal Agents

Avanafil* (*Stendra*)	Tadalafil* (eg, *Cialis*)	Itraconazole* (eg, *Sporanox*)	Posaconazole (*Noxafil*)
Sildenafil* (eg, *Viagra*)	Vardenafil* (eg, *Levitra*)	Ketoconazole* (eg, *Nizoral*)	Voriconazole (eg, *Vfend*)

Significance	Onset	Severity	Documentation
2	□ Rapid ■ **Delayed**	□ Major ■ **Moderate** □ Minor	□ Established □ Probable ■ **Suspected** □ Possible □ Unlikely

Effects PDE5 INHIBITOR plasma levels may be elevated, increasing the risk of adverse reactions.

Mechanism Inhibition of PDE5 INHIBITOR metabolism (CYP3A4) by certain AZOLE ANTIFUNGAL AGENTS may occur.

Management Administer PDE5 INHIBITORS with caution and in reduced doses to patients taking certain AZOLE ANTIFUNGAL AGENTS. In patients taking ITRACONAZOLE or KETOCONAZOLE, consider a starting dose of SILDENAFIL 25 mg[1] and do not exceed a single dose of TADALAFIL 10 mg in 72 hours.[2] For patients taking ITRACONAZOLE or KETOCONAZOLE 400 mg daily, do not exceed a single dose of VARDENAFIL 2.5 mg in 24 hours. For patients taking ITRACONAZOLE or KETOCONAZOLE 200 mg daily, do not exceed a single dose of VARDENAFIL 5 mg in 24 hours.[3] Avoid coadministration of AVANAFIL.[4]

Discussion

In patients receiving ketoconazole 400 mg daily, administration of a single dose of tadalafil 20 mg increased tadalafil AUC and C_{max} 312% and 22%, respectively, compared with giving tadalafil alone.[2] In patients receiving ketoconazole 200 mg daily, administration of a single dose of tadalafil 20 mg increased tadalafil AUC and C_{max} 107% and 15%, respectively, compared with giving tadalafil alone.[2] In healthy volunteers, ketoconazole 200 mg daily increased the AUC and C_{max} of vardenafil 10- and 4-fold, respectively.[3] Higher doses of ketoconazole (eg, 400 mg daily) can be expected to result in greater increases in the AUC and C_{max}. A 56-year-old man experienced painful erections repeatedly over 72 hours while receiving itraconazole 400 mg/day and tadalafil 10 mg.[5] The reaction did not occur with coadministration of itraconazole and sildenafil.

1 *Viagra* [package insert]. New York, NY: Pfizer Labs; September 2002.
2 *Cialis* [package insert]. Indianapolis, IN: Eli Lilly; November 2003.
3 *Levitra* [package insert]. West Haven, CT: Bayer Health Care; August 2003.
4 *Stendra* [package insert]. Mountain View, CA: Vivus Inc; April 2012.
5 Galatti L, et al. *Ann Pharmacother.* 2005;39(1):200.

* Asterisk indicates drugs cited in interaction reports. Based on pharmacologic and pharmacokinetic considerations, similar interactions may occur with other drugs that are listed.

Phosphodiesterase Type 5 Inhibitors — **Bosentan**

Avanafil (*Stendra*)
Sildenafil* (eg, *Viagra*)
Tadalafil* (eg, *Cialis*)
Vardenafil (eg, *Levitra*)

Bosentan* (*Tracleer*)

Significance	Onset	Severity	Documentation
4	□ Rapid	□ Major	□ Established
	■ **Delayed**	■ **Moderate**	□ Probable
		□ Minor	□ Suspected
			■ **Possible**
			□ Unlikely

Effects PDE5 INHIBITOR plasma concentrations may be reduced, decreasing efficacy. BOSENTAN plasma levels may be elevated, increasing the risk of toxicity.

Mechanism Induction of PDE5 INHIBITOR hepatic and/or gut wall metabolism (CYP3A4) by BOSENTAN. Inhibition of BOSENTAN metabolism by PDE5 INHIBITORS.

Management Coadminister these agents with caution and close monitoring of the clinical response and adverse reactions.

Discussion

Because both bosentan and sildenafil (*Revatio*) are indicated for the treatment of pulmonary arterial hypertension, their combined use can be anticipated in some patients. The effect of bosentan on the pharmacokinetics of sildenafil was studied in 10 patients with pulmonary arterial hypertension.[1] Each patient received bosentan 62.5 mg twice daily for 1 month, followed by 125 mg twice daily for the second month. Sildenafil 100 mg was administered as a single oral dose before starting bosentan and at the end of the first and second months of bosentan treatment. The first 4 weeks of bosentan therapy were associated with a 50% decrease in sildenafil AUC and a 2-fold increase in oral clearance, compared with giving sildenafil alone. When the bosentan dosage was increased to 125 mg twice daily, there was a further decrease in sildenafil AUC and an increase in oral clearance. The C_{max} decreased 56% from the first dose of sildenafil to the third dose. In addition, there was a decrease in the sildenafil $t_{½}$, while patients received the higher dose of bosentan. Also, bosentan treatment resulted in a dose-related decrease in the $t_{½}$ and AUC of the desmethylsildenafil metabolite. The potential for a 2-way pharmacokinetic interaction between sildenafil and bosentan was studied in 51 healthy men.[2] Bosentan 125 mg twice daily decreased the sildenafil AUC and C_{max} 62.6% and 55.4%, respectively. Sildenafil, titrated to 80 mg 3 times daily, increased the bosentan AUC and C_{max} 49.8% and 42%, respectively. In a study of healthy men, coadministration of bosentan 125 mg twice daily and tadalafil 40 mg once daily for 10 days reduced tadalafil exposure 41.5%, compared with administration of tadalafil alone.[3]

[1] Paul GA, et al. *Br J Clin Pharmacol.* 2005;60(1):107.
[2] Burgess G, et al. *Eur J Clin Pharmacol.* 2008;64(1):43.
[3] Wrishko RE, et al. *J Clin Pharmacol.* 2008;48(5):610.

* Asterisk indicates drugs cited in interaction reports. Based on pharmacologic and pharmacokinetic considerations, similar interactions may occur with other drugs that are listed.

Phosphodiesterase Type 5 Inhibitors × HCV Protease Inhibitors

Phosphodiesterase Type 5 Inhibitors		HCV Protease Inhibitors	
Sildenafil* (eg, *Viagra*)	Vardenafil* (eg, *Levitra*)	Boceprevir* (*Victrelis*)	Telaprevir* (*Incivek*)
Tadalafil* (eg, *Cialis*)			

Significance	Onset	Severity	Documentation
1	☐ Rapid ■ **Delayed**	■ **Major** ☐ Moderate ☐ Minor	☐ Established ☐ Probable ■ **Suspected** ☐ Possible ☐ Unlikely

Effects PDE5 INHIBITOR plasma concentrations may be elevated, increasing the pharmacologic effects and risk of adverse reactions (eg, visual abnormalities, hypotension, prolonged erection, syncope).

Mechanism Inhibition of PDE5 INHIBITOR metabolism (CYP3A4) by HEPATITIS C VIRUS (HCV) PROTEASE INHIBITORS.

Management Coadministration of PDE5 INHIBITORS for treatment of pulmonary arterial hypertension and HCV PROTEASE INHIBITORS is contraindicated. For the treatment of erectile dysfunction, coadminister PDE5 INHIBITORS and HCV PROTEASE INHIBITORS with caution and do not exceed a dose of sildenafil 25 mg every 48 hours, tadalafil 10 mg every 72 hours, or vardenafil 2.5 mg every 24 hours.[1,2]

Discussion

Boceprevir or telaprevir is contraindicated when coadministered with drugs that are highly dependent on CYP3A4 metabolism for clearance and for which elevated plasma concentrations are associated with serious and/or life-threatening adverse reactions (ie, drugs with a narrow therapeutic index). Coadministration of boceprevir or telaprevir is expected to increase PDE5 inhibitor plasma concentrations and may result in adverse reactions, including hypotension, visual disturbances, and prolonged erection. Coadministration of PDE5 inhibitors for the treatment of pulmonary arterial hypertension and boceprevir or telaprevir is contraindicated. For the treatment of erectile dysfunction, coadminister the PDE5 inhibitor in reduced dosages.[1,2]

The basis for this monograph is information on file with the manufacturer. Published clinical data are needed to further assess this interaction. Because of the seriousness of the interaction, clinical evaluation in humans is not likely to be forthcoming.

[1] *Victrelis* [package insert]. Whitehouse Station, NJ: Schering Corporation; May 2011.

[2] *Incivek* [package insert]. Cambridge, MA: Vertex Pharmaceuticals Incorporated; May 2011.

* Asterisk indicates drugs cited in interaction reports.

Phosphodiesterase Type 5 Inhibitors		**Macrolide & Related Antibiotics**	
Avanafil* (*Stendra*)	Tadalafil (eg, *Cialis*)	Clarithromycin* (eg, *Biaxin*)	Telithromycin (*Ketek*)
Sildenafil* (eg, *Viagra*)	Vardenafil (eg, *Levitra*)	Erythromycin* (eg, *Ery-Tab*)	

Significance	Onset	Severity	Documentation
2	☐ Rapid ■ **Delayed**	☐ Major ■ **Moderate** ☐ Minor	☐ Established ☐ Probable ■ **Suspected** ☐ Possible ☐ Unlikely

Effects PDE5 INHIBITOR plasma concentrations may be elevated, increasing the risk of adverse reactions.

Mechanism Inhibition of PDE5 INHIBITOR first-pass metabolism (CYP3A4) by certain MACROLIDE AND RELATED ANTIBIOTICS is suspected.

Management In patients receiving certain MACROLIDE AND RELATED ANTIBIOTICS, consider giving a lower PDE5 INHIBITOR dose. Administration of a MACROLIDE ANTIBIOTIC not metabolized by CYP3A4 (eg, azithromycin [eg, *Zithromax*]) may be a safer alternative. Avoid coadministration of AVANAFIL.[1]

Discussion

The effects of multiple doses of erythromycin and azithromycin on the pharmacokinetics of a single dose of sildenafil were investigated in 2 placebo-controlled, parallel-group studies.[2] In 1 study, 24 men received sildenafil 100 mg on day 1, then one-half of the subjects received placebo while the other half received erythromycin 500 mg twice daily on days 2 to 6. On day 6, each subject received a second dose of sildenafil 100 mg. In the second study, 24 men received sildenafil 100 mg on day 1, then one-half of the subjects received placebo while the other half received azithromycin 500 mg once daily on days 2 to 4. On day 4, each subject received a second dose of sildenafil 100 mg. Compared with placebo administration, erythromycin increased the sildenafil AUC 2.8-fold and the peak concentration 2.6-fold. T_{max}, elimination rate constant, and $t_{½}$ of sildenafil were not affected by erythromycin coadministration. The AUC of the UK-103,320 metabolite of sildenafil was increased, while the elimination $t_{½}$ was decreased. Despite the increase in the AUCs for sildenafil and its metabolite when erythromycin was coadministered, no subject experienced any serious adverse reaction. Azithromycin did not affect the pharmacokinetics of sildenafil or its metabolite. Twelve men received sildenafil 50 mg alone and 2 hours after a single dose of clarithromycin 500 mg.[3] Compared with taking sildenafil alone, clarithromycin increased sildenafil plasma levels with a nearly 2.3-fold increase in AUC. No adverse reactions were noted.

[1] *Stendra* [package insert]. Mountain View, CA: Vivus Inc; April 2012.
[2] Muirhead GJ, et al. *Br J Clin Pharmacol.* 2002;53(suppl 1):37S.
[3] Hedaya MA, et al. *Biopharm Drug Dispos.* 2006;27(2):103.

* Asterisk indicates drugs cited in interaction reports. Based on pharmacologic and pharmacokinetic considerations, similar interactions may occur with other drugs that are listed.

Phosphodiesterase Type 5 Inhibitors — *Quinolones*

Phosphodiesterase Type 5 Inhibitors		Quinolones
Avanafil (*Stendra*)	Tadalafil (eg, *Cialis*)	Ciprofloxacin* (eg, *Cipro*)
Sildenafil* (eg, *Viagra*)	Vardenafil (eg, *Levitra*)	

Significance	Onset	Severity	Documentation
4	☐ Rapid	☐ Major	☐ Established
	■ **Delayed**	■ **Moderate**	☐ Probable
		☐ Minor	☐ Suspected
			■ **Possible**
			☐ Unlikely

Effects PDE5 INHIBITOR plasma levels may be elevated, increasing the risk of adverse reactions.

Mechanism Inhibition of PDE5 metabolism (CYP3A4) by CIPROFLOXACIN is suspected.

Management In patients receiving CIPROFLOXACIN, consider a lower dose of the PDE5 INHIBITOR. Consider withholding PDE5 INHIBITORS in patients at high risk of developing PDE5 INHIBITOR adverse reactions during coadministration of CIPROFLOXACIN.

Discussion

The effects of ciprofloxacin on the pharmacokinetics of sildenafil were studied in 12 healthy men.[1] In a crossover study, each subject received sildenafil 50 mg alone and ciprofloxacin 500 mg plus sildenafil 50 mg. Compared with giving sildenafil alone, coadministration of ciprofloxacin and sildenafil increased the sildenafil AUC and C_{max} more than 2-fold and prolonged the elimination $t_{½}$ by 35%.

[1] Hedaya MA, et al. *Biopharm Drug Dispos*. 2006;27(2):103.

* Asterisk indicates drugs cited in interaction reports. Based on pharmacologic and pharmacokinetic considerations, similar interactions may occur with other drugs that are listed.

Phosphodiesterase Type 5 Inhibitors | **Serotonin Reuptake Inhibitors**

Avanafil (*Stendra*)	Tadalafil (eg, *Cialis*)	Fluoxetine (eg, *Prozac*)	Nefazodone
Sildenafil* (eg, *Viagra*)	Vardenafil (eg, *Levitra*)	Fluvoxamine* (eg, *Luvox CR*)	

Significance	Onset	Severity	Documentation
2	□ Rapid ■ **Delayed**	□ Major ■ **Moderate** □ Minor	□ Established □ Probable ■ **Suspected** □ Possible □ Unlikely

Effects PDE5 INHIBITOR plasma levels may be elevated, increasing the risk of adverse reactions.

Mechanism Inhibition of PDE5 INHIBITOR metabolism (CYP3A4) by certain SRIs.

Management Until more clinical data are available, administer PDE5 INHIBITORS with caution to patients receiving certain SRIs. Consider reducing the initial dose of the PDE5 INHIBITOR if coadministration cannot be avoided.

Discussion

The effects of fluvoxamine on the pharmacokinetics and pharmacodynamics of sildenafil were studied in 12 healthy men.[1] Using a randomized, double-blind, placebo-controlled, crossover design, each subject received oral fluvoxamine 50 mg/day on days 1 through 3 and 100 mg/day on days 4 through 10. On day 11, a single oral dose of sildenafil 50 mg was administered. The effect of sildenafil on sodium nitroprusside (*Nitropress*)-induced venodilation was evaluated by infusing a constant dose of nitroprusside into the dorsal hand vein. Compared with placebo, fluvoxamine administration increased sildenafil exposure 40%, as measured by the AUC, and increased the $t_{½}$ 19%. In addition, nitroprusside-induced venodilation was augmented 59% during fluvoxamine dosing compared with placebo.

[1] Hesse C, et al. *J Clin Psychopharmacol.* 2005;25(6):589.

* Asterisk indicates drugs cited in interaction reports. Based on pharmacologic and pharmacokinetic considerations, similar interactions may occur with other drugs that are listed.

Pimozide — *Aprepitant*

Pimozide* (*Orap*)	Aprepitant* (*Emend*)	Fosaprepitant* (*Emend*)

Significance	Onset	Severity	Documentation
1	☐ Rapid ■ **Delayed**	■ **Major** ☐ Moderate ☐ Minor	☐ Established ☐ Probable ■ **Suspected** ☐ Possible ☐ Unlikely

Effects The risk of life-threatening cardiac arrhythmias may be increased.

Mechanism APREPITANT may inhibit the metabolism (CYP3A4) of PIMOZIDE.

Management Coadministration of APREPITANT or FOSAPREPITANT and PIMOZIDE is contraindicated.

Discussion

Although not studied, coadministration of aprepitant with pimozide may increase pimozide plasma concentrations, resulting in QT prolongation and increased risk of cardiac arrhythmias. Coadministration of pimozide and aprepitant or fosaprepitant is contraindicated by the manufacturer.[1,2]

The basis for this monograph is information on file with the manufacturer. Published clinical data are needed to further assess this interaction. Because of the seriousness of the cardiac problem, clinical evaluation of this interaction in humans is not likely to be forthcoming. See Drug-Induced Prolongation of the QT Interval and Torsades de Pointes.

[1] *Emend* oral [package insert]. White House Station, NJ: Merck & Co, Inc; March 2003.

[2] *Emend* IV [package insert]. Whitehouse Station, NJ: Merck & Co, Inc; January 2008.

* Asterisk indicates drugs cited in interaction reports.

Pimozide — *Azole Antifungal Agents*

Pimozide*	Itraconazole*	Posaconazole*
(*Orap*)	(eg, *Sporanox*)	(*Noxafil*)
	Ketoconazole*	Voriconazole*
	(eg, *Nizoral*)	(*Vfend*)

Significance	Onset	Severity	Documentation
1	☐ Rapid	■ **Major**	☐ Established
	■ **Delayed**	☐ Moderate	☐ Probable
		☐ Minor	■ **Suspected**
			☐ Possible
			☐ Unlikely

Effects The risk of life-threatening cardiac arrhythmias may be increased.

Mechanism AZOLE ANTIFUNGAL AGENTS may inhibit the metabolism (CYP3A4) of PIMOZIDE.

Management Coadministration of AZOLE ANTIFUNGAL AGENTS and PIMOZIDE is contraindicated.

Discussion

Although not studied, coadministration of itraconazole or ketoconazole with pimozide may increase pimozide plasma concentrations, resulting in QT prolongation and increasing the risk of cardiac arrhythmias.[1] Coadministration of pimozide and azole antifungal agents is contraindicated by the manufacturer.[1-3]

The basis for this monograph is information on file with the manufacturer. Published clinical data are needed to further assess this interaction. Because of the seriousness of the cardiac problem, clinical evaluation of this interaction in humans is not likely to be forthcoming.

[1] *Orap* [package insert]. North Wales, PA: Teva Pharmaceuticals; August 1999.
[2] *Noxafil* [package insert]. Kenilworth, NJ: Schering Corporation; October 2006.
[3] *Vfend* [package insert]. New York, NY: Pfizer, Inc; November 2006.

* Asterisk indicates drugs cited in interaction reports.

Pimozide — *HCV Protease Inhibitors*

Pimozide* (*Orap*)	Boceprevir* (*Victrelis*)	Telaprevir* (*Incivek*)

Significance	Onset	Severity	Documentation
1	☐ Rapid ■ **Delayed**	■ **Major** ☐ Moderate ☐ Minor	☐ Established ☐ Probable ■ **Suspected** ☐ Possible ☐ Unlikely

Effects PIMOZIDE plasma concentrations may be elevated, increasing the pharmacologic effects and risk of life-threatening cardiac arrhythmias, including torsades de pointes.

Mechanism PIMOZIDE metabolism (CYP3A) may be inhibited by HEPATITIS C VIRUS (HCV) PROTEASE INHIBITORS.

Management Coadministration of PIMOZIDE and HCV PROTEASE INHIBITORS is contraindicated.[1,2]

Discussion

Concurrent use of strong CYP3A4 inhibitors, such as boceprevir, may elevate pimozide plasma concentrations, increasing the risk of serious adverse effects (eg, life-threatening cardiac arrhythmias).[1,2] Concomitant use of pimozide and boceprevir or telaprevir is contraindicated.

The basis for this monograph is information on file with the manufacturer. Published clinical data are needed to further assess this interaction. Because of the seriousness of the cardiac problem, clinical evaluation of the interaction in humans is not likely to be forthcoming.

[1] *Victrelis* [package insert]. Whitehouse Station, NJ: Schering Corporation; May 2011.

[2] *Incivek* [package insert]. Cambridge, MA: Vertex Pharmaceuticals Incorporated; May 2011.

* Asterisk indicates drugs cited in interaction reports.

Pimozide | Macrolide & Related Antibiotics

Pimozide	Macrolide & Related Antibiotics	
Pimozide* (*Orap*)	Azithromycin* (eg, *Zithromax*)	Erythromycin* (eg, *Ery-Tab*)
	Clarithromycin* (eg, *Biaxin*)	Telithromycin* (*Ketek*)
	Dirithromycin*†	

Significance	Onset	Severity	Documentation
1	☐ Rapid	■ **Major**	☐ Established
	■ **Delayed**	☐ Moderate	■ **Probable**
		☐ Minor	☐ Suspected
			☐ Possible
			☐ Unlikely

Effects Increased PIMOZIDE plasma concentrations with cardiotoxicity may occur.

Mechanism MACROLIDE AND RELATED ANTIBIOTICS may inhibit the hepatic metabolism (CYP3A4) of PIMOZIDE.

Management MACROLIDE AND RELATED ANTIBIOTICS are contraindicated in patients receiving PIMOZIDE.[1,2]

Discussion

In a randomized, double-blind, placebo-controlled, crossover study involving 12 healthy subjects, the effect of clarithromycin on pimozide pharmacokinetics and QTc interval was investigated.[3] Each subject received a single dose of pimozide 6 mg after 5 days of pretreatment with clarithromycin 500 mg twice daily or placebo. When compared with baseline measurements, pimozide administration prolonged the QTc interval in the first 20 hours in the clarithromycin- and placebo-treated patients. However, the QTc interval was greater in the subjects receiving pimozide with clarithromycin (23.8 msec) than when pimozide was given with placebo (16.8 msec). Compared with placebo, clarithromycin administration resulted in a 39% increase in the C_{max} (from 4.4 to 6.1 ng/mL), a 38% increase in elimination $t_{½}$, a 112% increase in AUC, and a 46% decrease in the clearance of pimozide. Neither the pharmacokinetics nor pharmacodynamics of pimozide were affected by gender or by subjects being poor or extensive metabolizers of CYP2D6. Death attributed to a pimozide-clarithromycin interaction was reported in a 27-year-old man.[4] He had been taking pimozide 14 mg/day and had a normal baseline ECG. Four days after starting clarithromycin 500 mg twice daily, he experienced syncopal episodes and a prolonged QT interval. The next day, he was found dead. His pimozide plasma level was 2.5 times the upper limit of the therapeutic range. Subsequently, the authors reviewed 39 reports of arrhythmia from pimozide, including 10 fatal cases. One was similar to the case presented. Coadministration of telithromycin and pimozide is contraindicated.[2]

[1] *Orap* [package insert]. Sellerville, PA: Teva Pharmaceuticals USA; June 2004.

[2] *Ketek* [package insert]. Kansas City, MO: Aventis Pharmaceuticals; June 2004.

[3] Desta Z, et al. *Clin Pharmacol Ther.* 1999;65(1):10.

[4] Flockhart DA, et al. *J Clin Psychopharmacol.* 2000;20(3):317.

* Asterisk indicates drugs cited in interaction reports.
† Not available in the United States.

Pimozide ✕ **Mifepristone**

Pimozide*
(*Orap*)

Mifepristone*
(eg, *Korlym*)

Significance	Onset	Severity	Documentation
1	□ Rapid ■ **Delayed**	■ **Major** □ Moderate □ Minor	□ Established □ Probable ■ **Suspected** □ Possible □ Unlikely

Effects PIMOZIDE plasma concentrations may be elevated, increasing the pharmacologic effects and risk of adverse reactions (eg, life-threatening cardiac arrhythmias).

Mechanism MIFEPRISTONE may inhibit PIMOZIDE metabolism (CYP3A4).

Management Coadministration of PIMOZIDE with MIFEPRISTONE is contraindicated.[1]

Discussion

Because mifepristone inhibits CYP3A4, coadministration of mifepristone with a drug that is metabolized mainly or solely by CYP3A4 (eg, pimozide) is likely to increase plasma concentrations of the drug.[1] Therefore, the concurrent use of drugs with a narrow therapeutic index that are CYP3A4 substrates, such as pimozide, is contraindicated. The risk of pimozide adverse reactions (eg, life-threatening arrhythmias, including torsades de pointes) may be increased.

[1] *Korlym* [package insert]. Menlo Park, CA: Corcept Therapeutics Incorporated; February 2012.

* Asterisk indicates drugs cited in interaction reports.

Pimozide — *Nefazodone*

Pimozide* (*Orap*)	Nefazodone*

Significance	Onset	Severity	Documentation
1	☐ Rapid ■ **Delayed**	■ **Major** ☐ Moderate ☐ Minor	☐ Established ☐ Probable ■ **Suspected** ☐ Possible ☐ Unlikely

Effects The risk of life-threatening cardiac arrhythmias may be increased.

Mechanism NEFAZODONE may inhibit the metabolism (CYP3A4) of PIMOZIDE.

Management Coadministration of NEFAZODONE and PIMOZIDE is contraindicated.

Discussion

Although not studied, coadministration of nefazodone and pimozide may increase pimozide plasma concentrations, resulting in QT prolongation and increasing the risk of cardiac arrhythmias.[1] Coadministration of pimozide and nefazodone is contraindicated by the manufacturer. See Pimozide-Serotonin Reuptake Inhibitors.

The basis for this monograph is information on file with the manufacturer. Published clinical data are needed to further assess this interaction. Because of the seriousness of the cardiac problem, clinical evaluation of this interaction in humans is not likely to be forthcoming.

[1] *Orap* [package insert]. North Wales, PA: Teva Pharmaceuticals USA; June 2004.

* Asterisk indicates drugs cited in interaction reports.

Pimozide — *NNRT Inhibitors*

Pimozide* (*Orap*)	Delavirdine* (*Rescriptor*)	Efavirenz* (*Sustiva*)

Significance	Onset	Severity	Documentation
1	☐ Rapid ■ **Delayed**	■ **Major** ☐ Moderate ☐ Minor	☐ Established ☐ Probable ■ **Suspected** ☐ Possible ☐ Unlikely

Effects Elevated PIMOZIDE plasma concentrations with increased risk of adverse reactions, including life-threatening cardiac arrhythmias (eg, torsades de pointes).

Mechanism Certain NNRT INHIBITORS may inhibit the hepatic metabolism (CYP3A4) of PIMOZIDE.

Management Coadministration of PIMOZIDE with DELAVIRDINE or EFAVIRENZ is contraindicated.

Discussion

Pimozide is metabolized by the CYP3A4 isozyme.[1] Drugs that inhibit this isozyme may cause increased pimozide plasma concentrations and increase the risk of QT prolongation and subsequent serious cardiac arrhythmias.[2] The manufacturers of delavirdine and efavirenz warn against coadministering these antiviral agents with pimozide because potentially serious and life-threatening adverse reactions (eg, cardiac arrhythmias) could occur.[3,4] See also Appendix: Drug-induced Prolongation of the QT Interval and Torsades de Pointes.

The basis for this monograph is information on file with the manufacturer. Because of the seriousness of the cardiac problems, clinical evaluation of this interaction in humans is not likely to be forthcoming.

[1] *Orap* [package insert]. Sellersville, PA: Teva Pharmaceuticals; June 2004.
[2] Thomas M, et al. *Br J Clin Pharmacol.* 1996;41(2):77.
[3] *Rescriptor* [package insert]. New York, NY: Pfizer Inc; June 2006.
[4] *Sustiva* [package insert]. Princeton, NJ: Bristol-Myers Squibb Company; March 2008.

* Asterisk indicates drugs cited in interaction reports.

Pimozide — *Protease Inhibitors*

Pimozide	Protease Inhibitors	
Pimozide* (*Orap*)	Amprenavir*†	Lopinavir/Ritonavir* (*Kaletra*)
	Atazanavir* (*Reyataz*)	Nelfinavir* (*Viracept*)
	Darunavir* (*Prezista*)	Ritonavir* (*Norvir*)
	Fosamprenavir* (*Lexiva*)	Saquinavir* (*Invirase*)
	Indinavir* (*Crixivan*)	

Significance	Onset	Severity	Documentation
1	☐ Rapid	■ **Major**	☐ Established
	■ **Delayed**	☐ Moderate	☐ Probable
		☐ Minor	■ **Suspected**
			☐ Possible
			☐ Unlikely

Effects The risk of life-threatening cardiac arrhythmias may be increased.

Mechanism PROTEASE INHIBITORS may inhibit the metabolism (CYP3A4) of PIMOZIDE.

Management Coadministration of PROTEASE INHIBITORS and PIMOZIDE is contraindicated.[1-5]

Discussion

Although not studied, coadministration of protease inhibitors and pimozide may increase pimozide plasma concentrations, resulting in QT prolongation and an increased risk of cardiac arrhythmias.[1] Coadministration of pimozide and protease inhibitors is contraindicated by the manufacturer.[1-5]

The basis for this monograph is information on file with the manufacturer. Published clinical data are needed to further assess this interaction. Because of the seriousness of the cardiac problem, clinical evaluation of this interaction in humans is not likely to be forthcoming.

1 *Orap* [package insert]. North Wales, PA: Teva Pharmaceuticals USA; June 2004.
2 *Reyataz* [package insert]. Princeton, NJ: Bristol-Myers Squibb Co; October 2004.
3 *Lexiva* [package insert]. Cambridge, MA: Vertex Pharmaceuticals, Inc; June 2005.
4 *Kaletra* [package insert]. North Chicago, IL: Abbott Laboratories; April 2005.
5 *Prezista* [package insert]. Raritan, NJ: Tibotec Therapeutics; June 2006.

* Asterisk indicates drugs cited in interaction reports.
†Not available in the US.

Pimozide — *Serotonin Reuptake Inhibitors*

Pimozide*
(*Orap*)

Citalopram*
(eg, *Celexa*)
Escitalopram*
(*Lexapro*)
Fluoxetine*
(eg, *Prozac*)
Fluvoxamine*
(eg, *Luvox CR*)
Paroxetine*
(eg, *Paxil*)
Sertraline*
(eg, *Zoloft*)

Significance	Onset	Severity	Documentation
1	□ Rapid ■ **Delayed**	■ **Major** □ Moderate □ Minor	□ Established □ Probable ■ **Suspected** □ Possible □ Unlikely

Effects The risk of life-threatening cardiac arrhythmias, including torsades de pointes, may be increased.

Mechanism Unknown.

Management Coadministration of PIMOZIDE and these SRIs is contraindicated.[1-6]

Discussion

In a controlled study of a single dose of pimozide 2 mg, coadministration of sertraline 200 mg/day to steady state was associated with a mean increase in pimozide AUC and C_{max} of approximately 40%[1] but was not associated with changes in the ECG. Because the highest recommended dose of pimozide (10 mg) has not been evaluated in combination with sertraline, the effect on the QT interval at doses greater than 2 mg are not known. In a controlled study, a single dose of pimozide 2 mg coadministered with citalopram 40 mg once daily for 11 days was associated with a mean increase in QTc values of approximately 10 msec compared with pimozide alone.[2] Pimozide AUC and C_{max} were not affected by citalopram. In a controlled study of healthy volunteers, coadministration of paroxetine (titrated to 60 mg/day) and a single dose of pimozide 2 mg increased the AUC and C_{max} of pimozide 151% and 62%, respectively, compared with giving pimozide alone.[5] A 77-year-old man experienced life-threatening sinus bradycardia (pulse, 35 to 45 bpm) on 2 occasions while receiving pimozide and fluoxetine.[7] His pulse rate increased when either drug was stopped.

The basis for this monograph is information on file with the manufacturer. Published clinical data are needed to further assess this interaction.

[1] *Zoloft* [package insert]. New York, NY: Pfizer, Inc; November 2002.
[2] *Celexa* [package insert]. St. Louis, MO: Forest Pharmaceuticals, Inc; August 2004.
[3] *Lexapro* [package insert]. St. Louis, MO: Forest Pharmaceuticals, Inc; May 2007.
[4] *Orap* [package insert]. Sellersville, PA: Teva Pharmaceuticals; August 2005.
[5] *Paxil* [package insert]. Research Triangle Park, NC: GlaxoSmithKline; June 2007.
[6] *Prozac* [package insert]. Indianapolis, IN: Eli Lilly and Company; June 21, 2007.
[7] Ahmed I, et al. *Can J Psychiatry*. 1993;38(1):62.

* Asterisk indicates drugs cited in interaction reports.

Pimozide — *Zileuton*

Pimozide* (*Orap*)	Zileuton* (*Zyflo*)

Significance	Onset	Severity	Documentation
1	☐ Rapid ■ **Delayed**	■ **Major** ☐ Moderate ☐ Minor	☐ Established ☐ Probable ■ **Suspected** ☐ Possible ☐ Unlikely

Effects The risk of life-threatening cardiac arrhythmias may be increased.

Mechanism ZILEUTON may inhibit the metabolism (CYP3A4) of PIMOZIDE.

Management Coadministration of ZILEUTON and PIMOZIDE is contraindicated.

Discussion

Although not studied, coadministration of zileuton and pimozide may increase pimozide plasma concentrations, resulting in QT prolongation and increasing the risk of cardiac arrhythmias.[1] Coadministration of pimozide and zileuton is contraindicated by the manufacturer.[1]

The basis for this monograph is information on file with the manufacturer. Published clinical data are needed to further assess this interaction. Because of the seriousness of the cardiac problem, clinical evaluation of this interaction in humans is not likely to be forthcoming.

[1] *Orap* [package insert]. North Wales, PA: Teva Pharmaceuticals; August 1999.

* Asterisk indicates drugs cited in interaction reports.

Pioglitazone — *Quinolones*

Pioglitazone* (*Actos*)	Gatifloxacin* (*Tequin*)

Significance	Onset	Severity	Documentation
4	■ **Rapid**	□ Major	□ Established
	□ Delayed	■ **Moderate**	□ Probable
		□ Minor	□ Suspected
			■ **Possible**
			□ Unlikely

Effects Severe and persistent hypoglycemia may occur.

Mechanism Unknown; however, GATIFLOXACIN does not affect glucose tolerance or pancreatic beta-cell function.[1]

Management Until more information is available, consider avoiding GATIFLOXACIN in patients receiving PIOGLITAZONE therapy. If therapy cannot be avoided, closely monitor blood glucose when starting GATIFLOXACIN. If hypoglycemia occurs, it may be necessary to discontinue both agents before resuming PIOGLITAZONE therapy.

Discussion

Severe and persistent hypoglycemia was reported in a 94-year-old woman with type 2 diabetes mellitus during administration of gatifloxacin and pioglitazone.[2] The patient was receiving glyburide 5 mg/day (eg, *DiaBeta*) and pioglitazone 30 mg/day for diabetes. Her blood glucose was 217 mg/dL 2 hours after the morning doses of hypoglycemic agents and 4 hours before the start of gatifloxacin (200 mg/day) therapy. The patient's blood glucose was measured at 42 mg/dL 45 minutes after gatifloxacin administration. Despite receiving orange juice and oral glucose 8 g, followed by IV dextrose 50 g, the blood glucose decreased to 33 mg/dL over a 9-hour period. Multiple boluses of IV dextrose 50 g followed by a dextrose 50% infusion were administered. The next day gatifloxacin, glyburide, and pioglitazone were withheld, and her blood glucose returned to between 100 and 200 mg/dL. Glyburide and pioglitazone were restarted 2 days later without further episodes of hypoglycemia.

Additional studies are needed to determine if this possible interaction occurs with other quinolone antibiotics or oral hypoglycemic agents. See also Repaglinide-Quinolones, Sulfonylureas-Quinolones.

[1] Gajjar DA, et al. *Pharmacotherapy*. 2000;20(6, pt 2):76S.

[2] Menzies DJ, et al. *Am J Med*. 2002;113(3):232.

* Asterisk indicates drugs cited in interaction reports.

Polypeptide Antibiotics		*Aminoglycosides*	
Bacitracin Capreomycin (*Capastat*) Colistimethate* (*Coly-Mycin M*)	Polymyxin B* (*Aerosporin*)	Amikacin (*Amikin*) Gentamicin (eg, *Garamycin*) Kanamycin* (eg, *Kantrex*) Neomycin* (*Mycifradin*)	Netilmicin (*Netromycin*) Paromomycin (*Humatin*) Streptomycin* Tobramycin (*Nebcin*)

Significance	Onset	Severity	Documentation
4	■ **Rapid** □ Delayed	■ **Major** □ Moderate □ Minor	□ Established □ Probable □ Suspected ■ **Possible** □ Unlikely

Effects Coadministration of POLYPEPTIDE ANTIBIOTICS and AMINOGLYCOSIDES may increase the risk of respiratory paralysis and renal dysfunction.

Mechanism Unknown.

Management Coadministration of these agents may require close monitoring of respiratory and renal function. If signs of respiratory arrest or renal dysfunction occur, this interaction should be suspected and at least colistimethate discontinued.

Discussion

There have been several cases of respiratory arrest or renal dysfunction development in patients who were receiving both a polypeptide antibiotic and an aminoglycoside, often along with other medications.[1-3] However, the data are insufficient to state that these reactions could not have occurred from a single agent rather than the combination.

[1] Lindesmith LA, et al. *Ann Intern Med.* 1968;68:318.
[2] Koch-Weser J, et al. *Ann Intern Med.* 1970;72:857.
[3] Lee C, et al. *Anesthesiology.* 1979;50:218.

* Asterisk indicates drugs cited in interaction reports. Based on pharmacologic and pharmacokinetic considerations, similar interactions may occur with other drugs that are listed.

Polypeptide Antibiotics | *Cephalosporins*

Colistimethate* (*Coly-Mycin M*)	Cephalothin* (eg, *Keflin*)

Significance	Onset	Severity	Documentation
4	■ **Rapid** □ Delayed	□ Major ■ **Moderate** □ Minor	□ Established □ Probable □ Suspected ■ **Possible** □ Unlikely

Effects Coadministration of COLISTIMETHATE and CEPHALOTHIN sodium may increase the risk of renal dysfunction.

Mechanism Unknown.

Management Coadministration of these agents requires close monitoring of kidney function. If signs of renal dysfunction occur, and the patient's situation allows, this interaction should be suspected and at least COLISTIMETHATE discontinued.

Discussion

A review of 317 active courses of colistimethate therapy revealed a 20.2% incidence of renal reactions (90% were renal insufficiency).[1] The only concomitant drug which altered this reaction rate was cephalothin sodium. Of 78 cases where cephalothin sodium and colistimethate were used concurrently, the incidence of renal reactions was 33.3%, which was significantly greater than in those patients who received colistimethate alone (15.9%).

A report of four cases of nonoliguric renal failure stated that sodium colistimethate and cephalothin sodium were used concurrently in three of the cases, and that colistimethate was started as cephalothin was discontinued in the other case.[2]

[1] Koch-Weser J, et al. *Ann Intern Med.* 1970;72:857. [2] Adler S, et al. *Am J Med Sci.* 1971;261:109.

* Asterisk indicates drugs cited in interaction reports.

Polypeptide Antibiotics — *Phenothiazines*

Polypeptide Antibiotics		Phenothiazines	
Bacitracin	Polymyxin B* (*Aerosporin*)	Acetophenazine (*Tindal*)	Promazine (eg, *Sparine*)
Capreomycin (*Capastat*)		Chlorpromazine (eg, *Thorazine*)	Promethazine* (eg, *Phenergan*)
Colistimethate (*Coly-Mycin M*)		Ethopropazine (*Parsidol*)	Propiomazine (*Largon*)
		Fluphenazine (eg, *Prolixin*)	Thiethylperazine (*Torecan*)
		Methdilazine (*Tacaryl*)	Thioridazine
		Methotrimeprazine (*Levoprome*)	Trifluoperazine
		Perphenazine	Triflupromazine (*Vesprin*)
		Prochlorperazine* (*Compazine*)	Trimeprazine (*Temaril*)

Significance	Onset	Severity	Documentation
5	■ **Rapid**	■ **Major**	□ Established
	□ Delayed	□ Moderate	□ Probable
		□ Minor	□ Suspected
			□ Possible
			■ **Unlikely**

Effects Coadministration of POLYPEPTIDE ANTIBIOTICS and PHENOTHIAZINES may increase the risk of respiratory paralysis.

Mechanism Unknown.

Management Coadministration of these agents may require close monitoring of respiratory function. If signs of respiratory arrest occur, this interaction should be suspected and the POLYPEPTIDE ANTIBIOTIC discontinued.

Discussion

A couple of case reports have demonstrated the possibility of respiratory arrest developing in patients who were receiving a polypeptide antibiotic and phenothiazine, often along with other medications.[2,3] An animal study suggests the possibility that these agents could produce the same effect when administered alone.[1]

[1] Sabawala PB, et al. *Anesthesiology*. 1959;20:659.
[2] Pohlmann G. *JAMA*. 1966;196:181.
[3] Anthony MA, et al. *Ohio State Med J*. 1966;62:336.

* Asterisk indicates drugs cited in interaction reports. Based on pharmacologic and pharmacokinetic considerations, similar interactions may occur with other drugs that are listed.

Posaconazole — *Metoclopramide*

Posaconazole* (*Noxafil*)	Metoclopramide* (eg, *Reglan*)

Significance	Onset	Severity	Documentation
4	☐ Rapid	☐ Major	☐ Established
	■ **Delayed**	■ **Moderate**	☐ Probable
		☐ Minor	☐ Suspected
			■ **Possible**
			☐ Unlikely

Effects POSACONAZOLE plasma concentrations may be reduced, decreasing the pharmacologic effects.

Mechanism Decreased GI absorption of POSACONAZOLE due to an increase in gastric motility and emptying time, resulting from METOCLOPRAMIDE administration.

Management A clinically important interaction is unlikely to occur. However, if an interaction is suspected, monitor the clinical status of the patient for any signs of a decrease in response to POSACONAZOLE. If an interaction is suspected, consider alternative therapy to METOCLOPRAMIDE.

Discussion

The pharmacokinetics of posaconazole were evaluated in 13 healthy subjects receiving metoclopramide.[1] Using an open-label, randomized, crossover design, each subject received a single dose of posaconazole 400 mg and a nutritional supplement or posaconazole 400 mg and a nutritional supplement on the second day of receiving metoclopramide 10 mg 3 times daily for 2 days. Compared with taking posaconazole without metoclopramide, coadministration of metoclopramide reduced the posaconazole C_{max} and AUC 21% and 19%, respectively. The posaconazole T_{max} was not affected.

[1] Krishna G, et al. *Antimicrob Agents Chemother.* 2009;53(3):958.

* Asterisk indicates drugs cited in interaction reports.

Potassium Chloride — *Anticholinergics*

Potassium Chloride	Anticholinergics	
Potassium Chloride*	Atropine* (eg, *Sal-Tropine*)	Methscopolamine* (eg, *Pamine*)
	Belladonna*	Orphenadrine* (eg, *Norflex*)
	Benztropine* (eg, *Cogentin*)	Oxybutynin* (eg, *Ditropan*)
	Biperiden*†	Procyclidine*†
	Clidinium*†	Propantheline* (eg, *Pro-Banthine*)
	Dicyclomine* (eg, *Bentyl*)	Scopolamine* (eg, *Scopace*)
	Glycopyrrolate* (eg, *Robinul*)	Trihexyphenidyl* (eg, *Trihexy-2*)
	Hyoscyamine* (eg, *Anaspaz*)	Trospium* (*Sanctura*)
	Mepenzolate* (*Cantil*)	

Significance

2

Onset
- ■ **Rapid**
- □ Delayed

Severity
- □ Major
- ■ **Moderate**
- □ Minor

Documentation
- □ Established
- □ Probable
- ■ **Suspected**
- □ Possible
- □ Unlikely

Effects Arrest or delay in POTASSIUM CHLORIDE tablet passage through the GI tract.

Mechanism ANTICHOLINERGICS may slow GI motility, delaying POTASSIUM CHLORIDE tablet passage through the GI tract.

Management Solid dosage forms of POTASSIUM CHLORIDE are contraindicated with ANTICHOLINERGICS. POTASSIUM CHLORIDE liquid may be a suitable alternative.

Discussion

All solid oral dosage forms of potassium chloride are contraindicated in any patient in whom there is pharmacologic cause for arrest or delay in tablet passage through the GI tract.[1] Pharmacologic causes include anticholinergic agents or other agents with anticholinergic properties at doses sufficient to exert anticholinergic effects.

The basis for this monograph is information on file with the manufacturer.[1]

[1] *K-Dur* [package insert]. Kenilworth, NJ: Key Pharmaceuticals Inc; April 2004.

* Asterisk indicates drugs cited in interaction reports.
† Not available in the United States.

Potassium Preparations		***ACE Inhibitors***	
Potassium Acetate Potassium Acid Phosphate (eg, *K-Phos*) Potassium Bicarbonate Potassium Chloride*	Potassium Citrate (eg, *Urocit-K*) Potassium Gluconate Potassium Phosphate	Benazepril (eg, *Lotensin*) Captopril* (eg, *Capoten*) Enalapril* (eg, *Vasotec*) Fosinopril Lisinopril* (eg, *Prinivil*)	Moexipril (eg, *Univasc*) Perindopril (eg, *Aceon*) Quinapril (eg, *Accupril*) Ramipril (eg, *Altace*) Trandolapril (eg, *Mavik*)

Significance	Onset	Severity	Documentation
4	☐ Rapid ■ **Delayed**	☐ Major ■ **Moderate** ☐ Minor	☐ Established ☐ Probable ☐ Suspected ■ **Possible** ☐ Unlikely

Effects ACE INHIBITORS plus POTASSIUM SUPPLEMENTATION may elevate serum potassium in certain patients, possibly resulting in severe hyperkalemia.

Mechanism ACE INHIBITORS decrease aldosterone secretion, possibly resulting in potassium retention.

Management Regularly measure serum potassium concentrations and adjust POTASSIUM SUPPLEMENTATION as needed.

Discussion

Captopril mildly increased serum potassium levels in patients with hypertension, especially those with high plasma renin activity or taking potassium supplementation.[1,2] In 7 case reports, serum potassium levels rose from 4.6 to 7 mEq/L.[3-5] Renal dysfunction was present in at least 3 patients. Potassium supplementation or a potassium-sparing diuretic was used in each case. In a patient on a potassium-rich diet taking lisinopril, serum potassium was 9.7 mEq/L.[6] In a study of 76 patients with end-stage chronic renal failure treated by hemodialysis containing potassium (1.5 mEq/L), captopril produced an increase in the mean serum potassium level.[7] The captopril group was compared with a normotensive control group and a hypertensive group receiving either methyldopa, clonidine (eg, *Catapres*), or a beta-blocker/hydralazine combination. After 1 month of treatment, 75% on captopril, 42% on other antihypertensives, and 29% without hypertension had serum potassium levels higher than 5.5 mEq/L. Hyperkalemia was reported with combined use of ACE inhibitors and potassium-containing salt substitutes.[8] A retrospective review of 127 hospitalized patients receiving captopril did not find captopril to increase serum potassium levels, even when potassium supplementation was used.[9] Likewise, in 6 volunteers with normal renal function, increases in plasma potassium levels were the same following an IV bolus of potassium, whether or not patients received enalapril.[10]

[1] Atlas SA, et al. *Hypertension*. 1979;1(3):274.
[2] Maslowski AH, et al. *Lancet*. 1981;1(8211):71.
[3] Warren SE, et al. *JAMA*. 1980;244(22):2551.
[4] Grossman A, et al. *Lancet*. 1980;1(8170):712.
[5] Burnakis TG, et al. *Arch Intern Med*. 1984;144(12):2371.
[6] Stoltz ML, et al. *JAMA*. 1990;264(21):2737.
[7] Papadimitriou M, et al. *Dial Transplant*. 1985;14:473.
[8] Ray K, et al. *J Hum Hypertens*. 1999;13(10):717.
[9] Schuna AA, et al. *Clin Pharm*. 1986;5(11):920.
[10] Scandling JD, et al. *J Clin Pharmacol*. 1989;29(10):916.

* Asterisk indicates drugs cited in interaction reports. Based on pharmacologic and pharmacokinetic considerations, similar interactions may occur with other drugs that are listed.

Potassium Preparations / Potassium-Sparing Diuretics

Potassium Preparations		Potassium-Sparing Diuretics	
Potassium Acetate	Potassium Gluconate (eg, *Kaon*)	Amiloride* (eg, *Midamor*)	Triamterene* (*Dyrenium*)
Potassium Acid Phosphate (eg, *K-Phos*)	Potassium Iodide (eg, *SSKI*)	Spironolactone* (eg, *Aldactone*)	
Potassium Bicarbonate	Potassium Phosphate		
Potassium Chloride*			
Potassium Citrate (eg, *Urocit-K*)			

Significance	Onset	Severity	Documentation
1	□ Rapid	■ **Major**	■ **Established**
	■ **Delayed**	□ Moderate	□ Probable
		□ Minor	□ Suspected
			□ Possible
			□ Unlikely

Effects POTASSIUM-SPARING DIURETICS will increase potassium retention and can produce severe hyperkalemia.

Mechanism A reduction in renal elimination of the potassium ion.

Management Do not use this combination without documented evidence that a patient has clinical symptoms of hypokalemia unresponsive to either agent alone. If the combination is required, the patient should have strict dietary counseling and close monitoring of serum potassium concentrations.

Discussion

Studies have shown that potassium-sparing diuretics enhance potassium retention.[1-3] Some studies and case reports have shown that hyperkalemia can develop from normal use of potassium-sparing diuretics and that severe disabilities, and death can develop in patients taking combinations of potassium supplementation and potassium-sparing diuretics.[4-7] One study shows death from hyperkalemia due to potassium supplementation is one of the more common causes of drug-related deaths.[4]

1 Hansen KB, et al. *Clin Pharmacol Ther.* 1967;8(3):392.
2 McNay JL, et al. *Metabolism.* 1970;19(1):58.
3 Walker BR, et al. *Clin Pharmacol Ther.* 1972;13(5):643.
4 Shapiro S, et al. *JAMA.* 1971;216(3):467.
5 Greenblatt DJ, et al. *JAMA.* 1973;225(1):40.
6 Kalbian VV. *South Med J.* 1974;67(3):342.
7 Simborg DW. *Johns Hopkins Med J.* 1976;139(1):23.

* Asterisk indicates drugs cited in interaction reports. Based on pharmacologic and pharmacokinetic considerations, similar interactions may occur with other drugs that are listed.

Potassium-Sparing Diuretics ✕ **ACE Inhibitors**

Potassium-Sparing Diuretics		ACE Inhibitors	
Amiloride* (*Midamor*)	Triamterene (*Dyrenium*)	Benazepril* (eg, *Lotensin*)	Moexipril* (*Univasc*)
Spironolactone* (eg, *Aldactone*)		Captopril* (eg, *Capoten*)	Perindopril* (*Aceon*)
		Enalapril* (eg, *Vasotec*)	Quinapril (*Accupril*)
		Fosinopril (eg, *Monopril*)	Ramipril* (*Altace*)
		Lisinopril* (eg, *Prinivil*)	Trandolapril (*Mavik*)

Significance	Onset	Severity	Documentation
1	☐ Rapid	■ **Major**	☐ Established
	■ **Delayed**	☐ Moderate	■ **Probable**
		☐ Minor	☐ Suspected
			☐ Possible
			☐ Unlikely

Effects Combining ACE INHIBITORS and POTASSIUM-SPARING DIURETICS may result in elevated serum potassium concentrations in certain high-risk (eg, renally impaired) patients.

Mechanism Unknown.

Management Regularly monitor renal function and serum potassium levels in patients receiving these agents concurrently. Be prepared to adjust therapy as needed.

Discussion

Captopril mildly increases serum potassium levels in patients with hypertension, especially those with high plasma renin activity or those on potassium supplementation.[1,2] In 7 case reports, serum potassium levels rose from 4.6 to 7 mEq/L.[3-5] Potassium supplements or a potassium-sparing diuretic was used in each case, and at least 3 patients had renal dysfunction. Two retrospective reviews found no association between captopril[6] or enalapril[7] use and serum potassium levels, even for patients taking potassium-sparing diuretics. In 5 diabetic patients taking enalapril or captopril, life-threatening hyperkalemia occurred 8 to 18 days after adding amiloride/hydrochlorothiazide (eg, *Moduretic*) to the regimen.[8] Four of the 5 patients had preexisting renal impairment (Ccr above 2), and 2 patients were taking NSAIDs. A retrospective review of 262 patients treated with an ACE inhibitor and spironolactone identified 25 high-risk patients who developed serious hyperkalemia (serum potassium greater than 6).[9] Another review identified patients who developed hyperkalemia while taking ACE inhibitors and spironolactone.[10] Risk factors included older age, decreased renal function, type 2 diabetes, and spironolactone doses greater than 25 mg/day.

1 Atlas SA, et al. *Hypertension.* 1979;1:274.
2 Maslowski AH, et al. *Lancet.* 1981;1:71.
3 Warren SE, et al. *JAMA.* 1980;244:2551.
4 Grossman A, et al. *Lancet.* 1980;1:712.
5 Burnakis TG, et al. *Arch Intern Med.* 1984;144:2371.
6 Schuna AA, et al. *Clin Pharm.* 1986;5:920.
7 Radley AS, et al. *J Clin Pharm Ther.* 1987;12:319.
8 Chiu TF, et al. *Ann Emerg Med.* 1997;30:612.
9 Schepkens H, et al. *Am J Med.* 2001;110:438.
10 Wrenger E, et al. *BMJ.* 2003;327:147.

* Asterisk indicates drugs cited in interaction reports. Based on pharmacologic and pharmacokinetic considerations, similar interactions may occur with other drugs that are listed.

Potassium-Sparing Diuretics / Angiotensin II Receptor Antagonists

Potassium-Sparing Diuretics		Angiotensin II Receptor Antagonists	
Amiloride (*Midamor*)	Triamterene (*Dyrenium*)	Candesartan* (*Atacand*)	Olmesartan (*Benicar*)
Spironolactone* (eg, *Aldactone*)		Eprosartan (*Teveten*)	Telmisartan* (*Micardis*)
		Irbesartan* (*Avapro*)	Valsartan (*Diovan*)
		Losartan* (*Cozaar*)	

Significance	Onset	Severity	Documentation
1	☐ Rapid	■ **Major**	☐ Established
	■ **Delayed**	☐ Moderate	☐ Probable
		☐ Minor	■ **Suspected**
			☐ Possible
			☐ Unlikely

Effects Combining ANGIOTENSIN II RECEPTOR ANTAGONISTS and POTASSIUM-SPARING DIURETICS may result in elevated serum potassium concentrations in certain high-risk patients (eg, renal impairment, type 2 diabetes).

Mechanism ANGIOTENSIN II RECEPTOR ANTAGONISTS and POTASSIUM-SPARING DIURETICS may increase serum potassium levels, leading to additive or synergistic effects.

Management Regularly monitor serum potassium concentrations and renal function in patients receiving these agents concurrently. Consider estimating Ccr in elderly patients and high-risk patients. Adjust therapy as needed.

Discussion

Six patients with congestive heart failure who were taking spironolactone and an angiotensin II receptor antagonist were admitted to the nephrology unit for treatment of life-threatening hyperkalemia.[1] Patients had received spironolactone 50, 100, or 150 mg daily. In addition, 4 patients received losartan 50 mg/day, 1 patient received telmisartan 80 mg/day plus captopril, and 1 patient received candesartan 16 mg/day. All patients had type 2 diabetes mellitus. Their serum potassium concentration on admission ranged from 6.2 to 9.65 mEq/L, and serum creatinine concentration ranged from 1.2 to 10.7 mg/dL. An 88-year-old woman developed life-threatening hyperkalemia during coadministration of spironolactone 25 mg/day and irbesartan 150 mg/day. In addition, she was receiving potassium chloride 20 mEq/day. Her serum potassium and serum creatinine concentrations on admission were 7.2 mEq/L and 3.1 mg/dL, respectively. She developed cardiac arrest and died. All patients had several risk factors that could contribute to the development of hyperkalemia (eg, diabetes mellitus and/or decreased renal perfusion). See also Potassium-Sparing Diuretics-ACE Inhibitors.

[1] Wrenger E, et al. *BMJ.* 2003;327:147.

[2] Blaustein DA, et al. *Am J Cardiol.* 2002;90:662.

* Asterisk indicates drugs cited in interaction reports. Based on pharmacologic and pharmacokinetic considerations, similar interactions may occur with other drugs that are listed.

Pravastatin — *Protease Inhibitors*

Pravastatin* (eg, *Pravachol*)	Nelfinavir* (*Viracept*) Ritonavir* (*Norvir*)	Saquinavir* (*Invirase*)

Significance	Onset	Severity	Documentation
1	☐ Rapid ■ **Delayed**	■ **Major** ☐ Moderate ☐ Minor	☐ Established ☐ Probable ■ **Suspected** ☐ Possible ☐ Unlikely

Effects PRAVASTATIN plasma levels may be reduced, decreasing the efficacy.

Mechanism Increased metabolism (glucuronidation) of PRAVASTATIN is suspected.

Management Carefully monitor patients receiving PRAVASTATIN for a decrease in clinical effect when starting therapy with certain PROTEASE INHIBITORS.

Discussion

The effects of ritonavir coadministered with saquinavir on the pharmacokinetics of pravastatin, as well as the effect of pravastatin on the pharmacokinetics of nelfinavir, were evaluated in 27 HIV-seronegative volunteers.[1] Using a randomized, open-label design, 13 patients were administered pravastatin 40 mg/day from days 1 through 4 and 15 through 18. Subjects received ritonavir (300 mg twice daily from days 4 to 8 and 400 mg twice daily from days 8 through 18) plus saquinavir (400 mg twice daily from days 4 through 18). A second group of 14 patients received nelfinavir 1,250 mg twice daily from days 1 through 14 and pravastatin 40 mg/day from days 15 through 18. Administration of ritonavir plus saquinavir decreased the pravastatin AUC 50%. In another study, nelfinavir reduced the pravastatin AUC 46.5%.[2] See Atorvastatin-Protease Inhibitors and Simvastatin-Protease Inhibitors.

[1] Fichtenbaum CJ, et al. *AIDS*. 2002;16(4):569.

[2] Aberg JA, et al. *AIDS*. 2006;20(5):725.

* Asterisk indicates drugs cited in interaction reports.

Praziquantel | **Azole Antifungal Agents**

Praziquantel* (*Biltricide*)	Itraconazole (eg, *Sporanox*)	Posaconazole (*Noxafil*)
	Ketoconazole* (eg, *Nizoral*)	Voriconazole (*Vfend*)

Significance	Onset	Severity	Documentation
4	☐ Rapid	☐ Major	☐ Established
	■ **Delayed**	■ **Moderate**	☐ Probable
		☐ Minor	☐ Suspected
			■ **Possible**
			☐ Unlikely

Effects PRAZIQUANTEL plasma concentration may be elevated, increasing the pharmacologic effect and adverse reactions.

Mechanism Inhibition of PRAZIQUANTEL metabolism (CYP3A4) by AZOLE ANTIFUNGAL AGENTS is suspected.

Management Observe patients for increased adverse reactions during coadministration of PRAZIQUANTEL and AZOLE ANTIFUNGAL AGENTS. If an interaction is suspected, reduce the dose of PRAZIQUANTEL.

Discussion

The effects of ketoconazole on the pharmacokinetics of praziquantel were studied in 10 healthy men.[1] In an open-label, randomized, crossover study, each subject received a single dose of praziquantel 20 mg/kg alone and after 5 days of pretreatment with ketoconazole 400 mg. Compared with administration of praziquantel alone, pretreatment with ketoconazole increased the mean AUC and C_{max} of praziquantel 93% and 102%, respectively, while decreasing the mean total clearance of praziquantel 58%. No adverse reactions occurred after praziquantel was taken alone; however, when ketoconazole and praziquantel were coadministered, mild GI discomfort occurred in 1 subject, mild nausea and vomiting occurred in 2 subjects, and mild headache was reported in 4 subjects. It was suggested that the dose of praziquantel be reduced by 50% when coadministered with ketoconazole.

[1] Ridtitid W, et al. *J Clin Pharm Ther.* 2007;32(6):585.

* Asterisk indicates drugs cited in interaction reports. Based on pharmacologic and pharmacokinetic considerations, similar interactions may occur with other drugs that are listed.

Praziquantel — *Carbamazepine*

Praziquantel* (*Biltricide*)	Carbamazepine* (eg, *Tegretol*)

Significance	Onset	Severity	Documentation
4	■ **Rapid**	□ Major	□ Established
	□ Delayed	■ **Moderate**	□ Probable
		□ Minor	□ Suspected
			■ **Possible**
			□ Unlikely

Effects Serum PRAZIQUANTEL concentrations may be reduced, possibly leading to treatment failures.

Mechanism Unknown.

Management Observe the clinical response of the patient. It may be necessary to increase the dose of PRAZIQUANTEL during concurrent use of CARBAMAZEPINE. Serum PRAZIQUANTEL concentrations may be useful in managing the patient.

Discussion

The effects of carbamazepine on the pharmacokinetics of a single dose of praziquantel were evaluated in an open, controlled, prospective study.[1] The AUC of praziquantel in healthy subjects receiving concurrent carbamazepine was 9.7% of that obtained in individuals receiving praziquantel alone. In addition, the maximum concentration of praziquantel with coadministration of carbamazepine was 7.9% of that obtained in subjects given only praziquantel. The $t_{1/2}$ of praziquantel and time to reach the maximum concentration were not affected by carbamazepine administration.

[1] Bittencourt PR, et al. *Neurology*. 1992;42:492.

* Asterisk indicates drugs cited in interaction reports.

Praziquantel — *Food*

Praziquantel*
(*Biltricide*)

Grapefruit Juice*

Significance	Onset	Severity	Documentation
5	☐ Rapid ■ **Delayed**	☐ Major ☐ Moderate ■ **Minor**	☐ Established ☐ Probable ☐ Suspected ■ **Possible** ☐ Unlikely

Effects PRAZIQUANTEL plasma concentrations may be elevated, increasing the pharmacologic and adverse effects.

Mechanism Inhibition of intestinal first-pass metabolism (CYP3A4) of PRAZIQUANTEL by GRAPEFRUIT JUICE is suspected.

Management Patients should avoid taking PRAZIQUANTEL with GRAPEFRUIT products. Advise patients to take PRAZIQUANTEL with a liquid other than GRAPEFRUIT JUICE.

Discussion

The effects of grapefruit juice on the pharmacokinetics of praziquantel were studied in 18 healthy men.[1] Using a randomized, crossover design, each subject received a single dose of praziquantel 1,800 mg with 250 mL of water or grapefruit juice. Compared with water, administration of praziquantel with grapefruit juice increased the peak plasma concentration and AUC of praziquantel 63% (from 638 to 1,038 ng/mL) and 90%, respectively. Grapefruit juice did not prolong the $t_{½}$ of praziquantel.

[1] Castro N, et al. *Antimicrob Agents Chemother.* 2002;46:1614.

* Asterisk indicates drugs cited in interaction reports.

Praziquantel	***Histamine H_2 Antagonists***
Praziquantel* (*Biltricide*)	Cimetidine* (eg, *Tagamet*)

Significance	Onset	Severity	Documentation
2	☐ Rapid	☐ Major	☐ Established
	■ **Delayed**	■ **Moderate**	■ **Probable**
		☐ Minor	☐ Suspected
			☐ Possible
			☐ Unlikely

Effects Plasma concentrations of PRAZIQUANTEL may be elevated, increasing the effectiveness and risk of adverse reactions.

Mechanism CIMETIDINE may inhibit the first-pass metabolism of PRAZIQUANTEL.

Management Observe patients for increased adverse reactions during coadministration of PRAZIQUANTEL and CIMETIDINE. Other HISTAMINE H_2 ANTAGONISTS (eg, ranitidine [eg, *Zantac*]) are less likely to interact and may be suitable alternatives.

Discussion

Increased praziquantel plasma levels have been reported following coadministration of cimetidine.[1-3] In a patient with neurocysticerosis in whom previous treatment with praziquantel had failed, cimetidine was given with praziquantel to achieve higher levels of praziquantel.[1] Coadministration of cimetidine 1,600 mg daily increased the peak plasma levels of praziquantel 136%, elimination $t_{½}$ 94%, and AUC 4-fold. Although the patient made slow improvement during coadministration of the drugs, it could not be determined that the improvement was caused by the drug interaction. Two studies in healthy volunteers also found peak concentrations,[2,3] $t_{½}$,[3] and AUC[3] of praziquantel increased with coadministration of cimetidine.

[1] Dachman WD, et al. *J Infect Dis.* 1994;169(3):689.
[2] Metwally A, et al. *Arzneimittelforschung.* 1995; 45(4):516.
[3] Castro N, et al. *Proc West Pharmacol Soc.* 1997;40:33.

* Asterisk indicates drugs cited in interaction reports.

Praziquantel — *Hydantoins*

Praziquantel* (*Biltricide*)	Ethotoin (*Peganone*)	Phenytoin* (eg, *Dilantin*)
	Fosphenytoin (*Cerebyx*)	

Significance	Onset	Severity	Documentation
4	■ **Rapid**	□ Major	□ Established
	□ Delayed	■ **Moderate**	□ Probable
		□ Minor	□ Suspected
			■ **Possible**
			□ Unlikely

Effects Serum PRAZIQUANTEL concentrations may be reduced, possibly leading to treatment failures.

Mechanism Unknown.

Management Observe the clinical response of patients. It may be necessary to increase the dose of PRAZIQUANTEL during concurrent use of HYDANTOINS. Serum PRAZIQUANTEL concentrations may be useful in managing patients.

Discussion

The effects of phenytoin on the pharmacokinetics of a single dose of praziquantel were evaluated in an open, controlled, prospective study.[1] The AUC of praziquantel in healthy subjects receiving concurrent phenytoin was 26% of that obtained in subjects receiving praziquantel alone. In addition, the maximum concentration of praziquantel with coadministration of phenytoin was 24% of that obtained in subjects given only praziquantel. The $t_{½}$ of praziquantel and time to reach the maximum concentration were not affected by phenytoin administration.

[1] Bittencourt PR, et al. *Neurology*. 1992;42(3)(pt 1):492.

* Asterisk indicates drugs cited in interaction reports. Based on pharmacologic and pharmacokinetic considerations, similar interactions may occur with other drugs that are listed.

Praziquantel — *Rifamycins*

Praziquantel* (*Biltricide*)	Rifabutin (*Mycobutin*)	Rifapentine (*Priftin*)
	Rifampin* (eg, *Rifadin*)	

Significance	Onset	Severity	Documentation
2	☐ Rapid	☐ Major	☐ Established
	■ **Delayed**	■ **Moderate**	☐ Probable
		☐ Minor	■ **Suspected**
			☐ Possible
			☐ Unlikely

Effects PRAZIQUANTEL plasma levels may be greatly reduced, possibly producing a loss in therapeutic effect.

Mechanism Increased hepatic metabolism (CYP3A4) of PRAZIQUANTEL by RIFAMYCINS may occur.

Management Avoid administration of PRAZIQUANTEL to patients receiving RIFAMYCINS.

Discussion

The effects of rifampin on the pharmacokinetics of single- or multiple-dose administration of praziquantel were investigated in 10 healthy men.[1] Subjects received a single dose of praziquantel 40 mg/kg alone and after pretreatment with rifampin 600 mg/day for 5 days. Compared with administration of praziquantel alone, pretreatment with rifampin resulted in praziquantel levels that were undetectable in 7 subjects. In 3 subjects in which praziquantel levels were measurable, the C_{max}, AUC, and $t_{1/2}$ were decreased 81%, 85%, and 45%, respectively. In the multiple-dose investigation, subjects received praziquantel 25 mg/kg for 3 doses (spaced at 8-hr intervals) alone and after 5 days of rifampin 600 mg daily administration. Compared with giving praziquantel alone, pretreatment with rifampin resulted in undetectable levels of praziquantel in 5 subjects. In the 5 subjects with measurable praziquantel levels, the C_{max}, AUC, and $t_{1/2}$ were reduced 74%, 80%, and 41%, respectively.

[1] Ridtitid W, et al. *Clin Pharmacol Ther.* 2002;72:505.

* Asterisk indicates drugs cited in interaction reports. Based on pharmacologic and pharmacokinetic considerations, similar interactions may occur with other drugs that are listed.

Prazosin — *Beta-Blockers*

Prazosin	Beta-Blockers	
Prazosin* (eg, *Minipress*)	Acebutolol (eg, *Sectral*)	Nadolol (eg, *Corgard*)
	Atenolol (eg, *Tenormin*)	Penbutolol (*Levatol*)
	Betaxolol (*Kerlone*)	Pindolol (eg, *Visken*)
	Bisoprolol (eg, *Zebeta*)	Propranolol* (eg, *Inderal*)
	Carteolol (*Cartrol*)	Sotalol (eg, *Betapace*)
	Esmolol (eg, *Brevibloc*)	Timolol (eg, *Timoptic*)
	Metoprolol (eg, *Lopressor*)	

Significance	Onset	Severity	Documentation
2	■ **Rapid**	□ Major	□ Established
	□ Delayed	■ **Moderate**	■ **Probable**
		□ Minor	□ Suspected
			□ Possible
			□ Unlikely

Effects Postural hypotension may be increased.

Mechanism Unknown.

Management Advise patients that symptomatic postural hypotension may occur in the early stages of concurrent therapy.

Discussion

Well-controlled trials have demonstrated a reduction in standing BP with the combination of prazosin and propranolol.[1,2] In 1 study of 8 healthy normotensive men, the duration of a pronounced hypotensive effect (arbitrarily defined as a fall in standing BP of greater than 20 mm Hg) was 2.8 hours on prazosin 1 mg, 3.4 hours on prazosin 1 mg and propranolol 80 mg, and 6.3 hours on prazosin 1 mg and primidolol 100 mg (not available in the US).[2] In the other study, 4 healthy volunteers who had syncopal episodes on prazosin alone experienced similar episodes on the combination of prazosin 1 mg and propranolol 80 mg twice daily.[1] Propranolol had no effect on the total drop in BP, but reduced the accompanying increase in heart rate. A study combining prazosin and alprenolol (not available in the US) in patients with essential hypertension reported symptoms of orthostatic hypotension in 4 patients.[3]

[1] Rubin P, et al. *Br J Clin Pharmacol.* 1980;10:33.
[2] Elliot HL, et al. *Clin Pharmacol Ther.* 1981;29:303.
[3] Seideman P, et al. *Br J Clin Pharmacol.* 1982;13:865.

* Asterisk indicates drugs cited in interaction reports. Based on pharmacologic and pharmacokinetic considerations, similar interactions may occur with other drugs that are listed.

Prazosin — *Indomethacin*

Prazosin* (eg, *Minipress*)	Indomethacin* (eg, *Indocin*)

Significance	Onset	Severity	Documentation
5	☐ Rapid	☐ Major	☐ Established
	■ **Delayed**	☐ Moderate	☐ Probable
		■ **Minor**	☐ Suspected
			■ **Possible**
			☐ Unlikely

Effects INDOMETHACIN may attenuate PRAZOSIN-induced postural hypotension.

Mechanism Unknown.

Management None required.

Discussion

In a study of 9 subjects, the addition of indomethacin to prazosin therapy reduced the maximum decrease in standing blood pressure by 20 mmHg.[1] Postural symptoms were experienced by 4 subjects on prazosin alone but by no subjects on combination therapy. A comparison of the mean blood pressures of the 2 groups showed no significant difference. See also Hydralazine-Indomethacin.

[1] Rubin P, et al. *Br J Clin Pharmacol.* 1980;10:33.

* Asterisk indicates drugs cited in interaction reports.

Prazosin		***Verapamil***
Prazosin* (eg, *Minipress*)		Verapamil* (eg, *Calan*)

Significance	Onset	Severity	Documentation
2	■ **Rapid**	□ Major	□ Established
	□ Delayed	■ **Moderate**	□ Probable
		□ Minor	■ **Suspected**
			□ Possible
			□ Unlikely

Effects VERAPAMIL appears to increase serum prazosin concentrations and may increase the sensitivity to PRAZOSIN-induced postural hypotension.

Mechanism Unknown.

Management When these drugs are to be used in combination, advise the patient to take precautions regarding postural hypotension when beginning PRAZOSIN therapy.

Discussion

A series of studies from the same researchers demonstrate an increase in both hypotensive episodes and serum prazosin concentrations when prazosin is administered with verapamil.[1-3] The largest trial evaluated 12 patients with essential hypertension.[3] Each patient was randomly assigned in a single-blind fashion to complete one of two treatment regimens (verapamil followed by prazosin, or vice-versa) and subsequently crossed over to the alternate regimen. The addition of verapamil to prazosin therapy produced a significant increase in both the area under the plasma concentration-time curve (84%), and the peak prazosin concentrations (103%). There was no significant change in the elimination half-life. When prazosin was added to verapamil therapy, no significant changes in verapamil pharmacokinetic parameters were noted. There also were no significant differences in the incidence of symptomatic postural hypotension, with four reports on prazosin only, two on verapamil only, and two on both drugs concurrently. The other two studies demonstrated a similar pattern with prazosin concentration changes.[1,2] One trial also showed a difference in the degree of postural hypotension produced by combination therapy over that of either agent alone.[2] By application of concentration-effect modeling, this interaction is the result of both pharmacokinetic and pharmacodynamic components.[4]

[1] Pasanisi F, et al. *Clin Pharmacol Ther.* 1984;36:716.
[2] Meredith PA, et al. *Br J Clin Pharmacol.* 1986;21:85P.
[3] Elliott HL, et al. *Clin Pharmacol Ther.* 1988;43:554.
[4] Meredith PA, et al. *Clin Pharmacol Ther.* 1992;51:708.

* Asterisk indicates drugs cited in interaction reports.

Primaquine ✕ ***Food***

Primaquine*	Grapefruit Juice*

Significance	Onset	Severity	Documentation
4	☐ Rapid ■ **Delayed**	☐ Major ■ **Moderate** ☐ Minor	☐ Established ☐ Probable ☐ Suspected ■ **Possible** ☐ Unlikely

Effects PRIMAQUINE plasma concentrations may be elevated, increasing the pharmacologic and toxic effects.

Mechanism Inhibition of gut wall metabolism (CYP3A4) or intestinal transport (eg, P-glycoprotein) is suspected.

Management Caution patients to avoid GRAPEFRUIT products while taking PRIMAQUINE. Advise patients to take PRIMAQUINE with a liquid other than GRAPEFRUIT JUICE.

Discussion

The effects of grapefruit juice on the pharmacokinetics of primaquine were studied in 20 healthy subjects.[1] Each subject received primaquine 30 mg with 300 mL of grapefruit juice 50% concentration or in the fasting state with 300 mL of water. Grapefruit juice increased the C_{max} and AUC of primaquine 23% and 19%, respectively, compared with fasting state values. Because there was marked interindividual variability, the quantitative effects of grapefruit juice on the pharmacokinetics of primaquine are not predictable at an individual level.

[1] Cuong BT, et al. *Br J Clin Pharmacol.* 2006;61:682.

* Asterisk indicates drugs cited in interaction reports.

Primidone — **Carbamazepine**

Primidone* (eg, *Mysoline*)	Carbamazepine* (eg, *Tegretol*)

Significance	Onset	Severity	Documentation
2	☐ Rapid	☐ Major	☐ Established
	■ **Delayed**	■ **Moderate**	☐ Probable
		☐ Minor	■ **Suspected**
			☐ Possible
			☐ Unlikely

Effects Concomitant PRIMIDONE and CARBAMAZEPINE administration may result in decreased PRIMIDONE, its metabolite phenobarbital, and CARBAMAZEPINE serum concentrations.

Mechanism Possibly due to an alteration in hepatic metabolism.

Management In a patient who requires both PRIMIDONE and CARBAMAZEPINE, monitor serum concentrations of both drugs regularly, and adjust their dosages appropriately.

Discussion

In a study of chronically treated epileptic patients, 523 taking primidone alone and 155 taking primidone combined with carbamazepine, the carbamazepine-treated group had a significantly lower serum primidone concentration/dose ratio and serum phenobarbital concentration/dose ratio, and a higher phenobarbital/primidone concentration ratio than the non-carbamazepine-treated group.[2] The significance in the differences of the 2 former ratios was seen in patients 0 to 9 years of age and for the latter ratio in patients 0 to 60 years of age.

Another study of 3- to 15-year-old patients receiving 14.9 mg/kg/day or less of carbamazepine noted a decrease in serum primidone concentrations.[1] A small group of patients in the study who received 15 mg/kg/day or more had a slight increase in serum primidone concentrations.

In 1 case report of a 15-year-old male receiving carbamazepine and primidone, phenobarbital and carbamazepine serum concentrations were monitored for 16 months.[3] At 2 months before withdrawal of primidone 12 mg/kg/day, carbamazepine clearance was 3.99 mL/kg/min, and the serum carbamazepine concentration was 3.5 mcg/mL on carbamazepine 10 mg/kg/day. An increase to carbamazepine 30 mg/kg/day increased the serum carbamazepine concentration to 4.8 mcg/mL. At 14 months, primidone was discontinued, carbamazepine clearance decreased to 1.63 mL/kg/min, and serum concentration increased to 12 mcg/mL.

[1] Windorfer A Jr, et al. *Neuropaediatie.* 1977;8:29.
[2] Battino D, et al. *Ther Drug Monit.* 1983;5:73.
[3] Benetello P, et al. *Int J Clin Pharmacol Res.* 1987;7:165.

* Asterisk indicates drugs cited in interaction reports.

Primidone / *Carbonic Anhydrase Inhibitors*

Primidone* (eg, *Mysoline*)	Acetazolamide* (eg, *Diamox*)	Methazolamide (eg, *Neptazane*)

Significance	Onset	Severity	Documentation
4	☐ Rapid ■ **Delayed**	☐ Major ■ **Moderate** ☐ Minor	☐ Established ☐ Probable ☐ Suspected ■ **Possible** ☐ Unlikely

Effects Concomitant administration of ACETAZOLAMIDE may alter PRIMIDONE serum and urine concentrations.

Mechanism Unknown.

Management If a patient is receiving both PRIMIDONE and ACETAZOLAMIDE, and PRIMIDONE and its metabolite phenobarbital concentrations are lower than expected, this interaction should be suspected. Consider separating the times of administration or discontinuing agents.

Discussion

In 3 patients who received primidone 500 mg alone and in combination with acetazolamide 250 mg, 2 had signs of altered primidone metabolism.[1] In 1 patient, only trace amounts of serum and urine primidone (and no phenobarbital or phenylethylmalonamide) concentrations were detected with combination therapy. In the remaining 2 patients, normal concentrations of primidone, phenylethylmalonamide, and phenobarbital were detected in both, but the peak serum primidone concentration and the urinary excretion of primidone and phenylethylmalonamide were delayed in 1 of the patients.

[1] Syversen GB, et al. *Arch Neurol.* 1977;34:80.

* Asterisk indicates drugs cited in interaction reports. Based on pharmacologic and pharmacokinetic considerations, similar interactions may occur with other drugs that are listed.

Primidone | *Hydantoins*

Primidone* (eg, *Mysoline*)	Ethotoin (*Peganone*)	Phenytoin* (eg, *Dilantin*)
	Fosphenytoin (*Cerebyx*)	

Significance	Onset	Severity	Documentation
2	□ Rapid	□ Major	□ Established
	■ **Delayed**	■ **Moderate**	■ **Probable**
		□ Minor	□ Suspected
			□ Possible
			□ Unlikely

Effects HYDANTOINS may increase the serum PRIMIDONE, phenobarbital, and phenylethylmalonomide concentrations in patients receiving PRIMIDONE.

Mechanism Unknown. Probable alteration in hepatic metabolism.

Management In patients requiring both PRIMIDONE and a HYDANTOIN, closely monitor serum concentrations of PRIMIDONE and PRIMIDONE metabolites following any alteration in HYDANTOIN therapy.

Discussion

A study of 9 patients who were receiving primidone and 31 who were receiving both primidone and phenytoin demonstrated a significant increase in the mean phenobarbital/primidone and phenylethylmalonomide/primidone ratios with combination therapy.[1] Another study had similar results and showed a 51% increase in the serum phenobarbital concentration when phenytoin was added to primidone therapy.[2] Several studies and cases support these results.[3-7]

A case report of severe phenobarbital intoxication was reported in a 6-month-old child treated with oral primidone 200 mg 3 times daily and phenytoin 23 mg/day.[8] After chronic therapy, the patient presented as semicomatose with a serum phenobarbital concentration of 202 mcg/mL.

1 Lambie DG, et al. *J Neurol Neurosurg Psychiatry.* 1981;44(2):148.
2 Schmidt D, et al. *J Neurol.* 1975;209(2):115.
3 Gallagher BB, et al. *Neurology.* 1973;23(2):145.
4 Reynolds EH, et al. *Br Med J.* 1975;2(5971):594.
5 Callaghan N, et al. *Acta Neurol Scand.* 1977;56(1):1.
6 Garrettson LK, et al. *Br J Clin Pharmacol.* 1977; 4(6):693.
7 Porro MG, et al. *Br J Clin Pharmacol.* 1982;14(2):294.
8 Wilson JT, et al. *J Pediatr.* 1973;83(3):484.

* Asterisk indicates drugs cited in interaction reports. Based on pharmacologic and pharmacokinetic considerations, similar interactions may occur with other drugs that are listed.

Primidone — *Isoniazid*

Primidone* (eg, *Mysoline*)	Isoniazid* (eg, *Nydrazid*)

Significance	Onset	Severity	Documentation
4	☐ Rapid ■ **Delayed**	☐ Major ■ **Moderate** ☐ Minor	☐ Established ☐ Probable ☐ Suspected ■ **Possible** ☐ Unlikely

Effects ISONIAZID may increase PRIMIDONE serum concentrations.

Mechanism Unknown.

Management Suspect this interaction in patients taking PRIMIDONE and ISONIAZID if elevated PRIMIDONE and phenobarbital serum concentrations occur unexpectedly.

Discussion

A 46-year-old woman had a primidone elimination $t_{1/2}$ of 8.7 hours while taking primidone alone and 14 hours while taking primidone and long-term isoniazid. Similarly, the mean serum primidone concentration increased 83% and the mean serum phenobarbital and phenylethylmalonamide concentrations decreased 12% and 29%, respectively. There was no change in seizure activity throughout the 21-month evaluation.[1]

[1] Sutton G, et al. *Neurology*. 1975;25(12):1179.

* Asterisk indicates drugs cited in interaction reports.

Primidone — *Nicotinamide*

Primidone* (eg, *Mysoline*)	Nicotinamide*

Significance	Onset	Severity	Documentation
4	☐ Rapid ■ **Delayed**	☐ Major ■ **Moderate** ☐ Minor	☐ Established ☐ Probable ☐ Suspected ■ **Possible** ☐ Unlikely

Effects NICOTINAMIDE may decrease the clearance rate of PRIMIDONE.

Mechanism Unknown.

Management If a patient has unexpectedly elevated PRIMIDONE concentrations while receiving both PRIMIDONE and NICOTINAMIDE, this interaction should be suspected. If necessary, the dose of PRIMIDONE could be decreased or NICOTINAMIDE discontinued.

Discussion

The addition of nicotinamide 41 to 178 mg/kg/day in three patients receiving primidone produced an increase in the serum primidone/phenobarbital concentration ratio and a decrease in primidone clearance.[1] The effect of the presence of carbamazepine in two of the patient's regimens was unaccounted for, but the carbamazepine and primidone doses were not changed throughout the study. The authors speculated the interaction may be a positive one, but more clinical data are required.

[1] Bourgeois BFD, et al. *Neurology*. 1982;32:1122.

* Asterisk indicates drugs cited in interaction reports.

Primidone — *Succinimides*

Primidone		Succinimides	
Primidone* (eg, *Mysoline*)		Ethosuximide* (*Zarontin*)	Phensuximide (*Milontin*)
		Methsuximide* (*Celontin*)	

Significance	Onset	Severity	Documentation
2	☐ Rapid	☐ Major	☐ Established
	■ **Delayed**	■ **Moderate**	☐ Probable
		☐ Minor	■ **Suspected**
			☐ Possible
			☐ Unlikely

Effects Coadministration of PRIMIDONE and a SUCCINIMIDE may result in lower PRIMIDONE and phenobarbital serum concentrations.

Mechanism Unknown.

Management A patient who requires both PRIMIDONE and a SUCCINIMIDE should have serum PRIMIDONE and phenobarbital concentrations monitored whenever a change is made in the SUCCINIMIDE therapy.

Discussion

A study of 121 patients on primidone and 15 patients on primidone and ethosuximide found that the ethosuximide group had a significantly lower phenobarbital concentration/dose ratio.[2] This was noted in patients in the 4- to 15-year-old age bracket only.

Another study of 4 patients on methsuximide and primidone had a significant increase in phenobarbital serum concentrations but not in serum primidone concentrations.[3]

A study of 9 patients on primidone and ethosuximide found no significant differences in the mean serum primidone or phenobarbital concentrations when compared with the results from a group of 28 patients on primidone alone.[1]

[1] Schmidt D. *J Neurol.* 1975;209:115.
[2] Battino D, et al. *Ther Drug Monitor.* 1983;5:73.
[3] Browne TR, et al. *Neurology.* 1983;33:414.

* Asterisk indicates drugs cited in interaction reports. Based on pharmacologic and pharmacokinetic considerations, similar interactions may occur with other drugs that are listed.

Probenecid — Salicylates

Probenecid	Salicylates	
Probenecid*	Aspirin* (eg, *Bayer*)	Salsalate (eg, *Disalcid*)
	Choline Salicylate (*Arthropan*)	Sodium Salicylate* (eg, *Uracel 5*)
	Magnesium Salicylate (eg, *Doan's*)	Sodium Thiosalicylate (eg, *Tusal*)

Significance	Onset	Severity	Documentation
2	☐ Rapid	☐ Major	☐ Established
	■ **Delayed**	■ **Moderate**	■ **Probable**
		☐ Minor	☐ Suspected
			☐ Possible
			☐ Unlikely

Effects Coadministration of PROBENECID and ASPIRIN may inhibit the uricosuric action of either drug alone.

Mechanism Unknown. Possibly due to an alteration in the renal filtration of uric acid.

Management Avoiding coadministration should allow maximum uricosuria to be attained. ASPIRIN therapy that keeps the serum concentration at non-anti-inflammatory concentrations may be acceptable in patients who require both agents.

Discussion

Early case reports demonstrate that coadministration of probenecid 2 g daily and aspirin 5.2 g daily prevented a decrease in serum uric acid concentrations.[2,3] One report says that this occurs no matter which agent is started first.[1] Interestingly, one group of patients had a gradual, limited return to baseline in uric acid concentrations when coadministration was continued for 3 weeks.[2] One analysis noted that serum salicylate concentrations at which uricosuria inhibition was seen were at least 5 to 10 mcg/mL on the morning after the evening dose of aspirin.[3] All reports had insufficient standards for patient selection, dosing, placebo controls, pharmacokinetic and laboratory techniques.

A study of six subjects demonstrated a mean 24-hour urinary uric acid excretion of 566 mg on no drug, 779 mg on probenecid only and 530 mg on probenecid and aspirin together in multiple doses.[4] When two subjects were studied following a single dose of aspirin 300 mg, the maximal urate excretion was decreased by 63% following the addition of aspirin to probenecid but was still 105% above the excretion rate without medication.

A single-dose study of probenecid and aspirin in eight healthy volunteers suggested that the probenecid-induced increase in uric acid clearance is inhibited between two and four hours after a dose of aspirin, but not between four and six hours after the dose.[5]

[1] Gutman AB, et al. *Trans Assoc Am Physicians.* 1951;64:279.
[2] Pascale LR, et al. *JAMA.* 1952;149:1188.
[3] Pascale LR, et al. *J Lab Clin Med.* 1955;45:771.
[4] Diamond HS, et al. *J Clin Invest.* 1973;52:1491.
[5] Brooks CD, et al. *J Int Med Res.* 1980;8:283.

* Asterisk indicates drugs cited in interaction reports. Based on pharmacologic and pharmacokinetic considerations, similar interactions may occur with other drugs that are listed.

Procainamide — *Amiodarone*

Procainamide* (eg, *Pronestyl*)	Amiodarone* (*Cordarone*)

Significance	Onset	Severity	Documentation
2	■ **Rapid** □ Delayed	□ Major ■ **Moderate** □ Minor	□ Established ■ **Probable** □ Suspected □ Possible □ Unlikely

Effects AMIODARONE may increase PROCAINAMIDE serum concentrations.

Mechanism Unknown.

Management A patient who requires AMIODARONE and PROCAINAMIDE should have close monitoring of serum procainamide and N-acetylprocainamide concentrations following an alteration in amiodarone therapy.

Discussion

A study was conducted in 23 patients, 12 with stable procainamide concentrations, who were started on amiodarone therapy.[1] The mean serum procainamide concentration increased by 57%, and the mean serum N-acetylprocainamide (NAPA) concentration increased by 32% following one week of amiodarone 800 to 1200 mg/day. A 20% decrease in the dose of procainamide was required in 65% of patients. In another study of 8 patients, pharmacokinetic and electrophysiologic parameters were monitored following IV procainamide alone and IV procainamide added to a 7 to 11 day regimen of amiodarone (not steady state). In the presence of amiodarone, the clearance of procainamide was reduced by a mean of 23%, while the half-life was prolonged by approximately 40%. The drug combination showed additive effects on a number of electrophysiologic parameters.[2]

Another study of 35 patients used procainamide and amiodarone concurrently to evaluate their electrophysiologic effects in sustained ventricular arrhythmias.[3] The study noted an additive effect on electrocardiographic changes but no significant change in mean procainamide serum concentrations for the group. The study did note, however, that three patients required a 10 to 25% reduction in the procainamide dose due to symptoms of transient hypotension or severe nausea.

[1] Saal AK, et al. *Am J Cardiol.* 1984;53:1264.
[2] Windle J, et al. *Clin Pharmacol Ther.* 1987;41:603.
[3] Marchlinski FE, et al. *Circulation.* 1988;78:583

* Asterisk indicates drugs cited in interaction reports.

Procainamide — *Beta-Blockers*

Procainamide* (eg, *Pronestyl*)	Metoprolol* (eg, *Lopressor*)	Propranolol* (eg, *Inderal*)

Significance	Onset	Severity	Documentation
5	☐ Rapid ■ **Delayed**	☐ Major ■ **Moderate** ☐ Minor	☐ Established ☐ Probable ☐ Suspected ☐ Possible ■ **Unlikely**

Effects PROPRANOLOL may alter procainamide serum concentrations.

Mechanism Unknown.

Management No adjustments are necessary. If procainamide serum concentrations are unexpectedly elevated, this interaction should be suspected.

Discussion

A study of six male patients reported an increase in the elimination half-life by 56% and volume of distribution by 51%, as well as a decrease in the plasma clearance by 19% of IV procainamide infused during long-term propranolol therapy.[1] A subsequent study found no changes in procainamide volume of distribution, elimination half-life or total clearance by either propranolol or metoprolol.[2] The study also found no pharmacologic interactions.

[1] Weidler DJ, et al. *Clin Pharmacol Ther.* 1981;29:289. [2] Ochs HR, et al. *J Cardiovasc Pharmacol.* 1983;5:392.

* Asterisk indicates drugs cited in interaction reports.

Procainamide — *Cimetidine*

Procainamide*
(eg, *Pronestyl*)

Cimetidine*
(eg, *Tagamet*)

Significance	Onset	Severity	Documentation
2	■ **Rapid**	□ Major	■ **Established**
	□ Delayed	■ **Moderate**	□ Probable
		□ Minor	□ Suspected
			□ Possible
			□ Unlikely

Effects Increased serum procainamide concentrations may occur.

Mechanism Probably reduced procainamide renal clearance.

Management Avoid this combination if possible. If cimetidine is necessary, closely monitor serum procainamide concentrations and adjust the dose as needed.

Discussion

Individual cases and controlled studies support an interaction between cimetidine and procainamide.[1-7] A study of six healthy, young, male subjects indicates that oral cimetidine produces a significant (44%) increase in the area under the concentration-time curve (AUC) and in the elimination half-life (by 26%), as well as a 42% reduction in the renal clearance of procainamide.[1] The N-acetylprocainamide (NAPA) AUC was increased by 25% and renal clearance was decreased by 24%. Another study demonstrated a 36% reduction in renal clearance of procainamide in healthy subjects who were receiving cimetidine.[3] The procainamide elimination half-life increased by 24% and the volume of distribution decreased by 12%. The renal clearance of NAPA was not altered. In 36 elderly patients receiving stable sustained-release procainamide doses, addition of cimetidine 300 mg every 6 hours for 3 days increased procainamide concentrations by 55% and NAPA levels by 36%.[7] Severe toxicity occurred in three patients and mild toxicity in nine patients. Symptoms included ECG abnormalities, nausea, malaise and weakness. Toxicity resolved within 1 day of stopping cimetidine. A 71-year-old man with a long-standing history of cardiac dysfunction treated with procainamide developed congestive heart failure 10 weeks after initiating cimetidine therapy.[2] His serum procainamide and NAPA concentrations increased 300% and 114%, respectively. When cimetidine was discontinued, the concentrations returned to baseline. See also Procainamide-Ranitidine.

1 Somogyi A, et al. *Eur J Clin Pharmacol.* 1983;25:339.
2 Higbee MD, et al. *J Am Geriatr Soc.* 1984;32:162.
3 Christian CD, Jr., et al. *Clin Pharmacol Ther.* 1984;36:221.
4 Paloucek F, et al. *J Clin Pharmacol.* 1986;26;541.
5 Rodvold KA, et al. *Ther Drug Monitor.* 1987;9:378.
6 Lai MY, et al. *Int J Clin Pharmacol Ther Toxicol.* 1988;26:118.
7 Bauer LA, et al. *J Am Geriatr Soc.* 1990;38:467.

* Asterisk indicates drugs cited in interaction reports.

Procainamide ✕ *Ciprofloxacin*

Procainamide* (eg, *Procanbid*)	Ciprofloxacin* (eg, *Cipro*)

Significance	Onset	Severity	Documentation
4	■ **Rapid**	□ Major	□ Established
	□ Delayed	■ **Moderate**	□ Probable
		□ Minor	□ Suspected
			■ **Possible**
			□ Unlikely

Effects PROCAINAMIDE plasma concentrations may be increased.

Mechanism Reduced active renal tubular secretion of PROCAINAMIDE.

Management Monitor PROCAINAMIDE plasma concentrations and observe patients for symptoms of PROCAINAMIDE toxicity. Adjust the dose as indicated.

Discussion

The effects of levofloxacin or ciprofloxacin on procainamide pharmacokinetics were evaluated in 10 healthy volunteers.[1] Levofloxacin reduced procainamide clearance 17% and clearance of the active metabolite of procainamide, N-acetyl procainamide (NAPA), 21%. Ciprofloxacin decreased procainamide renal clearance 15% but did not affect NAPA clearance. See also Antiarrhythmic Agents-Quinolones and Drug-Induced Prolongation of the QT Interval and Torsades de Pointes.

[1] Bauer LA, et al. *Antimicrob Agents Chemother.* 2005;49(4):1649.

* Asterisk indicates drugs cited in interaction reports.

Procainamide — *Ethanol*

Procainamide* (eg, *Procanbid*)	Ethanol*

Significance	Onset	Severity	Documentation
5	☐ Rapid ■ **Delayed**	☐ Major ☐ Moderate ■ **Minor**	☐ Established ☐ Probable ☐ Suspected ■ **Possible** ☐ Unlikely

Effects The actions of PROCAINAMIDE may be altered. Because its main metabolite (N-acetyl procainamide [NAPA]) is also an antiarrhythmic, specific effects are unclear.

Mechanism The liver degradation of PROCAINAMIDE, particularly NAPA, appears to be altered by ETHANOL.

Management No clinical interventions appear required.

Discussion

The effect of ethanol 0.73 g/kg on procainamide 10 mg/kg pharmacokinetics was studied in 19 volunteers.[1] Eleven of the volunteers were given procainamide, 6 of whom ingested ethanol 1.5 hours (0.11 g/kg) post drug ingestion and then hourly for 6 hours. In another study design, 8 subjects were given procainamide 2 hours after an initial ethanol dose, followed by hourly ethanol doses. There were 11 rapid acetylators in the 2 groups. Ethanol caused a significant reduction in the procainamide $t_{½}$ (13% to 25%) and a significant increase in total clearance (20% to 25%). The apparent volume of distribution and renal clearance of procainamide were unaffected. Ethanol increased the percentage of NAPA in blood and urine. The $t_{½}$ and total clearance of procainamide were significantly higher (18%) and lower (28%), respectively, in slow versus rapid acetylators.

This study measured pharmacokinetic parameters in healthy subjects; therefore, clinical ramifications remain unknown.

[1] Olsen H, et al. *Br J Clin Pharmacol.* 1982;13(2):203.

* Asterisk indicates drugs cited in interaction reports.

Procainamide — *Quinidine*

Procainamide* (eg, *Procanbid*)	Quinidine*

Significance	Onset	Severity	Documentation
4	■ **Rapid**	□ Major	□ Established
	□ Delayed	■ **Moderate**	□ Probable
		□ Minor	□ Suspected
			■ **Possible**
			□ Unlikely

Effects The pharmacologic effects of PROCAINAMIDE may be increased. Elevated PROCAINAMIDE and N-acetyl procainamide (NAPA) plasma levels with toxicity characterized by GI disturbances, weakness, hypotension, cardiac conduction abnormalities, and arrhythmias may occur.

Mechanism A probable explanation is competition by QUINIDINE for normal secretion of PROCAINAMIDE, via the organic base transport pathway.

Management Use with caution. If an interaction is suspected, measure PROCAINAMIDE plasma levels, assess the cardiac status of the patient, and adjust the dose accordingly.

Discussion

Increased plasma procainamide levels were observed in a 53-year-old man receiving concurrent quinidine gluconate.[1] The patient was treated with both drugs for sustained ventricular tachycardia. After an electrophysiologic study indicated that the patient's arrhythmia was suppressed by high-dose IV procainamide, sustained-release procainamide was administered orally. The dose was progressively increased to 3 g every 6 hours. Because of concern for drug toxicity, the dose of procainamide was decreased to 2 g every 6 hours, and quinidine gluconate 324 mg every 8 hours was added. When compared with the levels resulting from procainamide administration alone, addition of quinidine to the patient's treatment regimen was associated with increases in both procainamide and NAPA levels. Steady-state levels of procainamide increased 70% with a corresponding prolongation of $t_{1/2}$ and decrease in clearance. Because plasma levels were determined at a similar time after the oral dose and after steady-state was reached, no concurrent drugs were added or deleted from the regimen, and no physiologic changes known to affect procainamide elimination rate (eg, alterations in renal function) were present, the increased procainamide plasma levels were attributed to an interaction between procainamide and quinidine.

[1] Hughes B, et al. *Am Heart J.* 1987;114(4 pt 1):908.

* Asterisk indicates drugs cited in interaction reports.

Procainamide — *Ranitidine*

Procainamide* (eg, *Procanbid*)	Ranitidine* (eg, *Zantac*)

Significance	Onset	Severity	Documentation
4	■ **Rapid**	■ **Major**	□ Established
	□ Delayed	□ Moderate	□ Probable
		□ Minor	□ Suspected
			■ **Possible**
			□ Unlikely

Effects RANITIDINE may alter the bioavailability and renal clearance of PROCAINAMIDE, perhaps precipitating PROCAINAMIDE toxicity.

Mechanism Unknown.

Management Closely monitor serum PROCAINAMIDE concentrations. Adjust the PROCAINAMIDE dose as needed for patients requiring RANITIDINE.

Discussion

One controlled study of 6 healthy volunteers demonstrated that oral ranitidine 150 mg every 12 hours increased the AUC of oral procainamide 14%, reduced the renal clearance of procainamide 19%, and reduced the hepatic clearance 22%.[1,2] A higher dose of ranitidine (750 mg administered over 13 hours) in 3 of the subjects produced a 21% increase in the AUC and a 35% decrease in renal clearance. N-acetyl procainamide (NAPA) had a 12% increase in the AUC and a 38% reduction in renal clearance. The impaired-bioavailability hypothesis of this study has been criticized as lacking sufficient controls.[3] Another controlled study produced no alteration in procainamide pharmacokinetics when ranitidine 150 mg was given every 12 hours to 6 healthy volunteers.[4] An open, randomized, crossover study of 13 volunteers also found no change in the mean pharmacokinetic values for the group.[5] However, differences among individuals occurred. One group of patients had a 23% decrease in procainamide, while the other group had a 21% increase in renal clearance. These changes correlated with a 45% increase and a 41% decrease, respectively, in metabolic clearance for the 2 groups. There was a strong linear relationship in the negative correlation of these 2 changes for these subjects. Similar results were seen for NAPA. See also Procainamide-Cimetidine.

[1] Somogyi A, et al. *Br J Clin Pharmacol.* 1984;18(2):175.
[2] Somogyi A, et al. *Br J Clin Pharmacol.* 1985;20(2):182.
[3] Martin BK. *Br J Clin Pharmacol.* 1985;19(6):858.
[4] Rodvold KA, et al. *Ther Drug Monit.* 1987;9(4):378.
[5] Rocci ML Jr, et al. *J Pharmacol Exp Ther.* 1989;248(3):923.

* Asterisk indicates drugs cited in interaction reports.

Procainamide — *Trimethoprim*

Procainamide* (eg, *Pronestyl*)	Trimethoprim* (eg, *Proloprim*)

Significance	Onset	Severity	Documentation
2	■ **Rapid** □ Delayed	□ Major ■ **Moderate** □ Minor	□ Established □ Probable ■ **Suspected** □ Possible □ Unlikely

Effects Elevated PROCAINAMIDE and N-acetylprocainamide (NAPA) serum levels may produce an increase in the pharmacologic effects of PROCAINAMIDE.

Mechanism Competition for renal tubular cationic secretion between PROCAINAMIDE and TRIMETHOPRIM may be responsible.

Management Monitor PROCAINAMIDE and NAPA plasma levels and cardiac function of the patient. Adjust the dose accordingly.

Discussion

In an open, randomized, placebo-controlled, crossover study involving 10 healthy male volunteers, trimethoprim significantly ($P < 0.05$) increased the mean area under the plasma concentration-time curve (AUC) for both procainamide and its active metabolite, NAPA; decreased the oral plasma clearance of procainamide ($P < 0.05$); prolonged the mean plasma half-life of procainamide ($P < 0.05$); and decreased the mean renal clearance of procainamide and NAPA ($P < 0.01$ and 0.05, respectively).[2] Each subject received procainamide 1 g orally with either placebo or trimethoprim 200 mg, which followed 3 days of pretreatment with 100 mg twice daily. Blood and urine samples were collected at various intervals 24 hours or less after procainamide administration. Trimethoprim increased the mean AUC for procainamide 39% (from 19.8 to 27.6 mg•hr/L) and NAPA 25% (from 9.1 to 11.4 mg•hr/L) compared with placebo. The oral plasma clearance of procainamide decreased 32% (from 42 to 28.6 L/hr) when administered with trimethoprim, resulting in a 30% prolongation in the mean plasma half-life of procainamide (from 3.3 to 4.3 hours). Compared with placebo, trimethoprim decreased the mean renal clearance of procainamide 45% (from 487 to 267 mL/min) and the mean renal clearance of NAPA 26% (from 275 to 203 mL/min). The corrected QT interval, 2 hours after the procainamide dose, was 0.4 seconds with placebo and 0.43 seconds with trimethoprim ($P < 0.05$).

Similar results were found in a second study in which 8 healthy males received sustained-release procainamide 500 mg every 6 hours for 3 days alone or in combination with trimethoprim 200 mg/day for 4 days.[1] During concurrent administration of trimethoprim, the AUC of procainamide and NAPA increased by 63% and 52%, respectively, while renal clearance decreased by 47% and 13%, respectively. Coadministration of trimethoprim increased the urinary recovery of NAPA by 39%. There was a small but significant increase in the corrected QT interval.

[1] Kosoglou T, et al. *Clin Pharmacol Ther.* 1988;44:467. [2] Vlasses PH, et al. *Arch Intern Med.* 1989;149:1350.

* Asterisk indicates drugs cited in interaction reports.

Progestins — *Aminoglutethimide*

Progestins	Aminoglutethimide
Medroxyprogesterone* (eg, *Provera*)	Aminoglutethimide* (*Cytadren*)

Significance	Onset	Severity	Documentation
5	☐ Rapid ■ **Delayed**	☐ Major ☐ Moderate ■ **Minor**	☐ Established ☐ Probable ☐ Suspected ■ **Possible** ☐ Unlikely

Effects AMINOGLUTETHIMIDE may decrease MEDROXYPROGESTERONE ACETATE serum concentrations and perhaps its effectiveness.

Mechanism Unknown.

Management If MEDROXYPROGESTERONE ACETATE is ineffective in a patient who also is receiving AMINOGLUTETHIMIDE, this interaction should be suspected.

Discussion

A metabolic study of 7 women with metastatic carcinoma of the breast demonstrated an alteration in medroxyprogesterone acetate serum concentrations by aminoglutethimide.[1] Each patient received oral medroxyprogesterone acetate 500 mg 3 times daily for 8 weeks. Two weeks after starting medroxyprogesterone, oral aminoglutethimide 250 mg twice daily was started and increased 2 weeks later to 250 mg 4 times daily. A 50% decrease in the mean plasma medroxyprogesterone acetate concentration was noted 2 weeks after starting aminoglutethimide; this reduction was maintained throughout the study. In contrast, a study of 5 women receiving oral medroxyprogesterone acetate 10 mg twice daily for 5 weeks demonstrated that oral aminoglutethimide 250 mg 4 times daily for 3 to 6 weeks had no effect on the metabolic clearance rate or the volume of distribution of medroxyprogesterone acetate.[2] The lack of change in the metabolic clearance rate was noted in another study as well.[3]

[1] Van Deijk WA, et al. *Cancer Treat Rep.* 1985;69:85.
[2] Gupta C, et al. *J Clin Endocrinol Metab.* 1979;48:816.
[3] Santen RJ, et al. *Cancer Res.* 1982;42:3353S.

* Asterisk indicates drugs cited in interaction reports.

Progestins | **Barbiturates**

Levonorgestrel* (eg, *Mirena*)	Norgestrel (eg, *Ovral*)	Amobarbital (*Amytal*)	Phenobarbital* (eg, *Solfoton*)
		Butabarbital (eg, *Butisol*)	Primidone (eg, *Mysoline*)
		Mephobarbital (*Mebaral*)	Secobarbital (*Seconal*)
		Pentobarbital	

Significance	Onset	Severity	Documentation
1	☐ Rapid ■ **Delayed**	■ **Major** ☐ Moderate ☐ Minor	☐ Established ☐ Probable ■ **Suspected** ☐ Possible ☐ Unlikely

Effects Loss of contraceptive efficacy, possibly leading to pregnancy.

Mechanism Both BARBITURATE induction of PROGESTIN metabolism (CYP3A4) and sex hormone–binding globulin synthesis may reduce PROGESTIN concentrations.[1]

Management Inform women of the increased risk of contraceptive failure. Consider alternative or additional nonhormonal methods.

Discussion

Pregnancy occurred in a 21-year-old woman with levonorgestrel implants who also took phenobarbital 180 mg/day for a seizure disorder.[2] She had a history of irregular menses. Three months prior to levonorgestrel implantation, she received medroxyprogesterone acetate (eg, *Provera*) for contraception, which was stopped because of breakthrough bleeding. Six months after levonorgestrel implantation, increased partial seizure activity was diagnosed, and her phenobarbital dose was increased to 210 mg/day. For several months, she did not experience breakthrough bleeding. She was found to be 6 weeks pregnant, the implants were removed, and she gave birth to a healthy boy. One month after giving birth, she was started on a triphasic oral contraceptive containing ethinyl estradiol 35 mcg plus norgestimate (eg, *Ortho Tri-Cyclen*). She became pregnant again and gave birth to healthy twin boys. See Contraceptives, Hormonal-Barbiturates.

Levonorgestrel implants were not a reliable contraceptive in epileptic patients taking anticonvulsants known to induce liver enzymes, such as phenytoin (eg, *Dilantin*) alone or in combination with other anticonvulsants.[3] Two of 9 patients became pregnant. Six patients had decreased plasma concentrations of levonorgestrel compared with 10 subjects receiving levonorgestrel alone. See Progestins-Hydantoins.

[1] Back DJ, et al. *Contraception*. 1980;22(5):495.
[2] Shane-McWhorter L, et al. *Pharmacotherapy*. 1998;18(6):1360.
[3] Haukkamaa M. *Contraception*. 1986;33(6):559.

* Asterisk indicates drugs cited in interaction reports. Based on pharmacologic and pharmacokinetic considerations, similar interactions may occur with other drugs that are listed.

Progestins — *Bosentan*

Progestins		Bosentan
Medroxyprogesterone* (eg, *Depo-Provera*)	Norethindrone* (eg, *Ortho Micronor*)	Bosentan* (*Tracleer*)

Significance	Onset	Severity	Documentation
1	☐ Rapid ■ **Delayed**	■ **Major** ☐ Moderate ☐ Minor	☐ Established ☐ Probable ■ **Suspected** ☐ Possible ☐ Unlikely

Effects The efficacy of NORETHINDRONE may be reduced.

Mechanism Increased hepatic metabolism (CYP3A4) of NORETHINDRONE is suspected.

Management Monitor patients receiving BOSENTAN and NORETHINDRONE for a decrease in NORETHINDRONE efficacy. Adjust therapy as needed.

Discussion

The effect of bosentan on the pharmacokinetics of an oral contraceptive containing ethinyl estradiol 35 mcg plus norethindrone 1 mg was evaluated in 19 healthy women.[1] Using a randomized, crossover design, each woman received a single dose of the oral contraceptive alone and after 7 days of pretreatment with bosentan 125 mg twice daily. Compared with taking the oral contraceptive alone, bosentan administration reduced the AUC of norethindrone nearly 14% and ethinyl estradiol 31%. The maximum decreases in AUC of norethindrone and ethinyl estradiol in an individual subject were 56% and 66%, respectively. In the subject with the largest decrease in norethindrone AUC, ethinyl estradiol levels could not be measured. The C_{max} of the oral contraceptive components was not affected by bosentan. An in vitro study using human liver microsomes indicates that CYP3A4 is the isozyme mainly involved in the overall metabolism of medroxyprogesterone.[2]

[1] van Giersbergen PL, et al. *Int J Clin Pharmacol Ther.* 2006;44(3):113.

[2] Kobayashi K, et al. *Clin Cancer Res.* 2000;6(8):3297.

* Asterisk indicates drugs cited in interaction reports.

Progestins | **Hydantoins**

Levonorgestrel* (*Mirena*)	Norgestrel* (eg, *Ovrette*)	Ethotoin (*Peganone*) Fosphenytoin (*Cerebyx*)	Phenytoin* (eg, *Dilantin*)

Significance	Onset	Severity	Documentation
2	□ Rapid ■ **Delayed**	□ Major ■ **Moderate** □ Minor	□ Established □ Probable ■ **Suspected** □ Possible □ Unlikely

Effects PHENYTOIN may decrease the efficacy of ORAL CONTRACEPTIVE STEROIDS.

Mechanism Both HYDANTOIN induction of PROGESTIN metabolism (CYP3A4) and sex hormone–binding globulin synthesis may reduce PROGESTIN concentrations.[1,2]

Management Inform women of the increased risk of contraceptive failure. Consider alternative or additional nonhormonal methods.

Discussion

A 26-year-old woman with a levonorgestrel subdermal implant demonstrated an alteration in sex hormone serum concentrations during phenytoin therapy.[2] She had been receiving phenytoin 300 mg/day for 10 years when the implant was inserted. Her regular menses continued, and 9 months after levonorgestrel implantation she became pregnant. The pregnancy was terminated, and phenytoin was discontinued; her menses became irregular and erratic. Blood samples taken after phenytoin discontinuation indicated a 53% increase in serum levonorgestrel concentrations, a 44% decrease in serum sex hormone–binding globulin concentrations, and a 172% increase in the ratio of levonorgestrel to sex hormone–binding globulin. Levonorgestrel implants were not a reliable contraceptive in epileptic patients taking anticonvulsants known to induce liver enzymes, such as phenytoin alone or in combination with other anticonvulsants.[3] Two of 9 patients became pregnant. Six patients had decreased plasma concentrations of levonorgestrel compared with 10 subjects receiving levonorgestrel alone.

[1] Back DJ, et al. *Contraception*. 1980;22:495.
[2] Odlind V, et al. *Contraception*. 1986;33:257.
[3] Haukkamaa M. *Contraception*. 1986;33:559.

* Asterisk indicates drugs cited in interaction reports. Based on pharmacologic and pharmacokinetic considerations, similar interactions may occur with other drugs that are listed.

Progestins		*NNRT Inhibitors*
Norethindrone* (eg, *Micronor*)	Delavirdine (*Rescriptor*) Efavirenz (*Sustiva*)	Nevirapine* (*Viramune*)

Significance	Onset	Severity	Documentation
4	☐ Rapid ■ **Delayed**	☐ Major ■ **Moderate** ☐ Minor	☐ Established ☐ Probable ☐ Suspected ■ **Possible** ☐ Unlikely

Effects The efficacy of NORETHINDRONE may be reduced.

Mechanism Increased hepatic metabolism of NORETHINDRONE by NONNUCLEOSIDE REVERSE TRANSCRIPTASE (NNRT) INHIBITORS is suspected.

Management Monitor patients receiving NNRT inhibitors and NORETHINDRONE for a decrease in NORETHINDRONE efficacy. Adjust therapy as needed.

Discussion

The effects of nevirapine on the pharmacokinetics of ethinyl estradiol 1 mg plus norethindrone 35 mcg (*Ortho-Novum 1/35*) were evaluated in 10 HIV-1-infected women.[1] Each patient received 200 mg of nevirapine once daily on days 2 to 15 followed by 200 mg twice daily on days 16 through 29. On days 0 and 30, single doses of ethinyl estradiol/norethindrone (EE/NET) were administered. Nevirapine decreased the AUC of norethindrone 18%. In addition, coadministration of nevirapine with EE/NET reduced the median AUC of ethinyl estradiol 29%, decreased the terminal $t_{½}$ (from 15.7 to 11.6 hr), and reduced the mean residence time (from 16.1 to 11.7 hr). The steady-state pharmacokinetics of nevirapine were not altered by EE/NET administration.

[1] Mildvan D, et al. *J Acquir Immune Defic Syndr.* 2002;29:471.

* Asterisk indicates drugs cited in interaction reports. Based on pharmacologic and pharmacokinetic considerations, similar interactions may occur with other drugs that are listed.

Progestins			*Rifamycins*
Ethynodiol (eg, *Demulen*)	Norethindrone* (eg, *Aygestin*)	Rifabutin* (*Mycobutin*)	Rifapentine (*Priftin*)
Hydroxyprogesterone	Norethynodrel	Rifampin* (eg, *Rifadin*)	
Medroxyprogesterone (eg, *Provera*)	Progesterone (eg, *Prochieve*)		

Significance	Onset	Severity	Documentation
1	□ Rapid ■ **Delayed**	■ **Major** □ Moderate □ Minor	□ Established □ Probable ■ **Suspected** □ Possible □ Unlikely

Effects RIFAMPIN may increase the elimination rate of PROGESTIN-containing oral contraceptive steroids.

Mechanism Probable induction of metabolism (CYP3A4) by RIFAMYCINS.

Management Patients who require concurrent contraception and antitubercular therapy should avoid use of either oral contraceptives or RIFAMPIN.

Discussion

A study of 9 women with tuberculosis demonstrated an effect on norethindrone pharmacokinetics by rifampin.[1] In 8 women who were not on contraceptive therapy, a single dose of norethindrone acetate 1 mg and ethinyl estradiol 50 mcg was administered near the end of 1 year of rifampin therapy and again 1 month after rifampin was discontinued. In the patient concurrently receiving oral contraceptive therapy, daily blood samples were obtained for the last 2 weeks of each contraceptive cycle, for the last 2 months of rifampin therapy, and again for 2 months subsequent to rifampin therapy. The AUC of norethindrone increased 73% after rifampin was discontinued. A similar increase (94%) was seen in the elimination $t_{½}$. The multiple-dose study demonstrated a 435% increase in the mean steady-state plasma norethindrone concentration once rifampin was discontinued. Two studies compared the effects of rifampin and rifabutin on the pharmacokinetics of ethinyl estradiol-norethindrone (*Ortho-Novum 1/35*).[2,3] The AUC and $t_{½}$ of ethinyl estradiol and norethindrone were decreased by both drugs, but rifampin had a greater effect. Spotting and menstrual irregularities were reported more often with rifampin.

[1] Back DJ, et al. *Eur J Clin Pharmacol.* 1979;15:193.
[2] Barditch-Crovo P, et al. *Clin Pharmacol Ther.* 1999;65:428.
[3] LeBel M, et al. *J Clin Pharmacol.* 1998;38:1042.

* Asterisk indicates drugs cited in interaction reports. Based on pharmacologic and pharmacokinetic considerations, similar interactions may occur with other drugs that are listed.

Propafenone — *Cimetidine*

Propafenone* (eg, *Rythmol*)	Cimetidine* (eg, *Tagamet*)

Significance	Onset	Severity	Documentation
5	■ **Rapid**	□ Major	□ Established
	□ Delayed	■ **Moderate**	□ Probable
		□ Minor	□ Suspected
			□ Possible
			■ **Unlikely**

Effects The pharmacologic effects of PROPAFENONE may be increased.

Mechanism Inhibition of PROPAFENONE metabolism.

Management Based upon currently available data, no special precautions other than usual monitoring of cardiac function are needed.

Discussion

In a single-blind, 3-phase study involving 12 healthy volunteers, the pharmacokinetic and pharmacodynamic effects of propafenone 225 mg every 8 hours were investigated alone and during coadministration of cimetidine 400 mg every 8 hours.[1] Each subject received propafenone plus placebo, cimetidine plus placebo, and coadministration of propafenone and cimetidine. The maximum concentration of propafenone increased from 993 to 1,230 ng/mL (approximately 24%; $P = 0.0622$) during coadministration of cimetidine, compared with administration of propafenone alone. In addition, there was a slight increase in the electrocardiographic wave duration with coadministration of both drugs (103 msec), compared with propafenone administration alone (98 msec). The mean steady-state plasma concentration, time-to-peak plasma concentration, $t_{½}$, and PR interval were not different when propafenone was given alone, compared with coadministration with cimetidine. The pharmacokinetic and pharmacodynamic changes observed during coadministration of propafenone and cimetidine were slight and are not be expected to be clinically important.

Additional studies are needed.

[1] Pritchett EL, et al. *J Clin Pharmacol.* 1988;28:619.

* Asterisk indicates drugs cited in interaction reports.

Propafenone — *Food*

Propafenone* (*Rythmol*)	Food*

Significance	Onset	Severity	Documentation
4	■ **Rapid**	□ Major	□ Established
	□ Delayed	■ **Moderate**	□ Probable
		□ Minor	□ Suspected
			■ **Possible**
			□ Unlikely

Effects FOOD may increase the effects of PROPAFENONE in certain patients.

Mechanism Enhanced bioavailability.

Management Consider giving PROPAFENONE in a consistent manner relative to meals to help assure uniform bioavailability.

Discussion

In a randomized, 2-way crossover study involving 24 healthy volunteers, the effect of food on the bioavailability of a single dose of propafenone was investigated in a fasted state and after a standard breakfast.[1] Each subject received 300 mg propafenone orally during fasting and with a standard breakfast containing 20 g protein, 17 g fat, and 50 g carbohydrate. When data from the 4 patients who were slow metabolizers of propafenone were excluded, food produced an average increase of 147% (638% in 1 patient) in the area under the concentration-time curve. In slow metabolizers, food did not affect the bioavailability of propafenone, implying that food may diminish the first-pass effect. Although the clinical significance of administration of propafenone with meals needs to be determined, giving the drug in a consistent manner relative to meals may help assure uniform bioavailability.

Additional multiple-dose studies are needed to determine the clinical significance of this possible interaction.

[1] Axelson JE, et al. *Br J Clin Pharmacol.* 1987;23:735.

* Asterisk indicates drugs cited in interaction reports.

Propafenone — *Quinidine*

Propafenone* (*Rythmol*)	Quinidine* (eg, *Quinidex*)

Significance	Onset	Severity	Documentation
2	☐ Rapid	☐ Major	☐ Established
	■ **Delayed**	■ **Moderate**	☐ Probable
		☐ Minor	■ **Suspected**
			☐ Possible
			☐ Unlikely

Effects Serum propafenone levels may be increased in rapid, extensive metabolizers of the drug (approximately 90% of the patients), increasing the pharmacologic effects of PROPAFENONE.

Mechanism The hepatic hydroxylation metabolic pathway of PROPAFENONE is inhibited by QUINIDINE. PROPAFENONE is metabolized by cytochrome P450IID6 and QUINIDINE is a specific and potent inhibitor of that enzyme.

Management Monitor cardiac function. It may be necessary to lower the dose or reduce the dosing frequency of PROPAFENONE.

Discussion

Combined use of quinidine and propafenone may be beneficial.[1,2] Administration of propafenone 300 to 600 mg daily with quinidine sulfate (maximum dose of 1200 mg daily) for treating ventricular arrhythmias were studied in patients in whom quinidine monotherapy had failed to suppress ectopy.[1] Propafenone produced a reduction in the frequency of premature ventricular contractions compared to quinidine therapy alone. Higher doses of propafenone were needed during monotherapy compared to administration with quinidine. In another report, the effect of quinidine sulfate on the pharmacologic activity of propafenone was studied in extensive and poor metabolizers who were being treated for ventricular arrhythmias.[2] Patients were admitted to the study while receiving 450 to 900 mg propafenone daily. However, all patients received 450 mg propafenone daily during the study. In extensive metabolizers, quinidine increased the mean steady-state plasma propafenone concentration from 408 to 1096 ng/mL, decreased the concentration of the 5-hydroxy metabolite (5-hydroxypropafenone) from 242 to 125 ng/mL, and reduced propafenone oral clearance by 58%. Despite changes in the plasma concentration of propafenone, electrocardiographic and ventricular arrhythmia frequency were not altered by concomitant quinidine, indicating that, in extensive metabolizers, 5-hydroxypropafenone may contribute to the pharmacologic activity of propafenone. In the two poor metabolizers, plasma concentrations of propafenone and 5-hydroxypropafenone were unaffected by quinidine. In extensive metabolizers, quinidine increased the beta blocking activity of propafenone (a property of the parent drug but not the metabolite).[3]

[1] Klein RC, et al. *Am Heart J.* 1987;114:551.
[2] Funck-Brentano C, et al. *Br J Clin Pharmacol.* 1989;27:435.
[3] Morike KE, et al. *Clin Pharmacol Ther.* 1994;55:28.

* Asterisk indicates drugs cited in interaction reports.

Propafenone — *Rifamycins*

Propafenone* (eg, *Rythmol*)	Rifabutin (eg, *Mycobutin*)	Rifapentine (*Priftin*)
	Rifampin* (eg, *Rifadin*)	

Significance	Onset	Severity	Documentation
2	☐ Rapid	☐ Major	☐ Established
	■ **Delayed**	■ **Moderate**	■ **Probable**
		☐ Minor	☐ Suspected
			☐ Possible
			☐ Unlikely

Effects Increased PROPAFENONE clearance producing a decrease in plasma levels and a possible loss of therapeutic effects.

Mechanism RIFAMYCINS may induce the hepatic microsomal enzymes responsible for metabolizing PROPAFENONE.[2]

Management Consider an alternative anti-infective agent for patients stabilized on PROPAFENONE. If coadministration can not be avoided, monitor PROPAFENONE serum levels and observe the patient for loss of therapeutic effect. Adjust the PROPAFENONE dose accordingly.

Discussion

A possible interaction has been reported in a 42-year-old man with complex ventricular arrhythmias during coadministration of propafenone and rifampin.[1] The patient's arrhythmias had been treated successfully for 5 months with propafenone 300 mg 3 times a day. Treatment for recurrent staphylococcal epididymitis was started with the nonsteroidal anti-inflammatory drug, nimesulide (not available in US) and rifampin 450 mg twice daily. On the third day of therapy, serum levels of propafenone and its 2 active metabolites, 5-hydroxypropafenone (5OHP) and N-depropylpropafenone (NDPP), were 993, 195, and 110 ng/mL, respectively. On the day 12 of rifampin treatment, 1 week after nimesulide had been discontinued, plasma levels of propafenone and the 5OHP metabolite were decreased to 176 and 64 ng/mL, respectively, while the level of the NDPP metabolite increased to 192 ng/mL. Ventricular arrhythmias recurred. The infection resolved, and rifampin was discontinued. Two weeks later, no arrhythmias were present, and serum levels of propafenone and the metabolites were at acceptable levels of 1411, 78, and 158 ng/mL, respectively. The effect of rifampin on the pharmacokinetics of propafenone was studied in 6 elderly extensive metabolizers of CYP2D6.[2] Each subject received single doses of 70 mg of propafenone IV and 300 mg orally before and after 9 days of rifampin (600 mg/day). No pharmacokinetic or pharmacodynamic changes were noted for IV propafenone. However, oral propafenone bioavailability decreased from 30% to 4%, N-dealkylation increased 433%, glucuronidation increased 415% and maximum QRS prolongation decreased 33%.

[1] Castel JM, et al. *Br J Clin Pharmacol.* 1990;30:155.
[2] Dilger K, et al. *Clin Pharmacol Ther.* 2000;67:512.

* Asterisk indicates drugs cited in interaction reports. Based on pharmacologic and pharmacokinetic considerations, similar interactions may occur with other drugs that are listed.

Propafenone — *Ritonavir*

Propafenone* (*Rythmol*)	Ritonavir* (*Norvir*)

Significance	Onset	Severity	Documentation
1	☐ Rapid	■ **Major**	☐ Established
	■ **Delayed**	☐ Moderate	☐ Probable
		☐ Minor	■ **Suspected**
			☐ Possible
			☐ Unlikely

Effects Large increases in serum PROPAFENONE concentrations may occur, increasing the risk of PROPAFENONE toxicity.

Mechanism RITONAVIR may inhibit the metabolism (cytochrome P450 2D6) of PROPAFENONE.

Management RITONAVIR is contraindicated in patients receiving PROPAFENONE.

Discussion

In patients with ventricular tachycardia, propafenone prolongs atrioventricular (AV) conduction. Ritonavir is expected to produce large increases in propafenone plasma concentrations, increasing the risk of toxicity.[1] Cardiovascular adverse reactions reported with propafenone include new or worsened arrhythmias. These proarrhythmic effects range from an increase in frequency of premature ventricular contractions to more severe ventricular tachycardia, ventricular fibrillation, or torsades de pointes. Propafenone causes first degree AV block. The average PR interval prolongation and increases in QRS duration are correlated with dosage increases and concurrent increases in propafenone plasma concentration.[1] Second and third degree AV block, bundle branch block, and intraventricular conduction delay have also been reported.

The basis for this monograph is information on file with the manufacturer. Published clinical data are needed to further assess this interaction. However, because of the seriousness of the cardiac problems, clinical evaluation of this interaction in humans is not likely to be forthcoming.

[1] Product Information. Ritonavir (*Norvir*). Abbott Laboratories. February 1996.

* Asterisk indicates drugs cited in interaction reports.

Propafenone — *Serotonin Reuptake Inhibitors*

Propafenone* (eg, *Rythmol*)	Duloxetine (*Cymbalta*)	Paroxetine (eg, *Paxil*)
	Fluoxetine* (eg, *Prozac*)	Sertraline (*Zoloft*)

Significance	Onset	Severity	Documentation
2	☐ Rapid	☐ Major	☐ Established
	■ **Delayed**	■ **Moderate**	☐ Probable
		☐ Minor	■ **Suspected**
			☐ Possible
			☐ Unlikely

Effects Plasma PROPAFENONE levels may be elevated, increasing the pharmacologic and adverse reactions.

Mechanism Certain SRIs may inhibit the metabolism (CYP2D6) of PROPAFENONE.

Management Carefully monitor cardiac function if certain SRIs are coadministered with PROPAFENONE. Citalopram (eg, *Celexa*) does not inhibit CYP2D6 and may be a safer alternative.

Discussion

The effects of fluoxetine on the pharmacokinetics of propafenone enantiomers (ie, S- and R-propafenone) were studied in 9 healthy volunteers phenotyped with dextromethorphan as CYP2D6 extensive metabolizers.[1] Each subject received a single oral dose of propafenone 400 mg before and after pretreatment with fluoxetine (20 mg/day for 10 days). Compared with baseline, fluoxetine increased the elimination $t_{1/2}$, peak concentration, and AUC of the 2 propafenone enantiomers, while decreasing the oral clearance. The peak concentration of R- and S-propafenone were increased 71% and 39%, respectively. The time to reach the peak concentration was increased only for R-propafenone. Compared with baseline, there were no percentage changes in the PR and QRS intervals.

[1] Cai WM, et al. *Clin Pharmacol Ther.* 1999;66:516.

* Asterisk indicates drugs cited in interaction reports. Based on pharmacologic and pharmacokinetic considerations, similar interactions may occur with other drugs that are listed.

Propofol	***Benzodiazepines***	
Propofol* (eg, *Diprivan*)	Diazepam* (eg, *Valium*)	Midazolam*

Significance	Onset	Severity	Documentation
4	■ **Rapid** □ Delayed	□ Major ■ **Moderate** □ Minor	□ Established □ Probable □ Suspected ■ **Possible** □ Unlikely

Effects The pharmacologic effects of PROPOFOL and certain BENZODIAZEPINES may be synergistic, which may be beneficial in some cases.

Mechanism Unknown.

Management Based on currently available documentation, no special precautions appear necessary. Assess the clinical status of the patient and provide supportive therapy if needed.

Discussion

Prolonged sleep has been reported with coadministration of propofol and diazepam.[1] Two patients, 18 and 22 years of age, undergoing sedation with diazepam 15 and 20 mg, respectively, received propofol 100 and 150 mg, respectively, as an adjunct. Both patients were asleep, and gastroscopy proceeded without difficulty; however, neither patient was arousable for 3 to 4 hours, and no response to painful stimuli occurred. Excessive sedation was not reported in another patient receiving propofol, aminophylline, and bolus doses of midazolam 2.5 mg concurrently.[2] (See Propofol-Theophyllines.) In 92 patients given midazolam and propofol at various doses, synergism was demonstrated on 3 induction variables when both drugs were given concurrently compared with values for either drug alone.[3] Synergy was also demonstrated in a prospective study of 75 mechanically ventilated patients randomly assigned to receive propofol or midazolam alone or in combination.[4] Coadministration of both drugs achieved equal sedation with lower doses and fewer adverse effects than either agent alone.[4,5] In addition to similar pharmacodynamic effects, midazolam levels may be increased.[4] In a study of 24 patients, propofol reduced midazolam clearance 37% and prolonged the $t_{½}$ 61%,[6] while another study reported a 26.9% increase in midazolam concentrations.[7]

Additional studies are needed to determine the clinical importance of this possible interaction.

1 Gademsetty MK. *Anaesthesia.* 1988;43(7):611.
2 Taylor BL, et al. *Anaesthesia.* 1988;43(6):508.
3 McClune S, et al. *Br J Anaesth.* 1992;69(3):240.
4 Carrasco G, et al. *Crit Care Med.* 1998;26(5):844.
5 Reimann FM, et al. *Endoscopy.* 2000;32(3):239.
6 Hamaoka N, et al. *Clin Pharmacol Ther.* 1999;66(2):110.
7 Lichtenbelt BJ, et al. *Anesth Analg.* 2010;110(6):1597.

* Asterisk indicates drugs cited in interaction reports.

Propofol | **Droperidol**

Propofol*
(eg, *Diprivan*)

Droperidol*
(eg, *Inapsine*)

Significance	Onset	Severity	Documentation
4	■ **Rapid** ☐ Delayed	☐ Major ■ **Moderate** ☐ Minor	☐ Established ☐ Probable ☐ Suspected ■ **Possible** ☐ Unlikely

Effects Increased frequency of postoperative nausea and vomiting during coadministration of PROPOFOL and DROPERIDOL.

Mechanism Unknown.

Management The antiemetic properties of PROPOFOL alone are not enhanced by coadministration of DROPERIDOL. Use PROPOFOL alone.

Discussion

A retrospective review of 266 records was conducted to determine whether the antiemetic activity of propofol would be enhanced by coadministration of small doses of droperidol.[1] The medical records reviewed were selected from patients who underwent laparoscopic operations. All patients received nitrous oxide anesthesia with either thiopental (eg, *Pentothal*) or propofol induction, with or without droperidol for antiemetic prophylaxis. Patients were categorized into 4 groups based on having received propofol alone, thiopental alone, or droperidol combined with thiopental or propofol. The frequency of postoperative nausea and vomiting was significantly less with coadministration of droperidol plus thiopental (10.5%; $P = 0.0001$) than with droperidol plus propofol (16%). However, propofol alone (7.9%) was more effective than thiopental alone (23.9%) in preventing postoperative nausea and vomiting and was more effective than coadministration of droperidol and propofol. Although the findings are limited by the retrospective nature of the investigation, it is not recommended that droperidol be added to propofol anesthesia for prophylaxis of postoperative nausea and vomiting.

[1] Wagner BK, et al. *Pharmacotherapy*. 1994;14(5):586.

* Asterisk indicates drugs cited in interaction reports.

Propofol — *Methylene Blue*

Propofol* (eg, *Diprivan*)	Methylene Blue* (eg, *Urolene Blue*)

Significance	Onset	Severity	Documentation
4	■ **Rapid** □ Delayed	□ Major ■ **Moderate** □ Minor	□ Established □ Probable □ Suspected ■ **Possible** □ Unlikely

Effects The anesthetic requirements of PROPOFOL may be reduced and the time to awakening may be prolonged.

Mechanism Unknown. However, METHYLENE BLUE may have additive or synergistic effects with PROPOFOL.

Management Coadminister with caution. Take care to ensure an adequate depth of anesthesia by using brain monitoring devices (eg, bispectral index, cerebral state index) to titrate PROPOFOL administration. Neurological examination within 4 hours after surgery, whenever METHYLENE BLUE has been infused perioperatively, is recommended.

Discussion

In a case-control study, propofol requirements were assessed during phases of anesthesia induction and maintenance in 2 groups of patients undergoing parathyroid or thyroid surgery.[1] One group of 11 patients received methylene blue 5 mg/kg approximately 60 minutes before propofol induction. A second group of 11 patients received propofol without methylene blue pretreatment. In patients pretreated with methylene blue, the mean propofol dose was 50% lower compared with patients receiving propofol alone. In addition, the time to anesthesia emergence was prolonged in the patients receiving methylene blue.

[1] Licker M, et al. *Anaesthesia.* 2008;63(4):352.

* Asterisk indicates drugs cited in interaction reports.

Propofol — *Theophyllines*

Propofol* (eg, *Diprivan*)	Aminophylline*	Theophylline (eg, *Theochron*)
	Dyphylline (eg, *Lufyllin*)	

Significance	Onset	Severity	Documentation
5	■ **Rapid**	□ Major	□ Established
	□ Delayed	□ Moderate	□ Probable
		■ **Minor**	□ Suspected
			■ **Possible**
			□ Unlikely

Effects THEOPHYLLINES may antagonize the sedative effects of PROPOFOL.

Mechanism The general cerebral excitatory effect produced by therapeutic THEOPHYLLINE levels may be a contributing factor.

Management Based on currently available documentation, no special precautions are necessary. Assess the clinical status of the patient, and adjust the PROPOFOL dose as needed.

Discussion

Possible antagonism of propofol sedation has been reported in a 24-year-old woman during coadministration of aminophylline.[1] The patient was receiving respiratory support for treatment of status asthmaticus and persistent intense bronchospasms. She received nebulized albuterol (eg, *Proventil*), IV antibiotics, and steroids, as well as infusions of terbutaline (eg, *Brethine*), ipratropium (eg, *Atrovent*), and aminophylline. Sedation was difficult, and the patient eventually received propofol 400 to 500 mg/hour. After discontinuation of aminophylline and a reduction in the steroid dosage, the infusion requirement of propofol decreased. During coadministration of aminophylline, the patient required a total of propofol 6,950 mg in a 12-hour period. However, 36 hours after aminophylline was withdrawn, the patient required only propofol 3,900 mg over a 12-hour period, although boluses of midazolam 2.5 mg (eg, *Versed*) were also administered. Eight healthy men received propofol anesthesia with saline or an aminophylline infusion.[2] Coadministration of aminophylline increased the mean propofol dose from 1.4 to 2.2 ng/kg and prolonged the time to loss of consciousness from 5.1 to 7.7 minutes compared with saline administration. See Propofol-Benzodiazepines.

Additional studies are needed to determine the clinical importance of this interaction.

[1] Taylor BL, et al. *Anaesthesia.* 1988;43(6):508.

[2] Turan A, et al. *Anesth Analg.* 2010;110(2):449.

* Asterisk indicates drugs cited in interaction reports. Based on pharmacologic and pharmacokinetic considerations, similar interactions may occur with other drugs that are listed.

Propoxyphene — *Ritonavir*

Propoxyphene* (eg, *Darvon*)	Ritonavir* (*Norvir*)

Significance	Onset	Severity	Documentation
1	☐ Rapid ■ **Delayed**	■ **Major** ☐ Moderate ☐ Minor	☐ Established ☐ Probable ■ **Suspected** ☐ Possible ☐ Unlikely

Effects Large increases in serum PROPOXYPHENE concentrations may occur, increasing the risk of PROPOXYPHENE toxicity.

Mechanism RITONAVIR may inhibit the metabolism (cytochrome P450 2D6) of PROPOXYPHENE.

Management RITONAVIR is contraindicated in patients receiving PROPOXYPHENE.

Discussion

Ritonavir is expected to produce large increases in propoxyphene plasma concentrations, increasing the risk of toxicity.[1] Toxic effects of propoxyphene include convulsions, respiratory depression, and apnea, as well as cardiac arrhythmias, pulmonary edema, and circulatory collapse.

The basis for this monograph is information on file with the manufacturer. Published clinical data are needed to further assess this information.

[1] *Norvir* [package insert]. Abbott Park, IL: Abbott Laboratories; February 1996.

* Asterisk indicates drugs cited in interaction reports.

Protease Inhibitors — *Ascorbic Acid*

Indinavir* (*Crixivan*)	Ascorbic Acid* (eg, *Vitamin C*)

Significance	Onset	Severity	Documentation
4	☐ Rapid ■ **Delayed**	☐ Major ■ **Moderate** ☐ Minor	☐ Established ☐ Probable ☐ Suspected ■ **Possible** ☐ Unlikely

Effects INDINAVIR plasma concentrations may be reduced, decreasing the efficacy.

Mechanism Unknown.

Management Avoid concurrent use if possible. However, if ASCORBIC ACID is considered necessary, monitor patients for a decrease in antiretroviral activity. Be prepared to adjust the dosage of INDINAVIR if needed. Caution patients to consult their health care provider before using nonprescription or herbal products.

Discussion

The effects of daily, high-dose vitamin C on the steady-state pharmacokinetics of indinavir were studied in 7 healthy volunteers.[1] In a prospective, open-label, longitudinal, 2-period investigation, each subject received indinavir 800 mg alone every 8 hours for 4 doses and again starting on day 6 of a 7-day course of vitamin C 1,000 mg/day. Compared with administration of indinavir alone, pretreatment with vitamin C decreased the mean steady-state plasma concentration of indinavir 20% (from 10.3 to 8.2 mcg/mL) and the AUC 14%. The $t_{½}$ and oral clearance of indinavir were not altered.

The clinical importance of this interaction is not established.

[1] Slain D, et al. *Pharmacotherapy*. 2005;25:165.

* Asterisk indicates drugs cited in interaction reports.

Protease Inhibitors — Azole Antifungal Agents

Protease Inhibitors		Azole Antifungal Agents	
Amprenavir*†	Nelfinavir (*Viracept*)	Fluconazole* (eg, *Diflucan*)	Ketoconazole* (eg, *Nizoral*)
Atazanavir* (*Reyataz*)	Ritonavir* (*Norvir*)	Itraconazole* (eg, *Sporanox*)	Posaconazole* (*Noxafil*)
Darunavir* (*Prezista*)	Saquinavir* (*Invirase*)		
Fosamprenavir* (*Lexiva*)	Tipranavir* (*Aptivus*)		
Indinavir* (*Crixivan*)			
Lopinavir/Ritonavir (*Kaletra*)			

Significance	Onset	Severity	Documentation
2	☐ Rapid	☐ Major	☐ Established
	■ **Delayed**	■ **Moderate**	■ **Probable**
		☐ Minor	☐ Suspected
			☐ Possible
			☐ Unlikely

Effects Plasma PROTEASE INHIBITOR and AZOLE ANTIFUNGAL AGENT levels may be elevated, increasing the risk of toxicity.

Mechanism AZOLE ANTIFUNGAL AGENT and PROTEASE INHIBITOR metabolism may be inhibited.

Management It may be necessary to reduce the dose of either agent. Monitor patients for toxicity and adjust the dose as needed.

Discussion

Because administration of ketoconazole 400 mg with indinavir 400 mg produced a 68% increase in the indinavir AUC,[1] the manufacturer recommends considering a dosage of indinavir 600 mg every 8 h instead of 800 mg every 8 h when starting indinavir in patients receiving ketoconazole or starting both drugs at the same time. Ketoconazole increased the saquinavir AUC 190%.[2] However, when ketoconazole was given with ritonavir-boosted saquinavir, neither ritonavir nor saquinavir levels changed, but the ketoconazole AUC increased 2.68-fold.[3] A patient taking ritonavir 600 mg and saquinavir 400 mg twice daily developed protease inhibitor toxicity 1 wk after itraconazole was increased from 100 to 200 mg twice daily.[4] The itraconazole level was markedly elevated, with a $t_{1/2}$ of 216 h. Two of 4 patients receiving indinavir developed hyperbilirubinemia and slightly elevated transaminase levels while receiving itraconazole. Levels returned to pretreatment values after discontinuing itraconazole. Similarly, elevated itraconazole levels were reported in a 54-year-old HIV-infected man receiving lopinavir/ritonavir.[5] In 7 patients, ketoconazole had no effect on saquinavir levels.[6] In other studies, ketoconazole increased the AUC of amprenavir 31%,[7] ritonavir 29%, darunavir 155%, ritonavir-boosted darunavir 42%,[8] and saquinavir 37%[9]; while fluconazole increased the AUC of ritonavir 12%,[10] tipranavir 50%,[11] and saquinavir 50%.[12] The ritonavir cerebrospinal fluid level was markedly elevated. In healthy subjects, fosamprenavir/ritonavir increased ketoconazole levels nearly 2.7-fold.[13] In an open-label, randomized, crossover study in 12 healthy adults, posaconazole increased the atazanavir C_{max} and AUC by 2.6- and 3.7-fold, respectively.[14] When atazanavir was given with ritonavir, posaconazole administration increased the atazanavir C_{max} and AUC by 1.5- and 2.5-fold, respectively. Most subjects receiving atazanavir (with or without ritonavir) and posaconazole experienced clinically important increases in total bilirubin. In an open-label, crossover study in healthy volunteers, coadministration of fosamprenavir with posaconazole decreased the posaconazole AUC 23% and the amprenavir AUC 65% compared with ritonavir-boosted fosamprenavir.[15] It was concluded that unboosted fosamprenavir should not be given with posaconazole. See also Voriconazole-Ritonavir.

1 *Crixivan* [package insert]. White House Station, NJ: Merck & Co Inc; 1996.
2 Grub S, et al. *Eur J Clin Pharmacol.* 2001;57(2):115.
3 Kaeser B, et al. *Antimicrob Agents Chemother.* 2009; 53(2):609.
4 MacKenzie-Wood AR, et al. *Med J Aust.* 1999; 170(1):46.
5 Crommentuyn KM, et al. *Clin Infect Dis.* 2004; 38(8):e73.
6 Collazos J, et al. *J Antimicrob Chemother.* 2000; 46(1):151.
7 Polk RE, et al. *Pharmacotherapy.* 1999;19(12):1378.
8 Sekar VJ, et al. *Br J Clin Pharmacol.* 2008;66(2):215.
9 Khaliq Y, et al. *Clin Pharmacol Ther.* 2000;68(6):637.
10 Cato A 3rd, et al. *Drug Metab Dispos.* 1997; 25(9):1104.
11 la Porte CJ, et al. *Antimicrob Agents Chemother.* 2009;53(1):162.
12 Koks CH, et al. *Br J Clin Pharmacol.* 2001;51(6):631.
13 Wire MB, et al. *Antimicrob Agents Chemother.* 2007; 51(8):2982.
14 Krishna G, et al. *J Acquir Immune Defic Syndr.* 2009; 51(4):437.
15 Brüggemann RJ, et al. *J Antimicrob Chemother.* 2010; 65(10):2188.

* Asterisk indicates drugs cited in interaction reports. Based on pharmacologic and pharmacokinetic considerations, similar interactions may occur with other drugs that are listed.
† Not available in the United States.

Protease Inhibitors — *Cat's Claw*

Atazanavir* (*Reyataz*)	Nelfinavir (*Viracept*)	Cat's Claw* (*Uncaria tomentosa*)
Fosamprenavir (*Lexiva*)	Ritonavir* (*Norvir*)	
Indinavir (*Crixivan*)	Saquinavir* (*Invirase*)	
Lopinavir/Ritonavir (*Kaletra*)		

Significance	Onset	Severity	Documentation
4	□ Rapid	□ Major	□ Established
	■ **Delayed**	■ **Moderate**	□ Probable
		□ Minor	□ Suspected
			■ **Possible**
			□ Unlikely

Effects PROTEASE INHIBITOR trough plasma concentrations may be elevated, increasing the risk of toxicity.

Mechanism Inhibition of PROTEASE INHIBITOR metabolism (CYP3A4) by CAT'S CLAW is suspected.

Management Patients receiving PROTEASE INHIBITORS should avoid use of the herbal product CAT'S CLAW. Caution patients receiving PROTEASE INHIBITORS to consult their health care provider before using nonprescription or herbal products.

Discussion

Elevated atazanavir, ritonavir, and saquinavir plasma trough concentrations were observed in a 45-year-old woman who was HIV-positive.[1] While she was receiving atazanavir 300 mg daily, ritonavir 100 mg daily, and saquinavir 2,000 mg daily, trough concentrations were 1.22, 6.13, and 3.4 mcg/mL, respectively. No signs or symptoms of protease inhibitor overdosage were observed. Questioning of the patient revealed she had been taking a cat's claw preparation for the previous 2 months. She was asked to stop taking cat's claw, and 15 days later, plasma trough concentrations had normalized to atazanavir 0.3 mcg/mL, ritonavir 0.92 mcg/mL, and saquinavir 0.64 mcg/mL.

[1] López Galera RM, et al. *Eur J Clin Pharmacol.* 2008;64(12):1235.

* Asterisk indicates drugs cited in interaction reports. Based on pharmacologic and pharmacokinetic considerations, similar interactions may occur with other drugs that are listed.

Protease Inhibitors — *Enfuvirtide*

Ritonavir* (*Norvir*)	Tipranavir* (*Aptivus*)	Enfuvirtide* (*Fuzeon*)

Significance	Onset	Severity	Documentation
4	□ Rapid ■ **Delayed**	□ Major ■ **Moderate** □ Minor	□ Established □ Probable □ Suspected ■ **Possible** □ Unlikely

Effects PROTEASE INHIBITOR concentrations may be elevated, increasing the risk of adverse reactions.

Mechanism Unknown.

Management It may be necessary to adjust the PROTEASE INHIBITOR dose when ENFUVIRTIDE is started or stopped.

Discussion

Ritonavir and tipranavir plasma concentrations were measured in a cohort study of 55 AIDS patients who received tipranavir 500 mg and ritonavir 200 mg twice daily plus 2 nucleoside reverse transcriptase inhibitors.[1] In addition, 27 patients received subcutaneous enfuvirtide 90 mg twice daily while 28 patients did not receive enfuvirtide. Tipranavir and ritonavir trough concentrations were elevated in patients receiving enfuvirtide compared with patients not receiving enfuvirtide. The increase in tipranavir exposure was approximately 50%. In 2 patients who discontinued enfuvirtide, tipranavir trough concentrations decreased approximately 51% and 26%, respectively, while in 1 patient who added enfuvirtide to the drug regimen, the tipranavir trough concentration increased approximately 72%.

[1] González de Requena D, et al. *AIDS*. 2006;20(15):1977.

* Asterisk indicates drugs cited in interaction reports.

Protease Inhibitors — *Evening Primrose Oil*

Protease Inhibitors	Evening Primrose Oil
Lopinavir/Ritonavir* (*Kaletra*)	Evening Primrose Oil*

Significance	Onset	Severity	Documentation
4	□ Rapid	□ Major	□ Established
	■ **Delayed**	■ **Moderate**	□ Probable
		□ Minor	□ Suspected
			■ **Possible**
			□ Unlikely

Effects LOPINAVIR plasma concentrations may be elevated, increasing the pharmacologic effects and risk of adverse reactions (eg, diarrhea).

Mechanism Unknown.

Management Patients receiving LOPINAVIR should avoid EVENING PRIMROSE OIL. Caution patients taking PROTEASE INHIBITORS to consult their health care provider before using nonprescription or herbal products.

Discussion

Lopinavir 533 mg/ritonavir 133 mg twice daily was included in the antiretroviral regimen of a 47-year-old man diagnosed with HIV.[1] Lopinavir plasma concentrations ranged between 4 and 9 mg/L (normal, 5 to 10 mg/L). While taking herbal products, one of which contained evening primrose oil (eg, *Efamol*), the patient developed persistent diarrhea that was severe enough to interfere with his daily life. At that time, the lopinavir concentration was 15.2 mg/L. Six weeks after discontinuing the herbal products, including evening primrose oil, the lopinavir plasma concentration was 5.3 mg/L, and the patient no longer had diarrhea. One week after rechallenge with the evening primrose oil-containing product, the lopinavir trough plasma concentration increased from 6.69 to 8.11 mg/L. The herbal product was discontinued and lopinavir concentrations remained within the normal range at successive visits.[1]

[1] van den Bout-van den Beukel CJ, et al. *AIDS*. 2008;22(10):1243.

* Asterisk indicates drugs cited in interaction reports.

Protease Inhibitors — Food

Indinavir* (*Crixivan*)	Orange Juice, Seville*

Significance	Onset	Severity	Documentation
3	☐ Rapid	☐ Major	☐ Established
	■ **Delayed**	☐ Moderate	☐ Probable
		■ **Minor**	■ **Suspected**
			☐ Possible
			☐ Unlikely

Effects The time to reach INDINAVIR C_{max} may be prolonged.

Mechanism Unknown.

Management Based on available data, no special precautions are needed.

Discussion

The effects of Seville orange juice on the pharmacokinetics of indinavir were studied in 13 healthy volunteers.[1] In an open-label, crossover investigation, each subject received indinavir 800 mg every 8 hours for 1 day and a single 800 mg dose the next morning with 8 oz of water or Seville orange juice. Compared with water, taking indinavir with Seville orange juice prolonged the T_{max} 50% (from 1.25 to 1.87 hours). Other pharmacokinetic values of indinavir were not altered by Seville orange juice.

[1] Penzak SR, et al. *J Clin Pharmacol.* 2002;42(10):1165.

* Asterisk indicates drugs cited in interaction reports.

Protease Inhibitors — *Garlic*

Atazanavir (*Reyataz*)	Nelfinavir (*Viracept*)	Garlic*
Darunavir (*Prezista*)	Ritonavir (*Norvir*)	
Fosamprenavir (*Lexiva*)	Saquinavir* (*Invirase*)	
Indinavir (*Crixivan*)	Tipranavir (*Aptivus*)	
Lopinavir/Ritonavir (*Kaletra*)		

Significance	Onset	Severity	Documentation
2	□ Rapid	□ Major	□ Established
	■ **Delayed**	■ **Moderate**	□ Probable
		□ Minor	■ **Suspected**
			□ Possible
			□ Unlikely

Effects PROTEASE INHIBITOR plasma concentrations may be reduced, decreasing the pharmacologic effect.

Mechanism Inhibition of CYP3A4 metabolism of PROTEASE INHIBITORS by GARLIC is suspected.

Management Caution patients receiving PROTEASE INHIBITORS to avoid GARLIC.

Discussion

Data are conflicting. The effects of garlic on the pharmacokinetics of ritonavir were studied in 10 healthy volunteers.[1] In a randomized, crossover investigation, each subject received ritonavir 400 mg alone or with 10 mg of odorless garlic extract. Subjects received garlic extract twice daily for 4 days. A single dose of ritonavir was administered simultaneously with the seventh dose of garlic. Short-term administration of garlic did not affect the ritonavir C_{max} or AUC compared with taking ritonavir alone. The effect of garlic supplements on the pharmacokinetics of saquinavir was studied in 10 healthy subjects.[2] Data were analyzed for 9 of the subjects. The investigation was a 2-treatment, 3-period, longitudinal design. Subjects received saquinavir (1,200 mg 3 times daily for 10 doses) alone, then following pretreatment with garlic 2 caplets twice daily, garlic caplets and saquinavir were coadministered. After a 10-day washout period, saquinavir was administered. Compared with administration of saquinavir alone, coadministration with garlic supplements decreased the saquinavir AUC 51%, decreased trough levels 8 hours after saquinavir administration 49%, and decreased the mean peak concentration 54%. After the washout period, the AUC, trough and peak level values returned to 65%, 70%, and 61% of their baseline values, respectively. A crossover study in 10 healthy men found that administration of garlic extract 1,200 mg daily for 3 weeks did not affect CYP3A4 hepatic function or the pharmacokinetics of single-dose administration of saquinavir 1,200 mg.[3]

[1] Gallicano K, et al. *Br J Clin Pharmacol.* 2003;55(2):199.

[2] Piscitelli SC, et al. *Clin Infect Dis.* 2002;34(2):234.

[3] Jacek H, et al. *Clin Pharmacol Ther.* 2004;75(2):P80.

* Asterisk indicates drugs cited in interaction reports. Based on pharmacologic and pharmacokinetic considerations, similar interactions may occur with other drugs that are listed.

Protease Inhibitors		*Interleukins*
Indinavir* (*Crixivan*)	Ritonavir (*Norvir*)	Aldesleukin* (Interleukin [IL]-2; *Proleukin*)
Nelfinavir (*Viracept*)	Saquinavir (*Invirase*)	

Significance	Onset	Severity	Documentation
2	☐ Rapid ■ **Delayed**	☐ Major ■ **Moderate** ☐ Minor	☐ Established ☐ Probable ■ **Suspected** ☐ Possible ☐ Unlikely

Effects PROTEASE INHIBITOR concentrations may be elevated, increasing the risk of toxicity.

Mechanism ALDESLEUKIN (IL-2) may induce the formation of IL-6, which may inhibit PROTEASE INHIBITOR metabolism (CYP3A4).

Management It may be necessary to adjust the PROTEASE INHIBITOR dose when INTERLEUKINS are started or stopped.

Discussion

Coadministration of interleukins and protease inhibitors may be beneficial in the treatment of HIV. The effect of aldesleukin on the pharmacokinetics of indinavir was studied in patients infected with HIV.[1] All subjects had been receiving oral indinavir 800 mg every 8 hours for at least 4 weeks when a 5-day continuous infusion of aldesleukin 3 to 12 million units/day was coadministered. Phase 1 consisted of an observational, noncontrolled trial in which data were collected from 8 patients during inpatient visits for an indinavir/IL-2 clinical trial. Phase 2 was a prospective study in which a separate group of 9 patients had serial pharmacokinetics sampling conducted on days 1 and 5 of aldesleukin therapy. During the observational phase, the mean trough concentrations of indinavir increased 154% (from 264 to 670 ng/mL) by day 5 of concurrent therapy. Concentrations increased in 7 of the 8 patients, and decreased 35% in 1 patient. In the prospective study phase, there was an 88% (range, 27% to 215%) increase in indinavir AUC in 8 of the 9 patients. One patient had a 29% decrease in the AUC. The oral clearance of indinavir decreased 56% (from 57.1 to 25.3 L/hr) by day 5 of concomitant therapy. During the 5 days of aldesleukin administration, there was a 20-fold increase in the mean level of the cytokine IL-6.

[1] Piscitelli SC, et al. *Pharmacotherapy*. 1998;18(6):1212.

* Asterisk indicates drugs cited in interaction reports. Based on pharmacologic and pharmacokinetic considerations, similar interactions may occur with other drugs that are listed.

Protease Inhibitors — *Loperamide*

Saquinavir* (*Invirase*)	Loperamide* (eg, *Imodium*)

Significance	Onset	Severity	Documentation
4	☐ Rapid ■ **Delayed**	☐ Major ■ **Moderate** ☐ Minor	☐ Established ☐ Probable ☐ Suspected ■ **Possible** ☐ Unlikely

Effects SAQUINAVIR plasma concentrations and clinical efficacy may be reduced, while LOPERAMIDE levels may be increased.

Mechanism Unknown. However, impaired SAQUINAVIR absorption caused by LOPERAMIDE administration is suspected.

Management Until more clinical data are available, avoid LOPERAMIDE therapy in patients receiving SAQUINAVIR. If LOPERAMIDE and SAQUINAVIR are coadministered, closely monitor the patient for a decrease in antiretroviral activity.

Discussion

In a single-dose, randomized, double-blind, 3-way, crossover study, the pharmacokinetic effects of loperamide and saquinavir on each other were investigated in 12 healthy volunteers.[1] Each subject received saquinavir 600 mg or placebo, loperamide 16 mg or placebo, or saquinavir plus loperamide. Coadministration of saquinavir and loperamide increased loperamide plasma concentrations, resulting in a 40% increase in the AUC of loperamide. The metabolic clearance of loperamide to the desmethylloperamide metabolite was decreased 20%. The $t_{½}$ of loperamide was unchanged. Loperamide administration decreased the C_{max} and AUC of saquinavir 46.3% and 53.7%, respectively. The renal clearance of saquinavir was not affected by loperamide administration.

[1] Mikus G, et al. *Clin Pharmacokinet.* 2004;43(14):1015.

* Asterisk indicates drugs cited in interaction reports.

Protease Inhibitors		Macrolide & Related Antibiotics	
Amprenavir*†	Ritonavir* (*Norvir*)	Clarithromycin* (eg, *Biaxin*)	Telithromycin (*Ketek*)
Atazanavir (*Reyataz*)	Saquinavir (*Invirase*)	Erythromycin (eg, *Ery-Tab*)	
Darunavir* (*Prezista*)	Tipranavir* (*Aptivus*)		
Fosamprenavir (*Lexiva*)			
Lopinavir/Ritonavir (*Kaletra*)			

Significance	Onset	Severity	Documentation
2	☐ Rapid	☐ Major	☐ Established
	■ **Delayed**	■ **Moderate**	☐ Probable
		☐ Minor	■ **Suspected**
			☐ Possible
			☐ Unlikely

Effects AMPRENAVIR and TIPRANAVIR plasma concentrations may be elevated, increasing the risk of adverse reactions. CLARITHROMYCIN plasma levels may be increased by DARUNAVIR and TIPRANAVIR.

Mechanism Inhibition of MACROLIDE AND RELATED ANTIBIOTICS and PROTEASE INHIBITOR metabolism (CYP3A4) may occur.

Management Based on available data, no dosage adjustment of either drug is needed. Be prepared to make appropriate changes in dosage if an interaction is suspected.

Discussion

Coadministration of amprenavir and clarithromycin was assessed for a possible pharmacokinetic interaction in 12 healthy men.[1] In an open-label, randomized, crossover study, each subject received amprenavir 1,200 mg twice daily for 4 days, clarithromycin 500 mg twice daily for 4 days, and both drugs concurrently for 4 days. Compared with administration of amprenavir or clarithromycin alone, coadministration of both agents increased the mean AUC of amprenavir 18%, the peak plasma concentration 15%, and the trough concentration 39%. For clarithromycin, the T_{max} was increased 2 hours, the renal clearance was increased 34%, and the AUC for the 14-R-hydroxyclarithromycin metabolite was decreased 35%. Coadministration of darunavir 400 mg and ritonavir 100 mg with clarithromycin 500 mg twice daily for 7 days decreased the darunavir AUC 13% and increased the clarithromycin AUC 57%.[2] Neither change was considered clinically important. Twenty-four healthy subjects received clarithromycin alone for 5 days and with tipranavir/ritonavir for 7 days.[3] Tipranavir/ritonavir increased clarithromycin AUC and C_{max} 19% and 68%, respectively, compared with giving clarithromycin alone. In addition, clarithromycin increased the tipranavir C_{max} 66%. The tipranavir concentration was increased 2-fold at 12 hours.

[1] Brophy DF, et al. *Antimicrob Agents Chemother.* 2000;44(4):978.
[2] Sekar VJ, et al. *J Clin Pharmacol.* 2008;48(1):60.
[3] la Porte CJ, et al. *Antimicrob Agents Chemother.* 2009;53(1):162.

* Asterisk indicates drugs cited in interaction reports. Based on pharmacologic and pharmacokinetic considerations, similar interactions may occur with other drugs that are listed.
† Not available in the United States.

Protease Inhibitors — *NNRT Inhibitors*

Protease Inhibitors		NNRT Inhibitors	
Atazanavir* (*Reyataz*)	Nelfinavir* (*Viracept*)	Efavirenz* (*Sustiva*)	Nevirapine* (eg, *Viramune*)
Darunavir* (*Prezista*)	Ritonavir* (*Norvir*)		
Fosamprenavir* (*Lexiva*)	Saquinavir (*Invirase*)		
Indinavir* (*Crixivan*)	Tipranavir (*Aptivus*)		
Lopinavir/Ritonavir* (*Kaletra*)			

Significance	Onset	Severity	Documentation
2	☐ Rapid	☐ Major	☐ Established
	■ **Delayed**	■ **Moderate**	■ **Probable**
		☐ Minor	☐ Suspected
			☐ Possible
			☐ Unlikely

Effects PROTEASE INHIBITOR plasma levels and clinical efficacy may be reduced.

Mechanism Increased hepatic metabolism (CYP3A4) of the PROTEASE INHIBITOR is suspected.

Management Monitor PROTEASE INHIBITOR levels and clinical response when EFAVIRENZ or NEVIRAPINE is started or stopped. Adjust PROTEASE INHIBITOR dosage as needed. In children, EFAVIRENZ may result in suboptimal AMPRENAVIR[†] levels.

Discussion

In a study of 7 patients with advanced HIV, nevirapine reduced nelfinavir AUC and plasma levels 50%, C_{max} 43%, and trough levels 53%, and shortened the T_{max} from 4 to 2 hr.[1] In a study of 21 patients, nevirapine decreased trough levels of indinavir and ritonavir.[2] In patients infected with HIV, nevirapine and fosamprenavir coadministration reduced amprenavir exposure 25% to 35%.[3] No change in amprenavir exposure occurred when nevirapine was given to patients receiving ritonavir-boosted fosamprenavir. Coadministration of amprenavir and efavirenz to children infected with HIV resulted in undetectable amprenavir levels within 4 hr of ingestion. In contrast, amprenavir and delavirdine (*Rescriptor*) coadministration resulted in amprenavir C_{max} levels approximately 3-fold higher and trough levels 5- to 10-fold higher than with amprenavir alone.[4] In patients infected with HIV-1, coadministration of nevirapine and lopinavir plus ritonavir resulted in a 50% increase in lopinavir clearance and a corresponding decrease in trough levels.[5] The AUC of ritonavir-boosted lopinavir was reduced 51% and 44% by efavirenz and nevirapine, respectively.[6] These effects were reversed by increasing the lopinavir/ritonavir dose 50%. In a study of healthy adults, administration of a lopinavir/ritonavir dose of lopinavir 500 mg/ritonavir 125 mg twice daily with efavirenz closely approximates the pharmacokinetic exposure of a lopinavir/ritonavir dose of lopinavir 400 mg/ritonavir 100 mg twice daily given alone.[7] In patients receiving ritonavir-boosted atazanavir, administration of nevirapine or efavirenz decreased atazanavir levels.[8,9] In a study of patients infected with HIV, there was no pharmacokinetic interaction between the NNRT inhibitor etravirine (*Intelence*) and darunavir.[10] There was a small and clinically unimportant increase in nevirapine concentrations when nevirapine was administered with ritonavir-boosted darunavir.[11] Efavirenz reduced the $t_{½}$ of ritonavir-boosted darunavir from 15.3 to 8.5 hr, leading to a 45% reduction in trough levels.[12] However, these levels were still above the effective concentrations. In healthy volunteers, efavirenz did not have a clinically important effect on the pharmacokinetics of tipranavir-ritonavir.[13]

1 Merry C, et al. *AIDS.* 1998;12(10):1163.
2 Burger DM, et al. *J Acquir Immune Defic Syndr.* 2004;35(1):97.
3 DeJesus E, et al. *Antimicrob Agents Chemother.* 2006;50(9):3157.
4 Wintergerst U, et al. *AIDS.* 2000;14(12):1866.
5 Dailly E, et al. *Eur J Clin Pharmacol.* 2005;61(2):153.
6 Kityo C, et al. *Antimicrob Agents Chemother.* 2010;54(7):2965.
7 NG J, et al. *J Clin Pharmacol.* 2012;52(8):1248.
8 Dailly E, et al. *Eur J Clin Pharmacol.* 2006;62(7):523.
9 Moltó J, et al. *Ther Drug Monit.* 2010;32(1):93.
10 Boffito M, et al. *AIDS.* 2007;21(11):1449.
11 Sekar V, et al. *Br J Clin Pharmacol.* 2009;68(1):116.
12 Soon GH, et al. *Antimicrob Agents Chemother.* 2010;54(7):2775.
13 la Porte CJ, et al. *Antimicrob Agents Chemother.* 2009;53(11):4840.

* Asterisk indicates drugs cited in interaction reports. Based on pharmacologic and pharmacokinetic considerations, similar interactions may occur with other drugs that are listed.
† Not available in the United States.

Protease Inhibitors — Nucleotide Analog Reverse Transcriptase Inhibitors

Atazanavir* (*Reyataz*)	Tenofovir* (*Viread*)

Significance	Onset	Severity	Documentation
2	☐ Rapid	☐ Major	☐ Established
	■ **Delayed**	■ **Moderate**	☐ Probable
		☐ Minor	■ **Suspected**
			☐ Possible
			☐ Unlikely

Effects ATAZANAVIR plasma concentrations may be reduced, decreasing the antiviral effect.

Mechanism Unknown.

Management In patients receiving ATAZANAVIR, monitor ATAZANAVIR plasma concentrations and response to therapy if TENOFOVIR is coadministered.

Discussion

The effects of tenofovir on the pharmacokinetics of atazanavir/ritonavir were studied in 10 patients infected with HIV.[1,2] In patients receiving atazanavir 300 mg plus ritonavir 100 mg daily, administration of tenofovir 300 mg daily for 4 weeks decreased atazanavir C_{max} 34% and AUC 27%, and increased the clearance 33%.[1] In 40 patients receiving nucleoside reverse transcriptase inhibitors in addition to atazanavir 300 mg plus ritonavir 100 mg daily, tenofovir administration reduced the atazanavir trough plasma concentration 27% and increased the clearance 19%, compared with patients receiving the same regimen without tenofovir.[2] Darunavir (*Prezista*) plus ritonavir (*Norvir*) increased the AUC of tenofovir 22%,[3] while lopinavir/ritonavir (*Kaletra*) increased the AUC of tenofovir 13%.[4] Neither of these changes is considered clinically important.

1 Taburet AM, et al. *Antimicrob Agents Chemother.* 2004;48(6):2091.
2 Dailly E, et al. *Eur J Clin Pharmacol.* 2006;62(7):523.
3 Hoetelmans RM, et al. *Br J Clin Pharmacol.* 2007;64(5):655.
4 Kiser JJ, et al. *Clin Pharmacol Ther.* 2008;83(2):265.

* Asterisk indicates drugs cited in interaction reports.

Protease Inhibitors — Proton Pump Inhibitors

Protease Inhibitors		Proton Pump Inhibitors	
Atazanavir* (*Reyataz*)	Nelfinavir* (*Viracept*)	Esomeprazole* (*Nexium*)	Pantoprazole* (eg, *Protonix*)
Indinavir* (*Crixivan*)	Saquinavir* (*Invirase*)	Lansoprazole* (eg, *Prevacid*)	Rabeprazole* (*Aciphex*)
Lopinavir/Ritonavir* (*Kaletra*)		Omeprazole* (eg, *Prilosec*)	

Significance	Onset	Severity	Documentation
1	☐ Rapid ■ **Delayed**	■ **Major** ☐ Moderate ☐ Minor	☐ Established ☐ Probable ■ **Suspected** ☐ Possible ☐ Unlikely

Effects The antiviral activity of certain PROTEASE INHIBITORS may be reduced. SAQUINAVIR and LOPINAVIR plasma levels may be increased.

Mechanism PROTON PUMP INHIBITORS may decrease the dissolution of certain PROTEASE INHIBITORS, reducing GI absorption.

Management Monitor patients for a decrease in antiviral activity if INDINAVIR or NELFINAVIR and a PROTON PUMP INHIBITOR are coadministered. Monitor for SAQUINAVIR adverse reactions. Adjust the PROTEASE INHIBITOR dose as needed. Concomitant use of ATAZANAVIR and PROTON PUMP INHIBITORS is not recommended.[1]

Discussion

Plasma indinavir levels in 9 patients receiving indinavir 800 mg 3 times daily plus omeprazole 20 to 40 mg daily were compared with those of 15 patients receiving the same dose of indinavir alone.[2] Four of the 9 patients on combined indinavir and omeprazole therapy had indinavir plasma levels less than 95% confidence interval (CI) of the 15 patients receiving indinavir alone. The indinavir level was higher than 95% CI in 1 patient. In another patient, the reference value of indinavir decreased from 96% to 38% after he began taking omeprazole. In 2 other patients, increasing the dosage of indinavir to 1,000 mg 3 times daily during concurrent omeprazole therapy produced indinavir plasma levels that were no different than those of patients receiving indinavir alone. This interaction was not seen in all patients. The effects of omeprazole on a single dose of indinavir 800 mg alone or with ritonavir 200 mg were evaluated in 14 healthy volunteers.[3] Administration of omeprazole 20 or 40 mg/day for 7 days decreased the indinavir AUC approximately 34% and 47%, respectively. After pretreatment with omeprazole 40 mg daily for 7 days, the addition of ritonavir 200 mg to indinavir 800 mg increased the indinavir AUC approximately 53%. In a study of 12 healthy volunteers, omeprazole 40 mg/day reduced the nelfinavir AUC 36%.[4] A population-based study of viral loads in patients taking nelfinavir-based HIV regimens plus proton pump inhibitors did not find a loss of virologic control but found a 50% increase in the risk of virologic rebound.[5] In healthy volunteers given ritonavir (*Norvir*)–boosted darunavir (*Prezista*), neither ritonavir nor darunavir pharmacokinetics were affected by omeprazole.[6] In a study utilizing retrospective chart review, 9 patients receiving atazanavir and a proton pump inhibitor achieved successful viral outcomes (undetectable viral load).[7] However, in a study in healthy volunteers, atazanavir AUC decreased 62% when ritonavir-boosted atazanavir was coadministered with omeprazole.[8] Low dose omeprazole (20 mg daily) decreased atazanavir AUC 42%.[9] In a study of 18 healthy subjects receiving saquinavir 1,000 mg plus ritonavir 100 mg twice daily, omeprazole 40 mg/day increased the AUC of saquinavir 82%.[10] Separating the administration times of omeprazole and saquinavir/ritonavir by 2 hours did not make a difference.[11] Lopinavir and ritonavir AUCs were increased 23% and 27%, respectively, during coadministration with omeprazole 40 mg daily.[12]

[1] *Reyataz* [package insert]. Princeton, NJ: Bristol-Myers Squibb Company; October 2004.
[2] Burger DM, et al. *AIDS*. 1998;12(15):2080.
[3] Tappouni HL, et al. *Am J Health Syst Pharm*. 2008;65(5):422.
[4] Fang AF, et al. *Pharmacotherapy*. 2008;28(1):42.
[5] Saberi P, et al. *Pharmacotherapy*. 2011;31(3):253.
[6] Sekar VJ, et al. *Antimicrob Agents Chemother*. 2007;51(3):958.
[7] Sahloff EG, et al. *Ann Pharmacother*. 2006;40(10):1731.
[8] Klein CE, et al. *J Clin Pharmacol*. 2008;48(5):553.
[9] Zhu L, et al. *J Clin Pharmacol*. 2011;51(3):368.
[10] Winston A, et al. *AIDS*. 2006;20(10):1401.
[11] Singh K, et al. *Clin Pharmacol Ther*. 2008;83(6):867.
[12] Overton ET, et al. *J Clin Pharmacol*. 2010;50(9):1050.

* Asterisk indicates drugs cited in interaction reports.

Protease Inhibitors — *St. John's Wort*

Atazanavir* (*Reyataz*)	Nelfinavir* (*Viracept*)	St. John's Wort*
Darunavir* (*Prezista*)	Ritonavir* (*Norvir*)	
Fosamprenavir* (*Lexiva*)	Saquinavir* (*Invirase*)	
Indinavir* (*Crixivan*)		

Significance	Onset	Severity	Documentation
1	□ Rapid	■ **Major**	□ Established
	■ **Delayed**	□ Moderate	□ Probable
		□ Minor	■ **Suspected**
			□ Possible
			□ Unlikely

Effects Plasma PROTEASE INHIBITOR concentrations and clinical efficacy may be decreased.

Mechanism Increased hepatic metabolism (CYP3A4) of the PROTEASE INHIBITOR is suspected.

Management Coadministration of FOSAMPRENAVIR and ST. JOHN'S WORT is contraindicated.[1] Caution patients receiving a PROTEASE INHIBITOR to consult their health care provider before using nonprescription or herbal products. Do not coadminister PROTEASE INHIBITORS with ST. JOHN'S WORT.[2-6]

Discussion

In an open-label study, the effect of St. John's wort on indinavir plasma concentrations was evaluated in 8 healthy volunteers.[7] Each subject received indinavir 800 mg every 8 hours for 3 doses alone and again starting on day 14 of receiving St. John's wort 300 mg 3 times daily (standardized to hypericin 0.3%). Taking indinavir with St. John's wort resulted in a 54% decrease in the AUC of indinavir, a 28% reduction in indinavir C_{max}, and a 49% to 99% decrease in indinavir concentration 8 hours after taking indinavir. Concurrent use of saquinavir and St. John's wort or products containing St. John's wort is not recommended by the manufacturer of saquinavir.[5] Administration of protease inhibitors, including saquinavir, with St. John's wort is expected to substantially decrease protease inhibitor concentrations. It also may result in suboptimal levels of saquinavir and lead to loss of virologic response and possible resistance to saquinavir or to the class of protease inhibitors.

The ingredients of many herbal products are not standardized. It is unclear if herbal products contain ingredients other than those listed on the label or purported to be present that could interact with protease inhibitor therapy.

[1] *Lexiva* [package insert]. Research Triangle Park, NC: GlaxoSmithKline; April 2010.
[2] *Norvir* [package insert]. Abbott Park, IL: Abbott Laboratories; September 2001.
[3] *Viracept* [package insert]. La Jolla, CA: Agouron Pharmaceuticals Inc; December 2002.
[4] *Reyataz* [package insert]. Princeton, NJ: Bristol-Myers Squibb; June 2003.
[5] *Fortovase* [package insert]. Nutley, NJ: Roche Laboratories Inc; July 2002.
[6] *Prezista* [package insert]. Raritan, NJ: Tibotec Therapeutics; June 2006.
[7] Piscitelli SC, et al. *Lancet.* 2000;355(9203):547.

* Asterisk indicates drugs cited in interaction reports.

Proton Pump Inhibitors — *Fluvoxamine*

Proton Pump Inhibitors		Fluvoxamine
Esomeprazole (*Nexium*)	Pantoprazole (eg, *Protonix*)	Fluvoxamine* (eg, *Luvox CR*)
Lansoprazole* (eg, *Prevacid*)	Rabeprazole* (*Aciphex*)	
Omeprazole (eg, *Prilosec*)		

Significance	Onset	Severity	Documentation
4	□ Rapid	□ Major	□ Established
	■ **Delayed**	■ **Moderate**	□ Probable
		□ Minor	□ Suspected
			■ **Possible**
			□ Unlikely

Effects Plasma concentrations of certain PROTON PUMP INHIBITORS may be elevated, increasing the pharmacologic and adverse reactions.

Mechanism Inhibition of certain PROTON PUMP INHIBITOR metabolism (CYP2C19) in extensive metabolizers.

Management Monitor for increased adverse reactions in patients receiving certain PROTON PUMP INHIBITORS.

Discussion

The effects of fluvoxamine on the metabolism of lansoprazole in relation to CYP2C19 genotypes were studied in 18 healthy volunteers[1] consisting of 6 homozygous extensive metabolizers (EMs), 6 heterozygous EMs, and 6 poor metabolizers (PMs) for CYP2C19. Each subject received fluvoxamine 25 mg or matching placebo twice daily for 6 days. On day 6, they received a single oral dose of lansoprazole 60 mg. Compared with placebo, fluvoxamine administration increased the AUC of lansoprazole in homozygous and heterozygous EMs 3.8- and 2.5-fold, respectively, and prolonged the elimination $t_{½}$ 3- and 1.7-fold, respectively. The pharmacokinetics of lansoprazole were not changed in PMs. Fluvoxamine decreased the C_{max} of 5-hydroxylansoprazole and the AUC ratios of the 5-hydroxy metabolite to lansoprazole in both groups of EMs. In addition, fluvoxamine increased the C_{max} of lansoprazole sulfone in homozygous EMs and the AUC of the sulfone metabolite in homozygous and heterozygous EMs. In a similar study, comparable results occurred in healthy volunteers receiving fluvoxamine 50 mg/day and a single dose of omeprazole 40 mg.[2] Fluvoxamine 10 mg/day for 7 days has been reported to increase omeprazole levels.[3] In another study, the effects of fluvoxamine on the metabolism of rabeprazole were studied in 21 healthy subjects.[4] Compared with placebo, fluvoxamine prolonged the $t_{½}$ and increased the AUC of rabeprazole 2.8- and 1.7-fold in homozygous and heterozygous EMs, respectively. The $t_{½}$ was prolonged and the AUC of the rabeprazole thioether metabolite was increased 5.1- and 2.6-fold in homozygous and heterozygous EMs, respectively. No difference in pharmacokinetic parameters occurred in PMs.

1 Yasui-Furukori N, et al. *J Clin Pharmacol.* 2004;44(11):1223.
2 Yasui-Furukori N, et al. *Br J Clin Pharmacol.* 2004;57(4):487.
3 Christensen M, et al. *Clin Pharmacol Ther.* 2002;71(3):141.
4 Uno T, et al. *Br J Clin Pharmacol.* 2006;61(3):309.

* Asterisk indicates drugs cited in interaction reports. Based on pharmacologic and pharmacokinetic considerations, similar interactions may occur with other drugs that are listed.

Proton Pump Inhibitors — Food

Lansoprazole* (*Prevacid*)	Grapefruit Juice*

Significance	Onset	Severity	Documentation
5	☐ Rapid	☐ Major	☐ Established
	■ **Delayed**	☐ Moderate	☐ Probable
		■ **Minor**	☐ Suspected
			☐ Possible
			■ **Unlikely**

Effects LANSOPRAZOLE plasma concentrations may be elevated in some patients. However, it is unlikely that the effects will be clinically important.

Mechanism Inhibition of sulfoxidation of LANSOPRAZOLE metabolism (CYP3A4) by GRAPEFRUIT JUICE is suspected.

Management Based on available data, no special precautions are needed.

Discussion

The effects of grapefruit juice on the pharmacokinetics of lansoprazole were studied in 21 healthy Japanese volunteers.[1] Subjects had been genotyped for CYP2C19 and consisted of 7 homozygous extensive metabolizers (EMs), 7 heterozygous EMs, and 7 poor metabolizers (PMs). All subjects ingested 200 mL of water or fresh-squeezed grapefruit juice 30 minutes before taking lansoprazole 60 mg with 200 mL of water. Compared with water, the mean total AUC of lansoprazole was slightly decreased after grapefruit ingestion. There was no difference in the AUC of the 5-hydroxylansoprazole or lansoprazole sulfone metabolites. In addition, the plasma C_{max}, time to reach the C_{max}, and the elimination $t_{½}$ of lansoprazole or its metabolites were not different when lansoprazole was taken after water or grapefruit juice. Grapefruit juice increased the AUC of lansoprazole in PMs and decreased the AUC ratio of lansoprazole sulfone to lansoprazole in heterozygous EMs. The data suggest that grapefruit juice partially inhibits formation of lansoprazole sulfone catalyzed by CYP3A4. This interaction is not likely to be clinically important because the bioavailability of lansoprazole is 80% to 90%, CYP3A4 inhibition by grapefruit juice is only in the small intestine, and the CYP2C19 genotype is the major determinant of lansoprazole clearance.

[1] Uno T, et al. *J Clin Pharmacol.* 2005;45(6):690.

* Asterisk indicates drugs cited in interaction reports.

Proton Pump Inhibitors — *Ginkgo biloba*

Omeprazole* (eg, *Prilosec*)	Ginkgo biloba*

Significance	Onset	Severity	Documentation
2	□ Rapid ■ **Delayed**	□ Major ■ **Moderate** □ Minor	□ Established □ Probable ■ **Suspected** □ Possible □ Unlikely

Effects OMEPRAZOLE plasma concentrations may be reduced, decreasing the pharmacologic effect.

Mechanism Increased metabolism (CYP2C19) of OMEPRAZOLE by GINKGO BILOBA.

Management Avoid coadministration of OMEPRAZOLE and GINKGO BILOBA. If coadministration cannot be avoided, monitor patients for OMEPRAZOLE effectiveness.

Discussion

The effects of *Ginkgo biloba* on the pharmacokinetics of omeprazole were studied in 18 healthy Chinese subjects previously genotyped for CYP2C19.[1] Subjects consisted of 6 homozygous extensive metabolizers (EMs), 5 heterozygous EMs, and 7 poor metabolizers (PMs). All subjects received omeprazole 40 mg at baseline and after 12 days of treatment with *Ginkgo biloba* 140 mg twice daily. Compared with receiving omeprazole alone, pretreatment with *Ginkgo biloba* decreased the AUC of omeprazole in homozygous EMs, heterozygous EMs, and PMs 41.5%, 27.2%, and 40.4%, respectively. The decreases in the omeprazole sulfone metabolite AUC were 41.2%, 36%, and 36%, respectively. In contrast, plasma concentrations of the 5-hydroxyomeprazole metabolite were increased 37.5%, 100.7%, and 232.4% in homozygous EMs, heterozygous EMs, and PMs, respectively. The ratio of the omeprazole AUC to the 5-hydroxyl metabolite AUC was decreased in each genotype; however, the decrease was greater in PMs than the other 2 genotypes. Therefore, *Ginkgo biloba* induces omeprazole hydroxylation in a CYP2C19 genotype–dependent manner. In addition, renal clearance of 5-hydroxyomeprazole was decreased after *Ginkgo biloba*, compared with baseline, but was not different among the 3 genotypes.

[1] Yin OQ, et al. *Pharmacogenetics*. 2004;14(12):841.

* Asterisk indicates drugs cited in interaction reports.

Proton Pump Inhibitors — *Lopinavir/Ritonavir*

Proton Pump Inhibitors		Lopinavir/Ritonavir
Esomeprazole (*Nexium*)	Omeprazole* (eg, *Prilosec*)	Lopinavir/Ritonavir* (*Kaletra*)
Lansoprazole (*Prevacid*)	Pantoprazole (eg, *Protonix*)	

Significance	Onset	Severity	Documentation
4	☐ Rapid ■ **Delayed**	☐ Major ■ **Moderate** ☐ Minor	☐ Established ☐ Probable ☐ Suspected ■ **Possible** ☐ Unlikely

Effects PROTON PUMP INHIBITOR plasma concentrations may be reduced, decreasing the efficacy.

Mechanism Induction of certain PROTON PUMP INHIBITOR metabolism (CYP2C19) by LOPINAVIR/RITONAVIR is suspected.

Management If an interaction is suspected, it may be necessary to increase the PROTON PUMP INHIBITOR dose.

Discussion

In an open-label study, 14 healthy HIV-negative subjects received a single oral dose of omeprazole 40 mg alone and after receiving lopinavir 400 mg/ritonavir 100 mg twice daily for 14 days.[1] The ratio of omeprazole to its 5-hydroxy metabolite was reduced 53%, indicating an increase in CYP2C19 activity. The possibility of subtherapeutic omeprazole plasma concentrations should be considered. See also Protease Inhibitors-Proton Pump Inhibitors.

[1] Yeh RF, et al. *J Acquir Immune Defic Syndr.* 2006;42(1):52.

* Asterisk indicates drugs cited in interaction reports. Based on pharmacologic and pharmacokinetic considerations, similar interactions may occur with other drugs that are listed.

Proton Pump Inhibitors | **Macrolide Antibiotics**

Esomeprazole* (*Nexium*)	Lansoprazole* (*Prevacid*)	Clarithromycin* (eg, *Biaxin*)

Significance	Onset	Severity	Documentation
2	☐ Rapid ■ **Delayed**	☐ Major ■ **Moderate** ☐ Minor	☐ Established ☐ Probable ■ **Suspected** ☐ Possible ☐ Unlikely

Effects Plasma levels of certain PROTON PUMP INHIBITORS may be elevated, increasing the pharmacologic effects and adverse reactions.

Mechanism Inhibition of the metabolism of certain PROTON PUMP INHIBITORS (CYP3A) by CLARITHROMYCIN is suspected, and, to a lesser degree, bioavailability may be increased by inhibition of P-glycoprotein.

Management In patients receiving LANSOPRAZOLE or ESOMEPRAZOLE, monitor for an increase in adverse reactions during coadministration of CLARITHROMYCIN.

Discussion

In vitro data indicate that sulfoxidation of lansoprazole is catalyzed by the CYP3A isozyme, and that hydroxylation is catalyzed by CYP2C19 at low concentrations and CYP3A at high concentrations.[1] In 12 patients treated for *Helicobacter pylori*, clarithromycin 400 or 800 mg/day inhibited the clearance and increased lansoprazole levels in a dose-dependent manner.[2] The effects of clarithromycin on the metabolism of lansoprazole among CYP2C19 genotypes were studied in 18 healthy Japanese volunteers.[1] Of the 18 subjects, 6 were homozygous extensive metabolizers, 6 heterozygous extensive metabolizers, and 6 poor metabolizers for CYP2C19. Using a double-blind, placebo-controlled design, each subject received clarithromycin 400 mg twice daily or placebo twice daily for 6 days. On day 6, they received a single oral dose of lansoprazole 60 mg. Compared with placebo, clarithromycin administration increased the lansoprazole C_{max} in homozygous, heterozygous, and poor metabolizers 1.47-, 1.71-, and 1.52-fold, respectively. In these genotype groups, the AUC was increased 1.55-, 1.74-, and 1.8-fold, respectively. The elimination $t_{1/2}$ was prolonged only in poor metabolizers. The percent increase in the pharmacokinetic parameters resulting from clarithromycin administration did not differ among the 3 CYP2C19 subgroups. S-lansoprazole levels were affected more than R-lansoprazole levels in all 3 genotype groups.[3] Coadministration of esomeprazole and clarithromycin increased the esomeprazole AUC between 1.7- and 2.3-fold in patients who were poor or extensive CYP2C19 metabolizers.[4] Clarithromycin did not affect rabeprazole pharmacokinetics.[5]

1 Saito M, et al. *Br J Clin Pharmacol.* 2005;59(3):302.
2 Ushiama H, et al. *Clin Pharmacol Ther.* 2002;72(1):33.
3 Miura M, et al. *Chirality.* 2005;17(6):338.
4 Hassan-Alin M, et al. *Int J Clin Pharmacol Ther.* 2006;44(3):119.
5 Shimizu M, et al. *Eur J Clin Pharmacol.* 2006;62(8):597.

* Asterisk indicates drugs cited in interaction reports.

Proton Pump Inhibitors — *St. John's Wort*

Omeprazole* (eg, *Prilosec*)	St. John's Wort*

Significance	Onset	Severity	Documentation
2	☐ Rapid ■ **Delayed**	☐ Major ■ **Moderate** ☐ Minor	☐ Established ☐ Probable ■ **Suspected** ☐ Possible ☐ Unlikely

Effects OMEPRAZOLE plasma concentrations may be reduced, decreasing the pharmacologic effect.

Mechanism Increased metabolism (CYP2C19 and CYP3A4) of OMEPRAZOLE by ST. JOHN'S WORT.

Management Avoid coadministration of OMEPRAZOLE and ST. JOHN'S WORT. If concurrent use cannot be avoided, carefully monitor the patient's clinical response and adjust the dose of OMEPRAZOLE as needed.

Discussion

The effects of St. John's wort on the pharmacokinetics of omeprazole and its metabolites were studied in 12 healthy men.[1] Using a 2-phase, crossover design, each subject received St. John's wort 300 mg or placebo 3 times daily for 14 days. On day 15, all subjects received omeprazole 20 mg after an overnight fast. Compared with placebo, St. John's wort administration decreased the AUC and C_{max} of omeprazole approximately 50% and 38%, respectively. In addition, the AUC and C_{max} of the omeprazole sulfone metabolite increased nearly 137% and 160%, respectively, while the AUC and C_{max} of the 5-hydroxyomeprazole metabolite increased approximately 37% and 38%, respectively. The metabolites of omeprazole were increased in a CYP2C19 genotype–dependent manner.

[1] Wang LS, et al. *Clin Pharmacol Ther*. 2004;75(3):191.

* Asterisk indicates drugs cited in interaction reports.

Quetiapine | *Azole Antifungal Agents*

Quetiapine	Azole Antifungal Agents	
Quetiapine* (*Seroquel*)	Fluconazole (eg, *Diflucan*)	Posaconazole (*Noxafil*)
	Itraconazole (eg, *Sporanox*)	Voriconazole (eg, *Vfend*)
	Ketoconazole* (eg, *Nizoral*)	

Significance	Onset	Severity	Documentation
2	□ Rapid ■ **Delayed**	□ Major ■ **Moderate** □ Minor	□ Established □ Probable ■ **Suspected** □ Possible □ Unlikely

Effects QUETIAPINE plasma levels may be elevated, increasing the pharmacologic and adverse effects.

Mechanism AZOLE ANTIFUNGAL AGENTS inhibit the metabolism (CYP3A4) of QUETIAPINE.[1]

Management Closely monitor patients receiving QUETIAPINE when AZOLE ANTIFUNGAL AGENTS are started or stopped. Be prepared to change the QUETIAPINE dose as needed.

Discussion

The effects of ketoconazole on the pharmacokinetics of quetiapine were studied in 12 healthy men.[1] In an open-label, crossover study, each subject received quetiapine 25 mg before and after 4 days of treatment with ketoconazole 200 mg daily. Compared with taking quetiapine alone, pretreatment with ketoconazole increased the quetiapine mean C_{max} 3.35-fold (from 45 to 150 ng/mL) and the AUC 6.2-fold, and decreased the clearance 84% (from 138 to 22 L/hr). An in vitro portion of the study demonstrated that the interaction is mediated via inhibition of the CYP3A4 isozyme by ketoconazole.

[1] Grimm SW, et al. *Br J Clin Pharmacol.* 2006;61(1):58.

* Asterisk indicates drugs cited in interaction reports. Based on pharmacologic and pharmacokinetic considerations, similar interactions may occur with other drugs that are listed.

Quetiapine — *Hydantoins*

Quetiapine* (*Seroquel*)	Fosphenytoin Phenytoin* (eg, *Dilantin*)

Significance	Onset	Severity	Documentation
2	☐ Rapid ■ **Delayed**	☐ Major ■ **Moderate** ☐ Minor	☐ Established ☐ Probable ■ **Suspected** ☐ Possible ☐ Unlikely

Effects QUETIAPINE plasma concentrations and pharmacologic effects may be decreased.

Mechanism Increased metabolism (CYP3A4) of QUETIAPINE is suspected.

Management In patients receiving QUETIAPINE, monitor clinical response when starting, stopping, or changing the dose of PHENYTOIN. Be prepared to change the dose of QUETIAPINE as needed.

Discussion

In an open-label, nonrandomized, multiple-dose study, the effects of phenytoin on the pharmacokinetics of quetiapine were evaluated in 10 men with schizophrenia, schizoaffective disorder, or bipolar disorder.[1] Each patient received escalating doses of quetiapine from 25 to 250 mg over a 10-day period 3 times daily followed by a maintenance dose of quetiapine 250 mg 3 times daily from days 11 to 22. Phenytoin 100 mg 3 times daily was administered between days 13 and 22. Compared with administration of quetiapine alone, coadministration of phenytoin decreased the mean steady-state AUC of quetiapine 80%, the steady-state peak plasma concentration 66% (from 1,048 to 359 ng/mL), the steady-state trough plasma concentration 89% (from 224 to 24 ng/mL), and increased the mean oral clearance 5.5-fold (from 80.3 to 440 L/h). No serious adverse reactions were reported after administration of quetiapine alone or with phenytoin.

[1] Wong YW, et al. *J Clin Psychopharmacol.* 2001;21(1):89.

* Asterisk indicates drugs cited in interaction reports. Based on pharmacologic and pharmacokinetic considerations, similar interactions may occur with other drugs that are listed.

Quetiapine — *Macrolide & Related Antibiotics*

Quetiapine	Macrolide & Related Antibiotics	
Quetiapine* (*Seroquel*)	Clarithromycin* (eg, *Biaxin*)	Telithromycin (*Ketek*)
	Erythromycin* (eg, *Ery-Tab*)	

Significance	Onset	Severity	Documentation
2	☐ Rapid	☐ Major	☐ Established
	■ **Delayed**	■ **Moderate**	☐ Probable
		☐ Minor	■ **Suspected**
			☐ Possible
			☐ Unlikely

Effects QUETIAPINE plasma concentrations may be elevated, increasing the pharmacologic effects and adverse reactions.

Mechanism Certain MACROLIDE AND RELATED ANTIBIOTICS may inhibit the metabolism (CYP3A4) of QUETIAPINE.

Management Closely monitor patients receiving QUETIAPINE when certain MACROLIDE AND RELATED ANTIBIOTICS are started or stopped. Be prepared to change the QUETIAPINE dose as needed.

Discussion

The effect of erythromycin on the metabolism of quetiapine was studied in 19 patients suffering from schizophrenia.[1] Each patient was started on quetiapine 25 mg twice daily, reaching a dosage of 200 mg twice daily by day 4. Patients continued to receive quetiapine 200 mg twice daily through day 12. On days 9 through 12, erythromycin 500 mg 3 times daily was coadministered with quetiapine. Compared with giving quetiapine alone, coadministration of erythromycin increased quetiapine C_{max}, AUC, and elimination $t_{½}$ 68%, 129%, and 92%, respectively. The clearance and elimination rate constant decreased 52% and 55%, respectively. The C_{max}, AUC, and AUC ratio (AUC of the metabolite to the AUC of quetiapine) for the inactive quetiapine sulfoxide metabolite decreased 64%, 23%, and 70%, respectively, while the $t_{½}$ increased 211%. For the active metabolite 7-hydroxy-quetiapine, the elimination rate constant and AUC ratio decreased 61% and 45%, respectively, and the $t_{½}$ increased 203%. For the active 7-hydroxy-N-desalkyl-quetiapine metabolite, the C_{max}, AUC, and AUC ratio decreased 36%, 40%, and 71%, respectively. Psychiatric symptoms had resolved in a 32-year-old man with schizo-affective disorder while receiving quetiapine 700 mg daily.[2] After receiving 2 doses of clarithromycin 500 mg, the patient became markedly somnolent and was transferred to the intensive care unit. His quetiapine blood concentration was 827 mcg/L (therapeutic range, 70 to 170 mcg/L).

[1] Li KY, et al. *Eur J Clin Pharmacol.* 2005;60(11):791.

[2] Schulz-Du Bois C, et al. *Pharmacopsychiatry.* 2008;41(6):258.

* Asterisk indicates drugs cited in interaction reports. Based on pharmacologic and pharmacokinetic considerations, similar interactions may occur with other drugs that are listed.

Quetiapine — *Protease Inhibitors*

Quetiapine	Protease Inhibitors	
Quetiapine* (eg, *Seroquel*)	Atazanavir* (*Reyataz*)	Nelfinavir* (*Viracept*)
	Darunavir* (*Prezista*)	Ritonavir* (*Norvir*)
	Fosamprenavir* (*Lexiva*)	Saquinavir* (*Invirase*)
	Indinavir* (*Crixivan*)	Tipranavir* (*Aptivus*)
	Lopinavir/Ritonavir* (*Kaletra*)	

Significance	Onset	Severity	Documentation
2	☐ Rapid	☐ Major	☐ Established
	■ **Delayed**	■ **Moderate**	☐ Probable
		☐ Minor	■ **Suspected**
			☐ Possible
			☐ Unlikely

Effects QUETIAPINE plasma concentrations may be elevated, increasing the pharmacologic effects and risk of toxicity.

Mechanism PROTEASE INHIBITORS may inhibit the metabolism (CYP3A4) of QUETIAPINE.

Management Use with caution. Closely monitor patients receiving QUETIAPINE when PROTEASE INHIBITORS are started or stopped. Be prepared to adjust the QUETIAPINE dose as needed.

Discussion

A 32-year-old woman with HIV and an anxiety disorder developed increased sedation and mental confusion when ritonavir-boosted atazanavir was added to her antianxiety regimen that included quetiapine.[1] Her symptoms resolved quickly after quetiapine was discontinued. Caution is recommended when administering quetiapine with CYP3A4 inhibitors, including protease inhibitors.[2]

[1] Pollack TM, et al. *Pharmacotherapy*. 2009; 29(11):1386.

[2] *Seroquel* [package insert]. Wilmington, DE: AstraZeneca Pharmaceuticals LP; November 2009.

* Asterisk indicates drugs cited in interaction reports.

Quetiapine — *Valproic Acid*

Quetiapine	Valproic Acid
Quetiapine* (*Seroquel*)	Divalproex Sodium* (eg, *Depakote*)
	Valproate Sodium (eg, *Depacon*)
	Valproic Acid* (eg, *Depakene*)

Significance	Onset	Severity	Documentation
2	□ Rapid	□ Major	□ Established
	■ **Delayed**	■ **Moderate**	□ Probable
		□ Minor	■ **Suspected**
			□ Possible
			□ Unlikely

Effects QUETIAPINE plasma concentrations may be elevated, increasing the pharmacologic effects and adverse reactions. An increased risk of neutropenia has been reported in children.

Mechanism Inhibition of QUETIAPINE metabolism (CYP3A4) by VALPROIC ACID is suspected.

Management Closely monitor patients receiving QUETIAPINE when the VALPROIC ACID dose is started, stopped, or changed. Be prepared to change the QUETIAPINE dose as needed.

Discussion

Severe cervical dystonia was reported in a 60-year-old woman receiving quetiapine after valproic acid was added to her treatment regimen.[1] The patient was receiving quetiapine 800 mg daily for acute schizoaffective disorder with symptoms of psychosis and mania. Valproic acid 900 mg/day was started for generalized seizures and as an additional mood stabilizer. The dosage of quetiapine was reduced to 600 mg/day. Four days later, she developed acute anterocollis, and quetiapine plasma concentrations were elevated (increased from 0.15 to 0.24 mg/L). The cervical dystonia improved when biperiden† was administered and disappeared when the dosages of quetiapine and valproic acid were reduced. The potential for a 2-way pharmacokinetic interaction between divalproex sodium (either 500 or 1,000 mg daily) and quetiapine (300 mg daily) was investigated in 33 patients.[2] The addition of divalproex sodium did not affect the quetiapine AUC, but increased the C_{max} 17%. The addition of quetiapine decreased the valproic acid AUC and C_{max} 11%. The magnitude of these changes is not likely to be clinically important. In a retrospective analysis of 133 children admitted to a psychiatric hospital, coadministration of quetiapine and valproic acid was associated with a 44% incidence of neutropenia, compared with 26% or 6% for administration of valproic acid or quetiapine alone, respectively.[3]

[1] Habermeyer B, et al. *J Clin Psychopharmacol.* 2007;27(4):396.
[2] Winter HR, et al. *Hum Psychopharmacol.* 2007; 22(7):469.
[3] Rahman A, et al. *Ann Pharmacother.* 2009;43(5):822.

* Asterisk indicates drugs cited in interaction reports. Based on pharmacologic and pharmacokinetic considerations, similar interactions may occur with other drugs that are listed.
† Not available in the United States.

Quinidine — *Amiloride*

Quinidine*	Amiloride* (*Midamor*)

Significance	Onset	Severity	Documentation
1	□ Rapid ■ **Delayed**	■ **Major** □ Moderate □ Minor	□ Established □ Probable ■ **Suspected** □ Possible □ Unlikely

Effects Combined treatment with AMILORIDE and QUINIDINE may contribute to proarrhythmia and reversal of the antiarrhythmic effects of QUINIDINE.

Mechanism Possible synergistic increase in myocardial sodium channel blockade is suspected.

Management Avoid this drug combination. If coadministration of AMILORIDE and QUINIDINE cannot be avoided, closely monitor the ECG.

Discussion

The antiarrhythmic and electrophysiologic effects of quinidine alone and in combination with amiloride were evaluated in 10 patients with inducible sustained ventricular tachycardia.[1] Therapy was instituted with oral quinidine, and the dose was increased gradually until a trough serum concentration of 10 mcmol/L was obtained or a maximum well-tolerated dose was reached. After performing an electrophysiologic study at steady-state quinidine therapy, oral amiloride was started at 5 mg twice daily and increased to 10 mg twice daily if serum potassium remained within normal limits. During treatment with quinidine alone, no patient experienced adverse reactions. In contrast, during coadministration of amiloride and quinidine, 7 of the 10 patients had adverse reactions. Three patients, who had experienced suppression of inducible ventricular tachycardia while on quinidine alone, experienced sustained ventricular tachycardia induced by the addition of amiloride. Three other patients experienced somatic adverse reactions that resulted in discontinuation of combined therapy, and 1 patient had 12 episodes of sustained ventricular tachycardia during coadministration of quinidine and amiloride. Surface electrocardiographic wave duration was more prolonged during combined therapy than during treatment with quinidine alone.

[1] Wang L, et al. *Clin Pharmacol Ther.* 1994;56(6 pt 1):659.

* Asterisk indicates drugs cited in interaction reports.

Quinidine — *Amiodarone*

Quinidine*	Amiodarone* (eg, *Cordarone*)

Significance	Onset	Severity	Documentation
1	■ **Rapid** □ Delayed	■ **Major** □ Moderate □ Minor	□ Established ■ **Probable** □ Suspected □ Possible □ Unlikely

Effects The addition of AMIODARONE to QUINIDINE therapy may increase QUINIDINE serum concentrations and produce potentially fatal cardiac dysrhythmias.

Mechanism Unknown.

Management If the combination is necessary, monitor QUINIDINE serum concentrations, and observe patients for signs and symptoms of QUINIDINE toxicity. Adjust the QUINIDINE dose as needed.

Discussion

A study of 11 patients receiving quinidine for supraventricular or ventricular arrhythmias demonstrated that amiodarone 600 mg every 12 hours for 5 to 7 days can increase quinidine serum concentrations.[1] The mean quinidine serum concentration increased 32%. Because of occasional evidence of clinical toxicity (eg, arrhythmias, GI irritation, hypotension, rash, vertigo), the daily quinidine dose was decreased by a mean of 37% in 9 patients. Even with this downward adjustment, the mean quinidine serum concentration increased from 4.4 mcg/mL before amiodarone to 5.2 mcg/mL after the addition of amiodarone and the reduction in quinidine dosage.

There also have been 4 case reports of torsades de pointes in patients who had amiodarone added to existing quinidine therapy.[2,3] An increase in quinidine serum concentration and a prolongation of the electrocardiographic QT interval was noted; 1 patient required cardiopulmonary resuscitation. Conversely, addition of quinidine for up to 48 hours in patients on long-term amiodarone therapy was well tolerated and helped convert those with atrial fibrillation to normal sinus rhythm.[4] See Drug-Induced Prolongation of the QT Interval and Torsades de Pointes.

[1] Saal AK, et al. *Am J Cardiol.* 1984;53(9):1264.
[2] Tartini R, et al. *Lancet.* 1982;1(8285):1327.
[3] Tartini R, et al. *Schweiz Med Wochenschr.* [in German]. 1982;112(45):1585.
[4] Kerin NZ, et al. *Am Heart J.* 1993;125(4):1017.

* Asterisk indicates drugs cited in interaction reports.

Quinidine — *Antacids*

Quinidine*	Aluminum Hydroxide* (eg, *Amphojel*)	Magnesium Hydroxide* (eg, *Milk of Magnesia*)
	Aluminum/Magnesium Hydroxide* (eg, *Maalox*)	Sodium Bicarbonate*

Significance	Onset	Severity	Documentation
2	☐ Rapid	☐ Major	☐ Established
	■ **Delayed**	■ **Moderate**	☐ Probable
		☐ Minor	■ **Suspected**
			☐ Possible
			☐ Unlikely

Effects Certain ANTACIDS may increase serum QUINIDINE concentrations, which may result in toxicity.

Mechanism Possibly caused by a pH-related decrease in the urinary excretion of QUINIDINE.

Management Monitor serum QUINIDINE concentrations throughout the ANTACID therapy. An aluminum-only ANTACID may be preferable for initial therapy.

Discussion

Oral quinidine sulfate 200 mg every 6 hours was administered to 4 men for 5 days.[1] The urine was then alkalinized by a combination of acetazolamide (eg, *Diamox* 500 mg every 12 hours and sodium bicarbonate. As the urine pH increased from 6 to 7.5, the urine quinidine concentration decreased 88.5%, and the urine quinidine excretion rate decreased 69.9%. Similarly, the serum quinidine concentration increased, and the electrocardiographic QT interval lengthened.

One case of quinidine intoxication was reported in a patient on oral quinidine 300 mg daily who had taken 8 tablets of magnesium hydroxide 200 mg/aluminum hydroxide 200 mg/simethicone 20 mg (eg, *Mylanta*) daily for 8 days.[2] A single-dose study of 4 healthy volunteers demonstrated that the coadministration of quinidine sulfate 200 mg and aluminum hydroxide 30 mL gel had no effect on serum quinidine concentrations compared with quinidine administration alone.[3] Similarly, in 8 volunteers, the pharmacokinetics of a single dose of quinidine gluconate 684 mg was not affected by aluminum hydroxide gel; changes in 2 of the subjects may have been significant.[4]

[1] Gerhardt RE, et al. *Ann Intern Med.* 1969;71(5):927.
[2] Zinn MB. *Tex Med.* 1970;66(12):64.
[3] Romankiewicz JA, et al. *Am Heart J.* 1978;96(4):518.
[4] Mauro VF, et al. *DICP.* 1990;24(3):252.

* Asterisk indicates drugs cited in interaction reports.

Quinidine — *Azole Antifungal Agents*

Quinidine	Azole Antifungal Agents	
Quinidine*	Itraconazole* (eg, *Sporanox*)	Voriconazole* (*Vfend*)
	Posaconazole* (*Noxafil*)	

Significance	Onset	Severity	Documentation
1	☐ Rapid	■ **Major**	☐ Established
	■ **Delayed**	☐ Moderate	■ **Probable**
		☐ Minor	☐ Suspected
			☐ Possible
			☐ Unlikely

Effects Plasma QUINIDINE concentrations may be elevated, increasing the risk of serious cardiovascular events.

Mechanism Certain AZOLE ANTIFUNGAL AGENTS may inhibit the metabolism (CYP-450 3A4) and active renal secretion of QUINIDINE.

Management Certain AZOLE ANTIFUNGAL AGENTS are contraindicated in patients receiving QUINIDINE.[1-3]

Discussion

The effects of oral itraconazole on the pharmacokinetics and pharmacodynamics of oral quinidine were evaluated in 9 healthy volunteers.[4] Using a randomized, double-blind, crossover design, each subject received either itraconazole 200 mg or placebo once daily for 4 days. On the fourth day, each subject was given a single dose of quinidine sulfate 100 mg. During administration of itraconazole and quinidine, plasma quinidine concentrations increased 59%, the time to reach the maximum plasma concentration increased 67% (from 3 to 5 hours), the AUC increased 142%, and the $t_{½}$ of quinidine increased 58% (from 7.4 to 11.7 hours), compared with giving quinidine with placebo. The area under the 3-hydroxyquinidine metabolite/quinidine ratio–time curve decreased 78%, and the renal clearance of quinidine decreased 49%. There were large interindividual differences in the extent of the interaction (a 10% to 170% range in peak quinidine concentration). The QT, but not the QTc, interval was prolonged significantly ($P < 0.05$) during the itraconazole phase compared with the placebo phase.

[1] *Sporanox* [package insert]. Titusville, NJ: Janssen Pharmaceutica, LP; January 2004.
[2] *Noxafil* [package insert]. Kenilworth, NJ: Schering Corporation; October 2006.
[3] *Vfend* [package insert]. New York, NY: Pfizer Inc.; November 2006.
[4] Kaukonen KM, et al. *Clin Pharmacol Ther.* 1997;62(5):510.

* Asterisk indicates drugs cited in interaction reports.

Quinidine — *Barbiturates*

Quinidine	Barbiturates	
Quinidine* (eg, *Quinidex Extentabs*)	Amobarbital (*Amytal*)	Pentobarbital* (eg, *Nembutal*)
	Aprobarbital (*Alurate*)	Phenobarbital* (eg, *Solfoton*)
	Butabarbital (eg, *Butisol*)	Primidone* (eg, *Mysoline*)
	Butalbital	Secobarbital (eg, *Seconal*)
	Mephobarbital (*Mebaral*)	

Significance	Onset	Severity	Documentation
2	☐ Rapid	☐ Major	☐ Established
	■ **Delayed**	■ **Moderate**	■ **Probable**
		☐ Minor	☐ Suspected
			☐ Possible
			☐ Unlikely

Effects BARBITURATES appear to produce decreased QUINIDINE serum concentrations and a decreased QUINIDINE elimination half-life.

Mechanism Possibly because of an increased metabolic clearance of QUINIDINE.

Management Closely monitor serum concentrations in a patient who requires QUINIDINE if BARBITURATE therapy is added to or removed from the patient's therapy.

Discussion

Several case reports have suggested that the coadministration of quinidine and phenobarbital results in a shortened elimination half-life and decreased serum concentrations for quinidine.[1-4] In most cases, the half-life was reduced by approximately 50%. Other barbiturates also noted as potentially interacting drugs include pentobarbital[2] and primidone.[1-3]

1 Data JL, et al. *N Engl J Med.* 1976;294:699.
2 Chapron DJ, et al. *Arch Intern Med.* 1979;139:363.
3 Kroboth FJ, et al. *N Engl J Med.* 1983;308:725.
4 Rogers GC, et al. *DICP.* 1983;17:819.

* Asterisk indicates drugs cited in interaction reports. Based on pharmacologic and pharmacokinetic considerations, similar interactions may occur with other drugs that are listed.

Quinidine — *Carbamazepine*

Quinidine*	Carbamazepine* (eg, *Tegretol*)

Significance	Onset	Severity	Documentation
4	☐ Rapid ■ **Delayed**	☐ Major ■ **Moderate** ☐ Minor	☐ Established ☐ Probable ☐ Suspected ■ **Possible** ☐ Unlikely

Effects QUINIDINE plasma concentrations may be reduced, decreasing the therapeutic effect.

Mechanism CARBAMAZEPINE increased the metabolism (CYP3A4) of QUINIDINE.

Management Monitor QUINIDINE plasma concentrations and the clinical response of the patient when starting, stopping, or changing the CARBAMAZEPINE dose. Adjust the QUINIDINE dose as needed.

Discussion

The effects of carbamazepine on the pharmacokinetics of quinidine were evaluated in 8 healthy men.[1] In an open-label study, each subject received carbamazepine, which was titrated to 800 mg daily, for 17 days. In addition, subjects received a single dose of quinidine 200 mg before and after the course of carbamazepine. Compared with giving quinidine alone, carbamazepine increased the formation of the 3-hydroxyquinidine metabolite 181%, decreased the mean quinidine C_{max} 33%, and decreased the mean $t_{½}$ of quinidine 32%.

[1] Andreasen AH, et al. *Epilepsia*. 2007;48(3):490.

* Asterisk indicates drugs cited in interaction reports.

Quinidine | **Carbonic Anhydrase Inh.**

Quinidine*	Acetazolamide* (eg, *Diamox*)	Methazolamide

Significance	Onset	Severity	Documentation
4	☐ Rapid ■ **Delayed**	☐ Major ■ **Moderate** ☐ Minor	☐ Established ☐ Probable ☐ Suspected ■ **Possible** ☐ Unlikely

Effects A possible increase in the pharmacologic and toxicologic effects of QUINIDINE may occur. It is unclear how soon this effect is reversed once ACETAZOLAMIDE is discontinued.

Mechanism An increase in urine pH secondary to ACETAZOLAMIDE results in an increased renal tubular reabsorption of QUINIDINE and, consequently, decreased urinary excretion.

Management Frequent monitoring of QUINIDINE concentrations may be required to guide a reduction in QUINIDINE dosage.

Discussion

A single study documents this interaction.[1] In this trial, 4 subjects were dosed to steady state with oral quinidine. An alkaline urine was then produced with a combination of acetazolamide and sodium bicarbonate. A study of the quinidine urinary excretion rate revealed a mean decrease of 69.9% with urinary alkalinization. In these subjects, the quinidine urine concentration was 115 mg/L for a urine pH of less than 6, but decreased to 13 mg/L when the urine pH increased to more than 7.5. Another 6 subjects studied demonstrated increases in serum quinidine concentrations and lengthening of ECG QT intervals during urinary alkalinization. Because sodium bicarbonate was also utilized to produce urinary alkalinization, it is unclear how much of this interaction is due to acetazolamide.

[1] Gerhardt RE, et al. *Ann Intern Med.* 1969;71(5):927.

* Asterisk indicates drugs cited in interaction reports. Based on pharmacologic and pharmacokinetic considerations, similar interactions may occur with other drugs that are listed.

Quinidine — *Cimetidine*

Quinidine* | Cimetidine* (eg, *Tagamet*)

Significance	Onset	Severity	Documentation
2	☐ Rapid	☐ Major	☐ Established
	■ **Delayed**	■ **Moderate**	■ **Probable**
		☐ Minor	☐ Suspected
			☐ Possible
			☐ Unlikely

Effects An increase in the pharmacologic and toxicologic effects of QUINIDINE may occur secondary to increased QUINIDINE concentrations. The QUINIDINE concentrations appear to return to pretreatment values approximately 48 hours after CIMETIDINE is discontinued.

Mechanism It is unclear if this interaction is due to increased QUINIDINE absorption, decreased QUINIDINE metabolism, or a combination of the two.

Management Frequent monitoring of QUINIDINE concentrations is necessary to guide QUINIDINE dosage reductions. If possible, avoid this combination.

Discussion

Two well-controlled human pharmacokinetic studies exist to support this interaction.[1-3] In a study of 9 volunteers, a dosage of cimetidine 1.2 g/day for 4 days resulted in an average increase in the oral quinidine AUC by 14.5% and a mean 22.6% increase in the quinidine $t_{1/2}$.[3] They found no significant differences in the peak quinidine concentration or in ECG parameters, but failed to conduct their ECG measurements when the difference in quinidine concentrations was maximized. A similar study in 6 volunteers revealed a mean 55% increase in quinidine half-life, a mean 37% decrease in oral quinidine clearance, and a mean 21% increase in the quinidine peak concentration after 7 days of cimetidine therapy at 1.2 g/day. This study also monitored the subjects with ECGs and noted an increase in the QTc interval, although this was not a statistically significant change.[4]

A single case report also documents this interaction.[2] A patient receiving quinidine was treated on 2 different occasions with cimetidine 1.2 g/day. On both occasions, quinidine trough concentrations increased by approximately 50% within 48 hours after cimetidine initiation and reversed within 48 hours after cimetidine discontinuation. The patient experienced no adverse effects secondary to this interaction. Although no reports exist documenting adverse reactions in patients due to this interaction, the potential for an adverse effect is high because quinidine is known to have a narrow therapeutic index and may produce severe toxicities.

[1] Hardy BG, et al. *Am J Cardiol.* 1983;52(1):172.
[2] Farringer JA, et al. *Clin Pharm.* 1984;3(1):81.
[3] Kolb KW, et al. *Ther Drug Monit.* 1984;6(3):306.
[4] Fruncillo RJ, et al. *J Pharm Sci.* 1983;72(7):826.

* Asterisk indicates drugs cited in interaction reports.

Quinidine — *Diltiazem*

Quinidine*	Diltiazem* (eg, *Cardizem*)

Significance	Onset	Severity	Documentation
2	☐ Rapid ■ **Delayed**	☐ Major ■ **Moderate** ☐ Minor	☐ Established ☐ Probable ■ **Suspected** ☐ Possible ☐ Unlikely

Effects The therapeutic and adverse effects of QUINIDINE may be increased.

Mechanism DILTIAZEM may inhibit the hepatic metabolism of QUINIDINE by competition for the same isozyme.

Management Closely monitor serum quinidine concentrations and cardiovascular function when starting, stopping or changing the dose of DILTIAZEM. Adjust the QUINIDINE dose as needed.

Discussion

The pharmacokinetic and pharmacodynamic consequences of concomitant administration of quinidine and diltiazem were investigated in 12 healthy male volunteers.[1] To determine the effects of diltiazem on the pharmacokinetics and pharmacodynamics of quinidine, each subject was given a single oral dose of 200 mg of quinidine sulfate with and without pretreatment with oral diltiazem. Pretreatment consisted of administering 90 mg of sustained release diltiazem twice daily for 5 doses. The last dose was given 1½ hours before quinidine. To determine the effects of quinidine on the pharmacokinetics and pharmacodynamics of diltiazem, each subject was given a single oral dose of 60 mg of diltiazem with and without pretreatment with oral quinidine. Pretreatment consisted of administering 100 mg of quinidine twice daily for 5 doses. The last dose was given 1½ hours before diltiazem. Diltiazem pretreatment increased the area under the plasma concentration-time curve by 51%, prolonged the elimination half-life from 6.8 to 9.3 hours and decreased the oral clearance by 33%. In addition, diltiazem pretreatment prolonged the QTc and PR intervals, and decreased the heart rate and diastolic blood pressure observed after a single dose of quinidine. Pretreatment with quinidine did not affect the pharmacokinetics or pharmacodynamics of diltiazem.

See also, Quinidine-Nifedipine and Quinidine-Verapamil.

[1] Lagani `ere S, et al. *Clin Pharmacol Ther.* 1996;60:255.

* Asterisk indicates drugs cited in interaction reports.

Quinidine — *Diphenoxylate*

Quinidine*	Diphenoxylate-Atropine* (eg, *Lomotil*)

Significance	Onset	Severity	Documentation
5	☐ Rapid ■ **Delayed**	☐ Major ☐ Moderate ■ **Minor**	☐ Established ☐ Probable ☐ Suspected ■ **Possible** ☐ Unlikely

Effects Peak serum QUINIDINE concentrations and the time to reach the peak concentration may be decreased. Bioavailability is not affected.

Mechanism DIPHENOXYLATE may slow the rate of QUINIDINE absorption.

Management Based on available data, no alterations in therapy appear to be necessary.

Discussion

Using a randomized, crossover design, the effect of diphenoxylate with atropine on the single-dose bioavailability of quinidine sulfate was studied in eight healthy volunteers.[1] Each subject received 300 mg of quinidine sulfate on the morning of the study day. Quinidine was either taken alone (controls) or with diphenoxylate 2.5 mg in combination with atropine 0.025 mg at midnight before the study day and on the morning of the study day, approximately 1 hour before quinidine was administered. When diphenoxylate was administered, the time to reach peak quinidine concentrations was 1.21 hours compared with 0.89 hours for the controls (a 30 minute difference) and the mean maximum concentration was 1.65 mcg/mL in the treatment group versus 2.10 mcg/mL in the controls (a 21% decrease). There was no difference between the treatment and control groups in area under the plasma concentration-time curve (bioavailability) of quinidine. Controlled studies are needed to determine the clinical importance of multiple dose administration of these agents in patients.

[1] Ponzillo JJ, et al. *Clin Pharm.* 1988;7:139.

* Asterisk indicates drugs cited in interaction reports.

Quinidine — *Fluvoxamine*

Quinidine* | Fluvoxamine*

Significance	Onset	Severity	Documentation
4	□ Rapid ■ **Delayed**	□ Major ■ **Moderate** □ Minor	□ Established □ Probable □ Suspected ■ **Possible** □ Unlikely

Effects QUINIDINE levels may be elevated, increasing the therapeutic and adverse effects.

Mechanism Inhibition of QUINIDINE metabolism (CYP3A4) is suspected.

Management Carefully monitor QUINIDINE levels and observe the clinical response of the patient when starting, stopping, or changing the dose of FLUVOXAMINE. Adjust the QUINIDINE dose as needed.

Discussion

In an open-label study, the effects of fluvoxamine on the pharmacokinetics of quinidine were assessed in 6 healthy volunteers.[1] Each subject received a single dose of quinidine 200 mg alone and on the fifth day of fluvoxamine 100 mg/day administration. Fluvoxamine administration decreased the total apparent oral clearance of quinidine 29%. In addition, quinidine clearance by N-oxidation and 3-hydroxylation was decreased 33% and 44%, respectively. Fluvoxamine did not affect the renal clearance or peak concentration of quinidine.

Additional studies are needed to determine the clinical importance of this interaction.

[1] Damkier P, et al. *Eur J Clin Pharmacol.* 1999;55:451.

* Asterisk indicates drugs cited in interaction reports.

Quinidine — *Food*

Quinidine*	Grapefruit Juice*

Significance	Onset	Severity	Documentation
5	■ **Rapid**	□ Major	□ Established
	□ Delayed	□ Moderate	□ Probable
		■ **Minor**	□ Suspected
			■ **Possible**
			□ Unlikely

Effects The onset of QUINIDINE action may be delayed.

Mechanism Delayed absorption of QUINIDINE and inhibition of metabolism (cytochrome P450 3A4) of QUINIDINE to its major metabolite.

Management Until there are more clinical data, patients taking QUINIDINE should avoid GRAPEFRUIT products.

Discussion

Using an open-labeled, randomized, crossover design, the effects of grapefruit juice on the pharmacokinetics of quinidine and QT interval changes were studied in 12 healthy men.[1] Each subject received 2 oral doses of quinidine sulfate 400 mg with water or grapefruit juice. Compared with water, grapefruit juice prolonged the time to reach maximum plasma quinidine concentrations 106% (from 1.6 to 3.3 hr) and decreased the AUC and peak concentrations of the major metabolite of quinidine, 3-hydroxyquinidine, thus reducing the conversion of quinidine to the 3-hydroxy-metabolite. The AUC of quinidine was not affected. Administration of quinidine with grapefruit juice delayed the maximal effect on QT_c and reduced the maximum effect. In vitro data indicate that the flavonoids in grapefruit juice have the potential to inhibit quinidine metabolism.[2] It has been recommended that grapefruit juice be avoided in patients receiving quinidine.[3]

Controlled clinical studies are needed to determine the clinical importance of this possible drug interaction.

[1] Min DI, et al. *J Clin Pharmacol.* 1996;36:469.
[2] Ha HR, et al. *Eur J Clin Pharmacol.* 1995;48:367.
[3] *Quinidex Extentabs* [package insert]. A.H. Robins. September 2000.

* Asterisk indicates drugs cited in interaction reports.

Quinidine — *Hydantoins*

Quinidine*	Fosphenytoin Phenytoin* (eg, *Dilantin*)

Significance	Onset	Severity	Documentation
2	☐ Rapid ■ **Delayed**	☐ Major ■ **Moderate** ☐ Minor	☐ Established ☐ Probable ■ **Suspected** ☐ Possible ☐ Unlikely

Effects A decrease in the therapeutic effect of QUINIDINE may occur.

Mechanism Appears to be due to PHENYTOIN stimulation of the hepatic microsomal enzyme system, resulting in an increase in QUINIDINE metabolism.

Management Frequent monitoring of serum QUINIDINE concentrations is recommended; an increase in the QUINIDINE dose may be required.

Discussion

Three case reports document increased quinidine requirements during concomitant phenytoin therapy.[1-3] In one case, the quinidine concentration decreased by almost 50%, and the clinical condition worsened after the addition of phenytoin.[2] In the second case, a patient treated with phenytoin required massive doses of oral quinidine to obtain therapeutic plasma concentrations.[1] Once phenytoin was discontinued, this patient manifested clinical quinidine toxicity, necessitating dosage reduction. This interaction was also studied in 2 volunteers.[1] Findings included a reduction in quinidine $t_{½}$ by 50% and a decrease in quinidine AUC by 60% after 2 weeks of phenytoin. In the third case, the quinidine/3-hydroxyquinidine ratio decreased from 4:1 to 1.7:1 during 1 week of combination therapy.[3] This suggests an increase in quinidine metabolism secondary to phenytoin. Two additional cases demonstrate this interaction, but these patients were treated with other hepatic microsomal enzyme inducers in combination with phenytoin.[4,5] A study with dogs found a similar effect of phenytoin on quinidine pharmacokinetics using both IV and oral quinidine.[6] This study documented a marked decrease in quinidine volume of distribution during concomitant phenytoin therapy.

1 Data JL, et al. *N Engl J Med.* 1976;294(13):699.
2 Urbano AM. *N Engl J Med.* 1983;308(4):225.
3 Farringer JA, et al. *Drug Intell Clin Pharm.* 1985;19(6):461.
4 Kroboth FJ, et al. *N Engl J Med.* 1983;308:725.
5 Rodgers GC, et al. *Drug Intell Clin Pharm.* 1983;17(11):819.
6 Jaillon P, et al. *J Pharmacol Exp Ther.* 1980;213(1):33.

* Asterisk indicates drugs cited in interaction reports. Based on pharmacologic and pharmacokinetic considerations, similar interactions may occur with other drugs that are listed.

Quinidine ✕ *Mifepristone*

Quinidine*	Mifepristone* (eg, *Korlym*)

Significance	Onset	Severity	Documentation
1	□ Rapid ■ **Delayed**	■ **Major** □ Moderate □ Minor	□ Established □ Probable ■ **Suspected** □ Possible □ Unlikely

Effects QUINIDINE plasma concentrations may be elevated, increasing the pharmacologic effects and risk of adverse reactions (eg, serious cardiovascular events).

Mechanism MIFEPRISTONE may inhibit QUINIDINE metabolism (CYP3A4).

Management Coadministration of QUINIDINE with MIFEPRISTONE is contraindicated.[1]

Discussion

Because mifepristone inhibits CYP3A4, coadministration of mifepristone with a drug that is metabolized mainly or solely by CYP3A4 (eg, quinidine) is likely to increase plasma concentrations of the drug.[1] Therefore, the concurrent use of drugs with a narrow therapeutic index that are CYP3A4 substrates, such as quinidine, is contraindicated. The risk of quinidine adverse reactions (eg, hypotension, heart failure) may be increased.

[1] *Korlym* [package insert]. Menlo Park, CA: Corcept Therapeutics Incorporated; February 2012.

* Asterisk indicates drugs cited in interaction reports.

Quinidine — *Nifedipine*

Quinidine*	Nifedipine* (eg, *Procardia*)

Significance	Onset	Severity	Documentation
2	☐ Rapid ■ **Delayed**	☐ Major ■ **Moderate** ☐ Minor	☐ Established ☐ Probable ■ **Suspected** ☐ Possible ☐ Unlikely

Effects Serum levels and actions of QUINIDINE may be lower than predicted by the dosage. Serum concentrations and actions of NIFEDIPINE may be increased.

Mechanism Unknown.

Management No special precautions other than routine clinical monitoring are necessary. Check serum levels of QUINIDINE after NIFEDIPINE therapy is started or stopped; tailor dosage as needed.

Discussion

Several case reports describe a possible interference with the pharmacokinetics of quinidine due to concomitant therapy with nifedipine.[1-3] One patient's serum quinidine level decreased from 2.4 to 1.6 mcg/mL after starting nifedipine. Despite increases up to a maximum of quinidine gluconate 2,592 mg daily, levels were still less than 2 mcg/mL, and the patient's arrhythmia was not controlled. In 2 patients, marked increases in serum quinidine levels occurred after discontinuation of nifedipine. The increases were transient and, in 1 patient, returned to baseline within 10 days of stopping nifedipine.[2] Another patient required a 50% increase in quinidine levels to produce a modest increase in levels.[3] All patients in these studies had left ventricular dysfunction, with ejection fractions of 25% to 41%; 1 patient developed transient hypotension during initiation of nifedipine therapy. To investigate a possible relationship between depressed left ventricular function and this interaction, 2 groups of 6 patients with normal and depressed ejection fractions were studied.[4] One patient with normal ejection fraction demonstrated a 41% decrease in steady-state serum quinidine levels. More data are needed to identify which patient characteristics may predispose to this low frequency interaction. In a study involving 10 volunteers, the elimination $t_{1/2}$ of nifedipine was prolonged from 1.9 to 2.8 hours during coadministration of quinidine.[5] Nifedipine clearance and AUC were unaffected. In 10 healthy subjects, administration of quinidine and nifedipine produced a 37% increase in the nifedipine AUC.[6] A slight increase in heart rate was noted within the first 2 hours compared with either drug alone. In 12 volunteers, the pharmacokinetics of quinidine were unaffected by 3 days of pretreatment with nifedipine or felodipine (*Plendil*).[7]

[1] Green JA, et al. *Clin Pharm.* 1983;2(5):461.
[2] Farringer JA, et al. *Am Heart J.* 1984;108(6):1570.
[3] Van Lith RM, et al. *Drug Intell Clin Pharm.* 1985;19(11):829.
[4] Munger MA, et al. *Clin Pharmacol Ther.* 1989; 45(4):411.
[5] Schellens JH, et al. *Clin Pharmacol Ther.* 1991;50(5)(pt 1):520.
[6] Bowles SK, et al. *J Clin Pharmacol.* 1993;33(8):727.
[7] Bailey DG, et al. *Clin Pharmacol Ther.* 1993;53(3):354.

* Asterisk indicates drugs cited in interaction reports.

Quinidine — *Oxcarbazepine*

Quinidine*	Oxcarbazepine* (eg, *Trileptal*)

Significance	Onset	Severity	Documentation
4	□ Rapid	□ Major	□ Established
	■ **Delayed**	■ **Moderate**	□ Probable
		□ Minor	□ Suspected
			■ **Possible**
			□ Unlikely

Effects QUINIDINE plasma concentrations may be reduced, decreasing the therapeutic effect.

Mechanism OXCARBAZEPINE increased the metabolism (CYP3A4) of QUINIDINE.

Management Monitor QUINIDINE plasma concentrations and the clinical response of the patient when starting, stopping, or changing the OXCARBAZEPINE dose. Adjust the QUINIDINE dose as needed.

Discussion

The effects of oxcarbazepine on the pharmacokinetics of quinidine were evaluated in 8 healthy men.[1] In an open-label study, each subject received oxcarbazepine, which was titrated to 1,200 mg daily, for 17 days. In addition, subjects received a single dose of quinidine 200 mg before and after the course of oxcarbazepine. Compared with giving quinidine alone, oxcarbazepine increased the formation of the 3-hydroxyquinidine metabolite 89%, decreased the mean quinidine C_{max} 29%, and decreased the mean $t_{½}$ of quinidine 12%.[1]

[1] Andreasen AH, et al. *Epilepsia.* 2007;48(3):490.

* Asterisk indicates drugs cited in interaction reports.

Quinidine — *Protease Inhibitors*

Quinidine*	Nelfinavir* (*Viracept*)	Ritonavir* (*Norvir*)

Significance	Onset	Severity	Documentation
1	☐ Rapid ■ **Delayed**	■ **Major** ☐ Moderate ☐ Minor	☐ Established ☐ Probable ■ **Suspected** ☐ Possible ☐ Unlikely

Effects Large increases in serum QUINIDINE concentrations may occur, increasing the risk of QUINIDINE toxicity.

Mechanism RITONAVIR may inhibit the metabolism (CYP3A4) of QUINIDINE.

Management RITONAVIR and NELFINAVIR are contraindicated in patients receiving QUINIDINE.

Discussion

Ritonavir[1] and nelfinavir [2] are expected to produce increases in quinidine plasma concentrations, increasing the risk of toxicity. Elevated serum concentrations of quinidine may cause QT prolongation and subsequent serious cardiac arrhythmias.[3] Quinidine is metabolized by the CYP3A4 isozyme, and drugs that block the metabolism of quinidine may produce an increase in plasma concentrations of quinidine. Studies using human liver microsomes have demonstrated that CYP3A is a major isoform in ritonavir metabolism.[1] Therefore, coadministration of ritonavir and quinidine is contraindicated.

The basis for this monograph is information on file with the manufacturer. Published clinical data are needed to further assess this interaction. However, because of the seriousness of the cardiac problems, clinical evaluation of this interaction in humans is not likely to be forthcoming.

[1] *Norvir* [package insert]. Abbott Park, IL: Abbott Laboratories; September 2001.

[2] *Viracept* [package insert]. La Jolla, CA: Agouron Pharmaceuticals Inc; December 2002.

[3] Thomas M, et al. *Br J Clin Pharmacol.* 1996;41(2):77.

* Asterisk indicates drugs cited in interaction reports.

Quinidine — *Sucralfate*

Quinidine*	Sucralfate* (eg, *Carafate*)

Significance	Onset	Severity	Documentation
4	☐ Rapid ■ **Delayed**	☐ Major ■ **Moderate** ☐ Minor	☐ Established ☐ Probable ☐ Suspected ■ **Possible** ☐ Unlikely

Effects Serum QUINIDINE levels may be reduced, decreasing the therapeutic effects.

Mechanism Possibly, QUINIDINE binds to SUCRALFATE, decreasing GI absorption.

Management Monitor serum QUINIDINE levels. If a decrease in clinical response occurs, it may be necessary to discontinue SUCRALFATE.

Discussion

Coadministration of sucralfate produced subtherapeutic levels of quinidine in 1 patient.[1] A 71-year-old woman with a 3-day history of intermittent chest pain, shortness of breath, and fatigue was admitted to the hospital to rule out MI. The patient had a history of atrial fibrillation, recurrent deep venous thrombosis, pulmonary embolism, peptic ulcer disease, degenerative joint disease, and right total knee replacement; she was receiving digoxin (eg, *Lanoxin*) 0.125 mg/day, sustained-release quinidine 300 mg twice daily, warfarin (eg, *Coumadin*) 7.5 mg/day, and sucralfate 2 g twice daily. Administration of sucralfate was separated from her other medications by 2 hours. Upon admission, the doses of digoxin, quinidine, and warfarin were not changed, and they were coadministered with sucralfate. In addition, she was prescribed nitroglycerin paste (eg, *Nitrostat*), diltiazem (eg, *Cardizem*, subcutaneous heparin, meperidine (eg, *Demerol*) with promethazine (eg, *Phenergan*) for chest pain unrelieved by 3 sublingual nitroglycerin tablets, and acetaminophen (eg, *Tylenol*). On the evening of admission, the patient had an episode of atrial flutter with a rapid ventricular response accompanied by chest pain and shortness of breath. The patient was given IV digoxin 0.25 mg on 2 consecutive days. Her symptoms resolved and the serum digoxin level increased from 0.13 to 1.9 nmol/L. On the same day, sucralfate administration was changed to be given 4 hours apart from her other medication. On the next day, sucralfate was discontinued. One day later, the patient's digoxin level was 1.15 nmol/L. Her quinidine level increased from 0.31 mcmol/L at the time of hospitalization to 5.55 mcmol/L the day after sucralfate was discontinued. Except for sucralfate, the patient was maintained on her initial drug regimen.

[1] Rey AM, et al. *DICP*. 1991;25(7-8):745.

* Asterisk indicates drugs cited in interaction reports.

Quinidine / *Urinary Alkalinizers*

Quinidine	Urinary Alkalinizers	
Quinidine*	Potassium Citrate (eg, *Urocit-K*)	Sodium Citrate
	Sodium Acetate	Sodium Lactate
	Sodium Bicarbonate*	Tromethamine (*Tham*)

Significance	Onset	Severity	Documentation
4	☐ Rapid	☐ Major	☐ Established
	■ **Delayed**	■ **Moderate**	☐ Probable
		☐ Minor	☐ Suspected
			■ **Possible**
			☐ Unlikely

Effects Urinary elimination of QUINIDINE is reduced. Serum QUINIDINE concentrations may increase accompanied by increased QUINIDINE effect on the heart, such as prolongation of the QRS duration or the Q-T interval.

Mechanism Unknown. Both QUINIDINE and quinine, the optical isomer of QUINIDINE, exhibit pH-dependent urinary elimination, probably due to increased tubular reabsorption of un-ionized drug with increasing urine pH.

Management Monitor serum QUINIDINE levels and the ECG if adding or removing URINARY ALKALINIZERS to a stable QUINIDINE regimen.

Discussion

The urinary excretion of quinidine was studied in 4 male volunteers under conditions of aciduria and alkaluria.[1] Subjects were given 200 mg of quinidine sulfate every 6 hours for 5 days. Urinary excretion of quinidine was inversely related to urine pH. At urine pH less than 6, quinidine elimination averaged 115 ± 84 mg/L; for pH more than 7.5, average excretion was 13 ± 8 mg/L. Mean renal clearance of quinidine was reduced by 50% at a urine pH of 7 to 8 when compared with a urine pH of 6 to 7. In contrast, there was no significant change in PAH or insulin clearances at the different pHs. Additional studies in 6 normal male volunteers using the same conditions showed that serum quinidine concentrations increased in 5 of the 6 under conditions of alkaline urine. An increase in the quinidine serum level was also associated with an increase in the QT-interval, a measure of quinidine effect on the heart, in the 3 subjects whose heart rates were stable enough to calculate the rate-corrected Q-T interval. Although dated and deficient in design, the study established the pH dependency of quinidine urinary elimination. Additional studies, using more sensitive and specific assays, and monitoring are needed to elaborate on this interaction. Less than 20% of administered quinidine is eliminated unchanged via urine; however, active metabolites also undergo urinary elimination (their pH dependency has not been studied). Urinary alkalinization of patients on quinidine could result in dose-dependent toxicity. Conversely, urine acidification could result in loss of arrhythmia control.

[1] Gerhardt RE, et al. *Ann Intern Med.* 1969;71:927.

* Asterisk indicates drugs cited in interaction reports. Based on pharmacologic and pharmacokinetic considerations, similar interactions may occur with other drugs that are listed.

Quinidine — *Verapamil*

Quinidine* (eg, *Quinidex Extentabs*)	Verapamil* (eg, *Calan*)

Significance	Onset	Severity	Documentation
1	■ **Rapid**	■ **Major**	□ Established
	□ Delayed	□ Moderate	□ Probable
		□ Minor	■ **Suspected**
			□ Possible
			□ Unlikely

Effects Hypotension, bradycardia, ventricular tachycardia and AV block may occur.

Mechanism VERAPAMIL appears to interfere with the clearance of QUINIDINE and prolong its half-life.

Management Use this combination when no other alternative exists. Monitor patients closely. Stop one or both of the drugs if the interaction is manifested and treat symptomatically.

Discussion

Although verapamil and quinidine have been used together successfully,[3] significant adverse reactions from the combination have been reported. When oral doses of both drugs were used, hypotension (systolic pressure of 50 mm Hg in one patient), pulmonary edema, ventricular tachycardia, bradycardia and atrioventricular block, along with diaphoresis, dizziness and blurred vision were recorded in four patients.[1,4] Three of the patients had hypertrophic cardiomyopathy. Complications were noted within 1 day of combination therapy and as late as 5 months. In three patients on long-term quinidine therapy, IV verapamil caused a rapid drop in blood pressure that responded to conventional therapy and discontinuation of the verapamil and sometimes quinidine.[2]

A competitive interaction between the two drugs at the alpha receptors has been described[2] and may contribute to the interaction. One case report,[4] however, described elevated trough levels of quinidine when verapamil was given, and a study[5] in six healthy males demonstrated the clearance of a single dose of quinidine was reduced by verapamil administration while the half-life was prolonged from 6.9 to 9 to 9.3 hours.

This interaction had potentially serious effects. More studies are needed to identify patients who may be at risk.

[1] Epstein SE, et al. *Circulation.* 1981;64:437.
[2] Maisel AS, et al. *N Engl J Med.* 1985;312:167.
[3] Ochs HR, et al. *J Clin Pharmacol.* 1985;25:204.
[4] Trohman RG, et al. *Am J Cardiol.* 1986;57:706.
[5] Edwards DJ, et al. *Clin Pharmacol Ther.* 1987;41:68.

* Asterisk indicates drugs cited in interaction reports.

Quinine — *Cimetidine*

Quinine*	Cimetidine* (eg, *Tagamet*)

Significance	Onset	Severity	Documentation
5	☐ Rapid ■ **Delayed**	☐ Major ☐ Moderate ■ **Minor**	☐ Established ☐ Probable ☐ Suspected ■ **Possible** ☐ Unlikely

Effects The oral clearance of QUININE may be reduced, and the mean elimination t½ may be increased.

Mechanism CIMETIDINE may reduce the metabolism of QUININE by inhibiting the hepatic microsomal mixed-function oxidase enzyme system.

Management Monitor for dose-dependent toxicity such as cinchonism if CIMETIDINE is added to a stable regimen of QUININE, particularly in patients receiving antimalarial doses of QUININE. No special precautions appear necessary in patients receiving lower doses.

Discussion

The pharmacokinetics of a single dose of oral quinine sulfate 600 mg, equivalent to 497 mg of the base, were determined in 6 healthy volunteers before and after a 7-day course of cimetidine or ranitidine (eg, *Zantac*).[1] Subjects were studied on 3 occasions, separated by at least 3 weeks. In a randomized fashion, subjects received no pretreatment, cimetidine 200 mg 3 times daily plus 400 mg at bedtime, or ranitidine 150 mg twice daily. Cimetidine pretreatment produced a 27% reduction in the apparent oral clearance of quinine. This was associated with a 49% increase (range, 17% to 90%) in the mean elimination t½ from 7.6 to 11.3 hours. Peak plasma quinine concentrations and the time to peak were not altered after cimetidine pretreatment. Ranitidine had no effect on any of the measured pharmacokinetic parameters.

No assessment of the therapeutic or toxic implications of this interaction could be made from this single-dose study. However, a sustained increase in the elimination t½ of quinine could predispose patients receiving antimalarial doses of quinine 650 mg 3 times daily to dose-dependent toxic effects or could allow the use of reduced doses of quinine when these 2 drugs are coadministered. See also Quinidine-Cimetidine.

[1] Wanwimolruk S, et al. *Br J Clin Pharmacol.* 1986;22(3):346.

* Asterisk indicates drugs cited in interaction reports.

Quinine — *Food*

Quinine* | Grapefruit Juice*

Significance	Onset	Severity	Documentation
4	☐ Rapid	■ **Major**	☐ Established
	■ **Delayed**	☐ Moderate	☐ Probable
		☐ Minor	☐ Suspected
			■ **Possible**
			☐ Unlikely

Effects The risk of life-threatening arrhythmias, including torsades de pointes, may be increased.

Mechanism Unknown.

Management Caution patients to avoid concurrent ingestion of GRAPEFRUIT products or GRAPEFRUIT JUICE and QUININE, especially patients with a history of long QT syndrome.

Discussion

A 31-year-old woman developed frequent, convulsive syncopes caused by torsades de pointes (QTc interval, 0.58 seconds).[1] Investigation revealed that she had been drinking large amounts of grapefruit juice and tonic water containing quinine. The torsades de pointes reversed 48 hours after the beverages were stopped (QTc interval, 0.45 seconds). The patient had a history of asymptomatic long QT syndrome and asymptomatic second-degree atrioventricular block. Her 2 older siblings died of sudden death when they were about 30 years of age.

[1] Hermans K, et al. *Am J Med.* 2003;114(6):511.

* Asterisk indicates drugs cited in interaction reports.

Quinine — *Ritonavir*

Quinine*

Ritonavir* (*Norvir*)

Significance	Onset	Severity	Documentation
2	□ Rapid	□ Major	□ Established
	■ **Delayed**	■ **Moderate**	□ Probable
		□ Minor	■ **Suspected**
			□ Possible
			□ Unlikely

Effects QUININE plasma concentrations may be elevated, increasing the pharmacologic effects and risk of adverse reactions, while RITONAVIR plasma concentrations may be modestly increased.

Mechanism Inhibition of QUININE metabolism (CYP3A4) by RITONAVIR and inhibition of RITONAVIR metabolism (CYP2D6) by QUININE are suspected.

Management Monitor the response of the patient to QUININE when RITONAVIR is started or stopped. Adjust the QUININE dose as needed.

Discussion

The possible pharmacokinetic interaction between quinine and ritonavir was evaluated in 10 healthy subjects.[1] Each subject received a single dose of quinine 600 mg alone, ritonavir 200 mg every 12 hours for 9 days, and a single dose of quinine 600 mg on day 8 of ritonavir administration. Compared with giving quinine alone, coadministration with ritonavir increased the quinine C_{max} and AUC approximately 4-fold and increased the $t_{½}$. The quinine oral clearance was decreased about 4.5-fold. In addition, there were modest increases in the ritonavir C_{max}, AUC, and $t_{½}$.

[1] Soyinka JO, et al. *Br J Clin Pharmacol.* 2010;69(3):262.

* Asterisk indicates drugs cited in interaction reports.

Quinine Derivatives — *Anticholinesterases*

Quinine Derivatives	Anticholinesterases	
Quinidine*	Ambenonium (*Mytelase*)	Physostigmine*
Quinine (*Qualaquin*)	Edrophonium (*Enlon*)	Pyridostigmine (eg, *Mestinon*)
	Neostigmine (eg, *Prostigmin*)	

Significance	Onset	Severity	Documentation
2	☐ Rapid	☐ Major	☐ Established
	■ **Delayed**	■ **Moderate**	☐ Probable
		☐ Minor	■ **Suspected**
			☐ Possible
			☐ Unlikely

Effects QUININE DERIVATIVES may reverse the effects of ANTICHOLINESTERASES and vice versa.

Mechanism ANTICHOLINESTERASES and QUININE DERIVATIVES may antagonize the CNS effects of each other.

Management Unless these agents are being coadministered for their antagonistic effects, avoid QUININE DERIVATIVES in patients receiving ANTICHOLINESTERASES for their therapeutic effects (eg, treatment of myasthenia gravis).

Discussion

Delirium in a 69-year-old man with quinidine intoxication was repeatedly and rapidly reversed by physostigmine administration.[1]

[1] Summers WK, et al. *West J Med.* 1981;135(5):411.

* Asterisk indicates drugs cited in interaction reports. Based on pharmacologic and pharmacokinetic considerations, similar interactions may occur with other drugs that are listed.

Quinine Derivatives — *Ketoconazole*

Quinine Derivatives	Ketoconazole
Quinidine*	Ketoconazole* (eg, *Nizoral*)
Quinine* (*Qualaquin*)	

Significance	Onset	Severity	Documentation
2	□ Rapid	□ Major	□ Established
	■ **Delayed**	■ **Moderate**	□ Probable
		□ Minor	■ **Suspected**
			□ Possible
			□ Unlikely

Effects QUININE DERIVATIVE serum levels may be elevated, increasing therapeutic and toxic effects.

Mechanism KETOCONAZOLE inhibits QUININE DERIVATIVE metabolism (CYP3A4).[1]

Management Consider monitoring serum QUININE DERIVATIVE levels when KETOCONAZOLE is started or stopped. Adjust the dose as needed.

Discussion

Coadministration of ketoconazole and quinidine sulfate resulted in elevated serum quinidine levels in a 68-year-old man with acute myelomonoblastic leukemia.[2] He had a medical history of chronic atrial fibrillation, chronic obstructive pulmonary disease, and mild renal function impairment. Upon admission, his medications included the following: digoxin (eg, *Lanoxin*); quinidine 300 mg 4 times daily; theophylline (eg, *Theo-24*); 2 courses of therapy with cytarabine (eg, *DepoCyt*); doxorubicin (eg, *Adriamycin*); vincristine (eg, *Vincasar*); and prednisone. Ketoconazole 200 mg/day was given for *Candida* esophagitis. Prior to the administration of ketoconazole, serum quinidine levels ranged from 1.4 to 2.7 mg/L. Approximately 1 week after starting ketoconazole treatment, serum quinidine levels increased to 6.9 mg/L and the elimination $t_{1/2}$ was 25 hours. Quinidine was stopped for 2 days and restarted at 200 mg twice daily. The serum quinidine level at this time had decreased to 2.2 mg/L. Over the following 4 weeks, the dose of quinidine was increased to 300 mg every 6 hours in order to maintain therapeutic levels of the drug. During this time, the patient continued to receive ketoconazole treatment. A study has shown that ketoconazole inhibits the metabolism of quinine, which is the stereoisomer of quinidine.[1]

[1] Mirghani RA, et al. *Clin Pharmacol Ther.* 1999;66(5):454.

[2] McNulty RM, et al. *Clin Pharm.* 1989;8(3):222.

* Asterisk indicates drugs cited in interaction reports.

Quinine Derivatives | *Rifamycins*

Quinine Derivatives		Rifamycins	
Quinidine*		Rifabutin (*Mycobutin*)	Rifapentine (*Priftin*)
Quinine* (*Qualaquin*)		Rifampin* (eg, *Rifadin*)	

Significance	Onset	Severity	Documentation
2	□ Rapid	□ Major	□ Established
	■ **Delayed**	■ **Moderate**	■ **Probable**
		□ Minor	□ Suspected
			□ Possible
			□ Unlikely

Effects Reduced therapeutic effects of QUININE DERIVATIVES may occur.

Mechanism RIFAMYCINS increase the hepatic metabolism of QUININE DERIVATIVES.

Management Addition of RIFAMYCINS to stable regimens of QUININE DERIVATIVES may require increased doses of QUININE DERIVATIVES to maintain the desired therapeutic effect. Withdrawal of RIFAMYCINS may result in QUININE DERIVATIVE dose-related toxicity. Monitor QUININE DERIVATIVE serum levels and ECG.

Discussion

Coadministration of rifampin with quinidine caused a reduction in quinidine C_{max} from 4 to less than 0.5 mcg/mL and a loss of arrhythmia control.[1] The pharmacokinetics of single doses of oral (4 subjects) and IV (4 subjects) quinidine were determined at baseline and after 7 days of oral rifampin 600 mg/day.[2] There was an average 3-fold reduction in the mean elimination $t_{½}$ and almost a 6-fold reduction in the mean AUC before rifampin administration. Subjects in the IV quinidine group showed similar increases in quinidine clearance without any change in quinidine distribution. A greater than predicted increase in apparent oral clearance compared with the AUC suggested that rifampin increased the first-pass metabolism of oral quinidine. Case reports have demonstrated the clinical importance of this interaction and documented its reversibility after rifampin is discontinued.[3-5] In 9 healthy volunteers, the pharmacokinetics of single doses of oral quinine were determined at baseline and after 14 days of oral rifampin 600 mg/day.[6] Compared with placebo, rifampin caused a 6.9-fold increase in unbound quinine clearance, which corresponded to a decrease in $t_{½}$ (from 11.1 to 5.5 hours). In addition, C_{max} and mean AUC of quinine were reduced. In patients with malaria, rifampin increased the metabolic clearance of quinine and reduced the cure rate.[7]

1 Ahmad D, et al. *Br J Dis Chest.* 1979;73(4):409.
2 Twum-Barima Y, et al. *N Engl J Med.* 1981;304(24):1466.
3 Bussey HI, et al. *Drug Intell Clin Pharm.* 1983;17(6):436.
4 Schwartz A, et al. *Am Heart J.* 1984;107(4):789.
5 Bussey HI, et al. *Arch Intern Med.* 1984;144(5):1021.
6 Wanwimolruk S, et al. *Br J Clin Pharmacol.* 1995;40(1):87.
7 Pukrittayakamee S, et al. *Antimicrob Agents Chemother.* 2003;47(5):1509.

* Asterisk indicates drugs cited in interaction reports. Based on pharmacologic and pharmacokinetic considerations, similar interactions may occur with other drugs that are listed.

Quinolones — *Aminoquinolines*

Ciprofloxacin* (eg, *Cipro*)	Chloroquine * (eg, *Aralen*)

Significance	Onset	Severity	Documentation
4	□ Rapid ■ **Delayed**	□ Major ■ **Moderate** □ Minor	□ Established □ Probable □ Suspected ■ **Possible** □ Unlikely

Effects CIPROFLOXACIN plasma concentrations may be reduced, decreasing the efficacy.

Mechanism Unknown.

Management When possible, consider avoiding concurrent use of CIPROFLOXACIN and CHLOROQUINE.

Discussion

The effect of chloroquine on ciprofloxacin plasma concentrations was studied in 5 healthy men.[1] Each subject received oral ciprofloxacin 500 mg alone and with chloroquine 600 mg. Compared with giving ciprofloxacin alone, coadministration of chloroquine decreased the AUC and C_{max} of ciprofloxacin 43% and 18% (from 3.42 to 2.8 mcg/mL), respectively.

[1] Ilo CE, et al. *Am J Ther.* 2006:13(5):432.

* Asterisk indicates drugs cited in interaction reports.

Quinolones — *Antacids*

Quinolones		Antacids	
Ciprofloxacin* (eg, *Cipro*)	Lomefloxacin* (*Maxaquin*)	Aluminum Hydroxide* (eg, *Amphojel*)	Calcium Carbonate* (eg, *Tums*)
Gatifloxacin* (*Zymar*)	Moxifloxacin* (*Avelox*)	Aluminum/ Magnesium Hydroxide* (eg, *Riopan*)	Magnesium Hydroxide* (eg, *Milk of Magnesia*)
Gemifloxacin* (*Factive*)	Norfloxacin* (*Noroxin*)	Calcium Acetate* (*PhosLo*)	
Levofloxacin* (*Levaquin*)	Ofloxacin* (eg, *Floxin*)		

Significance	Onset	Severity	Documentation
2	■ **Rapid**	□ Major	□ Established
	□ Delayed	■ **Moderate**	■ **Probable**
		□ Minor	□ Suspected
			□ Possible
			□ Unlikely

Effects Decreased pharmacologic effects of QUINOLONES.

Mechanism GI absorption of QUINOLONES may be decreased.

Management If concurrent use cannot be avoided, consult the package insert for QUINOLONE-specific guidelines.

Discussion

Coadministration of aluminum/magnesium hydroxide–containing antacids and quinolone antibacterial agents has resulted in the following pharmacokinetic changes: 1) ciprofloxacin C_{max} was decreased 17-fold, and AUC and unchanged drug in urine were markedly decreased[1]; 2) norfloxacin bioavailability was greatly reduced when taken 5 minutes after the antacid but increased 9-fold when taken 2 hours before the antacid[2]; urinary excretion was reduced 86% to 90%,[3] possibly leading to therapeutic failure[4]; 3) ofloxacin bioavailability was reduced 73%[5]; low-dose antacid (2 hours prior to ofloxacin) decreased the C_{max}, AUC, and relative bioavailability of ofloxacin, while giving ofloxacin 2 hours before the antacid circumvented the interaction,[6] and others found no interaction[5]; 4) lomefloxacin C_{max} and bioavailability were reduced 50% and 40%, respectively[7]; and 5) gatifloxacin absorption was decreased.[8] Calcium carbonate reduced norfloxacin bioavailability 37.5%[4] and lomefloxacin AUC 21%,[9] but other studies demonstrated no effect on lomefloxacin[10] or ofloxacin.[6] Aluminum phosphate did not affect ofloxacin,[11] while aluminum hydroxide decreased ofloxacin levels[12] and bioavailability of levofloxacin 45%.[13] Calcium acetate decreased gemifloxacin bioavailability 51%.[14] Because of the high magnesium content in quinapril tablets (eg, *Accupril*), this interaction may occur with quinapril and certain quinolones.

1 Lomaestro BM, et al. *DICP.* 1991;25(11):1249.
2 Nix DE, et al. *Antimicrob Agents Chemother.* 1990;34(3):432.
3 Campbell NR, et al. *Br J Clin Pharmacol.* 1992;33(1):115.
4 Noyes M, et al. *Ann Intern Med.* 1988;109(2):168.
5 Hoffken G, et al. *Rev Infect Dis.* 1988;10(suppl):5138.
6 Flor S, et al. *Antimicrob Agents Chemother.* 1990;34(12):2436.
7 Shimada J, et al. *Antimicrob Agents Chemother.* 1992;36(6):1219.
8 Lober S, et al. *Antimicrob Agents Chemother.* 1999;43(5):1067.
9 Pletz MW, et al. *Antimicrob Agents Chemother.* 2003; 47(7):2158.
10 Lehto P, et al. *Clin Pharmacol Ther.* 1994;56(5):477.
11 Martinez Cabarga M, et al. *Antimicrob Agents Chemother.* 1991;35(10):2102.
12 Akerele JO, et al. *J Antimicrob Chemother.* 1991;28(1):87.
13 Shiba K, et al. *Drugs.* 1995;49(suppl 2):360.
14 Kays MB, et al. *Am J Kidney Dis.* 2003;42(6):1253.

* Asterisk indicates drugs cited in interaction reports.

Quinolones		***Antineoplastic Agents***	
Ciprofloxacin* (*Cipro*)	Ofloxacin (*Floxin*)	Cyclophosphamide* (eg, *Cytoxan*)	Mitoxantrone* (*Novantrone*)
Levofloxacin (*Levaquin*)	Sparfloxacin (*Zagam*)	Cytarabine* (eg, *Cytosar-U*)	Prednisolone* (eg, *Prelone*)
Lomefloxacin (*Maxaquin*)	Trovafloxacin (*Trovan*)	Daunorubicin* (*DaunoXome*)	Vincristine* (eg, *Vincasar PFS*)
Norfloxacin (*Noroxin*)		Doxorubicin* (eg, *Adriamycin*)	

Significance	Onset	Severity	Documentation
4	☐ Rapid ■ **Delayed**	☐ Major ■ **Moderate** ☐ Minor	☐ Established ☐ Probable ☐ Suspected ■ **Possible** ☐ Unlikely

Effects The antimicrobial effect of QUINOLONES may be decreased.

Mechanism Chemotherapy with ANTINEOPLASTIC AGENTS may decrease QUINOLONE absorption by altering the intestinal mucosa.

Management Monitor the response of the patient to QUINOLONE therapy, and adjust the dose accordingly.

Discussion

The effect of cancer chemotherapy on the absorption of ciprofloxacin was studied in 5 patients with newly diagnosed acute myeloid leukemia and 1 patient with non-Hodgkin lymphoma.[1] Ciprofloxacin was administered throughout the chemotherapy and for a minimum of 21 days afterward. In 5 patients, the peak serum concentration of ciprofloxacin attained was higher before chemotherapy than after. Following 13 days of chemotherapy, the mean peak concentration of ciprofloxacin decreased from 3.3 to 2 mg/L. The mean peak concentration of ciprofloxacin achieved decreased from 3.7 to 2 mg/L by the thirteenth day of chemotherapy, and the mean time-to-reach peak concentration after an oral dose of ciprofloxacin decreased from 2.3 to 1.2 hr 13 days after chemotherapy. The AUC also decreased during chemotherapy. The decrease in AUC was greater from 2 to 4 hr (56%) than from 0 to 2 hr (37.5%).

Additional studies are warranted.

[1] Johnson EJ, et al. *J Antimicrob Chemother.* 1990;25:837.

* Asterisk indicates drugs cited in interaction reports. Based on pharmacologic and pharmacokinetic considerations, similar interactions may occur with other drugs that are listed.

Quinolones — *Cisapride*

Gatifloxacin* (*Tequin*)	Moxifloxacin* (*Avelox*)	Cisapride*† (*Propulsid*)
Levofloxacin* (*Levaquin*)	Sparfloxacin* (*Zagam*)	

Significance	Onset	Severity	Documentation
1	☐ Rapid ■ **Delayed**	■ **Major** ☐ Moderate ☐ Minor	☐ Established ☐ Probable ■ **Suspected** ☐ Possible ☐ Unlikely

Effects The risk of CV side effects may be increased. The pharmacologic effects of SPARFLOXACIN may be increased.

Mechanism Unknown.

Management CISAPRIDE is contraindicated in patients receiving other QTc-prolonging drugs or drugs reported to cause torsades de pointes, such as GATIFLOXACIN, LEVOFLOXACIN, MOXIFLOXACIN, and SPARFLOXACIN.[1-6]

Discussion

In an open, randomized, crossover design, the effects of cisapride on the pharmacokinetics of sparfloxacin were evaluated in 15 healthy volunteers.[7] In addition, the effects of coadministration of sparfloxacin and cisapride on the QTc interval were evaluated. Each subject received a single 400 mg dose of sparfloxacin 2 days after receiving cisapride 10 mg 3 times daily. Sparfloxacin was taken 15 minutes after cisapride. Cisapride administration increased peak serum sparfloxacin concentrations 37% and decreased the time to reach the peak serum concentration 54%. However, the bioavailability of sparfloxacin was not altered. During coadministration of cisapride and sparfloxacin, the QTc interval increased from 376 to 405 msec (7.7%). Rare cases of torsades de pointes have been reported in patients receiving gatifloxacin.[5] Moxifloxacin has prolonged the QT interval in some patients.[6] Because studies between gatifloxacin or moxifloxacin and drugs that prolong the QTc interval have not been performed, use gatifloxacin and moxifloxacin with caution when drugs that prolong the QT interval (eg, cisapride) are coadministered.[5,6] Levofloxacin has been associated with prolongation of the QT interval and infrequent cases of cardiac arrhythmias.[2] The risk of arrhythmias may be reduced by avoiding coadministration with other drugs that prolong the QT interval (eg, cisapride).[4]

1 *Zagam* [package insert]. Morgantown, WV: Bertek Pharmaceuticals, Inc; January 2004.
2 Thomas M, et al. *Br J Clin Pharmacol.* 1996;41:77.
3 *Propulsid* [package insert]. Titusville, NJ: Janssen Pharmaceutica; January 2000.
4 *Levaquin* [package insert]. Raritan, NJ: Ortho-McNeil Pharmaceutical, Inc; February 2004.
5 *Tequin* [package insert]. Princeton, NJ: Bristol-Myers Squibb Company; March 2004.
6 *Avelox* [package insert]. West Haven, CT: Bayer Health Care; April 2004.
7 Zix JA, et al. *Antimicrob Agents Chemother.* 1997;41:1668.

* Asterisk indicates drugs cited in interaction reports.
† Available from the manufacturer on a limited-access protocol.

Quinolones — *Didanosine*

Quinolones		Didanosine
Ciprofloxacin* (eg, *Cipro*)	Norfloxacin (*Noroxin*)	Didanosine* (eg, *Videx*)
Lomefloxacin (*Maxaquin*)	Ofloxacin (eg, *Floxin*)	

Significance	Onset	Severity	Documentation
2	■ **Rapid**	□ Major	□ Established
	□ Delayed	■ **Moderate**	□ Probable
		□ Minor	■ **Suspected**
			□ Possible
			□ Unlikely

Effects The pharmacologic effects of QUINOLONES may be decreased.

Mechanism The magnesium and aluminum cations in the buffers present in DIDANOSINE tablets decrease GI absorption of QUINOLONES via chelation.

Management If concurrent use cannot be avoided, give the QUINOLONE at least 2 hours before or 6 hours after DIDANOSINE chewable tablets.

Discussion

The bioavailability of ciprofloxacin was studied in 12 healthy volunteers during the coadministration of the buffer given with didanosine.[1] In a randomized, open, crossover trial, each subject received a single ciprofloxacin 750 mg tablet alone or with the didanosine-placebo tablet containing the magnesium-aluminum cation buffer. Each study period was separated by 7 days. During the didanosine phase, subjects received 2 didanosine-placebo tablets every 12 hours for 2 doses. On the second day, each subject chewed and swallowed the didanosine-placebo tablets and, within 1 minute, was given ciprofloxacin 750 mg. Compared with giving ciprofloxacin alone, didanosine-placebo administration resulted in a decrease in ciprofloxacin serum concentration from 3.38 to 0.25 mcg/mL, a decrease in AUC from 15.5 to 0.26 mcg•hr/mL, and a decrease in the mean time to maximum concentration from 1.56 to 0.75 hours. In 16 patients, concurrent use of didanosine and ciprofloxacin affected the pharmacokinetics of each agent.[2] Ciprofloxacin 750 mg every 12 hours was given 2 hours prior to didanosine 200 mg every 12 hours (as 100 mg chewable/dispersible tablets). The AUC of ciprofloxacin was decreased 26%, while the AUC of didanosine was decreased 16%. This change was not considered clinically important.

Administration of ciprofloxacin 2 hours before didanosine prevented the interaction in a healthy volunteer.[3] See Quinolones-Antacids.

[1] Sahai J, et al. *Clin Pharmacol Ther.* 1993;53:292.
[2] Knupp CA, et al. *Biopharm Drug Dispos.* 1997;18:65.
[3] Sahai J. *Ann Intern Med.* 1995;123:394.

* Asterisk indicates drugs cited in interaction reports. Based on pharmacologic and pharmacokinetic considerations, similar interactions may occur with other drugs that are listed.

Quinolones — *Enteral Nutrition*

Quinolones		Enteral Nutrition
Ciprofloxacin* (eg, *Cipro*)	Ofloxacin* (eg, *Floxin*)	Enteral Nutrition* (eg, *Ensure*)
Gatifloxacin* (*Tequin*)		

Significance	Onset	Severity	Documentation
4	☐ Rapid	☐ Major	☐ Established
	■ **Delayed**	■ **Moderate**	☐ Probable
		☐ Minor	☐ Suspected
			■ **Possible**
			☐ Unlikely

Effects Serum concentrations of certain QUINOLONES may be reduced, decreasing the efficacy.

Mechanism Decreased absorption of certain QUINOLONES.

Management In patients receiving ENTERAL NUTRITION, increased doses of GATIFLOXACIN and CIPROFLOXACIN may be needed. Monitor the clinical response of the patient and adjust the QUINOLONE dosage as needed.

Discussion

In 12 healthy volunteers, ingestion of gatifloxacin 400 mg crushed and mixed with *Ensure* decreased the gatifloxacin C_{max} 45% and AUC 26% and prolonged the median time to reach C_{max}, compared with crushing and administering gatifloxacin with water.[1] In 16 critically ill patients, enteral nutrition products (*Glucerna, Impact, Jevity, Promote, Pulmocare*) did not reduce the bioavailability of gatifloxacin 400 mg administered as a slurry via gastric tube.[2] In a study of 13 healthy volunteers, coadministration of ciprofloxacin with *Ensure* decreased the ciprofloxacin C_{max} 47% and AUC 27% and prolonged the median time to reach C_{max} 2.6-fold, compared with water.[3] In the same study, coadministration of ofloxacin with *Ensure* decreased the ofloxacin C_{max} 36% and AUC 10% and prolonged the median time to reach C_{max} 2.5-fold, compared with water. In 26 hospitalized patients, enteral feeding with *Sustacal*, given orally or via gastrectomy or jejunostomy tubes, decreased the ciprofloxacin (powder suspension) AUC 26% to 67% and C_{max} 39% to 67% and prolonged the median time to reach C_{max} 2- to 3-fold, compared with water.[4] Reductions in ciprofloxacin C_{max} as a result of feedings given via gastrectomy tube are similar to those following oral administration on an empty stomach. Although ciprofloxacin absorption following nasogastric (NG) tube administration was decreased by enteral feeding with *Pulmocare*, levels were above the minimum inhibitory concentration for many pathogenic bacteria.[5] In 6 healthy volunteers, administration of a ciprofloxacin crushed tablet suspension through an NG tube was not affected by enteral feeding with *Osmolite*.[6]

[1] Kays MB, et al. *Pharmacotherapy*. 2005;25:1530.
[2] Kanji S, et al. *Crit Care Med*. 2003;31:1347.
[3] Mueller BA, et al. *Antimicrob Agents Chemother*. 1994;38:2101.
[4] Healy DP, et al. *Antimicrob Agents Chemother*. 1996;40:6.
[5] Cohn SM, et al. *J Antimicrob Chemother*. 1996;38:871.
[6] Yuk JH, et al. *Antimicrob Agents Chemother*. 1989;33:1118.

* Asterisk indicates drugs cited in interaction reports.

Quinolones — *Food*

Ciprofloxacin* (eg, *Cipro*)	Norfloxacin* (*Noroxin*)	Food*

Significance	Onset	Severity	Documentation
2	■ **Rapid** □ Delayed	□ Major ■ **Moderate** □ Minor	□ Established □ Probable ■ **Suspected** □ Possible □ Unlikely

Effects Decreased pharmacologic effects of QUINOLONES.

Mechanism Decreased GI absorption of QUINOLONES.

Management If milk cannot be avoided, lengthen the interval between milk ingestion and QUINOLONE ingestion by as much as possible.

Discussion

Concurrent ingestion of milk and either ciprofloxacin or norfloxacin can reduce the bioavailability of the antibacterial agent.[1,2] The effects of milk on the absorption of norfloxacin were evaluated in a single-dose study involving 6 healthy volunteers.[2] In a 2-way crossover investigation, each subject received norfloxacin 200 mg with either 200 mL of tap water or 200 mL of milk (containing calcium 218 mg) after an overnight fast. When norfloxacin was coadministered with milk, the serum concentration 30 minutes after ingestion was 11% of the control value. Serum norfloxacin concentrations were decreased no more than 10 hours after concurrent ingestion with milk. The values for the AUC for norfloxacin were 62% of those obtained when the antibiotic was taken with water. Similarly, in a crossover investigation, the effects of milk and yogurt on the bioavailability of ciprofloxacin were studied in 7 healthy volunteers.[1] Thirty minutes after ingestion of milk or yogurt, serum ciprofloxacin concentrations were reduced 70% and 92%, respectively. Milk decreased the peak plasma ciprofloxacin concentration 36%, while yogurt reduced the level 47%. Both milk and yogurt decreased the bioavailability, as determined by total AUC, 30% to 36%. In contrast, neither milk,[3] a standard breakfast, nor a high-fat breakfast[4] had any effect on the bioavailability of lomefloxacin (*Maxaquin*), and neither milk nor breakfast affected the bioavailability of ofloxacin (eg, *Floxin*).[5] Milk does not affect the bioavailability of fleroxacin (not available in the US).[6] Similarly, breakfast foods (without milk) did not affect the bioavailability of enoxacin[7] or ciprofloxacin.[8] See also Quinolones-Antacids.

[1] Neuvonen PJ, et al. *Clin Pharmacol Ther.* 1991;50:498.
[2] Minami R, et al. *J Clin Pharmacol.* 1993;33:1238.
[3] Lehto P, et al. *Clin Pharmacol Ther.* 1994;56:477.
[4] Hooper WD, et al. *Antimicrob Agents Chemother.* 1990;34:1797.
[5] Dudley MN, et al. *Eur J Clin Pharmacol.* 1991;41:569.
[6] Hoogkamer JF, et al. *Drugs.* 1995;49(suppl 2):346.
[7] Somogyi AA, et al. *Antimicrob Agents Chemother.* 1987;31:638.
[8] Ledergerber B, et al. *Antimicrob Agents Chemother.* 1985;27:350.

* Asterisk indicates drugs cited in interaction reports.

Quinolones	*Histamine H_2 Antagonists*	
Enoxacin*†	Cimetidine* (eg, *Tagamet*)	Nizatidine (eg, *Axid*)
Lomefloxacin* (*Maxaquin*)	Famotidine (eg, *Pepcid*)	Ranitidine* (eg, *Zantac*)

Significance	Onset	Severity	Documentation
4	■ **Rapid** □ Delayed	□ Major ■ **Moderate** □ Minor	□ Established □ Probable □ Suspected ■ **Possible** □ Unlikely

Effects Variable, depending on the route of administration. The pharmacologic effects of orally administered ENOXACIN may be decreased by H_2 ANTAGONISTS, while CIMETIDINE may increase the effects of parenteral ENOXACIN.

Mechanism Possible decrease in the GI absorption of ENOXACIN caused by reduced gastric ENOXACIN solubility as a result of H_2 ANTAGONIST-induced decrease in gastric pH. The mechanism is unknown for parenterally administered ENOXACIN; however, CIMETIDINE may compete with ENOXACIN for active renal secretion.

Management Closely monitor the response to the QUINOLONE antibiotic or consider use of an antibacterial agent in another class.

Discussion

The effects of ranitidine administration on enoxacin absorption were investigated in a randomized, crossover study involving 10 healthy volunteers.[1] Subjects received IV ranitidine 50 mg 2 hr before an oral dose of enoxacin 400 mg. Ranitidine decreased enoxacin bioavailability 40% and the C_{max} 44%. In a randomized, crossover study in 12 healthy volunteers, oral administration of enoxacin 400 mg 2 hr after an IV dose of ranitidine 50 mg and repeated 6 and 14 hr after the enoxacin dose decreased the mean enoxacin C_{max} 38% and the bioavailability 26%.[2] In a nonblinded, randomized, crossover study, oral administration of ranitidine 150 mg twice daily did not alter the pharmacokinetics of IV administered enoxacin.[3] However, oral administration of cimetidine 300 mg twice daily decreased the renal clearance of enoxacin 26% and the systemic clearance 20%, while increasing the elimination $t_{½}$ 30%. Limited data suggest that ranitidine does not affect the bioavailability of orally administered ciprofloxacin (eg, *Cipro*) or ofloxacin (eg, *Floxin*).[1] While there is a statistical decrease in lomefloxacin clearance by ranitidine, the effect is small and not likely to be clinically important.[4]

1 Grasela, TH Jr, et al. *Antimicrob Agents Chemother.* 1989;33:615.
2 Lebsack ME, et al. *Clin Pharmacol Ther.* 1992;52:252.
3 Misiak PM, et al. *J Clin Pharmacol.* 1993;33:53.
4 Sudoh T, et al. *Eur J Clin Pharmacol.* 1996;51;95.

* Asterisk indicates drugs cited in interaction reports.
† Not available in the US.

Quinolones / Iron Salts

Quinolones		Iron Salts	
Ciprofloxacin* (eg, *Cipro*)	Lomefloxacin* (*Maxaquin*)	Ferrous Fumarate (eg, *Femiron*)	Polysaccharide-Iron Complex (eg, *Hytinic*)
Gatifloxacin (*Tequin*)	Moxifloxacin* (*Avelox*)	Ferrous Gluconate* (eg, *Fergon*)	
Gemifloxacin (*Factive*)	Norfloxacin* (*Noroxin*)	Ferrous Sulfate* (eg, *Feosol*)	
Levofloxacin (*Levaquin*)	Ofloxacin* (eg, *Floxin*)		

Significance	Onset	Severity	Documentation
2	■ **Rapid**	□ Major	□ Established
	□ Delayed	■ **Moderate**	■ **Probable**
		□ Minor	□ Suspected
			□ Possible
			□ Unlikely

Effects Decreased anti-infective response to QUINOLONES.

Mechanism GI absorption of QUINOLONES may be decreased by formation of an iron-quinolone complex.

Management Separate the administration of these agents by as much time as possible (at least 2 hr).

Discussion

In a crossover design, ciprofloxacin 500 mg was administered alone, prior to, and with the last dose of ferrous sulfate 325 mg 3 times daily for 7 days.[1] The AUC and the mean peak levels for the regimen containing iron were lower. Iron reduced the mean bioavailability of the antibiotic 64%. Similarly, during coadministration of ciprofloxacin and ferrous sulfate to a 68-year-old man, peak and trough antibiotic serum levels were 0.3 to 0.5 and 0.1 to 0.2 mg/L, respectively, compared with 5.2 and 1.2 mg/L, respectively, when ciprofloxacin was given without iron.[2] In a crossover study of 8 healthy volunteers, coadministration of ciprofloxacin with ferrous sulfate 300 mg, ferrous gluconate 600 mg, or a combination tablet containing 10 mg elemental iron reduced ciprofloxacin AUC (46%, 67%, 57%, respectively) and C_{max} (37%, 56%, 37%, respectively).[3] A study of 8 volunteers demonstrated a 55% decrease in urinary excretion of norfloxacin 400 mg when taken with ferrous sulfate 300 mg, suggesting a reduction in norfloxacin bioavailability.[4] In a randomized evaluation, coadministration of ferrous sulfate (100 mg elemental sustained-release iron) with norfloxacin 400 mg, ciprofloxacin 500 mg, or ofloxacin 400 mg, reduced the AUC 73%, 57%, and 25%, respectively.[5] The bioavailability of moxifloxacin was 61% when taken with ferrous sulfate compared with taking moxifloxacin alone.[6] By contrast, studies of healthy volunteers found a clinically insignificant decrease in ofloxacin bioavailability (10%)[7] or lomefloxacin bioavailability (13%)[8] when given with sustained-release ferrous sulfate.

[1] Polk RE, et al. *Antimicrob Agents Chemother.* 1989;33:1841.
[2] Le Pennec MP, et al. *J Antimicrob Chemother.* 1990;25:184.
[3] Kara M, et al. *Br J Clin Pharmacol.* 1991;31:257.
[4] Campbell NR, et al. *Br J Clin Pharmacol.* 1992;33:115.
[5] Lehto P, et al. *Br J Clin Pharmacol.* 1994;37:82.
[6] Stass H, et al. *Clin Pharmacokinet.* 2001;40(suppl1):57.
[7] Lomaestro BM, et al. *DICP.* 1991;25:1249.
[8] Lehto P, et al. *Clin Pharmacol Ther.* 1994;56:477.

* Asterisk indicates drugs cited in interaction reports. Based on pharmacologic and pharmacokinetic considerations, similar interactions may occur with other drugs that are listed.

Quinolones / *Loop Diuretics*

Quinolones		Loop Diuretics	
Ciprofloxacin (eg, *Cipro*)	Ofloxacin (*Floxin*)	Bumetanide	Torsemide (eg, *Demadex*)
Lomefloxacin*		Ethacrynic Acid (eg, *Edecrin*)	
Norfloxacin (*Noroxin*)		Furosemide* (eg, *Lasix*)	

Significance	Onset	Severity	Documentation
5	■ **Rapid**	□ Major	□ Established
	□ Delayed	□ Moderate	□ Probable
		■ **Minor**	□ Suspected
			■ **Possible**
			□ Unlikely

Effects The pharmacologic effects of LOMEFLOXACIN may be increased.

Mechanism At least in part, FUROSEMIDE decreases the renal clearance of LOMEFLOXACIN, possibly by competition for tubular secretion.

Management Based on currently available clinical data, no special precautions are necessary.

Discussion

The pharmacokinetic profiles of lomefloxacin and furosemide given alone and together were compared in 8 healthy subjects.[1] In an open, randomized, crossover study, each subject received single oral doses of lomefloxacin 200 mg and furosemide 40 mg separately and together. Plasma lomefloxacin concentrations tended to be or were significantly higher ($P < 0.05$) when administered with furosemide compared with giving lomefloxacin alone. The total clearance and renal clearance of lomefloxacin were significantly decreased by furosemide ($P < 0.05$). In addition, furosemide significantly increased the lomefloxacin AUC from 7.46 to 8.35 mg•hr/L ($P < 0.05$). However, the magnitude of these changes was small and may not be clinically important. In contrast, lomefloxacin did not affect any pharmacokinetic parameter of furosemide.

[1] Sudoh T, et al. *Eur J Clin Pharmacol.* 1994;46(3):267.

* Asterisk indicates drugs cited in interaction reports. Based on pharmacologic and pharmacokinetic considerations, similar interactions may occur with other drugs that are listed.

Quinolones — *Probenecid*

Ciprofloxacin* (eg, *Cipro*	Gemifloxacin* (*Factive*

Probenecid*

Significance	Onset	Severity	Documentation
4	□ Rapid	□ Major	□ Established
	■ **Delayed**	■ **Moderate**	□ Probable
		□ Minor	□ Suspected
			■ **Possible**
			□ Unlikely

Effects Plasma concentrations of certain QUINOLONES may be elevated, increasing the pharmacologic effects and adverse reactions.

Mechanism Decreased renal clearance of certain QUINOLONES as a result of inhibition of renal tubular secretion by PROBENECID is suspected.

Management Monitor the response of the patient. If an interaction is suspected, adjust the QUINOLONE dose as needed.

Discussion

The effects of probenecid on the pharmacokinetics of ciprofloxacin were studied in 12 healthy volunteers.[1] In a randomized, crossover study, each subject received a single IV dose of ciprofloxacin 200 mg with and without oral probenecid. Probenecid was given 10 hours (500 mg) and 2 hours (1,000 mg) before ciprofloxacin infusion, and probenecid 500 mg was given 4, 10, and 16 hours after the end of the infusion. Compared with giving ciprofloxacin alone, coadministration of probenecid increased the ciprofloxacin AUC and elimination $t_{1/2}$ 75% and 51%, respectively, and decreased urinary recovery, total clearance, and renal clearance 39%, 41%, and 64%, respectively. Probenecid inhibited the renal tubular secretion of ciprofloxacin.[2] In a study of 17 healthy subjects, each subject received a single oral dose of gemifloxacin 320 mg alone or with probenecid 4.5 g.[3] Coadministration of probenecid increased gemifloxacin plasma concentrations and decreased the amount excreted in the urine, compared with giving gemifloxacin alone. In these studies, probenecid was administered in doses greater than those usually given.

[1] Jaehde U, et al. *Clin Pharmacol Ther.* 1995;58(5):532.
[2] Landersdorfer CB, et al. *Br J Clin Pharmacol.* 2010;69(2):167.
[3] Landersdorfer CB, et al. *Antimicrob Agents Chemother.* 2009;53(9):3902.

* Asterisk indicates drugs cited in interaction reports.

Quinolones — *Proton Pump Inhibitors*

Quinolones	Proton Pump Inhibitors	
Trovafloxacin*†	Esomeprazole (*Nexium*)	Pantoprazole (eg, *Protonix*)
	Lansoprazole (eg, *Prevacid*)	Rabeprazole (*Aciphex*)
	Omeprazole* (eg, *Prilosec*)	

Significance	Onset	Severity	Documentation
5	☐ Rapid	☐ Major	☐ Established
	■ **Delayed**	☐ Moderate	☐ Probable
		■ **Minor**	☐ Suspected
			■ **Possible**
			☐ Unlikely

Effects Plasma TROVAFLOXACIN levels may be reduced, decreasing the pharmacologic effect.

Mechanism Decreased absorption of TROVAFLOXACIN, resulting from gastric acid suppression, is suspected.

Management Observe the clinical response of the patient to TROVAFLOXACIN.

Discussion

The effect of omeprazole on the bioavailability of trovafloxacin was investigated in a placebo-controlled, crossover study involving 12 healthy volunteers.[1] During each phase, subjects received placebo or trovafloxacin 300 mg the night before the study phase. The next morning, each subject received trovafloxacin 30 minutes after placebo or 2 hours after omeprazole 40 mg. Omeprazole did not affect the $t_{1/2}$ of trovafloxacin; however, omeprazole decreased the AUC and peak plasma level of trovafloxacin 18% and 32%, respectively. The mean relative bioavailability of trovafloxacin after omeprazole was 82% compared with placebo.

[1] Teng R, et al. *J Antimicrob Chemother.* 1997;39(suppl B):93.

* Asterisk indicates drugs cited in interaction reports. Based on pharmacologic and pharmacokinetic considerations, similar interactions may occur with other drugs that are listed.
† Not available in the United States.

Quinolones — *Rifamycins*

Quinolones		Rifamycins	
Moxifloxacin* (eg, *Avelox*)	Norfloxacin (*Noroxin*)	Rifabutin (*Mycobutin*) Rifampin* (eg, *Rifadin*)	Rifapentine* (*Priftin*)

Significance	Onset	Severity	Documentation
4	☐ Rapid ■ **Delayed**	☐ Major ■ **Moderate** ☐ Minor	☐ Established ☐ Probable ☐ Suspected ■ **Possible** ☐ Unlikely

Effects MOXIFLOXACIN plasma concentrations may be reduced, decreasing its efficacy.

Mechanism Increased MOXIFLOXACIN metabolism (glucuronidation or sulphation) by RIFAMYCINS is suspected.

Management Monitor the response of the patient. A higher dose of QUINOLONE ANTIBIOTIC may be needed during coadministration of RIFAMPIN.

Discussion

The effects of rifampin on the pharmacokinetics of moxifloxacin were studied in 19 patients with pulmonary tuberculosis.[1] In an open-label, crossover study, each subject received moxifloxacin 400 mg daily for 5 days with rifampin 450 mg and isoniazid 600 mg (eg, *Nydrazid*) 3 times/week or moxifloxacin 400 mg daily alone for 5 days. Compared with giving moxifloxacin alone, coadministration of rifampin plus isoniazid decreased the AUC and C_{max} of moxifloxacin 31% and 32%, respectively. In addition, the T_{max} for moxifloxacin was prolonged from 1 to 2.5 hours. In a similar study in 16 healthy volunteers, rifampin administration reduced the moxifloxacin AUC 27%, but did not affect the C_{max}.[2] Because rifampin induces phase 2 metabolism, the interaction was attributed to rifampin.[1] Rifapentine 3 times weekly coadministered with moxifloxacin daily reduced the moxifloxacin AUC 17.2%.[3] In contrast, ciprofloxacin 750 mg twice daily coadministered with rifampin 300 mg twice daily did not alter ciprofloxacin pharmacokinetics.[4]

[1] Nijland HM, et al. *Clin Infect Dis.* 2007;45(8):1001.
[2] Weiner M, et al. *Antimicrob Agents Chemother.* 2007;51(8):2861.
[3] Dooley K, et al. *Antimicrob Agents Chemother.* 2008;52(11):4037.
[4] Chandler MH, et al. *Antimicrob Agents Chemother.* 1990;34(3):442.

* Asterisk indicates drugs cited in interaction reports. Based on pharmacologic and pharmacokinetic considerations, similar interactions may occur with other drugs that are listed.

Quinolones — *Sevelamer*

Ciprofloxacin* (eg, *Cipro*)	Sevelamer* (*Renagel*)

Significance	Onset	Severity	Documentation
2	■ **Rapid** □ Delayed	□ Major ■ **Moderate** □ Minor	□ Established □ Probable ■ **Suspected** □ Possible □ Unlikely

Effects Bioavailability of CIPROFLOXACIN may be reduced, decreasing the clinical efficacy and promoting bacterial resistance to CIPROFLOXACIN.

Mechanism Decreased GI absorption of CIPROFLOXACIN is suspected.

Management If concurrent use cannot be avoided, separate the administration times by at least 4 hr.

Discussion

The effects of sevelamer on the bioavailability of ciprofloxacin were studied in 15 healthy volunteers.[1] In a randomized, crossover study, each subject received ciprofloxacin 750 mg alone and with 7 sevelamer 403 mg capsules. Sevelamer decreased the peak plasma concentration of ciprofloxacin 34% (from 3.77 to 2.49 mcg/mL) and the AUC 39%, compared with administering ciprofloxacin alone. However, 2 subjects had a larger AUC when ciprofloxacin was administered with sevelamer. The relative bioavailability of ciprofloxacin was decreased 48% by sevelamer.

The effect of sevelamer on the bioavailability of other quinolone antibiotics needs to be determined.

[1] Kays MB, et al. *Am J Kidney Dis*. 2003;42:1253.

* Asterisk indicates drugs cited in interaction reports.

Quinolones — *Sucralfate*

Quinolones		Sucralfate
Ciprofloxacin* (eg, *Cipro*)	Norfloxacin* (*Noroxin*)	Sucralfate* (eg, *Carafate*)
Lomefloxacin* (*Maxaquin*)	Ofloxacin* (eg, *Floxin*)	
Moxifloxacin* (*Avelox*)	Sparfloxacin* (*Zagam*)	

Significance	Onset	Severity	Documentation
2	■ **Rapid**	□ Major	□ Established
	□ Delayed	■ **Moderate**	■ **Probable**
		□ Minor	□ Suspected
			□ Possible
			□ Unlikely

Effects Decreased pharmacologic effects of QUINOLONES.

Mechanism Decreased GI absorption of the QUINOLONES.

Management If concurrent use cannot be avoided, give SUCRALFATE at least 6 hr after the QUINOLONE.

Discussion

In 8 healthy men, coadministration of norfloxacin 400 mg and sucralfate 1 g resulted in a decrease in the bioavailability of norfloxacin.[1] The relative bioavailability of norfloxacin was 1.8% when administered with sucralfate and 56.6% when taken 2 hr later. In addition, the concentration of norfloxacin in the urine decreased more than 90% when the antibiotic was administered with sucralfate. In 12 volunteers, a 30% reduction in ciprofloxacin bioavailability was measured.[2] Sucralfate 1 g was administered 2 and 6 hr prior to ciprofloxacin 750 mg. Four subjects experienced a greater than 50% decrease in ciprofloxacin bioavailability. Several studies and case reports demonstrated a 10-fold decrease in ciprofloxacin peak level, as well as a reduction in urinary excretion and AUC, when sucralfate was taken concurrently.[3-5] However, no change in ciprofloxacin pharmacokinetics was observed when the antibiotic was taken 2 or 6 hr before sucralfate.[6] This effect may be caused by complexation of ciprofloxacin by the aluminum contained in sucralfate. Ciprofloxacin failure has been attributed to this interaction.[5] Coadministration of lomefloxacin 400 mg with sucralfate 1 g to 8 volunteers caused a 51% reduction in bioavailability and a 64% decrease in peak levels.[7] Coadministration of sucralfate and moxifloxacin decreased the moxifloxacin AUC 60% and the peak plasma level 71%.[8] Sucralfate 1 g given 30 minutes prior to sparfloxacin 400 mg reduced the bioavailability of sparfloxacin 44%.[9] However, no effect was seen if sparfloxacin was given 4 hr before sucralfate.[10] Similarly, 6 healthy volunteers who received ofloxacin 200 mg with sucralfate 1 g exhibited a 61% reduction in bioavailability when fasting, compared with a 31% decrease after eating.[11] The bioavailability of levofloxacin (*Levaquin*) was not altered when taken 2 hr before sucralfate.[12] See also Quinolones-Antacids.

1 Parpia SH, et al. *Antimicrob Agents Chemother.* 1989;33:99.
2 Nix DE, et al. *Pharmacotherapy.* 1989;9:377.
3 Brouwers JR, et al. *Drug Invest.* 1990;2:197.
4 Lomaestro BM, et al. *DICP.* 1991;25:1249.
5 Spivey JM, et al. *Pharmacotherapy.* 1996;16:314.
6 Van Slooten AD, et al. *DICP.* 1991;25:578.
7 Lehto P, et al. *Clin Pharm Ther.* 1994;56:477.
8 Stass H, et al. *Clin Pharmacokinet.* 2001;40(suppl 1):49.
9 Zix JA, et al. *Antimicrob Agents Chemother.* 1997;41:1668.
10 Kamberi M, et al. *Br J Clin Pharmacol.* 2000;49:98.
11 Kawakami J, et al. *Eur J Clin Pharmacol.* 1994;47:67.
12 Lee LJ, et al. *Antimicrob Agents Chemother.* 1997;41:2196.

* Asterisk indicates drugs cited in interaction reports.

Quinolones — *Zinc Salts*

Quinolones		Zinc Salts	
Ciprofloxacin* (eg, *Cipro*)	Norfloxacin* (*Noroxin*)	Zinc Gluconate	Zinc Sulfate*
Lomefloxacin†	Ofloxacin		

Significance	Onset	Severity	Documentation
4	☐ Rapid	☐ Major	☐ Established
	■ **Delayed**	■ **Moderate**	☐ Probable
		☐ Minor	☐ Suspected
			■ **Possible**
			☐ Unlikely

Effects The anti-infective response to QUINOLONES may be decreased.

Mechanism The GI absorption of certain QUINOLONES may be decreased by ZINC SALTS.

Management Consider avoiding coadministration of oral QUINOLONES and ZINC SALTS.

Discussion

Using a crossover design, the effects of a multivitamin with zinc on the absorption of ciprofloxacin were studied in 12 healthy men.[1] Ciprofloxacin 500 mg was administered alone. Subjects then received a multivitamin with zinc (zinc 23.9 mg) once daily for 7 days. Ciprofloxacin 500 mg was administered with the last dose of the multivitamin preparation and again after a 7-day washout period. Compared with giving ciprofloxacin alone, pretreatment with the multivitamin with zinc significantly ($P < 0.01$) reduced the ciprofloxacin AUC and C_{max}. In addition, pretreatment with the multivitamin with zinc reduced ciprofloxacin bioavailability 24% and significantly ($P < 0.01$) reduced the 24-hour urinary excretion of ciprofloxacin. In a single-dose study of 8 volunteers, coadministration of norfloxacin 400 mg with zinc sulfate 200 mg caused a 56% decrease in 24-hour excretion of norfloxacin, suggesting a reduction in norfloxacin bioavailability.[2]

Additional multidose studies are needed to determine if the decreased ciprofloxacin levels are clinically important.

[1] Polk RE, et al. *Antimicrob Agents Chemother.* 1989;33(11):1841.

[2] Campbell NR, et al. *Br J Clin Pharmacol.* 1992;33(1):115.

* Asterisk indicates drugs cited in interaction reports. Based on pharmacologic and pharmacokinetic considerations, similar interactions may occur with other drugs that are listed.

† Not available in the United States.

Raltegravir — *Atazanavir*

Raltegravir* (*Isentress*)	Atazanavir* (*Reyataz*)

Significance	Onset	Severity	Documentation
4	☐ Rapid ■ **Delayed**	☐ Major ■ **Moderate** ☐ Minor	☐ Established ☐ Probable ☐ Suspected ■ **Possible** ☐ Unlikely

Effects RALTEGRAVIR plasma concentrations may be elevated, increasing the pharmacologic effects and risk of adverse reactions.

Mechanism Decreased RALTEGRAVIR metabolism due to inhibition of uridine diphosphate glucuronosyltransferase by ATAZANAVIR.

Management Monitor RALTEGRAVIR concentrations in patients receiving ATAZANAVIR and adjust the RALTEGRAVIR dose as needed.

Discussion

The effect of atazanavir on the pharmacokinetics of raltegravir was studied in 12 healthy men.[1] In a double-blind, randomized, 2-phase study, subjects received raltegravir 100 mg or placebo alone and on day 7 of a 9-day course of atazanavir 400 mg daily. Atazanavir increased raltegravir C_{max} and AUC approximately 53% and 72%, respectively, compared with giving raltegravir alone. A 45-year-old HIV-infected man experienced increased alkaline phosphatase during concurrent treatment with raltegravir and an antiretroviral regimen that contained atazanavir.[2] When raltegravir was discontinued, alkaline phosphatase normalized. Rechallenge with raltegravir resulted in an increase in alkaline phosphatase. Atazanavir was discontinued and alkaline phosphatase decreased slightly despite continued raltegravir administration. Two additional studies have shown that atazanavir increases raltegravir exposure.[3,4] However, there was considerable intersubject variability. See Raltegravir-Protease Inhibitors.[1]

[1] Iwamoto M, et al. *Clin Infect Dis.* 2008;47(1):137.
[2] Fleischbein E, et al. *AIDS.* 2008;22(17):2404.
[3] Cattaneo D, et al. *Ther Drug Monit.* 2010;32(6):782.
[4] Neely M, et al. *Antimicrob Agents Chemother.* 2010;54(11):4619.

* Asterisk indicates drugs cited in interaction reports.

Raltegravir — *NNRT Inhibitors*

Raltegravir* (*Isentress*)	Efavirenz (*Sustiva*)	Nevirapine (eg, *Viramune*)
	Etravirine* (*Intelence*)	

Significance	Onset	Severity	Documentation
4	☐ Rapid ■ **Delayed**	☐ Major ■ **Moderate** ☐ Minor	☐ Established ☐ Probable ☐ Suspected ■ **Possible** ☐ Unlikely

Effects RALTEGRAVIR trough concentrations may be reduced, decreasing the efficacy.

Mechanism Induction of RALTEGRAVIR metabolism (CYP3A4) by NNRT INHIBITORS is suspected.

Management Coadminister with caution. Close clinical and laboratory monitoring is warranted. Adjust the RALTEGRAVIR dose as needed.

Discussion

An open-label study was conducted in 19 healthy subjects to assess a 2-way interaction between etravirine and raltegravir.[1] Etravirine had a modest effect on the pharmacokinetics of raltegravir, reducing the raltegravir trough concentration approximately 34% and the C_{max} and AUC approximately 11% and 10%, respectively, compared with raltegravir alone. Coadministration of raltegravir and etravirine increased etravirine trough concentrations approximately 18% and the C_{max} and AUC approximately 4% and 10%, respectively, compared with etravirine alone. These changes are not expected to be clinically relevant. In contrast, more dramatic decreases in raltegravir trough concentrations were reported in 4 HIV-infected patients receiving etravirine and raltegravir as part of their antiretroviral therapy.[2] Raltegravir trough concentrations were decreased approximately 97% in 1 patient and were subtherapeutic in another.

Additional studies are needed to determine if this interaction is more clinically relevant in HIV-infected patients compared with healthy subjects.

[1] Anderson MS, et al. *Antimicrob Agents Chemother.* 2008;52(12):4228.

[2] Ménard A, et al. *AIDS.* 2009;23(7):869.

* Asterisk indicates drugs cited in interaction reports. Based on pharmacologic and pharmacokinetic considerations, similar interactions may occur with other drugs that are listed.

Raltegravir — *Protease Inhibitors*

Raltegravir* (*Isentress*)	Ritonavir* (*Norvir*)	Tipranavir* (*Aptivus*)

Significance	Onset	Severity	Documentation
4	☐ Rapid ■ **Delayed**	☐ Major ■ **Moderate** ☐ Minor	☐ Established ☐ Probable ☐ Suspected ■ **Possible** ☐ Unlikely

Effects RALTEGRAVIR trough concentrations may be reduced.

Mechanism Unknown.

Management Based on available data, no special precautions are needed. RALTEGRAVIR and TIPRANAVIR plus RITONAVIR may be given without dosage adjustment.

Discussion

The effects of tipranavir plus ritonavir administration on the pharmacokinetics of raltegravir were evaluated in 15 healthy subjects.[1] Using an open-label, 3-period, fixed-sequence design, each subject received raltegravir 400 mg twice daily for 4 days alone, tipranavir 500 mg plus ritonavir 200 mg twice daily for 7 days without raltegravir, and raltegravir 400 mg twice daily coadministered with tipranavir 500 mg plus ritonavir 200 mg twice daily for 4 days. Compared with administering raltegravir alone, the raltegravir trough concentration was decreased when administered with tipranavir-ritonavir. However, the raltegravir AUC and C_{max} were not substantially altered by tipranavir-ritonavir administration. There are sufficient clinical efficacy data available that demonstrate raltegravir and tipranavir-ritonavir can be coadministered without dose adjustment.[1] See Raltegravir-Atazanavir.

[1] Hanley WD, et al. *Antimicrob Agents Chemother.* 2009;53(7):2752.

* Asterisk indicates drugs cited in interaction reports.

Raltegravir — *Proton Pump Inhibitors*

Raltegravir	Proton Pump Inhibitors	
Raltegravir* (*Isentress*)	Esomeprazole (*Nexium*)	Pantoprazole (eg, *Protonix*)
	Lansoprazole (eg, *Prevacid*)	Rabeprazole (*Aciphex*)
	Omeprazole* (eg, *Prilosec*)	

Significance	Onset	Severity	Documentation
4	□ Rapid	□ Major	□ Established
	■ **Delayed**	■ **Moderate**	□ Probable
		□ Minor	□ Suspected
			■ **Possible**
			□ Unlikely

Effects RALTEGRAVIR plasma concentrations may be elevated, increasing the pharmacologic effects and risk of adverse reactions.

Mechanism Increased solubility and absorption of RALTEGRAVIR as a result of increased gastric pH due to PROTON PUMP INHIBITOR administration is suspected.

Management Monitor the patient for an increase in RALTEGRAVIR adverse reactions. If an interaction is suspected, adjust the raltegravir dose as needed.

Discussion

The effects of omeprazole on the pharmacokinetics of raltegravir were studied in 14 healthy subjects.[1] Using a randomized, crossover design, each subject received a single oral dose of raltegravir 400 mg alone and after 4 days of receiving omeprazole 20 mg once daily. Pretreatment with omeprazole increased the AUC and C_{max} of raltegravir approximately 3- and 4-fold, respectively, compared with giving raltegravir alone.

[1] Iwamoto M, et al. *Clin Infect Dis*. 2009;48(4):489.

* Asterisk indicates drugs cited in interaction reports. Based on pharmacologic and pharmacokinetic considerations, similar interactions may occur with other drugs that are listed.

Raltegravir | **Rifamycins**

Raltegravir* (*Isentress*)		Rifabutin (*Mycobutin*) Rifampin* (eg, *Rifadin*)	Rifapentine (*Priftin*)

Significance	Onset	Severity	Documentation
2	□ Rapid ■ **Delayed**	□ Major ■ **Moderate** □ Minor	□ Established □ Probable ■ **Suspected** □ Possible □ Unlikely

Effects RALTEGRAVIR plasma concentrations may be reduced, decreasing the pharmacologic effects.

Mechanism Increased RALTEGRAVIR metabolic elimination due to uridine diphosphate glucuronosyltransferase 1A1 induction by RIFAMPIN.

Management Coadminister with caution. Dosage escalation of RALTEGRAVIR to 800 mg twice daily is recommended if RIFAMPIN is coadministered.[1]

Discussion

In 2 open-label, 2-period, fixed-sequence studies, the effects of rifampin on the pharmacokinetics of raltegravir were assessed in 9 healthy subjects. In 1 study, subjects received a single dose of raltegravir 400 mg alone and after pretreatment with rifampin 600 mg for 14 days. Compared with taking raltegravir alone, rifampin decreased the raltegravir C_{max}, AUC, and trough concentration by approximately 38%, 40%, and 61%, respectively. In the second study, subjects received raltegravir 400 mg every 12 hours for 4 days. Subsequently, subjects received raltegravir 800 mg every 12 hours plus rifampin 600 mg once daily for 14 days. Compared with administration of raltegravir alone, coadministration of rifampin increased the raltegravir C_{max} and AUC approximately 62% and 27%, respectively; however, the trough concentration was decreased approximately 53%. These 2 studies indicate that coadministration of raltegravir and rifampin is likely to result in raltegravir trough concentrations that are at the lower limit of clinical experience.[2] In a study involving 19 healthy volunteers, rifabutin did not alter the pharmacokinetics of raltegravir.[3] In a case series of 8 HIV-infected patients with tuberculosis, coadministration of raltegravir 800 mg twice daily with an antitubercular regimen containing rifampin resulted in successful treatment of tuberculosis without impairing the antiretroviral effect of raltegravir.[4]

[1] *Isentress* [package insert]. Whitehouse Station, NJ: Merck & Co Inc; July 2009.

[2] Wenning LA, et al. *Antimicrob Agents Chemother.* 2009;53(7):2852.

[3] Brainard DM, et al. *J Clin Pharmacol.* 2011;51(6):943.

[4] Mena A, et al. *J Antimicrob Chemother.* 2011;66(4):951.

* Asterisk indicates drugs cited in interaction reports. Based on pharmacologic and pharmacokinetic considerations, similar interactions may occur with other drugs that are listed.

Ramelteon — *Fluvoxamine*

Ramelteon* (*Rozerem*)	Fluvoxamine* (eg, *Luvox CR*)

Significance	Onset	Severity	Documentation
2	☐ Rapid ■ **Delayed**	☐ Major ■ **Moderate** ☐ Minor	☐ Established ☐ Probable ■ **Suspected** ☐ Possible ☐ Unlikely

Effects RAMELTEON plasma concentrations may be greatly elevated, increasing the risk of adverse reactions.

Mechanism Inhibition of RAMELTEON metabolism (CYP1A2) by FLUVOXAMINE.

Management Do not coadminister RAMELTEON and FLUVOXAMINE. Other SSRIs (eg, citalopram [eg, *Celexa*], escitalopram [*Lexapro*], fluoxetine [eg, *Prozac*]) may be safer alternatives.

Discussion

Subjects received fluvoxamine 100 mg twice daily for 3 days prior to the administration of a single dose of ramelteon 16 mg with fluvoxamine.[1] Compared with ramelteon administered alone, pretreatment with fluvoxamine increased the AUC and C_{max} of ramelteon approximately 190- and 70-fold, respectively. Ramelteon and fluvoxamine should not be used concurrently.

The basis for this monograph is information on file with the manufacturer.

[1] *Rozerem* [package insert]. Deerfield, IL: Takeda Pharmaceuticals; April 2006.

* Asterisk indicates drugs cited in interaction reports.

Ranitidine — *Antacids*

Ranitidine	Antacids	
Ranitidine* (eg, *Zantac*)	Aluminum Hydroxide (eg, *Alternagel*)	Magnesium Hydroxide (eg, *Milk of Magnesia*)
	Aluminum/Magnesium Hydroxide* (eg, *Maalox*)	

Significance	Onset	Severity	Documentation
5	□ Rapid	□ Major	□ Established
	■ **Delayed**	□ Moderate	□ Probable
		■ **Minor**	□ Suspected
			■ **Possible**
			□ Unlikely

Effects The bioavailability of RANITIDINE may be reduced, decreasing the pharmacologic effect.

Mechanism Unknown.

Management Based on available data, no clinical intervention is needed.

Discussion

Studies of this interaction have produced conflicting results. Two crossover studies in healthy volunteers showed that coadministration of antacid reduced ranitidine bioavailability approximately one-third.[1,2] In 1 study, 6 subjects received ranitidine 150 mg orally alone or in combination with 30 mL of *Mylanta II* (magnesium/aluminum hydroxide plus simethicone), which has an acid neutralizing capacity of 125 mEq per 30 mL.[1] The C_{max} and AUC were reduced 30% and 33%, respectively. A similar study in 10 subjects using 11 g of aluminum phosphate gel reported reductions in C_{max} and AUC of 40% and 30%, respectively. A study in 12 subjects using 30 mL of *Maalox* (magnesium/aluminum hydroxide, 80 mEq per 30 mL neutralizing capacity) failed to show any significant effect on ranitidine absorption.[3] Another study of 11 volunteers also failed to show any effect on ranitidine absorption when antacid (approximately 48 mEq neutralizing capacity) was given 1 and 3 hours after oral ranitidine 150 mg.[4] Acid neutralizing capabilities of the antacids may account for the conflicting results.

The combination of antacids and ranitidine has been used clinically, with no apparent reduction in ulcer healing rates. Because the investigations that demonstrated an interaction did not determine the clinical practicality of the reduced bioavailability, the clinical significance of such an interaction cannot be assessed.

[1] Mihaly GW, et al. *Br Med J.* 1982;285(6347):998.
[2] Albin H, et al. *Eur J Clin Pharmacol.* 1987;32(1):97.
[3] Donn KH, et al. *Pharmacotherapy.* 1984;4(2):89.
[4] Frislid K, et al. *Br Med J.* 1983;286(6374):1358.

* Asterisk indicates drugs cited in interaction reports. Based on pharmacologic and pharmacokinetic considerations, similar interactions may occur with other drugs that are listed.

Ranolazine — *Aprepitant*

Ranolazine* (*Ranexa*)	Aprepitant* (*Emend*)

Significance	Onset	Severity	Documentation
2	☐ Rapid	☐ Major	☐ Established
	■ **Delayed**	■ **Moderate**	☐ Probable
		☐ Minor	■ **Suspected**
			☐ Possible
			☐ Unlikely

Effects RANOLAZINE plasma concentrations may be elevated, increasing the pharmacologic effects and risk of toxicity.

Mechanism APREPITANT inhibits the metabolism (CYP3A4) of RANOLAZINE.

Management Closely monitor patients for RANOLAZINE toxicity, including QT interval prolongation, during coadministration of APREPITANT. Limit the RANOLAZINE dosage to 500 mg twice daily.[1]

Discussion

Data from coadministration of ranolazine with diltiazem or verapamil indicate that moderate CYP3A inhibitors increase ranolazine steady-state plasma concentrations. It is recommended that the dosage of ranolazine be limited to 500 mg daily in patients receiving moderate CYP3A inhibitors (eg, aprepitant).[1]

Ranolazine prolongs the QTc interval in a dose-related manner. The relationship between the change in the QTc interval and ranolazine plasma concentrations is linear through doses that are several-fold higher than the maximum recommended dose of ranolazine (1,000 mg twice daily).[1]

The basis for this monograph is information on file with the manufacturer. Published clinical data are needed to further assess this interaction.

[1] *Ranexa* [package insert]. Palo Alto, CA: CV Therapeutics, Inc; November 2008.

* Asterisk indicates drugs cited in interaction reports.

Ranolazine — *Azole Antifungal Agents*

Ranolazine* (*Ranexa*)	Itraconazole* (eg, *Sporanox*)	Ketoconazole* (eg, *Nizoral*)

Significance	Onset	Severity	Documentation
1	☐ Rapid ■ **Delayed**	■ **Major** ☐ Moderate ☐ Minor	☐ Established ☐ Probable ■ **Suspected** ☐ Possible ☐ Unlikely

Effects RANOLAZINE plasma concentrations may be elevated, increasing the pharmacologic effects and risk of toxicity.

Mechanism AZOLE ANTIFUNGAL AGENTS inhibit the metabolism (CYP3A4) of RANOLAZINE.

Management Coadministration of RANOLAZINE and certain AZOLE ANTIFUNGAL AGENTS is contraindicated.[1]

Discussion

Ketoconazole 200 mg twice daily increased the average ranolazine steady-state plasma concentration 3.2-fold. Coadministration of ranolazine to patients receiving strong CYP3A inhibitors (eg, itraconazole, ketoconazole) is contraindicated. Ranolazine prolongs the QTc interval in a dose-related manner. The relationship between the change in the QTc interval and ranolazine plasma concentrations is linear through doses that are several-fold higher than the maximum recommended dose of ranolazine (1,000 mg twice daily). Coadministration of ranolazine with a strong CYP3A inhibitor may increase the risk of ranolazine-associated QT prolongation.[1]

The basis for this monograph is information on file with the manufacturer. Published clinical data are needed to further assess this interaction. See also Ranolazine-Fluconazole.

[1] *Ranexa* [package insert]. Palo Alto, CA: CV Therapeutics, Inc; November 2008.

* Asterisk indicates drugs cited in interaction reports.

Ranolazine — *Barbiturates*

Ranolazine* (*Ranexa*)	Phenobarbital* (eg, *Solfoton*)

Significance	Onset	Severity	Documentation
2	☐ Rapid ■ **Delayed**	☐ Major ■ **Moderate** ☐ Minor	☐ Established ☐ Probable ■ **Suspected** ☐ Possible ☐ Unlikely

Effects RANOLAZINE plasma concentrations may be reduced, decreasing the pharmacologic effect.

Mechanism PHENOBARBITAL may increase the metabolism (CYP3A4) of RANOLAZINE.

Management Coadministration of RANOLAZINE and CYP3A inducers such as PHENOBARBITAL is contraindicated.[1]

Discussion

Data from coadministration of ranolazine and rifampin indicate that CYP3A inducers decrease ranolazine plasma concentrations. Coadministration of ranolazine and CYP3A inducers (eg, phenobarbital) should be avoided.[1]

The basis for this monograph is information on file with the manufacturer. Published clinical data are needed to further assess this interaction.

[1] *Ranexa* [package insert]. Palo Alto, CA: CV Therapeutics, Inc; November 2008.

* Asterisk indicates drugs cited in interaction reports.

Ranolazine — *Carbamazepine*

Ranolazine* (*Ranexa*)	Carbamazepine* (eg, *Tegretol*)

Significance	Onset	Severity	Documentation
2	☐ Rapid ■ **Delayed**	☐ Major ■ **Moderate** ☐ Minor	☐ Established ☐ Probable ■ **Suspected** ☐ Possible ☐ Unlikely

Effects RANOLAZINE plasma concentrations may be reduced, decreasing the pharmacologic effect.

Mechanism CARBAMAZEPINE may increase the metabolism (CYP3A4) of RANOLAZINE.

Management Coadministration of RANOLAZINE and CYP3A inducers such as CARBAMAZEPINE is contraindicated.[1]

Discussion

Data from coadministration of ranolazine and rifampin indicate that CYP3A inducers decrease ranolazine plasma concentrations. Coadministration of ranolazine and CYP3A inducers (eg, carbamazepine) should be avoided.[1]

The basis for this monograph is information on file with the manufacturer. Published clinical data are needed to further assess this interaction.

[1] *Ranexa* [package insert]. Palo Alto, CA: CV Therapeutics, Inc; November 2008.

* Asterisk indicates drugs cited in interaction reports.

Ranolazine | *Diltiazem*

Ranolazine* (*Ranexa*)	Diltiazem* (eg, *Cardizem*)

Significance	Onset	Severity	Documentation
2	☐ Rapid ■ **Delayed**	☐ Major ■ **Moderate** ☐ Minor	☐ Established ☐ Probable ■ **Suspected** ☐ Possible ☐ Unlikely

Effects RANOLAZINE plasma concentrations may be elevated, increasing the pharmacologic effects and risk of toxicity.

Mechanism DILTIAZEM inhibits the metabolism (CYP3A4) of RANOLAZINE.

Management Closely monitor patients for RANOLAZINE toxicity, including QT interval prolongation, during coadministration of DILTIAZEM. Limit the RANOLAZINE dosage to 500 mg twice daily.[1]

Discussion

Diltiazem 180 to 360 mg daily increased the ranolazine steady-state plasma concentration approximately 2-fold. It is recommended that the dosage of ranolazine be limited to 500 mg daily in patients receiving moderate CYP3A inhibitors (eg, diltiazem). The pharmacokinetics of diltiazem are not affected by ranolazine.[1]

Ranolazine prolongs the QTc interval in a dose-related manner. The relationship between the change in the QTc interval and ranolazine plasma concentrations is linear through doses that are several-fold higher than the maximum recommended dose of ranolazine (1,000 mg twice daily).[1]

The basis for this monograph is information on file with the manufacturer. Published clinical data are needed to further assess this interaction.

[1] *Ranexa* [package insert]. Palo Alto, CA: CV Therapeutics, Inc; November 2008.

* Asterisk indicates drugs cited in interaction reports.

Ranolazine — *Erythromycin*

Ranolazine* (*Ranexa*)	Erythromycin* (eg, *Ery-Tab*)

Significance	Onset	Severity	Documentation
2	☐ Rapid ■ **Delayed**	☐ Major ■ **Moderate** ☐ Minor	☐ Established ☐ Probable ■ **Suspected** ☐ Possible ☐ Unlikely

Effects RANOLAZINE plasma concentrations may be elevated, increasing the pharmacologic effects and risk of toxicity.

Mechanism ERYTHROMYCIN inhibits the metabolism (CYP3A4) of RANOLAZINE.

Management Closely monitor patients for RANOLAZINE toxicity, including QT interval prolongation, during coadministration of ERYTHROMYCIN. Limit the RANOLAZINE dosage to 500 mg twice daily.[1]

Discussion

Data from coadministration of ranolazine with diltiazem or verapamil indicate that moderate CYP3A inhibitors increase ranolazine steady-state plasma concentrations. It is recommended that the dosage of ranolazine be limited to 500 mg daily in patients receiving moderate CYP3A inhibitors (eg, erythromycin).[1]

Ranolazine prolongs the QTc interval in a dose-related manner. The relationship between the change in the QTc interval and ranolazine plasma concentrations is linear through doses that are several-fold higher than the maximum recommended dose of ranolazine (1,000 mg twice daily).[1]

The basis for this monograph is information on file with the manufacturer. Published clinical data are needed to further assess this interaction. See also Ranolazine-Macrolide & Related Antibiotics.

[1] *Ranexa* [package insert]. Palo Alto, CA: CV Therapeutics, Inc; November 2008.

* Asterisk indicates drugs cited in interaction reports.

Ranolazine — *Fluconazole*

Ranolazine* (*Ranexa*)	Fluconazole* (eg, *Diflucan*)

Significance	Onset	Severity	Documentation
2	☐ Rapid ■ **Delayed**	☐ Major ■ **Moderate** ☐ Minor	☐ Established ☐ Probable ■ **Suspected** ☐ Possible ☐ Unlikely

Effects RANOLAZINE plasma concentrations may be elevated, increasing the pharmacologic effects and risk of toxicity.

Mechanism FLUCONAZOLE inhibits the metabolism (CYP3A4) of RANOLAZINE.

Management Closely monitor patients for RANOLAZINE toxicity, including QT interval prolongation, during coadministration of FLUCONAZOLE. Limit the RANOLAZINE dosage to 500 mg twice daily.[1]

Discussion

Data from coadministration of ranolazine with diltiazem or verapamil indicate that moderate CYP3A inhibitors increase ranolazine steady-state plasma concentrations. It is recommended that the dosage of ranolazine be limited to 500 mg daily in patients receiving moderate CYP3A inhibitors (eg, fluconazole).[1]

Ranolazine prolongs the QTc interval in a dose-related manner. The relationship between the change in the QTc interval and ranolazine plasma concentrations is linear through doses that are several-fold higher than the maximum recommended dose of ranolazine (1,000 mg twice daily).[1]

The basis for this monograph is information on file with the manufacturer. Published clinical data are needed to further assess this interaction. See also Ranolazine-Azole Antifungal Agents.

[1] *Ranexa* [package insert]. Palo Alto, CA: CV Therapeutics, Inc; November 2008.

* Asterisk indicates drugs cited in interaction reports.

Ranolazine — *Food*

Ranolazine* (*Ranexa*)	Grapefruit Juice*

Significance	Onset	Severity	Documentation
2	☐ Rapid ■ **Delayed**	☐ Major ■ **Moderate** ☐ Minor	☐ Established ☐ Probable ■ **Suspected** ☐ Possible ☐ Unlikely

Effects RANOLAZINE plasma concentrations may be elevated, increasing the pharmacologic effects and risk of toxicity.

Mechanism GRAPEFRUIT JUICE inhibits the metabolism (CYP3A4) of RANOLAZINE.

Management Caution patients to avoid GRAPEFRUIT products while taking RANOLAZINE. RANOLAZINE should be taken with a liquid other than GRAPEFRUIT JUICE.

Discussion

Data from coadministration of ranolazine with diltiazem or verapamil indicate that moderate CYP3A inhibitors increase ranolazine steady-state plasma concentrations. It is recommended that the dosage of ranolazine be limited to 500 mg daily in patients receiving moderate CYP3A inhibitors (eg, grapefruit-containing products).[1]

Ranolazine prolongs the QTc interval in a dose-related manner. The relationship between the change in the QTc interval and ranolazine plasma concentrations is linear through doses that are several-fold higher than the maximum recommended dose of ranolazine (1,000 mg twice daily).[1]

The basis for this monograph is information on file with the manufacturer. Published clinical data are needed to further assess this interaction.

[1] *Ranexa* [package insert]. Palo Alto, CA: CV Therapeutics, Inc; November 2008.

* Asterisk indicates drugs cited in interaction reports.

Ranolazine — *Hydantoins*

Ranolazine* (*Ranexa*)	Phenytoin* (eg, *Dilantin*)

Significance	Onset	Severity	Documentation
2	☐ Rapid ■ **Delayed**	☐ Major ■ **Moderate** ☐ Minor	☐ Established ☐ Probable ■ **Suspected** ☐ Possible ☐ Unlikely

Effects RANOLAZINE plasma concentrations may be reduced, decreasing the pharmacologic effect.

Mechanism PHENYTOIN may increase the metabolism (CYP3A4) of RANOLAZINE.

Management Coadministration of RANOLAZINE and CYP3A inducers such as PHENYTOIN is contraindicated.[1]

Discussion

Data from coadministration of ranolazine and rifampin indicate that CYP3A inducers decrease ranolazine plasma concentrations. Avoid coadministration of ranolazine and CYP3A inducers (eg, phenytoin).[1]

The basis for this monograph is information on file with the manufacturer. Published clinical data are needed to further assess this interaction.

[1] *Ranexa* [package insert]. Palo Alto, CA: CV Therapeutics, Inc; November 2008.

* Asterisk indicates drugs cited in interaction reports.

Ranolazine | **Macrolide & Related Antibiotics**

Ranolazine* (*Ranexa*)	Clarithromycin (eg, *Biaxin*)	Telithromycin* (*Ketek*)

Significance	Onset	Severity	Documentation
1	□ Rapid	■ **Major**	□ Established
	■ **Delayed**	□ Moderate	□ Probable
		□ Minor	■ **Suspected**
			□ Possible
			□ Unlikely

Effects RANOLAZINE plasma concentrations may be elevated, increasing the pharmacologic effects and risk of toxicity.

Mechanism MACROLIDE AND RELATED ANTIBIOTICS may inhibit the metabolism (CYP3A4) of RANOLAZINE.

Management Coadministration of RANOLAZINE and certain MACROLIDE AND RELATED ANTIBIOTICS is contraindicated.[1]

Discussion

Data from coadministration of ranolazine and ketoconazole indicate that strong CYP3A inhibitors increase ranolazine steady-state plasma concentrations. Coadministration of ranolazine to patients receiving strong CYP3A inhibitors (eg, clarithromycin) is contraindicated. Ranolazine prolongs the QTc interval in a dose-related manner. The relationship between the change in the QTc interval and ranolazine plasma concentrations is linear through doses that are several-fold higher than the maximum recommended dose of ranolazine (1,000 mg twice daily). Coadministration of ranolazine with a strong CYP3A inhibitor may increase the risk of ranolazine-associated QT prolongation.[1]

The basis for this monograph is information on file with the manufacturer. Published clinical data are needed to further assess this interaction. See also Ranolazine-Erythromycin.

1 *Ranexa* [package insert]. Palo Alto, CA: CV Therapeutics, Inc; November 2008.

* Asterisk indicates drugs cited in interaction reports. Based on pharmacologic and pharmacokinetic considerations, similar interactions may occur with other drugs that are listed.

Ranolazine ✕ *Nefazodone*

Ranolazine* (*Ranexa*)	Nefazodone*

Significance	Onset	Severity	Documentation
1	□ Rapid	■ **Major**	□ Established
	■ **Delayed**	□ Moderate	□ Probable
		□ Minor	■ **Suspected**
			□ Possible
			□ Unlikely

Effects RANOLAZINE plasma concentrations may be elevated, increasing the pharmacologic effects and risk of toxicity.

Mechanism NEFAZODONE may inhibit the metabolism (CYP3A4) of RANOLAZINE.

Management Coadministration of RANOLAZINE and NEFAZODONE is contraindicated.[1]

Discussion

Data from coadministration of ranolazine and ketoconazole indicate that strong CYP3A inhibitors may increase ranolazine steady-state plasma concentrations. Coadministration of ranolazine to patients receiving strong CYP3A inhibitors (eg, nefazodone) is contraindicated. Ranolazine prolongs the QTc interval in a dose-related manner. The relationship between the change in the QTc interval and ranolazine plasma concentrations is linear through doses that are several-fold higher than the maximum recommended dose of ranolazine (1,000 mg twice daily).[1] Coadministration of ranolazine with a strong CYP3A inhibitor may increase the risk of ranolazine-associated QT prolongation.

The basis for this monograph is information on file with the manufacturer. Published clinical data are needed to further assess this interaction.

[1] *Ranexa* [package insert]. Palo Alto, CA: CV Therapeutics, Inc; November 2008.

* Asterisk indicates drugs cited in interaction reports.

Ranolazine — *Protease Inhibitors*

Ranolazine	Protease Inhibitors	
Ranolazine* (*Ranexa*)	Atazanavir (*Reyataz*)	Nelfinavir* (*Viracept*)
	Fosamprenavir (*Lexiva*)	Ritonavir* (*Norvir*)
	Indinavir* (*Crixivan*)	Saquinavir* (*Invirase*)
	Lopinavir/Ritonavir (*Kaletra*)	

Significance	Onset	Severity	Documentation
1	☐ Rapid	■ **Major**	☐ Established
	■ **Delayed**	☐ Moderate	☐ Probable
		☐ Minor	■ **Suspected**
			☐ Possible
			☐ Unlikely

Effects RANOLAZINE plasma concentrations may be elevated, increasing the pharmacologic effects and risk of toxicity.

Mechanism Certain PROTEASE INHIBITORS may inhibit the metabolism (CYP3A4) of RANOLAZINE.

Management Coadministration of RANOLAZINE and certain PROTEASE INHIBITORS is contraindicated.[1]

Discussion

Data from coadministration of ranolazine and ketoconazole indicate that strong CYP3A inhibitors increase ranolazine steady-state plasma concentrations. Coadministration of ranolazine to patients receiving strong CYP3A inhibitors (eg, indinavir, nelfinavir, ritonavir, saquinavir) is contraindicated.[1] Ranolazine prolongs the QTc interval in a dose-related manner. The relationship between the change in the QTc interval and ranolazine plasma concentrations is linear through doses that are several-fold higher than the maximum recommended dose of ranolazine (1,000 mg twice daily).[1] Coadministration of ranolazine with a strong CYP3A inhibitor may increase the risk of ranolazine-associated QT prolongation.

The basis for this monograph is information on file with the manufacturer. Published clinical data are needed to further assess this interaction.

[1] *Ranexa* [package insert]. Palo Alto, CA: CV Therapeutics, Inc; November 2008.

* Asterisk indicates drugs cited in interaction reports. Based on pharmacologic and pharmacokinetic considerations, similar interactions may occur with other drugs that are listed.

Ranolazine — *Rifamycins*

Ranolazine	Rifamycins	
Ranolazine* (*Ranexa*)	Rifabutin* (*Mycobutin*) Rifampin* (eg, *Rifadin*)	Rifapentine* (*Priftin*)

Significance	Onset	Severity	Documentation
2	☐ Rapid ■ **Delayed**	☐ Major ■ **Moderate** ☐ Minor	☐ Established ☐ Probable ■ **Suspected** ☐ Possible ☐ Unlikely

Effects RANOLAZINE plasma concentrations may be reduced, decreasing the pharmacologic effect.

Mechanism RIFAMYCINS may increase the metabolism (CYP3A4) and P-glycoprotein expression of RANOLAZINE.

Management Coadministration of RANOLAZINE and CYP3A inducers such as RIFAMYCINS is contraindicated.[1]

Discussion

Rifampin 600 mg once daily decreased the plasma concentration of ranolazine 1,000 mg twice daily approximately 95%. Avoid coadministration of ranolazine and CYP3A inducers.[1]

The basis for this monograph is information on file with the manufacturer. Published clinical data are needed to further assess this interaction.

[1] *Ranexa* [package insert]. Palo Alto, CA: CV Therapeutics, Inc; November 2008.

* Asterisk indicates drugs cited in interaction reports.

Ranolazine — *St. John's Wort*

Ranolazine* (*Ranexa*)	St. John's Wort*

Significance	Onset	Severity	Documentation
2	☐ Rapid ■ **Delayed**	☐ Major ■ **Moderate** ☐ Minor	☐ Established ☐ Probable ■ **Suspected** ☐ Possible ☐ Unlikely

Effects RANOLAZINE plasma concentrations may be reduced, decreasing the pharmacologic effect.

Mechanism ST. JOHN'S WORT may increase the metabolism (CYP3A4) and P-glycoprotein expression of RANOLAZINE.

Management Coadministration of RANOLAZINE and CYP3A inducers such as ST. JOHN'S WORT is contraindicated.[1]

Discussion

Data from coadministration of ranolazine and rifampin indicate that CYP3A inducers decrease ranolazine plasma concentrations. Avoid coadministration of ranolazine and CYP3A inducers (eg, St. John's wort).[1]

The basis for this monograph is information on file with the manufacturer. Published clinical data are needed to further assess this interaction.

[1] *Ranexa* [package insert]. Palo Alto, CA: CV Therapeutics, Inc; November 2008.

* Asterisk indicates drugs cited in interaction reports.

Ranolazine — *Verapamil*

Ranolazine* (*Ranexa*)	Verapamil* (eg, *Calan*)

Significance	Onset	Severity	Documentation
2	☐ Rapid	☐ Major	☐ Established
	■ **Delayed**	■ **Moderate**	☐ Probable
		☐ Minor	■ **Suspected**
			☐ Possible
			☐ Unlikely

Effects RANOLAZINE plasma concentrations may be elevated, increasing the pharmacologic effects and risk of toxicity.

Mechanism VERAPAMIL inhibits the metabolism (CYP3A4) of RANOLAZINE.

Management Closely monitor patients for RANOLAZINE toxicity, including QT interval prolongation, during coadministration of VERAPAMIL. Limit the RANOLAZINE dosage to 500 mg twice daily.[1]

Discussion

Verapamil 120 mg 3 times daily increased the ranolazine steady-state plasma concentration approximately 2-fold. It is recommended that the dosage of ranolazine be limited to 500 mg daily in patients receiving moderate CYP3A inhibitors (eg, verapamil).[1]

Ranolazine prolongs the QTc interval in a dose-related manner. The relationship between the change in the QTc interval and ranolazine plasma concentrations is linear through doses that are several-fold higher than the maximum recommended dose of ranolazine (1,000 mg twice daily).[1]

The basis for this monograph is information on file with the manufacturer. Published clinical data are needed to further assess this interaction.

[1] *Ranexa* [package insert]. Palo Alto, CA: CV Therapeutics, Inc; November 2008.

* Asterisk indicates drugs cited in interaction reports.

Rasagiline — *St. John's Wort*

Rasagiline* (*Azilect*)	St. John's Wort*

Significance	Onset	Severity	Documentation
1	☐ Rapid	■ **Major**	☐ Established
	■ **Delayed**	☐ Moderate	☐ Probable
		☐ Minor	■ **Suspected**
			☐ Possible
			☐ Unlikely

Effects The risk of serotonin syndrome or hypertensive crisis may be increased.

Mechanism Unknown.

Management RASAGILINE is contraindicated in patients taking ST. JOHN'S WORT.[1]

Discussion

Rasagiline administration is contraindicated in patients receiving other MAOIs because of the increased risk of hypertensive crisis.[1] Allow at least 14 days to elapse between discontinuation of rasagiline and initiation of MAOI therapy. Also, do not coadminister rasagiline with SSRIs.[1] Hyperforin, a major constituent of St. John's wort, is a potent SRI.[2] In addition, there are conflicting data as to whether another component of St. John's wort, hypericin, has MAOI activity.[2] The potential for a serious interaction contraindicates the concurrent use of rasagiline with St. John's wort.

[1] *Azilect* [package insert]. Kansas City, MO: Teva Neuroscience, Inc; May 16, 2006.

[2] DerMarderosian A, Beutler JA, eds. *The Review of Natural Products.* 4th ed. St. Louis, MO: Wolters Kluwer Health, Inc; 2005:1083.

* Asterisk indicates drugs cited in interaction reports.

Rauwolfia Alkaloids ✕ *General Anesthetics*

Rauwolfia*	Reserpine*	General Anesthetics*

Significance	Onset	Severity	Documentation
4	■ **Rapid** □ Delayed	□ Major ■ **Moderate** □ Minor	□ Established □ Probable □ Suspected ■ **Possible** □ Unlikely

Effects Patients taking RAUWOLFIA ALKALOIDS may demonstrate cardiovascular instability, manifested mostly as hypotension, when subjected to GENERAL ANESTHESIA.

Mechanism Depletion of neurotransmitters by RAUWOLFIA ALKALOIDS is possible.

Management If hypotension occurs during GENERAL ANESTHESIA in a patient treated with RAUWOLFIA ALKALOIDS, look for causes other than the RAUWOLFIA. If a pressor drug is required, use a direct-acting sympathomimetic rather than a mixed-acting drug, thereby avoiding any effect of neurotransmitter depletion mediated by RAUWOLFIA ALKALOIDS.[1]

Discussion

Early literature consisting primarily of anecdotal reports indicated that patients treated with rauwolfia alkaloids were at an increased risk of developing hypotension and bradycardia when receiving general anesthesia.[2-4] However, other evaluations of this interaction indicate that rauwolfia-treated patients are not exposed to any special risk.[5-8] In one series, 22 of 42 patients on reserpine at the time of surgery demonstrated neurocirculatory instability compared with 7 of 16 patients who had been withdrawn from reserpine at least 8 days prior to surgery.[5] In a comparison of 100 reserpine-treated hypertensive patients with 100 non–reserpine-treated hypertensive patients receiving general anesthesia, 18 of the reserpine-treated patients demonstrated a 30% or greater reduction in systolic BP compared with 30 of the control patients.[8]

There is no evidence to support the routine discontinuation of rauwolfia alkaloids 1 to 2 weeks before general anesthesia or to delay necessary surgery because of therapy with these drugs.[1]

1 Ominsky AJ, et al. *Anesthesiology*. 1969;30(4):443.
2 Coakley CS, et al. *J Am Med Assoc*. 1956; 161(12):1143.
3 Ziegler CH, et al. *JAMA*. 1961;176:916.
4 Smessaert AA, et al. *N Y State J Med*. 1961;61:2399.
5 Munson WM, et al. *Anesthesiology*. 1962;23:741.
6 Morrow DH, et al. *Br J Anaesth*. 1963;35(5):313.
7 Alper MH, et al. *Anesthesiology*. 1963;24:524.
8 Katz RL, et al. *Anesthesiology*. 1964;25:142.

* Asterisk indicates drugs cited in interaction reports.

Red Yeast Rice — *Cyclosporine*

Red Yeast Rice*	Cyclosporine* (eg, *Neoral*)

Significance	Onset	Severity	Documentation
4	□ Rapid ■ **Delayed**	■ **Major** □ Moderate □ Minor	□ Established □ Probable □ Suspected ■ **Possible** □ Unlikely

Effects Risk of HMG-CoA reductase inhibitor–like adverse reactions (eg, rhabdomyolysis) may be increased.

Mechanism Elevated plasma concentrations of HMG-CoA reductase inhibitor–like component(s) of RED YEAST RICE caused by inhibition of metabolism by CYCLOSPORINE is suspected.

Management Caution patients receiving CYCLOSPORINE against ingesting RED YEAST RICE or other herbal products to lower cholesterol. Advise patients taking CYCLOSPORINE to inform their health care provider before using OTC or herbal products.

Discussion

A 28-year-old woman who received a live-donor allograft 6 years earlier for end-stage renal disease was receiving posttransplant medications, one of which was cyclosporine 300 mg/day.[1] Two months after starting an herbal preparation containing rice fermented with red yeast, the patient was diagnosed with rhabdomyolysis and her serum creatine phosphokinase (CPK) was 2,600 units/L. Two weeks after stopping the red yeast preparation, the patient was clinically well and her CPK was 600 units/L. Red yeast contains several naturally occurring mevinic acid compounds (eg, lovastatin [eg, *Mevacor*]), which possess HMG-CoA reductase inhibitor activity. It was postulated that cyclosporine inhibited the metabolism of these compounds, resulting in elevated plasma concentrations of the HMG-CoA reductase inhibitor and, subsequently, rhabdomyolysis. See also HMG-CoA Reductase Inhibitors-Cyclosporine.

[1] Prasad GV, et al. *Transplantation.* 2002;74(8):1200.

* Asterisk indicates drugs cited in interaction reports.

Repaglinide ✕ *Azole Antifungal Agents*

Repaglinide* (*Prandin*)	Itraconazole (eg, *Sporanox*)	Ketoconazole* (eg, *Nizoral*)

Significance	Onset	Severity	Documentation
4	☐ Rapid ■ **Delayed**	☐ Major ■ **Moderate** ☐ Minor	☐ Established ☐ Probable ☐ Suspected ■ **Possible** ☐ Unlikely

Effects Certain AZOLE ANTIFUNGAL AGENTS may elevate REPAGLINIDE plasma concentrations, increasing the pharmacologic effects.

Mechanism Inhibition of REPAGLINIDE metabolism (CYP3A4) by certain AZOLE ANTIFUNGAL AGENTS is suspected.

Management In patients receiving REPAGLINIDE, carefully monitor blood glucose levels when the AZOLE ANTIFUNGAL AGENT is started or stopped. Adjust the REPAGLINIDE dose as needed.

Discussion

The effects of ketoconazole on the pharmacokinetics, pharmacodynamics, and safety of repaglinide were studied in healthy volunteers.[1] Using an open-label, 2-period, randomized, crossover design, 8 healthy men received repaglinide 2 mg alone and on day 5 of ketoconazole (200 mg daily for 5 days) administration. Compared with administering repaglinide alone, administration after pretreatment with ketoconazole increased the mean bioavailability and C_{max} of repaglinide 15% and 7%, respectively. Ketoconazole administration altered the blood glucose profile of repaglinide less than 8%. The safety profile of repaglinide was not altered by ketoconazole administration.

[1] Hatorp V, et al. *J Clin Pharmacol.* 2003;43(6):649.

* Asterisk indicates drugs cited in interaction reports. Based on pharmacologic and pharmacokinetic considerations, similar interactions may occur with other drugs that are listed.

Repaglinide		***Colesevelam***
Repaglinide* (*Prandin*)		Colesevelam* (*Welchol*)

Significance	Onset	Severity	Documentation
3	☐ Rapid	☐ Major	☐ Established
	■ **Delayed**	☐ Moderate	☐ Probable
		■ **Minor**	■ **Suspected**
			☐ Possible
			☐ Unlikely

Effects REPAGLINIDE concentrations may be reduced; however, total exposure to repaglinide is not likely to be altered.

Mechanism COLESEVELAM may bind with REPAGLINIDE in the GI tract, decreasing REPAGLINIDE absorption.

Management Based on available data, no special precautions are needed.

Discussion

Using an open-label, randomized design, the effects of colesevelam on the pharmacokinetics of repaglinide were evaluated in 33 healthy volunteers.[1] Each subject received repaglinide 2 mg simultaneously with colesevelam 3,750 mg, repaglinide 2 mg 1 hour before colesevelam 3,750 mg, and repaglinide 2 mg alone. Coadministration of repaglinide and colesevelam decreased the maximum exposure to repaglinide (the geometric least square mean [LSM] ratio C_{max} 80.6%) compared with giving repaglinide alone. However, total repaglinide exposure was not affected. When repaglinide was administered 1 hour before colesevelam, the geometric LSM for all parameters was not affected.

[1] Brown KS, et al. *J Clin Pharmacol.* 2010;50(5):554.

* Asterisk indicates drugs cited in interaction reports.

Repaglinide — *Deferasirox*

Repaglinide* (*Prandin*)	Deferasirox* (*Exjade*)

Significance	Onset	Severity	Documentation
4	☐ Rapid ■ **Delayed**	☐ Major ■ **Moderate** ☐ Minor	☐ Established ☐ Probable ☐ Suspected ■ **Possible** ☐ Unlikely

Effects REPAGLINIDE plasma concentrations may be elevated, increasing the pharmacologic effects and risk of adverse reactions.

Mechanism DEFERASIROX may inhibit the metabolism (CYP2C8) of REPAGLINIDE.

Management Carefully monitor blood glucose when DEFERASIROX is started or stopped in patients receiving REPAGLINIDE.[1] Adjust the REPAGLINIDE dose as needed.

Discussion

The effects of deferasirox on the pharmacokinetics of repaglinide were studied in 24 healthy men.[2] Each subject received deferasirox 30 mg/kg/day or placebo for 4 days. On day 4, repaglinide 0.5 mg was administered. Compared with placebo, pretreatment with deferasirox increased both the repaglinide C_{max} and AUC 2.3-fold. There was little change in blood glucose measurements.

[1] *Exjade* [package insert]. East Hanover, NJ: Novartis Pharmaceuticals Corporation; January 2010.

[2] Skerjanec A, et al. *J Clin Pharmacol.* 2010;50(2):205.

* Asterisk indicates drugs cited in interaction reports.

Repaglinide | **Gemfibrozil**

Repaglinide* (*Prandin*)	Gemfibrozil* (eg, *Lopid*)

Significance	Onset	Severity	Documentation
1	□ Rapid ■ **Delayed**	■ **Major** □ Moderate □ Minor	□ Established ■ **Probable** □ Suspected □ Possible □ Unlikely

Effects REPAGLINIDE plasma concentrations may be greatly increased and prolonged, increasing the risk of severe and protracted hypoglycemia.

Mechanism Inhibition of REPAGLINIDE metabolism (CYP2C8) by GEMFIBROZIL.

Management Coadministration of REPAGLINIDE and GEMFIBROZIL is contraindicated.[1]

Discussion

The pharmacokinetics and pharmacodynamics of repaglinide were studied in 12 healthy volunteers administered gemfibrozil alone and in combination with itraconazole (eg, *Sporanox*).[2] In a randomized, crossover, placebo-controlled investigation, each subject received gemfibrozil 600 mg, both gemfibrozil and itraconazole, or placebo twice daily for 3 days. On day 3 of each phase, the subjects received repaglinide 0.25 mg. Gemfibrozil increased the repaglinide AUC 8.1-fold and prolonged the $t_{½}$ from 1.3 to 3.7 hours, compared with placebo. The combination of gemfibrozil and itraconazole increased the repaglinide AUC 19.4-fold and prolonged the $t_{½}$ to 6.1 hours. Seven hours after administration of repaglinide, gemfibrozil alone and the combination of gemfibrozil and itraconazole increased plasma concentrations of repaglinide 28.6- and 70.4-fold, respectively, compared with placebo. Although the blood glucose–lowering effect of repaglinide had almost subsided 7 hours after administration when given with the placebo, the effect was enhanced extensively by gemfibrozil and gemfibrozil plus itraconazole. Two subjects required carbohydrate supplementation for symptomatic hypoglycemia during the gemfibrozil-itraconazole phase. Other studies of healthy volunteers have confirmed these results.[3,4] The relationship between the time of gemfibrozil administration to that of repaglinide was studied in 10 healthy volunteers.[5] When repaglinide and gemfibrozil were given at the same time, the repaglinide AUC increased 6.1-fold. The repaglinide AUC increased 4.7-fold, even when repaglinide was administered 12 hours after gemfibrozil. Inhibition of repaglinide metabolism persisted up to 48 hours after the last dose of gemfibrozil.[6]

1 *Prandin* [package insert]. Princeton, NJ: Novo Nordisk Inc; March 2010.
2 Niemi M, et al. *Diabetologia.* 2003;46(3):347.
3 Kalliokoski A, et al. *Clin Pharmacol Ther.* 2008;84(4):488.
4 Honkalammi J, et al. *Clin Pharmacol Ther.* 2012;91(5):846.
5 Tornio A, et al. *Clin Pharmacol Ther.* 2008;84(3):403.
6 Backman JT, et al. *Drug Metab Dispos.* 2009;37(12):2359.

* Asterisk indicates drugs cited in interaction reports.

Repaglinide — HMG-CoA Reductase Inhibitors

Repaglinide* (*Prandin*)	Atorvastatin* (*Lipitor*)

Significance	Onset	Severity	Documentation
4	☐ Rapid ■ **Delayed**	☐ Major ■ **Moderate** ☐ Minor	☐ Established ☐ Probable ☐ Suspected ■ **Possible** ☐ Unlikely

Effects REPAGLINIDE plasma concentrations may be elevated, increasing the pharmacologic effects and adverse reactions.

Mechanism Inhibition of organic anion-transporting polypeptide 1B1 (OATP1B1) by ATORVASTATIN is suspected.

Management In patients receiving REPAGLINIDE, closely monitor blood glucose levels when ATORVASTATIN is started or stopped. Adjust the REPAGLINIDE dose as needed.

Discussion

The effects of atorvastatin on the pharmacokinetics of repaglinide were studied in 24 healthy, nondiabetic subjects.[1] Using a randomized, placebo-controlled, crossover design, each subject received atorvastatin 40 mg at 8 AM and placebo at 8 PM or placebo twice daily for 2 days. On day 3, repaglinide 0.25 mg was administered 1 hour after the dose of atorvastatin or placebo. Atorvastatin increased the repaglinide C_{max} and AUC 41% and 18%, respectively, compared with placebo.

Additional studies are needed to determine if other HMG-CoA reductase inhibitors interact similarly.

[1] Kalliokoski A, et al. *Clin Pharmacol Ther.* 2008;84(4):488.

* Asterisk indicates drugs cited in interaction reports.

Repaglinide ✕ **Macrolide & Related Antibiotics**

Repaglinide	Macrolide & Related Antibiotics	
Repaglinide* (*Prandin*)	Clarithromycin* (eg, *Biaxin*)	Telithromycin* (*Ketek*)
	Erythromycin (eg, *Ery-Tab*)	

Significance	Onset	Severity	Documentation
2	☐ Rapid ■ **Delayed**	☐ Major ■ **Moderate** ☐ Minor	☐ Established ☐ Probable ■ **Suspected** ☐ Possible ☐ Unlikely

Effects Certain MACROLIDE AND RELATED ANTIBIOTICS may elevate REPAGLINIDE plasma levels, increasing the pharmacologic effects and adverse reactions.

Mechanism Certain MACROLIDE AND RELATED ANTIBIOTICS may inhibit metabolism (CYP3A4) of REPAGLINIDE.

Management In patients receiving REPAGLINIDE, carefully monitor blood glucose levels when starting or stopping MACROLIDE AND RELATED ANTIBIOTIC therapy. Adjust the REPAGLINIDE dose as needed. Azithromycin (eg, *Zithromax*) does not inhibit CYP3A4 and may be a safer alternative.

Discussion

Severe hypoglycemia (blood glucose less than 30 mg/dL) was reported in an 80-year-old man receiving repaglinide 2 days after starting clarithromycin plus ampicillin (eg, *Principen*).[1] The effects of clarithromycin on the pharmacokinetics and pharmacodynamics of repaglinide were studied in 9 healthy volunteers.[2] Using a randomized, double-blind, 2-phase, crossover design, each subject was pretreated for 4 days with oral clarithromycin 250 mg or placebo twice daily. On day 5, each subject received clarithromycin 250 mg or placebo followed 1 hour later by a single oral dose of repaglinide 0.25 mg. Compared with placebo, clarithromycin administration increased the mean total AUC of repaglinide approximately 42% and the peak plasma concentration approximately 66% (from 4.4 to 7.3 ng/mL), and prolonged the elimination $t_{1/2}$ approximately 22% (from 1.4 to 1.7 hours). In addition, compared with placebo, clarithromycin increased the serum insulin mean incremental AUC (0 to 3) 51% and the maximum increase in serum insulin concentration 61%. The effect of telithromycin on the pharmacokinetics of repaglinide was studied in 12 healthy subjects.[3] Each subject received telithromycin 800 mg/day for 3 days and, on day 3, a single dose of repaglinide was administered. Compared with placebo, telithromycin increased the repaglinide C_{max} and AUC 38% and 77%, respectively, resulting in a decrease in blood glucose.

[1] Khamaisi M, et al. *Pharmacotherapy.* 2008;28(5):682.
[2] Niemi M, et al. *Clin Pharmacol Ther.* 2001;70(1):58.
[3] Kajosaari LI, et al. *Clin Pharmacol Ther.* 2006; 79(3):231.

* Asterisk indicates drugs cited in interaction reports. Based on pharmacologic and pharmacokinetic considerations, similar interactions may occur with other drugs that are listed.

Repaglinide | **_Quinolones_**

Repaglinide*
(*Prandin*)

Gatifloxacin*
(*Zymar*)

Significance	Onset	Severity	Documentation
4	■ **Rapid** ☐ Delayed	☐ Major ■ **Moderate** ☐ Minor	☐ Established ☐ Probable ☐ Suspected ■ **Possible** ☐ Unlikely

Effects Severe and persistent hypoglycemia may occur.

Mechanism Unknown; however, GATIFLOXACIN does not affect glucose tolerance or pancreatic beta-cell function.[1]

Management Until more information is available, consider avoiding GATIFLOXACIN in patients receiving REPAGLINIDE therapy. If therapy cannot be avoided, closely monitor blood glucose when starting GATIFLOXACIN. If hypoglycemia occurs, it may be necessary to discontinue both agents before resuming REPAGLINIDE therapy.

Discussion

Severe and persistent hypoglycemia was reported in a 74-year-old man with type 2 diabetes mellitus during administration of gatifloxacin and repaglinide.[2] The patient was receiving repaglinide 0.5 mg every 8 hours for diabetes. His blood glucose was 76 mg/dL prior to gatifloxacin 400 mg/day administration. Repaglinide was discontinued 6 hours after giving gatifloxacin because of a lack of appetite. Two hours after the second dose of gatifloxacin, the patient experienced a tonic-clonic seizure (blood glucose 27 mg/dL). The patient remained hypoglycemic for the next 32 hours. However, blood glucose returned to the normal range after administration of IV dextrose and discontinuation of gatifloxacin. Therapy with repaglinide was resumed 4 days later without further episodes of hypoglycemia.

Additional studies are needed to determine if this possible interaction occurs with other quinolone antibiotics or oral hypoglycemic agents. See also Pioglitazone-Quinolones, Sulfonylureas-Quinolones.

[1] Gajjar DA, et al. *Pharmacotherapy.* 2000;20(6, pt 2):76S.

[2] Menzies DJ, et al. *Am J Med.* 2002;113(3):232.

* Asterisk indicates drugs cited in interaction reports.

Repaglinide — *Trimethoprim*

Repaglinide* (*Prandin*)	Trimethoprim* (eg, *Primsol*)	Trimethoprim/ Sulfamethoxazole* (eg, *Bactrim*)

Significance	Onset	Severity	Documentation
4	□ Rapid	□ Major	□ Established
	■ **Delayed**	■ **Moderate**	□ Probable
		□ Minor	□ Suspected
			■ **Possible**
			□ Unlikely

Effects REPAGLINIDE plasma concentrations may be elevated, increasing the risk of hypoglycemia.

Mechanism Inhibition of REPAGLINIDE metabolism (CYP2C8) by TRIMETHOPRIM is suspected.

Management In patients receiving REPAGLINIDE, closely monitor blood glucose after TRIMETHOPRIM is started or stopped. Be prepared to adjust therapy as needed.

Discussion

The effects of trimethoprim on the pharmacokinetics and pharmacodynamics of repaglinide were studied in 9 healthy volunteers.[1] Using a randomized, double-blind, crossover design, each subject took trimethoprim 160 mg or placebo twice daily for 3 days. On day 3, subjects ingested repaglinide 0.25 mg 1 hour after the last dose of trimethoprim. Compared with placebo, trimethoprim increased the AUC and C_{max} of repaglinide 61% and 41%, respectively, while prolonging the $t_{½}$ from 0.9 to 1.1 hours. The blood glucose-lowering effect of repaglinide was not affected by trimethoprim. Severe symptomatic hypoglycemia (blood glucose 34 mg/dL) developed in a 76-year-old diabetic patient with mild renal function impairment 5 days after trimethoprim/sulfamethoxazole was added to the treatment regimen, which included repaglinide.[2] The patient had no previous hypoglycemic events while taking repaglinide.

[1] Niemi M, et al. *Br J Clin Pharmacol.* 2004;57(4):441. [2] Roustit M, et al. *Ann Pharmacother.* 2010;44(4):764.

* Asterisk indicates drugs cited in interaction reports.

Retinoids — *Tetracyclines*

Acitretin* (*Soriatane*)	Isotretinoin* (eg, *Accutane*)	Demeclocycline* Doxycycline* (eg, *Vibramycin*) Minocycline* (eg, *Minocin*)	Oxytetracycline*† Tetracycline*

Significance	Onset	Severity	Documentation
2	□ Rapid ■ **Delayed**	□ Major ■ **Moderate** □ Minor	□ Established □ Probable ■ **Suspected** □ Possible □ Unlikely

Effects Risk of pseudotumor cerebri (benign intracranial hypertension) may be increased.

Mechanism Additive or synergistic adverse effect.

Management Concomitant use of ACITRETIN or ISOTRETINOIN and TETRACYCLINES is not recommended.

Discussion

Isotretinoin use has been associated with a number of cases of pseudotumor cerebri, some of which involved coadministration of tetracyclines.[1] In the single case reported with acitretin, the patient was not taking tetracycline.[2] Various tetracyclines have been associated with pseudotumor cerebri.[3] This suggests the risk is increased if a tetracycline is taken with isotretinoin or acitretin. However, it remains to be determined if the reaction is caused by an additive or synergistic effect. Therefore, avoid concomitant use of isotretinoin or acitretin and tetracyclines. Early signs and symptoms of pseudotumor cerebri include headache, nausea, vomiting, visual disturbances, and papilledema.

The basis for this monograph is information on file with the manufacturer. Published clinical data are needed to further assess this interaction. However, because of the increased risk of benign intracranial hypertension, clinical evaluation of this interaction in humans is not likely to be forthcoming.

1 *Accutane* [package insert]. Nutley, NJ: Roche Pharmaceuticals Inc; 2001.
2 *Soriatane* [package insert]. Nutley, NJ: Roche Pharmaceuticals Inc; April 2003.
3 Lee AG. *Cutis*. 1995;55(3):165.

* Asterisk indicates drugs cited in interaction reports.
† Not available in the United States.

Rifamycins — *Pyrazinamide*

Rifamycins	Pyrazinamide
Rifampin* (eg, *Rifadin*)	Pyrazinamide*

Significance	Onset	Severity	Documentation
5	■ **Rapid**	□ Major	□ Established
	□ Delayed	□ Moderate	□ Probable
		■ **Minor**	□ Suspected
			□ Possible
			■ **Unlikely**

Effects Serum RIFAMPIN levels may be decreased, possibly reducing the clinical effect of RIFAMPIN.

Mechanism Unknown.

Management No action is required. If an interaction is suspected, consider increasing the dose of RIFAMPIN.

Discussion

A study was conducted in 16 patients with tuberculosis to assess if there is a drug interaction between rifampin and pyrazinamide.[1] Fourteen patients were given either single doses of isoniazid (eg, *Nydrazid*) 300 mg and rifampin 450 mg (phase 1), or isoniazid 300 mg, rifampin 450 mg, and pyrazinamide 1,500 mg (phase 2). Due to body weight, 2 patients received isoniazid 300 mg, rifampin 600 mg, and pyrazinamide 2,000 mg. The investigation was a crossover study with each patient serving as their own control after a 48-hour washout period between the 2 phases of the study. Serum rifampin concentrations at 0.5, 2, and 4 hours were not different in the 2 study phases. However, serum rifampin concentrations were significantly lower at 6 hours ($P < 0.01$) and 8 hours ($P < 0.05$) in patients also receiving pyrazinamide. The mean serum rifampin concentration at 6 hours in phase 1 was 3.81 mcg/mL compared with 3.61 mcg/mL in phase 2. The mean serum rifampin concentration at 8 hours in phase 1 was 2.57 mcg/mL compared with 2.39 mcg/mL in phase 2. The rifampin AUC was significantly less ($P < 0.05$) in phase 2 than in phase 1 (decreased from 52.14 to 49.6 mcg•h/mL), indicating that pyrazinamide reduced the bioavailability of rifampin. The elimination rate constant, elimination $t_{1/2}$, and volume of distribution of rifampin were not significantly different in the 2 phases of the study.

[1] Jain A, et al. *Tuber Lung Dis.* 1993;74(2):87.

* Asterisk indicates drugs cited in interaction reports.

Rilpivirine — *Carbamazepine*

Rilpivirine* (*Edurant*)	Carbamazepine* (eg, *Tegretol*)

Significance	Onset	Severity	Documentation
1	☐ Rapid	■ **Major**	☐ Established
	■ **Delayed**	☐ Moderate	☐ Probable
		☐ Minor	■ **Suspected**
			☐ Possible
			☐ Unlikely

Effects RILPIVIRINE plasma concentrations may be reduced, resulting in a loss of virologic response and possible resistance.

Mechanism RILPIVIRINE metabolism (CYP3A4) may be increased by CARBAMAZEPINE.

Management Coadministration of RILPIVIRINE with CARBAMAZEPINE is contraindicated.[1]

Discussion

Inducers of CYP3A4, such as carbamazepine, may reduce rilpivirine plasma concentrations, which may result in a loss of virologic response and possible resistance to rilpivirine and/or to the class of NNRT inhibitors.[1] Concomitant use of rilpivirine with carbamazepine is contraindicated.

The basis for this monograph is information on file with the manufacturer. Published clinical data are needed to further assess this interaction. Because of the seriousness of this interaction, clinical evaluation in humans is not likely to be forthcoming

[1] *Edurant* [package insert]. Raritan, NJ: Tibotec Therapeutics; May 2011.

* Asterisk indicates drugs cited in interaction reports.

Rilpivirine — *Dexamethasone*

Rilpivirine* (*Edurant*)	Dexamethasone* (eg, *Baycadron*)

Significance	Onset	Severity	Documentation
1	☐ Rapid ■ **Delayed**	■ **Major** ☐ Moderate ☐ Minor	☐ Established ☐ Probable ■ **Suspected** ☐ Possible ☐ Unlikely

Effects RILPIVIRINE plasma concentrations may be reduced, resulting in a loss of virologic response and possible resistance.

Mechanism RILPIVIRINE metabolism (CYP3A4) may be increased by DEXAMETHASONE.

Management Coadministration of RILPIVIRINE with more than 1 dose of DEXAMETHASONE is contraindicated.

Discussion

Inducers of CYP3A4, such as dexamethasone, may reduce rilpivirine plasma concentrations, which may result in a loss of virologic response and possible resistance to rilpivirine and/or to the class of NNRT inhibitors. Concomitant use of rilpivirine with more than 1 dose of dexamethasone is contraindicated.[1]

The basis for this monograph is information on file with the manufacturer. Published clinical data are needed to further assess this interaction. Because of the seriousness of this interaction, clinical evaluation in humans is not likely to be forthcoming.

[1] *Edurant* [package insert]. Raritan, NJ: Tibotec Therapeutics; May 2011.

* Asterisk indicates drugs cited in interaction reports.

Rilpivirine — *Hydantoins*

Rilpivirine* (*Edurant*)	Ethotoin (*Peganone*)	Phenytoin* (eg, *Dilantin*)
	Fosphenytoin	

Significance	Onset	Severity	Documentation
1	□ Rapid	■ **Major**	□ Established
	■ **Delayed**	□ Moderate	□ Probable
		□ Minor	■ **Suspected**
			□ Possible
			□ Unlikely

Effects RILPIVIRINE plasma concentrations may be reduced, resulting in a loss of virologic response and possible resistance.

Mechanism RILPIVIRINE metabolism (CYP3A4) may be increased by HYDANTOINS.

Management Coadministration of RILPIVIRINE with PHENYTOIN is contraindicated.[1]

Discussion

Inducers of CYP3A4, such as phenytoin, may reduce rilpivirine plasma concentrations, which may result in a loss of virologic response and possible resistance to rilpivirine and/or to the class of NNRT inhibitors.[1] Concomitant use of rilpivirine with phenytoin is contraindicated.

The basis for this monograph is information on file with the manufacturer. Published clinical data are needed to further assess this interaction. Because of the seriousness of this interaction, clinical evaluation in humans is not likely to be forthcoming.

[1] *Edurant* [package insert]. Raritan, NJ: Tibotec Therapeutics; May 2011.

* Asterisk indicates drugs cited in interaction reports. Based on pharmacologic and pharmacokinetic considerations, similar interactions may occur with other drugs that are listed.

Rilpivirine — *Oxcarbazepine*

Rilpivirine* (*Edurant*)	Oxcarbazepine* (eg, *Trileptal*)

Significance	Onset	Severity	Documentation
1	☐ Rapid ■ **Delayed**	■ **Major** ☐ Moderate ☐ Minor	☐ Established ☐ Probable ■ **Suspected** ☐ Possible ☐ Unlikely

Effects RILPIVIRINE plasma concentrations may be reduced, resulting in a loss of virologic response and possible resistance.

Mechanism RILPIVIRINE metabolism (CYP3A4) may be increased by OXCARBAZEPINE.

Management Coadministration of RILPIVIRINE with OXCARBAZEPINE is contraindicated.[1]

Discussion

Inducers of CYP3A4, such as oxcarbazepine, may reduce rilpivirine plasma concentrations, which may result in a loss of virologic response and possible resistance to rilpivirine and/or to the class of NNRT inhibitors.[1] Concomitant use of rilpivirine with oxcarbazepine is contraindicated.

The basis for this monograph is information on file with the manufacturer. Published clinical data are needed to further assess this interaction. Because of the seriousness of this interaction, clinical evaluation in humans is not likely to be forthcoming.

[1] *Edurant* [package insert]. Raritan, NJ: Tibotec Therapeutics; May 2011.

* Asterisk indicates drugs cited in interaction reports.

Rilpivirine — *Phenobarbital*

Rilpivirine* (*Edurant*)	Phenobarbital* (eg, *Luminal*)

Significance	Onset	Severity	Documentation
1	☐ Rapid ■ **Delayed**	■ **Major** ☐ Moderate ☐ Minor	☐ Established ☐ Probable ■ **Suspected** ☐ Possible ☐ Unlikely

Effects RILPIVIRINE plasma concentrations may be reduced, resulting in a loss of virologic response and possible resistance.

Mechanism RILPIVIRINE metabolism (CYP3A4) may be increased by PHENOBARBITAL.

Management Coadministration of RILPIVIRINE with PHENOBARBITAL is contraindicated.[1]

Discussion

Inducers of CYP3A4, such as phenobarbital, may reduce rilpivirine plasma concentrations, which may result in a loss of virologic response and possible resistance to rilpivirine and/or to the class of NNRT inhibitors.[1] Concomitant use of rilpivirine with phenobarbital is contraindicated.

The basis for this monograph is information on file with the manufacturer. Published clinical data are needed to further assess this interaction. Because of the seriousness of this interaction, clinical evaluation in humans is not likely to be forthcoming

[1] *Edurant* [package insert]. Raritan, NJ: Tibotec Therapeutics; May 2011.

* Asterisk indicates drugs cited in interaction reports.

Rilpivirine — *Proton Pump Inhibitors*

Rilpivirine	Proton Pump Inhibitors	
Rilpivirine* (*Edurant*)	Dexlansoprazole* (*Dexilant*)	Omeprazole* (eg, *Prilosec*)
	Esomeprazole* (*Nexium*)	Pantoprazole* (eg, *Protonix*)
	Lansoprazole* (eg, *Prevacid*)	Rabeprazole* (*AcipHex*)

Significance	Onset	Severity	Documentation
1	☐ Rapid	■ **Major**	☐ Established
	■ **Delayed**	☐ Moderate	☐ Probable
		☐ Minor	■ **Suspected**
			☐ Possible
			☐ Unlikely

Effects RILPIVIRINE plasma concentrations may be reduced, resulting in a loss of virologic response and possible resistance.

Mechanism PROTON PUMP INHIBITOR–induced increase in gastric pH may decrease absorption of RILPIVIRINE.

Management Coadministration of RILPIVIRINE with PROTON PUMP INHIBITORS is contraindicated.[1]

Discussion

Drugs that increase gastric pH, such as omeprazole, may reduce rilpivirine plasma concentrations, which may result in a loss of virologic response and possible resistance to rilpivirine and/or to the class of NNRT inhibitors.[1] In 16 subjects, coadministration of high-dose rilpivirine 150 mg daily with omeprazole 20 mg daily decreased the rilpivirine C_{max}, AUC, and C_{min} 40%, 40%, and 33%, respectively. Concomitant use of rilpivirine with proton pump inhibitors is contraindicated.

The basis for this monograph is information on file with the manufacturer. Published clinical data are needed to further assess this interaction. Because of the seriousness of this interaction, clinical evaluation in humans is not likely to be forthcoming.

[1] *Edurant* [package insert]. Raritan, NJ: Tibotec Therapeutics; May 2011.

* Asterisk indicates drugs cited in interaction reports.

Rilpivirine — *Rifamycins*

Rilpivirine*	Rifamycins
Rilpivirine* (*Edurant*)	Rifabutin* (*Mycobutin*) Rifampin* (eg, *Rifadin*) Rifapentine* (*Priftin*)

Significance	Onset	Severity	Documentation
1	☐ Rapid ■ **Delayed**	■ **Major** ☐ Moderate ☐ Minor	☐ Established ☐ Probable ■ **Suspected** ☐ Possible ☐ Unlikely

Effects RILPIVIRINE plasma concentrations may be reduced, resulting in a loss of virologic response and possible resistance.

Mechanism RILPIVIRINE metabolism (CYP3A4) may be increased by RIFAMYCINS.

Management Coadministration of RILPIVIRINE with RIFAMYCINS is contraindicated.[1]

Discussion

Inducers of CYP3A4, such as rifampin, may reduce rilpivirine plasma concentrations, which may result in a loss of virologic response and possible resistance to rilpivirine and/or to the class of NNRT inhibitors. In 16 subjects, coadministration of high-dose rilpivirine 150 mg daily with rifampin 600 mg daily decreased the C_{max}, AUC, and C_{min} of rilpivirine 69%, 80%, and 89%, respectively. Similarly, in 16 patients, high-dose rilpivirine 150 mg daily coadministered with rifabutin 300 mg daily decreased the rilpivirine C_{max}, AUC, and C_{min} 35%, 46%, and 49%, respectively.[1] Concomitant use of rilpivirine with rifamycins is contraindicated.

The basis for this monograph is information on file with the manufacturer. Published clinical data are needed to further assess this interaction. Because of the seriousness of this interaction, clinical evaluation in humans is not likely to be forthcoming.

[1] *Edurant* [package insert]. Raritan, NJ: Tibotec Therapeutics; May 2011.

* Asterisk indicates drugs cited in interaction reports.

Rilpivirine | **St. John's Wort**

Rilpivirine* (*Edurant*)

St. John's Wort*

Significance	Onset	Severity	Documentation
1	☐ Rapid ■ **Delayed**	■ **Major** ☐ Moderate ☐ Minor	☐ Established ☐ Probable ■ **Suspected** ☐ Possible ☐ Unlikely

Effects RILPIVIRINE plasma concentrations may be reduced, resulting in a loss of virologic response and possible resistance.

Mechanism RILPIVIRINE metabolism (CYP3A4) may be increased by ST. JOHN'S WORT.

Management Coadministration of RILPIVIRINE with ST. JOHN'S WORT is contraindicated.[1]

Discussion

Inducers of CYP3A4, such as St. John's wort, may reduce rilpivirine plasma concentrations, which may result in a loss of virologic response and possible resistance to rilpivirine and/or to the class of NNRT inhibitors.[1] Concomitant use of rilpivirine with St. John's wort is contraindicated.

The basis for this monograph is information on file with the manufacturer. Published clinical data are needed to further assess this interaction. Because of the seriousness of this interaction, clinical evaluation in humans is not likely to be forthcoming.

[1] *Edurant* [package insert]. Raritan, NJ: Tibotec Therapeutics; May 2011.

* Asterisk indicates drugs cited in interaction reports.

Rimantadine — *Cimetidine*

Rimantadine* (eg, *Flumadine*)	Cimetidine* (eg, *Tagamet*)

Significance	Onset	Severity	Documentation
5	☐ Rapid	☐ Major	☐ Established
	■ **Delayed**	☐ Moderate	☐ Probable
		■ **Minor**	☐ Suspected
			☐ Possible
			■ **Unlikely**

Effects Serum RIMANTADINE concentrations may be increased.

Mechanism CIMETIDINE may inhibit the metabolism of RIMANTADINE.

Management No clinical intervention appears necessary. Based on the magnitude of the interaction, a clinically important consequence is unlikely.

Discussion

Using an open-label, single-dose, sequential design, the effects of cimetidine on the pharmacokinetics of rimantadine were studied in 23 healthy subjects.[1] Each subject received a single oral dose of rimantadine 100 mg alone or after 6 days of cimetidine, 300 mg 4 times daily. When rimantadine was administered with cimetidine, there were no changes in the rate of absorption or renal clearance of rimantadine. However, there was a significant increase in the AUC (20%; $P < 0.01$), and a reduction in the total body clearance (18%; $P < 0.01$) of rimantadine compared with when the drug was taken alone.

Controlled studies in patients with influenza are needed to assess the clinical importance of this interaction.

[1] Holazo AA, et al. *Antimicrob Agents Chemother.* 1989;33(6):820.

* Asterisk indicates drugs cited in interaction reports.

Risperidone — *Azole Antifungal Agents*

Risperidone	Azole Antifungal Agents	
Risperidone* (eg, *Risperdal*)	Fluconazole (eg, *Diflucan*)	Ketoconazole (eg, *Nizoral*)
	Itraconazole* (eg, *Sporanox*)	

Significance	Onset	Severity	Documentation
2	☐ Rapid	☐ Major	☐ Established
	■ **Delayed**	■ **Moderate**	☐ Probable
		☐ Minor	■ **Suspected**
			☐ Possible
			☐ Unlikely

Effects RISPERIDONE plasma levels may be elevated, increasing the pharmacologic and adverse effects.

Mechanism Inhibition of RISPERIDONE metabolism (CYP3A4) by AZOLE ANTIFUNGAL AGENTS is suspected.

Management Monitor the clinical response to RISPERIDONE after starting or stopping an AZOLE ANTIFUNGAL AGENT. Observe the patient for RISPERIDONE adverse effects during concurrent therapy with an AZOLE ANTIFUNGAL AGENT. Adjust the RISPERIDONE dose as needed.

Discussion

The effect of itraconazole, a CYP3A4 inhibitor, on risperidone plasma concentrations was studied in 19 schizophrenic patients.[1] Patients who had been receiving risperidone 2 to 8 mg daily for more than 2 months were given itraconazole 200 mg daily for 1 week. Dose-normalized, steady-state mean plasma levels of risperidone and the active metabolite 9-hydroxyrisperidone, were increased 82% and 70%, respectively. The concentration of risperidone plus 9-hydroxyrisperidone increased 71%. However, the ratios of risperidone to 9-hydroxyrisperidone did not change during the study period. Risperidone plasma levels increased 69% and 75% in CYP2D6 extensive and poor metabolizers, respectively. There was a slight improvement in psychiatric scores as measured by the Brief Psychiatric Rating Scale.

[1] Jung SM, et al. *Clin Pharmacol Ther.* 2005;78(5):520.

* Asterisk indicates drugs cited in interaction reports. Based on pharmacologic and pharmacokinetic considerations, similar interactions may occur with other drugs that are listed.

Risperidone — *Carbamazepine*

Risperidone* (*Risperdal*)	Carbamazepine* (eg, *Tegretol*)

Significance	Onset	Severity	Documentation
4	☐ Rapid ■ **Delayed**	☐ Major ■ **Moderate** ☐ Minor	☐ Established ☐ Probable ☐ Suspected ■ **Possible** ☐ Unlikely

Effects The pharmacologic effects of RISPERIDONE may be decreased.

Mechanism CARBAMAZEPINE may increase RISPERIDONE metabolism.

Management Closely observe the clinical response to RISPERIDONE when starting, stopping, or changing the dose of CARBAMAZEPINE. Adjust the dose of RISPERIDONE as needed.

Discussion

Decreased plasma concentrations of the active metabolite of risperidone, 9-hydroxyrisperidone, were reported in a 22-year-old man with schizophrenia during coadministration of carbamazepine.[1] While the patient was receiving risperidone 4 mg/day and carbamazepine 600 mg/day, plasma concentrations of the active metabolite were less than 50% the expected level of 10 mcg/L. The dose of risperidone was increased to 8 mg/day, and the plasma concentration of the risperidone metabolite increased to 19 mcg/L. Subsequently, carbamazepine was gradually discontinued. The patient's 9-hydroxyrisperidone plasma concentration increased to 49 mcg/L 10 days later. A 50-year old man, who was characterized as a poor CYP2D6 metabolizer, was receiving a steady dose of risperidone 6 mg/day.[2] After 5 days of carbamazepine therapy, levels of risperidone and the active 9-hydroxyrisperidone metabolite decreased from 22 and 30 mg/mL to 6 and 11 mg/mL, respectively. The changes in level were associated with resurgence of schizophrenic symptoms. In a study involving 11 schizophrenic inpatients, plasma levels of risperidone and the 9-hydroxymetabolite were lower during carbamazepine administration than levels seen prior to carbamazepine administration.[3] Two men receiving risperidone and carbamazepine developed parkinsonian symptoms after stopping carbamazepine.[4] While no plasma levels were drawn, the symptoms were suggestive of high risperidone levels. In a study of 8 patients stabilized on carbamazepine, risperidone caused a modest, clinically insignificant increase in carbamazepine plasma levels.[5]

[1] de Leon J, et al. *J Clin Psychiatry*. 1997;58:450.
[2] Spina E, et al. *J Clin Psychopharmacol*. 2001;21:108.
[3] Ono S, et al. *Psychopharmacology*. 2002;162:50.
[4] Takahashi H, et al. *Clin Neuropharmacol*. 2001;24:358.
[5] Mula M, et al. *Clin Neuropharmacol*. 2002;25:97.

* Asterisk indicates drugs cited in interaction reports.

Risperidone — *Lamotrigine*

Risperidone* (*Risperdal*)	Lamotrigine* (*Lamictal*)

Significance	Onset	Severity	Documentation
4	☐ Rapid ■ **Delayed**	☐ Major ■ **Moderate** ☐ Minor	☐ Established ☐ Probable ☐ Suspected ■ **Possible** ☐ Unlikely

Effects RISPERIDONE plasma concentrations may be elevated, increasing the pharmacologic and adverse effects.

Mechanism Unknown.

Management In patients receiving RISPERIDONE, observe the clinical response to RISPERIDONE when starting, stopping, or changing the dose of LAMOTRIGINE. Be prepared to adjust the RISPERIDONE dose as needed.

Discussion

A possible drug interaction between lamotrigine and risperidone was reported in a 26-year-old woman with schizophrenia that included imperative auditory hallucinations.[1] The patient had been receiving clozapine (eg, *Clozaril*) 550 mg daily for 5 years and risperidone 8 mg daily for 4 weeks (plasma concentration 55 to 70 ng/mL). Because she had only a partial response, lamotrigine was added to her treatment regimen. The lamotrigine dose was titrated up to 250 mg daily in increments of 25 mg/week. While receiving lamotrigine 175 mg daily, her risperidone plasma level was 69 ng/mL. When the dose of lamotrigine was increased to 200 mg daily, the risperidone plasma level increased to 284 ng/mL. Following a further increase in the dose of lamotrigine to 225 mg daily, the risperidone plasma concentration increased to 412 ng/mL, and the patient complained of dizziness and tiredness. Subsequently, the dose of risperidone was reduced to 2 mg/day and then discontinued 1 week later.

[1] Bienentreu SD, et al. *Am J Psychiatry*. 2005;162:811.

* Asterisk indicates drugs cited in interaction reports.

Risperidone		***Phenothiazines***
Risperidone* (*Risperdal*)	Thioridazine*	

Significance	Onset	Severity	Documentation
4	☐ Rapid ■ **Delayed**	☐ Major ■ **Moderate** ☐ Minor	☐ Established ☐ Probable ☐ Suspected ■ **Possible** ☐ Unlikely

Effects RISPERIDONE plasma concentrations may be elevated, increasing the pharmacologic and adverse effects.

Mechanism Inhibition of RISPERIDONE metabolism (CYP2D6) by THIORIDAZINE is suspected.

Management In patients receiving RISPERIDONE, monitor the clinical response to RISPERIDONE when starting, stopping, or changing the dose of THIORIDAZINE. Observe patients for RISPERIDONE adverse effects and adjust the RISPERIDONE dose as needed.

Discussion

The effects of thioridazine on plasma concentrations of risperidone and its active metabolite, 9-hydroxyrisperidone, were studied in 12 schizophrenic inpatients with prevailing anxiety symptoms.[1] Subjects had received risperidone 3 mg twice daily for 4 to 54 weeks. Each subject received coadministration of thioridazine 25 mg twice daily for 2 weeks. During coadministration of thioridazine, mean plasma concentrations of risperidone were increased 5-fold compared with administration of risperidone alone (34.4 versus 6.9 ng/mL). Plasma concentrations of 9-hydroxyrisperidone decreased, while concentrations of risperidone plus 9-hydroxyrisperidone increased. The ratio of risperidone/9-hydroxyrisperidone was higher during thioridazine administration compared with administration of risperidone alone (1.11 versus 0.18). Three CYP2D6 genotypes were identified in the patients. There were no differences in clinical symptoms or side effects in any of the genotype subgroups.

[1] Nakagami T, et al. *J Clin Psychopharmacol.* 2005;25:89.

* Asterisk indicates drugs cited in interaction reports.

Risperidone — *Protease Inhibitors*

Risperidone	Protease Inhibitors	
Risperidone* (*Risperdal*)	Amprenavir (*Agenerase*)	Nelfinavir (*Viracept*)
	Atazanavir (*Reyataz*)	Ritonavir* (*Norvir*)
	Indinavir* (*Crixivan*)	Saquinavir (eg, *Fortovase*)
	Lopinavir/Ritonavir (*Kaletra*)	

Significance	Onset	Severity	Documentation
4	☐ Rapid	☐ Major	☐ Established
	■ **Delayed**	■ **Moderate**	☐ Probable
		☐ Minor	☐ Suspected
			■ **Possible**
			☐ Unlikely

Effects RISPERIDONE plasma concentrations may be elevated, increasing the risk of side effects.

Mechanism Inhibition of RISPERIDONE metabolism (CYP3A4; CYP2D6 [ritonavir]) by PROTEASE INHIBITORS is suspected.

Management Observe the clinical response to RISPERIDONE when starting or stopping PROTEASE INHIBITOR therapy. Adjust the RISPERIDONE dose as needed.

Discussion

A 48-year-old patient receiving risperidone developed a profound coma while receiving treatment with ritonavir and indinavir.[1] The patient had previously been diagnosed with AIDS and was receiving zidovudine (eg, *Retrovir*), didanosine (eg, *Videx*), and the protease inhibitors indinavir 400 mg twice daily and ritonavir 200 mg twice daily for HIV infection. He was admitted to the hospital psychiatric department for manic symptoms and treatment with risperidone 3 mg twice daily was started. After 2 doses of risperidone, he complained of ataxia and became drowsy, disoriented, lethargic, and comatose. His medications were discontinued. Twenty-four hours later, his neurologic status returned to baseline and, subsequently, the manic symptoms returned. A drug interaction between risperidone and the protease inhibitors ritonavir and indinavir was suspected.

[1] Jover F, et al. *Clin Neuropharmacol.* 2002;25:251.

* Asterisk indicates drugs cited in interaction reports. Based on pharmacologic and pharmacokinetic considerations, similar interactions may occur with other drugs that are listed.

Risperidone — *Rifamycins*

Risperidone	Rifamycins	
Risperidone* (eg, *Risperdal*)	Rifabutin (*Mycobutin*)	Rifapentine (*Priftin*)
	Rifampin* (eg, *Rifadin*)	

Significance	Onset	Severity	Documentation
4	☐ Rapid	☐ Major	☐ Established
	■ **Delayed**	■ **Moderate**	☐ Probable
		☐ Minor	☐ Suspected
			■ **Possible**
			☐ Unlikely

Effects Plasma concentrations of RISPERIDONE and 9-hydroxyrisperidone may be reduced, decreasing the pharmacologic effects of RISPERIDONE and 9-hydroxyrisperidone.

Mechanism Increased RISPERIDONE metabolism and decreased absorption of RISPERIDONE by induction of both CYP3A4 and P-glycoprotein, respectively, by RIFAMPIN is suspected.

Management If this combination cannot be avoided, monitor the clinical response to RISPERIDONE when RIFAMYCIN is started or stopped. Adjust the RISPERIDONE dose as needed.

Discussion

The effects of rifampin on the pharmacokinetics of risperidone were studied in 10 healthy men.[1] In a randomized, open-label, crossover study, each subject received rifampin 600 mg daily or a matched placebo for 7 days. On the morning of day 6, a single dose of risperidone 1 mg was administered. Compared with placebo, rifampin decreased the mean AUC and mean C_{max} of risperidone 51% and 38%, respectively. In addition, the mean AUC and C_{max} of the main active metabolite of risperidone, 9-hydroxyrisperidone, were decreased 43% and 46%, respectively. The apparent oral clearance of risperidone doubled after rifampin administration. In a similar study, pretreatment with rifampin 600 mg daily for 5 days decreased the AUC and C_{max} of risperidone 4 mg 72% and 50%, respectively, compared with giving risperidone alone.[2]

[1] Kim KA, et al. *J Clin Pharmacol.* 2008;48(1):66.

[2] Mahatthanatrakul W. *J Clin Pharm Ther.* 2007;32(2):161.

* Asterisk indicates drugs cited in interaction reports. Based on pharmacologic and pharmacokinetic considerations, similar interactions may occur with other drugs that are listed.

Risperidone / *Serotonin Reuptake Inhibitors*

Risperidone	Serotonin Reuptake Inhibitors	
Risperidone* (eg, *Risperdal*)	Fluoxetine* (eg, *Prozac*) Paroxetine* (eg, *Paxil*)	Sertraline* (eg, *Zoloft*)

Significance	Onset	Severity	Documentation
1	■ **Rapid** □ Delayed	■ **Major** □ Moderate □ Minor	□ Established ■ **Probable** □ Suspected □ Possible □ Unlikely

Effects RISPERIDONE plasma concentrations may be elevated, increasing the risk of adverse reactions. Serotonin syndrome (eg, altered consciousness, CNS irritability, increased muscle tone, myoclonus) may occur. Nasal bleeding has been reported.

Mechanism Inhibition of RISPERIDONE metabolism (CYP2D6) by FLUOXETINE and PAROXETINE is suspected; rapid accumulation of serotonin in the CNS may occur.

Management Observe the clinical response to RISPERIDONE when the dose of FLUOXETINE or PAROXETINE is started, stopped, or changed, or when giving high dosages of SERTRALINE (more than 100 mg/day). Adjust the RISPERIDONE dose as needed. If nasal bleeding occurs, consider alternative treatment for one of the agents.

Discussion

The effects of paroxetine 20 mg/day for 4 weeks on the steady-state plasma levels of risperidone 4 to 8 mg/day and its active metabolite, 9-hydroxyrisperidone, were studied in 10 patients with schizophrenia or schizoaffective disorder.[1] After receiving both drugs for 2 weeks, the mean plasma level of risperidone increased from 17 to 83 nmol/L (388%); after 4 weeks, risperidone levels increased to 94 nmol/L (453%). In addition, the mean plasma risperidone/9-hydroxyrisperidone ratio was increased. In the second week of concurrent therapy, 1 patient developed parkinsonism. The plasma levels of risperidone and 9-hydroxyrisperidone were increased 62% over baseline at week 4. In a similar study, risperidone levels increased from 12 to 56 ng/mL (367%) in patients stabilized on risperidone 4 to 6 mg/day during 4 weeks of concurrent fluoxetine 20 mg/day therapy.[2] Levels of the 9-hydroxyrisperidone metabolite were not affected. At least 3 patients experienced symptoms consistent with serotonin syndrome during coadministration of risperidone and paroxetine.[3,4] One patient died; however, serotonin syndrome was not implicated as the cause of death.[4] High dosages of sertraline (more than 100 mg/day) may elevate risperidone plasma levels.[5] Nasal bleeding was reported in a 22-year-old man after fluoxetine 20 mg daily was added to his risperidone regimen.[6] On 2 other occasions, rechallenge with coadministration of fluoxetine and risperidone resulted in nasal bleeding. Nasal bleeding did not occur when nortriptyine (eg, *Aventyl*) was substituted for fluoxetine.

1 Spina E, et al. *Ther Drug Monit.* 2001;23(3):223.
2 Spina E, et al. *J Clin Psychopharmacol.* 2002; 22(4):419.
3 Hamilton S, et al. *J Clin Psychopharmacol.* 2000;20(1):103.
4 Karki SD, et al. *Ann Pharmacother.* 2003;37(3):388.
5 Spina E, et al. *Ther Drug Monit.* 2004;26(4):386.
6 Mowla A, et al. *Pharmacopsychiatry.* 2009;42(5):204.

* Asterisk indicates drugs cited in interaction reports.

Risperidone — *Verapamil*

Risperidone* (eg, *Risperdal*)	Verapamil* (eg, *Calan*)

Significance	Onset	Severity	Documentation
4	□ Rapid	□ Major	□ Established
	■ **Delayed**	■ **Moderate**	□ Probable
		□ Minor	□ Suspected
			■ **Possible**
			□ Unlikely

Effects RISPERIDONE plasma concentrations may be elevated, increasing the pharmacologic and adverse reactions.

Mechanism Increased RISPERIDONE absorption because of suspected VERAPAMIL-induced inhibition of P-glycoprotein in the small intestine.

Management In patients receiving RISPERIDONE, monitor the response to RISPERIDONE after starting, stopping, or changing the VERAPAMIL dose. Adjust the RISPERIDONE dose as needed.

Discussion

The effects of verapamil on the pharmacokinetics of risperidone were studied in a randomized, crossover investigation.[1] Twelve healthy men received placebo or verapamil 240 mg/day for 6 days. On day 6, a single oral dose of risperidone 1 mg was administered. Compared with placebo, verapamil pretreatment increased the C_{max} and AUC of risperidone 1.8- and 2-fold, respectively, but did not affect the elimination $t_{½}$. The AUC of the risperidone metabolite, 9-hydroxyrisperidone, was increased approximately 1.5-fold.

[1] Nakagami T, et al. *Clin Pharmacol Ther.* 2005;78(1):43.

* Asterisk indicates drugs cited in interaction reports.

Ritonavir — *Fluoxetine*

Ritonavir* (*Norvir*)	Fluoxetine* (eg, *Prozac*)

Significance	Onset	Severity	Documentation
2	☐ Rapid	☐ Major	☐ Established
	■ **Delayed**	■ **Moderate**	☐ Probable
		☐ Minor	■ **Suspected**
			☐ Possible
			☐ Unlikely

Effects The AUC of RITONAVIR may be increased. Serotonin syndrome (eg, CNS irritability, increased muscle tone, myoclonus, altered consciousness) may occur.

Mechanism FLUOXETINE and RITONAVIR may inhibit the metabolism (CYP2D6) of each other.

Management Closely monitor for adverse effects. Serotonin syndrome requires immediate medical attention, including withdrawal of FLUOXETINE and supportive care.

Discussion

In an open-label investigation involving 16 healthy volunteers, the effect of fluoxetine on the pharmacokinetics of ritonavir was studied.[1] Each subject received single doses of ritonavir 600 mg on days 1 and 10. On study days 3 to 10, each subject received fluoxetine 30 mg every 12 hr for 16 doses. Fluoxetine administration increased the AUC of ritonavir 19%. There was little or no effect of fluoxetine on the peak serum concentration, time to reach peak serum concentration, or elimination rate constant of ritonavir. The magnitude of the increase in ritonavir AUC appeared to be related to the concentration of the active metabolite of fluoxetine (norfluoxetine) rather than to the concentration of fluoxetine. The pharmacokinetic changes were considered small and not clinically important. Three patients developed symptoms consistent with serotonin syndrome when ritonavir-containing anti-HIV regimens were added to fluoxetine.[2] Patients experienced nausea, diarrhea, altered mental status, fever, and muscle twitching.

[1] Ouellet D, et al. *Antimicrob Agents Chemother.* 1998;42:3107.

[2] DeSilva KE, et al. *AIDS.* 2001;15:1281.

* Asterisk indicates drugs cited in interaction reports.

Ritonavir		***Rifamycins***	
Ritonavir* (*Norvir*)		Rifabutin* (*Mycobutin*) Rifampin* (eg, *Rifadin*)	Rifapentine* (*Priftin*)

Significance	Onset	Severity	Documentation
1	□ Rapid	■ **Major**	□ Established
	■ **Delayed**	□ Moderate	■ **Probable**
		□ Minor	□ Suspected
			□ Possible
			□ Unlikely

Effects RIFAMYCINS may decrease RITONAVIR serum levels. RITONAVIR may elevate serum RIFABUTIN levels, increasing the risk of RIFABUTIN hematologic toxicity.

Mechanism RIFAMYCINS increase RITONAVIR metabolism (CYP3A4). RITONAVIR decreases RIFAMYCIN metabolism (CYP3A4).

Management Coadministration of RITONAVIR and RIFABUTIN is contraindicated. Carefully monitor the patient's response to RITONAVIR during coadministration of RIFAMPIN or RIFAPENTINE. If an interaction is suspected, it may be necessary to increase the dose of RITONAVIR.[1,2]

Discussion

Coadministration of rifampin 300 or 600 mg/day for 10 days and ritonavir 500 mg every 12 hr for 20 days decreased the ritonavir AUC and C_{max} 35% and 25%, respectively.[1] Healthy volunteers were given rifabutin 150 mg/day for 14 days. On the 15th day, subjects continued receiving rifabutin while being randomized to also receive placebo or ritonavir (escalating dosages up to 500 mg twice daily) for 10 days.[3] In 5 subjects completing the ritonavir phase, rifabutin AUC and C_{max} increased 4- and 2.5-fold, respectively. Similarly, C_{max} and AUC of the 25-*O*-desacetylrifabutin metabolite increased 16- and 35-fold, respectively. Conversely, ritonavir blunted the interaction between saquinavir (*Invirase*) and rifampin.[4] Three patients receiving ritonavir-boosted atazanavir (*Reyataz*) were given rifampin 600 mg/day for active tuberculosis.[5] The AUC of ritonavir was reduced 66%, and subtherapeutic concentrations of atazanavir occurred. In a study of 6 HIV-infected patients, rifampin 300 mg/day for 4 days decreased mean ritonavir levels 94%.[6] A study of HIV-infected patients receiving saquinavir and ritonavir, each at a dosage of 400 mg twice daily, demonstrated no pharmacokinetic changes when rifabutin 150 mg was taken every 3 days or once weekly.[7] The dose of rifabutin was intentionally reduced to one-seventh the usual dose to compensate for the known rifabutin and ritonavir interaction. In a study of 15 healthy volunteers, administration of fosamprenavir/ritonavir with a 75% reduced dosage of rifabutin (from 300 mg daily to 150 mg every other day) resulted in a comparable rifabutin AUC but an 11-fold increase in the active metabolite, 25-*O*-desacetylrifabutin.[8] In a study of 10 HIV-infected patients with tuberculosis, lopinavir/ritonavir decreased rifabutin clearance 71% and prolonged the $t_{½}$ 81%.[9] Despite the increase in concentration, the recommended dose of rifabutin 150 mg 3 times a week produced subtherapeutic rifabutin levels and the dose had to be increased in 8 patients. See also Indinavir-Rifamycins.

1 *Norvir* [package insert]. Abbott Park, IL: Abbott Laboratories; February 1996.
2 *Priftin* [package insert]. Kansas City, MO: Hoechst Marion Roussel; June 1998.
3 Cato A III, et al. *Clin Pharmacol Ther.* 1998;63(4):414.
4 Veldkamp AI, et al. *Clin Infect Dis.* 1999;29(6):1586.
5 Mallolas J, et al. *HIV Med.* 2007;8(2):131.
6 Justesen US, et al. *Clin Infect Dis.* 2004;38(3):426.
7 Gallicano K, et al. *Clin Pharmacol Ther.* 2001;70(2):149.
8 Ford SL, et al. *Antimicrob Agents Chemother.* 2008;52(2):534.
9 Boulanger C, et al. *Clin Infect Dis.* 2009;49(9):1305.

* Asterisk indicates drugs cited in interaction reports.

Rivaroxaban — *NSAIDs*

Rivaroxaban*
(*Xarelto*)

Diclofenac*
(eg, *Cataflam*)
Etodolac*
Fenoprofen*
(eg, *Nalfon*)
Flurbiprofen*
Ibuprofen*
(eg, *Motrin*)
Indomethacin*
(eg, *Indocin*)
Ketoprofen*
Ketorolac*
Meclofenamate*
Mefenamic Acid*
(eg, *Ponstel*)
Meloxicam*
(eg, *Mobic*)
Nabumetone*
Naproxen*
(eg, *Naprosyn*)
Oxaprozin*
(eg, *Daypro*)
Piroxicam*
(eg, *Feldene*)
Sulindac*
(eg, *Clinoril*)
Tolmetin*

Significance	Onset	Severity	Documentation
1	☐ Rapid	■ **Major**	☐ Established
	■ **Delayed**	☐ Moderate	☐ Probable
		☐ Minor	■ **Suspected**
			☐ Possible
			☐ Unlikely

Effects The risk of bleeding may be increased.

Mechanism Inhibition of the normal clotting mechanism may be increased.

Management Coadminister with caution. Promptly evaluate any signs or symptoms of blood loss.[1]

Discussion

The effects of naproxen on the pharmacokinetics and pharmacodynamics of rivaroxaban were evaluated in 11 healthy men.[2] Using an open-label, randomized, crossover design, each subject received naproxen alone (500 mg on 2 consecutive days), rivaroxaban 15 mg alone, or naproxen 500 mg on 2 consecutive days with rivaroxaban 15 mg on the second day. All treatments were well tolerated. Coadministration of rivaroxaban and naproxen increased bleeding time compared with rivaroxaban alone. However, except for 1 patient, the difference was small compared with the effect of naproxen alone. Coadministration of rivaroxaban and naproxen slightly increased the rivaroxaban C_{max} and AUC approximately 10%. Rivaroxaban inhibited Factor Xa activity, and prolonged prothrombin time and activated partial thrombin time. Coadministration of naproxen did not alter the effect of rivaroxaban on these parameters. In addition, concurrent use of rivaroxaban with naproxen did not alter platelet aggregation. The manufacturer of rivaroxaban cautions that NSAIDs are known to increase bleeding, and the risk of bleeding may be increased when rivaroxaban and NSAIDs are coadministered.[1]

[1] *Xarelto* [package insert]. Titusville, NJ: Janssen Pharmaceuticals Inc; July 2011.

[2] Kubitza D, et al. *B J Clin Pharmacol.* 2007;63(4):469.

* Asterisk indicates drugs cited in interaction reports.

Rivaroxaban — *Salicylates*

Rivaroxaban* (*Xarelto*)	Aspirin*

Significance	Onset	Severity	Documentation
1	☐ Rapid	■ **Major**	☐ Established
	■ **Delayed**	☐ Moderate	☐ Probable
		☐ Minor	■ **Suspected**
			☐ Possible
			☐ Unlikely

Effects The risk of bleeding may be increased.

Mechanism Inhibition of the normal clotting mechanism may be increased.

Management Coadminister with caution. Promptly evaluate any signs or symptoms of blood loss.[1]

Discussion

The effects of aspirin on the pharmacokinetics and pharmacodynamics of rivaroxaban were evaluated in 13 healthy men.[2] Using an open-label, randomized, crossover design, each subject received aspirin alone (500 mg the first day followed by 100 mg on the second day), rivaroxaban 15 mg alone, or aspirin 500 mg on the first day followed by aspirin 100 mg and rivaroxaban 15 mg on the second day. Coadministration of rivaroxaban with aspirin resulted in a slight increase in bleeding time (2.28 minutes) compared with aspirin alone. All treatments were well tolerated. Coadministration of aspirin with rivaroxaban did not alter the effect of rivaroxaban on Factor Xa activity or clotting tests. Rivaroxaban did not result in a clinically important effect of aspirin on platelet aggregation and bleeding time. Aspirin did not affect the pharmacokinetics of rivaroxaban. The manufacturer of rivaroxaban cautions that aspirin is known to increase bleeding, and the risk of bleeding may be increased when rivaroxaban and aspirin are coadministered.[1]

[1] *Xarelto* [package insert]. Titusville, NJ: Janssen Pharmaceuticals Inc; July 2011.

[2] Kubitza D, et al. *J Clin Pharmacol.* 2006;46(9):981.

* Asterisk indicates drugs cited in interaction reports.

Rivaroxaban — *St. John's Wort*

Rivaroxaban* (*Xarelto*)	St. John's Wort*

Significance	Onset	Severity	Documentation
1	☐ Rapid ■ **Delayed**	■ **Major** ☐ Moderate ☐ Minor	☐ Established ☐ Probable ■ **Suspected** ☐ Possible ☐ Unlikely

Effects RIVAROXABAN plasma concentrations may be reduced, decreasing the efficacy.

Mechanism ST. JOHN'S WORT may induce CYP3A4 and P-gp, resulting in decreased RIVAROXABAN systemic exposure.

Management If coadministration of RIVAROXABAN and ST. JOHN'S WORT cannot be avoided, consider increasing the RIVAROXABAN dose when ST. JOHN'S WORT is given concurrently.[1]

Discussion

Concurrent use of rivaroxaban with a combined P-gp and strong CYP3A4 inducer, such as St. John's wort, may reduce rivaroxaban plasma concentrations, resulting in a decrease in rivaroxaban exposure and efficacy. Avoid coadministration of rivaroxaban with agents that are combined P-gp and strong CYP3A4 inducers. If concomitant use cannot be avoided, consider increasing the rivaroxaban dose.[1]

The basis for this monograph is information on file with the manufacturer. Published clinical data are needed to further assess this interaction. Because of the seriousness of the interaction, clinical evaluation in humans is not likely to be forthcoming.

[1] *Xarelto* [package insert]. Titusville, NJ: Janssen Pharmaceuticals Inc; July 2011.

* Asterisk indicates drugs cited in interaction reports.

Rizatriptan — *Propranolol*

Rizatriptan* (*Maxalt*)	Propranolol* (eg, *Inderal*)

Significance	Onset	Severity	Documentation
2	☐ Rapid	☐ Major	☐ Established
	■ **Delayed**	■ **Moderate**	☐ Probable
		☐ Minor	■ **Suspected**
			☐ Possible
			☐ Unlikely

Effects RIZATRIPTAN plasma concentrations may be elevated, increasing the pharmacologic effects and adverse reactions.

Mechanism Inhibition of RIZATRIPTAN metabolism (MAO A) by PROPRANOLOL is suspected.

Management In patients receiving RIZATRIPTAN, consider administering a 5 mg dose during coadministration of PROPRANOLOL. Closely monitor the response to therapy if PROPRANOLOL is started or stopped. Be prepared to adjust the dose of RIZATRIPTAN as needed. Metoprolol (eg, *Lopressor*) and nadolol (eg, *Corgard*) do not appear to interact with RIZATRIPTAN and, when indicated, may be safer alternatives for PROPRANOLOL.

Discussion

The effects of metoprolol, nadolol, and propranolol on the pharmacokinetics and pharmacodynamics of rizatriptan were studied in 51 healthy subjects.[1] In 4 double-blind, randomized, placebo-controlled, crossover investigations, a single dose of rizatriptan 10 mg was administered after 7 days of metoprolol 100 mg 2 times per day, nadolol 80 mg 2 times per day, propranolol 60 and 120 mg 2 times per day, or placebo. Coadministration of rizatriptan with metoprolol or nadolol did not affect the pharmacokinetics of rizatriptan. Compared with placebo, coadministration of rizatriptan and propranolol (120 mg 2 times per day) increased the AUC of rizatriptan 67% and the peak plasma level 75%. Decreasing the dose of propranolol to 60 mg 2 times per day or separating the administration times of propranolol and rizatriptan by 1 or 2 hours did not change the effect of propranolol on the pharmacokinetics of rizatriptan. Coadministration of rizatriptan and any of the beta-adrenergic blocking agents did not quantitatively or qualitatively affect the adverse reactions of rizatriptan.

[1] Goldberg MR, et al. *Br J Clin Pharmacol.* 2001;52(1):69.

* Asterisk indicates drugs cited in interaction reports.

Roflumilast — *Rifamycins*

Roflumilast* (*Daliresp*)	Rifabutin (*Mycobutin*)	Rifapentine (*Priftin*)
	Rifampin* (eg, *Rifadin*)	

Significance	Onset	Severity	Documentation
2	□ Rapid	□ Major	□ Established
	■ **Delayed**	■ **Moderate**	□ Probable
		□ Minor	■ **Suspected**
			□ Possible
			□ Unlikely

Effects ROFLUMILAST plasma concentrations may be reduced, decreasing the pharmacologic effects.

Mechanism Increased ROFLUMILAST metabolism (CYP2C19 and/or CYP3A4) by RIFAMYCINS.

Management If coadministration cannot be avoided, closely monitor the clinical response to ROFLUMILAST and adjust the dose as needed.

Discussion

The effects of rifampin on the pharmacokinetics of roflumilast and the roflumilast N-oxide active metabolite were evaluated in 16 healthy men.[1] In an open-label, 3-period study, each subject received a single oral dose of roflumilast 500 mcg on days 1 and 12 and repeated oral doses of rifampin 600 mg once daily on days 5 to 15. Administration of roflumilast during steady-state administration of rifampin decreased roflumilast AUC and C_{max} 80% and 68%, respectively, compared with giving roflumilast alone. The roflumilast N-oxide AUC decreased 56% and the C_{max} increased 30%. The total phosphodiesterase 4 inhibitory activity of roflumilast and roflumilast N-oxide decreased 58%.

[1] Nassr N, et al. *Br J Clin Pharmacol.* 2009;68(4):580.

* Asterisk indicates drugs cited in interaction reports. Based on pharmacologic and pharmacokinetic considerations, similar interactions may occur with other drugs that are listed.

Romidepsin — *St. John's Wort*

Romidepsin* (*Istodax*)	St. John's Wort*

Significance	Onset	Severity	Documentation
2	☐ Rapid	☐ Major	☐ Established
	■ **Delayed**	■ **Moderate**	☐ Probable
		☐ Minor	■ **Suspected**
			☐ Possible
			☐ Unlikely

Effects ROMIDEPSIN plasma concentrations may be reduced, decreasing the efficacy.

Mechanism Induction of ROMIDEPSIN metabolism (CYP3A4) by ST. JOHN'S WORT.

Management Avoid coadministration of ROMIDEPSIN and ST. JOHN'S WORT.[1] Caution patients taking ROMIDEPSIN to inform their health care provider before taking ST. JOHN'S WORT.

Discussion

Because romidepsin is a substrate of CYP3A4, coadministration of a CYP3A4 inducer such as St. John's wort may decrease romidepsin plasma concentrations, resulting in a possible decrease in romidepsin efficacy. Therefore, it is recommended that coadministration of romidepsin and St. John's wort be avoided.[1]

The basis for this monograph is information on file with the manufacturer. Clinical evaluation of this interaction is needed to determine the consequences of coadministration of romidepsin and St. John's wort.

[1] *Istodax* [package insert]. Cambridge, MA: Gloucester Pharmaceuticals Inc; 2009.

* Asterisk indicates drugs cited in interaction reports.

Ropivacaine — *Azole Antifungal Agents*

Ropivacaine		Azole Antifungal Agents	
Ropivacaine* (*Naropin*)		Fluconazole (eg, *Diflucan*)	Itraconazole (eg, *Sporanox*)
		Ketoconazole* (eg, *Nizoral*)	

Significance	Onset	Severity	Documentation
5	☐ Rapid	☐ Major	☐ Established
	■ **Delayed**	☐ Moderate	☐ Probable
		■ **Minor**	☐ Suspected
			■ **Possible**
			☐ Unlikely

Effects ROPIVACAINE plasma levels may be elevated, increasing the pharmacologic effects and adverse reactions.

Mechanism Inhibition of ROPIVACAINE metabolism (CYP3A4) by AZOLE ANTIFUNGAL AGENTS is suspected. FLUCONAZOLE, especially 200 mg/day or more, may inhibit CYP3A4.

Management Based on available data, no special actions are needed. Consider the possibility of increased local anesthetic effect of ROPIVACAINE in patients receiving an AZOLE ANTIFUNGAL AGENT.

Discussion

In a randomized, crossover study, 12 healthy subjects received a single IV dose of ropivacaine 40 mg (infused over 20 minutes) alone and with oral ketoconazole 100 mg twice daily for 2 days.[1] The ropivacaine infusion was started 1 hour after taking the morning dose of ketoconazole on the second day of ketoconazole administration. Ketoconazole administration decreased the plasma clearance of ropivacaine 15% (from 354 to 302 mL/min). In a study of 8 healthy volunteers, itraconazole did not alter the pharmacokinetics of ropivacaine[2]; however, the formation of 1 metabolite was decreased.

Additional studies are needed to assess the clinical importance of this interaction.

[1] Arlander E, et al. *Clin Pharmacol Ther.* 1998; 64(5):484.

[2] Jokinen MJ, et al. *Pharmacol Toxicol.* 2001;88(4):187.

* Asterisk indicates drugs cited in interaction reports. Based on pharmacologic and pharmacokinetic considerations, similar interactions may occur with other drugs that are listed.

Ropivacaine — *Fluvoxamine*

Ropivacaine* (*Naropin*)	Fluvoxamine* (eg, *Luvox*)

Significance	Onset	Severity	Documentation
2	□ Rapid ■ **Delayed**	□ Major ■ **Moderate** □ Minor	□ Established □ Probable ■ **Suspected** □ Possible □ Unlikely

Effects ROPIVACAINE plasma concentrations may be elevated; the pharmacologic effects may be prolonged, increasing the risk of toxicity.

Mechanism Inhibition of ROPIVACAINE metabolism (CYP1A2) by FLUVOXAMINE.

Management In patients receiving FLUVOXAMINE, administer ROPIVACAINE with caution and monitor for ROPIVACAINE toxicity. Adjust the dose of ROPIVACAINE as needed.

Discussion

Ropivacaine is metabolized by CYP1A2 and CYP3A4. The coadministration effects of fluvoxamine, a CYP1A2 inhibitor, and erythromycin, a CYP3A4 inhibitor, on the pharmacokinetics of ropivacaine were studied in 8 healthy volunteers.[1] In a randomized, double-blind, 4-way crossover study, each subject received 500 mg of erythromycin 3 times/day for 6 days, 100 mg of fluvoxamine once daily for 5 days, both erythromycin and fluvoxamine, or placebo. On day 6 of each study period, ropivacaine 0.6 mg/kg was infused over a 30-minute period. Compared with placebo, administration of fluvoxamine without erythromycin increased the AUC and mean residence time (MRT) of ropivacaine 3.7-fold, prolonged the $t_{½}$ from 2.3 to 7.4 hr, and decreased the clearance 77%. Administration of erythromycin without fluvoxamine resulted in only minor effects on the pharmacokinetics of ropivacaine; however, compared with administration of fluvoxamine with ropivacaine, coadministration of fluvoxamine plus erythromycin with ropivacaine further increased the AUC of ropivacaine 50%, the MRT 64%, and prolonged the $t_{½}$ from 7.4 to 11.9 hr.

[1] Jokinen MJ, et al. *Anesth Analg.* 2000;91:1207.

* Asterisk indicates drugs cited in interaction reports.

Ropivacaine / *Quinolones*

Ropivacaine* (*Naropin*)	Ciprofloxacin* (eg, *Cipro*)	Norfloxacin (*Noroxin*)

Significance	Onset	Severity	Documentation
4	□ Rapid ■ **Delayed**	□ Major ■ **Moderate** □ Minor	□ Established □ Probable □ Suspected ■ **Possible** □ Unlikely

Effects ROPIVACAINE plasma concentrations may be elevated, increasing the pharmacologic and toxic effects.

Mechanism CIPROFLOXACIN inhibits the metabolism (CYP1A2) of ROPIVACAINE.

Management In patients receiving CIPROFLOXACIN, administer ROPIVACAINE with caution and closely monitor the patient. Adjust the dose of ROPIVACAINE as needed.

Discussion

Using a double-blind, randomized, crossover design, the effects of ciprofloxacin on the pharmacokinetics of ropivacaine were studied in 9 healthy volunteers.[1] Each subject received oral ciprofloxacin 500 mg or placebo every 12 hr for 2.5 days and, on the third day, 0.6 mg/kg of ropivacaine was given IV over 30 minutes. Compared with placebo, ciprofloxacin increased the AUC of ropivacaine 22% and decreased the clearance 31%. There was no change in the peak concentration, t½, or volume of distribution of ropivacaine. Ciprofloxacin decreased the AUC of the 3-hydroxyropivacaine (3-OH-R) metabolite 38% and the peak plasma concentration 53%, while increasing the t½ 46%. In addition, ciprofloxacin increased the AUC of the 2′,6′-pipecoloxylidide (PPX) metabolite of ropivacaine 71% and the peak plasma concentration 60%. The urinary excretion of ropivacaine was increased 79%, 3-OH-R was decreased 27%, and PPX was increased 97%.

[1] Jokinen MJ, et al. *Eur J Clin Pharmacol.* 2003;58:653.

* Asterisk indicates drugs cited in interaction reports. Based on pharmacologic and pharmacokinetic considerations, similar interactions may occur with other drugs that are listed.

Rosuvastatin — *Protease Inhibitors*

Rosuvastatin* (*Crestor*)	Lopinavir/Ritonavir* (*Kaletra*)

Significance	Onset	Severity	Documentation
1	☐ Rapid ■ **Delayed**	■ **Major** ☐ Moderate ☐ Minor	☐ Established ■ **Probable** ☐ Suspected ☐ Possible ☐ Unlikely

Effects ROSUVASTATIN plasma concentrations may be elevated, increasing the risk of adverse reactions (eg, rhabdomyolysis).

Mechanism Unknown.

Management Coadminister ROSUVASTATIN and LOPINAVIR/RITONAVIR with caution. Limit the dosage of ROSUVASTATIN to 10 mg once daily in patients receiving LOPINAVIR/RITONAVIR.[1]

Discussion

In an open-label study, the effects of lopinavir 400 mg/ritonavir 100 mg on the pharmacokinetics of rosuvastatin were evaluated in 15 healthy subjects.[2] Each subject received rosuvastatin 20 mg/day alone for 7 days, then lopinavir/ritonavir alone for 10 days, and finally the agents were coadministered for 7 days. Lopinavir/ritonavir increased the C_{max} and AUC of rosuvastatin 4.7- and 2.1-fold, respectively, compared with administration of rosuvastatin alone.

Additional studies are needed to determine the mechanism of this interaction and if other protease inhibitors interact similarly with rosuvastatin.

[1] *Crestor* [package insert]. Wilmington, DE: AstraZeneca Pharmaceuticals LP; November 2007.

[2] Kiser JJ, et al. *J Acquir Immune Defic Syndr.* 2008;47(5):570.

* Asterisk indicates drugs cited in interaction reports.

Rosuvastatin — *St. John's Wort*

Rosuvastatin* (*Crestor*)	St. John's Wort*

Significance	Onset	Severity	Documentation
4	☐ Rapid	☐ Major	☐ Established
	■ **Delayed**	■ **Moderate**	☐ Probable
		☐ Minor	☐ Suspected
			■ **Possible**
			☐ Unlikely

Effects The cholesterol-lowering effect of ROSUVASTATIN may be decreased.

Mechanism Unknown.

Management Advise patients receiving ROSUVASTATIN to avoid taking ST. JOHN'S WORT.

Discussion

A 59-year-old man showed marked improvement in his lipid profile after starting rosuvastatin 10 mg daily.[1] A routine lipid panel performed after 6 months demonstrated increases of total and LDL cholesterol. Subsequently, the patient started taking an herbal supplement for insomnia that contained St. John's wort 300 mg, rosemary 80 mg, and spirulina 40 mg. He stopped taking the herbal supplement and a repeat lipid panel 4 months later showed marked improvement in his lipid profile. See also HMG-CoA Reductase Inhibitors-St. John's Wort.

[1] Gordon RY, et al. *Am J Med.* 2009;122(2):e1.

* Asterisk indicates drugs cited in interaction reports.

Rufinamide — *Valproic Acid*

Rufinamide	Valproic Acid	
Rufinamide* (*Banzel*)	Divalproex Sodium (eg, *Depakote*)	Valproic Acid* (eg, *Depakene*)
	Valproate Sodium (eg, *Depacon*)	

Significance	Onset	Severity	Documentation
2	☐ Rapid	☐ Major	☐ Established
	■ **Delayed**	■ **Moderate**	☐ Probable
		☐ Minor	■ **Suspected**
			☐ Possible
			☐ Unlikely

Effects RUFINAMIDE plasma concentrations may be elevated, increasing the pharmacologic effects and risk of adverse reactions.

Mechanism Unknown.

Management Therapeutic drug monitoring is warranted. It is recommended that children receiving VALPROIC ACID start RUFINAMIDE at a dosage lower than 10 mg/kg/day and adults receiving RUFINAMIDE start RUFINAMIDE at a dosage lower than 400 mg/day.[1]

Discussion

The effects of valproic acid on the pharmacokinetics of rufinamide were studied retrospectively in epileptic patients.[2] Mean rufinamide plasma concentrations were 86.6% higher when valproic acid concentrations were greater than 90 mcg/mL and 45.4% higher when valproic acid concentrations were between 50 and 90 mcg/mL, compared with administering rufinamide with antiepileptic drugs but without valproic acid. However, rufinamide concentrations were not significantly different when valproic acid concentrations were less than 50 mcg/mL (4.4%, $P > 0.1$).

[1] *Banzel* [package insert]. Woodcliff Lake, NJ: Eisai Inc; March 2011.

[2] May TW, et al. *Ther Drug Monit.* 2011;33(2):214.

* Asterisk indicates drugs cited in interaction reports. Based on pharmacologic and pharmacokinetic considerations, similar interactions may occur with other drugs that are listed.

Ruxolitinib — *Azole Antifungal Agents*

Ruxolitinib	Azole Antifungal Agents	
Ruxolitinib* (*Jakafi*)	Itraconazole* (eg, *Sporanox*)	Posaconazole* (*Noxafil*)
	Ketoconazole* (eg, *Nizoral*)	Voriconazole* (eg, *Vfend*)

Significance	Onset	Severity	Documentation
2	☐ Rapid	☐ Major	☐ Established
	■ **Delayed**	■ **Moderate**	☐ Probable
		☐ Minor	■ **Suspected**
			☐ Possible
			☐ Unlikely

Effects RUXOLITINIB plasma concentrations may be elevated, increasing the pharmacologic effect and risk of adverse reactions.

Mechanism Inhibition of RUXOLITINIB metabolism (CYP3A4) by AZOLE ANTIFUNGAL AGENTS.

Management Close clinical and laboratory monitoring are warranted. A RUXOLITINIB dosage adjustment may be needed. A starting dose of RUXOLITINIB 10 mg twice daily is recommended in patients receiving a strong CYP3A4 inhibitor (eg, KETOCONAZOLE).[1] Avoid coadministration of RUXOLITINIB with strong CYP3A4 inhibitors in patients with a platelet count less than 100 x 10^9/L.

Discussion

The effects of ketoconazole on the pharmacokinetics and pharmacodynamics of ruxolitinib were studied in 16 healthy volunteers.[2] Each subject received ketoconazole 200 mg twice daily for 4 days. On the last day of ketoconazole administration, subjects received a single dose of ruxolitinib 10 mg. Compared with giving ruxolitinib alone, pretreatment with ketoconazole increased the ruxolitinib C_{max} and AUC 33% and 91%, respectively, and increased the ruxolitinib pharmacodynamic activity 2-fold. Coadministration of ketoconazole increased the $t_{1/2}$ of ruxolitinib from 3.5 to 5.6 hours. When administering ruxolitinib with strong CYP3A4 inhibitors (eg, itraconazole, ketoconazole, posaconazole, voriconazole), a dose reduction is recommended.[1] Closely monitor patients and the titrate dose based on safety and efficacy.

[1] *Jakafi* [package insert]. Wilmington, DE: Incyte Corporation; November 2011.

[2] Shi JG, et al. *J Clin Pharmacol.* 2012;52(6):809.

* Asterisk indicates drugs cited in interaction reports.

Ruxolitinib | **Macrolide & Related Antibiotics**

Ruxolitinib	Macrolide & Related Antibiotics	
Ruxolitinib* (*Jakafi*)	Azithromycin (eg, *Zithromax*)	Erythromycin* (eg, *Ery-Tab*)
	Clarithromycin* (eg, *Biaxin*)	Telithromycin* (*Ketek*)

Significance	Onset	Severity	Documentation
2	☐ Rapid	☐ Major	☐ Established
	■ **Delayed**	■ **Moderate**	☐ Probable
		☐ Minor	■ **Suspected**
			☐ Possible
			☐ Unlikely

Effects RUXOLITINIB plasma concentrations may be elevated, increasing the pharmacologic effect and risk of adverse reactions.

Mechanism Inhibition of RUXOLITINIB metabolism (CYP3A4) by MACROLIDE AND RELATED ANTIBIOTICS.

Management Close clinical and laboratory monitoring are warranted. RUXOLITINIB dosage adjustment may be needed. A starting dose of RUXOLITINIB 10 mg twice daily is recommended in patients receiving a strong CYP3A4 inhibitor (eg, CLARITHROMYCIN, TELITHROMYCIN).[1] Avoid coadministration of RUXOLITINIB with strong CYP3A4 inhibitors in patients with a platelet count less than 100×10^9/L. However, no dosage adjustment is recommended when a mild or moderate CYP3A4 inhibitor (eg, ERYTHROMYCIN) is coadministered with RUXOLITINIB.[1]

Discussion

When administering ruxolitinib with strong CYP3A4 inhibitors (eg, clarithromycin, telithromycin) a dose reduction is recommended. Closely monitor patients and titrate the dose based on safety and efficacy. However, no dosage adjustment is recommended when ruxolitinib is coadministered with mild or moderate CYP3A4 inhibitors (eg, erythromycin).[1] The effects of erythromycin on the pharmacokinetics and pharmacodynamics of ruxolitinib were studied in 14 healthy volunteers.[2] Each subject received erythromycin 500 mg twice daily for 4 days. On the last day of erythromycin administration, subjects received a single dose of ruxolitinib 10 mg. Pretreatment with erythromycin increased the ruxolitinib C_{max} and AUC 8% and 27%, respectively, compared with administration of ruxolitinib alone. Coadministration of erythromycin did not alter the $t_{½}$ of ruxolitinib appreciably. The magnitude of these changes is not likely to be clinically important.

[1] *Jakafi* [package insert]. Wilmington, DE: Incyte Corporation; November 2011.

[2] Shi JG, et al. *J Clin Pharmacol.* 2012;52(6):809.

* Asterisk indicates drugs cited in interaction reports. Based on pharmacologic and pharmacokinetic considerations, similar interactions may occur with other drugs that are listed.

Ruxolitinib — *Rifamycins*

Ruxolitinib	Rifamycins	
Ruxolitinib* (*Jakafi*)	Rifabutin (*Mycobutin*)	Rifapentine (*Priftin*)
	Rifampin* (eg, *Rifadin*)	

Significance	Onset	Severity	Documentation
4	☐ Rapid	☐ Major	☐ Established
	■ **Delayed**	■ **Moderate**	☐ Probable
		☐ Minor	☐ Suspected
			■ **Possible**
			☐ Unlikely

Effects RUXOLITINIB plasma concentrations may be reduced, decreasing the pharmacologic effect.

Mechanism Induction of RUXOLITINIB metabolism (CYP3A4) by RIFAMYCINS.

Management No dose adjustment is recommended when RUXOLITINIB is coadministered with RIFAMYCINS. Closely monitor patients and titrate the dose of RUXOLITINIB based on safety and efficacy.[1]

Discussion

The effects of the strong CYP3A4 inducer rifampin on the pharmacokinetics and pharmacodynamics of ruxolitinib were studied in 8 healthy volunteers.[2] Each subject received rifampin 600 mg once daily for 10 days. On the last day of rifampin administration, subjects received a single dose of ruxolitinib 50 mg. Compared with giving ruxolitinib alone, pretreatment with rifampin decreased the ruxolitinib C_{max} and AUC 52% and 71%, respectively. Coadministration of rifampin decreased the t½ of ruxolitinib from 3.2 to 1.6 hours. However, the ruxolitinib pharmacodynamic activity decreased only 10%.

[1] *Jakafi* [package insert]. Wilmington, DE: Incyte Corporation; November 2011.

[2] Shi JG, et al. *J Clin Pharmacol.* 2012;52(6):809.

* Asterisk indicates drugs cited in interaction reports. Based on pharmacologic and pharmacokinetic considerations, similar interactions may occur with other drugs that are listed.

Salicylates — *Antacids*

Salicylates		Antacids	
Aspirin* (eg, *Bayer*)	Salsalate (eg, *Disalcid*)	Aluminum Hydroxide (eg, *Amphojel*)	Magnesium Hydroxide (eg, *Milk of Magnesia*)
Choline Salicylate* (*Arthropan*)	Sodium Salicylate	Aluminum/Magnesium Hydroxide* (eg, *Maalox*)	
Magnesium Salicylate (eg, *Doan's*)	Sodium Thiosalicylate (eg, *Tusal*)		

Significance	Onset	Severity	Documentation
3	☐ Rapid	☐ Major	☐ Established
	■ **Delayed**	☐ Moderate	■ **Probable**
		■ **Minor**	☐ Suspected
			☐ Possible
			☐ Unlikely

Effects Serum SALICYLATE concentrations may be reduced.

Mechanism ANTACID-induced increase in urinary pH reduces the renal reabsorption of SALICYLATE, increasing SALICYLATE clearance.

Management Patients stabilized on large doses of SALICYLATES may require monitoring of serum SALICYLATE concentrations and tailoring of dosage when ANTACID therapy is either initiated or discontinued.

Discussion

While single doses of antacids are unlikely to have a significant effect,[2,5] chronic therapy with antacids can increase urinary pH in a dose-dependent manner.[1,2,4,5] This effect persists for at least 1 day after the last dose of antacid.[2] Three boys with rheumatic fever being treated with aspirin demonstrated 30% to 70% reductions in serum salicylate concentrations when a magnesium and aluminum hydroxide combination antacid was administered.[3] Similar, although less impressive, results were noted in nine healthy male adults receiving choline salicylate with or without *Maalox*, 120 mL/day. Six of the subjects achieved serum salicylate levels higher than 10 mg/dL while receiving choline salicylate alone. The mean serum salicylate concentration of these six subjects declined by 20% (from 19.8 to 15.8 mg/dL) during antacid administration.[6]

[1] Gibaldi M, et al. *Clin Pharmacol Ther.* 1974;16:520.
[2] Gibaldi M, et al. *J Pharm Sci.* 1975;64:2003.
[3] Levy G, et al. *N Engl J Med.* 1975;293:323.
[4] Muller FO, et al. *S Afr Med J.* 1977;51:379.
[5] Ayres JW, et al. *Eur J Clin Pharmacol.* 1977;12:415.
[6] Hansten PD, et al. *J Clin Pharmacol.* 1980;24:326.

* Asterisk indicates drugs cited in interaction reports. Based on pharmacologic and pharmacokinetic considerations, similar interactions may occur with other drugs that are listed.

Salicylates		***Carbonic Anhydrase Inh.***	
Aspirin* (eg, *Bayer*) Choline Salicylate (*Arthropan*) Magnesium Salicylate (eg, *Doan's*)	Salsalate* (eg, *Disalcid*) Sodium Salicylate* Sodium Thiosalicylate (eg, *Tusal*)	Acetazolamide* (eg, *Diamox*) Dichlorphenamide* (*Daranide*)	Methazolamide (*GlaucTabs*, *Neptazane*)

Significance	Onset	Severity	Documentation
2	☐ Rapid ■ **Delayed**	☐ Major ■ **Moderate** ☐ Minor	☐ Established ☐ Probable ■ **Suspected** ☐ Possible ☐ Unlikely

Effects Use of CARBONIC ANHYDRASE INHIBITORS (CAIs) and SALICYLATES may result in CAI accumulation and toxicity including CNS depression and metabolic acidosis.

Mechanism ASPIRIN (ASA) displaces ACETAZOLAMIDE from plasma protein binding sites and inhibits renal clearance. CAI-induced acidosis may allow increased CNS penetration by SALICYLATES.

Management Minimize or avoid SALICYLATE and CAI coadministration. Elderly patients and those with renal failure are predisposed to ACETAZOLAMIDE accumulation. When a CAI is required in a patient taking SALICYLATES, monitor plasma salicylate concentrations, acid-base parameters and CNS status.

Discussion

In 3 reports, 5 elderly patients taking ASA for arthritis and a CAI for glaucoma developed toxicity consisting of lethargy, confusion, fatigue, anorexia, urinary incontinence, tachypnea, and hyperchloremic metabolic acidosis.[1,3,4] Alterations of drug regimens preceded symptoms by days to weeks. Although these patients were elderly and received relatively high doses of ASA (up to 8 g/day) or salsalate (3 g/day), one study reported 2 young patients with normal renal and hepatic function who demonstrated toxic symptoms while using lower salicylate doses (up to 4 g/day) with CAIs.[2] Plasma salicylate values in 6 of the 7 cases ranged from 21.6 to 26.2 mg/dL; chronic concentrations greater than 15 mg/dL may produce toxicity. Studies using 4 healthy volunteers demonstrated salicylate dose-dependent displacement of acetazolamide from plasma proteins and inhibition of renal clearance of acetazolamide.[3] The acidosis accompanying CAI accumulation increases the potential for unionized salicylate penetration into the CNS. The relative contributions of CAI and salicylate toxicity to observed signs and symptoms remain unknown.

[1] Anderson CJ, et al. *Am J Ophthalmol.* 1978;86:516.
[2] Cowan RA, et al. *BMJ.* 1984;289:347.
[3] Sweeney KR, et al. *Clin Pharmacol Ther.* 1986;40:518.
[4] Rousseau P, et al. *J Am Geriatr Soc.* 1993;41:868.

* Asterisk indicates drugs cited in interaction reports. Based on pharmacologic and pharmacokinetic considerations, similar interactions may occur with other drugs that are listed.

Salicylates / *Contraceptives, Hormonal*

Salicylates		Contraceptives, Hormonal
Aspirin* (eg, *Bayer*)	Salsalate (eg, *Salflex*)	Contraceptives, Oral* (eg, *Ortho-Novum*)
Choline Salicylate	Sodium Salicylate	
Magnesium Salicylate (eg, *Doan's*)		

Significance	Onset	Severity	Documentation
5	☐ Rapid	☐ Major	☐ Established
	■ **Delayed**	☐ Moderate	☐ Probable
		■ **Minor**	☐ Suspected
			■ **Possible**
			☐ Unlikely

Effects SALICYLATE effectiveness may be impaired in women taking ORAL CONTRACEPTIVES (OCs). The interaction may not occur in chronic OC users.

Mechanism OCs induce the hepatic metabolism of SALICYLATES via glycine and glucuronic acid conjugation, resulting in lower plasma SALICYLATE levels, shorter $t_{1/2}$, and increased clearance.

Management Women taking OCs may require higher or more frequent ASPIRIN doses for desired clinical effects. When maintenance of a specific plasma concentration is crucial, monitor SALICYLATE levels when OCs are started or discontinued.

Discussion

The short-term use of a low-dose combination OC (ethinyl estradiol 30 mcg plus norethisterone 1 mg) on aspirin kinetics has been investigated.[1] Following a single dose of aspirin 300 or 600 mg, 10 subjects taking OCs for 2 menstrual cycles exhibited lowered salicylate plasma concentrations, $t_{1/2}$, and AUC. The values returned to previous levels within 3 to 5 months after OC discontinuation. Five women taking OCs for more than 2 years who received a dose of aspirin 600 mg demonstrated plasma salicylate levels and $t_{1/2}$ that were similar to controls. Thus, long-term OC use may not significantly affect aspirin kinetics.

Researchers demonstrated a 41% average increase in salicylic acid clearance in 8 women taking various combination OCs after a single dose of aspirin 900 mg, compared with controls.[2] Renal clearance of salicyluric acid and salicyl glucuronide was significantly greater in OC users, suggesting induction of hepatic glycine and glucuronic acid conjugation of aspirin. More study is required to evaluate the clinical importance of the observed interaction and the possible significance of chronic coadministration of OCs and salicylates.

[1] Gupta KC, et al. *Int J Clin Pharmacol Ther Toxicol.* 1982;20(11):511.

[2] Miners JO, et al. *Br J Clin Pharmacol.* 1986;22(2):135.

* Asterisk indicates drugs cited in interaction reports. Based on pharmacologic and pharmacokinetic considerations, similar interactions may occur with other drugs that are listed.

Salicylates — *Corticosteroids*

Salicylates		Corticosteroids	
Aspirin* (eg, *Bayer*)	Magnesium Salicylate (eg, *Doans*)	Betamethasone (eg, *Celestone*)	Methylprednisolone* (eg, *Medrol*)
Bismuth Subsalicylate (eg, *Pepto-Bismol*)	Salsalate	Budesonide (eg, *Pulmicort*)	Prednisolone* (eg, *Prelone*)
Choline Salicylate*	Sodium Salicylate*	Cortisone	Prednisone* (eg, *Sterapred*)
		Dexamethasone* (eg, *Baycadron*)	Triamcinolone* (eg, *Kenalog*)
		Fludrocortisone	
		Hydrocortisone* (eg, *Cortef*)	

Significance	Onset	Severity	Documentation
3	□ Rapid	□ Major	□ Established
	■ **Delayed**	□ Moderate	■ **Probable**
		■ **Minor**	□ Suspected
			□ Possible
			□ Unlikely

Effects CORTICOSTEROIDS will reduce serum SALICYLATE levels and may decrease SALICYLATE effectiveness; discontinuation of CORTICOSTEROIDS may increase SALICYLATE levels.

Mechanism CORTICOSTEROIDS probably stimulate liver metabolism of SALICYLATES and may also increase renal elimination.

Management Tailor SALICYLATE dosage as needed; monitor plasma SALICYLATE concentrations when CORTICOSTEROIDS are added or withdrawn.

Discussion

Studies show that administration of salicylates has no[1] or limited[2] effect on endogenous corticosteroid elimination. Conversely, corticosteroids enhance salicylate elimination.[3-8] Ten patients with rheumatoid arthritis taking enteric-coated aspirin 1.3 to 4.6 g/day for at least 4 weeks received intra-articular corticosteroid injections. Their calculated mean steady-state plasma salicylate levels decreased 29%, while their mean salicylate plasma clearances increased 39%.[3] Another study reported similar findings.[4] Administration of constant doses of aspirin or choline salicylate during tapering of corticosteroid dosage resulted in significant increases in serum salicylate concentrations in 5 patients, including salicylate intoxication in a 5-year-old boy whose serum salicylate level increased from less than 10 to 88 mg/dL.[3] While suggested that the increase is primarily renal,[3,5] evidence points to increased hepatic elimination as the mechanism,[6] but this has not been clearly established.[7] Men may be more affected than women.[6] Single doses of salicylates are probably not problematic.[9]

1 Peterson RE, et al. *Arthritis Rheum.* 1958;1(1):29.
2 Elliot HC. *Metabolism.* 1962;11:1015.
3 Edelman J, et al. *Br J Clin Pharmacol.* 1986;21(3):301.
4 Baer PA, et al. *Arthritis Rheum.* 1987;30(3):345.
5 Klinenberg JR, et al. *JAMA.* 1965;194(6):601.
6 Graham GG, et al. *Clin Pharmacol Ther.* 1977;22(4):410.
7 Koren G, et al. *Ther Drug Monit.* 1987;9(2):177.
8 Bardare M, et al. *Arch Dis Child.* 1978;53(5):381.
9 Day RO, et al. *Br J Clin Pharmacol.* 1988;26(3):334.

* Asterisk indicates drugs cited in interaction reports. Based on pharmacologic and pharmacokinetic considerations, similar interactions may occur with other drugs that are listed.

Salicylates | **Ethanol**

Aspirin* (eg, *Bayer*) | Ethanol*

Significance	Onset	Severity	Documentation
3	☐ Rapid	☐ Major	☐ Established
	■ **Delayed**	☐ Moderate	☐ Probable
		■ **Minor**	■ **Suspected**
			☐ Possible
			☐ Unlikely

Effects ETHANOL may potentiate ASPIRIN-induced GI blood loss and bleeding time prolongation. The latter may occur up to 36 hours after ASPIRIN (ASA) administration. Clinically significant bleeding is possible in predisposed patients.

Mechanism ASA and ETHANOL damage the gastric mucosal barrier. The production of gastric acid stimulated by ETHANOL promotes this damage.

Management Consider separating ASA and ETHANOL intake by 12 hours. GI blood loss is reduced with buffered aqueous solutions (eg, *Alka-Seltzer*) and enteric-coated or extended-release ASA tablets. Consider using a nonacetylated salicylate.

Discussion

Controlled studies in 35 healthy volunteers demonstrated that the combination of moderate amounts of ethanol with therapeutic ASA doses over 2 to 3 days caused greater fecal blood loss than ASA alone.[1-3] Gastroduodenal lesions visualized endoscopically in 60 subjects[4] were intensified by ethanol. Ethanol alone did not damage the gastric mucosa or cause GI blood loss. A retrospective study of 817 patients hospitalized for GI bleeding implied a possible synergistic effect of ethanol and ASA.[5] In controlled trials, neither buffered sodium acetylsalicylate 728 mg solution (eg, *Alka-Seltzer*)[6,7] nor diflunisal (eg, *Dolobid*) 500 mg/day,[2,3] with or without alcohol, increased occult fecal blood loss. Ethanol alone does not affect bleeding time or platelet aggregation. Administration of ethanol within 36 hours after an ASA 325 mg dose variably increased the magnitude and duration of ASA-induced bleeding time prolongation.[8,9] When ethanol was given 12 hours prior to ASA, no interaction occurred. Choline salicylate, with or without ethanol, did not affect bleeding time. While ASA increases the bioavailability and peak levels of ethanol when imbibed after meals, it is unknown if the change translates to a marked enhancement of ethanol effect.[10] Another study did not confirm that ASA increased ethanol levels.[11] Coadministration of ASA and ethanol to 12 volunteers reduced peak ASA concentrations by 25%.

[1] Goulston K, et al. *Br Med J.* 1968;4(5632):664.
[2] DeSchepper PJ, et al. *Clin Pharmacol Ther.* 1978;23(6):669.
[3] De Schepper PJ, et al. *Curr Med Res Opin.* 1978;5(7):520.
[4] Lanza FL, et al. *Am J Gastroenterol.* 1985;80(10):767.
[5] Needham CD, et al. *Gut.* 1971;12(10):819.
[6] Bouchier IA, et al. *Lancet.* 1969;1(7587):178.
[7] Leonards JR. *Lancet.* 1969;1(7601):943.
[8] Deykin D, et al. *N Engl J Med.* 1982;306(14):852.
[9] Rosove MH, et al. *Thromb Res.* 1983;31(3):525.
[10] Roine R, et al. *JAMA.* 1990;264(18):2406.
[11] Melander O, et al. *Eur J Clin Pharmacol.* 1995;48(2):151.

* Asterisk indicates drugs cited in interaction reports.

Salicylates | **Ginkgo biloba**

Aspirin*
(eg, *Bayer*)

Ginkgo biloba*

Significance	Onset	Severity	Documentation
4	□ Rapid ■ **Delayed**	□ Major ■ **Moderate** □ Minor	□ Established □ Probable □ Suspected ■ **Possible** □ Unlikely

Effects The risk of bleeding may be increased.

Mechanism Possible additive or synergistic inhibitory effect on platelet aggregation.

Management Caution patients to avoid concurrent use of ASPIRIN and GINKGO BILOBA because of potential serious bleeding complications.

Discussion

Spontaneous hemorrhage into the anterior chamber of the right eye was reported in a 70-year-old man while he was taking aspirin and *Ginkgo biloba*.[1] The patient had experienced recurrent blurred vision in his right eye, with each episode lasting 15 minutes. Gonioscopy revealed a layer of blood coming from a fine stream of blood oozing down the margin of the iris. Bleeding stopped spontaneously after 5 minutes. One week earlier, the patient had begun taking *Ginkgo biloba* tablets twice daily containing 40 mg of concentrate extract. The patient had been taking aspirin 325 mg/day for 3 years after coronary artery bypass surgery. He stopped taking the ginkgo extract but continued the daily aspirin. No further bleeding occurred over a 3-month follow-up period.

The ingredients of many herbal products are not standardized. It is unclear if herbal products contain ingredients other than those listed on the label or purported to be present that could affect coagulation. *Ginkgo biloba* extract may contain 1 or more components that affect platelet aggregation.[2] Therefore, patients may be at an increased risk of bleeding if they take aspirin, which has antiplatelet activity.

[1] Chung KF, et al. *Lancet*. 1987;1(8527):248.

[2] Rosenblatt M, et al. *N Engl J Med*. 1997;336(15):1108.

* Asterisk indicates drugs cited in interaction reports.

Salicylates / *Griseofulvin*

Salicylates	Griseofulvin
Aspirin* (eg, *Bayer*)	Griseofulvin* (eg, *Grisactin*)

Significance	Onset	Severity	Documentation
4	☐ Rapid ■ **Delayed**	☐ Major ■ **Moderate** ☐ Minor	☐ Established ☐ Probable ☐ Suspected ■ **Possible** ☐ Unlikely

Effects Serum SALICYLATE concentrations may be decreased.

Mechanism Unknown.

Management If there is no suitable alternative to ASPIRIN, such as a nonsteroidal anti-inflammatory drug (eg, ibuprofen [eg, *Advil*]), consider separating the doses of ASPIRIN and GRISEOFULVIN. Monitor SALICYLATE concentrations and adjust the dose of ASPIRIN as needed.

Discussion

Griseofulvin was reported to decrease serum salicylate levels in an 8-year-old boy with rheumatic heart disease.[1] The patient had a past medical history of acute rheumatic fever for which he was discharged from the hospital with an aluminum-magnesium hydroxide antacid (eg, *Maalox*), aspirin, captopril (eg, *Capoten*), digoxin (eg, *Lanoxin*), furosemide (eg, *Lasix*), iron, and potassium, as well as monthly benzathine penicillin (eg, *Permapen*). On this hospital admission, these medications were continued. On day 5 and 6, therapy with amoxicillin (eg, *Amoxil*) and griseofulvin was started for otitis media and tinea capitis, respectively. Because the serum salicylate concentration was 30.6 mg/dL (therapeutic, 15 to 30 mg/dL) on day 4, on day 6 the daily dose of aspirin was reduced from 147 to 110 mg/kg. On day 8, peak and trough salicylate concentrations were below detectable limits. A drug interaction between aspirin and griseofulvin was suspected, and the antifungal agent was discontinued the next day. Serum salicylate concentrations on the next 2 days were within the therapeutic range.

[1] Phillips KR, et al. *Pediatr Infect Dis J.* 1993;12:350.

* Asterisk indicates drugs cited in interaction reports.

Salicylates — *Kaolin-Pectin*

Aspirin* (eg, *Bayer*)	Kaolin-Pectin* (eg, *Kao-Spen*)

Significance	Onset	Severity	Documentation
5	■ **Rapid**	□ Major	□ Established
	□ Delayed	□ Moderate	□ Probable
		■ **Minor**	□ Suspected
			□ Possible
			■ **Unlikely**

Effects KAOLIN-PECTIN may decrease the bioavailability of ASPIRIN.

Mechanism Possibly due to reduced GI absorption of ASPIRIN.

Management Based on available data, no alterations in therapy appear to be necessary.

Discussion

The effects of kaolin-pectin suspension on the absorption of aspirin were studied in 10 volunteers.[1] When 30, 60, or 90 mL of kaolin-pectin suspension was administered with a 975 mg dose of aspirin, the recovery of salicylate in the urine was 90.6%, 94.6%, and 95.3%, respectively. Although the percent recovery in the urine for the 30 and 60 mL doses of kaolin-pectin was significantly less ($P < 0.05$) than the control (ie, no adsorbent), the 5% to 10% reduction in absorption would not be expected to be clinically important.

[1] Juhl RP. *Am J Hosp Pharm.* 1979;36:1097.

* Asterisk indicates drugs cited in interaction reports.

Salicylates — *Omega-3-Acid Ethyl Esters*

Salicylates	Omega-3-Acid Ethyl Esters
Aspirin* (eg, *Bayer*)	Omega-3-acid ethyl esters*

Significance	Onset	Severity	Documentation
4	☐ Rapid	■ **Major**	☐ Established
	■ **Delayed**	☐ Moderate	☐ Probable
		☐ Minor	☐ Suspected
			■ **Possible**
			☐ Unlikely

Effects OMEGA-3-ACID ETHYL ESTERS (OM3) in combination with ASPIRIN may increase the risk of serious bleeding.

Mechanism Unknown; however, additive platelet effects may be involved.

Management If coadministration of these agents cannot be avoided, use with caution and closely monitor patients. Advise patients of the possible risk of increased bleeding.

Discussion

A 75-year-old man experienced a minor fall when a stool on which he was sitting tipped.[1] He was brought to the emergency department (ED) after developing a headache and, later that day, experiencing decreased coordination, trouble walking, and slurred speech. Among the drugs he was taking were warfarin (7.5 mg 4 days/week and 5 mg 3 days/week) and aspirin 81 mg/day, as well as over-the-counter OM3 6 g/day. The patient's most recent INR was 2.8 (target range, 2 to 3), measured 1 month before the fall. At the time he was seen in the ED, his INR was 3.2. Results of a CT scan disclosed an acute large right subdural hematoma that measured 3 cm. The patient's coagulopathy was treated with fresh frozen plasma and vitamin K. He underwent a craniotomy for drainage and evacuation of the hematoma. He was discharged to a rehabilitation facility, and warfarin was restarted at 7.5 mg/day until the INR was above 2.5. Subsequently, he was placed on a maintenance dosage of warfarin 7.5 mg 3 days/week plus 5 mg 4 days/week. The patient was instructed not to resume taking OM3 or aspirin.

[1] McClaskey EM, et al. *Pharmacotherapy*. 2007;27(1):152.

* Asterisk indicates drugs cited in interaction reports.

Salicylates — *Proton Pump Inhibitors*

Salicylates		Proton Pump Inhibitors	
Aspirin* (eg, *Bayer*)	Sodium Salicylate*	Esomeprazole* (*Nexium*)	Pantoprazole* (eg, *Protonix*)
		Lansoprazole* (eg, *Prevacid*)	Rabeprazole* (*Aciphex*)
		Omeprazole* (eg, *Prilosec*)	

Significance	Onset	Severity	Documentation
3	☐ Rapid	☐ Major	☐ Established
	■ **Delayed**	☐ Moderate	☐ Probable
		■ **Minor**	■ **Suspected**
			☐ Possible
			☐ Unlikely

Effects Enteric-coated SALICYLATES may dissolve more rapidly, increasing gastric adverse effects. PROTON PUMP INHIBITORS may reduce the antiplatelet activity of low-dose aspirin.

Mechanism PROTON PUMP INHIBITOR–mediated increase in gastric pH results in a more rapid dissolution and release of SALICYLATE from the enteric-coated product.

Management Educate patients taking enteric-coated SALICYLATES and a PROTON PUMP INHIBITOR to monitor for increased gastric adverse effects. Patients at risk of serious gastric disorders due to the release of SALICYLATES in the stomach should avoid concurrent use of these agents.

Discussion

The effect of omeprazole-induced increase gastric pH on the release rate of salicylate from an enteric-coated formulation was investigated in a randomized, crossover design study of 8 healthy subjects.[1] Each subject received a single dose of uncoated aspirin 500 mg or enteric-coated sodium salicylate 500 mg alone or after 4 days of treatment with a dose of omeprazole 20 mg. Salicylate was absorbed rapidly from uncoated aspirin tablets, appearing in serum within 30 minutes. Omeprazole did not affect the absorption of aspirin from uncoated tablets. In 3 subjects, the enteric-coated formulation was absorbed almost as rapidly as from the uncoated preparation, and absorption was not affected by omeprazole administration. In 5 subjects, the enteric-coated formulation reduced the time to reach peak plasma concentrations from 4 to 2.7 hours compared with giving this formulation alone. In a case-control study of 418 patients with coronary artery disease taking aspirin 75 mg daily, those patients who received proton pump inhibitors concomitantly had a reduced platelet response.[2]

[1] Nefesoglu FZ, et al. *Int J Clin Pharmacol Ther.* 1998;36(10):549.

[2] Würtz M, et al. *Heart.* 2010;96(5):368.

* Asterisk indicates drugs cited in interaction reports.

Salicylates — *Urinary Alkalinizers*

Salicylates		Urinary Alkalinizers	
Aspirin* (eg, *Bayer*)	Salsalate (eg, *Salflex*)	Potassium Citrate (*Urocit-K*)	Sodium Lactate
Choline Salicylate*	Sodium Salicylate	Sodium Acetate	Tromethamine (*Tham*)
Magnesium Salicylate (eg, *Doan's*)		Sodium Bicarbonate*	
		Sodium Citrate (*Citra pH*)	

Significance	Onset	Severity	Documentation
3	☐ Rapid	☐ Major	■ **Established**
	■ **Delayed**	☐ Moderate	☐ Probable
		■ **Minor**	☐ Suspected
			☐ Possible
			☐ Unlikely

Effects Urine alkalinization leads to increased renal clearance and reduced serum levels of SALICYLATES. SALICYLATE therapeutic and toxic effects may be diminished.

Mechanism When urine pH rises, SALICYLATE excretion is promoted by the process of ion-trapping in tubular fluid. Renal clearance of SALICYLATES increases dramatically above urine pH 7.

Management The patient receiving concurrent URINARY ALKALINIZER and anti-inflammatory SALICYLATE therapy may require higher than expected SALICYLATE doses. Monitor plasma SALICYLATE levels and perform home urine pH testing to determine dosage.

Discussion

Alkalinization of the urine results in increased renal salicylate clearance and decreased plasma salicylate levels.[1-7] This effect may be pronounced in patients taking regular anti-inflammatory doses of salicylates. Urine alkalinization is an accepted therapy in cases of acute and chronic salicylate poisoning.[7,8] The impact of alkalinization on salicylate excretion is greatest above pH 7, although significant effects may be seen in the physiologic (acidic) range of urine pH. It is estimated that lowering urine pH from 6.5 to 5.5 in a patient maintained at plasma salicylate levels of 20 to 30 mg/dL would result in a 2-fold increase in those levels.[6] Elimination of diflunisal is not affected by urinary alkalinization.[9] Caution patients on chronic anti-inflammatory salicylate therapy about the agents that alter urinary pH, and instruct them to report loss of salicylate effectiveness or evidence of toxicity (eg, confusion, fever, tinnitus, vomiting). See also Salicylates-Antacids and Salicylates-Carbonic Anhydrase Inhibitors.

1 Smull K, et al. *J Am Med Assoc.* 1944;125(17):1173.
2 Smith PK, et al. *J Pharmacol Exp Ther.* 1946;87:237.
3 Hoffman WS, et al. *J Lab Clin Med.* 1950;35(2):237.
4 Gutman A, et al. *J Clin Invest.* 1955;34(5):711.
5 MacPherson CR, et al. *Br J Pharmacol Chemother.* 1955;10(4):484.
6 Levy G, et al. *JAMA.* 1971;217(1):81.
7 Prescott LF, et al. *Br Med J (Clin Res Ed).* 1982;285(6352):1383.
8 Berg KJ. *Eur J Clin Pharmacol.* 1977;11(2):111.
9 Balali-Mood M, et al. *Br J Clin Pharmacol.* 1980;10(2):163.

* Asterisk indicates drugs cited in interaction reports. Based on pharmacologic and pharmacokinetic considerations, similar interactions may occur with other drugs that are listed.

Saquinavir — *Food*

Saquinavir* (*Invirase*)	Grapefruit Juice*

Significance	Onset	Severity	Documentation
2	☐ Rapid ■ **Delayed**	☐ Major ■ **Moderate** ☐ Minor	☐ Established ☐ Probable ■ **Suspected** ☐ Possible ☐ Unlikely

Effects Plasma SAQUINAVIR levels may be elevated, increasing the pharmacologic effects and adverse reactions.

Mechanism Inhibition of SAQUINAVIR gut wall metabolism (CYP3A4) and, to a minor extent, increased SAQUINAVIR bioavailability because of modulation of P-glycoprotein function.[1]

Management Avoid coadministration of SAQUINAVIR and GRAPEFRUIT products. Caution patients to take SAQUINAVIR with a liquid other than GRAPEFRUIT JUICE.

Discussion

The effect of grapefruit juice on the bioavailability of saquinavir mesylate was investigated in an open-label, crossover study involving 8 healthy volunteers.[2] Each subject was pretreated with water or single-strength grapefruit juice before administration of IV saquinavir (12 mg) or oral (600 mg). Grapefruit juice did not affect the distribution or elimination of IV saquinavir. In contrast, the AUC and the bioavailability of oral saquinavir increased 50% and 100%, respectively. The clearance of saquinavir was not affected by grapefruit juice. The interindividual variability in the bioavailability of saquinavir was high. Grapefruit juice ingestion increased saquinavir bioavailability in 7 of the 8 subjects. The subject who did not show an increase in saquinavir bioavailability also had a high bioavailability when pretreated with water.

[1] Eagling VA, et al. *Br J Clin Pharmacol.* 1999;48(4):543.

[2] Kupferschmidt HH, et al. *Br J Clin Pharmacol.* 1998;45(4):355.

* Asterisk indicates drugs cited in interaction reports.

Saquinavir — *Histamine H_2 Antagonists*

Saquinavir	Histamine H_2 Antagonists	
Saquinavir* (*Invirase*)	Cimetidine* (eg, *Tagamet*)	Nizatidine (eg, *Axid*)
	Famotidine (eg, *Pepcid*)	Ranitidine* (eg, *Zantac*)

Significance	Onset	Severity	Documentation
4	☐ Rapid ■ **Delayed**	☐ Major ■ **Moderate** ☐ Minor	☐ Established ☐ Probable ☐ Suspected ■ **Possible** ☐ Unlikely

Effects SAQUINAVIR plasma concentrations may be elevated, increasing the therapeutic effect and adverse reactions.

Mechanism Unknown.

Management In patients receiving SAQUINAVIR, monitor the patient's clinical response when HISTAMINE H_2 ANTAGONISTS are started or stopped. Be prepared to adjust the SAQUINAVIR dose as needed.

Discussion

The effect of cimetidine on the steady-state pharmacokinetics of saquinavir soft-gelatin capsules was investigated in 12 healthy volunteers.[1] Using an open-label, 2-stage design, each subject received saquinavir 1,200 mg 3 times daily for 13 days. From day 14 to 26, subjects received saquinavir 1,200 mg twice daily with cimetidine 400 mg twice daily. The pharmacokinetics of saquinavir on days 13 and 26 were compared. Taking saquinavir twice daily with cimetidine increased the AUC and C_{max} of saquinavir 120% and 179%, respectively, compared with taking saquinavir alone 3 times daily. Although there was marked interindividual variability in the AUC of saquinavir during both phases of the study, all but 1 subject experienced an increase in AUC after coadministration of cimetidine, compared with administering saquinavir alone. There was no statistically significant difference in saquinavir trough levels during the 2 phases and no substantial differences in adverse reactions. In a single-dose study of 12 healthy men, when saquinavir was taken with ranitidine plus a meal, the relative bioavailability and C_{max} of saquinavir were 167% and 212% higher, respectively, compared with taking saquinavir with a meal only.[2] However, there was considerable intersubject variability.

[1] Boffito M, et al. *J Antimicrob Chemother.* 2002;50(6):1081.

[2] Kakuda TN, et al. *Pharmacotherapy.* 2006;26(8):1060.

* Asterisk indicates drugs cited in interaction reports. Based on pharmacologic and pharmacokinetic considerations, similar interactions may occur with other drugs that are listed.

Saquinavir — *Rifamycins*

Saquinavir* (*Invirase*)		Rifabutin* (*Mycobutin*) Rifampin (eg, *Rifadin*)	Rifapentine (*Priftin*)

Significance	Onset	Severity	Documentation
1	☐ Rapid	■ **Major**	☐ Established
	■ **Delayed**	☐ Moderate	■ **Probable**
		☐ Minor	☐ Suspected
			☐ Possible
			☐ Unlikely

Effects RIFAMYCINS may decrease SAQUINAVIR serum concentrations. In addition, SAQUINAVIR may elevate RIFAMYCIN serum concentrations, increasing the risk of adverse reactions.

Mechanism RIFAMYCINS may increase SAQUINAVIR metabolism (CYP3A4), while SAQUINAVIR may decrease the metabolism of RIFAMYCINS by inhibiting the enzyme.

Management Administer SAQUINAVIR with caution and monitor carefully in patients receiving RIFAMYCINS.

Discussion

In an open-label, partially randomized, 3-way crossover study, the effects of rifabutin and saquinavir soft gelatin capsules on the pharmacokinetics of each other were investigated in 14 HIV-infected patients.[1] Each subject received rifabutin 300 mg/day alone for 10 days, saquinavir 1,200 mg 3 times daily alone for 10 days, and saquinavir 1,200 mg 3 times daily plus rifabutin 300 mg once daily for 10 days. Coadministration of saquinavir and rifabutin reduced the AUC of saquinavir 47% and the C_{max} 39%, compared with giving saquinavir alone. Coadministration of saquinavir and rifabutin increased the AUC of rifabutin an average of 44% and the C_{max} 45%, compared with giving rifabutin alone. The only adverse reactions observed were GI intolerance and asymptomatic increases in liver enzymes. In an open-label study, 22 patients with treatment-naive HIV infection and active tuberculosis received rifampin and isoniazid plus 1 or 2 other antituberculosis agents for 2 months followed by rifampin and isoniazid only for an additional 2 months.[2] At 2 months, antiretroviral therapy, including saquinavir, was started. Antiretroviral therapy did not affect the pharmacokinetics of rifampin; however, the AUC and C_{max} of saquinavir were reduced 41% and 36%, respectively, during coadministration of rifampin and isoniazid. See also Indinavir-Rifamycins and Ritonavir-Rifamycins.

[1] Moyle GJ, et al. *Br J Clin Pharmacol.* 2002;54(2):178.
[2] Ribera E, et al. *J Antimicrob Chemother.* 2007;59(4):690.

* Asterisk indicates drugs cited in interaction reports. Based on pharmacologic and pharmacokinetic considerations, similar interactions may occur with other drugs that are listed.

Saquinavir — *Ritonavir*

Saquinavir Mesylate* (*Invirase*)	Ritonavir* (*Norvir*)

Significance	Onset	Severity	Documentation
3	■ **Rapid**	□ Major	□ Established
	□ Delayed	□ Moderate	□ Probable
		■ **Minor**	■ **Suspected**
			□ Possible
			□ Unlikely

Effects Plasma SAQUINAVIR concentrations may be elevated. Adverse effects may be increased.

Mechanism Possibly decreased first-pass metabolism (CYP3A4) and postabsorptive clearance of SAQUINAVIR.

Management Based on available data, no interventions, other than routine monitoring, are necessary. If adverse effects occur, it may be necessary to adjust the dose of SAQUINAVIR.

Discussion

The pharmacokinetic interaction between 2 protease inhibitors, saquinavir and ritonavir, and the safety of combination regimens were evaluated in 57 healthy volunteers.[1] Single doses of saquinavir and ritonavir were administered in a randomized, open-label, 2-way (groups 1 through 5) and 3-way (group 6) crossover design. Saquinavir did not affect the pharmacokinetics of ritonavir. However, coadministration of saquinavir and ritonavir increased peak plasma levels of saquinavir 22-fold and increased the AUC of saquinavir more than 50-fold. For a constant dose of ritonavir, the saquinavir pharmacokinetics were proportional to the dose. For a constant dose of saquinavir, the increase in concentration of saquinavir was less than proportional to the ritonavir dose. Intersubject variability in the pharmacokinetics of saquinavir was reduced from 70% to approximately 30% to 40% by ritonavir coadministration. Adverse effects were mild.

This interaction is based on administration of saquinavir mesylate soft gelatin capsules (*Fortorase*)[†]. The relative bioavailability of saquinavir soft gelatin capsules is approximately 331% greater than that of *Invirase*. In a study of 66 volunteers, administration of saquinavir soft gelatin capsules (400 to 800 mg twice daily) with ritonavir (200 to 400 mg twice daily) increased saquinavir plasma levels at all ritonavir doses tested (eg, ritonavir 200 mg twice daily increased the AUC of saquinavir 800 mg twice daily by 17-fold).[2] The inhibition of saquinavir metabolism by ritonavir is of such a magnitude that it reverses induction of saquinavir metabolism by rifampin (eg, *Rifadin*).[3] This reversal of effect on saquinavir metabolism has been used therapeutically to treat tuberculosis in HIV-infected patients.

[1] Hsu A, et al. *Clin Pharmacol Ther.* 1998;63(4):453.
[2] Buss N, et al. *Br J Clin Pharmacol.* 2001;52(3):255.
[3] Veldkamp AI, et al. *Clin Infect Dis.* 1999;29(6):1586.

* Asterisk indicates drugs cited in interaction reports.
† = not available in the United States.

Saxagliptin — *Rifamycins*

Saxagliptin* (*Onglyza*)	Rifabutin (*Mycobutin*) Rifapentine (*Priftin*)	Rifampin* (eg, *Rifadin*)

Significance	Onset	Severity	Documentation
4	☐ Rapid	☐ Major	☐ Established
	■ **Delayed**	■ **Moderate**	☐ Probable
		☐ Minor	☐ Suspected
			■ **Possible**
			☐ Unlikely

Effects SAXAGLIPTIN plasma concentrations may be reduced, decreasing the pharmacologic effect.

Mechanism Increased SAXAGLIPTIN metabolism (CYP3A4) and/or P-gp–mediated efflux in the intestine is suspected.

Management Monitor blood glucose in patients receiving SAXAGLIPTIN when a RIFAMYCIN is started or stopped. Adjust the SAXAGLIPTIN dose as needed.

Discussion

The effect of rifampin on the pharmacokinetics of saxagliptin was evaluated in 13 healthy subjects.[1] Using a nonrandomized, open-label, single sequence design, each subject received a single dose of saxagliptin 5 mg alone and after receiving rifampin 600 mg once daily for 6 days. Compared with giving saxagliptin alone, pretreatment with rifampin decreased the saxagliptin mean C_{max} and AUC approximately 53% and 76%, respectively, while increasing the mean C_{max} of the active metabolite, 5-hydroxy saxagliptin, 39% with no change in the AUC. Saxagliptin administration with or without rifampin was generally well tolerated.

[1] Upreti VV, et al. *Br J Clin Pharmacol.* 2011;72(1):92.

* Asterisk indicates drugs cited in interaction reports. Based on pharmacologic and pharmacokinetic considerations, similar interactions may occur with other drugs that are listed.

Scopolamine — *Food*

Scopolamine* (eg, *Scopace*)	Grapefruit Juice*

Significance	Onset	Severity	Documentation
5	□ Rapid ■ **Delayed**	□ Major □ Moderate ■ **Minor**	□ Established □ Probable □ Suspected ■ **Possible** □ Unlikely

Effects SCOPOLAMINE absorption may be delayed and bioavailability may be increased.

Mechanism Increased bioavailability of SCOPOLAMINE because inhibition of intestinal first-pass metabolism (CYP3A4) is suspected.

Management Based on available data, no special precautions are needed.

Discussion

The effects of grapefruit juice on the bioavailability of scopolamine were investigated in 14 healthy subjects.[1] Each subject received scopolamine 0.5 mg by IV and oral administration. Fresh-squeezed grapefruit juice (150 mL) or water (150 mL) was ingested 60 minutes before, 15 minutes before, and concomitantly with oral scopolamine. Compared with water, grapefruit juice increased the bioavailability of scopolamine 30% and increased the time to reach peak scopolamine plasma concentrations 188%.

[1] Ebert U, et al. *Int J Clin Pharmacol Ther.* 2000;38(11):523.

* Asterisk indicates drugs cited in interaction reports.

Selective 5-HT$_1$ Receptor Agonists — *Azole Antifungal Agents*

Selective 5-HT$_1$ Receptor Agonists		Azole Antifungal Agents	
Almotriptan* (*Axert*)	Eletriptan* (*Relpax*)	Fluconazole* (eg, *Diflucan*) Itraconazole* (eg, *Sporanox*)	Ketoconazole* (eg, *Nizoral*)

Significance	Onset	Severity	Documentation
2	☐ Rapid ■ **Delayed**	☐ Major ■ **Moderate** ☐ Minor	☐ Established ☐ Probable ■ **Suspected** ☐ Possible ☐ Unlikely

Effects Plasma concentrations of certain SELECTIVE 5-HT$_1$ RECEPTOR AGONISTS may be elevated, increasing the pharmacologic effects and adverse reactions.

Mechanism Inhibition of certain SELECTIVE 5-HT$_1$ RECEPTOR AGONISTS' gut wall and first-pass metabolism (CYP3A4) or decreased renal clearance by certain AZOLE ANTIFUNGAL AGENTS is suspected.

Management ELETRIPTAN should not be taken within 72 hours of ITRACONAZOLE or KETOCONAZOLE,[1] and ALMOTRIPTAN should not be taken within 7 days of ITRACONAZOLE or KETOCONAZOLE.[2]

Discussion

In a randomized, open-label, crossover investigation, the effects of ketoconazole on the pharmacokinetics and pharmacodynamics of almotriptan were studied in 16 healthy volunteers.[3] Each subject received almotriptan 12.5 mg alone and ketoconazole 400 mg daily for 3 days with 1 almotriptan 12.5 mg tablet administered on day 2. Compared with giving almotriptan alone, coadministration of ketoconazole increased the mean AUC of almotriptan 57% and the C_{max} 61% (from 52.6 to 84.5 ng/mL), while decreasing the mean oral clearance 36% (from 40.7 to 26.2 L/hr) and renal clearance 16% (from 16.4 to 13.8 L/hr). The time to reach the peak concentration and $t_{1/2}$ of almotriptan were not affected. There were no statistically significant differences in diastolic BP or heart rate. It has been reported that coadministration of eletriptan and fluconazole increased C_{max} and AUC of eletriptan approximately 1.4- and 2-fold, respectively.[1]

[1] *Relpax* [package insert]. New York, NY: Pfizer Inc; April 2006.
[2] *Axert* [package insert]. Raritan, NJ: Ortho-McNeil Pharmaceuticals Inc; May 2003.
[3] Fleishaker JC, et al. *J Clin Pharmacol*. 2003;43(4):423.

* Asterisk indicates drugs cited in interaction reports.

Selective 5-HT₁ Receptor Agonists × *Ergot Derivatives*

Selective 5-HT1 Receptor Agonists		Ergot Derivatives	
Eletriptan* (*Relpax*)	Rizatriptan* (*Maxalt*)	Dihydroergotamine* (eg, *D.H.E. 45*)	Methysergide*†
Frovatriptan* (*Frova*)	Sumatriptan* (eg, *Imitrex*)	Ergotamine* (*Ergomar*)	
Naratriptan* (eg, *Amerge*)	Zolmitriptan* (*Zomig*)		

Significance	Onset	Severity	Documentation
1	■ **Rapid**	■ **Major**	□ Established
	□ Delayed	□ Moderate	□ Probable
		□ Minor	■ **Suspected**
			□ Possible
			□ Unlikely

Effects The risk of vasospastic reactions may be increased.[1-6]

Mechanism Possibly additive vasospastic effects.

Management Use of SELECTIVE 5-HT_1 RECEPTOR AGONISTS within 24 hours of treatment with an ERGOT-containing medication is contraindicated. Similarly, coadministration of two 5-HT_1 RECEPTOR AGONISTS within 24 hours of each other is contraindicated.

Discussion

A case of MI caused by the combined use of sumatriptan and methysergide was reported in a 43-year-old woman.[7] The patient had taken 2 doses of methysergide 2 mg 12 hours apart. Her migraine continued, and she injected sumatriptan 6 mg. Severe chest pain developed 10 to 15 minutes after the injection. Upon admission to a hospital, an anterior MI was confirmed. Cardiac catheterization revealed a 50% stenosis of the proximal left anterior descending coronary artery, suggesting the infarction was the result of sustained vasospasm.

1 *Imitrex* [package insert]. Shawnee Mission, KS: Cerenex Pharmaceuticals; June 1995.
2 *Zomig* [package insert]. Wilmington, DE: Zeneca Pharmaceuticals; November 1997.
3 *Maxalt* [package insert]. West Point, PA: Merck & Co Inc; June 1998.
4 *Amerge* [package insert]. Philadelphia, PA: Glaxo-Wellcome Inc; February 1998.
5 *Frova* [package insert]. Iselin, NJ: Elan Pharmaceuticals; November 2001.
6 *Relpax* [package insert]. New York, NY: Pfizer Inc; December 2002.
7 Liston H, et al. *Arch Intern Med.* 1999;159(5):511.

* Asterisk indicates drugs cited in interaction reports.
† Not available in the United States.

Selective 5-HT$_1$ Receptor Agonists | *Linezolid*

Selective 5-HT$_1$ Receptor Agonists		Linezolid
Almotriptan* (*Axert*)	Rizatriptan* (*Maxalt*)	Linezolid* (*Zyvox*)
Eletriptan* (*Relpax*)	Sumatriptan* (eg, *Imitrex*)	
Frovatriptan* (*Frova*)	Zolmitriptan* (*Zomig*)	
Naratriptan* (eg, *Amerge*)		

Significance	Onset	Severity	Documentation
1	■ **Rapid**	■ **Major**	☐ Established
	☐ Delayed	☐ Moderate	☐ Probable
		☐ Minor	■ **Suspected**
			☐ Possible
			☐ Unlikely

Effects Serotonin syndrome (eg, agitation, altered consciousness, ataxia, myoclonus, overactive, reflexes, shivering) may occur in some patients.

Mechanism Accumulation of serotonin in the CNS.

Management Unless patients are carefully observed for signs and symptoms of serotonin syndrome, LINEZOLID should not be coadministered with SELECTIVE 5-HT$_1$ RECEPTOR AGONISTS.[1]

Discussion

Unless patients are carefully observed for signs and symptoms of serotonin syndrome, linezolid should not be coadministered with serotonin 5-HT$_1$ receptor agonists.[1]

The basis for this monograph is information on file with the manufacturer. Published clinical data are needed to further assess this interaction. However, due to the seriousness of this interaction, clinical evaluation in humans is not likely to be forthcoming.

[1] *Zyvox* [package insert]. New York, NY: Pharmacia & Upjohn Company; December 2009.

* Asterisk indicates drugs cited in interaction reports.

Selective 5-HT$_1$ Receptor Agonists — *Macrolide & Related Antibiotics*

Selective 5-HT$_1$ Receptor Agonists	Macrolide & Related Antibiotics	
Eletriptan* (*Relpax*)	Clarithromycin* (eg, *Biaxin*)	Telithromycin (*Ketek*)
	Erythromycin* (eg, *Ery-Tab*)	

Significance	Onset	Severity	Documentation
4	☐ Rapid	■ **Major**	☐ Established
	■ **Delayed**	☐ Moderate	☐ Probable
		☐ Minor	☐ Suspected
			■ **Possible**
			☐ Unlikely

Effects Plasma levels of certain SELECTIVE 5-HT$_1$ RECEPTOR AGONISTS may be elevated, increasing the pharmacologic and toxic effects.

Mechanism Inhibition of metabolism (CYP3A4) of certain SELECTIVE 5-HT$_1$ RECEPTOR AGONISTS by certain MACROLIDE & RELATED ANTIBIOTICS is suspected.

Management ELETRIPTAN should not be taken within 72 hours of potent CYP3A4 inhibitors (eg, CLARITHROMYCIN).[1]

Discussion

In a clinical study, coadministration of eletriptan and erythromycin increased the C_{max} and AUC of eletriptan approximately 2- and 4-fold, respectively.[1] Based on these results, it is recommended that eletriptan not be taken within at least 72 hours of treatment with potent CYP3A4 inhibitors (eg, clarithromycin).[1]

The basis for this monograph is information on file with the manufacturer. Additional studies are needed to determine if other selective-5HT[1] receptor agonists interact similarly and the magnitude of the interaction between members of these classes of agents.

[1] *Relpax* [package insert]. New York, NY: Pfizer Inc.; April 2006.

* Asterisk indicates drugs cited in interaction reports. Based on pharmacologic and pharmacokinetic considerations, similar interactions may occur with other drugs that are listed.

Selective 5-HT$_1$ Receptor Agonists — *MAOIs*

Selective 5-HT$_1$ Receptor Agonists		MAOIs	
Rizatriptan* (*Maxalt*)	Zolmitriptan* (*Zomig*)	Isocarboxazid* (*Marplan*)	Tranylcypromine* (eg, *Parnate*)
Sumatriptan* (*Imitrex*)		Phenelzine* (*Nardil*)	

Significance	Onset	Severity	Documentation
1	■ **Rapid** □ Delayed	■ **Major** □ Moderate □ Minor	□ Established □ Probable ■ **Suspected** □ Possible □ Unlikely

Effects Serum concentrations of certain SELECTIVE 5-HT$_1$ RECEPTOR AGONISTS may be elevated, increasing the risk of cardiac toxicity (eg, coronary artery vasospasm, transient myocardial ischemia).

Mechanism Inhibition of metabolism via monoamine oxidase, subtype A (MAO-A).

Management Use of certain SELECTIVE 5-HT$_1$ RECEPTOR AGONISTS concomitantly or within 2 weeks following the discontinuation of an MAOI is contraindicated. If it is necessary to use these agents together, naratriptan (*Amerge*) appears to be less likely to interact with MAOIs.[1]

Discussion

In 12 subjects, administration of rizatriptan 10 mg with the selective MAO-A inhibitor moclobemide† resulted in a mean increase of 119% in the AUC of rizatriptan and a 41% increase in the C_{max}.[2] The AUC of the active N-monodesmethyl metabolite of rizatriptan was increased more than 400%. Following 1 week of administration of moclobemide 150 mg twice daily, the AUC and C_{max} of zolmitriptan increased approximately 25%,[3] and the AUC and C_{max} of the active N-desmethyl metabolite of zolmitriptan increased 3-fold. In women pretreated with an MAO-A inhibitor, subcutaneous administration of sumatriptan resulted in a marked increase in sumatriptan AUC and t½.[4] This drug interaction may be greatest with irreversible MAOIs (eg, phenelzine). No pharmacokinetic interaction is expected in patients receiving selective MAO-B inhibitors (eg, selegiline [eg, *Eldepryl*]) and rizatriptan, sumatriptan, or zolmitriptan.[2-4] Because naratriptan does not inhibit MAO, an interaction between naratriptan and drugs metabolized by MAO is unlikely.[1]

The basis for this monograph is information on file with the manufacturers. Published clinical data are needed to further assess this interaction. However, because of the seriousness of the cardiac events, clinical evaluation of this interaction in humans is not likely.

[1] *Amerge* [package insert]. Philadelphia, PA: GlaxoSmithKline; February 1998.

[2] *Maxalt* [package insert]. White House Station, NJ: Merck and Co., Inc.; June 1998.

[3] *Zomig* [package insert]. Wilmington, DE: AstraZeneca; November 1997.

[4] *Imitrex* [package insert]. Philadelphia, PA: GlaxoSmithKline; June 1995.

* Asterisk indicates drugs cited in interaction reports.

† Not available in the United States.

Selective 5-HT₁ Receptor Agonists — *Serotonin Reuptake Inhibitors*

Selective 5-HT$_1$ Receptor Agonists		Serotonin Reuptake Inhibitors	
Almotriptan (*Axert*)	Rizatriptan (*Maxalt*)	Citalopram (eg, *Celexa*)	Milnacipran (*Savella*)
Eletriptan (*Relpax*)	Sumatriptan* (eg, *Imitrex*)	Duloxetine (*Cymbalta*)	Nefazodone
Frovatriptan (*Frova*)	Zolmitriptan (*Zomig*)	Escitalopram (*Lexapro*)	Paroxetine (eg, *Paxil*)
Naratriptan (*Amerge*)		Fluoxetine* (eg, *Prozac*)	Sertraline* (eg, *Zoloft*)
		Fluvoxamine (eg, *Luvox*)	Venlafaxine (eg, *Effexor*)

Significance	Onset	Severity	Documentation
2	■ **Rapid**	□ Major	□ Established
	□ Delayed	■ **Moderate**	□ Probable
		□ Minor	■ **Suspected**
			□ Possible
			□ Unlikely

Effects Serotonin syndrome (eg, agitation, altered consciousness, ataxia, myoclonus, overactive reflexes, shivering) may occur in some patients.

Mechanism Rapid accumulation of serotonin in the CNS may occur.

Management If coadministration of these agents is indicated, start with low dosages and closely monitor patients. Be prepared to provide supportive care, stop the serotonergic agent, and give an antiserotonergic agent (eg, cyproheptadine).

Discussion

After starting fluoxetine, a 30-year-old woman with migraine attacks previously responsive to oral sumatriptan 100 mg experienced an increase in migraine frequency and reduced efficacy of sumatriptan in providing symptom relief.[1] Transient neurologic symptoms suggestive of serotonin syndrome occurred in 2 patients taking sumatriptan and sertraline.[2] One patient also was taking methysergide[†] and lithium (eg, *Lithobid*). Of the 22 adverse reactions voluntarily reported during postmarketing surveillance of fluoxetine, 6 were judged to provide some evidence (2 provided good evidence) of an interaction with sumatriptan.[3] Symptoms were consistent with serotonin syndrome. Twelve patients using sumatriptan and an SRI did not experience adverse reactions during coadministration of these agents for 103 episodes of migraine.[4] No apparent adverse reactions occurred in 6 patients receiving sumatriptan and an SRI for 3 to 18 months[5] or in 11 healthy men receiving paroxetine 20 mg/day for 16 days and subcutaneous sumatriptan 6 mg.[6] In 12 healthy subjects, coadministration of paroxetine and rizatriptan was well tolerated.[7] Adverse reactions were similar to those with coadministration of rizatriptan and placebo.

[1] Szabo CP. *J Clin Psychiatry*. 1995;56(1):37.
[2] Mathew NT, et al. *Cephalalgia*. 1996;16(5):323.
[3] Joffe RT, et al. *Acta Psychiatr Scand*. 1997;95(6):551.
[4] Blier P, et al. *J Clin Psychopharmacol*. 1995;15(2):106.
[5] Leung M, et al. *Headache*. 1995;35(8):488.
[6] Wing YK, et al. *Psychopharmacology (Berl)*. 1996;124(4):377.
[7] Goldberg MR, et al. *J Clin Pharmacol*. 1999;39(2):192.

* Asterisk indicates drugs cited in interaction reports. Based on pharmacologic and pharmacokinetic considerations, similar interactions may occur with other drugs that are listed.
† Not available in the United States.

Selective 5-HT$_1$ Receptor Agonists — *Verapamil*

Almotriptan* (*Axert*)	Verapamil* (eg, *Calan*)

Significance	Onset	Severity	Documentation
4	□ Rapid	□ Major	□ Established
	■ **Delayed**	■ **Moderate**	□ Probable
		□ Minor	□ Suspected
			■ **Possible**
			□ Unlikely

Effects ALMOTRIPTAN plasma concentrations may be elevated slightly, increasing the pharmacologic effects and adverse reactions.

Mechanism Inhibition of ALMOTRIPTAN metabolism (CYP3A4) by VERAPAMIL is suspected.

Management In patients taking ALMOTRIPTAN, observe the clinical response when VERAPAMIL is started or stopped. Be prepared to adjust the therapy as needed.

Discussion

The effects of verapamil on the pharmacokinetics of almotriptan were evaluated in 12 healthy volunteers.[1] Using a randomized, open-label, crossover design, each subject received almotriptan 12.5 mg alone after receiving sustained-release verapamil 120 mg for 7 days. Compared with receiving almotriptan alone, pretreatment with verapamil increased almotriptan C_{max} and AUC, while the volume of distribution and oral clearance were decreased. The magnitude of these changes was approximately 20%. Except for sitting systolic BP at 2 hours, BP and pulse were not altered.

[1] Fleishaker JC, et al. *Clin Pharmacol Ther.* 2000;67(5):498.

* Asterisk indicates drugs cited in interaction reports.

Selegiline — *Contraceptives, Hormonal*

Selegiline* (eg, *Eldepryl*)	Contraceptives, Oral* (eg, *Nordette*)

Significance	Onset	Severity	Documentation
2	☐ Rapid	☐ Major	☐ Established
	■ **Delayed**	■ **Moderate**	☐ Probable
		☐ Minor	■ **Suspected**
			☐ Possible
			☐ Unlikely

Effects Plasma SELEGILINE concentrations may be elevated, causing a loss of selective inhibition of MAO-type B and increasing the risk of SELEGILINE adverse reactions.

Mechanism ORAL CONTRACEPTIVES may inhibit the metabolism of SELEGILINE.

Management It may be necessary to reduce the SELEGILINE dose if concurrent use of these agents cannot be avoided. Closely monitor the clinical response of the patient; be prepared to alter therapy as needed.

Discussion

In a pharmacokinetic study of the dose relationship of selegiline and its metabolite, desmethylselegiline, in 8 women (4 taking oral contraceptives), oral contraceptive use was found to increase the bioavailability of selegiline.[1] In an open, 4-period, randomized study, 8 women received a single dose of selegiline 5, 10, 20, or 40 mg. In the 4 women taking oral contraceptives (gestodene plus ethinyl estradiol or levonorgestrel plus ethinyl estradiol), there was a dramatic increase in selegiline plasma concentrations. The total AUC of selegiline increased 20-fold, and the peak concentration increased more than 10-fold in the subjects taking oral contraceptives. The AUC of desmethylselegiline increased in a dose-related manner in subjects who were not taking the oral contraceptive but not in the contraceptive users. The metabolic ratio (AUC [desmethylselegiline]/AUC [selegiline]) was several-fold lower in the oral contraceptive users compared with the nonusers.

[1] Laine K, et al. *Br J Clin Pharmacol.* 1999;47(3):249.

* Asterisk indicates drugs cited in interaction reports.

Serotonin Reuptake Inhibitors | **Azole Antifungal Agents**

Paroxetine*
(eg, *Paxil*)

Itraconazole*
(eg, *Sporanox*)

Significance	Onset	Severity	Documentation
4	☐ Rapid ■ **Delayed**	☐ Major ■ **Moderate** ☐ Minor	☐ Established ☐ Probable ☐ Suspected ■ **Possible** ☐ Unlikely

Effects PAROXETINE plasma concentrations may be elevated, increasing pharmacologic and adverse effects.

Mechanism Increased absorption or decreased clearance of PAROXETINE by inhibition of the P-glycoprotein efflux pump in the intestine or liver is suspected

Management If an interaction is suspected, it may be necessary to adjust the PAROXETINE dose when starting or stopping ITRACONAZOLE.

Discussion

The effects of itraconazole on the pharmacokinetics of paroxetine were studied in 13 healthy volunteers.[1] In a randomized, crossover study, each subject received itraconazole 100 mg twice daily or a matching placebo for 6 days. On day 6, subjects received a single dose of paroxetine 20 mg. Compared with placebo, pretreatment with itraconazole increased the C_{max} and AUC of paroxetine approximately 34% and 45%, respectively. Following the single dose of paroxetine, there was no relationship between observed adverse reactions and AUC.

[1] Yasui-Furukori N, et al. *Ther Drug Monit.* 2007;29(1):45.

* Asterisk indicates drugs cited in interaction reports.

Serotonin Reuptake Inhibitors × Cimetidine

Serotonin Reuptake Inhibitors		Cimetidine
Citalopram* (eg, *Celexa*)	Nefazodone	Cimetidine* (eg, *Tagamet*)
Duloxetine (*Cymbalta*)	Paroxetine* (eg, *Paxil*)	
Escitalopram* (*Lexapro*)	Sertraline (eg, *Zoloft*)	
Fluoxetine (eg, *Prozac*)	Venlafaxine* (eg, *Effexor*)	
Fluvoxamine (eg, *Luvox*)		

Significance	Onset	Severity	Documentation
	□ Rapid	□ Major	□ Established
	■ **Delayed**	■ **Moderate**	□ Probable
		□ Minor	□ Suspected
			■ **Possible**
			□ Unlikely

Effects Serum levels and the pharmacologic effects of certain SRIs may be increased.

Mechanism CIMETIDINE may inhibit first-pass metabolism.

Management If an interaction is suspected, it may be necessary to adjust the SRI dose after the dose of CIMETIDINE is started, stopped, or changed. Other H_2-antagonists (eg, famotidine [eg, *Pepcid*]) may be less likely to interact and are possible alternatives to CIMETIDINE.

Discussion

The effects of multiple-dose administration of cimetidine on the pharmacokinetics of a single oral dose of paroxetine 30 mg were studied in 10 healthy subjects.[1] Based on the group mean values for the AUC, C_{max}, and $t_{½}$ achieved for paroxetine, there were no statistically significant differences between administration of paroxetine alone and with cimetidine. However, on a patient-by-patient basis, individual differences in AUC, C_{max}, and $t_{½}$ of paroxetine were observed. The AUC of paroxetine increased in 6 subjects after treatment with cimetidine. In another study, 11 healthy men received paroxetine 30 mg alone for 21 days followed by a combination of paroxetine 30 mg/day and cimetidine 300 mg 3 times/day for 7 days.[2] Peak levels of paroxetine increased 45%, and the AUC increased 51%. A possible increase in diastolic BP was observed during coadministration of cimetidine and paroxetine. Twelve volunteers received citalopram 40 mg/day for 21 days followed by citalopram and cimetidine 400 mg 2 times/day for 7 days.[3] Cimetidine reduced the oral clearance of citalopram, producing a 43% increase in the AUC. Similarly, cimetidine increased the escitalopram AUC 72%.[4] In a study of 18 healthy subjects, 5 days of venlafaxine and cimetidine coadministration increased the sum of venlafaxine plus the active O-desmethyl-venlafaxine metabolite plasma levels 13% compared with giving venlafaxine alone.[5]

[1] G reb WH, et al. *Acta Psychiatr Scand Suppl.* 1989;350:95.
[2] Bannister SJ, et al. *Acta Psychiatr Scand Suppl.* 1989;350:102.
[3] Priskorn M, et al. *Eur J Clin Pharmacol.* 1997;52(3);241.
[4] Malling D, et al. *Br J Clin Pharmacol.* 2005;60(3):287.
[5] Troy SM, et al. *J Clin Pharmacol.* 1998;38(5);467.

* Asterisk indicates drugs cited in interaction reports. Based on pharmacologic and pharmacokinetic considerations, similar interactions may occur with other drugs that are listed.

Serotonin Reuptake Inhibitors / *Cyclobenzaprine*

Citalopram (eg, *Celexa*)	Milnacipran (*Savella*)	Cyclobenzaprine* (eg, *Flexeril*)
Duloxetine* (*Cymbalta*)	Nefazodone	
Escitalopram (*Lexapro*)	Paroxetine (eg, *Paxil*)	
Fluoxetine (eg, *Prozac*)	Sertraline (eg, *Zoloft*)	
Fluvoxamine (eg, *Luvox*)	Venlafaxine (eg, *Effexor*)	

Significance	Onset	Severity	Documentation
4	■ **Rapid**	■ **Major**	□ Established
	□ Delayed	□ Moderate	□ Probable
		□ Minor	□ Suspected
			■ **Possible**
			□ Unlikely

Effects Serotonin syndrome (eg, agitation, altered consciousness, ataxia, myoclonus, overactive reflexes, shivering) may occur.

Mechanism The serotonergic effects of these agents may be additive.

Management Closely monitor patients for adverse reactions. Serotonin syndrome requires immediate medical attention, including withdrawal of the serotonergic agents and supportive care. Administration of an antiserotonergic agent (eg, cyproheptadine) may be helpful.

Discussion

A 53-year-old man with a history of chronic pain and depression had been receiving duloxetine 60 mg/day.[1] Shortly after starting cyclobenzaprine 10 mg 3 times daily, he became confused and experienced hallucinations. Three days later, he became diaphoretic, tachycardic, and agitated. In addition, pronounced tremors, spontaneous sustained clonus, and multifocal myoclonus were present. Cyclobenzaprine and duloxetine were discontinued, and cyproheptadine was administered. His clinical status improved over several days. The patient had received other drugs (eg, opiates, bupropion [eg, *Wellbutrin*]) that may have contributed to development of serotonin syndrome.

[1] Keegan MT, et al. *Anesth Analg.* 2006;103(6):1466.

* Asterisk indicates drugs cited in interaction reports. Based on pharmacologic and pharmacokinetic considerations, similar interactions may occur with other drugs that are listed.

Serotonin Reuptake Inhibitors — *Cyproheptadine*

Serotonin Reuptake Inhibitors		Cyproheptadine
Citalopram (eg, *Celexa*)	Nefazodone	Cyproheptadine*
Escitalopram (*Lexapro*)	Paroxetine* (eg, *Paxil*)	
Fluoxetine* (eg, *Prozac*)	Sertraline (eg, *Zoloft*)	
Fluvoxamine (eg, *Luvox*)	Venlafaxine (*Effexor*)	

Significance	Onset	Severity	Documentation
2	■ **Rapid**	□ Major	□ Established
	□ Delayed	■ **Moderate**	□ Probable
		□ Minor	■ **Suspected**
			□ Possible
			□ Unlikely

Effects Decreased pharmacologic effects of SRIs.

Mechanism Because CYPROHEPTADINE is a serotonin antagonist, the interaction may occur at the receptor level.

Management If a loss of the antidepressant efficacy occurs, consider discontinuing CYPROHEPTADINE.

Discussion

Coadministration of cyproheptadine and fluoxetine reversed the antidepressant activity of fluoxetine in 3 depressed men.[1] Also, 3 patients receiving fluoxetine for depression experienced difficulty in ejaculation.[2] Because reversal of fluoxetine-induced anorgasmia by cyproheptadine has been reported without loss of antidepressant efficacy, cyproheptadine was prescribed. In each patient, depression recurred during administration of cyproheptadine. One patient experienced depressive symptoms within 4 hours of the first dose of cyproheptadine. Upon discontinuation of cyproheptadine, symptoms of depression decreased; however, ejaculatory difficulty persisted. A 54-year-old woman receiving paroxetine experienced reemergence of depression with psychotic symptoms within 2 days of adding cyproheptadine for the treatment of anorgasmia.[3] Her psychotic symptoms resolved within 2 days of stopping cyproheptadine. Two women receiving fluoxetine for bulimia nervosa reported anorgasmia after 1 to 3 months of therapy.[4] Cyproheptadine was added to their fluoxetine regimens, and both patients experienced reemergence of binge-eating episodes. After discontinuation of cyproheptadine, the binge eating remitted. A 54-year-old woman receiving fluoxetine experienced recurrence of depressive symptoms within 36 hours of taking cyproheptadine.[5] Symptoms resolved within 5 days of stopping cyproheptadine but returned and resolved within 36 hours following a rechallenge. A 17-year-old adolescent girl, successfully treated for depression with fluoxetine 20 mg/day, experienced recurrence of depression after cyproheptadine was started for migraine prevention.[6]

[1] Feder R. *J Clin Psychiatry.* 1991;52(4):163.
[2] McCormick S, et al. *J Clin Psychiatry.* 1990;51(9):383.
[3] Christensen RC. *J Clin Psychiatry.* 1995;56(9):433.
[4] Goldbloom DS, et al. *J Clin Psychiatry.* 1991;52(6):261.
[5] Katz RJ, et al. *J Clin Psychiatry.* 1994;55(7):314.
[6] Boon F. *J Am Acad Child Adolesc Psychiatry.* 1999;38(2):112.

* Asterisk indicates drugs cited in interaction reports. Based on pharmacologic and pharmacokinetic considerations, similar interactions may occur with other drugs that are listed.

Serotonin Reuptake Inhibitors — *Fluvoxamine*

Duloxetine* (*Cymbalta*)	Fluvoxamine* (eg, *Luvox*)

Significance	Onset	Severity	Documentation
2	□ Rapid	□ Major	□ Established
	■ **Delayed**	■ **Moderate**	□ Probable
		□ Minor	■ **Suspected**
			□ Possible
			□ Unlikely

Effects DULOXETINE plasma concentrations may be elevated, increasing the pharmacologic effects and adverse reactions.

Mechanism Inhibition of DULOXETINE metabolism (CYP1A2) by FLUVOXAMINE.

Management Avoid coadministration of DULOXETINE with potent CYP1A2 inhibitors (eg, FLUVOXAMINE).[1] If both agents are coadministered, monitor the clinical response and observe the patient for DULOXETINE adverse reactions.

Discussion

In a study involving 14 men, coadministration of duloxetine 60 mg with fluvoxamine 100 mg increased the duloxetine AUC and C_{max} approximately 6- and 2.5-fold, respectively, while increasing the $t_{½}$ approximately 3-fold.[1] In an open-label study, a single dose of duloxetine (either as a 10 mg IV infusion over 30 minutes or 60 mg orally) was administered to healthy subjects who received duloxetine alone and with oral fluvoxamine (100 mg once daily) at steady state.[2] Following oral administration of duloxetine, fluvoxamine increased the duloxetine AUC and C_{max} approximately 460% and 141%, respectively, compared with taking duloxetine alone. In addition, fluvoxamine increased the bioavailability of duloxetine from approximately 43% to 82%. With IV administration of duloxetine, fluvoxamine increased the duloxetine AUC 170%, but decreased the C_{max} 16%.

[1] *Cymbalta* [package insert]. Indianapolis, IN: Eli Lilly and Company; June 2007.

[2] Lobo ED, et al. *Clin Pharmacokinet.* 2008;47(3):191.

* Asterisk indicates drugs cited in interaction reports.

Serotonin Reuptake Inhibitors ✕ Linezolid

Serotonin Reuptake Inhibitors		Linezolid
Citalopram* (eg, *Celexa*)	Nefazodone	Linezolid* (*Zyvox*)
Duloxetine (*Cymbalta*)	Paroxetine* (eg, *Paxil*)	
Escitalopram* (*Lexapro*)	Sertraline* (eg, *Zoloft*)	
Fluoxetine* (eg, *Prozac*)	Venlafaxine* (*Effexor*)	
Fluvoxamine (eg, *Luvox*)		

Significance	Onset	Severity	Documentation
1	□ Rapid	■ **Major**	□ Established
	■ **Delayed**	□ Moderate	□ Probable
		□ Minor	■ **Suspected**
			□ Possible
			□ Unlikely

Effects Serotonin syndrome (eg, agitation, altered consciousness, ataxia, myoclonus, overactive reflexes, shivering) may occur.

Mechanism Possible excessive accumulation of serotonin.

Management Coadminister LINEZOLID and SRIs with caution. Because LINEZOLID has MAOI activity, allow at least 2 weeks between stopping LINEZOLID and starting an SRI.

Discussion

Serotonin syndrome, possibly from administration of linezolid shortly after the discontinuation of paroxetine, was reported in a 56-year-old woman.[1] She was admitted for elective laminectomy. In addition to paroxetine, she was receiving numerous other preoperative medications. On postoperative day 11, the dose of paroxetine was tapered for 3 days and then discontinued. The patient developed a grossly infected surgical wound, and vancomycin (eg, *Vancocin*) was started. Because of suspected drug fever, linezolid was substituted for vancomycin on postoperative day 17. Within 24 hours, the patient developed anger, delirium, hostility, hypertension, and tremors. A psychiatric consultant attributed the symptoms to serotonin syndrome. Linezolid was discontinued, vancomycin was restarted, and the patient's mental status returned to baseline within 48 hours. Because linezolid has MAOI activity and was the only new drug started before the onset of serotonin syndrome, the reaction was attributed to a potential interaction with paroxetine. Five additional cases of serotonin syndrome were reported after starting linezolid therapy in patients receiving citalopram,[2] fluoxetine,[3] sertraline,[4] or venlafaxine.[5] In 1 case, symptoms resolved after decreasing the venlafaxine dosage from 300 to 150 mg/day.[5] In a retrospective review of 52 hospitalized patients treated with linezolid plus an SRI or venlafaxine, 2 patients were categorized as having a high probability of exhibiting serotonin syndrome.[6] In a retrospective chart review of 53 patients receiving linezolid and an SRI. Serotonin syndrome occurred in 2 patients receiving linezolid with either citalopram or escitalopram.[7]

[1] Wigen CL, et al. *Clin Infect Dis.* 2002;34(12):1651.
[2] Jones SL, et al. *J Antimicrob Chemother.* 2004;54(1):289.
[3] Steinberg M, et al. *Am J Health Syst Pharm.* 2007;64(1):59.
[4] Clark DB, et al. *Pharmacotherapy.* 2006;26(2):269.
[5] Bergeron L, et al. *Ann Pharmacother.* 2005;39(5):956.
[6] Taylor JJ, et al. *Clin Infect Dis.* 2006;43(2):180.
[7] Lorenz RA, et al. *Int J Psychiatry Med.* 2008;38(1):81.

* Asterisk indicates drugs cited in interaction reports. Based on pharmacologic and pharmacokinetic considerations, similar interactions may occur with other drugs that are listed.

Serotonin Reuptake Inhibitors / Macrolide & Related Antibiotics

Serotonin Reuptake Inhibitors		Macrolide & Related Antibiotics	
Citalopram (eg, *Celexa*)	Paroxetine (eg, *Paxil*)	Clarithromycin* (eg, *Biaxin*)	Telithromycin (*Ketek*)
Fluoxetine* (eg, *Prozac*)	Sertraline* (eg, *Zoloft*)	Erythromycin* (eg, *Ery-Tab*)	

Significance	Onset	Severity	Documentation
4	☐ Rapid ■ **Delayed**	■ **Major** ☐ Moderate ☐ Minor	☐ Established ☐ Probable ☐ Suspected ■ **Possible** ☐ Unlikely

Effects Serotonin syndrome (eg, agitation, altered consciousness, ataxia, myoclonus, overactive reflexes, shivering) may occur.

Mechanism Possible inhibition of FLUOXETINE or SERTRALINE metabolism.

Management If administration of this combination cannot be avoided, it may be necessary to adjust the dose of FLUOXETINE or SERTRALINE when the dose of the MACROLIDE ANTIBIOTIC is started, stopped, or changed. Closely monitor patients.

Discussion

A possible case of serotonin syndrome resulting from coadministration of sertraline and erythromycin was reported in a 12-year-old boy.[1] The boy had been taking sertraline 37.5 mg in the morning for 5 weeks for severe obsessive-compulsive disorder with simple phobia. The dose of sertraline had been administered in the morning at 12.5 mg and titrated to 37.5 mg over 12 weeks. When a presumed infection provoked an autoimmune neuropsychiatric disorder, he was started on erythromycin 200 mg twice daily. Within 4 days of erythromycin therapy, the boy began to feel mildly nervous. Over the next 10 days, he developed symptoms of confusion, decreased concentration, intermittent agitation, irritability, panic, paresthesias, restlessness, and tremulousness. Both drugs were discontinued, and within 72 hours, the boy reported feeling more calm and was less irritable and confused. A causal relationship between drug coadministration and occurrence of the syndrome cannot be established because plasma levels were not measured, rechallenge was not performed, and sertraline alone can cause serotonin syndrome. However, the temporal relationship between the onset of the syndrome and initiation of erythromycin therapy implicates the antibiotic as precipitating the reaction.

Delirium was reported in a 53-year-old man during coadministration of fluoxetine, nitrazepam,† and clarithromycin.[2] The delirium subsided after drug therapy was discontinued and did not recur when the patient was treated with fluoxetine and nitrazepam without antibiotics or with erythromycin alone.

[1] Lee DO, et al. *Pharmacotherapy*. 1999;19(7):894.

[2] Pollak PT, et al. *Ann Pharmacother*. 1995;29(5):486.

* Asterisk indicates drugs cited in interaction reports. Based on pharmacologic and pharmacokinetic considerations, similar interactions may occur with other drugs that are listed.

† Not available in the United States.

Serotonin Reuptake Inhibitors | MAOIs

Citalopram* (eg, *Celexa*)
Duloxetine* (*Cymbalta*)
Escitalopram (*Lexapro*)
Fluoxetine* (eg, *Prozac*)
Fluvoxamine (eg, *Luvox CR*)
Milnacipran* (*Savella*)
Nefazodone
Paroxetine (eg, *Paxil*)
Sertraline* (eg, *Zoloft*)
Venlafaxine* (eg, *Effexor*)
Vilazodone* (*Viibryd*)

Isocarboxazid* (*Marplan*)
Phenelzine* (eg, *Nardil*)
Rasagiline (*Azilect*)
Selegiline* (eg, *Eldepryl*)
Tranylcypromine* (eg, *Parnate*)

Significance	Onset	Severity	Documentation
	■ **Rapid** □ Delayed	■ **Major** □ Moderate □ Minor	□ Established ■ **Probable** □ Suspected □ Possible □ Unlikely

Effects Serotonin syndrome (eg, agitation, altered consciousness, ataxia, myoclonus, overactive reflexes, shivering) may occur.

Mechanism Possible rapid, excessive accumulation of serotonin.[1]

Management Do not coadminister. Allow at least 5 days after stopping DULOXETINE or MILNACIPRAN; 1 week after stopping NEFAZODONE or VENLAFAXINE; 2 weeks after stopping CITALOPRAM, ESCITALOPRAM, FLUVOXAMINE, PAROXETINE, SERTRALINE, or VILAZODONE; and 5 weeks after stopping FLUOXETINE before giving an MAOI. After stopping an MAOI, allow at least 14 days before giving any SRI.

Discussion

Serotonin syndrome has been reported in patients who stopped fluoxetine and received an MAOI shortly thereafter.[1-3] This syndrome was reported during administration of sertraline and tranylcypromine or phenelzine,[4-6] and when taking venlafaxine with isocarboxazid, phenelzine, or tranylcypromine.[7-12] Several deaths have been reported by the manufacturer.[13] In a retrospective study, patients treated with fluoxetine and an MAOI (together or at least 10 days after stopping fluoxetine) had a high incidence of adverse reactions, particularly serotonin syndrome.[14] These patients also were taking other medications. Similar reactions were reported with the selective MAO type B inhibitor selegiline.[15,16] A similar reaction may occur with duloxetine,[17] milnacipran,[18] or vilazodone.[19] In patients with Parkinson disease, selegiline given with sertraline, paroxetine, or fluoxetine was well tolerated.[20,21] In a study of 12 healthy men, coadministration of escitalopram and rasagiline was well tolerated.[22]

1 Kline SS, et al. *Clin Pharm.* 1989;8(7):510.
2 Sternbach H. *Lancet.* 1988;2(8615):850.
3 Ooi TK. *Anaesthesia.* 1991;46(6):507.
4 Bhatara VS, et al. *Clin Pharm.* 1993;12(3):222.
5 Brannan SK, et al. *J Clin Psychopharmacol.* 1994;14(2):144.
6 Graber MA, et al. *Ann Pharmacother.* 1994;28(6):732.
7 Phillips SD, et al. *Am J Psychiatry.* 1995;152(9):1400.
8 Klysner R, et al. *Lancet.* 1995;346(8985):1298.
9 Brubacher JF, et al. *J Toxicol Clin Toxicol.* 1995;33(5):523.
10 Hodgman M, et al. *J Toxicol Clin Toxicol.* 1995;33(5):554.
11 Heisler MA, et al. *Ann Pharmacother.* 1996;30(1):84.
12 Weiner LA, et al. *Pharmacotherapy.* 1998;18(2):399.
13 Beasley CM Jr, et al. *J Clin Psychopharmacol.* 1993;13(5):312.
14 Feighner JP, et al. *J Clin Psychiatry.* 1990;51(6):222.
15 Suchowersky O, et al. *Can J Psychiatry.* 1990;35(6):571.
16 Shad MU, et al. *J Clin Psychopharmacol.* 2001;21(1):119.
17 *Cymbalta* [package insert]. Indianapolis, IN: Eli Lilly and Company; 2004.
18 *Savella* [package insert]. New York, NY: Forest Laboratories Inc; January 2009.
19 Waters CH. *Can J Neurol Sci.* 1994;21(3):259.
20 Toyama SC, et al. *Ann Pharmacother.* 1994;28(3):405.
21 Hilli J, et al. *Prog Neuropsychopharmacol Biol Psychiatry.* 2009;33(8):1526.
22 *Viibryd* [package insert]. New Haven, CT: Trovis Pharmaceuticals LLC; January 2011.

* Asterisk indicates drugs cited in interaction reports. Based on pharmacologic and pharmacokinetic considerations, similar interactions may occur with other drugs that are listed.

Serotonin Reuptake Inhibitors — Methylene Blue

Serotonin Reuptake Inhibitors		Methylene Blue
Citalopram* (eg, *Celexa*)	Milnacipran (*Savella*)	Methylene Blue*
Duloxetine (*Cymbalta*)	Nefazodone	
Escitalopram (*Lexapro*)	Paroxetine* (eg, *Paxil*)	
Fluoxetine* (eg, *Prozac*)	Sertraline (eg, *Zoloft*)	
Fluvoxamine (eg, *Luvox*)	Venlafaxine* (eg, *Effexor*)	

Significance	Onset	Severity	Documentation
1	■ **Rapid** ☐ Delayed	■ **Major** ☐ Moderate ☐ Minor	☐ Established ■ **Probable** ☐ Suspected ☐ Possible ☐ Unlikely

Effects Neurologic adverse reactions, including symptoms consistent with serotonin syndrome (eg, agitation, altered consciousness, ataxia, myoclonus, overactive reflexes, shivering), may occur.

Mechanism Unknown. METHYLENE BLUE has been shown to have monoamine oxidase inhibitory properties.[1] CNS serotonin activity may be increased.

Management Avoid use of METHYLENE BLUE in patients receiving SRIs.

Discussion

A 58-year-old woman receiving paroxetine was given methylene blue for visualization of the parathyroid gland.[2] Postoperatively, she exhibited symptoms consistent with serotonin syndrome. Symptoms resolved without treatment over the next 48 hours. Similar reactions have occurred in other patients receiving methylene blue for parathyroid gland localization and citalopram,[3,4] fluoxetine,[5] paroxetine,[6,7] or venlafaxine.[8] Complete recovery occurred within 2 to 14 days.[2,3,5-8] However, some patients required reintubation[3,5,6] and admission to the intensive care unit.[3-5] Hemodialysis was started in 1 patient with end-stage renal failure to remove the methylene blue.[3]

1 Ramsay RR, et al. *Br J Pharmacol.* 2007;152(6):946.
2 Ng BK, et al. *Can J Anaesth.* 2008;55(1):36.
3 Mathew S, et al. *Anaesthesia.* 2006;61(6):580.
4 Khavandi A, et al. *Med J Aust.* 2008;189(9):534.
5 Martindale SJ, et al. *Anaesthesia.* 2003;58(10):1041.
6 Mihai R, et al. *Can J Anaesth.* 2007;54(1):79.
7 Bach KK, et al. *Anesth Analg.* 2004;99(5):1573.
8 Majithia A, et al. *J Laryngol Otol.* 2006;120(2):138.

* Asterisk indicates drugs cited in interaction reports. Based on pharmacologic and pharmacokinetic considerations, similar interactions may occur with other drugs that are listed.

Serotonin Reuptake Inhibitors — *Metoclopramide*

Serotonin Reuptake Inhibitors		Metoclopramide
Citalopram (eg, *Celexa*)	Paroxetine (eg, *Paxil*)	Metoclopramide* (eg, *Reglan*)
Fluoxetine (eg, *Prozac*)	Sertraline* (eg, *Zoloft*)	
Fluvoxamine (eg, *Luvox*)	Venlafaxine* (*Effexor*)	
Nefazodone		

Significance	Onset	Severity	Documentation
1	■ **Rapid**	■ **Major**	□ Established
	□ Delayed	□ Moderate	□ Probable
		□ Minor	■ **Suspected**
			□ Possible
			□ Unlikely

Effects Serotonin syndrome (eg, agitation, altered consciousness, ataxia, myoclonus, overactive reflexes, shivering) may occur. METOCLOPRAMIDE plasma levels may be elevated, increasing the risk of adverse reactions.

Mechanism Inhibition of METOCLOPRAMIDE metabolism (CYP2D6) by SRIs is suspected.

Management Closely monitor patients for adverse reactions when METOCLOPRAMIDE is coadministered with an SRI. Serotonin syndrome requires immediate medical attention, including supportive care and withdrawal of the serotonergic agent. Administration of an antiserotonergic agent (eg, cyproheptadine) may be helpful.

Discussion

Two cases of serotonin syndrome with extrapyramidal reactions were reported with coadministration of IV metoclopramide 10 mg and sertraline or venlafaxine.[1] When metoclopramide was started, 1 patient had been receiving sertraline 100 mg/day for 18 mo, while the second patient had been receiving venlafaxine 150 mg in the morning and 75 mg at bedtime for 3 years. Within hours of metoclopramide administration, 1 patient developed involuntary twitching; tremors of the arms, shoulders, and neck; twitching of the lips; stiffness of the jaw and tongue; and difficulties in controlling tongue movements. Metoclopramide administration in the second patient produced generalized shaking, jerking movements of the limbs, twitching of the jaw, and clenching of the teeth. After a subsequent dose of metoclopramide, the second patient experienced myoclonic jerks and muscle rigidity, involuntary twitching of the face, horizontal nystagmus, dilated pupils, confusion, agitation, and diaphoresis. Both patients improved following administration of IV diazepam 5 mg.

The effects of fluoxetine on metoclopramide pharmacokinetics were studied in 24 healthy subjects.[2] Each subject received a single dose of metoclopramide 20 mg alone and after 8 days of pretreatment with fluoxetine 60 mg daily. Compared with administering metoclopramide alone, coadministration of fluoxetine increased the metoclopramide mean C_{max} 42% (from 44.02 to 62.72 ng/mL) and AUC 89%, and prolonged the $t_{½}$ from 5.52 to 8.47 hours.

[1] Fisher AA, et al. *Ann Pharmacother.* 2002;36(1):67.

[2] Vlase L, et al. *Biopharm Drug Dispos.* 2006;27(6):285.

* Asterisk indicates drugs cited in interaction reports. Based on pharmacologic and pharmacokinetic considerations, similar interactions may occur with other drugs that are listed.

Serotonin Reuptake Inhibitors / Opioid Analgesics

Serotonin Reuptake Inhibitors		Opioid Analgesics	
Citalopram* (eg, *Celexa*)	Paroxetine (eg, *Paxil*)	Meperidine* (eg, *Demerol*)	Oxycodone* (eg, *Roxicodone*)
Fluoxetine* (eg, *Prozac*)	Sertraline* (eg, *Zoloft*)		
Fluvoxamine (eg, *Luvox*)			

Significance	Onset	Severity	Documentation
2	■ **Rapid** □ Delayed	□ Major ■ **Moderate** □ Minor	□ Established □ Probable ■ **Suspected** □ Possible □ Unlikely

Effects The risk of serotonin syndrome (eg, agitation, altered consciousness, ataxia, myoclonus, overactive reflexes, shivering) may be increased.

Mechanism Unknown.

Management Closely monitor patients for adverse reactions. Serotonin syndrome requires immediate medical attention, including withdrawal of the serotonergic agent and supportive care. Administration of an antiserotonergic agent (eg, cyproheptadine) may be helpful.

Discussion

A possible serotonin-like syndrome was reported in a 34-year-old man during coadministration of sertraline and oxycodone.[1] The patient, with a stable drug regimen, had undergone an allogenic bone marrow transplant and was receiving sertraline 50 mg/day and oxycodone 10 mg as needed. The dosage of oxycodone was increased from 10 to 20 mg/day to twenty 10 mg tablets in 48 hours after the patient experienced severe pain. Following the increase in oxycodone, the patient began to experience severe tremors and visual hallucinations. Because he had experienced similar tremors a year earlier when cyclosporine therapy was initiated, cyclosporine and oxycodone were withheld. The visual hallucinations decreased but still were present, and he continued to have severe tremors. At this point, serotonin syndrome was considered; sertraline was discontinued, and cyproheptadine was administered. The patient did not immediately respond to cyproheptadine. However, 12 hours later, his hallucinations resolved, and the tremors lessened. He was discharged the following morning. In another case, a 43-year-old man experienced diaphoresis, confusion, agitation, diarrhea, hypertension, and tachycardia shortly after meperidine 50 mg IV was started.[2] The patient had been taking fluoxetine and took the last dose approximately 2 weeks prior to the event. Symptoms consistent with serotonin syndrome occurred in a 44-year-old woman receiving citalopram 40 mg/day 10 hours after meperidine was added to her pain control regimen.[3] Symptoms subsided 12 hours after discontinuing meperidine. Pretreatment with paroxetine did not affect the pharmacokinetics of single-dose administration of oxycodone.[4]

[1] Rosebraugh CJ, et al. *J Clin Pharmacol.* 2001;41(2):224.
[2] Tissot TA. *Anesthesiology.* 2003;98(6):1511.
[3] Altman EM, et al. *Psychosomatics.* 2007;48(4):361.
[4] Kummer O, et al. *Eur J Clin Pharmacol.* 2011;67(1):63.

* Asterisk indicates drugs cited in interaction reports. Based on pharmacologic and pharmacokinetic considerations, similar interactions may occur with other drugs that are listed.

Serotonin Reuptake Inhibitors × *Proton Pump Inhibitors*

Serotonin Reuptake Inhibitors		Proton Pump Inhibitors
Citalopram (eg, *Celexa*)	Sertraline (eg, *Zoloft*)	Omeprazole* (eg, *Prilosec*)
Escitalopram* (*Lexapro*)		

Significance	Onset	Severity	Documentation
4	□ Rapid	□ Major	□ Established
	■ **Delayed**	■ **Moderate**	□ Probable
		□ Minor	□ Suspected
			■ **Possible**
			□ Unlikely

Effects Serum concentrations and the pharmacologic effects of certain SRIs may be increased.

Mechanism Inhibition of metabolism is suspected.

Management If an interaction is suspected, it may be necessary to adjust the dose of the SRI when OMEPRAZOLE is started or stopped.

Discussion

The effects of omeprazole on the pharmacokinetics of escitalopram were studied in 16 healthy subjects.[1] In a randomized, double-blind, crossover study, subjects received omeprazole 30 mg daily or placebo for 6 days. On day 5, each subject received a single dose of escitalopram 20 mg. Omeprazole increased the escitalopram AUC 51% and prolonged the $t_{½}$ from 26.5 to 34.8 hours, compared with placebo. No increase in adverse reactions occurred. The pharmacokinetics of racemic citalopram were studied in 9 healthy volunteers before and after administration of omeprazole 20 mg for 7 days.[2] Subjects were phenotyped as CYP2C19 and CYP2D6 extensive metabolizers. The AUC of both (R)- and (S)-citalopram increased; however, the effect was greatest for (S)-citalopram.

[1] Malling D, et al. *Br J Clin Pharmacol.* 2005;60(3):287. [2] Rocha A, et al. *Br J Clin Pharmacol.* 2010;70(1):43.

* Asterisk indicates drugs cited in interaction reports. Based on pharmacologic and pharmacokinetic considerations, similar interactions may occur with other drugs that are listed.

Serotonin Reuptake Inhibitors — *Quetiapine*

Fluvoxamine* (eg, *Luvox*)

Quetiapine* (*Seroquel*)

Significance	Onset	Severity	Documentation
4	☐ Rapid ■ **Delayed**	■ **Major** ☐ Moderate ☐ Minor	☐ Established ☐ Probable ☐ Suspected ■ **Possible** ☐ Unlikely

Effects The risk of neuroleptic malignant syndrome (NMS) may be increased. QUETIAPINE levels may be elevated.

Mechanism A dopamine-serotonin disequilibrium may be involved. In addition, FLUVOXAMINE inhibits QUETIAPINE metabolism (CYP3A4).

Management Closely monitor patients for adverse reactions. NMS requires immediate medical attention, including withdrawal of therapy, treatment with dantrolene (eg, *Dantrium*), and supportive care.

Discussion

NMS was reported in a 57-year-old man during coadministration of fluvoxamine and quetiapine.[1] The patient had been receiving fluvoxamine 150 mg/day for 1 year for major depression. During that time, no clinically important adverse reactions were noted. When his condition remitted, fluvoxamine treatment was tapered off. Five months later, risperidone (eg, *Risperdal*) was started for irritation and agitation. When the patient developed drug-induced extrapyramidal effects, risperidone was replaced with quetiapine 150 mg/day. Two months later, the patient developed a depressive mood and inhibition. Fluvoxamine 50 mg/day was started and increased to 100 mg/day after 1 week. He stopped eating and drinking and developed muscle rigidity on day 10 of therapy. Three days later, he was admitted to the hospital with a high fever, elevated BP, tachycardia, and severe extrapyramidal symptoms. In addition, he was falling into a stupor. His creatine phosphokinase and leukocyte levels were elevated. He was diagnosed with NMS and treated with dantrolene infusion. Gradually, his symptoms improved, and he recovered; his laboratory values returned to baseline. In a retrospective study of 11 patients receiving fluvoxamine and quetiapine, the quetiapine concentration-to-dose ratio was increased 159%.[2]

[1] Matsumoto R, et al. *Am J Psychiatry.* 2005;162(4):812.

[2] Castberg I, et al. *J Clin Psychiatry.* 2007;68(10):1540.

* Asterisk indicates drugs cited in interaction reports.

Serotonin Reuptake Inhibitors — Rifamycins

Citalopram* (eg, *Celexa*)	Sertraline* (*Zoloft*)	Rifabutin (*Mycobutin*) Rifampin* (eg, *Rifadin*)	Rifapentine (*Priftin*)

Significance	Onset	Severity	Documentation
4	□ Rapid ■ **Delayed**	□ Major ■ **Moderate** □ Minor	□ Established □ Probable □ Suspected ■ **Possible** □ Unlikely

Effects The therapeutic effect of certain SRIs may be decreased, resulting in withdrawal-type symptoms (eg, dizziness, lethargy).

Mechanism Induction of the hepatic metabolism (CYP3A4) of certain SRIs is suspected.

Management Carefully monitor clinical response to certain SRIs when starting, stopping, or changing the dose of the RIFAMYCIN.

Discussion

A worsening of previously controlled anxiety symptoms and symptoms of SRI withdrawal were reported in a 34-year-old man previously controlled on sertraline following the addition of rifampin to his treatment regimen.[1] The patient was receiving sertraline 200 mg at bedtime. He was started on rifampin 300 mg twice daily and sulfamethoxazole plus trimethoprim (eg, *Bactrim DS*) for a methicillin-resistant *Staphylococcus aureus* skin infection. Seven days later, the patient presented at the outpatient clinic reporting a decrease in the efficacy of sertraline. He was beginning to experience anxiety, excessive worry, and poor energy. In addition, he was feeling “spaced out” and reported dizziness, lethargy, and insomnia. A sertraline-rifampin interaction was suspected; the antianxiety medication was changed. The dose of sertraline was slowly tapered over 8 days. During antibiotic treatment, sertraline and the N-desmethyl metabolite of sertraline concentrations were decreased 67% and 54%, respectively, compared with giving sertraline alone. After rifampin was discontinued, the concentrations of sertraline and its metabolite increased. A 55-year-old man receiving citalopram 20 mg/day for panic disorder experienced a decrease in citalopram's therapeutic effect when rifampin 600 mg twice daily was started.[2] When rifampin was discontinued, his condition improved.

[1] Markowitz JS, et al. *J Clin Psychopharmacol.* 2000;20:109.

[2] Kukoyi O, et al. *Pharmacotherapy.* 2005;25:435.

* Asterisk indicates drugs cited in interaction reports. Based on pharmacologic and pharmacokinetic considerations, similar interactions may occur with other drugs that are listed.

Serotonin Reuptake Inhibitors — *St. John's Wort*

Serotonin Reuptake Inhibitors		St. John's Wort
Citalopram (eg, *Celexa*)	Nefazodone*	St. John's Wort*
Duloxetine (*Cymbalta*)	Paroxetine* (eg, *Paxil*)	
Fluoxetine (eg, *Prozac*)	Sertraline* (eg, *Zoloft*)	
Fluvoxamine (eg, *Luvox CR*)	Venlafaxine (*Effexor*)	

Significance	Onset	Severity	Documentation
2	■ **Rapid**	□ Major	□ Established
	□ Delayed	■ **Moderate**	□ Probable
		□ Minor	■ **Suspected**
			□ Possible
			□ Unlikely

Effects Increased sedative-hypnotic effects.

Mechanism Possible additive serotonin reuptake inhibition.

Management Caution patients who are taking an SRI to inform their health care provider before taking ST. JOHN'S WORT. Avoid concurrent use.

Discussion

A possible interaction was reported in a 50-year-old woman following concurrent ingestion of paroxetine and an herbal preparation of St. John's wort.[1] The patient had been taking paroxetine 40 mg/day for 8 months for depression. She stopped paroxetine and began taking powdered St. John's wort 600 mg/day, apparently without problems. She self-administered paroxetine 20 mg 11 days later because she was having trouble sleeping. The next day, she had difficulty getting out of bed; she was arousable but incoherent, groggy, and slow-moving. Approximately 2 hours later, she complained of nausea, weakness, and fatigue. Within 24 hours, her status returned to baseline. Five elderly patients on stable SRI regimens (4 on sertraline 50 to 75 mg/day and 1 on nefazodone 200 mg/day) developed symptoms consistent with serotonin syndrome (eg, anxiety, dizziness, nausea, restlessness, vomiting) within 2 to 4 days of starting St. John's wort 600 mg/day.[2] Symptoms resolved in all patients taking sertraline when sertraline and St. John's wort were discontinued and did not recur when sertraline alone was resumed. In the nefazodone-treated patient, symptoms resolved when nefazodone, but not St. John's wort, was discontinued.

The ingredients of herbal products are not standardized. It is unclear whether herbal products contain ingredients other than those listed on the label or purported to be present that could cause CNS adverse reactions.

[1] Gordon JB. *Am Fam Physician.* 1998;57(5):950.

[2] Lantz MS, et al. *J Geriatr Psychiatry Neurol.* 1999;12(1):7.

* Asterisk indicates drugs cited in interaction reports. Based on pharmacologic and pharmacokinetic considerations, similar interactions may occur with other drugs that are listed.

Serotonin Reuptake Inhibitors — Terbinafine

Paroxetine* (eg, *Paxil*)	Venlafaxine* (*Effexor*)	Terbinafine* (eg, *Lamisil*)

Significance	Onset	Severity	Documentation
2	☐ Rapid ■ **Delayed**	☐ Major ■ **Moderate** ☐ Minor	☐ Established ☐ Probable ■ **Suspected** ☐ Possible ☐ Unlikely

Effects SRI plasma concentrations may be elevated, increasing the pharmacologic effects and adverse reactions.

Mechanism Inhibition of SRI metabolism (CYP2D6) by TERBINAFINE is suspected.

Management In patients receiving PAROXETINE or VENLAFAXINE, monitor the clinical response and observe patients for adverse reactions when starting or stopping TERBINAFINE. Adjust the SRI dose as needed.

Discussion

The effects of terbinafine on the pharmacokinetics of paroxetine were studied in 12 volunteers.[1] In a randomized, crossover study, each subject received 6 days of pretreatment with placebo or terbinafine 125 mg daily. On day 6, a single oral dose of paroxetine 20 mg was administered. Compared with placebo, terbinafine increased the C_{max} and AUC of paroxetine 1.9- and 2.5-fold, respectively. In addition, the elimination $t_{½}$ was increased from 15.3 to 22.7 hours. The effect of terbinafine on venlafaxine pharmacokinetics was studied in 12 healthy men.[2] Each subject received terbinafine 250 mg/day for 4 days followed by a single dose of venlafaxine 75 mg. Terbinafine increased the venlafaxine C_{max} and AUC 4.9-fold and 2.67-fold, respectively, compared with giving venlafaxine alone.

[1] Yasui-Furukori N, et al. *Eur J Clin Pharmacol.* 2007;63(1):51.

[2] Hynninen VV, et al. *Clin Phamacol Ther.* 2008:83(2):342.

* Asterisk indicates drugs cited in interaction reports.

Serotonin Reuptake Inhibitors ✕ Tramadol

Serotonin Reuptake Inhibitors		Tramadol
Citalopram* (eg, *Celexa*)	Milnacipran (*Savella*)	Tramadol* (eg, *Ultram*)
Duloxetine (*Cymbalta*)	Nefazodone	
Escitalopram (*Lexapro*)	Paroxetine* (eg, *Paxil*)	
Fluoxetine* (eg, *Prozac*)	Sertraline* (eg, *Zoloft*)	
Fluvoxamine (eg, *Luvox*)	Venlafaxine* (eg, *Effexor*)	

Significance	Onset	Severity	Documentation
1	☐ Rapid	■ **Major**	☐ Established
	■ **Delayed**	☐ Moderate	☐ Probable
		☐ Minor	■ **Suspected**
			☐ Possible
			☐ Unlikely

Effects Serotonin syndrome (eg, agitation, altered consciousness, ataxia, myoclonus, overactive reflexes, shivering) may occur. In addition, PAROXETINE may reduce the efficacy of TRAMADOL.

Mechanism The serotonergic effects of these agents may be additive. PAROXETINE may inhibit the metabolism (CYP2D6) of TRAMADOL to (+)-O-desmethyltramadol.

Management Closely monitor patients for adverse reactions. Serotonin syndrome requires immediate medical attention, including withdrawal of the serotonergic agent and supportive care.

Discussion

A 42-year-old woman taking sertraline 100 mg/day for more than 1 year developed symptoms typical of serotonin syndrome after starting tramadol 300 mg/day.[1] However, she was receiving other drugs that could have contributed to her symptoms. A 75-year-old woman taking tramadol 50 mg/day experienced serotonin syndrome following the first dose of sertraline 50 mg.[2] A 31-year-old woman receiving fluoxetine 20 mg/day for 3 years presented with serotonin syndrome 4 weeks after starting tramadol.[3] Both drugs were stopped, and she improved over 7 days. A 72-year-old woman receiving fluoxetine for 10 years presented with piloerection and muscle contractions 18 days after starting tramadol 150 mg/day.[4] After stopping both drugs, symptoms subsided within 21 days. In another patient, serotonin syndrome occurred with fluoxetine 80 mg/day and tramadol 800 mg/day.[5] A 70-year-old woman receiving citalopram 10 mg/day for 3 years developed serotonin syndrome symptoms after starting tramadol 50 mg/day. Symptoms subsided after tramadol was discontinued and recurred 1 year later when tramadol 20 mg/day was given while she was still taking citalopram.[6] Serotonin syndrome was reported in a 47-year-old man taking venlafaxine 300 mg/day after increasing the tramadol dosage from 300 to 400 mg/day.[7] Pretreatment with paroxetine increased the AUC of tramadol while inhibiting formation of the active metabolite (M1).[8] However, there was no change in the analgesic effect of tramadol. Similar effects of paroxetine on tramadol metabolism were seen in a study of 12 healthy CYP2D6 extensive metabolizers.[9]

1 Mason BJ, et al. *Ann Pharmacother.* 1997;31(2):175.
2 Mittino D, et al. *Clin Neuropharmacol.* 2004;27(3):150.
3 Kesavan S, et al. *J R Soc Med.* 1999;92(9):474.
4 Gonzalez-Pinto A, et al. *Am J Psychiatry.* 2001;158(6):964.
5 Lange-Asschenfeldt C, et al. *J Clin Psychopharmacol.* 2002;22(4):440.
6 Mahlberg R, et al. *Am J Psychiatry.* 2004;161(6):1129.
7 Houlihan DJ. *Ann Pharmacother.* 2004;38(3):411.
8 Laugesen S, et al. *Clin Pharmacol Ther.* 2005;77(4):312.
9 Nielsen AG, et al. *Eur J Clin Pharmacol.* 2010;66(7):655.

* Asterisk indicates drugs cited in interaction reports. Based on pharmacologic and pharmacokinetic considerations, similar interactions may occur with other drugs that are listed.

Serotonin Reuptake Inhibitors — *Trazodone*

Serotonin Reuptake Inhibitors		Trazodone
Citalopram (eg, *Celexa*)	Paroxetine* (eg, *Paxil*)	Trazodone* (eg, *Oleptro*)
Fluoxetine* (eg, *Prozac*)	Sertraline (eg, *Zoloft*)	
Fluvoxamine (eg, *Luvox*)	Venlafaxine* (eg, *Effexor*)	
Nefazodone*		

Significance	Onset	Severity	Documentation
1	■ **Rapid**	■ **Major**	□ Established
	□ Delayed	□ Moderate	□ Probable
		□ Minor	■ **Suspected**
			□ Possible
			□ Unlikely

Effects Plasma TRAZODONE levels may be elevated, resulting in increased pharmacologic and toxic effects with some SRIs. Serotonin syndrome (eg, agitation, altered consciousness, ataxia, myoclonus, overactive reflexes, shivering) may occur.

Mechanism Possible rapid serotonin accumulation in the CNS. Certain SRIs may inhibit TRAZODONE metabolism (CYP2D6).

Management If coadministration cannot be avoided, start with a low dose of the SRI or TRAZODONE, and closely monitor the patient.

Discussion

An early case report[1] and placebo-controlled study[2] document a pharmacokinetic and pharmacodynamic interaction between trazodone and fluoxetine. A 31% increase in the trazodone plasma level to dose ratio accompanied by sedation and unstable gait was reported in an 82-year-old woman following the addition of fluoxetine 40 mg/day to her regimen.[1] In 11 patients receiving trazodone 100 mg/day, the addition of fluoxetine 20 mg/day resulted in a 65% increase in trazodone levels, a 239% increase in the active metabolite of trazodone (meta-chlorophenylpiperzine), and an improvement in clinical outcome.[2] A 29-year-old woman taking trazodone 50 mg/day developed symptoms suggestive of serotonin syndrome (eg, agitation, difficulty with memory and concentration, increased reflexes, myoclonus, piloerection, shaking, shivering, sweating, teeth chattering) 24 hours after starting paroxetine 20 mg/day.[3] Symptoms resolved within 24 hours of discontinuation of the antidepressants. Symptoms consistent with serotonin syndrome were reported in all patients receiving nefazodone 500 mg/day plus trazodone 20 to 50 mg/day[4] and in a patient treated with venlafaxine 225 mg/day plus trazodone 100 mg/day.[5] Symptoms resolved within 1 day of drug discontinuation.

[1] Aranow AB, et al. *Am J Psychiatry*. 1989;146(7):911.
[2] Maes M, et al. *J Clin Psychopharmacol*. 1997;17(5):358
[3] Reeves RR, et al. *Psychosomatics*. 1995;36(2):159.
[4] Margolese HC, et al. *Am J Psychiatry*. 2000;157(6):1022.
[5] McCue RE, et al. *Am J Psychiatry*. 2001;158(12):2088.

* Asterisk indicates drugs cited in interaction reports. Based on pharmacologic and pharmacokinetic considerations, similar interactions may occur with other drugs that are listed.

Serotonin Reuptake Inhibitors — *L-Tryptophan*

Citalopram (eg, *Celexa*)	Fluvoxamine (eg, *Luvox CR*)	L-Tryptophan*†
Duloxetine (*Cymbalta*)	Paroxetine (eg, *Paxil*)	
Fluoxetine* (eg, *Prozac*)	Sertraline (eg, *Zoloft*)	

Significance	Onset	Severity	Documentation
4	☐ Rapid	☐ Major	☐ Established
	■ **Delayed**	■ **Moderate**	☐ Probable
		☐ Minor	☐ Suspected
			■ **Possible**
			☐ Unlikely

Effects The coadministration of L-TRYPTOPHAN and certain SRIs may produce symptoms related to central and peripheral toxicity.

Mechanism May be related to inhibition of serotonin reuptake by the SRIs, along with increased substrate availability from L-TRYPTOPHAN supplementation.

Management Monitor patients for symptoms of CNS and peripheral toxicity. If symptoms occur, discontinue L-TRYPTOPHAN.

Discussion

In a preliminary uncontrolled study of 5 patients with obsessive-compulsive disorder, L-tryptophan was added to fluoxetine treatment to augment the response of fluoxetine.[1] All patients had been unresponsive or previously intolerant to a number of psychotropic agents and antidepressants. Four of the patients had been treated with L-tryptophan without experiencing adverse reactions. In addition, 2 of these patients had received L-tryptophan concurrently with clomipramine (eg, *Anafranil*), a less potent SRI. In all 5 patients, no adverse reactions occurred while fluoxetine 50 to 100 mg/day was administered alone. Following the addition of small doses of L-tryptophan (1 to 4 g/day for 7 to 22 days), all patients experienced symptoms related to central and peripheral toxicity. All symptoms resolved when L-tryptophan was discontinued.

Additional controlled studies are necessary to confirm this potential interaction.

[1] Steiner W, et al. *Biol Psychiatry*. 1986;21(11):1067. [2] *FDA Drug Bull*. 1990;20:2.

* Asterisk indicates drugs cited in interaction reports. Based on pharmacologic and pharmacokinetic considerations, similar interactions may occur with other drugs that are listed.

† The FDA requested a nationwide recall of all nonprescription supplements that contain L-tryptophan as the sole major component because of a possible link with eosinophilia myalgia.[2] However, it may still be available in some supplements or natural products.

Sertraline / *Carbamazepine*

Sertraline* (eg, *Zoloft*)	Carbamazepine* (eg, *Tegretol*)

Significance	Onset	Severity	Documentation
2	☐ Rapid ■ **Delayed**	☐ Major ■ **Moderate** ☐ Minor	☐ Established ☐ Probable ■ **Suspected** ☐ Possible ☐ Unlikely

Effects The therapeutic effect of SERTRALINE may be decreased or reversed by CARBAMAZEPINE.

Mechanism Increased metabolism (CYP3A4) of SERTRALINE is suspected.

Management In patients receiving CARBAMAZEPINE, consider administration of an antidepressant that is not affected by CYP3A4 metabolism (eg, paroxetine [eg, *Paxil*]). In patients receiving SERTRALINE, closely monitor patient response and be prepared to adjust the dose of SERTRALINE when starting, stopping, or changing the dose of CARBAMAZEPINE.

Discussion

Lack of sertraline efficacy was noted in 2 patients during coadministration of carbamazepine.[1] The first patient, a 33-year-old woman with a diagnosis of bipolar-type schizoaffective disorder, had been successfully treated for 3 years with carbamazepine 1,000 mg/day and haloperidol (eg, *Haldol*). Sertraline 50 mg/day was started after she developed depression. Her depression did not respond to treatment, and the sertraline dose was slowly titrated to 300 mg/day. Within 2 weeks of taking sertraline 300 mg/day, the patient's appetite, concentration, energy, and sleep improved. The second patient, a 25-year-old man with post-traumatic stress disorder, had been successfully treated for 13 years with carbamazepine 400 mg/day. Sertraline 50 mg/day was added to his treatment regimen when he developed major depression. When the patient failed to respond, the dose of sertraline was slowly titrated to 300 mg/day. At this dose, his energy, interest, mood, and sleep improved. In a retrospective analysis, lower sertraline plasma levels, relative to the dose, were seen in patients taking either carbamazepine or phenytoin compared with patients taking sertraline without these drugs.[2]

[1] Khan A, et al. *J Clin Psychiatry*. 2000;61(7):526.

[2] Pihlsgard M, et al. *Eur J Clin Pharmacol*. 2002;57(12):915.

* Asterisk indicates drugs cited in interaction reports.

Sertraline | **Food**

Sertraline*
(*Zoloft*)

Grapefruit Juice*

Significance	Onset	Severity	Documentation
5	☐ Rapid ■ **Delayed**	☐ Major ☐ Moderate ■ **Minor**	☐ Established ☐ Probable ☐ Suspected ■ **Possible** ☐ Unlikely

Effects SERTRALINE plasma concentrations may be elevated, increasing the pharmacologic and adverse effects.

Mechanism Inhibition of SERTRALINE metabolism (CYP3A4) is suspected.

Management Based on available data, no special precautions are needed.

Discussion

The effect of grapefruit juice on sertraline plasma levels was evaluated in 5 patients receiving stable sertraline dosages 50 to 75 mg daily.[1] Subjects took their usual dose of sertraline for 7 days with 240 mL of water. For the next 7 days, they took their usual dose of sertraline with 240 mL of grapefruit juice. Compared with taking sertraline with water, ingestion with grapefruit juice increased mean trough levels of sertraline approximately 47% (from 13.7 to 20.2 mcg/L).

[1] Lee AJ, et al. *Clin Ther.* 1999;21:1890.

* Asterisk indicates drugs cited in interaction reports.

Sibutramine — *Dextromethorphan*

Sibutramine* (*Meridia*)	Dextromethorphan* (eg, *Robitussin*)

Significance	Onset	Severity	Documentation
1	■ **Rapid** □ Delayed	■ **Major** □ Moderate □ Minor	□ Established □ Probable ■ **Suspected** □ Possible □ Unlikely

Effects A "serotonin syndrome," including CNS irritability, motor weakness, shivering, myoclonus, and altered consciousness, may occur.

Mechanism The serotonergic effects of these agents may be additive.

Management Concomitant administration of these agents is not recommended by the manufacturer. If concurrent use cannot be avoided, carefully monitor the patient for adverse effects. The serotonin syndrome requires immediate medical attention.

Discussion

Although rare, the potentially fatal "serotonin syndrome" has been reported with use of agents that inhibit serotonin reuptake or have serotonergic activity, such as dextromethorphan.[1] Because sibutramine inhibits serotonin reuptake, it should not be administered with other serotonergic agents, such as dextromethorphan.

The basis for this monograph is information on file with the manufacturer. Published clinical data are needed to further assess this interaction. However, due to the seriousness of this interaction, clinical evaluation in humans is not likely to be forthcoming.

[1] *Meridia* [package insert]. Abbott Park, IL: Abbott Laboratories; November 1997.

* Asterisk indicates drugs cited in interaction reports.

Sibutramine		***Ergot Alkaloids***	
Sibutramine* (*Meridia*)		Dihydroergotamine* (*D.H.E. 45*)	Methysergide (*Sansert*)
		Ergotamine (eg, *Ergomar*)	

Significance	Onset	Severity	Documentation
1	■ **Rapid**	■ **Major**	□ Established
	□ Delayed	□ Moderate	□ Probable
		□ Minor	■ **Suspected**
			□ Possible
			□ Unlikely

Effects A "serotonin syndrome," including CNS irritability, motor weakness, shivering, myoclonus, and altered consciousness, may occur.

Mechanism The serotonergic effects of these agents may be additive.

Management Concomitant administration of these agents is not recommended by the manufacturer. If concurrent use cannot be avoided, carefully monitor the patient for adverse effects. The serotonin syndrome requires immediate medical attention.

Discussion

Although rare, the potentially fatal "serotonin syndrome" has been reported with use of agents that inhibit serotonin reuptake or have serotonergic activity, such as dihydroergotamine.[1] Since sibutramine inhibits serotonin reuptake, it should not be administered with other serotonergic agents, such as dihydroergotamine.

The basis for this monograph is information on file with the manufacturer. Published clinical data are needed to further assess this interaction. However, due to the seriousness of this interaction, clinical evaluation in humans is not likely to be forthcoming.

[1] *Meridia* [package insert]. Abbott Park, IL: Abbott Laboratories; November 1997.

* Asterisk indicates drugs cited in interaction reports. Based on pharmacologic and pharmacokinetic considerations, similar interactions may occur with other drugs that are listed.

Sibutramine — **Lithium**

Sibutramine*
(*Meridia*)

Lithium*
(eg, *Lithobid*)

Significance	Onset	Severity	Documentation
1	■ **Rapid**	■ **Major**	□ Established
	□ Delayed	□ Moderate	□ Probable
		□ Minor	■ **Suspected**
			□ Possible
			□ Unlikely

Effects Serotonin syndrome, including altered consciousness, CNS irritability, motor weakness, myoclonus, and shivering, may occur.

Mechanism The serotonergic effects of these agents may be additive.

Management Coadministration of these agents is not recommended. If concurrent use cannot be avoided, carefully monitor the patient for adverse effects. Serotonin syndrome requires immediate medical attention.

Discussion

Although rare, the potentially fatal serotonin syndrome has been reported with use of agents that inhibit serotonin reuptake or have serotonergic activity, such as lithium.[1] Because sibutramine inhibits serotonin reuptake, it should not be administered with other serotonergic agents, such as lithium.

The basis for this monograph is information on file with the manufacturer. Published clinical data are needed to further assess this interaction. However, due to the seriousness of this interaction, clinical evaluation in humans is not likely to be forthcoming.

[1] *Meridia* [package insert]. Abbott Park, IL: Abbott Laboratories; November 1997.

* Asterisk indicates drugs cited in interaction reports.

Sibutramine — *MAOIs*

Sibutramine	MAOIs	
Sibutramine* (*Meridia*)	Isocarboxazid* (*Marplan*)	Rasagiline* (*Azilect*)
	Linezolid* (*Zyvox*)	Selegiline* (eg, *Eldepryl*)
	Phenelzine* (*Nardil*)	Tranylcypromine* (eg, *Parnate*)

Significance	Onset	Severity	Documentation
1	■ **Rapid**	■ **Major**	□ Established
	□ Delayed	□ Moderate	□ Probable
		□ Minor	■ **Suspected**
			□ Possible
			□ Unlikely

Effects Serotonin syndrome, including altered consciousness, CNS irritability, motor weakness, myoclonus, and shivering, may occur.

Mechanism The serotonergic effects of these agents may be additive.

Management Coadministration of these agents is contraindicated.[1] Allow at least 2 weeks after stopping MAOI therapy before starting treatment with SIBUTRAMINE. Similarly, allow at least 2 weeks after stopping SIBUTRAMINE therapy before starting treatment with an MAOI.

Discussion

Serious, sometimes fatal reactions (ie, serotonin syndrome) have been reported with concomitant administration of MAOI and serotonergic agents.[1] Because sibutramine inhibits serotonin reuptake, it should not be administered with an MAOI.

The basis for this monograph is information on file with the manufacturer. Published clinical data are needed to further assess this interaction. However, due to the seriousness of this interaction, clinical evaluation in humans is not likely to be forthcoming.

[1] *Meridia* [package insert]. Abbott Park, IL; Abbott Laboratories; November 1997.

* Asterisk indicates drugs cited in interaction reports.

Sibutramine — **Meperidine**

Sibutramine*
(*Meridia*)

Meperidine*
(eg, *Demerol*)

Significance	Onset	Severity	Documentation
1	■ **Rapid**	■ **Major**	□ Established
	□ Delayed	□ Moderate	□ Probable
		□ Minor	■ **Suspected**
			□ Possible
			□ Unlikely

Effects A "serotonin syndrome," including CNS irritability, motor weakness, shivering, myoclonus, and altered consciousness, may occur.

Mechanism The serotonergic effects of these agents may be additive.

Management Concomitant administration of these agents is not recommended by the manufacturer. If concurrent use cannot be avoided, carefully monitor the patient for adverse effects. The serotonin syndrome requires immediate medical attention.

Discussion

Although rare, the potentially fatal "serotonin syndrome" has been reported with use of agents that inhibit serotonin reuptake or have serotonergic activity, such as meperidine.[1] Since sibutramine inhibits serotonin reuptake, it should not be administered with other serotonergic agents, such as meperidine.

The basis for this monograph is information on file with the manufacturer. Published clinical data are needed to further assess this interaction. However, due to the seriousness of this interaction, clinical evaluation in humans is not likely to be forthcoming.

[1] *Meridia*. [package insert]. Abbott Park, IL: Abbott Laboratories; November 1997.

* Asterisk indicates drugs cited in interaction reports.

Sibutramine		*Selective 5-HT$_1$ Receptor Agonists*	
Sibutramine* (*Meridia*)		Naratriptan (*Amerge*)	Sumatriptan* (*Imitrex*)
		Rizatriptan (*Maxalt*)	Zolmitriptan (*Zomig*)

Significance	Onset	Severity	Documentation
1	■ **Rapid**	■ **Major**	□ Established
	□ Delayed	□ Moderate	□ Probable
		□ Minor	■ **Suspected**
			□ Possible
			□ Unlikely

Effects A "serotonin syndrome," including CNS irritability, motor weakness, shivering, myoclonus, and altered consciousness, may occur.

Mechanism The serotonergic effects of these agents may be additive.

Management Concomitant administration of these agents is not recommended by the manufacturer. If concurrent use cannot be avoided, carefully monitor the patient for adverse effects. The serotonin syndrome requires immediate medical attention.

Discussion

Although rare, the potentially fatal "serotonin syndrome" has been reported with use of agents that inhibit serotonin reuptake or have serotonergic activity, such as sumatriptan.[1] Since sibutramine inhibits serotonin reuptake, it should not be administered with other serotonergic agents, such as sumatriptan.

The basis for this monograph is information on file with the manufacturer. Published clinical data are needed to further assess this interaction. However, due to the seriousness of this interaction, clinical evaluation in humans is not likely to be forthcoming.

[1] *Meridia.* [package insert]. Abbott Park, IL: Abbott Laboratories; November 1997.

* Asterisk indicates drugs cited in interaction reports. Based on pharmacologic and pharmacokinetic considerations, similar interactions may occur with other drugs that are listed.

Sibutramine — *Serotonin Reuptake Inhibitors*

Sibutramine	Serotonin Reuptake Inhibitors	
Sibutramine* (*Meridia*)	Fluoxetine* (eg, *Prozac*)	Sertraline* (eg, *Zoloft*)
	Fluvoxamine* (eg, *Luvox*)	Venlafaxine* (eg, *Effexor*)
	Nefazodone	
	Paroxetine* (eg, *Paxil*)	

Significance	Onset	Severity	Documentation
1	■ **Rapid**	■ **Major**	□ Established
	□ Delayed	□ Moderate	□ Probable
		□ Minor	■ **Suspected**
			□ Possible
			□ Unlikely

Effects Serotonin syndrome, including CNS irritability, motor weakness, shivering, myoclonus, and altered consciousness, may occur.

Mechanism The serotonergic effects of these agents may be additive.

Management Coadministration of these agents is not recommended by the manufacturer. If concurrent use cannot be avoided, carefully monitor the patient for adverse effects. The serotonin syndrome requires immediate medical attention.

Discussion

Although rare, the potentially fatal serotonin syndrome has been reported with use of agents that inhibit serotonin reuptake or have serotonergic activity, such as fluoxetine.[1] Because sibutramine inhibits serotonin reuptake, it should not be administered with other serotonergic agents, such as fluoxetine.

The basis for this monograph is information on file with the manufacturer. Published clinical data are needed to further assess this interaction. However, due to the seriousness of this interaction, clinical evaluation in humans is not likely to be forthcoming.

[1] *Meridia*. [package insert]. Abbott Park, IL: Abbott Laboratories; November 1997.

* Asterisk indicates drugs cited in interaction reports. Based on pharmacologic and pharmacokinetic considerations, similar interactions may occur with other drugs that are listed.

Sibutramine — *Tryptophan*

Sibutramine* (*Meridia*)	Tryptophan*

Significance	Onset	Severity	Documentation
1	■ **Rapid**	■ **Major**	□ Established
	□ Delayed	□ Moderate	□ Probable
		□ Minor	■ **Suspected**
			□ Possible
			□ Unlikely

Effects Serotonin syndrome, including CNS irritability, motor weakness, shivering, myoclonus, and altered consciousness, may occur.

Mechanism The serotonergic effects of these agents may be additive.

Management Coadministration of these agents is not recommended by the manufacturer. If concurrent use cannot be avoided, carefully monitor the patient for adverse effects. The serotonin syndrome requires immediate medical attention.

Discussion

Although rare, the potentially fatal serotonin syndrome has been reported with use of agents that inhibit serotonin reuptake or have serotonergic activity, such as tryptophan.[1] Because sibutramine inhibits serotonin reuptake, it should not be administered with other serotonergic agents, such as tryptophan.

The basis for this monograph is information on file with the manufacturer. Published clinical data are needed to further assess this interaction. However, due to the seriousness of this interaction, clinical evaluation in humans is not likely to be forthcoming.

[1] *Meridia.* [package insert]. Abbott Park, IL: Abbott Laboratories; November 1997.

* Asterisk indicates drugs cited in interaction reports.

Sildenafil — *Cimetidine*

Sildenafil* (eg, *Viagra*)	Cimetidine* (eg, *Tagamet*)

Significance	Onset	Severity	Documentation
4	☐ Rapid ■ **Delayed**	☐ Major ■ **Moderate** ☐ Minor	☐ Established ☐ Probable ☐ Suspected ■ **Possible** ☐ Unlikely

Effects SILDENAFIL plasma concentrations may be elevated, increasing the risk of adverse effects.

Mechanism Inhibition of SILDENAFIL gut wall and first-pass hepatic metabolism (CYP3A4) by CIMETIDINE is suspected.

Management Based on available clinical data, no dosage adjustments appear to be necessary.

Discussion

The effects of cimetidine coadministration on the pharmacokinetics of sildenafil were studied in healthy men.[1] Using a parallel-group design, 22 subjects received sildenafil 50 mg on days 1 and 5. On days 3 to 6, subjects received cimetidine 800 mg or placebo. Cimetidine did not affect the sildenafil T_{max} or the elimination rate constant. However, compared with placebo, cimetidine administration resulted in a 56% increase in the sildenafil AUC and a 54% increase in the C_{max}. Cimetidine treatment resulted in a 30% increase in the AUC of the sildenafil metabolite (UK-103,320). There were no serious adverse events or treatment-related laboratory test abnormalities observed for any subject.

[1] Wilner K, et al. *Br J Clin Pharmacol.* 2002;53(suppl 1):31S.

* Asterisk indicates drugs cited in interaction reports.

Sildenafil — *Food*

Sildenafil* (eg, *Viagra*)	Grapefruit Juice*

Significance	Onset	Severity	Documentation
5	■ **Rapid** □ Delayed	□ Major □ Moderate ■ **Minor**	□ Established □ Probable □ Suspected ■ **Possible** □ Unlikely

Effects SILDENAFIL plasma concentrations may be increased and absorption delayed.

Mechanism Inhibition of enteric metabolism (CYP3A4) is suspected.

Management Based on available data, no special precautions are needed.

Discussion

The effect of taking sildenafil with grapefruit juice was investigated in an open, randomized, balanced, 2-period crossover study.[1] Twenty-four healthy men received sildenafil 50 mg with grapefruit juice or water. Each subject ingested 250 mL of grapefruit juice or water 1 hour before and concurrently with the sildenafil dose. Compared with water, taking sildenafil with grapefruit juice increased the AUC 23%. The AUC of the primary metabolite of sildenafil, N-desmethylsildenafil, was increased 24%. C_{max} of sildenafil and N-desmethylsildenafil were unchanged; however, the T_{max} of sildenafil was prolonged 0.25 hours. There were no differences in hemodynamic or other effects between either study period. In a case report involving a 70-year-old man, taking sildenafil 100 mg with grapefruit juice increased the peak concentration of sildenafil 42% without altering the AUC, compared with water.[2]

Additional studies are needed to clarify these conflicting data.

[1] Jetter A, et al. *Clin Pharmacol Ther.* 2002;71(1):21. [2] Lee M, et al. *Ther Drug Monit.* 2001;23(1):21.

* Asterisk indicates drugs cited in interaction reports.

Sildenafil — *Opioid Analgesics*

Sildenafil	Opioid Analgesics	
Sildenafil* (eg, *Viagra*)	Codeine	Morphine (eg, *Roxanol*)
	Dihydrocodeine*	Oxycodone (eg, *OxyContin*)
	Hydrocodone (eg, *Hycodan*)	Oxymorphone (eg, *Opana*)
	Hydromorphone (eg, *Dilaudid*)	
	Levorphanol	

Significance	Onset	Severity	Documentation
4	■ **Rapid**	□ Major	□ Established
	□ Delayed	■ **Moderate**	□ Probable
		□ Minor	□ Suspected
			■ **Possible**
			□ Unlikely

Effects Pharmacologic effects of SILDENAFIL may be prolonged.

Mechanism DIHYDROCODEINE produced high cyclic guanosine monophosphate levels at peripheral nerve endings, resulting in prolonged erections following orgasm in patients receiving SILDENAFIL.

Management Caution patients receiving SILDENAFIL and DIHYDROCODEINE about the possibility of prolonged erections following orgasm.

Discussion

Two patients were reported to have experienced prolonged erections during coadministration of sildenafil and dihydrocodeine.[1] The first patient was a 49-year-old man who experienced erectile dysfunction after a fall that caused thoracic vertebral fractures. Sildenafil 100 mg produced hard erections that detumesced immediately after orgasm. When the patient took sildenafil with dihydrocodeine (30 mg every 6 hours), which was prescribed for soft tissue injury pain, he was able to have an erection, orgasm, and ejaculate; however, his erection did not subside for 5 hours. A similar experience occurred on a second occasion, during which time his erection persisted for 4 hours. After stopping dihydrocodeine, sildenafil produced erections that subsided immediately after orgasm. The second patient was a 37-year-old man with HIV. The patient was diagnosed with psychogenic erectile dysfunction. While taking sildenafil 100 mg, the patient experienced hard erections that subsided after orgasm. On 3 occasions while taking sildenafil and dihydrocodeine (30 to 60 mg every 6 hours), he experienced erections that persisted for 2 to 3 hours after orgasm. The prolonged erections occurred during the first 7 days of his analgesic treatment. Subsequently, he took dihydrocodeine regularly for 2 weeks, and the erections he experienced when he took sildenafil detumesced immediately after orgasm.

[1] Goldmeier D, et al. *BMJ.* 2002;324(7353):1555.

* Asterisk indicates drugs cited in interaction reports. Based on pharmacologic and pharmacokinetic considerations, similar interactions may occur with other drugs that are listed.

Sildenafil — *Pomelo*

Sildenafil* (eg, *Viagra*)	Pomelo* (*Citrus Grandis*; pummelo)

Significance	Onset	Severity	Documentation
4	■ **Rapid**	□ Major	□ Established
	□ Delayed	■ **Moderate**	□ Probable
		□ Minor	□ Suspected
			■ **Possible**
			□ Unlikely

Effects SILDENAFIL plasma concentrations may be reduced, decreasing the effectiveness.

Mechanism Unknown.

Management Advise patients not to drink POMELO JUICE before or immediately after taking SILDENAFIL.

Discussion

The effect of pomelo juice on the pharmacokinetics of sildenafil was studied in 6 healthy men.[1] Using a randomized, single dose, crossover design, each subject drank 250 mL of freshly squeezed pomelo juice or 250 mL of water with sildenafil 50 mg. Compared with water, taking sildenafil with pomelo juice decreased the sildenafil C_{max} and AUC approximately 60% and 40%, respectively.

[1] Al-Ghazawi MA, et al. *Eur J Clin Pharmacol.* 2010;66(2):159.

* Asterisk indicates drugs cited in interaction reports.

Sildenafil — *Protease Inhibitors*

Sildenafil*
(eg, *Viagra*)

Fosamprenavir*
(*Lexiva*)
Indinavir*
(*Crixivan*)
Nelfinavir
(*Viracept*)
Ritonavir*
(*Norvir*)
Saquinavir*
(*Invirase*)

Significance	Onset	Severity	Documentation
1	■ **Rapid**	■ **Major**	□ Established
	□ Delayed	□ Moderate	■ **Probable**
		□ Minor	□ Suspected
			□ Possible
			□ Unlikely

Effects Plasma concentrations of SILDENAFIL may be elevated, resulting in severe and potentially fatal hypotension.

Mechanism Inhibition of SILDENAFIL metabolism (CYP3A4).

Management Administer SILDENAFIL with extreme caution and in reduced dosage to patients taking PROTEASE INHIBITORS. In patients taking RITONAVIR[1] or FOSAMPRENAVIR,[2] do not exceed a maximum single SILDENAFIL dose of 25 mg in a 48-hour period.[1] A starting dose of SILDENAFIL 25 mg is recommended in patients taking SAQUINAVIR.[1] When SILDENAFIL is used for the treatment of pulmonary arterial hypertension, coadministration with FOSAMPRENAVIR is contraindicated.[2]

Discussion

Death was reported in a 47-year-old man following concurrent use of ritonavir, saquinavir, and sildenafil.[3] The patient took sildenafil on 8 occasions without experiencing adverse reactions. On the ninth occasion, he experienced chest pain 1 hour after taking sildenafil 25 mg. He smoked 1½ packs of cigarettes daily for 30 years. An ECG showed an extensive anterolateral MI. He was given alteplase (eg, *Activase*) 100 mg. After initial improvement, his condition deteriorated and he died from cardiac arrest. In healthy volunteers not infected with HIV, administration of ritonavir 500 mg twice daily at steady state, with a single sildenafil 100 mg dose, increased peak sildenafil plasma levels 4-fold and AUC 11-fold.[1] At 24 hours, sildenafil plasma levels were still approximately 200 ng/mL, compared with approximately 5 ng/mL when sildenafil was given alone. In healthy men, administration of saquinavir 1,200 mg 3 times daily at steady state resulted in a 210% increase in sildenafil AUC.[1] In 2 groups of 28 healthy volunteers, sildenafil AUC was increased 11- and 3.9-fold by ritonavir and saquinavir, respectively.[4] In 6 patients infected with HIV and treated with indinavir, the AUC of sildenafil was increased 4.4-fold by indinavir compared with historical controls.[5] The AUC and $t_{½}$ of sildenafil were approximately doubled in a patient infected with HIV receiving lopinavir, ritonavir, and indinavir, compared with control subjects.[6]

1 *Viagra* [package insert]. New York, NY; January 2011.
2 *Lexiva* [package insert]. Research Triangle Park, NC: GlaxoSmithKline; April 2011.
3 Hall MC, et al. *Lancet.* 1999;353(9169):2071.
4 Muirhead GJ, et al. *Br J Clin Pharmacol.* 2000;50(2):99.
5 Merry C, et al. *AIDS.* 1999;13(15):F101.
6 Aschmann YZ, et al. *Ther Drug Monit.* 2008;30(1):130.

* Asterisk indicates drugs cited in interaction reports. Based on pharmacologic and pharmacokinetic considerations, similar interactions may occur with other drugs that are listed.

Sildenafil — *Tacrolimus*

Sildenafil* (eg, *Viagra*)	Tacrolimus* (eg, *Prograf*)

Significance	Onset	Severity	Documentation
4	□ Rapid ■ **Delayed**	□ Major ■ **Moderate** □ Minor	□ Established □ Probable □ Suspected ■ **Possible** □ Unlikely

Effects SILDENAFIL plasma concentrations may be elevated, increasing the risk of adverse reactions.

Mechanism Inhibition of SILDENAFIL metabolism (CYP3A4) by TACROLIMUS is suspected.

Management Consider starting with the lowest dose (25 mg) of SILDENAFIL.

Discussion

The pharmacokinetics of tacrolimus and sildenafil coadministration were studied in 10 male kidney transplant recipients with erectile dysfunction.[1] Because subjects were transplant patients, other medications remained unchanged during the study. Therefore, it was necessary to compare sildenafil data from this investigation with results from previous studies. On day 1, routine tacrolimus was administered. On day 2, a single dose of sildenafil 50 mg was added to the drug regimen. Sildenafil administration did not affect the pharmacokinetics of tacrolimus. Compared with results of previous studies, tacrolimus administration increased sildenafil mean peak concentrations 44% and the AUC 90%, while the $t_{½}$ was prolonged from 3 (in healthy volunteers) to 4.7 hours. Compared with results in healthy subjects, the AUC for the sildenafil metabolite UK-103,320 was increased 3-fold, and the $t_{½}$ was prolonged from 3.8 to 11.4 hours. In addition, pronounced decreases in BP were observed. Sildenafil 25 mg daily for 9 days did not affect tacrolimus $t_{½}$ in kidney transplant patients.[2] Additional studies are needed to assess if the changes in the pharmacokinetics of sildenafil were caused by an interaction with tacrolimus, other concurrent medications, or the underlying disease.

[1] Christ B, et al. *Urology*. 2001;58(4):589.

[2] Christ B, et al. *Int J Clin Pharmacol Ther*. 2004;42(3):149.

* Asterisk indicates drugs cited in interaction reports.

Simvastatin — *Amlodipine*

Simvastatin* (eg, *Zocor*)	Amlodipine* (eg, *Norvasc*)

Significance	Onset	Severity	Documentation
1	☐ Rapid	■ **Major**	☐ Established
	■ **Delayed**	☐ Moderate	☐ Probable
		☐ Minor	■ **Suspected**
			☐ Possible
			☐ Unlikely

Effects SIMVASTATIN plasma concentrations may be elevated, increasing the risk of toxicity (eg, myositis, rhabdomyolysis).

Mechanism Unknown.

Management Do not exceed a dosage of SIMVASTATIN 20 mg daily in patients receiving AMLODIPINE.[1]

Discussion

The effects of amlodipine on the pharmacokinetics and pharmacodynamics of simvastatin were studied in 8 patients with hypercholesterolemia and hypertension.[2] Each patient received oral simvastatin 5 mg daily for 4 weeks followed by coadministration of simvastatin 5 mg daily with amlodipine 5 mg daily for 4 weeks. Coadministration of simvastatin with amlodipine increased the C_{max} and AUC of simvastatin approximately 43% and 28%, respectively, compared with simvastatin administered alone. The cholesterol-lowering effect of simvastatin was not altered. No serious clinical or laboratory effects or adverse reactions were reported. When a single dose of simvastatin 80 mg was administered after pretreatment with amlodipine 10 mg daily for 10 days, the simvastatin acid C_{max} and AUC increased 56% and 58%, respectively.[1]

[1] *Zocor* [package insert]. Whitehouse Station, NJ: Merck & Co; June 2011.

[2] Nishio S, et al. *Hypertens Res.* 2005;28(3):223.

* Asterisk indicates drugs cited in interaction reports.

Simvastatin — *Ezetimibe*

Simvastatin* (eg, *Zocor*)	Ezetimibe* (*Zetia*)

Significance	Onset	Severity	Documentation
4	☐ Rapid	☐ Major	☐ Established
	■ **Delayed**	■ **Moderate**	☐ Probable
		☐ Minor	☐ Suspected
			■ **Possible**
			☐ Unlikely

Effects SIMVASTATIN plasma concentrations may be elevated, increasing the pharmacologic effects and adverse reactions.

Mechanism EZETIMIBE inhibition of SIMVASTATIN metabolism via uridine diphosphate glucuronosyltransferase enzymes is suspected.

Management Monitor patients receiving SIMVASTATIN/EZETIMIBE combination therapy (or if EZETIMIBE is added to SIMVASTATIN therapy) for hepatotoxicity, and monitor serum aminotransferase levels while increasing the dose.

Discussion

Liver failure necessitating liver transplant was reported in a 70-year-old woman during administration of ezetimibe/simvastatin (*Vytorin*).[1] The patient had been receiving simvastatin 40 mg daily for hyperlipidemia for more than 1 year before being switched to simvastatin 40 mg/ezetimibe 10 mg daily combination therapy. Ten weeks later, the patient had elevated serum aminotransferase levels without clinical symptoms. Ezetimibe/simvastatin was discontinued; however, subsequent laboratory tests revealed further elevated aminotransferase levels, and she was admitted to the hospital for progressive liver failure. She later exhibited signs of fulminant hepatic failure, including encephalopathy and severe coagulopathy. She received a liver transplant and was clinically stable at her 2-year follow-up. The patient had been receiving other drugs that rarely have been associated with hepatotoxicity. However, she had been taking them for more than 1 year without evidence of hepatocellular damage.

[1] Tuteja S, et al. *Pharmacotherapy*. 2008;28(9):1188.

* Asterisk indicates drugs cited in interaction reports.

Simvastatin — *Protease Inhibitors*

Simvastatin* (eg, *Zocor*)	Atazanavir (*Reyataz*)	Lopinavir/Ritonavir (*Kaletra*)
	Darunavir* (*Prezista*)	Nelfinavir* (*Viracept*)
	Fosamprenavir* (*Lexiva*)	Ritonavir* (*Norvir*)
	Indinavir (*Crixivan*)	Saquinavir* (*Invirase*)

Significance	Onset	Severity	Documentation
1	☐ Rapid	■ **Major**	☐ Established
	■ **Delayed**	☐ Moderate	☐ Probable
		☐ Minor	■ **Suspected**
			☐ Possible
			☐ Unlikely

Effects SIMVASTATIN plasma levels may be elevated, increasing the risk of adverse reactions (eg, rhabdomyolysis).

Mechanism Inhibition of SIMVASTATIN first-pass metabolism (CYP3A4) in the GI tract is suspected.

Management SIMVASTATIN is contraindicated in patients receiving DARUNAVIR,[1] FOSAMPRENAVIR,[2] or NELFINAVIR[3]; avoid RITONAVIR coadministration.[4]

Discussion

The effects of ritonavir plus saquinavir on the pharmacokinetics of simvastatin were evaluated in 14 volunteers seronegative for HIV.[5] Using a randomized, open-label design, patients were administered simvastatin 40 mg/day on days 1 through 4 and 15 through 18. Subjects received ritonavir (300 mg twice daily on days 4 through 8 and 400 mg twice daily on days 8 through 18) plus saquinavir (400 mg twice daily on days 4 through 18). Ritonavir plus saquinavir increased the AUC of simvastatin 3,124%. Rhabdomyolysis was reported in a 51-year-old woman during coadministration of simvastatin 20 mg twice daily and ritonavir.[6] The patient had been receiving indinavir, zidovudine (eg, *Retrovir*), and lamivudine (eg, *Epivir*) for more than 2 years. One week prior to admission, ritonavir 100 mg twice daily was added to the drug regimen. Three days before hospital admission, the patient noticed body aches and weakness of her lower extremities that gradually extended to her upper extremities. Creatine kinase and liver function tests were markedly elevated. Antiviral medications and simvastatin were stopped, and within 6 days, she was able to walk again and move her upper extremities. See Atorvastatin-Protease Inhibitors and Pravastatin-Protease Inhibitors.

1 *Prezista* [package insert]. Raritan, NJ: Tibotec Therapeutics; October 2008.
2 *Lexiva* [package insert]. Research Triangle Park, NC: GlaxoSmithKline; April 2010.
3 *Viracept* [package insert]. New York, NY: Agouron Pharmaceuticals Inc; December 2002.
4 *Norvir* [package insert]. Abbott Park, IL: Abbott Laboratories; September 2001.
5 Fichtenbaum CJ, et al. *AIDS*. 2002;16(4):569.
6 Cheng CH, et al. *Am J Health Syst Pharm*. 2002;59(8):728.

* Asterisk indicates drugs cited in interaction reports. Based on pharmacologic and pharmacokinetic considerations, similar interactions may occur with other drugs that are listed.

Sirolimus | **Amiodarone**

Sirolimus*
(*Rapamune*)

Amiodarone*
(eg, *Cordarone*)

Significance	Onset	Severity	Documentation
4	☐ Rapid ■ **Delayed**	■ **Major** ☐ Moderate ☐ Minor	☐ Established ☐ Probable ☐ Suspected ■ **Possible** ☐ Unlikely

Effects SIROLIMUS concentrations may be elevated, increasing the risk of adverse reactions.

Mechanism Inhibition of SIROLIMUS metabolism (CYP3A4) and P-gp expression by AMIODARONE is suspected.

Management If AMIODARONE cannot be avoided in patients receiving SIROLIMUS, consider decreasing the SIROLIMUS dose and frequently monitoring SIROLIMUS blood concentrations. Adjust the SIROLIMUS dose as needed.

Discussion

A 2-year-old girl who received a heart transplant at 4 months of age was admitted to the hospital with unexplained anemia, renal dysfunction, and moderate liver dysfunction.[1] As part of her maintenance immunosuppressive therapy, the patient was receiving tacrolimus. Because of elevated trough blood levels, tacrolimus was withheld on day 2 for 5 days. Amiodarone 75 mg every 12 hours was started on day 7 to control ventricular arrhythmias. On day 11, oral sirolimus 1 mg daily was started. Because tacrolimus was going to be discontinued, the dosage of sirolimus was increased to 2 mg daily with a target sirolimus trough concentration of 10 mcg/L. However, 3 days after the increase in the sirolimus dosage, the trough concentration was 52.7 mcg/L and sirolimus was withheld. Sirolimus blood levels remained above the target range for an additional 14 days despite dose manipulations. Ultimately, the patient was maintained on sirolimus 0.3 mg daily with a trough concentration of 13.4 mcg/L. See Cyclosporine-Amiodarone and Tacrolimus-Amiodarone.

[1] Nalli N, et al. *Pediatr Transplant.* 2006;10(6):736.

* Asterisk indicates drugs cited in interaction reports.

Sirolimus — *Azole Antifungal Agents*

Sirolimus	Azole Antifungal Agents	
Sirolimus* (*Rapamune*)	Fluconazole (eg, *Diflucan*)	Ketoconazole* (eg, *Nizoral*)
	Itraconazole* (eg, *Sporanox*)	Posaconazole* (*Noxafil*)

Significance	Onset	Severity	Documentation
2	☐ Rapid ■ **Delayed**	☐ Major ■ **Moderate** ☐ Minor	☐ Established ■ **Probable** ☐ Suspected ☐ Possible ☐ Unlikely

Effects Plasma SIROLIMUS concentrations may be elevated, increasing the risk of toxicity.

Mechanism Possible inhibition of SIROLIMUS gut metabolism or intestinal P-gp activity.

Management Monitor SIROLIMUS plasma concentrations, and observe the patient for toxicity when an AZOLE ANTIFUNGAL AGENT is started or stopped. Adjust the dose of SIROLIMUS as needed. Coadministration of POSACONAZOLE and SIROLIMUS is contraindicated.[1]

Discussion

Markedly elevated sirolimus blood levels were reported in 2 transplant patients treated with itraconazole.[2,3] The effect of ketoconazole on the pharmacokinetics of sirolimus was evaluated in 23 healthy volunteers.[4] Each patient received sirolimus 5 mg alone and with ketoconazole at steady state (following 10 days of ketoconazole 200 mg/day). Compared with giving sirolimus alone, coadministration with ketoconazole increased the sirolimus AUC 11-fold, C_{max} increased 4.4-fold, and T_{max} and mean residence time increased 1.4-fold. The $t_{½}$ was unchanged. The pharmacokinetic effect of ketoconazole was on bioavailability rather than elimination of sirolimus. Ketoconazole has been coadministered with sirolimus to reduce the sirolimus dose and associated drug cost.[5] See Cyclosporine-Azole Antifungal Agents and Tacrolimus-Azole Antifungal Agents.

1 *Noxafil* [package insert]. Kenilworth, NJ: Schering Corporation; September 2010.
2 Kuypers DR, et al. *Transplantation*. 2005;79(6):737.
3 Said A, et al. *Pharmacotherapy*. 2006;26(2):289.
4 Floren LC, et al. *Clin Pharmacol Ther*. 1999;65(2):159.
5 Thomas PP, et al. *Transplantation*. 2004;77(3):474.

* Asterisk indicates drugs cited in interaction reports. Based on pharmacologic and pharmacokinetic considerations, similar interactions may occur with other drugs that are listed.

Sirolimus | **Cyclosporine**

Sirolimus* (*Rapamune*)	Cyclosporine* (eg, *Neoral*)

Significance	Onset	Severity	Documentation
2	□ Rapid	□ Major	□ Established
	■ **Delayed**	■ **Moderate**	■ **Probable**
		□ Minor	□ Suspected
			□ Possible
			□ Unlikely

Effects SIROLIMUS plasma concentrations may be increased, resulting in increased toxicity.

Mechanism Increased bioavailability of SIROLIMUS, resulting from inhibition of P-gp expression by CYCLOSPORINE, is suspected.

Management Administer SIROLIMUS 4 hours after CYCLOSPORINE to prevent variations in SIROLIMUS concentrations. Monitor SIROLIMUS blood levels and adjust the dose as needed.

Discussion

The effect of the timing of cyclosporine and sirolimus administration on the bioavailability of both drugs was studied in a randomized, crossover trial involving 24 stable kidney transplant patients.[1] Following transplantation, patients received individualized doses of cyclosporine microemulsion formulation (mean dose, 3.6 mg/kg divided twice daily) and sirolimus (mean dose, 2.7 mg/m^2 once daily). In 1 dosing schedule, patients received morning doses of cyclosporine and sirolimus simultaneously for 7 days; in a second dosing schedule, patients received sirolimus 4 hours after cyclosporine for 7 days. Simultaneous administration of the 2 drugs increased sirolimus C_{max} 72%, AUC 45%, and trough levels 49%, compared with giving the drugs 4 hours apart. In addition, sirolimus C_{max} was reached earlier with simultaneous administration. Timing of administration did not affect cyclosporine pharmacokinetics. A similar study was conducted in 21 healthy subjects.[2] When sirolimus and cyclosporine were given jointly, sirolimus AUC and C_{max} increased 230% and 116%, respectively. However, when sirolimus was given 4 hours after cyclosporine, the AUC and C_{max} increased 80% and 37%, respectively. In a study of 495 kidney transplant recipients receiving sirolimus with various other immunosuppressants, sirolimus trough levels were higher in patients who also received cyclosporine.[3] A study in 53 kidney transplant patients reported that coadministration of cyclosporine and sirolimus increased the AUC of both drugs.[4] The extent of the interaction may differ depending on the cyclosporine formulation administered.[5]

[1] Kaplan B, et al. *Clin Pharmacol Ther.* 1998;63(1):48.
[2] Zimmerman JJ, et al. *J Clin Pharmacol.* 2003;43(10):1168.
[3] Cattaneo D, et al. *Am J Transplant.* 2004;4(8):1345.
[4] Felipe CR, et al. *Fundam Clin Pharmacol.* 2009;23(5):625.
[5] Kovarik JM, et al. *Eur J Clin Pharmacol.* 2006;62(5):361.

* Asterisk indicates drugs cited in interaction reports.

Sirolimus — *Diltiazem*

Sirolimus* (*Rapamune*)	Diltiazem* (eg, *Cardizem*)

Significance	Onset	Severity	Documentation
2	☐ Rapid	☐ Major	☐ Established
	■ **Delayed**	■ **Moderate**	☐ Probable
		☐ Minor	■ **Suspected**
			☐ Possible
			☐ Unlikely

Effects SIROLIMUS plasma levels may be elevated, increasing the risk of adverse reactions.

Mechanism Inhibition of SIROLIMUS first-pass metabolism (CYP3A4) by DILTIAZEM is suspected.

Management Closely monitor SIROLIMUS concentrations when the DILTIAZEM dose is started, stopped, or changed. Adjust the SIROLIMUS dose as needed.

Discussion

The effects of diltiazem on the pharmacokinetics of sirolimus were investigated in an open-label, 3-phase, randomized, crossover investigation involving 18 healthy subjects.[1] Each subject received a single oral dose of sirolimus 10 mg, a single oral dose of diltiazem 120 mg, and both drugs together. Compared with giving sirolimus alone, coadministration with diltiazem increased the whole-blood sirolimus AUC 60% (range, 35% to 90%) and C_{max} 43% (range, 14% to 81%), while decreasing the elimination $t_{½}$ from 79 to 67 hours and the apparent oral clearance and volume of distribution 38% and 45%, respectively. Sirolimus did not affect the pharmacokinetics of diltiazem.

[1] Böttiger Y, et al. *Clin Pharmacol Ther.* 2001;69(1):32.

* Asterisk indicates drugs cited in interaction reports.

Sirolimus — *Dronedarone*

Sirolimus* (*Rapamune*)	Dronedarone* (*Multaq*)

Significance	Onset	Severity	Documentation
4	□ Rapid	□ Major	□ Established
	■ **Delayed**	■ **Moderate**	□ Probable
		□ Minor	□ Suspected
			■ **Possible**
			□ Unlikely

Effects SIROLIMUS plasma concentrations may be elevated, increasing the risk of toxicity.

Mechanism Inhibition of SIROLIMUS metabolism (CYP3A4) and P-gp expression by DRONEDARONE is suspected.

Management If DRONEDARONE cannot be avoided in patients receiving SIROLIMUS, a lower SIROLIMUS dose may be needed at the start of therapy. Closely monitor SIROLIMUS blood concentrations and adjust the SIROLIMUS dose as needed.

Discussion

Following a kidney transplant, a 67-year-old man was on a stable immunosuppressive regimen that contained sirolimus 5 mg daily for more than 1 year.[1] Sirolimus trough concentrations ranged between 5 and 13.5 ng/mL. Three days after the start of dronedarone 400 mg twice daily for atrial fibrillation, the sirolimus concentration increased to 38.6 ng/mL. Sirolimus was held for 6 days and the trough concentrations decreased to 7.8 ng/mL. The sirolimus dose was reduced to 1 mg daily without need for further dose adjustments.

[1] Tichy EM, et al. *Ann Pharmacother.* 2010;44(7-8):1338.

* Asterisk indicates drugs cited in interaction reports.

Sirolimus — *Food*

Sirolimus*
(*Rapamune*)

Grapefruit Juice*

Significance	Onset	Severity	Documentation
2	☐ Rapid ■ **Delayed**	☐ Major ■ **Moderate** ☐ Minor	☐ Established ☐ Probable ■ **Suspected** ☐ Possible ☐ Unlikely

Effects SIROLIMUS concentrations may be elevated, increasing the risk of toxicity.

Mechanism Inhibition of metabolism (CYP3A4) of SIROLIMUS in the jejunal mucosa.

Management Advise patients taking SIROLIMUS to avoid GRAPEFRUIT JUICE and to not use GRAPEFRUIT JUICE for dilution of oral solution. Caution patients not to coadminister herbal products and SIROLIMUS without consulting their health care provider.

Discussion

Although there is no report of an interaction with concurrent ingestion of grapefruit juice and sirolimus administration, the manufacturer of sirolimus warns that grapefruit juice inhibits CYP3A4. Sirolimus is a substrate for CYP3A4. Therefore, there is potential that ingestion of grapefruit juice in patients receiving sirolimus could cause an increase in sirolimus concentrations.[1] See Cyclosporine-Food.

[1] *Rapamune* [package insert]. Philadelphia, PA: Wyeth Pharmaceuticals Inc; November 2010.

* Asterisk indicates drugs cited in interaction reports.

Sirolimus | **HMG-CoA Reductase Inhibitors**

Sirolimus* (*Rapamune*)	Atorvastatin* (*Lipitor*)	Fluvastatin* (*Lescol*)

Significance	Onset	Severity	Documentation
4	☐ Rapid ■ **Delayed**	■ **Major** ☐ Moderate ☐ Minor	☐ Established ☐ Probable ☐ Suspected ■ **Possible** ☐ Unlikely

Effects SIROLIMUS trough concentrations may be elevated, increasing the risk of adverse reactions. Rhabdomyolysis has been reported with coadministration of SIROLIMUS and FLUVASTATIN.

Mechanism Decreased metabolism (CYP3A4) of SIROLIMUS by ATORVASTATIN is suspected.

Management Closely monitor SIROLIMUS concentrations when the ATORVASTATIN dose is started, stopped, or changed. Adjust the SIROLIMUS dose as needed.

Discussion

A possible drug interaction was reported in a 36-year-old woman during coadministration of sirolimus and atorvastatin.[1] The patient was a pancreatic islet transplant recipient who was receiving numerous other drugs when sirolimus was started. For the first 5 postoperative months, the sirolimus dosage was between 8 and 11 mg/day, resulting in trough levels between 6.1 and 20.5 ng/mL. Six months after starting sirolimus therapy, atorvastatin was started for hypercholesterolemia. Six weeks after starting atorvastatin, the sirolimus trough concentrations were 20.5 ng/mL, and the dose of sirolimus was reduced. After 3 months of atorvastatin therapy, the sirolimus dose had been reduced 50%, resulting in sirolimus trough levels ranging between 8.3 and 34.3 ng/mL. No adverse reactions were reported with the increased sirolimus concentrations. A 66-year-old woman with a renal transplant who was receiving sirolimus was hospitalized with rhabdomyolysis 2 weeks after fluvastatin 80 mg daily was added to her treatment regimen.[2]

Additional studies are needed to determine the clinical importance of this interaction and to assess the risk of adverse reactions.

[1] Barshes NR, et al. *Transplantation.* 2003; 76(11):1649.

[2] Basic-Jukic N, et al. *Nephrol Dial Transplant.* 2010;25(6):2036.

* Asterisk indicates drugs cited in interaction reports.

Sirolimus — *Hydantoins*

Sirolimus* (*Rapamune*)	Fosphenytoin Phenytoin* (eg, *Dilantin*)

Significance	Onset	Severity	Documentation
4	☐ Rapid ■ **Delayed**	☐ Major ■ **Moderate** ☐ Minor	☐ Established ☐ Probable ☐ Suspected ■ **Possible** ☐ Unlikely

Effects SIROLIMUS concentrations may be decreased by PHENYTOIN administration, resulting in a decrease in the immunosuppressive effect of SIROLIMUS. This may increase the chance of transplant rejection.

Mechanism PHENYTOIN may increase the metabolism (CYP3A4) of SIROLIMUS.

Management Closely monitor SIROLIMUS blood concentrations when the PHENYTOIN dose is started, stopped, or changed. Adjust the SIROLIMUS dose as needed.

Discussion

A 62-year-old woman with diabetes developed a seizure disorder approximately 1 week after undergoing orthotopic liver transplant and was started on phenytoin 100 mg IV twice daily.[1] At that time, the patient was receiving tacrolimus (eg, *Prograf*), which was replaced by cyclosporine (eg, *Neoral*). Subsequently, cyclosporine was stopped, and sirolimus 5 mg/day was started and then increased to 15 mg/day. The pharmacokinetics of sirolimus were evaluated during and 10 days after phenytoin therapy was discontinued. After phenytoin was discontinued, sirolimus C_{max} increased from 44.6 to 51 ng/mL, $t_{½}$ increased from 10.2 to 22.4 hours, and AUC increased 65%.

[1] Fridell JA, et al. *Ther Drug Monit.* 2003;25(1):117.

* Asterisk indicates drugs cited in interaction reports. Based on pharmacologic and pharmacokinetic considerations, similar interactions may occur with other drugs that are listed.

Sirolimus ✕ **Mifepristone**

Sirolimus* (*Rapamune*)	Mifepristone* (eg, *Korlym*)

Significance	Onset	Severity	Documentation
1	☐ Rapid ■ **Delayed**	■ **Major** ☐ Moderate ☐ Minor	☐ Established ☐ Probable ■ **Suspected** ☐ Possible ☐ Unlikely

Effects SIROLIMUS plasma concentrations may be elevated, increasing the pharmacologic effects and risk of adverse reactions (eg, thrombocytopenia).

Mechanism MIFEPRISTONE may inhibit SIROLIMUS metabolism (CYP3A4).

Management Coadministration of SIROLIMUS with MIFEPRISTONE is contraindicated.[1]

Discussion

Because mifepristone inhibits CYP3A4, coadministration of mifepristone with a drug that is metabolized mainly or solely by CYP3A4 (eg, sirolimus) is likely to increase plasma concentrations of the drug.[1] Therefore, the concurrent use of drugs with a narrow therapeutic index that are CYP3A4 substrates, such as sirolimus, is contraindicated. The risk of sirolimus adverse reactions (eg, hypertension, thrombocytopenia) may be increased.

[1] *Korlym* [package insert]. Menlo Park, CA: Corcept Therapeutics Incorporated; February 2012.

* Asterisk indicates drugs cited in interaction reports.

Sirolimus — *St. John's Wort*

Sirolimus* (*Rapamune*)	St. John's Wort*

Significance	Onset	Severity	Documentation
1	☐ Rapid ■ **Delayed**	■ **Major** ☐ Moderate ☐ Minor	☐ Established ☐ Probable ■ **Suspected** ☐ Possible ☐ Unlikely

Effects SIROLIMUS concentrations may be reduced, resulting in organ transplant rejection.

Mechanism Increased hepatic metabolism (CYP3A4) of SIROLIMUS and activation of P-gp efflux.

Management Advise patients taking SIROLIMUS to avoid ST. JOHN'S WORT. Caution patients not to coadminister herbal products and SIROLIMUS without consulting their health care provider.

Discussion

Although there is no report of an interaction with concurrent use of St. John's wort and sirolimus, the manufacturer of sirolimus warns that St. John's wort induces CYP3A4 and P-gp. Sirolimus is a substrate for both CYP3A4 and P-gp. Therefore, there is a potential that use of St. John's wort in patients receiving sirolimus could cause a decrease in sirolimus concentrations.[1] See Cyclosporine-St. John's Wort, Tacrolimus-St. John's Wort.

[1] *Rapamune* [package insert]. Philadelphia, PA: Wyeth Pharmaceuticals Inc; November 2010.

* Asterisk indicates drugs cited in interaction reports.

Sirolimus — *Voriconazole*

Sirolimus*	Voriconazole*
(*Rapamune*)	(eg, *Vfend*)

Significance	Onset	Severity	Documentation
2	☐ Rapid	☐ Major	☐ Established
	■ **Delayed**	■ **Moderate**	☐ Probable
		☐ Minor	■ **Suspected**
			☐ Possible
			☐ Unlikely

Effects SIROLIMUS plasma concentrations may be elevated, increasing the risk of adverse reactions.

Mechanism VORICONAZOLE may inhibit the metabolism (CYP3A4) of SIROLIMUS.

Management Coadministration of VORICONAZOLE and SIROLIMUS is contraindicated.

Discussion

In healthy subjects, repeat dose administration of voriconazole 400 mg oral every 12 hours for 1 day followed by 200 mg every 12 hours for 8 days increased the AUC and C_{max} of a single dose of sirolimus 2 mg by an average of 11- and 7-fold, respectively.[1] In a case series, 11 patients with allogenic stem-cell transplantation received sirolimus and voriconazole for treatment or prevention of aspergillosis.[2] Eight patients had an empiric sirolimus dose reduction to 10% of the dose they were receiving prior to voriconazole initiation. One additional patient had the same 90% dose reduction after 6 days of concurrent voriconazole. Sirolimus trough concentrations were similar to those levels prior to voriconazole coadministration and were within the therapeutic range. In contrast, 2 patients did not have their sirolimus dose reduced and had markedly elevated sirolimus levels and toxicity. A review of 31 cases of coadministration of sirolimus and voriconazole in 23 patients supports the occurrence of this interaction.[3] Two cases of adverse reactions (renal dysfunction, thrombocytopenia) occurred, possibly attributable to elevated sirolimus concentrations.

[1] *Vfend* [package insert]. New York, NY: Pfizer Labs; May 2002.
[2] Marty FM, et al. *Biol Blood Marrow Transplant.* 2006;12(5):552.
[3] Surowiec D, et al. *Pharmacotherapy.* 2008;28(6):719.

* Asterisk indicates drugs cited in interaction reports.

Sodium Polystyrene Sulfonate ✕ *Antacids*

Sodium Polystyrene Sulfonate* (eg, *Kayexalate*)	Aluminum/ Magnesium Hydroxide* (eg, *Maalox*)	Calcium Carbonate* (eg, *Tums*)

Significance	Onset	Severity	Documentation
2	☐ Rapid	☐ Major	■ **Established**
	■ **Delayed**	■ **Moderate**	☐ Probable
		☐ Minor	☐ Suspected
			☐ Possible
			☐ Unlikely

Effects Concomitant therapy with SODIUM POLYSTYRENE SULFONATE and ANTACIDS in patients with renal impairment may result in unanticipated metabolic alkalosis and a reduction of the resin's binding of potassium.

Mechanism The cations of the ANTACID usually neutralize bicarbonate secreted into the small intestine, preventing its reabsorption. However, in the presence of SODIUM POLYSTYRENE SULFONATE, they may preferentially bind to the resin, resulting in bicarbonate reabsorption and metabolic alkalosis.

Management Separate doses of ANTACID and SODIUM POLYSTYRENE SULFONATE by several hours.[1]

Discussion

Eleven patients (9 with renal impairment) received either antacid or sodium polystyrene sulfonate or antacid plus sodium polystyrene sulfonate.[2] Each segment of the study lasted 5 days. Potassium supplementation was provided during the resin phases of the study. The combination of antacid and sodium polystyrene sulfonate resulted in a significant increase in plasma carbon monoxide[2] content not encountered in the other phases of the study. This effect was noted in patients receiving a magnesium-aluminum combination and calcium-containing antacids, but not in those receiving aluminum hydroxide products. A subsequent case report showed the development of metabolic alkalosis in an anephric child receiving aluminum carbonate.[3] In another case, a hypocalcemic patient received sodium polystyrene sulfonate and antacids and experienced metabolic acidosis and a tonic-clonic seizure.[4] The antacid may have interfered with the resin's ability to bind potassium. Additionally, the combination of sodium polystyrene sulfonate and magnesium hydroxide reversed metabolic acidosis in a patient with renal impairment.[5]

[1] Madias NE, et al. *Am J Med.* 1983;74(1):155.
[2] Schroeder ET. *Gastroenterology.* 1969;56(5):868.
[3] Baluarte HJ, et al. *J Pediatr.* 1978;92(2):237.
[4] Ziessman HA. *South Med J.* 1976;69(4):497.
[5] Fernandez PC, et al. *N Engl J Med.* 1972;286(1):23.

* Asterisk indicates drugs cited in interaction reports.

Solifenacin — *Azole Antifungal Agents*

Solifenacin* (*Vesicare*)	Ketoconazole* (eg, *Nizoral*)

Significance	Onset	Severity	Documentation
2	☐ Rapid ■ **Delayed**	☐ Major ■ **Moderate** ☐ Minor	☐ Established ☐ Probable ■ **Suspected** ☐ Possible ☐ Unlikely

Effects SOLIFENACIN plasma concentrations may be elevated, increasing the pharmacological and adverse effects.

Mechanism Inhibition of SOLIFENACIN metabolism (CYP3A4) by KETOCONAZOLE.

Management When administered with KETOCONAZOLE, it is recommended that the dose of SOLIFENACIN not exceed 5 mg daily.[1]

Discussion

Administration of solifenacin 10 mg and ketoconazole 400 mg increased the mean C_{max} and AUC of solifenacin 1.5- and 2.7-fold, respectively.[1]

[1] *Vesicare* [package insert]. Paramus, NJ: Yamanouchi Pharma Technologies Inc; November 2004.

* Asterisk indicates drugs cited in interaction reports.

Sotalol — *Oseltamivir*

Sotalol*	Oseltamivir*
(eg, *Betapace*)	(*Tamiflu*)

Significance	Onset	Severity	Documentation
4	☐ Rapid	■ **Major**	☐ Established
	■ **Delayed**	☐ Moderate	☐ Probable
		☐ Minor	☐ Suspected
			■ **Possible**
			☐ Unlikely

Effects The risk of life-threatening arrhythmias, including torsades de pointes, may be increased.

Mechanism Unknown.

Management Closely monitor the ECG during coadministration of SOTALOL and OSELTAMIVIR. Be prepared to discontinue one or both drugs if QTc prolongation occurs.

Discussion

A 63-year-old woman was admitted to the hospital after 1 week of fever.[1] She had a history of paroxysmal atrial fibrillation and had been maintained on a stable dose of sotalol 80 mg twice daily for 1 year. On admission, the QTc was 506 ms. She was treated with oseltamivir 75 mg twice daily for presumed influenza. Approximately 2 hours after her sixth dose of oseltamivir, the patient was unresponsive. The initial rhythm was ventricular fibrillation. Sinus rhythm was restored with multiple shocks and IV magnesium. The QTc was 521 ms and sotalol was discontinued. That night, the patient developed typical symptomatic torsades de pointes and the QTc was 598 ms. Oseltamivir was discontinued. The QT interval gradually shortened and there were no further cardiac arrests.

[1] Wells Q, et al. *Heart Rhythm.* 2010;7(10):1454.

* Asterisk indicates drugs cited in interaction reports.

Spironolactone | **Salicylates**

Spironolactone* (eg, *Aldactone*)

Aspirin* (eg, *Bayer*)
Bismuth Subsalicylate (eg, *Pepto-Bismol*)
Choline Salicylate (*Arthropan*)
Magnesium Salicylate (eg, *Novasal*)
Salsalate (eg, *Amigesic*)
Sodium Salicylate
Sodium Thiosalicylate (eg, *Rexolate*)

Significance	Onset	Severity	Documentation
3	☐ Rapid ■ **Delayed**	☐ Major ☐ Moderate ■ **Minor**	☐ Established ☐ Probable ■ **Suspected** ☐ Possible ☐ Unlikely

Effects SALICYLATES block SPIRONOLACTONE-induced natriuresis. Limited data suggest that SALICYLATES do not compromise the antihypertensive effects of SPIRONOLACTONE.

Mechanism ASPIRIN appears to block the renal tubular secretion of canrenone, the principal unconjugated metabolite of SPIRONOLACTONE.

Management Monitor BP and serum sodium in patients chronically receiving SPIRONOLACTONE and SALICYLATES. Increasing the SPIRONOLACTONE dose may reverse the effects of the interaction.

Discussion

Single doses of aspirin 600 mg to 5 g promote sodium retention[1-3] and interfere with the natriuretic action of spironolactone.[2,4,5] Administration of a single dose of aspirin 600 mg to 7 subjects receiving spironolactone 100 mg/day for 7 days reduced mean urine sodium content 30%.[5] One study found that a single aspirin dose diminished the urinary excretion of canrenone, spironolactone's principal active metabolite, 26%.[6] The renal antimineralocorticoid activity of spironolactone is closely related to canrenone concentration in tubular fluid. Salicylates may compete with canrenone for renal tubular secretion. Animal studies suggest that increasing the spironolactone dose may overcome the effects of salicylates.[4] Seven hypertensive patients with mineralocorticoid excess syndromes (low-renin essential hypertension or primary aldosteronism) stabilized on spironolactone 100 to 300 mg/day received aspirin 2.4 to 4.8 g/day for several weeks in a placebo-controlled study.[7] No changes in BP or serum electrolytes were observed.

[1] Hetzel BS, et al. *Metabolism.* 1959;8:205.
[2] Elliott HC. *Metabolism.* 1962;11:1015.
[3] Elliott HC, et al. *Proc Soc Exp Biol Med.* 1962;109:333.
[4] Hofmann LM, et al. *J Pharmacol Exp Ther.* 1972; 180:1.
[5] Tweeddale MG, et al. *N Engl J Med.* 1973;289:198.
[6] Ramsey LE, et al. *Eur J Clin Pharmacol.* 1976;10:43.
[7] Hollifield JW. *South Med J.* 1976;69:1034.

* Asterisk indicates drugs cited in interaction reports. Based on pharmacologic and pharmacokinetic considerations, similar interactions may occur with other drugs that are listed.

St. John's Wort — *Carbamazepine*

St. John's Wort*	Carbamazepine* (eg, *Tegretol*)

Significance	Onset	Severity	Documentation
5	☐ Rapid	☐ Major	☐ Established
	■ **Delayed**	☐ Moderate	☐ Probable
		■ **Minor**	☐ Suspected
			■ **Possible**
			☐ Unlikely

Effects CARBAMAZEPINE may decrease the AUC of pseudohypericin, an ingredient of ST. JOHN'S WORT extract.

Mechanism Unknown.

Management Based on available data, no special precautions are needed.

Discussion

The effects of carbamazepine on the pharmacokinetics of the St. John's wort extract ingredients hypericin and pseudohypericin were studied in healthy volunteers.[1] Compared with administration of St. John's wort alone, coadministration of carbamazepine decreased the AUC of pseudohypericin 29%. St. John's wort does not appear to affect the pharmacokinetics of carbamazepine.[2]

[1] Johne A, et al. *Eur J Clin Pharmacol.* 2004;60:617.

[2] Burstein AH, et al. *Clin Pharmacol Ther.* 2000;68:605.

* Asterisk indicates drugs cited in interaction reports.

St. John's Wort — Cimetidine

St. John's Wort*	Cimetidine* (eg, *Tagamet*)

Significance	Onset	Severity	Documentation
5	☐ Rapid	☐ Major	☐ Established
	■ **Delayed**	☐ Moderate	☐ Probable
		■ **Minor**	☐ Suspected
			■ **Possible**
			☐ Unlikely

Effects CIMETIDINE may increase the AUC of hypericin.

Mechanism Unknown.

Management Based on available data, no special precautions are needed.

Discussion

The effects of cimetidine on the pharmacokinetics of the St. John's wort extract (hypericin 92 mcg and pseudohypericin 262 mcg) were studied in healthy volunteers.[1] All subjects received St. John's wort extract alone for 11 days, and starting with day 12, placebo or cimetidine (200 mg twice daily and 400 mg once daily) was administered with St. John's wort for 7 days. Eleven subjects received St. John's wort extract and placebo, and 11 subjects received St. John's wort extract and cimetidine. Compared with administration of St. John's wort alone, cimetidine increased the AUC of hypericin 25%.

[1] Johne A, et al. *Eur J Clin Pharmacol.* 2004;60(9):617.

* Asterisk indicates drugs cited in interaction reports.

Succinimides — *Carbamazepine*

Succinimides		Carbamazepine
Ethosuximide* (eg, *Zarontin*)	Methsuximide (*Celontin*)	Carbamazepine* (eg, *Tegretol*)

Significance	Onset	Severity	Documentation
5	☐ Rapid ■ **Delayed**	☐ Major ☐ Moderate ■ **Minor**	☐ Established ☐ Probable ☐ Suspected ☐ Possible ■ **Unlikely**

Effects SUCCINIMIDE drug serum levels may be decreased.

Mechanism CARBAMAZEPINE stimulation of the liver microsomal enzyme system resulting in enhanced breakdown of SUCCINIMIDES.

Management No clinical interventions are required.

Discussion

Six healthy adult volunteers received 250 mg ethosuximide twice daily for 28 days. On the eleventh through the twenty–seventh study days, they also received 200 mg carbamazepine. A comparison of mean ethosuximide plasma concentrations from days 10 and 28 showed a 17% reduction. Mean ethosuximide clearance was increased 20% while the mean half-life declined 17%. There was considerable interpatient variability in the results.[1] Whether these results could be expected in epileptic patients who are likely to be already receiving hepatic enzyme-inducing drugs remains to be determined.

[1] Warren JW Jr, et al. *Clin Pharmacol Ther*. 1980;28:646.

* Asterisk indicates drugs cited in interaction reports. Based on pharmacologic and pharmacokinetic considerations, similar interactions may occur with other drugs that are listed.

Succinimides — *Valproic Acid*

Ethosuximide* (eg, *Zarontin*)	Methsuximide* (*Celontin*)	Valproic Acid* (eg, *Depakene*)

Significance	Onset	Severity	Documentation
5	☐ Rapid ■ **Delayed**	☐ Major ☐ Moderate ■ **Minor**	☐ Established ☐ Probable ☐ Suspected ■ **Possible** ☐ Unlikely

Effects Increases and decreases in ETHOSUXIMIDE blood levels and decreases in VALPROIC ACID levels have been reported.

Mechanism Increases in ETHOSUXIMIDE level are probably caused by VALPROIC ACID inhibition of ETHOSUXIMIDE metabolism.

Management Measure SUCCINIMIDE and valproate serum levels and adjust the dose as needed if there is a change in patient response.

Discussion

The effects of this interaction are varied. Some studies have found no net effect,[1-4] others found either increased or decreased ethosuximide levels. In 1 report in 5 patients, the addition of valproic acid increased the mean ethosuximide serum level 39%. This increase resulted in sedation, necessitating a reduction in ethosuximide dose. One of the patients did not demonstrate a rise in ethosuximide level. This patient was the only one not receiving antiepileptic drugs other than ethosuximide and valproic acid.[5] In 6 healthy volunteers given 500 mg ethosuximide before and after 9 days of valproic acid administration, the mean ethosuximide serum half-lives increased 23% and the mean clearance of ethosuximide decreased 15% during valproic acid administration. No interaction occurred in 2 subjects.[6] Five patients receiving ethosuximide and valproic acid were found to have lower serum ethosuximide levels than 39 patients receiving ethosuximide alone.[7] The pharmacokinetics of ethosuximide (750 mg initially followed by 250 mg every 12 hours for 10 days) were studied in 6 healthy volunteers. This same regimen plus valproic acid was repeated for an additional 14 days. Chronic administration of ethosuximide reduced ethosuximide clearance 15%, but addition of valproic acid had no further effect.[3] Inhibition of ethosuximide metabolism by valproic acid may only be a problem when other antiepileptic drugs are being used, competing for the enzyme systems.[4,5] Ethosuximide has been reported to decrease valproic acid levels.[8] In 4 children, valproic acid levels were 28% lower during coadministration of ethosuximide than during valproic acid monotherapy. In 9 other children, valproic acid levels increased when ethosuximide was stopped. Valproic acid levels declined 32% in 17 patients after starting methosuximide (2.4 to 22.2 mg/kg/day).[9]

1 Gram L, et al. *Epilepsia.* 1977;18:141.
2 Wilder BJ, et al. *Neurology.* 1978;28:892.
3 Bauer LA, et al. *Clin Pharmacol Ther.* 1982;31:741.
4 Bourgeois BF. *Am J Med.* 1988;84 (1A):29.
5 Mattson RH, et al. *Ann Neurol.* 1980;7:583.
6 Pisani F, et al. *Epilepsia.* 1984;25:229.
7 Battino D, et al. *Clin Pharmacokinet.* 1982;7:176.
8 Sälke-Kellermann RA, et al. *Epilepsy Res.* 1997;26:345.
9 Besag FM, et al. *Ther Drug Monit.* 2001;23:694.

* Asterisk indicates drugs cited in interaction reports.

Succinylcholine ✕ *Aminoglycosides*

Succinylcholine	Aminoglycosides	
Succinylcholine* (eg, *Anectine*)	Amikacin (*Amikin*)	Netilmicin (*Netromycin*)
	Gentamicin (eg, *Garamycin*)	Paromomycin (*Humatin*)
	Kanamycin (eg, *Kantrex*)	Streptomycin*
	Neomycin* (*Mycifradin*)	Tobramycin (*Nebcin*)

Significance	Onset	Severity	Documentation
2	■ **Rapid**	□ Major	□ Established
	□ Delayed	■ **Moderate**	■ **Probable**
		□ Minor	□ Suspected
			□ Possible
			□ Unlikely

Effects AMINOGLYCOSIDES potentiate the neuromuscular effects of SUCCINYLCHOLINE.

Mechanism AMINOGLYCOSIDES may be additive or synergistic with SUCCINYLCHOLINE secondary to their ability to stabilize the postjunctional membrane and impair prejunctional calcium influx and acetylcholine output.

Management Undertake coadministration cautiously, particularly in patients vulnerable to the development of high AMINOGLYCOSIDE plasma levels (eg, patients with renal impairment; peritoneal instillation). Delay administration of AMINOGLYCOSIDES as long as possible after recovery of adequate spontaneous respiration. If respiratory depression occurs, support patients with mechanical ventilation. The IV administration of calcium or the administration of anticholinesterases have shown promise.

Discussion

Numerous reports are documented in the literature which suggest that IV, IM or intraperitoneal administration of aminoglycoside antibiotics to patients who have received succinylcholine may result in prolonged neuromuscular blockade.[1-4,6] One report describes a case in which adequate spontaneous respiration did not resume until 4.5 hours after intraperitoneal administration of 3.5 g of neomycin to a patient who had received succinylcholine during surgery.[5]

[1] Jones WPG, et al. *JAMA.* 1959;170:943.
[2] Blake-Knox PEA. *Br Med J.* 1961;1:1319.
[3] Benz HG, et al. *Br Med J.* 1961;2:241.
[4] Foldes FF, et al. *JAMA.* 1963;183:146.
[5] Warner WA, et al. *JAMA.* 1971;215:1153.
[6] Levanen J, et al. *Ann Clin Res.* 1975;7:47.
[7] Burkett L, et al. *Anesth Analg.* 1979;58:107.
[8] Lippmann M, et al. *Anesth Analg.* 1982;61:767.

* Asterisk indicates drugs cited in interaction reports. Based on pharmacologic and pharmacokinetic considerations, similar interactions may occur with other drugs that are listed.

Succinylcholine | **Anticholinesterases**

Succinylcholine	Anticholinesterases	
Succinylcholine* (eg, *Anectine*)	Ambenonium Chloride (*Mytelase*)	Neostigmine* (eg, *Prostigmin*)
	Demecarium (*Humorsol*)	Physostigmine* (eg, *Antilirium*)
	Edrophonium* (*Tensilon*)	Pyridostigmine* (*Mestinon, Regonol*)

Significance	Onset	Severity	Documentation
2	■ **Rapid**	□ Major	□ Established
	□ Delayed	■ **Moderate**	■ **Probable**
		□ Minor	□ Suspected
			□ Possible
			□ Unlikely

Effects The neuromuscular blockade produced by SUCCINYLCHOLINE may be prolonged or antagonized by ANTICHOLINESTERASE agents.

Mechanism Inhibition of plasma cholinesterase by ANTICHOLINESTERASES may delay hydrolysis of SUCCINYLCHOLINE. After prolonged depolarization produced by SUCCINYLCHOLINE the endplates are refractory. Thus, increased levels of acetylcholine may further contribute to the neuromuscular blockade.[1-3]

Management Use this combination with caution. The patient should have evidence of spontaneous muscle activity and edrophonium administration should result in normalization of respiration for at least 5 minutes before longer acting agents are administered.[4]

Discussion

Numerous cases in the literature document the potentiation of succinylcholine-induced neuromuscular blockade by anticholinesterases.[1-3,5-10] Anticholinesterases potentiate the depolarizing neuromuscular blockade that occurs when succinylcholine is initially administered. However, anticholinesterases can either potentiate or antagonize the desensitizing blockade that may also be produced in certain patients. Patients who are most likely to exhibit such desensitization blockade are those who receive succinylcholine by continuous infusion, repeatedly receive large bolus doses or have atypical pseudocholinesterase.[2,4,5,7]

1 Vickers MDA. *Br J Anaesth.* 1963;35:260.
2 Gissen AJ, et al. *Anesthesiology.* 1966;27:242.
3 Manoguerra AS, et al. *Clin Toxicol.* 1981;18:803.
4 Miller RD, et al. *Anesthesiology.* 1972;36:511.
5 Baraka A. *Br J Anaesth.* 1975;47:416.
6 Bentz EW, et al. *Anesthesiology.* 1976;44:258.
7 Baraka A. *Br J Anaesth.* 1977;49:479.
8 Kopman AF, et al. *Anesthesiology.* 1978;49:142.
9 Sunew KY, et al. *Anesthesiology.* 1978;49:188.
10 James MFM, et al. *Br J Anaesth.* 1990;65:430.

* Asterisk indicates drugs cited in interaction reports. Based on pharmacologic and pharmacokinetic considerations, similar interactions may occur with other drugs that are listed.

Succinylcholine — *Benzodiazepines*

Succinylcholine* (eg, *Anectine*)	Diazepam* (eg, *Valium*)	Oxazepam* (eg, *Serax*)

Significance	Onset	Severity	Documentation
5	■ **Rapid** ☐ Delayed	☐ Major ☐ Moderate ■ **Minor**	☐ Established ☐ Probable ☐ Suspected ☐ Possible ■ **Unlikely**

Effects Both antagonism and potentiation of the pharmacologic effects of SUCCINYLCHOLINE may occur.

Mechanism Unknown.

Management Present data does not indicate that any change in therapy is necessary.

Discussion

One study that involved human subjects reported the IV administration of diazepam 0.15 to 0.2 mg/kg decreased the duration of the neuromuscular blockade produced by 25 mg of succinylcholine.[1] Two studies which involved laboratory animals reported potentiation of the succinylcholine-induced neuromuscular blockade by diazepam administration.[2,3] Additional studies reported no significant interaction between succinylcholine and benzodiazepines.[4-7] The present data does not confirm the presence of a clinically significant drug interaction.

[1] Feldman SA, et al. *BMJ.* 1970;2:336.
[2] Sharma KK, et al. *J Pharm Pharmacol.* 1978;30:64.
[3] Driessen JJ, et al. *Br J Anaesth.* 1984;56:1131.
[4] Dretchen K, et al. *Anesthesiology.* 1971;34:463.
[5] Fahmy NR, et al. *Clin Pharmacol Ther.* 1979;26:395.
[6] Bradshaw EG, et al. *Br J Anaesth.* 1979;51:955.
[7] Eisenberg M, et al. *Anesth Analg.* 1979;58:314.

* Asterisk indicates drugs cited in interaction reports.

Succinylcholine — *Cimetidine*

Succinylcholine* (eg, *Anectine*)	Cimetidine* (*Tagamet*)

Significance	Onset	Severity	Documentation
4	■ **Rapid**	☐ Major	☐ Established
	☐ Delayed	■ **Moderate**	☐ Probable
		☐ Minor	☐ Suspected
			■ **Possible**
			☐ Unlikely

Effects Possible prolongation of the neuromuscular blocking effects of SUCCINYLCHOLINE.

Mechanism CIMETIDINE inhibition of liver microsomal enzyme systems resulting in slower metabolism of SUCCINYLCHOLINE.

Management Present data suggest that no action other than normal patient monitoring is necessary.

Discussion

Conflicting data have been reported concerning the existence of this drug interaction.[1-4] Although one study reported a 2 to 2.5 times increase in the duration of succinylcholine-induced neuromuscular blockade after patients were pretreated with cimetidine, another study reported no significant change in succinylcholine duration of action.[1-4] Further studies are needed to clarify this conflict in the present data.

[1] Kambam JR, et al. *Anesth Analg.* 1987;66:191.
[2] Ramzan IM, et al. *Anesth Analg.* 1987;66:1346.
[3] Kao YJ, et al. *Anesth Analg.* 1988;67:802.
[4] Stirt JA, et al. *Anesthesiology.* 1988;69:607.

* Asterisk indicates drugs cited in interaction reports.

Succinylcholine — *Cyclophosphamide*

Succinylcholine* (eg, *Anectine*)	Cyclophosphamide* (eg, *Cytoxan*)

Significance	Onset	Severity	Documentation
2	■ **Rapid**	□ Major	□ Established
	□ Delayed	■ **Moderate**	■ **Probable**
		□ Minor	□ Suspected
			□ Possible
			□ Unlikely

Effects The neuromuscular blockade produced by SUCCINYLCHOLINE may be prolonged.

Mechanism CYCLOPHOSPHAMIDE inhibits plasma cholinesterase (pseudocholinesterase) activity resulting in a decreased metabolic rate for SUCCINYLCHOLINE.

Management If SUCCINYLCHOLINE must be administered to a patient who has been receiving CYCLOPHOSPHAMIDE, measure plasma cholinesterase levels and if they are decreased, consider a reduction in SUCCINYLCHOLINE dosage.

Discussion

Both laboratory studies and case reports support that concomitant administration of succinylcholine and cyclophosphamide may prolong the succinylcholine-induced neuromuscular blockade.[1-6] One study documented a 50% decline in plasma cholinesterase activity in a patient receiving cyclophosphamide orally 50 mg per day.[2] In vitro studies of this decline in enzyme activity suggest that cyclophosphamide effects on plasma cholinesterase is dose dependent.

1 Wang RIH, et al. *Anesthesiology*. 1963;24:363.
2 Mone JG, et al. *Anaesthesia*. 1967;22:55.
3 Walker IR, et al. *Aust NZ J Med*. 1972;3:247.
4 Gurman GM. *Anesth Analg*. 1972;51:761.
5 Zsigmond EK, et al. *Can Anaesth Soc J*. 1972;19:75.
6 Dillman JB. *Anesth Analg*. 1987;66:351.

* Asterisk indicates drugs cited in interaction reports.

Succinylcholine — *Echothiophate*

Succinylcholine* (eg, *Anectine*) | Echothiophate* (*Phospholine Iodide*)

Significance	Onset	Severity	Documentation
2	■ **Rapid**	□ Major	■ **Established**
	□ Delayed	■ **Moderate**	□ Probable
		□ Minor	□ Suspected
			□ Possible
			□ Unlikely

Effects The neuromuscular blocking effects of SUCCINYLCHOLINE may be prolonged.

Mechanism The systemic absorption of ECHOTHIOPHATE ophthalmic solutions results in reduced levels of plasma cholinesterase (pseudocholinesterase) which is the enzyme responsible for SUCCINYLCHOLINE metabolism resulting in prolongation of succinylcholine-induced neuromuscular blockade.

Management If patients currently using ECHOTHIOPHATE ophthalmic drops must receive SUCCINYLCHOLINE, measure plasma cholinesterase activity first to identify any patient who might be at higher risk for prolonged neuromuscular blockade due to decreased metabolic rate of succinylcholine secondary to low plasma cholinesterase activity. After discontinuation of echothiophate therapy plasma cholinesterase activity does not immediately normalize, so use a cautious approach to this combination for several weeks after discontinuation.

Discussion

It has been well documented that local application of echothiophate to the eye results in significant systemic absorption. After absorption echothiophate exerts its anticholinesterase activity systemically.[1-8] A decrease in enzyme activity is reported to be significant as early as one week after initiation of therapy and by the third week of therapy a profound effect is apparent.[2,7] One study involving 72 patients treated with echothiophate for 2 months to 7 years reported a 50% reduction in plasma cholinesterase activity in 37% of the subjects and a 75% reduction in 14% of the subjects.[6] A reduction of enzyme activity of greater than 95% has been reported.[2] These reductions in plasma cholinesterase activity result in impaired metabolism of succinylcholine. Several reports of prolonged neuromuscular blockade resulting in prolonged respiratory depression are documented after administration of succinylcholine to patients using echothiophate ophthalmic solution.[3-5]

[1] Leopold IH, et al. *Trans Am Ophthalmol Soc.* 1959;57:63.
[2] De Roetth A Jr, et al. *Am J Ophthalmol.* 1965;59:586.
[3] Pantuck EJ. *Br J Anaesth.* 1966;38:406.
[4] Gesztes T. *Br J Anaesth.* 1966;38:408.
[5] Mone JG, et al. *Anaesthesia.* 1967;22:55.
[6] Eilderton TE, et al. *Can Anaesth Soc J.* 1968;15:291.
[7] Cavallaro RJ, et al. *Anesth Analg.* 1968;47:570.
[8] Donati F, et al. *Can Anaesth Soc J.* 1981;28:488.

* Asterisk indicates drugs cited in interaction reports.

Succinylcholine — *Estrogens*

Succinylcholine	Estrogens	
Succinylcholine* (eg, *Anectine*)	Chlorotrianisene (*Tace*)	Estrogenic Substance (eg, *Gynogen*)
	Conjugated Estrogens (eg, *Premarin*)	Estrone (eg, *Theelin*)
	Diethylstilbestrol* (DES)	Estropipate (*Ogen*)
	Esterified Estrogens (*Estratab, Menest*)	Ethinyl Estradiol (*Estinyl, Feminone*)
	Estradiol (eg, *Estrace*)	Mestranol (eg, *Enovid*)
		Quinestrol (*Estrovis*)

Significance	Onset	Severity	Documentation
4	☐ Rapid	☐ Major	☐ Established
	■ **Delayed**	■ **Moderate**	☐ Probable
		☐ Minor	☐ Suspected
			■ **Possible**
			☐ Unlikely

Effects Prolongation of SUCCINYLCHOLINE activity is possible.

Mechanism A decrease in serum cholinesterase which could result in a decreased metabolic rate of SUCCINYLCHOLINE.

Management The present data do not suggest that any change in therapy is necessary.

Discussion

A significant decrease in serum cholinesterase and pseudocholinesterase has been measured in patients receiving oral contraceptives or diethylstilbesterol, respectively.[1-3] This may result from steroid-induced depression of the liver's ability to synthesize protein or to secrete it into the circulation.[1] Only one case has been reported of a patient who had a clinically significant reaction, and the complicated nature of the patient's condition makes it difficult to establish that the prolonged respiratory depression reported was due to a diethylstilbestrol-succinylcholine interaction.[3]

[1] Robertson GS. *Lancet.* 1967;1:232.

[2] Sidell FR, et al. *Clin Chem.* 1975;21:1393.

[3] Archer TL, et al. *Anesth Analg.* 1978;57:726.

* Asterisk indicates drugs cited in interaction reports. Based on pharmacologic and pharmacokinetic considerations, similar interactions may occur with other drugs that are listed.

Succinylcholine — *Ketamine*

Succinylcholine* (eg, *Anectine*)	Ketamine* (*Ketalar*)

Significance	Onset	Severity	Documentation
4	■ **Rapid**	□ Major	□ Established
	□ Delayed	■ **Moderate**	□ Probable
		□ Minor	□ Suspected
			■ **Possible**
			□ Unlikely

Effects Prolongation of SUCCINYLCHOLINE-induced neuromuscular blockade may occur.

Mechanism Postulated mechanisms include a KETAMINE-induced depression of end-plate sensitivity and/or a KETAMINE-induced decrease in presynaptic release of acetylcholine.[2,4,5]

Management Observe patients receiving these medications concurrently for the possible occurrence of prolongation of neuromuscular blockade.

Discussion

Studies involving laboratory animals have reported a prolongation of neuromuscular blockade produced by succinylcholine when ketamine is administered concurrently.[2,4,5] Although one study involving human subjects supported this animal data, the other published study based on the evaluation of 38 surgical patients reported no change in succinylcholine-induced neuromuscular blockade during ketamine administration.[1,3] Additional studies are necessary to clarify the significance of this possible drug interaction.

[1] Bovill JG, et al. *Lancet.* 1971;1:1285.
[2] Cronnelly R, et al. *Eur J Pharmacol.* 1973;22:17.
[3] Johnston RR, et al. *Anesth Analg.* 1974;53:496.
[4] Kraunak P, et al. *Br J Anaesth.* 1977;49:765.
[5] Amaki Y, et al. *Anesth Analg.* 1978;57:238.

* Asterisk indicates drugs cited in interaction reports.

Succinylcholine | *Lidocaine*

Succinylcholine*	Lidocaine*
(eg, *Anectine*)	(eg, *Xylocaine*)

Significance	Onset	Severity	Documentation
2	■ **Rapid**	□ Major	□ Established
	□ Delayed	■ **Moderate**	□ Probable
		□ Minor	■ **Suspected**
			□ Possible
			□ Unlikely

Effects Prolongation of neuromuscular blockade produced by SUCCINYLCHOLINE may occur.

Mechanism Unknown.

Management Present data suggest no change in therapy is generally necessary. However, monitor patients receiving high dose LIDOCAINE infusions, patients who may achieve higher than anticipated lidocaine levels secondary to reduced cardiac output or patients receiving prolonged lidocaine infusions more closely. Have mechanical respiratory support available in case prolonged respiratory depression occurs.

Discussion

Experimental studies involving both human subjects and laboratory animals have reported that the coadministration of IV lidocaine and succinylcholine may result in a prolongation of succinylcholine-induced neuromuscular blockade and, therefore, prolongation of respiratory depression.[1-5] It has been hypothesized that lidocaine may block conduction of the nonmyelinated terminal motor nerve fiber, interfere with release of acetylcholine from presynaptic sites and/or inhibit depolarization of the postjunctional membrane by blocking the Na^+ and K^+ channels.[6] More clinical trials are necessary to establish the significance of this interaction.

[1] De Clive-Lowe SG, et al. *Anaesthesia.* 1954;9:96.
[2] DeKornfeld TJ, et al. *Anesth Analg.* 1959;38:173.
[3] Usubiaga JE, et al. *Anesth Analg.* 1967;46:39.
[4] Matsuo S, et al. *Anesth Analg.* 1978;57:580.
[5] Fukuda S, et al. *Anesth Analg.* 1987;66:325.
[6] Bruckner J, et al. *Anesth Analg.* 1980;59:678.

* Asterisk indicates drugs cited in interaction reports.

Succinylcholine — *Lincosamides*

Succinylcholine* (eg, *Anectine*)	Clindamycin* (*Cleocin*)	Lincomycin (*Lincocin*)

Significance	Onset	Severity	Documentation
5	■ **Rapid**	□ Major	□ Established
	□ Delayed	■ **Moderate**	□ Probable
		□ Minor	□ Suspected
			□ Possible
			■ **Unlikely**

Effects SUCCINYLCHOLINE'S action to inhibit neuromuscular transmissions may be prolonged.

Mechanism Unknown.

Management Present data do not indicate that any change in therapy is necessary.

Discussion

One case is reported in the literature which describes prolonged apnea lasting 5 minutes in a patient receiving both succinylcholine and clindamycin.[1] However, there is insufficient data to establish that the apneic episode was secondary to a succinylcholine-clindamycin interaction.

[1] Avery D, et al. *Dis Nerv Syst.* 1977;38:473.

* Asterisk indicates drugs cited in interaction reports. Based on pharmacologic and pharmacokinetic considerations, similar interactions may occur with other drugs that are listed.

Succinylcholine — *Lithium*

Succinylcholine* (eg, *Anectine*)	Lithium* (eg, *Eskalith*)

Significance	Onset	Severity	Documentation
4	■ **Rapid**	□ Major	□ Established
	□ Delayed	■ **Moderate**	□ Probable
		□ Minor	□ Suspected
			■ **Possible**
			□ Unlikely

Effects Coadministration of LITHIUM may potentiate the neuromuscular blocking effects of SUCCINYLCHOLINE.

Mechanism Possible reversible inhibition of serum cholinesterase activity.

Management Observe the patient carefully for any signs of enhanced neuromuscular blockade.

Discussion

Several reports associate lithium coadministration with enhancing the pharmacologic activity of succinylcholine.[1-4] However, these reports involved either animal subjects or complex clinical situations which made a definitive conclusion impossible. One study reported no interaction in 17 patients who received succinylcholine for electroconvulsive therapy (ECT) and whose lithium levels were within the therapeutic range.[5] This would suggest that lithium therapy should not be considered a contraindication to the use of succinylcholine during ECT.

[1] Hill GE, et al. *Anesthesiology*. 1976;44:439.
[2] Hill GE, et al. *Anesthesiology*. 1977;46:122.
[3] Reimherr FW, et al. *Am J Psychiatry*. 1977;134:205.
[4] Choi SJ, et al. *Prog Neuropsychopharmacol*. 1980;4:107.
[5] Martin BA, et al. *Am J Psychiatry*. 1982;139:1326.

* Asterisk indicates drugs cited in interaction reports.

Succinylcholine		***Metoclopramide***
Succinylcholine* (eg, *Anectine*)		Metoclopramide* (eg, *Reglan*)

Significance	Onset	Severity	Documentation
2	■ **Rapid** □ Delayed	□ Major ■ **Moderate** □ Minor	□ Established □ Probable ■ **Suspected** □ Possible □ Unlikely

Effects The neuromuscular blocking effects of SUCCINYLCHOLINE may be increased, producing prolonged respiratory depression and apnea.

Mechanism METOCLOPRAMIDE may inhibit plasma cholinesterase, interfering with the inactivation of SUCCINYLCHOLINE.

Management Use this combination with caution. Closely monitor neuromuscular function and provide mechanical respiratory support as necessary.

Discussion

In a blind, randomized study, the effects of preoperative IV administration of metoclopramide 10 mg on the duration of neuromuscular blockade produced by an intubating dose of succinylcholine 1 mg/kg were investigated in 70 postpartum patients.[1] The time from onset of 95% block to 25% recovery was measured. Metoclopramide prolonged the neuromuscular blockade produced by succinylcholine by 23% (from 8 to 9.83 minutes; $P < 0.05$). Although this effect would not be expected to be clinically significant at intubation doses, it could be significant if larger doses were used in rapid sequence induction. In a second study, 22 patients undergoing elective gynecological surgery were randomly divided into two groups.[2] In both groups, tracheal intubation followed IV succinylcholine and patients received 20 mg of succinylcholine for the determination of duration of neuromuscular blockade. The time from onset of 95% block to 25% recovery was measured. Patients in one group received metoclopramide 10 mg IV followed by succinylcholine 20 mg IV, while the second group of patients received only succinylcholine 20 mg IV. Following coadministration of metoclopramide and succinylcholine, the time to recovery was 135% to 228% greater than after succinylcholine alone.

[1] Turner DR, et al. *Br J Anaesth.* 1989;63:348.

[2] Kao YJ, et al. *Anesthesiology.* 1989;70:905.

* Asterisk indicates drugs cited in interaction reports.

Succinylcholine — *Phenothiazines*

Succinylcholine* (eg, *Anectine*)	Promazine* (eg, *Sparine*)

Significance	Onset	Severity	Documentation
5	■ **Rapid**	□ Major	□ Established
	□ Delayed	■ **Moderate**	□ Probable
		□ Minor	□ Suspected
			□ Possible
			■ **Unlikely**

Effects SUCCINYLCHOLINE's action to inhibit neuromuscular transmissions may be prolonged.

Mechanism Unknown.

Management Present data does not indicate that any change in therapy is necessary.

Discussion

One case is reported in the literature which describes prolonged neuromuscular blockade (4 hours) in a patient who received promazine 25 mg intravenously after a total of 550 mg of succinylcholine was administered over a period of 5 hours and 40 minutes.[1] However, there is insufficient data to establish that this was secondary to a succinylcholine-promazine interaction.

[1] Regan AG, et al. *Anesth Analg.* 1967;46:315.

* Asterisk indicates drugs cited in interaction reports.

Succinylcholine — *Procainamide*

Succinylcholine* (eg, *Anectine*)	Procainamide* (eg, *Pronestyl*)

Significance	Onset	Severity	Documentation
4	■ **Rapid**	□ Major	□ Established
	□ Delayed	■ **Moderate**	□ Probable
		□ Minor	□ Suspected
			■ **Possible**
			□ Unlikely

Effects Potentiation of the neuromuscular blockade produced by SUCCINYLCHOLINE could theoretically manifest.

Mechanism Unknown.

Management Present data do not suggest that any therapeutic modifications are necessary.

Discussion

One study reported that in laboratory cats, procainamide infused IV either just prior to the injection of succinylcholine or during neuromuscular blockade enhanced the succinylcholine-induced neuromuscular blockade. The authors of this study proposed three possible mechanisms for this effect: Procainamide inhibition of plasma cholinesterase (pseudocholinesterase), procainamide interference with release of acetylcholine from preganglionic sites, or procainamide interference with cation transport at the neuromuscular junction.[1] No reports of this interaction in human subjects has been documented in the literature. See also Succinylcholine-Procaine.

[1] Cuthbert MF. *Br J Anaesth.* 1966;38:775.

* Asterisk indicates drugs cited in interaction reports.

Succinylcholine — *Procaine*

Succinylcholine* (eg, *Anectine*)	Procaine* (eg, *Novocain*)

Significance	Onset	Severity	Documentation
2	■ **Rapid**	□ Major	□ Established
	□ Delayed	■ **Moderate**	■ **Probable**
		□ Minor	□ Suspected
			□ Possible
			□ Unlikely

Effects The neuromuscular blockade produced by SUCCINYLCHOLINE may be prolonged.

Mechanism Since both PROCAINE and SUCCINYLCHOLINE are hydrolyzed by plasma cholinesterase (pseudocholinesterase), competition for the enzyme may result in slowed succinylcholine metabolism and, therefore, prolonged activity.[1,2] Additional mechanisms have also been postulated.[3]

Management Observe patients receiving this combination carefully. Have mechanical respiratory support available if prolonged respiratory depression occurs.

Discussion

Prolongation of succinylcholine-induced neuromuscular blockade by administration of procaine has been documented in both human studies and in laboratory animals.[1-4] However, this interaction appears to be most significant at procaine doses not usually administered in clinical anesthesia (11 mg/kg).[2,4]

[1] Foldes FF, et al. *Science.* 1953;117:383.
[2] Usubiaga JE, et al. *Anesth Analg.* 1967;46:39.
[3] Matsuo S, et al. *Anesth Analg.* 1978;57:580.
[4] Salgado AS. *Anesthesiology.* 1961;22:897.

* Asterisk indicates drugs cited in interaction reports.

Succinylcholine — *Propofol*

Succinylcholine* (eg, *Anectine*)	Propofol* (*Diprivan*)

Significance	Onset	Severity	Documentation
4	■ **Rapid** □ Delayed	□ Major ■ **Moderate** □ Minor	□ Established □ Probable □ Suspected ■ **Possible** □ Unlikely

Effects Severe bradycardia has occurred during coadministration of PROPOFOL and SUCCINYLCHOLINE.

Mechanism Unknown. However, PROPOFOL appears to exaggerate the muscarinic effects of SUCCINYLCHOLINE.

Management If an alternative agent is not suitable, consider atropine premedication when PROPOFOL administration precedes SUCCINYLCHOLINE.

Discussion

Coadministration of propofol and succinylcholine has been reported to produce severe bradycardia.[1] Two unpremedicated outpatients undergoing laparoscopy received propofol 2.5 mg/kg IV for induction anesthesia. While asleep, succinylcholine 1.5 mg/kg was administered and was promptly followed by severe sinus bradycardia (heart rate decreased from 70 to 80 bpm to less than 30 to 40 bpm). The heart rate increased after the administration of 0.6 mg atropine IV. The next four patients undergoing laparoscopy were premedicated with atropine 0.6 mg IM prior to anesthesia, which was induced with propofol and succinylcholine. Bradycardia did not occur in these four patients.[1] In another report, a 42-year-old woman received fentanyl (*Sublimaze*), propofol and succinylcholine.[2] She developed asystole 20 seconds after administration of succinylcholine. Although the contribution of each drug to the asystole cannot be ascertained, the patient had previously received fentanyl-succinylcholine anesthesia uneventfully.

Additional studies are needed to confirm this possible interaction and to determine the clinical significance.

[1] Baraka A. *Br J Anaesth.* 1988;61:482.

[2] Egan TD, et al. *Anesth Analg.* 1991;73:818.

* Asterisk indicates drugs cited in interaction reports.

Succinylcholine ✕ *Quinine Derivatives*

Succinylcholine	Quinine Derivatives	
Succinylcholine* (eg, *Anectine*)	Quinidine* (eg, *Quinidex*)	Quinine (eg, *Quinamm*)

Significance	Onset	Severity	Documentation
2	■ **Rapid**	□ Major	□ Established
	□ Delayed	■ **Moderate**	□ Probable
		□ Minor	■ **Suspected**
			□ Possible
			□ Unlikely

Effects The neuromuscular blockade produced by SUCCINYLCHOLINE may be prolonged.

Mechanism QUINIDINE may produce a decrease in plasma cholinesterase activity resulting in a slowed metabolic rate for succinylcholine.[4]

Management Use this combination with caution.

Discussion

The concomitant administration of quinidine and succinylcholine has been reported to prolong succinylcholine-induced neuromuscular blockade in both human subjects and laboratory animals.[1-4] One study reported a 75% decrease in plasma cholinesterase activity in a patient who received quinidine sulfate orally 300 mg 4 times a day. Further studies are necessary to establish the significance of this potential interaction.

[1] Schmidt JL, et al. *JAMA*. 1963;183:669.
[2] Grogono AW. *Lancet*. 1963;2:1039.
[3] Cuthbert MF. *Br J Anaesth*. 1966;38:775.
[4] Kambam JR, et al. *Anesthesiology*. 1987;67:858.

* Asterisk indicates drugs cited in interaction reports. Based on pharmacologic and pharmacokinetic considerations, similar interactions may occur with other drugs that are listed.

Succinylcholine — *Trimethaphan*

Succinylcholine* (eg, *Anectine*)	Trimethaphan* (*Arfonad*)

Significance	Onset	Severity	Documentation
2	■ **Rapid** □ Delayed	□ Major ■ **Moderate** □ Minor	□ Established ■ **Probable** □ Suspected □ Possible □ Unlikely

Effects The neuromuscular blockade induced by SUCCINYLCHOLINE may be prolonged.

Mechanism TRIMETHAPHAN is a potent noncompetitive inhibitor of pseudocholinesterase which may result in a decreased rate of SUCCINYLCHOLINE metabolism. TRIMETHAPHAN may also directly decrease the sensitivity of the respiratory center contributing to prolongation of apnea.

Management Avoid this drug combination. Nitroprusside (eg, *Nipride*) has been suggested as an appropriate alternative to trimethaphan.

Discussion

Trimethaphan administration prolonged the duration of apnea induced by succinylcholine.[1-3] A study that examined pseudocholinesterase activity in vitro suggests that trimethaphan could double the duration of succinylcholine activity.[4] The same study reported that nitroprusside showed no inhibitory effect on pseudocholinesterase activity.[4]

[1] Tewfik GI, et al. *Anaesthesia.* 1957;12:326.
[2] Wilson SL, et al. *Anesth Analg.* 1976;55:353.
[3] Poulton TJ, et al. *Anesthesiology.* 1979;50:54.
[4] Sklar GS, et al. *Anesthesiology.* 1977;47:31.

* Asterisk indicates drugs cited in interaction reports.

Succinylcholine — *Vancomycin*

Succinylcholine* (eg, *Anectine*)	Vancomycin* (eg, *Vancocin*)

Significance	Onset	Severity	Documentation
4	■ **Rapid**	■ **Major**	□ Established
	□ Delayed	□ Moderate	□ Probable
		□ Minor	□ Suspected
			■ **Possible**
			□ Unlikely

Effects VANCOMYCIN may potentiate the neuromuscular blocking effects of SUCCINYLCHOLINE.

Mechanism Unknown. However, potentiation of succinylcholine-induced neuromuscular block by VANCOMYCIN in the presence of residual Phase II block is suspected.

Management Consider avoiding VANCOMYCIN administration during the post-anesthetic period in patients who have received SUCCINYLCHOLINE-induced neuromuscular block, particularly during Phase II block.

Discussion

Neuromuscular paralysis and respiratory collapse occurred in an 82-year-old patient recovering from succinylcholine-induced neuromuscular paralysis within 30 minutes of starting a vancomycin infusion.[1] The patient was scheduled for general anesthesia for removal of scar tissue within the larynx. He was sedated with fentanyl (eg, *Sublimaze*) and midazolam (*Versed*). Anesthesia was accomplished with propofol (*Diprivan*), while paralysis was provided with succinylcholine. The patient received 2.8 mg/kg of succinylcholine during 45 minutes of anesthesia. Near the completion of surgery, succinylcholine and propofol infusions were decreased and ultimately discontinued. Before transporting the patient to the post-anesthetic care unit (PACU), an IV infusion of vancomycin was started. The patient appeared to be comfortable and ventilation was normal for the first 10 minutes in the PACU. Approximately 20 minutes after admission to the PACU, the patient's condition deteriorated and he experienced near-complete neuromuscular block and respiratory collapse. The vancomycin infusion was discontinued and return of neuromuscular function began within 30 minutes.

[1] Albrecht RF II, et al. *Anesth Analg.* 1993;77:1300.

* Asterisk indicates drugs cited in interaction reports.

Sulfinpyrazone	***Niacin***
Sulfinpyrazone* (eg, *Anturane*)	Niacin* (eg, *Nicobid*)

Significance	Onset	Severity	Documentation
5	□ Rapid ■ **Delayed**	□ Major □ Moderate ■ **Minor**	□ Established □ Probable □ Suspected ■ **Possible** □ Unlikely

Effects NIACIN may reduce SULFINPYRAZONE'S uricosuric effect.

Mechanism The inhibition of renal tubular reabsorption of uric acid by SULFINPYRAZONE is reduced by NIACIN (nicotinic acid). The precise mechanism is unknown.

Management When SULFINPYRAZONE is being used for its uricosuric actions, consider using an alternative to NIACIN.

Discussion

Administration of sulfinpyrazone produced increased fractional uric acid excretion of 140% and 686% in two patients.[1] When nicotinic acid was administered with sulfinpyrazone, the increase in fractional uric acid excretion decreased from 140% to −15% in one patient and from 686% to 275% in the other patient. Acute episodes of gout as a result of adding niacin to sulfinpyrazone therapy have not been reported; however, it may be prudent to use an alternative to niacin in patients treated with sulfinpyrazone for conditions related to hyperuricemia.

[1] Gershon SL, et al. *J Lab Clin Med.* 1974;84:179.

* Asterisk indicates drugs cited in interaction reports.

Sulfinpyrazone — *Salicylates*

Sulfinpyrazone	Salicylates	
Sulfinpyrazone* (eg, *Anturane*)	Aspirin (eg, *Bayer*)	Salsalate (eg, *Disalcid*)
	Bismuth Subsalicylate (*Pepto-Bismol*)	Sodium Salicylate* (eg, *Uracel 5*)
	Choline Salicylate (*Arthropan*)	Sodium Thiosalicylate (eg, *Tusal*)
	Magnesium Salicylate (eg, *Doan's*)	

Significance	Onset	Severity	Documentation
2	□ Rapid	□ Major	■ **Established**
	■ **Delayed**	■ **Moderate**	□ Probable
		□ Minor	□ Suspected
			□ Possible
			□ Unlikely

Effects

The uricosuria produced by SULFINPYRAZONE may be suppressed by coadministration of SALICYLATES.

Mechanism

SULFINPYRAZONE is displaced from plasma protein binding sites by SALICYLATES which results in a fall in plasma concentration of total SULFINPYRAZONE in the absence of increased excretion which implies an expansion of sulfinpyrazone distribution. SALICYLATE also blocks the inhibitory effect of SULFINPYRAZONE on tubular reabsorption of uric acid.[3]

Management

Counsel patients receiving SULFINPYRAZONE as a uricosuric not to take salicylate-containing products, including combination products containing SALICYLATES, on a regular or extended basis.

Discussion

The addition of a uricosuric dose of salicylate to a uricosuric dose of sulfinpyrazone resulted in a decrease in uric acid excretion to a rate below that in untreated controls and a corresponding increase in serum uric acid to a level above those in untreated controls.[1,2] One study reported only 700 mg of aspirin added to sulfinpyrazone therapy resulted in a reduction of uric acid excretion to control values in two out of the three patients studied.[1] The available data suggest that salicylates and sulfinpyrazone impair each other's uricosuric activity.[1-3]

[1] Kersley GD, et al. *Ann Rheum Dis.* 1958;17:326.
[2] Seegmiller JE, et al. *JAMA.* 1960;173:1076.
[3] Yu TF, et al. *J Clin Invest.* 1963;42:1330.

* Asterisk indicates drugs cited in interaction reports. Based on pharmacologic and pharmacokinetic considerations, similar interactions may occur with other drugs that are listed.

Sulfonamides — *MAOIs*

Sulfisoxazole*	Phenelzine* (*Nardil*)

Significance	Onset	Severity	Documentation
4	☐ Rapid	☐ Major	☐ Established
	■ **Delayed**	■ **Moderate**	☐ Probable
		☐ Minor	☐ Suspected
			■ **Possible**
			☐ Unlikely

Effects SULFONAMIDE or MAOI toxicity.

Mechanism Competitive inhibition for hepatic metabolism leading to accumulation of either SULFONAMIDES or MAOIs has been proposed.

Management Observe for SULFONAMIDE or MAOI toxicity. If signs of toxicity appear, consider an alternative to either the SULFONAMIDE or MAOI

Discussion

Extreme weakness, ataxia, vertigo, tinnitus, muscle pain, and parathesias were reported in a patient maintained on phenylzine 1 week after initiation of sulfisoxazole for a urinary tract infection.[1] Symptoms resolved after discontinuation of sulfisoxazole. Because both sulfonamides and MAOIs are associated with these adverse reactions, it is not possible to discern which was the causative agent in this case.

[1] Boyer WF, et al. *Am J Psychiatry*. 1983;140(2):264.

* Asterisk indicates drugs cited in interaction reports.

Sulfonamides — *Methenamine*

Sulfonamides		Methenamine
Sulfadiazine*	Sulfasalazine* (eg, *Azulfidine*)	Methenamine* (eg, *Hiprex*)
Sulfamethoxazole/ Trimethoprim* (eg, *Septra*)	Sulfisoxazole*	

Significance	Onset	Severity	Documentation
4	☐ Rapid	☐ Major	☐ Established
	■ **Delayed**	■ **Moderate**	☐ Probable
		☐ Minor	☐ Suspected
			■ **Possible**
			☐ Unlikely

Effects The risk of formation of insoluble precipitates in the urine is increased.

Mechanism METHENAMINE is hydrolyzed to formaldehyde in acid urine. Insoluble precipitates may form when certain SULFONAMIDES are exposed to formaldehyde.

Management Coadministration of METHENAMINE and SULFONAMIDES is contraindicated.

Discussion

Methenamine is hydrolyzed to formaldehyde in the urine. Methenamine preparations should not be administered to patients taking sulfonamides.[1] Some sulfonamides may form an insoluble precipitate with formaldehyde in the urine.

The basis for this monograph is information on file with the manufacturer. Published clinical data are needed to further assess this interaction.

[1] *Hiprex* [package insert]. Cincinnati, OH: Patheon Pharmaceuticals Inc; February 2004.

* Asterisk indicates drugs cited in interaction reports.

Sulfones — *Para-Aminobenzoic Acid*

Dapsone*	Para-Aminobenzoic Acid* (eg, *Potaba*)

Significance	Onset	Severity	Documentation
4	☐ Rapid	☐ Major	☐ Established
	■ **Delayed**	■ **Moderate**	☐ Probable
		☐ Minor	☐ Suspected
			■ **Possible**
			☐ Unlikely

Effects SULFONE suppression of clinical *Plasmodium* infections (malaria) can be reversed by PARA-AMINOBENZOIC ACID (PABA).

Mechanism The antimalarial action of SULFONES has been attributed to interference with the causative organism's conversion of PABA to folic acid. Sufficient amounts of exogenous PABA can overcome this interference and reverse the antimalarial action of SULFONES.

Management Attempt to avoid the use of PABA in combination with SULFONES when they are being used for their antimicrobial activity.

Discussion

PABA has been shown to reverse the anti-infective actions of sulfones in both animals and humans.[1,2] *Plasmodium gallinaceum* sensitivity to dapsone was reversed by coadministration of PABA in chicks.[1] In a study involving (prison) volunteers exposed to infected mosquitos,[2] signs of clinical malaria were suppressed in 19 of 23 volunteers treated with either 25 or 50 mg of dapsone daily 1 day before exposure and for 30 days after. In contrast, all 5 volunteers treated with dapsone 25 mg plus PABA 4,000 mg daily 1 day before exposure and for 30 days after manifested signs of clinical malaria.

[1] Bishop A. *Parasitology*. 1965;55(3):407.

[2] Degowin RL, et al. *Bull World Health Organ*. 1966;34(5):671.

* Asterisk indicates drugs cited in interaction reports.

Sulfones — *Probenecid*

Dapsone* | Probenecid*

Significance	Onset	Severity	Documentation
4	☐ Rapid	☐ Major	☐ Established
	■ **Delayed**	■ **Moderate**	☐ Probable
		☐ Minor	☐ Suspected
			■ **Possible**
			☐ Unlikely

Effects The pharmacologic and toxic effects of DAPSONE may be increased.

Mechanism Competitive inhibition of renal tubular secretion by PROBENECID, leading to accumulation of DAPSONE and its metabolites, has been proposed.

Management Observe for DAPSONE toxicity; consider lowering the dose of DAPSONE or discontinuing PROBENECID.

Discussion

The effect of probenecid on dapsone excretion was studied in 12 Ethiopian men.[1] Probenecid inhibited renal excretion of acid-labile dapsone metabolites and free drug by nearly 40% during the first 8 hours after drug administration compared with giving dapsone alone. Serum dapsone concentrations were correspondingly higher when probenecid was administered with dapsone. The clinical importance of this interaction is unclear because of the higher than usual doses of dapsone used (300 mg).

Additional studies are needed.

[1] Goodwin CS, et al. *Lancet.* 1969;2:884.

* Asterisk indicates drugs cited in interaction reports.

Sulfones — *Rifamycins*

Dapsone*	Rifabutin* (*Mycobutin*)	Rifampin* (eg, *Rifadin*)

Significance	Onset	Severity	Documentation
2	☐ Rapid ■ **Delayed**	☐ Major ■ **Moderate** ☐ Minor	☐ Established ☐ Probable ■ **Suspected** ☐ Possible ☐ Unlikely

Effects The pharmacologic effect of DAPSONE may be decreased.

Mechanism Increased clearance of DAPSONE. RIFAMYCINS may increase the metabolism of DAPSONE.

Management Monitor for clinical failure of DAPSONE when administered with a RIFAMYCIN. Higher doses of DAPSONE may be necessary. Consider alternative *Pneumocystis carinii* pneumonia prophylaxis when a RIFAMYCIN is used.

Discussion

In studies involving patients infected with *Mycobacterium leprae* (leprosy), dapsone clearance was greater when it was administered with rifampin.[1-3] This may result from an increase in the rate of metabolism induced by rifampin.[1] Markedly reduced dapsone levels have been reported.[2] A study of 12 HIV-infected patients demonstrated a reduction in dapsone AUC of 36% when rifabutin 300 mg/day was started 2 weeks before dapsone.[4] Higher doses of dapsone may be necessary when it is administered with rifampin, particularly in the prophylaxis of *Pneumocystis carinii* pneumonia.[5]

[1] Gelber RH, et al. *Am J Trop Med Hyg.* 1975;24:963.
[2] Peters JH, et al. *Fed Proc.* 1977;36:996.
[3] Krishna DR, et al. *Drug Develop Indust Pharm.* 1986;12:443.
[4] Winter HR, et al. *Clin Pharmacol Ther.* 2004;76:579.
[5] Horowitz HW, et al. *Lancet.* 1992;339:747.

* Asterisk indicates drugs cited in interaction reports.

Sulfones — *Trimethoprim*

Sulfones	Trimethoprim	
Dapsone*	Trimethoprim* (eg, *Proloprim*)	Trimethoprim/Sulfamethoxazole* (eg, *Bactrim*)

Significance	Onset	Severity	Documentation
2	☐ Rapid ■ **Delayed**	☐ Major ■ **Moderate** ☐ Minor	☐ Established ☐ Probable ■ **Suspected** ☐ Possible ☐ Unlikely

Effects Increased serum levels of dapsone and trimethoprim may occur, possibly increasing the pharmacologic and toxic effects of each drug.

Mechanism Unknown; however, possibly caused by DAPSONE and TRIMETHOPRIM decreasing the elimination of one another.

Management Monitor patients receiving both drugs for DAPSONE toxicity (eg, methemoglobinemia).

Discussion

The potential for a drug interaction between dapsone and trimethoprim was evaluated in 78 patients with AIDS.[1] In the open-labeled phase of the study, 18 patients were treated with dapsone 100 mg/day alone for 21 days. In the double-blind prospective study, 30 patients received dapsone 100 mg/day plus trimethoprim 20 mg/kg/day for 21 days while a second group of 30 patients were given trimethoprim 20 mg/kg/day plus sulfamethoxazole 100 mg/kg/day for 21 days. The concentration of dapsone was 40% higher (increased from 1.5 to 2.1 mcg/mL; $P < 0.05$) in patients treated with dapsone plus trimethoprim compared with dapsone alone. Although patients receiving trimethoprim plus dapsone experienced fewer treatment failures, more adverse reactions (eg, methemoglobinemia) and discontinuations of therapy because of toxicity occurred with the combination compared with dapsone alone. The serum trimethoprim level was 48% higher (increased from 12.4 to 18.4 mcg/mL; $P < 0.05$) in the group receiving trimethoprim plus dapsone than in those patients receiving trimethoprim plus sulfamethoxazole. However, no adverse reactions were attributed to the increased trimethoprim levels. Discontinuation of therapy because of toxicity occurred more frequently in the trimethoprim plus sulfamethoxazole group (57% compared with 30%), which presumably implicates sulfamethoxazole as causing greater toxicity than dapsone alone or dapsone plus trimethoprim.

[1] Lee BL, et al. *Ann Intern Med.* 1989;110:606.

* Asterisk indicates drugs cited in interaction reports.

Sulfonylureas — *ACE Inhibitors*

Sulfonylureas		ACE Inhibitors	
Chlorpropamide (eg, *Diabinese*)	Glyburide* (eg, *DiaBeta*)	Benazepril (eg, *Lotensin*)	Moexipril (*Univasc*)
Glimepiride (eg, *Amaryl*)	Tolazamide	Captopril (eg, *Capoten*)	Perindopril (*Aceon*)
Glipizide (eg, *Glucotrol*)	Tolbutamide (eg, *Orinase*)	Enalapril* (eg, *Vasotec*)	Quinapril (eg, *Accupril*)
		Enalaprilat	Ramipril (*Altace*)
		Fosinopril (eg, *Monopril*)	Trandolapril (*Mavik*)
		Lisinopril (eg, *Prinivil*)	

Significance	Onset	Severity	Documentation
2	■ **Rapid**	□ Major	□ Established
	□ Delayed	■ **Moderate**	□ Probable
		□ Minor	■ **Suspected**
			□ Possible
			□ Unlikely

Effects Risk of hypoglycemia may be increased.

Mechanism Temporary increase in insulin sensitivity by ACE INHIBITORS is suspected.

Management Carefully observe for symptoms of hypoglycemia when initiating ACE INHIBITOR therapy in patients receiving SULFONYLUREA therapy.

Discussion

The effects of enalapril on the pharmacokinetics and pharmacodynamics of glyburide were studied in 9 healthy volunteers.[1] In a randomized, double-blind, crossover investigation, each subject received 3 days of treatment with either enalapril 5 mg or placebo. On the morning of day 4, glyburide 3.5 mg was administered with either enalapril 10 mg or placebo. Compared with placebo, enalapril administration transiently increased the metabolic effect of glyburide 67%, which persisted for 120 to 240 minutes after enalapril administration. The total metabolic effect of glyburide was nearly the same between subjects taking enalapril or placebo. Serum insulin concentrations and serum glyburide profiles did not differ with enalapril compared with placebo.

Expect a similar interaction with other oral hypoglycemic agents (eg, metformin [eg, *Glucophage*], nateglinide [*Starlix*], pioglitazone [*Actos*], repaglinide [*Prandin*], rosiglitazone [*Avandia*]).

[1] Rave K, et al. *Diabetes Metab Res Rev.* 2005;21:459.

* Asterisk indicates drugs cited in interaction reports. Based on pharmacologic and pharmacokinetic considerations, similar interactions may occur with other drugs that are listed.

Sulfonylureas — *Androgens*

Sulfonylureas		Androgens
Acetohexamide (eg, *Dymelor*)	Glyburide (*DiaBeta*, *Micronase*)	Methandrostenolone*
Chlorpropamide (eg, *Diabinese*)	Tolazamide (eg, *Tolinase*)	
Glipizide (*Glucotrol*)	Tolbutamide* (eg, *Orinase*)	

Significance	Onset	Severity	Documentation
4	☐ Rapid	☐ Major	☐ Established
	■ **Delayed**	■ **Moderate**	☐ Probable
		☐ Minor	☐ Suspected
			■ **Possible**
			☐ Unlikely

Effects Hypoglycemic actions of SULFONYLUREAS may be enhanced.

Mechanism Unknown.

Management Monitor blood glucose concentrations and observe for clinical signs of hypoglycemia during coadministration of a SULFONYLUREA hypoglycemic agent and an ANDROGEN, particularly methandrostenolone.

Discussion

Plasma insulin response to tolbutamide injections was greater and fasting blood glucose concentrations were lower in volunteer subjects during methandrostenolone coadministration.[3] The mechanism by which methandrostenolone may augment the hypoglycemic action of tolbutamide is not clear. Androgens have separate effects on carbohydrate metabolism. In the absence of a sulfonylurea hypoglycemic agent, androgens (methandrostenolone) can lower fasting blood glucose concentrations.[1,2] Although there have been no reports of clinical hypoglycemia as a result of the combined use of an androgen and a sulfonylurea, blood glucose concentrations should be monitored during coadministration.

[1] Landon J, et al. *Metabolism.* 1962;11:501.
[2] Landon J, et al. *Metabolism.* 1962;11:513.
[3] Landon J, et al. *Metabolism.* 1963;12:924.

* Asterisk indicates drugs cited in interaction reports. Based on pharmacologic and pharmacokinetic considerations, similar interactions may occur with other drugs that are listed.

Sulfonylureas — **Anticoagulants**

Sulfonylureas		Anticoagulants
Chlorpropamide* (eg, *Diabinese*)	Tolbutamide* (eg, *Orinase*)	Dicumarol*

Significance	Onset	Severity	Documentation
2	☐ Rapid	☐ Major	☐ Established
	■ **Delayed**	■ **Moderate**	■ **Probable**
		☐ Minor	☐ Suspected
			☐ Possible
			☐ Unlikely

Effects A greater than expected hypoglycemic response that can extend to clinical hypoglycemia.

Mechanism Metabolic degradation (hepatic) of SULFONYLUREA is slowed by the oral ANTICOAGULANT (DICUMAROL) leading to SULFONYLUREA accumulation.

Management Perform blood glucose monitoring and observe for signs of clinical hypoglycemia. Tailor dosages as needed.

Discussion

Clinical hypoglycemia has been reported in patients receiving dicumarol with either tolbutamide or chlorpropamide.[2,4,6] Pharmacokinetic investigations have revealed that the plasma elimination half-lives of tolbutamide and chlorpropamide can prolong by as much as three-fold when coadministered with dicumarol.[4-6,8] A similar effect on tolbutamide elimination has not been associated with other oral anticoagulants such as warfarin, phenprocoumon, or phenindione,[8] suggesting that warfarin may be a safer alternative when tolbutamide or chlorpropamide are used concurrently with an oral anticoagulant.

A temporal relationship between the addition of tolbutamide and excessive prolongations of prothrombin time was observed in two patients maintained on dicumarol.[1] Subsequent investigations, however, failed to confirm an effect of sulfonylureas on oral anticoagulant action.[1,3,7,9,10] Although tolbutamide can increase the clearance of dicumarol, the clinical effects appear to be offset by tolbutamide displacement of dicumarol from its protein binding sites.[7,10]

1 Chaplin H, et al. *Am J Med Sci.* 1958;235:706.
2 Spurny OM, et al. *Arch Intern Med.* 1965;115:53.
3 Poucher RL, et al. *JAMA.* 1966;197:1069.
4 Kristensen M, et al. *Diabetes.* 1967;16:211.
5 Solomon HM, et al. *Metabolism.* 1967;16:1029.
6 Kristensen M, et al. *Acta Med Scand.* 1968;183:83.
7 Welch RM, et al. *Clin Pharmacol Ther.* 1969;10:817.
8 Skovsted L, et al. *Acta Med Scand.* 1976;199:513.
9 Heine P, et al. *Eur J Clin Pharmacol.* 1976;10:31.
10 Jahnchen E, et al. *Eur J Clin Pharmacol.* 1976;10:349.

* Asterisk indicates drugs cited in interaction reports.

Sulfonylureas — *Beta-Blockers*

Sulfonylureas		Beta-Blockers	
Chlorpropamide* (eg, *Diabinese*)	Glyburide (eg, *DiaBeta*)	Carteolol (eg, *Cartrol*)	Propranolol* (eg, *Inderal*)
Glimepiride (eg, *Amaryl*)	Tolazamide	Nadolol (eg, *Corgard*)	Sotalol (eg, *Betapace*)
Glipizide (eg, *Glucotrol*)	Tolbutamide* (eg, *Orinase*)	Penbutolol (*Levatol*)	Timolol (eg, *Blocadren*)
		Pindolol (eg, *Visken*)	

Significance	Onset	Severity	Documentation
5	☐ Rapid	☐ Major	☐ Established
	■ **Delayed**	☐ Moderate	☐ Probable
		■ **Minor**	☐ Suspected
			■ **Possible**
			☐ Unlikely

Effects Hypoglycemic effects of SULFONYLUREAS may be attenuated.

Mechanism Unknown.

Management Perform blood glucose monitoring, and observe patients for clinical signs of hyperglycemia.

Discussion

Results of studies investigating the effect of beta-blockers on the hypoglycemic actions of sulfonylureas have been equivocal. Some studies showed that beta-blockers attenuated the hypoglycemic actions of sulfonylureas,[1-3] while others did not demonstrate an effect.[4,5] An epidemiologic study of the risk of hypoglycemia in patients receiving sulfonylureas who were also taking a cardioselective or nonselective beta-blocker did not find an increased risk with 20,774 person-years of exposure.[6] Two cases have attributed hyperglycemia to coadministration of a sulfonylurea (tolbutamide, chlorpropamide) and propranolol.[2,7]

Hypoglycemia can be prolonged, and the tachycardic response may be blunted. This may be more likely with nonselective beta-blockers.[8]

1 De Divitiis O, et al. *Lancet.* 1968;1:749.
2 Podolsky S, et al. *Metabolism.* 1973;22:685.
3 Scandellari C, et al. *Diabetologia.* 1978;15:297.
4 Massara F, et al. *Diabetologia.* 1971;7:287.
5 Totterman KJ, et al. *Ann Clin Res.* 1982;14:190.
6 Shorr RI, et al. *JAMA.* 1997;278:40.
7 Holt RJ, et al. *DICP.* 1981;15:599.
8 Ostman J. *Acta Med Scand.* Suppl. 1983;672:69. Review.

* Asterisk indicates drugs cited in interaction reports. Based on pharmacologic and pharmacokinetic considerations, similar interactions may occur with other drugs that are listed.

Sulfonylureas — *Chloramphenicol*

Sulfonylureas		Chloramphenicol
Chlorpropamide* (eg, *Diabinese*)	Glyburide (eg, *DiaBeta*)	Chloramphenicol* (eg, *Chloromycetin*)
Glimepiride (eg, *Amaryl*)	Tolazamide	
Glipizide (eg, *Glucotrol*)	Tolbutamide* (eg, *Orinase*)	

Significance	Onset	Severity	Documentation
2	□ Rapid ■ **Delayed**	□ Major ■ **Moderate** □ Minor	□ Established □ Probable ■ **Suspected** □ Possible □ Unlikely

Effects Hypoglycemia may occur.

Mechanism Proposed reduction in SULFONYLUREA hepatic clearance by CHLORAMPHENICOL, leading to SULFONYLUREA accumulation.

Management Monitor blood glucose concentrations and observe patients for symptoms of hypoglycemia when initiating CHLORAMPHENICOL therapy in patients maintained on a SULFONYLUREA hypoglycemic agent.

Discussion

Clinical hypoglycemia has occurred during chloramphenicol therapy in patients maintained on tolbutamide.[1-3] A causal relationship between this interaction and the occurrence of hypoglycemia has not been established. However, pharmacokinetic investigations have shown that administration of chloramphenicol with either tolbutamide or chlorpropamide results in prolongation of the sulfonylurea elimination $t_{1/2}$ by as much as 3-fold. As a result, serum sulfonylurea concentrations increase, and blood glucose concentrations may decrease.[2-4]

[1] Soeldner JS, et al. *JAMA.* 1965;193:398.
[2] Christensen LK, et al. *Lancet.* 1969;2:1397.
[3] Brunova E, et al. *Int J Clin Pharmacol Biopharm.* 1977;15:7.
[4] Petitpierre B, et al. *Lancet.* 1970;1:789.

* Asterisk indicates drugs cited in interaction reports. Based on pharmacologic and pharmacokinetic considerations, similar interactions may occur with other drugs that are listed.

Sulfonylureas		*Cholestyramine*
Glipizide* (*Glucotrol*)		Cholestyramine* (eg, *Questran*)

Significance	Onset	Severity	Documentation
4	☐ Rapid ■ **Delayed**	☐ Major ■ **Moderate** ☐ Minor	☐ Established ☐ Probable ☐ Suspected ■ **Possible** ☐ Unlikely

Effects Serum glipizide levels may be decreased, producing a decrease in the hypoglycemic effects.

Mechanism Administration of GLIPIZIDE with CHOLESTYRAMINE may impair the absorption of the hypoglycemic agent.

Management Consider having the patient ingest GLIPIZIDE 1 to 2 hours prior to CHOLESTYRAMINE. Monitor serum glucose levels and observe the patient for signs of hyperglycemia.

Discussion

The effect of cholestyramine on the GI absorption of glipizide was studied in six healthy male volunteers.[1] In a crossover study, subjects received 5 mg glipizide with water or cholestyramine 8 g. There were significant ($P < 0.001$) differences in the area under the glipizide concentration-time curve (AUC) and maximum glipizide serum concentration. Cholestyramine decreased the glipizide AUC by 29% ($P < 0.01$) and the peak plasma concentration by 33% ($P < 0.01$). During the control period, patients experienced symptoms of hypoglycemia, including palpitations, sweating and hand tremor. However, most patients were symptom-free with coadministration of cholestyramine and glipizide.

Additional studies are needed to confirm the clinical significance of this possible interaction.

[1] Kivisto KT, et al. *Br J Clin Pharmacol.* 1990;30:733.

* Asterisk indicates drugs cited in interaction reports.

Sulfonylureas — *Clofibrate*

Sulfonylureas		Clofibrate
Chlorpropamide* (eg, *Diabinese*)	Glyburide* (eg, *DiaBeta*)	Clofibrate*†
Glimepiride (eg, *Amaryl*)	Tolazamide*	
Glipizide (eg, *Glucotrol*)	Tolbutamide* (eg, *Orinase*)	

Significance	Onset	Severity	Documentation
2	☐ Rapid	☐ Major	☐ Established
	■ **Delayed**	■ **Moderate**	☐ Probable
		☐ Minor	■ **Suspected**
			☐ Possible
			☐ Unlikely

Effects SULFONYLUREA hypoglycemic actions may be amplified. The antidiuretic action of CLOFIBRATE in patients with diabetes insipidus can be antagonized by glyburide.[1]

Mechanism Unknown.

Management Monitor blood glucose concentrations and observe patients for signs of hypoglycemia. Adjust the SULFONYLUREA dose accordingly.

Discussion

A hypoglycemic response has been associated with the addition of clofibrate to a sulfonylurea regimen, although this has not been a consistent observation.[2-9] The mechanism by which this may occur is not clear. Clofibrate can reduce the clearance of chlorpropamide, leading to its accumulation.[10] However, clofibrate may have additive hypoglycemic effects.[6]

1 Rado JP, et al. *J Clin Pharmacol.* 1974;14:290.
2 Jain AK, et al. *N Engl J Med.* 1975;293:1283.
3 Daubresse JC, et al. *N Engl J Med.* 1976;294:613.
4 Ferrari C, et al. *N Engl J Med.* 1976;294:1184.
5 Barnett D, et al. *Br J Clin Pharmacol.* 1977;4:455.
6 Ferrari C, et al. *Metabolism.* 1977;26:129.
7 Kudzma DJ, et al. *Diabetes.* 1977;26:291.
8 Daubresse JC, et al. *Br J Clin Pharmacol.* 1979;7:599.
9 Calvert GD, et al. *Eur J Clin Pharmacol.* 1980;17:355.
10 Petitpierre B, et al. *Int J Clin Pharmacol.* 1972;6:120.

* Asterisk indicates drugs cited in interaction reports. Based on pharmacologic and pharmacokinetic considerations, similar interactions may occur with other drugs that are listed.

† Not available in the United States.

Sulfonylureas — *Diazoxide*

Sulfonylureas		Diazoxide
Chlorpropamide* (eg, *Diabinese*)	Glyburide (eg, *DiaBeta*)	Diazoxide* (eg, *Hyperstat IV*)
Glimepiride (eg, *Amaryl*)	Tolazamide	
Glipizide (eg, *Glucotrol*)	Tolbutamide* (eg, *Orinase*)	

Significance	Onset	Severity	Documentation
2	☐ Rapid	☐ Major	☐ Established
	■ **Delayed**	■ **Moderate**	■ **Probable**
		☐ Minor	☐ Suspected
			☐ Possible
			☐ Unlikely

Effects The addition of DIAZOXIDE to the regimen of a non-insulin-dependent diabetic patient stabilized on SULFONYLUREA therapy may result in hyperglycemia.

Mechanism Postulated mechanisms; decreased insulin release secondary to DIAZOXIDE'S effect on cell membrane calcium flux or stimulation of alpha-adrenergic receptor sites in the beta cell, and DIAZOXIDE stimulation of the release of catecholamines may occur, resulting in increased glucose and free fatty acids.[1-8]

Management If DIAZOXIDE is coadministered with a SULFONYLUREA, monitor blood glucose and adjust the dosage of each drug as needed.

Discussion

There are no studies reported in the literature that specifically investigated the clinical implications of the addition of diazoxide to the therapy of a non-insulin-dependent diabetic patient stabilized on a sulfonylurea. However, a number of cases have been documented that report the successful treatment of chlorpropamide-induced hypoglycemia with diazoxide.[8-10] Conversely, 2 studies document that tolbutamide can correct diazoxide-induced hyperglycemia.[11,12]

1 Graber AL, et al. *Diabetes.* 1966;15:143.
2 Fajans SS, et al. *Ann N Y Acad Sci.* 1968;150:261.
3 Porte D Jr. *Ann N Y Acad Sci.* 1968;150:281.
4 Field JB, et al. *Ann N Y Acad Sci.* 1968;150:415.
5 Seltzer HS, et al. *Diabetes.* 1969;18:19.
6 Greenwood RH, et al. *Lancet.* 1976;1:444.
7 Jacobs RF, et al. *J Pediatr.* 1978;93:801.
8 Pfeifer MA, et al. *South Med J.* 1978;71:606.
9 Johnson SF, et al. *Am J Med.* 1977;63:799.
10 Jeffery WH, et al. *Drug Intell Clin Pharm.* 1983;17:372.
11 Wolff F. *Lancet.* 1964;13:309.
12 Wales JK, et al. *Lancet.* 1967;1:1137.

* Asterisk indicates drugs cited in interaction reports. Based on pharmacologic and pharmacokinetic considerations, similar interactions may occur with other drugs that are listed.

Sulfonylureas | **Echinacea**

Tolbutamide*
(eg, *Orinase*)

Echinacea*

Significance	Onset	Severity	Documentation
5	□ Rapid ■ **Delayed**	□ Major □ Moderate ■ **Minor**	□ Established □ Probable □ Suspected □ Possible ■ **Unlikely**

Effects TOLBUTAMIDE plasma concentrations may be increased, enhancing the effect.

Mechanism ECHINACEA may inhibit the metabolism (CYP2C9) of TOLBUTAMIDE.

Management Based on available clinical data, no special precautions are necessary.

Discussion

The effects of echinacea (*Echinacea purpurea* root) on cytochrome P450 (CYP) activity were assessed when administering the probe drug tolbutamide (CYP2C9).[1] Twelve subjects received tolbutamide 500 mg alone and after 8 days of pretreatment with echinacea 400 mg 4 times daily. Oral clearance of tolbutamide was decreased 11% by echinacea administration. This change was not considered to be clinically important.

The ingredients of many herbal products are not standardized. It is unclear if herbal products contain ingredients other than those listed on the label or purported to be present that could interact with tolbutamide.

[1] Gorski JC, et al. *Clin Pharmacol Ther.* 2004;75:89.

* Asterisk indicates drugs cited in interaction reports.

Sulfonylureas — *Ethanol*

Sulfonylureas		Ethanol
Chlorpropamide* (eg, *Diabinese*)	Glyburide (eg, *DiaBeta*)	Ethanol* (Alcohol, Ethyl Alcohol)
Glimepiride (eg, *Amaryl*)	Tolazamide	
Glipizide* (eg, *Glucotrol*)	Tolbutamide* (eg, *Orinase*)	

Significance	Onset	Severity	Documentation
2	■ **Rapid**	□ Major	■ **Established**
	□ Delayed	■ **Moderate**	□ Probable
		□ Minor	□ Suspected
			□ Possible
			□ Unlikely

Effects Three effects of ETHANOL have been identified with SULFONYLUREAS. ETHANOL may prolong, but not augment, GLIPIZIDE-induced reductions in blood glucose.[1] Chronic use of ETHANOL may decrease TOLBUTAMIDE $t_{½}$.[2-4] ETHANOL ingestion by patients taking CHLORPROPAMIDE may result in a disulfiram-like reaction.[5-7]

Mechanism ETHANOL prolongs GLIPIZIDE activity by delaying GLIPIZIDE absorption and elimination.[1] ETHANOL decreases TOLBUTAMIDE $t_{½}$ by causing a decrease in absorption of the active drug and a more rapid metabolism by the liver.[8] The mechanism for the ALCOHOL-CHLORPROPAMIDE disulfiram-like reaction has not been elucidated.

Management Counsel patients receiving SULFONYLUREAS to avoid ETHANOL intake in excess of an occasional, single drink.

Discussion

Alcohol inhibits gluconeogenesis, so hypoglycemia may occur whenever gluconeogenesis is required to maintain glucose levels.[9-11] However, hyperglycemia may occur in non-insulin-dependent diabetic patients stabilized on tolbutamide when alcohol is used chronically because of a subsequent 2-fold reduction in tolbutamide $t_{½}$.[4-6] The disulfiram-like reaction that may occur when alcohol is ingested with chlorpropamide is characterized by facial flushing that may spread to the neck and, occasionally, a burning sensation, headache, nausea, and tachycardia. Typically, the flush starts 10 to 20 minutes after alcohol ingestion, peaks at 30 to 40 minutes, and persists for 1 to 2 hours.[5-7] Naloxone (eg, *Narcan*) has been shown to antagonize this reaction.[12] It is not known which, if any, of these interactions may occur with other sulfonylureas.

[1] Hartling SG, et al. *Diabetes Care.* 1987;10:683.
[2] Kater RM, et al. *JAMA.* 1969;207:363.
[3] Carulli N, et al. *Eur J Clin Invest.* 1971;1:421.
[4] Shah MN, et al. *Am J Clin Nutr.* 1972;25:135.
[5] Johnston C, et al. *Diabetologia.* 1984;26:1.
[6] Hillson RM, et al. *Diabetologia.* 1984;26:6.
[7] Wolfsthal SD, et al. *Ann Intern Med.* 1985;103:158.
[8] Horowitz SH, et al. *Am J Med Sci.* 1972;264:395.
[9] Field JB, et al. *J Clin Invest.* 1963;42:497.
[10] Freinkel N, et al. *J Clin Invest.* 1963;42:1112.
[11] Arky RA, et al. *JAMA.* 1968;206:575.
[12] Baraniuk JN, et al. *Alcohol: Clin Exp Res.* 1987;11:518.

* Asterisk indicates drugs cited in interaction reports. Based on pharmacologic and pharmacokinetic considerations, similar interactions may occur with other drugs that are listed.

Sulfonylureas — *Fenfluramine*

Sulfonylureas		Fenfluramine
Chlorpropamide* (eg, *Diabinese*)	Glyburide* (eg, *DiaBeta*)	Fenfluramine*†
Glimepiride (eg, *Amaryl*)	Tolazamide	
Glipizide* (eg, *Glucotrol*)	Tolbutamide (eg, *Orinase*)	

Significance	Onset	Severity	Documentation
3	☐ Rapid	☐ Major	☐ Established
	■ **Delayed**	☐ Moderate	☐ Probable
		■ **Minor**	■ **Suspected**
			☐ Possible
			☐ Unlikely

Effects An increase in hypoglycemia, above that achievable with SULFONYLUREAS alone, may occur. The blood sugar appears to return to pretreatment values weeks after FENFLURAMINE is discontinued.

Mechanism FENFLURAMINE appears to increase glucose uptake by skeletal muscle tissue, thus augmenting the hypoglycemic activity of SULFONYLUREAS.

Management This interaction may be used as a therapeutic advantage in achieving normoglycemia in diabetic patients refractory to SULFONYLUREAS and diet therapy.

Discussion

Several studies support the synergistic hypoglycemic activity of fenfluramine and sulfonylureas. In a study of 11 diabetic patients with inadequate control using diet and tolbutamide, fenfluramine 40 mg twice daily for 3 months improved glucose control as measured with an oral glucose tolerance test.[1] An additional 21 patients in this trial, all with diabetes and receiving treatment with diet or diet and tolbutamide, were also examined for their response to a single dose of fenfluramine 40 mg prior to a standard breakfast. Fenfluramine resulted in a 35% decrease in blood glucose compared with control at 1 hour and a similar decrease at 2 hours after the standard breakfast. In a separate trial of 10 obese patients with diabetes being treated with both diet and various sulfonylureas, the addition of sustained-release fenfluramine 60 mg each morning for 3 months resulted in a 25% decrease in the glucose tolerance test AUC compared with that achieved with their previous regimen.[2] Further studies have obtained similar results and suggest that the hypoglycemic effect of fenfluramine is dose related[3] and unrelated to changes in insulin concentrations.[4] These combinations have been well tolerated.

[1] Turtle JR, et al. *Diabetes.* 1973;22:858.
[2] Wales JK. *Curr Med Res Opin.* 1979;6(suppl 1):226.
[3] Salmela PI, et al. *Diabetes Care.* 1981;4:535.
[4] Verdy M, et al. *Int J Obes.* 1983;7:289.

* Asterisk indicates drugs cited in interaction reports. Based on pharmacologic and pharmacokinetic considerations, similar interactions may occur with other drugs that are listed.
† Not available in the United States.

Sulfonylureas — *Fluconazole*

Glimepiride* (*Amaryl*)	Fluconazole* (*Diflucan*)
Tolbutamide* (eg, *Orinase*)	

Significance	Onset	Severity	Documentation
2	□ Rapid	□ Major	□ Established
	■ **Delayed**	■ **Moderate**	□ Probable
		□ Minor	■ **Suspected**
			□ Possible
			□ Unlikely

Effects The hypoglycemic effects of certain SULFONYLUREAS may be increased.

Mechanism Inhibition of SULFONYLUREA metabolism (CYP2C9) by FLUCONAZOLE is suspected.

Management Consider monitoring blood glucose levels during coadministration of certain SULFONYLUREAS and FLUCONAZOLE.

Discussion

The effect of fluconazole on tolbutamide plasma levels was studied in 19 healthy men.[1] Compared with placebo, coadministration of a single 500 mg dose of tolbutamide, 2 hr after a single 150 mg dose of fluconazole, produced a statistically significant ($P < 0.01$) increase in the peak plasma concentration of tolbutamide (from 51.7 to 56.2 mcg/mL). In addition, coadministration of a single 500 mg dose of tolbutamide after a 6-day course of fluconazole (100 mg/day) resulted in a statistically significant ($P < 0.01$) increase in tolbutamide peak plasma levels (from 51.7 to 57.4 mcg/mL). For both study regimens, there were also statistically significant ($P < 0.01$) increases in the AUCs of 43% and 59%, respectively. There were no clinically important effects on blood glucose levels in any of the subjects receiving both fluconazole and tolbutamide. In a study of 12 volunteers, administration of fluconazole, 200 mg/day for 4 days, increased the AUC of a test dose of glimepiride (0.5 mg) 139% and the peak level 48% (from 33 to 49 ng/mL).[2]

Additional studies are needed to substantiate this possible interaction.

[1] Lazar JD, et al. *Rev Infect Dis.* 1990;12(suppl 3):S327. [2] Niemi M, et al. *Clin Pharmacol Ther.* 2001;69:194.

* Asterisk indicates drugs cited in interaction reports.

Sulfonylureas — *Fluvoxamine*

Glimepiride* (*Amaryl*)	Tolbutamide* (eg, *Orinase*)	Fluvoxamine* (eg, *Luvox*)

Significance	Onset	Severity	Documentation
4	□ Rapid ■ **Delayed**	□ Major ■ **Moderate** □ Minor	□ Established □ Probable □ Suspected ■ **Possible** □ Unlikely

Effects The pharmacologic and adverse effects of certain SULFONYLUREAS may be increased.

Mechanism Inhibition of SULFONYLUREA metabolism (CYP2C9) by FLUVOXAMINE.

Management In patients receiving certain SULFONYUREAS, carefully monitor blood glucose levels when FLUVOXAMINE is started or stopped. Be prepared to adjust the SULFONYLUREA dose as needed.

Discussion

Using an open, randomized, crossover design, the effect of fluvoxamine on the metabolism of tolbutamide was studied in 14 healthy volunteers.[1] Each subject took a single oral dose of tolbutamide 500 mg alone and then was randomly assigned to receive 75 or 150 mg fluvoxamine daily for 5 days. Each group then received a single oral dose of 500 mg tolbutamide. In subjects receiving 75 mg fluvoxamine, there was a 19% decrease in the median total clearance of tolbutamide (from 845 to 688 mL/hr). There was also a reduction in total tolbutamide clearance in subjects receiving 150 mg fluvoxamine; however, the decrease did not reach statistical significance. The clearances of the 2 metabolites of tolbutamide, 4-hydroxytolbutamide and carboxytolbutamide, were reduced 37% and 65% in subjects receiving 75 or 150 mg fluvoxamine, respectively. The effects of fluvoxamine on the pharmacokinetics and pharmacodynamics of glimepiride were investigated in 12 healthy volunteers. Fluvoxamine increased the peak plasma concentration of glimepiride 43% (from 32.7 to 46.7 ng/mL) and prolonged the elimination $t_{½}$ from 2 to 2.3 hr, compared with placebo.[2]

[1] Madsen H, et al. *Clin Pharmacol Ther.* 2001;69:41.
[2] Niemi M, et al. *Clin Pharmacol Ther.* 2001;69:194.

* Asterisk indicates drugs cited in interaction reports.

Sulfonylureas — *Gemfibrozil*

Glimepiride* (eg, *Amaryl*)	Glyburide* (eg, *DiaBeta*)	Gemfibrozil* (eg, *Lopid*)

Significance	Onset	Severity	Documentation
4	☐ Rapid ■ **Delayed**	☐ Major ■ **Moderate** ☐ Minor	☐ Established ☐ Probable ☐ Suspected ■ **Possible** ☐ Unlikely

Effects The hypoglycemic effects of certain SULFONYLUREAS may be increased.

Mechanism Inhibition of SULFONYLUREA metabolism (CYP2C9) by GEMFIBROZIL is suspected.

Management In patients receiving certain SULFONYLUREAS, closely monitor blood glucose levels when GEMFIBROZIL is added or discontinued. Adjust the dose of the SULFONYLUREA accordingly.

Discussion

A 53-year-old patient with diabetes mellitus that was well controlled with glyburide 5 mg/day for 9 months developed hypoglycemia following the addition of gemfibrozil 1,200 mg/day to her treatment regimen.[1] Three weeks later, the patient's blood glucose levels were low, and she stated that she had been experiencing hypoglycemic attacks since beginning treatment with gemfibrozil. On 2 occasions, she had fallen. The dose of glyburide was decreased to 1.25 mg/day. No additional episodes of hypoglycemia occurred, and her blood glucose levels were adequately controlled. The triglyceride level decreased to 140 mg/dL, and gemfibrozil was discontinued. Because the blood glucose levels increased to 240 mg/dL over the next 2 weeks, the dose of glyburide was increased to 5 mg/day with good control of the patient's diabetes. Two months later, the patient's triglyceride levels were once again elevated, and gemfibrozil was restarted at 1,200 mg/day. After 3 days, severe hypoglycemia occurred (blood glucose ranged from 50 to 70 mg/dL), and the dose of glyburide was reduced to 1.25 mg/day. For the next 4 weeks, no hypoglycemic attacks were noted, and the diabetes remained under satisfactory control. In a randomized, crossover study, 10 volunteers received glimepiride before and after treatment with gemfibrozil.[2] Glimepiride AUC increased 23%, but there were no changes in insulin levels or blood glucose responses.

[1] Ahmad S. *South Med J.* 1991;84(1):102.

[2] Niemi M, et al. *Clin Pharmacol Ther.* 2001;70(5):439.

* Asterisk indicates drugs cited in interaction reports.

Sulfonylureas — *Ginkgo biloba*

Tolbutamide* (eg, *Orinase*)	Ginkgo biloba*

Significance	Onset	Severity	Documentation
4	☐ Rapid ■ **Delayed**	☐ Major ■ **Moderate** ☐ Minor	☐ Established ☐ Probable ☐ Suspected ■ **Possible** ☐ Unlikely

Effects TOLBUTAMIDE plasma concentrations may be reduced, decreasing the hypoglycemic effect.

Mechanism Unknown.

Management Caution patients to avoid concurrent use of GINKGO BILOBA and TOLBUTAMIDE.

Discussion

The effects of *Ginkgo biloba* extract on the pharmacokinetics and pharmacodynamics of tolbutamide were studied in 10 healthy men.[1] Each subject received tolbutamide 125 mg alone and after taking *Ginkgo biloba* extract 120 mg 3 times daily for 28 days. Compared with taking tolbutamide alone, pretreatment with *Ginkgo biloba* reduced the tolbutamide AUC 16% and tended to attenuate the blood glucose–lowering effect of tolbutamide. In an open-label, randomized, crossover study in healthy volunteers receiving *Ginkgo biloba* and tolbutamide, *Ginkgo biloba* did not inhibit or induce CYP2C9 activity.[2]

[1] Uchida S, et al. *J Clin Pharmacol.* 2006;46(11):1290.

[2] Zadoyan G, et al. *Eur J Clin Pharmacol.* 2012;68(5):553.

* Asterisk indicates drugs cited in interaction reports.

Sulfonylureas — *Histamine H_2 Antagonists*

Chlorpropamide	Glyburide* (eg, *DiaBeta*)	Cimetidine* (eg, *Tagamet*)	Ranitidine* (eg, *Zantac*)
Glimepiride (eg, *Amaryl*)	Tolazamide		
Glipizide* (eg, *Glucotrol*)	Tolbutamide*		

Significance	Onset	Severity	Documentation
4	☐ Rapid	☐ Major	☐ Established
	■ **Delayed**	■ **Moderate**	☐ Probable
		☐ Minor	☐ Suspected
			■ **Possible**
			☐ Unlikely

Effects Reduced clearance of SULFONYLUREAS that may result in hypoglycemia.

Mechanism H_2 ANTAGONIST inhibition of SULFONYLUREA hepatic metabolism, resulting in an accumulation of SULFONYLUREA.

Management Monitor blood glucose and observe for signs of clinical hypoglycemia after initiation of H_2 ANTAGONIST therapy in patients maintained on a SULFONYLUREA. Adjust the SULFONYLUREA dosage as necessary.

Discussion

Pharmacokinetic investigations of this interaction have been equivocal. In 1 study involving 6 diabetic patients, glipizide clearance was reduced by cimetidine, and postprandial blood glucose concentrations were reduced 40%.[1] In 2 groups of 6 diabetic patients, cimetidine and ranitidine increased the AUC. This was associated with a decrease in postprandial glucose values and asymptomatic hypoglycemia.[2] In other studies involving healthy volunteers, tolbutamide and glyburide clearances were also decreased when administered with cimetidine.[3-5] In contrast, other investigations did not confirm the altered tolbutamide pharmacokinetics as a result of coadministration of cimetidine.[6,7] These discrepancies can only be partially explained by methodological differences.

In 6 non–insulin-dependent patients, ranitidine potentiated the hypoglycemic response to glipizide.[8]

1 Feely J, et al. *Br J Clin Pharmacol.* 1983;15:607P.
2 Feely J, et al. *Br J Clin Pharmacol.* 1993;35(3):321.
3 Kubacka RT, et al. *Drug Intell Clin Pharm.* 1985;19(6):461.
4 Cate EW, et al. *J Clin Pharmacol.* 1986;26(5):372.
5 Toon S, et al. *J Pharm Pharmacol.* 1995;47(1):85.
6 Stockley C, et al. *Eur J Clin Pharmacol.* 1986;31(2):235.
7 Dey NG, et al. *Br J Clin Pharmacol.* 1983;16(4):438.
8 MacWalter RS, et al. *Br J Clin Pharmacol.* 1985;19:121P.

* Asterisk indicates drugs cited in interaction reports. Based on pharmacologic and pharmacokinetic considerations, similar interactions may occur with other drugs that are listed.

Sulfonylureas | **HMG-CoA Reductase Inhibitors**

Glimepiride (*Amaryl*)	Tolbutamide*	Fluvastatin* (*Lescol*)	Simvastatin* (eg, *Zocor*)
Glyburide* (eg, *DiaBeta*)			

Significance	Onset	Severity	Documentation
5	☐ Rapid ■ **Delayed**	☐ Major ☐ Moderate ■ **Minor**	☐ Established ☐ Probable ☐ Suspected ☐ Possible ■ **Unlikely**

Effects SULFONYLUREA concentrations may be elevated, increasing the hypoglycemic effect.

Mechanism Unknown.

Management Based on available data, no special precautions are necessary. Decreasing the dose of the SULFONYLUREA may be necessary if an interaction is suspected.

Discussion

In a randomized, open-label, placebo-controlled study, 3 groups of 16 healthy subjects received once-daily administration of fluvastatin 40 mg, simvastatin 20 mg, or placebo for 15 days.[1] A single oral dose of tolbutamide 1 g or glyburide 3.5 mg was given on days 1, 8, and 15. Fluvastatin increased the C_{max} and AUC of tolbutamide 10% and 23%, respectively. Compared with placebo, simvastatin did not affect the peak concentration or AUC of tolbutamide. Fluvastatin increased the C_{max} and AUC of glyburide 21% and 19%, respectively, while simvastatin increased these values 21% and 28%, respectively. Neither fluvastatin nor simvastatin affected the hypoglycemic action of tolbutamide or glyburide. A further study, involving 32 patients with type 2 diabetes mellitus, investigated the effects of single and multiple dosing of fluvastatin (40 mg given in the evening) on the pharmacokinetics and hypoglycemic action of glyburide (5 to 20 mg given the following morning). Fluvastatin had no effects on either the pharmacokinetics or the hypoglycemic action of glyburide. Neither glyburide nor tolbutamide affected fluvastatin or simvastatin plasma levels.

[1] Appel S, et al. *Am J Cardiol.* 1995;76(2):29A.

* Asterisk indicates drugs cited in interaction reports. Based on pharmacologic and pharmacokinetic considerations, similar interactions may occur with other drugs that are listed.

Sulfonylureas | **Hydantoins**

Acetohexamide (eg, *Dymelor*) Chlorpropamide (eg, *Diabinese*) Glimepiride (eg, *Amaryl*) Glipizide (eg, *Glucotrol*)	Glyburide (eg, *DiaBeta*) Tolazamide Tolbutamide* (eg, *Orinase*)	Ethotoin (*Peganone*) Fosphenytoin (*Cerebyx*)	Phenytoin* (eg, *Dilantin*)

Significance	Onset	Severity	Documentation
5	☐ Rapid ■ **Delayed**	☐ Major ☐ Moderate ■ **Minor**	☐ Established ☐ Probable ☐ Suspected ■ **Possible** ☐ Unlikely

Effects PHENYTOIN may cause an increase in blood glucose levels, necessitating a higher dose of SULFONYLUREAS for control of hyperglycemia.

Mechanism Unknown.

Management The available data do not suggest that any change in therapy is necessary.

Discussion

Elevation of blood sugar has been reported in patients receiving phenytoin.[1-5] Two of these reports involve patients who experienced phenytoin toxicity.[1,3] No cases have been reported of patients with type 2 diabetes mellitus becoming hyperglycemic after phenytoin administration when controlled with sulfonylurea therapy.

[1] Peters BH, et al. *N Engl J Med.* 1969;281(2):91.
[2] Fariss BL, et al. *Diabetes.* 1971;20(3):177.
[3] Treasure T, et al. *Arch Dis Child.* 1971;46(248):563.
[4] Malherbe C, et al. *N Engl J Med.* 1972;286(7):339.
[5] Stambaugh JE, et al. *Diabetes.* 1974;23(8):679.

* Asterisk indicates drugs cited in interaction reports. Based on pharmacologic and pharmacokinetic considerations, similar interactions may occur with other drugs that are listed.

Sulfonylureas — *Ketoconazole*

Acetohexamide (eg, *Dymelor*)	Glyburide (eg, *DiaBeta*)	Ketoconazole* (eg, *Nizoral*)
Chlorpropamide (eg, *Diabinese*)	Tolazamide	
Glimepiride (eg, *Amaryl*)	Tolbutamide* (eg, *Orinase*)	
Glipizide (eg, *Glucotrol*)		

Significance	Onset	Severity	Documentation
2	□ Rapid	□ Major	□ Established
	■ **Delayed**	■ **Moderate**	□ Probable
		□ Minor	■ **Suspected**
			□ Possible
			□ Unlikely

Effects Serum SULFONYLUREA concentrations may be elevated, increasing the hypoglycemic effect.

Mechanism Possibly inhibition of TOLBUTAMIDE metabolism.

Management In patients receiving TOLBUTAMIDE, consider monitoring blood glucose concentrations and observing the patient for symptoms of hypoglycemia when KETOCONAZOLE is added to or discontinued from the treatment regimen. Adjust the dose of TOLBUTAMIDE accordingly.

Discussion

The effects of ketoconazole on the pharmacokinetics of tolbutamide were studied in 7 healthy men.[1] After an overnight fast, each volunteer received oral tolbutamide 500 mg. Starting the next day, for 7 consecutive days, subjects received ketoconazole 200 mg orally. Following an overnight fast and 30 minutes after administration of the last dose of ketoconazole, each volunteer was given tolbutamide 500 mg. Fasting blood glucose was not altered by ketoconazole treatment. However, during coadministration of ketoconazole, tolbutamide produced mild symptoms of hypoglycemia (eg, weakness, sweating, reeling sensations) in 5 of the subjects. Ketoconazole administration potentiated the blood glucose reduction produced by tolbutamide at 1.5, 2, 3, 4, and 8 hours by a maximum of an additional 15%. The maximum effect occurred at 2 hours. In addition, ketoconazole treatment increased tolbutamide serum concentration, $t_{1/2}$ (from 3.7 to 12.3 hours), and AUC (from 309 to 546 mcg•hr/mL). Hydroxylation clearance of tolbutamide was decreased following ketoconazole administration. See also Sulfonylureas-Fluconazole.

Controlled studies are needed to determine the clinical importance of this possible interaction in diabetic patients.

[1] Krishnaiah YS, et al. *Br J Clin Pharmacol*. 1994;37(2):205.

* Asterisk indicates drugs cited in interaction reports. Based on pharmacologic and pharmacokinetic considerations, similar interactions may occur with other drugs that are listed.

Sulfonylureas | **Loop Diuretics**

Sulfonylureas		Loop Diuretics	
Chlorpropamide (eg, *Diabinese*)	Glyburide (eg, *DiaBeta*)	Bumetanide (eg, *Bumex*)	Furosemide (eg, *Lasix*)
Glimepiride (eg, *Amaryl*)	Tolazamide	Ethacrynic Acid (eg, *Edecrin*)	
Glipizide (eg, *Glucotrol*)	Tolbutamide (eg, *Orinase*)		

Significance	Onset	Severity	Documentation
5	☐ Rapid	☐ Major	☐ Established
	■ **Delayed**	☐ Moderate	☐ Probable
		■ **Minor**	☐ Suspected
			■ **Possible**
			☐ Unlikely

Effects LOOP DIURETICS may decrease glucose tolerance, resulting in hyperglycemia in patients previously well controlled on SULFONYLUREAS.

Mechanism Unknown.

Management The present data do not suggest that any alteration in therapy is necessary.

Discussion

Although some data suggest that loop diuretics are capable of causing hyperglycemia or altered carbohydrate metabolism, other studies report no significant alteration in blood sugar or carbohydrate metabolism.[1-9]

No studies have been published that specifically examine the effect of the addition of a loop diuretic to the regimen of a non-insulin-dependent diabetic patient controlled on a sulfonylurea. Such controlled trials are necessary to clarify the importance of this interaction.

1 Jackson WP, et al. *Br Med J.* 1966;2:333.
2 Toivonen S, et al. *Br Med J.* 1966;1:920.
3 Weller JM, et al. *Metabolism.* 1967;16:532.
4 Andersen OO, et al. *Br Med J.* 1968;2:798.
5 Russell RP, et al. *JAMA.* 1968;205:81.
6 Kohner EM, et al. *Lancet.* 1971;1:986.
7 Giugliano D, et al. *Diabetologia.* 1980;18:293.
8 Robinson DS, et al. *J Clin Pharmacol.* 1981;21:637.
9 Oli JM, et al. *Curr Ther Res.* 1983;34:537.

* Asterisk indicates drugs cited in interaction reports. Based on pharmacologic and pharmacokinetic considerations, similar interactions may occur with other drugs that are listed.

Sulfonylureas | **Macrolide Antibiotics**

Glipizide* (eg, *Glucotrol*)	Glyburide* (eg, *DiaBeta*)	Clarithromycin* (eg, *Biaxin*)

Significance	Onset	Severity	Documentation
4	□ Rapid ■ **Delayed**	□ Major ■ **Moderate** □ Minor	□ Established □ Probable □ Suspected ■ **Possible** □ Unlikely

Effects Hypoglycemic action of SULFONYLUREAS may be increased.

Mechanism Unknown.

Management Monitor blood glucose concentrations and observe patients for signs of hypoglycemia after starting CLARITHROMYCIN.

Discussion

Severe hypoglycemia during coadministration of clarithromycin and sulfonylurea therapy was reported in 2 elderly men.[1] Both patients had type 2 diabetes mellitus that was well controlled in 1 patient by glyburide 5 mg/day and glipizide 15 mg/day in the other individual. Both patients were older than 70 years of age and had moderately impaired renal function, hypertension, atherosclerotic heart disease, and mildly decreased albumin levels. Both patients were diagnosed with bronchitis and were started on clarithromycin 1,000 mg/day. Within 48 hours of starting clarithromycin therapy, the patients developed severe hypoglycemia (*Accu-Chek* reading of 20 mg/dL in 1 patient and 24 mg/dL in the other) and profound mental status changes. Administration of IV dextrose resolved the problem. However, 1 patient experienced a second episode of hypoglycemia 12 hours later that was resolved by administration of IV dextrose. After discontinuing the sulfonylureas, no further episodes of hypoglycemia occurred.

[1] Bussing R, et al. *Diabetes Care*. 2002;25:1659.

* Asterisk indicates drugs cited in interaction reports.

Sulfonylureas — *Magnesium Salts*

Sulfonylureas		Magnesium Salts	
Chlorpropamide* (eg, *Diabinese*)	Glyburide* (eg, *DiaBeta*)	Aluminum Hydroxide/ Magnesium Hydroxide* (eg, *Maalox*)	Magnesium Hydroxide* (eg, *Milk of Magnesia*)
Glipizide* (eg, *Glucotrol*)	Tolbutamide* (eg, *Orinase*)		

Significance	Onset	Severity	Documentation
5	■ **Rapid** □ Delayed	□ Major □ Moderate ■ **Minor**	□ Established □ Probable □ Suspected ■ **Possible** □ Unlikely

Effects Hypoglycemic effects of SULFONYLUREAS increased.

Mechanism Increased or more rapid absorption of SULFONYLUREAS.

Management If an interaction is suspected, measure blood glucose and adjust the SULFONYLUREA dose accordingly.

Discussion

In a single-dose, randomized, crossover study, 8 healthy volunteers received 2.5 mg glyburide with and without an antacid (3.65 g magnesium hydroxide plus 3.25 g aluminum hydroxide).[1] Compared with taking glyburide alone, coadministration of the drugs increased the AUC, peak concentration, and time to reach peak levels. Bioavailability of glyburide was increased 33%. No clinically significant effect was observed. In 7 volunteers, magnesium hydroxide caused similar changes in subjects receiving nonmicronized glyburide compared with the micronized formulation.[2] The effect on the micronized product was less. In another report, magnesium hydroxide caused more rapid absorption of chlorpropamide or tolbutamide.[3] The pharmacologic effect of tolbutamide was increased, but hypoglycemia did not occur. The effects of magnesium hydroxide on the pharmacokinetics and pharmacodynamics of a rapidly absorbed glipizide preparation (*Melizid*; Leiras, Finland) were investigated in a randomized, crossover trial involving 8 healthy volunteers.[4] Each subject received 5 mg glipizide either alone or with 150 mL water containing 850 mg magnesium hydroxide. Compared with the control period, magnesium hydroxide administration significantly increased the AUC of glipizide within the first hour (from 155 to 262 ng•hr/mL). Within this time period, the pharmacologic actions of glipizide were increased. The peak plasma glipizide concentration, time to peak level, total AUC, elimination $t_{1/2}$, and mean residence time were not significantly affected by magnesium hydroxide. The clinical significance of this possible interaction remains to be determined.

[1] Zuccaro P, et al. *Drugs Exp Clin Res.* 1989;15:165.
[2] Neuvonen PJ, et al. *Br J Clin Pharmacol.* 1991;32:215.
[3] Kivisto KT, et al. *Eur J Clin Pharmacol.* 1992;42:675.
[4] Kivisto KT, et al. *Clin Pharmacol Ther.* 1991;49:39.

* Asterisk indicates drugs cited in interaction reports.

Sulfonylureas			*MAOIs*
Chlorpropamide* (eg, *Diabinese*)	Glyburide (eg, *DiaBeta*)	Isocarboxazid (*Marplan*)	Tranylcypromine* (eg, *Parnate*)
Glimepiride (eg, *Amaryl*)	Tolazamide	Phenelzine* (*Nardil*)	
Glipizide (eg, *Glucotrol*)	Tolbutamide* (eg, *Orinase*)		

Significance	Onset	Severity	Documentation
2	■ **Rapid**	□ Major	□ Established
	□ Delayed	■ **Moderate**	□ Probable
		□ Minor	■ **Suspected**
			□ Possible
			□ Unlikely

Effects MAOIs enhance the SULFONYLUREA hypoglycemic action.

Mechanism Unknown.

Management If a patient develops hypoglycemia while taking both medications, tailor the doses to achieve euglycemia.

Discussion

Several case reports suggest that mebanazine, an MAOI, enhances the hypoglycemic action of sulfonylureas and insulin.[1-3] One case report indicates no change in blood glucose concentrations when a patient who was receiving chronic tranylcypromine 90 mg/day and glyburide 5 mg/day had the tranylcypromine discontinued.[4] A study of mebanazine, phenelzine, and tranylcypromine in rabbits indicated that the effect of insulin on blood glucose concentrations was enhanced when mebanazine and phenelzine, but not tranylcypromine, were added.[5]

[1] Cooper AJ. *Int J Neuropsychiatry.* 1966;2:342.
[2] Cooper AJ, et al. *Diabetes.* 1967;16:272.
[3] Adnitt PI. *Diabetes.* 1968;17:628.
[4] Absher JR, et al. *J Clin Psychopharmacol.* 1988;8:379.
[5] Cooper AJ, et al. *Lancet.* 1966;1:407.

* Asterisk indicates drugs cited in interaction reports. Based on pharmacologic and pharmacokinetic considerations, similar interactions may occur with other drugs that are listed.

Sulfonylureas — *Methyldopa*

Sulfonylureas		Methyldopa
Chlorpropamide (eg, *Diabinese*)	Tolazamide	Methyldopa* (eg, *Aldomet*)
Glipizide (eg, *Glucotrol*)	Tolbutamide* (eg, *Orinase*)	
Glyburide (eg, *DiaBeta*)		

Significance	Onset	Severity	Documentation
5	☐ Rapid	☐ Major	☐ Established
	■ **Delayed**	☐ Moderate	☐ Probable
		■ **Minor**	☐ Suspected
			■ **Possible**
			☐ Unlikely

Effects The biologic $t_{½}$ of TOLBUTAMIDE may be prolonged. The hypoglycemic effect may be enhanced if the drug accumulates.

Mechanism METHYLDOPA may impair the metabolic breakdown of TOLBUTAMIDE.

Management Monitor the blood sugar of patients receiving this combination. Reduce the dose of TOLBUTAMIDE if necessary.

Discussion

In 10 patients (3 men, 7 women), tolbutamide $t_{½}$ and its apparent volume of distribution were determined before and after a 1-week course of methyldopa 1 g/day.[1] The $t_{½}$ of tolbutamide increased from 7.18 ± 0.52 to 8.87 ± 0.69 hours. Volume of distribution and metabolic clearance rate were unchanged. Serum glucose concentrations were not measured.

The clinical effect of this interaction and the effect of methyldopa on other sulfonylureas have not been determined.

[1] Gachalyi B, et al. *Int J Clin Pharmacol Ther Toxicol.* 1980;18:133.

* Asterisk indicates drugs cited in interaction reports. Based on pharmacologic and pharmacokinetic considerations, similar interactions may occur with other drugs that are listed.

Sulfonylureas — *Omeprazole*

Chlorpropamide	Tolazamide	Omeprazole* (eg, *Prilosec*)
Glipizide (eg, *Glucotrol*)	Tolbutamide*	
Glyburide (eg, *DiaBeta*)		

Significance	Onset	Severity	Documentation
4	☐ Rapid	☐ Major	☐ Established
	■ **Delayed**	■ **Moderate**	☐ Probable
		☐ Minor	☐ Suspected
			■ **Possible**
			☐ Unlikely

Effects Serum SULFONYLUREA concentrations may be elevated, increasing the hypoglycemic effects.

Mechanism Possible inhibition of SULFONYLUREA metabolism.

Management Based on available information, no special precautions are needed. If an interaction is suspected, adjust the dose of the SULFONYLUREA as indicated.

Discussion

The effects of omeprazole on the pharmacokinetics of tolbutamide were investigated in a placebo-controlled, crossover study involving 16 healthy men.[1] Each subject received either placebo or omeprazole 40 mg/day after breakfast for 7 days. On day 4, a single oral dose of tolbutamide 500 mg was administered 1 hour after omeprazole. Omeprazole administration resulted in a 10% increase in the AUC for tolbutamide.

Although the available data do not indicate that a clinically important interaction will occur with coadministration of tolbutamide and omeprazole, controlled studies are needed in diabetic patients receiving these agents long term to assess the clinical importance of this drug interaction.

[1] Toon S, et al. *J Pharm Pharmacol.* 1995;47(1):85.

* Asterisk indicates drugs cited in interaction reports. Based on pharmacologic and pharmacokinetic considerations, similar interactions may occur with other drugs that are listed.

Sulfonylureas — *Probenecid*

Sulfonylureas		Probenecid
Chlorpropamide*	Glyburide (eg, *DiaBeta*)	Probenecid*
Glimepiride (eg, *Amaryl*)	Tolazamide	
Glipizide (eg, *Glucotrol*)	Tolbutamide*	

Significance	Onset	Severity	Documentation
4	☐ Rapid	☐ Major	☐ Established
	■ **Delayed**	■ **Moderate**	☐ Probable
		☐ Minor	☐ Suspected
			■ **Possible**
			☐ Unlikely

Effects The actions of CHLORPROPAMIDE may be enhanced.

Mechanism It has been postulated that PROBENECID may compete with CHLORPROPAMIDE for renal tubular excretion, resulting in CHLORPROPAMIDE accumulation.

Management Monitor blood glucose levels and decrease the dose of CHLORPROPAMIDE if indicated.

Discussion

Only 1 study, which included 6 patients, has documented this interaction.[1] The study reported a mean chlorpropamide $t_{1/2}$ of 35.6 ± 11.8 hours in controls and a mean $t_{1/2}$ of 50 ± 27 hours in patients treated concurrently with probenecid 1 to 2 g/day. No information was reported concerning any correlation between the increase in chlorpropamide $t_{1/2}$ and changes in the clinical condition of the patients.

A preliminary report described a prolongation of the plasma $t_{1/2}$ of tolbutamide in 2 patients who were administered probenecid.[2] However, a subsequent controlled trial in 8 healthy volunteers refuted these earlier findings.[3] Additional clinical studies are required to evaluate the clinical importance of this possible interaction.

[1] Petitpierre B, et al. *Int J Clin Pharmacol.* 1972;6(2):120.

[2] Stowers JM, et al. *Lancet.* 1958;1(7015):278.

[3] Brook R, et al. *Clin Pharmacol Ther.* 1968;9(3):314.

* Asterisk indicates drugs cited in interaction reports. Based on pharmacologic and pharmacokinetic considerations, similar interactions may occur with other drugs that are listed.

Sulfonylureas		*Quinolones*	
Glimepiride* (eg, *Amaryl*)	Glyburide* (eg, *DiaBeta*)	Ciprofloxacin* (eg, *Cipro*) Gatifloxacin* (eg, *Zymar*)	Levofloxacin (eg, *Levaquin*)

Significance	Onset	Severity	Documentation
1	■ **Rapid** ☐ Delayed	■ **Major** ☐ Moderate ☐ Minor	☐ Established ☐ Probable ■ **Suspected** ☐ Possible ☐ Unlikely

Effects Severe and persistent hypoglycemia may occur.

Mechanism Unknown; however, GATIFLOXACIN does not affect glucose tolerance or pancreatic beta-cell function.[1]

Management Avoid certain QUINOLONES in patients receiving SULFONYLUREA therapy. If therapy cannot be avoided, closely monitor blood glucose when starting certain QUINOLONES. If hypoglycemia occurs, it may be necessary to discontinue both agents before resuming SULFONYLUREA therapy.

Discussion

Severe and persistent hypoglycemia was reported in 2 patients with type 2 diabetes mellitus during administration of gatifloxacin and oral sulfonylurea hypoglycemic agents.[2] One patient was receiving glyburide 5 mg/day and pioglitazone (*Actos*) 30 mg/day for diabetes. Her blood glucose was 217 mg/dL 2 hours after the morning doses of hypoglycemic agents and 4 hours before the start of gatifloxacin 200 mg/day. The patient's blood glucose was measured at 42 mg/dL 45 min after gatifloxacin administration. When gatifloxacin, glyburide, and pioglitazone were withheld, her blood glucose returned to between 100 and 200 mg/dL. Glyburide and pioglitazone were restarted 2 days later without further episodes of hypoglycemia. The second patient was receiving glimepiride 2 mg before breakfast and 1 mg before dinner. Her blood glucose levels ranged from 150 to 250 mg/dL. Glimepiride was withheld when IV gatifloxacin 400 mg/day and clindamycin (eg, *Cleocin*) were started. Her blood glucose levels ranged from 75 to 150 mg/dL. The patient became diaphoretic and clammy (blood glucose, 22 mg/dL) 12 hours after gatifloxacin was given. The next day, gatifloxacin and glimepiride were discontinued. Her blood glucose returned to the 150 to 250 mg/dL range. Subsequently, glimepiride was restarted without further episodes of hypoglycemia. Hypoglycemia and an elevated plasma glyburide level were reported in a patient 1 wk after starting ciprofloxacin.[3] The patient had been receiving long-term therapy with glyburide. Severe, life-threatening hypoglycemia precipitated by ciprofloxacin was reported in a 65-year-old woman receiving glipizide.[4] Although hypoglycemia has been reported in patients receiving quinolones alone, avoid coadministration of quinolones and sulfonylureas until additional data are available. See also Pioglitazone-Quinolones, Repaglinide-Quinolones.

[1] Gajjar DA, et al. *Pharmacotherapy*. 2000;20(6, pt 2):76S.
[2] Menzies DJ, et al. *Am J Med*. 2002;113(3):232.
[3] Roberge RJ, et al. *Ann Emerg Med*. 2000;36(2):160.
[4] Kelesidis T, et al. *Am J Med*. 2010;123(2):e5.

* Asterisk indicates drugs cited in interaction reports. Based on pharmacologic and pharmacokinetic considerations, similar interactions may occur with other drugs that are listed.

Sulfonylureas — *Rifamycins*

Sulfonylureas		Rifamycins	
Chlorpropamide*	Glyburide* (eg, *DiaBeta*)	Rifabutin (*Mycobutin*)	Rifapentine (*Priftin*)
Glimepiride* (eg, *Amaryl*)	Tolazamide	Rifampin* (eg, *Rifadin*)	
Glipizide (eg, *Glucotrol*)	Tolbutamide* (eg, *Orinase*)		

Significance	Onset	Severity	Documentation
2	□ Rapid	□ Major	□ Established
	■ **Delayed**	■ **Moderate**	■ **Probable**
		□ Minor	□ Suspected
			□ Possible
			□ Unlikely

Effects RIFAMYCINS may decrease the $t_{1/2}$ and serum levels while increasing the clearance of some SULFONYLUREAS, possibly resulting in hyperglycemia.

Mechanism The hepatic metabolism of certain SULFONYLUREAS may be increased by RIFAMYCINS.

Management Closely monitor blood glucose. The dose of the SULFONYLUREA may need to be increased.

Discussion

Three studies have shown that the administration of a single dose of tolbutamide after rifampin therapy results in a decreased tolbutamide $t_{1/2}$ of 43% to 56% and an increased plasma clearance of 55% to 76%.[1-3] In 1 investigation, the serum level of tolbutamide was decreased (30% 3 hr after the dose, 49% 6 hr after the dose).[2] However, there was no difference in blood glucose values following coadministration compared with pretreatment values.[2] In a study of healthy volunteers, rifampin reduced the AUC of glimepiride 34% and the $t_{1/2}$ 25% (from 2.6 to 2 hr).[4] Rifampin 600 mg/day for 5 days decreased the $t_{1/2}$ of glyburide from 2 to 1.7 hr and glipizide from 3 to 1.9 hr.[5] The effect on the AUC and blood glucose response was statistically significant only for glyburide. Another study in which healthy volunteers received oral rifampin and glyburide reported that rifampin administration resulted in a 63% decrease in glyburide AUC.[6] In a case report, a patient maintained on chlorpropamide 250 mg/day for 6 years started therapy with isoniazid 300 mg/day and rifampin 600 mg/day.[7] Within 1 month, the chlorpropamide dosage was increased to 400 mg/day because of an increase in blood glucose; the serum chlorpropamide level was decreased 66%. When rifampin was discontinued, the patient's chlorpropamide concentration increased, and the blood glucose level decreased. In another case report, a 67-year-old woman taking glyburide 5 mg/day required increased doses of glyburide and the addition of insulin after starting treatment with isoniazid and rifampin 600 mg/day. Upon discontinuing rifampin, serum glyburide levels increased markedly.[8]

[1] Zilly W, et al. *Eur J Clin Pharmacol.* 1975;9(2-3):219.
[2] Syvälahti E, et al. *Int J Clin Pharmacol Biopharm.* 1976;13(2):83.
[3] Zilly W, et al. *Eur J Clin Pharmacol.* 1977;11(4):287.
[4] Niemi M, et al. *Br J Clin Pharmacol.* 2000;50(6):591.
[5] Niemi M, et al. *Clin Pharmacol Ther.* 2001;69(6):400.
[6] Zheng HX, et al. *Clin Pharmacol Ther.* 2009;85(1):78.
[7] Self TH, et al. *Chest.* 1980;77(6):800.
[8] Self TH, et al. *Chest.* 1989;96(6):1443.

* Asterisk indicates drugs cited in interaction reports. Based on pharmacologic and pharmacokinetic considerations, similar interactions may occur with other drugs that are listed.

Sulfonylureas — *Salicylates*

Sulfonylureas		Salicylates	
Chlorpropamide*	Tolazamide	Aspirin* (eg, *Bayer*)	Salsalate (eg, *Amigesic*)
Glimepiride (eg, *Amaryl*)	Tolbutamide* (eg, *Orinase*)	Magnesium Salicylate (eg, *Doan's*)	Sodium Salicylate*†
Glipizide (eg, *Glucotrol*)			
Glyburide* (eg, *DiaBeta*)			

Significance	Onset	Severity	Documentation
2	☐ Rapid	☐ Major	☐ Established
	■ **Delayed**	■ **Moderate**	■ **Probable**
		☐ Minor	☐ Suspected
			☐ Possible
			☐ Unlikely

Effects Increased hypoglycemic effect of SULFONYLUREAS.

Mechanism SALICYLATES reduce basal plasma glucose levels and enhance insulin secretion. Inhibition of prostaglandin synthesis may inhibit acute insulin responses to glucose. Displaced SULFONYLUREA protein binding has been suggested.

Management Monitor the patient's blood glucose. If hypoglycemia develops, consider decreasing the SULFONYLUREA dose. Consider alternative therapy with acetaminophen (eg, *Tylenol*) or an NSAID (eg, sulindac [eg, *Clinoril*]).[1]

Discussion

Many studies show that salicylates reduce basal plasma glucose levels, increase glucose tolerance, and augment acute insulin response.[2-19] When salicylates are coadministered with sulfonylureas, the hypoglycemic effect may be increased. In 2 reports, salicylates had no effect on nondiabetic subjects.[4,6] In 1 study in healthy volunteers, the coadministration of single doses of chlorpropamide 200 mg and sodium salicylate 3 g was additive in reducing blood glucose.[16] When the dose of each drug was halved, the response was no different than the response to either agent alone at the higher dose. In 21 healthy volunteers, aspirin 3.2 g/day for 3 days enhanced basal insulin levels, arginine-stimulated insulin secretion, and tolbutamide-stimulated insulin secretion with corresponding decreases in glycemia.[18]

1 Tatro DS. *Pharm Pract News.* 1996;23:6.
2 Stowers JM, et al. *Ann N Y Acad Sci.* 1959;74(3):689.
3 Hecht A, et al. *Metabolism.* 1959;8(4, pt 1):418.
4 Gilgore SG, et al. *Metabolism.* 1961;10:419.
5 Wishinsky H, et al. *Diabetes.* 1962;11(suppl):18.
6 Field JB, et al. *Lancet.* 1967;1(7501):1191.
7 Peaston MJ, et al. *Br J Clin Pract.* 1968;22:30.
8 Schulz E. *Arch Klin Med.* 1968;214(2):135.
9 Robertson RP, et al. *J Clin Invest.* 1977;60(3):747.
10 Giugliano D, et al. *Diabetologia.* 1978;14(6):359.
11 Chen M, et al. *Diabetes.* 1978;27(7):750.
12 Torella R, et al. *Metabolism.* 1979;28(9):887.
13 Micossi P, et al. *Diabetes.* 1978;27(12):1196.
14 Prince RL, et al. *Metabolism.* 1981;30(3):293.
15 Giugliano D, et al. *J Clin Endocrinol Metab.* 1985;61(1):160.
16 Richardson T, et al. *Br J Clin Pharmacol.* 1986;22(1):43.
17 Giugliano D, et al. *Diabete Metab.* 1988;14(4):431.
18 Cattaneo AG, et al. *Int J Clin Pharmacol Ther Toxicol.* 1990;28(6):229.
19 Kubacka RT, et al. *Ann Pharmacother.* 1996;30(1):20.

* Asterisk indicates drugs cited in interaction reports. Based on pharmacologic and pharmacokinetic considerations, similar interactions may occur with other drugs that are listed.
† Not available in the United States.

Sulfonylureas — *Sulfinpyrazone*

Tolbutamide*	Sulfinpyrazone*†

Significance	Onset	Severity	Documentation
2	☐ Rapid	☐ Major	☐ Established
	■ **Delayed**	■ **Moderate**	☐ Probable
		☐ Minor	■ **Suspected**
			☐ Possible
			☐ Unlikely

Effects SULFINPYRAZONE may decrease the clearance and increase the $t_{1/2}$ of TOLBUTAMIDE; hypoglycemia may result.

Mechanism SULFINPYRAZONE impairs the hepatic metabolic conversion of TOLBUTAMIDE.

Management Monitor blood glucose during concurrent TOLBUTAMIDE and SULFINPYRAZONE therapy. The dose of TOLBUTAMIDE may need to be decreased.

Discussion

In 6 healthy subjects, the coadministration of a single dose of IV tolbutamide 500 mg and a dose of oral sulfinpyrazone 400 mg was followed by 7 days of sulfinpyrazone 200 mg every 6 hours and another IV dose of tolbutamide 24 hours after the last sulfinpyrazone dose.[1] When the 2 agents were administered simultaneously, the mean $t_{1/2}$ of tolbutamide increased 80% and its mean clearance decreased 40% compared with tolbutamide alone. When tolbutamide was administered 24 hours after 7 days of sulfinpyrazone, its $t_{1/2}$ increased 19% and its plasma clearance increased 30%; no sulfinpyrazone was detected in the plasma of the subjects at this time. In vitro studies indicated that sulfinpyrazone displaces tolbutamide from protein-binding sites, but is concentration-dependent; therefore, it is only apparent at high sulfinpyrazone concentrations. However, sulfinpyrazone had a negligible effect on protein binding of tolbutamide in vivo.

In a study of 19 patients with diabetes, sulfinpyrazone had no effect on glyburide.[2] It is not known whether sulfinpyrazone would interact with the other sulfonylureas.

[1] Miners JO, et al. *Eur J Clin Pharmacol.* 1982;22(4):321.

[2] Kritz H, et al. *Wien Med Wochenschr.* 1983;133(9):237.

* Asterisk indicates drugs cited in interaction reports.
† Not available in the United States.

Sulfonylureas | **Sulfonamides**

Chlorpropamide*	Tolazamide	Multiple Sulfonamides	Sulfasalazine (eg, *Azulfidine*)
Glimepiride (eg, *Amaryl*)	Tolbutamide*	Sulfamethizole*†	Sulfisoxazole*
Glipizide* (eg, *Glucotrol*)		Sulfamethoxazole*†	

Significance	Onset	Severity	Documentation
2	□ Rapid	□ Major	□ Established
	■ **Delayed**	■ **Moderate**	□ Probable
		□ Minor	■ **Suspected**
			□ Possible
			□ Unlikely

Effects The coadministration of SULFONAMIDES and SULFONYLUREAS may increase the $t_{½}$ of the SULFONYLUREA; hypoglycemia may occur.

Mechanism SULFONAMIDES may impair hepatic metabolism of SULFONYLUREAS or alter plasma protein binding.

Management Monitor blood glucose. The SULFONYLUREA dose may need to be decreased. Glyburide may be a noninteracting alternative.

Discussion

Administration of a sulfonamide with tolbutamide or chlorpropamide may result in hypoglycemia. In volunteers given a single IV dose of tolbutamide after trimethoprim/sulfamethoxazole (TMP/SMZ) or either component alone for 7 days, the total clearance of tolbutamide was affected most by the combination.[1] Sulfamethizole increased the $t_{½}$ of tolbutamide 54% to 61% in several patients.[2,3] Hypoglycemia occurred in 1 patient receiving tolbutamide and sulfisoxazole.[4] In several patients, sulfaphenazole† prolonged the $t_{½}$ of tolbutamide 3- to 6-fold.[5-7] In contrast, the $t_{½}$ of tolbutamide was not prolonged or affected by other sulfonamides.[3] In 2 case reports, concurrent chlorpropamide and TMP/SMZ or sulfisoxazole caused hypoglycemia.[8,9] In a hospitalized elderly patient taking glipizide, TMP/SMZ produced symptomatic hypoglycemia.[10] In contrast, a study in 8 healthy volunteers failed to detect a pharmacokinetic interaction or an altered hypoglycemic response with glipizide when TMP/SMZ was given.[11] In 8 patients, the plasma levels or bioavailability of glyburide (eg, *DiaBeta*) were not affected by TMP/SMZ.[12]

1 Christensen LK, et al. *Lancet.* 1963;2(7321):1298.
2 Soeldner JS, et al. *JAMA.* 1965;193(5):398.
3 Dubach VC, et al. *Schweiz Med Wochenschr.* 1966;96:1483.
4 Tucker HS Jr, et al. *N Engl J Med.* 1972;286(2):110.
5 Siersbaek-Nielsen K, et al. *Clin Pharmacol Ther.* 1973;14:148.
6 Lumholtz B, et al. *Clin Pharmacol Ther.* 1975;17(6):731.
7 Pond SM, et al. *Clin Pharmacol Ther.* 1977;22(5, pt 1):573.
8 Baciewicz AM, et al. *Drug Intell Clin Pharm.* 1984;18(4):309.
9 Wing LM, et al. *Br J Clin Pharmacol.* 1985;20(5):482.
10 Sjöberg S, et al. *Diabet Med.* 1987;4(3):245.
11 Johnson JF, et al. *DICP.* 1990;24(3):250.
12 Kradjan WA, et al. *J Clin Pharmacol.* 1994;34(10):997.

* Asterisk indicates drugs cited in interaction reports. Based on pharmacologic and pharmacokinetic considerations, similar interactions may occur with other drugs that are listed.
† Not available in the United States.

Sulfonylureas / *Thiazide Diuretics*

Sulfonylureas		Thiazide Diuretics	
Chlorpropamide* (eg, *Diabinese*)	Glyburide (eg, *DiaBeta*)	Bendroflumethiazide (*Naturetin*)	Hydroflumethiazide*†
Glimepiride (eg, *Amaryl*)	Tolazamide	Chlorothiazide* (eg, *Diuril*)	Indapamide (eg, *Lozol*)
Glipizide (eg, *Glucotrol*)	Tolbutamide* (eg, *Orinase*)	Chlorthalidone (eg, *Hygroton*)	Methyclothiazide (eg, *Enduron*)
		Hydrochlorothiazide* (eg, *HydroDIURIL*)	Metolazone (eg, *Zaroxolyn*)

Significance	Onset	Severity	Documentation
2	□ Rapid	□ Major	□ Established
	■ **Delayed**	■ **Moderate**	■ **Probable**
		□ Minor	□ Suspected
			□ Possible
			□ Unlikely

Effects THIAZIDE DIURETICS increase fasting blood glucose and may decrease SULFONYLUREA hypoglycemia. This effect may occur after several days to many months of THIAZIDE therapy. Hyponatremia also may occur.

Mechanism THIAZIDE DIURETICS may decrease insulin tissue sensitivity, decrease insulin secretion, or increase potassium loss, causing hyperglycemia.

Management Closely monitor blood glucose. If hyperglycemia develops, possibly increase the SULFONYLUREA dose.

Discussion

Many studies have shown that thiazide and related diuretics increase fasting blood glucose, possibly decreasing the hypoglycemic effect of coadministered sulfonylureas.[1-13] The effects of this interaction may occur within days or months of initiating therapy. When the thiazide diuretic is discontinued, a decrease in blood glucose levels occurs, indicating thiazide-induced hyperglycemia is reversible. Hyperosmolar nonketotic coma also has been associated with the use of thiazide diuretics.[14] Symptoms are often not severe enough to warrant drug discontinuation. This interaction appears more likely to occur in diabetic patients or those with a predisposition to diabetes.[1-3] Hyponatremia also has occurred.[15,16]

1 Goldner MG, et al. *N Engl J Med.* 1960;262:403.
2 Shapiro AP, et al. *N Engl J Med.* 1961;265:1028.
3 Runyan JW Jr. *N Engl J Med.* 1962;267:541.
4 Samaan N, et al. *Lancet.* 1963;47:1244.
5 Carliner NH, et al. *JAMA.* 1965;191:535.
6 Fajans SS, et al. *J Clin Invest.* 1966;45:481.
7 Breckenridge A, et al. *Lancet.* 1967;1:61.
8 Malins JM. *Practitioner.* 1968;201:357.
9 Tranquada RE. *JAMA.* 1968;206:1580.
10 Kansal PC, et al. *South Med J.* 1969;62:1372.
11 Lewis PJ, et al. *Lancet.* 1976;1:564.
12 Amery A, et al. *Lancet.* 1978;1:681.
13 Murphy MB, et al. *Lancet.* 1982;2:1293.
14 Gerich JE, et al. *Diabetes.* 1971;20:228.
15 Fichman MP, et al. *Ann Intern Med.* 1971;75:853.
16 Zalin AM, et al. *Br Med J (Clin Res Ed).* 1984;289:659.

* Asterisk indicates drugs cited in interaction reports. Based on pharmacologic and pharmacokinetic considerations, similar interactions may occur with other drugs that are listed.
† Not available in the United States.

Sulfonylureas — *Tricyclic Antidepressants*

Chlorpropamide* (eg, *Diabinese*)	Tolazamide*	Doxepin* (eg, *Sinequan*)	Nortriptyline* (eg, *Pamelor*)

Significance	Onset	Severity	Documentation
4	☐ Rapid	☐ Major	☐ Established
	■ **Delayed**	■ **Moderate**	☐ Probable
		☐ Minor	☐ Suspected
			■ **Possible**
			☐ Unlikely

Effects The pharmacologic effects of SULFONYLUREAS may be increased.

Mechanism Unknown.

Management If an interaction is suspected, measure blood glucose and adjust the dose accordingly.

Discussion

Two cases of severe hypoglycemia have been reported following coadministration of sulfonylurea oral hypoglycemic agents and tricyclic antidepressants.[1] One patient, a 71-year-old woman, had stable but elevated blood glucose while receiving tolazamide 1 g/day for at least 6 months prior to the addition of doxepin to her regimen. Eleven days after the start of doxepin therapy, the patient experienced a dramatic decrease in blood glucose. After improvement, the patient was restarted on doxepin and tolazamide 100 mg/day without further episodes of hypoglycemia. The second patient, a 59-year-old woman receiving chronic treatment with chlorpropamide, experienced hypoglycemia 4 days after the start of nortriptyline therapy.

A causal relationship cannot be established in these cases. Additional studies are needed to determine the clinical importance of this potential interaction.

[1] True BL, et al. *Am J Psychiatry*. 1987;144:1220.

* Asterisk indicates drugs cited in interaction reports.

Sulfonylureas	***Urinary Acidifiers***
Chlorpropamide* (eg, *Diabinese*)	Ammonium Chloride* Potassium Acid Phosphate (*K-Phos Original*) Sodium Acid Phosphate

Significance	Onset	Severity	Documentation
3	☐ Rapid ■ **Delayed**	☐ Major ☐ Moderate ■ **Minor**	☐ Established ☐ Probable ■ **Suspected** ☐ Possible ☐ Unlikely

Effects Acidification of the urine by agents such as AMMONIUM CHLORIDE may increase the bioavailability of CHLORPROPAMIDE; hypoglycemic actions may be enhanced.

Mechanism Urinary pH appears to determine the relative contribution of metabolic and renal clearance of CHLORPROPAMIDE; with an acidic urine, metabolic clearance dominates elimination and renal clearance is decreased.

Management Monitor patient's blood glucose during coadministration of CHLORPROPAMIDE and a URINARY ACIDIFIER; a lower CHLORPROPAMIDE dose may be necessary.

Discussion

Six subjects were given a single 250 mg dose of chlorpropamide, and the urine was acidified to pH 4.7 to 5.5 with ammonium chloride.[1] The amount of ammonium chloride taken between 1 and 64 hours after chlorpropamide to keep the urine acidic was 21.2 g. Compared to controls, the chlorpropamide half-life increased from 49.7 to 68.5 hours (38%), the AUC increased by 41%, and total clearance was reduced by 28%. The cumulative 72 hour urinary excretion of chlorpropamide was decreased from 50.9 to 3.5 mg, which accounted for less than 1.5% of the dose.

It is not known if other sulfonylureas would be similarly affected. See also Sulfonylureas-Urinary Alkalinizers.

[1] Neuvonen PJ, et al. *Clin Pharmacol Ther.* 1983;33:386.

* Asterisk indicates drugs cited in interaction reports. Based on pharmacologic and pharmacokinetic considerations, similar interactions may occur with other drugs that are listed.

Sulfonylureas		***Urinary Alkalinizers***	
Chlorpropamide* (eg, *Diabinese*)		Potassium Citrate (*Urocit-K*)	Sodium Citrate
		Sodium Acetate	Sodium Lactate
		Sodium Bicarbonate*	Tromethamine (*Tham, Tham-E*)

Significance	Onset	Severity	Documentation
2	☐ Rapid	☐ Major	☐ Established
	■ **Delayed**	■ **Moderate**	☐ Probable
		☐ Minor	■ **Suspected**
			☐ Possible
			☐ Unlikely

Effects Alkalinization of the urine by an agent such as SODIUM BICARBONATE may increase the elimination of CHLORPROPAMIDE. This may be useful in the treatment of CHLORPROPAMIDE intoxication; however, patients taking SODIUM BICARBONATE for other reasons may have a decreased therapeutic response to CHLORPROPAMIDE.

Mechanism The renal clearance of CHLORPROPAMIDE increases as urinary pH increases. It appears that urinary pH affects the ratio of renal and metabolic clearance.

Management Alkalinization of the urine may be useful in the treatment of CHLORPROPAMIDE toxicity. However, the dose of CHLORPROPAMIDE may need to be increased in a patient routinely taking SODIUM BICARBONATE. Monitor the patient's blood glucose during coadministration.

Discussion

In a study of six subjects, a single dose of chlorpropamide 250 mg was followed by sodium bicarbonate starting 1 hour after chlorpropamide to keep the urine alkaline at pH 7.1 to 8.2 (mean sodium bicarbonate dose between 1 and 64 hours: 41.5 g).[1] The absorption of chlorpropamide was increased by sodium bicarbonate based on a decreased time to peak concentration of 42.5% (from 4.7 to 2.7 hours). The elimination half-life of chlorpropamide decreased from 49.7 to 12.8 hours (74.2%) with an alkaline urine, and total clearance increased approximately 400%. Cumulative 72 hour urinary excretion was 85% of the dose, which is approximately 4 times that during the control phase.

Sodium bicarbonate appears useful in the treatment of chlorpropamide intoxication. It is not known if alkalinization of the urine would affect the elimination of the other sulfonylureas.

[1] Neuvonen PJ, et al. *Clin Pharmacol Ther.* 1983;33:386.

* Asterisk indicates drugs cited in interaction reports. Based on pharmacologic and pharmacokinetic considerations, similar interactions may occur with other drugs that are listed.

Sulindac — *Dimethyl Sulfoxide (DMSO)*

Sulindac* (eg, *Clinoril*)	Dimethyl Sulfoxide (DMSO)* (*Rimso-50*)

Significance	Onset	Severity	Documentation
4	☐ Rapid ■ **Delayed**	☐ Major ■ **Moderate** ☐ Minor	☐ Established ☐ Probable ☐ Suspected ■ **Possible** ☐ Unlikely

Effects The administration of DIMETHYL SULFOXIDE (DMSO) may decrease the formation of the active metabolite of SULINDAC, possibly resulting in a decreased therapeutic effect. Severe peripheral neuropathy also has occurred when topical DMSO was used concurrently with SULINDAC.

Mechanism DMSO appears to competitively inhibit SULINDAC reductase, thereby decreasing the formation of the active sulfide metabolite. The mechanism for the occurrence of peripheral neuropathy is unknown.

Management Because the therapeutic effect of SULINDAC may be decreased and because peripheral neuropathy may develop with concurrent DMSO, consider avoiding coadministration.

Discussion

In a study of 8 healthy volunteers, the administration of a single dose of sulindac 400 mg 60 minutes after DMSO 70% oral solution resulted in lower plasma concentrations of the active sulfide metabolite of sulindac.[1] The mean AUC of the metabolite was decreased 30%. Similarly, in an animal study, DMSO decreased the formation of the sulfide metabolite.[2]

In 2 case reports, concurrent use of sulindac 150 to 200 mg twice daily and topical application of DMSO (90% in 1 patient) resulted in peripheral neuropathy that manifested slowly and became more severe as coadministration continued.[3,4] Symptoms included progressive loss of normal gait, myalgia, cramps, fasciculations, wasting of thigh and leg muscles, and difficulty in standing and walking. One patient gradually improved over 1 year following the discontinuation of DMSO; sulindac therapy was continued.

[1] Swanson BN, et al. *J Lab Clin Med.* 1983;102(1):95.
[2] Swanson BN, et al. *Drug Metab Dispos.* 1981;9(6):499.
[3] Reinstein L, et al. *Arch Phys Med Rehabil.* 1982;63(11):581.
[4] Swanson BN, et al. *Arthritis Rheum.* 1983;26(6):791.

* Asterisk indicates drugs cited in interaction reports.

Sunitinib — **Food**

Sunitinib*
(*Sutent*)

Grapefruit Juice*

Significance	Onset	Severity	Documentation
3	☐ Rapid	☐ Major	☐ Established
	■ **Delayed**	☐ Moderate	☐ Probable
		■ **Minor**	■ **Suspected**
			☐ Possible
			☐ Unlikely

Effects SUNITINIB plasma concentrations may be slightly elevated, increasing the risk of adverse reactions.

Mechanism Inhibition of SUNITINIB metabolism (CYP3A4) by GRAPEFRUIT products.

Management Based on available data, no special precautions are needed.

Discussion

The manufacturer of sunitinib states that grapefruit ingestion may increase sunitinib plasma concentrations.[1] The effect of grapefruit juice on steady-state sunitinib pharmacokinetics was studied in 8 cancer patients receiving sunitinib monotherapy.[2] Taking sunitinib with grapefruit juice increased the bioavailability of sunitinib 11% compared with taking sunitinib without grapefruit juice.

[1] *Sutent* [package insert]. New York, NY: Pfizer Labs; May 2011.

[2] van Erp NP, et al. *Cancer Chemother Pharmacol.* 2011;67(3):695.

* Asterisk indicates drugs cited in interaction reports.

Sympathomimetics (Beta-Agonists) — *Beta-Blockers*

Sympathomimetics (Beta-Agonists)		Beta-Blockers	
Albuterol* (eg, *Proventil*)	Levalbuterol* (eg, *Xopenex*)	Carteolol*	Propranolol* (eg, *Inderal*)
Arformoterol* (*Brovana*)	Salmeterol* (*Serevent*)	Nadolol* (eg, *Corgard*)	Sotalol* (eg, *Betapace*)
Bitolterol*†	Terbutaline*	Penbutolol* (*Levatol*)	Timolol*
Formoterol* (eg, *Foradil*)		Pindolol*	

Significance	Onset	Severity	Documentation
1	■ **Rapid**	■ **Major**	□ Established
	□ Delayed	□ Moderate	□ Probable
		□ Minor	■ **Suspected**
			□ Possible
			□ Unlikely

Effects Pharmacologic effects of SYMPATHOMIMETIC BETA-AGONISTS may be antagonized by BETA-BLOCKERS. Bronchospasm may occur.

Mechanism Pharmacologic effects of SYMPATHOMIMETIC BETA-AGONISTS may be antagonized by noncardioselective BETA-BLOCKERS.

Management If possible, avoid coadministration of these agents. If a BETA-BLOCKER is necessary, consider cautiously using a cardioselective BETA-BLOCKER.

Discussion

Beta-adrenergic receptor blocking agents (eg, propranolol) may block the pulmonary effect of beta-agonists (eg, albuterol) and may produce severe bronchospasm in asthmatic patients.[1] Usually, patients with asthma should not be treated with beta-blockers. Although, under certain circumstances (eg, prophylaxis after MI), there may not be a suitable alternative to beta-adrenergic blocking agents in asthma patients. In this situation, consider administering cardioselective beta-blockers; however, use cardioselective agents with caution. In a study of 6 healthy men, propranolol 40 mg was more effective than the cardioselective agent atenolol (eg, *Tenormin*) 100 mg in reversing symptomatic salmeterol overdose.[2]

[1] *Proventil HFA* [package insert]. Kenilworth, NJ: Key Pharmaceuticals Inc; October 2001.

[2] Minton NA, et al. *Eur J Clin Pharmacol.* 1989;36(5):449.

* Asterisk indicates drugs cited in interaction reports.
† Not available in the United States.

Sympathomimetics — *Desflurane*

Dobutamine*	Dopamine*	Desflurane* (*Suprane*)

Significance	Onset	Severity	Documentation
4	■ **Rapid** □ Delayed	■ **Major** □ Moderate □ Minor	□ Established □ Probable □ Suspected ■ **Possible** □ Unlikely

Effects Death associated with cardiac ischemia has been reported.

Mechanism Unknown.

Management This drug interaction has not been proven; however, because of its severity, consider the possibility of this drug interaction.

Discussion

In 21 consecutive patients undergoing advanced head and neck reconstructive surgery, 4 deaths associated with cardiac ischemia were reported.[1] The fatalities occurred in patients receiving desflurane inhalation anesthesia plus dobutamine or dopamine 5 to 10 mcg•kg/min. All patients experienced sudden bradycardia or tachycardia associated with ST-segment ECG changes. The 4 patients who died had a history of coronary artery disease. One patient died during surgery and the other 3 patients died 1, 2, and 12 days after surgery. A causal relationship has not been proven between coadministration of desflurane anesthesia with dobutamine or dopamine and fatal cardiac outcomes.

Because of the seriousness of the cardiac outcomes, clinical evaluation of this interaction in humans is not likely to be forthcoming.

[1] Murray JM, et al. *Can J Anaesth.* 1998;45(12):1200.

* Asterisk indicates drugs cited in interaction reports.

Sympathomimetics — *Furazolidone*

Sympathomimetics		Furazolidone
Dobutamine (eg, *Dobutrex*)	Metaraminol (*Aramine*)	Furazolidone*†
Dopamine (eg, *Intropin*)	Norepinephrine (eg, *Levophed*)	
Ephedrine	Phenylephrine (eg, *Neo-Synephrine*)	
Epinephrine (eg, *Adrenalin*)	Pseudoephedrine (eg, *Sudafed*)	
Mephentermine (*Wyamine*)		

Significance	Onset	Severity	Documentation
1	■ **Rapid**	■ **Major**	□ Established
	□ Delayed	□ Moderate	□ Probable
		□ Minor	■ **Suspected**
			□ Possible
			□ Unlikely

Effects

FURAZOLIDONE may increase the pressor sensitivity to mixed and indirect-acting SYMPATHOMIMETICS possibly resulting in hypertension. Direct-acting SYMPATHOMIMETICS (eg, dobutamine [eg, *Dobutrex*]) are not affected.

Mechanism

SYMPATHOMIMETICS with mixed and indirect-acting activity liberate large amounts of norepinephrine during MAO inhibition; FURAZOLIDONE inhibits MAO inhibitors.

Management

Avoid the coadministration of FURAZOLIDONE and mixed or indirect-acting SYMPATHOMIMETICS. If these agents are used concurrently, monitor the patient; if a hypertensive crisis results, consider using phentolamine (eg, *Regitine*).

Discussion

Furazolidone, an antibacterial agent with MAO inhibitory activity, may increase the pressor response of mixed or indirect-acting sympathomimetics in a manner similar to the other MAO inhibitors, which would result in hypertension.[1-3] In 1 study, 10 patients received tyramine (indirect-acting, metabolized by MAO), dextroamphetamine (indirect-acting, not a substrate for MAO), and norepinephrine (direct-acting) IV until the systolic pressure was 25 mm Hg for norepinephrine or at least 30 mm Hg for the other 2 agents.[3] Furazolidone 400 to 800 mg/day increased the sensitivity to tyramine and dextroamphetamine approximately 2- to 4-fold. When furazolidone was administered for at least 2 weeks, the pressor sensitivity increased to a greater extent.[2] The pressor sensitivity to norepinephrine was not affected. See also Sympathomimetics-MAO Inhibitors.

[1] Stern IJ, et al. *J Pharmacol Exp Ther.* 1967;156:492.
[2] Pettinger WA, et al. *Clin Pharmacol Ther.* 1968;9:341.
[3] Pettinger WA, et al. *Clin Pharmacol Ther.* 1968;9:442.

* Asterisk indicates drugs cited in interaction reports. Based on pharmacologic and pharmacokinetic considerations, similar interactions may occur with other drugs that are listed.
† Not available in the United States.

Sympathomimetics ✕ *Histamine H_2 Antagonists*

Dobutamine*	Cimetidine* (eg, *Tagamet*)

Significance	Onset	Severity	Documentation
4	■ **Rapid** ☐ Delayed	☐ Major ■ **Moderate** ☐ Minor	☐ Established ☐ Probable ☐ Suspected ■ **Possible** ☐ Unlikely

Effects The pressor effects of DOBUTAMINE may be increased, resulting in hypertension.

Mechanism Unknown.

Management Monitor blood pressure. Adjust the DOBUTAMINE dose as needed.

Discussion

Severe hypertension occurred in a 55-year-old man receiving cimetidine during infusion of dobutamine.[1] The patient had coronary artery disease and was scheduled for a coronary artery bypass graft. He had a peptic ulcer and was receiving cimetidine 1 g/day in divided doses. Prior to surgery, the patient was treated with atenolol (eg, *Tenormin*) 25 mg twice daily. Preoperatively, the patient received morphine (eg, *MS Contin*) 10 mg, promethazine (eg, *Phenergan*) 25 mg, and scopolamine (eg, *Scopace*) 0.4 mg. Anesthesia was induced with midazolam, fentanyl (eg, *Sublimaze*), and vecuronium (eg, *Norcuron*). Following induction, his arterial blood pressure was 80/40 mm Hg, and a dobutamine infusion at a rate of 5 mcg/kg/min was initiated. Within 2 minutes, the arterial blood pressure increased to 210/100 mm Hg with a heart rate of 75 bpm. Dobutamine was stopped immediately, which was followed by a decrease in arterial pressure to 90/50 mm Hg over 15 minutes. Subsequently, the blood pressure was maintained at 125/80 mm Hg when a new preparation of dobutamine was infused at a rate of 1 mcg/kg/min.

Additional studies are needed to confirm this possible interaction.

[1] Baraka A, et al. *Anaesthesia.* 1992;47(11):965.

* Asterisk indicates drugs cited in interaction reports.

Sympathomimetics	*Hydantoins*	
Dopamine*	Fosphenytoin (*Cerebyx*)	Phenytoin* (eg, *Dilantin*)

Significance	Onset	Severity	Documentation
1	■ **Rapid** □ Delayed	■ **Major** □ Moderate □ Minor	□ Established □ Probable ■ **Suspected** □ Possible □ Unlikely

Effects The administration of PHENYTOIN during a DOPAMINE infusion may result in profound hypotension and possible cardiac arrest.

Mechanism Unknown. Possible depletion of catecholamines by DOPAMINE in combination with a myocardial depressant effect of PHENYTOIN.

Management Use PHENYTOIN with extreme caution in patients receiving a DOPAMINE infusion. If PHENYTOIN must be administered, carefully monitor BP and discontinue the PHENYTOIN infusion if hypotension occurs.

Discussion

In several case reports, 5 patients were receiving dopamine infusions to maintain systolic BP above 100 mm Hg.[1] When seizures developed in each patient, phenytoin infusions were started. Two of the patients suffered cardiac arrest and died; the other 3 patients developed profound hypotension that resolved in 2 of the patients when the phenytoin was discontinued. These effects occurred within minutes of beginning the phenytoin infusion.

It is not known if a similar interaction would occur between phenytoin and the other sympathomimetics.

[1] Bivins BA, et al. *Arch Surg.* 1978;113(3):245.

* Asterisk indicates drugs cited in interaction reports.

Sympathomimetics — *Lithium*

Epinephrine (eg, *Adrenalin*)	Phenylephrine* (eg, *Neo-Synephrine*)	Lithium* (eg, *Lithobid*)
Norepinephrine* (eg, *Levophed*)		

Significance	Onset	Severity	Documentation
5	☐ Rapid	☐ Major	☐ Established
	■ **Delayed**	☐ Moderate	☐ Probable
		■ **Minor**	☐ Suspected
			■ **Possible**
			☐ Unlikely

Effects The coadministration of LITHIUM and direct-acting SYMPATHOMIMETICS may decrease the pressor sensitivity of the SYMPATHOMIMETIC.

Mechanism Unknown.

Management Monitor patients for a decreased response to direct-acting SYMPATHOMIMETICS during concurrent LITHIUM therapy. An increased SYMPATHOMIMETIC dose may be necessary.

Discussion

Lithium carbonate administration may decrease the pressor sensitivity to the direct-acting sympathomimetics.[1,2] In 1 study, 17 patients receiving lithium carbonate for 4 or more weeks were administered tyramine, norepinephrine, and phenylephrine.[2] Lithium decreased the pressor sensitivities of norepinephrine and phenylephrine (direct-acting agents) but had no effect on tyramine sensitivity (indirect-acting agent). In another study, 8 hypomanic patients received 7 to 10 days of lithium therapy (1.2 g/day) followed by a single IV infusion of tyramine and norepinephrine.[1] The pressor effect of norepinephrine was decreased by 22%; the pressor effect of tyramine was not affected.

Other studies have reported that lithium attenuates the effect of amphetamine, an indirect-acting sympathomimetic.[3,4]

[1] Fann WE, et al. *Clin Pharmacol Ther.* 1972;13(1):71.
[2] Ghose K. *Eur J Clin Pharmacol.* 1980;17(4):233.
[3] Flemenbaum A. *Am J Psychiatry.* 1974;131(7):820.
[4] Van Kammen DP, et al. *Psychopharmacologia.* 1975;44(3):215.

* Asterisk indicates drugs cited in interaction reports. Based on pharmacologic and pharmacokinetic considerations, similar interactions may occur with other drugs that are listed.

Sympathomimetics — *MAOIs*

Sympathomimetics		MAOIs	
Brimonidine* (eg, *Alphagan P*)	Metaraminol*†	Isocarboxazid* (*Marplan*)	Rasagiline* (*Azilect*)
Dopamine*	Norepinephrine* (eg, *Levophed*)	Linezolid* (*Zyvox*)	Selegiline* (eg, *Eldepryl*)
Ephedrine*	Phenylephrine* (eg, *Neo-Synephrine*)	Phenelzine* (*Nardil*)	Tranylcypromine* (eg, *Parnate*)
Epinephrine* (eg, *Adrenalin*)	Pseudoephedrine* (eg, *Sudafed*)		
Isometheptene Mucate*†			

Significance	Onset	Severity	Documentation
1	■ **Rapid**	■ **Major**	■ **Established**
	□ Delayed	□ Moderate	□ Probable
		□ Minor	□ Suspected
			□ Possible
			□ Unlikely

Effects Coadministration of an MAOI and an indirect- or mixed-acting SYMPATHOMIMETIC may cause hypertensive crisis.[1-14] Direct-acting agents may interact minimally.[15]

Mechanism When MAO is inhibited, NOREPINEPHRINE accumulates and is released by indirect- and mixed-acting SYMPATHOMIMETICS, producing an increased pressor response at receptor sites.

Management Avoid coadministration. If used together, closely monitor for increases in blood pressure. If hypertension develops, administer phentolamine (eg, *OraVerse*). RASAGILINE is contraindicated in patients receiving SYMPATHOMIMETICS.[13] BRIMONIDINE is contraindicated in patients receiving MAOIs.[16]

Discussion

A patient receiving pargyline† for more than 1 month was given metaraminol IM to increase his BP (80/60 mm Hg).[5] Within 10 min, his systolic BP was more than 300 mm Hg, severe generalized headache and chest pain developed, and he lost consciousness. His BP was 150/110 mm Hg 2 hr later; within several days, it was 120/70 mm Hg. In 1 report, MAOIs caused a 2- to 2.5-fold potentiation of the pressor effect of phenylephrine, a direct-acting agent with some indirect activity.[10] Isometheptene mucate also has been associated with hypertensive crisis when given with phenelzine.[17] Do not overlook nonprescription products (eg, decongestants) as a source of sympathomimetics.[18,19] Linezolid should not be coadministered with sympathomimetics (eg, epinephrine, norepinephrine) unless patients are monitored for increases in blood pressure.[20] See Anorexiants-MAOIs.

1 Horwitz D, et al. *J Lab Clin Med.* 1960;56:747.
2 Stark DC. *Lancet.* 1962;279(7244):1405.
3 Goldberg LI. *JAMA.* 1964;190:456.
4 Sjöqvist F. *Proc R Soc Med.* 1965;58(11, part 2):967.
5 Horler AR, et al. *Br Med J.* 1965;2(5459):460.
6 Elis J, et al. *Br Med J.* 1967;2(5544):75.
7 Cuthbert MF, et al. *Br Med J.* 1969;1(5641):404.
8 Humberstone PM. *Br Med J.* 1969;1(5647):846.
9 Cuthbert MF, et al. *Br J Pharmacol.* 1971;43(3):639.
10 Boakes AJ, et al. *Br Med J.* 1973;1(5849):311.
11 Davies B, et al. *Lancet.* 1978;1(8057):172.
12 Smookler S, et al. *Ann Emerg Med.* 1982;11(9):482.
13 *Azilect* [package insert]. Kansas City, MO: Teva Neuroscience Inc; May 2006.
14 *Eldepryl* [package insert]. Tampa, FL: Somerset Pharmaceuticals Inc; February 1997.
15 Thompson DS, et al. *J Clin Psychopharmacol.* 1997;17(4):322.
16 *Alphagan* [package insert]. Irvine, CA: Allergan Inc; December 2001.
17 Kraft KE, et al. *JAMA.* 1996;275(14):1087.
18 Harrison WM, et al. *J Clin Psychiatry.* 1989;50(2):64.
19 Dawson JK, et al. *Accid Emerg Med.* 1995;12(1):49.
20 *Zyvox* [package insert]. New York, NY: Pharmacia & Upjohn Co; December 2009.

* Asterisk indicates drugs cited in interaction reports.
† Not available in the United States.

Sympathomimetics | **Maprotiline**

Dopamine*	Metaraminol*	Maprotiline*
Ephedrine	(*Aramine*)	

Significance	Onset	Severity	Documentation
5	■ **Rapid**	☐ Major	☐ Established
	☐ Delayed	☐ Moderate	☐ Probable
		■ **Minor**	☐ Suspected
			■ **Possible**
			☐ Unlikely

Effects MAPROTILINE may decrease the pressor response of the indirect- or mixed-acting SYMPATHOMIMETICS but have no effect on the direct-acting agents.

Mechanism Unknown.

Management No special precautions appear necessary. Observe patients for a decreased pressor response to the SYMPATHOMIMETIC during concurrent MAPROTILINE therapy.

Discussion

Three subjects received 75 mg/day of maprotiline, a tetracyclic antidepressant, for 10 to 14 days.[1] Following rapid IV injection of tyramine (0.1 to 5 mg per dose), a 3-fold reduction in the response to tyramine was observed. However, there was no potentiation of the pressor effect of norepinephrine (eg, *Levophed*) following a 0.07 to 7.76 mcg/min infusion of norepinephrine. This indicates that maprotiline may decrease the pressor response of indirect- or mixed-acting sympathomimetics but have no effect on direct-acting agents.

Tricyclic antidepressants have also been shown to interact with sympathomimetics. See Sympathomimetics-Tricyclic Antidepressants.

[1] Briant RH, et al. *Br J Clin Pharmacol.* 1974;1:113.

* Asterisk indicates drugs cited in interaction reports. Based on pharmacologic and pharmacokinetic considerations, similar interactions may occur with other drugs that are listed.

Sympathomimetics — *Methyldopa*

Sympathomimetics		Methyldopa
Dobutamine	Norepinephrine* (eg, *Levophed*)	Methyldopa*
Dopamine	Phenylephrine (eg, *Neo-Synephrine*)	
Ephedrine	Pseudoephedrine (eg, *Sudafed*)	
Epinephrine (eg, *Adrenalin*)		
Metaraminol (*Aramine*)		

Significance	Onset	Severity	Documentation
2	■ **Rapid**	□ Major	□ Established
	□ Delayed	■ **Moderate**	□ Probable
		□ Minor	■ **Suspected**
			□ Possible
			□ Unlikely

Effects The coadministration of METHYLDOPA and SYMPATHOMIMETICS may result in an increased pressor response, possibly resulting in hypertension.

Mechanism Unknown.

Management Monitor patient's BP during coadministration of METHYLDOPA and a SYMPATHOMIMETIC. Discontinuation of the SYMPATHOMIMETIC or administration of phentolamine may be necessary.

Discussion

Methyldopa may increase the pressor response to sympathomimetics, resulting in hypertension.[1-4] However, the effect of this interaction may depend on the degree of direct-, mixed-, or indirect-acting activity of the sympathomimetic. In 10 patients, a slight increase in the pressor response to a single IV dose of norepinephrine occurred following 10 days of methyldopa therapy.[2] The rise in BP with a norepinephrine 2 or 4 mcg dose alone was 27/15 and 35/20 mm Hg, respectively; with concurrent methyldopa, it was 35/19 and 48/25 mm Hg, respectively. The duration of the pressor action was increased 2- to 5-fold with concurrent methyldopa, compared with norepinephrine alone. Similar results were reported in 2 other studies.[1,3] In a case report, a patient maintained on methyldopa 250 mg twice daily and oxprenolol[†] received a combination product containing phenylpropanolamine 12.5 mg and acetaminophen (eg, *Tylenol*) 500 mg (2 tablets 3 times/day).[4] Within 2 days, the patient's BP increased from 140/80 to 200/150 mm Hg. The BP decreased to 140/110 mm Hg within 1 day of discontinuing the phenylpropanolamine combination.

[1] Pettinger W, et al. *Nature*. 1963;200:1107.
[2] Dollery CT, et al. *Br Heart J*. 1963;25:670.
[3] Dollery CT. *Proc R Soc Med*. 1965;58(11 pt 2):983.
[4] McLaren EH. *Br Med J*. 1976;2(6030):283.

* Asterisk indicates drugs cited in interaction reports. Based on pharmacologic and pharmacokinetic considerations, similar interactions may occur with other drugs that are listed.
† Not available in the United States.

Sympathomimetics — *Oxytocic Drugs*

Sympathomimetics		Oxytocic Drugs	
Dobutamine (*Dobutrex*)	Metaraminol (*Aramine*)	Ergonovine* (eg, *Ergotrate*)	Oxytocin* (eg, *Pitocin*, *Syntocinon*)
Dopamine* (eg, *Intropin*)	Methoxamine* (*Vasoxyl*)	Methylergonovine* (*Methergine*)	
Ephedrine	Norepinephrine (*Levophed*)		
Epinephrine (eg, *Adrenalin*)	Phenylephrine (*Neo-Synephrine*)		
Mephentermine (*Wyamine*)			

Significance	Onset	Severity	Documentation
4	■ **Rapid**	□ Major	□ Established
	□ Delayed	■ **Moderate**	□ Probable
		□ Minor	□ Suspected
			■ **Possible**
			□ Unlikely

Effects The coadministration of a SYMPATHOMIMETIC and an OXYTOCIC may result in hypertension.

Mechanism A synergistic and additive vasoconstrictive effect may occur.

Management The incidence of hypertension decreases when the SYMPATHOMIMETIC is not used prior to the administration of the OXYTOCIC DRUG. Also, chlorpromazine (eg, *Thorazine*) was shown to reverse the hypertension that occurred when both drugs were coadministered.

Discussion

In a retrospective study, 741 women received methoxamine 8 to 12 mg at initiation of caudal block and an oxytocic drug at the time of placental delivery.[2] Of the 741 patients, 34 (4.6%) developed postpartum hypertension; the systolic blood pressure was 140 mm Hg or more, 14 patients had diastolic blood pressure of approximately 90 mm Hg and 20 had diastolic pressure of 100 mm Hg or more. Hypertension developed in an average of 39.5 minutes after administration of the oxytocic (range, 10 to 80 minutes). Severe headache developed in 80% of the patients. One patient developed a subarachnoid hemorrhage. Chlorpromazine (eg, *Thorazine*) 12.5 to 15 mg appears to decrease the blood pressure that develops during concurrent use. In a single case report, a patient received ergotamine 0.8 mg IV to control uterine bleeding.[2] The patient became hypotensive; a dopamine infusion was started at 10 mg/kg/min and increased to 20 mg/kg/min over the next 12 hours. The patient subsequently developed symmetrical incipient gangrene of both the hands and feet. Although the dopamine was discontinued, the gangrene became demarcated and the patient died. Either agent alone may produce gangrene; however, it was suggested that the coadministration of these agents had a synergistic effect.

[1] Casady GN, et al. *JAMA*. 1960;172:1011.
[2] Buchanan N, et al. *Intens Care Med*. 1977; 3:55.

* Asterisk indicates drugs cited in interaction reports. Based on pharmacologic and pharmacokinetic considerations, similar interactions may occur with other drugs that are listed.

Sympathomimetics — *Rauwolfia Alkaloids*

Sympathomimetics		Rauwolfia Alkaloids	
Dobutamine (*Dobutrex*)	Metaraminol (*Aramine*)	Alseroxylon (*Rauwiloid*)	Rescinnamine (*Moderil*)
Dopamine (eg, *Intropin*)	Methoxamine (*Vasoxyl*)	Deserpidine (*Harmonyl*)	Reserpine* (eg, *Serpasil*)
Ephedrine*	Norepinephrine* (*Levophed*)	Rauwolfia (*Raudixin*)	
Epinephrine (eg, *Adrenalin*)	Phenylephrine (*Neo-Synephrine*)		
Mephentermine (*Wyamine*)			

Significance	Onset	Severity	Documentation
2	■ **Rapid**	□ Major	□ Established
	□ Delayed	■ **Moderate**	□ Probable
		□ Minor	■ **Suspected**
			□ Possible
			□ Unlikely

Effects RESERPINE potentiates the pressor response of the direct-acting SYMPATHOMIMETICS which may result in hypertension. The pressor response of the indirect-acting agents is decreased by RESERPINE.

Mechanism RESERPINE depletes stores of catecholamines, increasing the receptor sensitivity to the direct-acting SYMPATHOMIMETICS while antagonizing the effects of the indirect-acting agents which release norepinephrine from the neurons.

Management If these agents must be used together, monitor blood pressure. Depending on the SYMPATHOMIMETIC used, the dose may need to be increased or decreased.

Discussion

Reserpine appears to increase the pressor response to direct-acting sympathomimetics and decrease the sensitivity to the indirect-acting agents.[1-7] This interaction is mainly based on animal studies.[1-3,5,6]

In a case report, a patient receiving reserpine for 8 months developed hypotension during surgery.[4] In an attempt to increase the blood pressure, ephedrine was administered; however, this was unsuccessful. Norepinephrine administration resulted in an immediate rise in blood pressure to preoperative levels. In a study of seven subjects, reserpine administration significantly reduced ephedrine mydriasis following the ophthalmic instillation of ephedrine.[7]

[1] Burn JH, et al. *J Physiol.* 1958;144:314.
[2] Eger EI, et al. *Anesthesiology.* 1959;20:641.
[3] Maxwell RA, et al. *J Pharmacol Exp Ther.* 1959;125:178.
[4] Ziegler CH, et al. *JAMA.* 1961;176:916.
[5] Stone CA, et al. *J Pharmacol Exp Ther.* 1962;136:80.
[6] Moore JI, et al. *J Pharmacol Exp Ther.* 1962;136:89.
[7] Sneddon JM, et al. *Clin Pharmacol Ther.* 1969;10:64.

* Asterisk indicates drugs cited in interaction reports. Based on pharmacologic and pharmacokinetic considerations, similar interactions may occur with other drugs that are listed.

Sympathomimetics — Serotonin Reuptake Inhibitors

Sympathomimetics		Serotonin Reuptake Inhibitors	
Amphetamine*	Lisdexamfetamine (*Vyvanse*)	Citalopram* (eg, *Celexa*)	Milnacipran (*Savella*)
Amphetamine/ Dextroamphetamine (eg, *Adderall*)	Methamphetamine (*Desoxyn*)	Duloxetine (*Cymbalta*)	Nefazodone
Benzphetamine (eg, *Didrex*)	Phendimetrazine (eg, *Prelu-2*)	Escitalopram (*Lexapro*)	Paroxetine (eg, *Paxil*)
Dextroamphetamine* (eg, *Dexedrine*)	Phentermine* (eg, *Ionamin*)	Fluoxetine* (eg, *Prozac*)	Sertraline (eg, *Zoloft*)
Diethylpropion		Fluvoxamine (eg, *Luvox*)	Venlafaxine* (eg, *Effexor*)

Significance	Onset	Severity	Documentation
2	■ **Rapid**	□ Major	□ Established
	□ Delayed	■ **Moderate**	□ Probable
		□ Minor	■ **Suspected**
			□ Possible
			□ Unlikely

Effects Increased sensitivity to SYMPATHOMIMETIC effects and increased risk of serotonin syndrome.

Mechanism Unknown.

Management If these agents must be used concurrently, monitor for increased CNS effects. Adjust therapy as needed.

Discussion

Following the ingestion of phentermine, a toxic reaction was reported in a 22-year-old woman who had been taking fluoxetine 20 mg/day for major depression.[1] After 3 months of treatment, the patient's depression resolved, and she decided to stop taking fluoxetine. The patient had been taking phentermine, which she stopped before starting fluoxetine. Eight days after stopping fluoxetine, the patient took 1 phentermine 30 mg tablet. Within several hours, she complained of jitteriness and that her thoughts were "going too fast." In addition, she reported stomach cramps, dry eyes, palpitations, and tremors. When she sat, she rhythmically jiggled her feet and repeatedly sprang to her feet to pace. Lorazepam (eg, *Ativan*) 1.5 mg was prescribed to be taken that evening. When she returned to the clinic the next morning, her symptoms had resolved. Two cases of excessive amphetamine effects (eg, agitation, anxiety, restlessness) have been reported during concomitant use of fluoxetine and illicit amphetamine ingestion.[2] A 32-year-old man receiving dextroamphetamine for attention deficit hyperactivity disorder experienced symptoms consistent with serotonin syndrome 2 weeks after starting venlafaxine.[3] Symptoms resolved when all drugs were discontinued, and he was treated with cyproheptadine. Citalopram was started 1 week after discharge, and serotonin syndrome symptoms recurred.

[1] Bostwick JM, et al. *J Clin Psychopharmacol.* 1996;16(2):189.

[2] Barrett J, et al. *Br J Psychiatry.* 1996;168(2):253.

[3] Prior FH, et al. *Med J Aust.* 2002;176(5):240.

* Asterisk indicates drugs cited in interaction reports. Based on pharmacologic and pharmacokinetic considerations, similar interactions may occur with other drugs that are listed.

Sympathomimetics — *Tricyclic Antidepressants*

Sympathomimetics		Tricyclic Antidepressants	
Dobutamine Dopamine Ephedrine Epinephrine* (eg, *Adrenalin*)	Metaraminol (*Aramine*) Norepinephrine* (*Levophed*) Phenylephrine* (eg, *Neo-Synephrine*)	Amitriptyline* Amoxapine Desipramine* (eg, *Norpramin*) Doxepin (eg, *Sinequan*) Imipramine* (eg, *Tofranil*)	Nortriptyline* (eg, *Pamelor*) Protriptyline* (eg, *Vivactil*) Trimipramine (*Surmontil*)

Significance	Onset	Severity	Documentation
2	■ **Rapid** □ Delayed	□ Major ■ **Moderate** □ Minor	■ **Established** □ Probable □ Suspected □ Possible □ Unlikely

Effects TRICYCLIC ANTIDEPRESSANTS potentiate the pressor response of the direct-acting SYMPATHOMIMETICS; dysrhythmias have occurred. The pressor response to the indirect-acting SYMPATHOMIMETICS is decreased by the TRICYCLIC ANTIDEPRESSANTS.

Mechanism TRICYCLIC ANTIDEPRESSANTS inhibit the reuptake of the SYMPATHOMIMETICS in the neuron, increasing or decreasing their sensitivity at the receptor, depending on the agent.

Management If these agents must be used concurrently, a dosage adjustment of the SYMPATHOMIMETIC may be necessary. Closely monitor patients for dysrhythmias and hypertension.

Discussion

Tricyclic antidepressants appear to increase the pressor response to direct-acting sympathomimetics and decrease the sensitivity to the indirect-acting agents.[1-6] In 1 study, protriptyline potentiated the effects of norepinephrine approximately 9-fold and those of epinephrine approximately 3-fold.[1] In another study, the pressor effects of norepinephrine, epinephrine, and phenylephrine were reduced 4- to 8-fold, 2- to 4-fold, and 2- to 3-fold, respectively, by imipramine.[3] Dysrhythmias also occurred in the patients receiving epinephrine. Amitriptyline and protriptyline increased the pressor response to norepinephrine.[2,5]

In contrast, the tricyclic antidepressants blocked the pressor effects of tyramine and indirect-acting sympathomimetics.[2,4-6] In 1 study, the pressor effects of phenylephrine were decreased by amitriptyline.[6]

1 Svedmyr N. *Life Sci.* 1968;7:77.
2 Mitchell JR, et al. *J Clin Invest.* 1970;49:1596.
3 Boakes AJ, et al. *Br Med J.* 1973;1:311.
4 Ghose K, et al. *Br J Clin Pharmacol.* 1976;3:334.
5 Ghose K, et al. *Psychopharmacology (Berl).* 1978;57:109.
6 Ghose K. *Eur J Clin Pharmacol.* 1980;17:233.

* Asterisk indicates drugs cited in interaction reports. Based on pharmacologic and pharmacokinetic considerations, similar interactions may occur with other drugs that are listed.

Sympathomimetics — *Urinary Acidifiers*

Sympathomimetics	Urinary Acidifiers
Ephedrine*	Ammonium Chloride*
Pseudoephedrine (eg, *Sudafed*)	Potassium Phosphate
	Sodium Acid Phosphate

Significance	Onset	Severity	Documentation
3	■ **Rapid**	☐ Major	☐ Established
	☐ Delayed	☐ Moderate	☐ Probable
		■ **Minor**	■ **Suspected**
			☐ Possible
			☐ Unlikely

Effects Acidification of the urine may decrease the t½ and increase the elimination of EPHEDRINE or PSEUDOEPHEDRINE. The therapeutic effects of the SYMPATHOMIMETIC may be decreased.

Mechanism The tubular reabsorption of the SYMPATHOMIMETIC may be decreased because of a decreased urinary pH by URINARY ACIDIFIERS.

Management An increased dose of the SYMPATHOMIMETIC may be necessary during coadministration of a URINARY ACIDIFIER. Acidification of the urine may be useful in the treatment of SYMPATHOMIMETIC intoxication.

Discussion

Urinary pH appears to alter the elimination of ephedrine and pseudoephedrine; alkalinization decreases their elimination, and acidification increases their elimination.[1-3]

In 1 study, 8 subjects received a single dose of pseudoephedrine and ammonium chloride to maintain urine pH in the desired acidic range.[3] The elimination t½ at a pH of approximately 5.6 was 1.9 hours compared with 21 hours with an alkaline urine. In another study, the t½ of pseudoephedrine decreased 20% to 42% when the urinary pH was decreased to approximately 5 with ammonium chloride.[2] Alkaline urine markedly increased the t½. Another study reported that the amount of ephedrine excreted in 24 hours ranged from 73.8% to 99% with an acidic urine compared with a 24-hour urinary excretion of 21.8% to 34.7% with an alkaline urine.[1] The clinical importance was not determined in any of the studies.

[1] Wilkinson GR, et al. *J Pharmacol Exp Ther.* 1968;162:139.
[2] Kuntzman RG, et al. *Clin Pharmacol Ther.* 1971;12:62.
[3] Brater DC, et al. *Clin Pharmacol Ther.* 1980;28:690.

* Asterisk indicates drugs cited in interaction reports. Based on pharmacologic and pharmacokinetic considerations, similar interactions may occur with other drugs that are listed.

Sympathomimetics — *Urinary Alkalinizers*

Sympathomimetics	Urinary Alkalinizers	
Ephedrine*	Potassium Citrate (*Urocit-K*)	Sodium Citrate (*Citra pH*)
Pseudoephedrine* (eg, *Sudafed*)	Sodium Acetate	Sodium Lactate
	Sodium Bicarbonate* (eg, *Neut*)	Tromethamine (*Tham*)

Significance	Onset	Severity	Documentation
2	☐ Rapid ■ **Delayed**	☐ Major ■ **Moderate** ☐ Minor	☐ Established ☐ Probable ■ **Suspected** ☐ Possible ☐ Unlikely

Effects Urinary alkalinization may increase the half-life and decrease the elimination of EPHEDRINE or PSEUDOEPHEDRINE. The therapeutic or toxic effects of the SYMPATHOMIMETIC may be increased.

Mechanism The tubular reabsorption of the SYMPATHOMIMETIC may be increased because of an increased urinary pH by URINARY ALKALINIZERS.

Management The SYMPATHOMIMETIC dose may need to be decreased during coadministration of a URINARY ALKALINIZER.

Discussion

Urinary pH appears to alter the elimination of ephedrine and pseudoephedrine, with alkalinization decreasing their elimination and acidification increasing their elimination.[1-3]

In 1 study, 8 subjects received a single dose of pseudoephedrine and sodium bicarbonate to maintain urinary pH in the desired alkaline range (higher than 7).[3] The elimination half-life of pseudoephedrine increased from 1.9 hours with an acidic urine to 21 hours following sodium bicarbonate administration. In another study, the half-life of pseudoephedrine increased 71% to 110% when the urinary pH was increased to approximately 8 with sodium bicarbonate.[2] Acidic urine markedly decreased the pseudoephedrine half-life. Another study reported that the amount of ephedrine excreted in 24 hours ranged from 21.8% to 34.7% in 3 subjects when the urinary pH was increased with sodium bicarbonate, compared with a 24-hour urinary excretion of 73.8% to 99% with an acidic urine.[1] The clinical significance was not determined in any of the studies.

[1] Wilkinson GR, et al. *J Pharmacol Exp Ther.* 1968;162:139.
[2] Kuntzman RG, et al. *Clin Pharmacol Ther.* 1971;12:62.
[3] Brater DC, et al. *Clin Pharmacol Ther.* 1980;28:690.

* Asterisk indicates drugs cited in interaction reports. Based on pharmacologic and pharmacokinetic considerations, similar interactions may occur with other drugs that are listed.

Tacrine — *Cimetidine*

Tacrine* (*Cognex*)	Cimetidine* (eg, *Tagamet*)

Significance	Onset	Severity	Documentation
4	□ Rapid ■ **Delayed**	□ Major ■ **Moderate** □ Minor	□ Established □ Probable □ Suspected ■ **Possible** □ Unlikely

Effects Serum TACRINE concentrations may be elevated, increasing the pharmacologic and adverse effects of TACRINE.

Mechanism Possible inhibition of first-pass hepatic metabolism of TACRINE.

Management When possible, administer an alternative H_2 antagonist. If CIMETIDINE is given when TACRINE is started or if treatment with both drugs is initiated concurrently, administer a conservative dose of TACRINE, and monitor serum transaminase levels frequently.

Discussion

Concurrent administration of tacrine and cimetidine has been associated with a 64% increase in the area under the tacrine plasma concentration-time curve (AUC) and a 54% increase in the maximum serum tacrine concentration.[1,2] Because tacrine administration may be associated with abnormal liver function tests (eg, increases in serum bilirubin, transaminase, gamma-glutamyl transpeptidase levels), and because serum transaminase levels nearly 20 times the upper limit of normal have been reported, monitor serum transaminase levels (specifically ALT) weekly for at least 12 weeks if cimetidine is started in a patient who is receiving tacrine. In addition, observe the patient's clinical response, and adjust the tacrine dose as indicated. In 10 healthy volunteers, administration of cimetidine 1,200 mg/day for 3 days before a 40 mg test dose of tacrine decreased the apparent tacrine clearance by 30%, leading to a 40% increase in AUC.[3] The elimination rate was unchanged, suggesting an inhibition of tacrine first-pass hepatic metabolism.

[1] Product Information. Tacrine (*Cognex*). Parke-Davis. May 1993.
[2] Personal Communications. Parke-Davis. October 1993.
[3] Forgue ST, et al. *Clin Pharmacol Ther.* 1996;59:444.

* Asterisk indicates drugs cited in interaction reports.

Tacrine — *Fluvoxamine*

Tacrine*	Fluvoxamine*
(*Cognex*)	(*Luvox*)

Significance	Onset	Severity	Documentation
2	☐ Rapid	☐ Major	☐ Established
	■ **Delayed**	■ **Moderate**	☐ Probable
		☐ Minor	■ **Suspected**
			☐ Possible
			☐ Unlikely

Effects Plasma TACRINE concentrations may be elevated, increasing the pharmacologic and adverse effects.

Mechanism Possibly inhibition of TACRINE metabolism (cytochrome P450 1A2) by FLUVOXAMINE.

Management If this combination cannot be avoided, monitor for side effects, including hepatotoxicity, when FLUVOXAMINE is initiated in patients receiving TACRINE or if both drugs are started concomitantly. Other selective serotonin reuptake inhibitors that are not metabolized by cytochrome P450 1A2 (eg, fluoxetine [*Prozac*]) may be safer alternatives.

Discussion

In a double-blind, randomized, crossover trial, the influence of fluvoxamine on single-dose tacrine pharmacokinetics was evaluated in 13 healthy male volunteers.[1] Each subject received a single dose of tacrine 40 mg with placebo or fluvoxamine 100 mg daily for 6 days, with tacrine given on the sixth day of fluvoxamine administration. Fluvoxamine increased the tacrine area under the plasma concentration-time curve (AUC) 8-fold and peak plasma concentrations of tacrine 5-fold and decreased the oral clearance of tacrine 88%. Fluvoxamine administration caused a 2- to 5-fold increase in the three monohydroxylated tacrine metabolites. There was a 7-fold increase in the urinary recovery of tacrine during concurrent fluvoxamine administration. No side effects were observed during the tacrine plus placebo period; however, 5 subjects experienced adverse reactions during concomitant tacrine and fluvoxamine administration. These side effects included nausea, vomiting, sweating, and diarrhea.

[1] Becquemont L, et al. *Clin Pharmacol Ther.* 1997;61:619.

* Asterisk indicates drugs cited in interaction reports.

Tacrine | **NSAIDs**

Tacrine*
(*Cognex*)

Ibuprofen*
(eg, *Motrin*)

Significance	Onset	Severity	Documentation
4	☐ Rapid ■ **Delayed**	☐ Major ■ **Moderate** ☐ Minor	☐ Established ☐ Probable ☐ Suspected ■ **Possible** ☐ Unlikely

Effects Delirium was reported during concurrent administration of IBUPROFEN and TACRINE.

Mechanism Unknown.

Management Observe the patient for signs and symptoms of delirium. If an interaction is suspected, adjust therapy as needed.

Discussion

Delirium developed in a 71-year-old woman during concurrent administration of ibuprofen and tacrine.[1] Eight months prior to receiving ibuprofen, tacrine 40 mg 4 times a day was started for probable Alzheimer's disease. After several weeks of therapy, the patient experienced delusions, hallucinations, and fluctuating awareness, which were worse at night, as well as bradycardia, diaphoresis, and dizziness. Her symptoms gradually resolved after the dose of tacrine was decreased to 20 mg 4 times a day. Her status remained stable over the next 8 months. Ibuprofen 600 mg daily was started for shoulder pain, and, within 2 weeks, her delirium returned. Both drugs were discontinued, and the delirium resolved.

[1] Hooten WM, et al. *Am J Psychiatry.* 1996;153:842.

* Asterisk indicates drugs cited in interaction reports.

Tacrolimus — *Amiodarone*

Tacrolimus* (eg, *Prograf*)	Amiodarone* (eg, *Cordarone*)

Significance	Onset	Severity	Documentation
4	■ **Rapid**	■ **Major**	□ Established
	□ Delayed	□ Moderate	□ Probable
		□ Minor	□ Suspected
			■ **Possible**
			□ Unlikely

Effects TACROLIMUS plasma concentrations may be elevated, increasing the risk of adverse reactions and QT interval prolongation.

Mechanism Inhibition of TACROLIMUS metabolism (CYP3A4) and P-glycoprotein expression by AMIODARONE is suspected. QT interval prolongation may be additive.

Management If coadministration cannot be avoided, consider decreasing the initial TACROLIMUS dose and closely monitoring TACROLIMUS blood concentrations. Adjust the TACROLIMUS dose as needed.

Discussion

A 65-year-old man was receiving amiodarone 200 mg daily for 5 years for atrial fibrillation.[1] He was started on an immunosuppressant regimen that contained tacrolimus 3 mg twice daily following renal transplantation. The initial tacrolimus dose had been reduced approximately 50% because of an anticipated interaction with amiodarone. On postoperative day 1, his ECG showed normal sinus rhythm, but his QTc interval was prolonged to 535 msec. When treatment with IV magnesium did not improve the QTc interval prolongation, amiodarone was discontinued on postoperative day 2. Subsequently, the QTc interval slowly decreased, reaching 493 on postoperative day 5. See Cyclosporine-Amiodarone and Sirolimus-Amiodarone.

[1] Burger CI, et al. *Transplantation.* 2010;89(9):1166.

* Asterisk indicates drugs cited in interaction reports.

Tacrolimus — *Androgens*

Tacrolimus*
(eg, *Prograf*)

Danazol*

Significance	Onset	Severity	Documentation
4	☐ Rapid ■ **Delayed**	☐ Major ■ **Moderate** ☐ Minor	☐ Established ☐ Probable ☐ Suspected ■ **Possible** ☐ Unlikely

Effects Trough TACROLIMUS concentrations may be elevated, increasing the risk of adverse reactions (eg, nephrotoxicity).

Mechanism Possible inhibition of the hepatic metabolism of TACROLIMUS.

Management Monitor TACROLIMUS concentrations and renal function during coadministration of DANAZOL. Adjust the dose of TACROLIMUS as needed.

Discussion

Increased tacrolimus concentrations were reported in a 34-year-old woman following initiation of danazol treatment.[1] The patient received a cadaveric renal transplant for end-stage renal failure secondary to interstitial nephritis. She was maintained on oral tacrolimus 5 mg twice daily. Her serum creatinine was 1.8 mg/dL, and the trough tacrolimus concentration was 0.5 to 0.7 ng/mL. Nine months later, she developed idiopathic thrombocytopenic purpura. After failing to respond to prednisone, she was given danazol 400 mg 3 times daily. Within 4 days, tacrolimus concentrations increased from 0.7 to 2.7 ng/mL (286%). Serum creatinine increased from 1.4 to 2.4 mg/dL (71%) over the next month. The tacrolimus dosage was decreased to 6 mg/day, then to 4 mg/day, and the danazol dosage was reduced to 600 mg/day, then to 400 mg/day; however, tacrolimus and serum creatinine concentrations remained elevated. The patient's platelet count responded to danazol and returned to normal. After discontinuing danazol, trough tacrolimus and serum creatinine concentrations returned to baseline values.

Additional studies are needed to assess the importance of this drug interaction and to determine if other 17-alkyl androgens interact similarly. See also Cyclosporine-Androgens.

[1] Shapiro R, et al. *Lancet.* 1993;341(8856):1344.

* Asterisk indicates drugs cited in interaction reports.

Tacrolimus — *Azole Antifungal Agents*

Tacrolimus	Azole Antifungal Agents	
Tacrolimus* (eg, *Prograf*)	Fluconazole* (eg, *Diflucan*)	Ketoconazole* (eg, *Nizoral*)
	Itraconazole* (eg, *Sporanox*)	Posaconazole* (*Noxafil*)

Significance	Onset	Severity	Documentation
2	☐ Rapid	☐ Major	■ **Established**
	■ **Delayed**	■ **Moderate**	☐ Probable
		☐ Minor	☐ Suspected
			☐ Possible
			☐ Unlikely

Effects TACROLIMUS levels and toxicity may be increased.

Mechanism Inhibition of TACROLIMUS gut and hepatic metabolism.

Management Monitor renal function and TACROLIMUS plasma levels during coadministration of TACROLIMUS and AZOLE ANTIFUNGAL AGENTS. Adjust the dose of TACROLIMUS as needed.

Discussion

Elevated tacrolimus levels and toxicity occurred in 2 patients after starting itraconazole therapy.[1,2] In another patient, tacrolimus levels more than doubled after the addition of itraconazole.[3] A 17.5-fold reduction in tacrolimus dose was needed in a patient taking itraconazole 400 mg/day.[4] Renal function worsened, despite a reduction in the tacrolimus dose. Fluconazole 100 or 200 mg/day was given to 12 and 8 transplant patients, respectively,[5] and corresponding median plasma trough tacrolimus levels increased 1.4- and 3.1-fold. The highest tacrolimus levels occurred within 3 days of starting fluconazole. To maintain tacrolimus levels less than 2 ng/mL, the median dose was reduced 56%. The initial increase in tacrolimus serum levels was associated with acute renal dysfunction in 3 patients and acute mental status changes in 2 patients. In 1 patient, discontinuation of fluconazole produced a decrease in the AUC, $t_{½}$, and trough plasma levels of tacrolimus. In a case report, discontinuation of itraconazole decreased tacrolimus trough levels.[6] In 15 patients, the addition of IV fluconazole to IV tacrolimus changed tacrolimus steady-state levels and clearance.[7] Oral ketoconazole increased tacrolimus levels from 11.1 to 27.9 ng/mL despite empiric dose reduction.[8] Compared with tacrolimus alone, the bioavailability of oral tacrolimus increased from 14% to 30% during ketoconazole administration.[9] There was no consistent change in hepatic clearance, implicating inhibition of intestinal tacrolimus metabolism. In a retrospective review of 14 lung transplant patients with cystic fibrosis, pharmacokinetic adjustment of the tacrolimus dose during posaconazole therapy reduced the tacrolimus dose by a factor of 3, allowing safe treatment during this interaction.[10] In 2 studies, low-dose itraconazole[11] or ketoconazole[12] was given to reduce tacrolimus doses and associated costs without increasing adverse reactions. In a 21-year-old woman, successful coadministration of tacrolimus with itraconazole was achieved by frequent tacrolimus blood level measurement and dose adjustments.[13] The tacrolimus maintenance dose, when coadministered with itraconazole, was 0.1 mg daily compared with 4 mg daily when tacrolimus was given alone. In a study in lung transplant patients, the tacrolimus dose was reduced more with itraconazole than with voriconazole, without increased rejection rate and with preserved renal function.[14] See Tacrolimus-Voriconazole.

[1] Furlan V, et al. *Transplant Proc.* 1998;30(1):187.
[2] Capone D, et al. *Ann Pharmacother.* 1999;33(10):1124.
[3] Ideura T, et al. *Nephrol Dial Transplant.* 2000;15(10):1721.
[4] Cervelli MJ, et al. *Ther Drug Monit.* 2003;25(4):483.
[5] Mañez R, et al. *Transplantation.* 1994;57(10):1521.
[6] Outeda Macías M, et al. *Ann Pharmacother.* 2000;34(4):536.
[7] Osowski CL, et al. *Transplantation.* 1996;61(8):1268.
[8] Moreno M, et al. *Transplant Proc.* 1999;31(6):2252.
[9] Floren LC, et al. *Clin Pharmacol Ther.* 1997;62(1):41.
[10] Berge M, et al. *Ther Drug Monit.* 2009;31(3):396.
[11] Shitrit D, et al. *J Heart Lung Transplant.* 2005;24(12):2148.
[12] Soltero L, et al. *Transplant Proc.* 2003;35(4):1319.
[13] Nara M, et al. *Am J Hematol.* 2010;85(8):634.
[14] Kramer MR, et al. *Clin Transplant.* 2011;25(2):E163.

* Asterisk indicates drugs cited in interaction reports.

Tacrolimus — *Barbiturates*

Tacrolimus		Barbiturates	
Tacrolimus* (*Prograf*)		Amobarbital (*Amytal*)	Phenobarbital* (eg, *Solfoton*)
		Butabarbital (eg, *Butisol*)	Primidone (eg, *Mysoline*)
		Butalbital	Secobarbital (*Seconal*)
		Pentobarbital	

Significance	Onset	Severity	Documentation
2	☐ Rapid	☐ Major	☐ Established
	■ **Delayed**	■ **Moderate**	☐ Probable
		☐ Minor	■ **Suspected**
			☐ Possible
			☐ Unlikely

Effects TACROLIMUS concentrations may be reduced.

Mechanism Increased hepatic metabolism (CYP3A4) of TACROLIMUS by BARBITURATES.

Management Monitor TACROLIMUS whole-blood concentrations and observe the clinical response of the patient when starting, stopping, or changing the BARBITURATE dose. Adjust the TACROLIMUS dose as needed.

Discussion

At least 3 cases have been reported in which IV phenobarbital was administered in the management of pediatric patients with acute elevations in tacrolimus whole-blood concentrations following liver transplantation.[1,2] In 2 patients, tacrolimus whole-blood concentrations decreased approximately 83% within approximately 60 hours after starting phenobarbital 5 mg/kg IV every 12 hours.[1] In the third patient, a 73% reduction in tacrolimus whole-blood concentrations occurred with administration of phenobarbital 5 mg/kg/day IV divided twice daily.[1]

[1] Quirós-Tejeira RE, et al. *Pediatr Transplant.* 2005;9(6):792.

[2] McLaughlin GE, et al. *Transplant Proc.* 2000;32(3):665.

* Asterisk indicates drugs cited in interaction reports. Based on pharmacologic and pharmacokinetic considerations, similar interactions may occur with other drugs that are listed.

Tacrolimus — *Chloramphenicol*

Tacrolimus* (*Prograf*)	Chloramphenicol* (eg, *Chloromycetin*)

Significance	Onset	Severity	Documentation
4	☐ Rapid ■ **Delayed**	☐ Major ■ **Moderate** ☐ Minor	☐ Established ☐ Probable ☐ Suspected ■ **Possible** ☐ Unlikely

Effects TACROLIMUS concentrations may be elevated, increasing the risk of toxicity.

Mechanism Inhibition of hepatic metabolism of TACROLIMUS is suspected.

Management Carefully monitor renal function in renal transplant patients and TACROLIMUS whole blood trough concentrations when starting or stopping CHLORAMPHENICOL.

Discussion

Elevated tacrolimus concentrations occurred in a 13-year-old girl during coadministration of chloramphenicol.[1] The patient developed severe abdominal pain 12 days after an uncomplicated renal transplantation. Based on the results of cultures and sensitivities, treatment for vancomycin (eg, *Vancocin*)-resistant *Enterococcus peritonitis* was initiated with chloramphenicol 600 mg every 6 hours. At the time chloramphenicol therapy was initiated, medications the patient was receiving included tacrolimus 6 mg every 12 hours, mycophenolate mofetil (eg, *CellCept*), prednisone (eg, *Sterapred*), acyclovir (eg, *Zovirax*), amlodipine (eg, *Norvasc*), trimethoprim/sulfamethoxazole (eg, *Bactrim*), ranitidine (eg, *Zantac*), phosphorus, and insulin. On day 2 of chloramphenicol therapy, tacrolimus whole blood trough concentrations increased to toxic levels. To maintain acceptable tacrolimus trough concentrations, the dose of tacrolimus had to be reduced 83%. The dose-adjusted AUC for tacrolimus was 7.5-fold higher during coadministration of chloramphenicol. A 47-year-old liver transplant patient, with stable tacrolimus levels (between 9 and 11 ng/mL) while receiving 5 mg twice daily, developed a vancomycin-resistant enterococcal urinary tract infection and was treated with high-dose IV chloramphenicol.[2] Three days later, his tacrolimus level was greater than 60 ng/mL, and he experienced symptoms of tacrolimus toxicity, including fatigue, headache, lethargy, and tremors. These symptoms resolved when both drugs were discontinued.

[1] Schulman SL, et al. *Transplantation.* 1998;65(10):1397.

[2] Taber DJ, et al. *Transplant Proc.* 2000;32(3):660.

* Asterisk indicates drugs cited in interaction reports.

Tacrolimus — *Cinacalcet*

Tacrolimus* (*Prograf*)	Cinacalcet* (*Sensipar*)

Significance	Onset	Severity	Documentation
4	□ Rapid	□ Major	□ Established
	■ **Delayed**	■ **Moderate**	□ Probable
		□ Minor	□ Suspected
			■ **Possible**
			□ Unlikely

Effects TACROLIMUS serum concentrations may be reduced, decreasing the pharmacologic effect.

Mechanism Unknown.

Management Closely monitor TACROLIMUS concentrations when starting or stopping CINACALCET. Adjust the TACROLIMUS dose as needed.

Discussion

A 48-year-old female renal transplant recipient who was receiving tacrolimus 4 mg twice daily was started on cinacalcet 30 mg/day.[1] Tacrolimus concentrations ranged from 4 to 8 mcg/L prior to starting cinacalcet. One week after starting cinacalcet therapy, tacrolimus concentrations decreased to 2.6 mcg/L. In addition, serum creatinine increased from 3.9 to 4.9 mg/dL. Cinacalcet was discontinued after 19 days of therapy, and tacrolimus levels increased immediately. However, serum creatinine did not decrease.

[1] Maass E, et al. *Transplant Proc.* 2007;39(10):3468.

* Asterisk indicates drugs cited in interaction reports.

Tacrolimus — *Clotrimazole*

Tacrolimus* (eg, *Prograf*)	Clotrimazole* (eg, *Mycelex*)

Significance	Onset	Severity	Documentation
2	☐ Rapid ■ **Delayed**	☐ Major ■ **Moderate** ☐ Minor	☐ Established ■ **Probable** ☐ Suspected ☐ Possible ☐ Unlikely

Effects Plasma TACROLIMUS levels may be elevated, increasing the risk of toxicity.

Mechanism Inhibition of TACROLIMUS metabolism (CYP3A4) in the gut wall is suspected.

Management Monitor TACROLIMUS blood levels during use of these agents, and adjust the TACROLIMUS dose accordingly.

Discussion

A 55-year-old male liver transplant patient receiving clotrimazole troches for oropharyngeal moniliasis experienced an increase in plasma tacrolimus concentrations.[1] To confirm the possibility of a drug interaction, 2 pharmacokinetic studies were conducted while the patient was receiving a fixed dose of tacrolimus. Addition of clotrimazole to the patient's medication schedule resulted in an increase in trough plasma tacrolimus concentrations from 3.5 to 5.6 ng/mL within 1 day and to more than 9 ng/mL within 8 days. During clotrimazole use, there was a 2-fold increase in the AUC of tacrolimus; however, the $t_{½}$ of tacrolimus was not changed. During a second trial, tacrolimus concentrations increased during clotrimazole use. In another study, 35 renal transplant patients receiving tacrolimus were randomly allocated to receive clotrimazole troches or nystatin (eg, *Mycostatin*) suspension for oral thrush prophylaxis immediately after surgery.[2] Compared with nystatin, tacrolimus trough levels were higher in patients treated with clotrimazole. In addition, by day 7, the average tacrolimus dose was lower in clotrimazole-treated patients. The effect of clotrimazole troches on the pharmacokinetics of tacrolimus was studied in 6 renal transplant patients.[3] Administration of clotrimazole for 6 days increased the tacrolimus AUC 147%. Peak and trough tacrolimus blood levels increased more than 2-fold.

[1] Mieles L, et al. *Transplantation.* 1991;52(6):1086.
[2] Vasquez E, et al. *Clin Transplant.* 2001;15(2):95.
[3] Vasquez EM, et al. *Ther Drug Monit.* 2005;27(5):587.

* Asterisk indicates drugs cited in interaction reports.

Tacrolimus — *Corticosteroids*

Tacrolimus* (eg, *Prograf*)	Prednisolone* (eg, *Prelone*)	Prednisone*

Significance	Onset	Severity	Documentation
2	☐ Rapid ■ **Delayed**	☐ Major ■ **Moderate** ☐ Minor	☐ Established ☐ Probable ■ **Suspected** ☐ Possible ☐ Unlikely

Effects TACROLIMUS plasma concentrations may be decreased, increasing the risk of rejection.

Mechanism Unknown.

Management In patients receiving TACROLIMUS, closely monitor TACROLIMUS concentrations when the dose of CORTICOSTEROIDS is started, stopped, or changed. Adjust the TACROLIMUS dose as needed.

Discussion

The effects of prednisolone/prednisone on the pharmacokinetics of tacrolimus were studied in 65 kidney transplant recipients.[1] All patients received tacrolimus (twice daily to achieve trough concentrations of 15 to 20 ng/mL during the first 2 weeks, 10 to 15 ng/mL between weeks 3 and 6, and 5 to 10 ng/mL thereafter) and mycophenolate mofetil (eg, *CellCept*) in combination with daclizumab† or prednisolone 100 mg IV on the first 3 postoperative days and oral prednisone, dosed to body weight, thereafter for 3 months. Tacrolimus dose adjustment was 30% lower at month 1 in the corticosteroid group compared with the daclizumab group. Within the corticosteroid group, statistically significant differences in the tacrolimus dose adjustments were observed before and after withdrawal of prednisone. The incidence of acute kidney rejection was comparable in the corticosteroid and daclizumab group (5 vs 3, respectively). In another study of 83 kidney transplant patients, a dose-related pharmacokinetic interaction was found between prednisone and tacrolimus.[2] The larger the prednisone dose, the greater the tacrolimus dose needed to achieve target trough levels. In renal transplant patients receiving tacrolimus and sirolimus, administration of decreasing dosages of prednisone (tapered from 0.46 to 0.1 mg/kg/day over several months) resulted in dose corrected increases in tacrolimus AUC.[3]

[1] Hesselink DA, et al. *Br J Clin Pharmacol.* 2003;56(3):327.
[2] Anglicheau D, et al. *Nephrol Dial Transplant.* 2003;18(11):2409.
[3] Park SI, et al. *Fundam Clin Pharmacol.* 2009;23(1):137.

* Asterisk indicates drugs cited in interaction reports.
†Not available in the United States.

Tacrolimus — *Cyclosporine*

Tacrolimus* (eg, *Prograf*)	Cyclosporine* (eg, *Neoral*)

Significance	Onset	Severity	Documentation
4	☐ Rapid ■ **Delayed**	☐ Major ■ **Moderate** ☐ Minor	☐ Established ☐ Probable ☐ Suspected ■ **Possible** ☐ Unlikely

Effects The risk of nephrotoxicity may be increased.

Mechanism Additive or synergistic toxicity.

Management Do not use TACROLIMUS simultaneously with CYCLOSPORINE. When switching patients from CYCLOSPORINE to TACROLIMUS, do not administer the first dose of TACROLIMUS sooner than 24 hours after the last dose of CYCLOSPORINE.

Discussion

The pharmacokinetics of cyclosporine before and during tacrolimus administration and changes in serum creatinine were studied in 7 orthotopic liver transplant patients.[1] The $t_{½}$ of IV cyclosporine before and during tacrolimus administration was unchanged. In addition, no other pharmacokinetic parameters of cyclosporine were altered when measured by high-pressure liquid chromatography. However, this does not rule out the possibility that cyclosporine may affect the pharmacokinetics of tacrolimus, or that coadministration of cyclosporine and tacrolimus may result in renal impairment caused by additive or synergistic nephrotoxicity. In patients who had experienced nephrotoxicity while taking cyclosporine, administration of tacrolimus after cyclosporine was stopped resulted in renal function deterioration.[2] This was initially associated with elevated cyclosporine concentrations in most patients; however, serum creatinine remained elevated even after plasma cyclosporine concentrations were no longer detectable.

[1] Jain AB, et al. *Transplant Proc.* 1991;23(6):2777.

[2] McCauley J, et al. *Transplant Proc.* 1990;22(1):17.

* Asterisk indicates drugs cited in interaction reports.

Tacrolimus — *Diltiazem*

Tacrolimus* (eg, *Prograf*)	Diltiazem* (eg, *Cardizem*)

Significance	Onset	Severity	Documentation
2	□ Rapid ■ **Delayed**	□ Major ■ **Moderate** □ Minor	□ Established □ Probable ■ **Suspected** □ Possible □ Unlikely

Effects TACROLIMUS levels may be elevated, increasing toxicity.

Mechanism Inhibition of TACROLIMUS hepatic metabolism (CYP3A4).

Management Closely monitor TACROLIMUS concentrations when starting, stopping, or changing the DILTIAZEM dose. Adjust the TACROLIMUS dose as needed.

Discussion

Elevated tacrolimus whole blood trough concentrations and neurotoxicity were reported in a 68-year-old man after the addition of diltiazem to his multiple-drug regimen.[1] Four months after liver transplantation, he was admitted to the intensive care unit with diarrhea, dehydration, and atrial fibrillation. Tacrolimus 8 mg twice daily resulted in levels of 12.9 ng/mL on admission. He was treated with IV hydration and continuous infusion of diltiazem 5 to 10 mg/h, which was changed the next day to 30 mg orally every 8 hours. Three days after admission, the patient developed delirium, confusion, and agitation. His tacrolimus level was 55 ng/mL. Tacrolimus was withheld and diltiazem was discontinued, while labetalol (eg, *Trandate*), hydralazine, nitroglycerin ointment (eg, *Nitro-Bid*), furosemide (eg, *Lasix*), and potassium chloride were added. Over the next 3 days, the patient's tacrolimus level decreased to 6.7 ng/mL, and his mental status improved. Tacrolimus was resumed at 3 mg twice daily and gradually increased to 5 mg twice daily (levels were between 9 and 10 ng/mL). Diltiazem and protease inhibitors may have contributed to markedly elevated tacrolimus levels (up to 202 ng/mL) in a kidney transplant patient with HIV.[2]

The dose-response relationship of the interaction between tacrolimus and diltiazem was studied in 2 stable renal transplant recipients.[3] Patients received diltiazem 0, 10, 20, 30, or 60 mg in the morning followed by 60 or 90 mg twice daily with the tacrolimus doses. The AUC of tacrolimus increased even with diltiazem 20 mg. The greatest increase occurred with diltiazem 90 mg twice daily. Another report found that a single daily dose of diltiazem 10, 20, 30, or 60 mg with the morning dose of tacrolimus resulted in a larger AUC of tacrolimus measured in the evening.[3] In a retrospective study, renal transplant patients who expressed the CYP3A5 genotype were more susceptible to diltiazem-induced inhibition of tacrolimus metabolism compared with CYP3A5 nonexpressers.[4] See also Cyclosporine-Diltiazem, Sirolimus-Diltiazem, Tacrolimus-Protease Inhibitors.

[1] Hebert MF, et al. *Ann Pharmacother.* 1999;33(6):680.
[2] Hardy G, et al. *Eur J Clin Pharmacol.* 2004;60(8):603.
[3] Jones TE, et al. *Clin Pharmacokinet.* 2002;41(5):381.
[4] Li JL, et al. *Pharmacogenomics J.* 2011;11(4):300.

* Asterisk indicates drugs cited in interaction reports.

Tacrolimus — *Felodipine*

Tacrolimus* (eg, *Prograf*)	Felodipine*

Significance	Onset	Severity	Documentation
4	☐ Rapid ■ **Delayed**	☐ Major ■ **Moderate** ☐ Minor	☐ Established ☐ Probable ☐ Suspected ■ **Possible** ☐ Unlikely

Effects TACROLIMUS trough plasma levels may be elevated, increasing the risk of toxicity.

Mechanism Unknown.

Management Closely monitor TACROLIMUS trough plasma levels when FELODIPINE is started or stopped. Adjust the TACROLIMUS dose as needed.

Discussion

A possible drug interaction was reported during coadministration of tacrolimus and felodipine in a 13-year-old boy with renal dysplasia.[1] The patient had received a living-related renal transplant at 12 years of age from his mother. On postoperative day 15, the patient was started on felodipine 2.5 mg/day for hypertension. His other medications consisted of tacrolimus (4 mg twice daily), fluconazole (eg, *Diflucan* [100 mg once daily]), prednisolone (eg, *Orapred*), mycophenolate mofetil (eg, *CellCept*), ganciclovir (eg, *Cytovene*), and trimethoprim-sulfamethoxazole (eg, *Bactrim*). At this time, his 12-hour tacrolimus trough levels ranged from 10.6 to 20 ng/mL. Two weeks after starting felodipine, the tacrolimus trough level was higher than 30 ng/mL. The tacrolimus dose was reduced incrementally to 0.5 mg twice daily, resulting in stable target tacrolimus trough levels of 8.9 to 9.4 ng/mL. Three months after renal transplantation, fluconazole was discontinued, and it was necessary to increase the dose of tacrolimus to 1.5 mg twice daily to maintain target trough levels. Eight months after transplantation, felodipine was discontinued, and 1 week later, the tacrolimus trough level decreased to 5.1 ng/mL. The dose of tacrolimus was increased to 2.5 mg twice daily. The tacrolimus trough level continued to drift down, and 1 month later, the dose of tacrolimus was increased to 3 mg twice daily. The patient was maintained on this dose for 1 month, at which time a 12-hour AUC was obtained and compared with one taken after fluconazole was discontinued. The 2 AUC measurements were similar.

[1] Butani L, et al. *Transplantation.* 2002;73(1):159.

* Asterisk indicates drugs cited in interaction reports.

Tacrolimus | **Food**

Tacrolimus* (eg, *Prograf*)	Grapefruit Juice*

Significance	Onset	Severity	Documentation
2	☐ Rapid ■ **Delayed**	☐ Major ■ **Moderate** ☐ Minor	☐ Established ☐ Probable ■ **Suspected** ☐ Possible ☐ Unlikely

Effects TACROLIMUS concentrations may be elevated, increasing the risk of toxicity.

Mechanism Inhibition of metabolism (CYP3A4) of TACROLIMUS in the jejunal mucosa.

Management Advise patients taking TACROLIMUS to avoid GRAPEFRUIT products and to take TACROLIMUS with a liquid other than GRAPEFRUIT JUICE. Caution patients not to use herbal products and TACROLIMUS without consulting their health care provider.

Discussion

Tacrolimus trough blood concentrations were increased in a 28-year-old female liver transplant recipient after ingestion of grapefruit juice (250 mL 4 times daily for 3 days).[1] Tacrolimus blood concentrations were not changed during or immediately after repeated grapefruit juice ingestion. However, approximately one week after the final ingestion of grapefruit juice, tacrolimus blood concentrations increased 10-fold (from 4.7 to 47.4 ng/mL). The increase resulted in a profound reduction of calcineurin phosphate activity in peripheral blood mononuclear cells. In addition, headache and nausea, but not nephrotoxicity or hyperglycemia, occurred throughout the period of elevated blood concentrations. In a prospective study of liver transplant recipients, coadministration of tacrolimus with grapefruit juice increased the bioavailability of tacrolimus.[2] Compared with tacrolimus values at the beginning of the study, ingestion of tacrolimus with fresh grapefruit juice (250 mL twice daily for 7 days) increased tacrolimus trough concentrations approximately 110 mg (from 9.34 to 19.66 ng/mL).

[1] Fukatsu S, et al. *Drug Metab Pharmacokinet.* 2006;21(2):122.

[2] Liu C, et al. *Eur J Clin Pharmacol.* 2009;65(9):881.

* Asterisk indicates drugs cited in interaction reports.

Tacrolimus — *HCV Protease Inhibitors*

Tacrolimus* (eg, *Prograf*)	Boceprevir* (*Victrelis*)	Telaprevir* (*Incivek*)

Significance	Onset	Severity	Documentation
1	☐ Rapid ■ **Delayed**	■ **Major** ☐ Moderate ☐ Minor	☐ Established ☐ Probable ■ **Suspected** ☐ Possible ☐ Unlikely

Effects TACROLIMUS plasma concentrations may be elevated, increasing the pharmacologic effects and risk of adverse reactions (including QT prolongation).

Mechanism TACROLIMUS metabolism (CYP3A) may be inhibited by HEPATITIS C VIRUS (HCV) PROTEASE INHIBITORS.

Management Closely monitor TACROLIMUS blood concentrations as well as renal function and TACROLIMUS-related adverse reactions (including QT interval) when an HCV PROTEASE INHIBITOR is coadministered.[1,2] Adjust the TACROLIMUS dose and dosing interval as needed. TACROLIMUS blood concentration monitoring may be needed for approximately 2 weeks after stopping TELAPREVIR.[3]

Discussion

The effects of telaprevir on the pharmacokinetics of a single oral dose of tacrolimus were evaluated in 9 healthy volunteers.[3] Using an open-label, randomized design, each subject received a single dose of tacrolimus 2 mg, followed by a minimum 14-day washout period, and subsequent administration of a single dose of tacrolimus 0.5 mg with steady-state telaprevir (750 mg every 8 hours). Steady-state telaprevir increased the tacrolimus dose-normalized AUC approximately 70-fold and prolonged the terminal elimination $t_{1/2}$ from a mean of 40.7 hours to 196 hours compared with giving tacrolimus alone.

1 *Victrelis* [package insert]. Whitehouse Station, NJ: Schering Corporation; May 2011.
2 *Incivek* [package insert]. Cambridge, MA: *Vertex Pharmaceuticals Incorporated*; May 2011.
3 Garg V, et al. *Hepatology*. 2011;54(1):20.

* Asterisk indicates drugs cited in interaction reports.

Tacrolimus — *Hydantoins*

Tacrolimus* (eg, *Prograf*)	Fosphenytoin (eg, *Cerebyx*)	Phenytoin* (eg, *Dilantin*)

Significance	Onset	Severity	Documentation
2	☐ Rapid	☐ Major	☐ Established
	■ **Delayed**	■ **Moderate**	☐ Probable
		☐ Minor	■ **Suspected**
			☐ Possible
			☐ Unlikely

Effects TACROLIMUS serum concentrations may be decreased by PHENYTOIN, while PHENYTOIN serum concentrations may be increased by TACROLIMUS.

Mechanism PHENYTOIN may increase the metabolism (CYP3A4) of TACROLIMUS.

Management Monitor serum concentrations of TACROLIMUS and PHENYTOIN. Observe the clinical response of the patient during coadministration of these drugs. Adjust the doses as needed.

Discussion

A possible drug interaction was reported in a 43-year-old male renal transplant patient receiving phenytoin and tacrolimus concomitantly.[1] He was hospitalized following an episode of syncope in his physician's office. The patient had a history of hypertension, generalized seizures, and diabetes. His prehospitalization medications consisted of phenytoin 600 and 500 mg/day on alternate days, azathioprine (eg, *Imuran*), bumetanide, digoxin (eg, *Lanoxin*), diltiazem (eg, *Cardizem*), heparin, insulin, prednisone, and tacrolimus 14 mg twice daily. One month prior to admission, serum tacrolimus concentrations were low (10.8 ng/mL), and the dose of the drug was increased to 16 mg twice daily. Upon hospitalization, the dose of tacrolimus was increased to 17 mg twice daily. In addition, after tacrolimus therapy was initiated, serum phenytoin concentrations increased from 18.4 to 36.2 mcg/mL. Upon hospitalization, phenytoin therapy was withheld and restarted 9 days later at 500 and 400 mg/day on alternate days. The patient did not experience further syncope. After discharge, the patient was maintained on phenytoin 500 and 400 mg/day on alternate days (phenytoin concentrations, 19.9 to 22.4 mcg/mL) and tacrolimus 16 mg twice daily (tacrolimus concentrations, 8 to 11.1 ng/mL). In another renal transplant patient, the tacrolimus dosage was decreased from 0.25 to 0.16 mg/day after discontinuing phenytoin.[2]

[1] Thompson PA, et al. *Ann Pharmacother.* 1996;30(5):544.

[2] Moreno M, et al. *Transplant Proc.* 1999;31(6):2252.

* Asterisk indicates drugs cited in interaction reports. Based on pharmacologic and pharmacokinetic considerations, similar interactions may occur with other drugs that are listed.

Tacrolimus | **Macrolide & Related Antibiotics**

Tacrolimus*
(eg, *Prograf*)

Azithromycin*
(eg, *Zithromax*)

Clarithromycin*
(eg, *Biaxin*)

Erythromycin*
(eg, *Ery-Tab*)

Telithromycin
(*Ketek*)

Significance	Onset	Severity	Documentation
2	☐ Rapid ■ **Delayed**	☐ Major ■ **Moderate** ☐ Minor	☐ Established ☐ Probable ■ **Suspected** ☐ Possible ☐ Unlikely

Effects Plasma TACROLIMUS levels may be elevated, increasing the risk of toxicity.

Mechanism Inhibition of TACROLIMUS hepatic metabolism (CYP3A4).

Management Monitor renal function and TACROLIMUS blood levels during coadministration of MACROLIDE AND RELATED ANTIBIOTICS. Adjust the TACROLIMUS dose as needed. Consider another antibiotic class.

Discussion

Increased tacrolimus plasma levels and renal toxicity have been reported in adults[1-8] and children[9] after the introduction of macrolides to stable tacrolimus regimens. In a 34-year-old man receiving tacrolimus 6 mg twice daily, serum creatinine increased from 190 to 330 mcmol/L, and tacrolimus plasma levels increased from 1.4 to 8.4 nmol/L after receiving erythromycin 250 mg every 6 hours for 4 days.[1] In a 62-year-old man, serum tacrolimus levels increased from 1.3 to 8.5 ng/mL within 48 hours of starting erythromycin.[2] Serum creatinine increased from 318 to more than 530 mcmol/L, and serum potassium increased from within the normal range (3.5 to 5 mmol/L) to 6.4 mmol/L. The tacrolimus dosage was decreased from 10 mg twice daily to 6 mg twice daily, then increased to 10 mg twice daily when erythromycin was discontinued. In a 45-year-old renal transplant patient, tacrolimus plasma levels increased despite a 64% decrease in the dose after clarithromycin was added to the treatment regimen.[3] Elevated tacrolimus levels and serum creatinine were reported in 2 patients after the addition of clarithromycin to their treatment regimen.[4] Elevated tacrolimus concentrations were reported in a patient following IV administration of azithromycin and ceftriaxone (eg, *Rocephin*).[10]

[1] Shaeffer MS, et al. *Ann Pharmacother.* 1994;28(2):280.
[2] Jensen C, et al. *Lancet.* 1994;344(8925):825.
[3] Wolter K, et al. *Eur J Clin Pharmacol.* 1994;47(2):207.
[4] Gómez G, et al. *Transplant Proc.* 1999;31(6):2250.
[5] Moreno M, et al. *Transplant Proc.* 1999;31(6):2252.
[6] Lauzurica R, et al. *Transplantation.* 2002;73(6):1006.
[7] Ibrahim RB, et al. *Ann Pharmacother.* 2002;36(12):1971.
[8] Kunicki PK, et al. *Ther Drug Monit.* 2005;27(1):107.
[9] Furlan V, et al. *Transplantation.* 1995;59(8):1217.
[10] Shullo MA, et al. *Transplant Proc.* 2010;42(5):1870.

* Asterisk indicates drugs cited in interaction reports. Based on pharmacologic and pharmacokinetic considerations, similar interactions may occur with other drugs that are listed.

Tacrolimus — *Metoclopramide*

Tacrolimus* (eg, *Prograf*)	Metoclopramide* (eg, *Reglan*)

Significance	Onset	Severity	Documentation
4	☐ Rapid	☐ Major	☐ Established
	■ **Delayed**	■ **Moderate**	☐ Probable
		☐ Minor	☐ Suspected
			■ **Possible**
			☐ Unlikely

Effects An increase in the immunosuppressive and toxic effects of TACROLIMUS may result with METOCLOPRAMIDE coadministration.

Mechanism Accelerated gastric emptying secondary to METOCLOPRAMIDE may improve delivery of TACROLIMUS to the small intestine, which may allow for an increase in TACROLIMUS absorption, especially in patients with gastric dysmotility.

Management In patients receiving TACROLIMUS, closely monitor the patient when METOCLOPRAMIDE is started or stopped. Be prepared to adjust the TACROLIMUS dose as needed.

Discussion

A 52-year-old woman who had undergone liver transplantation 11.5 years earlier experienced a dramatic increase in tacrolimus trough levels and evidence of tacrolimus toxicity after metoclopramide was added to her regimen.[1] She was admitted to a hospital with suspected acute graft rejection and undetectable tacrolimus levels while taking tacrolimus 14 mg twice daily. Her tacrolimus dose was increased to 28 mg twice daily on day 5. On day 11, ketoconazole was added. Metoclopramide 10 mg 4 times daily was added for suspected gastric dysmotility on day 14. When GI symptoms did not improve, tacrolimus was increased to 20 mg 4 times daily on day 19. She was discharged on day 20 with a tacrolimus trough level of 5.6 ng/mL. The next day, her tacrolimus level was greater than 30 ng/mL, and the tacrolimus dosage was reduced to 20 mg twice daily. Two days later, she returned with signs and symptoms suggesting tacrolimus toxicity (eg, neurotoxicity, acute renal failure), and she was readmitted. Tacrolimus was held, but trough levels remained greater than 30 ng/mL for 2 days before beginning a downward trend. Improvement in renal function was noted. She was discharged on tacrolimus 4 mg twice daily. The dose of metoclopramide was reduced, then discontinued. About 4 months later, she was being maintained on tacrolimus 1 mg twice daily with stable trough levels of 6.8 ng/mL. The reason the patient could be maintained on the low tacrolimus dose was not determined. See Cyclosporine-Metoclopramide.

[1] Prescott WA Jr, et al. *Pharmacotherapy*. 2004;24(4):532.

* Asterisk indicates drugs cited in interaction reports.

Tacrolimus — *Metronidazole*

Tacrolimus* (eg, *Prograf*)	Metronidazole* (eg, *Flagyl*)

Significance	Onset	Severity	Documentation
4	☐ Rapid ■ **Delayed**	☐ Major ■ **Moderate** ☐ Minor	☐ Established ☐ Probable ☐ Suspected ■ **Possible** ☐ Unlikely

Effects TACROLIMUS blood concentrations and the risk of toxicity may be increased.

Mechanism Possible inhibition of TACROLIMUS hepatic metabolism (CYP3A4).

Management It may be necessary to adjust the dose of TACROLIMUS when starting, stopping, or changing the dose of METRONIDAZOLE. Closely monitor TACROLIMUS blood concentrations and adjust the dose as needed.

Discussion

A possible drug interaction with coadministration of tacrolimus and metronidazole was reported in a 69-year-old man who underwent renal transplantation.[1] The patient's immunosuppressive therapy consisted of cyclosporine (eg, *Neoral*), prednisolone, and sirolimus (*Rapamune*). The patient developed acute vascular rejection that responded to 3 days of treatment with IV methylprednisolone (eg, *Solu-Medrol*) plus the conversions of cyclosporine to tacrolimus and sirolimus to mycophenolate (eg, *CellCept*). On a daily dose of tacrolimus 5 mg (3 mg every morning plus 2 mg every evening), plasma creatinine stabilized at 21 mmol/L, and mean trough blood tacrolimus concentrations stabilized at 10.4 mcg/L. Two months later, the patient was treated with a 2-wk course of metronidazole 400 mg 3 times daily for *Clostridium difficile*. During metronidazole therapy, the patient's tacrolimus concentrations rose from 9 to 17.9 mcg/L over 9 days that was accompanied by an increase in plasma creatinine from 0.15 to 0.21 mmol/L. After a decrease in the dose of tacrolimus to 1 mg twice daily, the tacrolimus concentration fell to 8.1 mcg/L, and the creatinine concentration fell to 0.16 mmol/L. Metronidazole was discontinued at the conclusion of the 2-wk course of therapy, and tacrolimus levels decreased to 5.2 mcg/L. The dose of tacrolimus was increased to 2 mg twice daily, resulting in a blood concentration of 8.8 mcg/L. See also Cyclosporine-Metronidazole.

Like tacrolimus, sirolimus is a substrate for CYP3A4. Therefore, metronidazole also may inhibit the metabolism of sirolimus, resulting in a similar interaction as occurs with tacrolimus.

[1] Herzig K, et al. *Nephrol Dial Transplant.* 1999;14(2):521.

* Asterisk indicates drugs cited in interaction reports.

Tacrolimus — *Mifepristone*

Tacrolimus* (eg, *Prograf*)	Mifepristone* (eg, *Korlym*)

Significance	Onset	Severity	Documentation
1	□ Rapid ■ **Delayed**	■ **Major** □ Moderate □ Minor	□ Established □ Probable ■ **Suspected** □ Possible □ Unlikely

Effects TACROLIMUS plasma concentrations may be elevated, increasing the pharmacologic effects and risk of adverse reactions (eg, thrombocytopenia).

Mechanism MIFEPRISTONE may inhibit TACROLIMUS metabolism (CYP3A4).

Management Coadministration of TACROLIMUS with MIFEPRISTONE is contraindicated.[1]

Discussion

Because mifepristone inhibits CYP3A4, coadministration of mifepristone with a drug that is metabolized mainly or solely by CYP3A4 (eg, tacrolimus) is likely to increase plasma concentrations of the drug.[1] Therefore, the concurrent use of drugs with a narrow therapeutic index that are CYP3A4 substrates, such as tacrolimus, is contraindicated. The risk of tacrolimus adverse reactions (eg, hypertension, thrombocytopenia) may be increased.

[1] *Korlym* [package insert]. Menlo Park, CA: Corcept Therapeutics Incorporated; February 2012.

* Asterisk indicates drugs cited in interaction reports.

Tacrolimus — *Nefazodone*

Tacrolimus* (eg, *Prograf*)	Nefazodone*

Significance	Onset	Severity	Documentation
4	☐ Rapid ■ **Delayed**	☐ Major ■ **Moderate** ☐ Minor	☐ Established ☐ Probable ☐ Suspected ■ **Possible** ☐ Unlikely

Effects TACROLIMUS concentrations and toxicity may be increased.

Mechanism NEFAZODONE may inhibit the metabolism (CYP3A4) of TACROLIMUS.

Management Closely monitor TACROLIMUS concentrations when NEFAZODONE is started or stopped. Adjust the dose of TACROLIMUS as needed. Antidepressants that do not inhibit the CYP3A4 isozyme or that are metabolized primarily by other isozymes (eg, paroxetine [eg, *Paxil*], sertraline [eg, *Zoloft*]) may be safer alternatives.

Discussion

In several case reports, nefazodone use in tacrolimus-treated transplant patients resulted in increased tacrolimus levels and toxicity.[1-3] In a 16-year-old boy who received a cadaveric renal transplant, tacrolimus toxicity occurred during coadministration of nefazodone.[1] He was taking tacrolimus 5 mg/day when nefazodone therapy 150 mg/day was started for depression with suicidal ideation. Four weeks after starting nefazodone, he was hospitalized with delirium and renal failure. Tacrolimus levels were 46.4 ng/mL compared with a baseline value of 9.4 ng/mL (approximately 3 months earlier while taking 6 mg/day). His creatinine level had increased from 106.1 to 212.2 mcmol/L. The tacrolimus dose was decreased to 2 mg/day. Nefazodone was discontinued, and paroxetine 20 mg/day was started. Less than 3 days after discontinuing nefazodone, the tacrolimus level was 10.2 ng/mL. The tacrolimus dose was increased to 5 mg/day, and within 2 days, the level of tacrolimus was 12.4 ng/mL. A 57-year-old woman with end-stage renal disease received a living, related renal allograft transplantation.[2] After receiving cyclosporine (eg, *Neoral*) for 3 months, tacrolimus 5 mg/day was substituted. She was maintained on prednisone, azathioprine (eg, *Imuran*), and tacrolimus for 2 years when nefazodone 50 mg twice daily was started for depression. After 1 week of nefazodone therapy, the patient experienced headache, confusion, and gray areas in her vision. Trough tacrolimus levels were considerably elevated (30 ng/mL), and her serum creatinine increased from a baseline of 132 to 194 mcmol/L. Nefazodone was discontinued, and within 36 hours there were no signs or symptoms of tacrolimus neurotoxicity. Sertraline was substituted for nefazodone. See also Cyclosporine-Nefazodone.

[1] Campo JV, et al. *Arch Gen Psychiatry.* 1998;55(11):1050.

[2] Olyaei AJ, et al. *Pharmacotherapy.* 1998;18(6):1356.

[3] Garton T. *Transplantation.* 2002;74(5):745.

* Asterisk indicates drugs cited in interaction reports.

Tacrolimus | **Nifedipine**

Tacrolimus* (eg, *Prograf*)	Nifedipine* (eg, *Procardia*)

Significance	Onset	Severity	Documentation
2	□ Rapid ■ **Delayed**	□ Major ■ **Moderate** □ Minor	□ Established □ Probable ■ **Suspected** □ Possible □ Unlikely

Effects TACROLIMUS whole blood trough concentrations may be elevated, increasing the risk of toxicity.

Mechanism Possible inhibition of the hepatic metabolism of TACROLIMUS by NIFEDIPINE.

Management Monitor renal function and TACROLIMUS whole blood trough concentrations during coadministration of NIFEDIPINE and TACROLIMUS and when NIFEDIPINE is discontinued. Adjust the TACROLIMUS dose as needed.

Discussion

In a retrospective investigation, the effects of nifedipine on tacrolimus whole blood trough concentrations were studied in 50 liver transplant patients.[1] The patients were divided into 2 comparable groups. One group was composed of 22 liver transplant recipients who received nifedipine for hypertension and tacrolimus concurrently, while the second group was composed of 28 liver transplant patients who received tacrolimus without nifedipine. The 2 groups were compared over a 1-year period. The daily doses, cumulative doses, and whole blood trough concentrations of tacrolimus were compared between the 2 groups at 5 time periods (immediately before nifedipine was started, then at 1-, 3-, 6-, and 12-month intervals). The daily tacrolimus dosages were calculated as the exact daily dose of tacrolimus the patient was receiving at the end of each time period. The mean onset of hypertension was 5.9 months after liver transplant. There was a difference between daily dosage requirements of tacrolimus at 3, 6, and 12 months in patients receiving concomitant nifedipine, compared with patients not receiving nifedipine. For these time periods, the daily doses of tacrolimus were decreased 26%, 29%, and 38%, respectively. Compared with the non-nifedipine group, there were 25% and 31% reductions in tacrolimus cumulative doses at 6 and 12 months, respectively. Tacrolimus whole blood trough concentrations increased 55% in the nifedipine group. Tacrolimus doses were reduced to keep the whole blood trough concentration within the therapeutic range (5 to 10 ng/mL). The group receiving concomitant tacrolimus and nifedipine showed improved kidney function as measured by serum creatinine.

Controlled retrospective studies are needed to further assess this drug interaction.

[1] Seifeldin RA, et al. *Ann Pharmacother.* 1997;31(5):571.

* Asterisk indicates drugs cited in interaction reports.

Tacrolimus	**Protease Inhibitors**
Tacrolimus* (eg, *Prograf*)	Atazanavir* (*Reyataz*) Darunavir* (*Prezista*) Indinavir* (*Crixivan*) Lopinavir/Ritonavir* (*Kaletra*) Nelfinavir* (*Viracept*) Ritonavir* (*Norvir*) Saquinavir* (*Invirase*)

Significance	Onset	Severity	Documentation
2	□ Rapid ■ **Delayed**	□ Major ■ **Moderate** □ Minor	□ Established ■ **Probable** □ Suspected □ Possible □ Unlikely

Effects TACROLIMUS levels may be elevated, increasing the risk of toxicity.

Mechanism Inhibition of hepatic metabolism (CYP3A4) of TACROLIMUS is suspected.

Management Closely monitor renal function and TACROLIMUS whole blood concentrations when the dose of the PROTEASE INHIBITOR is started, stopped, or changed. Adjust the TACROLIMUS dose as needed. Consider reducing the TACROLIMUS dose when starting concurrent PROTEASE INHIBITOR therapy.

Discussion

A possible drug interaction occurred in a 49-year-old man during coadministration of nelfinavir and tacrolimus after an orthoptic liver transplant caused by hepatitis C virus with decompensated cirrhosis.[1] The patient also was infected with HIV and had severe hemophilia A. Shortly after tacrolimus therapy was started, high blood concentrations were noted. Although he was receiving other medications, the increase in tacrolimus concentration was observed on 3 separate occasions after initiation of nelfinavir therapy. Over the next 3 months, the patient was treated with nelfinavir 1.5 g daily, while the dosage of tacrolimus was gradually reduced to 0.5 mg weekly to maintain a tacrolimus concentration between 5 and 15 ng/mL. The dose requirement of tacrolimus was 1.4% of the usual dose. Markedly elevated tacrolimus blood levels occurred in a liver transplant patient 3 days after starting lopinavir/ritonavir treatment.[2] The presumed suppression of tacrolimus metabolism was long-lasting, with an eventual dosage stabilization at tacrolimus 0.5 mg once weekly. Markedly elevated tacrolimus levels (up to 202 ng/mL) occurred in a kidney transplant patient who was receiving saquinavir and ritonavir.[3] The interaction may have been caused, in part, by residual effects from diltiazem, which was stopped postoperatively. Markedly elevated tacrolimus concentrations were reported in a renal transplant patient after ritonavir-boosted darunavir was added to his treatment regimen.[4] It was necessary to decrease his tacrolimus dose to 3.5% of the usual dose to maintain stable tacrolimus trough levels. Low tacrolimus dosages (0.03 to 0.08 mg/day) were given to manage the interaction in 3 patients receiving ritonavir-boosted fosamprenavir, lopinavir, or saquinavir treatment[5] and in 1 patient receiving atazanavir.[6]

1 Schvarcz R, et al. *Transplantation.* 2000;69(10):2194.
2 Schonder KS, et al. *Ann Pharmacother.* 2003;37(12):1793.
3 Hardy G, et al. *Eur J Clin Pharmacol.* 2004;60(8):603.
4 Mertz D, et al. *Am J Kidney Dis.* 2009;54(1):e1.
5 Bickel M, et al. *J Antimicrob Chemother.* 2010;65(5):999.
6 Tsapepas DS, et al. *Am J Health Syst Pharm.* 2011;68(2):138.

* Asterisk indicates drugs cited in interaction reports.

Tacrolimus — *Proton Pump Inhibitors*

Tacrolimus* (eg, *Prograf*)	Esomeprazole (*Nexium*)	Omeprazole* (eg, *Prilosec*)
	Lansoprazole* (eg, *Prevacid*)	Rabeprazole* (*Aciphex*)

Significance	Onset	Severity	Documentation
2	□ Rapid	□ Major	□ Established
	■ **Delayed**	■ **Moderate**	□ Probable
		□ Minor	■ **Suspected**
			□ Possible
			□ Unlikely

Effects Increased TACROLIMUS plasma levels and toxicity.

Mechanism Inhibition of TACROLIMUS hepatic metabolism (CYP3A4) by LANSOPRAZOLE is suspected, while OMEPRAZOLE may increase intestinal CYP3A4 metabolism.

Management Closely monitor TACROLIMUS trough concentrations when LANSOPRAZOLE or OMEPRAZOLE is started or stopped. Adjust the TACROLIMUS dose as needed.

Discussion

Elevated tacrolimus blood levels were reported in a 34-year-old man during administration of lansoprazole.[1] The patient was receiving tacrolimus 17 mg/day, and his tacrolimus trough level was 15.6 ng/mL on posttransplantation day 3. Lansoprazole 30 mg/day was started on posttransplantation day 4. The next day, the tacrolimus trough level increased to 20.4 ng/mL. The dosage of tacrolimus was decreased gradually; however, the trough level continued to increase, reaching 25.6 ng/mL in 10 days. Lansoprazole was discontinued, and famotidine (eg, *Pepcid*) was started 2 days later. The next day, the tacrolimus trough level decreased to 11.7 ng/mL. Tacrolimus trough levels increased 52% in a 57-year-old renal transplant patient 3 days after starting lansoprazole.[2] Tacrolimus levels decreased when lansoprazole was changed to famotidine, and levels did not increase when famotidine was switched to rabeprazole. In renal transplant recipients receiving tacrolimus, converting therapy from cimetidine (eg, *Tagamet*) to omeprazole decreased dose/weight-normalized tacrolimus trough levels by 15%.[3] In a 13-year-old liver transplant patient, omeprazole treatment resulted in an increase in tacrolimus trough levels associated with a rise in serum creatinine.[4] When omeprazole was discontinued, tacrolimus blood levels decreased, and serum creatinine values returned to normal. In a review of 51 cases, omeprazole withdrawal resulted in a small decrease in tacrolimus levels but no change in the level-to-dose ratio.[5] Rabeprazole does not appear to affect tacrolimus levels.[6-9] In contrast, rabeprazole (and lansoprazole) may inhibit tacrolimus metabolism in poor CYP2C19 metabolizers with a specific CYP3A5 genotype.[10,11]

[1] Takahashi K, et al. *Ann Pharmacother.* 2004;38(5):791.
[2] Homma M, et al. *Transplantation.* 2002;73(2):303.
[3] Lemahieu WP, et al. *Kidney Int.* 2005;67(3):1152.
[4] Moreau C, et al. *Transplantation.* 2006;81(3):487.
[5] Pascual J, et al. *Transplant Proc.* 2005;37(9):3752.
[6] Itagaki F, et al. *Transplant Proc.* 2002;34(7):2777.
[7] Takahashi K, et al. *Drug Metab Pharmacokinet.* 2007;22(6):441.
[8] Hosohata K, et al. *Drug Metab Pharmacokinet.* 2008;23(2):134.
[9] Hosohata K, et al. *Drug Metab Pharmacokinet.* 2009;24(5):458.
[10] Miura M, et al. *Biopharm Drug Dispos.* 2007;28(4):167.
[11] Miura M, et al. *J Clin Pharm Ther.* 2011;36(2):208.

* Asterisk indicates drugs cited in interaction reports. Based on pharmacologic and pharmacokinetic considerations, similar interactions may occur with other drugs that are listed.

Tacrolimus — *Quinolones*

Tacrolimus* (eg, *Prograf*)	Levofloxacin* (eg, *Levaquin*)

Significance	Onset	Severity	Documentation
4	☐ Rapid ■ **Delayed**	☐ Major ■ **Moderate** ☐ Minor	☐ Established ☐ Probable ☐ Suspected ■ **Possible** ☐ Unlikely

Effects TACROLIMUS concentrations may be elevated, increasing the risk of toxicity.

Mechanism Inhibition of TACROLIMUS metabolism (CYP3A4) by LEVOFLOXACIN is suspected.

Management In patients receiving TACROLIMUS, closely monitor renal function and TACROLIMUS whole blood concentrations when LEVOFLOXACIN is started or stopped. Based on clinical and laboratory signs, be prepared to adjust the TACROLIMUS dose as needed.

Discussion

The effects of levofloxacin on the pharmacokinetics of tacrolimus were studied in 5 renal transplant patients with urinary tract infections receiving stable doses of tacrolimus.[1] Tacrolimus blood concentrations were measured before and at day 6 of levofloxacin (500 mg twice daily) administration. Compared with taking tacrolimus alone, levofloxacin increased tacrolimus average blood concentration and mean AUC approximately 25%. Other tacrolimus pharmacokinetic parameters were not altered.

[1] Federico S, et al. *Clin Pharmacokinet.* 2006;45(2):169.

* Asterisk indicates drugs cited in interaction reports.

Tacrolimus — *Ranolazine*

Tacrolimus* (eg, *Prograf*)	Ranolazine* (*Ranexa*)

Significancea	Onset	Severity	Documentation
4	■ **Rapid**	□ Major	□ Established
	□ Delayed	■ **Moderate**	□ Probable
		□ Minor	□ Suspected
			■ **Possible**
			□ Unlikely

Effects TACROLIMUS blood concentrations may be elevated, increasing the risk of toxicity.

Mechanism Inhibition of CYP3A4 metabolism and P-gp in the intestine by RANOLAZINE, resulting in decreased gut metabolism and increased GI absorption of TACROLIMUS, is suspected.

Management Closely monitor TACROLIMUS blood concentrations and the patient for toxicity when initiating RANOLAZINE therapy. Anticipate TACROLIMUS dosage adjustment when starting or stopping RANOLAZINE.

Discussion

Increased tacrolimus plasma concentrations were reported in a 64-year-old woman within 24 hours of starting ranolazine.[1] The patient, a kidney allograft recipient, was admitted to the hospital for worsening chronic angina pain. She was receiving a stable dose of tacrolimus 10 mg twice daily when ranolazine 500 mg twice daily was started. Tacrolimus trough concentrations rose from 8.1 ng/mL preadmission to 17.8 ng/mL within 24 hours of starting ranolazine. The dose of tacrolimus was reduced 70% to 3 mg twice daily to maintain steady-state trough concentrations between 6.6 and 7.9 ng/mL during concomitant ranolazine therapy. On a subsequent hospital admission, ranolazine was discontinued and resulted in subtherapeutic tacrolimus trough concentrations, which necessitated a tacrolimus dosage increase.

[1] Pierce DA, et al. *Ann Pharmacother.* 2010;44(11):1844.

* Asterisk indicates drugs cited in interaction reports.

Tacrolimus | **Rifamycins**

Tacrolimus*
(eg, *Prograf*)

Rifabutin
(*Mycobutin*)
Rifampin*
(eg, *Rifadin*)

Rifapentine
(*Priftin*)

Significance	Onset	Severity	Documentation
1	☐ Rapid ■ **Delayed**	■ **Major** ☐ Moderate ☐ Minor	☐ Established ■ **Probable** ☐ Suspected ☐ Possible ☐ Unlikely

Effects The immunosuppressive effects of TACROLIMUS may be reduced as early as 2 days after starting a RIFAMYCIN.

Mechanism Induced TACROLIMUS hepatic and intestinal metabolism (CYP3A4) by RIFAMYCINS.

Management Closely monitor TACROLIMUS whole blood concentrations when a RIFAMYCIN is started or stopped. Adjust the dose of TACROLIMUS as indicated.

Discussion

The need to markedly increase tacrolimus doses during rifampin therapy has been reported in multiple cases.[1-6] A 10-year-old boy who received a liver transplant was administered tacrolimus 4 mg twice daily to control chronic rejection.[1] Tacrolimus trough whole blood levels were approximately 10 ng/mL. Rifampin 150 mg twice daily was started 15 days later to relieve pruritus. Two days later, tacrolimus whole blood trough levels were undetectable. The dosage of tacrolimus was increased to 8 mg twice daily. When rifampin therapy was discontinued, it was necessary to decrease the tacrolimus dosage to 3 mg twice daily to maintain tacrolimus trough levels at approximately 10 ng/mL. A 10-month-old liver transplant patient was started on rifampin.[2] Over several weeks, tacrolimus dose requirements increased to 30 to 40 mg/day in order to maintain adequate blood levels. In a study of 6 healthy volunteers, rifampin increased the clearance of tacrolimus 47% and decreased the bioavailability from 14.4% to 7%.[3] There was substantial intersubject variability (up to a 203% increase in clearance and a 69% decrease in bioavailability). In a 25-year-old man, tacrolimus levels decreased from 9.2 to 1.7 ng/mL 2 days after starting rifampin.[4] Despite doubling the tacrolimus dose, levels only increased to 2.8 ng/mL 2 days later, and rifampin was discontinued. Tacrolimus levels decreased 12 days after starting rifampin in a 61-year-old man.[5] Subsequently, serum creatinine increased and oliguria ensued. To maintain therapeutic tacrolimus levels, it was necessary to increase the tacrolimus dose 10-fold over several months. In 1 report, it took 14 days following rifampin discontinuation before the enzyme induction effects were sufficiently reduced and the enzyme inhibition effects of other drugs (eg, diltiazem [eg, *Cardizem*]) were apparent.[6]

[1] Furlan V, et al. *Transplantation.* 1995;59(8):1217.
[2] Kiuchi T, et al. *Transplant Proc.* 1996;28(6):3171.
[3] Hebert MF, et al. *J Clin Pharmacol.* 1999;39(1):91.
[4] Moreno M, et al. *Transplant Proc.* 1999;31(6):2252.
[5] Chenhsu RY, et al. *Ann Pharmacother.* 2000;34(1):27.
[6] Bhaloo S, et al. *Transplant Proc.* 2003;35(7):2449.

* Asterisk indicates drugs cited in interaction reports. Based on pharmacologic and pharmacokinetic considerations, similar interactions may occur with other drugs that are listed.

Tacrolimus — *Schisandra*

Tacrolimus*
(eg, *Prograf*)

Schisandra*

Significance	Onset	Severity	Documentation
2	☐ Rapid ■ **Delayed**	☐ Major ■ **Moderate** ☐ Minor	☐ Established ☐ Probable ■ **Suspected** ☐ Possible ☐ Unlikely

Effects Bioavailability of TACROLIMUS may be increased by SCHISANDRA.

Mechanism SCHISANDRA may inhibit CYP3A4 and P-glycoprotein in the intestine, resulting in decreased gut metabolism and increased GI absorption of TACROLIMUS.

Management Avoid concurrent use of SCHISANDRA in patients receiving TACROLIMUS. If coadministration of SCHISANDRA and TACROLIMUS cannot be avoided, closely monitor TACROLIMUS blood concentrations and adjust the dosage accordingly.

Discussion

Schisandra sphenanthera has been used medicinally in China to treat viral and drug-induced hepatitis.[1] The effects of schisandra extract on the pharmacokinetics of tacrolimus were studied in 12 healthy men.[1] One day prior to starting schisandra, each subject received an oral dose of tacrolimus 2 mg, followed by 3 capsules of schisandra extract (deoxyschizandrin 11.25 mg/capsule) twice daily for 13 days. The next day, subjects were administered another single oral dose of tacrolimus 2 mg followed by 3 schisandra capsules. Compared with administration of tacrolimus alone, schisandra administration increased the tacrolimus AUC and C_{max} approximately 164% and 227%, respectively, and increased the time to reach the C_{max} 36.8%. In addition, the average decreases in oral clearance and apparent oral volume of distribution were 49% and 53.7%, respectively.

[1] Xin HW, et al. *Br J Clin Pharmacol.* 2007;64(4):469.

* Asterisk indicates drugs cited in interaction reports.

Tacrolimus — *Sevelamer*

Tacrolimus* (eg, *Prograf*)	Sevelamer* (eg, *Renagel*)

Significance	Onset	Severity	Documentation
4	☐ Rapid ■ **Delayed**	☐ Major ■ **Moderate** ☐ Minor	☐ Established ☐ Probable ☐ Suspected ■ **Possible** ☐ Unlikely

Effects TACROLIMUS concentrations may be reduced, decreasing the immunosuppressive effect and increasing the risk of transplant rejection.

Mechanism Unknown. However, decreased absorption of TACROLIMUS is suspected.

Management In patients receiving TACROLIMUS, closely monitor TACROLIMUS concentrations when SEVELAMER is coadministered. If an interaction is suspected, consider separating the administration times of TACROLIMUS and SEVELAMER as much as possible; give TACROLIMUS at least 1 hour before or 3 hours after SEVELAMER.

Discussion

In a 55-year-old male kidney transplant patient, a progressive decline in tacrolimus blood levels occurred after starting sevelamer.[1] Tacrolimus target levels were only temporarily measurable in spite of increasing the tacrolimus dose. Compared with tacrolimus C_{max} and AUC 3 days after sevelamer was discontinued, coadministration of sevelamer reduced the tacrolimus C_{max} and AUC approximately 24% and 59%, respectively. See Cyclosporine-Sevelamer.

[1] Merkle M, et al. *Transplantation*. 2005;80(5):707.

* Asterisk indicates drugs cited in interaction reports.

Tacrolimus — *Sirolimus*

Tacrolimus*
(eg, *Prograf*)

Sirolimus*
(*Rapamune*)

Significance	Onset	Severity	Documentation
1	☐ Rapid ■ **Delayed**	■ **Major** ☐ Moderate ☐ Minor	☐ Established ☐ Probable ■ **Suspected** ☐ Possible ☐ Unlikely

Effects TACROLIMUS trough plasma concentrations may be reduced, decreasing the pharmacologic effect.

Mechanism Unknown; however, TACROLIMUS oral bioavailability is reduced.

Management In patients receiving TACROLIMUS, frequently monitor trough levels after starting, stopping, or changing the SIROLIMUS dose. Adjust the TACROLIMUS dose as needed. SIROLIMUS as immunosuppressive therapy is not recommended in liver or lung transplant patients.[1]

Discussion

The effects of adding sirolimus to a tacrolimus-based immunosuppressive protocol were studied in 8 pediatric renal transplant recipients.[2] Each patient was converted to tacrolimus- and sirolimus-based immunosuppression as rescue therapy for chronic allograft nephropathy. Tacrolimus 0.14 mg/kg/day was administered and produced trough levels of 6.3 ng/mL. After starting sirolimus 0.13 mg/kg/day in 2 divided doses, the median dose required to maintain tacrolimus blood trough concentrations within the target range increased 71%. Dose-normalized tacrolimus AUC decreased to 67% and the dose-normalized C_{max} decreased to 54%, with no change in the terminal $t_{½}$. There was considerable interindividual variability. Sixteen adult patients receiving tacrolimus after renal transplantation were studied before and after discontinuation of concurrent sirolimus therapy.[3] Tacrolimus AUC increased between 15% and 32% 15 days after discontinuing sirolimus. In studies in de novo liver transplant patients, the use of sirolimus in combination with tacrolimus has been associated with an increase in hepatic artery thrombosis.[1] Most cases led to graft loss or death. Death related to bronchial anastomotic dehiscence has been reported in de novo lung transplant patients receiving sirolimus as part of an immunosuppressive regimen.[1] Sirolimus as immunosuppressive therapy is not recommended in liver or lung transplant patients.

[1] *Rapamune* [package insert]. Philadelphia, PA: Wyeth Pharmaceuticals, Inc; July 2005.
[2] Filler G, et al. *Am J Transplant.* 2005;5(8):2005.
[3] Baldan N, et al. *Pharmacol Res.* 2006;54(3):181.

* Asterisk indicates drugs cited in interaction reports.

Tacrolimus	***St. John's Wort***
Tacrolimus* (eg, *Prograf*)	St. John's Wort*

Significance	Onset	Severity	Documentation
1	☐ Rapid ■ **Delayed**	■ **Major** ☐ Moderate ☐ Minor	☐ Established ■ **Probable** ☐ Suspected ☐ Possible ☐ Unlikely

Effects TACROLIMUS concentrations may be reduced, increasing the risk of organ transplant rejection.

Mechanism Increased hepatic metabolism (CYP3A4) of TACROLIMUS induced by ST. JOHN'S WORT is suspected.

Management Avoid concurrent use of TACROLIMUS and ST. JOHN'S WORT. Caution patients not to use herbal products and TACROLIMUS without consulting their health care provider or pharmacist.

Discussion

A possible drug interaction was reported in a 65-year-old renal transplant patient during coadministration of tacrolimus and St. John's wort (*Hypericum perforatum*).[1] The patient was receiving tacrolimus 2 mg/day and mycophenolate mofetil (eg, *CellCept*) as immunosuppressive therapy. During long-term treatment with tacrolimus, the patient's tacrolimus whole-blood trough concentrations were stable, ranging from 6 to 10 mcg/L. The patient began self-medicating with St. John's wort 600 mg/day for a depressive mood state. Subsequently, his tacrolimus level decreased to a minimum of 1.6 mcg/L. Unexpectedly, the decrease in tacrolimus concentrations was associated with decreases in serum creatinine concentrations from approximately 1.6 to a nadir of 0.8 mg/dL. The patient stopped taking St. John's wort, and tacrolimus concentrations returned to the 6 to 10 mcg/L range without a change in the tacrolimus dose. Over the next month, serum creatinine concentrations gradually increased to 1.3 mg/dL. Administration of St. John's wort to healthy volunteers decreased the tacrolimus C_{max} 23% and AUC in 9 of 10 subjects (range, 15% to 64%); the AUC was increased 31% in 1 subject.[2] In addition, the apparent oral clearance and volume of distribution were increased. In 10 renal transplant patients, pretreatment with St. John's wort extract (600 mg/day for 14 days) decreased the AUC of tacrolimus 58% compared with giving tacrolimus alone.[3] It was necessary to increase the median tacrolimus doses 78% (from 4.5 to 8 mg/day) to maintain therapeutic levels. Two weeks after discontinuing St. John's wort, the median doses of tacrolimus were decreased to 6.5 mg/day.

[1] Bolley R, et al. *Transplantation.* 2002;73(6):1009.
[2] Hebert MF, et al. *J Clin Pharmacol.* 2004;44(1):89.
[3] Mai I, et al. *Nephrol Dial Transplant.* 2003;18(4):819.

* Asterisk indicates drugs cited in interaction reports.

Tacrolimus — *Theophyllines*

Tacrolimus* (eg, *Prograf*)	Theophylline* (eg, *Theochron*)

Significance	Onset	Severity	Documentation
4	☐ Rapid ■ **Delayed**	☐ Major ■ **Moderate** ☐ Minor	☐ Established ☐ Probable ☐ Suspected ■ **Possible** ☐ Unlikely

Effects Elevated serum creatinine and TACROLIMUS trough blood concentrations, increasing the risk of toxicity.

Mechanism Unknown.

Management Closely monitor TACROLIMUS trough blood concentrations and renal function when starting, stopping, or changing the THEOPHYLLINE dose.

Discussion

An interaction between tacrolimus and theophylline was reported in a 33-year-old man who received a cadaveric kidney transplant.[1] Posttransplantation, the patient received immunosuppressive therapy with tacrolimus 7 mg/day, azathioprine (eg, *Imuran*), and prednisone (eg, *Sterapred*). Tacrolimus trough blood concentrations were stable at 5 to 15 ng/mL. In order to reduce the increased serum erythropoietin level, enalapril (eg, *Vasotec*) was administered. Subsequently, theophylline 600 mg/day was added to reduce the need for phlebotomies. After 1 month, serum creatinine and tacrolimus trough blood concentrations increased. The theophylline dosage was decreased to 300 mg 4 times/week. However, 1 month later, serum creatinine and tacrolimus trough blood concentrations continued to increase; theophylline was discontinued and enalapril was replaced with losartan (*Cozaar*). Serum creatinine and tacrolimus levels returned to baseline values. Theophylline was reintroduced at a lower dosage (125 mg/day for 4 days). Tacrolimus trough blood concentrations increased without any change in serum creatinine. Theophylline was subsequently discontinued because of gastric discomfort.

[1] Boubenider S, et al. *Nephrol Dial Transplant.* 2000;15(7):1066.

* Asterisk indicates drugs cited in interaction reports.

Tacrolimus | **_Voriconazole_**

Tacrolimus*
(eg, *Prograf*)

Voriconazole*
(eg, *Vfend*)

Significance	Onset	Severity	Documentation
2	☐ Rapid ■ **Delayed**	☐ Major ■ **Moderate** ☐ Minor	☐ Established ■ **Probable** ☐ Suspected ☐ Possible ☐ Unlikely

Effects TACROLIMUS blood concentrations may be elevated, increasing the risk of toxicity.

Mechanism VORICONAZOLE inhibits the hepatic metabolism (CYP3A4) of TACROLIMUS.

Management When VORICONAZOLE is started or stopped in patients receiving TACROLIMUS, closely monitor TACROLIMUS blood levels and adjust the dose as needed.

Discussion

The effect of voriconazole on tacrolimus blood concentrations was assessed in 2 liver transplant recipients.[1] The study design was an open-label, randomized, 2-period, 2-treatment, placebo-controlled investigation. Prior to the study, patients were stabilized for at least 1 week on their present tacrolimus dose. One patient was randomized to receive voriconazole 200 mg oral twice daily for 5 days, and the second was randomized to receive placebo. During voriconazole administration, the tacrolimus trough blood concentration increased nearly 10-fold. The mechanism of the interaction was investigated in vitro using human liver microsomes. At a voriconazole concentration of 10.4 mcg/mL, tacrolimus metabolism was inhibited 50%. A 44-year-old woman with a liver transplant was admitted to the hospital for weakness and loss of balance.[2] Voriconazole 400 mg twice daily was given for presumed reactivation of coccidioidomycosis and for empiric reduction of the tacrolimus dosage. The tacrolimus dosage had to be lowered to 0.15 mg/day (a 90% reduction) to maintain therapeutic tacrolimus levels. Markedly elevated tacrolimus levels (25 ng/mL after 17 days) occurred in a 55-year-old male kidney transplant recipient after he was switched from itraconazole to voriconazole.[3] The tacrolimus dosage was reduced and then withheld for 3 days before it was restarted at 0.5 mg every other day. Painful neuromuscular disorders were reported following lung transplantation in 9 of 27 patients treated with voriconazole and tacrolimus concurrently.[4] The onset of symptoms varied from 2 weeks after treatment to more than 1 year. Complete recovery occurred within approximately 1 week after discontinuing voriconazole. In a 44-year-old kidney transplant patient, greatly elevated tacrolimus levels occurred within 1 day of starting voriconazole despite an empiric reduction in the tacrolimus dose of 50%.[5] In a 43-year-old kidney transplant patient, tacrolimus trough concentrations markedly increased and hyponatremia developed 6 days after starting voriconazole.[6] In a study in lung-transplant patients, the tacrolimus dose was reduced more with itraconazole than with voriconazole, without increasing the rejection rate and with preserving renal function.[7] See Tacrolimus-Azole Antifungal Agents.

[1] Venkataramanan R, et al. *Antimicrob Agents Chemother.* 2002;46(9):3091.
[2] Pai MP, et al. *Clin Infect Dis.* 2003;36(8):1089.
[3] Tintillier M, et al. *Nephrol Dial Transplant.* 2005;20(3):664.
[4] Boussaud V, et al. *J Heart Lung Transplant.* 2008; 27(2):229.
[5] Capone D, et al. *J Clin Pharm Ther.* 2010;35(1):121.
[6] Chang HH, et al. *Int J Infect Dis.* 2010;14(4):e348.
[7] Kramer MR, et al. *Clin Transplant.* 2011;25(2):E163

* Asterisk indicates drugs cited in interaction reports.

Tamoxifen — *Rifamycins*

Tamoxifen	Rifamycins	
Tamoxifen* (eg, *Soltamox*)	Rifabutin (*Mycobutin*)	Rifapentine (*Priftin*)
	Rifampin* (eg, *Rifadin*)	

Significance	Onset	Severity	Documentation
4	☐ Rapid	☐ Major	☐ Established
	■ **Delayed**	■ **Moderate**	☐ Probable
		☐ Minor	☐ Suspected
			■ **Possible**
			☐ Unlikely

Effects TAMOXIFEN plasma concentrations may be reduced, while those of its active metabolite, endoxifen, are increased or decreased.

Mechanism RIFAMYCINS increase TAMOXIFEN metabolism (CYP3A4) to its active metabolite, endoxifen.

Management Monitor the clinical response of patients and monitor for TAMOXIFEN adverse reactions resulting from the active metabolite.

Discussion

In a randomized, placebo-controlled, crossover trial, the effects of rifampin on the pharmacokinetics of tamoxifen were studied in 10 healthy men.[1] Each subject received rifampin 600 mg or placebo once daily for 5 days. On day 6, patients were given tamoxifen 80 mg. Pretreatment with rifampin reduced the C_{max} of tamoxifen 56% (from 145 to 64 ng/mL) and increased plasma levels of its active N-demethyltamoxifen metabolite 46% (from 41 to 60 ng/mL), which is hydroxylated to endoxifen. In addition, rifampin administration decreased the AUC of tamoxifen 86% and the elimination $t_{½}$ 42% (from 118 to 68 hours). However, in a report involving 4 patients, both tamoxifen and endoxifen concentrations were decreased by rifampin administration, suggesting a reduced therapeutic effect.[2]

[1] Kivistö KT, et al. *Clin Pharmacol Ther.* 1998;64(6):648.
[2] Binkhorst L, et al. *Clin Pharmacol Ther.* 2012;92(1):62.

* Asterisk indicates drugs cited in interaction reports. Based on pharmacologic and pharmacokinetic considerations, similar interactions may occur with other drugs that are listed.

Tamoxifen — *Serotonin Reuptake Inhibitors*

Tamoxifen	Serotonin Reuptake Inhibitors	
Tamoxifen* (eg, *Soltamox*)	Fluoxetine* (eg, *Prozac*)	Sertraline* (eg, *Zoloft*)
	Paroxetine* (eg, *Paxil*)	

Significance	Onset	Severity	Documentation
1	☐ Rapid	■ **Major**	☐ Established
	■ **Delayed**	☐ Moderate	■ **Probable**
		☐ Minor	☐ Suspected
			☐ Possible
			☐ Unlikely

Effects Clinical response to TAMOXIFEN may be reduced, increasing the risk of death from breast cancer.

Mechanism Inhibition of TAMOXIFEN metabolism (CYP2D6) by certain SRIs may reduce the conversion of TAMOXIFEN to its active metabolite, endoxifen.

Management Based on available information, avoid coadministration of TAMOXIFEN and FLUOXETINE or PAROXETINE in women with breast cancer.[1,2] When coadministration of TAMOXIFEN and an antidepressant is needed, give an antidepressant with little or no CYP2D6 inhibition (eg, citalopram [eg, *Celexa*], venlafaxine [eg, *Effexor*]).[3]

Discussion

The effects of CYP2D6 inhibitors on the metabolism of tamoxifen were evaluated in 78 women with newly diagnosed breast cancer.[3] Metabolism of tamoxifen by CYP2D6 is responsible for the formation of endoxifen, 1 of the active metabolites of tamoxifen. After 4 months of tamoxifen therapy, patients who carried 1 mutant CYP2D6 allele had a 55% decrease in endoxifen concentrations compared with patients who were homozygous for the wild-type CYP2D6 genotype. In patients with 2 mutant alleles, endoxifen concentrations were 26% of the wild-type patients. When drugs known to inhibit CYP2D6 (eg, citalopram, fluoxetine, paroxetine, sertraline) were given to patients who were extensive metabolizers, endoxifen concentrations were decreased 58% compared with patients not taking a CYP2D6 inhibitor. The outcome for women with breast cancer who were treated with tamoxifen and an SRI was studied in women who were at least 66 years of age. The risk of death from breast cancer increased in proportion to the overlapping time of tamoxifen and paroxetine coadministration.[1] Other antidepressants were not associated with death from breast cancer.

[1] Kelly CM, et al. *BMJ*. 2010;340:c693.
[2] Andersohn F, et al. *BMJ*. 2010;340:c783.
[3] Jin Y, et al. *J Natl Cancer Inst*. 2005;97(1):30.

* Asterisk indicates drugs cited in interaction reports.

Taxoids		**Azole Antifungal Agents**	
Docetaxel* (*Taxotere*)	Paclitaxel (eg, *Abraxane*)	Ketoconazole* (eg, *Nizoral*)	
Significance	Onset	Severity	Documentation
1	☐ Rapid ■ **Delayed**	■ **Major** ☐ Moderate ☐ Minor	☐ Established ☐ Probable ■ **Suspected** ☐ Possible ☐ Unlikely

Effects TAXOID plasma concentrations may be elevated, increasing the pharmacologic effects and risk of toxicity (eg, neutropenia).

Mechanism Inhibition of TAXOID hepatic metabolism (CYP3A4) by KETOCONAZOLE is suspected.

Management If coadministration of these agents cannot be avoided, give the TAXOID with caution and reduce the TAXOID dose as needed.

Discussion

The effects of ketoconazole on the pharmacokinetics of docetaxel were evaluated in 7 patients with a histologically or cytologically confirmed cancer diagnosis.[1] In a randomized, crossover design, each subject received 2 courses of docetaxel IV. One course consisted of docetaxel 100 mg/m^2 alone, while the second course involved administration of docetaxel 10 mg/m^2 plus ketoconazole 200 mg once daily for 3 days beginning 1 hour before docetaxel infusion started. Compared with giving docetaxel alone, coadministration of ketoconazole decreased the clearance of docetaxel 49%. However, there was large interindividual variability in the reduction in clearance. The clearance ratio of docetaxel was weakly related to the ketoconazole AUC. A study evaluating coadministration of docetaxel and ketoconazole showed a dose-dependent increase in docetaxel AUC from 1.3- to 2.6-fold with increasing doses of ketoconazole (300, 600, and 1,200 mg daily).[2]

[1] Engels FK, et al. *Clin Pharmacol Ther.* 2004;75(5):448. [2] Figg WD, et al. *J Urol.* 2010;183(6):2219.

* Asterisk indicates drugs cited in interaction reports. Based on pharmacologic and pharmacokinetic considerations, similar interactions may occur with other drugs that are listed.

Temsirolimus — *Azole Antifungal Agents*

Temsirolimus	Azole Antifungal Agents	
Temsirolimus* (*Torisel*)	Itraconazole* (eg, *Sporanox*) Ketoconazole* (eg, *Nizoral*)	Voriconazole* (eg, *Vfend*)

Significance	Onset	Severity	Documentation
2	□ Rapid ■ **Delayed**	□ Major ■ **Moderate** □ Minor	□ Established □ Probable ■ **Suspected** □ Possible □ Unlikely

Effects SIROLIMUS plasma concentrations may be elevated, increasing the risk of SIROLIMUS toxicity.

Mechanism AZOLE ANTIFUNGAL AGENTS inhibit the metabolism (CYP3A4) of TEMSIROLIMUS to its active metabolite, sirolimus.

Management Avoid coadministration of TEMSIROLIMUS and AZOLE ANTIFUNGAL AGENTS. If these agents must be used concurrently, consider a dosage reduction of TEMSIROLIMUS to 12.5 mg/wk and monitor SIROLIMUS levels.[1] If the AZOLE ANTIFUNGAL AGENT is discontinued, allow a washout period of approximately 1 week before the TEMSIROLIMUS dose is adjusted upward to the indicated dose.

Discussion

CYP3A4 is the major isozyme responsible for the formation of 5 temsirolimus metabolites.[1] The principle metabolite is sirolimus, an active metabolite of temsirolimus. Because sirolimus has a longer $t_{1/2}$ than temsirolimus, coadministration of strong inhibitors of CYP3A4 (eg, ketoconazole) is expected to increase sirolimus plasma concentrations. Coadministration of IV temsirolimus and oral ketoconazole had no effect on temsirolimus C_{max} or AUC.[1,2] However, sirolimus AUC and C_{max} increased 3.1- and 2.2-fold, respectively, compared with administration of temsirolimus alone.[1,2] Therefore, if alternative treatment cannot be given, consider temsirolimus dosage adjustments for patients receiving a strong CYP3A4 inhibitor concurrently.

The basis for this monograph is information on file with the manufacturer.[1] There are no clinical data with dose adjustments in patients receiving temsirolimus and a strong CYP3A4 inhibitor. Studies are needed to determine the clinical importance of this interaction and the effect of other azole antifungal agents on temsirolimus metabolism.

[1] *Torisel* [package insert]. Philadelphia, PA: Wyeth Pharmaceuticals Inc; May 2007.

[2] Boni JP, et al. *Br J Cancer*. 2008;98(11):1797.

* Asterisk indicates drugs cited in interaction reports.

Temsirolimus — Barbiturates

Temsirolimus* (*Torisel*)	Phenobarbital* (eg, *Solfoton*)	Primidone (eg, *Mysoline*)

Significance	Onset	Severity	Documentation
2	☐ Rapid ■ **Delayed**	☐ Major ■ **Moderate** ☐ Minor	☐ Established ☐ Probable ■ **Suspected** ☐ Possible ☐ Unlikely

Effects Plasma concentrations of SIROLIMUS (a major metabolite of TEMSIROLIMUS) may be reduced, decreasing the efficacy.

Mechanism Induction of TEMSIROLIMUS metabolism (CYP3A4) by PHENOBARBITAL.

Management Avoid coadministration of TEMSIROLIMUS and PHENOBARBITAL. If these agents must be used concurrently, consider increasing the dosage to TEMSIROLIMUS 50 mg/wk and monitor SIROLIMUS levels.[1] If PHENOBARBITAL is discontinued, reduce TEMSIROLIMUS to the indicated dose.

Discussion

CYP-450 3A4 is the major isozyme responsible for the formation of 5 temsirolimus metabolites.[1] The principle metabolite is sirolimus, an active metabolite of temsirolimus. Coadministration of strong inducers of CYP3A4 (eg, phenobarbital) is expected to decrease sirolimus plasma concentrations. Therefore, if alternative treatment cannot be given, consider temsirolimus dosage adjustments when phenobarbital is started or stopped.

The basis for this monograph is information on file with the manufacturer.[1] There are no clinical data with dosage adjustments in patients receiving temsirolimus and phenobarbital. Studies are needed to determine the clinical importance of this interaction and the effect of other barbiturates on temsirolimus metabolism.

[1] *Torisel* [package insert]. Philadelphia, PA: Wyeth Pharmaceuticals, Inc; May 2007.

* Asterisk indicates drugs cited in interaction reports. Based on pharmacologic and pharmacokinetic considerations, similar interactions may occur with other drugs that are listed.

Temsirolimus — *Carbamazepine*

Temsirolimus* (*Torisel*)	Carbamazepine* (eg, *Tegretol*)

Significance	Onset	Severity	Documentation
2	☐ Rapid	☐ Major	☐ Established
	■ **Delayed**	■ **Moderate**	☐ Probable
		☐ Minor	■ **Suspected**
			☐ Possible
			☐ Unlikely

Effects Plasma concentrations of SIROLIMUS (a major metabolite of TEMSIROLIMUS) may be reduced, decreasing the efficacy.

Mechanism Induction of TEMSIROLIMUS metabolism (CYP3A4) by CARBAMAZEPINE.

Management Avoid TEMSIROLIMUS and CARBAMAZEPINE coadministration. If these agents must be used concurrently, consider increasing the dosage to TEMSIROLIMUS 50 mg/wk and monitor SIROLIMUS levels.[1] If CARBAMAZEPINE is discontinued, reduce TEMSIROLIMUS to the indicated dose.

Discussion

CYP-450 3A4 is the major isozyme responsible for the formation of 5 temsirolimus metabolites.[1] The principle metabolite is sirolimus, an active metabolite of temsirolimus. Coadministration of strong inducers of CYP3A4 (eg, carbamazepine) is expected to decrease sirolimus plasma concentrations. Therefore, if alternative treatment cannot be given, consider temsirolimus dosage adjustments when carbamazepine is started or stopped.

The basis for this monograph is information on file with the manufacturer.[1] There are no clinical data with dosage adjustments in patients receiving temsirolimus and carbamazepine. Studies are needed to determine the clinical importance of this interaction.

[1] *Torisel* [package insert]. Philadelphia, PA: Wyeth Pharmaceuticals, Inc; May 2007.

* Asterisk indicates drugs cited in interaction reports.

Temsirolimus — *Corticosteroids*

Temsirolimus* (*Torisel*)	Dexamethasone* (eg, *Decadron*)

Significance	Onset	Severity	Documentation
2	☐ Rapid	☐ Major	☐ Established
	■ **Delayed**	■ **Moderate**	☐ Probable
		☐ Minor	■ **Suspected**
			☐ Possible
			☐ Unlikely

Effects Plasma concentrations of SIROLIMUS (a major metabolite of TEMSIROLIMUS) may be reduced, decreasing the efficacy.

Mechanism Induction of TEMSIROLIMUS metabolism (CYP3A4) by DEXAMETHASONE.

Management Avoid TEMSIROLIMUS and DEXAMETHASONE coadministration. If these agents must be used concurrently, consider increasing the dosage to TEMSIROLIMUS 50 mg/wk and monitor SIROLIMUS levels.[1] If DEXAMETHASONE is discontinued, reduce TEMSIROLIMUS to the indicated dose.

Discussion

CYP-450 3A4 is the major isozyme responsible for the formation of 5 temsirolimus metabolites.[1] The principle metabolite is sirolimus, an active metabolite of temsirolimus. Coadministration of strong inducers of CYP3A4 (eg, dexamethasone) is expected to decrease sirolimus plasma concentrations. Therefore, if alternative treatment cannot be given, consider temsirolimus dosage adjustments when dexamethasone is started or stopped.

The basis for this monograph is information on file with the manufacturer.[1] There are no clinical data with dosage adjustments in patients receiving temsirolimus and dexamethasone. Studies are needed to determine the clinical importance of this interaction and the effect of other corticosteroids on temsirolimus metabolism.

[1] *Torisel* [package insert]. Philadelphia, PA: Wyeth Pharmaceuticals, Inc; May 2007.

* Asterisk indicates drugs cited in interaction reports.

Temsirolimus — *Food*

Temsirolimus* (*Torisel*)	Grapefruit Juice*

Significance	Onset	Severity	Documentation
2	☐ Rapid ■ **Delayed**	☐ Major ■ **Moderate** ☐ Minor	☐ Established ☐ Probable ■ **Suspected** ☐ Possible ☐ Unlikely

Effects SIROLIMUS plasma concentrations may be elevated, increasing the risk of SIROLIMUS toxicity.

Mechanism GRAPEFRUIT inhibits the metabolism (CYP3A4) of TEMSIROLIMUS to its active metabolite, sirolimus.

Management Patients receiving TEMSIROLIMUS should avoid GRAPEFRUIT PRODUCTS.

Discussion

CYP-450 3A4 is the major isozyme responsible for the formation of 5 temsirolimus metabolites.[1] The principle metabolite is sirolimus, an active metabolite of temsirolimus. Because sirolimus has a longer $t_{1/2}$ than temsirolimus, ingestion of temsirolimus and grapefruit juice, an inhibitor of CYP3A4, is expected to increase sirolimus plasma concentrations. Therefore, patients taking temsirolimus should avoid grapefruit.[1]

The basis for this monograph is information on file with the manufacturer.[1] There are no clinical data with dose adjustments in patients receiving temsirolimus and grapefruit. Studies are needed to determine the clinical importance of this interaction.

[1] *Torisel* [package insert]. Philadelphia, PA: Wyeth Pharmaceuticals, Inc; May 2007.

* Asterisk indicates drugs cited in interaction reports.

Temsirolimus — *Hydantoins*

Temsirolimus* (*Torisel*)	Fosphenytoin (*Cerebyx*)	Phenytoin* (eg, *Dilantin*)

Significance	Onset	Severity	Documentation
2	☐ Rapid ■ **Delayed**	☐ Major ■ **Moderate** ☐ Minor	☐ Established ☐ Probable ■ **Suspected** ☐ Possible ☐ Unlikely

Effects Plasma concentrations of SIROLIMUS (a major metabolite of TEMSIROLIMUS) may be reduced, decreasing the efficacy.

Mechanism Induction of TEMSIROLIMUS metabolism (CYP3A4) by HYDANTOINS.

Management Avoid TEMSIROLIMUS and HYDANTOIN coadministration. If these agents must be used concurrently, consider increasing the dosage to TEMSIROLIMUS 50 mg/wk and monitor SIROLIMUS levels.[1] If the HYDANTOIN is discontinued, reduce TEMSIROLIMUS to the indicated dose.

Discussion

CYP-450 3A4 is the major isozyme responsible for the formation of 5 temsirolimus metabolites.[1] The principle metabolite is sirolimus, an active metabolite of temsirolimus. Coadministration of strong inducers of CYP3A4 (eg, phenytoin) is expected to decrease sirolimus plasma concentrations. Therefore, if alternative treatment cannot be given, consider temsirolimus dosage adjustments when phenytoin is started or stopped.

The basis for this monograph is information on file with the manufacturer.[1] There are no clinical data with dosage adjustments in patients receiving temsirolimus and phenytoin. Studies are needed to determine the clinical importance of this interaction and the effect of other hydantoins on temsirolimus metabolism.

[1] *Torisel* [package insert]. Philadelphia, PA: Wyeth Pharmaceuticals, Inc; May 2007.

* Asterisk indicates drugs cited in interaction reports. Based on pharmacologic and pharmacokinetic considerations, similar interactions may occur with other drugs that are listed.

Temsirolimus — *Macrolide & Related Antibiotics*

Temsirolimus* (*Torisel*)	Clarithromycin* (eg, *Biaxin*)	Telithromycin* (*Ketek*)

Significance	Onset	Severity	Documentation
2	☐ Rapid	☐ Major	☐ Established
	■ **Delayed**	■ **Moderate**	☐ Probable
		☐ Minor	■ **Suspected**
			☐ Possible
			☐ Unlikely

Effects SIROLIMUS plasma concentrations may be elevated, increasing the risk of TEMSIROLIMUS toxicity.

Mechanism MACROLIDE AND RELATED ANTIBIOTICS inhibit the metabolism (CYP3A4) of TEMSIROLIMUS to its active metabolite, SIROLIMUS.

Management Avoid coadministration of TEMSIROLIMUS and MACROLIDE AND RELATED ANTIBIOTICS. If these agents must be used concurrently, consider a dose reduction of TEMSIROLIMUS to 12.5 mg/wk and monitor SIROLIMUS levels.[1] If the MACROLIDE OR RELATED ANTIBIOTIC is discontinued, allow a washout period of approximately 1 week before the TEMSIROLIMUS dose is adjusted upward to the indicated dose.

Discussion

CYP-450 3A4 is the major isozyme responsible for the formation of 5 temsirolimus metabolites.[1] The principle metabolite is sirolimus, an active metabolite of temsirolimus. Because sirolimus has a longer $t_{½}$ than temsirolimus, coadministration of strong inhibitors of CYP3A4 (eg, clarithromycin) is expected to increase sirolimus plasma concentrations. Therefore, if alternative treatment cannot be given, consider temsirolimus dosage adjustments in patients receiving a strong CYP3A4 inhibitor concurrently.

The basis for this monograph is information on file with the manufacturer.[1] There are no clinical data with dose adjustments in patients receiving temsirolimus and a strong CYP3A4 inhibitor. Studies are needed to determine the clinical importance of this interaction and the effect of other macrolide and related antibiotics on temsirolimus metabolism.

[1] *Torisel* [package insert]. Philadelphia, PA: Wyeth Pharmaceuticals, Inc; May 2007.

* Asterisk indicates drugs cited in interaction reports.

Temsirolimus — *Nefazodone*

Temsirolimus* (*Torisel*)	Nefazodone*

Significance	Onset	Severity	Documentation
2	☐ Rapid	☐ Major	☐ Established
	■ **Delayed**	■ **Moderate**	☐ Probable
		☐ Minor	■ **Suspected**
			☐ Possible
			☐ Unlikely

Effects SIROLIMUS plasma concentrations may be elevated, increasing the risk of SIROLIMUS toxicity.

Mechanism NEFAZODONE inhibits the metabolism (CYP3A4) of TEMSIROLIMUS to its active metabolite, SIROLIMUS.

Management Avoid coadministration of TEMSIROLIMUS and NEFAZODONE. If these agents must be used concurrently, consider a dosage reduction of TEMSIROLIMUS to 12.5 mg/wk and monitor SIROLIMUS levels.[1] If NEFAZODONE is discontinued, allow a washout period of approximately 1 week before the TEMSIROLIMUS dose is adjusted upward to the indicated dose.

Discussion

CYP-450 3A4 is the major isozyme responsible for the formation of 5 temsirolimus metabolites.[1] The principle metabolite is sirolimus, an active metabolite of temsirolimus. Because sirolimus has a longer $t_{½}$ than temsirolimus, coadministration of strong inhibitors of CYP3A4 (eg, nefazodone) is expected to increase sirolimus plasma concentrations. Therefore, if alternative treatment cannot be given, consider temsirolimus dosage adjustments for patients receiving a strong CYP3A4 inhibitor concurrently.

The basis for this monograph is information on file with the manufacturer.[1] There are no clinical data with dose adjustments in patients receiving temsirolimus and a strong CYP3A4 inhibitor. Studies are needed to determine the clinical importance of this interaction.

[1] *Torisel* [package insert]. Philadelphia, PA: Wyeth Pharmaceuticals, Inc; May 2007.

* Asterisk indicates drugs cited in interaction reports.

Temsirolimus — *Protease Inhibitors*

Temsirolimus	Protease Inhibitors	
Temsirolimus* (*Torisel*)	Atazanavir* (*Reyataz*)	Ritonavir* (*Norvir*)
	Indinavir* (*Crixivan*)	Saquinavir* (*Invirase*)
	Nelfinavir* (*Viracept*)	

Significance	Onset	Severity	Documentation
2	☐ Rapid ■ **Delayed**	☐ Major ■ **Moderate** ☐ Minor	☐ Established ☐ Probable ■ **Suspected** ☐ Possible ☐ Unlikely

Effects SIROLIMUS plasma concentrations may be elevated, increasing the risk of TEMSIROLIMUS toxicity.

Mechanism PROTEASE INHIBITORS inhibit the metabolism (CYP3A4) of TEMSIROLIMUS to its active metabolite, SIROLIMUS.

Management Avoid coadministration of TEMSIROLIMUS and PROTEASE INHIBITORS. If these agents must be used concurrently, consider a dosage reduction of TEMSIROLIMUS to 12.5 mg/wk and monitor SIROLIMUS levels.[1] If the PROTEASE INHIBITOR is discontinued, allow a washout period of approximately 1 week before the TEMSIROLIMUS dose is adjusted upward to the indicated dose.

Discussion

CYP-450 3A4 is the major isozyme responsible for the formation of 5 temsirolimus metabolites.[1] The principle metabolite is sirolimus, an active metabolite of temsirolimus. Because sirolimus has a longer $t_{1/2}$ than temsirolimus, coadministration of strong inhibitors of CYP3A4 (eg, indinavir) is expected to increase sirolimus plasma concentrations. Therefore, if alternative treatment cannot be given, consider temsirolimus dosage adjustments for patients receiving a strong CYP3A4 inhibitor concurrently.

The basis for this monograph is information on file with the manufacturer.[1] There are no clinical data with dose adjustments in patients receiving temsirolimus and a strong CYP3A4 inhibitor. Studies are needed to determine the clinical importance of this interaction and the effect of other protease inhibitors on temsirolimus metabolism.[1]

[1] *Toreisel* [package insert]. Philadelphia, PA: Wyeth Pharmaceuticals, Inc; May 2007.

* Asterisk indicates drugs cited in interaction reports.

Temsirolimus — *Rifamycins*

Temsirolimus* (*Torisel*)	Rifabutin* (*Mycobutin*)	Rifampin* (eg, *Rifadin*)

Significance	Onset	Severity	Documentation
2	□ Rapid ■ **Delayed**	□ Major ■ **Moderate** □ Minor	□ Established □ Probable ■ **Suspected** □ Possible □ Unlikely

Effects Plasma concentrations of SIROLIMUS (a major metabolite of TEMSIROLIMUS) may be reduced, decreasing the efficacy.

Mechanism Induction of TEMSIROLIMUS metabolism (CYP3A4) by RIFAMYCINS.

Management Avoid TEMSIROLIMUS and RIFAMYCINS coadministration. If these agents must be used concurrently, consider increasing the dosage to TEMSIROLIMUS 50 mg/wk and monitor SIROLIMUS levels.[1] If the RIFAMYCIN is discontinued, reduce TEMSIROLIMUS to the indicated dose.

Discussion

CYP-450 3A4 is the major isozyme responsible for the formation of 5 temsirolimus metabolites.[1] The principle metabolite is sirolimus, an active metabolite of temsirolimus. Coadministration of strong inducers of CYP3A4 (eg, rifampin) is expected to decrease sirolimus plasma concentrations. Coadministration of IV temsirolimus and rifampin had no effect on temsirolimus C_{max} or AUC.[1] However, sirolimus AUC and C_{max} decreased 56% and 65%, respectively, compared with administration of temsirolimus alone. Therefore, if alternative treatment cannot be given, consider temsirolimus dosage adjustments when a strong CYP3A4 inducer is started or stopped.

The basis for this monograph is information on file with the manufacturer.[1] There are no clinical data with dosage adjustments in patients receiving temsirolimus and a strong CYP3A4 inducer. Studies are needed to determine the clinical importance of this interaction and the effect of other rifamycins on temsirolimus metabolism.

[1] *Torisel* [package insert]. Philadelphia, PA: Wyeth Pharmaceuticals, Inc; May 2007.

* Asterisk indicates drugs cited in interaction reports.

Temsirolimus — *St. John's Wort*

Temsirolimus* (*Torisel*)	St. John's Wort*

Significance	Onset	Severity	Documentation
2	☐ Rapid	☐ Major	☐ Established
	■ **Delayed**	■ **Moderate**	☐ Probable
		☐ Minor	■ **Suspected**
			☐ Possible
			☐ Unlikely

Effects Plasma concentrations of SIROLIMUS (a major metabolite of TEMSIROLIMUS) may be reduced, decreasing the efficacy.

Mechanism Induction of TEMSIROLIMUS metabolism (CYP3A4) by ST. JOHN'S WORT.

Management Avoid coadministration of TEMSIROLIMUS and ST. JOHN'S WORT. Caution patients taking TEMSIROLIMUS to inform their health care provider before taking nonprescription or herbal products.

Discussion

CYP-450 3A4 is the major isozyme responsible for the formation of 5 temsirolimus metabolites.[1] The principle metabolite is sirolimus, an active metabolite of temsirolimus. Coadministration of strong inducers of CYP3A4 (eg, St. John's wort) is expected to decrease sirolimus plasma concentrations. Therefore, avoid St. John's wort in patients taking temsirolimus.

The basis for this monograph is information on file with the manufacturer.[1] There are no clinical data with dosage adjustments in patients receiving temsirolimus and St. John's wort. Studies are needed to determine the clinical importance of this interaction.

[1] *Torisel* [package insert]. Philadelphia, PA: Wyeth Pharmaceuticals, Inc; May 2007.

* Asterisk indicates drugs cited in interaction reports.

Teniposide — *Barbiturates*

Teniposide* (*Vumon*)	Butabarbital (eg, *Butisol*)	Phenobarbital* (eg, *Solfoton*)
	Butalbital	Primidone (eg, *Mysoline*)
	Mephobarbital (*Mebaral*)	Secobarbital (*Seconal*)
	Pentobarbital	

Significance	Onset	Severity	Documentation
4	☐ Rapid	■ **Major**	☐ Established
	■ **Delayed**	☐ Moderate	☐ Probable
		☐ Minor	☐ Suspected
			■ **Possible**
			☐ Unlikely

Effects TENIPOSIDE plasma concentrations may be reduced, decreasing the efficacy.

Mechanism Increased hepatic metabolism of TENIPOSIDE by PHENOBARBITAL is suspected.

Management Closely monitor the clinical response to TENIPOSIDE when starting, stopping, or changing the dose of PHENOBARBITAL. Be prepared to adjust the TENIPOSIDE dose as needed.

Discussion

The effects of phenobarbital on the pharmacokinetics of teniposide were studied in 2 children with acute lymphocytic leukemia.[1] Teniposide clearance in these patients was compared with clearance in matched controls who were receiving teniposide but not phenobarbital. Compared with the control patients, phenobarbital administration increased teniposide clearance 2- to 3-fold. In a retrospective study of 716 children with acute lymphoblastic leukemia, coadministration of teniposide and anticonvulsant therapy (including phenobarbital) was related to worse event-free survival, hematologic relapse, and CNS relapse compared with children who were receiving teniposide but who were not receiving anticonvulsants.[2]

[1] Baker DK, et al. *J Clin Oncol.* 1992;10(2):311.

[2] Relling MV, et al. *Lancet.* 2000;356(9226):285.

* Asterisk indicates drugs cited in interaction reports. Based on pharmacologic and pharmacokinetic considerations, similar interactions may occur with other drugs that are listed.

Teniposide — *Hydantoins*

Teniposide* (*Vumon*)	Fosphenytoin (*Cerebyx*)	Phenytoin* (eg, *Dilantin*)

Significance	Onset	Severity	Documentation
4	☐ Rapid ■ **Delayed**	■ **Major** ☐ Moderate ☐ Minor	☐ Established ☐ Probable ☐ Suspected ■ **Possible** ☐ Unlikely

Effects TENIPOSIDE plasma concentrations may be reduced, decreasing the efficacy.

Mechanism Increased hepatic metabolism of TENIPOSIDE by PHENYTOIN is suspected.

Management Closely monitor the clinical response to TENIPOSIDE when starting, stopping, or changing the dose of PHENYTOIN. Be prepared to adjust the TENIPOSIDE dose as needed.

Discussion

The effects of phenytoin on the pharmacokinetics of teniposide were studied in 4 children with acute lymphocytic leukemia.[1] Teniposide clearance in these patients was compared with clearance in matched control patients who were receiving teniposide but not phenytoin. Compared with the control patients, phenytoin administration increased teniposide clearance 2- to 3-fold.

[1] Baker DK, et al. *J Clin Oncol.* 1992;10(2):311.

* Asterisk indicates drugs cited in interaction reports. Based on pharmacologic and pharmacokinetic considerations, similar interactions may occur with other drugs that are listed.

Tenofovir — *Protease Inhibitors*

Tenofovir* (*Viread*)	Amprenavir*†

Significance	Onset	Severity	Documentation
4	☐ Rapid	☐ Major	☐ Established
	■ **Delayed**	■ **Moderate**	☐ Probable
		☐ Minor	☐ Suspected
			■ **Possible**
			☐ Unlikely

Effects Risk of kidney dysfunction may be increased.

Mechanism Unknown.

Management If coadministration of these agents cannot be avoided, carefully monitor renal function and adjust therapy as needed.

Discussion

The effect of antiviral agents and clinical factors on the development of tenofovir-associated renal dysfunction was investigated in an observational cohort study of HIV-infected patients.[1] Using glomerular filtration rate (GFR) as estimated by the Cockcroft-Gault (CG) equation (which incorporates patient weight), renal function was assessed prior to initiating tenofovir therapy and during tenofovir administration. A secondary analysis used the simplified Modification of Diet in Renal Disease (MDRD) equation, which does not incorporate patient weight. Among 445 patients starting tenofovir, 51 (11%) developed a decrease in renal function. Using a multivariate analysis, the decrease in kidney function was associated with concurrent use of amprenavir or didanosine (eg, *Videx*), patients being older than 50 years of age, and lower baseline weight. Patients receiving amprenavir-based regimens and tenofovir were at least 3 times more likely to develop a decline in GFR than patients receiving efavirenz (*Sustiva*) with tenofovir. Patients receiving didanosine with tenofovir were 3 times more likely to develop a decline in GFR than patients receiving lamivudine (*Epivir*) with tenofovir. Patients older than 50 years of age were 4 times more likely to develop a decline in GFR compared with patients younger than 30 years of age. At the start of therapy, patients with lower baseline weight (ie, less than 70 kg) were more likely to develop a decline in GFR compared with patients with a higher weight (ie, greater than 70 kg). Kidney dysfunction identified in patients by the MDRD equation did not fully overlap with those identified by the CG equation, emphasizing the effect of including patient weight in the estimation of GFR in HIV-infected patients.

Additional studies are needed to further define the clinical and treatment factors affecting renal function of HIV-infected patients taking tenofovir regimens. See Didanosine-Tenofovir.

[1] Crane HM, et al. *AIDS*. 2007;21(11):1431.

* Asterisk indicates drugs cited in interaction reports.
† Not available in the United States.

Tetanus Toxoid ✕ *Tetanus Immune Globulin*

Tetanus Toxoid*	Tetanus Immune Globulin* (*Bay Tet*)

Significance	Onset	Severity	Documentation
4	☐ Rapid	☐ Major	☐ Established
	■ **Delayed**	■ **Moderate**	☐ Probable
		☐ Minor	☐ Suspected
			■ **Possible**
			☐ Unlikely

Effects TETANUS IMMUNE GLOBULIN (TIG) may interfere with the immune response to TETANUS TOXOID.

Mechanism Unknown.

Management In subjects with low prevaccination tetanus antibody titers, coadministration of TIG and TETANUS TOXOID still may result in low tetanus antibody titers. In these subjects, further immunization may be warranted.

Discussion

A clinical trial was conducted in adults to determine whether the simultaneous administration of tetanus-diphtheria (Td) and TIG could interfere with the immune response to Td.[1] In a randomized, open, controlled trial, 119 subjects received Td vaccine alone or Td vaccine plus TIG. The Td vaccine was formulated to contain 1 Lf units adsorbed tetanus toxoid and 1.5 Lf units adsorbed diphtheria toxoid. Each ampule of TIG contained the equivalent of tetanus antitoxin 500 units. The 2 preparations were injected IM; the Td vaccine was given in the right arm, and the TIG was administered in the left arm. Four weeks after giving the Td vaccine, the mean titers obtained for tetanus and diphtheria antitoxins were significantly higher ($P = 0.02$ and $P = 0.03$, respectively) in subjects who received Td vaccine alone compared with those subjects receiving Td vaccine plus TIG. TIG interfered with immune response to Td only in those subjects who had low prevaccination antibody titers (basal titers less than 0.1 units/mL). In these subjects, the tetanus antibody titers were still less than 0.1 units/mL at 4 weeks and 4 months. This level is considered too low to provide these subjects with enough circulating tetanus antibody to protect them in the short- or medium-term.

The conclusion of this study may be limited because the subset of subjects receiving Td vaccine and TIG who had prevaccination tetanus titers less than 0.1 units/mL at 4 weeks and 4 months were not defined prior to the start of the study. Additional studies are needed.

[1] Dal-Ré R, et al. *J Clin Pharmacol.* 1995;35(4):420.

* Asterisk indicates drugs cited in interaction reports.

Tetrabenazine — *Reserpine*

Tetrabenazine*
(*Xenazine*)

Reserpine*

Significance	Onset	Severity	Documentation
2	☐ Rapid ■ **Delayed**	☐ Major ■ **Moderate** ☐ Minor	☐ Established ☐ Probable ■ **Suspected** ☐ Possible ☐ Unlikely

Effects The pharmacologic effects of RESERPINE and TETRABENAZINE may be decreased.

Mechanism TETRABENAZINE and RESERPINE bind to vesicular monoamine transporter type 2 (VMAT2).

Management Coadministration of TETRABENAZINE and RESERPINE is contraindicated.

Discussion

Tetrabenazine reversibly inhibits VMAT2.[1] Reserpine binds irreversibly to VMAT2 and the duration of its effect is several days. Therefore, caution is advised when switching a patient from reserpine to tetrabenazine. To avoid overdosage and major depletion of serotonin and norepinephrine in the CNS, wait for chorea to re-emerge after stopping reserpine and before starting tetrabenazine. At least 20 days should elapse after stopping reserpine before starting tetrabenazine.[1]

[1] *Xenazine* [package insert]. Washington, DC: Prestwick Pharmaceuticals; May 2008.

* Asterisk indicates drugs cited in interaction reports.

Tetracyclines — *Aluminum Salts*

Tetracyclines		Aluminum Salts	
Demeclocycline* (eg, *Declomycin*)	Oxytetracycline*†	Aluminum Carbonate*	Magaldrate (eg, *Riopan*)
Doxycycline* (eg, *Vibramycin*)	Tetracycline* (eg, *Sumycin*)	Aluminum Hydroxide* (eg, *Amphojel*)	
Minocycline (eg, *Minocin*)			

Significance	Onset	Severity	Documentation
2	☐ Rapid	☐ Major	☐ Established
	■ **Delayed**	■ **Moderate**	■ **Probable**
		☐ Minor	☐ Suspected
			☐ Possible
			☐ Unlikely

Effects Reduced serum levels of TETRACYCLINE, possibly decreasing the anti-infective response.

Mechanism TETRACYCLINES form an insoluble chelate with ALUMINUM SALTS, decreasing absorption.

Management Avoid simultaneous administration of TETRACYCLINES and ALUMINUM SALTS; separate the administration of these agents by 3 to 4 hours.

Discussion

Many studies show that tetracyclines form insoluble chelates with polyvalent metal cations, including aluminum salts.[1-9] This results in a decrease in absorption (50% to more than 90%) and serum levels of tetracyclines, possibly resulting in a decreased therapeutic effect. In 5 subjects, single doses of tetracycline 250 mg and a magnesium-aluminum hydroxide gel reduced the bioavailability of tetracycline 90%, and serum levels were decreased. In 4 volunteers, coadministration of single doses of demeclocycline 300 mg and aluminum hydroxide resulted in reduced demeclocycline C_{max}.[5] In another study, the absorption of single doses of demeclocycline and doxycycline was negligible when aluminum hydroxide was coadministered in 4 subjects.[6] Similarly, in 10 volunteers, aluminum-magnesium hydroxide reduced the bioavailability of doxycycline 85%.[10] In another study, aluminum hydroxide decreased the $t_{1/2}$ and the AUC of doxycycline IV by interfering with enterohepatic circulation.[11] Five subjects taking oxytetracycline 1 g/day for 4 days were given an aluminum salt on days 3 and 4.[3] A reduction in oxytetracycline serum levels occurred, preventing a satisfactory therapeutic response in 1 patient.

1 Seed JC, et al. *Bull Johns Hopkins Hosp.* 1950;86(6):415.
2 Waisbren BA, et al. *Proc Soc Exp Biol Med.* 1950;73(1):73.
3 Michel JC, et al. *J Lab Clin Med.* 1950;36(4):632.
4 Albert A, et al. *Nature.* 1956;177(4505):433.
5 Scheiner J, et al. *Surg Gynecol Obstet.* 1962;114:9.
6 Rosenblatt JE, et al. *Antimicrob Agents Chemother (Bethesda).* 1966;6:134.
7 Neuvonen PJ. *Drugs.* 1976;11(1):45.
8 Garty M, et al. *Clin Pharmacol Ther.* 1980;28(2):203.
9 D'Arcy PF, et al. *Drug Intell Clin Pharm.* 1987;21(7-8):607.
10 Deppermann KM, et al. *Antimicrob Agents Chemother.* 1989;33(11):1901.
11 Nguyen VX, et al. *Antimicrob Agents Chemother.* 1989;33(4):434.

* Asterisk indicates drugs cited in interaction reports. Based on pharmacologic and pharmacokinetic considerations, similar interactions may occur with other drugs that are listed.
† Not available in the United States.

Tetracyclines — *Bismuth Salts*

Tetracyclines		Bismuth Salts	
Demeclocycline (*Declomycin*)	Oxytetracycline (eg, *Terramycin*)	Bismuth Subgallate (*Devrom*)	Bismuth Subsalicylate* (eg, *Pepto-Bismol*)
Doxycycline* (eg, *Vibramycin*)	Tetracycline* (eg, *Sumycin*)		
Minocycline (*Minocin*)			

Significance	Onset	Severity	Documentation
2	☐ Rapid ■ **Delayed**	☐ Major ■ **Moderate** ☐ Minor	☐ Established ☐ Probable ■ **Suspected** ☐ Possible ☐ Unlikely

Effects Coadministration of BISMUTH SALTS in liquid formulations may decrease the serum levels of TETRACYCLINES, resulting in a decreased therapeutic response to the antibiotic.

Mechanism TETRACYCLINES appear to adsorb to the suspending agent (Mg-Al silicate) present in most liquid formulations of BISMUTH SALTS, reducing the absorption of TETRACYCLINES.

Management Give the BISMUTH SALT 2 hours after the TETRACYCLINE.

Discussion

Fifteen healthy volunteers received a single dose of tetracycline 250 mg with and without a single dose of bismuth subsalicylate 60 mL.[1] Tetracycline serum levels were lower when bismuth subsalicylate was coadministered. The average decrease in individual peak serum levels was 27%, the area under the plasma concentration-time curve (AUC) decreased 33%, and the 72-hour urinary recovery of tetracycline decreased 33%. The average times of individual peak serum levels did not differ, indicating that absorption rates were similar. Six healthy subjects received a single dose of doxycycline 200 mg simultaneously with bismuth subsalicylate 60 mL, bismuth subsalicyclate 2 hours before or after doxycycline, or bismuth subsalicylate every 6 hours for 5 doses followed by doxycycline.[2] Doxycycline peak serum levels decreased with every regimen except bismuth subsalicylate given after doxycycline. When doxycycline was given after multiple bismuth subsalicylate doses, the peak serum levels decreased 58%. The doxycycline AUC was decreased following simultaneous administration or after multiple dosing (63% and 49%, respectively).

In vitro studies have not demonstrated chelation of bismuth subsalicylate with tetracycline. Instead, tetracycline adsorbed to the suspending agent (Mg-Al silicate [*Veegum*]).[3] In 12 volunteers given a special bismuth salicylate formulation without *Veegum*, a 13% reduction in bioavailability occurred, compared with 27% when *Veegum* was present.[3] The importance of a bismuth-tetracycline interaction has been questioned because these drugs are used to eradicate *Helicobacter pylori*.[4] The intraluminal nature of the infection allows antibacterial action even though chelation may be occurring.

[1] Albert KS, et al. *J Pharm Sci.* 1979;68:586.
[2] Ericsson CD, et al. *JAMA.* 1982;247:2266.
[3] Healy DP, et al. *Ann Pharmacother.* 1997;31:1460.
[4] Tkach CL, et al. *Ann Pharmacother.* 1998;32:387.

* Asterisk indicates drugs cited in interaction reports. Based on pharmacologic and pharmacokinetic considerations, similar interactions may occur with other drugs that are listed.

Tetracyclines — *Calcium Salts*

Tetracyclines		Calcium Salts	
Demeclocycline (*Declomycin*)	Oxytetracycline* (eg, *Terramycin*)	Calcium Carbonate (eg, *Oscal-500*)	Calcium Gluconate
Methacycline*†	Tetracycline* (eg, *Sumycin*)	Calcium Citrate (*Citracal*)	Calcium Lactate
Minocycline (*Minocin*)		Calcium Glubionate (*Neo-Calglucon*)	Tricalcium Phosphate* (*Posture*)

Significance	Onset	Severity	Documentation
2	☐ Rapid	☐ Major	☐ Established
	■ **Delayed**	■ **Moderate**	■ **Probable**
		☐ Minor	☐ Suspected
			☐ Possible
			☐ Unlikely

Effects Coadministration of TETRACYCLINES and CALCIUM SALTS decreases the absorption and serum levels of the TETRACYCLINES; a decreased anti-infective response may occur.

Mechanism TETRACYCLINES form an insoluble chelate with CALCIUM SALTS, decreasing absorption and serum levels of the TETRACYCLINES.

Management Avoid simultaneous administration of TETRACYCLINES and CALCIUM SALTS; separate administration of these agents by 3 to 4 hours.

Discussion

Many studies have shown that tetracyclines form insoluble chelates with polyvalent cations, including calcium salts.[1-5] This results in a decrease in absorption (50% to more than 90%) and serum levels of the tetracyclines, possibly resulting in a decreased therapeutic effect. The ingestion of milk and other dairy products containing calcium also reduces the absorption of tetracyclines;[6-9] however, the absorption of doxycycline is affected to a smaller extent.[7] Other studies have shown that the use of a dicalcium phosphate excipient in a tetracycline capsule formulation decreases the absorption of the tetracycline, compared with the use of other fillers, decreasing its serum levels.[10,11]

[1] Albert A, et al. *Nature.* 1956;177:433.
[2] Chin T-F, et al. *Am J Hosp Pharm.* 1975;32:625.
[3] Newman EC, et al. *J Pharm Sci.* 1976;65:1728.
[4] Neuvonen PJ. *Drugs.* 1976;11:45.
[5] D'Arcy PF, et al. *DICP.* 1987;21:607.
[6] Scheiner J, et al. *Surg Gynecol Obstet.* 1962;114:9.
[7] Rosenblatt JE, et al. *Antimicrob Agents Chemother.* 1966;134.
[8] Neuvonen P, et al. *Scand J Clin Lab Invest.* 1971; 116(Suppl 27):76.
[9] Poiger H, et al. *Eur J Clin Pharmacol.* 1978;14:129.
[10] Sweeney WM, et al. *Antibiot Med.* 1957;4:642.
[11] Boger WP, et al. *N Engl J Med.* 1959;261:828.

* Asterisk indicates drugs cited in interaction reports. Based on pharmacologic and pharmacokinetic considerations, similar interactions may occur with other drugs that are listed.
†Not available in the United States.

Tetracyclines — *Cimetidine*

Tetracyclines		Cimetidine
Demeclocycline (*Declomycin*)	Minocycline (*Minocin*)	Cimetidine* (*Tagamet*)
Doxycycline (eg, *Vibramycin*)	Oxytetracycline (eg, *Terramycin*)	
Methacycline (*Rondomycin*)	Tetracycline* (eg, *Achromycin V*)	

Significance	Onset	Severity	Documentation
5	☐ Rapid	☐ Major	☐ Established
	■ **Delayed**	■ **Moderate**	☐ Probable
		☐ Minor	☐ Suspected
			☐ Possible
			■ **Unlikely**

Effects CIMETIDINE may decrease the absorption of TETRACYCLINE. However, documentation is conflicting. A clinically significant interaction appears unlikely.

Mechanism Unknown. Decreased gastric acidity may play a role, although this has been questioned.

Management No clinical interventions appear required. Routinely monitor the patient and increase the TETRACYCLINE dose if the patient's infection does not respond as expected.

Discussion

The effects of cimetidine on tetracycline absorption are inconsistent.[1-3] In 1 study, 5 patients received cimetidine 1 g/day for 3 days beginning the day before a single 500 mg dose of tetracycline.[3] The same drugs were administered in a second phase of the study, except the tetracycline was dissolved in 200 mL of water. Cimetidine decreased the absorption of tetracycline when administered as a capsule; the mean cumulative amount of tetracycline excreted was decreased approximately 30% during cimetidine coadministration. However, when tetracycline was given as a solution, cimetidine had no effect. In another study involving 6 healthy subjects, a single dose of cimetidine 400 mg decreased the tetracycline area-under-the-curve (AUC) 40% following a single dose of tetracycline 500 mg.[1] The mean peak plasma concentration was reduced 40% and the 72-hour urinary tetracycline excretion was decreased approximately 30%. In contrast, cimetidine 400 mg 3 times daily and at bedtime for 6 days had no effect on tetracycline when the antibiotic was administered as a tablet or solution on the fifth day of cimetidine administration. Another single-dose study in 5 subjects showed that cimetidine 300 mg had no effect on the AUC, peak serum level, or urinary elimination of tetracycline following a 250 mg dose.[2]

[1] Fisher P, et al. *Br J Clin Pharmacol.* 1980;9:153.
[2] Garty M, et al. *Clin Pharmacol Ther.* 1980;28:203.
[3] Cole JJ, et al. *Lancet.* 1980;2:536.

* Asterisk indicates drugs cited in interaction reports. Based on pharmacologic and pharmacokinetic considerations, similar interactions may occur with other drugs that are listed.

Tetracyclines — *Colestipol*

Demeclocycline (*Declomycin*)	Minocycline (*Minocin*)	Colestipol* (*Colestid*)
Doxycycline (eg, *Vibramycin*)	Oxytetracycline (eg, *Terramycin*)	
Methacycline (*Rondomycin*)	Tetracycline* (eg, *Achromycin V*)	

Significance	Onset	Severity	Documentation
4	☐ Rapid	☐ Major	☐ Established
	■ **Delayed**	■ **Moderate**	☐ Probable
		☐ Minor	☐ Suspected
			■ **Possible**
			☐ Unlikely

Effects Coadministration of COLESTIPOL may decrease the serum levels of TETRACYCLINES, resulting in a decreased therapeutic response to the antibiotic.

Mechanism COLESTIPOL appears to decrease the absorption of TETRACYCLINES.

Management Based on currently available documentation, no special precautions are necessary. Observe the clinical response of the patient and adjust the dose of the TETRACYCLINE if needed.

Discussion

The extent to which coadministration of citric acid affects the ability of colestipol to impair tetracycline hydrochloride bioavailability was investigated in 9 healthy male volunteers.[1] The study was a single-dose three-way crossover design, in which subjects received a 500 mg dose of tetracycline on 3 occasions, each separated by 1 week. Tetracycline was given with 180 mL water, 30 g colestipol mixed with 180 mL water (usual dose of colestipol is 15 to 30 g daily in 2 to 4 divided doses), or 30 g colestipol mixed with 180 mL orange juice, containing approximately 1 g citric acid per 100 mL juice. All subjects completed the 3 phases. When administered with water, more than 50% of the tetracycline dose was recovered in the urine compared to 23% to 24% when administered with colestipol or colestipol plus citric acid. The mean 48-hour excretion of tetracycline when administered with water was 237 mg compared to 109 and 104 mg when administered with colestipol or colestipol plus citric acid. Although the results from the 2 trials in which tetracycline was administered with colestipol were not significantly different from each other, they were significantly reduced compared to the values obtained following administration with water alone ($P < 0.05$).

Additional multi-dose studies utilizing the usual dose of colestipol are needed to determine the extent and clinical significance of this possible interaction.

[1] Friedman H, et al. *J Clin Pharmacol.* 1989;29:748.

* Asterisk indicates drugs cited in interaction reports. Based on pharmacologic and pharmacokinetic considerations, similar interactions may occur with other drugs that are listed.

Tetracyclines — *Diuretics*

Tetracyclines		Diuretics	
Demeclocycline (eg, *Declomycin*)	Minocycline (eg, *Minocin*)	Bendroflumethiazide	Furosemide (eg, *Lasix*)
Doxycycline (eg, *Vibramycin*)	Tetracycline* (eg, *Sumycin*)	Bumetanide (eg, *Bumex*)	Hydrochlorothiazide (eg, *HydroDiuril*)
		Chlorothiazide (eg, *Diuril*)	Indapamide
		Chlorthalidone (eg, *Hygroton*)	Methyclothiazide (eg, *Enduron*)
		Ethacrynic Acid (*Edecrin*)	Metolazone (eg, *Zaroxolyn*)

Significance	Onset	Severity	Documentation
5	☐ Rapid	☐ Major	☐ Established
	■ **Delayed**	☐ Moderate	☐ Probable
		■ **Minor**	☐ Suspected
			☐ Possible
			■ **Unlikely**

Effects The coadministration of TETRACYCLINE with a diuretic may result in a significant increase in serum urea nitrogen (SUN), possibly resulting in uremia.

Mechanism Unknown. TETRACYCLINE alone may cause an increase in SUN.

Management No clinical interventions appear to be required. If the SUN levels begin to indicate dysfunction, consider halting one, or perhaps both, of the agents.

Discussion

In a detailed screening analysis from a drug surveillance program, it was determined that a clinically significant rise in SUN levels occurred more frequently (3-fold) in 20 patients receiving diuretics (specific diuretics not stated) and concurrent tetracycline compared with patients receiving diuretics alone.[1] A rise in SUN has been reported as an adverse reaction to tetracycline. Eighteen of the 20 patients received tetracycline within 1 week prior to the rise in SUN. Uremia was not reported in any of the patients.

The conclusions of this study have been questioned.[2] Further study is needed.

[1] Tetracycline and drug-attributed rises in blood urea nitrogen. A report from the Boston Collaborative drug surveillance program. *JAMA*. 1972;220(3):377.

[2] Tetracycline and rises in urea nitrogen. *JAMA*. 1972;221(7):713.

* Asterisk indicates drugs cited in interaction reports. Based on pharmacologic and pharmacokinetic considerations, similar interactions may occur with other drugs that are listed.

Tetracyclines — *Ethanol*

Doxycycline* (eg, *Vibramycin*)	Tetracycline* (eg, *Sumycin*)	Ethanol* (Alcohol, Ethyl Alcohol)

Significance	Onset	Severity	Documentation
5	□ Rapid ■ **Delayed**	□ Major □ Moderate ■ **Minor**	□ Established □ Probable □ Suspected ■ **Possible** □ Unlikely

Effects

Chronic ALCOHOL consumption results in faster DOXYCYCLINE clearance. Acute ALCOHOL consumption may increase TETRACYCLINE absorption.

Mechanism

Sustained ALCOHOL consumption possibly increases hepatic drug clearance. Acute ALCOHOL consumption may delay gastric emptying, increasing TETRACYCLINE dissolution and subsequent intestinal absorption.

Management

Observe response. It may be necessary to increase the DOXYCYCLINE dose, especially in patients receiving other drugs that induce hepatic metabolism. No special precautions are needed with TETRACYCLINE and ALCOHOL ingestion.

Discussion

The pharmacokinetics of doxycycline were compared in 6 alcoholic and 6 healthy volunteers.[1] The alcoholic patients had sustained ethanol use in amounts of 100 to 200 g/day, but had not been drinking for up to 30 days before this study. Doxycycline was given as an initial 200 mg dose followed by 100 mg every morning for an additional 2 days. The $t_{1/2}$ of doxycycline was 10.5 hours in the alcoholic patients compared with 14.7 hours in healthy volunteers. In addition, doxycycline trough serum concentrations were 0.5 mcg/mL or less in 4 of the 6 patients. A parallel study with oral tetracycline showed no pharmacokinetic differences between the volunteers and alcoholic subjects. In a study in 9 healthy volunteers, coadministration of tetracycline 500 mg with alcohol 270 mL/kg (blood alcohol level approximately 0.4 g/L 15 minutes after ingestion) produced a 32% increase in peak tetracycline levels and a 50% increase in the AUC when compared with water ingestion.[2] Given the magnitude of the increase in tetracycline levels, the interaction is not likely to be toxic and may be minimally beneficial.

It is not known if the alterations in doxycycline pharmacokinetics induced by alcohol result in impairment of therapeutic efficacy.

[1] Neuvonen PJ, et al. *Int J Clin Pharmacol Biopharm.* 1976;14(4):303.

[2] Seitz C, et al. *Int J Clin Pharmacol Ther.* 1995;33(8):462.

* Asterisk indicates drugs cited in interaction reports.

Tetracyclines — *Food*

Demeclocycline* (eg, *Declomycin*)	Oxytetracycline*	Food*
Methacycline*	Tetracycline* (eg, *Sumycin*)	

Significance	Onset	Severity	Documentation
2	☐ Rapid	☐ Major	☐ Established
	■ **Delayed**	■ **Moderate**	■ **Probable**
		☐ Minor	☐ Suspected
			☐ Possible
			☐ Unlikely

Effects Antimicrobial effectiveness of TETRACYCLINES may be reduced by food.

Mechanism Foods such as milk and dairy products contain calcium, which forms poorly absorbed chelates with the TETRACYCLINES.

Management Administer the interacting TETRACYCLINES at least 1 hour before or 2 hours after meals.

Discussion

A number of studies have reported the serum levels of demeclocycline, methacycline, oxytetracycline, and tetracycline to be 50% to 80% lower when administered in the presence of milk products.[1-4]

The inhibitory effect of food and milk on the absorption of doxycycline (eg, *Vibramycin*) and minocycline (eg, *Minocin*) is considerably less than that observed with other tetracycline derivatives. This may be due to a lower binding affinity to calcium ions. In 1 study, serum levels of tetracycline were reduced approximately 50% by test meals, whereas serum levels of doxycycline were reduced 20%.[5] In another study, the absorption of tetracycline was inhibited 46% by food (compared with 13% for minocycline) and 65% by milk (compared with 27% for minocycline).[6] Although food may inhibit the absorption of doxycycline and minocycline to some extent, these changes are not likely to be of clinical significance. Accordingly, these 2 agents are often administered without regard to meals. Administering doxycycline with food may reduce the occurrence of GI adverse reactions sometimes experienced with this antibiotic. Milk may inhibit the absorption of doxycycline and minocycline to a greater extent than other foods. Although these changes are not of clinical importance in most individuals, it is preferable to avoid the administration of milk with all tetracycline derivatives.

1 Scheiner J, et al. *Surg Gynecol Obstet.* 1962;114:9.
2 Rosenblatt JE, et al. *Antimicrob Agents Chemother.* 1966;6:134.
3 Neuvonen P, et al. *Scand J Clin Lab Invest.* 1971; 116(suppl 27):76
4 Mattila MJ, et al. *Excerpta Med Int Cong Series.* 1972;254:128.
5 Welling PG, et al. *Antimicrob Agents Chemother.* 1977;11(3):462.
6 Leyden JJ. *J Am Acad Dermatol.* 1985;12(2, pt 1):308.

* Asterisk indicates drugs cited in interaction reports.

Tetracyclines — *Iron Salts*

Tetracyclines		Iron Salts	
Demeclocycline (eg, *Declomycin*)	Minocycline (eg, *Minocin*)	Ferrous Fumarate* (eg, *Hemocyte*)	Ferrous Sulfate* (eg, *Feosol*)
Doxycycline* (eg, *Vibramycin*)	Oxytetracycline*	Ferrous Gluconate* (eg, *Fergon*)	Iron Polysaccharide (eg, *Niferex*)
Methacycline*	Tetracycline* (eg, *Sumycin*)		

Significance	Onset	Severity	Documentation
2	□ Rapid	□ Major	□ Established
	■ **Delayed**	■ **Moderate**	■ **Probable**
		□ Minor	□ Suspected
			□ Possible
			□ Unlikely

Effects Coadministration may decrease absorption and serum levels of TETRACYCLINES; a decreased anti-infective response may occur. Absorption of IRON SALTS may also be decreased.

Mechanism TETRACYCLINES form insoluble chelates with IRON SALTS, decreasing absorption and serum levels of either.

Management Avoid coadministration of TETRACYCLINES and IRON SALTS. This interaction may be minimized by separating administration by 3 to 4 hours, or by using an enteric-coated or sustained-release formulation of the IRON SALT.

Discussion

Many studies have shown that tetracyclines form insoluble chelates with polyvalent metal cations including iron salts.[1,2] This results in decreased absorption (50% to more than 90%) and serum levels of the tetracyclines, possibly resulting in a decreased therapeutic effect.[3-6] This may depend on the iron salt and the use of a tablet or capsule formulation.[7] Several studies show that the absorption and serum levels of doxycycline, methacycline, minocycline, and oxytetracycline are decreased by the coadministration of iron salts.[3,6,8,9] Even parenteral doxycycline may be affected.[10] In 1 study, inhibition of tetracycline absorption by ferrous sulfate, ferrous gluconate, or ferrous fumarate was 85%, 70%, and 80%, respectively.[11] Capsule formulations of ferrous sulfate may reduce the absorption of tetracycline to a greater extent than tablet formulations, and enteric-coated iron preparations inhibit absorption to a lesser extent than regular tablets[1]; interaction is also reduced with a sustained-release formulation of iron. The absorption of the iron salts may also be decreased during tetracycline coadministration.[11,12]

1 Neuvonen PJ. *Drugs.* 1976;11(1):45.
2 D'Arcy PF, et al. *Drug Intell Clin Pharm.* 1987;21(7-8):607.
3 Neuvonen PJ, et al. *Br Med J.* 1970;4(5734):532.
4 Greenberger NJ. *Ann Intern Med.* 1971;74(5):792.
5 Gothoni G, et al. *Acta Med Scand.* 1972;191(5):409.
6 Mattila MJ, et al. *Excerpta Med Int Cong Series.* 1972;254:128.
7 Neuvonen PJ, et al. *Eur J Clin Pharmacol.* 1974;7(5):357.
8 Neuvonen PJ, et al. *Eur J Clin Pharmacol.* 1974;7(5):361.
9 Leyden JJ. *J Am Acad Dermatol.* 1985;12(2, pt 1):308.
10 Venho VM, et al. *Eur J Clin Pharmacol.* 1978;14(4):277.
11 Heinrich HC, et al. *Klin Wochenschr.* 1974;52(10):493.
12 Heinrich HC, et al. *Naturwissenschaften.* 1973;60(11):524.

* Asterisk indicates drugs cited in interaction reports. Based on pharmacologic and pharmacokinetic considerations, similar interactions may occur with other drugs that are listed.

Tetracyclines			*Magnesium Salts*
Demeclocycline (eg, *Declomycin*)	Minocycline (eg, *Minocin*)	Magaldrate (eg, *Riopan*)	Magnesium Hydroxide* (eg, Milk of Magnesia)
Doxycycline (eg, *Vibramycin*)	Tetracycline* (eg, *Sumycin*)	Magnesium Carbonate (eg, *Marblen*)	Magnesium Oxide (eg, *Mag-Ox*)
		Magnesium Citrate	Magnesium Sulfate*
		Magnesium Gluconate (eg, *Magtrate*)	

Significance	Onset	Severity	Documentation
2	□ Rapid	□ Major	□ Established
	■ **Delayed**	■ **Moderate**	■ **Probable**
		□ Minor	□ Suspected
			□ Possible
			□ Unlikely

Effects Coadministration of TETRACYCLINES and MAGNESIUM SALTS decreases the absorption and serum levels of the TETRACYCLINES; a decreased antimicrobial response may occur.

Mechanism TETRACYCLINES form an insoluble chelate with MAGNESIUM SALTS, decreasing absorption and serum levels of the TETRACYCLINES.

Management Avoid simultaneous administration of TETRACYCLINES and MAGNESIUM SALTS; separate the administration of these agents by 3 to 4 hours.

Discussion

Many studies have shown that tetracyclines form insoluble chelates with polyvalent metal cations including magnesium salts.[1-6] This results in a significant decrease in absorption (50% to more than 90%) and serum levels of the tetracyclines, possibly resulting in a decreased therapeutic effect. In 1 study, 5 patients were given single doses of tetracycline 250 mg and a magnesium-aluminum hydroxide gel.[5] The bioavailability of tetracycline was reduced 90%, and serum levels were decreased. In a study involving 10 volunteers, the coadministration of single doses of tetracycline 300 to 1,000 mg and oral magnesium sulfate decreased the serum levels of tetracycline 4-fold compared with tetracycline alone or with castor oil.[2]

[1] Albert A, et al. *Nature.* 1956;177(4505):433.
[2] Harcourt RS, et al. *J Lab Clin Med.* 1957;50(3):464.
[3] Chin TF, et al. *Am J Hosp Pharm.* 1975;32(6):625.
[4] Neuvonen PJ. *Drugs.* 1976;11(1):45.
[5] Garty M, et al. *Clin Pharmacol Ther.* 1980;28(2):203.
[6] D'Arcy PF, et al. *Drug Intell Clin Pharm.* 1987;21(7-8):607.

* Asterisk indicates drugs cited in interaction reports. Based on pharmacologic and pharmacokinetic considerations, similar interactions may occur with other drugs that are listed.

Tetracyclines		Urinary Alkalinizers	
Demeclocycline (*Declomycin*)	Minocycline (*Minocin*)	Potassium Citrate (*Urocit-K*)	Sodium Citrate
Doxycycline* (eg, *Vibramycin*)	Oxytetracycline (eg, *Terramycin*)	Sodium Acetate	Sodium Lactate*
Methacycline (*Rondomycin*)	Tetracycline* (eg, *Achromycin V*)	Sodium Bicarbonate*	Tromethamine (*Tham, Tham-E*)

Significance	Onset	Severity	Documentation
2	☐ Rapid ■ **Delayed**	☐ Major ■ **Moderate** ☐ Minor	☐ Established ☐ Probable ■ **Suspected** ☐ Possible ☐ Unlikely

Effects

Coadministration of TETRACYCLINES with URINARY ALKALINIZERS may result in increased excretion of the TETRACYCLINES and decreased serum levels. A decreased therapeutic response could occur. Other reports conflict.

Mechanism

Possibly altered tubular reabsorption of the TETRACYCLINES due to the alkaline urine. Increased gastric pH may decrease TETRACYCLINE absorption. This may only be significant with formulations having poor bioavailability.

Management

Separate use of these agents by 3 to 4 hours. However, if the pH of the urine is increased by URINARY ALKALINIZERS, this may not be effective in minimizing the interaction. Increased doses of TETRACYCLINE may be necessary.

Discussion

In 2 studies, alkalinization of the urine with sodium lactate increased the cumulative urinary excretion of tetracycline 500 mg (24%) and doxycycline 200 mg (54% to 65%) compared with controls or acidic urine.[1,2] Doxycycline serum levels also decreased, and the half-life decreased 30.5% to 32%. In another study, sodium bicarbonate given simultaneously with tetracycline decreased the cumulative amount of unchanged tetracycline in the urine, indicating a 50% reduction in tetracycline absorption.[3] This study suggested that a low gastric pH is necessary for the dissolution and absorption of tetracycline; therefore, the increased gastric pH by sodium bicarbonate decreased tetracycline's absorption. However, other reports suggest that the increased gastric pH only plays a role when tetracycline capsules with poor bioavailability are used.[4,5] The bioavailability of the tetracycline capsule in the previous study was only 61.5%. In contrast, 2 other studies reported that sodium bicarbonate administration did not affect the absorption of tetracycline.[5,6] Further studies are needed.

[1] Jaffe JM, et al. *J Pharmacokinet Biopharm.* 1973;1:267.
[2] Jaffe JM, et al. *J Pharm Sci.* 1974;63:1256.
[3] Barr WH, et al. *Clin Pharmacol Ther.* 1971;12:779.
[4] Elliott GR, et al. *Clin Pharmacol Ther.* 1972;13:459.
[5] Kramer PA, et al. *Clin Pharmacol Ther.* 1978;23:467.
[6] Garty M, et al. *Clin Pharmacol Ther.* 1980;28:203.

* Asterisk indicates drugs cited in interaction reports. Based on pharmacologic and pharmacokinetic considerations, similar interactions may occur with other drugs that are listed.

Tetracyclines — *Zinc Salts*

Tetracyclines		Zinc Salts
Demeclocycline (*Declomycin*)	Oxytetracycline (eg, *Terramycin*)	Zinc Gluconate
Methacycline (*Rondomycin*)	Tetracycline* (eg, *Achromycin V*)	Zinc Sulfate* (eg, *Orazinc*)
Minocycline (*Minocin*)		

Significance	Onset	Severity	Documentation
2	☐ Rapid	☐ Major	☐ Established
	■ **Delayed**	■ **Moderate**	■ **Probable**
		☐ Minor	☐ Suspected
			☐ Possible
			☐ Unlikely

Effects Coadministration of TETRACYCLINES and ZINC SALTS decreases the absorption and serum levels of the TETRACYCLINES; a decreased anti-infective response may occur.

Mechanism TETRACYCLINES form an insoluble chelate with ZINC SALTS, decreasing absorption and serum levels of the TETRACYCLINES.

Management Avoid coadministration of TETRACYCLINES and ZINC SALTS; separate the administration of these agents by 3 to 4 hours. Doxycycline may be a non-interacting alternative to TETRACYCLINE, although further study is needed.

Discussion

Many studies have shown that tetracyclines form insoluble chelates with polyvalent metal cations, including zinc salts.[1-3] This results in a significant decrease in absorption (50% to more than 90%) and serum levels of the tetracyclines, possibly resulting in a decreased therapeutic effect. In 1 study, 4 subjects received single doses of tetracycline 250 mg and zinc sulfate 220 mg; the mean cumulative amount of tetracycline excreted was decreased 75% compared with tetracycline alone.[4] In another study, 7 subjects were given single doses of tetracycline 500 mg and zinc sulfate.[5] Compared with tetracycline alone, coadministration with zinc sulfate resulted in a 53% decrease in mean maximum tetracycline serum levels. Seven healthy volunteers received a single dose of either tetracycline 500 mg or doxycycline 200 mg with zinc sulfate.[6] Zinc reduced tetracycline's serum concentration, AUC, and excretion approximately 30% to 40%. However, doxycycline was not affected by concurrent zinc administration.

[1] Albert A, et al. *Nature.* 1956;177:433.
[2] Neuvonen PJ. *Drugs.* 1976;11:45.
[3] D'Arcy PF, et al. *Drug Intell Clin Pharm.* 1987;21:607.
[4] Mapp RK, et al. *S Afr Med J.* 1976;50:1829.
[5] Anderson K-E, et al. *Eur J Clin Pharmacol.* 1976;10:59.
[6] Penttila O, et al. *Eur J Clin Pharmacol.* 1975;9:131.

* Asterisk indicates drugs cited in interaction reports. Based on pharmacologic and pharmacokinetic considerations, similar interactions may occur with other drugs that are listed.

Theophyllines — *Acyclovir*

Aminophylline*	Theophylline* (eg, *Theo-Dur*)	Acyclovir* (*Zovirax*)
Oxtriphylline†		

Significance	Onset	Severity	Documentation
2	☐ Rapid	☐ Major	☐ Established
	■ **Delayed**	■ **Moderate**	☐ Probable
		☐ Minor	■ **Suspected**
			☐ Possible
			☐ Unlikely

Effects Plasma THEOPHYLLINE concentrations may be elevated, increasing the pharmacologic and adverse effects.

Mechanism Possible inhibition of oxidative metabolism of THEOPHYLLINE.

Management Carefully monitor plasma THEOPHYLLINE concentrations and observe the patient for side effects during concurrent administration of ACYCLOVIR. Adjust the THEOPHYLLINE dose as needed.

Discussion

As the result of the occurrence of theophylline side effects and increased plasma theophylline concentrations in a patient after starting acyclovir, a study of the effects of acyclovir on the pharmacokinetics of theophylline was conducted in 5 healthy male volunteers.[1] In a crossover design, with each subject serving as his own control, each individual initially received a single dose of aminophylline 400 mg. After a washout period of 13 days, acyclovir 800 mg 5 times daily was administered. Following 2 days of acyclovir administration, each subject received 400 mg aminophylline. Acyclovir administration increased the area under the theophylline plasma concentration-time curve 45%, increased plasma theophylline concentrations 54%, and decreased the total body clearance of theophylline 30%.

[1] Maeda Y, et al. *Biol Pharm Bull.* 1996;19:1591.

* Asterisk indicates drugs cited in interaction reports. Based on pharmacologic and pharmacokinetic considerations, similar interactions may occur with other drugs that are listed.
† Not available in the United States.

Theophyllines — *Allopurinol*

Theophyllines	Allopurinol
Aminophylline	Allopurinol* (eg, *Zyloprim*)
Theophylline* (eg, *Theo-24*)	

Significance	Onset	Severity	Documentation
4	☐ Rapid	☐ Major	☐ Established
	■ **Delayed**	■ **Moderate**	☐ Probable
		☐ Minor	☐ Suspected
			■ **Possible**
			☐ Unlikely

Effects THEOPHYLLINE clearance may be decreased with large dosages of ALLOPURINOL (600 mg/day), leading to increased plasma THEOPHYLLINE levels and possible toxicity.

Mechanism ALLOPURINOL 600 mg/day or more may impair liver degradation of THEOPHYLLINE.

Management No problems should occur when ALLOPURINOL is given in normal therapeutic amounts (300 mg/day). With larger ALLOPURINOL doses, monitor THEOPHYLLINE levels and tailor dosages as needed to avoid toxicity.

Discussion

Two investigations in healthy men determined theophylline clearance before and after pretreatment with allopurinol 300 mg/day for 7 days.[1,2] No significant difference was found in theophylline clearance during concomitant allopurinol use.

In a separate study involving 12 healthy men, theophylline kinetics were determined before and after pretreatment with allopurinol 600 mg/day for 14 and 28 days.[3] The mean theophylline AUC was significantly increased (27%), the mean $t_{½}$ was significantly increased (25%), and the mean clearance was significantly decreased (21%) at 14 days. After 28 consecutive days of allopurinol therapy, theophylline disposition was not significantly different than at day 14.

Additional studies are needed to determine the actual clinical significance of this interaction. Of interest, allopurinol can interfere with the spectrophotometric assay for theophylline in biological fluids.[4] If unusual results are obtained from a theophylline assay, consider this source of possible interference and use an alternate method to analyze theophylline levels. See also Theophyllines-Febuxostat.

[1] Grygiel JJ, et al. *Clin Pharmacol Ther.* 1979;26(5):660.
[2] Vozeh S, et al. *Clin Pharmacol Ther.* 1980;27(2):194.
[3] Manfredi RL, et al. *Clin Pharmacol Ther.* 1981;29(2):224.
[4] Woodman TF, et al. *Am J Hosp Pharm.* 1977;34(9):984.

* Asterisk indicates drugs cited in interaction reports. Based on pharmacologic and pharmacokinetic considerations, similar interactions may occur with other drugs that are listed.

Theophyllines — *Amiodarone*

Theophylline* (eg, *Theo-24*)	Amiodarone* (eg, *Cordarone*)

Significance	Onset	Severity	Documentation
4	☐ Rapid	☐ Major	☐ Established
	■ **Delayed**	■ **Moderate**	☐ Probable
		☐ Minor	☐ Suspected
			■ **Possible**
			☐ Unlikely

Effects Increased THEOPHYLLINE levels with toxicity may occur. Because of the long $t_{1/2}$ of AMIODARONE, effects may not be seen for at least 1 week and may persist for an extended period of time after discontinuation of AMIODARONE.

Mechanism Inhibition of the THEOPHYLLINE metabolism by AMIODARONE is suspected.

Management Consider monitoring serum THEOPHYLLINE levels and observing the patient for signs of toxicity. Adjust the dose of THEOPHYLLINE if needed.

Discussion

An 86-year-old patient with a history of chronic obstructive pulmonary disease and atrial fibrillation experienced increased theophylline levels during coadministration of amiodarone.[1] The patient was receiving furosemide (eg, *Lasix*) 40 mg daily, digoxin (eg, *Lanoxin*) 0.25 mg 5 days per week, domperidone† 10 mL 3 times daily, and sustained-release theophylline 300 mg twice daily. Physical examination disclosed signs of nausea, biventricular failure with an arrhythmic pulse rate of 110 beats/min, and respirations of 28 breaths/min. His serum theophylline and digoxin levels obtained 12 and 24 hours after the last dose were 93.24 mcmol/L (therapeutic range, 55 to 110 mcmol/L) and 3.07 nmol/L (therapeutic range, 0.6 to 2.8 nmol/L), respectively. Digoxin was discontinued because of suspected toxicity. After 2 days, his nausea improved but he remained tachycardic. Digoxin was reinstated at 0.125 mg 5 times per week, and amiodarone 600 mg daily was initiated. Nine days later, the patient's heart rate increased to 130 beats/min, and he had symptoms of nervousness and hand tremors. Theophylline and digoxin concentrations were 194.2 mcmol/L and 2.2 nmol/L, respectively. Theophylline toxicity was suspected, and the drug was discontinued. Within 48 hours, the patient's heart rate was 90 beats/min, and symptoms of theophylline toxicity were no longer present. Theophylline was reintroduced at a dose of 150 mg twice daily. Four days later, the patient experienced cardiorespiratory arrest and died.

Additional studies are needed to confirm this possible interaction because this case may have been secondary to congestive heart failure.

[1] Soto J, et al. *DICP*. 1990;24(11):1115.

* Asterisk indicates drugs cited in interaction reports.
† Not available in the United States.

Theophyllines — Barbiturates

Theophyllines		Barbiturates	
Aminophylline*	Theophylline* (eg, *Bronkodyl*)	Amobarbital (eg, *Amytal*)	Pentobarbital* (eg, *Nembutal*)
Oxtriphylline*†		Aprobarbital (*Alurate*)	Phenobarbital*
		Butabarbital (eg, *Butisol*)	Primidone (eg, *Mysoline*)
		Butalbital	Secobarbital* (eg, *Seconal*)
		Mephobarbital (*Mebaral*)	

Significance	Onset	Severity	Documentation
2	☐ Rapid	☐ Major	☐ Established
	■ **Delayed**	■ **Moderate**	☐ Probable
		☐ Minor	■ **Suspected**
			☐ Possible
			☐ Unlikely

Effects Decreased THEOPHYLLINE levels, possibly resulting in reduced therapeutic effects.

Mechanism BARBITURATES may induce cytochrome P450, stimulating THEOPHYLLINE metabolism and increasing clearance.

Management Increased THEOPHYLLINE dosages may be required with use of a BARBITURATE. Closely monitor plasma levels of THEOPHYLLINE when BARBITURATES are added to or removed from a patient's drug regimen; tailor dosage as needed.

Discussion

Data indicate that barbiturates stimulate the metabolism of theophylline.[1-9] Single-dose studies in healthy subjects describe theophylline clearance increases of 17%,[1] 11% to 60%,[2] and 4% to 79%.[10] Similar effects have been reported in children[6] and premature infants,[8,9] although 1 study in premature neonates showed phenobarbital had little effect on theophylline clearance.[11] Barbiturates were also found to affect theophylline disposition in pulmonary patients, pediatric patients, and healthy subjects.[3] In 1 case, phenobarbital appeared to be additive to phenytoin in stimulating theophylline clearance.[12] While little data from controlled trials are available, barbiturates appear to alter theophylline kinetics. Aminophylline and oxtriphylline have also been implicated. Dyphylline (eg, *Lufyllin*), which undergoes renal elimination, would not be expected to be affected.

[1] Piafsky KM, et al. *Clin Pharmacol Ther.* 1977;22:336.
[2] Landay RA, et al. *J Allergy Clin Immunol.* 1978;62:27.
[3] Jusko WJ, et al. *J Pharm Sci.* 1979;68:1358.
[4] Paladino JA, et al. *Ther Drug Monit.* 1983;5:135.
[5] Gibson GA, et al. *Ther Drug Monit.* 1985;7:181.
[6] Saccar CL, et al. *J Allergy Clin Immunol.* 1985;75:716.
[7] Lhermitte M, et al. *J Pediatr.* 1987;11:667.
[8] Yazdani M, et al. *Am J Dis Child.* 1987;141:97.
[9] Wilschanski M, et al. *Am J Dis Child.* 1988;142:122.
[10] Dahlquist R, et al. *Ther Drug Monit.* 1989;11:408.
[11] Kandrotas RJ, et al. *Ther Drug Monit.* 1990;12:139.
[12] Nicholson JP, et al. *Ann Pharmacother.* 1992;26:334.

* Asterisk indicates drugs cited in interaction reports. Based on pharmacologic and pharmacokinetic considerations, similar interactions may occur with other drugs that are listed.
† Not available in the United States.

Theophyllines — *Beta-Blockers, Non-Selective*

Theophyllines		Beta-Blockers, Non-Selective	
Aminophylline*†	Oxtriphylline†	Carteolol (*Cartrol*)	Propranolol* (eg, *Inderal*)
Dyphylline (eg, *Lufyllin*)	Theophylline* (eg, *Bronkodyl*)	Penbutolol (*Levatol*)	Timolol (eg, *Blocadren*)
		Pindolol (eg, *Visken*)	

Significance	Onset	Severity	Documentation
2	■ **Rapid**	□ Major	□ Established
	□ Delayed	■ **Moderate**	■ **Probable**
		□ Minor	□ Suspected
			□ Possible
			□ Unlikely

Effects Reduced elimination of THEOPHYLLINE has been noted in the presence of certain BETA-BLOCKERS. Pharmacologic antagonism can also be expected, thus reducing the effects of one or both medications.

Mechanism Pharmacologic antagonism. BETA-BLOCKERS may reduce the n-demethylation of THEOPHYLLINE.

Management Monitor patients for clinical changes. Monitor plasma THEOPHYLLINE levels when a BETA-BLOCKER is added or deleted from a regimen. Beta-selective agents may be preferred.

Discussion

Pharmacologic antagonism can be expected between theophylline and beta-blockers, particularly non-selective beta-blockers.[1,2] Beta-blockers have stimulated airway resistance in patients.[1] Resistance has been reversed successfully with a beta-agonist when selective beta-blockers were present.[1] When necessary, selective beta-blockers are preferred in patients on theophylline. However, selectivity is lost with high doses of the beta-blocker.

Propranolol is thought to inhibit n-demethylation of theophylline. Clearance of theophylline has been reduced 30% to 50% by propranolol.[3-5] Altered clearance may be dose dependent but requires further evaluation. A study evaluating metoprolol's effect on theophylline clearance noted a dramatic change in smokers whose clearance was initially high.[3] Conversely, in 6 volunteer smokers neither atenolol (a cardioselective agent) nor nadolol significantly altered theophylline kinetics.[6] Propranolol's usefulness in theophylline overdosage has been suggested.[7,8] Caution is warranted because propranolol may alter theophylline metabolism.[9] Beta-blockers that affect the hepatic mixed oxidase system would be expected to act similarly.

[1] Horvath JS, et al. *Aust NZ J Med.* 1978;8:1.
[2] Mue S, et al. *Int J Clin Pharmacol Biopharm.* 1979; 17:346.
[3] Conrad KA, et al. *Clin Pharmacol Ther.* 1980;28:463.
[4] Miners JO, et al. *Br J Clin Pharmacol.* 1985;20:219.
[5] Lombardi TP, et al. *J Clin Pharmacol.* 1987;27:523.
[6] Corsi CM, et al. *Br J Clin Pharmac.* 1990;29:265.
[7] Amin DN, et al. *Lancet.* 1985;1:520.
[8] Kearney TE, et al. *Ann Intern Med.* 1985;102:766.
[9] Farrar KT, et al. *Lancet.* 1985;1:983.

* Asterisk indicates drugs cited in interaction reports. Based on pharmacologic and pharmacokinetic considerations, similar interactions may occur with other drugs that are listed.
† Not available in the United States.

Theophyllines			*Caffeine*
Aminophylline* Oxtriphylline†	Theophylline (eg, *Bronkodyl*)	Caffeine*	

Significance	Onset	Severity	Documentation
5	■ **Rapid** □ Delayed	□ Major □ Moderate ■ **Minor**	□ Established □ Probable □ Suspected ■ **Possible** □ Unlikely

Effects Serum THEOPHYLLINE concentrations may be increased.

Mechanism Unknown. However, interference with THEOPHYLLINE metabolism appears to be involved, as well as the derivation of additional THEOPHYLLINE from caffeine metabolism.

Management In most patients, the effect will be minimal. Inform patients of the effect of CAFFEINE ingestion on THEOPHYLLINE therapy and advise them to avoid drastic changes in their daily intake of CAFFEINE.

Discussion

In an open crossover trial, the effects of dietary caffeine (coffee) on the pharmacokinetics of theophylline, following a single oral dose of aminophylline 400 mg, were studied in 6 healthy volunteers.[1] Each subject consumed 2 to 7 cups of regular instant coffee (120 to 630 mg caffeine) during a 24-hour period. Subsequently, each subject received 400 mg aminophylline before breakfast. Three to 24 hours after theophylline administration, the serum drug concentration was greater following caffeine intake compared with when the same subjects had not drunk coffee. In addition, in subjects having caffeine, the half-life of theophylline was prolonged 32% ($P < 0.01$), and the clearance was decreased 23% ($P < 0.001$). The peak serum concentration, the time to reach the peak serum concentration, and the volume of distribution of theophylline were not changed significantly.

[1] Sato J, et al. *Eur J Clin Pharmacol.* 1993;44:295.

* Asterisk indicates drugs cited in interaction reports. Based on pharmacologic and pharmacokinetic considerations, similar interactions may occur with other drugs that are listed.
† Not available in the United States.

Theophyllines — *Carbamazepine*

Aminophylline	Theophylline* (eg, *Bronkodyl*)	Carbamazepine* (eg, *Tegretol*)
Oxtriphylline†		

Significance	Onset	Severity	Documentation
4	☐ Rapid	☐ Major	☐ Established
	■ **Delayed**	■ **Moderate**	☐ Probable
		☐ Minor	☐ Suspected
			■ **Possible**
			☐ Unlikely

Effects THEOPHYLLINE levels may be increased or decreased. CARBAMAZEPINE levels may be decreased.

Mechanism Possibly mutual induction of hepatic metabolism.

Management Monitor THEOPHYLLINE and CARBAMAZEPINE levels. Adjust the dosages accordingly.

Discussion

In a case report, an 11-year-old girl was treated with theophylline 23 mg/kg/day and phenobarbital.[1] Substitution of carbamazepine for phenobarbital resulted in subtherapeutic theophylline concentrations and intermittent wheezing. After 3 weeks of carbamazepine therapy, the elimination $t_{1/2}$ of theophylline had decreased from 5.25 to 2.75 hours. Carbamazepine was changed to ethotoin (*Peganone*) and in 3 weeks the patient's asthma was controlled. Theophylline elimination $t_{1/2}$ increased to 6.5 hours.

Another case report involving a 10-year-old girl suggests that theophylline reduces carbamazepine levels.[2] The patient was stabilized on carbamazepine 10 mg/kg daily when she suffered a grand mal seizure after receiving theophylline 14 mg/kg/day for 8 days. She had received theophylline on 3 prior occasions with no adverse effect. To determine whether a drug interaction was responsible, the patient's carbamazepine level was measured daily. The trough levels were between 27 to 30 mcmol/L and the $t_{1/2}$ was 11.9 hours. Theophylline 20 mg/kg daily was added, and after 7 doses, the patient had a grand mal seizure. The serum theophylline level was 142 mcmol/L and the serum carbamazepine level was 19 mcmol/L with a decrease in carbamazepine $t_{1/2}$ to 10.5 hours. Theophylline was stopped and, after 2 days, trough levels of carbamazepine remained below baseline.

[1] Rosenberry KR, et al. *J Pediatr.* 1983;102:472.

[2] Mitchell EA, et al. *NZ Med J.* 1986;1:69.

* Asterisk indicates drugs cited in interaction reports. Based on pharmacologic and pharmacokinetic considerations, similar interactions may occur with other drugs that are listed.

† Not available in the United States.

Theophyllines — *Cimetidine*

Aminophylline*	Theophylline* (eg, *Theolair*)	Cimetidine* (eg, *Tagamet*)
Oxtriphylline*†		

Significance	Onset	Severity	Documentation
2	□ Rapid	□ Major	■ **Established**
	■ **Delayed**	■ **Moderate**	□ Probable
		□ Minor	□ Suspected
			□ Possible
			□ Unlikely

Effects Increased THEOPHYLLINE levels with toxicity may occur.

Mechanism Inhibition of the hepatic metabolism of THEOPHYLLINES.

Management Monitor THEOPHYLLINE levels. Adding CIMETIDINE may necessitate a 20% to 40% reduction in THEOPHYLLINE dose.

Discussion

Data from case reports,[1-5] trials in healthy subjects,[6-20] and those with pulmonary disease[21-23] found a decrease in theophylline clearance of approximately 33%, an increase in $t_{1/2}$ of approximately 50%, and increases in plasma levels of 33% to 50%. No changes in volume of distribution were noted. Smaller changes were noted when using nonprescription doses of cimetidine 200 mg twice daily.[24] One study described kinetic changes within 24 hours[8]; however, maximal changes usually occur within 72 hours.[21] Age has no effect.[15,16,25] Smoking, while stimulating theophylline clearance, has not consistently altered cimetidine's effect on theophylline.[12,13,16] Protein deficient diets have increased kinetic changes.[26] A genetic resistance to the interaction has been proposed.[17] The demethylation pathway may be saturable[4,15] and dose-dependent, so patients with theophylline levels greater than 15 mcg/mL are at highest risk for toxicity. Patients with fast basal theophylline metabolic rates show a greater decrease in clearance.[17] IV administration of cimetidine may not alter IV theophylline kinetics.[27] Hospitalizations from theophylline toxicity in patients receiving both drugs were 5 times greater than with theophylline use alone.[28] Seizures have been reported.[3,4] Coadministration of cimetidine and ciprofloxacin reduced theophylline clearance more than either drug alone.[25,26] See Theophylline-Famotidine and Theophylline-Ranitidine.

1 Weinberger MM, et al. *N Engl J Med.* 1981;304:672.
2 Campbell MA, et al. *Ann Intern Med.* 1981;95:68.
3 Lofgren RP, et al. *Ann Intern Med.* 1982;96:378.
4 Bauman JH, et al. *Ann Allergy.* 1982;48:100.
5 Pride M, et al. *Am Fam Phy.* 1995;52:2180.
6 Roberts RK, et al. *Gastroenterology.* 1981;81:19.
7 Jackson JE, et al. *Am Rev Respir Dis.* 1981;123:615.
8 Reitberg DP, et al. *Ann Intern Med.* 1981;95:582.
9 Breen KJ, et al. *Clin Pharmacol Ther.* 1982;31:297.
10 Schwartz JI, et al. *Clin Pharm.* 1982;1:534.
11 DeAngelis C, et al. *Clin Pharm.* 1983;2:563.
12 Grygiel JJ, et al. *Eur J Clin Pharmacol.* 1984;26:335.
13 Cusack BJ, et al. *Clin Pharmacol Ther.* 1985;37:330.
14 Dal Negro R, et al. *Int J Clin Pharmacol Ther Toxicol.* 1985;23:329.
15 Cohen IA, et al. *Ther Drug Monit.* 1985;7:426.
16 Vestal RE, et al. *J Pharmacol Exp Ther.* 1987;241:488.
17 Cremer KF, et al. *J Clin Pharmacol.* 1989;29:451.
18 Yoshimura N, et al. *Int J Clin Pharmacol Ther Tox.* 1989;27:308.
19 Krstenansky PM, et al. *Clin Pharm.* 1989;8:206.
20 Adebyo GI. *Biopharm Drug Disp.* 1989;10:77.
21 Vestal RE, et al. *Br J Clin Pharmacol.* 1983;15:411.
22 Boehning W. *Eur J Clin Pharmacol.* 1990;38:43.
23 Bachmann K, et al. *J Clin Pharmacol.* 1995;35:529.
24 Nix DE, et al. *J Clin Pharmacol.* 1999;39:855.
25 Loi CM, et al. *Br J Clin Pharmacol.* 1993;36:195.
26 Dean M, et al. *Drug Intell Clin Pharm.* 1986;20:470.
27 Gaska JA, et al. *J Clin Pharmacol.* 1991;31:668.
28 Derby LE, et al. *Pharmacotherapy.* 1990;10:112.
29 Loi CM, et al. *J Pharmacol Exp Ther.* 1997;280:627.

* Asterisk indicates drugs cited in interaction reports.
† Not available in the United States.

Theophyllines / *Contraceptives, Hormonal*

Aminophylline*	Contraceptives, Oral*
Theophylline	(eg, *Ortho-Novum*)
(eg, *Theochron*)	

Significance	Onset	Severity	Documentation
2	□ Rapid	□ Major	□ Established
	■ **Delayed**	■ **Moderate**	□ Probable
		□ Minor	■ **Suspected**
			□ Possible
			□ Unlikely

Effects Possible THEOPHYLLINE toxicity because of decreased elimination.

Mechanism ORAL CONTRACEPTIVES decrease the oxidative degradation of THEOPHYLLINE by cytochrome P-448.

Management Clinical assessment and periodic determinations of THEOPHYLLINE serum level are advocated in patients receiving concomitant therapy. Tailor THEOPHYLLINE dosage as needed.

Discussion

Five published studies have evaluated the effect of oral contraceptives on theophylline kinetics. Decreased total theophylline clearance and increased theophylline $t_{1/2}$ have been noted.[1-3] One study also noted similar findings but only in smokers.[4] Contrary to the previous information, another study of adolescent girls found no alterations in theophylline kinetics between the test group and controls.[5] Differences have been attributed to age of the study group (women vs adolescents), use of oral vs IV theophylline, and length of time on oral contraceptives. Until further information is available to delineate true dependent variables, caution is advised.

[1] Tornatore KM, et al. *Eur J Clin Pharmacol.* 1982;23(2):129.
[2] Gardner MJ, et al. *Br J Clin Pharmacol.* 1983;16(3):271.
[3] Roberts RK, et al. *J Lab Clin Med.* 1983;101(6):821.
[4] Jusko WJ, et al. *J Pharm Sci.* 1979;68(11):1358.
[5] Koren G, et al. *Clin Invest Med.* 1985;8(3):222.

* Asterisk indicates drugs cited in interaction reports. Based on pharmacologic and pharmacokinetic considerations, similar interactions may occur with other drugs that are listed.

Theophyllines | *Corticosteroids*

Theophyllines	Corticosteroids	
Aminophylline*	Hydrocortisone* (eg, *Cortef*)	Prednisone* (eg, *Sterapred*)
Theophylline* (eg, *Theochron*)		

Significance	Onset	Severity	Documentation
4	■ **Rapid**	□ Major	□ Established
	□ Delayed	■ **Moderate**	□ Probable
		□ Minor	□ Suspected
			■ **Possible**
			□ Unlikely

Effects Alterations in pharmacologic activity of THEOPHYLLINE as well as PREDNISONE may occur.

Mechanism Unknown.

Management If signs of THEOPHYLLINE intoxication appear, monitor serum levels and tailor dosage as needed.

Discussion

A rise in theophylline levels during hydrocortisone administration occurred in 3 patients experiencing status asthmaticus.[1] Plasma concentrations were elevated and caused nausea and headache in 2 patients. Decreased bioavailability of prednisolone from prednisone in the presence of theophylline (administered as aminophylline) has been reported.[2] Unfortunately, neither of these interactions is supported by other research.[3-6] In fact, a 21% increase in theophylline clearance was noted in 7 healthy subjects stabilized on theophylline who received methylprednisolone or hydrocortisone IV.[5] Many of these studies are single dose in healthy volunteers with small sample sizes. This makes clinical interpretation difficult. Alterations in patient response may occur and should be monitored, but no clinical interventions seem warranted until further research delineates the significance of this interaction.

[1] Buchanan N, et al. *S Afr Med J.* 1979;56(27):1147.
[2] Anderson JL, et al. *Clin Pharm.* 1984;3(2):187.
[3] Brooks SM, et al. *J Clin Pharmacol.* 1977;17(5-6):308.
[4] Jusko WJ, et al. *J Pharm Sci.* 1979;68(11):1358.
[5] Leavengood DC, et al. *Ann Allergy.* 1983;50(4):249.
[6] Fergusson RJ, et al. *Thorax.* 1987;42(3):195.

* Asterisk indicates drugs cited in interaction reports.

Theophyllines — *Daidzein*

Aminophylline	Oxtriphylline†	Daidzein*
Dyphylline (eg, *Lufyllin*)	Theophylline* (eg, *Theolair*)	

Significance	Onset	Severity	Documentation
4	□ Rapid	□ Major	□ Established
	■ **Delayed**	■ **Moderate**	□ Probable
		□ Minor	□ Suspected
			■ **Possible**
			□ Unlikely

Effects THEOPHYLLINE serum concentrations may be elevated and the t½ may be prolonged, increasing the risk of side effects.

Mechanism Inhibition of THEOPHYLLINE metabolism (CYP1A2) by DAIDZEIN is suspected.

Management Patients taking THEOPHYLLINE should avoid eating large quantities of foods containing DAIDZEIN.

Discussion

The effects of daidzein, an isoflavone found in numerous edible plants (eg, soybeans, celery, puerarin, trefoil), on the pharmacokinetics of theophylline were studied in 20 healthy volunteers.[1] Using a single-blind, placebo-controlled, parallel design, each subject received 100 mg theophylline on day 3. Afterward, subjects were divided into 2 groups and received either 200 mg daidzein twice daily for 10 days or placebo. On day 12, the test group received 100 mg theophylline with 200 mg daidzein, and the other group received 100 mg theophylline with water. Daidzein increased the AUC, peak plasma concentration, and t½ of theophylline approximately 34%, 24%, and 41%, respectively, compared with placebo.

[1] Peng WX, et al. *Eur J Clin Pharmacol.* 2003;59:237.

* Asterisk indicates drugs cited in interaction reports. Based on pharmacologic and pharmacokinetic considerations, similar interactions may occur with other drugs that are listed.
† Not available in the United States.

Theophyllines — *Diltiazem*

Aminophylline* Oxtriphylline†	Theophylline* (eg, *Bronkodyl*)	Diltiazem* (eg, *Cardizem*)

Significance	Onset	Severity	Documentation
2	☐ Rapid ■ **Delayed**	☐ Major ■ **Moderate** ☐ Minor	☐ Established ☐ Probable ■ **Suspected** ☐ Possible ☐ Unlikely

Effects The pharmacologic and toxic effects of THEOPHYLLINES may be increased.

Mechanism May be due to inhibition of metabolism of THEOPHYLLINE by DILTIAZEM.

Management Monitor THEOPHYLLINE plasma concentrations and the patient for toxicity; adjust the dose accordingly.

Discussion

The effects of diltiazem on the pharmacokinetics of theophylline (IV infusion of aminophylline 6 mg/kg over 20 minutes) were studied in 9 healthy men (4 smokers and 5 nonsmokers). There was a decrease in total body clearance and an increase in the $t_{1/2}$ of theophylline after diltiazem therapy.[1] No change was observed in the volume of distribution at steady state. In the smokers, there was a greater increase in theophylline $t_{1/2}$ than that found in nonsmokers. Similarly, total body clearance decreased approximately 22% in smokers. In a single-dose study of healthy volunteers, 7 days of pretreatment with diltiazem decreased total theophylline clearance 11% and increased the $t_{1/2}$.[2] In 9 healthy nonsmoking volunteers, diltiazem 60 mg 3 times daily for 3 days prolonged theophylline (oral) $t_{1/2}$ from 7.58 to 8.59 hr as a result of reduction in total plasma clearance.[3] In a preliminary report, 18 patients with chronic asthma stabilized on theophylline received short-term administration of concurrent diltiazem. Only 4 patients demonstrated an increase in theophylline $t_{1/2}$ greater than 25%.[4] Similarly, a study of 8 patients with asthma or chronic obstructive pulmonary disease given IV aminophylline demonstrated an average 22% decrease in theophylline clearance following 5 days of diltiazem therapy.[5]

[1] Nafziger AN, et al. *J Clin Pharmacol.* 1987;27:862.
[2] Sirmans SM, et al. *Clin Pharmacol Ther.* 1988;44:29.
[3] Ohashi K, et al. *J Clin Pharmacol.* 1993; 33:1233.
[4] Christopher MA, et al. *Drug Intell Clin Pharm.* 1987;21:4A.
[5] Soto J, et al. *Ther Drug Monit.* 1994;16:49.

* Asterisk indicates drugs cited in interaction reports. Based on pharmacologic and pharmacokinetic considerations, similar interactions may occur with other drugs that are listed.
† Not available in the United States.

Theophyllines — *Disulfiram*

Aminophylline*	Theophylline	Disulfiram*
Oxtriphylline†	(eg, *Bronkodyl*)	(*Antabuse*)

Significance	Onset	Severity	Documentation
2	☐ Rapid	☐ Major	☐ Established
	■ **Delayed**	■ **Moderate**	☐ Probable
		☐ Minor	■ **Suspected**
			☐ Possible
			☐ Unlikely

Effects The pharmacologic and toxic effects of THEOPHYLLINES may be increased.

Mechanism DISULFIRAM inhibits both the hydroxylation and demethylation pathways of THEOPHYLLINE metabolism.

Management Consider monitoring serum THEOPHYLLINE levels and observing the patient for THEOPHYLLINE toxicity or a decrease in THEOPHYLLINE activity if DISULFIRAM is added to or discontinued from the treatment regimen. Adjust the THEOPHYLLINE dosage accordingly.

Discussion

In a study involving 20 recovering alcoholics, disulfiram administration impaired theophylline metabolism.[1] One group of 10 patients received 250 mg disulfiram daily while the second group of 10 patients was administered 500 mg daily. Theophylline kinetics were investigated in 2 single-dose theophylline studies, 1 evaluation as a baseline and the other following 1 week of disulfiram therapy. Each treatment group consisted of 8 smokers and 2 nonsmokers. During coadministration of theophylline and disulfiram, theophylline metabolism was reduced. The clearance of theophylline decreased from a mean of 106 to 83 mL/kg/hr and from 94 to 65 mL/kg/hr in the 250 and 500 mg disulfiram groups, respectively. Reciprocally, the elimination $t_{1/2}$ of theophylline was prolonged from 4.2 to 5.4 hr and from 5.1 to 7.1 hr in the 2 groups, respectively. Treatment with disulfiram 500 mg was associated with a greater than proportionate decrease in elimination of theophylline compared with the 250 mg dose, indicating that therapeutic doses of disulfiram exert dose-dependent inhibition of theophylline metabolism. In both groups, disulfiram decreased the formation of all theophylline metabolites in smokers; however, hydroxylation was affected more than demethylation.

[1] Loi CM, et al. *Clin Pharmacol Ther.* 1989;45:476.

* Asterisk indicates drugs cited in interaction reports. Based on pharmacologic and pharmacokinetic considerations, similar interactions may occur with other drugs that are listed.
† Not available in the United States.

Theophyllines — Ephedrine

Theophyllines		Ephedrine
Aminophylline	Oxtriphylline†	Ephedrine*
Dyphylline (eg, *Lufyllin*)	Theophylline* (eg, *Bronkodyl*)	

Significance	Onset	Severity	Documentation
5	□ Rapid	□ Major	□ Established
	■ **Delayed**	□ Moderate	□ Probable
		■ **Minor**	□ Suspected
			■ **Possible**
			□ Unlikely

Effects EPHEDRINE may cause THEOPHYLLINE toxicity.

Mechanism Unknown.

Management Dosage of THEOPHYLLINE may need to be decreased if signs or symptoms of toxicity occur. Monitor response to THEOPHYLLINE when EPHEDRINE is added to or withdrawn from a patient's regimen.

Discussion

The efficacy of theophylline-ephedrine combinations in asthmatics is controversial. A double-blind study in 12 asthmatic children showed no added therapeutic benefit of ephedrine.[1] Side effects were more common with the combination. A subsequent double-blind trial advocated avoidance of theophylline-ephedrine combinations that are no more effective than single-agent therapy and present more side effects.[2] Contrary to this, enhanced effects of theophylline-ephedrine combinations have been reported using lower doses of ephedrine.[4,5] An improvement in pulmonary function, although not statistically significant, was noted for theophylline-ephedrine-phenobarbital treatment vs theophylline alone.

Use of theophylline-ephedrine-phenobarbital combinations is widespread for treatment of asthma. While noted to be successful,[6] doses are often less than the recommended dosages of each agent alone. Definitive information is needed regarding the efficacy of combination therapy vs single agent therapy; combination therapy should be used cautiously.

[1] Weinberger M, et al. *J Pediatr.* 1974;84:421.
[2] Weinberger M, et al. *Clin Pharmacol Ther.* 1975;17:585.
[3] Badiei B, et al. *Ann Allergy.* 1975;35:32.
[4] Tinkelman DG, et al. *JAMA.* 1977;237:553.
[5] Sims JA, et al. *J Allergy Clin Immunol.* 1978;62:15.
[6] Direkwattanachai C, et al. *J Med Assoc Thailand.* 1986;69(suppl 2):31.

* Asterisk indicates drugs cited in interaction reports. Based on pharmacologic and pharmacokinetic considerations, similar interactions may occur with other drugs that are listed.
† Not available in the United States.

Theophyllines | *Famotidine*

Aminophylline Theophylline* (eg, *Theo-Dur*)	Famotidine* (eg, *Pepcid*)

Significance	Onset	Severity	Documentation
5	☐ Rapid ■ **Delayed**	☐ Major ■ **Moderate** ☐ Minor	☐ Established ☐ Probable ☐ Suspected ☐ Possible ■ **Unlikely**

Effects Increased THEOPHYLLINE concentrations, possibly producing toxicity.

Mechanism Unknown.

Management Monitor THEOPHYLLINE concentrations and observe the patient for THEOYPHYLLINE toxicity. Adjust the THEOPHYLLINE dose as needed.

Discussion

The effects of famotidine on the pharmacokinetics of theophylline were studied in 7 patients with chronic obstructive pulmonary disease and peptic ulcer.[1] Each patient received a single 3.4 mg/kg theophylline infusion administered over 5 minutes before and after treatment with famotidine 40 mg daily at bedtime for 8 days. The half-life of theophylline was prolonged from 5.3 to 8.6 hours while clearance was reduced from 1.13 to 0.73 mL/min/kg. The results of this study are unexpected because famotidine is cleared from the body primarily by renal excretion and is not known to interact with the cytochrome P450 enzyme system responsible for theophylline metabolism. The amount of decrease in theophylline clearance (36%) was enough to potentially produce toxicity in some patients maintained at the upper end of the theophylline plasma therapeutic range. A potential methodological problem of this study is that theophylline concentrations were only measured for 8 hours (approximately 1 half-life). In patients receiving 80 mg famotidine or 1,600 mg cimetidine (eg, *Tagamet*) per day for 9.5 days, famotidine did not affect theophylline pharmacokinetics following a 5 mg/kg IV dose.[2] In contrast, cimetidine decreased the clearance and prolonged the half-life of theophylline (See Theophylline-Cimetidine). Others have found that famotidine does not affect theophylline levels.[3]

[1] Dal Negro R, et al. *Clin Pharmacokinet.* 1993;24:255.
[2] Bachmann K, et al. *J Clin Pharmacol.* 1995;35:529.
[3] Verdiani P, et al. *Chest.* 1988;94:807.

* Asterisk indicates drugs cited in interaction reports. Based on pharmacologic and pharmacokinetic considerations, similar interactions may occur with other drugs that are listed.

Theophyllines — *Febuxostat*

Aminophylline	Febuxostat*
Theophylline*	(*Uloric*)
(eg, *Theo-24*)	

Significance	Onset	Severity	Documentation
2	□ Rapid	□ Major	□ Established
	■ **Delayed**	■ **Moderate**	□ Probable
		□ Minor	■ **Suspected**
			□ Possible
			□ Unlikely

Effects Plasma concentrations of THEOPHYLLINES may be elevated, increasing the risk of toxicity.

Mechanism FEBUXOSTAT may inhibit hepatic metabolism of THEOPHYLLINES by xanthine oxidase.

Management Coadministration of FEBUXOSTAT and THEOPHYLLINES is contraindicated.

Discussion

Although not studied, theophylline is metabolized by xanthine oxidase.[1] Because febuxostat inhibits xanthine oxidase, increased plasma concentrations of theophylline may occur, resulting in theophylline toxicity. Because theophylline has a narrow therapeutic index, coadministration of febuxostat and theophylline is contraindicated.[1]

The basis for this monograph is information on file with the manufacturer. Studies are needed to determine the clinical importance of this interaction. See also Theophyllines-Allopurinol.

[1] *Uloric* [package insert]. Deerfield, IL: Takeda Pharmaceuticals America Inc; February 2009.

* Asterisk indicates drugs cited in interaction reports. Based on pharmacologic and pharmacokinetic considerations, similar interactions may occur with other drugs that are listed.

Theophyllines — *Felodipine*

Aminophylline	Felodipine*
Theophylline* (eg, *Theo-24*)	

Significance	Onset	Severity	Documentation
4	☐ Rapid	☐ Major	☐ Established
	■ **Delayed**	■ **Moderate**	☐ Probable
		☐ Minor	☐ Suspected
			■ **Possible**
			☐ Unlikely

Effects Serum THEOPHYLLINE levels may be decreased, producing a decrease in the pharmacologic effects of THEOPHYLLINES. The decrease in THEOPHYLLINE levels appears to be slight. If a clinically important effect occurs, it would be expected mainly in patients whose THEOPHYLLINE levels are high in the therapeutic range when FELODIPINE treatment is discontinued or those who are in the low therapeutic range when FELODIPINE is added.

Mechanism Decreased GI absorption of THEOPHYLLINES is suspected.

Management Consider monitoring serum THEOPHYLLINE levels and observing patients for changes in clinical status. Adjust the dose of THEOPHYLLINES as needed.

Discussion

The possibility of an interaction between felodipine and theophylline was studied in 10 healthy men.[1] Each subject received theophylline aminopropanol† 200 mg (equivalent to anhydrous theophylline 141 mg) every 8 hours for 4 days, followed by felodipine 5 mg every 8 hours for 6 days. Subsequently, subjects received the combination of felodipine and theophylline for 4 days. Theophylline administration had no effect on serum felodipine levels. However, during coadministration, serum theophylline levels were decreased at all time points during the dosing interval. The AUC decreased 19% ($P < 0.01$). In addition, the mean peak serum theophylline concentration decreased from 44.3 to 38.4 mcmol/L ($P < 0.05$), while the mean minimum serum level decreased from 25.4 to 19.4 mcmol/L ($P < 0.01$).

[1] Bratel T, et al. *Eur J Clin Pharmacol.* 1989;36(5):481.

* Asterisk indicates drugs cited in interaction reports. Based on pharmacologic and pharmacokinetic considerations, similar interactions may occur with other drugs that are listed.
† Not available in the United States.

Theophyllines	***Fluvoxamine***
Aminophylline Theophylline* (eg, *Theo-24*)	Fluvoxamine* (eg, *Luvox*)

Significance	Onset	Severity	Documentation
2	□ Rapid ■ **Delayed**	□ Major ■ **Moderate** □ Minor	□ Established □ Probable ■ **Suspected** □ Possible □ Unlikely

Effects Increased THEOPHYLLINE serum concentrations with possible toxicity.

Mechanism FLUVOXAMINE inhibits the hepatic metabolism (CYP1A2) of THEOPHYLLINE.

Management Monitor THEOPHYLLINE levels when FLUVOXAMINE therapy is started or stopped and adjust the THEOPHYLLINE dosage as needed. A 33% reduction in THEOPHYLLINE dose has been recommended when starting THEOPHYLLINE in patients receiving FLUVOXAMINE.

Discussion

During coadministration of fluvoxamine, a 3-fold increase in serum theophylline levels was reported in a 78-year-old woman with a long history of chronic bronchitis.[1] For years, the patient had been receiving sustained-release theophylline 400 mg twice daily without problems (serum theophylline range, 55 to 110 mmol/L). In the hospital, the patient was started on fluvoxamine 50 mg/day for major depression. By the second day of concomitant fluvoxamine therapy, clinical symptoms of theophylline toxicity were evident; by day 6, serum theophylline concentrations had tripled. When the patient developed persistent nausea, it was attributed to fluvoxamine, and the drug was discontinued. The next day before the morning theophylline dose, the serum theophylline concentration was 197 mmol/L, and theophylline was discontinued. Seven hours later, the patient had a generalized tonic-clonic seizure and became comatose. An ECG showed supraventricular tachycardia at a rate of 200 bpm. She was transferred to the intensive care unit and treated with digoxin (eg, *Lanoxin*) and verapamil (eg, *Calan*) to control her heart rate. Three days later, the patient's theophylline concentration was less than 6 mmol/L. When theophylline was restarted and cautiously titrated to 400 mg twice daily, her condition remained stable. Fluvoxamine 75 mg/day increased the $t_{1/2}$ of theophylline from 7.6 to 19.2 hours and the AUC 138% in 9 healthy volunteers.[2] In another study, coadministration of fluoxetine reduced theophylline clearance 62% in 10 healthy subjects, compared with a 52% and 12% reduction in patients with mild or severe cirrhosis, respectively.[3]

[1] van den Brekel AM, et al. *CMAJ.* 1994;151(9):1289.
[2] Yao C, et al. *Clin Pharmacol Ther.* 2001;70(5):415.
[3] Orlando R, et al. *Clin Pharmacol Ther.* 2006;79(5):489.

* Asterisk indicates drugs cited in interaction reports. Based on pharmacologic and pharmacokinetic considerations, similar interactions may occur with other drugs that are listed.

Theophyllines — *Food*

Theophylline*
(eg, *Theolair*)

Food*

Significance	Onset	Severity	Documentation
2	■ **Rapid**	□ Major	□ Established
	□ Delayed	■ **Moderate**	□ Probable
		□ Minor	■ **Suspected**
			□ Possible
			□ Unlikely

Effects Effects of certain slow-release forms of THEOPHYLLINE may be altered by FOOD.

Mechanism Complex (see Discussion).

Management See Discussion.

Discussion

In 1 study, mean theophylline clearance increased 26% with a high-protein diet and decreased 21% with a low-protein diet.[1] These changes may be the result of altered hepatic clearance and are consistent with other studies.[2-4] Metabolism of theophylline is also increased by consumption of large amounts of charcoal-broiled beef. This has been attributed to the enzyme-induction effect of polycyclic hydrocarbons introduced in this cooking process.[5] Dietary changes represent significant departures from a typical diet.

Food does not alter the activity of theophylline when administered in an immediate-release formulation. Many controlled-release products also can be given with food without interaction; however, they must be considered on an individual basis. For example, food has little effect on the absorption of *Slo-bid Gyrocaps*.[6,7] *Theo-24*, taken less than 1 hour before a high-fat meal, undergoes increased theophylline absorption and C_{max}, increasing the risk of toxicity when compared with taking the drug while fasting.[6,8] Patients receiving doses of at least 900 mg or 13 mg/kg, whichever is less, should avoid eating a high-fat breakfast, take the dose at least 1 hour before eating, or be placed on a twice-daily dosage regimen. When *Theolair* was ingested immediately after a high-fat breakfast, serum theophylline levels, C_{max}, and AUC were decreased.[9] Food-induced increases in the absorption from *Uniphyl* also have been suggested.[6,10] Conversely, when *Theo-Dur Sprinkle* is administered with food, the extent of absorption and C_{max} are reduced.[6,10,11] Administer this product at least 1 hour before or 2 hours after a meal on a spoonful of soft food such as applesauce or pudding; this will not alter bioavailability.

1 Juan D, et al. *Clin Pharmacol Ther.* 1986;40:187.
2 Feldman CH, et al. *Pediatrics.* 1980;66:956.
3 Thompson PJ, et al. *Br J Clin Pharmacol.* 1983;16:267.
4 Juan D, et al. *Ther Drug Monit.* 1990;12:111.
5 Kappas A, et al. *Clin Pharmacol Ther.* 1978;23:445.
6 Jonkman JH. *Clin Pharmacokinet.* 1989;16:162.
7 Hendeles L, et al. *Chest.* 1985;87:758.
8 Vaughan L, et al. *Drug Intell Clin Pharm.* 1984;18:510.
9 Lefebvre RA, et al. *Int J Clin Pharmacol Ther Toxicol.* 1988;26:375.
10 Karim A, et al. *Clin Pharmacol Ther.* 1985;38:77.
11 Birkett DJ, et al. *Clin Pharmacol Ther.* 1989;45:305.

* Asterisk indicates drugs cited in interaction reports.

Theophyllines — *Halothane*

Aminophylline*	Oxtriphylline†
Dyphylline (eg, *Lufyllin*)	Theophylline* (eg, *Theolair*)

Halothane*

Significance	Onset	Severity	Documentation
1	■ **Rapid**	■ **Major**	□ Established
	□ Delayed	□ Moderate	■ **Probable**
		□ Minor	□ Suspected
			□ Possible
			□ Unlikely

Effects Catecholamine-induced arrhythmias have been reported when HALOTHANE was administered after THEOPHYLLINE.

Mechanism Unknown.

Management Avoid administration of HALOTHANE to patients taking THEOPHYLLINE. Consider the use of a noninteracting anesthetic such as enflurane.[1,2]

Discussion

Data from animal models[2-5] and several case reports[6,7] describe ventricular arrhythmias in subjects exposed to halothane after receiving theophylline. In animal models, administration of aminophylline after halothane did not produce cardiac arrhythmias.[8,9] The interaction is not believed to influence theophylline kinetics,[2,10] and anesthetic requirements are not altered.[11] Although this interaction has been well documented in animal models, the scarcity of reports in humans is probably because of lack of concurrent use. Although further research is needed to determine the mechanism, concurrent use is not recommended.

[1] Stirt JA, et al. *Anesth Analg.* 1981;60:871.
[2] Berger JM, et al. *Anesth Analg.* 1983;62:733.
[3] Takaori M, et al. *Can Anaesth Soc J.* 1965;12:275.
[4] Takaori M, et al. *Can Anaesth Soc J.* 1967;14:79.
[5] Stirt JA, et al. *Anesth Analg.* 1981;60:517.
[6] Roizen MF, et al. *Anesth Analg.* 1978;57:738.
[7] Richards W, et al. *Ann Allergy.* 1988;61:83.
[8] Stirt JA, et al. *Anesth Analg.* 1980;59:186.
[9] Stirt JA, et al. *Anesth Analg.* 1980;59:410.
[10] Nakatsu K, et al. *Anesth Analg.* 1986;65:423.
[11] Nicholls EA, et al. *Anesthesiology.* 1986;65:637.

* Asterisk indicates drugs cited in interaction reports. Based on pharmacologic and pharmacokinetic considerations, similar interactions may occur with other drugs that are listed.

† Not available in the United States.

Theophyllines — *Hydantoins*

Theophyllines	Hydantoins	
Aminophylline*	Fosphenytoin (*Cerebyx*)	Phenytoin* (eg, *Dilantin*)
Theophylline* (eg, *Theochron*)		

Significance	Onset	Severity	Documentation
2	☐ Rapid	☐ Major	☐ Established
	■ **Delayed**	■ **Moderate**	■ **Probable**
		☐ Minor	☐ Suspected
			☐ Possible
			☐ Unlikely

Effects Decrease or loss of pharmacological effects of THEOPHYLLINES or HYDANTOINS.

Mechanism It appears that phenytoin metabolism is enhanced by THEOPHYLLINE[1]; likewise, THEOPHYLLINE metabolism is increased by PHENYTOIN.[2-4]

Management When either medication is added to or deleted from a patient's regimen, monitor the plasma levels of each. Tailor dosages as needed.

Discussion

A 10- to 15-day course of phenytoin decreased the $t_{1/2}$ of theophylline (administered as aminophylline) and increased the clearance a mean of 2-fold in 10 healthy subjects.[2] Phenytoin dosages necessary to achieve therapeutic levels were administered but not discussed in detail. Similar findings were reported in a second study.[3] In 6 healthy subjects, a 31% to 65% increase in theophylline clearance was reported when phenytoin was added to the regimen.[5] Similar results have been reported in 46 additional subjects,[6,7] including 20 smokers in whom hepatic enzyme induction by phenytoin was additive to that of cigarette smoking.[6] In 1 case, phenobarbital appeared additive to phenytoin and cigarette smoking.[8] Subsequent case reports note that the interaction onset is within 5 days and warn of possible exacerbation of pulmonary symptoms.[7,9]

Limited data suggest that theophylline alters the metabolism and clearance of phenytoin.[1] Five of 14 healthy subjects exhibited a 40% mean increase in phenytoin serum concentration following discontinuation of theophylline.[1] Similar interactions with other hydantoin derivatives have not been documented. Ethotoin was reported not to exhibit this effect in 1 patient.[10]

1 Taylor JW, et al. *Drug Intell Clin Pharm* 1980;14(4):638.
2 Marquis JF, et al. *N Engl J Med* 1982;307(19):1189.
3 Reed RC, et al. *N Engl J Med* 1983;308:724.
4 Sklar SJ, et al. *Drug Intell Clin Pharm* 1985;19(1):34.
5 Miller M, et al. *Clin Pharmacol Ther* 1984;35(5):666.
6 Crowley JJ, et al. *J Pharmacol Exp Ther* 1988;245(2):513.
7 Adebayo GI. *Clin Exp Pharmacol Physiol* 1988;15(11):883.
8 Nicholson JP, et al. *Ann Pharmacother* 1992;26(3):334.
9 Landsberg K, et al. *Can J Hosp Pharm* 1988;41:31.
10 Rosenberry KR, et al. *J Pediatr* 1983;102(3):472.

* Asterisk indicates drugs cited in interaction reports. Based on pharmacologic and pharmacokinetic considerations, similar interactions may occur with other drugs that are listed.

Theophyllines — *Influenza Virus Vaccine*

Aminophylline* Oxtriphylline*†	Theophylline* (eg, *Theochron*)	Influenza Virus Vaccine* (eg, *Fluzone*)

Significance	Onset	Severity	Documentation
4	☐ Rapid	☐ Major	☐ Established
	■ **Delayed**	■ **Moderate**	☐ Probable
		☐ Minor	☐ Suspected
			■ **Possible**
			☐ Unlikely

Effects Elevation in THEOPHYLLINE serum levels and increase in THEOPHYLLINE $t_{1/2}$, possibly causing toxicity.

Mechanism Possible vaccine-induced depression of hepatic microsomal enzymes.[1]

Management Consider monitoring the patient closely for possible signs of THEOPHYLLINE toxicity for the first 24 hours after vaccination. Tailor the THEOPHYLLINE dosage if necessary.

Discussion

Theophylline toxicity has been reported in association with the influenza virus vaccine[2-4] as well as during an outbreak of influenza.[5] Patients have manifested signs of toxicity, including seizures, headache, nausea, and vomiting.[2,3,5] One study reported a mean increase in $t_{1/2}$ of 122% and increases in plasma concentrations exceeding 85%.[2] It has been recommended that theophylline doses be decreased for the first 24 hours after vaccination.[3] Subsequent reports have failed to confirm this interaction when evaluated in healthy subjects,[4,6-9] COPD/asthma patients,[1,6,10-12] elderly patients,[13,14] and pediatric patients.[15] This suggests that the interaction is unpredictable. Until further information is available, caution is warranted for the first 24 hours after vaccination.

1 Stults BM, et al. *West J Med.* 1983;139(5):651.
2 Renton KW, et al. *Can Med Assoc J.* 1980;123(4):288.
3 Walker S, et al. *Can Med Assoc J.* 1981;125(3):243.
4 Meredith CG, et al. *Clin Pharmacol Ther.* 1985;37(4):396.
5 Kraemer MJ, et al. *Pediatrics.* 1982;69(4):476.
6 Bukowskyj M, et al. *Am Rev Resp Dis.* 1984;129(5):672.
7 Winstanley PA, et al. *Br J Clin Pharmacol.* 1985;20(1):47.
8 Grabowski N, et al. *Am Rev Respir Dis.* 1985;131(6):934.
9 Jonkman JH, et al. *Ther Drug Monit.* 1988;10(3):345.
10 Goldstein RS, et al. *Can Med Assoc J.* 1982;126(5):470.
11 Britton L, et al. *Can Med Assoc J.* 1982;126(12):1375.
12 Fischer RG, et al. *Can Med Assoc J.* 1982;126(11):1312.
13 Patriarca PA, et al. *N Engl J Med.* 1983;308(26):1601.
14 Gomolin IH, et al. *J Am Geriatr Soc.* 1985;33(4):269.
15 San Joaquin VH, et al. *Clin Pediatr.* 1982;21:724.

* Asterisk indicates drugs cited in interaction reports. Based on pharmacologic and pharmacokinetic considerations, similar interactions may occur with other drugs that are listed.

† Not available in the United States.

Theophyllines — *Interferon*

Theophyllines		Interferon
Aminophylline*	Theophylline (eg, *Bronkodyl*)	Interferon alfa-2a* (*Roferon-A*)
Oxtriphylline†		

Significance	Onset	Severity	Documentation
4	■ **Rapid**	□ Major	□ Established
	□ Delayed	■ **Moderate**	□ Probable
		□ Minor	□ Suspected
			■ **Possible**
			□ Unlikely

Effects The pharmacologic effects of THEOPHYLLINES may be increased.

Mechanism Unknown.

Management If an interaction is suspected, measure plasma THEOPHYLLINE levels and adjust the dose accordingly.

Discussion

The effect of interferon on theophylline kinetics was studied in 4 healthy volunteers and in 5 patients with chronic active hepatitis B.[1] Theophylline clearance was determined 1 to 2 weeks before and 20 hours following a single IM injection of interferon alfa-2a. Aminophylline was administered IV in a dose of 5 mg/kg over 20 minutes. Interferon administration resulted in reduced theophylline clearance, ranging from 33% to 81%, in 8 of the 9 subjects. The remaining participant showed no change in theophylline clearance. During coadministration of these drugs, there was a significant reduction in median theophylline clearance from 0.7 to 0.36 mL/kg/min and a significant increase in the elimination half-life from 6.3 to 10.7 hours. These effects appear to be greatest in individuals who are fast metabolizers of theophylline (eg, smokers).

[1] Williams SJ, et al. *Lancet*. 1987;2:939.

* Asterisk indicates drugs cited in interaction reports. Based on pharmacologic and pharmacokinetic considerations, similar interactions may occur with other drugs that are listed.
† Not available in the United States.

Theophyllines — *Iodine[131]*

Aminophylline*	Theophylline	Iodine131*
Oxtriphylline†	(eg, *Bronkodyl*)	(I^{131})

Significance	Onset	Severity	Documentation
4	☐ Rapid	☐ Major	☐ Established
	■ **Delayed**	■ **Moderate**	☐ Probable
		☐ Minor	☐ Suspected
			■ **Possible**
			☐ Unlikely

Effects Serum THEOPHYLLINE levels may be increased if hypothyroidism is induced, producing toxicity.

Mechanism THEOPHYLLINE clearance may be decreased in patients with hypothyroidism. Patients treated with I^{131} can become hypothyroid. THEOPHYLLINE clearance returns to normal when a euthyroid state is achieved.

Management Monitor serum THEOPHYLLINE levels and observe the patient for symptoms of THEOPHYLLINE toxicity if I^{131} is administered. Adjust the THEOPHYLLINE dose accordingly.

Discussion

Theophylline toxicity was reported in a 39-year-old man after treatment with I^{131} for hyperthyroidism.[1] The patient had a 17-year history of asthma, which was well controlled with albuterol (eg, *Proventil*) 2 inhalations 4 times daily and aminophylline 400 mg 4 times daily. Following a diagnosis of Graves' disease, the patient received I^{131}. Three months after I^{131} treatment, thyroid function tests indicated hypothyroidism. His serum theophylline levels increased from 15.2 to 30.9 mcg/mL and the half-life increased from 4.95 to 10.04 hours. In addition, the patient complained of symptoms that were consistent with theophylline toxicity (eg, diarrhea, nausea, cramping). Treatment with levothyroxine (eg, *Synthroid*) 0.15 mg daily was started, and the aminophylline dosage was decreased to 200 mg every 6 hours. Two months later, the patient was euthyroid and his serum theophylline levels were subtherapeutic. The aminophylline dose was returned to 400 mg 4 times daily. Concomitant with the euthyroid state, the half-life of theophylline decreased to the previous value of about 5 hours. Six months later, the patient remained euthyroid and his asthma continued to be well controlled on sustained-release theophylline.

Similar effects may occur with the antithyroid drugs methimazole (*Tapazole*) and propylthiouracil (PTU). See also Theophyllines-Thioamines.

[1] Johnson CE, et al. *Clin Pharm.* 1988;7:620.

* Asterisk indicates drugs cited in interaction reports. Based on pharmacologic and pharmacokinetic considerations, similar interactions may occur with other drugs that are listed.
† Not available in the United States.

Theophyllines — *Isoniazid*

Aminophylline*	Theophylline* (eg, *Theo-Dur*)	Isoniazid* (eg, *Nydrazid*)
Oxtriphylline†		

Significance	Onset	Severity	Documentation
4	☐ Rapid	☐ Major	☐ Established
	■ **Delayed**	■ **Moderate**	☐ Probable
		☐ Minor	☐ Suspected
			■ **Possible**
			☐ Unlikely

Effects Mild reductions and elevations in THEOPHYLLINE plasma levels have occurred with this drug combination.

Mechanism ISONIAZID may induce and inhibit the hepatic enzymes responsible for THEOPHYLLINE metabolism.

Management Monitor THEOPHYLLINE levels routinely; tailor the dosage if necessary.

Discussion

In 4 healthy male subjects pretreated with isoniazid 300 mg/day for 6 days, the clearance of a single oral dose of theophylline 400 mg (*Slo-Phyllin*) was increased 16% over the same theophylline dose given alone.[1] There was little difference found in the maximum plasma concentration, time of maximum plasma concentration, elimination half-life, absorption rate constant, elimination rate constant, area under the plasma concentration-time curve, or the apparent volume of distribution. In contrast, 7 healthy adults received IV aminophylline (5 mg/kg over 1 hour followed by 0.5 mg/kg/hour for 5 hours) after pretreatment with isoniazid (10 mg/kg/day) for 10 days.[2] The plasma clearance of theophylline was significantly decreased after isoniazid pretreatment compared with when aminophylline was dosed alone, regardless of acetylator phenotype. As a result, theophylline plasma levels were significantly increased. In 13 healthy volunteers, isoniazid 400 mg daily for 14 days decreased theophylline clearance 21%.[4] In a case report, a woman demonstrated progressively higher theophylline levels (up to 25 mg/L) and experienced toxicity during concurrent isoniazid administration.[3] The interaction developed over several weeks, indicating that previous studies may not have been for a sufficient duration. This effect may be dose-dependent.[5]

Additional studies are needed to determine the clinical significance of this interaction.

[1] Thompson JR, et al. *Curr Ther Res.* 1982;32:921.
[2] Hoglund P, et al. *Eur J Resp Dis.* 1987;70:110.
[3] Torrent J, et al. *DICP Ann Pharmacother.* 1989;23:143.
[4] Samigun M, et al. *Br J Clin Pharmacol.* 1990;29:570.
[5] Thompson JR, et al. *Br J Clin Pharmacol.* 1990;30:909.

* Asterisk indicates drugs cited in interaction reports. Based on pharmacologic and pharmacokinetic considerations, similar interactions may occur with other drugs that are listed.
† Not available in the United States.

Theophyllines — *Ketamine*

Aminophylline*	Oxtriphylline†	Ketamine*
Dyphylline (eg, *Lufyllin*)	Theophylline (eg, *Bronkodyl*)	(*Ketalar*)

Significance	Onset	Severity	Documentation
4	■ **Rapid**	□ Major	□ Established
	□ Delayed	■ **Moderate**	□ Probable
		□ Minor	□ Suspected
			■ **Possible**
			□ Unlikely

Effects Unexpected and unpredictable adverse effects in the form of extensor-type seizures have been reported with the coadministration of THEOPHYLLINES and KETAMINE.

Mechanism Unknown.

Management Use this combination with caution.

Discussion

Four isolated cases of extensor-type seizures have been reported in patients given theophylline preparations and ketamine anesthesia.[1] The same research group determined in a laboratory experiment with mice that there appeared to be a lowering of the seizure threshold with the drug combination, not present with either drug alone. Conversely, ketamine has been used, with no adverse sequelae, in status asthmaticus unresponsive to conventional therapy.[2]

A causal relationship has not been established; however, data from well-designed human trials are necessary to give substance to this interaction.

[1] Hirshman CA, et al. *Anesthesiology.* 1982;56:464. [2] Rock MJ, et al. *Crit Care Med.* 1986;14:514.

* Asterisk indicates drugs cited in interaction reports. Based on pharmacologic and pharmacokinetic considerations, similar interactions may occur with other drugs that are listed.
† Not available in the United States.

Theophyllines — *Ketoconazole*

Aminophylline* Oxtriphylline†	Theophylline* (eg, *Uniphyl*)	Ketoconazole* (*Nizoral*)

Significance	Onset	Severity	Documentation
4	■ **Rapid** □ Delayed	□ Major ■ **Moderate** □ Minor	□ Established □ Probable □ Suspected ■ **Possible** □ Unlikely

Effects The pharmacologic effects of THEOPHYLLINES may be decreased.

Mechanism Possible decreased THEOPHYLLINE absorption when coadministered with KETOCONAZOLE.

Management If an interaction is suspected (eg, deterioration of pulmonary function) during coadministration of THEOPHYLLINES and KETOCONAZOLE, measure THEOPHYLLINE plasma levels and adjust the dose accordingly.

Discussion

Coadministration of ketoconazole and a slow-release theophylline preparation to a 45-year-old male asthmatic patient was associated with a decrease in serum theophylline levels.[1] The patient's drug regimen consisted of albuterol (*Proventil, Ventolin*) aerosol 4 times daily, prednisolone 5 mg daily, slow-release theophylline 600 mg at 10 p.m. and 200 mg at 10 a.m., and ketoconazole 200 mg daily. Peak expiratory flow rates fell after ketoconazole ingestion. The serum theophylline level at noon was significantly lower during ketoconazole administration than when the antifungal agent was omitted. The serum theophylline level fell below the lower limit of the therapeutic range (10 mg/L) for the first 2 hours following ketoconazole administration. In 2 other reports, the effect of single and multiple ketoconazole doses on the elimination of theophylline was evaluated in healthy, nonsmoking subjects.[2,3] Each subject received IV aminophylline and oral ketoconazole. No statistically significant difference in theophylline half-life or clearance was observed during ketoconazole coadministration. Thus, based on available information, if an interaction is to occur it would only be expected with oral dosing. Additional studies are needed.

[1] Murphy E, et al. *Irish Med J.* 1987;80:123.
[2] Brown MW, et al. *Clin Pharmacol Ther.* 1985;37:290.
[3] Heusner JJ, et al. *Drug Intell Clin Pharm.* 1987;21:514.

* Asterisk indicates drugs cited in interaction reports. Based on pharmacologic and pharmacokinetic considerations, similar interactions may occur with other drugs that are listed.
† = Not available in the United States.

Theophyllines — *Lansoprazole*

Aminophylline Oxtriphylline†	Theophylline* (eg, *Theo-Dur*)	Lansoprazole* (*Prevacid*)

Significance	Onset	Severity	Documentation
5	□ Rapid ■ **Delayed**	□ Major □ Moderate ■ **Minor**	□ Established □ Probable □ Suspected □ Possible ■ **Unlikely**

Effects Serum THEOPHYLLINE concentrations may be decreased.

Mechanism LANSOPRAZOLE may increase the hepatic metabolism of THEOPHYLLINES.

Management Based on available data, no special precautions are needed. If an interaction is suspected, it may be necessary to increase the dose of the THEOPHYLLINE.

Discussion

The interaction potential of lansoprazole and theophylline was assessed in 14 healthy male volunteers using a double-blind, 2-period, multiple-dose crossover design.[1] Each subject received 200 mg of anhydrous theophylline 4 times daily on study days 1 through 10. In addition, all subjects received placebo once daily at 8 am on study days 1 through 3 and then lansoprazole 60 mg or placebo once daily at 8 am on study days 4 through 13. Compared with placebo, lansoprazole administration produced decreases in the area under the plasma concentration-time curve (AUC) of theophylline on day 4 (from 49.54 to 46.59 mcg•hr/mL; $P = 0.04$), in the trough serum concentration (from 5.88 to 4.87 mcg/mL; $P = 0.037$), and AUC (from 50.64 to 43.94 mcg•hr/mL; $P = 0.02$) of theophylline on day 10. The terminal half-life and peak serum concentrations of theophylline were unaffected by lansoprazole. Similar results were found in a second study with administration of 30 mg of lansoprazole daily[2] and in another study with lansoprazole 60 mg/day.[3] Because the extent of decrease in steady-state serum theophylline concentrations is small, this interaction is not likely to be clinically important.

[1] Granneman GR, et al. *Ther Drug Monit.* 1995;17:460.
[2] Kokufu T, et al. *Eur J Clin Pharmacol.* 1995;48:391.
[3] Dilger K, et al. *Br J Clin Pharmacol.* 1999;48:438.

* Asterisk indicates drugs cited in interaction reports. Based on pharmacologic and pharmacokinetic considerations, similar interactions may occur with other drugs that are listed.

† Not available in the United States.

Theophyllines			***Loop Diuretics***
Aminophylline* Oxtriphylline†	Theophylline* (eg, *Theo-Dur*)	Furosemide* (eg, *Lasix*)	
Significance	Onset	Severity	Documentation
5	■ **Rapid** □ Delayed	□ Major □ Moderate ■ **Minor**	□ Established □ Probable □ Suspected ■ **Possible** □ Unlikely

Effects The actions of THEOPHYLLINES may be altered, enhanced, or inhibited by LOOP DIURETICS, although not reported.

Mechanism Undetermined.

Management No clinical interventions are required; however, monitor serum THEOPHYLLINE concentrations and tailor THEOPHYLLINE dosage as needed if unexpected events occur.

Discussion

Ten patients stabilized on continuous IV aminophylline for various respiratory problems received furosemide 40 mg IV.[1] The bolus furosemide injection caused an average increase in the serum theophylline concentration of 2.9 mcg/mL (range, 0.5 to 5.5 mcg/mL) and an increase in urine output of 995 mL above baseline over 4 hours. The most plausible mechanism appeared to be a constriction of theophylline's volume of distribution through hemoconcentration and reduced extravascular volume. The clinical importance of this study has been disputed.[2]

The opposite effect has also been reported.[3,4] Four premature neonates experienced decreases in serum theophylline concentration (at steady state) from 8 mcg/mL to 2 to 3 mcg/mL when furosemide was administered; 2 patients received both drugs orally and 2 patients received both drugs IV.[3] When the drug administrations were separated by 2 hours, serum theophylline concentrations returned to previous values. An additional study of 12 healthy volunteers reported no changes in steady-state serum theophylline concentration after two 20 mg oral doses of furosemide.[5]

[1] Conlon PF, et al. *Am J Hosp Pharm.* 1981;38:1345.
[2] Nakagawa RS. *Am J Hosp Pharm.* 1982;39:242.
[3] Toback JW, et al. *Pediatrics.* 1983;71:140.
[4] Carpentiere G, et al. *Ann Intern Med.* 1985;103:957.
[5] Janicke UA, et al. *Eur J Clin Pharmacol.* 1987;33:487.

* Asterisk indicates drugs cited in interaction reports. Based on pharmacologic and pharmacokinetic considerations, similar interactions may occur with other drugs that are listed.
Not available in the United States.

Theophyllines | *Macrolide Antibiotics*

Theophyllines		Macrolide Antibiotics	
Aminophylline*	Theophylline* (eg, *Theo-Dur*)	Azithromycin* (*Zithromax*)	Erythromycin* (eg, *E-Mycin*)
Oxtriphylline*†		Clarithromycin (*Biaxin*)	Troleandomycin*† (*Tao*)
		Dirithromycin* (*Dynabac*)	

Significance	Onset	Severity	Documentation
2	□ Rapid	□ Major	■ **Established**
	■ **Delayed**	■ **Moderate**	□ Probable
		□ Minor	□ Suspected
			□ Possible
			□ Unlikely

Effects Increased THEOPHYLLINE serum levels with toxicity may occur. Decreased ERYTHROMYCIN levels have been noted.

Mechanism Certain MACROLIDES inhibit the metabolism of THEOPHYLLINE; THEOPHYLLINE reduces the bioavailability and increases renal clearance of oral ERYTHROMYCIN.

Management Monitor THEOPHYLLINE levels when starting or stopping MACROLIDES. Tailor dosages as needed. Consider using an anti-infective agent that is unlikely to interact.

Discussion

Erythromycin inhibits the clearance and increases the half-life and plasma levels of theophylline in healthy adult subjects,[4-10,18-20] patients with pulmonary disease,[1,9,11,17] and pediatric patients.[3,21] Several reports suggesting no interaction between erythromycin and theophylline[3,8,14] have been criticized for design and drug usage.[13] Troleandomycin may inhibit theophylline metabolism, even when low doses are administered.[2,15,16,24] Patients with theophylline plasma levels in the upper therapeutic range are at greatest risk of toxicity. Studies have found a decrease in the area under the plasma erythromycin concentration-time curve and a 30% decrease in plasma levels.[10,18] This effect occurs with oral, and not IV, erythromycin, suggesting an alteration in bioavailability.[19,20] Increases in renal clearance have been noted.[18-20] Dirithromycin was reported to produce small decreases (18%) in average theophylline levels.[23] In a study of 5 patients, clarithromycin did not affect theophylline pharmacokinetics.[25] Transient decreases in theophylline levels were repeatedly noted in a 68-year-old man after stopping azithromycin therapy.[26]

[1] Kozak PP, et al. *J Allergy Clin Immunol.* 1977;60:149.
[2] Weinberger M, et al. *J Allergy Clin Immunol.* 1977;59:228.
[3] Pfeifer HJ, et al. *Clin Pharmacol Ther.* 1979;26:36.
[4] Zarowitz BJM, et al. *Clin Pharmacol Ther.* 1981;29:601.
[5] LaForce CF, et al. *J Pediatr.* 1981;99:153.
[6] Prince RA, et al. *J Allergy Clin Immunol.* 1981;68:427.
[7] Renton KW, et al. *Clin Pharmacol Ther.* 1981;30:422.
[8] May DC, et al. *J Clin Pharmacol.* 1982;22:125.
[9] Maddux MS, et al. *Chest.* 1982;81:563.
[10] Richer C, et al. *Clin Pharmacol Ther.* 1982;31:579.
[11] Iliopoulou A, et al. *Br J Clin Pharmacol.* 1982;14:495.
[12] Parish RA, et al. *Pediatrics.* 1983;72:828.
[13] Reisz G, et al. *Am Rev Respir Dis.* 1983;127:581.
[14] Kurisu S, et al. *DICP.* 1984;18:390.
[15] Hildebrandt R, et al. *Eur J Clin Pharmacol.* 1984;26:485.
[16] Descotes J, et al. *J Antimicrob Chemother.* 1985;15:659. Review.
[17] Ludden TM. *Clin Pharmacokinet.* 1985;10:63.
[18] Wiggins J, et al. *Eur J Resp Dis.* 1986;68:298.
[19] Paulsen O, et al. *Eur J Clin Pharmacol.* 1987;32:493.
[20] Pasic J, et al. *Xenobiotica.* 1987;17:493.
[21] Hildebrandt R, et al. *Int J Clin Pharmacol Ther Toxicol.* 1987;25:601.
[22] Tenenbein M, et al. *J Emerg Med.* 1989;7/3:249.
[23] Bachman K, et al. *J Clin Pharmacol.* 1990;30:1001.
[24] Kamada AK, et al. *Pharmacother.* 1992;12:98.
[25] Gillum JG, et al. *Antimicrob Agents Chemother.* 1996;40:1715.
[26] Pollak PT, et al. *Pharmacother.* 1997;17:827.

* Asterisk indicates drugs cited in interaction reports. Based on pharmacologic and pharmacokinetic considerations, similar interactions may occur with other drugs that are listed.
† Not available in the United States.

Theophyllines — *Mexiletine*

Aminophylline*	Theophylline* (eg, *Theo-Dur*)	Mexiletine* (eg, *Mexitil*)
Oxtriphylline†		

Significance	Onset	Severity	Documentation
2	☐ Rapid	☐ Major	■ **Established**
	■ **Delayed**	■ **Moderate**	☐ Probable
		☐ Minor	☐ Suspected
			☐ Possible
			☐ Unlikely

Effects Serum THEOPHYLLINE levels may be increased, resulting in an increase in the pharmacologic and toxic effects.

Mechanism The hepatic metabolism of THEOPHYLLINES via the cytochrome P450 oxidase system is inhibited by MEXILETINE.

Management Measure THEOPHYLLINE plasma levels and adjust the dose accordingly.

Discussion

Several cases of elevated serum theophylline levels have been reported.[1-4] Typically, patients had been on a stable theophylline dose and their serum level approximately doubled within days of starting mexiletine therapy. In some cases, toxic symptoms occurred (eg, nausea, vomiting, anorexia,[1] ventricular tachycardia[2]). In a randomized, crossover study of 12 healthy volunteers, concurrent administration of mexiletine and sustained-release theophylline resulted in a 58% increase in the area under the plasma concentration-time curve of theophylline and a 43% decrease in clearance.[5] Single-dose IV theophylline pharmacokinetic studies were performed in 15 healthy volunteers before and after 7 days of mexiletine 200 mg every 8 hours.[6] Theophylline clearance was reduced by 45% and 39% in female and male subjects, respectively. Another study established a correlation between baseline theophylline clearance and degree of metabolic inhibition in 8 healthy volunteers given sustained-release theophylline and mexiletine together for 2 days.[7] A 60% reduction in clearance occurred in a subject whose baseline theophylline clearance was 70 mL/hr/kg, while a 25% decrease occurred in the subject with 30 mL/hr/kg baseline clearance. The theophylline clearance in 6 elderly patients (average age, 73 years) also taking mexiletine was 27.8 mL/hr/kg, compared with an average clearance of 44.1 mL/hr/kg in 16 controls (average age, 61 years) not receiving mexiletine.[8] A reduction in the N-demethylation metabolite has been demonstrated,[6-8] indicating that mexiletine interferes with theophylline metabolism via cytochrome P450-mediated N-demethylation pathways.

1 Katz A, et al. *Int J Cardiol.* 1987;17:227.
2 Kessler KM, et al. *Am Heart J.* 1989;117:964.
3 Stanley R, et al. *Am J Med.* 1989;86:733.
4 Ueno K, et al. *DICP, Ann Pharmacother.* 1990;24:471.
5 Stoysich AM, et al. *J Clin Pharmacol.* 1991;31:354.
6 Loi C, et al. *Clin Pharmacol Ther.* 1991;49:571.
7 Hurwitz A, et al. *Clin Pharmacol Ther.* 1991;50:299.
8 Ueno, K, et al. *DICP, Ann Pharmacother.* 1991;25:727.

* Asterisk indicates drugs cited in interaction reports. Based on pharmacologic and pharmacokinetic considerations, similar interactions may occur with other drugs that are listed.
† Not available in the United States.

Theophyllines | **Moricizine**

Aminophylline*	Theophylline*	Moricizine*
Oxtriphylline†	(eg, *Theolair*)	(*Ethmozine*)

Significance	Onset	Severity	Documentation
4	☐ Rapid	☐ Major	☐ Established
	■ **Delayed**	■ **Moderate**	☐ Probable
		☐ Minor	☐ Suspected
			■ **Possible**
			☐ Unlikely

Effects MORICIZINE may cause decreased THEOPHYLLINE concentrations and exacerbation of pulmonary symptoms.

Mechanism Unknown. However, possibly caused by increased hepatic metabolism of THEOPHYLLINE.

Management Consider observing the patient's therapeutic response to THEOPHYLLINE and monitoring serum THEOPHYLLINE concentrations when MORICIZINE is started or stopped in a patient receiving THEOPHYLLINE.

Discussion

The effects of chronic oral administration of the antiarrhythmic agent moricizine on the pharmacokinetics of 2 oral forms of theophylline were studied in 12 healthy, nonsmoking subjects.[1] In an open-labeled, nonrandomized trial, patients were started on an 18-day course of moricizine 250 mg every 8 hr. On day 14 of moricizine administration, each subject received a single oral dose of immediate-release aminophylline (two 200 mg tablets), while on day 16 of moricizine administration, the subjects received a single dose of 300 mg controlled-release theophylline. Compared with plasma theophylline concentrations determined prior to moricizine administration, theophylline levels were measurably lower after moricizine was given. The mean AUC decreased for both the immediate- and controlled-release forms of theophylline, 32% and 36%, respectively. Clearance of the 2 forms of oral theophylline increased 44% and 66%, respectively. In addition, coadministration of moricizine decreased the mean $t_{1/2}$ of immediate- and controlled-release theophylline 33% and 20%, respectively.

[1] Pieniaszek HJ Jr., et al. *Ther Drug Monit.* 1993;15:199.

* Asterisk indicates drugs cited in interaction reports. Based on pharmacologic and pharmacokinetic considerations, similar interactions may occur with other drugs that are listed.

† Not available in the United States.

Theophyllines — *Nifedipine*

Aminophylline Oxtriphylline†	Theophylline* (eg, *Theolair*)	Nifedipine* (eg, *Procardia*)

Significance	Onset	Severity	Documentation
5	☐ Rapid ■ **Delayed**	☐ Major ■ **Moderate** ☐ Minor	☐ Established ☐ Probable ☐ Suspected ☐ Possible ■ **Unlikely**

Effects The actions of THEOPHYLLINES, particularly drug intoxication, may be enhanced.

Mechanism Unknown.

Management No clinical interventions appear necessary. If adverse events warrant, monitor serum THEOPHYLLINE concentrations and tailor the THEOPHYLLINE dosage as needed.

Discussion

Conflicting data exist. In 9 subjects, nifedipine did not affect theophylline steady-state trough serum concentrations, $t_{1/2}$, or AUC.[1] In addition, in 2 controlled studies involving healthy volunteers, slow-release nifedipine did not alter theophylline disposition,[2] clearance, AUC, or $t_{1/2}$.[3] Conversely, 2 patients exhibited elevated theophylline levels to the point of toxicity. This was correlated with coadministration of these drugs.[4,5] In addition, 1 study in 8 patients with stable symptomatic asthma receiving theophylline demonstrated a decrease in theophylline serum levels after slow-release nifedipine was added to their regimen.[6] No changes in asthma control occurred. In a single-dose study in healthy volunteers, 7 days of pretreatment with nifedipine produced no change in theophylline $t_{1/2}$.[7] In a preliminary report, 16 patients with chronic asthma stabilized on theophylline were given a short-term course of nifedipine. Only 1 of the 16 patients demonstrated an increase in theophylline $t_{1/2}$ greater than 25%.[8]

Preliminary data in 2 patients indicate that aminophylline may reverse the hemodynamic effects of nifedipine.[9] Additional studies are needed to confirm this finding. See Theophyllines-Verapamil and Theophyllines-Diltiazem.

1 Garty M, et al. *Clin Pharmacol Ther.* 1986;40:195.
2 Robson RA, et al. *Br J Clin Pharmacol.* 1988;25:397.
3 Jackson SH, et al. *Br J Clin Pharmacol.* 1986;21:389.
4 Parrillo SJ, et al. *Ann Emerg Med.* 1984;13:216.
5 Harrod CS. *Ann Intern Med.* 1987;106:480.
6 Smith SR, et al. *Thorax.* 1987;42:794.
7 Sirmans SM, et al. *Clin Pharmacol Ther.* 1988;44:29.
8 Christopher MA, et al. *Drug Intell Clin Pharm.* 1987;21:4A.
9 Kalra L, et al. *J Clin Pharmacol.* 1988;28:1056.

* Asterisk indicates drugs cited in interaction reports. Based on pharmacologic and pharmacokinetic considerations, similar interactions may occur with other drugs that are listed.
† Not available in the United States.

Theophyllines — *NSAIDs*

Aminophylline Oxtriphylline†	Theophylline* (eg, *Theolair*)	Rofecoxib* (*Vioxx*)

Significance	Onset	Severity	Documentation
4	□ Rapid ■ **Delayed**	□ Major ■ **Moderate** □ Minor	□ Established □ Probable □ Suspected ■ **Possible** □ Unlikely

Effects Increased THEOPHYLLINE serum concentrations with possible increased adverse reactions.

Mechanism ROFECOXIB inhibits the hepatic metabolism (CYP1A2) of THEOPHYLLINE.

Management In patients receiving THEOPHYLLINE, monitor THEOPHYLLINE levels and observe the patient for adverse effects when starting, stopping, or changing the dose of ROFECOXIB.

Discussion

The effects of rofecoxib on theophylline as a CYP1A2 probe were studied in 36 healthy men, divided into 3 panels of 12 subjects.[1] Using a randomized, 3-phase, placebo-controlled, 2-way, crossover design, each subject in a panel received 12.5, 25, or 50 mg of rofecoxib for 7 days. During each phase, subjects received a single 300 mg dose of theophylline on the morning of day 6. The geometric mean ratios (rofecoxib/placebo) for the theophylline AUC were 1.38, 1.51, and 1.6 with daily rofecoxib doses of 12.5, 25, and 50 mg, respectively. The mean values of the corresponding theophylline half-lives were increased from 7.2 to 10.1 hr, 6.9 to 10.9 hr and 7.6 to 13.1 hr, respectively, by administration of the 3 doses of rofecoxib. In addition, for each strength of rofecoxib, the apparent oral clearance of theophylline was decreased. Neither the theophylline peak plasma concentrations nor the times to reach the peak concentration were altered by any of the rofecoxib doses.

[1] Bachmann K, et al. *J Clin Pharmacol.* 2003;43:1082.

* Asterisk indicates drugs cited in interaction reports. Based on pharmacologic and pharmacokinetic considerations, similar interactions may occur with other drugs that are listed.
† Not available in the United States.

Theophyllines — *Omeprazole*

Theophylline* (eg, *Theo-Dur*)	Omeprazole* (*Prilosec*)

Significance	Onset	Severity	Documentation
4	■ **Rapid**	□ Major	□ Established
	□ Delayed	■ **Moderate**	□ Probable
		□ Minor	□ Suspected
			■ **Possible**
			□ Unlikely

Effects The rate of THEOPHYLLINE absorption from slow-release forms of THEOPHYLLINE may be increased.

Mechanism Hypochlorhydria induced by OMEPRAZOLE may amplify peristalsis in the small intestine and antiperistalsis in the proximal colon, resulting in increased THEOPHYLLINE absorption from sustained-release formulations.

Management Observe the clinical response of the patient and adjust the dose of THEOPHYLLINE as indicated.

Discussion

In a randomized, crossover study, the effects of increased intragastric pH on the absorption of theophylline from a sustained-release formulation was evaluated in 6 healthy male volunteers.[1] Each subject was pretreated with 240 mg omeprazole administered in 3 divided doses over a period of 22 hours preceding theophylline administration. Gastric hypoacidity produced by omeprazole increased the cumulative fractions of theophylline absorbed during a 3.5-hour period, starting 3.5 hours after dosing (0.5 hours after breakfast). The mean percentage of theophylline available for absorption after the formulation reached the large bowel was less during hypochlorhydria than under control conditions (ie, normochlorhydria). Despite the apparent acceleration of theophylline absorption with omeprazole administration, absorption was essentially complete at 24 hours and serum drug concentrations were not statistically different. Similarly, minor and clinically unimportant reductions in theophylline levels occurred in 20 healthy volunteers during coadministration of omeprazole 40 mg/day and sustained-release theophylline.[2]

[1] Sommers DK, et al. *Eur J Clin Pharmacol.* 1992;43:141.

[2] Dilger K, et al. *Br J Clin Pharmacol.* 1999;48:438.

* Asterisk indicates drugs cited in interaction reports.

Theophyllines			***Propafenone***
Aminophylline Oxtriphylline†	Theophylline* (eg, *Theo-Dur*)	Propafenone* (eg, *Rythmol*)	

Significance	Onset	Severity	Documentation
4	☐ Rapid ■ **Delayed**	☐ Major ■ **Moderate** ☐ Minor	☐ Established ☐ Probable ☐ Suspected ■ **Possible** ☐ Unlikely

Effects Increased THEOPHYLLINE serum levels with possible toxicity.

Mechanism Inhibition of THEOPHYLLINE metabolism is suspected.

Management Consider monitoring serum THEOPHYLLINE levels. Adjust the THEOPHYLLINE dosage as needed.

Discussion

Increased plasma theophylline levels with accompanying toxicity were reported in a 71-year-old man during concurrent administration of propafenone.[1] The patient had a history of chronic obstructive pulmonary disease, chronic bronchitis, angina pectoris, and nonsustained ventricular tachycardia with recurrent syncope. He had been smoking 1 pack of cigarettes daily for 50 years. The patient had been receiving theophylline 300 mg twice daily for 6 years and theophylline levels were stable during that time, ranging from 10.2 to 12.8 mcg/mL. Six weeks after the start of propafenone 150 mg 3 times daily, the theophylline concentration was 19 mcg/mL. The patient complained of poor appetite. Propafenone was discontinued because of symptoms of weakness and an increase in heart rate from 95 to 120 bpm. Within 24 hours of stopping propafenone, the serum theophylline concentration was 10.8 mcg/mL. Propafenone 150 mg 3 times daily was restarted. One week later, the theophylline level had increased from 12.8 to 17.5 mcg/mL. Decreasing the theophylline dosage to 200 mg twice daily produced a plasma theophylline level of 11.9 mcg/mL while the patient continued receiving 150 mg propafenone 3 times daily. In another case, administration of propafenone 150 to 300 mg 3 times daily decreased theophylline clearance 25% to 69%.[2] Although theophylline concentrations increased despite a reduction in theophylline dose, levels did not reach toxic values.

[1] Lee BL, et al. *Clin Pharmacol Ther.* 1992;51:353.

[2] Spinler SA, et al. *Pharmacotherapy.* 1993;13:68.

* Asterisk indicates drugs cited in interaction reports. Based on pharmacologic and pharmacokinetic considerations, similar interactions may occur with other drugs that are listed.

† Not available in the United States.

Theophyllines — *Quinolones*

Theophyllines	Quinolones	
Aminophylline*	Ciprofloxacin* (eg, *Cipro*)	Norfloxacin* (*Noroxin*)
Theophylline* (eg, *Theochron*)	Enoxacin*†	

Significance	Onset	Severity	Documentation
1	☐ Rapid	■ **Major**	■ **Established**
	■ **Delayed**	☐ Moderate	☐ Probable
		☐ Minor	☐ Suspected
			☐ Possible
			☐ Unlikely

Effects Increased THEOPHYLLINE levels with toxicity can occur.[1,2]

Mechanism Inhibition of the hepatic metabolism of THEOPHYLLINE.

Management If these agents must be given, monitor THEOPHYLLINE levels and observe for toxicity; adjust THEOPHYLLINE dosage as needed.

Discussion

Administration of theophylline with ciprofloxacin,[3-5] enoxacin,[3,4,6-12] or pefloxacin[†3] has decreased theophylline clearance[2-5,7,8,11-13] and increased plasma levels[3-8,11] and symptoms of toxicity,[3-6,9-11,14] including seizures.[2,13] Administration of theophylline and ciprofloxacin resulted in significant increases in theophylline $t_{1/2}$, volume of distribution, and serum levels; decreases in clearance have also occurred.[15-21] Ciprofloxacin further reduced the metabolism of theophylline in patients receiving cimetidine and theophylline.[21,22] Other data conflict.[23,24] While some suggest that norfloxacin,[25-28] ofloxacin,[29] and lomefloxacin[†30] do not interact, other studies show a decrease in theophylline clearance by norfloxacin.[4,11,31,32] Theophylline does not appear to alter quinolone kinetics.[33]

1 Green L, et al. *JAMA.* 1989;262(17):2383.
2 Grasela TH Jr, et al. *Arch Intern Med.* 1992;152(3):617.
3 Wijnands WJ, et al. *Br J Clin Pharmacol.* 1986;22(6):677.
4 Prince RA, et al. *J Clin Pharmacol.* 1989;29(7):650.
5 Richardson JP. *J Am Geriatr Soc.* 1990;38(3):236.
6 Wijnands WJ, et al. *Lancet.* 1984;2(8394):108.
7 Wijnands WJ, et al. *Br J Clin Pharmacol.* 1985;20(6):583.
8 Takagi K, et al. *Int J Clin Pharmacol Ther Toxicol.* 1988;26(6):288.
9 Duraski RM. *South Med J.* 1988;81(9):1206.
10 Holden R. *BMJ.* 1988;297(6659):1339.
11 Sano M, et al. *Eur J Clin Pharmacol.* 1989;36(3):323.
12 Koup JR, et al. *Antimicrob Agents Chemother.* 1990;34(5):803.
13 Semel JD, et al. *South Med J.* 1991;84(4):465.
14 Antoniou T, et al. *Eur J Clin Pharmacol.* 2011;67(5):521.
15 Raoof S, et al. *Am J Med.* 1987;82(4A):115.
16 Rybak MJ, et al. *Drug Intell Clin Pharm.* 1987;21(11):879.
17 Nix DE, et al. *J Antimicrob Chemother.* 1987;19(2):263.
18 Thomson AH, et al. *Eur J Clin Pharmacol.* 1987;33(4):435.
19 Bachmann KA, et al. *Br J Clin Pharmacol.* 1988;26(2):191.
20 Robson RA, et al. *Br J Clin Pharmacol.* 1990;29(4):491.
21 Davis RL, et al. *Ann Pharmacother.* 1992;26(1):11.
22 Loi CM, et al. *Br J Clin Pharmacol.* 1993;36(3):195.
23 Maesen FP, et al. *Lancet.* 1984;2(8401):530.
24 Fourtillan JB, et al. *Infection.* 1986;14(suppl 1):S67.
25 Niki Y, et al. *Chest.* 1987;92(4):663.
26 Sano M, et al. *Eur J Clin Pharmacol.* 1987;32(4):431.
27 Sano M, et al. *Eur J Clin Pharmacol.* 1988;35(2):161.
28 Davis RL, et al. *Antimicrob Agents Chemother.* 1989;33(2):212.
29 Wijnands WJ, et al. *Antimicrob Chemother.* 1988;22(suppl C):109.
30 Van Slooten A, et al. *Clin Pharmacol Ther.* 1992;51:160.
31 Bowles SK, et al. *Antimicrob Agents Chemother.* 1988;32(4):510.
32 Ho G, et al. *Clin Pharmacol Ther.* 1988;44(1):35.
33 Wijnands WJ, et al. *Drugs.* 1987;34(suppl 1):159.

* Asterisk indicates drugs cited in interaction reports. Based on pharmacologic and pharmacokinetic considerations, similar interactions may occur with other drugs that are listed.
† Not available in the United States.

Theophyllines — *Ranitidine*

Aminophylline	Theophylline* (eg, *Theo-24*)	Ranitidine* (eg, *Zantac*)
Dyphylline (eg, *Lufyllin*)		

Significance	Onset	Severity	Documentation
5	☐ Rapid	☐ Major	☐ Established
	■ **Delayed**	■ **Moderate**	☐ Probable
		☐ Minor	☐ Suspected
			☐ Possible
			■ **Unlikely**

Effects Elevated plasma THEOPHYLLINE levels have been described in case reports. However, controlled trials have not substantiated an interaction.

Mechanism Unknown.

Management No special precautions are necessary. Consider usual monitoring of serum levels and observe patients for signs of THEOPHYLLINE toxicity. Tailor the dosage as needed.

Discussion

Elevated plasma theophylline levels and signs of toxicity have occurred in some patients.[1-6] Patients taking theophylline have experienced nausea, vomiting, anxiety, tachycardia, and confusion 36 to 48 hours after the initiation of ranitidine. Some patients exhibited the same signs when rechallenged with ranitidine.[3,5] The documentation presented in the case reports has been questioned[7-12]; however, some patients may experience this interaction for unclear reasons. Controlled trials have not substantiated this interaction.[2,13-21]

1 Fernandes E, et al. *Ann Intern Med.* 1984;100(3):459.
2 Dal Negro R, et al. *Int J Clin Pharmacol Ther Toxicol.* 1985;23(6):329.
3 Roy AK, et al. *Am J Med.* 1988;85(4):525 [published correction appears in: Roy AK. *Am J Med.* 1989;86(4):513].
4 Skinner MH, et al. *Am J Med.* 1989;86(1):129.
5 Hegman GW, et al. *DICP.* 1991;25(1):21.
6 Gardner ME, et al. *Ann Intern Med.* 1985;102(4):559.
7 Dobbs JH, et al. *Ann Intern Med.* 1984;100(5):769.
8 Fernandes E, et al. *Ann Intern Med.* 1984;101(2):279.
9 Kelly HW. *Am J Med.* 1989;86(5):629.
10 Comment: Ranitidine does not inhibit theophylline metabolism. *DICP.* 1991;25(10):1139.
11 Williams DM, et al. *DICP.* 1991;25:1140.
12 Hegman GW. *DICP.* 1991;25(1):21.
13 Breen KJ, et al. *Clin Pharmacol Ther.* 1982;31(3):297.
14 Dal Negro R, et al. *Int J Clin Pharmacol Ther Toxicol.* 1984;22(4):221.
15 Powell JR, et al. *Arch Intern Med.* 1984;144(3):484.
16 Kelly HW, et al. *Clin Pharmacol Ther.* 1986;39(5):577.
17 Seggev JS, et al. *Arch Intern Med.* 1987;147(1):179.
18 Adebayo GI. *Biopharm Drug Dispos.* 1989;10(1):77.
19 Boehning W. *Eur J Clin Pharmacol.* 1990;38(1):43.
20 Wilson CG, et al. *Arzneimittelforschung.* 1991;41(11):1154.
21 Kehoe WA, et al. *Ann Pharmacother.* 1996;30(2):133.

* Asterisk indicates drugs cited in interaction reports. Based on pharmacologic and pharmacokinetic considerations, similar interactions may occur with other drugs that are listed.

Theophyllines — *Rifamycins*

Aminophylline*	Theophylline* (eg, *Theolair*)	Rifabutin (*Mycobutin*)	Rifapentine (*Priftin*)
Oxtriphylline*†		Rifampin* (eg, *Rifadin*)	

Significance	Onset	Severity	Documentation
2	□ Rapid	□ Major	■ **Established**
	■ **Delayed**	■ **Moderate**	□ Probable
		□ Minor	□ Suspected
			□ Possible
			□ Unlikely

Effects The addition of a RIFAMYCIN may cause decreased THEOPHYLLINE levels and exacerbation of pulmonary symptoms.

Mechanism RIFAMYCINS appears to induce the hepatic metabolism of THEOPHYLLINE.

Management In patients receiving THEOPHYLLINE, monitor THEOPHYLLINE levels and the patient's response when starting or stopping a RIFAMYCIN. Adjust the dose as needed.

Discussion

Investigators have documented an interaction between rifampin and theophylline.[1,2] Healthy volunteers given theophylline or aminophylline after 7 to 14 days of rifampin exhibited increased theophylline clearance[1-7] and elimination rate constant[2,4,6] and decreased plasma $t_{1/2}$ and AUC.[4-6] Increases in the volume of distribution (Vd) have also been reported,[1,5] although the reports are inconsistent.[4,6] The increase in Vd has been postulated to be a result of increased enterohepatic circulation.[5] A similar interaction has been documented in a pediatric patient.[8] In most instances, theophylline was added to rifampin; however, when rifampin was added to an existing theophylline regimen, a similar increase (82% ± 18%) in theophylline clearance occurred.[3]

[1] Hauser AR, et al. *Clin Pharmacol Ther.* 1983;33:254.
[2] Straughn AB, et al. *Ther Drug Monit.* 1984;6:153.
[3] Robson RA, et al. *Br J Clin Pharmacol.* 1984;18:445.
[4] Boyce EG, et al. *Clin Pharmacol Ther.* 1985;37:183.
[5] Powell-Jackson PR, et al. *Am Rev Respir Dis.* 1985;131:939.
[6] Boyce EG, et al. *J Clin Pharmacol.* 1986;26:696.
[7] Adebayo GI, et al. *Eur J Clin Pharmacol.* 1989;37:127.
[8] Brocks DR, et al. *Clin Pharm.* 1986;5:602.

* Asterisk indicates drugs cited in interaction reports. Based on pharmacologic and pharmacokinetic considerations, similar interactions may occur with other drugs that are listed.
† Not available in the United States.

Theophyllines — *St. John's Wort*

Aminophylline Oxtriphylline†	Theophylline* (eg, *Theolair*)	St. John's Wort*

Significance	Onset	Severity	Documentation
4	☐ Rapid ■ **Delayed**	☐ Major ■ **Moderate** ☐ Minor	☐ Established ☐ Probable ☐ Suspected ■ **Possible** ☐ Unlikely

Effects Plasma THEOPHYLLINE concentrations may be decreased.

Mechanism Increased hepatic metabolism (CYP1A2) of THEOPHYLLINES is suspected.

Management Because THEOPHYLLINE has a narrow therapeutic index, caution patients to consult their health care provider before using nonprescription or herbal products. If ST. JOHN'S WORT cannot be avoided, assess the patient's response to THEOPHYLLINE when ST. JOHN'S WORT is started or stopped. Monitoring THEOPHYLLINE plasma concentrations may be useful in adjusting the dose.

Discussion

A possible interaction between theophylline and St. John's wort was reported in a 42-year-old woman.[1] The patient had been stabilized on theophylline 300 mg twice daily for several months. After a hospital discharge, her theophylline levels were lower than desired, resulting in theophylline dosage increases of up to 800 mg twice daily. At this dose, the patient's theophylline concentration was 9.2 mcg/mL. Although the patient was receiving other medications, she stated that the only addition to her regimen was St. John's wort 300 mg/day (standardized to 0.3% hypericin), which she had been taking for 2 months. On her own initiative, the patient stopped taking the St. John's wort. One week later, her theophylline level was 19.6 mcg/mL; the theophylline dosage was then reduced. In an open-label, crossover study, in 12 healthy volunteers, St. John's wort 300 mg 3 times daily for 14 days did not affect the pharmacokinetics of theophylline (400 mg single dose).[2]

The ingredients of many herbal products are not standardized. It is unclear whether herbal products contain ingredients other than those listed on the label or purported to be present that could interact with theophylline.

[1] Nebel A, et al. *Ann Pharmacother.* 1999;33:502.

[2] Morimoto T, et al. *J Clin Pharmacol.* 2004;44:95.

* Asterisk indicates drugs cited in interaction reports. Based on pharmacologic and pharmacokinetic considerations, similar interactions may occur with other drugs that are listed.

† Not available in the United States.

Theophyllines — **Sulfinpyrazone**

Aminophylline
Theophylline*
(eg, *Theochron*)

Sulfinpyrazone*
(eg, *Anturane*)

Significance	Onset	Severity	Documentation
5	☐ Rapid ■ **Delayed**	☐ Major ☐ Moderate ■ **Minor**	☐ Established ☐ Probable ☐ Suspected ■ **Possible** ☐ Unlikely

Effects THEOPHYLLINE clearance may be increased, thus lowering plasma levels.

Mechanism The hepatic metabolism of THEOPHYLLINES may be increased; renal clearance may be decreased.

Management Monitor THEOPHYLLINE serum concentrations if there is an exacerbation in the patient's condition; adjust dosage as needed.

Discussion

In 6 nonsmoking men, sulfinpyrazone produced a 22% increase in total plasma theophylline clearance.[1] It is believed that sulfinpyrazone influenced demethylation and oxidative pathways. Although a minor component, renal clearance was decreased by 27%. See also Theophyllines-Probenecid.

[1] Birkett DJ, et al. *Br J Clin Pharmacol.* 1983;15(5):567.

* Asterisk indicates drugs cited in interaction reports. Based on pharmacologic and pharmacokinetic considerations, similar interactions may occur with other drugs that are listed.

Theophyllines | Sympathomimetics (Beta-Agonists)

Theophyllines		Sympathomimetics (Beta-Agonists)	
Aminophylline*	Theophylline* (eg, *Theochron*)	Albuterol* (eg, *Proventil*)	Metaproterenol (eg, *Alupent*)
Dyphylline (eg, *Lufyllin*)		Bitolterol (*Tornalate*)	Pirbuterol (*Maxair*)
		Isoetharine	Terbutaline* (eg, *Brethine*)
		Isoproterenol* (eg, *Isuprel*)	

Significance	Onset	Severity	Documentation
5	■ **Rapid**	□ Major	□ Established
	□ Delayed	□ Moderate	□ Probable
		■ **Minor**	□ Suspected
			■ **Possible**
			□ Unlikely

Effects Enhanced toxicity, particularly cardiotoxicity, has been noted. Decreased THEOPHYLLINE concentrations may occur.

Mechanism Unknown; see Discussion.

Management Monitor serum THEOPHYLLINE and potassium concentrations. Monitor patients for clinical signs of improvement or toxicity. Adjust the THEOPHYLLINE dose as needed.

Discussion

Traditionally, combination therapy with theophyllines and beta-agonists has been accepted practice and proven effective in patients.[1-3] Additive[4-6] or synergistic[7] effects have been reported. However, some data indicate that beta-agonists decrease theophylline levels, possibly by increasing clearance.[8-14] Hypokalemia potentiated by beta-agonists has been observed.[4,15] Also, 1 report of lactic acidosis secondary to aminophylline/beta-agonist therapy has been reported.[16] An important concern is the cardiotoxicity of combination therapy. One review highlights the problems with published trials.[17] More definitive data are needed.[18] Cardiotoxicity is a concern most associated with isoproterenol; bitolterol is believed to induce fewer arrhythmias compared with isoproterenol.[19]

Controlled studies are needed to clarify the clinical importance of this interaction.

[1] Hemstreet MP, et al. *J Allergy Clin Immunol.* 1982;69(4):360.
[2] Guyatt GH, et al. *Am Rev Respir Dis.* 1987;135(5):1069.
[3] Lombardi TP, et al. *J Clin Pharmacol.* 1987;27(7):523.
[4] Smith SR, et al. *Br J Clin Pharmacol.* 1986;21(4):451.
[5] Billing B, et al. *Eur J Respir Dis.* 1987;70(1):35.
[6] Cusack BJ, et al. *Clin Pharmacol Ther.* 1987;41(3):289.
[7] Abdallah AH, et al. *Drug Devel Res.* 1987;10:85.
[8] Roddick LG, et al. *Med J Aust.* 1979;2:153.
[9] Dawson KP, et al. *Arch Dis Child.* 1982;57(9):674.
[10] O'Rourke PP, et al. *Crit Care Med.* 1984;12(4):373.
[11] Danziger Y, et al. *Clin Pharmacol Ther.* 1985;37(4):469.
[12] Garty M, et al. *Clin Pharmacol Ther.* 1988;43:150.
[13] Griffith JA, et al. *Clin Pharm.* 1990;9(1):54.
[14] Amitai Y, et al. *Chest.* 1992;102(3):786.
[15] Whyte KF, et al. *Br J Clin Pharmacol.* 1988;25(5):571.
[16] Braden GL, et al. *N Engl J Med.* 1985;313(14):890.
[17] Kelly HW. *Clin Pharm.* 1984;3(4):386.
[18] Nicklas RA, et al. *J Allergy Clin Immunol.* 1984;73(1, pt 1):20.
[19] Walker SB, et al. *Pharmacotherapy.* 1985;5(3):127.

* Asterisk indicates drugs cited in interaction reports. Based on pharmacologic and pharmacokinetic considerations, similar interactions may occur with other drugs that are listed.

Theophyllines — *Tacrine*

Aminophylline*	Theophylline* (eg, *Theolair*)	Tacrine* (*Cognex*)
Oxtriphylline†		

Significance	Onset	Severity	Documentation
4	☐ Rapid	☐ Major	☐ Established
	■ **Delayed**	■ **Moderate**	☐ Probable
		☐ Minor	☐ Suspected
			■ **Possible**
			☐ Unlikely

Effects Increased THEOPHYLLINE concentrations with toxicity may occur.

Mechanism Possibly inhibition of the hepatic metabolism of THEOPHYLLINE.

Management Monitor serum THEOPHYLLINE concentrations and observe the patient for signs and symptoms of THEOPHYLLINE toxicity when initiating TACRINE therapy. If treatment with both drugs is started at the same time or if THEOPHYLLINE is initiated in a patient receiving TACRINE, reduce the dose of THEOPHYLLINE 25% to 50% and monitor serum THEOPHYLLINE concentrations. Adjust the dose of THEOPHYLLINE as indicated.

Discussion

Coadministration of tacrine and theophylline has been associated with a 2-fold increase in the elimination half-life and average plasma concentration of theophylline.[1-3] Data from a small study presented in an abstract reported a 50% reduction in theophylline oral clearance when tacrine, 20 mg every 6 hours, was given concurrently.[4]

Additional published clinical data are needed to assess the importance of this possible interaction. The effect of theophylline on tacrine pharmacokinetics has not been examined.

1 Madden S, et al. *Biochem Pharmacol.* 1993;46:13.
2 *Cognex* [package insert]. New York, NY: Parke-Davis; May 1993.
3 Personal communications. Parke-Davis. October 1993.
4 de Vries TM, et al. *Pharm Res.* 1993;10:S-333.

* Asterisk indicates drugs cited in interaction reports. Based on pharmacologic and pharmacokinetic considerations, similar interactions may occur with other drugs that are listed.
† Not available in the United States.

Theophyllines — *Terbinafine*

Aminophylline* Oxtriphylline†	Theophylline (eg, *Bronkodyl*)	Terbinafine* (*Lamisil*)

Significance	Onset	Severity	Documentation
4	☐ Rapid ■ **Delayed**	☐ Major ■ **Moderate** ☐ Minor	☐ Established ☐ Probable ☐ Suspected ■ **Possible** ☐ Unlikely

Effects Plasma THEOPHYLLINE levels may be elevated, increasing the pharmacologic and adverse effects.

Mechanism Unknown.

Management When starting TERBINAFINE in a patient receiving THEOPHYLLINE therapy, monitor plasma THEOPHYLLINE levels and observe the clinical response of the patients, especially those individuals at the upper end of the therapeutic range. Adjust the THEOPHYLLINE dose as needed.

Discussion

The effects of multiple oral doses of terbinafine (250 mg/day for 4 days) on the pharmacokinetics of a single dose of aminophylline oral solution (5 mg/kg) were evaluated in an open-labeled, randomized, crossover study involving 12 healthy volunteers.[1] Aminophylline was administered 2 hours after the final dose of terbinafine. Compared with administration of aminophylline alone, coadministration of terbinafine increased the area under the plasma concentration-time curve of theophylline 16%, decreased oral clearance 14%, and increased the half-life 24%.

[1] Trepanier EF, et al. *Antimicrob Agents Chemother.* 1998;42:695.

* Asterisk indicates drugs cited in interaction reports. Based on pharmacologic and pharmacokinetic considerations, similar interactions may occur with other drugs that are listed.

† Not available in the United States.

Theophyllines — *Tetracyclines*

Aminophylline	Oxtriphylline†	Demeclocycline (*Declomycin*)	Oxytetracycline (eg, *Terramycin*)
Dyphylline (eg, *Lufyllin*)	Theophylline* (eg, *Bronkodyl*)	Doxycycline* (eg, *Vibramycin*)	Tetracycline* (eg, *Achromycin V*)
		Minocycline* (*Minocin*)	

Significance	Onset	Severity	Documentation
4	☐ Rapid	☐ Major	☐ Established
	■ **Delayed**	■ **Moderate**	☐ Probable
		☐ Minor	☐ Suspected
			■ **Possible**
			☐ Unlikely

Effects The incidence of adverse reactions to THEOPHYLLINE may be increased.

Mechanism Unknown.

Management Until further definitive information is available, it is advisable to monitor THEOPHYLLINE levels and tailor dosages as needed when starting or stopping any TETRACYCLINE product.

Discussion

The Boston Collaborative Drug Surveillance[1] program reported that adverse reactions (ADRs) occurred more frequently in patients receiving theophylline and tetracycline than in those taking theophylline alone. While the number of ADRs was higher for concomitant use, the overall percentage was lower. In reports with 5 patients[2] and 6 patients[3] who received concomitant theophylline and tetracycline, no pharmacokinetic differences in theophylline were noted prior to tetracycline compared with after tetracycline. Each group had 1 smoker; when data for nonsmokers were evaluated separately, a slight inhibition of theophylline clearance was noted with concomitant tetracycline use.[2,3] In 10 asthmatic patients, theophylline concentrations were inconsistently affected by doxycycline.[4] Similar trials have failed to confirm alterations in theophylline pharmacokinetics by tetracycline.[5-7] A case report indicates that minocycline 100 mg IV twice daily for 6 days produced asymptomatic elevation of serum theophylline concentration (from 9.9 to 15.5 mcg/mL).[8] However, a number of other possible factors that could have altered theophylline concentrations were not discussed. This study does serve as a reminder to monitor patients closely. No symptoms of theophylline toxicity were apparent.

1 Pfeifer HJ, et al. *Chest.* 1978;73:455.
2 Gotz VP, et al. *Drug Intell Clin Pharm.* 1985;19:463.
3 Gotz VP, et al. *Drug Intell Clin Pharm.* 1986;20:694.
4 Seggev JS, et al. *Ann Allergy.* 1986;56:156.
5 Pfeifer HJ, et al. *Clin Pharmacol Ther.* 1979;26:36.
6 Mathis JW, et al. *Clin Pharm.* 1982;1:446.
7 Jonkman JHG, et al. *Ther Drug Monit.* 1985;7:92.
8 Kawai M, et al. *Ann Pharmacother.* 1992;26:1300.

* Asterisk indicates drugs cited in interaction reports. Based on pharmacologic and pharmacokinetic considerations, similar interactions may occur with other drugs that are listed.
† Not available in the United States.

Theophyllines — *Thiabendazole*

Aminophylline*	Theophylline* (eg, *Bronkodyl*)	Thiabendazole* (*Mintezol*)
Oxtriphylline†		

Significance	Onset	Severity	Documentation
2	☐ Rapid	☐ Major	☐ Established
	■ **Delayed**	■ **Moderate**	☐ Probable
		☐ Minor	■ **Suspected**
			☐ Possible
			☐ Unlikely

Effects Increased THEOPHYLLINE serum levels with possible toxicity.

Mechanism Unknown. However, metabolic inhibition is suspected.

Management Consider monitoring serum THEOPHYLLINE levels; tailor the dosage as needed.

Discussion

A 71-year-old male patient exhibited signs of theophylline toxicity when started on thiabendazole 4 g/day.[1] The theophylline level increased from 21 to 46 mcg/mL. A second case report indicated a greater than 50% reduction in theophylline clearance secondary to thiabendazole.[2] The patient received thiabendazole 1800 mg twice daily for 6 doses. In anticipation of an interaction, the dose of theophylline was reduced from 300 mg twice daily to 200 mg twice daily; however, by the third day of concurrent administration, the theophylline level had increased from a baseline of 14 to 15 mcg/mL to 22 mcg/mL. In a third case report of a 64-year-old man receiving an aminophylline infusion, the serum theophylline level increased from 19 to 26 mcg/mL after approximately 4 doses of thiabendazole 1.5 g twice daily, prompting a randomized crossover study in 6 healthy volunteers.[3] During concurrent administration of thiabendazole, theophylline half-life increased, clearance decreased, and the elimination rate constant decreased. Two subjects experienced nausea and vomiting during administration of both drugs.

[1] Sugar AM, et al. *Am Rev Resp Dis.* 1980;122:501.
[2] Lew G, et al. *Clin Pharm.* 1989;8:225.
[3] Schneider D, et al. *Chest.* 1990;97:84.

* Asterisk indicates drugs cited in interaction reports. Based on pharmacologic and pharmacokinetic considerations, similar interactions may occur with other drugs that are listed.
† Not available in the United States.

Theophyllines — *Thioamines*

Aminophylline*	Theophylline* (eg, *Bronkodyl*)	Methimazole* (*Tapazole*)	Propylthiouracil (PTU)
Oxtriphylline†			

Significance	Onset	Severity	Documentation
2	☐ Rapid	☐ Major	☐ Established
	■ **Delayed**	■ **Moderate**	☐ Probable
		☐ Minor	■ **Suspected**
			☐ Possible
			☐ Unlikely

Effects Increases in THEOPHYLLINE clearance can be expected in hyperthyroid patients. Clearance returns to normal when euthyroid state is achieved.

Mechanism There appears to be a positive correlation or a direct relationship between plasma thyroxine levels and THEOPHYLLINE clearance.[3] Hyperthyroid[2] and hypothyroid[1] patients have manifested alterations in THEOPHYLLINE clearance.

Management Achieving a euthyroid state is critical in controlling THEOPHYLLINE clearance. Monitor THEOPHYLLINE and tailor dosages as needed.

Discussion

It is known that thyroid disease affects drug metabolism. In general, hypothyroidism causes decreased elimination, whereas hyperthyroidism causes increased elimination of drugs.

In hypothyroid patients theophylline elimination is prolonged. A 70-year-old male hypothyroid patient manifested life-threatening theophylline intoxication. Theophylline plasma half-life was 29.5 hours prior to achieving a euthyroid state in which half-life was 5.7 hours.[1] In a similar case, theophylline clearance doubled (0.5 to 1.2 mL/min/kg) as the patient was brought to a euthyroid state.[4]

Hyperthyroid patients manifest increased theophylline clearance which returns to normal in the euthyroid state.[2,3] The pharmacokinetics of theophylline were evaluated in 5 hyperthyroid patients prior to and following carbimazole administration. While theophylline clearance fell after carbimazole, volume of distribution did not change.[3] Thyroxine concentration and theophylline clearance appeared to be associated in 15 subjects.[3] See also Theophylline-Thyroid Hormones.

[1] Aderka D, et al. *Respiration.* 1983;44:77.
[2] Bauman JH, et al. *Ann Allergy.* 1984;52:94.
[3] Vozeh S, et al. *Clin Pharmacol Ther.* 1984;36:634.
[4] Seifert CF, et al. *Drug Intell Clin Pharm.* 1987;21:442.

* Asterisk indicates drugs cited in interaction reports. Based on pharmacologic and pharmacokinetic considerations, similar interactions may occur with other drugs that are listed.
† Not available in the United States.

Theophyllines / *Thyroid Hormones*

Theophyllines		Thyroid Hormones	
Aminophylline*	Theophylline* (eg, *Bronkodyl*)	Dextrothyroxine (*Choloxin*)	Liotrix (*Euthroid, Thyrolar*)
Oxtriphylline†		Levothyroxine* (eg, *Synthroid*)	Thyroglobulin (*Proloid*)
		Liothyronine (eg, *Cytomel*)	Thyroid (eg, *Armour Thyroid*)

Significance	Onset	Severity	Documentation
2	☐ Rapid	☐ Major	☐ Established
	■ **Delayed**	■ **Moderate**	☐ Probable
		☐ Minor	■ **Suspected**
			☐ Possible
			☐ Unlikely

Effects Decreased THEOPHYLLINE clearance can be expected in hypothyroid patients. Clearance returns to normal when euthyroid state is achieved.

Mechanism There appears to be a positive correlation or a direct relationship between plasma thyroxine levels and THEOPHYLLINE clearance.[1] Hyperthyroid[2] and hypothyroid[3] patients have manifested alterations in THEOPHYLLINE clearance.

Management Achieving a euthyroid state is critical in controlling THEOPHYLLINE clearance. Monitor THEOPHYLLINE and tailor dosages as needed.

Discussion

It is known that thyroid disease affects drug metabolism. In general, hypothyroidism causes decreased elimination, whereas hyperthyroidism causes increased elimination of drugs.

In hypothyroid patients, theophylline elimination is prolonged. A 70-year-old male hypothyroid patient manifested life-threatening theophylline intoxication. Theophylline plasma half-life was 29.5 hours prior to achieving a euthyroid state in which half-life was 5.7 hours.[3] In a similar case, theophylline clearance doubled (from 0.5 to 1.0 mL/min/kg) with aggressive IV levothyroxine as the patient was brought to a euthyroid state.[4]

Hyperthyroid patients manifest increased theophylline clearance which returns to normal in the euthyroid state.[1,2] Theophylline kinetics were evaluated in 5 hyperthyroid patients before and after treatment with carbimazole. While theophylline clearance fell after carbimazole, volume of distribution did not change.[1] A positive correlation between thyroxine concentration and theophylline clearance was noted in 15 subjects.[1] See also Theophyllines-Thioamines.

[1] Vozeh S, et al. *Clin Pharmacol Ther.* 1984;36:634.
[2] Bauman JH, et al. *Ann Allergy.* 1984;52:94.
[3] Aderka D, et al. *Respiration.* 1983;44:77.
[4] Seifert CF, et al. *Drug Intell Clin Pharm.* 1987;21:442.

* Asterisk indicates drugs cited in interaction reports. Based on pharmacologic and pharmacokinetic considerations, similar interactions may occur with other drugs that are listed.
† Not available in the United States.

Theophyllines — *Ticlopidine*

Aminophylline Oxtriphylline†	Theophylline* (eg, *Slo-Phyllin*)	Ticlopidine* (*Ticlid*)

Significance	Onset	Severity	Documentation
2	☐ Rapid ■ **Delayed**	☐ Major ■ **Moderate** ☐ Minor	☐ Established ☐ Probable ■ **Suspected** ☐ Possible ☐ Unlikely

Effects Increased THEOPHYLLINE levels have been noted with the addition of TICLOPIDINE to regimen. THEOPHYLLINE toxicity in the form of nausea, vomiting, seizures, and arrhythmias may manifest.

Mechanism TICLOPIDINE impairs THEOPHYLLINE elimination.

Management Monitor THEOPHYLLINE serum levels when TICLOPIDINE is added or withdrawn from a patient's regimen; tailor dosages as needed.

Discussion

Pharmacokinetic parameters of theophylline were evaluated in 10 healthy male patients before, during, and 30 days after 10 days of ticlopidine treatment. All subjects illustrated significant decreases in theophylline clearance and increases in serum half-life. Kinetic parameters had returned to normal 30 days after ticlopidine. Caution is warranted until further information on this interaction is available.

[1] Colli A, et al. *Clin Pharmacol Ther.* 1987;41:358.

* Asterisk indicates drugs cited in interaction reports. Based on pharmacologic and pharmacokinetic considerations, similar interactions may occur with other drugs that are listed.
† Not available in the United States.

Theophyllines — *Verapamil*

Aminophylline*	Theophylline* (eg, *Slo-Phyllin*)	Verapamil* (eg, *Calan*)
Oxtriphylline†		

Significance	Onset	Severity	Documentation
4	□ Rapid	□ Major	□ Established
	■ **Delayed**	■ **Moderate**	□ Probable
		□ Minor	□ Suspected
			■ **Possible**
			□ Unlikely

Effects The effects of THEOPHYLLINES may be increased.

Mechanism Inhibition of hepatic metabolism of THEOPHYLLINES.[5]

Management Monitor serum THEOPHYLLINE concentrations and the patient for signs of THEOPHYLLINE toxicity. Adjust dosages as needed.

Discussion

An elderly woman was admitted to the hospital for evaluation and treatment of paroxysmal supraventricular tachycardia.[1] She was taking digoxin (eg, *Lanoxin*) and theophylline. Verapamil 240 mg/day was initiated, but 2 days later her heart rate had increased and remained so, despite increases in verapamil (360 mg/day) and digoxin. She also complained of nausea and vomiting; theophylline levels on day 6 were 27.9 mcg/mL, and theophylline was discontinued. Symptoms resolved, and the patient was maintained on lower doses of all 3 drugs. Conversely, verapamil interactions may be used therapeutically.[2] A 75-year-old female patient hospitalized for pneumonia experienced paroxysmal episodes of supraventricular tachycardia with elevated theophylline concentrations (serum concentrations, 16.5 to 22.1 mcg/mL).[3] She was converted to a normal sinus rhythm on 2 separate occasions by IV administration of verapamil 5 mg. In a study involving 9 healthy volunteers, verapamil 80 mg every 8 hours for 4 days did not significantly change theophylline disposition.[4] In a single oral-dose study in healthy volunteers, 7 days of pretreatment with verapamil caused an 18% decrease in total theophylline clearance and an increase in theophylline half-life.[5] Similarly, a study of 12 healthy volunteers given verapamil 40, 80, or 120 mg 3 times daily for 4 days found a dose-dependent decrease in theophylline clearance ranging from 8% to 18%.[6] The magnitude of these changes is small but could cause toxicity in patients maintained in the upper therapeutic range of theophylline.

[1] Burnakis TG, et al. *Clin Pharm.* 1983;2:458.
[2] Fuhr U, et al. *Eur J Clin Pharmacol.* 1992;42:463.
[3] Marchlinski FE, et al. *Chest.* 1985;88:931.
[4] Robson RA, et al. *Br J Clin Pharmacol.* 1988;25:397.
[5] Sirmans SM, et al. *Clin Pharmacol Ther.* 1988;44:29.
[6] Stringer KA, et al. *Eur J Clin Pharmacol.* 1992;43:35.

* Asterisk indicates drugs cited in interaction reports. Based on pharmacologic and pharmacokinetic considerations, similar interactions may occur with other drugs that are listed.
† Not available in the United States.

Theophyllines — *Zafirlukast*

Aminophylline Oxtriphylline†	Theophylline* (eg, *Slo-bid*)	Zafirlukast* (*Accolate*)

Significance	Onset	Severity	Documentation
4	☐ Rapid ■ **Delayed**	☐ Major ■ **Moderate** ☐ Minor	☐ Established ☐ Probable ☐ Suspected ■ **Possible** ☐ Unlikely

Effects THEOPHYLLINE serum levels may be elevated, resulting in an increase in the pharmacologic and toxic effects. ZAFIRLUKAST plasma levels may decrease.

Mechanism Unknown.

Management Observe the clinical response of the patient and carefully monitor THEOPHYLLINE serum concentrations when starting or stopping ZAFIRLUKAST.

Discussion

A marked increase in theophylline serum concentrations was reported in a 15-year-old female patient with asthma following the addition of zafirlukast to her treatment regimen.[1] The patient had been receiving theophylline 300 mg twice daily, fluticasone propionate (*Flovent*), salmeterol (*Serevent*), prednisone (eg, *Deltasone*), and albuterol (eg, *Proventil*) for several years. During that period, theophylline concentrations were approximately 11 mcg/mL. Shortly after zafirlukast was added to her treatment regimen, the patient complained of nausea, and her theophylline concentration was measured at 24 mcg/mL. Attempts to stop and resume theophylline therapy at a lower dose resulted in rapid development of increased serum theophylline levels (18 to 27 mcg/mL). To further assess the possible drug interaction, both drugs were discontinued for 1 week. The patient was admitted to the hospital, and treatment with theophylline 75 mg twice daily was started. On the third day of treatment, zafirlukast 20 mg twice daily was added. On the fifth day, theophylline serum concentrations increased 7-fold, and there was a 572% increase in the area under the plasma concentration-time curve of theophylline. Both drugs were discontinued, and 1 week later, theophylline 300 mg twice daily was started. She was maintained on that dose of theophylline with serum concentrations ranging from 10 to 11 mcg/mL. Other cases of increased theophylline serum concentrations during concomitant administration of zafirlukast have been reported to the FDA.[1]

In contrast to this case, the manufacturer of zafirlukast reports that at steady state, a single dose of liquid theophylline 6 mg/kg to asthmatic patients decreased mean plasma levels of zafirlukast by approximately 30% but had no effect on serum theophylline levels.[2]

[1] Katial RK, et al. *Arch Intern Med.* 1998;158:1713.

[2] *Accolate* [package insert]. Wilmington, DE: Astra Zeneca; September 1996.

* Asterisk indicates drugs cited in interaction reports. Based on pharmacologic and pharmacokinetic considerations, similar interactions may occur with other drugs that are listed.

† Not available in the United States.

Theophyllines | **Zileuton**

Aminophylline Oxtriphylline†	Theophylline* (eg, *Slo-Phyllin*)	Zileuton* (*Zyflo*)

Significance	Onset	Severity	Documentation
2	☐ Rapid ■ **Delayed**	☐ Major ■ **Moderate** ☐ Minor	☐ Established ■ **Probable** ☐ Suspected ☐ Possible ☐ Unlikely

Effects THEOPHYLLINE plasma concentrations may be elevated, increasing the pharmacologic and adverse effects.

Mechanism Possibly inhibition of THEOPHYLLINE metabolism.

Management Monitor THEOPHYLLINE concentrations and observe the patient for signs of toxicity. Adjust the THEOPHYLLINE dosage as needed. When starting ZILEUTON in patients who are receiving THEOPHYLLINE, reduce the THEOPHYLLINE dose approximately 50% and monitor plasma THEOPHYLLINE concentrations.

Discussion

The effects of zileuton on the pharmacokinetics of theophylline were evaluated in a randomized, double-blind, placebo-controlled, crossover study.[1] Sixteen healthy, nonsmoking male volunteers received theophylline 200 mg every 6 hours for 5 days. Each subject was assigned to receive either zileuton 800 mg twice daily or placebo. After a 15-day washout period, theophylline was resumed, and the study drugs were reversed. Zileuton administration increased peak and trough plasma theophylline concentrations approximately 75% and 125%, respectively, and decreased the plasma clearance 49% compared with placebo. Zileuton administration delayed the time to reach peak theophylline concentration 0.5 hours and increased the half-life of theophylline nearly 1.5 hours. When taking theophylline with placebo, 8 subjects reported a single adverse event compared with 44 adverse events in 14 volunteers receiving theophylline and zileuton concomitantly. Headache was the most common complaint in both groups. Three subjects receiving theophylline with zileuton withdrew from the study.

[1] Granneman GR, et al. *Clin Pharmacokinet.* 1995;29(Suppl 2):77.

* Asterisk indicates drugs cited in interaction reports. Based on pharmacologic and pharmacokinetic considerations, similar interactions may occur with other drugs that are listed.
† Not available in the United States.

Thiazide Diuretics — *Anticholinergics*

Bendroflumethiazide (*Naturetin*)
Benzthiazide (*Exna*)
Chlorothiazide* (eg, *Diuril*)
Chlorthalidone (eg, *Hygroton*)
Hydrochlorothiazide* (eg, *HydroDiuril*)
Hydroflumethiazide (eg, *Saluron*)
Indapamide (eg, *Lozol*)
Methyclothiazide (eg, *Enduron*)
Metolazone (*Mykrox*, *Zaroxolyn*)
Polythiazide (*Renese*)
Quinethazone (*Hydromox*)
Trichlormethiazide (eg, *Naqua*)

Anisotropine
Atropine
Belladonna
Benztropine (eg, *Cogentin*)
Biperiden (*Akineton*)
Clidinium (*Quarzan*)
Dicyclomine (eg, *Bentyl*)
Glycopyrrolate (eg, *Robinul*)
Hyoscyamine (eg, *Anaspaz*)
Isopropamide
Mepenzolate (*Cantil*)
Methantheline (*Banthine*)
Methscopolamine (*Pamine*)
Orphenadrine (eg, *Norflex*)
Oxybutynin (eg, *Ditropan*)
Procyclidine (*Kemadrin*)
Propantheline* (eg, *Pro-Banthine*)
Scopolamine
Tridihexethyl (*Pathilon*)
Trihexyphenidyl (eg, *Artane*)

Significance	Onset	Severity	Documentation
	☐ Rapid ■ **Delayed**	☐ Major ☐ Moderate ■ **Minor**	☐ Established ☐ Probable ☐ Suspected ■ **Possible** ☐ Unlikely

Effects THIAZIDE DIURETIC action may be stimulated, leading to altered diuresis patterns.

Mechanism ANTICHOLINERGICS increase oral THIAZIDE absorption by delaying GI motility and decreasing the stomach-emptying rate. The rate at which THIAZIDES pass the optimal absorption region in the small intestine is reduced.

Management No clinical interventions appear necessary.

Discussion

Six healthy adult male patients were given hydrochlorothiazide 75 mg alone or after pretreatment with propantheline 60 mg.[1] The peak hydrochlorothiazide plasma concentration did not differ between groups; however, propantheline pretreatment delayed the peak plasma levels of hydrochlorothiazide from 2.4 to 4.8 hours. The area under the concentration-time curve was greater when hydrochlorothiazide was preceded by propantheline. The 48-hour urinary recovery of hydrochlorothiazide was greater with propantheline. A study involving 8 healthy adult male patients found a greater 72-hour cumulative percentage urinary recovery of chlorothiazide (56.4%) when a single oral dose of chlorothiazide 500 mg solution was given 45 minutes after propantheline 30 mg. The 72-hour urine volume was not different between the 2 groups.[2]

[1] Beermann B, et al. *Eur J Clin Pharmacol.* 1978;13:385.

[2] Osman MA, et al. *Curr Ther Res.* 1983;34:404.

* Asterisk indicates drugs cited in interaction reports. Based on pharmacologic and pharmacokinetic considerations, similar interactions may occur with other drugs that are listed.

Thiazide Diuretics — *Cholestyramine*

Bendroflumethiazide (*Naturetin*)	Indapamide (*Lozol*)	Cholestyramine* (*Questran*)
Benzthiazide (eg, *Aquatag*)	Methyclothiazide (eg, *Enduron*)	
Chlorothiazide* (eg, *Diuril*)	Metolazone (*Diulo, Zaroxolyn*)	
Chlorthalidone (eg, *Hygroton*)	Polythiazide (*Renese*)	
Cyclothiazide (*Anhydron*)	Quinethazone (*Hydromox*)	
Hydrochlorothiazide* (eg, *HydroDiuril*)	Trichlormethiazide (eg, *Naqua*)	
Hydroflumethiazide (eg, *Saluron*)		

Significance	Onset	Severity	Documentation
3	☐ Rapid	☐ Major	☐ Established
	■ **Delayed**	☐ Moderate	■ **Probable**
		■ **Minor**	☐ Suspected
			☐ Possible
			☐ Unlikely

Effects Absorption of HYDROCHLOROTHIAZIDE is decreased by CHOLESTYRAMINE. A decrease in pharmacologic effect may be expected.

Mechanism As an anion-exchange resin, CHOLESTYRAMINE binds THIAZIDE DIURETICS.

Management CHOLESTYRAMINE should be taken at least 2 hours, and longer if possible, after a THIAZIDE DIURETIC. An increased dose of THIAZIDE may still be needed.

Discussion

Studies in animals[2] and humans[3-5] have illustrated a decreased absorption of thiazide diuretics by cholestyramine. Multiple doses of cholestyramine decreased hydrochlorothiazide absorption 85%.[3] Another multiple dose study showed a 35% decrease in absorption and 32% decrease in area under the curve.[4] Data indicate that cholestyramine given after hydrochlorothiazide has less influence on absorption than cholestyramine given before hydrochlorothiazide.[3-5] However, a 4-hour interval between hydrochlorothiazide and cholestyramine still decreased hydrochlorothiazide absorption 30% to 35%.[4]

[1] Kauffman RE, et al. *Clin Pharmacol Ther.* 1973;14:886.
[2] Phillips WA, et al. *J Pharm Sci.* 1976;65:1285.
[3] Hunninghake DB, et al. *Pharmacologist.* 1978;20:220.
[4] Hunninghake DB, et al. *Int J Clin Pharmacol Ther Toxicol.* 1982;20:151.
[5] Hunninghake DB, et al. *Clin Pharmacol Ther.* 1986;39:329.

* Asterisk indicates drugs cited in interaction reports. Based on pharmacologic and pharmacokinetic considerations, similar interactions may occur with other drugs that are listed.

Thiazide Diuretics — *Colestipol*

Bendroflumethiazide (*Naturetin*)
Benzthiazide (eg, *Aquatag*)
Chlorothiazide* (eg, *Diuril*)
Chlorthalidone (eg, *Hygroton*)
Cyclothiazide (*Anhydron*)
Hydrochlorothiazide* (eg, *HydroDiuril*)
Hydroflumethiazide (eg, *Saluron*)
Indapamide (*Lozol*)
Methyclothiazide (eg, *Enduron*)
Metolazone (*Diulo, Zaroxolyn*)
Polythiazide (*Renese*)
Quinethazone (*Hydromox*)
Trichlormethiazide (eg, *Naqua*)

Colestipol* (*Colestid*)

Significance	Onset	Severity	Documentation
3	☐ Rapid ■ **Delayed**	☐ Major ☐ Moderate ■ **Minor**	☐ Established ☐ Probable ■ **Suspected** ☐ Possible ☐ Unlikely

Effects The actions of oral THIAZIDE DIURETICS may be reduced when coadministered with COLESTIPOL.

Mechanism COLESTIPOL binds THIAZIDE DIURETICS in vitro. In vivo, this combination leads to decreased thiazide plasma levels and reduced cumulative urinary excretion of the diuretic.

Management Separate ingestion of COLESTIPOL from oral THIAZIDE DIURETICS as much as possible. Monitor patients closely because an increased diuretic dose may be necessary.

Discussion

Colestipol, an anion-exchange resin, can bind hydrochlorothiazide and chlorothiazide in vitro.[1,2] In vivo, this binding is believed to take place primarily in the small intestine.[1] In a study involving 10 hyperlipoproteinemic adult patients, 4 g colestipol was administered simultaneously and 1 hour after 1 g chlorothiazide.[1] A 24-hour urinary excretion of chlorothiazide was decreased 58% when the drug was ingested simultaneously with colestipol and 54% when the drugs were administered 1 hour apart.

In a separate study involving 6 healthy adults, 10 g colestipol was administered 2 minutes before 75 mg hydrochlorothiazide.[3] A 43% decrease in the total urinary excretion of hydrochlorothiazide was reported. Colestipol reduced hydrochlorothiazide serum levels beginning at 4 hours and continuing throughout the study. The mean peak hydrochlorothiazide plasma levels following colestipol were less than those seen with control; however, the difference was not significant. Similar results were reported by the same investigators in another study.[4]

[1] Kauffman RE, et al. *Clin Pharmacol Ther.* 1973;14:886.
[2] Phillips WA, et al. *J Pharm Sci.* 1976;65:1285.
[3] Hunninghake DB, et al. *Int J Clin Pharmacol Ther Toxicol.* 1982;20:151.
[4] Hunninghake DB, et al. *Pharmacologist.* 1978;20:220.

* Asterisk indicates drugs cited in interaction reports. Based on pharmacologic and pharmacokinetic considerations, similar interactions may occur with other drugs that are listed.

Thiazide-Type Diuretics — *NSAIDs*

Thiazide-Type Diuretics		NSAIDs	
Bendroflumethiazide*†	Indapamide	Diclofenac (eg, *Voltaren*)	Meclofenamic Acid (eg, *Ponstel*)
Chlorothiazide (eg, *Diuril*)	Methyclothiazide	Etodolac	Meloxicam (eg, *Mobic*)
Chlorthalidone* (eg, *Thalitone*)	Metolazone* (eg, *Zaroxolyn*)	Fenoprofen (eg, *Nalfon*)	Nabumetone
Hydrochlorothiazide* (eg, *Microzide*)		Flurbiprofen	Naproxen (eg, *Naprosyn*)
		Ibuprofen (eg, *Motrin*)	Oxaprozin (eg, *Daypro*)
		Indomethacin* (eg, *Indocin*)	Piroxicam (eg, *Feldene*)
		Ketoprofen	Sulindac* (eg, *Clinoril*)
		Ketorolac (eg, *Toradol*)	Tolmetin
		Meclofenamate	

Significance	Onset	Severity	Documentation
5	☐ Rapid	☐ Major	☐ Established
	■ **Delayed**	☐ Moderate	☐ Probable
		■ **Minor**	☐ Suspected
			■ **Possible**
			☐ Unlikely

Effects Decreased antihypertensive and, possibly, diuretic effects of THIAZIDE-TYPE DIURETICS may occur.

Mechanism Inhibition of renal prostaglandin synthesis by INDOMETHACIN and induction of sodium/water retention antagonizes the actions of THIAZIDE-TYPE DIURETICS.

Management Consider monitoring BP regularly. Adjust the diuretic dose accordingly.

Discussion

Indomethacin can elevate BP and decrease plasma renin in healthy and hypertensive subjects.[1,2] Indomethacin also induces transient sodium and water retention in subjects with normal[3,4] or reduced kidney function.[3] A 75% decrease in renin secretion occurred in patients treated with a thiazide diuretic and indomethacin.[2] Indomethacin seemed to blunt the antihypertensive effect, but little change in BP was noted in untreated patients. In a double-blind study, indomethacin increased BP in patients receiving thiazides.[5] Studies in healthy subjects indicate little effect of indomethacin on the diuretic action of thiazides.[6-8] However, indomethacin and, to a lesser extent, sulindac impaired the diuretic effect of a single metolazone dose in healthy volunteers.[9]

Conflicting data exist. Sulindac, which does not inhibit renal prostaglandins, also has been reported to enhance the diuretic effect of thiazides.[10-12] Naproxen (eg, *Naprosyn*) also has been implicated in enhancing the diuretic actions of thiazides.[11]

[1] Patak RV, et al. *Prostaglandins.* 1975;10(4):649.
[2] Lopez-Ovejero JA, et al. *Clin Sci Mol Med Suppl.* 1978;4:203s.
[3] Donker AJ, et al. *Nephron.* 1976;17(4):288.
[4] Brater DC. *Clin Pharmacol Ther.* 1979;25(3):322.
[5] Watkins J, et al. *Br Med J.* 1980;281(6242):702.
[6] Kramer HJ, et al. *Clin Sci.* 1980;59(1):67.
[7] Williams RL, et al. *J Clin Pharmacol.* 1982;22(1):32.
[8] Dusing R, et al. *Br J Clin Pharmacol.* 1983;16(4):377.
[9] Ripley EB, et al. *Int J Clin Pharmacol Ther.* 1994;32(1):12.
[10] Koopmans PP, et al. *Br Med J (Clin Red Ed).* 1984;289(6457):1492.
[11] Koopmans PP, et al. *Clin Pharmacol Ther.* 1985;37(6):625.
[12] Steiness E, et al. *Br Med J (Clin Res Ed).* 1982;285(6356):1702.

* Asterisk indicates drugs cited in interaction reports. Based on pharmacologic and pharmacokinetic considerations, similar interactions may occur with other drugs that are listed.
† Not available in the United States.

Thiazolidinediones		*Azole Antifungal Agents*	
Pioglitazone (*Actos*)	Rosiglitazone* (*Avandia*)	Fluconazole (eg, *Diflucan*) Itraconazole (eg, *Sporanox*)	Ketoconazole* (eg, *Nizoral*)

Significance	Onset	Severity	Documentation
4	☐ Rapid ■ **Delayed**	☐ Major ■ **Moderate** ☐ Minor	☐ Established ☐ Probable ☐ Suspected ■ **Possible** ☐ Unlikely

Effects Plasma concentrations of THIAZOLIDINEDIONE antidiabetic agents may be elevated, increasing the pharmacologic and adverse effects (eg, edema).

Mechanism Inhibition of THIAZOLIDINEDIONE metabolism (CYP2C8 and/or CYP2C9) by AZOLE ANTIFUNGAL AGENTS is suspected.

Management In patients receiving THIAZOLIDINEDIONE therapy, closely monitor blood glucose when starting or stopping an AZOLE ANTIFUNGAL AGENT and monitor patients for THIAZOLIDINEDIONE adverse effects (eg, edema) when starting the AZOLE ANTIFUNGAL AGENT.

Discussion

The effects of ketoconazole on the pharmacokinetics of rosiglitazone were investigated in 10 healthy men.[1] Using a randomized, open-label, 2-way crossover design, each subject received ketoconazole 200 mg twice daily or a matching placebo for 5 days. On day 5, a single oral dose of rosiglitazone 8 mg was administered. Compared with placebo administration, ketoconazole increased the rosiglitazone mean AUC 47%, prolonged the mean elimination $t_{½}$ 55% (from 3.55 to 5.5 hours), increased the C_{max} 17%, and decreased the apparent oral clearance of rosiglitazone 28%. The changes in oral clearance, $t_{½}$, and AUC occurred in all subjects receiving ketoconazole and rosiglitazone.

[1] Park JY, et al. *Br J Clin Pharmacol.* 2004;58(4):397.

* Asterisk indicates drugs cited in interaction reports. Based on pharmacologic and pharmacokinetic considerations, similar interactions may occur with other drugs that are listed.

Thiazolidinediones — *Gemfibrozil*

Thiazolidinediones		Gemfibrozil
Pioglitazone* (*Actos*)	Rosiglitazone* (*Avandia*)	Gemfibrozil* (eg, *Lopid*)

Significance	Onset	Severity	Documentation
2	☐ Rapid ■ **Delayed**	☐ Major ■ **Moderate** ☐ Minor	☐ Established ☐ Probable ■ **Suspected** ☐ Possible ☐ Unlikely

Effects Plasma concentrations of THIAZOLIDINEDIONE antidiabetic agents may be elevated, increasing hypoglycemic and other adverse effects (eg, peripheral and pulmonary edema) of these agents.

Mechanism Inhibition of THIAZOLIDINEDIONE metabolism (CYP2C8) by GEMFIBROZIL is suspected.

Management If coadministration of a THIAZOLIDINEDIONE and GEMFIBROZIL cannot be avoided, consider initiating therapy at a reduced THIAZOLIDINEDIONE dose, possibly as much as 50% to 70%. Closely monitor blood glucose, glycosolated hemoglobin, and THIAZOLIDINEDIONE adverse effects when starting or stopping GEMFIBROZIL therapy.

Discussion

The effects of gemfibrozil on the pharmacokinetics of rosiglitazone were investigated in a randomized, crossover study.[1] Ten healthy volunteers received oral gemfibrozil 600 mg or placebo twice daily for 4 days. On day 3, each subject took a single dose of rosiglitazone 4 mg. Compared with placebo, gemfibrozil administration increased the mean rosiglitazone AUC 2.3-fold, prolonged the elimination $t_{1/2}$ from 3.6 to 7.6 hours, and increased the plasma concentration of rosiglitazone measured 24 hours after dosing 9.8-fold. Gemfibrozil had a minor effect on rosiglitazone peak plasma levels (1.2-fold increase). In a study of 12 healthy volunteers, administration of gemfibrozil 600 mg twice daily for 4 days increased the pioglitazone AUC 3.2-fold and $t_{1/2}$ from 8.3 to 22.7 hours.[2] In a crossover study, 10 healthy men received gemfibrozil 600 mg twice daily for 1 week and, on day 3, they received gemfibrozil 600 mg followed 1 hour later by pioglitazone 30 mg.[3] Compared with placebo, gemfibrozil administration increased the pioglitazone AUC 3.4-fold. See also Repaglinide-Gemfibrozil and Sulfonylureas-Gemfibrozil.

[1] Niemi M, et al. *Diabetologia.* 2003;46:1319.
[2] Jaakkola T, et al. *Clin Pharmacol Ther.* 2005;77:404.
[3] Deng LJ, et al. *Eur J Clin Pharmacol.* 2005;61:831.

* Asterisk indicates drugs cited in interaction reports. Based on pharmacologic and pharmacokinetic considerations, similar interactions may occur with other drugs that are listed.

Thiazolidinediones — *Insulin*

Pioglitazone* (*Actos*)	Rosiglitazone* (*Avandia*)	Insulin*

Significance	Onset	Severity	Documentation
4	□ Rapid	□ Major	□ Established
	■ **Delayed**	■ **Moderate**	□ Probable
		□ Minor	□ Suspected
			■ **Possible**
			□ Unlikely

Effects Incidence of edema may be increased. Edema may occur after several months of combined therapy.

Mechanism Unknown. Possible additive or synergistic pharmacologic effects.

Management Monitor patients for development of edema during combined therapy with these agents.

Discussion

The incidence of edema in patients receiving either pioglitazone or rosiglitazone alone, or in combination with insulin was investigated using retrospective chart review.[1] Of 79 patients selected, 71 initially were receiving insulin alone, and 8 were taking rosiglitazone or pioglitazone. All patients later were changed to insulin plus rosiglitazone or pioglitazone. Seven patients developed edema while receiving insulin alone, compared with 18 who later received insulin plus a thiazolidinedione. One patient developed edema while receiving only a thiazolidinedione, compared with 2 patients who later received 1 of these agents plus insulin. The mean time to the onset of edema was 135 days of combination therapy. Of the 20 patients who developed edema on the combination, 14 were receiving insulin plus pioglitazone and 6 were taking insulin plus rosiglitazone. Other studies have reported a higher incidence of mild to moderate edema in patients receiving insulin plus a thiazolidinedione.[2,3] In 1 study, edema was reported in 12.6% of patients receiving insulin plus pioglitazone 15 mg and 17.6% of patients receiving insulin plus pioglitazone 30 mg, compared with 7% of patients receiving insulin plus placebo.[2] In another report, in patients receiving insulin plus rosiglitazone 4 mg or insulin plus rosiglitazone 8 mg, edema was reported in 13.1% and 16.2% of patients, respectively, compared with 4.7% of patients receiving insulin plus placebo.[3]

Because edema may occur with insulin or a thiazolidinedione alone, additional controlled studies are needed to determine the actual difference in the incidence of edema with combined therapy.

[1] King KA, et al. *Am J Health Syst Pharm.* 2004; 61:390.
[2] Rosenstock J, et al. *Int J Clin Pract.* 2002; 56:251.
[3] Raskin P, et al. *Diabetes Care.* 2001; 24:1226.

* Asterisk indicates drugs cited in interaction reports.

Thiazolidinediones — *Rifamycins*

Pioglitazone* (*Actos*)	Rosiglitazone* (*Avandia*)	Rifabutin (*Mycobutin*)	Rifapentine (*Priftin*)
		Rifampin* (eg, *Rifadin*)	

Significance	Onset	Severity	Documentation
2	☐ Rapid	☐ Major	☐ Established
	■ **Delayed**	■ **Moderate**	☐ Probable
		☐ Minor	■ **Suspected**
			☐ Possible
			☐ Unlikely

Effects RIFAMYCINS may reduce plasma concentrations and t½ while increasing the clearance of THIAZOLIDINEDIONES, possibly resulting in decreased glycemic control.

Mechanism Hepatic metabolism of THIAZOLIDINEDIONES (CYP2C8) may be increased by RIFAMYCINS.

Management In patients receiving THIAZOLIDINEDIONES, closely monitor blood glucose and glycosylated hemoglobin when starting or stopping RIFAMYCIN therapy.

Discussion

The effects of rifampin on the pharmacokinetics of rosiglitazone were studied in 10 healthy men.[1] Using an open-label, randomized, 2-way crossover design, each subject received rifampin 600 mg daily for 6 days or placebo. On day 7, a single oral dose of rosiglitazone 8 mg was administered. Compared with placebo, rifampin administration decreased the rosiglitazone AUC 65%, the C_{max} 31%, and the mean elimination t½ from 3.9 to 1.5 hours. In addition, rifampin increased the apparent oral clearance of rosiglitazone 3-fold. Ten healthy volunteers received rifampin 600 mg daily for 6 days.[2] On day 6, each subject received a single dose of pioglitazone 30 mg. Rifampin reduced the pioglitazone AUC 54%, and the t½ from 4.9 to 2.3 hours. See also Repaglinide-Rifamycins and Sulfonylureas-Rifamycins.

[1] Park JY, et al. *Clin Pharmacol Ther.* 2004;75(3):157.
[2] Jaakkola T, et al. *Br J Clin Pharmacol.* 2006;61(1):70.

* Asterisk indicates drugs cited in interaction reports. Based on pharmacologic and pharmacokinetic considerations, similar interactions may occur with other drugs that are listed.

Thiazolidinediones / *Serotonin Reuptake Inhibitors*

Thiazolidinediones		Serotonin Reuptake Inhibitors
Pioglitazone (*Actos*)	Rosiglitazone* (*Avandia*)	Fluvoxamine*

Significance	Onset	Severity	Documentation
4	☐ Rapid ■ **Delayed**	☐ Major ■ **Moderate** ☐ Minor	☐ Established ☐ Probable ☐ Suspected ■ **Possible** ☐ Unlikely

Effects Plasma concentrations of THIAZOLIDINEDIONE antidiabetic agents may be elevated, increasing hypoglycemic and other adverse reactions.

Mechanism Inhibition of THIAZOLIDINEDIONE metabolism (CYP2C8) by FLUVOXAMINE is suspected.

Management Closely monitor blood glucose and for THIAZOLIDINEDIONE adverse reactions when starting FLUVOXAMINE. The effect of FLUVOXAMINE on blood glucose may reverse when FLUVOXAMINE is discontinued.

Discussion

In an open-label, crossover study, the effects of fluvoxamine on the pharmacokinetics of rosiglitazone were evaluated in 21 healthy subjects.[1] In the first phase, each subject was given a single dose of rosiglitazone 4 mg alone. In the second phase, each patient was given fluvoxamine 50 mg twice daily for 3 days and then fluvoxamine 50 mg plus rosiglitazone 4 mg on the fourth day. Compared with administration of rosiglitazone alone, pretreatment with fluvoxamine moderately increased the rosiglitazone AUC (range, 12% to 25%) in 17 of the 21 subjects studied. In addition, fluvoxamine prolonged the $t_{1/2}$ of rosiglitazone from approximately 6 to 8 hours.

[1] Pedersen RS, et al. *Br J Clin Pharmacol.* 2006;62(6):682.

* Asterisk indicates drugs cited in interaction reports. Based on pharmacologic and pharmacokinetic considerations, similar interactions may occur with other drugs that are listed.

Thiazolidinediones — *Trimethoprim*

Pioglitazone* (*Actos*)	Rosiglitazone* (*Avandia*)	Trimethoprim* (eg, *Proloprim*)	Trimethoprim/ Sulfamethoxazole (eg, *Bactrim*)

Significance	Onset	Severity	Documentation
4	□ Rapid	□ Major	□ Established
	■ **Delayed**	■ **Moderate**	□ Probable
		□ Minor	□ Suspected
			■ **Possible**
			□ Unlikely

Effects Plasma concentrations of THIAZOLIDINEDIONE antidiabetic agents may be elevated, increasing the hypoglycemic effects and other adverse reactions.

Mechanism Inhibition of THIAZOLIDINEDIONE metabolism (CYP2C8) by TRIMETHOPRIM may occur.

Management Closely monitor blood glucose and for THIAZOLIDINEDIONE adverse reactions when starting TRIMETHOPRIM. The effect of TRIMETHOPRIM on blood glucose levels may reverse when TRIMETHOPRIM is discontinued.

Discussion

The effects of trimethoprim on the pharmacokinetics of rosiglitazone were studied in a randomized, crossover investigation.[1] Ten healthy volunteers received oral trimethoprim 160 mg or placebo twice daily for 4 days. On day 3, a single dose of rosiglitazone 4 mg was taken. Compared with placebo, trimethoprim administration increased the rosiglitazone AUC 37%, the C_{max} 14%, and prolonged the elimination $t_{½}$ from 3.8 to 4.8 hours. The formation of the rosiglitazone metabolite *N*-desmethylrosiglitazone was decreased. The effects of trimethoprim on the pharmacokinetics of pioglitazone were studied in 16 healthy volunteers.[2] Trimethoprim twice daily for 16 days increased the pioglitazone AUC 42% and prolonged the $t_{½}$ from 3.9 to 5.1 hours compared with placebo.

[1] Niemi M, et al. *Clin Pharmacol Ther.* 2004;76(3):239. [2] Tornio A, et al. *Drug Metab Dispos.* 2008;36(1):73.

* Asterisk indicates drugs cited in interaction reports. Based on pharmacologic and pharmacokinetic considerations, similar interactions may occur with other drugs that are listed.

Thiopurines — *Febuxostat*

Azathioprine (eg, *Imuran*)	Mercaptopurine* (eg, *Purinethol*)	Febuxostat* (*Uloric*)

Significance	Onset	Severity	Documentation
1	☐ Rapid ■ **Delayed**	■ **Major** ☐ Moderate ☐ Minor	☐ Established ☐ Probable ■ **Suspected** ☐ Possible ☐ Unlikely

Effects Plasma concentrations of THIOPURINES may be elevated, increasing the risk of toxicity.

Mechanism FEBUXOSTAT may inhibit hepatic metabolism of THIOPURINES by xanthine oxidase.

Management Coadministration of FEBUXOSTAT and THIOPURINES is contraindicated.

Discussion

Although not studied, azathioprine and mercaptopurine are metabolized by xanthine oxidase. Because febuxostat inhibits xanthine oxidase, increased plasma concentrations of azathioprine and mercaptopurine may occur, resulting in azathioprine or mercaptopurine toxicity. Coadministration of febuxostat and azathioprine or mercaptopurine is contraindicated.[1]

The basis for this monograph is information on file with the manufacturer. Studies are needed to further assess this interaction. However, because of the seriousness of this interaction, clinical evaluation in humans is not likely to be forthcoming.

[1] *Uloric* [package insert]. Deerfield, IL: Takeda Pharmaceuticals America Inc; February 2009.

* Asterisk indicates drugs cited in interaction reports. Based on pharmacologic and pharmacokinetic considerations, similar interactions may occur with other drugs that are listed.

Thiopurines			***Mesalamine***
Azathioprine* (eg, *Imuran*)	Mercaptopurine* (eg, *Purinethol*)	Mesalamine* (eg, *Pentasa*)	

Significance	Onset	Severity	Documentation
4	☐ Rapid ■ **Delayed**	☐ Major ■ **Moderate** ☐ Minor	☐ Established ☐ Probable ☐ Suspected ■ **Possible** ☐ Unlikely

Effects The risk of leukopenia may be increased.

Mechanism Inhibition of the thiopurine-metabolizing enzyme, thiopurine methyltransferase, by MESALAMINE is suspected.

Management In patients receiving THIOPURINES, closely monitor leukocyte counts when starting or stopping MESALAMINE. Be prepared to adjust therapy as needed.

Discussion

In Crohn disease patients receiving azathioprine or mercaptopurine, administration of mesalamine produced a high rate of leukopenia and an increase in whole blood 6-thioguanine nucleotide concentrations.[1] In a nonrandomized, parallel group study, patients being treated with stable doses of azathioprine or mercaptopurine for at least 16 weeks were given mesalamine 4 g/day. Leukopenia was defined separately during the study as a total leukocyte count of less than 3×10^9/L and less than or equal to 3.5×10^9/L at any time. A total leukocyte count of less than 3×10^9/L occurred in 1 of the 10 patients while receiving mesalamine. A total leukocyte count of less than or equal to 3.5×10^9/L occurred in 5 of the 10 patients while they were receiving mesalamine. Compared with baseline values, there were increases in the mean whole blood 6-thioguanine nucleotide concentrations at most of the timepoints during coadministration of mesalamine and azathioprine or mercaptopurine. Conversely, in a patient being treated with azathioprine and mesalamine, interruption of mesalamine therapy resulted in a relapse of the disease and a decrease in the active metabolite of azathioprine.[2]

[1] Lowry PW, et al. *Gut.* 2001;49(5):656.

[2] Stocco G, et al. *Dig Dis Sci.* 2008;53(12):3246.

* Asterisk indicates drugs cited in interaction reports.

Thiopurines — *Methotrexate*

Thiopurines		Methotrexate
Azathioprine (eg, *Imuran*)	Mercaptopurine* (eg, *Purinethol*)	Methotrexate* (eg, *Rheumatrex*)

Significance	Onset	Severity	Documentation
4	☐ Rapid	☐ Major	☐ Established
	■ **Delayed**	■ **Moderate**	☐ Probable
		☐ Minor	☐ Suspected
			■ **Possible**
			☐ Unlikely

Effects The actions of THIOPURINES may be enhanced.

Mechanism METHOTREXATE inhibits the first-pass metabolism of the THIOPURINES by inhibiting xanthine oxidase. The bioavailability of THIOPURINES may be enhanced when given concurrently with METHOTREXATE.

Management Increased THIOPURINE plasma levels may not be clinically important with standard low oral doses of METHOTREXATE. Reduced THIOPURINE dosage may be used during coadministration of METHOTREXATE.

Discussion

A thiopurine and methotrexate may be intentionally administered together to obtain added benefit in the treatment of acute lymphoblastic leukemia (ALL). Fourteen children with average-risk ALL were studied after an oral dose of mercaptopurine 75 mg/m^2 alone or with oral methotrexate 20 mg/m^2.[1] During coadministration, a 26% increase in peak mercaptopurine plasma levels was reported with a 31% increase in the AUC.[1] When dosed alone, mercaptopurine produced greater intrapatient variability in some pharmacokinetic parameters than when dosed with methotrexate.[1] In 10 children with ALL in remission, coadministration of mercaptopurine 25 mg/m^2/day with methotrexate 2 or 5 g/m^2 every other week increased mercaptopurine peak levels 108% to 121% and AUC 69% to 93%.[2] This interaction may be of greater magnitude in individuals with thiopurine-methyltransferase deficiency caused by genetic polymorphism.[3] Two such children developed severe pancytopenia during treatment for ALL with standard doses of mercaptopurine and methotrexate.

Additional studies are needed to determine the clinical importance of these findings.

[1] Balis FM, et al. *Clin Pharmacol Ther.* 1987;41(4):384.
[2] Innocenti F, et al. *Cancer Chemother Pharmacol.* 1996;37(5):409.
[3] Andersen JB, et al. *Acta Paediatr.* 1998;87(1):108.

* Asterisk indicates drugs cited in interaction reports. Based on pharmacologic and pharmacokinetic considerations, similar interactions may occur with other drugs that are listed.

Thiopurines — *Olsalazine*

Azathioprine (eg, *Imuran*) | Mercaptopurine* (eg, *Purinethol*) | Olsalazine* (*Dipentum*)

Significance	Onset	Severity	Documentation
4	□ Rapid ■ **Delayed**	■ **Major** □ Moderate □ Minor	□ Established □ Probable □ Suspected ■ **Possible** □ Unlikely

Effects The pharmacologic and toxic effects of THIOPURINES may be increased.

Mechanism Possible accumulation of THIOPURINES caused by inhibition of THIOPURINE methyltransferase activity in red blood cells.

Management Closely monitor hematologic function and adjust therapy as needed.

Discussion

Two episodes of reversible bone marrow suppression were reported in a 16-year-old girl with Crohn disease during coadministration of 6-mercaptopurine, olsalazine, and corticosteroids.[1] On initial presentation, the patient had normal bone marrow function. She first experienced leukopenia while receiving oral 6-mercaptopurine 75 mg/day, oral olsalazine 1,000 mg/day, prednisone (eg, *Sterapred*), fluoxetine (eg, *Prozac*), codeine, and diphenhydramine (eg, *Benadryl*). The dosage of 6-mercaptopurine was reduced to 25 mg/day while she continued to receive olsalazine 1,000 mg/day. The granular leukocyte count gradually recovered. Approximately 4 months later, a second, more severe episode of bone marrow suppression (leukopenia and anemia) occurred while the patient was receiving 6-mercaptopurine 50 mg/day and olsalazine 1,750 mg/day. Hematologic function recovered after stopping mercaptopurine and olsalazine.

Because monotherapy with 6-mercaptopurine or olsalazine may cause hematologic toxicity, additional documentation is needed to assess this possible drug interaction.

[1] Lewis LD, et al. *Clin Pharmacol Ther.* 1997;62(4):464.

* Asterisk indicates drugs cited in interaction reports. Based on pharmacologic and pharmacokinetic considerations, similar interactions may occur with other drugs that are listed.

Thiopurines — *Ribavirin*

Azathioprine* (eg, *Imuran*)	Mercaptopurine (eg, *Purinethol*)	Ribavirin* (eg, *Rebetol*)

Significance	Onset	Severity	Documentation
4	□ Rapid ■ **Delayed**	■ **Major** □ Moderate □ Minor	□ Established □ Probable □ Suspected ■ **Possible** □ Unlikely

Effects Risk of THIOPURINE-related myelosuppression (eg, pancytopenia) may be increased.

Mechanism RIBAVIRIN may block the enzyme inosine monophosphate dehydrogenase, which may increase concentrations of THIOPURINE methylated metabolites. Myelotoxicity appears to be associated with the elevated total methyl metabolite concentrations.

Management If coadministration of these agents cannot be avoided, closely monitor for myelotoxicity. Be prepared to discontinue one or both agents.

Discussion

The medical records of 8 patients, who developed severe pancytopenia after coadministration of azathioprine 2 mg/kg daily and ribavirin 1 to 1.2 g daily, were retrospectively reviewed.[1] Seven of the patients were receiving long-term treatment with azathioprine (11 months to 7 years) when ribavirin plus peginterferon were added to their treatment. Pancytopenia occurred 3 to 7 weeks after ribavirin was started. One patient was receiving ribavirin plus peginterferon for 8 weeks when azathioprine was started. Pancytopenia occurred 3 weeks after starting azathioprine. Azathioprine and ribavirin were stopped. After blood counts returned to normal, no hematologic toxicity occurred subsequent to restarting ribavirin plus peginterferon or azathioprine alone.

[1] Peyrin-Biroulet L, et al. *Aliment Pharmacol Ther.* 2008;28(8):984.

* Asterisk indicates drugs cited in interaction reports. Based on pharmacologic and pharmacokinetic considerations, similar interactions may occur with other drugs that are listed.

Thiopurines — *Sulfonamides*

Azathioprine* (eg, *Imuran*)	Mercaptopurine* (eg, *Purinethol*)	Sulfasalazine* (eg, *Azulfidine*)

Significance	Onset	Severity	Documentation
4	□ Rapid	□ Major	□ Established
	■ **Delayed**	■ **Moderate**	□ Probable
		□ Minor	□ Suspected
			■ **Possible**
			□ Unlikely

Effects The risk of leukopenia may be increased.

Mechanism Inhibition of the THIOPURINE-metabolizing enzyme, THIOPURINE methyltransferase, by SULFASALAZINE is suspected.

Management In patients receiving THIOPURINES, closely monitor leukocyte counts when SULFASALAZINE is started or stopped. Be prepared to adjust therapy as needed.

Discussion

In patients with Crohn disease receiving azathioprine or mercaptopurine, administration of sulfasalazine produced a high rate of leukopenia and an increase in whole blood 6-thioguanine nucleotide concentrations.[1] In a nonrandomized, parallel group study, patients being treated with stable doses of azathioprine or mercaptopurine for at least 16 weeks were given sulfasalazine 4 g/day. Leukopenia was defined separately during the study as a total leukocyte count of less than 3×10^9/L and less than or equal to 3.5×10^9/L at any time. A total leukocyte count of less than 3×10^9/L occurred in 1 of the 11 patients receiving sulfasalazine. A total leukocyte count of less than or equal to 3.5×10^9/L occurred in 6 of the 11 patients receiving sulfasalazine. Compared with baseline values, there were increases in the mean whole blood 6-thioguanine nucleotide concentrations at most of the time points during coadministration of sulfasalazine and azathioprine or mercaptopurine.

[1] Lowry PW, et al. *Gut*. 2001;49(5):656.

* Asterisk indicates drugs cited in interaction reports.

Thiopurines | **Xanthine Oxidase Inhibitors**

Azathioprine* (eg, *Imuran*)	Mercaptopurine* (eg, *Purinethol*)	Allopurinol* (eg, *Zyloprim*)	Febuxostat* (*Uloric*)

Significance	Onset	Severity	Documentation
1	☐ Rapid ■ **Delayed**	■ **Major** ☐ Moderate ☐ Minor	■ **Established** ☐ Probable ☐ Suspected ☐ Possible ☐ Unlikely

Effects

Increases in pharmacologic and toxic effects of orally administered THIOPURINES have occurred with coadministration of ALLOPURINOL.

Mechanism

Inhibition of xanthine oxidase by ALLOPURINOL reduces the rate at which MERCAPTOPURINE is converted to inactive 6-thiouric acid.[1] ALLOPURINOL inhibits the first-pass metabolism of oral MERCAPTOPURINE.

Management

Reduced dosages of THIOPURINES are necessary when ALLOPURINOL is administered. It is suggested that the initial THIOPURINE doses be reduced to 25% or 33% of the recommended initial dose during coadministration and that hematologic function be closely monitored. Coadministration of FEBUXOSTAT and AZATHIOPRINE or MERCAPTOPURINE is contraindicated.

Discussion

Azathioprine is converted to mercaptopurine, which is metabolized by xanthine oxidase to 6-thiouric acid. By inhibiting this enzyme, allopurinol increases the toxicity of the thiopurines. The interaction was first noted when coadministration of thiopurine and allopurinol necessitated a 25% decrease from the initial thiopurine dose.[2] Other reports have verified the importance of this interaction.[1,3-14] IV administration of 6-mercaptopurine was not affected by concomitant allopurinol therapy in 11 patients.[15] A comparative trial of oral and IV mercaptopurine showed that allopurinol pretreatment affected only the orally administered drug.[16] Another report described a similar lack of effect of allopurinol on IV mercaptopurine.[17] Febuxostat is contraindicated in patients receiving drugs metabolized by xanthine oxidase (eg, azathioprine, mercaptopurine).[18]

Thioguanine is not metabolized by xanthine oxidase and, therefore, would not be expected to interact with allopurinol.[15]

1 Elion GB, et al. *Biochem Pharmacol.* 1963;12(1):85.
2 Rundles RW, et al. *Trans Assoc Am Physicians.* 1963;76:126.
3 Elion GB, et al. *Cancer Res.* 1963;23:1207.
4 Levine AS, et al. *Cancer Chemother Rep.* 1969;53(1):53.
5 Nies AS, et al. *Am J Med.* 1971;51(6):812.
6 Berns A, et al. *N Engl J Med.* 1972;286(13):730.
7 Zazgornik J, et al. *Int J Clin Pharmacol Ther Toxicol.* 1981;19(3):96.
8 Brooks RJ, et al. *Biomed Pharmacother.* 1982;36(4):217.
9 Krowka MJ, et al. *Chest.* 1983;83(4):696.
10 Cox GJ, et al. *Arch Dermatol.* 1986;122(12):1413.
11 Boyd IW. *J Intern Med.* 1991;229(4):386.
12 Garcia-Ortiz RE, et al. *J Pharm Technol.* 1991;7:224.
13 Kennedy DT, et al. *Ann Pharmacother.* 1996;30(9):951.
14 Cummins D, et al. *Transplantation.* 1996;61(11):1661.
15 Coffey JJ, et al. *Cancer Res.* 1972;32(6):1283.
16 Zimm S, et al. *Clin Pharmacol Ther.* 1983;34(6):810.
17 Zimm S, et al. *Cancer Res.* 1985;45(4):1869.
18 *Uloric* [package insert]. Deerfield, IL: Takeda Pharmaceuticals America Inc; February 2009.

* Asterisk indicates drugs cited in interaction reports.

Thiotepa — *Carbamazepine*

Thiotepa* (eg, *Thioplex*)	Carbamazepine* (eg, *Tegretol*)

Significance	Onset	Severity	Documentation
4	■ **Rapid** □ Delayed	□ Major ■ **Moderate** □ Minor	□ Established □ Probable □ Suspected ■ **Possible** □ Unlikely

Effects Exposure to the active metabolite of THIOTEPA, tepa, may be increased, increasing the risk of toxicity.

Mechanism CARBAMAZEPINE may increase the metabolism (CYP3A4) of THIOTEPA.

Management Consider reducing the initial dose of THIOTEPA and monitoring the concentrations of the tepa metabolite as a guide to THIOTEPA dosing. Gabapentin (eg, *Neurontin*) or valproic acid derivatives (eg, *Depakote*) may be safer alternative anticonvulsant agents.

Discussion

A 52-year-old woman with metastatic breast cancer received a chemotherapy regimen that included thiotepa with and without coadministration of carbamazepine.[1] Each chemotherapy cycle lasted 4 days. On the first day of the cycles in which thiotepa was given with carbamazepine, exposure to the active metabolite of thiotepa, tepa, was increased 75%, while exposure to thiotepa was reduced 43%, compared with not administering carbamazepine. The effect of carbamazepine diminished over the 4-day course of treatment, being most pronounced during the first day of the cycle. Therefore, the clinical importance of this interaction appears to be of greatest consequences with single-dose administration of thiotepa.

[1] Ekhart C, et al. *Cancer Chemother Pharmacol.* 2009;63(3):543.

* Asterisk indicates drugs cited in interaction reports.

Thiotepa — *Hydantoins*

Thiotepa* (eg, *Thioplex*)	Phenytoin* (eg, *Dilantin*)

Significance	Onset	Severity	Documentation
4	☐ Rapid	☐ Major	☐ Established
	■ **Delayed**	■ **Moderate**	☐ Probable
		☐ Minor	☐ Suspected
			■ **Possible**
			☐ Unlikely

Effects Exposure to the active THIOTEPA metabolite may be increased, which increases the risk of toxicity.

Mechanism Induction of THIOTEPA metabolism (CYP2B6 and CYP3A4) by PHENYTOIN is suspected.

Management If PHENYTOIN administration cannot be avoided, consider reducing the initial dose of THIOTEPA and monitoring the concentration of the tepa metabolite as a guide to THIOTEPA dosing. Valproic acid derivatives (eg, *Depakote*) or gabapentin (eg, *Neurontin*) may be safer anticonvulsant agents.

Discussion

The effect of phenytoin on the metabolism of thiotepa was assessed during high-dose chemotherapy with cyclophosphamide, thiotepa 120 mg/m^2 daily, and carboplatin in a 42-year-old man with relapsing germ-cell cancer.[1] Five days prior to the second course of chemotherapy, the patient received phenytoin for generalized epileptic seizures that developed 3 weeks after the first course of chemotherapy. Blood samples were analyzed for thiotepa and the main active metabolite, tepa. Compared with the first course of chemotherapy, the AUC of tepa during the second course of chemotherapy was increased 115%. The AUC of thiotepa was reduced 29%. Because increased exposure to the active metabolite correlates with higher toxicity, the dose of thiotepa was reduced on day 3 of the second course of chemotherapy.

[1] de Jonge ME, et al. *Cancer Chemother Pharmacol.* 2005;55(5):507.

* Asterisk indicates drugs cited in interaction reports.

Thiothixene — *Lithium*

Thiothixene*
(eg, *Navane*)

Lithium*
(eg, *Lithobid*)

Significance	Onset	Severity	Documentation
4	☐ Rapid	☐ Major	☐ Established
	■ **Delayed**	■ **Moderate**	☐ Probable
		☐ Minor	☐ Suspected
			■ **Possible**
			☐ Unlikely

Effects The risk of neurotoxicity, including extrapyramidal symptoms, may be increased.

Mechanism Unknown.

Management Closely monitor patients for neurotoxicity. If an interaction is suspected, consider reducing the dose of one or both agents or discontinuing one of the drugs.

Discussion

In a survey of reports, 39 patients developed neurotoxicity while receiving lithium and a neuroleptic agent.[1] The most frequent symptoms were psychopathological (81.5%) and consisted of confusion, disorientation, and unconsciousness. Extrapyramidal symptoms occurred in approximately 74% of the patients. The majority of patients (91%) had serum lithium levels within the therapeutic range. One patient was receiving lithium and thiothixene. A single-blind study of 10 patients receiving neuroleptic agents assessed whether lithium exacerbates neuroleptic-induced extrapyramidal symptoms.[2] Six patients were receiving thiothixene. Nine additional patients were treated with neuroleptic agents alone in order to keep the evaluators blind regarding the treatment modalities. Patients receiving a neuroleptic agent plus lithium experienced an increase in extrapyramidal symptom scores, while those receiving only a neuroleptic agent did not show a change in extrapyramidal symptom scores. Lithium levels were within the nontoxic range.[1]

[1] Prakash R, et al. *Compr Psychiatry*. 1982;23(6):567. [2] Addonizio G, et al. *J Nerv Ment Dis*. 1988;176(11):682.

* Asterisk indicates drugs cited in interaction reports.

Thyroid Hormones — *Antacids*

Levothyroxine*
(eg, *Synthroid*)

Aluminum Hydroxide*
(eg, *Amphojel*)
Aluminum/Magnesium Hydroxide*
(eg, *Riopan*)
Calcium Carbonate*
(eg, *Tums*)
Magnesium Oxide*
(eg, *Maox*)

Significance	Onset	Severity	Documentation
2	☐ Rapid ■ **Delayed**	☐ Major ■ **Moderate** ☐ Minor	☐ Established ☐ Probable ■ **Suspected** ☐ Possible ☐ Unlikely

Effects Possible decreased effect of LEVOTHYROXINE. Increased serum thyroid-stimulating hormone.

Mechanism Decreased LEVOTHYROXINE bioavailability because of suspected interference with absorption.

Management Consider monitoring serum TSH levels in patients receiving oral LEVOTHYROXINE replacement if therapy with an ANTACID is started. Separating the administration times by 4 hours may minimize this interaction.[1]

Discussion

Elevated serum thyrotropin levels developed in a 60-year-old man after the addition of an aluminum hydroxide–containing antacid to his long-term maintenance treatment with levothyroxine.[2] The patient was euthyroid for approximately 5 years while taking a daily maintenance dose of levothyroxine sodium 0.15 mg. He then became a subject in a clinical trial and was administered an antacid containing aluminum hydroxide, simethicone, and co-dried aluminum-magnesium hydroxide 4 times/day for 4 months. At the conclusion of the study, the patient's serum thyrotropin level was 36 milliunits/L, with a serum T_4 level of 103 nmol/L. Two weeks after the antacid trial had been completed, his thyrotropin level decreased to 1.1 milliunits/L, and his serum T_4 level increased to 121 nmol/L. The patient was rechallenged with 2 antacid tablets 3 times/day (at least 3 hours after taking the levothyroxine) for 2 weeks, and the thyrotropin level increased to 4.63 milliunits/L. Following discontinuation of the antacid, the thyrotropin level decreased to 1 milliunit/L. Similar results occurred after another rechallenge. Throughout the study, the patient was asymptomatic. Increased TSH, suggesting decreased levothyroxine effect, also has been reported with an aluminum-magnesium antacid, a magnesium oxide laxative formulation,[3] and calcium carbonate[1,4,5] (used for calcium supplementation). In 20 patients on stable levothyroxine regimens, administration of calcium carbonate (elemental calcium 1,200 mg) daily for 3 months decreased T_3 and T_4 levels and increased thyrotropin levels (from 1.6 to 2.7 milliunits/L).[6] No patient exhibited symptoms of hypothyroidism.

1 Csako G, et al. *Ann Pharmacother.* 2001;35(12):1578.
2 Sperber AD, et al. *Arch Intern Med.* 1992;152(1):183.
3 Mersebach H, et al. *Pharmacol Toxicol.* 1999;84(3):107.
4 Schneyer CR. *JAMA.* 1998;279(10):750.
5 Mazokopakis EE, et al. *Can Fam Physician.* 2008;54(1):39.
6 Singh N, et al. *JAMA.* 2000;283(21):2822.

* Asterisk indicates drugs cited in interaction reports.

Thyroid Hormones		*Cholestyramine*
Levothyroxine* (eg, *Synthroid*)	Liotrix (*Thyrolar*)	Cholestyramine* (eg, *Questran*)
Liothyronine (eg, *Cytomel*)	Thyroid	

Significance	Onset	Severity	Documentation
2	☐ Rapid ■ **Delayed**	☐ Major ■ **Moderate** ☐ Minor	☐ Established ☐ Probable ■ **Suspected** ☐ Possible ☐ Unlikely

Effects Possible loss of efficacy of exogenously administered THYROID HORMONE and potential hypothyroidism.

Mechanism Probable binding of THYROID hormone in the GI tract by CHOLESTYRAMINE, preventing absorption.

Management If CHOLESTYRAMINE must be used in patients taking THYROID hormones, separate the administration by 6 hours.

Discussion

In hamsters, cholestyramine prevented the effect of exogenous thyroxine on the thyroid gland.[1] Studies with radioactive thyroxine indicated the hormone remains within the GI tract when given with cholestyramine,[1,2] and in vitro studies demonstrated that small amounts of cholestyramine tightly bind thyroxine.[2] If the 2 drugs were administered 4 to 5 hours apart, 70% of the absorption was restored. A case has been reported in which the patient's hypothyroidism returned when she was started on cholestyramine despite continued thyroid replacement therapy.[2] In another case, hypothyroidism returned when cholestyramine and levothyroxine were given concurrently.[3] The patient became euthyroid on the same dose of levothyroxine when cholestyramine was discontinued.

[1] Bergman F, et al. *Acta Endocrinol (Copenh).* 1966;53(2):256.

[2] Northcutt RC, et al. *JAMA.* 1969;208(10):1857.

[3] Harmon SM, et al. *Ann Intern Med.* 1991;115(8):658.

* Asterisk indicates drugs cited in interaction reports. Based on pharmacologic and pharmacokinetic considerations, similar interactions may occur with other drugs that are listed.

Thyroid Hormones — *Coffee*

Levothyroxine* (eg, *Synthroid*)	Liotrix (*Thyrolar*)	Coffee*
Liothyronine (eg, *Cytomel*)	Thyroid	

Significance	Onset	Severity	Documentation
4	☐ Rapid	☐ Major	☐ Established
	■ **Delayed**	■ **Moderate**	☐ Probable
		☐ Minor	☐ Suspected
			■ **Possible**
			☐ Unlikely

Effects The absorption of the THYROID HORMONE may be decreased by concurrently drinking COFFEE.

Mechanism Unknown.

Management THYROID HORMONES should be taken consistently with water, with COFFEE, or at least 1 hour before drinking COFFEE.

Discussion

The effect of drinking coffee/espresso on the intestinal absorption of levothyroxine was studied in 8 patients and 9 healthy volunteers.[1] Levothyroxine 200 mcg was administered with coffee, water, or water followed 60 minutes later by coffee. Compared with water, concurrent ingestion of levothyroxine and coffee decreased the intestinal absorption of levothyroxine. Coffee lowered the levothyroxine AUC 36% compared with 27% with water. However, when levothyroxine was administered 1 hour before drinking coffee, levothyroxine absorption was not affected.

The ingredient in coffee interfering with levothyroxine absorption was not identified.

[1] Benvenga S, et al. *Thyroid*. 2008;18(3):293.

* Asterisk indicates drugs cited in interaction reports. Based on pharmacologic and pharmacokinetic considerations, similar interactions may occur with other drugs that are listed.

Thyroid Hormones — *Colesevelam*

Thyroid Hormones		Colesevelam
Levothyroxine* (eg, *Synthroid*)	Liotrix (*Thyrolar*)	Colesevelam* (*Welchol*)
Liothyronine (eg, *Cytomel*)		

Significance	Onset	Severity	Documentation
2	☐ Rapid	☐ Major	☐ Established
	■ **Delayed**	■ **Moderate**	☐ Probable
		☐ Minor	■ **Suspected**
			☐ Possible
			☐ Unlikely

Effects THYROID HORMONE plasma concentrations may be decreased, reducing efficacy.

Mechanism THYROID HORMONES may bind to COLESEVELAM in the GI tract, decreasing absorption.

Management Administer the THYROID HORMONE at least 4 hours prior to COLESEVELAM.[1] Monitor TSH levels and be prepared to adjust the THYROID HORMONE dose as needed.

Discussion

The effects of colesevelam on the pharmacokinetics of levothyroxine were studied in 6 healthy, euthyroid volunteers.[2] Each subject received levothyroxine 1 mg alone with 240 mL of water and concurrently with colesevelam 3.75 g and 240 mL of water. Serum thyroxine (T_4) levels increased following administration of levothyroxine alone; however, the increase in T_4 was blunted by coadministration of colesevelam. The reduction in levothyroxine absorption may have been as much as 96%. None of the subjects experienced symptoms of thyrotoxicosis. In another study, healthy subjects were administered levothyroxine 0.6 mg alone, simultaneously with colesevelam 3,750 mg, and 1 and 4 hours before colesevelam.[3] Simultaneous administration of levothyroxine and colesevelam decreased the levothyroxine AUC and C_{max}. When levothyroxine was given 4 hours before colesevelam, no interaction was observed. The manufacturer of colesevelam recommends administering levothyroxine at least 4 hours prior to colesevelam.[1]

[1] *Welchol* [package insert]. Parsippany, NJ: Daiichi Sankyo Inc; January 2008.

[2] Weitzman SP, et al. *Thyroid.* 2009;19(1):77.

[3] Brown KS, et al. *J Clin Pharmacol.* 2010;50(5):554.

* Asterisk indicates drugs cited in interaction reports. Based on pharmacologic and pharmacokinetic considerations, similar interactions may occur with other drugs that are listed.

Thyroid Hormones		*Estrogens*	
Levothyroxine (eg, *Synthroid*) Liotrix (*Thyrolar*)	Thyroid	Conjugated Estrogens* (*Premarin*) Esterified Estrogens (*Menest*) Estradiol (eg, *Estrace*)	Estropipate (eg, *Ogen*) Ethinyl Estradiol Mestranol†

Significance	Onset	Severity	Documentation
2	☐ Rapid ■ **Delayed**	☐ Major ■ **Moderate** ☐ Minor	☐ Established ■ **Probable** ☐ Suspected ☐ Possible ☐ Unlikely

Effects Serum-free thyroxine concentration may be decreased, increasing serum thyrotropin concentration and the need for THYROID HORMONE.

Mechanism Changes in serum thyroxine and thyrotropin concentrations induced by ESTROGEN administration may result from the increase in serum thyroxine-binding globulin concentrations in hypothyroid women.

Management In women with hypothyroidism, measure serum thyrotropin concentrations approximately 12 weeks after starting ESTROGEN and adjust the THYROID HORMONE dose as needed.

Discussion

The effects of estrogen administration on pituitary-thyroid function were studied in 11 women with normal thyroid function and 25 women receiving thyroxine therapy for chronic hypothyroidism.[1] All women were started on conjugated estrogens 0.625 mg/day. The dosage was decreased to 0.3 mg/day in 1 woman because of breast tenderness and increased to 1.25 mg/day in another because of persistent menopausal symptoms. In women with normal thyroid function, serum-free thyroxine and thyrotropin levels did not change; however, at 12 weeks, the mean serum thyroxine level increased 30%, and serum thyroxine-binding globulin level increased 54%. In the women with hypothyroidism, the increases in serum thyroxine and thyroxine-binding globulin levels during estrogen administration were similar to the increases in women with normal thyroid function. However, the serum-free thyroxine level decreased 18%, and the serum thyrotropin level increased 256%. Serum thyrotropin levels increased to more than 7 microunits/mL in 7 of the women receiving thyroid replacement and to more than 1 microunit/mL in 3 women receiving thyrotropin-suppression, necessitating increases in thyroxine doses.

[1] Arafah BM. *N Engl J Med.* 2001;344(23):1743.

* Asterisk indicates drugs cited in interaction reports. Based on pharmacologic and pharmacokinetic considerations, similar interactions may occur with other drugs that are listed.
†Not available in the United States.

Thyroid Hormones — *Food*

Levothyroxine* (eg, *Synthroid*)	Grapefruit Juice*

Significance	Onset	Severity	Documentation
3	☐ Rapid	☐ Major	☐ Established
	■ **Delayed**	☐ Moderate	☐ Probable
		■ **Minor**	■ **Suspected**
			☐ Possible
			☐ Unlikely

Effects GRAPEFRUIT JUICE may delay the absorption of LEVOTHYROXINE slightly.

Mechanism Interference with LEVOTHYROXINE absorption from the intestinal lumen by GRAPEFRUIT JUICE is suspected.

Management Based on available data, no special precautions are needed.

Discussion

The effect of grapefruit juice on the pharmacokinetics of levothyroxine was studied in 10 healthy subjects.[1] Using a randomized, crossover design, each subject ingested 200 mL of grapefruit juice or water 3 times daily for 2 days. On day 3, a single dose of levothyroxine 0.6 mg was taken with grapefruit juice or water. Compared with taking levothyroxine with water, grapefruit juice ingestion decreased the total thyroxine (T_4) concentration 11%. In addition, the incremental serum T_4 and AUC during the first 4 and 6 hours was decreased 13% and 9%, respectively. The TSH serum concentration measured 24 hours after levothyroxine ingestion was not altered by grapefruit juice. Based on the small delay in absorption and the slight effect on bioavailability of levothyroxine, this interaction is not likely to be clinically important.

[1] Lilja JJ, et al. *Br J Clin Pharmacol.* 2005;60(3):337.

* Asterisk indicates drugs cited in interaction reports.

Thyroid Hormones | *HMG-CoA Reductase Inhibitors*

Thyroid Hormones	HMG-CoA Reductase Inhibitors	
Levothyroxine* (eg, *Synthroid*)	Lovastatin* (eg, *Mevacor*)	Simvastatin* (eg, *Zocor*)

Significance	Onset	Severity	Documentation
4	☐ Rapid ■ **Delayed**	☐ Major ■ **Moderate** ☐ Minor	☐ Established ☐ Probable ☐ Suspected ■ **Possible** ☐ Unlikely

Effects Possible increased or decreased effects of THYROID HORMONE.

Mechanism Unknown.

Management Monitor response to THYROID HORMONE therapy when treatment with certain HMG-CoA REDUCTASE INHIBITORS is started or stopped.

Discussion

Hypothyroidism was reported in an 18-year-old woman with type 1 diabetes, Hashimoto thyroiditis, and type IIA hyperlipoproteinemia.[1] Prior to starting treatment with lovastatin, the patient was euthyroid while receiving thyroxine 0.125 mg daily. She became hypothyroid during coadministration of thyroxine and lovastatin. Lovastatin was discontinued, and she became euthyroid again. When lovastatin treatment was resumed, her thyroid function test became abnormal and returned to normal after stopping lovastatin. A second patient, a 54-year-old man with Hashimoto thyroiditis and type 1 diabetes who was receiving levothyroxine as well as a number of other medications, developed hyperthyroidism after lovastatin was added to his treatment regimen.[2] Other patients have received coadministration of thyroid hormone and lovastatin without alteration of their thyroid function.[3] In addition, lovastatin has no effect on serum thyroid concentrations in patients with no thyroid disease. Two patients receiving levothyroxine experienced an increase in TSH after starting simvastatin.[4] When simvastatin was discontinued, TSH levels returned to the normal range and hypothyroid symptoms resolved in 1 patient.

Controlled studies are needed to assess the clinical importance of this possible drug interaction.

[1] Demke DM. *N Engl J Med.* 1989;321(19):1341.
[2] Lustgarten BP. *Ann Intern Med.* 1988;109(2):171.
[3] Gormley GJ, et al. *N Engl J Med.* 1989;321(19):1342.
[4] Kisch E, et al. *Ann Intern Med.* 2005;143(7):547.

* Asterisk indicates drugs cited in interaction reports.

Thyroid Hormones		***Hydantoins***
Levothyroxine* (eg, *Synthroid*)	Liotrix (*Thyrolar*)	Phenytoin* (eg, *Dilantin*)
Liothyronine (eg, *Cytomel*)	Thyroid (eg, *Armour Thyroid*)	

Significance	Onset	Severity	Documentation
5	■ **Rapid**	□ Major	□ Established
	□ Delayed	■ **Moderate**	□ Probable
		□ Minor	□ Suspected
			□ Possible
			■ **Unlikely**

Effects The effects of THYROID HORMONES may be decreased.

Mechanism Unknown.

Management Based on present evidence, no specific recommendations can be made.

Discussion

Coadministration of phenytoin to 2 patients receiving levothyroxine was associated with the necessity to increase the thyroid dose in 1 patient and with the development of supraventricular tachycardia in the other.[1,2] The former patient received IV phenytoin and did not have an intact pituitary-thyroid axis, indicating that initiation of phenytoin may increase thyroxine replacement requirements in primary hypothyroidism and, possibly, precipitating hypothyroidism in patients with diminished thyroid reserve.[2]

A causal relationship cannot be established in these cases. Controlled studies are needed to determine the importance of this potential interaction.

[1] Fulop M, et al. *JAMA*. 1966;196:454.
[2] Blackshear JL, et al. *Ann Intern Med*. 1983;99:341.

* Asterisk indicates drugs cited in interaction reports. Based on pharmacologic and pharmacokinetic considerations, similar interactions may occur with other drugs that are listed.

Thyroid Hormones — *Imatinib*

Levothyroxine* (eg, *Synthroid*)	Imatinib* (*Gleevec*)

Significance	Onset	Severity	Documentation
2	☐ Rapid	☐ Major	☐ Established
	■ **Delayed**	■ **Moderate**	☐ Probable
		☐ Minor	■ **Suspected**
			☐ Possible
			☐ Unlikely

Effects TSH levels may be increased, and symptoms of hypothyroidism may be evident.

Mechanism IMATINIB may increase LEVOTHYROXINE hepatic clearance.

Management Monitor thyroid function during coadministration of IMATINIB. Be prepared to adjust the LEVOTHYROXINE dosage when starting or stopping IMATINIB treatment.

Discussion

A potential interaction between levothyroxine and imatinib was reported in patients after thyroidectomy.[1] The effect of imatinib on levothyroxine therapy was reported in 8 patients who had undergone thyroidectomy and were receiving levothyroxine 100 to 200 mcg daily. Findings were compared with those of 3 patients receiving imatinib who had not undergone thyroidectomy. Thyroid function was measured before, during, and within 2 weeks after changes in imatinib or levothyroxine dosage. Symptoms of hypothyroidism occurred in all patients who had undergone thyroidectomy, while patients with their thyroid remained euthyroid. There was an average increase in TSH levels to 384% of the upper limit of normal (ULN) in patients after thyroidectomy. Free thyroxine (T_4) and free triiodothyronine (T_3) values remained within the reference range (within 59% and 63% of the ULN for free T_4 and free T_3, respectively). Despite an incremental levothyroxine dose increase to a mean of 206% of the dose before imatinib treatment in patients who had undergone thyroidectomy, hypothyroidism was reversed in only 3 patients before discontinuation of imatinib.

[1] de Groot JW, et al. *Clin Pharmacol Ther.* 2005;78:433.

* Asterisk indicates drugs cited in interaction reports.

Thyroid Hormones — *Iron Salts*

Thyroid Hormones	Iron Salts	
Levothyroxine* (eg, *Synthroid*)	Ferrous Fumarate (eg, *Hemocyte*)	Polysaccharide Iron Complex (eg, *Ferrex 150*)
	Ferrous Gluconate (eg, *Fergon*)	
	Ferrous Sulfate* (eg, *Feosol*)	

Significance	Onset	Severity	Documentation
2	□ Rapid	□ Major	□ Established
	■ **Delayed**	■ **Moderate**	□ Probable
		□ Minor	■ **Suspected**
			□ Possible
			□ Unlikely

Effects The efficacy of LEVOTHYROXINE may be decreased, resulting in hypothyroidism.

Mechanism Unknown. Probably decreased absorption of LEVOTHYROXINE caused by complex formation with the IRON SALT.

Management Separate the administration times of LEVOTHYROXINE and the IRON SALT by as much as possible. Monitor thyroid function during coadministration of these agents. Adjust the dose of LEVOTHYROXINE as necessary.

Discussion

The effects of simultaneous administration of levothyroxine and ferrous sulfate on thyroid hormone were studied in an uncontrolled clinical trial involving 14 patients with primary hypothyroidism.[1] Patients had varying degrees of hypothyroidism caused by Hashimoto thyroiditis or radioiodine therapy for hyperthyroidism. All patients were receiving oral levothyroxine 0.075 to 0.15 mg daily. The patients were given a 7-week supply of ferrous sulfate 300 mg and their usual dose of levothyroxine at weeks 0 and 6. The patients were instructed to take the ferrous sulfate and levothyroxine simultaneously each morning 30 to 60 minutes before breakfast. Compared with week 0, 11 patients had increased serum TSH at week 12 (increased from 1.6 to 5.4 milliunits/L). In 2 patients, TSH serum concentrations were indicative of hypothyroidism. In 1 patient, TSH levels increased from 2.6 to 40.8 milliunits/L. Nine patients with an increase in serum TSH also had an increase in their clinical hypothyroidism score. Three patients had a decrease in serum TSH. Ferrous sulfate did not significantly reduce free serum thyroxine index or total serum thyroxine ($P = 0.12$ and $P = 0.16$, respectively).

[1] Campbell NR, et al. *Ann Intern Med.* 1992;117(12):1010.

* Asterisk indicates drugs cited in interaction reports. Based on pharmacologic and pharmacokinetic considerations, similar interactions may occur with other drugs that are listed.

Thyroid Hormones — *Lanthanum*

Levothyroxine* (eg, *Synthroid*)	Liotrix (*Thyrolar*)	Lanthanum* (*Fosrenol*)
Liothyronine (eg, *Cytomel*)	Thyroid	

Significance	Onset	Severity	Documentation
4	☐ Rapid	☐ Major	☐ Established
	■ **Delayed**	■ **Moderate**	☐ Probable
		☐ Minor	☐ Suspected
			■ **Possible**
			☐ Unlikely

Effects THYROID HORMONE plasma concentrations may be decreased, reducing the efficacy.

Mechanism Decreased absorption of THYROID HORMONES caused by complex formation with LANTHANUM is suspected.

Management Separate the administration times of the THYROID HORMONE and LANTHANUM by as much as possible. Monitor TSH levels during coadministration of these agents and be prepared to adjust the THYROID HORMONE dose as needed.

Discussion

The effects of lanthanum on the pharmacokinetics of levothyroxine were studied in 6 healthy euthyroid volunteers.[1] Each subject received 1 mg of levothyroxine alone with 240 mL of water and concurrently with 500 mg of lanthanum and 240 mL of water. Serum thyroxine (T_4) levels increased following administration of levothyroxine alone; however, the increase in T_4 was blunted by coadministration of lanthanum. None of the subjects experienced symptoms of thyrotoxicosis.

[1] Weitzman SP, et al. *Thyroid.* 2009;19(1):77.

* Asterisk indicates drugs cited in interaction reports. Based on pharmacologic and pharmacokinetic considerations, similar interactions may occur with other drugs that are listed.

Thyroid Hormones — *Protease Inhibitors*

Thyroid Hormones	Protease Inhibitors	
Levothyroxine (eg, *Synthroid*)	Fosamprenavir (*Lexiva*)	Nelfinavir* (*Viracept*)
	Indinavir* (*Crixivan*)	Ritonavir (*Norvir*)
	Lopinavir/Ritonavir* (*Kaletra*)	Saquinavir (*Invirase*)

Significance	Onset	Severity	Documentation
4	☐ Rapid	☐ Major	☐ Established
	■ **Delayed**	■ **Moderate**	☐ Probable
		☐ Minor	☐ Suspected
			■ **Possible**
			☐ Unlikely

Effects Thyroxine serum concentrations may be increased or decreased, resulting in hyperthyroidism or hypothyroidism.

Mechanism Unknown.

Management Carefully monitor patients receiving LEVOTHYROXINE when PROTEASE INHIBITOR therapy is started or stopped.

Discussion

Hyperthyroidism was reported in a 36-year-old woman infected with HIV and taking levothyroxine for hypothyroidism after indinavir was added to her treatment regimen.[1] The patient had been taking levothyroxine 0.75 mg/day. During levothyroxine therapy, she was asymptomatic, with serum thyroid tests demonstrating euthyroidism. Approximately 7 weeks after starting indinavir, stavudine (eg, *Zerit*), and lamivudine (*Epivir*), the patient presented with nervousness, palpitations, restlessness with weakness, and a slight decrease in body weight. Serum thyroid tests showed complete suppression of TSH and increased plasma concentrations of free T_4 and T_3. One month after the levothyroxine dosage was decreased to 0.12 mg daily, the patient reported feeling well and her thyroid indices returned to baseline. Conversely, severe hypothyroidism was reported in a 58-year-old woman receiving levothyroxine after starting lamivudine, lopinavir/ritonavir, and zidovudine (eg, *Retrovir*).[2] Hypothyroidism persisted after 8 months despite a dosage of 225 mcg/day. Antiretroviral therapy was discontinued and the hypothyroidism resolved. When lopinavir/ritonavir was reintroduced, hypothyroidism recurred and persisted even after lopinavir/ritonavir was changed to nelfinavir. Additional studies are needed to clarify this interaction.

[1] Lanzafame M, et al. *Infection.* 2002;30(1):54.

[2] Touzot M, et al. *AIDS.* 2006;20(8):1210.

* Asterisk indicates drugs cited in interaction reports. Based on pharmacologic and pharmacokinetic considerations, similar interactions may occur with other drugs that are listed.

Thyroid Hormones — *Quinolones*

Thyroid Hormones	Quinolones
Levothyroxine* (eg, *Synthroid*)	Ciprofloxacin* (eg, *Cipro*)

Significance	Onset	Severity	Documentation
4	☐ Rapid	☐ Major	☐ Established
	■ **Delayed**	■ **Moderate**	☐ Probable
		☐ Minor	☐ Suspected
			■ **Possible**
			☐ Unlikely

Effects Possible loss of efficacy of exogenously administered LEVOTHYROXINE and potential hypothyroidism.

Mechanism Decreased absorption of LEVOTHYROXINE by CIPROFLOXACIN is suspected.

Management Monitor plasma TSH levels in patients receiving oral LEVOTHYROXINE replacement if CIPROFLOXACIN is coadministered for 3 weeks or more. If both agents are used, separate the administration times by at least 6 hours.

Discussion

Hypothyroidism was reported in 2 patients taking levothyroxine and ciprofloxacin.[1] One patient, an 80-year-old woman, had maintained suppressed TSH concentrations while taking levothyroxine 125 mcg daily. After 4 weeks of treatment with ciprofloxacin 750 mg twice daily, she complained of tiredness and her laboratory tests were consistent with hypothyroidism. Increasing the dosage of levothyroxine to 200 mcg daily had no effect. Thyroid function tests rapidly returned to normal when the levothyroxine dosage was reduced to 125 mcg daily and ciprofloxacin was discontinued. The second patient, a 79-year-old woman, had maintained stable thyroid function tests while taking levothyroxine 150 mcg daily. After 3 weeks of treatment with ciprofloxacin 500 mg twice daily, her thyroid function tests were consistent with hypothyroidism. Switching from coadministration of levothyroxine and ciprofloxacin to giving the drugs 6 hours apart resulted in rapid normalization of thyroid function tests.

[1] Cooper JG, et al. *BMJ.* 2005;330(7498):1002.

* Asterisk indicates drugs cited in interaction reports.

Thyroid Hormones		*Raloxifene*	
Levothyroxine* (eg, *Synthroid*)		Raloxifene* (*Evista*)	
Significance	Onset	Severity	Documentation
4	☐ Rapid ■ **Delayed**	☐ Major ■ **Moderate** ☐ Minor	☐ Established ☐ Probable ☐ Suspected ■ **Possible** ☐ Unlikely

Effects LEVOTHYROXINE levels may be delayed and decreased, reducing the pharmacologic effect.

Mechanism Unknown; however, simultaneous administration of these agents appears to decrease LEVOTHYROXINE absorption.

Management Separate the administration times of LEVOTHYROXINE and RALOXIFENE by at least 12 hours. Monitor thyroid function during administration of these agents and adjust the LEVOTHYROXINE dosage as needed.

Discussion

A 79-year-old woman with chronic primary hypothyroidism experienced an increase in her levothyroxine requirement while simultaneously taking raloxifene.[1] The patient was prescribed levothyroxine following a subtotal thyroidectomy. For several years, she maintained normal TSH levels while receiving levothyroxine 0.15 mg in the morning. Raloxifene 60 mg daily was prescribed for osteopenia and taken in the morning with levothyroxine. Within 2 to 3 months, the patient experienced symptoms of hypothyroidism with an elevated TSH level. The dosage of levothyroxine was increased to 0.2 mg daily. Because of continued TSH elevation and symptoms of hypothyroidism over the next 6 months, the levothyroxine dosage was increased to 0.3 mg daily. Nine months after starting raloxifene, the patient's TSH level remained elevated. It was suspected that raloxifene was interfering with levothyroxine absorption. Subsequently, on 2 occasions (lasting 6 to 8 weeks), the administration times of levothyroxine and raloxifene were separated by about 12 hours. Thyroid function tests revealed hypothyroidism when both drugs were taken simultaneously and improvement or resolution when the administration times were separated. An absorption study demonstrated lower levels of total thyroxine (T_4) at all study points when levothyroxine and raloxifene were administered simultaneously, compared with levothyroxine taken alone. In a similar case, a 47-year-old woman with primary hypothyroidism became slightly hyperthyroid when the levothyroxine and raloxifene administration times were separated by 12 hours, and it became necessary to reduce the levothyroxine dose.[2]

[1] Siraj ES, et al. *Arch Intern Med.* 2003;163(11):1367.
[2] Garwood CL, et al. *Pharmacotherapy.* 2006;26(6):881.

* Asterisk indicates drugs cited in interaction reports.

Thyroid Hormones — *Rifamycins*

Thyroid Hormones	Rifamycins	
Levothyroxine* (eg, *Synthroid*)	Rifabutin (*Mycobutin*)	Rifapentine (*Priftin*)
	Rifampin* (eg, *Rifadin*)	

Significance	Onset	Severity	Documentation
4	☐ Rapid	☐ Major	☐ Established
	■ **Delayed**	■ **Moderate**	☐ Probable
		☐ Minor	☐ Suspected
			■ **Possible**
			☐ Unlikely

Effects TSH levels may be increased, resulting in hypothyroidism.

Mechanism The data suggest that RIFAMYCINS may increase LEVOTHYROXINE hepatic clearance, producing a return to the hypothyroid state and a compensatory increase in TSH levels.[1,2]

Management Monitor thyroid status in patients receiving LEVOTHYROXINE when RIFAMYCIN therapy is started or stopped. Adjust the dose of LEVOTHYROXINE as needed.

Discussion

Elevated TSH levels were reported in 2 patients stable on levothyroxine after starting rifampin therapy.[1,2] The first patient, a 50-year-old man, had a history of hypothyroidism, idiopathic thrombocytopenia purpura, coronary artery disease, and non-insulin–dependent diabetes mellitus.[2] The patient was receiving levothyroxine 0.025 mg/day, docusate (eg, *Colace*), ferrous sulfate (eg, *Feosol*), metoprolol (eg, *Lopressor*), omeprazole (eg, *Prilosec*), and procainamide (eg, *Procanbid*), in additon to vancomycin (eg, *Vancocin*) for methicillin-resistant *Staphylococcus aureus*. Rifampin 600 mg/day for 14 days was added to the patient's drug regimen for synergy. After starting rifampin, the patient's TSH level increased, reaching a peak of 202% of the pretreatment level 3 days after the discontinuation of rifampin. Nine days after stopping rifampin, the TSH level had returned to baseline. A similar interaction occurred in the second patient, a 31-year-old woman with Turner syndrome and hypertension who had had a total thyroidectomy for a rapidly enlarging goiter.[2] The patient had been stable on levothyroxine 0.1 mg/day. Her serum thyroxine levels and free thyroxine index decreased, and her TSH levels increased during coadministration of rifampin 300 mg every 12 hours. These levels partially returned to baseline when rifampin therapy was discontinued. However, abnormal levels recurred when rifampin therapy was reinstated.

[1] Isley WL. *Ann Intern Med.* 1987;107(4):517.

[2] Nolan SR, et al. *South Med J.* 1999;92(5):529.

* Asterisk indicates drugs cited in interaction reports. Based on pharmacologic and pharmacokinetic considerations, similar interactions may occur with other drugs that are listed.

Thyroid Hormones | *Sertraline*

Levothyroxine* (eg, *Synthroid*)	Liotrix (*Thyrolar*)	Sertraline* (eg, *Zoloft*)
Liothyronine (eg, *Cytomel*)	Thyroid (eg, *Westhroid*)	

Significance	Onset	Severity	Documentation
4	□ Rapid	□ Major	□ Established
	■ **Delayed**	■ **Moderate**	□ Probable
		□ Minor	□ Suspected
			■ **Possible**
			□ Unlikely

Effects The effects of THYROID HORMONES may be decreased.

Mechanism Unknown.

Management Monitor thyroid function during coadministration of THYROID HORMONES and SERTRALINE. Be prepared to adjust the THYROID HORMONE dosage when starting, stopping, or changing the SERTRALINE dose.

Discussion

In 11 patients receiving levothyroxine, increased thyrotropin concentrations and decreased free thyroxine index occurred after starting sertraline.[1] No patient experienced symptoms of hypothyroidism. The dose of levothyroxine was increased in all patients, and thyrotropin concentrations returned to baseline. In another report, 14 patients experienced hypothyroidism while taking sertraline.[2] Seven of these patients were taking thyroxine concurrently. The sertraline product information lists hypothyroidism as an adverse reaction that was observed during postmarketing experience.[3]

[1] McCowen KC, et al. *N Engl J Med.* 1997;337(14):1010.
[2] Clary CM, et al. *N Engl J Med.* 1997;337(14):1011.
[3] *Zoloft* [package insert]. New York, NY: Pfizer, Inc; January 2008.

* Asterisk indicates drugs cited in interaction reports. Based on pharmacologic and pharmacokinetic considerations, similar interactions may occur with other drugs that are listed.

Thyroid Hormones		**Sevelamer**
Levothyroxine* (eg, *Synthroid*) Liothyronine (eg, *Cytomel*)	Liotrix (*Thyrolar*) Thyroid	Sevelamer* (eg, *Renagel*)

Significance	Onset	Severity	Documentation
4	☐ Rapid ■ **Delayed**	☐ Major ■ **Moderate** ☐ Minor	☐ Established ☐ Probable ☐ Suspected ■ **Possible** ☐ Unlikely

Effects The efficacy of THYROID HORMONES may be decreased, resulting in hypothyroidism.

Mechanism Decreased THYROID HORMONE absorption due to binding to SEVELAMER is suspected.

Management Separate the administration times of the THYROID HORMONE and SEVELAMER by as much as possible, but by at least 4 hours. Monitor thyroid function during coadministration of these agents. Adjust the THYROID HORMONE dose as needed. In patients receiving THYROID HORMONES, calcium acetate may be less likely to interact.

Discussion

The medical records of 13 patients receiving levothyroxine and sevelamer were reviewed to assess the effects of sevelamer on levothyroxine bioavailability.[1] Levothyroxine doses were higher in patients concomitantly receiving sevelamer compared with patients receiving levothyroxine and calcium carbonate or calcium acetate concurrently. In addition, after coadministration of levothyroxine and sevelamer for 6 months, the levothyroxine dose was higher than in patients receiving calcium carbonate or calcium acetate concurrently. Over time, compared with calcium acetate, calcium carbonate and sevelamer were associated with increased TSH levels in patients receiving levothyroxine. A 62-year-old woman with hypothyroidism and tubulointerstitial nephritis was receiving levothyroxine (dosage gradually titrated to 150 mcg/day) and sevelamer 3,200 mg with breakfast.[2] After 3 months of treatment, the patient was still hypothyroid and TSH levels were elevated. The patient was instructed to take levothyroxine at night (at least 4 hours after sevelamer). The patient felt much better 3 weeks later, and the TSH level had decreased from 196 to 19 milliunits/L. Nine months later, while levothyroxine and sevelamer were being coadministered in the morning, TSH levels were elevated. The TSH levels rapidly normalized when the levothyroxine administration time was changed back to the evening.

[1] Diskin CJ, et al. *Int Urol Nephrol.* 2007;39(2):599.

[2] Arnadottir M, et al. *Nephrol Dial Transplant.* 2008;23(1):420.

* Asterisk indicates drugs cited in interaction reports. Based on pharmacologic and pharmacokinetic considerations, similar interactions may occur with other drugs that are listed.

Thyroid Hormones — *Sucralfate*

Levothyroxine* (eg, *Synthroid*)	Sucralfate* (eg, *Carafate*)

Significance	Onset	Severity	Documentation
2	☐ Rapid ■ **Delayed**	☐ Major ■ **Moderate** ☐ Minor	☐ Established ☐ Probable ■ **Suspected** ☐ Possible ☐ Unlikely

Effects The effects of LEVOTHYROXINE may be decreased.

Mechanism Interference with intraluminal or transintestinal transport of LEVOTHYROXINE is suspected.

Management Monitor patients treated concurrently with SUCRALFATE and LEVOTHYROXINE for decreased LEVOTHYROXINE absorption. If an interaction is suspected, increase the dose of LEVOTHYROXINE or separate the administration times of SUCRALFATE and LEVOTHYROXINE by at least 8 hours.

Discussion

Suspected levothyroxine malabsorption in a 46-year-old woman being treated concurrently with sucralfate prompted a study of the effects of sucralfate on the absorption of levothyroxine in 5 healthy volunteers.[1] Each subject ingested levothyroxine 1,000 mcg without sucralfate, with sucralfate 1 g, and 8 hours after sucralfate. When levothyroxine was ingested with sucralfate, sucralfate 1 g was taken every 6 hours beginning at 8:00 AM. On the next morning, levothyroxine and sucralfate were ingested simultaneously. In the final phase of the study, each subject received sucralfate 2 g every 12 hours starting at noon; then on the subsequent day, levothyroxine was administered 8 hours after the final dose of sucralfate. When levothyroxine was taken alone, serum total T_4 concentrations began to increase within 30 minutes of levothyroxine ingestion, mean time to peak serum T_4 level was 180 minutes, and the mean maximum quantity of levothyroxine absorbed was 796 mcg. When administration of sucralfate and levothyroxine was separated by 8 hours, maximum levothyroxine absorption (777 mcg) occurred at 162 minutes. These values were not significantly different from administration of levothyroxine alone. However, when levothyroxine and sucralfate were taken simultaneously, the mean maximum T_4 absorption was 225 mcg ($P = 0.0029$) and occurred at 300 minutes. Serum TSH concentration decreased from a baseline value of 2.1 million units/L to 0.8 million units/L 24 hours after levothyroxine was ingested alone ($P = 0.003$) and to 1.3 million units/L when sucralfate and levothyroxine were coadministered ($P = 0.009$). In contrast, only a slight decrease in serum T_4 index was reported when levothyroxine 75 to 200 mcg was administered to 9 patients receiving sucralfate 1 g 4 times daily.[2]

[1] Sherman SI, et al. *Am J Med.* 1994;96(6):531.

[2] Campbell JA, et al. *Ann Intern Med.* 1994;121(2):152.

* Asterisk indicates drugs cited in interaction reports.

Tiagabine — *Gemfibrozil*

Tiagabine* (*Gabitril*)	Gemfibrozil* (eg, *Lopid*)

Significance	Onset	Severity	Documentation
4	■ **Rapid**	□ Major	□ Established
	□ Delayed	■ **Moderate**	□ Probable
		□ Minor	□ Suspected
			■ **Possible**
			□ Unlikely

Effects TIAGABINE plasma concentrations may be elevated, increasing the risk of toxicity.

Mechanism Unknown. However, displacement of TIAGABINE from protein-binding sites may be a factor.

Management Avoid this combination if possible. If concurrent use cannot be avoided, closely monitor the patient when TIAGABINE and GEMFIBROZIL are coadministered. Advise the patient of the possible interaction.

Discussion

A 39-year-old man taking tiagabine 16 mg 3 times daily and carbamazepine (eg, *Tegretol*) experienced generalized weakness and confusion and then fainted within 1 hour of taking the first dose of gemfibrozil 600 mg.[1] The patient was rechallenged under controlled conditions. The patient continued receiving tiagabine and carbamazepine. A one-time dose of gemfibrozil 300 mg was administered with the morning doses of tiagabine and carbamazepine. After administration of gemfibrozil, the patient experienced light-headedness, which resolved after several hours. However, approximately 7 hours after coadministration of gemfibrozil and tiagabine, the patient experienced 2 brief seizures. Tiagabine plasma concentrations 2 and 5 hours after taking gemfibrozil were increased 59% and 75%, respectively. The tiagabine AUC was increased approximately 61% following gemfibrozil administration. In addition, the unbound fraction of tiagabine increased from concentrations that were not quantifiable prior to gemfibrozil administration to 11.4% and 13.6% at 2 and 5 hours after gemfibrozil dosing, respectively. Gemfibrozil administration did not affect carbamazepine concentrations.

[1] Burstein AH, et al. *Ann Pharmacother.* 2009;43(2):379.

* Asterisk indicates drugs cited in interaction reports.

Ticlopidine — *Antacids*

Ticlopidine* (eg, *Ticlid*)	Aluminum Hydroxide (eg, *Amphojel*)	Magnesium Hydroxide (eg, *Milk of Magnesia*)
	Aluminum/Magnesium Hydroxide* (eg, *Maalox*)	

Significance	Onset	Severity	Documentation
4	■ **Rapid**	□ Major	□ Established
	□ Delayed	■ **Moderate**	□ Probable
		□ Minor	□ Suspected
			■ **Possible**
			□ Unlikely

Effects Serum TICLOPIDINE levels may be decreased. Because TICLOPIDINE is a potent inhibitor of platelet aggregation, the clinical effect of this decrease cannot be determined.

Mechanism Unknown. However, the absorption of TICLOPIDINE is decreased.

Management Based on available data, no special precautions appear necessary.

Discussion

The effect of food or aluminum-magnesium hydroxide antacid on the bioavailability of ticlopidine was studied in 12 healthy volunteers.[1] In a 4-way, crossover evaluation, each subject fasted beginning at midnight the evening before administration of the study drug. During the treatment periods, each subject received a single dose of ticlopidine 250 mg. One group ate a high-fat breakfast, which comprised approximately 69 g of protein, 32 g of fat, and 45 g of carbohydrate. The other (antacid) group received aluminum hydroxide 30 mL (225 mg per 5 mL)/magnesium hydroxide (200 mg per 5 mL) immediately before administration of ticlopidine. Plasma ticlopidine concentrations were significantly different ($P < 0.05$) between the groups. Serum ticlopidine levels were higher after the administration of food. Administration of ticlopidine with food produced an increase in the maximum ticlopidine serum concentration from 0.573 to 0.695 mcg/mL, a decrease in the time to reach the maximum serum level from 1.917 to 1.708 hours, and an increase in the ticlopidine AUC from 1.808 to 2.164 mcg•hr/mL compared with administration to fasting patients. Antacid treatment with aluminum/magnesium hydroxide, when compared with fasting, resulted in a decrease in the maximum serum concentration of ticlopidine from 0.573 to 0.375 mcg/mL and a decrease in the AUC from 1.808 to 1.484 mcg•hr/mL. Although ticlopidine was reasonably well tolerated by all subjects, the number of GI complaints was lowest when the drug was taken after the test meal.

Additional studies are needed to assess the clinical importance of this possible interaction.

[1] Shah J, et al. *J Clin Pharmacol.* 1990;30(8):733.

* Asterisk indicates drugs cited in interaction reports. Based on pharmacologic and pharmacokinetic considerations, similar interactions may occur with other drugs that are listed.

Ticlopidine — *Ergot Derivatives*

Ticlopidine	Ergot Derivatives	
Ticlopidine* (eg, *Ticlid*)	Dihydroergotamine (eg, *D.H.E. 45*)	Ergotamine (*Ergomar*)
	Ergoloid Mesylates*	Methylergonovine (*Methergine*)
	Ergonovine (*Ergotrate*)	

Significance	Onset	Severity	Documentation
4	☐ Rapid	☐ Major	☐ Established
	■ **Delayed**	■ **Moderate**	☐ Probable
		☐ Minor	☐ Suspected
			■ **Possible**
			☐ Unlikely

Effects TICLOPIDINE plasma concentrations may be reduced, decreasing the efficacy.

Mechanism Inhibition of organic anion transporting polypeptide–mediated uptake of TICLOPIDINE during the intestinal absorption phase by the ERGOT DERIVATIVE is suspected.

Management Until more clinical data are available, avoid concurrent use of ERGOT DERIVATIVES and TICLOPIDINE. If an alternative to TICLOPIDINE is not available, discontinue ERGOT DERIVATIVE therapy. Do not start ERGOT DERIVATIVE therapy in patients receiving TICLOPIDINE.

Discussion

The effects of ergoloid mesylates on the pharmacokinetics of ticlopidine were studied in 8 healthy volunteers.[1] Each subject received a single dose of ticlopidine 250 mg alone, followed by a 3-week washout period. Then each subject received ergoloid mesylates 1.5 mg 3 times daily for 4 days with ticlopidine 250 mg given concomitantly on day 4. Compared with administration of ticlopidine alone, pretreatment with ergoloid mesylates decreased the ticlopidine AUC and C_{max} 30% and 29%, respectively.

[1] Lu WJ, et al. *J Clin Pharmacol.* 2006;46:628.

* Asterisk indicates drugs cited in interaction reports. Based on pharmacologic and pharmacokinetic considerations, similar interactions may occur with other drugs that are listed.

Tizanidine		*Fluvoxamine*
Tizanidine* (eg, *Zanaflex*)		Fluvoxamine*

Significance	Onset	Severity	Documentation
2	☐ Rapid ■ **Delayed**	☐ Major ■ **Moderate** ☐ Minor	☐ Established ☐ Probable ■ **Suspected** ☐ Possible ☐ Unlikely

Effects TIZANIDINE plasma concentrations may be elevated, increasing the pharmacologic and adverse reactions (eg, hypotension).

Mechanism Inhibition of TIZANIDINE metabolism (CYP1A2) by FLUVOXAMINE is suspected.

Management Coadministration of TIZANIDINE and FLUVOXAMINE is contraindicated.

Discussion

The effects of fluvoxamine on the pharmacokinetics and pharmacodynamics of tizanidine were studied in 10 healthy subjects.[1] In a randomized, double-blind, crossover study, each subject received fluvoxamine 100 mg or placebo once daily for 4 days. On day 4, a single dose of tizanidine 4 mg was administered. Compared with placebo, pretreatment with fluvoxamine increased the tizanidine peak plasma concentration 12-fold, increased the AUC 33-fold, and prolonged the elimination $t_{½}$ from 1.5 to 4.3 hours. In addition, compared with placebo, there was a decrease in systolic BP (−35 mm Hg), diastolic BP (−20 mm Hg), and heart rate (−4 bpm). Subjective drowsiness was increased. All subjects reported somnolence, dizziness, and difficulty fixating their eyes and concentrating on psychomotor tests. Muscle weakness and dry mouth were reported. A 70-year-old woman taking fluvoxamine 150 mg/day experienced anuresis, dry mouth, low body temperature, and low heart rate (56 to 60 bpm) after taking tizanidine 3 mg/day.[2] After stopping tizanidine, symptoms improved immediately. In a retrospective survey of the medical records of 913 patients, adverse reactions (eg, dizziness, drowsiness, hypotension, low body temperature, low heart rate, speech disorder) occurred in 26% of patients receiving fluvoxamine and tizanidine, compared with 5% of patients taking tizanidine alone.[2]

[1] Granfors MT, et al. *Clin Pharmacol Ther.* 2004;75:331.

[2] Momo K, et al. *Clin Pharmacol Ther.* 2004;76:509.

* Asterisk indicates drugs cited in interaction reports.

Tizanidine — *Mexiletine*

Tizanidine* (eg, *Zanaflex*)	Mexiletine*

Significance	Onset	Severity	Documentation
1	☐ Rapid ■ **Delayed**	■ **Major** ☐ Moderate ☐ Minor	☐ Established ☐ Probable ■ **Suspected** ☐ Possible ☐ Unlikely

Effects TIZANIDINE plasma concentrations may be elevated, increasing the pharmacologic effects and risk of adverse reactions (eg, severe hypotension).

Mechanism Inhibition of TIZANIDINE metabolism (CYP1A2) by MEXILETINE.

Management If coadministration cannot be avoided, closely monitor for adverse reactions to TIZANIDINE (eg, hypotension).

Discussion

The effects of mexiletine on the pharmacokinetics and pharmacodynamics of tizanidine were studied in 12 healthy men.[1] Using an open-label design, each subject received a single dose of tizanidine 2 mg alone and after pretreatment with mexiletine 50 mg 3 times a day for 1 day and 2 times on the second day. Compared with taking tizanidine alone, coadministration of mexiletine increased the tizanidine C_{max} and AUC approximately 194% and 242%, respectively, and prolonged the $t_{½}$ from 1.3 to 1.8 hours. In addition, the systolic and diastolic blood pressure after tizanidine administration was increased by giving mexiletine concurrently.[1]

[1] Momo K, et al. *J Clin Pharmacol.* 2010;50(3):331.

* Asterisk indicates drugs cited in interaction reports.

Tizanidine — *Quinolones*

Tizanidine	Quinolones	
Tizanidine* (eg, *Zanaflex*)	Ciprofloxacin* (eg, *Cipro*)	Norfloxacin (*Noroxin*)

Significance	Onset	Severity	Documentation
1	■ **Rapid**	■ **Major**	□ Established
	□ Delayed	□ Moderate	□ Probable
		□ Minor	■ **Suspected**
			□ Possible
			□ Unlikely

Effects TIZANIDINE plasma concentrations may be elevated, increasing the pharmacologic and adverse reactions (eg, dizziness, hypotension).

Mechanism Suspected inhibition of TIZANIDINE metabolism (CYP1A2) by certain QUINOLONES.

Management Coadministration of TIZANIDINE and CIPROFLOXACIN is contraindicated.[1]

Discussion

Using a double-blind, randomized, 2-phase, crossover design, the effects of ciprofloxacin on the pharmacokinetics and pharmacodynamics of tizanidine were studied in 10 healthy men.[2] Each subject received ciprofloxacin 500 mg or matching placebo twice daily for 3 days. On day 3, a single oral dose of tizanidine 4 mg was taken 1 hour after ciprofloxacin. Compared with placebo, ciprofloxacin increased the AUC of tizanidine 10-fold (range, 6- to 24-fold) and the C_{max} 7-fold (range, 4- to 21-fold). The mean elimination $t_{½}$ of tizanidine was prolonged slightly (from 1.5 to 1.8 hours). Compared with placebo, ciprofloxacin administration resulted in an increase in tizanidine plasma concentrations. The increased tizanidine levels were associated with a decrease in BP within 1 hour after tizanidine was taken that lasted for several hours. In addition, subjects were somnolent and dizzy, and experienced a decrease in psychomotor performance that persisted for approximately 3 hours after tizanidine was taken. Lowered heart rate, BP, and body temperature were reported in a 45-year-old woman on long-term tizanidine therapy soon after she began taking ciprofloxacin.[3] These symptoms improved immediately after she stopped taking ciprofloxacin.

[1] *Cipro* [package insert]. Kenilworth, NJ: Schering Corporation; February 2011.
[2] Granfors MT, et al. *Clin Pharmacol Ther.* 2004;76(6):598.
[3] Momo K, et al. *Clin Pharmacol Ther.* 2006;80(6):717.

* Asterisk indicates drugs cited in interaction reports. Based on pharmacologic and pharmacokinetic considerations, similar interactions may occur with other drugs that are listed.

Tizanidine — *Rifampin*

Tizanidine*
(eg, *Zanaflex*)

Rifampin*
(eg, *Rifadin*)

Significance	Onset	Severity	Documentation
5	☐ Rapid ■ **Delayed**	☐ Major ☐ Moderate ■ **Minor**	☐ Established ☐ Probable ☐ Suspected ■ **Possible** ☐ Unlikely

Effects TIZANIDINE plasma concentrations may be reduced, decreasing the efficacy.

Mechanism Induction of first-pass metabolism (CYP1A2) of TIZANIDINE by RIFAMPIN is suspected.

Management Based on available data, the effect of RIFAMPIN on TIZANIDINE is weak and not likely to be clinically important. However, in patients receiving TIZANIDINE, monitor clinical response (eg, spasticity) more closely when RIFAMPIN is started or stopped; be prepared to adjust the TIZANIDINE dose as needed.

Discussion

The effects of rifampin on the pharmacokinetics and pharmacodynamics of tizanidine were studied in 10 healthy subjects.[1] Using a randomized, crossover design, each subject received rifampin 600 mg or placebo once daily. On day 6, tizanidine 4 mg was administered. Compared with placebo, rifampin reduced the tizanidine C_{max} and AUC 51% and 54%, respectively, and had no effect on tizanidine $t_{½}$. Rifampin slightly reduced the C_{max} and AUC of 2 tizanidine metabolites. During the placebo phase, tizanidine reduced systolic BP, diastolic BP, and heart rate from baseline values by −17 mm Hg, −13 mm Hg, and −12 bpm, respectively, compared with reductions of −10 mm Hg, −9 mm Hg, and −7 bpm, respectively, during the rifampin phase.

[1] Backman JT, et al. *Eur J Clin Pharmacol.* 2006;62(6):451.

* Asterisk indicates drugs cited in interaction reports.

Tocainide — *Cimetidine*

Tocainide* (*Tonocard*) | Cimetidine* (*Tagamet*)

Significance	Onset	Severity	Documentation
4	■ **Rapid**	□ Major	□ Established
	□ Delayed	■ **Moderate**	□ Probable
		□ Minor	□ Suspected
			■ **Possible**
			□ Unlikely

Effects The pharmacologic effects of TOCAINIDE may be decreased.

Mechanism Unknown; possible decrease in bioavailability of TOCAINIDE.

Management Based on current information, no specific recommendations can be made. Monitor plasma TOCAINIDE levels and adjust the dose accordingly.

Discussion

Seven healthy volunteers participated in a randomized, double-blind, placebo-controlled, crossover study evaluating the effects of cimetidine and ranitidine (*Zantac*) on the disposition of tocainide.[1] The dosage regimens were cimetidine 300 mg 4 times daily, ranitidine 150 mg twice daily with 1 placebo twice daily, and placebo 4 times daily. Following 48 hours of blinded medication administration and a 12-hour fast, a single oral dose of 400 mg tocainide was administered to each subject. While patients were receiving cimetidine concurrently, the area under the tocainide plasma concentration-time curve decreased in all subjects by an average of 23% ($P < 0.05$), the peak tocainide concentration was decreased 42% ($P < 0.05$), and the amount of unchanged tocainide excreted in the urine up to 58 hours decreased 14.4% ($P < 0.05$). There were no changes in the above values during ranitidine or placebo administration. When compared to placebo, the terminal half-life and the renal clearance of tocainide were not affected by either cimetidine or ranitidine administration.

These results suggest that cimetidine decreases the bioavailability of tocainide. Ranitidine appears to have little or no effect on tocainide bioavailability. Additional studies are needed to determine the precise mechanism and clinical significance of the observed interaction.

[1] North DS, et al. *J Clin Pharmacol.* 1988;28:640.

* Asterisk indicates drugs cited in interaction reports.

Tocainide — *Rifampin*

Tocainide*	Rifampin*
(*Tonocard*)	(eg, *Rimactane*)

Significance	Onset	Severity	Documentation
2	☐ Rapid	☐ Major	☐ Established
	■ **Delayed**	■ **Moderate**	☐ Probable
		☐ Minor	■ **Suspected**
			☐ Possible
			☐ Unlikely

Effects The pharmacologic effects of TOCAINIDE may be decreased.

Mechanism Unknown. However, hepatic metabolism of TOCAINIDE is believed to be increased by RIFAMPIN.

Management Based on current information, no specific recommendations can be made. Monitor plasma TOCAINIDE levels and adjust the dose accordingly.

Discussion

In an open, unrandomized study, the effects of metabolic enzyme induction by rifampin on the pharmacokinetics of tocainide were studied in 8 healthy volunteers.[1] Each subject received tocainide 600 mg orally after an overnight fast. Following a 4-week washout period, they then started rifampin 300 mg orally every 12 hours. After 10 doses, each volunteer received a second oral dose of tocainide 600 mg. Subjects continued to ingest rifampin during the period when blood and urine samples were obtained. Significant differences in elimination rate constant (increased from 0.0545 to 0.0748 per hour, $P = 0.002$), elimination half-life (decreased from 13.2 to 9.4 hours, $P = 0.003$), area under the concentration-time curve (decreased from 76.8 to 55.0 mg/hr/L, $P = 0.018$), and oral clearance (increased from 122.2 to 164.1 mL/min, $P = 0.009$) were observed during concurrent administration of rifampin compared to the control period. Rifampin treatment did not alter the renal clearance or volume of distribution of tocainide. The mechanism of this interaction appears to be rifampin-mediated metabolic enzyme induction.

Additional studies are needed to determine the clinical significance of this potential interaction.

[1] Rice TL, et al. *Clin Pharm.* 1989;8:200.

* Asterisk indicates drugs cited in interaction reports.

Tolterodine — Azole Antifungal Agents

Tolterodine*	Fluconazole	Ketoconazole*
(*Detrol*)	(eg, *Diflucan*)	(eg, *Nizoral*)
	Itraconazole	Posaconazole
	(eg, *Sporanox*)	(*Noxafil*)

Significance	Onset	Severity	Documentation
2	□ Rapid	□ Major	□ Established
	■ **Delayed**	■ **Moderate**	□ Probable
		□ Minor	■ **Suspected**
			□ Possible
			□ Unlikely

Effects TOLTERODINE plasma concentrations may be elevated, increasing the pharmacologic and adverse effects of TOLTERODINE.

Mechanism Possible inhibition of TOLTERODINE metabolism (CYP3A4). In addition, FLUCONAZOLE may inhibit CYP2D6 metabolism of TOLTERODINE and possibly CYP3A4 when administered in dosages of at least 200 mg/day.

Management Closely monitor the patient's clinical response and adjust the dose of TOLTERODINE as needed. The manufacturer of TOLTERODINE states that patients receiving AZOLE ANTIFUNGAL AGENTS (ie, KETOCONAZOLE, ITRACONAZOLE, or MICONAZOLE IV†) should not receive more than 1 mg of TOLTERODINE twice daily.[1]

Discussion

The effect of ketoconazole on the pharmacokinetics of tolterodine was investigated in 8 healthy subjects who were deficient in CYP2D6 activity.[2] In an open, nonrandomized, crossover study divided into 2 phases, participants received single-dose (8 subjects) and multiple-dose (6 subjects) administration of tolterodine with and without ketoconazole. Each subject received a single 2 mg dose of tolterodine at least 4 days prior to ketoconazole administration. Then, each subject received ketoconazole 200 mg once daily for 4 consecutive days in the single-dose phase and for 5 consecutive days in the multiple-dose phase. Tolterodine was given as a single 2 mg dose on day 2 of the single-dose phase and 1 mg twice daily for 4.5 days during the multiple-dose phase. Ketoconazole administration resulted in a decrease in the oral clearance of tolterodine from 10 to 12 L/hr to 4.3 to 4.7 L/hr, which produced an at least 2-fold increase in the AUC after both single- and multiple-dose administration of tolterodine. The mean terminal $t_{1/2}$ of tolterodine was increased 55% (from 9.7 to 15 hours) when it was given with ketoconazole.

[1] *Detrol* [package insert]. New York, NY: Pharmacia & Upjohn Company; March 1998.

[2] Brynne N, et al. *Br J Clin Pharmacol.* 1999;48(4):564.

* Asterisk indicates drugs cited in interaction reports. Based on pharmacologic and pharmacokinetic considerations, similar interactions may occur with other drugs that are listed.

† Not available in the United States.

Tolterodine — *Fluoxetine*

Tolterodine* (*Detrol*)	Fluoxetine* (eg, *Prozac*)

Significance	Onset	Severity	Documentation
5	☐ Rapid	☐ Major	☐ Established
	■ **Delayed**	☐ Moderate	☐ Probable
		■ **Minor**	☐ Suspected
			☐ Possible
			■ **Unlikely**

Effects The pharmacologic and adverse effects of TOLTERODINE may be increased.

Mechanism Inhibition of TOLTERODINE metabolism (CYP2D6) by FLUOXETINE.

Management Based on available data, the magnitude of the effect of the interaction is not likely to be clinically important.

Discussion

The effect of fluoxetine on the pharmacokinetics of tolterodine was assessed in 9 psychiatric patients with subjective symptoms of urinary incontinence.[1] The study was an open-label, nonrandomized, crossover design. Patients were treated with tolterodine 2 mg twice daily for 2.5 days, followed by fluoxetine 20 mg/day for 3 weeks, then concurrent administration of fluoxetine for an additional 2.5 days. Each patient was genotyped with respect to the CYP2D6 isozyme. Three patients were extensive metabolizers with 1 functional CYP2D6 gene (EM1), 4 patients were extensive metabolizers with 2 functional CYP2D6 genes (EM2), and 2 patients had no functional CYP2D6 genes (ie, poor metabolizers). The AUC of tolterodine was 4.4 times higher in EM1 patients and 30 times higher in poor metabolizers than in EM2 individuals. The AUC of the active 5-hydroxymethyl metabolite could not be measured in the poor metabolizers. Fluoxetine decreased the oral clearance of tolterodine 93% and 80% in EM2 and EM1 patients, respectively. The AUC of the 5-hydroxymethyl metabolite decreased in EM1 and increased in EM2 patients. Because the active moiety is equal to the unbound tolterodine plus the 5-hydroxymethyl metabolite and neither exhibited a large change, a clinically important interaction is unlikely.

[1] Brynne N, et al. *Br J Clin Pharmacol.* 1999;48(4):553.

* Asterisk indicates drugs cited in interaction reports.

Tolterodine — *Proton Pump Inhibitors*

Tolterodine	Proton Pump Inhibitors	
Tolterodine* (eg, *Detrol*)	Esomeprazole (*Nexium*)	Pantoprazole (eg, *Protonix*)
	Lansoprazole (eg, *Prevacid*)	Rabeprazole (*Aciphex*)
	Omeprazole* (eg, *Prilosec*)	

Significance	Onset	Severity	Documentation
4	□ Rapid	□ Major	□ Established
	■ **Delayed**	■ **Moderate**	□ Probable
		□ Minor	□ Suspected
			■ **Possible**
			□ Unlikely

Effects Plasma concentrations of TOLTERODINE and its active metabolite may be elevated, increasing the pharmacologic effects and adverse reactions.

Mechanism Increased rate of drug release from TOLTERODINE extended-release capsules caused by an increase in gastric pH associated with PROTON PUMP INHIBITOR administration.

Management Monitor the clinical response and adjust the TOLTERODINE dose as needed.

Discussion

Using an open-label, randomized, single-dose, crossover design, the effects of omeprazole on the bioavailability of tolterodine were studied in healthy volunteers.[1] Each subject received tolterodine 4 mg/day for 4 days and omeprazole 20 mg/day for 4 days, followed by tolterodine 4 mg 1.5 hours after the last dose of omeprazole. Compared with administration of tolterodine alone, the ratio of the AUC of tolterodine to its active metabolite, 5-hydroxymethyltolterodine, was within the accepted range for bioequivalence (80% to 125%) when administered after pretreatment with omeprazole. However, the peak concentration ratios for tolterodine and its active metabolite exceeded the 80% to 125% acceptable range for pharmacokinetic bioequivalence. The C_{max} values for tolterodine, the active metabolite, and the calculated active moiety were 40% to 45% greater when tolterodine administration was preceded by omeprazole.

[1] Dmochowski R, et al. *J Clin Pharmacol.* 2005;45(8):961.

* Asterisk indicates drugs cited in interaction reports. Based on pharmacologic and pharmacokinetic considerations, similar interactions may occur with other drugs that are listed.

Tolvaptan — *Azole Antifungal Agents*

Tolvaptan* (*Samsca*)	Itraconazole* (eg, *Sporanox*)	Ketoconazole* (eg, *Nizoral*)

Significance	Onset	Severity	Documentation
1	☐ Rapid ■ **Delayed**	■ **Major** ☐ Moderate ☐ Minor	☐ Established ☐ Probable ■ **Suspected** ☐ Possible ☐ Unlikely

Effects TOLVAPTAN plasma concentrations may be elevated, increasing the pharmacologic effects and risk of adverse reactions.

Mechanism AZOLE ANTIFUNGAL AGENTS may inhibit the metabolism (CYP3A4) of TOLVAPTAN.

Management Coadministration of TOLVAPTAN and ITRACONAZOLE or KETOCONAZOLE is contraindicated.[1]

Discussion

Because tolvaptan is a substrate of CYP3A4, coadministration of itraconazole or ketoconazole may increase tolvaptan plasma concentrations. The effect of ketoconazole on the pharmacokinetics of tolvaptan was evaluated in 22 healthy subjects.[2] Coadministration of tolvaptan 30 mg daily with ketoconazole 200 mg daily for 3 days increased the tolvaptan C_{max} and AUC approximately 3.5- and 5.4-fold, respectively, compared with placebo. Because there is not adequate experience to determine the tolvaptan dose adjustment that would be needed to allow safe use with strong CYP3A4 inhibitors, coadministration of tolvaptan with itraconazole or ketoconazole is contraindicated.[1]

[1] *Samsca* [package insert]. Rockville, MD: Otsuka America Pharmaceutical Inc; February 2012.

[2] Shoaf SE, et al. *Br J Clin Pharmacol.* 2012;73(4):579.

* Asterisk indicates drugs cited in interaction reports.

Tolvaptan — *Food*

Tolvaptan*
(*Samsca*)

Grapefruit Juice*

Significance	Onset	Severity	Documentation
2	☐ Rapid ■ **Delayed**	☐ Major ■ **Moderate** ☐ Minor	☐ Established ☐ Probable ■ **Suspected** ☐ Possible ☐ Unlikely

Effects TOLVAPTAN plasma concentrations may be elevated, increasing the pharmacologic effects and risk of adverse reactions.

Mechanism Inhibition of TOLVAPTAN metabolism (CYP3A4) in the small intestine by GRAPEFRUIT.

Management Avoid coadministration of TOLVAPTAN and GRAPEFRUIT. Administer TOLVAPTAN with a liquid other than GRAPEFRUIT JUICE.

Discussion

Because tolvaptan is a substrate of CYP3A4, consumption of grapefruit juice may increase tolvaptan plasma concentrations. The effects of grapefruit juice on the pharmacokinetics of tolvaptan were studied in 20 healthy subjects.[1] Using an open-label, randomized, crossover design, each subject received a single oral dose of tolvaptan 60 mg with 240 mL of water or grapefruit juice. Compared with water, grapefruit juice increased the mean C_{max} and AUC of tolvaptan 1.86- and 1.56-fold, respectively. Avoid coadministration of tolvaptan with moderate or strong CYP3A4 inhibitors.[2]

[1] Shoaf SE, et al. *Eur J Clin Pharmacol.* 2012;68(2):207.

[2] *Samsca* [package insert]. Rockville, MD: Otsuka America Pharmaceutical Inc; May 2009.

* Asterisk indicates drugs cited in interaction reports.

Tolvaptan — *Macrolide & Related Antibiotics*

Tolvaptan* (*Samsca*)	Clarithromycin* (eg, *Biaxin*)	Telithromycin* (*Ketek*)

Significance	Onset	Severity	Documentation
1	☐ Rapid ■ **Delayed**	■ **Major** ☐ Moderate ☐ Minor	☐ Established ☐ Probable ■ **Suspected** ☐ Possible ☐ Unlikely

Effects TOLVAPTAN plasma concentrations may be elevated, increasing the pharmacologic effects and risk of adverse reactions.

Mechanism Certain MACROLIDE AND RELATED ANTIBIOTICS may inhibit the metabolism (CYP3A4) of TOLVAPTAN.

Management Coadministration of TOLVAPTAN and CLARITHROMYCIN or TELITHROMYCIN is contraindicated.[1]

Discussion

Because tolvaptan is a substrate of CYP3A4, coadministration of clarithromycin or telithromycin may increase tolvaptan plasma concentrations. Although this interaction has not been evaluated, coadministration of ketoconazole 200 mg daily (a strong CYP3A4 inhibitor) and tolvaptan produced a 5-fold increase in tolvaptan exposure. Because there is not adequate experience to determine the tolvaptan dose adjustment needed to allow safe use with strong CYP3A4 inhibitors, coadministration of tolvaptan with strong CYP3A4 inhibitors, such as clarithromycin or telithromycin, is contraindicated.[1]

The basis for this monograph is information on file with the manufacturer. Clinical evaluation of this interaction is needed to determine the consequences of coadministration of tolvaptan and macrolide and related antibiotics.

[1] *Samsca* [package insert]. Rockville, MD: Otsuka America Pharmaceutical Inc; May 2009.

* Asterisk indicates drugs cited in interaction reports.

Tolvaptan	*Nefazodone*
Tolvaptan* (*Samsca*)	Nefazodone*

Significance	Onset	Severity	Documentation
1	☐ Rapid ■ **Delayed**	■ **Major** ☐ Moderate ☐ Minor	☐ Established ☐ Probable ■ **Suspected** ☐ Possible ☐ Unlikely

Effects TOLVAPTAN plasma concentrations may be elevated, increasing the pharmacologic effects and risk of adverse reactions.

Mechanism NEFAZODONE may inhibit the metabolism (CYP3A4) of TOLVAPTAN.

Management Coadministration of TOLVAPTAN and NEFAZODONE is contraindicated.[1]

Discussion

Because tolvaptan is a substrate of CYP3A4, coadministration of nefazodone may increase tolvaptan plasma concentrations. Although this interaction has not been evaluated, coadministration of ketoconazole 200 mg daily, a strong CYP3A4 inhibitor, and tolvaptan produced a 5-fold increase in tolvaptan exposure. Because there is not adequate experience to determine the tolvaptan dose adjustment that would be needed to allow safe use with strong CYP3A4 inhibitors, coadministration of tolvaptan with strong CYP3A4 inhibitors, such as nefazodone, is contraindicated.[1]

The basis for this monograph is information on file with the manufacturer. Clinical evaluation of this interaction is needed to determine the consequences of coadministration of tolvaptan and nefazodone.

[1] *Samsca* [package insert]. Rockville, MD: Otsuka America Pharmaceutical Inc; May 2009.

* Asterisk indicates drugs cited in interaction reports.

Tolvaptan	*Protease Inhibitors*	
Tolvaptan* (*Samsca*)	Indinavir* (*Crixivan*)	Ritonavir* (*Norvir*)
	Nelfinavir* (*Viracept*)	Saquinavir* (*Invirase*)

Significance	Onset	Severity	Documentation
1	□ Rapid	■ **Major**	□ Established
	■ **Delayed**	□ Moderate	□ Probable
		□ Minor	■ **Suspected**
			□ Possible
			□ Unlikely

Effects TOLVAPTAN plasma concentrations may be elevated, increasing the pharmacologic effects and risk of adverse reactions.

Mechanism PROTEASE INHIBITORS may inhibit the metabolism (CYP3A4) of TOLVAPTAN.

Management Coadministration of TOLVAPTAN and INDINAVIR, NELFINAVIR, RITONAVIR, or SAQUINAVIR is contraindicated.[1]

Discussion

Because tolvaptan is a substrate of CYP3A4, coadministration of indinavir, nelfinavir, ritonavir, or saquinavir may increase tolvaptan plasma concentrations.[1] Although this interaction has not been evaluated, coadministration of ketoconazole 200 mg daily, a strong CYP3A4 inhibitor, and tolvaptan produced a 5-fold increase in tolvaptan exposure. Because there is not adequate experience to determine the tolvaptan dose adjustment that would be needed to allow safe use with strong CYP3A4 inhibitors, coadministration of tolvaptan with strong CYP3A4 inhibitors (eg, indinavir, nelfinavir, ritonavir, saquinavir) is contraindicated.

The basis for this monograph is information on file with the manufacturer. Clinical evaluation of this interaction is needed to determine the consequences of coadministration of tolvaptan and protease inhibitors.

[1] *Samsca* [package insert]. Rockville, MD: Otsuka America Pharmaceutical Inc; May 2009.

* Asterisk indicates drugs cited in interaction reports.

Tolvaptan — *St. John's Wort*

Tolvaptan* (*Samsca*)	St. John's Wort*

Significance	Onset	Severity	Documentation
2	□ Rapid ■ **Delayed**	□ Major ■ **Moderate** □ Minor	□ Established □ Probable ■ **Suspected** □ Possible □ Unlikely

Effects TOLVAPTAN plasma concentrations may be reduced, decreasing efficacy.

Mechanism Induction of TOLVAPTAN metabolism (CYP3A4) by ST. JOHN'S WORT.

Management Avoid coadministration of TOLVAPTAN and ST. JOHN'S WORT.[1] If coadministration cannot be avoided, TOLVAPTAN dosage adjustments may be needed when ST. JOHN'S WORT is started or stopped. Caution patients taking TOLVAPTAN to ask their health care provider before taking St. JOHN'S WORT.

Discussion

Because tolvaptan is a substrate of CYP3A4, coadministration of a CYP3A4 inducer, such as St. John's wort, may decrease tolvaptan plasma concentrations, resulting in a possible decrease in efficacy. Therefore, it is recommended that coadministration of tolvaptan and St. John's wort be avoided.[1]

The basis for this monograph is information on file with the manufacturer. Clinical evaluation of this interaction is needed to determine the consequences of coadministration of tolvaptan and St. John's wort.

[1] *Samsca* [package insert]. Rockville, MD: Otsuka America Pharmaceutical Inc; May 2009.

* Asterisk indicates drugs cited in interaction reports.

Topiramate — *Carbamazepine*

Topiramate* (*Topamax*)	Carbamazepine* (eg, *Tegretol*)

Significance	Onset	Severity	Documentation
2	☐ Rapid	☐ Major	☐ Established
	■ **Delayed**	■ **Moderate**	☐ Probable
		☐ Minor	■ **Suspected**
			☐ Possible
			☐ Unlikely

Effects CARBAMAZEPINE may decrease the pharmacologic effects of TOPIRAMATE.

Mechanism CARBAMAZEPINE may increase the metabolism of TOPIRAMATE.

Management Monitor the clinical response to TOPIRAMATE when starting, stopping, or changing the dose of CARBAMAZEPINE. Adjust the dose as needed.

Discussion

The effects of topiramate 800 mg/day or less on the pharmacokinetics of carbamazepine were studied in 12 patients with epilepsy stabilized on carbamazepine monotherapy 900 to 2,400 mg/day.[1,2] The addition of topiramate therapy did not change plasma concentrations of carbamazepine or its active epoxide metabolite. When carbamazepine was discontinued in 3 patients, the clearance of topiramate was reduced nearly 48%, compared with concurrent carbamazepine treatment. This reduction in clearance was accompanied by an increase in topiramate peak plasma concentrations, time to reach peak concentration, and AUC. Plasma and urine topiramate and topiramate metabolite concentrations were evaluated in patients receiving topiramate alone and in combination with carbamazepine.[3,4] Compared with taking topiramate alone, coadministration of carbamazepine increased clearance from 1.2 to 2.2 L/hr.

[1] Doose DR, et al. *Epilepsia.* 1994;35(suppl 8):54.
[2] Sachdeo RC, et al. *Epilepsia.* 1996;37(8):774.
[3] Mimrod D, et al. *Epilepsia.* 2005;46(7):1046.
[4] Britzi M, et al. *Epilepsia.* 2005;46(3):378.

* Asterisk indicates drugs cited in interaction reports.

Topiramate		*Hydantoins*
Topiramate* (*Topamax*)	Ethotoin (*Peganone*) Fosphenytoin (*Cerebyx*)	Phenytoin* (eg, *Dilantin*)

Significance	Onset	Severity	Documentation
4	☐ Rapid ■ **Delayed**	☐ Major ■ **Moderate** ☐ Minor	☐ Established ☐ Probable ☐ Suspected ■ **Possible** ☐ Unlikely

Effects HYDANTOINS may decrease the pharmacologic effects of TOPIRAMATE, while TOPIRAMATE may increase the effects of HYDANTOINS.

Mechanism HYDANTOINS may increase the metabolism of TOPIRAMATE, while TOPIRAMATE may decrease the metabolism of HYDANTOINS.

Management Monitor clinical response when starting, stopping, or changing the dose of either agent. Monitor plasma HYDANTOIN levels and observe clinical response when TOPIRAMATE is started or stopped in patients receiving HYDANTOIN therapy. However, it is unlikely that resulting changes in HYDANTOIN plasma levels warrant dosage adjustments in most patients.

Discussion

The effects of topiramate 800 mg/day or less on the pharmacokinetics of phenytoin were studied in 12 patients stabilized on phenytoin monotherapy 260 to 600 mg/day.[1,2] In 6 patients, there were no changes in either total or unbound plasma phenytoin concentrations when topiramate was added to their regimen; however, in the other 6 patients, the AUC of phenytoin was approximately 25% greater during concurrent therapy with topiramate than during phenytoin monotherapy. It was not necessary to adjust the phenytoin dose in these patients. When phenytoin was discontinued, the plasma clearance of topiramate decreased 59% compared with its clearance during coadministration with phenytoin. This reduction in clearance was accompanied by increases in topiramate peak and average plasma concentrations, time to reach peak concentrations, and AUC. Similar results were noted in a study of 10 patients.[3] In addition, phenytoin increased the clearance of topiramate from 26.6 mL/min to a range of 55 to 65 mL/min, which resulted in a decrease in the AUC, C_{max}, and time to peak concentration.

[1] Bourgeois BF. *Epilepsia.* 1996;37(suppl 2):S14.
[2] Gisclon LG, et al. *Epilepsia.* 1994;35(suppl 8):54.
[3] Sachdeo RC, et al. *Epilepsia.* 2002;43(7):691.

* Asterisk indicates drugs cited in interaction reports. Based on pharmacologic and pharmacokinetic considerations, similar interactions may occur with other drugs that are listed.

Topiramate — *Posaconazole*

Topiramate* (eg, *Topamax*)	Posaconazole* (*Noxafil*)

Significance	Onset	Severity	Documentation
4	☐ Rapid	☐ Major	☐ Established
	■ **Delayed**	■ **Moderate**	☐ Probable
		☐ Minor	☐ Suspected
			■ **Possible**
			☐ Unlikely

Effects TOPIRAMATE plasma concentrations may be elevated, increasing the pharmacologic effects and adverse reactions.

Mechanism Inhibition of TOPIRAMATE metabolism (CYP3A4) by POSACONAZOLE is suspected.

Management Monitor the clinical response of the patient and adjust the TOPIRAMATE dose as needed.

Discussion

Topiramate toxicity was reported in a 48-year-old man during coadministration of posaconazole.[1] The patient had a long-standing history of epilepsy that had been stabilized on a regimen that included topiramate 100 mg twice daily. After being treated in the hospital for invasive aspergillosis, the patient was discharged on posaconazole 200 mg 4 times daily. The patient was hospitalized again 14 days later because of a 10-day progressive stupor, daytime somnolence, anorexia, decreased oral intake, and weight loss. Posaconazole was discontinued 2 days prior to hospital admission. At the time of hospitalization, topiramate plasma concentrations were grossly elevated (27.34 mcmol/L). Eleven days after posaconazole discontinuation, topiramate concentration was 11.51 mcmol/L and coincided with partial resolution of the patient's symptoms. Posaconazole treatment was replaced with voriconazole (*Vfend*) without further complications.[1]

[1] Marriott D, et al. *Ann Intern Med.* 2009;151(2):143.

* Asterisk indicates drugs cited in interaction reports.

Topiramate — *Valproic Acid*

Topiramate* (*Topamax*)	Divalproex Sodium (*Depakote*)	Valproic Acid* (eg, *Depakene*)
	Valproate Sodium (eg, *Depacon*)	

Significance	Onset	Severity	Documentation
4	□ Rapid	□ Major	□ Established
	■ **Delayed**	■ **Moderate**	□ Probable
		□ Minor	□ Suspected
			■ **Possible**
			□ Unlikely

Effects VALPROIC ACID may decrease the pharmacologic effects of TOPIRAMATE. Similarly, TOPIRAMATE may decrease the pharmacologic effects of VALPROIC ACID.

Mechanism Possible increased metabolism of both agents.

Management Monitor clinical response when concurrent therapy with either agent is started, stopped, or changed in dosage. However, it is unlikely that resulting changes in VALPROIC ACID or TOPIRAMATE plasma concentrations would warrant dosage adjustments in most patients. Adjust dose as needed.

Discussion

The effects of topiramate (doses up to 800 mg/day) on the pharmacokinetics of valproic acid were studied in 12 patients stabilized on valproic acid monotherapy (1,000 to 4,500 mg/day).[1] Addition of topiramate to the valproic acid regimen increased the clearance of valproic acid approximately 13%, producing an 11% decrease in the AUC of valproic acid. When valproic acid was discontinued, topiramate peak plasma concentrations and AUC increased approximately 18%. In contrast, valproic acid did not affect the clearance of topiramate compared with control patients.[2]

[1] Rosenfeld WE, et al. *Epilepsia*. 1997;38:324.

[2] Mimrod D, et al. *Epilepsia*. 2005;46:1046.

* Asterisk indicates drugs cited in interaction reports. Based on pharmacologic and pharmacokinetic considerations, similar interactions may occur with other drugs that are listed.

Topotecan		*Hydantoins*	
Topotecan* (*Hycamitin*)		Fosphenytoin (*Cerebyx*)	Phenytoin* (eg, *Dilantin*)

Significance	Onset	Severity	Documentation
4	☐ Rapid ■ **Delayed**	☐ Major ■ **Moderate** ☐ Minor	☐ Established ☐ Probable ☐ Suspected ■ **Possible** ☐ Unlikely

Effects TOPOTECAN plasma levels may be reduced, decreasing the pharmacologic effects.

Mechanism Increased hepatic metabolism of TOPOTECAN by PHENYTOIN is suspected.

Management In patients receiving TOPOTECAN, carefully monitor clinical response when PHENYTOIN is started or stopped. Adjust the TOPOTECAN dose as needed.

Discussion

The effects of phenytoin on topotecan pharmacokinetics were studied in a 5-year-old child with high-risk medulloblastoma.[1] Phenytoin oral suspension (5.2 mg/kg/day) was started as seizure prophylaxis 4 weeks prior to giving the first cycle of topotecan and was stopped 17 days prior to the second cycle. Compared with administration of topotecan alone, coadministration of phenytoin increased the lactone and total topotecan clearance 45% and 47%, respectively. Phenytoin increased the AUC of total N-desmethyl topotecan (an active metabolite) 117%. Although plasma levels of the active metabolite were increased, this increase in exposure is less than the decrease in exposure to topotecan lactone. Thus, an increase in topotecan dose may be necessary.

[1] Zamboni WC, et al. *Clin Cancer Res.* 1998;4:783.

* Asterisk indicates drugs cited in interaction reports. Based on pharmacologic and pharmacokinetic considerations, similar interactions may occur with other drugs that are listed.

Toremifene — *Rifamycins*

Toremifene* (*Fareston*)	Rifabutin (*Mycobutin*)	Rifapentine (*Priftin*)
	Rifampin* (eg, *Rifadin*)	

Significance	Onset	Severity	Documentation
2	□ Rapid	□ Major	□ Established
	■ **Delayed**	■ **Moderate**	□ Probable
		□ Minor	■ **Suspected**
			□ Possible
			□ Unlikely

Effects Plasma concentrations of TOREMIFENE may be reduced, decreasing the antiestrogenic effect.

Mechanism RIFAMYCINS increase TOREMIFENE metabolism by inducing CYP3A4.

Management Monitor the clinical response of the patient. It may be necessary to increase the dose of TOREMIFENE during coadministration of a RIFAMYCIN.

Discussion

In a randomized, placebo-controlled, crossover trial, the effects of rifampin on the pharmacokinetics of toremifene were studied in 9 healthy men.[1] Each subject received rifampin 600 mg or placebo once daily for 5 days. On day 6, toremifene 120 mg was taken. Pretreatment with rifampin reduced the peak plasma levels of toremifene 55% (from 722 to 322 ng/mL) and increased peak plasma levels of its active N-demethyltoremifene metabolite 46% (from 267 to 391 ng/mL). In addition, rifampin administration decreased the toremifene AUC 87% and the $t_{1/2}$ 46% (from 99 to 53 hours).

[1] Kivistö KT, et al. *Clin Pharmacol Ther.* 1998;64(6):648.

* Asterisk indicates drugs cited in interaction reports. Based on pharmacologic and pharmacokinetic considerations, similar interactions may occur with other drugs that are listed.

Tramadol — *MAOIs*

Tramadol	MAOIs	
Tramadol* (eg, *Ultram*)	Isocarboxazid* (*Marplan*)	Rasagiline* (*Azilect*)
	Linezolid* (*Zyvox*)	Selegiline* (eg, *Eldepryl*)
	Phenelzine* (eg, *Nardil*)	Tranylcypromine* (eg, *Parnate*)

Significance	Onset	Severity	Documentation
1	☐ Rapid	■ **Major**	☐ Established
	■ **Delayed**	☐ Moderate	☐ Probable
		☐ Minor	■ **Suspected**
			☐ Possible
			☐ Unlikely

Effects Potentially life-threatening serotonin syndrome (eg, agitation, altered consciousness, ataxia, myoclonus, overactive reflexes, shivering) may occur. In addition, the risk of seizures may be increased.

Mechanism Unknown.

Management Coadministration of TRAMADOL and RASAGILINE is contraindicated.[1] Use TRAMADOL with other MAOIs with extreme caution, especially when starting therapy or increasing the dose.[2] Be prepared to provide supportive care.

Discussion

Coadministration of rasagiline and tramadol is contraindicated because of possible serious adverse reactions.[1] Potentially life-threatening serotonin syndrome may occur with concurrent use of tramadol with MAOIs.[2] This may occur within the recommended dose of tramadol.

[1] *Azilect* [package insert]. North Wales, PA: Teva Pharmaceuticals Inc; December 2009.

[2] *Ultram* [package insert]. Raritan, NJ: Ortho-McNeil Pharmaceuticals Inc; March 2008.

* Asterisk indicates drugs cited in interaction reports.

Trazodone — *Carbamazepine*

Trazodone* (eg, *Oleptro*)	Carbamazepine* (eg, *Tegretol*)

Significance	Onset	Severity	Documentation
4	☐ Rapid ■ **Delayed**	☐ Major ■ **Moderate** ☐ Minor	☐ Established ☐ Probable ☐ Suspected ■ **Possible** ☐ Unlikely

Effects Plasma levels of TRAZODONE and its active metabolite may be decreased, producing a decrease in therapeutic effect, while CARBAMAZEPINE levels may be elevated, increasing therapeutic and adverse effects.

Mechanism Possibly increased metabolism (cytochrome P450 3A4) of TRAZODONE and m-chlorophenylpiperazine, and inhibition of CARBAMAZEPINE metabolism.

Management Monitor the clinical response of the patient when starting or stopping either agent and adjust therapy as needed.

Discussion

The effects of carbamazepine administration on plasma concentrations of trazodone and its active metabolite, m-chlorophenylpiperazine, were studied in 6 depressed patients being treated with trazodone.[1] Carbamazepine administration decreased plasma concentrations of trazodone and its active metabolite. Compared with trazodone alone, 4 weeks of concomitant administration of carbamazepine and trazodone decreased the plasma concentration of trazodone from 911 to 208 ng/mL, and the m-chlorophenylpiperazine concentration decreased from 106 to 44 ng/mL. The m-chlorophenylpiperazine/trazodone ratio increased from 0.128 to 0.221. There was no change in the clinical status of the patients with the lower trazodone plasma concentrations.

Elevated carbamazepine levels were reported in a 53-year-old man after adding trazodone to his treatment regimen.[2] Two months after starting trazodone, the patient's carbamazepine level increased from a range of 7.2 to 7.9 mg/L to a level of 10 mg/L. No toxicity was reported. The magnitude of the change is small. In a 77-year-old woman, the carbamazepine concentration increased from 8.4 to 11.6 mg/L (38%) 4 days after starting trazodone.[3] She experienced ataxia and tremor.

Additional studies are needed to determine the clinical importance of these findings.

[1] Otani K, et al. *Ther Drug Monit.* 1996;18(2):164.
[2] Romero AS, et al. *Ann Pharmacother.* 1999;33(12):1370.
[3] Sánchez-Romero A, et al. *Pharmacopsychiatry.* 2011;44(4):158.

* Asterisk indicates drugs cited in interaction reports.

Trazodone — *Ginkgo biloba*

Trazodone* (eg, *Oleptro*)	Ginkgo biloba*

Significance	Onset	Severity	Documentation
4	☐ Rapid	☐ Major	☐ Established
	■ **Delayed**	■ **Moderate**	☐ Probable
		☐ Minor	☐ Suspected
			■ **Possible**
			☐ Unlikely

Effects The sedative effects of TRAZODONE may be increased.

Mechanism Unknown.

Management Avoid the use of GINKGO BILOBA in patients treated with TRAZODONE. If GINKGO BILOBA cannot be avoided, assess the patient's response to TRAZODONE treatment when GINKGO BILOBA is started or stopped. If an interaction is suspected, it may be necessary to stop one or both agents.

Discussion

Coma was reported in an 80-year-old woman with Alzheimer disease during coadministration of trazodone and *Ginkgo biloba*. [1] Prior to receiving *Ginkgo biloba*, other medications the patient was receiving were discontinued. *Ginkgo biloba* 80 mg twice daily was started. To control behavioral disturbances, bromazepam† was replaced with trazodone 20 mg twice daily. Over the next 2 days, the patient's behavioral disturbances improved. On the third day, the patient became drowsy and developed instability of her gait. That evening, she fell asleep and her caregiver was unable to arouse her. The patient was taken to the hospital, where she received the benzodiazepine antagonist flumazenil (eg, *Romazicon*) 1 mg IV. The patient regained consciousness immediately. Trazodone and *Ginkgo biloba* were discontinued and bromazepam was restarted.

The ingredients of most herbal products are not standardized. It is unclear whether herbal products contain ingredients other than those listed on the label or purported to be present that could interact with trazodone.

[1] Galluzzi S, et al. *J Neurol Neurosurg Psychiatry*. 2000;68(5):679.

* Asterisk indicates drugs cited in interaction reports.
† Not available in the United States.

Trazodone ✕ *Macrolide & Related Antibiotics*

Trazodone	Macrolide & Related Antibiotics	
Trazodone* (eg, *Oleptro*)	Clarithromycin* (eg, *Biaxin*)	Telithromycin (*Ketek*)
	Erythromycin (eg, *Ery-Tab*)	

Significance	Onset	Severity	Documentation
4	☐ Rapid	☐ Major	☐ Established
	■ **Delayed**	■ **Moderate**	☐ Probable
		☐ Minor	☐ Suspected
			■ **Possible**
			☐ Unlikely

Effects TRAZODONE plasma concentrations may be elevated, increasing the pharmacologic effects and adverse reactions.

Mechanism Inhibition of TRAZODONE metabolism (CYP3A4) is suspected.

Management Monitor the clinical response of the patient to TRAZODONE and advise the patient of possible increased and prolonged sedation when certain MACROLIDE AND RELATED ANTIBIOTICS are started.

Discussion

The potential for a 2-way pharmacokinetic and pharmacodynamic interaction between trazodone and clarithromycin was evaluated in 10 healthy subjects.[1] In a randomized, double-blind, crossover study, each subject received clarithromycin 500 mg or a matching placebo 1 hour, 8 hours, and 24 hours prior to administration as well as 8 hours after administration of trazodone 50 mg, or a placebo. Compared with placebo, clarithromycin administration increased the trazodone C_{max} and AUC 35% and 99%, respectively, prolonged the $t_{1/2}$ from 7.1 to 13.9 hours, and reduced the oral clearance 46%. In addition, clarithromycin enhanced the sedative effects of trazodone. Trazodone did not affect the pharmacokinetics of clarithromycin.

[1] Farkas D, et al. *Clin Pharmacol Ther.* 2009;85(6):644.

* Asterisk indicates drugs cited in interaction reports. Based on pharmacologic and pharmacokinetic considerations, similar interactions may occur with other drugs that are listed.

Trazodone		*Phenothiazines*	
Trazodone* (eg, *Desyrel*)		Chlorpromazine (eg, *Thorazine*)	Promethazine (eg, *Phenergan*)
		Fluphenazine (eg, *Prolixin*)	Thiethylperazine (*Torecan*)
		Perphenazine	Thioridazine*
		Prochlorperazine (eg, *Compazine*)	Trifluoperazine
		Promazine (eg, *Sparine*)	

Significance	Onset	Severity	Documentation
4	☐ Rapid	☐ Major	☐ Established
	■ **Delayed**	■ **Moderate**	☐ Probable
		☐ Minor	☐ Suspected
			■ **Possible**
			☐ Unlikely

Effects Elevated TRAZODONE serum concentrations, increasing the pharmacologic and toxic effects.

Mechanism Possible inhibition of TRAZODONE hepatic metabolism (cytochrome P450 2D6) by THIORIDAZINE.

Management Consider monitoring the patient for a change in TRAZODONE activity if THIORIDAZINE is started or stopped. Adjust the dose of TRAZODONE as indicated.

Discussion

The effects of thioridazine on trazodone and its active metabolite, m-chlorophenylpiperazine (CPP), were studied in 11 depressed patients.[1] Ten patients received trazodone 150 mg at bedtime, and 1 received 300 mg for 18 weeks. Seven patients were also receiving a benzodiazepine. Thioridazine 20 mg twice daily was administered concurrently for 1 week. Thioridazine increased plasma concentrations of trazodone 36% (from 713 to 969 ng/mL) and CPP 54% (from 61 to 94 ng/mL).

[1] Yasui N, et al. *Ther Drug Monit.* 1995;17:333.

* Asterisk indicates drugs cited in interaction reports. Based on pharmacologic and pharmacokinetic considerations, similar interactions may occur with other drugs that are listed.

Trazodone | *Protease Inhibitors*

Trazodone	Protease Inhibitors	
Trazodone* (eg, *Desyrel*)	Amprenavir (*Agenerase*)	Lopinavir/Ritonavir (*Kaletra*)
	Atazanavir (*Reyataz*)	Nelfinavir (*Viracept*)
	Fosamprenavir (*Lexiva*)	Ritonavir* (*Norvir*)
	Indinavir (*Crixivan*)	Saquinavir (eg, *Fortovase*)

Significance	Onset	Severity	Documentation
2	□ Rapid ■ **Delayed**	□ Major ■ **Moderate** □ Minor	□ Established □ Probable ■ **Suspected** □ Possible □ Unlikely

Effects TRAZODONE plasma concentrations may be elevated, increasing the pharmacologic and adverse effects.

Mechanism Inhibition of TRAZODONE metabolism (CYP3A4) by PROTEASE INHIBITORS is suspected.

Management Monitor the patient for a change in TRAZODONE effect if a PROTEASE INHIBITOR is started or stopped. Adjust the dose of TRAZODONE as needed.

Discussion

The effects of short-term, low-dose administration of ritonavir (4 doses of 200 mg) on the pharmacokinetics and pharmacodynamics of trazodone were evaluated in 10 healthy volunteers.[1] Using a randomized, 4-way crossover design, each subject received a placebo to match trazodone plus a placebo to match ritonavir, trazodone (50 mg) plus ritonavir placebo, trazodone placebo plus ritonavir (4 doses of 200 mg), and trazodone (50 mg) plus ritonavir (4 doses of 200 mg). Compared with ritonavir placebo, ritonavir administration reduced the apparent oral clearance of trazodone 52% (from 155 to 75 mL/minute), prolonged the elimination $t_{1/2}$ 122% (from 6.7 to 14.9 hr), and increased the peak plasma concentration 34% (from 842 to 1125 ng/mL). Coadministration of ritonavir and trazodone impaired psychomotor performance as measured by the digital symbol substitution test. In addition, 3 subjects experienced nausea, dizziness, or hypotension; 1 of these subjects also experienced syncope.

[1] Greenblatt DJ, et al. *J Clin Pharmacol.* 2003;43:414.

* Asterisk indicates drugs cited in interaction reports. Based on pharmacologic and pharmacokinetic considerations, similar interactions may occur with other drugs that are listed.

Tretinoin — *Azole Antifungal Agents*

Tretinoin		Azole Antifungal Agents	
Tretinoin* (*Vesanoid*)		Fluconazole* (eg, *Diflucan*) Itraconazole (*Sporanox*)	Ketoconazole (eg, *Nizoral*)

Significance	Onset	Severity	Documentation
4	☐ Rapid ■ **Delayed**	■ **Major** ☐ Moderate ☐ Minor	☐ Established ☐ Probable ☐ Suspected ■ **Possible** ☐ Unlikely

Effects TRETINOIN plasma concentrations may be elevated, increasing the risk of neurotoxicity, including pseudotumor cerebri.

Mechanism Inhibition of TRETINOIN metabolism (CYP2C9 and CYP3A4) by AZOLE ANTIFUNGAL AGENTS is suspected.

Management If coadministration cannot be avoided, closely monitor for TRETINOIN side effects. Be prepared to change the TRETINOIN dose when an AZOLE ANTIFUNGAL AGENT is started or stopped.

Discussion

Pseudotumor cerebri was reported in a 4-year-old boy receiving tretinoin (45 mg/m^2/day) after fluconazole (100 mg/day) was added to his treatment regimen.[1] One day after starting fluconazole, the patient complained of headaches. By day 7, the patient had headaches, vomiting, and papilledema. A diagnosis of pseudotumor cerebri was made. When tretinoin was stopped, symptoms of increased intracranial pressure resolved within 24 hr. When tretinoin was restarted at 75% of the therapeutic dose, headache and vomiting recurred. When tretinoin was administered at 30% of the therapeutic dose, headaches and 1 episode of vomiting occurred over a 3-day period. Discontinuation of fluconazole resulted in complete resolution of his headache and vomiting within 24 hr, and the patient was able to tolerate the full dose of tretinoin (45 mg/m^2/day). Other medications the patient received that have been associated with pseudotumor cerebri were amphotericin B (discontinued 2 days prior to the development of any headache), cytarabine (discontinued 14 days prior to the headaches), and sulfamethoxazole (continued without adverse effects).

[1] Vanier KL, et al. *J Pediatr Hematol Oncol.* 2003;25:403.

* Asterisk indicates drugs cited in interaction reports. Based on pharmacologic and pharmacokinetic considerations, similar interactions may occur with other drugs that are listed.

Triamterene — *Cimetidine*

Triamterene* (*Dyrenium*)	Cimetidine* (eg, *Tagamet*)

Significance	Onset	Severity	Documentation
5	□ Rapid ■ **Delayed**	□ Major □ Moderate ■ **Minor**	□ Established □ Probable □ Suspected ■ **Possible** □ Unlikely

Effects CIMETIDINE increases the AUC and decreases the renal clearance and hydroxylation of TRIAMTERENE.

Mechanism Multiple mechanisms may be involved. CIMETIDINE may inhibit the oxidative metabolism of TRIAMTERENE and the renal tubular secretion of TRIAMTERENE.

Management If specific problems arise from the concomitant use of the 2 drugs, decrease the TRIAMTERENE dose or discontinue CIMETIDINE.

Discussion

In a single study of 6 healthy men after 4 days of combination therapy, cimetidine increased the AUC an average of 22% and decreased the renal clearance and hydroxylation of triamterene 28% and 32%, respectively.[1] Because of the large interindividual variation in the magnitude of change for the pharmacokinetic parameters and because a therapeutic range of serum concentrations for triamterene has not been established, it is unclear how clinically important this interaction is. If an individual patient does exhibit the interaction, it may be more useful to decrease the dose of triamterene than to change H_2 receptor antagonists because ranitidine (eg, *Zantac*) also alters the pharmacokinetics of triamterene.[2]

[1] Muirhead M, et al. *Clin Pharmacol Ther.* 1986;40:400.

[2] Muirhead M, et al. *J Pharmacol Exp Ther.* 1988;244:734.

* Asterisk indicates drugs cited in interaction reports.

Triamterene — *NSAIDs*

Triamterene	NSAIDs	
Triamterene* (*Dyrenium*)	Diclofenac* (eg, *Voltaren*)	Meclofenamic Acid (eg, *Ponstel*)
	Etodolac	Meloxicam (eg, *Mobic*)
	Fenoprofen (eg, *Nalfon*)	Nabumetone
	Flurbiprofen	Naproxen (eg, *Naprosyn*)
	Ibuprofen* (eg, *Motrin*)	Oxaprozin (eg, *Daypro*)
	Indomethacin* (eg, *Indocin*)	Piroxicam (eg, *Feldene*)
	Ketoprofen	Sulindac (eg, *Clinoril*)
	Ketorolac (eg, *Toradol*)	Tolmetin
	Meclofenamate	

Significance	Onset	Severity	Documentation
2	■ **Rapid**	□ Major	□ Established
	□ Delayed	■ **Moderate**	□ Probable
		□ Minor	■ **Suspected**
			□ Possible
			□ Unlikely

Effects Acute renal failure may occur.

Mechanism Possible NSAID inhibition of prostaglandins unmasks TRIAMTERENE nephrotoxicity.

Management Use the combination only when clearly needed; monitor closely. If renal failure occurs, stop both drugs and treat this complication. Recovery will begin within a few days, but full recovery may take weeks.

Discussion

Acute renal failure (oliguria, increased serum creatinine and serum urea nitrogen, decreased CrCl) was reported in patients and in 2 of 4 healthy subjects taking triamterene and indomethacin[1-4]; however, 3 patients[1,4] were hypovolemic and taking diuretics. Investigation into the possible mechanism suggests that triamterene increases prostaglandins E and F, which induce local vasodilation in the renal vasculature that mitigates nephrotoxic effects of triamterene.[5] When NSAIDs inhibit the prostaglandins, the toxicity of triamterene may be expressed. A survey of patients taking potassium-sparing diuretics has implicated these agents as a cause of renal failure in 19 patients.[6] Eight were taking triamterene/hydrochlorothiazide and 5 others were taking NSAIDs in addition to amiloride. NSAIDs may pose a risk as a similar picture has been seen in a patient using diclofenac and triamterene[7] and in 1 of 9 healthy subjects receiving ibuprofen and triamterene plus hydrochlorothiazide.[8]

[1] McCarthy JT, et al. *Mayo Clin Proc.* 1982;57(5):289.
[2] Favre L, et al. *Ann Intern Med.* 1982;96(3):317.
[3] Weinberg MS, et al. *Nephron.* 1985;40(2):216.
[4] Mathews A, et al. *Vet Hum Toxicol.* 1986;28(3):224.
[5] Favre L, et al. *Clin Sci.* 1983;64(4):407.
[6] Lynn KL, et al. *N Z Med J.* 1985;98(784):629.
[7] Harkonen M, et al. *Br Med J.* 1986;293:698.
[8] Gehr TW, et al. *Clin Pharmacol Ther.* 1990;47:200.

* Asterisk indicates drugs cited in interaction reports. Based on pharmacologic and pharmacokinetic considerations, similar interactions may occur with other drugs that are listed.

Tricyclic Antidepressants — *Androgens*

Imipramine* (eg, *Tofranil*)	Methyltestosterone* (eg, *Android*)

Significance	Onset	Severity	Documentation
5	□ Rapid ■ **Delayed**	□ Major □ Moderate ■ **Minor**	□ Established □ Probable □ Suspected ■ **Possible** □ Unlikely

Effects Administration of TRICYCLIC ANTIDEPRESSANTS and ANDROGENS may cause CNS effects (eg, paranoia).

Mechanism Unknown.

Management If an interaction is suspected, discontinue the ANDROGEN and reassess the status of the patient. Alternative therapy may be needed.

Discussion

Five men with primary unipolar depression were treated in a single-blind study with oral imipramine 75 to 150 mg/day and oral methyltestosterone 15 mg/day to determine if coadministration of the male hormone resulted in a more prompt response to the tricyclic antidepressant.[1] Within 1 to 4 days, 4 of the 5 patients exhibited a dramatic paranoid response that cleared rapidly upon hormone withdrawal.

More clinical data are needed to confirm this possible interaction.

[1] Wilson IC, et al. *Am J Psychiatry.* 1974;131(1):21.

* Asterisk indicates drugs cited in interaction reports.

Tricyclic Antidepressants — *Anorexiants*

Tricyclic Antidepressants		Anorexiants
Amitriptyline*	Imipramine* (eg, *Tofranil*)	Fenfluramine*†
Amoxapine	Nortriptyline (eg, *Pamelor*)	
Clomipramine (eg, *Anafranil*)	Protriptyline (eg, *Vivactil*)	
Desipramine* (eg, *Norpramin*)	Trimipramine (*Surmontil*)	
Doxepin (eg, *Sinequan*)		

Significance	Onset	Severity	Documentation
3	☐ Rapid	☐ Major	☐ Established
	■ **Delayed**	☐ Moderate	☐ Probable
		■ **Minor**	■ **Suspected**
			☐ Possible
			☐ Unlikely

Effects Serum concentrations of TRICYCLIC ANTIDEPRESSANTS (TCAs) may be increased.

Mechanism Possible inhibition of TCA metabolism by FENFLURAMINE.

Management Observe the patient's clinical response when starting or stopping FENFLURAMINE. Adjust the dose of TCA as needed.

Discussion

A possible drug interaction has been reported during coadministration of imipramine and fenfluramine.[1] The patient was a 55-year-old woman with a 5-year history of generalized anxiety disorder that had remained in remission while she was being treated with imipramine 350 mg/day. Other medications the patient had received during this time were hyoscyamine and levothyroxine. Her imipramine plus desipramine plasma levels, measured at the end of each year, ranged from 145 to 218 mcg/L. Four weeks after starting fenfluramine 20 mg 3 times daily for imipramine-related weight gain, the patient complained of momentarily falling asleep while driving. Her imipramine plus desipramine concentration was 704 mcg/L. Fenfluramine was discontinued, and she did not report any further episodes of daytime sleepiness. Her imipramine plus desipramine plasma concentration was 252 mcg/L. In an investigation of fenfluramine augmentation of desipramine in patients with depression refractory to desipramine, fenfluramine administration more than doubled steady-state plasma desipramine concentrations.[2] Steady-state plasma amitriptyline concentrations also have been found to increase after starting fenfluramine.[3]

[1] Fogelson DL. *Am J Psychiatry.* 1997;154(3):436.
[2] Price LH, et al. *J Clin Psychopharmacol.* 1990;10(5):312.
[3] Gunne LM, et al. *Postgrad Med J.* 1975;51(suppl 1):117.

* Asterisk indicates drugs cited in interaction reports. Based on pharmacologic and pharmacokinetic considerations, similar interactions may occur with other drugs that are listed.
† Not available in the United States.

Tricyclic Antidepressants — *Azole Antifungal Agents*

Amitriptyline* Imipramine* (eg, *Tofranil*)	Nortriptyline* (eg, *Pamelor*)	Fluconazole* (eg, *Diflucan*)	Ketoconazole* (eg, *Nizoral*)

Significance	Onset	Severity	Documentation
2	☐ Rapid ■ **Delayed**	☐ Major ■ **Moderate** ☐ Minor	☐ Established ☐ Probable ■ **Suspected** ☐ Possible ☐ Unlikely

Effects Serum TRICYCLIC ANTIDEPRESSANT (TCA) levels may be elevated, resulting in an increase in therapeutic and adverse effects, including cardiac arrhythmias.

Mechanism Inhibition of TCA metabolism is suspected (CYP2C9 by fluconazole; CYP3A4 by ketoconazole).

Management Monitor the patient's clinical response and TCA serum concentrations when starting or stopping AZOLE ANTIFUNGAL AGENTS. Adjust the dose of the TCA as needed.

Discussion

Drug interactions have been reported during coadministration of amitriptyline or nortriptyline with fluconazole[1-3] and imipramine with ketoconazole.[4] Toxicity has occurred.[1-3] In 4 patients, serum amitriptyline levels increased during coadministration of fluconazole.[2,3] Three of the 4 patients experienced signs of CNS toxicity associated with serum amitriptyline levels between 724 and 1,464 ng/mL (therapeutic levels, 150 to 250 ng/mL) after starting fluconazole therapy. There was a documented 89% increase in the serum amitriptyline level (from 185 to 349 ng/mL) in the fourth patient, who did not experience toxicity after 33 days of combined therapy with the TCA and fluconazole. Torsades de pointes, possibly caused by coadministration of amitriptyline and fluconazole, was reported in a 57-year-old woman.[5] Use of amitriptyline in combination with fluconazole has been reported to cause repeated syncopal episodes[5] and prolongation of the QT interval with torsades de pointes.[6] In a 65-year-old woman, the trough steady-state serum concentration of nortriptyline increased approximately 70% (from 149 to 252 ng/mL) 12 days after fluconazole treatment was started.[1] In a randomized controlled investigation, the effects of ketoconazole on the pharmacokinetics of single doses of imipramine and desipramine were studied in 2 groups of 6 healthy patients.[4] Ketoconazole did not affect the pharmacokinetics of desipramine or the 2-hydroxydesipramine metabolite of desipramine. However, ketoconazole administration decreased the oral clearance of imipramine 17%, prolonged the $t_{1/2}$ 15% (from 16.7 to 19.2 hours), increased the AUC 20%, and decreased the AUC of the desipramine metabolite of imipramine 9%.

1 Gannon RH, et al. *Ann Pharmacother.* 1992;26(11):1456.
2 Newberry DL, et al. *Clin Infect Dis.* 1997;24(2):270.
3 Duggal HS. *Gen Hosp Psychiatry.* 2003;25(4):297.
4 Spina E, et al. *Br J Clin Pharmacol.* 1997;43(3):315.
5 Dorsey ST, et al. *Am J Emerg Med.* 2000;18(2):227.
6 Robinson RF, et al. *Ann Pharmacother.* 2000;34(12):1406.

* Asterisk indicates drugs cited in interaction reports.

Tricyclic Antidepressants — *Barbiturates*

Tricyclic Antidepressants		Barbiturates	
Amitriptyline*	Nortriptyline* (eg, *Aventyl*)	Amobarbital* (*Amytal*)	Phenobarbital* (eg, *Solfoton*)
Amoxapine	Protriptyline* (eg, *Vivactil*)	Butabarbital (eg, *Butisol*)	Primidone (eg, *Mysoline*)
Clomipramine (eg, *Anafranil*)	Trimipramine (*Surmontil*)	Butalbital	Secobarbital (*Seconal*)
Desipramine* (eg, *Norpramin*)		Mephobarbital (*Mebaral*)	
Doxepin (eg, *Sinequan*)		Pentobarbital (eg, *Nembutal*)	
Imipramine* (eg, *Tofranil*)			

Significance	Onset	Severity	Documentation
5	☐ Rapid	☐ Major	☐ Established
	■ **Delayed**	☐ Moderate	☐ Probable
		■ **Minor**	☐ Suspected
			■ **Possible**
			☐ Unlikely

Effects BARBITURATES may lower serum concentrations of TRICYCLIC ANTIDEPRESSANTS (TCAs). CNS and respiratory depressant effects may be additive.

Mechanism Enhanced metabolism of TCAs is suspected. Possible additive or synergistic pharmacologic actions.

Management Adjust the dose of the TCA based upon patient response. Benzodiazepines may be alternatives to BARBITURATES. Separating the administration times of the 2 drugs may diminish the additive sedative effects.

Discussion

Although barbiturates are known enzyme-inducers, there are only a few reports of decreased serum concentrations of TCAs when these agents are used concurrently.[1-8] In most patients, adverse clinical effects were not noted.[5] Given the wide interindividual variation in response and serum concentration after a specific dose of TCA, the effect of the combination may be difficult to predict.[5,6] Because TCAs can cause toxicity and depression is not adequately treated by low serum concentrations, patients should be monitored when barbiturates are started or stopped.[9,10] Because benzodiazepines have been reported not to alter serum concentrations of TCAs, they might be an alternative to barbiturates.[4,5,11] There have been some reports of possible additive pharmacologic effects. Studies in rats described an increase in phenobarbital-induced sleep time when concomitant TCAs were used.[6,12] Two reviews of TCA toxicity indicated that phenobarbital can accentuate associated respiratory depression.[9,10]

[1] Hammer W, et al. *Int Congr Ser.* 1966;122:301.
[2] Alexanderson B, et al. *Br Med J.* 1969;4:764.
[3] Burrows GD, et al. *Br Med J.* 1971;4:113.
[4] Silverman G, et al. *Br Med J.* 1972;4:111.
[5] Ballinger BR, et al. *Psychopharmacol.* 1974;39:267.
[6] Moody JP, et al. *Eur J Clin Pharmacol.* 1977;11:51.
[7] Spina E, et al. *Ther Drug Monit.* 1996;18:60.
[8] von Bahr C, et al. *Clin Pharmacol Ther.* 1998;64:18.
[9] Crocker J, et al. *Clin Toxicol.* 1969;2:397.
[10] Noble J, et al. *Clin Toxicol.* 1969;2:403.
[11] Silverman G, et al. *Br Med J.* 1973;3:18.
[12] Liu SJ, et al. *Biochem Pharmacol.* 1976;25:2211.

* Asterisk indicates drugs cited in interaction reports. Based on pharmacologic and pharmacokinetic considerations, similar interactions may occur with other drugs that are listed.

Tricyclic Antidepressants ╳ *Benzodiazepines*

Desipramine* (eg, *Norpramin*)	Clonazepam* (eg, *Klonopin*)

Significance	Onset	Severity	Documentation
5	☐ Rapid ■ **Delayed**	☐ Major ☐ Moderate ■ **Minor**	☐ Established ☐ Probable ☐ Suspected ■ **Possible** ☐ Unlikely

Effects The pharmacologic effects of DESIPRAMINE may be decreased.

Mechanism Unknown.

Management Observe the patient's condition and monitor plasma DESIPRAMINE levels. Adjust the DESIPRAMINE dose as needed.

Discussion

After the addition of clonazepam to the therapeutic regimen, decreased serum desipramine levels occurred in a 34-year-old male psychiatric inpatient being treated for major depression with panic attacks.[1] The patient was treated with desipramine 200 mg daily, yielding a serum level of 99 ng/mL. Because of continuing depressive symptoms and panic attacks, the desipramine dose was increased to 300 mg daily (serum level, 171 ng/mL). During the fourth month of outpatient treatment, the patient experienced reemergence of panic attacks and was started on adjunctive clonazepam, which was titrated to a dose of 3 mg/day. Two weeks after being stabilized on 3 mg/day clonazepam and 300 mg/day desipramine, serum concentrations of desipramine were 90 ng/mL. As a result of the lower desipramine serum concentrations the dose was increased to 350 mg daily, resulting in serum concentrations of 180 ng/mL. The patient was maintained on both drugs for 3 months, at which time the clonazepam dose was tapered and discontinued. One week after stopping clonazepam treatment, the serum desipramine level increased to 280 ng/mL. The dose of desipramine was decreased to 300 mg daily, resulting in a serum concentration of 175 ng/mL. The patient remained free of depressive symptoms and panic attacks at this dosage. In a retrospective study, nortriptyline plasma levels were not affected by oxazepam (eg, *Serax*), alprazolam (eg, *Xanax*), or flunitrazepam (not available in the United States).[2] Whether nortriptyline was given by itself or derived from amitriptyline was not noted.

Additional controlled studies are needed to determine the clinical importance of this possible drug interaction.

[1] Deicken RF. *J Clin Psychopharmacol.* 1988;8:71.

[2] Jerling M, et al. *Ther Drug Monit.* 1994;16:1.

* Asterisk indicates drugs cited in interaction reports.

Tricyclic Antidepressants — *Beta-Blockers*

Imipramine* (eg, *Tofranil*)	Labetalol* (eg, *Normodyne*)

Significance	Onset	Severity	Documentation
4	☐ Rapid ■ **Delayed**	☐ Major ■ **Moderate** ☐ Minor	☐ Established ☐ Probable ☐ Suspected ■ **Possible** ☐ Unlikely

Effects The pharmacologic and toxic effects of IMIPRAMINE may be increased.

Mechanism Inhibition of IMIPRAMINE metabolism by the cytochrome P450 2D6 isozyme is suspected. In addition, more IMIPRAMINE is metabolized to the active metabolite, desipramine, so that desipramine serum levels are also higher.

Management Monitor patients for signs of IMIPRAMINE toxicity if LABETALOL is coadministered.

Discussion

In a placebo-controlled, 4-period crossover study, the effect of diltiazem (eg, *Cardizem*), verapamil (eg, *Calan*,) and labetalol on the bioavailability and metabolism of imipramine was investigated in 13 healthy subjects.[1] During 4 separate 7-day periods, subjects were randomly assigned to receive diltiazem 90 mg every 8 hours, verapamil 120 mg every 8 hours, labetalol 200 mg every 12 hours, or a placebo tablet every 12 hours. Each phase was separated by a minimum of 1 week. Imipramine 100 mg was administered 1 hour after the morning dose on the fourth day of the randomized treatment. Twelve subjects completed all 4 treatment periods. Compared with placebo, the AUC of imipramine was significantly increased by labetalol 53% ($P < 0.01$). The peak imipramine concentration was increased by labetalol (from 65 to 83 ng/mL). In addition, during labetalol administration, the amounts of imipramine metabolized to 2-hydroxyimipramine and from desipramine to 2-hydroxydesipramine were decreased.

[1] Hermann DJ, et al. *J Clin Pharmacol.* 1992;32:176.

* Asterisk indicates drugs cited in interaction reports.

Tricyclic Antidepressants		*Bupropion*
Amitriptyline Amoxapine Clomipramine (eg, *Anafranil*) Desipramine (eg, *Norpramine*) Doxepin (eg, *Sinequan*)	Imipramine* (eg, *Tofranil*) Nortriptyline* (eg, *Aventyl*) Protriptyline (*Vivactil*) Trimipramine* (eg, *Surmontil*)	Bupropion* (eg, *Wellbutrin*)

Significance	Onset	Severity	Documentation
4	☐ Rapid ■ **Delayed**	☐ Major ■ **Moderate** ☐ Minor	☐ Established ☐ Probable ☐ Suspected ■ **Possible** ☐ Unlikely

Effects Plasma concentrations of TRICYCLIC ANTIDEPRESSANTS (TCAs) may be elevated, producing an increase in pharmacologic and adverse effects.

Mechanism Possible inhibition of TCA metabolism by BUPROPION.

Management Observe the clinical response of the patient to the TCA when BUPROPION therapy is started or stopped.

Discussion

Increases in plasma levels of imipramine and the desipramine metabolite of imipramine were reported in a 64-year-old woman during coadministration of bupropion.[1] During an 8-year period, 10 plasma levels of imipramine were measured while the patient was receiving imipramine (150 or 200 mg/day) alone, and 4 levels were measured while she was receiving bupropion (225 mg/day) concurrently. Compared with administration of imipramine alone, coadministration of bupropion decreased the clearance of imipramine and desipramine 57% and 82%, respectively. In an 83-year-old woman, addition of bupropion to nortriptyline (75 mg/day) resulted in an increase in nortriptyline levels (from 96 to 274 ng/mL).[2] The patient became lethargic and confused and had fallen several times. Similarly, in a 62-year-old woman receiving trimipramine (100 mg/day), the addition of bupropion resulted in a generalized tonic-clonic seizure and trimipramine plasma levels in the toxic range.[3]

[1] Shad MU, et al. *J Clin Psychopharmacol.* 1997;17:118.
[2] Weintraub D. *Depress Anxiety.* 2001;13:50.
[3] Enns MW. *J Clin Psychiatry.* 2001;62:476.

* Asterisk indicates drugs cited in interaction reports. Based on pharmacologic and pharmacokinetic considerations, similar interactions may occur with other drugs that are listed.

Tricyclic Antidepressants — *Cholestyramine*

Doxepin* (eg, *Sinequan*)	Imipramine* (eg, *Tofranil*)	Cholestyramine* (eg, *Questran*)

Significance	Onset	Severity	Documentation
4	☐ Rapid ■ **Delayed**	☐ Major ■ **Moderate** ☐ Minor	☐ Established ☐ Probable ☐ Suspected ■ **Possible** ☐ Unlikely

Effects Serum TRICYCLIC ANTIDEPRESSANT (TCA) concentrations may be decreased, resulting in a decrease in therapeutic effects.

Mechanism Probable decreased bioavailability of the TCA caused by decreased absorption.

Management If both agents are coadministered, separate the administration times by as much time as possible and monitor patient response. Adjust the dose of TCA as indicated.

Discussion

Cholestyramine has been reported to decrease serum concentrations of TCAs.[1,2] The effect of cholestyramine on the steady-state plasma concentrations of imipramine and its metabolite, desipramine, was studied in 6 depressed patients.[2] Each patient was receiving chronic treatment with imipramine 75 to 150 mg/day in divided doses. All patients were receiving cholestyramine 4 g dissolved in fruit juice 3 times daily for 5 days. Steady-state plasma concentrations of imipramine and desipramine were estimated on 2 occasions the week before cholestyramine was started, on days 4 and 5 of treatment with the resin, and on 2 occasions after stopping cholestyramine. Imipramine was taken simultaneously with cholestyramine, and the dosage remained unchanged throughout the study. Coadministration of cholestyramine and imipramine produced a decrease in plasma concentrations of the TCA from 211 to 159 nmol/L (25%; range, 11% to 30%). The effect was observed in all patients. Plasma concentrations of the desipramine metabolite were only marginally decreased. Plasma imipramine levels returned to baseline after cholestyramine administration was discontinued. In addition to this study, a case of decreased therapeutic effects of doxepin was described in a 69-year-old depressed man who was psychiatrically stable while receiving doxepin 300 mg at bedtime.[1] The patient was subsequently placed on cholestyramine 6 g 3 times daily prior to meals for the treatment of severe diarrhea. Three days later, his diarrhea was controlled and the dosage of cholestyramine was reduced to 6 g twice daily at 7 a.m. and 5 p.m. Within 2 weeks after starting cholestyramine, his affective symptoms recurred. The return of depression correlated with low serum doxepin concentrations. Cholestyramine appeared to decrease serum doxepin concentrations, even when the administration times of the drugs were separated by 6 hours.

[1] Geeze DS, et al. *Psychosomatics.* 1988;29(2):233.
[2] Spina E, et al. *Ther Drug Monit.* 1994;16(4):432.

* Asterisk indicates drugs cited in interaction reports.

Tricyclic Antidepressants — *Cinacalcet*

Amitriptyline	Imipramine (eg, *Tofranil*)	Cinacalcet* (*Sensipar*)
Amoxapine	Nortriptyline (eg, *Pamelor*)	
Clomipramine (eg, *Anafranil*)	Protriptyline (eg, *Vivactil*)	
Desipramine* (eg, *Norpramin*)	Trimipramine (*Surmontil*)	
Doxepin (eg, *Sinequan*)		

Significance	Onset	Severity	Documentation
4	☐ Rapid	☐ Major	☐ Established
	■ **Delayed**	■ **Moderate**	☐ Probable
		☐ Minor	☐ Suspected
			■ **Possible**
			☐ Unlikely

Effects Elevated plasma concentrations of certain TRICYCLIC ANTIDEPRESSANTS may be elevated, increasing the pharmacologic and toxic effects.

Mechanism Inhibition of certain TRICYCLIC ANTIDEPRESSANT metabolism (CYP2D6) by CINACALCET is suspected.

Management In patients receiving TRICYCLIC ANTIDEPRESSANTS, monitor the clinical response when CINACALCET is started or stopped. Plasma levels of TRICYCLIC ANTIDEPRESSANTS may be useful in managing these patients. Be prepared to adjust TRICYCLIC ANTIDEPRESSANT therapy as needed.

Discussion

The effects of cinacalcet on the pharmacokinetics of desipramine were evaluated in 14 healthy subjects.[1] Using a randomized, open-label, crossover design, each subject received a single dose of desipramine 50 mg alone and after a 7-day course of cinacalcet 90 mg daily. Compared with giving desipramine alone, coadministration of cinacalcet increased the desipramine AUC and C_{max} 3.6- and 1.8-fold, respectively, and prolonged the desipramine t½ from 21 to 43.3 hours. Adverse reactions occurred in 33% of subjects receiving desipramine alone compared with 86% when cinacalcet was coadministered with desipramine. All adverse reactions were mild to moderate severity.

[1] Harris RZ, et al. *Eur J Clin Pharmacol.* 2007;63(2):159.

* Asterisk indicates drugs cited in interaction reports. Based on pharmacologic and pharmacokinetic considerations, similar interactions may occur with other drugs that are listed.

Tricyclic Antidepressants — *Contraceptives, Hormonal*

Amitriptyline*	Imipramine (eg, *Tofranil*)	Contraceptives, Oral* (eg, *Ortho-Novum*)
Amoxapine	Nortriptyline (eg, *Pamelor*)	
Clomipramine (eg, *Anafranil*)	Protriptyline (*Vivactil*)	
Desipramine (eg, *Norpramin*)	Trimipramine (*Surmontil*)	
Doxepin (eg, *Sinequan*)		

Significance	Onset	Severity	Documentation
5	■ **Rapid**	□ Major	□ Established
	□ Delayed	□ Moderate	□ Probable
		■ **Minor**	□ Suspected
			■ **Possible**
			□ Unlikely

Effects Bioavailability and serum concentrations of the TRICYCLIC ANTIDEPRESSANTS (TCAs) may be increased in women taking ORAL CONTRACEPTIVES (OCs).

Mechanism Inhibition of hepatic metabolism of TCAs by OCs.

Management Monitor patient clinical response and serum TCA concentration, and decrease the TCA dose if needed.

Discussion

One study of healthy women found that the bioavailability of oral imipramine was increased by concurrent OC use, while clearance decreased and $t_{1/2}$ did not change.[1] The only change in the pharmacokinetic parameters after IV imipramine was an increase in $t_{1/2}$. These results are consistent with a decrease in hepatic oxidative metabolizing ability and a reduction in first-pass metabolism of the TCA. Bulimic women taking oral contraceptives had higher serum concentrations of amitriptyline compared with women who did not take OCs.[2] OCs had no effect on serum levels of clomipramine,[3] nor did they appear to alter the final response to clomipramine.[4] Although there is a potential for an interaction and TCAs are potent drugs with significant adverse reactions, no clinically important adverse reactions have been reported to date.

[1] Abernethy DR, et al. *Clin Pharmacol Ther.* 1984;35(6):792.
[2] Edelbroek PM, et al. *Clin Chim Acta.* 1987;165(2-3):177.
[3] John VA, et al. *J Int Med Res.* 1980;8(suppl 3):88.
[4] Gringas M, et al. *J Int Med Res.* 1980;8(suppl 3):76.

* Asterisk indicates drugs cited in interaction reports. Based on pharmacologic and pharmacokinetic considerations, similar interactions may occur with other drugs that are listed.

Tricyclic Antidepressants — *Diltiazem*

Imipramine* (eg, *Tofranil*)	Nortriptyline* (eg, *Pamelor*)	Diltiazem* (eg, *Cardizem*)

Significance	Onset	Severity	Documentation
4	☐ Rapid ■ **Delayed**	☐ Major ■ **Moderate** ☐ Minor	☐ Established ☐ Probable ☐ Suspected ■ **Possible** ☐ Unlikely

Effects The pharmacologic and adverse effects of certain TRICYCLIC ANTIDEPRESSANTS may be increased.

Mechanism Metabolism of imipramine or nortriptyline may be decreased.

Management Consider monitoring patients for signs of TRICYCLIC ANTIDEPRESSANTS toxicity if DILTIAZEM is coadministered.

Discussion

In a placebo-controlled, 4-period crossover study, the effect of diltiazem, verapamil (eg, *Calan*), and labetalol (eg, *Normodyne*, *Trandate*) on the bioavailability and metabolism of imipramine was investigated in 13 healthy subjects.[1] During 4 separate 7-day periods, subjects were randomly assigned to receive diltiazem 90 mg every 8 hours, verapamil 120 mg every 8 hours, labetalol 200 mg every 12 hours, or a placebo tablet every 12 hours. Each phase was separated by a minimum of 1 week. Imipramine 100 mg was administered 1 hour after the morning dose on the fourth day of the randomized treatment. Twelve subjects completed all 4 treatment periods. Compared with placebo, the AUC of imipramine was significantly increased by diltiazem 30% ($P < 0.01$). The peak imipramine concentration was increased by diltiazem (from 65 to 88 ng/mL). In a case report, nortriptyline serum levels increased from 58 to 167 mcg/L after addition of diltiazem (240 mg/day).[2]

[1] Hermann DJ, et al. *J Clin Pharmacol.* 1992;32:176.
[2] Krähenbühl S, et al. *Eur J Clin Pharmacol.* 1996;49:417.

* Asterisk indicates drugs cited in interaction reports.

Tricyclic Antidepressants — *Estrogens*

Tricyclic Antidepressants		Estrogens	
Amitriptyline*	Imipramine* (eg, *Tofranil*)	Conjugated Estrogens* (eg, *Premarin*)	Estrogenic Substance (eg, *Gynogen*)
Amoxapine	Nortriptyline (eg, *Pamelor*)	Diethylstilbestrol (DES)	Estrone (eg, *Theelin*)
Clomipramine (eg, *Anafranil*)	Protriptyline (*Vivactil*)	Esterified Estrogens (eg, *Estratab*)	Estropipate
Desipramine (eg, *Norpramin*)	Trimipramine (eg, *Surmontil*)	Estradiol (*Estrace*)	Ethinyl Estradiol* (*Estinyl*)
Doxepin* (eg, *Sinequan*)			

Significance	Onset	Severity	Documentation
5	☐ Rapid	☐ Major	☐ Established
	■ **Delayed**	☐ Moderate	☐ Probable
		■ **Minor**	☐ Suspected
			■ **Possible**
			☐ Unlikely

Effects ESTROGENS may augment the effects, both beneficial and adverse, of TRICYCLIC ANTIDEPRESSANTS (TCAs).

Mechanism Possible inhibition of TCA metabolism.

Management If adverse effects of TCAs occur, discontinue or lower the ESTROGEN dose or lower the ANTIDEPRESSANT dose.

Discussion

An early report described a beneficial effect on depression when low-dose (25 mcg) ethinyl estradiol was given with imipramine.[1,2] Higher doses caused toxicity (eg, drowsiness, hypotension) and others have noted adverse effects (eg, lethargy, headache, nausea, hypotension, akathisias) from the combination;[3,4] however, a beneficial effect from a high dose (15 mg) of conjugated estrogens was observed in 1 patient.[5] In contrast, no benefit from coadministration of imipramine and conjugated estrogen was seen in 11 patients resistant to tricyclic antidepressant therapy, and there was no change in total imipramine-desipramine concentrations.[6] It has been suggested that estrogens inhibit tricyclic antidepressant metabolism,[7] and a study in rats[8] demonstrated such an effect.

[1] Anon. *JAMA*. 1972;219:143.
[2] Prange AJ. *Excerpta Med Int Cong Series*. 1973;274:1023.
[3] Khurana RC. *JAMA*. 1972;222:702.
[4] Krishnan KR, et al. *Am J Psychiatry*. 1984;141:696.
[5] Berlanga C. *J Clin Psychiatry*. 1988;49:504.
[6] Shapira B, et al. *Biol Psychiatry*. 1985;20:570.
[7] Somani SM, et al. *JAMA*. 1973;223:560.
[8] Kok EC, et al. *Prog Neuropsychopharmacol Biol Psychiatry*. 1986;10:49.

* Asterisk indicates drugs cited in interaction reports. Based on pharmacologic and pharmacokinetic considerations, similar interactions may occur with other drugs that are listed.

Tricyclic Antidepressants — *Fluoxetine*

Amitriptyline*	Imipramine* (eg, *Tofranil*)	Fluoxetine* (eg, *Prozac*)
Amoxapine	Nortriptyline* (eg, *Pamelor*)	
Clomipramine (eg, *Anafranil*)	Protriptyline* (eg, *Vivactil*)	
Desipramine* (eg, *Norpramin*)	Trimipramine (*Surmontil*)	
Doxepin* (eg, *Sinequan*)		

Significance	Onset	Severity	Documentation
2	☐ Rapid ■ **Delayed**	☐ Major ■ **Moderate** ☐ Minor	☐ Established ■ **Probable** ☐ Suspected ☐ Possible ☐ Unlikely

Effects The pharmacologic and toxic effects of TRICYCLIC ANTIDEPRESSANTS (TCAs) may be increased.

Mechanism FLUOXETINE may inhibit TCA hepatic metabolism.

Management Observe the patient for signs of TCA toxicity and monitor TCA levels. Adjust the dose as necessary. When adding FLUOXETINE, it may be necessary to decrease the TCA dose as much as 75%. Start with lower than usual TCA doses when giving the drugs together or even several weeks after FLUOXETINE is discontinued.

Discussion

Healthy volunteers and patients treated for depression with desipramine, imipramine, or nortriptyline exhibited 37% to 250% increases in TCA levels after fluoxetine was added to their regimen.[1-10] Elevated blood levels and adverse reactions developed in 5 days to more than 5 weeks. In 5 patients, the reaction occurred despite a reduction in the TCA dose. Delirium was reported in a patient after 5 days of accidental ingestion of protriptyline while receiving fluoxetine.[11] Symptoms and elevated TCA levels may persist for several weeks after stopping fluoxetine.[1,2,4,6,7,12] In 2 groups of 6 patients receiving desipramine and imipramine 50 mg before and after giving fluoxetine 60 mg/day for 8 days, the oral clearance of both TCAs was decreased, $t_{1/2}$ was prolonged, and plasma levels elevated.[10] Compared with patients receiving amitriptyline alone, patients concurrently receiving fluoxetine had elevated amitriptyline and metabolite (nortriptyline) levels.[13] A patient died 6 weeks after starting amitriptyline 150 mg/day and fluoxetine 40 mg/day.[14] Death was caused by long-term amitriptyline intoxication secondary to fluoxetine-induced reduction in clearance.

1 Vaughan DA. *Am J Psychiatry.* 1988;145(11):1478.
2 Bell IR, et al. *J Clin Psychopharmacol.* 1988;8(6):447.
3 Downs JM, et al. *J Clin Psychiatry.* 1989;50(6):226.
4 Goodnick PJ. *Am J Psychiatry.* 1989;146(4):552.
5 Aranow AB, et al. *Am J Psychiatry.* 1989;146(7):911.
6 Schraml F, et al. *Am J Psychiatry.* 1989;146(12):1636.
7 Kahn DG. *J Clin Psychiatry.* 1990;51(1):36.
8 Downs JM, et al. *Am J Psychiatry.* 1990;147(9):1251.
9 Westermeyer J. *J Clin Pharmacol.* 1991;31(4):388.
10 Bergstrom RF, et al. *Clin Pharmacol Ther.* 1992;51(3):239.
11 Paul KL, et al. *Ann Pharmacother.* 1997;31(10):1260.
12 Rosenstein DL, et al. *Am J Psychiatry.* 1991;148(6):807.
13 el-Yazigi A, et al. *J Clin Pharmacol.* 1995;35(1):17.
14 Preskorn SH, et al. *JAMA.* 1997;277(21):1682.

* Asterisk indicates drugs cited in interaction reports. Based on pharmacologic and pharmacokinetic considerations, similar interactions may occur with other drugs that are listed.

Tricyclic Antidepressants — *Fluvoxamine*

Amitriptyline*	Trimipramine* (*Surmontil*)	Fluvoxamine* (eg, *Luvox*)
Clomipramine* (eg, *Anafranil*)		
Imipramine* (eg, *Tofranil*)		

Significance	Onset	Severity	Documentation
2	□ Rapid	□ Major	□ Established
	■ **Delayed**	■ **Moderate**	■ **Probable**
		□ Minor	□ Suspected
			□ Possible
			□ Unlikely

Effects The pharmacologic and toxic effects of TRICYCLIC ANTIDEPRESSANTS (TCAs) may be increased.

Mechanism FLUVOXAMINE may inhibit the oxidative metabolism (CYP2D6) of TCA.

Management If this combination cannot be avoided, the dose of the TCA may need to be reduced during coadministration of FLUVOXAMINE. Carefully observe the clinical response of the patient and monitor serum TCA concentrations when concurrent FLUVOXAMINE therapy is started or stopped. Using a TCA that does not undergo oxidation, such as desipramine (eg, *Pertofrane*), may avoid this interaction.

Discussion

Coadministration of amitriptyline, clomipramine, imipramine, or trimipramine with fluvoxamine has resulted in increased serum concentrations of these drugs, increasing the risk of toxicity.[1-5] One report involving 3 patients with major depression found a marked change in the parent TCA drug/metabolite ratio (6- to 9-fold increase).[1] The effect of fluvoxamine 100 mg daily for 10 days on the kinetics of a single oral dose of imipramine 50 mg was investigated in 12 healthy subjects.[3] Fluvoxamine treatment prolonged the $t_{1/2}$ of imipramine (from 22.8 to 40.5 hours) and decreased imipramine clearance (from 1.02 to 0.28 L/hr/kg). The inhibitory effects of fluvoxamine on the metabolism of the TCA dissipated 1 to 2 weeks after stopping concurrent fluvoxamine treatment.[2] The pharmacokinetics of the TCA desipramine, which is metabolized by hydroxylation, were not affected by concomitant administration of fluvoxamine.[3,4] The results of at least 1 investigation indicate that the drug interaction may be bidirectional, with plasma fluvoxamine concentrations increasing after administration of a TCA.[2]

[1] Bertschy G, et al. *Eur J Clin Pharmacol.* 1991;40(1):119.
[2] Härtter S, et al. *Psychopharmacology (Berl).* 1993;110(3):302.
[3] Spina E, et al. *Ther Drug Monit.* 1993;15(3):243.
[4] Spina E, et al. *Int J Clin Pharmacol Res.* 1993;13(3):167.
[5] Szegedi A, et al. *J Clin Psychiatry.* 1996; 57(6):257.

* Asterisk indicates drugs cited in interaction reports.

Tricyclic Antidepressants — *Food*

Amitriptyline*	Imipramine (eg, *Tofranil*)	High-Fiber Diet*
Amoxapine	Nortriptyline (eg, *Pamelor*)	
Clomipramine (eg, *Anafranil*)	Protriptyline (eg, *Vivactil*)	
Desipramine* (eg, *Norpramin*)	Trimipramine (*Surmontil*)	
Doxepin* (eg, *Sinequan*)		

Significance	Onset	Severity	Documentation
4	☐ Rapid	☐ Major	☐ Established
	■ **Delayed**	■ **Moderate**	☐ Probable
		☐ Minor	☐ Suspected
			■ **Possible**
			☐ Unlikely

Effects TRICYCLIC ANTIDEPRESSANT (TCA) serum levels may be reduced, decreasing the therapeutic effects.

Mechanism A HIGH-FIBER DIET may decrease TCA absorption.

Management Observe the patient's response to the TCA during ingestion of a HIGH-FIBER DIET. Adjust the diet as needed.

Discussion

Three patients with major depression successfully treated with TCAs experienced loss of therapeutic effect after adding high fiber to their diet.[1] A 43-year-old man was treated successfully on 6 occasions with doxepin 300 mg daily. Total serum doxepin levels (doxepin plus desmethyldoxepin levels) measured between 145 and 154 ng/mL during successful treatment (therapeutic range, 135 to 250 ng/mL). Six months after changing to a high-fiber diet, he was again treated for depression. He did not respond to doxepin 300 mg daily (total level, 114 ng/mL), and the dose was increased to 450 mg daily (total level, 116 ng/mL). The patient felt worse and lost 3 pounds. One month after stopping the high-fiber diet, he was no longer depressed, and his total serum doxepin level was 353 ng/mL. The dose of doxepin was reduced to 300 mg daily (total level, 154 ng/mL). A 42-year-old woman had been treated successfully on 4 occasions with desipramine 75 mg. Her serum levels ranged between 239 and 262 ng/mL (therapeutic range, 125 to 300 ng/mL). After she started eating a bran muffin for breakfast and lunch, an episode of depression failed to respond to a 3-week course of desipramine 75 mg daily (serum level, 114 ng/mL). She stopped eating the muffins and within 2 wk her depression was relieved (serum level, 245 ng/mL). A 52-year-old woman had previously been successfully treated with doxepin 225 mg daily (total serum doxepin level ranged from 155 to 176 ng/mL). After changing her diet to include fiber with each meal, a subsequent episode of depression failed to respond to doxepin 225 mg daily. The dose was increased to 350 mg daily. After 12 wk, the total serum doxepin level was 112 ng/mL. Within 3 wk of decreasing her fiber intake, her depression subsided and her total serum doxepin level increased to 166 ng/mL.

[1] Stewart DE. *J Clin Psychopharmacol.* 1992;12:438.

* Asterisk indicates drugs cited in interaction reports. Based on pharmacologic and pharmacokinetic considerations, similar interactions may occur with other drugs that are listed.

Tricyclic Antidepressants — *Furazolidone*

Amitriptyline*	Imipramine (eg, *Tofranil*)	Furazolidone*†
Amoxapine	Nortriptyline (eg, *Pamelor*)	
Clomipramine (eg, *Anafranil*)	Protriptyline (eg, *Vivactil*)	
Desipramine (eg, *Norpramin*)	Trimipramine (*Surmontil*)	
Doxepin (eg, *Sinequan*)		

Significance	Onset	Severity	Documentation
4	☐ Rapid	☐ Major	☐ Established
	■ **Delayed**	■ **Moderate**	☐ Probable
		☐ Minor	☐ Suspected
			■ **Possible**
			☐ Unlikely

Effects Variable. Acute psychosis has been noted.

Mechanism Possible release or augmentation of amines in the CNS.

Management Avoid this combination if possible. If concurrent use is necessary, follow all the precautions of MAO inhibitor and TRICYCLIC ANTIDEPRESSANT (TCA) combination therapy, such as using low doses, implementing dietary restrictions, and warning patients about potential side effects.

Discussion

A variety of effects have been attributed to this interaction including hypertension, hyperpyrexia, excitability, seizures, delirium, tachycardia, and tachypnea. The mechanism is presumed to be an intensification of amine action in the CNS.[1] Furazolidone has MAO inhibitor activity[2,3] and thus it may interact with the TCAs. One case report described a potential interaction between furazolidone and amitriptyline in a patient who developed blurred vision, diaphoresis, chills and hot flashes, hyperactivity, delusions, and hallucinations 3 days after beginning the combination.[4] In 1 study, the full MAO inhibitor activity of furazolidone was delayed for a few days after starting furazolidone and continued for several days after it was discontinued.[3] Thus, wait at least 2 wk after stopping furazolidone if a TCA is to be added. See also Tricyclic Antidepressants-MAO Inhibitors.

[1] Ponto LB, et al. *Am J Hosp Pharm.* 1977;34:954.
[2] Pettinger WA, et al. *Clin Pharmacol Ther.* 1968;9:341.
[3] Pettinger WA, et al. *Clin Pharmacol Ther.* 1968;9:442.
[4] Aderhold RM, et al. *JAMA.* 1970;213:2080.

* Asterisk indicates drugs cited in interaction reports. Based on pharmacologic and pharmacokinetic considerations, similar interactions may occur with other drugs that are listed.
† Not available in the United States.

Tricyclic Antidepressants — *Haloperidol*

Amitriptyline	Imipramine* (eg, *Tofranil*)	Haloperidol* (eg, *Haldol*)
Amoxapine (eg, *Asendin*)	Nortriptyline* (eg, *Pamelor*)	
Clomipramine (*Anafranil*)	Protriptyline (*Vivactil*)	
Desipramine (eg, *Norpramin*)	Trimipramine (eg, *Surmontil*)	
Doxepin (eg, *Sinequan*)		

Significance	Onset	Severity	Documentation
5	☐ Rapid	☐ Major	☐ Established
	■ **Delayed**	☐ Moderate	☐ Probable
		■ **Minor**	☐ Suspected
			■ **Possible**
			☐ Unlikely

Effects Increased serum concentration of the TRICYCLIC ANTIDEPRESSANT. A tonic-clonic seizure was seen in 1 patient.

Mechanism Possibly decreased metabolism of the TRICYCLIC ANTIDEPRESSANT.

Management Monitor serum concentrations and effects of the ANTIDEPRESSANT when HALOPERIDOL is started or stopped. Adjust the dose of the ANTIDEPRESSANT as needed.

Discussion

In 5 patients, higher serum concentrations or decreased urinary excretion of the tricyclic antidepressant was noted while the patient was taking haloperidol.[1-3] In 1 study, haloperidol was given to only 2 of 15 patients on neuroleptics and the effect of the haloperidol was not separated out.[2] Although no clinically significant effects were noted in these patients, 1 patient did have a single tonic-clonic seizure after more than 2 weeks of haloperidol and desipramine.[4] At the time, her serum concentration of desipramine was 610 ng/mL.

[1] Gram LF, et al. *BMJ.* 1972;1:463.
[2] Gram LF, et al. *Am J Psychiatry.* 1974;131:863.
[3] Nelson JC, et al. *Am J Psychiatry.* 1980;137:1232.
[4] Mahr GC, et al. *Can J Psychiatry.* 1987;32:463.

* Asterisk indicates drugs cited in interaction reports. Based on pharmacologic and pharmacokinetic considerations, similar interactions may occur with other drugs that are listed.

Tricyclic Antidepressants — *Histamine H_2 Antagonists*

Tricyclic Antidepressants		Histamine H_2 Antagonists
Amitriptyline*	Imipramine* (eg, *Tofranil*)	Cimetidine* (*Tagamet*)
Amoxapine (eg, *Asendin*)	Nortriptyline* (eg, *Pamelor*)	
Clomipramine (*Anafranil*)	Protriptyline (*Vivactil*)	
Desipramine* (eg, *Norpramin*)	Trimipramine (eg, *Surmontil*)	
Doxepin* (eg, *Sinequan*)		

Significance	Onset	Severity	Documentation
2	■ **Rapid**	□ Major	□ Established
	□ Delayed	■ **Moderate**	■ **Probable**
		□ Minor	□ Suspected
			□ Possible
			□ Unlikely

Effects Increased serum concentrations of the TRICYCLIC ANTIDEPRESSANT (TCA); mild symptoms have been noted.

Mechanism Interference with the metabolism of the TCA and decreased first-pass effect resulting in increased bioavailability and higher serum concentrations.

Management Monitor patient status and serum concentrations of TCAs when CIMETIDINE is used, particularly for several days after CIMETIDINE is started or stopped. Decrease the TCA dose as needed. Ranitidine may be substituted.

Discussion

Numerous controlled pharmacokinetic studies, mostly in healthy volunteers, have demonstrated that cimetidine increases the serum concentrations of TCAs when used concurrently.[1-7] Pharmacokinetic alterations include increased area under the concentration-time curve,[1,4,5,7,8] increased half-life,[2,5-7,9] decreased clearance,[1,2,5,7,9] and decreased volume of distribution.[1] Cimetidine also decreased the metabolism (hydroxylation and demethylation) of the TCA.[1-3,10,11] This effect was also seen as a decreased first-pass effect resulting in higher bioavailability.[1,2,8,4] The interaction was noted in a few cases clinically[3,6,9,10,12,13] and some patients reported adverse effects including anticholinergic effects, dizziness, drowsiness, and psychosis.[3,6,9,12-14] Thus, caution, and probably lower doses of TCAs, are necessary if the combination is used. Several researchers have found ranitidine to have no effect on the TCA.[5,6,11,15]

[1] Henauer SA, et al. *Clin Pharmacol Ther.* 1984;35:183.
[2] Abernethy DR, et al. *J Pharmacol Exper Ther.* 1984;229:702.
[3] Amsterdam JD, et al. *Psychopharmacology.* 1984;83:373.
[4] Abernethy DR, et al. *J Clin Psychopharmacol.* 1986;6:8.
[5] Wells BG, et al. *Eur J Clin Pharmacol.* 1986;31:285.
[6] Sutherland DL, et al. *Eur J Clin Pharmacol.* 1987;32:159.
[7] Steiner E, et al. *Clin Pharmacol Ther.* 1987;42:278.
[8] Curry SH, et al. *Eur J Clin Pharmacol.* 1985;29:429.
[9] Miller DD, et al. *Am J Psychiatry.* 1983;140:351.
[10] Brown MA, et al. *J Clin Psychopharmacol.* 1985;5:245.
[11] Spina E, et al. *Eur J Clin Pharmacol.* 1986;30:239.
[12] Miller DD, et al. *Drug Intell Clin Pharm.* 1983;17:904.
[13] Shapiro PA. *Am J Psychiatry.* 1984;141:152.
[14] Miller ME, et al. *Psychosomatics.* 1987;28:217.
[15] Curry SH, et al. *Eur J Clin Pharmacol.* 1987;32:317.

* Asterisk indicates drugs cited in interaction reports. Based on pharmacologic and pharmacokinetic considerations, similar interactions may occur with other drugs that are listed.

Tricyclic Antidepressants — *Lithium*

Tricyclic Antidepressants		Lithium
Amitriptyline	Imipramine* (eg, *Tofranil*)	Lithium* (eg, *Lithobid*)
Amoxapine	Nortriptyline* (eg, *Pamelor*)	
Clomipramine (eg, *Anafranil*)	Protriptyline (eg, *Vivactil*)	
Desipramine (eg, *Norpramin*)	Trimipramine (*Surmontil*)	
Doxepin (eg, *Sinequan*)		

Significance	Onset	Severity	Documentation
4	☐ Rapid	☐ Major	☐ Established
	■ **Delayed**	■ **Moderate**	☐ Probable
		☐ Minor	☐ Suspected
			■ **Possible**
			☐ Unlikely

Effects Neurotoxicity and psychotic symptoms have been reported, despite therapeutic LITHIUM levels.

Mechanism Unknown.

Management If an interaction is suspected, discontinue LITHIUM or the TRICYCLIC ANTIDEPRESSANT. Measure LITHIUM blood levels and adjust the dose accordingly.

Discussion

A 39-year-old woman was receiving imipramine when lithium 300 mg 3 times daily was initiated to reduce the risk of inducing mania before increasing the imipramine dosage for persistent depression.[1] Over the next few days, the patient became manic. Imipramine was discontinued and the lithium dosage was increased to 600 mg 3 times daily. The manic symptoms resolved over a 3-week period, with the patient remaining euthymic. This effect was attributed to lithium augmentation of the antidepressant effects of imipramine.[2,3] In 2 patients, high-dose administration of lithium carbonate produced myoclonic jerks when added to nortriptyline. Myoclonic jerking disappeared after the reduction or discontinuation of lithium therapy.[4] A 65-year-old woman taking nortriptyline 50 mg/day developed tremor, memory difficulties, distraction, and disorganized thinking 4 days after starting lithium 300 mg twice daily.[5] Her lithium concentration was 0.82 mEq/L. Symptoms resolved when the lithium was discontinued and haloperidol was started. Amitriptyline has been studied in combination with lithium in bipolar patients.[6] No change in lithium levels was noted, and adverse reactions were those seen with amitriptyline alone. No manic episodes were seen in the 23 patients treated for 6 weeks.[6] In a study of lithium augmentation of nortriptyline, no increase in adverse reactions or benefit occurred in depressed patients.[7]

1 Delisle JD. *Am J Psychiatry.* 1986;143(10):1326.
2 Dé Montigny C, et al. *Br J Psychiatry.* 1981;138:252.
3 Heninger GR, et al. *Arch Gen Psychiatry.* 1983;40(12):1335.
4 Devanand DP, et al. *J Clin Psychopharmacol.* 1988;8(6):446.
5 Austin LS, et al. *J Clin Psychiatry.* 1990;51(8):344.
6 Bauer M, et al. *J Clin Psychopharmacol.* 1999;19(2):164.
7 Nierenberg AA, et al. *J Clin Psychopharmacol.* 2003;23(1):92.

* Asterisk indicates drugs cited in interaction reports. Based on pharmacologic and pharmacokinetic considerations, similar interactions may occur with other drugs that are listed.

Tricyclic Antidepressants — *MAOIs*

Tricyclic Antidepressants		MAOIs	
Amitriptyline*	Imipramine* (eg, *Tofranil*)	Isocarboxazid* (*Marplan*)	Rasagiline (*Azilect*)
Amoxapine	Nortriptyline (eg, *Pamelor*)	Linezolid (*Zyvox*)	Selegiline (eg, *Eldepryl*)
Clomipramine* (eg, *Anafranil*)	Protriptyline (eg, *Vivactil*)	Phenelzine* (*Nardil*)	Tranylcypromine* (eg, *Parnate*)
Desipramine* (eg, *Norpramin*)	Trimipramine (*Surmontil*)		
Doxepin (eg, *Sinequan*)			

Significance	Onset	Severity	Documentation
1	■ **Rapid**	■ **Major**	■ **Established**
	□ Delayed	□ Moderate	□ Probable
		□ Minor	□ Suspected
			□ Possible
			□ Unlikely

Effects Hyperpyretic crises, convulsions, and death have occurred.

Mechanism Unknown.

Management Do not administer TCAs with or within 2 weeks of MAOI treatment.

Discussion

MAOIs and TCAs have been used together safely.[1-6] However, case reports have described adverse reactions from the combination,[7-20] including confusion, hyperexcitability, rigidity, seizures, increased temperature, pulse, respiration, sweating, mydriasis, flushing, headache, coma, disseminated intravascular coagulation, and death. Many reports are complicated by drug overdose, use of other drugs, underlying medical conditions, or food reactions.[4,21] Often, either the TCA or MAOI was given after the patient had been taking the other class of drugs for some time. Occasionally the reaction occurred when the drug was added 3 to 4 days after stopping the first agent.[12,14] Imipramine and clomipramine may be more likely to cause the reaction.[4,21]

1 Spiker DG, et al. *Arch Gen Psychiatry.* 1976;33(7):828.
2 Young JP, et al. *Br Med J.* 1979;2(6201):1315.
3 White K, et al. *Am J Psychiatry.* 1980;137(11):1422.
4 White K, et al. *J Clin Psychopharmacol.* 1981;1(5):264.
5 Razani J, et al. *Arch Gen Psychiatry.* 1983;40(6):657.
6 O'Brien S, et al. *J Clin Psychopharmacol.* 1992;12(2):104.
7 Davies G. *Br Med J.* 1960;2(5204):1019.
8 Singh H. *Am J Psychiatry.* 1960;117(4):360.
9 Howarth E. *J Ment Sci.* 1961;107:100.
10 Ayd FJ Jr. *J Neuropsychiatr.* 1961;2(suppl 1):119.
11 Kane FJ Jr, et al. *Am J Psychiatry.* 1963;120:79.
12 Brachfeld J, et al. *JAMA.* 1963;186:1172.
13 McCurdy RL, et al. *Am J Psychiatry.* 1964;121:397.
14 Ciocatto E, et al. *Resuscitation.* 1972;1(1):69.
15 Rom WN, et al. *Calif Med.* 1972;117(6):65.
16 Graham PM, et al. *Lancet.* 1982;2(8295):440.
17 de la Fuente JR, et al. *J Clin Psychiatry.* 1986;47(1):40.
18 Pascual J, et al. *Clin Neuropharmacol.* 1987;10(6):565.
19 Richards GA, et al. *J Neurol Neurosurg Psychiatry.* 1987;50(9):1240.
20 Tackley RM, et al. *Anaesthesia.* 1987;42(7):760.
21 Ponto LB, et al. *Am J Hosp Pharm.* 1977;34(9):954.

* Asterisk indicates drugs cited in interaction reports. Based on pharmacologic and pharmacokinetic considerations, similar interactions may occur with other drugs that are listed.

Tricyclic Antidepressants — *Methylphenidate*

Amitriptyline	Imipramine* (eg, *Tofranil*)	Methylphenidate* (eg, *Ritalin*)
Amoxapine	Nortriptyline (eg, *Aventyl*)	
Clomipramine (eg, *Anafranil*)	Protriptyline (eg, *Vivactil*)	
Desipramine (eg, *Norpramin*)	Trimipramine (eg, *Surmontil*)	
Doxepin (eg, *Sinequan*)		

Significance	Onset	Severity	Documentation
5	□ Rapid ■ **Delayed**	□ Major □ Moderate ■ **Minor**	□ Established □ Probable □ Suspected ■ **Possible** □ Unlikely

Effects Increased serum concentration of TRICYCLIC ANTIDEPRESSANTS.

Mechanism Inhibition of TRICYCLIC ANTIDEPRESSANT metabolism.

Management Consider monitoring for clinical symptoms. Decrease the dose of ANTIDEPRESSANT or stop either drug if adverse effects are noted.

Discussion

Initial reports indicated that methylphenidate improved the clinical response to imipramine.[1,2] Although in vitro studies[2] demonstrated that methylphenidate inhibits metabolism of imipramine, there is considerable interindividual variation. In addition, serum levels of methylphenidate and imipramine are frequently not reported. Two other case reports confirm a beneficial effect from the combination.[3,4] One report noted that serum antidepressant concentrations increased and then decreased when methylphenidate was started and stopped, respectively.[3] However, the second report may represent a natural time course in tricyclic antidepressant response;[4] methylphenidate was added 4 weeks after starting imipramine and no deterioration in clinical status was noted when methylphenidate was discontinued 2 weeks later. Significant adverse effects (eg, progressive dysfunctional behavior including violence, suicidal ideation, and depression) were seen in 2 adolescents given the combination, which improved when the 2 drugs were stopped.[5] High imipramine concentrations or additive pharmacologic actions may have been the cause.

Although the combination may prove beneficial in some patients, further data on the pharmacokinetic effects are needed.

1 Zeidenberg P, et al. *Am J Psychiatry.* 1971;127:1321.
2 Wharton RN, et al. *Am J Psychiatry.* 1971;127:1619.
3 Cooper TB, et al. *Am J Psychiatry.* 1973;130:721.
4 Meyers B. *Am J Psychiatry.* 1978;135:1420.
5 Grob CS, et al. *J Dev Behav Pediatr.* 1986;7:265.

* Asterisk indicates drugs cited in interaction reports. Based on pharmacologic and pharmacokinetic considerations, similar interactions may occur with other drugs that are listed.

Tricyclic Antidepressants — *NSAIDs*

Desipramine* (eg, *Norpramin*)	Ibuprofen* (eg, *Motrin*)

Significance	Onset	Severity	Documentation
4	☐ Rapid ■ **Delayed**	☐ Major ■ **Moderate** ☐ Minor	☐ Established ☐ Probable ☐ Suspected ■ **Possible** ☐ Unlikely

Effects Serum concentrations of DESIPRAMINE may be elevated, increasing the risk of adverse effects.

Mechanism Unknown.

Management Observe the clinical status of the patient when IBUPROFEN is started, stopped, or changed in dosage. Serum levels of DESIPRAMINE may be useful in managing the patient. Adjust the dose of DESIPRAMINE as needed.

Discussion

Tricyclic antidepressant toxicity was reported in a 15-year-old boy during coadministration of desipramine and ibuprofen.[1] The patient was receiving desipramine 50 mg every morning and 100 mg at bedtime for attention deficit disorder, major depressive disorder, and dysthymia. With this regimen, the desipramine serum concentration was 40 ng/mL. He had some periods of poor medication compliance and breakthrough symptoms and was placed on 300 mg of desipramine at bedtime (desipramine level 164 ng/mL). Because the patient would forget to take his medicine once or twice a week, the desipramine dose was increased to 375 mg at bedtime. One week later, he presented with chest wall pain and was treated with ibuprofen 600 mg 3 times daily. Seven days later, he experienced blurred vision, clouding of consciousness, 2 grand mal seizures, and ECG abnormalities (including prolongation of the QT_c interval). Medication counts ruled out overdose. His consciousness cleared with administration of IV physostigmine (*Antilirium*). Tricyclic antidepressant toxicity was confirmed when the desipramine concentration was measured to be 657 ng/mL.

[1] Gillette DW. *J Am Acad Child Adolesc Psychiatry*. 1998;37:1129.

* Asterisk indicates drugs cited in interaction reports.

Tricyclic Antidepressants — *Olanzapine*

Clomipramine*
(eg, *Anafranil*)

Olanzapine*
(eg, *Zyprexa*)

Significance	Onset	Severity	Documentation
4	☐ Rapid ■ **Delayed**	☐ Major ■ **Moderate** ☐ Minor	☐ Established ☐ Probable ☐ Suspected ■ **Possible** ☐ Unlikely

Effects Plasma CLOMIPRAMINE concentrations may be elevated, increasing the pharmacologic and adverse effects (eg, increased risk of seizures).

Mechanism Unknown.

Management Carefully monitor the clinical response of the patient during coadministration of CLOMIPRAMINE and OLANZAPINE.

Discussion

Seizures were reported in a 34-year-old man with schizophrenia complicated by obsessive-compulsive disorder during concurrent treatment with olanzapine and clomipramine.[1] Olanzapine 20 mg/day was started on an inpatient basis. The patient's psychotic symptoms, including thought disorganization, resolved, and he was discharged on olanzapine monotherapy. Subsequently, the patient was readmitted because of obsessive-compulsive hand washing. Clomipramine 50 mg/day was started and gradually increased to 250 mg/day. One week later, the patient reported myoclonic jerks of his right arm in association with dizziness. Generalized motor seizures were witnessed 11 days later, and electroencephalogram (EEG) findings were consistent with seizure activity. In addition, plasma clomipramine levels were elevated. Both drugs were withheld, and the seizures were treated with diazepam (eg, *Valium*). The patient's obsessive-compulsive symptoms persisted, and clomipramine was restarted with gradual increases in dose to 300 mg/day. When the patient later complained of auditory hallucinations, olanzapine was restarted at 15 mg/day. One week later, the patient experienced myoclonic jerks and an abnormal EEG. Both drugs were once again discontinued, and the seizures were managed with diazepam.

[1] Deshauer D, et al. *J Clin Psychopharmacol.* 2000;20(2):283.

* Asterisk indicates drugs cited in interaction reports.

Tricyclic Antidepressants — Paroxetine

Amitriptyline*	Nortriptyline* (eg, *Pamelor*)	Paroxetine* (eg, *Paxil*)
Desipramine* (eg, *Norpramin*)		
Imipramine* (eg, *Tofranil*)		

Significance	Onset	Severity	Documentation
2	☐ Rapid	☐ Major	☐ Established
	■ **Delayed**	■ **Moderate**	☐ Probable
		☐ Minor	■ **Suspected**
			☐ Possible
			☐ Unlikely

Effects The pharmacologic and toxic effects of certain TRICYCLIC ANTIDEPRESSANTS (TCAs) may be increased.

Mechanism PAROXETINE may inhibit the metabolism of certain TCAs (eg, DESIPRAMINE) in some patients (eg, extensive metabolizers of sparteine†) and may increase metabolism in some patients (eg, poor metabolizers of sparteine†).

Management Observe the patient for signs of TCA toxicity and monitor TCA plasma levels. Adjust the TCA dose as necessary when PAROXETINE is started or stopped. Be alert for signs of serotonin syndrome (eg, altered mental status, autonomic dysfunction, neuromuscular abnormalities) and be prepared to discontinue TCA therapy and treat as indicated.

Discussion

The effects of paroxetine 20 mg/day on the metabolism of a single dose of desipramine 100 mg were studied in 9 extensive and 8 poor metabolizers of sparteine. Paroxetine administration resulted in a 5-fold decrease in desipramine clearance in extensive metabolizers. Prior to giving paroxetine, desipramine metabolic clearance to 2-hydroxy desipramine was 40 times higher in extensive metabolizers than in poor metabolizers, compared with 2 times higher during paroxetine coadministration, suggesting that paroxetine increases formation of 2-hydroxydesipramine in poor metabolizers. Paroxetine increased the metabolism of desipramine to 2-hydroxydesipramine glucuronide in extensive and poor metabolizers, indicating paroxetine is also an inducer of glucuronidation.[1] Paroxetine increased the AUC of desipramine 5.2-fold.[2] In rapid metabolizers of nortriptyline, paroxetine 20 and 40 mg/day increased nortiptyline levels 3- and 5-fold, respectively.[3] Increases in amitriptyline levels have also been reported when paroxetine was added.[4] In 9 volunteers, pretreatment with paroxetine 30 mg/day for 4 days impaired the clearance of a single 50 mg dose of imipramine, resulting in an increase in peak levels and half-life of about 50%.[5] The half-life and AUC of the metabolite of imipramine (desipramine) were increased 150% and 300%, respectively. Serotonin syndrome symptoms (eg, bizarre movements, delirium, tachycardia) were reported in a patient receiving paroxetine 30 mg/day about 2 hours after taking imipramine 50 mg.[6] Symptoms resolved within 24 hours of discontinuing antidepressant therapy and starting a short course of cyproheptadine.

[1] Brøsen K, et al. *Eur J Clin Pharmacol.* 1993;44(4):349.
[2] Nichols AI, et al. *J Clin Pharmacol.* 2009;49(2):219.
[3] Laine K, et al. *Clin Pharmacol Ther.* 2001;70(4):327.
[4] Leucht S, et al. *Psychopharmacology.* 2000;147(4):378.
[5] Albers LJ, et al. *Psychiatry Res.* 1996;59(3):189.
[6] Weiner AL, et al. *Conn Med.* 1997;61(11):717.

* Asterisk indicates drugs cited in interaction reports.
† Not available in the United States.

Tricyclic Antidepressants — *Phenothiazines*

Tricyclic Antidepressants		Phenothiazines	
Amitriptyline	Imipramine* (eg, *Tofranil*)	Chlorpromazine* (eg, *Thorazine*)	Prochlorperazine (eg, *Compazine*)
Amoxapine	Nortriptyline* (eg, *Aventyl*)	Fluphenazine* (eg, *Prolixin*)	Thioridazine*
Clomipramine (*Anafranil*)	Protriptyline (eg, *Vivactil*)	Perphenazine*	Trifluoperazine
Desipramine* (eg, *Norpramin*)	Trimipramine (*Surmontil*)		
Doxepin (eg, *Sinequan*)			

Significance	Onset	Severity	Documentation
3	☐ Rapid	☐ Major	☐ Established
	■ **Delayed**	☐ Moderate	■ **Probable**
		■ **Minor**	☐ Suspected
			☐ Possible
			☐ Unlikely

Effects Increased serum concentrations of the TRICYCLIC ANTIDEPRESSANTS (TCAs).

Mechanism Possibly competitive inhibition of TCA metabolism.

Management Decrease the ANTIDEPRESSANT dose if adverse effects are noted.

Discussion

Several studies comparing groups of patients[1-4] or using the patient as his own control[5-10] have demonstrated that phenothiazines (PTZs) can increase the serum concentrations or decrease urinary excretion of TCAs. In 1 study,[11] there was no change in the TCA; however, this study used a single dose of PTZ with an established TCA regimen, whereas the other studies used multiple doses of PTZs. Studies with depot preparations of PTZs[12-14] indicate this might have the same effect as oral preparations; however, these studies used literature values of TCA concentrations as a comparison. It is probable that PTZs inhibit the metabolism of TCAs, perhaps competitively.[1,5,6,15] Studies with amitriptyline[15,16] have shown no change in amitriptyline concentration but have shown an increase in its metabolite nortriptyline, indicating that metabolic inhibition is related to specific pathways.[3,7,14,15] Only 1 study looked at the effect of TCAs on PTZs and found an increase in chlorpromazine concentration with concomitant use.[17] Although TCAs have significant adverse effects at higher concentrations, no toxicities were reported from the combination.

[1] Bock JL, et al. *Clin Pharmacol Ther.* 1983;33:322.
[2] Hirschowitz J, et al. *J Clin Psychopharmacol.* 1983;3:376.
[3] Jarling M, et al. *Ther Drug Monit.* 1994;16:1.
[4] Linnet K. *Ther Drug Monit.* 1995;17:308.
[5] Gram LF, et al. *Br Med J.* 1972;1:463.
[6] Gram LF, et al. *Am J Psychiatry.* 1974;131:863.
[7] Gram LF, et al. *Psychopharmacol Comm.* 1975;1:165.
[8] Overo KF, et al. *Acta Pharmacol Toxicol.* 1977;40:97.
[9] Maynard GL, et al. *Ther Drug Monit.* 1996;18:729.
[10] Mulsant BH, et al. *J Clin Psychopharmacol.* 1997;17:318.
[11] Kragh-Sorensen P, et al. *Eur J Clin Pharmacol.* 1977;11:479.
[12] Siris SG, et al. *Am J Psychiatry.* 1982;139:104.
[13] Siris SG, et al. *J Clin Psychiatry.* 1988;49:64.
[14] Siris SG, et al. *Clin Chem.* 1988;34:837.
[15] Vandel S, et al. *Neuropsychobiology.* 1986;15:15.
[16] Vandel B, et al. *Psychopharmacol.* 1979;65:187.
[17] Loga S, et al. *Clin Pharmacokinet.* 1981;6:454.

* Asterisk indicates drugs cited in interaction reports. Based on pharmacologic and pharmacokinetic considerations, similar interactions may occur with other drugs that are listed.

Tricyclic Antidepressants ✕ Propafenone

Tricyclic Antidepressants		Propafenone
Amitriptyline	Imipramine (eg, *Tofranil*)	Propafenone* (eg, *Rythmol*)
Amoxapine	Nortriptyline (eg, *Aventyl*)	
Clomipramine (eg, *Anafranil*)	Protriptyline (eg, *Vivactil*)	
Desipramine* (eg, *Norpramin*)	Trimipramine (*Surmontil*)	
Doxepin (eg, *Sinequan*)		

Significance	Onset	Severity	Documentation
4	☐ Rapid ■ **Delayed**	☐ Major ■ **Moderate** ☐ Minor	☐ Established ☐ Probable ☐ Suspected ■ **Possible** ☐ Unlikely

Effects The pharmacologic and toxic effects of TRICYCLIC ANTIDEPRESSANTS (TCAs) may be increased.

Mechanism Possibly inhibition of TCA metabolism.

Management Consider measuring serum TCA levels when the patient is receiving PROPAFENONE and when unexpected side effects or other findings suggest a possible interaction. Adjust the dose accordingly.

Discussion

Increased serum desipramine levels occurred in a 68-year-old man when the TCA was added to a treatment schedule that included digoxin (eg, *Lanoxin*) and propafenone.[1] The patient was hospitalized and started on desipramine 125 mg daily for an agitated major depression. The patient continued to feel depressed. His plasma desipramine level was 442 nmol/L (therapeutic range, 500 to 1,000 nmol/L), and the dosage was increased to 175 mg daily, which produced an excellent clinical response without side effects. The patient complained of palpitations, and a 24-hr Holter monitor disclosed paroxysmal atrial fibrillation and flutter. His cardiac rhythm did not improve with digoxin 0.25 mg daily; desipramine therapy was tapered then stopped. Several weeks later, his arrhythmia was suppressed when propafenone 150 mg twice daily and 300 mg at bedtime was added to the digoxin regimen. Following a relapse of major depression, desipramine was restarted and the dose was gradually increased to 150 mg daily. Although the patient's mood improved, he complained of dry mouth, sedation, and shakiness. Serum desipramine levels were 2,092 nmol/L. Desipramine was discontinued and restarted 5 days later at 75 mg daily. Plasma desipramine levels were still elevated (1,130 nmol/L) at this dose.

[1] Katz MR. *J Clin Psychiatry*. 1991;52:432.

* Asterisk indicates drugs cited in interaction reports. Based on pharmacologic and pharmacokinetic considerations, similar interactions may occur with other drugs that are listed.

Tricyclic Antidepressants — *Propoxyphene*

Doxepin* (eg, *Silenor*)	Nortriptyline* (eg, *Pamelor*)	Propoxyphene* (eg, *Darvon*)

Significance	Onset	Severity	Documentation
5	☐ Rapid ■ **Delayed**	☐ Major ☐ Moderate ■ **Minor**	☐ Established ☐ Probable ☐ Suspected ■ **Possible** ☐ Unlikely

Effects Increased serum concentrations of TRICYCLIC ANTIDEPRESSANTS. Clinical symptoms of CNS depression may be noted.

Mechanism Inhibition of TRICYCLIC ANTIDEPRESSANT metabolism.

Management If an interaction is suspected, decrease the dose of the TRICYCLIC ANTIDEPRESSANT or discontinue PROPOXYPHENE.

Discussion

Doxepin serum concentrations approximately doubled when propoxyphene was added to the drug regimen of an 89-year-old man.[1] The man became lethargic but gradually improved when propoxyphene was stopped. In rats, the combination of doxepin and propoxyphene produced a level of analgesia greater than propoxyphene alone, while doxepin alone produced no analgesia.[2] No measurements of serum concentrations were made. Studies with antipyrine indicate that propoxyphene can inhibit oxidative metabolism.[1] In a retrospective study, 10 patients at least 60 years of age receiving nortriptyline and propoxyphene had a higher concentration/dose ratio than patients receiving nortriptyline monotherapy.[3] The average propoxyphene dosage was 210 mg/day. Average nortriptyline concentrations were 405 nM with both drugs and 350 nM with monotherapy, indicating that the magnitude of the interaction is small and may not be clinically important.

Controlled studies are needed.

[1] Abernethy DR, et al. *Ann Intern Med.* 1982;97(2):223.
[2] Tofanetti O, et al. *Psychopharmacology (Berl).* 1977;51(2):213.
[3] Jerling M, et al. *Ther Drug Monit.* 1994;16(1):1.

* Asterisk indicates drugs cited in interaction reports.

Tricyclic Antidepressants — *Protease Inhibitors*

Tricyclic Antidepressants		Protease Inhibitors	
Amitriptyline	Nortriptyline (eg, *Pamelor*)	Atazanavir (*Reyataz*)	Ritonavir* (*Norvir*)
Clomipramine (eg, *Anafranil*)	Trimipramine (eg, *Surmontil*)	Fosamprenavir (*Lexiva*)	Tipranavir (*Aptivus*)
Desipramine* (eg, *Norpramin*)		Lopinavir/Ritonavir (*Kaletra*)	
Imipramine (eg, *Tofranil*)			

Significance	Onset	Severity	Documentation
4	☐ Rapid	☐ Major	☐ Established
	■ **Delayed**	■ **Moderate**	☐ Probable
		☐ Minor	☐ Suspected
			■ **Possible**
			☐ Unlikely

Effects TRICYCLIC ANTIDEPRESSANT (TCA) plasma concentrations may be elevated, increasing the pharmacologic effects and adverse reactions.

Mechanism Inhibition of TCA metabolism (CYP2D6) by PROTEASE INHIBITORS.

Management Consider monitoring TCA plasma concentrations. Observe the response of the patient when PROTEASE INHIBITOR therapy is started or stopped. Adjust the TCA dose as needed.

Discussion

In an open-label study, the effects of low-dose ritonavir (100 mg twice daily) on the pharmacokinetics of desipramine were investigated in 13 healthy men.[1] Each subject took a single dose of desipramine 50 mg alone and after 14 days of receiving ritonavir 100 mg twice daily. Compared with taking desipramine alone, pretreatment with low-dose ritonavir increased desipramine geometric mean AUC 26% and prolonged the $t_{1/2}$ from 17.1 to 22.3 hours. Coadministration of desipramine and ritonavir was well tolerated without any serious adverse reactions.

Additional studies are needed to determine the magnitude of the interaction with other TCAs and larger doses of ritonavir or other protease inhibitors.

[1] Aarnoutse RE, et al. *Clin Pharmacol Ther.* 2005;78(6):664.

* Asterisk indicates drugs cited in interaction reports. Based on pharmacologic and pharmacokinetic considerations, similar interactions may occur with other drugs that are listed.

Tricyclic Antidepressants — *Quinidine*

Desipramine* (eg, *Norpramin*)	Imipramine* (eg, *Tofranil*)	Quinidine*

Significance	Onset	Severity	Documentation
4	☐ Rapid ■ **Delayed**	☐ Major ■ **Moderate** ☐ Minor	☐ Established ☐ Probable ☐ Suspected ■ **Possible** ☐ Unlikely

Effects The pharmacologic effects of certain TRICYCLIC ANTIDEPRESSANTS (TCAs) may be increased.

Mechanism Competitive inhibition of the P450 isozyme responsible for 2-hydroxylation of DESIPRAMINE and IMIPRAMINE.

Management Consider observing the clinical response of the patient to TCAs and adjusting the dosage as needed.

Discussion

In 6 healthy volunteers, administration of quinidine significantly reduced the clearance of desipramine and imipramine via 2-hydroxylation but not via demethylation.[1] In 2 study periods of 12 days, patients ingested single oral doses of 200 mg sustained-release quinidine sulfate in the evening. At 8 AM on the fourth day, each subject received a single oral dose of 100 mg desipramine or imipramine. During coadministration of quinidine, the average total clearance of desipramine was reduced 85%, and that of imipramine 35%. Although quinidine administration did not significantly reduce the clearance of imipramine by demethylation, clearance by other pathways, primarily 2-hydroxylation, was reduced more than 50% ($P < 0.05$). Neither 2-hydroxyimipramine nor 2-hydroxydesipramine was detected in the plasma during coadministration of quinidine, but both were measurable in the absence of quinidine. These results were confirmed in another study of 10 volunteers in whom urinary excretion of 2-hydroxydesipramine was reduced during coadministration of quinidine.[2]

Controlled studies are needed to determine the clinical relevance and long-term effects of these observations.

[1] Brosen K, et al. *Eur J Clin Pharmacol.* 1989;37:155. [2] Steiner E, et al. *Clin Pharmacol Ther.* 1987;43:577.

* Asterisk indicates drugs cited in interaction reports.

Tricyclic Antidepressants ✕ *Quinolones*

Tricyclic Antidepressants		Quinolones	
Amitriptyline	Imipramine* (eg, *Tofranil*)	Gatifloxacin* (*Tequin*)	Moxifloxacin* (*Avelox*)
Amoxapine	Nortriptyline (eg, *Aventyl*)	Levofloxacin* (*Levaquin*)	Sparfloxacin* (*Zagam*)
Clomipramine (eg, *Anafranil*)	Protriptyline (eg, *Vivactil*)		
Desipramine (eg, *Norpramin*)	Trimipramine (*Surmontil*)		
Doxepin (eg, *Sinequan*)			

Significance	Onset	Severity	Documentation
1	□ Rapid	■ **Major**	□ Established
	■ **Delayed**	□ Moderate	□ Probable
		□ Minor	■ **Suspected**
			□ Possible
			□ Unlikely

Effects The risk of life-threatening cardiac arrhythmias, including torsades de pointes, may be increased.

Mechanism Unknown.

Management SPARFLOXACIN is contraindicated in patients receiving drugs that prolong the QTc interval (eg, TRICYCLIC ANTIDEPRESSANTS [TCAs]).[1] LEVOFLOXACIN should be avoided,[2] while GATIFLOXACIN[3] and MOXIFLOXACIN[4] should be used with caution. Other quinolone antibiotics that do not prolong the QTc interval or are not metabolized by the CYP3A4 isozyme may be suitable alternatives.

Discussion

Because torsades de pointes has been reported in patients receiving sparfloxacin concomitantly with amiodarone (eg, *Cordarone*) and disopyramide (eg, *Norpace*), sparfloxacin is contraindicated in patients receiving these antiarrhythmic agents or other QTc-prolonging drugs (eg, TCAs) or drugs known to cause torsades de pointes.[1,5] Rare cases of torsades de pointes have been reported in patients receiving gatifloxacin.[3] Moxifloxacin has prolonged the QT interval in some patients.[4] Because studies between gatifloxacin or moxifloxacin and drugs that prolong the QTc interval have not been performed, gatifloxacin and moxifloxacin should be used with caution when drugs that prolong the QT interval (eg, TCAs) are coadministered.[3,4] Levofloxacin has been associated with prolongation of the QT interval and infrequent cases of cardiac arrhythmias.[2] The risk of arrhythmias may be reduced by avoiding coadministration with other drugs that prolong the QT interval.[2]

[1] Thomas M, et al. *Br J Clin Pharmacol.* 1996;41:77.
[2] *Levaquin* [package insert]. Raritan, NJ: Ortho-McNeil Pharmaceuticals, Inc; February 2004.
[3] *Zagam* [package insert]. Collegeville, PA: Rhone-Poulenc Rorer Pharmaceuticals, Inc; November 1996.
[4] *Tequin* [package insert]. Princeton, NJ: Bristol-Myers Squibb Co; March 2004.
[5] *Avelox* [package insert]. West Haven, CT: Bayer Health Care; April 2004.

* Asterisk indicates drugs cited in interaction reports. Based on pharmacologic and pharmacokinetic considerations, similar interactions may occur with other drugs that are listed.

Tricyclic Antidepressants — *Rifamycins*

Tricyclic Antidepressants		Rifamycins	
Amitriptyline	Imipramine (eg, *Tofranil*)	Rifabutin (*Mycobutin*)	Rifampin* (eg, *Rifadin*)
Amoxapine (eg, *Asendin*)	Nortriptyline* (eg, *Pamelor*)		
Clomipramine (eg, *Anafranil*)	Protriptyline (eg, *Vivactil*)		
Desipramine (eg, *Norpramin*)	Trimipramine (*Surmontil*)		
Doxepin (eg, *Sinequan*)			

Significance	Onset	Severity	Documentation
2	☐ Rapid	☐ Major	☐ Established
	■ **Delayed**	■ **Moderate**	☐ Probable
		☐ Minor	■ **Suspected**
			☐ Possible
			☐ Unlikely

Effects TRICYCLIC ANTIDEPRESSANT (TCA) levels may be decreased, resulting in a decrease in pharmacologic effects.

Mechanism Hepatic metabolism of TCAs may be increased.

Management Consider monitoring TCA concentrations when starting, discontinuing, or altering the dose of RIFAMPIN. Adjust the TCA dose accordingly.

Discussion

During concurrent administration of rifampin and nortriptyline, higher-than-expected doses of the TCA were required to achieve therapeutic drug levels.[1] Following a diagnosis of pulmonary tuberculosis, a 51-year-old male patient was started on a regimen of isoniazid (eg, *Nydrazid*) 300 mg/day, rifampin 600 mg/day, pyrazinamide 500 mg 3 times daily, and pyridoxine (eg, *Nestrex*) 25 mg/day. In addition, a diagnosis of organic mood disorder with depressed mood was made, and nortriptyline 10 mg/day was initiated. The dose of nortriptyline was gradually titrated to 175 mg/day. While the dose of the TCA was being increased, pyrazinamide was discontinued without any effect on serum nortriptyline levels. Within 1 month of reaching a therapeutic serum level, the patient's depression improved. After 10 months of treatment, isoniazid, rifampin, and pyridoxine were discontinued. At this time, the serum nortriptyline level was 193 nmol/L (therapeutic, 150 to 500 nmol/L). Three weeks later, the patient suddenly became drowsy. The serum nortriptyline levels measured on 2 occasions were 562 and 671 nmol/L. The dose of nortriptyline was gradually decreased to 75 mg/day, resulting in a return of serum levels to the therapeutic range. A patient receiving nortriptyline (75 mg/day) had undetectable nortriptyline levels during concurrent administration of rifampin.[2] The serum nortriptyline concentration was 140 ng/mL 27 days after stopping rifampin.

Controlled studies are needed to determine the importance of this possible interaction.

[1] Bebchuk JM, et al. *Int J Psychiatry Med.* 1991;21:183.

[2] Self T, et al. *Am J Med Sci.* 1996;311:80.

* Asterisk indicates drugs cited in interaction reports. Based on pharmacologic and pharmacokinetic considerations, similar interactions may occur with other drugs that are listed.

Tricyclic Antidepressants — *Sertraline*

Amitriptyline*	Imipramine* (eg, *Tofranil*)	Sertraline* (*Zoloft*)
Amoxapine (eg, *Asendin*)	Nortriptyline* (eg, *Pamelor*)	
Clomipramine (eg, *Anafranil*)	Protriptyline (eg, *Vivactil*)	
Desipramine* (eg, *Norpramin*)	Trimipramine (*Surmontil*)	
Doxepin (eg, *Sinequan*)		

Significance	Onset	Severity	Documentation
2	☐ Rapid ■ **Delayed**	☐ Major ■ **Moderate** ☐ Minor	☐ Established ☐ Probable ■ **Suspected** ☐ Possible ☐ Unlikely

Effects The pharmacologic and toxic effects of TRICYCLIC ANTIDEPRESSANTS (TCAs) may be increased. "Serotonin syndrome" has been reported.

Mechanism Probable inhibition of TCA hepatic metabolism (CYP2D6).

Management If this combination cannot be avoided, observe the patient for signs of TCA toxicity and monitor TCA plasma levels. Adjust the TCA dose as needed when starting or stopping SERTRALINE. Be alert for signs of the serotonin syndrome (eg, altered mental status, autonomic dysfunction, neuromuscular abnormalities) and be prepared to discontinue the antidepressants and treat as needed.

Discussion

Desipramine plasma levels increased 60% in a 40-year-old man after starting sertraline 50 mg/day.[1] No adverse effects were noted. The effects of sertraline on the pharmacokinetics of desipramine were assessed in 18 healthy male volunteers who were extensive metabolizers of dextromethorphan.[2] Each subject received desipramine 50 mg/day for 49 days. Nine subjects received sertraline 50 mg/day for 3 weeks, starting on the eighth day of desipramine administration. Sertraline increased the mean peak plasma level of desipramine 34% and the area under the plasma concentration-time curve (AUC) 26%. After 3 weeks of sertraline and desipramine co-administration, desipramine values had reached steady state. Desipramine trough levels approached baseline values within 1 week of stopping sertraline. Elevations in plasma nortriptyline levels ranging from 2% to 117% were reported in 14 elderly depressed patients when sertraline was added to stable nortriptyline regimens.[4] Sertraline 150 mg/day to 12 healthy males resulted in a 22% increase in peak plasma levels, a 54% increase in the AUC of a single dose of desipramine 50 mg, a 39% increase in peak plasma levels, and a 68% increase in AUC of imipramine.[5]

Serotonin syndrome symptoms (eg, fever, diaphoresis, and hyperreflexia) were reported in a 40-year-old woman receiving 50 mg/day of sertraline 3 days after adding amitriptyline to her regimen.[3] The symptoms resolved within 24 hours of stopping both drugs.

See also Tricyclic Antidepressants-Fluoxetine and Tricyclic Antidepressants-Paroxetine.

[1] Lydiard RB, et al. *Am J Psychiatry.* 1993;150:1125.
[2] Preskorn SH, et al. *J Clin Psychopharmacol.* 1994;14:90.
[3] Alderman CP, et al. *Ann Pharmacother.* 1996;30:1499.
[4] Solai LKK, et al. *J Clin Psychiatry.* 1997;58:440.
[5] Kurtz DL, et al. *Clin Pharmacol Ther.* 1997;62:145.

* Asterisk indicates drugs cited in interaction reports. Based on pharmacologic and pharmacokinetic considerations, similar interactions may occur with other drugs that are listed.

Tricyclic Antidepressants — St. John's Wort

Tricyclic Antidepressants		St. John's Wort
Amitriptyline*	Imipramine (eg, *Tofranil*)	St. John's Wort*
Amoxapine	Nortriptyline* (eg, *Pamelor*)	
Clomipramine (eg, *Anafranil*)	Protriptyline (eg, *Vivactil*)	
Desipramine (eg, *Norpramin*)	Trimipramine (*Surmontil*)	
Doxepin (eg, *Sinequan*)		

Significance	Onset	Severity	Documentation
4	☐ Rapid	☐ Major	☐ Established
	■ **Delayed**	■ **Moderate**	☐ Probable
		☐ Minor	☐ Suspected
			■ **Possible**
			☐ Unlikely

Effects TRICYCLIC ANTIDEPRESSANT (TCA) concentrations may be reduced, resulting in a decrease in the pharmacologic effects.

Mechanism Increased hepatic metabolism or drug transporters of TCAs induced by ST. JOHN'S WORT are suspected.

Management Avoid the use of ST. JOHN'S WORT in patients treated with a TCA unless recommended and monitored by the patient's physician. Assess response to TCA treatment when ST. JOHN'S WORT is started or stopped. Adjust the TCA dose as needed.

Discussion

In an open-label investigation, the effect of St. John's wort extract (*Hypericum perforatum*) on the steady-state pharmacokinetics of amitriptyline was studied in 12 depressed patients.[1] Each subject received hypericum extract 900 mg/day concomitantly with amitriptyline 75 mg twice daily for at least 14 days. Coadministration of amitriptyline and St. John's wort resulted in a 21.7% decrease in the AUC of amitriptyline and a 40.6% decrease in the AUC of the nortriptyline metabolite of amitriptyline.

The ingredients of most herbal products are not standardized. It is unclear whether herbal products contain ingredients other than those listed on the label or purported to be present that could interact with TCAs.

[1] Johne A, et al. *J Clin Psychopharmacol.* 2002;22:46.

* Asterisk indicates drugs cited in interaction reports. Based on pharmacologic and pharmacokinetic considerations, similar interactions may occur with other drugs that are listed.

Amitriptyline*	Nortriptyline* (eg, *Pamelor*)	Terbinafine* (*Lamisil*)
Desipramine* (eg, *Norpramin*)		
Imipramine* (eg, *Tofranil*)		

Significance	Onset	Severity	Documentation
2	☐ Rapid	☐ Major	☐ Established
	■ **Delayed**	■ **Moderate**	☐ Probable
		☐ Minor	■ **Suspected**
			☐ Possible
			☐ Unlikely

Effects The pharmacologic and toxic effects of TRICYCLIC ANTIDEPRESSANTS (TCAs) may be increased.

Mechanism Inhibition of TCA metabolism (CYP2D6) by TERBINAFINE is suspected.

Management Monitor patients for signs of TCA toxicity if TERBINAFINE is coadministered. Adjust the TCA dose as needed.

Discussion

A 74-year-old man developed nortriptyline toxicity after terbinafine was added to his treatment regimen.[1] His serum nortriptyline level had been maintained at 200 ng/mL (therapeutic range, 75 to 150 ng/mL) for 3 months. After terbinafine was started, he experienced increasing fatigue and vertigo, as well as loss of energy and appetite. A few days later, he fell down a flight of stairs. His nortriptyline level was 366 ng/mL and increased to 450 ng/mL 7 days later. Terbinafine had been started 14 days previously for the treatment of onychomycosis. Because terbinafine was suspected to be the cause of the patient's reaction, the drug was discontinued. The dose of nortriptyline was reduced to 75 mg/day, and nortriptyline levels decreased to 125 ng/mL over a 3-week period. A rechallenge test was performed with terbinafine 250 mg/day. Nortriptyline levels increased to 200 ng/mL by day 7, and on day 8 he reported symptoms of nortriptyline toxicity again. Fifteen days after discontinuing terbinafine, nortriptyline levels decreased to 150 ng/mL. A similar report in a 48-year-old woman cited an increase in nortriptyline levels from 125 to 365 ng/mL.[2] In a 52-year-old man, terbinafine caused an increase in desipramine levels from 116 to 580 ng/mL and was associated with toxicity (eg, ataxia, difficulty swallowing, dizziness).[3] In 12 volunteers, terbinafine increased the AUC of desipramine nearly 5-fold.[4] A 51-year-old patient on stable imipramine doses developed toxicity (eg, muscle twitching) after receiving terbinafine.[5] Imipramine levels increased to 530 ng/mL from a baseline of 100 to 200 ng/mL. A 37-year-old woman experienced increased amitriptyline and nortriptyline levels as well as dizziness, dry mouth, and nausea after receiving terbinafine 250 mg/day for 1 month.[6] Despite discontinuation of terbinafine, the interaction appeared to persist for 6 months.

[1] van der Kuy PH, et al. *BMJ*. 1998;316:441.
[2] van der Kuy PH, et al. *Ann Pharmacother*. 2002;36:1712.
[3] O'Reardon JP, et al. *Am J Psychiatry*. 2002;159:492.
[4] Madani S, et al. *J Clin Pharmacol*. 2002;42:1211.
[5] Teitelbaum ML, et al. *Am J Psychiatry*. 2001;158:2086.
[6] Castberg I, et al. *Ther Drug Monit*. 2005;27:680.

* Asterisk indicates drugs cited in interaction reports.

Tricyclic Antidepressants ✕ *Thyroid Hormones*

Tricyclic Antidepressants		Thyroid Hormones	
Amitriptyline*	Imipramine* (eg, *Tofranil*)	Levothyroxine (eg, *Synthroid*)	Liotrix (*Thyrolar*)
Amoxapine	Nortriptyline (eg, *Pamelor*)	Liothyronine* (eg, *Cytomel*)	Thyroid* (eg, *Armour Thyroid*)
Clomipramine (eg, *Anafranil*)	Protriptyline (eg, *Vivactil*)		
Desipramine (eg, *Norpramin*)	Trimipramine (*Surmontil*)		
Doxepin (eg, *Sinequan*)			

Significance	Onset	Severity	Documentation
5	☐ Rapid	☐ Major	☐ Established
	■ **Delayed**	☐ Moderate	☐ Probable
		■ **Minor**	☐ Suspected
			■ **Possible**
			☐ Unlikely

Effects Acceleration of the onset of ANTIDEPRESSANT action. Increased adverse reactions of either agent.

Mechanism Unknown.

Management If adverse reactions are noted, discontinue one of the drugs.

Discussion

In controlled studies, the addition of small doses of thyroid accelerated the onset of action of the tricyclic antidepressant without effect on the ultimate response to the tricyclic antidepressant.[1-3] One study demonstrated a beneficial effect only when patients taking imipramine and liothyronine were compared with all other treatment groups combined.[4] When compared with patients taking imipramine alone, there were no differences. Two case reports have described potential toxicity from the combination. One patient developed dizziness, nausea, and paroxysmal tachycardia 21 days after beginning combination therapy.[5] A child developed thyrotoxicosis 5 months after starting combination therapy. She had remained euthyroid while taking thyroid supplements for almost 9 years.[6] A variety of mechanisms have been proposed for the interaction, but none have been demonstrated.[2]

[1] Wheatley D. *Arch Gen Psychiatry.* 1972;26(3):229.
[2] Prange AJ Jr, et al. *Am J Psychiatry.* 1969;126(4):457.
[3] Wilson IC, et al. *N Engl J Med.* 1970;282(19):1063.
[4] Coppen A, et al. *Arch Gen Psychiatry.* 1972;26(3):234.
[5] Prange AJ Jr. *Am J Psychiatry.* 1963;119:994.
[6] Colantonio LA, et al. *Am J Dis Child.* 1974;128(3):396.

* Asterisk indicates drugs cited in interaction reports. Based on pharmacologic and pharmacokinetic considerations, similar interactions may occur with other drugs that are listed.

Tricyclic Antidepressants — *Tramadol*

Amitriptyline*	Imipramine (eg, *Tofranil*)	Tramadol* (eg, *Ultram*)
Amoxapine	Nortriptyline (eg, *Pamelor*)	
Clomipramine (eg, *Anafranil*)	Protriptyline (eg, *Vivactil*)	
Cyclobenzaprine (eg, *Flexeril*)	Trimipramine (*Surmontil*)	
Desipramine (eg, *Norpramin*)		
Doxepin (eg, *Sinequan*)		

Significance	Onset	Severity	Documentation
2	☐ Rapid	☐ Major	☐ Established
	■ **Delayed**	■ **Moderate**	☐ Probable
		☐ Minor	■ **Suspected**
			☐ Possible
			☐ Unlikely

Effects Serotonin syndrome (eg, agitation, altered consciousness, ataxia, myoclonus, overactive reflexes, shivering) may occur.

Mechanism The serotonergic effects of these agents may be additive.

Management If coadministration of these agents cannot be avoided, closely monitor for symptoms of serotonin syndrome. Serotonin syndrome requires immediate medical attention, including withdrawal of the serotonergic agents and supportive care. Administration of an antiserotonergic agent (eg, cyproheptadine) may be helpful.

Discussion

A 79-year-old woman who had been taking amitriptyline 75 mg/day for a number of years developed symptoms consistent with serotonin syndrome after starting tramadol.[1,2] The day after starting tramadol, the patient experienced confusion and collapsed. Upon admission to the hospital, 3 days after starting tramadol, she was delirious and hallucinating. Over the next 2 days, her condition worsened and she became confused and sweaty, with pyrexia and muscular rigidity. Two days later, she experienced frequent seizures, increasing pyrexia and rigidity, deepening coma, tachycardia, sweating, and diaphoresis. Subsequently, the patient became unresponsive, hypotensive, and bradycardic, with poor respiratory effort, and died, despite intubation, fluid loading, and high-dose epinephrine.

Cyclobenzaprine is structurally related to TCAs and may interact similarly.

[1] Kitson R, et al. *Anaesthesia.* 2005;60(9):934.
[2] Kitson R. *Anaesthesia.* 2006;61(1):76.

* Asterisk indicates drugs cited in interaction reports. Based on pharmacologic and pharmacokinetic considerations, similar interactions may occur with other drugs that are listed.

Tricyclic Antidepressants — *Valproic Acid*

Tricyclic Antidepressants		Valproic Acid	
Amitriptyline*	Imipramine (eg, *Tofranil*)	Divalproex Sodium* (eg, *Depakote*)	Valproic Acid* (eg, *Depakene*)
Amoxapine	Nortriptyline (eg, *Aventyl*)	Valproate Sodium* (eg, *Depacon*)	
Clomipramine* (eg, *Anafranil*)	Protriptyline (eg, *Vivactil*)		
Desipramine (eg, *Norpramin*)	Trimipramine (*Surmontil*)		
Doxepin (eg, *Sinequan*)			

Significance	Onset	Severity	Documentation
2	☐ Rapid ■ **Delayed**	☐ Major ■ **Moderate** ☐ Minor	☐ Established ☐ Probable ■ **Suspected** ☐ Possible ☐ Unlikely

Effects Plasma concentrations and adverse reactions of the TRICYCLIC ANTIDEPRESSANT (TCA) may be increased.

Mechanism Decreased first-pass metabolism and inhibition of hepatic metabolism of the TCA.

Management Monitor plasma TCA concentrations and observe the clinical response of the patient when VALPROIC ACID is started or stopped. In patients stabilized on VALPROIC ACID, start with a conservative dose of the TCA when possible. Adjust the TCA dose as needed.

Discussion

The effect of divalproex sodium administration on the pharmacokinetics of amitriptyline and its active metabolite, nortriptyline, was studied in 15 healthy subjects.[1] Each subject received an oral dose of amitriptyline 50 mg alone. After the ninth dose, divalproex sodium 500 mg was administered once every 12 hours. Divalproex administration resulted in a 17% increase in the peak plasma concentration of amitriptyline and a 31% elevation in the AUC. The peak plasma concentration and AUC of nortriptyline were increased 28% and 55%, respectively. Coadministration of divalproex resulted in a 19% increase in the sum of the peak plasma concentrations of amitriptyline and nortriptyline, as well as a 42% increase in the sum of the AUCs. In a case report, clomipramine 75 mg/day was added to the treatment of a patient who was well controlled on valproic acid 750 mg 3 times daily.[2] Twelve days after the initiation of clomipramine, the patient developed status epilepticus, which was subsequently attributed to extremely high clomipramine serum levels (342 ng/mL) despite the low clomipramine dose. Similarly, clomipramine levels increased 142% (from 185 to 447 ng/mL) 5 days after starting valproate 1 g/day in a 46-year-old woman.[3]

[1] Wong SL, et al. *Clin Pharmacol Ther.* 1996;60(1):48.
[2] DeToledo JC, et al. *Ther Drug Monit.* 1997;19(1):71.
[3] Fehr C, et al. *J Clin Psychopharmacol.* 2000;20(4):493.

* Asterisk indicates drugs cited in interaction reports. Based on pharmacologic and pharmacokinetic considerations, similar interactions may occur with other drugs that are listed.

Tricyclic Antidepressants ✕ *Venlafaxine*

Tricyclic Antidepressants		Venlafaxine
Amitriptyline	Imipramine* (eg, *Tofranil*)	Venlafaxine* (eg, *Effexor*)
Amoxapine	Nortriptyline (eg, *Pamelor*)	
Clomipramine (eg, *Anafranil*)	Protriptyline (eg, *Vivactil*)	
Desipramine* (eg, *Norpramin*)	Trimipramine* (*Surmontil*)	
Doxepin (eg, *Sinequan*)		

Significance	Onset	Severity	Documentation
4	☐ Rapid	☐ Major	☐ Established
	■ **Delayed**	■ **Moderate**	☐ Probable
		☐ Minor	☐ Suspected
			■ **Possible**
			☐ Unlikely

Effects TRICYCLIC ANTIDEPRESSANT plasma levels may be elevated, increasing the pharmacologic effects and adverse reactions.

Mechanism VENLAFAXINE inhibits the hepatic metabolism (CYP2D6) of TRICYCLIC ANTIDEPRESSANTS.

Management In patients receiving TRICYCLIC ANTIDEPRESSANTS, observe the clinical response when VENLAFAXINE is started or stopped. TRICYCLIC ANTIDEPRESSANT plasma levels may be useful in managing the patient. Adjust TRICYCLIC ANTIDEPRESSANT therapy as needed. Desvenlafaxine (*Pristiq*) may be a safer alternative.[1]

Discussion

The effect of venlafaxine on the metabolism of imipramine was studied in 6 men.[2] Two additional patients were excluded from the study after being phenotyped as poor metabolizers of dextromethorphan. Each subject received imipramine 100 mg alone and after 3 days of treatment with venlafaxine 50 mg 3 times daily. Compared with taking imipramine alone, venlafaxine coadministration increased the imipramine AUC 28%. Venlafaxine increased the AUC of the metabolite of imipramine, desipramine, 40%; increased the peak concentration 41%; and decreased the clearance and volume of distribution of desipramine 20% and 25%, respectively. In a study of 20 healthy subjects, desvenlafaxine had a minimal impact on desipramine pharmacokinetics compared with duloxetine (*Cymbalta*).[1] Seizures, possibly associated with coadministration of trimipramine and venlafaxine, have been reported in a 25-year-old woman.[3] However, other causes could not be excluded.

[1] Patroneva A, et al. *Drug Metab Dispos.* 2008;36(12):2484.
[2] Albers LJ, et al. *Psychiatry Res.* 2000;96(3):235.
[3] Schlienger RG, et al. *Ann Pharmacother.* 2000;34(12):1402.

* Asterisk indicates drugs cited in interaction reports. Based on pharmacologic and pharmacokinetic considerations, similar interactions may occur with other drugs that are listed.

Tricyclic Antidepressants — *Verapamil*

Imipramine* (eg, *Tofranil*)	Verapamil* (eg, *Calan*)

Significance	Onset	Severity	Documentation
4	☐ Rapid ■ **Delayed**	☐ Major ■ **Moderate** ☐ Minor	☐ Established ☐ Probable ☐ Suspected ■ **Possible** ☐ Unlikely

Effects The pharmacologic and toxic effects of IMIPRAMINE may be increased.

Mechanism IMIPRAMINE clearance may be decreased.

Management Monitor patients for signs of IMIPRAMINE toxicity if VERAPAMIL is coadministered.

Discussion

In a placebo-controlled, 4-period crossover study, the effect of diltiazem (eg, *Cardizem*), verapamil, and labetalol (eg, *Trandate*) on the bioavailability and metabolism of imipramine was investigated in 13 healthy subjects.[1] During 4 separate 7-day periods, subjects were randomly assigned to receive diltiazem 90 mg every 8 hours, verapamil 120 mg every 8 hours, labetalol 200 mg every 12 hours, or a placebo tablet every 12 hours. Each phase was separated by a minimum of 1 week. Imipramine 100 mg was administered 1 hour after the morning dose on the fourth day of the randomized treatment. Twelve subjects completed all 4 treatment periods. Compared with placebo, the AUC of imipramine was significantly increased by verapamil 15% ($P < 0.05$). The peak imipramine concentration was increased by verapamil (from 65 to 76 ng/mL). Two subjects developed second-degree heart block during coadministration of imipramine and verapamil. Effects on the active metabolite of imipramine, desipramine, were not reported.

[1] Hermann DJ, et al. *J Clin Pharmacol.* 1992;32:176.

* Asterisk indicates drugs cited in interaction reports.

Trimethoprim — *Rifamycins*

Trimethoprim (eg, *Trimpex*)	Trimethoprim/ Sulfamethoxazole* (eg, *Bactrim*)	Rifampin* (eg, *Rifadin*)

Significance	Onset	Severity	Documentation
4	☐ Rapid	☐ Major	☐ Established
	■ **Delayed**	■ **Moderate**	☐ Probable
		☐ Minor	☐ Suspected
			■ **Possible**
			☐ Unlikely

Effects TRIMETHOPRIM/SULFAMETHOXAZOLE (TMP-SMZ) serum levels may be reduced, decreasing the therapeutic effect.

Mechanism Induction of TMP-SMZ metabolism by RIFAMPIN is suspected.

Management In patients receiving TMP-SMZ, monitor for a decrease in therapeutic effect during coadministration of RIFAMPIN.

Discussion

The effect of rifampin on the pharmacokinetics of trimethoprim-sulfamethoxazole was studied in 10 adult HIV-infected patients who were admitted to the hospital with tuberculosis.[1] Prior to hospitalization, all subjects had taken 1 double-strength tablet of TMP-SMZ (containing 160 mg TMP and 800 mg SMZ) once daily for more than 1 month for *Pneumocystis carinii* prophylaxis. Antituberculosis treatment, started in the hospital, consisted of rifampin (600 mg/day), isoniazid (eg, *Nydrazid*), pyrazinamide, and ethambutol (*Myambutol*). During treatment with rifampin, serum TMP-SMZ concentrations were lower compared with giving TMP-SMZ alone. Rifampin administration produced a 47% decrease in TMP area under the plasma concentration-time curve. There was a decrease in the TMP serum concentration from 2 hours postdosing with rifampin. In addition, rifampin reduced SMZ AUC 23% and there was a decrease in SMZ serum concentration from 4 hours postdosing.

[1] Ribera E, et al. *Antimicrob Agents Chemother.* 2001;45:3238.

* Asterisk indicates drugs cited in interaction reports. Based on pharmacologic and pharmacokinetic considerations, similar interactions may occur with other drugs that are listed.

Troglitazone | *Bile Acid Sequestrants*

Troglitazone*† (*Rezulin*) | Cholestyramine* (eg, *Questran*)

Significance	Onset	Severity	Documentation
2	☐ Rapid	☐ Major	☐ Established
	■ **Delayed**	■ **Moderate**	■ **Probable**
		☐ Minor	☐ Suspected
			☐ Possible
			☐ Unlikely

Effects The pharmacologic effect of TROGLITAZONE may be decreased.

Mechanism TROGLITAZONE probably binds to CHOLESTYRAMINE in the GI tract, decreasing TROGLITAZONE absorption.

Management Avoid concurrent use of TROGLITAZONE and CHOLESTYRAMINE.

Discussion

Using an open-labeled, 2-way crossover design, the effects of cholestyramine on the pharmacokinetics of troglitazone were studied in 12 healthy volunteers.[1] Each subject received a single oral dose of troglitazone (400 mg) alone and with cholestyramine (12 g in an aqueous solution) in random order. Troglitazone was taken 30 minutes after a standardized breakfast and cholestyramine was administered 1 hour after troglitazone ingestion. Compared with taking troglitazone alone, coadministration of troglitazone and cholestyramine resulted in a decrease in the mean AUC of troglitazone and its 2 main metabolites (ie, sulfate and quinone). The percentage decreases in the AUC for troglitazone and the sulfate and quinone metabolites were 71%, 80%, and 86%, respectively. The peak concentration of the sulfate metabolite was decreased 72%.

[1] Young MA, et al. *Br J Clin Pharmacol.* 1998;45:37.

* Asterisk indicates drugs cited in interaction reports.
† Not available in the United States.

Valproic Acid — *Acyclovir*

Divalproex Sodium* (*Depakote*)	Valproic Acid* (eg, *Depakene*)	Acyclovir* (eg, *Zovirax*)

Significance	Onset	Severity	Documentation
4	☐ Rapid	☐ Major	☐ Established
	■ **Delayed**	■ **Moderate**	☐ Probable
		☐ Minor	☐ Suspected
			■ **Possible**
			☐ Unlikely

Effects Serum VALPROIC ACID concentrations may be decreased, resulting in a decrease in activity.

Mechanism Unknown.

Management Consider monitoring the patient for a change in VALPROIC ACID activity if ACYCLOVIR is started or stopped. Adjust the dose of VALPROIC ACID as indicated.

Discussion

Decreased antiepileptic activity occurred in a 7-year-old boy with severe symptomatic partial epilepsy receiving phenytoin, valproic acid, and nitrazepam† several days after starting treatment with acyclovir.[1] Prior to receiving acyclovir, the patient's clinical status had been stable for the preceding 2 years while he was receiving phenytoin and valproic acid 1,000 mg twice daily. Plasma phenytoin concentrations were 18 and 19 mcg/mL, while his trough and peak valproic acid concentrations were 35 and 70 mcg/mL, respectively. The boy's pediatrician prescribed acyclovir 1 g daily for throat and mouth lesions suspected to be due to a virus. Ten days prior to starting acyclovir treatment, phenytoin and valproic acid concentrations were 17 and 32 mcg/mL, respectively. Seizure frequency was less than 1/month. Four days after the start of acyclovir treatment, the patient was admitted to the hospital for previously scheduled verification of his antiepileptic regimen. At this time, his trough and peak concentrations of phenytoin were 5 and 7.1 mcg/mL, respectively, while valproic acid concentrations were 22 and 50 mcg/mL. Acyclovir treatment was discontinued 2 days after hospitalization. Six days later, phenytoin and valproic acid concentrations were still low, and the next day the patient had 25 serial partial seizures. The phenytoin dose was increased, and plasma concentrations increased to values of 23 to 24 mcg/mL after 10 days. Valproic acid concentrations returned to initial values without dose modification. Seizure frequency was 2 to 3/week. The phenytoin dose was reduced, and plasma trough and peak concentrations decreased to 14 and 15 mcg/mL, respectively. The patient's clinical status, electroencephalogram, and antiepileptic drug status remained stable over the next 10 months.

[1] Parmeggiani A, et al. *Ther Drug Monit.* 1995;17:312.

* Asterisk indicates drugs cited in interaction reports.
† Not available in the United States.

Valproic Acid — *Antacids*

Valproic Acid		Antacids	
Divalproex Sodium* (*Depakote*)	Valproic Acid* (eg, *Depakene*)	Aluminum Hydroxide* (eg, *Amphojel*)	Calcium Carbonate* (eg, *Tums*)
		Aluminum/ Magnesium Hydroxide* (eg, *Riopan*)	Magnesium Hydroxide* (eg, *Milk of Magnesia*)

Significance	Onset	Severity	Documentation
5	□ Rapid	□ Major	□ Established
	■ **Delayed**	□ Moderate	□ Probable
		■ **Minor**	□ Suspected
			■ **Possible**
			□ Unlikely

Effects Increased AUC for VALPROIC ACID when given with ANTACIDS.

Mechanism Increased bioavailability of VALPROIC ACID.

Management Separate the dose of VALPROIC ACID and ANTACID if possible. If not, monitor seizure activity and serum concentrations of VALPROIC ACID. Use food to minimize GI symptoms associated with VALPROIC ACID therapy.

Discussion

Aluminum-magnesium hydroxide increased the AUC of valproic acid by a mean of 12% (range, 3% to 28%), and there was a trend for a similar effect with calcium carbonate and aluminum-magnesium trisilicate.[1] Although the clearance decreased, this is attributable to a mathematical artifact because volume of distribution and t½ were not changed. Increased bioavailability was the probable cause. No clinical problems were noted in this single-dose study of healthy individuals, and the magnitude of change was small. If valproic acid bioavailability increases, there is a potential for valproic acid toxicity, alterations in seizure control, and alterations in the serum concentrations of other anticonvulsants. Monitor patients if antacids are given at the same time as valproic acid.

[1] May CA, et al. *Clin Pharm.* 1982;1:244.

* Asterisk indicates drugs cited in interaction reports.

Valproic Acid — *Antineoplastic Agents*

Valproic Acid* (eg, *Depakene*)	Cisplatin*

Significance	Onset	Severity	Documentation
4	☐ Rapid ■ **Delayed**	☐ Major ■ **Moderate** ☐ Minor	☐ Established ☐ Probable ☐ Suspected ■ **Possible** ☐ Unlikely

Effects VALPROIC ACID serum concentrations may be decreased, leading to loss of seizure control.

Mechanism Unknown.

Management Carefully monitor VALPROIC ACID plasma concentrations and observe the patient for seizure activity when starting CISPLATIN-based chemotherapy. Be prepared to adjust the VALPROIC ACID dosage or administer additional anticonvulsant therapy.

Discussion

A 34-year-old man receiving valproic acid 1,200 mg daily for symptomatic epilepsy had steady valproic acid serum concentrations for about 1 year.[1] He experienced severe seizures 7 weeks after his first chemotherapeutic cycle with a regimen containing bleomycin (eg, *Blenoxane*), etoposide (eg, *VePesid*), and cisplatin. Serum valproic acid concentrations decreased 50%. Subsequently, the patient underwent 3 chemotherapy cycles with the same agents and 3 cycles with a regimen of paclitaxel (eg, *Taxol*), ifosfamide (eg, *Ifex*), and cisplatin. In all cycles, the patient experienced seizures and a decrease in valproic acid concentrations. Because cisplatin was in both regimens, it was considered the main drug interacting with valproic acid. It was not determined if the other chemotherapy agents caused or contributed to the interaction.

[1] Ikeda H, et al. *Br J Clin Pharmacol.* 2005;59:593.

* Asterisk indicates drugs cited in interaction reports.

Valproic Acid | **Carbamazepine**

Divalproex Sodium* (eg, *Depakote*)	Valproic Acid* (eg, *Depakene*)	Carbamazepine* (eg, *Tegretol*)
Valproate Sodium* (eg, *Depacon*)		

Significance	Onset	Severity	Documentation
2	☐ Rapid ■ **Delayed**	☐ Major ■ **Moderate** ☐ Minor	■ **Established** ☐ Probable ☐ Suspected ☐ Possible ☐ Unlikely

Effects Decreased VALPROIC ACID (VPA) levels with possible loss of seizure control. Variable changes in CARBAMAZEPINE (CBZ) levels.

Mechanism Multiple mechanisms are probably involved.

Management Monitor serum levels and observe patients for seizure activity and toxicity for at least 1 month after either drug is started or stopped. Alter the dosage as needed.

Discussion

CBZ can decrease serum levels and increase the clearance of VPA.[1-8] In 1 study, VPA concentrations did not plateau until 4 weeks after stopping CBZ.[7] One case of VPA toxicity occurred after stopping CBZ,[9] probably caused by an alteration of VPA metabolism by enzyme induction.[4,5] CBZ may increase the metabolic conversion of VPA to a teratogenic and hepatotoxic metabolite.[10] CBZ does not appear to alter VPA protein binding.[11,12] Reports of toxicity are rare. The effects of VPA on CBZ are complex.[13] VPA displaces CBZ from protein-binding sites in a dose-related manner.[12-14] Serum CBZ levels are inconsistently and unpredictably altered.[3,7,14-20] However, VPA may increase serum levels of the active CBZ metabolite, carbamazepine 10,11-epoxide,[13,17-23] possibly by inhibiting the metabolism.[13,17-19,24,25] The final CBZ concentration depends on these factors (and the sampling procedures) because CBZ levels can fluctuate daily.[18] Pancreatitis associated with increased VPA levels after stopping CBZ[7] and acute psychosis occurred 8 days after CBZ was added to long-term VPA[26] therapy. Conversely, VPA and CBZ have been used safely together in the management of epilepsy and psychiatric disorders.[27]

1 Bowdle TA, et al. *Clin Pharmacol Ther.* 1979;26(5):629.
2 Mihaly GW, et al. *Eur J Clin Pharmacol.* 1979;16(1):23.
3 Reunanen MI, et al. *Curr Ther Res Clin Exp.* 1980;28(3):456.
4 Schapel GJ, et al. *Eur J Clin Pharmacol.* 1980;17(1):71.
5 Hoffmann F, et al. *Eur J Clin Pharmacol.* 1981;19(5):383.
6 May T, et al. *Ther Drug Monit.* 1985;7(4):387.
7 Jann MW, et al. *Epilepsia.* 1988;29(5):578.
8 Panesar SK, et al. *Br J Clin Pharmacol.* 1989;27(3):323.
9 McKee RJ, et al. *Lancet.* 1989;1(8630):167.
10 Kondo T, et al. *Br J Clin Pharmacol.* 1990;29(1):116.
11 Fleitman JS, et al. *J Clin Pharmacol.* 1980;20(8-9):514.
12 Mattson GF, et al. *Ther Drug Monit.* 1982;4(2):181.
13 Liu H, et al. *Clin Neuropharmacol.* 1995;18(1):1.
14 Redenbaugh JE, et al. *Neurology.* 1980;30(1):1.
15 Adams DJ, et al. *Neurology.* 1978;28(2):152.
16 Wilder BJ, et al. *Neurology.* 1978;28(9, pt 1):892.
17 Brodie MJ, et al. *Br J Clin Pharmacol.* 1983;16(6):747.
18 Levy RH, et al. *Epilepsia.* 1984;25(3):338.
19 Pisani F, et al. *Epilepsia.* 1986;27(5):548.
20 Macphee GJ, et al. *Br J Clin Pharmacol.* 1988;25(1):59.
21 Ramsay RE, et al. *Ther Drug Monit.* 1990;12(3):235.
22 Johnsen SD, et al. *Ann Neurol.* 1991;30(3):491.
23 Svinarov DA, et al. *Ther Drug Monit.* 1995;17(3):217.
24 Robbins DK, et al. *Br J Clin Pharmacol.* 1990;29(6):759.
25 Bernus I, et al. *Br J Clin Pharmacol.* 1997;44(1):21.
26 Sovner R. *J Clin Psychopharmacol.* 1988;8(6):448.
27 Ketter TA, et al. *J Clin Psychopharmacol.* 1992;12(4):276.

* Asterisk indicates drugs cited in interaction reports.

Valproic Acid — *Carbapenem Antibiotics*

Divalproex Sodium (eg, *Depakote*)	Valproic Acid* (eg, *Stavzor*)	Doripenem (*Doribax*)	Imipenem/Cilastatin* (eg, *Primaxin*)
Valproate Sodium* (eg, *Depacon*)		Ertapenem* (*Invanz*)	Meropenem* (eg, *Merrem*)

Significance	Onset	Severity	Documentation
1	☐ Rapid ■ **Delayed**	■ **Major** ☐ Moderate ☐ Minor	☐ Established ■ **Probable** ☐ Suspected ☐ Possible ☐ Unlikely

Effects

VALPROIC ACID (VPA) plasma levels may be decreased, leading to loss of seizure control.

Mechanism

Inhibition of the hydrolysis of VPA glucuronide to VPA and reduced VPA plasma levels from shifts in distribution by CARBAPENEM ANTIBIOTICS.

Management

Monitor VPA plasma concentrations and observe patients for seizure activity when starting a CARBAPENEM ANTIBIOTIC. If an interaction is suspected, it may be necessary to use alternative antibiotic therapy. If the CARBAPENEM ANTIBIOTIC is stopped, the VPA dose may need to be reduced.

Discussion

Greatly reduced VPA levels have been reported in patients treated with meropenem[1-9] and ertapenem.[10,11] A 21-year-old woman had a recurrence of epileptic seizures during coadministration of VPA 1,920 mg as a continuous IV infusion over 24 h and IV meropenem 1 g 3 times daily.[1] Prior to initiation of meropenem therapy, VPA plasma levels were 52.5 mcg/mL. Two days after coadministration of VPA and meropenem, VPA levels decreased to 42 mcg/mL, and the patient experienced myoclonic seizures. The IV dose of VPA was increased to 2,880 mg over 24 h. Two days later, another generalized tonic-clonic seizure occurred. The VPA plasma level was 7 mcg/mL, and the daily dose was increased to 3,600 mg. The plasma concentration of VPA remained below 10 mcg/mL. An interaction with meropenem was suspected, and meropenem was discontinued. Ceftazidime (eg, *Fortaz*) plus ciprofloxacin (eg, *Cipro*) was started, and over the next few days, VPA levels increased to therapeutic levels. Seizures did not recur. Approximately 10 days later, the patient was asymptomatic and was discharged from the hospital on VPA 500 mg orally every 8 h. Six months later, she had not reported any further seizures. A retrospective review of 39 patients receiving valproate and meropenem revealed a 66% reduction in VPA levels.[6] Similarly, imipenem treatment reduced VPA levels 43% to 51% in 2 patients.[12] A 9.5-year-old girl with infantile neuroaxonal dystrophy and epilepsy experienced a rapid decrease in valproate serum levels and exacerbation of seizures 5 days after IV meropenem was started.[3] Similarly, valproic acid concentrations were undetectable in a 46-year-old man after starting meropenem.[13] A marked reduction in VPA levels leading to seizure activity was reported in a 41-year-old man 7 days after starting ertapenem.[7] After starting ertapenem, greatly decreased VPA concentrations occurred in 2 patients receiving valproate sodium.[11] In a 49-year-old woman, therapeutic valproate plasma concentrations were achieved and maintained despite coadministration with meropenem.[14]

1 Coves-Orts FJ, et al. *Ann Pharmacother.* 2005;39(3):533.
2 Clause D, et al. *Intensive Care Med.* 2005;31(9):1293.
3 Santucci M, et al. *J Child Neurol.* 2005;20(5):456.
4 Fudio S, et al. *J Clin Pharm Ther.* 2006;31(4):393.
5 Spriet I, et al. *Am J Health Syst Pharm.* 2007;64(1):54.
6 Spriet I, et al. *Ann Pharmacother.* 2007;41(7/8):1130.
7 Harotiunian S, et al. *J Clin Pharmacol.* 2009;49(11):1363.
8 Mancl EE, et al. *Ann Pharmacother.* 2009;43(12):2082.
9 Mink S, et al. *Clin Neurol Neurosurg.* 2011;113(8):644.
10 Lunde JL, et al. *Pharmacotherapy.* 2007;27(8):1202.
11 Liao FF, et al. *Am J Health Syst Pharm.* 2010;67(15):1260.
12 Omoda K, et al. *J Pharm Sci.* 2005;94(8):1685.
13 Muzyk AJ, et al. *Gen Hosp Psychiatry.* 2010;32(5):560.e1.
14 Spriet I, et al. *Ann Pharmacother.* 2011;45(9):1167.

* Asterisk indicates drugs cited in interaction reports. Based on pharmacologic and pharmacokinetic considerations, similar interactions may occur with other drugs that are listed.

Valproic Acid | **Chitosan**

Divalproex Sodium (eg, *Depakote*)	Valproic Acid* (eg, *Depakene*)	Chitosan*
Valproate Sodium (eg, *Depacon*)		

Significance	Onset	Severity	Documentation
2	☐ Rapid	☐ Major	☐ Established
	■ **Delayed**	■ **Moderate**	☐ Probable
		☐ Minor	■ **Suspected**
			☐ Possible
			☐ Unlikely

Effects VALPROATE serum concentrations may be reduced, increasing the risk of seizures.

Mechanism CHITOSAN contains positively charged amino groups that may bind to the anionic carboxyl group of the lipophilic VALPROATE, decreasing GI absorption.

Management Patients receiving VALPROIC ACID should avoid CHITOSAN. Caution patients taking VALPROIC ACID to consult their health care provider before using nonprescription or herbal products.

Discussion

Chitin is a cellulose-like biopolymer found mainly in exoskeletons of marine invertebrates and arthropods, such as shrimp, crabs, or lobsters.[1] Chitosan is deacetylated chitin. Decreased valproate concentrations and reappearance of seizures were reported in 2 patients taking chitosan.[2] A 35-year-old woman with idiopathic generalized epilepsy was seizure free for 3 years while taking valproate 500 mg twice daily and phenobarbital. A few days after she started taking a dietary supplement containing chitosan, she experienced a sudden reappearance of myoclonic jerks, absences, and tonic-clonic seizures. Seizures subsided after stopping chitosan. Three months later, she restarted chitosan, and within 5 days, her seizures reappeared. Valproate serum concentrations were undetectable. Chitosan was discontinued and her seizures remitted. The valproate concentrations returned to baseline within 4 days. A 29-year-old woman with idiopathic generalized epilepsy had been seizure free while being treated with valproate 1,250 mg daily. She experienced 2 tonic-clonic seizures and daily absences 1 week after starting chitosan supplementation. Valproate serum concentrations were undetectable. Her seizures promptly disappeared after discontinuing chitosan.

[1] DerMarderosian A, Beutler JA, eds. Chitosan. *The Review of Natural Products*. 6th ed. St. Louis, MO: Wolters Kluwer Health: 2010.

[2] Striano P, et al. *BMJ*. 2009;339:b3751.

* Asterisk indicates drugs cited in interaction reports. Based on pharmacologic and pharmacokinetic considerations, similar interactions may occur with other drugs that are listed.

Valproic Acid — *Cholestyramine*

Divalproex Sodium (*Depakote*)	Valproic Acid* (eg, *Depakene*)	Cholestyramine* (eg, *Questran*)

Significance	Onset	Severity	Documentation
2	■ **Rapid** □ Delayed	□ Major ■ **Moderate** □ Minor	□ Established □ Probable ■ **Suspected** □ Possible □ Unlikely

Effects Serum concentrations and bioavailability of VALPROIC ACID may be reduced, resulting in a decrease in therapeutic effects.

Mechanism CHOLESTYRAMINE interferes with the GI absorption of VALPROIC ACID.

Management Administer VALPROIC ACID at least 3 hours before but not within 3 hours following CHOLESTYRAMINE. Monitor the patient's clinical response and adjust the dose of VALPROIC ACID as needed.

Discussion

The effects of cholestyramine on the pharmacokinetics of valproic acid were investigated in 6 healthy volunteers.[1] Using an open-label, 3-way crossover design, each subject received the following: 1) A single dose of valproic acid 250 mg alone, 2) cholestyramine 4 g twice daily for 24 hours before the study day, then valproic acid 250 mg with the morning dose of cholestyramine, and 3) cholestyramine 4 g twice daily for 24 hours before the study day, then valproic acid 250 mg 3 hours before the morning dose of cholestyramine. Compared with valproic acid given alone, coadministration of cholestyramine and valproic acid resulted in a 21% decrease in peak serum valproic acid concentrations ($P < 0.05$) and a 15% decrease in the AUC of valproic acid ($P < 0.05$). When the administration times of the drugs were staggered by administering valproic acid 3 hours prior to cholestyramine, there was no decrease in the AUC or C_{max} of valproic acid compared with valproic acid given alone. Relative to taking valproic acid alone, the bioavailability of valproic acid was 86.2% when given concomitantly with cholestyramine and 95.3% when staggered with cholestyramine.

[1] Malloy MJ, et al. *Int J Clin Pharmacol Ther.* 1996;34:208.

* Asterisk indicates drugs cited in interaction reports. Based on pharmacologic and pharmacokinetic considerations, similar interactions may occur with other drugs that are listed.

Valproic Acid — Cimetidine

Divalproex Sodium (*Depakote*)	Valproic Acid* (eg, *Depakene*)	Cimetidine* (eg, *Tagamet*)
Valproate Sodium (eg, *Depacon*)		

Significance	Onset	Severity	Documentation
4	☐ Rapid	☐ Major	☐ Established
	■ **Delayed**	■ **Moderate**	☐ Probable
		☐ Minor	☐ Suspected
			■ **Possible**
			☐ Unlikely

Effects CIMETIDINE may decrease the clearance and increase the t½ of VALPROIC ACID.

Mechanism CIMETIDINE may alter the metabolism of VALPROIC ACID.

Management In patients receiving VALPROIC ACID, monitor serum VALPROIC ACID levels when treatment with CIMETIDINE is instituted, increased, decreased, or discontinued. Adjust the dose of VALPROIC ACID accordingly.

Discussion

Single doses of valproate sodium tablets were given to 12 patients taking either cimetidine 1 g/day in divided doses or ranitidine 150 mg twice daily for peptic ulcer.[1] A small but potentially clinically important decrease in valproate clearance was measured in the patients taking cimetidine (5 of 6 patients had a 2% to 17% decrease). The t½ was increased from an average of 9.6 hours to 11 hours.

Although the changes are small, they may be important in patients with serum valproic acid levels near the upper limit of the therapeutic range.

[1] Webster LK, et al. *Eur J Clin Pharmacol.* 1984;27:341.

* Asterisk indicates drugs cited in interaction reports. Based on pharmacologic and pharmacokinetic considerations, similar interactions may occur with other drugs that are listed.

Valproic Acid — *Contraceptives, Hormonal*

Valproic Acid		Contraceptives, Hormonal
Divalproex Sodium* (eg, *Depakote*)	Valproic Acid (eg, *Depakene*)	Contraceptives, Oral* (eg, *Kelnor*)
Valproate Sodium (eg, *Depacon*)		

Significance	Onset	Severity	Documentation
2	☐ Rapid	☐ Major	☐ Established
	■ **Delayed**	■ **Moderate**	☐ Probable
		☐ Minor	■ **Suspected**
			☐ Possible
			☐ Unlikely

Effects Decreased VALPROIC ACID serum concentrations and exacerbation of seizures may occur.

Mechanism Induction of hepatic glucuronidation by HORMONAL CONTRACEPTIVES is suspected.

Management Monitor VALPROIC ACID serum concentrations and clinical effects. Adjust the dosage as needed.

Discussion

A possible drug interaction between oral contraceptives and divalproex sodium was reported in a 26-year-old woman with a history of suspected mixed-type epilepsy, beginning with absence seizures at 7 years of age.[1] The patient had been treated with ethosuximide (eg, *Zarontin*); she had no seizures after 9 years of age and ethosuximide was discontinued. She did well until 13 years of age, when she experienced her first generalized convulsive seizure. Her seizures continued, despite trials with a number of antiepileptic drugs. While taking valproic acid, she had her last generalized seizure at 23 years of age. Subsequently, she developed partial seizures with onset in close proximity to the initiation of oral contraceptive treatment (ethynodiol diacetate 1 mg and ethinyl estradiol 35 mcg), which was started for management of irregular menstrual cycles and menorrhagia. Seizure charting revealed that the seizures occurred with a greater frequency while the patient was taking active, rather than inactive, tablets. Over a 5-month period, she had 12 seizures during 105 days of active tablet use and none during 35 days of inactive tablet ingestion. The morning valproic acid trough serum concentration was 53.6 mcg/mL during the third week of active drug use and 139 mcg/mL between days 5 and 7 of inactive tablet use. Trough concentrations during subsequent cycles were 70 mcg/mL total, with 6.9 mcg/mL of free valproic acid on active drug and 110 mcg/mL total with 12.8 mcg/mL of free valproic acid during inactive tablet administration. Nine women with epilepsy taking valproic acid and an estrogen-progestin–containing oral contraceptive were studied at the end of the hormone-containing portion of the oral contraceptive regimen and after the 4- to 7-day, hormone-free period.[2] Valproic acid levels increased from 350 to 425 mcmol/L during the hormone-free period compared with the hormone-containing period, indicating that oral contraceptive hormones increased total valproic acid clearance. Compared with taking valproic acid alone, coadministration of oral contraceptives decreased valproic acid levels 23.4%.[3]

[1] Herzog AG, et al. *Epilepsia.* 2005;46(6):970.
[2] Galimberti CA, et al. *Epilepsia.* 2006;47(9):1569.
[3] Herzog AG, et al. *Neurology.* 2009;72(10):911.

* Asterisk indicates drugs cited in interaction reports. Based on pharmacologic and pharmacokinetic considerations, similar interactions may occur with other drugs that are listed.

Valproic Acid — *Efavirenz*

Divalproex Sodium (eg, *Depakote*)	Valproate Sodium (eg, *Depakene*)	Efavirenz* (*Sustiva*)
Valproic Acid* (eg, *Depacon*)		

Significance	Onset	Severity	Documentation
4	☐ Rapid	☐ Major	☐ Established
	■ **Delayed**	■ **Moderate**	☐ Probable
		☐ Minor	☐ Suspected
			■ **Possible**
			☐ Unlikely

Effects VALPROATE plasma concentrations may be reduced, decreasing the pharmacologic effect.

Mechanism Unknown.

Management Closely monitor VALPROATE plasma concentrations and the clinical response. Adjust the VALPROIC ACID dose as needed.

Discussion

A 30-year-old man with bipolar disorder who was HIV-positive for years and had a 10-year history of cocaine and heroin abuse was treated with valproic acid 1.5 g daily.[1] His valproate plasma concentration was 70 mg/dL. Two months later, he was started on an antiretroviral regimen that contained efavirenz 600 mg daily. Three months later, he was admitted to a psychiatric hospital because of intense cocaine ingestion. At the time, he was manic and his valproate plasma concentration was 29 mg/dL. Only after increasing the valproic acid dose to 4 g daily were valproate target concentrations (52 mg/dL) obtained. After 2 months, the dose of valproic acid was reduced to 1.5 g daily. Despite this reduction, a month later the valproate concentration was measured at 52 mg/dL.

[1] Saraga M, et al. *Bipolar Disord.* 2006;8(4):415.

* Asterisk indicates drugs cited in interaction reports. Based on pharmacologic and pharmacokinetic considerations, similar interactions may occur with other drugs that are listed.

Valproic Acid — *Erythromycin*

Divalproex Sodium* (eg, *Depakote*)	Valproic Acid* (eg, *Depakene*)	Erythromycin* (eg, *Ery-Tab*)
Valproate Sodium (eg, *Depacon*)		

Significance	Onset	Severity	Documentation
4	☐ Rapid	☐ Major	☐ Established
	■ **Delayed**	■ **Moderate**	☐ Probable
		☐ Minor	☐ Suspected
			■ **Possible**
			☐ Unlikely

Effects ERYTHROMYCIN may increase serum VALPROIC ACID concentrations, producing VALPROIC ACID toxicity.

Mechanism Possible inhibition of VALPROIC ACID metabolism.

Management Consider monitoring serum VALPROIC ACID concentrations when the dose of ERYTHROMYCIN is started, stopped, or changed. Adjust the dose of VALPROIC ACID accordingly.

Discussion

A 38-year-old woman was admitted to the hospital with symptoms of valproic acid toxicity following the addition of erythromycin to her treatment regimen.[1] She had been receiving valproic acid 3,500 mg daily and clorazepate (eg, *Tranxene*) 3.75 mg 4 times daily for an idiopathic disorder involving complex partial and generalized seizures. In addition, she was receiving lithium carbonate (eg, *Lithobid*) 300 mg twice daily for bipolar affective disorder. Two months prior to hospitalization, the valproic acid concentration was 88.8 mcg/mL (therapeutic, 50 to 100 mcg/mL). One week prior to admission, erythromycin 250 mg 4 times daily was prescribed for an upper respiratory tract infection. The next day, the patient experienced fatigue and difficulty walking, which progressed to slurred speech, confusion, lethargy, difficulty concentrating, and a worsening gait over the next week. At the time of admission, the patient was anxious, confused, inattentive, incoherent, and unable to perform simple memory tests. Marked asterixis of both upper extremities was present. The patient was unable to stand steadily without falling. Her valproic acid concentration was 260.4 mcg/mL, and her lithium concentration was in the lower therapeutic range. Valproic acid and erythromycin were withheld; 15 hours later, the valproic acid level was 94.6 mcg/mL. Valproic acid was restarted at the previous dosage. The patient's confusion and ataxia improved slowly, while her dysarthria resolved over the next 24 hours.

[1] Redington K, et al. *Ann Intern Med.* 1992;116(10):877.

* Asterisk indicates drugs cited in interaction reports. Based on pharmacologic and pharmacokinetic considerations, similar interactions may occur with other drugs that are listed.

Valproic Acid — *Felbamate*

Divalproex Sodium* (*Depakote*)	Valproic Acid* (eg, *Depakene*)	Felbamate* (eg, *Felbatol*)
Valproate Sodium (eg, *Depacon*)		

Significance	Onset	Severity	Documentation
2	□ Rapid	□ Major	□ Established
	■ **Delayed**	■ **Moderate**	■ **Probable**
		□ Minor	□ Suspected
			□ Possible
			□ Unlikely

Effects Serum VALPROIC ACID concentrations may be increased, possibly producing toxicity.

Mechanism Inhibition of VALPROIC ACID metabolism.

Management Consider titrating the dose of FELBAMATE slowly or decreasing the dose of VALPROIC ACID during rapid titration of FELBAMATE therapy. Monitor VALPROIC ACID concentrations when starting, stopping, or altering the dose of FELBAMATE.

Discussion

The effects of felbamate administration on the pharmacokinetics of valproic acid were studied in a randomized, 3-period, crossover design.[1] Ten patients with epilepsy were previously stabilized on 9.5 to 31.7 mg/kg daily of valproic acid. Concurrent administration of felbamate 1,200 or 2,400 mg daily increased the mean valproic acid AUC by 28% and 54%, respectively, peak concentration (from 86.1 to 115.1 and 133.4 mcg/mL, respectively) and average steady-state concentration (from 66.9 to 85.4 and 103 mcg/mL, respectively). However, data were presented on only 4 patients who completed both felbamate dosage levels. The effects of various doses of felbamate were studied in 18 healthy volunteers taking valproic acid 400 mg daily for 21 days. Felbamate was given from day 8 to day 21 in doses ranging from 1,200 to 3,600 mg/day. Peak valproic acid levels and AUC were increased as a result of decreasing clearance to approximately half with the various felbamate doses.[2] The same investigators reported on the effect of felbamate on plasma protein binding of valproic acid.[3] The protein binding effect is minor. Consequently, the interaction is the result of inhibition of valproic acid metabolism.

[1] Wagner ML, et al. *Clin Pharmacol Ther.* 1994;56(5):494.
[2] Hooper WD, et al. *Epilepsia.* 1996;37(1):91.
[3] Bernus I, et al. *Clin Drug Invest.* 1995;10:288.

* Asterisk indicates drugs cited in interaction reports. Based on pharmacologic and pharmacokinetic considerations, similar interactions may occur with other drugs that are listed.

Valproic Acid — *Fluoxetine*

Divalproex Sodium* (*Depakote*)	Valproic Acid* (eg, *Depakene*)	Fluoxetine* (eg, *Prozac*)
Valproate Sodium (eg, *Depacon*)		

Significance	Onset	Severity	Documentation
4	☐ Rapid	☐ Major	☐ Established
	■ **Delayed**	■ **Moderate**	☐ Probable
		☐ Minor	☐ Suspected
			■ **Possible**
			☐ Unlikely

Effects Serum VALPROIC ACID concentrations may be elevated, increasing the risk of side effects.

Mechanism FLUOXETINE may inhibit the hepatic metabolism of VALPROIC ACID.

Management Monitor VALPROIC ACID levels and observe the clinical response of the patient when starting, stopping, or altering the dose of FLUOXETINE.

Discussion

Fluoxetine has been reported to increase serum valproic acid concentrations.[1] A 26-year-old obese woman was receiving valproic acid 2,000 mg daily for generalized seizures and pseudoseizures. Valproic acid levels (78 mg/L) were within the therapeutic range (50 to 120 mg/L). After receiving valproic acid for 1 year, fluoxetine (20 mg daily increased to 40 mg after 1 week) was added to her treatment regimen for the treatment of major depression with binge eating. Over the next 20 days, valproic acid levels increased to 131 mg/L. When fluoxetine was withdrawn, her valproic acid concentrations gradually decreased, reaching 87 mg/L after 3 weeks. At least 2 other patients have been reported to have experienced increased valproic acid serum levels (range, 27% to 52% increase) within 2 weeks of initiating treatment with fluoxetine for depression.[2,3] In both patients, valproic acid concentrations decreased to within acceptable levels when the doses of valproic acid (in 1 patient) and divalproex sodium (in 1 patient) were reduced.

[1] Lucena MI, et al. *Am J Psychiatry*. 1998;155(4):575.
[2] Sovner R, et al. *J Clin Psychopharmacol.* 1991;11(6):389.
[3] Cruz-Flores S, et al. *MO Med.* 1995;92(6):296.

* Asterisk indicates drugs cited in interaction reports. Based on pharmacologic and pharmacokinetic considerations, similar interactions may occur with other drugs that are listed.

Valproic Acid — *Oxcarbazepine*

Valproic Acid		Oxcarbazepine
Divalproex Sodium (eg, *Depakote*)	Valproic Acid* (eg, *Depakene*)	Oxcarbazepine* (eg, *Trileptal*)
Valproate Sodium (eg, *Depacon*)		

Significance	Onset	Severity	Documentation
4	☐ Rapid	☐ Major	☐ Established
	■ **Delayed**	■ **Moderate**	☐ Probable
		☐ Minor	☐ Suspected
			■ **Possible**
			☐ Unlikely

Effects VALPROIC ACID serum concentrations may be elevated, increasing the risk of toxicity.

Mechanism Unknown.

Management In patients receiving VALPROIC ACID and OXCARBAZEPINE concurrently, closely observe the clinical response of the patient and monitor VALPROIC ACID serum concentrations, including free VALPROIC ACID levels. Be prepared to adjust the VALPROIC ACID dose, if needed.

Discussion

Valproic acid toxicity was reported in a 51-year-old woman with a history of schizoaffective disorder during coadministration of valproic acid and oxcarbazepine.[1] When the patient was admitted to the psychiatric unit, she was receiving valproic acid 1,500 mg twice daily and her total valproic acid level was 105.1 mcg/mL (reference range, 50 to 125 mcg/mL). Because of increasing mania, oxcarbazepine was started and titrated to 600 mg twice daily, while the valproic acid dose was decreased to 1,000 mg twice daily. Oxcarbazepine was discontinued when she developed symptoms consistent with valproic acid toxicity with total valproic acid level of 115.6 mcg/mL and free valproic acid levels of 47.8 mcg/mL (reference range, 6 to 20 mcg/mL). Five days later, total valproic acid and free valproic acid were 108.5 and 26.8 mcg/mL, respectively. One week later, manic symptoms reappeared and oxcarbazepine 300 mg twice daily was restarted. Five days later, total valproic acid and free valproic acid were 119.6 mcg/mL and 39.1 mcg/mL, respectively. Oxcarbazepine was discontinued, and quetiapine (eg, *Seroquel*) was started. The patient's condition returned to baseline, and she was discharged 2 weeks later.

[1] Xiong GL, et al. *J Clin Psychopharmacol.* 2008;28(4):472.

* Asterisk indicates drugs cited in interaction reports. Based on pharmacologic and pharmacokinetic considerations, similar interactions may occur with other drugs that are listed.

Valproic Acid — *Phenothiazines*

Valproic Acid* (eg, *Depakene*)	Chlorpromazine* (eg, *Thorazine*)

Significance	Onset	Severity	Documentation
4	☐ Rapid	☐ Major	☐ Established
	■ **Delayed**	■ **Moderate**	☐ Probable
		☐ Minor	☐ Suspected
			■ **Possible**
			☐ Unlikely

Effects The clearance of VALPROIC ACID was decreased and the $t_{½}$ and trough concentrations were increased in a patient receiving CHLORPROMAZINE.

Mechanism Possibly inhibition of VALPROIC ACID metabolism.

Management Monitor valproic acid serum concentrations and effects and tailor the dosage if needed.

Discussion

A single study of 11 patients noted a 14% decrease in valproic acid clearance during coadministration of chlorpromazine.[1] The $t_{½}$ was prolonged and trough concentrations of valproic acid increased from 27.1 to 33.2 mcg/mL. It was postulated that chlorpromazine inhibited valproic acid metabolism. Although decreased clearance of valproic acid could potentially lead to toxic serum concentrations, the magnitude of the change was relatively small, and no clinically adverse effects were noted. Coadministration of sodium valproate and chlorpromazine, both known to cause hepatotoxicity, may have had a synergistic adverse effect, producing prolonged and severe hepatic dysfunction, bile duct injury, cholestasis, and fibrosis in a 45-year-old man being treated for persistent hiccoughs.[2]

Additional studies are warranted.

[1] Ishizaki T, et al. *J Clin Psychopharmacol.* 1984;4:254. [2] Bach N, et al. *Dig Dis Sci.* 1989;34:1303.

* Asterisk indicates drugs cited in interaction reports.

Valproic Acid — *Risperidone*

Divalproex Sodium (*Depakote*)	Valproate Sodium (eg, *Depacon*)	Risperidone* (*Risperdal*)
Valproic Acid* (eg, *Depakene*)		

Significance	Onset	Severity	Documentation
4	☐ Rapid	☐ Major	☐ Established
	■ **Delayed**	■ **Moderate**	☐ Probable
		☐ Minor	☐ Suspected
			■ **Possible**
			☐ Unlikely

Effects VALPROIC ACID serum levels may be elevated, increasing the risk of side effects.

Mechanism Unknown.

Management In patients receiving VALPROIC ACID, closely observe the clinical response and monitor serum concentrations when starting or stopping RISPERIDONE. Adjust therapy as needed.

Discussion

Elevated valproic acid serum concentrations occurred in a 10-year-old boy receiving valproic acid after risperidone was added to his treatment regimen.[1] Treatment with valproic acid, titrated to 1750 mg/day, was started in the patient because of mood swings with increasingly aggressive behavior. Valproic acid was well tolerated and valproate serum levels (143 mg/L) remained in the therapeutic range (50 to 150 mg/L). Because there was only mild improvement of symptoms after he was treated for 10 days with 1750 mg/day of valproic acid, risperidone 2 mg/day was started and increased to 3 mg/day on day 4. On the fifth day of risperidone treatment, the patient's symptoms improved; however, the valproic acid level had increased by approximately 34% (to 191 mg/L). The dose of valproic acid was decreased to 1000 mg/day and the serum level decreased to 108 mg/L within 3 days. Valproic acid and risperidone were continued and good behavior control was achieved.

[1] van Wattum PJ. *J Am Acad Child Adolesc Psychiatry*. 2001;40:866.

* Asterisk indicates drugs cited in interaction reports. Based on pharmacologic and pharmacokinetic considerations, similar interactions may occur with other drugs that are listed.

Valproic Acid — *Salicylates*

Valproic Acid	Salicylates	
Valproic Acid* (eg, *Depakene*)	Aspirin* (eg, *Bayer*)	Magnesium Salicylate (eg, *Doan's*)
	Bismuth Subsalicylate (eg, *Pepto-Bismol*)	Salsalate (eg, *Amigesic*)

Significance	Onset	Severity	Documentation
2	☐ Rapid	☐ Major	☐ Established
	■ **Delayed**	■ **Moderate**	☐ Probable
		☐ Minor	■ **Suspected**
			☐ Possible
			☐ Unlikely

Effects Increased free fraction of VALPROIC ACID, possibly leading to toxic effects of VALPROIC ACID.

Mechanism Displacement of VALPROIC ACID from protein binding sites by ASPIRIN. ASPIRIN may also alter the metabolic pathways of VALPROIC ACID.

Management When ASPIRIN is given to a patient taking VALPROIC ACID, monitor serum VALPROIC ACID concentrations (including free fraction if readily available), symptoms of VALPROIC ACID toxicity, and liver enzymes.

Discussion

In vitro, salicylic acid can displace valproic acid from albumin binding sites.[1,2] A series of studies in 6 epileptic children (plus 1 adult in 1 study)[2-4] demonstrated that aspirin increased the free fraction of valproic acid an average of 49% (range, 31% to 66%) and decreased free valproic acid clearance 28%. Total valproic acid concentration and clearance were also increased and decreased, respectively. The changes did not reach significance when mid-dosing concentrations were compared, but were significant when trough concentrations were compared. Aspirin also altered the pathways by which valproic acid is metabolized, leading to a greater formation of the potentially hepatotoxic metabolites.[2,5] Three cases of probable valproic acid toxicity (eg, ataxia, drowsiness, nystagmus, personality changes, tremor) have been described when aspirin was given,[6] though the third patient in the series had reduced concentrations of valproic acid when measured 2 and 3 days after stopping the aspirin. A 76-year-old man receiving valproic acid experienced elevated free valproic acid levels and toxicity during coadministration of aspirin 325 mg/day.[7] Total valproic acid concentrations were normal.

1 Fleitman JS, et al. *J Clin Pharmacol.* 1980;20(8-9):514.
2 Abbott FS, et al. *Clin Pharmacol Ther.* 1986;40(1):94.
3 Orr JM, et al. *Clin Pharmacol Ther.* 1982;31(5):642.
4 Farrell K, et al. *J Pediatr.* 1982;101(1):142.
5 Rettenmeier AW, et al. *Drug Metab Dispos.* 1985;13(1):81.
6 Goulden KJ, et al. *Neurology.* 1987;37(8):1392.
7 Sandson NB, et al. *Am J Psychiatry.* 2006;163(11):1891.

* Asterisk indicates drugs cited in interaction reports. Based on pharmacologic and pharmacokinetic considerations, similar interactions may occur with other drugs that are listed.

Vardenafil	*Alpha-1 Adrenergic Blockers*	
Vardenafil* (*Levitra*)	Alfuzosin* (*Uroxatral*)	Silodosin* (*Rapaflo*)
	Doxazosin* (eg, *Cardura*)	Tamsulosin* (*Flomax*)
	Prazosin* (eg, *Minipress*)	Terazosin* (eg, *Hytrin*)

Significance	Onset	Severity	Documentation
2	■ **Rapid**	☐ Major	☐ Established
	☐ Delayed	■ **Moderate**	☐ Probable
		☐ Minor	■ **Suspected**
			☐ Possible
			☐ Unlikely

Effects Risk of hypotension is increased.

Mechanism Additive or synergistic pharmacologic action.

Management Caution is advised when VARDENAFIL and an ALPHA-1 ADRENERGIC BLOCKER are coadministered.[1]

Discussion

Coadministration of vardenafil and an alpha-1 adrenergic blocking agent can produce hypotension. It is recommended that patients be stable on alpha-blocker therapy prior to starting a phosphodiesterase type 5 (PDE5) inhibitor (eg, vardenafil). Patients who demonstrate hemodynamic instability on alpha-blocker therapy alone are at an increased risk of symptomatic hypotension with concurrent use of PDE5 inhibitors. In patients on stable alpha-blocker therapy, vardenafil should be initiated at the lowest recommended starting dose. In patients already taking an optimized dose of vardenafil, alpha-blocker therapy should be started at the lowest dose.[1]

The basis for this monograph is information on file with the manufacturer. Published clinical data are needed to further assess this interaction.

[1] *Levitra* [package insert]. West Haven, CT: Bayer Pharmaceuticals Corporation; March 2008.

* Asterisk indicates drugs cited in interaction reports.

Vardenafil	*Antiarrhythmic Agents*	
Vardenafil* (*Levitra*)	Amiodarone* (eg, *Cordarone*) Bretylium* Disopyramide* (eg, *Norpace*) Moricizine* (*Ethmozine*)	Procainamide* (eg, *Procanbid*) Sotalol* (eg, *Betapace*)

Significance	Onset	Severity	Documentation
1	■ **Rapid** □ Delayed	■ **Major** □ Moderate □ Minor	□ Established □ Probable ■ **Suspected** □ Possible □ Unlikely

Effects The risk of life-threatening cardiac arrhythmias, including torsades de pointes, may be increased.

Mechanism Unknown.

Management Avoid use of VARDENAFIL in patients receiving class IA or class III ANTIARRHYTHMIC AGENTS.

Discussion

In a study of the effect of vardenafil on QT intervals in 59 healthy men, therapeutic (10 mg) and supratherapeutic (80 mg) doses of vardenafil produced increases in the QTc intervals similar to those of the active control (moxifloxacin [*Avelox*]). Thus, patients with congenital QT prolongation and those taking class IA or class III antiarrhythmic agents should avoid taking vardenafil.[1]

The basis for this monograph is information on file with the manufacturer of vardenafil.[1] Because of the seriousness of the cardiac problems, clinical evaluation of this interaction in humans is not likely to be forthcoming.

[1] *Levitra* [package insert]. West Haven, CT: Bayer Pharmaceuticals Corporation; August 2003.

* Asterisk indicates drugs cited in interaction reports.

Venlafaxine — *Azole Antifungal Agents*

Venlafaxine*	Fluconazole	Ketoconazole*
(*Effexor*)	(eg, *Diflucan*)	(eg, *Nizoral*)
	Itraconazole	Voriconazole
	(eg, *Sporanox*)	(*Vfend*)

Significance	Onset	Severity	Documentation
2	☐ Rapid	☐ Major	☐ Established
	■ **Delayed**	■ **Moderate**	☐ Probable
		☐ Minor	■ **Suspected**
			☐ Possible
			☐ Unlikely

Effects VENLAFAXINE plasma levels may be elevated, increasing the adverse effects.

Mechanism While CYP2D6 is the major pathway for VENLAFAXINE metabolism, CYP3A4 inhibition by AZOLE ANTIFUNGAL AGENTS may be an important factor in poor metabolizers.

Management In patients receiving VENLAFAXINE, closely observe the clinical response when starting or stopping AZOLE ANTIFUNGAL AGENTS. Be prepared to adjust therapy as needed.

Discussion

The effect of CYP3A4 inhibition by ketoconazole on the pharmacokinetics of venlafaxine with different CYP2D6 pheno- and genotypes was evaluated in 20 healthy volunteers (14 extensive metabolizers and 6 poor metabolizers).[1] Extensive metabolizers were given venlafaxine 50 mg and poor metabolizers were administered 25 mg before and after a third dose of ketoconazole 100 mg twice daily. Compared with taking venlafaxine alone, ketoconazole increased the venlafaxine AUC 36% (70% in poor metabolizers and 21% in extensive metabolizers). Venlafaxine C_{max} was increased 32% (48% in poor metabolizers and 26% in extensive metabolizers).

[1] Lindh JD, et al. *Eur J Clin Pharmacol.* 2003;59:401.

* Asterisk indicates drugs cited in interaction reports. Based on pharmacologic and pharmacokinetic considerations, similar interactions may occur with other drugs that are listed.

Venlafaxine — *Bupropion*

Venlafaxine* (eg, *Effexor XR*)	Bupropion* (eg, *Wellbutrin*)

Significance	Onset	Severity	Documentation
2	☐ Rapid ■ **Delayed**	☐ Major ■ **Moderate** ☐ Minor	☐ Established ☐ Probable ■ **Suspected** ☐ Possible ☐ Unlikely

Effects VENLAFAXINE plasma concentrations may be elevated, increasing the pharmacologic effects and risk of adverse reactions.

Mechanism Inhibition of VENLAFAXINE metabolism (CYP2D6) by the BUPROPION metabolite, hydroxybupropion, is suspected.

Management Coadminister with caution. Clinical and therapeutic drug monitoring are warranted. Adjust the VENLAFAXINE dose as needed.

Discussion

In an open-label pharmacokinetic study in patients with a major depressive episode, the addition of bupropion sustained-release 150 mg daily to venlafaxine ER monotherapy increased venlafaxine steady-state concentrations 2.5-fold.[1] At least 3 cases of increased venlafaxine plasma concentrations have been reported.[2] Symptoms consistent with serotonin syndrome occurred in 1 patient, while another patient reported mild adverse reactions. It was necessary to reduce the venlafaxine dose to avoid serotonergic adverse effects.

[1] Kennedy SH, et al. *J Clin Psychiatry.* 2002;63(3):181.
[2] Paslakis G, et al. *J Clin Psychopharmacol.* 2010;30(4):473.

* Asterisk indicates drugs cited in interaction reports.

Venlafaxine — *Propafenone*

Venlafaxine* (eg, *Effexor XR*)	Propafenone* (eg, *Rythmol*)

Significance	Onset	Severity	Documentation
4	☐ Rapid	☐ Major	☐ Established
	■ **Delayed**	■ **Moderate**	☐ Probable
		☐ Minor	☐ Suspected
			■ **Possible**
			☐ Unlikely

Effects VENLAFAXINE serum levels may be elevated, increasing the pharmacologic effects and adverse reactions.

Mechanism Inhibition of VENLAFAXINE metabolism (CYP2D6) by PROPAFENONE is suspected.

Management In patients receiving VENLAFAXINE, closely observe the clinical response when starting, stopping, or changing the dose of PROPAFENONE. Monitoring VENLAFAXINE serum levels may be useful in patient management.

Discussion

Organic psychosis was reported in a 67-year-old woman during coadministration of venlafaxine and propafenone.[1] The patient had bipolar affective disorder of several years' duration and had been treated with venlafaxine 225 mg/day. Because of a new depressive disorder, she was referred to the hospital. The dose of venlafaxine was increased to 300 mg/day. After admission, the patient developed intermittent atrial fibrillation that was treated with propafenone 600 mg/day. After approximately 2 weeks of treatment, the patient became paranoid and exhibited delusions with varying themes. Upon investigation, it was determined that the patient's venlafaxine serum concentration had increased from 85 to 520 ng/mL (upper therapeutic level, 150 ng/mL), and the level of the O-desmethylvenlafaxine metabolite increased from less than 10 to 165 ng/mL (upper therapeutic level, 325 ng/mL). Venlafaxine therapy was withheld for several days and resumed at 75 mg/day. Her mental condition improved but was impeded by the development of orthostatic hypotension. Her mental status remained unstable for several weeks. Minor changes in the treatment regimen were instituted. When the dosage of propafenone was reduced to 300 mg/day to improve orthostatic hypotension, venlafaxine serum levels decreased. Following an increase in the propafenone dosage to 600 mg/day, venlafaxine concentrations increased. The venlafaxine dosage was decreased to 50 mg/day in order to maintain therapeutic serum levels. Agitation and visual hallucinations were reported in an 85-year-old woman taking propafenone 150 mg twice daily after her venlafaxine dosage was increased to 150 mg/day.[2] Symptoms resolved 4 days after stopping venlafaxine.

[1] Pfeffer F, et al. *Int J Psychiatry Med.* 2001;31(4):427. [2] Gareri P, et al. *Ann Pharmacother.* 2008;42(3):434.

* Asterisk indicates drugs cited in interaction reports.

Verapamil — *Barbiturates*

Verapamil* (eg, *Calan*)

Amobarbital (*Amytal*)
Aprobarbital (*Alurate*)
Butabarbital (eg, *Butisol*)
Butalbital
Mephobarbital (*Mebaral*)
Pentobarbital (eg, *Nembutal*)
Phenobarbital*
Primidone (eg, *Mysoline*)
Secobarbital (eg, *Seconal*)

Significance	Onset	Severity	Documentation
4	■ **Rapid**	□ Major	□ Established
	□ Delayed	■ **Moderate**	□ Probable
		□ Minor	□ Suspected
			■ **Possible**
			□ Unlikely

Effects The pharmacologic effects of VERAPAMIL may be decreased.

Mechanism BARBITURATES may decrease the oral bioavailability of VERAPAMIL by increasing first-pass hepatic metabolism.

Management If an interaction is suspected, consider increasing the dose of VERAPAMIL during concurrent use of BARBITURATES.

Discussion

In a randomized, crossover study, the effects of phenobarbital on the disposition of verapamil were studied in 7 healthy male volunteers.[1] The subjects received 3 verapamil regimens that were administered before and after phenobarbital treatment: 1) A single oral dose of 80 mg; 2) a single IV dose of 0.15 mg/kg infused over 3 minutes; 3) multiple oral doses of 80 mg every 6 hours for 5 days. Each regimen was separated by 5 days. Following phenobarbital treatment 100 mg daily for 3 weeks, mean total oral clearance of the single dose of verapamil was increased 5-fold ($P < 0.05$) and the volume of distribution for both total and free drug was significantly elevated ($P < 0.05$). Free oral clearance of verapamil increased, resulting in a 4-fold and 3-fold decrease in AUC after phenobarbital treatment for total and free verapamil, respectively ($P < 0.05$). Following administration of IV verapamil, mean total systemic clearance of verapamil was increased from 9.95 ± 1.3 to 18.9 ± 8.7 mL/min/kg ($P < 0.05$) by phenobarbital; and total verapamil AUC decreased from 255.6 ± 36.5 to 169.8 ± 94.2 ng•hr/mL ($P < 0.05$). Other parameters for verapamil were not significantly altered. After multiple doses of oral verapamil, mean total oral clearance increased 4-fold ($P < 0.05$) and free oral clearance increased more than 3-fold ($P < 0.05$).

Additional studies are needed to determine the clinical relevance of this possible interaction.

[1] Rutledge DR, et al. *J Pharmacol Exp Ther.* 1988;246:7.

* Asterisk indicates drugs cited in interaction reports. Based on pharmacologic and pharmacokinetic considerations, similar interactions may occur with other drugs that are listed.

Verapamil — *Calcium Salts*

Verapamil	Calcium Salts	
Verapamil* (eg, *Calan*)	Ca Acetate (eg, *PhosLo*)	Calcium Gluconate*
	Calcium Carbonate (eg, *Os-Cal 500*)	Calcium Glycerophosphate
	Calcium Chloride*	Calcium Lactate
	Calcium Citrate (*Citracal*)	Calcium Levulinate
	Calcium Glubionate (*Neo-Calglucon*)	Tricalcium Phosphate (*Posture*)
	Calcium Gluceptate	

Significance	Onset	Severity	Documentation
2	■ **Rapid**	□ Major	□ Established
	□ Delayed	■ **Moderate**	□ Probable
		□ Minor	■ **Suspected**
			□ Possible
			□ Unlikely

Effects Clinical effects and toxicities of VERAPAMIL may be reversed by CALCIUM.

Mechanism Pharmacologic antagonism.

Management CALCIUM may be used therapeutically to reverse VERAPAMIL actions. For stabilized patients use adjunct CALCIUM carefully and monitor for loss of VERAPAMIL effectiveness.

Discussion

In dogs, calcium can reverse some verapamil effects in a dose-related manner.[1] Verapamil-induced changes in cardiac output, blood pressure, and AH intervals were all reduced by calcium, but slowing of sinus rate and atrioventricular block were not. This antagonism has been used advantageously in clinical situations. Calcium salts have been used successfully to treat verapamil overdose,[2-5] treat acute hypotension from verapamil,[6-8] and prevent initial hypotension in patients requiring verapamil for whom decreases in blood pressure could be detrimental.[9,10] In 1 case oral calcium salts reversed the beneficial effect verapamil had on atrial fibrillation.[11] However, in 2 cases of severe verapamil poisoning, calcium gluconate improved arrhythmias but did not reverse hypotension or bradycardia.[12,13] A single dose of calcium gluconate had no effect on mean heart rate or blood pressure of patients on chronic (4 weeks) verapamil therapy. Individual patients, however, had large increases or decreases in blood pressure.[14] Studies in isolated rabbit hearts indicate calcium may potentiate verapamil.[15] While calcium seems useful (eg, verapamil overdose, reversing/preventing hypotension) the effectiveness may depend on factors such as dose of each drug and chronicity of verapamil dosing.

1 Hariman RJ, et al. *Circulation.* 1979;59:797.
2 Perkins CM. *Br Med J.* 1978;2:1127.
3 Woie L, et al. *Eur Heart J.* 1981;2:239.
4 Chimienti M, et al. *Clin Cardiol.* 1982;5:219.
5 Luscher TF, et al. *N Engl J Med.* 1994; 330:718.
6 Lipman J, et al. *Intensive Care Med.* 1982;8:55.
7 Morris DL, et al. *JAMA.* 1983;249:3212.
8 Guadagnino V, et al. *J Clin Pharmacol.* 1987;27:407.
9 Weiss AT, et al. *Int J Cardiol.* 1983;4:275.
10 Salerno DM, et al. *Ann Intern Med.* 1987;107:623.
11 David BO, et al. *Br Med J.* 1981;282:1585.
12 Crump BJ, et al. *Lancet.* 1982;2:939.
13 Orr GM, et al. *Lancet.* 1982;2:1218.
14 Midtbo K, et al. *Pharmacol Toxicol.* 1987;60:330.
15 Watanabe Y, et al. *Int J Cardiol.* 1984;6:275.

* Asterisk indicates drugs cited in interaction reports. Based on pharmacologic and pharmacokinetic considerations, similar interactions may occur with other drugs that are listed.

Verapamil — Cimetidine

Verapamil* (*Calan*) | Cimetidine* (*Tagamet*)

Significance	Onset	Severity	Documentation
5	■ **Rapid**	□ Major	□ Established
	□ Delayed	■ **Moderate**	□ Probable
		□ Minor	□ Suspected
			□ Possible
			■ **Unlikely**

Effects Oral bioavailability and half-life of VERAPAMIL were increased while clearance was decreased by CIMETIDINE in some studies. Others refute this finding.

Mechanism Inhibition of VERAPAMIL metabolism.

Management Because no significant clinical effects were noted, no special clinical interventions appear necessary; monitor patients.

Discussion

Verapamil clearance was decreased 21% and half-life was increased 50% by cimetidine without any changes in other pharmacokinetic parameters or in hepatic blood flow.[1] Verapamil bioavailability nearly doubled when cimetidine was given, however, this was due to small changes in the area under the curve (AUC) after oral and intravenous dosing leading to a larger change in the ratio.[2] No other changes in pharmacokinetic parameters were noted and other investigators were unable to demonstrate an interaction.[3,4] No changes in verapamil-induced ECG alterations have been recorded.[2,3] Thus, there does not appear to be a significant interaction between these two drugs.

[1] Loi CM, et al. *Clin Pharmacol Ther.* 1985;37:654.
[2] Smith MS, et al. *Clin Pharmacol Ther.* 1984;36:551.
[3] Abernethy DR, et al. *Clin Pharmacol Ther.* 1985;38:342.
[4] Wing LMH, et al. *Br J Clin Pharmacol.* 1985;19:385.

* Asterisk indicates drugs cited in interaction reports.

Verapamil — *Clonidine*

Verapamil* (eg, *Calan*)	Clonidine* (eg, *Catapres*)

Significance	Onset	Severity	Documentation
4	■ **Rapid**	■ **Major**	□ Established
	□ Delayed	□ Moderate	□ Probable
		□ Minor	□ Suspected
			■ **Possible**
			□ Unlikely

Effects Synergistic pharmacologic and toxic effects, possibly causing atrioventricular block and severe hypotension.

Mechanism Unknown.

Management Use extreme caution when administering these drugs concurrently, even in patients who do not have sinus or atrioventricular node dysfunction.

Discussion

Atrioventricular block in two patients and severe hypotension in one of the patients occurred during concurrent administration of clonidine and verapamil.[1] The first patient, a 54-year-old female with hyperaldosteronism and refractory hypertension of 240/140 mm Hg associated with hypokalemia was started on verapamil 160 mg 3 times daily and spironolactone (eg, *Aldactone*) 100 mg daily. After 10 days of treatment, clonidine 0.15 mg twice daily was added. Following the first dose of clonidine, her BP was 180/100 mm Hg. The second dose was given 12 hours later. The patient became confused and arterial BP could not be measured by a cuff sphygmomanometer. After insertion of an intra-arterial cannula, her BP was 90/70 mm Hg and an ECG displayed a nodal rhythm of 50 bpm. Within 8 hours of stopping all antihypertensive medication and administration of IV fluids, her BP returned to previous levels and normal sinus rhythm was restored. The second patient, a 65-year-old female patient, had persistent hypertension that did not respond to captopril (*Capoten*) 50 mg 3 times daily or to the addition of extended-release verapamil 240 mg daily. Her BP was 165/100 mm Hg and her heart rate was 76 bpm. Clonidine 0.15 mg twice daily was added to her antihypertensive regimen. A routine ECG the day after starting clonidine revealed a nodal rhythm of 80 bpm while her BP was 130/80 mm Hg. Antihypertensive therapy was withdrawn and, within 4 hours, returning to normal sinus rhythm after an additional 24 hours.

[1] Jaffe R, et al. *Ann Pharmacother.* 1994;28:881.

* Asterisk indicates drugs cited in interaction reports.

Verapamil	*Dantrolene*
Verapamil* (eg, *Calan*)	Dantrolene* (eg, *Dantrium*)

Significance	Onset	Severity	Documentation
4	■ **Rapid** □ Delayed	■ **Major** □ Moderate □ Minor	□ Established □ Probable □ Suspected ■ **Possible** □ Unlikely

Effects Hyperkalemia and myocardial depression may occur with administration of VERAPAMIL and DANTROLENE.

Mechanism Bradycardia and myocardial depression are likely caused by additive effects of VERAPAMIL and the hyperkalemia; the mechanism for hyperkalemia is unknown.

Management Consider monitoring serum potassium and hemodynamic function when VERAPAMIL and DANTROLENE are coadministered. Alternatively, use a dihydropyridine calcium antagonist (eg, nifedipine [eg, *Procardia*]) in patients who are receiving DANTROLENE.

Discussion

A 60-year-old man experienced hyperkalemia and myocardial depression during coadministration of dantrolene and verapamil.[1] The patient was being treated with transdermal nitroglycerin (eg, *Nitro-Dur*), verapamil 80 mg 3 times daily, neutral protamine Hagedorn insulin, and regular insulin every morning. One hour prior to arrival in the operating room he received ranitidine (eg, *Zantac*), diazepam (eg, *Valium*), metoclopramide (eg, *Reglan*), verapamil 80 mg, morphine, and transdermal nitroglycerin. Because the patient was susceptible to malignant hyperthermia, IV dantrolene 2.4 mg/kg (220 mg total) was infused over 30 minutes. After completion of the dantrolene infusion, anesthesia was induced with fentanyl (eg, *Sublimaze*) and atracurium (eg, *Tracrium*). Subsequently, serum potassium increased from 4.7 mmol/L prior to the dantrolene infusion and reached a peak of 7.1 mmol/L 2.5 hours after the dantrolene was infused (5 hours following verapamil administration). No further episodes of hyperkalemia or myocardial depression were observed when verapamil was withheld for 24 hours after the last dose of dantrolene. Six months later, the patient required extensive oral surgery. Two weeks prior to surgery, verapamil was discontinued and nifedipine 10 mg 3 times daily was substituted. Prior to surgery, serum potassium was 4.1 mmol/L and increased to a peak of 5.4 mmol/L 3 hours after the dantrolene infusion (5 hours after nifedipine); however, there was no evidence of myocardial depression.

Because dantrolene alone may cause hyperkalemia, additional studies are needed to determine the clinical importance of this possible drug interaction.

[1] Rubin AS, et al. *Anesthesiology*. 1987;66(2):246.

* Asterisk indicates drugs cited in interaction reports.

Verapamil — *Food*

Verapamil*
(eg, *Calan*)

Grapefruit Juice*

Significance	Onset	Severity	Documentation
2	■ **Rapid**	□ Major	□ Established
	□ Delayed	■ **Moderate**	□ Probable
		□ Minor	■ **Suspected**
			□ Possible
			□ Unlikely

Effects VERAPAMIL plasma concentrations may be elevated, increasing the pharmacologic effects and adverse reactions.

Mechanism Inhibition of gut wall metabolism (CYP3A4) of VERAPAMIL by GRAPEFRUIT JUICE is suspected.

Management Avoid coadministration of VERAPAMIL with GRAPEFRUIT products. Caution patients to take VERAPAMIL with a liquid other than GRAPEFRUIT JUICE.

Discussion

The effect of grapefruit juice on the pharmacokinetics and pharmacodynamics of racemic verapamil (S- and R-verapamil) was studied in 9 healthy men.[1] Using a randomized, crossover design, each subject received 200 mL of orange juice (control) or grapefruit juice twice daily for 5 days (study days 1 through 5) and oral verapamil 120 mg twice daily for 3 days (study days 3 through 5). On day 6, subjects received the morning dose of verapamil with orange juice or grapefruit juice. Compared with orange juice, grapefruit juice increased the AUC of S- and R-verapamil 36% and 28%, respectively, the steady-state peak concentrations 57% and 40%, respectively, and the trough levels 16.7% and 13%, respectively. Grapefruit juice did not affect the $t_{½}$ or renal clearance of S- or R-verapamil. There were no differences in systolic or diastolic BP, heart rate, or PR interval when verapamil was taken with grapefruit juice compared with orange juice. There was considerable intersubject variability. Because verapamil is a substrate for P-glycoprotein, investigation of the effect of grapefruit juice in activating P–glycoprotein–mediated efflux of verapamil as part of the overall mechanism for this interaction is warranted. In an open-label, crossover study, 24 healthy volunteers received prolonged-release verapamil 120 mg for 7 days with 250 mL of water or grapefruit juice. Compared with water, grapefruit juice increased the AUC of verapamil at steady-state 1.45-fold and the peak plasma level 1.63-fold.[2] During administration of verapamil with grapefruit juice, the PR interval was prolonged above 350 msec in 2 subjects. Complete heart block with hypoxia and severe hypotension in association with markedly elevated verapamil blood concentrations (2,772 mg/mL; therapeutic range, 100 to 600 mg/mL) occurred in a patient taking sustained-release verapamil 360 mg daily who consumed 3 to 4 L of grapefruit juice over the week preceding hospitalization.[3]

[1] Ho PC, et al. *Eur J Clin Pharmacol.* 2000;56(9-10):693.
[2] Fuhr U, et al. *Eur J Clin Pharmacol.* 2002;58(1):45.
[3] Pillai V, et al. *South Med J.* 2009;102(3):308.

* Asterisk indicates drugs cited in interaction reports.

Verapamil — *Hydantoins*

Verapamil		Hydantoins	
Verapamil* (eg, *Calan*)		Ethotoin (*Peganone*)	Phenytoin* (eg, *Dilantin*)
		Fosphenytoin (*Cerebyx*)	

Significance	Onset	Severity	Documentation
4	☐ Rapid	☐ Major	☐ Established
	■ **Delayed**	■ **Moderate**	☐ Probable
		☐ Minor	☐ Suspected
			■ **Possible**
			☐ Unlikely

Effects Serum VERAPAMIL levels may be decreased, reducing the pharmacologic effects of VERAPAMIL.

Mechanism HYDANTOINS may induce the hepatic enzymes responsible for the metabolism of VERAPAMIL.

Management Monitor cardiovascular status. If an interaction is suspected, consider increasing the dose of VERAPAMIL during coadministration with HYDANTOINS.

Discussion

Coadministration of verapamil and phenytoin may decrease serum verapamil levels.[1] A 28-year-old woman with presumed epilepsy had been receiving phenytoin 100 mg twice daily for 10 years. The patient experienced dyspnea while climbing stairs and episodes of syncope; she was diagnosed with hypertrophic obstructive cardiomyopathy. She was started on verapamil 80 mg twice daily. The patient had consistently low serum verapamil levels of less than 50 ng/mL, and the dosage was increased to 160 mg twice daily after 2 months. After 17 months, the dosage was increased to 160 mg 3 times daily. Despite increases in the verapamil dose, serum verapamil concentrations never exceeded 44 ng/mL. After 12 months, phenytoin treatment was discontinued, and trough plasma verapamil levels increased to 50 ng/mL. In addition, the concentration of verapamil at 1 and 4 hours after ingestion increased to 320 and 195 ng/mL, respectively.

Controlled clinical studies are needed to assess the clinical importance of this possible interaction.

[1] Woodcock BG, et al. *N Engl J Med.* 1991;325(16):1179.

* Asterisk indicates drugs cited in interaction reports. Based on pharmacologic and pharmacokinetic considerations, similar interactions may occur with other drugs that are listed.

Verapamil		Macrolide & Related Antibiotics	
Verapamil* (eg, *Calan*)		Clarithromycin* (eg, *Biaxin*) Erythromycin* (eg, *Ery-Tab*)	Telithromycin* (*Ketek*)

Significance	Onset	Severity	Documentation
1	☐ Rapid ■ **Delayed**	■ **Major** ☐ Moderate ☐ Minor	☐ Established ☐ Probable ■ **Suspected** ☐ Possible ☐ Unlikely

Effects Increased risk of VERAPAMIL adverse reactions (eg, hypotension).

Mechanism Increased ERYTHROMYCIN absorption, resulting from inhibition of P-gp and ERYTHROMYCIN metabolism (CYP3A4) by VERAPAMIL. Inhibition of VERAPAMIL metabolism (CYP3A4) by certain MACROLIDE AND RELATED ANTIBIOTICS.

Management Closely monitor patients for VERAPAMIL adverse reactions when VERAPAMIL and certain MACROLIDE AND RELATED ANTIBIOTICS are coadministered.

Discussion

Ferythromycin were discontinued, and IV fluids, dopamine, and calcium were administered. BP increased to 110/70 mm Hg, and heart rate increased to 64 bpm. Two days after admission, ECG showed normal sinus rhythm at 72 bpm, with a PR interval within normal limits. Four days after admission, the QT interval prolongation resolved completely. Besides a possible drug interaction, the patient had other risk factors for QT prolongation (eg, slow baseline heart rate). A 76-year-old woman receiving verapamil 180 mg/day for hypertension developed a sudden onset of shortness of breath, weakness, profound hypotension (systolic BP 50 to 60 mm Hg), and a heart rate of 30 bpm 2 days after starting telithromycin 800 mg/day.[2] She was treated with crystalloids, vasopressors, and transvenous pacing. Her BP and heart rate returned to normal within 72 hours. Additional reports document this interaction.[3,4] See also Diltiazem-Macrolide and Related Antibiotics.

[1] Goldschmidt N, et al. *Ann Pharmacother.* 2001;35(11):1396.

[2] Reed M, et al. *Ann Pharmacother.* 2005;39(2):357.

[3] Kaeser YA, et al. *Am J Health Syst Pharm.* 1998;55(22):2417.

[4] Wright AJ, et al. *CMAJ.* 2011;183(3):303.

* Asterisk indicates drugs cited in interaction reports.

Verapamil — *Rifampin*

Verapamil*
(eg, *Calan*)

Rifampin*
(eg, *Rifadin*)

Significance	Onset	Severity	Documentation
2	■ **Rapid**	□ Major	□ Established
	□ Delayed	■ **Moderate**	□ Probable
		□ Minor	■ **Suspected**
			□ Possible
			□ Unlikely

Effects Loss of clinical effectiveness of oral VERAPAMIL.

Mechanism Increased first-pass hepatic metabolism resulting in lowered bioavailability of oral VERAPAMIL.

Management Use IV VERAPAMIL or substitute another agent for VERAPAMIL or RIFAMPIN. If RIFAMPIN is stopped, lower the dose of VERAPAMIL and monitor closely.

Discussion

Two case reports described a lack of therapeutic efficacy for oral verapamil when given to patients taking rifampin.[1,2] IV verapamil was effective in one instance.[2] Subsequent pharmacokinetic studies have demonstrated minimal effects of rifampin on IV verapamil.[3,4] However, with oral verapamil, serum concentrations were less than5 ng/mL in 2 patients[3] and area under the plasma concentration-time curve, peak serum concentration, and bioavailability were reduced 93%, 96%, and 92%, respectively, in 6 volunteers.[4] Rifampin probably induced the enzymes metabolizing verapamil. Because verapamil is highly extracted, this is manifested by an increase in first-pass extraction and a significant decrease in bioavailability after oral dosing.[4] In a study involving 8 healthy volunteers, rifampin induced the prehepatic clearance of verapamil.[5] The study used IV radio-labeled verapamil to elucidate hepatic clearance at the same time as oral drugs. Clearance of both S- and R-sterioisomers of verapamil increased after IV verapamil, indicating an inducing effect of rifampin on hepatic clearance. However, the clearance of oral verapamil was greatly affected with S- and R-verapamil clearance increasing by a factor of 32 and 57, respectively. This suggests that intestinal enzyme (cytochrome P450 3A4) inhibition is much more important than hepatic and largely explains the magnitude of this interaction.

1 Rahn KH, et al. *N Engl J Med.* 1985;312:920.
2 Barbarash RA. *DICP.* 1985;19:559.
3 Mooy J, et al. *Eur J Clin Pharmacol.* 1987;32:107.
4 Barbarash RA, et al. *Chest.* 1988;94:954.
5 Fromm MF, et al. *Hepatology.* 1996;24:796.

* Asterisk indicates drugs cited in interaction reports.

Verapamil / Serotonin Reuptake Inhibitors

Verapamil* (eg, *Calan SR*)		Fluoxetine* (eg, *Prozac*)	Nefazodone (*Serzone*)

Significance	Onset	Severity	Documentation
4	☐ Rapid	☐ Major	☐ Established
	■ **Delayed**	■ **Moderate**	☐ Probable
		☐ Minor	☐ Suspected
			■ **Possible**
			☐ Unlikely

Effects Pharmacologic and adverse effects of VERAPAMIL may be increased.

Mechanism Certain SEROTONIN REUPTAKE INHIBITORS (SRIs) may inhibit the metabolism (CYP3A4) of VERAPAMIL.

Management In patients receiving VERAPAMIL, closely observe the clinical response when starting or stopping a SRI.

Discussion

Potentiation of the effects of verapamil was reported in 2 patients during coadministration of fluoxetine.[1] One patient developed pedal edema 6 weeks after fluoxetine (20 mg every other day) and trazodone (eg, *Desyrel*) were added to her treatment regimen, which consisted of verapamil 240 mg/day, aspirin (eg, *Bayer*), and chlorpropamide (eg, *Diabinese*). The dose of verapamil was reduced to 120 mg/day and the edema resolved within 3 weeks. The second patient started verapamil (240 mg at bedtime) 2 weeks after the dose of fluoxetine was decreased from 40 to 20 mg/day. Two weeks after starting verapamil, the dose of fluoxetine was increased to 40 mg/day. One week later, the patient began awakening in the morning with a mild to moderate dull, throbbing headache. After stopping verapamil, the morning headaches subsided; however, the patient suffered 2 moderate to severe migraines over the next week.

Additional studies are needed to determine the clinical importance of this possible interaction.

[1] Sternbach H. *J Clin Psychopharmacol*. 1991;11:390.

* Asterisk indicates drugs cited in interaction reports. Based on pharmacologic and pharmacokinetic considerations, similar interactions may occur with other drugs that are listed.

Verapamil — *St. John's Wort*

Verapamil* (eg, *Calan*)	St. John's Wort

Significance	Onset	Severity	Documentation
2	☐ Rapid	☐ Major	☐ Established
	■ **Delayed**	■ **Moderate**	☐ Probable
		☐ Minor	■ **Suspected**
			☐ Possible
			☐ Unlikely

Effects VERAPAMIL plasma concentrations may be reduced, decreasing the pharmacologic effects.

Mechanism Increased first-pass metabolism (CYP3A4) of VERAPAMIL in the gut resulting from ST. JOHN'S WORT is suspected.

Management Advise patients to avoid use of ST. JOHN'S WORT while taking VERAPAMIL. If use of ST. JOHN'S WORT cannot be avoided, assess the patient's clinical response when ST. JOHN'S WORT is started or stopped. If an interaction is suspected, adjust the dose of VERAPAMIL as needed.

Discussion

The effects of repeated oral administration of St. John's wort on jejunal transport and presystemic extraction of the R- and S-verapamil enantiomers were studied in 8 healthy men.[1] Each subject received racemic verapamil 120 mg/L by jejunal infusion for 100 minutes before and after 14 days of treatment with St. John's wort (300 mg 3 times daily). Compared with administration of verapamil before St. John's wort, pretreatment with St. John's wort decreased the AUC of R- and S-verapamil 78% and 80%, respectively, and the peak concentrations decreased 76% and 78%, respectively. The AUC for R-verapamil was 6 times higher than S-verapamil in both the control and study phases. The AUCs for the R- and S-norverapamil metabolites of verapamil decreased 51% and 63%, respectively.

[1] Tannergren C, et al. *Clin Pharmacol Ther*. 2004;75:298.

* Asterisk indicates drugs cited in interaction reports.

Verapamil — *Sulfinpyrazone*

Verapamil* (*Calan, Isoptin*)	Sulfinpyrazone* (eg, *Anturane*)

Significance	Onset	Severity	Documentation
4	■ **Rapid**	□ Major	□ Established
	□ Delayed	■ **Moderate**	□ Probable
		□ Minor	□ Suspected
			■ **Possible**
			□ Unlikely

Effects VERAPAMIL'S therapeutic efficacy may be compromised.

Mechanism SULFINPYRAZONE may increase the metabolic clearance of VERAPAMIL, decreasing the oral bioavailability.

Management Consider monitoring the patient for a change in VERAPAMIL activity if SULFINPYRAZONE is added to or discontinued from the treatment regimen. Adjust the dose of VERAPAMIL accordingly.

Discussion

In a randomized investigation involving 8 healthy volunteers, sulfinpyrazone has been shown to interact with verapamil.[1] On 2 study days, single doses of verapamil were administered in randomized order, an 80 mg oral dose on one day and a 0.15 mg/kg IV dose on the other day. In the pretreatment phase, patients received 200 mg of oral sulfinpyrazone every 6 hours starting 7 days prior to the 2 verapamil study days. Following sulfinpyrazone pretreatment, apparent oral clearance increased by more than 220% (from 4.27 to 13.77 L $h^{-1}kg^{-1}$), systemic clearance increased by nearly 15% (from 1.05 to 1.2 L $h^{-1}kg^{-1}$), and oral bioavailability decreased from 27% to 10%. The volume of distribution and half-life were not affected.

More controlled data are needed to determine the clinical relevance of this possible interaction.

[1] Wing LMH, et al. *Br J Clin Pharmacol.* 1985;19:385.

* Asterisk indicates drugs cited in interaction reports.

Verapamil — *Vitamin D*

Verapamil	Vitamin D	
Verapamil* (*Calan, Isoptin*)	Calcifediol (*Calderol*)	Dihydrotachysterol (*DHT, Hytakerol*)
	Calcitriol (*Rocaltrol*)	Ergocalciferol* (eg, *Calciferol*)
	Cholecalciferol (eg, *Delta-D*)	

Significance	Onset	Severity	Documentation
4	□ Rapid	□ Major	□ Established
	■ **Delayed**	■ **Moderate**	□ Probable
		□ Minor	□ Suspected
			■ **Possible**
			□ Unlikely

Effects The therapeutic activity of VERAPAMIL may be reduced.

Mechanism VITAMIN D may counteract the activity of VERAPAMIL.

Management Monitor the cardiovascular status of patients receiving VERAPAMIL and VITAMIN D concomitantly.

Discussion

A 70-year-old woman, successfully treated with verapamil, reverted to atrial fibrillation after ingestion of calcium and ergocalciferol caused hypercalcemia.[1] Following the intravenous administration of verapamil, furosemide (eg, *Lasix*), and saline hydration, the patient reconverted to sinus rhythm.

Several case reports have demonstrated that the cardiac and hemodynamic effects of verapamil can be reversed by intravenous administration of calcium.[2-4] This antagonistic effect has been used clinically to treat verapamil toxicity. Well conducted investigations are necessary to adequately assess if a clinically significant interaction occurs with the administration of vitamin D alone and verapamil.

[1] Bar-Or D, et al. *Br Med J.* 1981;282:1585.
[2] Perkins CM. *Br Med J.* 1978;2:1127.
[3] Morris DL, et al. *JAMA.* 1983;249:3212.
[4] Guadagnino V, et al. *J Clin Pharmacol.* 1987;27:407.

* Asterisk indicates drugs cited in interaction reports. Based on pharmacologic and pharmacokinetic considerations, similar interactions may occur with other drugs that are listed.

Vinblastine — *Erythromycin*

Vinblastine*	Erythromycin* (eg, *Ery-Tab*)

Significance	Onset	Severity	Documentation
1	☐ Rapid ■ **Delayed**	■ **Major** ☐ Moderate ☐ Minor	☐ Established ☐ Probable ■ **Suspected** ☐ Possible ☐ Unlikely

Effects The risk of VINBLASTINE toxicity (eg, constipation, myalgia, neutropenia) may be increased.

Mechanism Possible inhibition of VINBLASTINE metabolism by ERYTHROMYCIN.

Management Avoid this drug combination. If VINBLASTINE and ERYTHROMYCIN must be given concurrently, administer a conservative dose of VINBLASTINE and closely monitor patients for VINBLASTINE adverse reactions.

Discussion

Severe vinblastine toxicity (eg, constipation, myalgia, neutropenia), typical of much higher doses of vinblastine than were given, was reported in 3 patients during coadministration of erythromycin.[1] All patients had metastatic renal cell carcinoma. Cyclosporine (eg, *Neoral*) was administered in 4 divided daily doses for 3 days, vinblastine 7 to 10 mg/m^2 was given by IV push on day 3, and oral erythromycin was started 24 hours before the first dose of cyclosporine. Erythromycin was given to increase cyclosporine serum concentrations and was administered until the evening of day 3, when cyclosporine was discontinued. During coadministration of erythromycin and vinblastine, each patient developed constipation, myalgia, and severe neutropenia. Neutropenia and myalgia either did not occur or were mild in 2 patients when erythromycin therapy was omitted, but they did recur in the third patient when erythromycin was administered without cyclosporine. See also Vinorelbine-Macrolide & Related Antibiotics.

[1] Tobe SW, et al. *Cancer Chemother Pharmacol.* 1995;35(3):188.

* Asterisk indicates drugs cited in interaction reports.

Vinca Alkaloids — *Azole Antifungal Agents*

Vinca Alkaloids		Azole Antifungal Agents	
Vinblastine*	Vinorelbine* (eg, *Navelbine*)	Fluconazole* (eg, *Diflucan*)	Posaconazole* (*Noxafil*)
Vincristine* (eg, *Vincasar PFS*)		Itraconazole* (eg, *Sporanox*)	Voriconazole* (*Vfend*)
		Ketoconazole (eg, *Nizoral*)	

Significance	Onset	Severity	Documentation
1	☐ Rapid	■ **Major**	☐ Established
	■ **Delayed**	☐ Moderate	■ **Probable**
		☐ Minor	☐ Suspected
			☐ Possible
			☐ Unlikely

Effects The risk of VINCA ALKALOID toxicity (eg, constipation, myalgia, neutropenia) may be increased.

Mechanism Possible inhibition of VINCA ALKALOID metabolism (CYP3A4) by the AZOLE ANTIFUNGAL AGENT.

Management Avoid coadministration of these agents whenever possible. If these agents must be coadministered, closely monitor the patient for VINCA ALKALOID toxicity. It may be necessary to discontinue the AZOLE ANTIFUNGAL AGENT.

Discussion

Vincristine neurotoxicity was reported in 2 patients with acute lymphoblastic leukemia (ALL) during itraconazole coadministration.[1] One patient developed vincristine toxicity (eg, abdominal pain and distention, hypertension, hyponatremia) 28 days into treatment, while a second patient developed similar symptoms 13 days into treatment. Itraconazole was discontinued in both patients. They recovered and chemotherapy was continued. Itraconazole 2.5 mg/kg/day was implicated in enhancing vincristine toxicity in 5 children with ALL.[2] Each child developed abdominal pain, constipation, hypertension, paralytic ileus, and hyponatremia (caused by inappropriate antidiuretic hormone secretion) while receiving itraconazole and vincristine. In adults with ALL, paresthesia, muscle weakness, and paralytic ileus occurred in 4 of 14 (29%) patients receiving vincristine plus itraconazole, compared with 6% of 460 patients receiving chemotherapy without itraconazole.[3] Severe neurotoxicity, including lower limb paralysis, was reported with coadministration of itraconazole and vincristine.[4] Severe bone marrow toxicity and mucositis were reported with coadministration of itraconazole and vinblastine.[5] A case series described severe neurotoxicity in 8 children given vincristine and itraconazole.[6] One patient also had perforation of the sigmoid colon associated with paralytic ileus. Arthralgia, ileus, and myalgia were reported in 5 children given itraconazole and vincristine.[7] A patient developed peripheral neuropathy when vincristine and voriconazole were coadministered but was able to tolerate vincristine therapy when voriconazole treatment was concluded.[8] Coadministration of posaconazole and vincristine has been reported to cause severe neurotoxicity.[9-11] In a retrospective review, 50% of adult patients receiving vincristine and fluconazole concurrently developed signs and symptoms of vincristine toxicity.[12] In a retrospective study of 20 children with acute lymphocytic leukemia, vincristine toxicity was increased by coadministration of azole antifungal agents.[13]

1 Gillies J, et al. *Clin Lab Haematol.* 1998;20(2):123.
2 Murphy JA, et al. *Lancet.* 1995;346(8972):443.
3 Böhme A, et al. *Ann Hematol.* 1995;71(6):311.
4 Bermúdez M, et al. *J Pediatr Hematol Oncol.* 2005;27(7):389.
5 Bashir H, et al. *J Pediatr Hematol Oncol.* 2006;28(1):33.
6 Kamaluddin M, et al. *Acta Paediatr.* 2001;90(10):1204.
7 Takahashi N, et al. *Intern Med.* 2008;47(7):651.
8 Porter CC, et al. *Pediatr Blood Cancer.* 2009;52(2):298.
9 Mantadakis E, et al. *J Pediatr Hematol Oncol.* 2007;29(2):130.
10 Eiden C, et al. *J Pediatr Hematol Oncol.* 2009;31(4):292.
11 Jain S, et al. *Pediatr Blood Cancer.* 2010;54(5):783.
12 Harnicar S, et al. *J Oncol Pharm Pract.* 2009;15(3):175.
13 van Schie RM, et al. *J Antimicrob Chemother.* 2011;66(8):1853.

* Asterisk indicates drugs cited in interaction reports. Based on pharmacologic and pharmacokinetic considerations, similar interactions may occur with other drugs that are listed.

Vinca Alkaloids — *Carbamazepine*

Vinblastine (*Velban*)	Vincristine* (eg, *Oncovin*)	Carbamazepine* (eg, *Tegretol*)

Significance	Onset	Severity	Documentation
4	☐ Rapid ■ **Delayed**	☐ Major ■ **Moderate** ☐ Minor	☐ Established ☐ Probable ☐ Suspected ■ **Possible** ☐ Unlikely

Effects VINCA ALKALOID plasma concentration and efficacy may be decreased.

Mechanism Increased metabolism (CYP3A4) of the VINCA ALKALOID by CARBAMAZEPINE is suspected.

Management In patients receiving VINCA ALKALOIDS, observe the clinical response when starting or stopping CARBAMAZEPINE. Be prepared to adjust the dose as needed.

Discussion

The effect of carbamazepine on the pharmacokinetics of vincristine was studied in 8 patients with brain tumors who were receiving chemotherapy with procarbazine, lomustine, and IV vincristine.[1] Compared with 6 patients who were not receiving an obvious CYP3A4-inducing medication, coadministration of carbamazepine increased the systemic clearance of vincristine 63%, decreased the elimination half-life 35%, and decreased the AUC 43%.

Additional studies are needed to determine the clinical importance of this interaction.

[1] Villikka K, et al. *Clin Pharmacol Ther*. 1999;66(6):589.

* Asterisk indicates drugs cited in interaction reports. Based on pharmacologic and pharmacokinetic considerations, similar interactions may occur with other drugs that are listed.

Vinca Alkaloids — *Protease Inhibitors*

Vinca Alkaloids		Protease Inhibitors	
Vinblastine*	Vinorelbine (eg, *Navelbine*)	Atazanavir (*Reyataz*)	Nelfinavir (*Viracept*)
Vincristine* (eg, *Vincasar*)		Darunavir (*Prezista*)	Ritonavir* (*Norvir*)
		Fosamprenavir (*Lexiva*)	Saquinavir (*Invirase*)
		Indinavir (*Crixivan*)	Tipranavir (*Aptivus*)
		Lopinavir/Ritonavir* (*Kaletra*)	

Significance	Onset	Severity	Documentation
1	☐ Rapid ■ **Delayed**	■ **Major** ☐ Moderate ☐ Minor	☐ Established ■ **Probable** ☐ Suspected ☐ Possible ☐ Unlikely

Effects Pharmacologic effects and toxicity of VINCA ALKALOIDS may be increased.

Mechanism Inhibition of VINCA ALKALOID metabolism (CYP3A4) and/or P-gp by PROTEASE INHIBITORS is suspected.

Management Closely monitor patients for VINCA ALKALOID toxicity. It may be necessary to temporarily stop PROTEASE INHIBITOR therapy in patients experiencing toxicity.

Discussion

A 55-year-old HIV-infected man experienced severe constipation and persistent pancytopenia while receiving vinblastine 6 mg/m^2 and a ritonavir-boosted lopinavir antiretroviral regimen.[1] Antiretroviral therapy was suspended and vinblastine 6 mg/m^2 was administered as monotherapy. Subsequently, the vinblastine dosage was reduced to 2 mg/m^2 every 3 weeks and antiretroviral therapy was resumed without toxicity. A 36-year-old HIV-infected man with Hodgkin lymphoma developed fever and neutropenia while receiving a ritonavir-boosted lopinavir-based antiretroviral regimen and vinblastine, doxorubicin, bleomycin, and dacarbazine.[2] The neutropenia was managed by withholding lopinavir/ritonavir for 48 hours before and after chemotherapy. Complete remission of the patient's Hodgkin lymphoma occurred. A 39-year-old HIV-infected man was receiving abacavir/lamivudine and lopinavir/ritonavir when he was treated with vincristine, cyclophosphamide, doxorubicin, and methotrexate for Burkitt lymphoma.[3] Four days after the second dose of vincristine he developed constipation. Paralytic ileus was diagnosed by imaging. Subsequently, vincristine was replaced with etoposide and was well tolerated. The toxicity was attributed to an interaction between lopinavir/ritonavir and vincristine. In a retrospective study involving 16 HIV-infected patients, coadministration of protease inhibitor therapy with vinblastine-containing chemotherapy for Hodgkin lymphoma was associated with a greater incidence of grade III-IV neutropenia compared with non–protease inhibitor therapy.[4] Two patients receiving lopinavir/ritonavir died from sepsis.

[1] Kotb R, et al. *Eur J Haematol.* 2006;76(3):269.
[2] Makinson A, et al. *Eur J Haematol.* 2007;78(4):358.
[3] Levêque D, et al. *Pharm World Sci.* 2009;31(6):619.
[4] Cingolani A, et al. *AIDS.* 2010;24(15):2408.

* Asterisk indicates drugs cited in interaction reports. Based on pharmacologic and pharmacokinetic considerations, similar interactions may occur with other drugs that are listed.

Vincristine	*Nifedipine*
Vincristine* (eg, *Oncovin*)	Nifedipine* (eg, *Procardia*)

Significance	Onset	Severity	Documentation
4	☐ Rapid ■ **Delayed**	☐ Major ■ **Moderate** ☐ Minor	☐ Established ☐ Probable ☐ Suspected ■ **Possible** ☐ Unlikely

Effects VINCRISTINE concentrations may be elevated, possibly increasing toxicity.

Mechanism Unknown.

Management Observe patients for an increase in VINCRISTINE adverse effects.

Discussion

Calcium channel blockers may reverse vincristine tumor cell resistance through enhanced intracellular vincristine retention.[1] A preliminary pharmacokinetic study was conducted in 26 patients receiving vincristine 2 mg IV.[2] Twelve patients were given nifedipine 10 mg 3 times daily beginning 3 days before vincristine and for 7 days thereafter. The remaining 14 patients served as controls. When examined as a 3-compartment model, nifedipine decreased the initial vincristine distribution half-life and markedly prolonged the terminal half-life from 22 to 86 hours. Because the AUC also increased while the volume of distribution remained the same, it appeared that clearance was reduced. Intracellular vincristine sequestration was considered as a possible explanation for the change in clearance. None of the patients given nifedipine experienced unexpected drug toxicity.

Additional clinical trials are needed to determine if the increased vincristine concentrations produce an increase in efficacy, particularly if the calcium channel blocker reverses or prevents tumor cell resistance phenomena. Increased toxicity may also occur.

[1] Tsuruo T, et al. *Cancer Res.* 1983;43(5):2267. [2] Fedeli L, et al. *Cancer.* 1989;64(9):1805.

* Asterisk indicates drugs cited in interaction reports.

Vinorelbine — Macrolide & Related Antibiotics

Vinorelbine	Macrolide & Related Antibiotics	
Vinorelbine* (eg, *Navelbine*)	Azithromycin (eg, *Zithromax*)	Erythromycin (eg, *Ery-Tab*)
	Clarithromycin* (eg, *Biaxin*)	Telithromycin (*Ketek*)

Significance	Onset	Severity	Documentation
4	☐ Rapid	■ **Major**	☐ Established
	■ **Delayed**	☐ Moderate	☐ Probable
		☐ Minor	☐ Suspected
			■ **Possible**
			☐ Unlikely

Effects VINORELBINE plasma concentrations may be elevated, increasing the pharmacologic effects and risk of toxicity (eg, neutropenia).

Mechanism Inhibition of VINORELBINE metabolism (CYP3A4) by MACROLIDE AND RELATED ANTIBIOTICS is suspected.

Management If coadministration of these agents cannot be avoided, closely monitor patients and adjust the VINORELBINE dose as needed.

Discussion

In a retrospective, cohort study, computerized medical records were reviewed to determine if patients who received vinorelbine were at increased risk of neutropenia with coadministration of clarithromycin.[1] Patients with non–small cell lung cancer were classified based on whether they received vinorelbine alone or in combination with clarithromycin. The incidence of grade 4 neutropenia was greater in patients receiving vinorelbine and clarithromycin concurrently (31.6%) compared with those receiving vinorelbine alone (2.5%).

Because of the uncontrolled nature of this investigation, additional studies are needed to establish this interaction. See also Vinblastine-Erythromycin.

[1] Yano R, et al. *Ann Pharmacother.* 2009;43(3):453.

* Asterisk indicates drugs cited in interaction reports. Based on pharmacologic and pharmacokinetic considerations, similar interactions may occur with other drugs that are listed.

Vitamin A		*Aminoglycosides*	
Vitamin A* (*Aquasol A*)		Kanamycin (*Kantrex*)	Paromomycin (*Humatin*)
		Neomycin* (eg, *Mycifradin*)	

Significance	Onset	Severity	Documentation
5	☐ Rapid	☐ Major	☐ Established
	■ **Delayed**	☐ Moderate	☐ Probable
		■ **Minor**	☐ Suspected
			■ **Possible**
			☐ Unlikely

Effects The biologic and therapeutic action of Vitamin A may be reduced.

Mechanism Orally administered AMINOGLYCOSIDES may decrease the GI absorption of VITAMIN A.

Management Based upon currently available documentation, no clinical interventions appear necessary.

Discussion

In a double-blind controlled study involving 5 healthy male subjects acting as their own controls, oral administration of a single 2 g dose of neomycin sulfate, given with a test meal containing 300,000 IU of retinyl palmitate, decreased the serum retinol levels measured over a 4-hour period following the meal.[1] In 6 patients receiving supplemental carotene, daily oral administration of 12 g of neomycin for 6 to 8 days markedly decreased plasma carotene concentrations.[2] When neomycin was discontinued, plasma carotene levels increased. Similarly, in 10 healthy volunteers, oral administration of 2 or 12 g daily of neomycin was associated with reversible decreases in plasma carotene.[3]

[1] Barrowman JA, et al. *Eur J Clin Pharmacol.* 1973;5:199.
[2] Jacobson ED, et al. *Am J Med.* 1960;28:524.
[3] Levine RA. *Gastroenterology.* 1967;52:685.

* Asterisk indicates drugs cited in interaction reports. Based on pharmacologic and pharmacokinetic considerations, similar interactions may occur with other drugs that are listed.

Vitamin A | **Mineral Oil**

Vitamin A*
(*Aquasol A*)

Mineral Oil*

Significance	Onset	Severity	Documentation
5	☐ Rapid ■ **Delayed**	☐ Major ☐ Moderate ■ **Minor**	☐ Established ☐ Probable ☐ Suspected ■ **Possible** ☐ Unlikely

Effects The biologic and therapeutic action of VITAMIN A may be reduced.

Mechanism MINERAL OIL may decrease GI absorption of VITAMIN A.

Management Consider separating the dose of VITAMIN A and MINERAL OIL by several hours. Consider also substituting an alternative therapy for MINERAL OIL.

Discussion

Administration of mineral oil decreases the absorption of carotene and vitamin A from the GI tract.[1-3] In 5 healthy male subjects receiving a controlled diet containing carotene and periodic supplements of 50,000 IU of vitamin A, mineral oil increased the fecal excretion of vitamin A.[3]

There are no recent studies evaluating the effects of mineral oil on vitamin A absorption.

[1] Curtis AC, et al. *JAMA*. 1939;113:1785.
[2] Curtis AC, et al. *Arch Intern Med*. 1939;63:54.
[3] Mahle AE, et al. *Gastroenterology*. 1947;9:44.

* Asterisk indicates drugs cited in interaction reports.

Vitamin B_{12} — *Aminosalicylic Acid*

Vitamin B_{12}*	Aminosalicylic Acid*

Significance	Onset	Severity	Documentation
3	☐ Rapid	☐ Major	☐ Established
	■ **Delayed**	☐ Moderate	☐ Probable
		■ **Minor**	■ **Suspected**
			☐ Possible
			☐ Unlikely

Effects The biologic and therapeutic action of VITAMIN B_{12} may be reduced. In addition, an abnormal Schilling test and symptoms of VITAMIN B_{12} deficiency may occur.

Mechanism AMINOSALICYLIC ACID may decrease GI absorption of VITAMIN B_{12}.

Management In patients requiring both drugs concurrently, administer the VITAMIN B_{12} parenterally.

Discussion

The association between aminosalicylic acid (PAS) administration and vitamin B_{12} malabsorption was first reported when it was observed that long-term administration of PAS in the treatment of tuberculosis decreased the Schilling test results in all 10 patients studied.[1] Two weeks after discontinuing PAS, the Schilling test values returned to the normal range. Several other investigators have reported vitamin B_{12} malabsorption during PAS therapy.[2-6] When the dose of PAS was stated, vitamin B_{12} malabsorption was observed with PAS doses of 8 to 12 g daily.[2,3,5,6] The effect of PAS on vitamin B_{12} absorption may occur within 5 days[5] but is usually not seen until several weeks into PAS therapy.[2,3] Absorption of vitamin B_{12} returns to normal following discontinuation of PAS administration. Not all investigations have found PAS administration to interfere with vitamin B_{12} absorption.[7]

[1] Heinivaara O, et al. *Acta Med Scand.* 1964;175:469.
[2] Akhtar AJ, et al. *Tubercle.* 1968;49:328.
[3] Coltart DJ. *Br Med J.* 1969;1:825.
[4] Palva IP, et al. *Scand J Haematol.* 1972:9:5.
[5] Toskes PP, et al. *Gastroenterology.* 1972;62:1232.
[6] Halsted CH, et al. *Arch Intern Med.* 1972;130:935.
[7] Paaby P, et al. *Acta Med Scand.* 1966;180:561.

* Asterisk indicates drugs cited in interaction reports.

Vitamin B_{12} — *Chloramphenicol*

Vitamin B_{12}* (eg, *Redisol*)	Chloramphenicol* (eg, *Chloromycetin*)

Significance	Onset	Severity	Documentation
3	☐ Rapid	☐ Major	☐ Established
	■ **Delayed**	☐ Moderate	☐ Probable
		■ **Minor**	■ **Suspected**
			☐ Possible
			☐ Unlikely

Effects The hematologic effects of VITAMIN B_{12} in patients with pernicious anemia may be decreased by concurrent administration of CHLORAMPHENICOL.

Mechanism Unknown.

Management Monitor the patient's clinical response to VITAMIN B_{12} during concomitant administration of CHLORAMPHENICOL. Consider alternative antibiotic therapy.

Discussion

In 4 patients with pernicious anemia, reticulocyte response to vitamin B_{12} administration was delayed or interrupted by concurrent treatment with chloramphenicol.[1] When coadministered with chloramphenicol, large doses of vitamin B complex, including folinic acid, vitamin B_6, and vitamin B_{12}, did not correct the erythropoietic lesion.[2] Normal marrow was established when the antibiotic was discontinued.

[1] Saidi P, et al. *J Lab Clin Med.* 1961;57:247.

[2] Jiji RM, et al. *Arch Intern Med.* 1963;111:70.

* Asterisk indicates drugs cited in interaction reports.

Vitamin B_{12} | **Omeprazole**

Vitamin B_{12}* (*Cyanocobalamin*) | Omeprazole* (*Prilosec*)

Significance	Onset	Severity	Documentation
5	☐ Rapid	☐ Major	☐ Established
	■ **Delayed**	☐ Moderate	☐ Probable
		■ **Minor**	☐ Suspected
			■ **Possible**
			☐ Unlikely

Effects The therapeutic action of VITAMIN B_{12} may be decreased.

Mechanism OMEPRAZOLE-induced hypohydria or achlorhydria may decrease the absorption of vitamin B_{12}.

Management If both drugs are to be given chronically, consider administering VITAMIN B_{12} parenterally.

Discussion

The effect of omeprazole on cyanocobalamin absorption was studied in 10 healthy men.[1] Five subjects received 20 mg omeprazole and the remaining 5 were given 40 mg omeprazole daily for 2 weeks. Each participant had a modified Schilling test (protein-bound cyanocobalamin) and gastric analysis as well as measurements of serum cyanocobalamin, gastrin, and folate concentrations before and after 2 weeks of omeprazole therapy. For individuals receiving omeprazole 20 mg daily, the mean basal acid output decreased from a baseline of 2.5 mEq/hr to 0.7 mEq/hr after 2 weeks of omeprazole therapy. In the 5 subjects receiving omeprazole 40 mg daily, the decrease in basal acid output was from 2.8 to 0.09 mEq/hr after 2 weeks of therapy. In the participants receiving 20 and 40 mg omeprazole, the mean absorption of protein-bound cyanocobalamin at baseline was 3.2% and 3.4%, respectively. Protein-bound cyanocobalamin absorption decreased to 0.9% and 0.4% after 2 weeks of receiving 20 or 40 mg omeprazole/day, respectively. After 20 and 40 mg omeprazole daily, the median values of protein-bound cyanocobalamin absorption decreased from 2.2% and 2.3% at baseline to 0.8% and 0.5%.

[1] Marcuard SP, et al. *Ann Intern Med.* 1994;120:211.

* Asterisk indicates drugs cited in interaction reports.

Vitamin D — *Thiazide Diuretics*

Vitamin D		Thiazide Diuretics	
Calcifediol (*Calderol*)	Dihydrotachysterol* (DHT; *Hytakerol*)	Bendroflumethiazide* (*Naturetin*)	Indapamide (*Lozol*)
Calcitriol (*Rocaltrol*)	Ergocalciferol* (eg, *Calciferol*)	Benzthiazide (eg, *Exna*)	Methyclothiazide* (eg, *Enduron*)
Cholecalciferol* (eg, *Delta-D*)		Chlorothiazide* (eg, *Diuril*)	Metolazone (*Mykrox*, *Zaroxolyn*)
		Chlorthalidone (eg, *Hygroton*)	Polythiazide (*Renese*)
		Hydrochlorothiazide (eg, *HydroDIURIL*)	Quinethazone (*Hydromox*)
		Hydroflumethiazide (eg, *Saluron*)	Trichlormethiazide (eg, *Naqua*)

Significance	Onset	Severity	Documentation
5	☐ Rapid ■ **Delayed**	☐ Major ☐ Moderate ■ **Minor**	☐ Established ☐ Probable ☐ Suspected ■ **Possible** ☐ Unlikely

Effects The biological actions of VITAMIN D may be enhanced. Hypercalcemia could manifest.

Mechanism Since THIAZIDE-TYPE DIURETICS may decrease urinary excretion of calcium, coadministration of VITAMIN D may potentiate the increase in serum calcium.

Management Consider monitoring serum calcium levels and, if necessary, discontinuing one or both drugs.

Discussion

Thiazide diuretics decreased the urinary excretion of calcium in normal subjects and in patients with various disorders.[1-8] In addition, thiazide diuretics may cause hypercalcemia to a greater extent than would be expected from decreased urinary calcium excretion alone. Both depletion of extracellular fluid volume and the presence of intact parathyroid glands appear required for a decrease in urinary calcium excretion in response to thiazides.[3] Administration of chlorothiazide to 1 patient was associated with symptomatic hypercalcemia and elevated BUN, while in 2 patients with primary hyperparathyroidism receiving chlorothiazide or methyclothiazide, preexisting hypercalcemia was exacerbated.[1] Plasma calcium levels returned to pretreatment values and symptoms disappeared following diuretic discontinuation. Twelve of 33 patients with chronic hypoparathyroidism receiving cholecalciferol, ergocalciferol, or DHT were given either bendroflumethiazide or methyclothiazide for edema or hypertension; 5 patients developed hypercalcemia.[5] However, in another study, hypoparathyroid patients receiving cholecalciferol and chlorothiazide did not experience increased serum calcium.[7]

1 Parfitt AM, et al. *N Engl J Med.* 1969;281:55.
2 Duarte CG, et al. *N Engl J Med.* 1971;284:828.
3 Brickman AS, et al. *J Clin Invest.* 1972;51:945.
4 Parfitt AM. *J Clin Invest.* 1972;51:1879.
5 Parfitt AM. *Ann Intern Med.* 1972;77:557.
6 Middler S, et al. *Metabolism.* 1973;22:139.
7 Popovtzer MM, et al. *J Clin Invest.* 1975;55:1295.
8 Riis B, et al. *Metabolism.* 1985;34:421.

* Asterisk indicates drugs cited in interaction reports. Based on pharmacologic and pharmacokinetic considerations, similar interactions may occur with other drugs that are listed.

Vitamin E — **Orlistat**

Vitamin E*	Orlistat* (*Xenical*)

Significance	Onset	Severity	Documentation
3	□ Rapid ■ **Delayed**	□ Major □ Moderate ■ **Minor**	□ Established □ Probable ■ **Suspected** □ Possible □ Unlikely

Effects The biologic and therapeutic actions of VITAMIN E may be reduced.

Mechanism ORLISTAT may decrease the GI absorption of VITAMIN E.

Management Based upon available information, no special precautions are needed. However, in patients with VITAMIN E deficiency who are undergoing ORLISTAT therapy, consider this interaction when implementing treatment.

Discussion

The effect of orlistat on vitamin E absorption was studied in an open-label, placebo-controlled, randomized crossover investigation involving 12 healthy volunteers.[1] Each subject received vitamin E (400 units alpha-tocopheryl acetate tablet) on the fourth day of treatment with orlistat (120 mg 3 times daily) or placebo. Compared with placebo, orlistat administration decreased peak plasma concentration and AUC of vitamin E approximately 43% and 60%, respectively.

[1] Melia AT, et al. *J Clin Pharmacol.* 1996;36:647.

* Asterisk indicates drugs cited in interaction reports.

Vitamin K — *Mineral Oil*

Vitamin K	Mineral Oil
Phytonadione* (*Mephyton*)	Mineral Oil*

Significance	Onset	Severity	Documentation
5	☐ Rapid	☐ Major	☐ Established
	■ **Delayed**	☐ Moderate	☐ Probable
		■ **Minor**	☐ Suspected
			■ **Possible**
			☐ Unlikely

Effects The effectiveness of VITAMIN K may be compromised. Prothrombin activity has been observed to be lessened.

Mechanism MINERAL OIL may decrease GI absorption of VITAMIN K.

Management Consider separating the dose of VITAMIN K and MINERAL OIL by several hours, or substitute an alternative therapy for MINERAL OIL. If MINERAL OIL must be continued, consider administering VITAMIN K parenterally.

Discussion

Prolonged oral ingestion of mineral oil has been associated with hypoprothrombinemia.[1] This effect was not reversed by the oral administration of vitamin K; however, prothrombin time returned to 100% of normal when vitamin K was administered parenterally, as well as when mineral oil was discontinued and vitamin K was given orally or parenterally.

[1] Javert CT, et al. *Am J Obstet Gynecol.* 1941;42:409.

* Asterisk indicates drugs cited in interaction reports.

Voriconazole — *Barbiturates*

Voriconazole* (*Vfend*)	Mephobarbital* (*Mebaral*)	Phenobarbital*

Significance	Onset	Severity	Documentation
1	□ Rapid ■ **Delayed**	■ **Major** □ Moderate □ Minor	□ Established □ Probable ■ **Suspected** □ Possible □ Unlikely

Effects VORICONAZOLE plasma concentrations may be reduced, decreasing the therapeutic effect.

Mechanism Certain BARBITURATES (ie, long-acting) may increase the metabolism (CYP3A4) of VORICONAZOLE.

Management Coadministration of VORICONAZOLE and long-acting BARBITURATES is contraindicated.

Discussion

Although not studied, coadministration of voriconazole with a long-acting barbiturate is likely to decrease voriconazole plasma concentrations, resulting in a decrease in therapeutic effect.[1] Coadministration of long-acting barbiturates and voriconazole is contraindicated by the manufacturer.[1]

The basis for this monograph is information on file with the manufacturer. Published clinical data are needed to further assess this interaction.

[1] Product information. Voriconazole (*Vfend*). Pfizer Labs. May 2002.

* Asterisk indicates drugs cited in interaction reports.

Voriconazole — *Carbamazepine*

Voriconazole* (eg, *Vfend*)	Carbamazepine* (eg, *Tegretol*)

Significance	Onset	Severity	Documentation
2	☐ Rapid	☐ Major	☐ Established
	■ **Delayed**	■ **Moderate**	☐ Probable
		☐ Minor	■ **Suspected**
			☐ Possible
			☐ Unlikely

Effects VORICONAZOLE plasma concentrations may be reduced, decreasing the therapeutic effect.

Mechanism CARBAMAZEPINE may increase the metabolism (CYP3A4) of VORICONAZOLE.

Management Coadministration of VORICONAZOLE and CARBAMAZEPINE is contraindicated.

Discussion

Although it has not been studied, coadministration of voriconazole with carbamazepine is likely to decrease voriconazole plasma concentrations, resulting in a decrease in therapeutic effect.[1] Coadministration of carbamazepine and voriconazole is contraindicated by the manufacturer. A 62-year-old woman receiving carbamazepine 400 mg daily was started on oral voriconazole.[2] Five days later, voriconazole concentrations were subtherapeutic and voriconazole treatment was changed to IV voriconazole 510 mg on day 1 followed by 425 mg twice daily. Despite the high dose of voriconazole, concentrations remained subtherapeutic and antifungal therapy was changed to caspofungin.[1]

[1] *Vfend* [package insert]. New York, NY: Pfizer Labs; May 2002.

[2] Malingré MM, et al. *Br J Clin Pharmcol.* 2011;74(1):205.

* Asterisk indicates drugs cited in interaction reports.

Voriconazole — *Chloramphenicol*

Voriconazole* (eg, *Vfend*)	Chloramphenicol*

Significance	Onset	Severity	Documentation
4	☐ Rapid ■ **Delayed**	☐ Major ■ **Moderate** ☐ Minor	☐ Established ☐ Probable ☐ Suspected ■ **Possible** ☐ Unlikely

Effects VORICONAZOLE plasma concentrations may be elevated, increasing the pharmacologic effects and adverse reactions.

Mechanism Unknown.

Management Closely monitor patients receiving VORICONAZOLE when CHLORAMPHENICOL is started or stopped. Adjust the VORICONAZOLE dose as needed.

Discussion

A 14-year-old boy with fulminant pneumococcal meningitis was receiving IV chloramphenicol and voriconazole as part of his treatment regimen.[1] During coadministration of chloramphenicol and voriconazole, voriconazole plasma trough concentrations ranged between 2.2 and 3.5 mcg/mL. After chloramphenicol was discontinued, voriconazole concentrations decreased to less than 1 mcg/mL. The voriconazole dose had to be almost doubled to keep concentrations in the range considered to be therapeutic for *Aspergillus fumigatus*. Subsequently, the patient died of cerebral aspergillosis.

[1] Hafner V, et al. *Antimicrob Agents Chemother.* 2008;52(11):4172.

* Asterisk indicates drugs cited in interaction reports.

Voriconazole — *Efavirenz*

Voriconazole* (eg, *Vfend*)	Efavirenz* (*Sustiva*)

Significance	Onset	Severity	Documentation
1	☐ Rapid ■ **Delayed**	■ **Major** ☐ Moderate ☐ Minor	☐ Established ☐ Probable ■ **Suspected** ☐ Possible ☐ Unlikely

Effects VORICONAZOLE plasma concentrations may be reduced, decreasing the therapeutic effect. EFAVIRENZ plasma levels may be elevated, increasing the risk of adverse reactions.

Mechanism EFAVIRENZ increases the metabolism (CYP2C9, CYP2C19) of VORICONAZOLE. VORICONAZOLE may inhibit the metabolism (CYP3A4) of EFAVIRENZ.

Management Coadministration of VORICONAZOLE and EFAVIRENZ is contraindicated at standard doses. When VORICONAZOLE is coadministered with EFAVIRENZ, increase the VORICONAZOLE maintenance dosage to 400 mg every 12 hours, and decrease the EFAVIRENZ dosage to 300 mg once daily using the capsule formulation.[1] Monitor the clinical response of the patient.

Discussion

In healthy subjects, steady-state efavirenz (400 mg/day) decreased the steady-state C_{max} and AUC of oral voriconazole (400 mg every 12 hours for 1 day, followed by 200 mg every 12 hours for 9 days) an average of 66% and 80%, respectively.[2] Steady-state voriconazole increased the steady-state C_{max} and AUC of efavirenz an average of 37% and 43%, respectively. In healthy men, coadministration of voriconazole 300 mg every 12 hours with efavirenz 300 mg every 24 hours decreased voriconazole AUC and C_{max} 55% and 36%, respectively, compared with voriconazole monotherapy.[3] In contrast, compared with monotherapy regimens, coadministration of voriconazole 400 mg every 12 hours with efavirenz 300 mg every 24 hours decreased voriconazole AUC 7% and increased the C_{max} 23%, while increasing efavirenz AUC 17%.

[1] *Sustiva* [package insert]. Princeton, NJ: Bristol-Myers Squibb Co; March 2009.
[2] Liu P, et al. *J Clin Pharmacol.* 2008;48(1):73.
[3] Damle B, et al. *Br J Clin Pharmacol.* 2008;65(4):523.

* Asterisk indicates drugs cited in interaction reports.

Voriconazole — *Erythromycin*

Voriconazole* (eg, *Vfend*)	Erythromycin* (eg, *Ery-Tab*)

Significance	Onset	Severity	Documentation
4	□ Rapid ■ **Delayed**	□ Major ■ **Moderate** □ Minor	□ Established □ Probable □ Suspected ■ **Possible** □ Unlikely

Effects VORICONAZOLE plasma concentrations may be increased in a CYP2C19 genotype–dependent manner.

Mechanism ERYTHROMYCIN may inhibit the metabolism (CYP2C19 and CYP3A4) of VORICONAZOLE.

Management Closely monitor for VORICONAZOLE adverse reactions. Lower VORICONAZOLE doses may be needed in CYP2C19 poor metabolizers and heterozygous extensive metabolizers.

Discussion

The effects of erythromycin on the pharmacokinetics of voriconazole with respect to CYP2C19 genotypes were studied in 18 healthy men.[1] Six CYP2C19 homozygous extensive metabolizer (EMs), 6 CYP2C19 heterozygous EMs (HEMs), and 6 CYP2C19 poor metabolizers (PMs) received a single dose of voriconazole 200 mg oral after 3 days of pretreatment with erythromycin 500 mg or placebo 3 times daily. Compared with placebo, pretreatment with erythromycin increased the voriconazole C_{max} and AUC and decreased the oral clearance. Increased voriconazole AUC and decreased oral clearance occurred after erythromycin pretreatment in HEMs and PMs but not in EMs. Both CYP2C19 and CYP3A4 inhibition by erythromycin influence voriconazole plasma concentration, and the effect of erythromycin with CYP2C19 polymorphism is in a genotype-dependent manner.

[1] Shi H, et al. *Eur J Clin Pharmacol.* 2010;66(11):1131.

* Asterisk indicates drugs cited in interaction reports.

Voriconazole		***Rifamycins***	
Voriconazole* (eg, *Vfend*)		Rifabutin* (*Mycobutin*)	Rifampin* (eg, *Rifadin*)

Significance	Onset	Severity	Documentation
1	☐ Rapid ■ **Delayed**	■ **Major** ☐ Moderate ☐ Minor	☐ Established ☐ Probable ■ **Suspected** ☐ Possible ☐ Unlikely

Effects VORICONAZOLE plasma concentrations may be reduced, decreasing the therapeutic effect. RIFABUTIN plasma levels may be elevated, increasing the risk of adverse reactions.

Mechanism RIFAMYCINS increase the metabolism (CYP3A4) of VORICONAZOLE. VORICONAZOLE inhibits the metabolism (CYP3A4) of RIFABUTIN.

Management Coadministration of VORICONAZOLE and RIFAMPIN or RIFABUTIN is contraindicated.[1]

Discussion

In healthy subjects, administration of rifampin 600 mg once daily decreased the steady-state AUC and peak plasma level of voriconazole (200 mg every 12 hours for 7 days) by an average of 96% and 93%, respectively.[1] During coadministration of rifampin, increasing the dosage of voriconazole to 400 mg every 12 hours did not restore adequate exposure to voriconazole. In healthy subjects, administration of rifabutin 300 mg once daily decreased the AUC and peak plasma level of voriconazole 200 mg twice daily by an average of 79% and 67%, respectively.[1] During coadministration of rifabutin 300 mg once daily and voriconazole 400 mg twice daily, the AUC and peak plasma level of voriconazole were, on average, approximately 2 times higher compared with giving voriconazole 200 mg twice daily alone. In addition, compared with administration of rifabutin 300 mg twice daily alone, coadministration of voriconazole 400 mg twice daily increased the AUC and peak plasma level of rifabutin 4- and 3-fold, respectively.[1] The C_{max} and AUC of voriconazole were markedly reduced in a patient who was given rifampin in error while participating in a long-term voriconazole pharmacokinetic study.[2] Subtherapeutic voriconazole concentrations and a lack of clinical response occurred in a 30-year-old woman receiving several drugs, including voriconazole and rifabutin.[3] Increasing the voriconazole dosage to 300 mg 3 times daily resulted in therapeutic drug levels.

[1] *Vfend* [package insert]. New York, NY: Pfizer Inc; May 2002.
[2] Geist MJ, et al. *Antimicrob Agents Chemother.* 2007;51(9):3455.
[3] Schwiesow JN, et al. *Pharmacotherapy.* 2008;28(8):1076.

* Asterisk indicates drugs cited in interaction reports.

Voriconazole | *Ritonavir*

Voriconazole* (eg, *Vfend*)	Ritonavir* (*Norvir*)

Significance	Onset	Severity	Documentation
1	□ Rapid ■ **Delayed**	■ **Major** □ Moderate □ Minor	□ Established □ Probable ■ **Suspected** □ Possible □ Unlikely

Effects VORICONAZOLE plasma concentrations may be reduced (decreasing the therapeutic effect) or elevated (increasing adverse reactions).

Mechanism RITONAVIR increases the metabolism (primarily CYP2C19 and CYP2C9) of VORICONAZOLE, although short-term exposure may cause inhibition of metabolism (CYP3A4).

Management Coadministration of VORICONAZOLE and RITONAVIR is contraindicated.[1]

Discussion

In healthy subjects, administration of ritonavir 400 mg every 12 hours for 9 days decreased the steady-state C_{max} and AUC of oral voriconazole (400 mg every 12 hours for 1 day, followed by 200 mg every 12 hours for 8 days) an average of 66% and 82%, respectively.[1] Voriconazole did not affect the pharmacokinetics of ritonavir. Twenty healthy volunteers received ritonavir 300 mg or placebo twice daily for 2 days.[2] Immediately thereafter, voriconazole 400 mg was administered. Study subjects consisted of all CYP2C19 genotypes. Ritonavir decreased voriconazole clearance, leading to a 4.5-fold increase in AUC. The decrease occurred in all genotypes, suggesting that ritonavir inhibited CYP3A4, the secondary pathway for voriconazole metabolism. In 2 parallel studies, the effects of ritonavir 400 and 100 mg twice daily on the pharmacokinetics of voriconazole 200 mg twice daily were evaluated in 51 patients.[3] Compared with giving voriconazole alone, ritonavir administration decreased voriconazole exposure in a dose-dependent manner. High-dose ritonavir reduced the voriconazole AUC 82%, while the low-dose ritonavir reduced the AUC 39%. One patient in each of the high- and low-dose groups experienced a 2.5- to 3-fold increase in voriconazole exposure and was excluded from the statistical analysis. See also Protease Inhibitors-Azole Antifungal Agents.

[1] *Vfend* [package insert]. New York, NY: Pfizer Inc; December 2003.
[2] Mikus G, et al. *Clin Pharmacol Ther.* 2006;80(2):126.
[3] Liu P, et al. *Antimicrob Agents Chemother.* 2007;51(10):3617.

* Asterisk indicates drugs cited in interaction reports.

Voriconazole — *St. John's Wort*

Voriconazole* (*Vfend*)	St. John's Wort*

Significance	Onset	Severity	Documentation
2	☐ Rapid ■ **Delayed**	☐ Major ■ **Moderate** ☐ Minor	☐ Established ☐ Probable ■ **Suspected** ☐ Possible ☐ Unlikely

Effects

Short-term administration of ST. JOHN'S WORT may produce a clinically unimportant increase in VORICONAZOLE levels, while long-term administration may reduce the bioavailability of VORICONAZOLE and its antifungal activity.

Mechanism

Short-term administration of ST. JOHN'S WORT may inhibit VORICONAZOLE metabolism, while long-term administration may increase VORICONAZOLE metabolism.

Management

Advise patients to avoid coadministration of VORICONAZOLE and ST. JOHN'S WORT. Caution patients receiving VORICONAZOLE to consult their health care provider before using nonprescription or herbal products.

Discussion

The effects of short- and long-term administration of St. John's wort on the pharmacokinetics of voriconazole were studied in 16 healthy men stratified for CYP2C19 genotype.[1] Using a controlled, open-label design, each subject received a single dose of oral voriconazole 400 mg before and on days 1 and 15 of St. John's wort extract administration (*Jarsin* 300 mg, Lichtwer Pharma, Berlin, Germany). During the first 10 hr of the first day of St. John's wort administration, the voriconazole AUC increased 22% compared with the control period. In contrast, after taking St. John's wort for 15 days, the voriconazole AUC decreased 59% compared with the control period, and the oral clearance of voriconazole increased 144%.

[1] Rengelshausen J, et al. *Clin Pharmacol Ther.* 2005;78:25.

* Asterisk indicates drugs cited in interaction reports.

Zidovudine — *Acetaminophen*

Zidovudine* (*Retrovir*)	Acetaminophen* (eg, *Tylenol*)

Significance	Onset	Severity	Documentation
4	☐ Rapid	☐ Major	☐ Established
	■ **Delayed**	■ **Moderate**	☐ Probable
		☐ Minor	☐ Suspected
			■ **Possible**
			☐ Unlikely

Effects The pharmacologic effects of ZIDOVUDINE may be decreased.

Mechanism Enhanced nonhepatic or renal clearance of ZIDOVUDINE appears to be involved.

Management If an interaction is suspected, consider increasing the dose of ZIDOVUDINE or avoiding ACETAMINOPHEN.

Discussion

The effect of acetaminophen on the clearance of zidovudine was studied in 27 patients with AIDS or advanced AIDS-related complex.[1] Each patient received zidovudine 200 mg and acetaminophen concurrently every 4 hr. Thirteen patients received acetaminophen 325 mg for 3 days, 8 patients received 650 mg for 3 days, and 6 patients received 650 mg for 7 days. The mean AUC of zidovudine decreased with each dosing regimen of acetaminophen. The magnitude of the change in AUC for each group and the cumulative dose of acetaminophen was linearly related, indicating an increase in total clearance of 5%, 11%, and 33%, respectively, for the 3 different acetaminophen dosing schedules. In addition, in the 6 patients receiving acetaminophen 650 mg for 7 days, the mean $t_{1/2}$ of zidovudine was different after acetaminophen administration compared with the other 2 acetaminophen dosing schedules. Other pharmacokinetic parameters were not different from baseline measurements.

A 31-year-old man with AIDS developed severe, reversible hepatotoxicity after taking acetaminophen 3.3 g over a 36-hr period.[2] He was malnourished and taking zidovudine and trimethoprim-sulfamethoxazole (eg, *Septra*). It could not be determined whether this reaction was caused by an interaction. Additional information is needed to substantiate this adverse effect. In 1 patient receiving acetaminophen 3 g/day chronically, the addition of zidovudine did not affect acetaminophen concentrations; however, zidovudine absorption may have been increased.[3]

[1] Sattler FR, et al. *Ann Intern Med.* 1991;114:937.
[2] Shriner K, et al. *Am J Med.* 1992;93:94.
[3] Burger DM, et al. *Ann Pharmacother.* 1994;28:327.

* Asterisk indicates drugs cited in interaction reports.

Zidovudine — *Atovaquone*

Zidovudine* (eg, *Retrovir*)	Atovaquone* (*Mepron*)

Significance	Onset	Severity	Documentation
2	☐ Rapid	☐ Major	☐ Established
	■ **Delayed**	■ **Moderate**	☐ Probable
		☐ Minor	■ **Suspected**
			☐ Possible
			☐ Unlikely

Effects Serum ZIDOVUDINE concentrations may be elevated, increasing the risk of ZIDOVUDINE toxicity.

Mechanism ATOVAQUONE appears to inhibit the glucuronidation of ZIDOVUDINE.

Management Monitor the effects of ZIDOVUDINE during coadministration of ATOVAQUONE. If an interaction is suspected, a lower dose of ZIDOVUDINE may be needed.

Discussion

Utilizing an open-label, randomized, crossover design, the pharmacokinetics of coadministration of oral atovaquone and zidovudine were studied in 14 patients infected with HIV.[1] Each patient received atovaquone 750 mg every 12 hours and zidovudine 200 mg every 8 hours, alone and in combination. Atovaquone significantly increased the AUC of zidovudine 31% ($P < 0.05$) and decreased the clearance of zidovudine from 2,029 to 1,512 mL/min ($P < 0.05$). At the same time, the AUC of the glucuronide metabolite of zidovudine was decreased 6% ($P < 0.1$) and the ratio between the AUC of the glucuronide metabolite of zidovudine and that of zidovudine decreased from 4.48 to 3.12 ($P < 0.05$). Zidovudine had no effect on the pharmacokinetics of atovaquone.

The clinical importance of this interaction may be increased in patients receiving other drugs that are toxic to the bone marrow.[1] It may be necessary to decrease the dose of zidovudine 33% in patients with evidence of bone marrow toxicity.

[1] Lee BL, et al. *Clin Pharmacol Ther.* 1996;59:14.

* Asterisk indicates drugs cited in interaction reports.

Zidovudine — *Benzodiazepines*

Zidovudine* (AZT; eg, *Retrovir*)	Oxazepam* (eg, *Serax*)

Significance	Onset	Severity	Documentation
4	☐ Rapid	☐ Major	☐ Established
	■ **Delayed**	■ **Moderate**	☐ Probable
		☐ Minor	☐ Suspected
			■ **Possible**
			☐ Unlikely

Effects The incidence of headache may be increased.

Mechanism Unknown.

Management If headache occurs, discontinue OXAZEPAM before concluding that the headache is due to ZIDOVUDINE or an HIV-related pathology.

Discussion

To determine whether a pharmacokinetic drug interaction exists between zidovudine and oxazepam, a study was conducted in 6 HIV-infected individuals.[1] No clinically important pharmacokinetic interaction occurred during coadministration of zidovudine and oxazepam. However, 5 of 6 participants receiving the drug combination experienced headache compared with 1 subject who experienced headache with oxazepam administration alone and none with zidovudine alone.

[1] Mole L, et al. *J Acquir Immune Defic Syndr.* 1993;6:56.

* Asterisk indicates drugs cited in interaction reports.

Zidovudine — *Clarithromycin*

Zidovudine* (AZT; eg, *Retrovir*)	Clarithromycin* (eg, *Biaxin*)

Significance	Onset	Severity	Documentation
4	☐ Rapid ■ **Delayed**	☐ Major ■ **Moderate** ☐ Minor	☐ Established ☐ Probable ☐ Suspected ■ **Possible** ☐ Unlikely

Effects Peak serum ZIDOVUDINE concentrations may be increased or decreased.

Mechanism CLARITHROMYCIN may alter the rate of absorption of ZIDOVUDINE.

Management Based on currently available data, no special considerations are necessary.

Discussion

The effects of clarithromycin on the pharmacokinetics of zidovudine were evaluated in 18 volunteers with AIDS who did not have a *Mycobacterium avium* complex infection or clinical evidence of gastroenteritis.[1] Each subject received zidovudine 200 mg every 8 hours either alone or with clarithromycin 1 g every 12 hours, separated by 2 hours from the zidovudine dose. The mean zidovudine C_{max} was significantly higher (949 vs 616.6 ng/mL; $P < 0.001$) and the mean time to reach the C_{max} was significantly shorter (1 vs 2.1 hours; $P = 0.005$) when zidovudine was administered with clarithromycin than when zidovudine was given alone. The zidovudine AUC and the minimum zidovudine serum concentration were not significantly different when zidovudine was administered alone or with clarithromycin. The results indicate that clarithromycin may increase the rate, but not the extent, of zidovudine absorption. These findings are in contrast to another report in which clarithromycin decreased zidovudine plasma concentrations in some patients.[2]

Additional studies are needed to clarify this drug interaction and to determine the clinical importance.

[1] Vance E, et al. *Antimicrob Agents Chemother.* 1995;39:1355.

[2] Gustavson LE, et al. *Clin Pharmacol Ther.* 1993;53:163.

* Asterisk indicates drugs cited in interaction reports.

Zidovudine — *Food*

Zidovudine* (*AZT; Retrovir*)	High-Fat Diet

Significance	Onset	Severity	Documentation
4	■ **Rapid**	□ Major	□ Established
	□ Delayed	■ **Moderate**	□ Probable
		□ Minor	□ Suspected
			■ **Possible**
			□ Unlikely

Effects The absorption of ZIDOVUDINE may be decreased.

Mechanism The rate and extent of ZIDOVUDINE absorption may be decreased by fatty meals.

Management Administer ZIDOVUDINE at least 1 hour before meals.

Discussion

The effects of food on the pharmacokinetics of zidovudine have been evaluated in several studies.[1,2] The systemic availability of oral zidovudine administered with breakfast or while fasting was investigated in 13 patients with AIDS.[1] After an overnight fast, 250 mg zidovudine was taken on an empty stomach or in the middle of a breakfast containing approximately 40 g of fat. Each subject participated in both phases of the investigation. Zidovudine concentrations were higher in fasting subjects compared with those taking the medication with breakfast. The maximum plasma concentration ranged from 3.7 to 19.4 mcmol/L in fasting patients compared with 1.5 to 6.5 mcmol/L when taken during the meal. When ingested by fasting subjects, the maximum zidovudine concentration achieved was 2.8 times higher than when taken with the meal ($P < 0.001$). The time to reach the peak concentration was significantly shorter in fasting subjects ($P < 0.001$). The area under the plasma concentration-time curve (AUC) for zidovudine (ie, systemic availability) when taken during the meal was 78% of the value when taken on an empty stomach ($P < 0.05$). The plasma half-life and duration of plasma zidovudine concentration more than 1 mcmol/L did not differ whether zidovudine was taken with the meal or while fasting. In contrast, protein-based meals may not alter zidovudine absorption.[2] In a randomized, 2-treatment, 2-period crossover study, the effects of a 25 g protein meal (*ProMod*) on zidovudine pharmacokinetics were studied in 11 HIV-infected patients. Following an overnight fast, each patient received 200 mg zidovudine with either 220 mL orange juice or immediately after a 25 g protein supplement diluted with 220 mL orange juice. The protein meal decreased the maximum zidovudine concentration and increased mean residence time ($P = 0.001$) but AUC, time to reach the maximum serum concentration, terminal half-life, and renal clearance of zidovudine were not affected.

[1] Lotterer E, et al. *Eur J Clin Pharmacol.* 1991;40:305. [2] Sahai J, et al. *Br J Clin Pharmacol.* 1992;33:657.

* Asterisk indicates drugs cited in interaction reports.

Zidovudine — *Histamine H_2 Antagonists*

Zidovudine	Histamine H_2 Antagonists
Zidovudine* (*Retrovir*)	Cimetidine* (eg, *Tagamet*)

Significance	Onset	Severity	Documentation
5	☐ Rapid	☐ Major	☐ Established
	■ **Delayed**	☐ Moderate	☐ Probable
		■ **Minor**	☐ Suspected
			☐ Possible
			■ **Unlikely**

Effects No change in ZIDOVUDINE serum concentration is expected.

Mechanism CIMETIDINE may reduce the renal clearance of ZIDOVUDINE, presumably by inhibiting renal tubular secretion.

Management Based on available data, no action is needed.

Discussion

Using a randomized, crossover design, the effects of cimetidine or ranitidine (eg, *Zantac*) on the pharmacokinetics of zidovudine were investigated in 6 HIV-infected patients.[1] Each subject received 600 mg/day of zidovudine alone, zidovudine with cimetidine 1,200 mg/day for 7 days, and zidovudine with ranitidine 300 mg/day for 7 days. Cimetidine reduced the renal clearance of zidovudine 56% and urinary excretion 40%. However, there were no changes in zidovudine serum concentrations. Ranitidine did not affect the pharmacokinetics of zidovudine. Neither famotidine (eg, *Pepcid*) nor nizatidine (*Axid*) would be expected to affect the pharmacokinetics of zidovudine.

[1] Fletcher CV, et al. *Pharmacotherapy*. 1995;15:701.

* Asterisk indicates drugs cited in interaction reports.

Zidovudine | **_Interferon Beta-1b_**

Zidovudine* (eg, *Retrovir*) | Interferon Beta-1b* (*Betaseron*)

Significance	Onset	Severity	Documentation
4	□ Rapid ■ **Delayed**	□ Major ■ **Moderate** □ Minor	□ Established □ Probable □ Suspected ■ **Possible** □ Unlikely

Effects Serum ZIDOVUDINE levels may be elevated, increasing the pharmacologic and toxic effects of ZIDOVUDINE.

Mechanism BETA INTERFERON may inhibit the glucuronidation of ZIDOVUDINE.

Management Closely monitor the effects of ZIDOVUDINE in patients receiving BETA INTERFERON concurrently. A lower dose of ZIDOVUDINE may be needed.

Discussion

The pharmacokinetics of zidovudine were studied in HIV-infected patients receiving concurrent recombinant beta interferon.[1] Zidovudine was administered in a dose of 200 mg every 4 hours orally for 8 weeks prior to the administration of subcutaneous beta interferon 90×10^6 units daily. Concomitant administration of zidovudine and beta interferon reduced the rate of metabolism of zidovudine from 1.18 hr^{-1} to 0.4 and 0.08 hr^{-1} at days 3 and 15, respectively; increased the volume of distribution from 2.7 L/kg to 7 and 5.8 L/kg on days 3 and 15, respectively; and increased the half-life 2- to 3-fold by day 15. In a second study, interleukin-2 (*Proleukin*), a compound that is believed to stimulate the production of gamma interferon, had no effect on the half-life of zidovudine or the area under the concentration-time curve.[2]

Documentation for this possible interaction consists of abstracts. More substantive data are needed to evaluate the clinical importance of this reported interaction.

[1] Nokta M, et al. *Fifth Int Conf AIDS.* 1989;278. Abstract.

[2] Skinner MH, et al. *Clin Pharmacol Ther.* 1989;45:128. Abstract.

* Asterisk indicates drugs cited in interaction reports.

Zidovudine — *Methadone*

Zidovudine* (eg, *Retrovir*)	Methadone* (eg, *Dolophine*)

Significance	Onset	Severity	Documentation
2	☐ Rapid ■ **Delayed**	☐ Major ■ **Moderate** ☐ Minor	☐ Established ■ **Probable** ☐ Suspected ☐ Possible ☐ Unlikely

Effects Serum ZIDOVUDINE concentrations may be elevated, increasing the risk of side effects.

Mechanism Unknown.

Management Monitor the effects of ZIDOVUDINE during concurrent use of METHADONE. If an interaction is suspected, a lower dose of ZIDOVUDINE may be needed.

Discussion

The pharmacokinetics of methadone and zidovudine, administered alone and in combination, were investigated in 14 HIV-infected patients.[1] Nine patients had been receiving a constant daily dose of 30 to 90 mg methadone for at least 9 months; 5 patients had not received methadone. All patients received zidovudine 200 mg every 4 hours. Coadministration of these drugs did not alter the pharmacokinetics of methadone. However, in patients receiving methadone, serum zidovudine concentrations were 43% higher than those seen in patients given zidovudine alone. The area under the plasma concentration-time curve (AUC) of zidovudine in 4 participants receiving concurrent methadone was approximately 2-fold higher than in patients receiving zidovudine monotherapy. Similar results were found in a study of 8 recently detoxified patients who were given acute methadone therapy and reevaluated after 2 months.[2] Acute methadone therapy increased the AUC of oral zidovudine 41% while chronic treatment increased the AUC 29%.

[1] Schwartz EL, et al. *J Acquir Immune Defic Syndr.* 1992;5:619.

[2] McCance-Katz EF, et al. *J Acquir Immune Defic Syndr Hum Retrovirol.* 1998;18:435.

* Asterisk indicates drugs cited in interaction reports.

Zidovudine — *Probenecid*

Zidovudine* (eg, *Retrovir*)	Probenecid*

Significance	Onset	Severity	Documentation
2	☐ Rapid ■ **Delayed**	☐ Major ■ **Moderate** ☐ Minor	☐ Established ☐ Probable ■ **Suspected** ☐ Possible ☐ Unlikely

Effects Cutaneous eruptions accompanied by systemic symptoms including malaise, myalgia, and fever have been reported.

Mechanism PROBENECID appears to inhibit ZIDOVUDINE glucuronidation; however, it is unclear whether this kinetic effect causes the observed toxicity.

Management Coadminister ZIDOVUDINE and PROBENECID with caution. Observe the patient for possible rash and systemic symptoms.

Discussion

In a preliminary report involving 12 patients with AIDS or AIDS-related complex (ARC), coadministration of zidovudine and probenecid increased the zidovudine area under the concentration-time curve 80% and the amount of unchanged zidovudine recovered in the urine.[1] These data suggested that in certain patients probenecid could be used to reduce the daily dose and the cost of zidovudine therapy by allowing the dosing interval to be doubled. However, due to the low therapeutic index of zidovudine, the combination of these 2 drugs could be difficult to manage clinically.[2] In a subsequent study, the effect of probenecid on zidovudine metabolism and the longer-term tolerance to the combination were assessed over a 28-day period vs the 6-day trials of the earlier report.[3] Eight male patients with HIV infection were given zidovudine 100 to 200 mg every 8 hours and probenecid 500 mg every 8 hours. During concomitant treatment with the 2 drugs, 6 patients developed a rash. Two had minor rashes during the first week of concurrent therapy. The rashes were localized to the trunk and resolved with continued administration of the drugs. Three patients experienced a widespread maculopapular erythematous eruption and systemic symptoms including myalgia, malaise, and fever. In these patients and in a fourth who did not experience symptoms, probenecid was discontinued after 10 to 13 days of therapy. A biopsy in 2 patients revealed intradermal lesions compatible with a diagnosis of drug eruption. Although probenecid appears to inhibit zidovudine glucuronidation and renal excretion of the metabolite,[2] this would not account for the rash. In a report involving 7 patients receiving zidovudine 600 mg/day and probenecid 500 mg 3 times daily, no rash was observed.[4]

Controlled studies are needed to determine the clinical importance of this interaction.

[1] Kornhauser DM, et al. *Lancet.* 1989;2:473.
[2] de Miranda P, et al. *Clin Pharmacol Ther.* 1989;46:494.
[3] Petty BG, et al. *Lancet.* 1990;335:1044.
[4] Duckworth AS, et al. *Lancet.* 1990;336:441.

* Asterisk indicates drugs cited in interaction reports.

Zidovudine — *Rifamycins*

Zidovudine	Rifamycins	
Zidovudine* (*Retrovir*)	Rifabutin* (*Mycobutin*)	Rifapentine (*Priftin*)
	Rifampin* (eg, *Rifadin*)	

Significance	Onset	Severity	Documentation
4	□ Rapid ■ **Delayed**	□ Major ■ **Moderate** □ Minor	□ Established □ Probable □ Suspected ■ **Possible** □ Unlikely

Effects The pharmacologic effects of ZIDOVUDINE may be decreased.

Mechanism Unknown.

Management If an interaction is suspected, consider increasing the dose of ZIDOVUDINE.

Discussion

The effects of rifampin on the pharmacokinetics of zidovudine were evaluated in patients infected with human immunodeficiency virus (HIV).[1] The results of 4 patients receiving long-term treatment with rifampin and zidovudine were compared with those of patients administered zidovudine without rifampin. The patients receiving both rifampin 600 mg/day and zidovudine had lower areas under the plasma concentration-time curve (AUC) for zidovudine and a correspondingly higher clearance than did patients who did not receive rifampin. In addition, in 1 patient followed for 2.5 months, the zidovudine AUC was approximately 50% lower while the patient was taking rifampin than after the rifampin was discontinued. No influence of rifampin administration on the half-life of zidovudine was detected. Although the patients in both groups had been receiving other medications, none of the other drugs were known to decrease zidovudine concentrations. A similar drug interaction has been observed with rifabutin, a drug structurally related to rifampin, and zidovudine. Concurrent administration of rifabutin and zidovudine decreased the AUC of zidovudine 32% and increased the clearance 43%. In a study of 8 asymptomatic HIV-infected patients, coadministration of zidovudine 200 mg every 8 hours and rifampin 600 mg/day resulted in a 43% decrease in the peak levels and a 47% decrease in the AUC of zidovudine.[2] These data suggest a decrease in zidovudine bioavailability.

Because resistance of the human immunodeficiency virus to zidovudine increases with prolonged administration, the clinical importance of the findings of this investigation needs to be further evaluated.

[1] Burger DM, et al. *Antimicrob Agents Chemother.* 1993;37:1426.

[2] Gallicano KD, et al. *Br J Clin Pharmacol.* 1999;48;168.

* Asterisk indicates drugs cited in interaction reports.

Zidovudine — *Trimethoprim*

Zidovudine	Trimethoprim	
Zidovudine* (eg, *Retrovir*)	Trimethoprim* (eg, *Proloprim*)	Trimethoprim/ Sulfamethoxazole* (eg, *Bactrim*)

Significance	Onset	Severity	Documentation
4	■ **Rapid** □ Delayed	□ Major ■ **Moderate** □ Minor	□ Established □ Probable □ Suspected ■ **Possible** □ Unlikely

Effects The pharmacologic effects of ZIDOVUDINE may be increased in patients with hepatic function impairment who receive TRIMETHOPRIM.

Mechanism The renal clearance of ZIDOVUDINE and its glucuronide metabolite appear to be decreased.

Management This interaction may only be important in patients with impaired hepatic glucuronidation from liver disease or drug inhibition. Monitor the effects of ZIDOVUDINE in patients with impaired hepatic glucuronidation receiving TRIMETHOPRIM concurrently. A lower dose of ZIDOVUDINE may be needed.

Discussion

In an open, randomized, 3-phase crossover trial, the effects of coadministration of trimethoprim or trimethoprim/sulfamethoxazole on the renal excretion and metabolism of zidovudine were studied in 9 patients with HIV infections.[1] During the study, patients received zidovudine 3 mg/kg as a 1-hour IV infusion with the oral administration of either trimethoprim 150 mg alone or trimethoprim 160 mg in combination with sulfamethoxazole 800 mg (TMP-SMZ). The metabolism of zidovudine was not affected by coadministration of trimethoprim or TMP-SMZ. However, the serum levels of zidovudine and its glucuronide metabolite were increased by administration of trimethoprim and TMP-SMZ. This change resulted from a decrease in renal clearance. Renal clearance of zidovudine was decreased 58% and 48% by TMP-SMZ and trimethoprim, respectively, while the renal clearance of the glucuronide metabolite was decreased 27% and 20%. The fraction of the dose excreted as zidovudine decreased, as did the metabolic ratio. None of the other pharmacokinetic parameters of zidovudine differed between administration of zidovudine alone or with trimethoprim or TMP-SMZ, suggesting an increase in the elimination of zidovudine by a nonrenal route (eg, biliary excretion). The magnitude of the decreases in renal clearance of zidovudine and its metabolite with both trimethoprim and TMP-SMZ indicate that the interaction is caused by the trimethoprim component.

[1] Chatton JY, et al. *Br J Clin Pharmacol.* 1992;34(6):551.

* Asterisk indicates drugs cited in interaction reports.

Zidovudine — *Valproic Acid*

Zidovudine* (eg, *Retrovir*)	Divalproex Sodium* (*Depakote*)	Valproic Acid* (eg, *Depakene*)

Significance	Onset	Severity	Documentation
2	☐ Rapid ■ **Delayed**	☐ Major ■ **Moderate** ☐ Minor	☐ Established ☐ Probable ■ **Suspected** ☐ Possible ☐ Unlikely

Effects ZIDOVUDINE AUC may be increased, leading to ZIDOVUDINE toxicity.

Mechanism First-pass glucuronide metabolism of ZIDOVUDINE may be decreased.

Management It may be necessary to adjust the dose of ZIDOVUDINE when starting, stopping, or changing the dose of VALPROIC ACID. Monitor hemoglobin and hematocrit.

Discussion

The effects of valproic acid administration on the pharmacokinetics of zidovudine were studied in 6 HIV-positive patients.[1] All patients had tolerated zidovudine at doses of 500 mg/day or more for 6 weeks prior to the investigation. During the study, patients received oral zidovudine 100 mg every 8 hours for 4 days. On day 5, each patient received zidovudine 100 mg, and blood samples were collected at varying intervals over a 12-hour period. On days 6 through 9, patients received zidovudine 100 mg every 8 hours; 5 patients received oral valproic acid 250 mg every 8 hours, while 1 patient was given valproic acid 500 mg every 8 hours. The zidovudine AUC increased 80% (from 0.65 to 1.17 mcg•hr/mL), while clearance and volume of distribution were decreased 38% (from 2,351 to 1,449 mL/min) and 36% (from 5.02 to 3.22 L/kg), respectively. Valproic acid administration caused a 57% decrease in the mean urinary excretion ratio of the zidovudine glucuronide metabolite to zidovudine; the systemic clearance of zidovudine was not changed, indicating an inhibition of zidovudine first-pass metabolism by valproic acid. In a 44-year-old HIV-positive man, coadministration of zidovudine and valproic acid produced a 2- to 3-fold increase in zidovudine levels and a 74% increase in zidovudine cerebral spinal fluid levels (from 27 to 47 ng/mL).[2] Severe anemia developed in a 42-year-old man receiving chronic zidovudine after starting valproic acid.[3]

[1] Lertora JJ, et al. *Clin Pharmacol Ther.* 1994;56(3):272.
[2] Akula SK, et al. *Am J Med Sci.* 1997;313(4):244.
[3] Antoniou T, et al. *Clin Infect Dis.* 2004;38(5):e38.

* Asterisk indicates drugs cited in interaction reports.

Ziprasidone — *Antiarrhythmic Agents*

Ziprasidone	Antiarrhythmic Agents	
Ziprasidone* (*Geodon*)	Amiodarone* (eg, *Cordarone*)	Quinidine* (eg, *Quinidex*)
	Bretylium*	Sotalol* (eg, *Betapace*)
	Disopyramide* (eg, *Norpace*)	
	Procainamide* (*Procanbid*)	

Significance	Onset	Severity	Documentation
1	☐ Rapid	■ **Major**	☐ Established
	■ **Delayed**	☐ Moderate	☐ Probable
		☐ Minor	■ **Suspected**
			☐ Possible
			☐ Unlikely

Effects The risk of life-threatening cardiac arrhythmias, including torsades de pointes, may be increased.

Mechanism Possibly synergistic or additive prolongation of the QT interval.

Management ZIPRASIDONE is contraindicated in patients receiving certain ANTIARRHYTHMIC AGENTS.[1]

Discussion

Do not use ziprasidone with other drugs that prolong the QT interval. Ziprasidone causes dose-related prolongation of the QT interval; other drugs that prolong the QT interval (eg, quinidine, sotalol)[2] have been associated with fatal arrhythmias.[1] Sudden, unexplained deaths have been reported in patients receiving ziprasidone at recommended doses. In addition to other agents that prolong the QT interval, certain factors may increase the risk of occurrence of torsades de pointes and sudden death in association with ziprasidone, including bradycardia, hypokalemia, hypomagnesemia, and congenital prolongation of the QT interval.

The basis for this monograph is information on file with the manufacturer. Because of the seriousness of the cardiac problems, clinical evaluation of this interaction in humans is not likely to be forthcoming.

[1] *Geodon* [package insert]. New York, NY: Pfizer Labs; 2001.

[2] Thomas M, et al. *Br J Clin Pharmacol.* 1996;41:77.

* Asterisk indicates drugs cited in interaction reports.

Ziprasidone — *Arsenic Trioxide*

Ziprasidone* (*Geodon*)	Arsenic Trioxide* (*Trisenox*)

Significance	Onset	Severity	Documentation
1	☐ Rapid	■ **Major**	☐ Established
	■ **Delayed**	☐ Moderate	☐ Probable
		☐ Minor	■ **Suspected**
			☐ Possible
			☐ Unlikely

Effects The risk of life-threatening cardiac arrhythmias, including torsades de pointes, may be increased.

Mechanism Possibly synergistic or additive prolongation of the QT interval.

Management ZIPRASIDONE is contraindicated in patients receiving ARSENIC TRIOXIDE.[1]

Discussion

Do not use ziprasidone with other drugs that prolong the QT interval. Neither pharmacokinetic nor pharmacodynamic studies between ziprasidone and other drugs that prolong the QT interval have been conducted. However, an additive effect of ziprasidone with coadministration of other drugs that prolong the QT interval (eg, arsenic trioxide) cannot be excluded. Therefore, ziprasidone should not be administered with other drugs that prolong the QT interval.[1] Sudden, unexplained deaths have been reported in patients receiving ziprasidone at recommended doses. In addition to other agents that prolong the QT interval, certain factors may increase the risk of occurrence of torsades de pointes and sudden death in association with ziprasidone, including bradycardia, hypokalemia, hypomagnesemia, and congenital prolongation of the QT interval.

The basis for this monograph is information on file with the manufacturer. Because of the seriousness of the cardiac problems, clinical evaluation of this interaction in humans is not likely to be forthcoming.

[1] *Geodon* [package insert]. New York, NY: Pfizer Labs; June 2002.

* Asterisk indicates drugs cited in interaction reports.

Ziprasidone — *Azole Antifungal Agents*

Ziprasidone	Azole Antifungal Agents	
Ziprasidone* (*Geodon*)	Fluconazole (eg, *Diflucan*)	Ketoconazole* (eg, *Nizoral*)
	Itraconazole (eg, *Sporanox*)	

Significance	Onset	Severity	Documentation
5	□ Rapid	□ Major	□ Established
	■ **Delayed**	□ Moderate	□ Probable
		■ **Minor**	□ Suspected
			■ **Possible**
			□ Unlikely

Effects ZIPRASIDONE plasma concentrations may be elevated, increasing side effects.

Mechanism Inhibition of ZIPRASIDONE metabolism (CYP3A4) by AZOLE ANTIFUNGAL AGENTS is suspected.

Management Observe the patient for ZIPRASIDONE side effects during coadministration of AZOLE ANTIFUNGAL AGENTS. Be prepared to decrease the ZIPRASIDONE dose if needed.

Discussion

The effects of multiple-dose ketoconazole administration (400 mg once daily for 6 days) on the pharmacokinetics of a single oral dose of ziprasidone 40 mg were evaluated in 13 healthy subjects.[1] In an open-label, randomized, crossover study, each subject received ziprasidone before and after 5 days of ketoconazole or placebo administration. Ziprasidone was administered immediately after consumption of a high-fat breakfast. Compared with placebo, administration of ziprasidone with ketoconazole increased the mean AUC of ziprasidone 33% and mean peak concentration 34%. Compared with ketoconazole plasma levels measured before ziprasidone dosing, ketoconazole plasma levels were increased 2-fold 1 day after ziprasidone administration. The increases in ketoconazole levels were attributed to the high-fat meal. However, the increase in ketoconazole levels may have increased the magnitude of the interaction with ziprasidone. Additional studies are needed to determine the clinical importance of this interaction and the contribution of the high-fat meal to the outcome of the investigation.

[1] Miceli JJ, et al. *Br J Clin Pharmacol.* 2000;49 (suppl 1):71S.

* Asterisk indicates drugs cited in interaction reports. Based on pharmacologic and pharmacokinetic considerations, similar interactions may occur with other drugs that are listed.

Ziprasidone — *Carbamazepine*

Ziprasidone* (*Geodon*)	Carbamazepine* (eg, *Tegretol*)

Significance	Onset	Severity	Documentation
2	☐ Rapid ■ **Delayed**	☐ Major ■ **Moderate** ☐ Minor	☐ Established ☐ Probable ■ **Suspected** ☐ Possible ☐ Unlikely

Effects ZIPRASIDONE plasma concentrations may be reduced, decreasing the therapeutic effect.

Mechanism Increased ZIPRASIDONE metabolism (CYP3A4), induced by CARBAMAZEPINE, is suspected.

Management Monitor the clinical response of the patient to ZIPRASIDONE when starting, stopping, or changing the dose of CARBAMAZEPINE. Be prepared to change the ZIPRASIDONE dose as needed.

Discussion

The effects of steady-state carbamazepine administration on the pharmacokinetics of ziprasidone were evaluated in 19 patients.[1] In an open-label, randomized, placebo-controlled, parallel group investigation, subjects received ziprasidone on days 1, 2, and 3 as well as on days 26, 27, and 28 of the study. On days 5 through 29, subjects received carbamazepine or placebo. Compared with placebo, carbamazepine administration decreased the mean AUC of ziprasidone 36% and the mean peak plasma concentration 27%. Additional studies are needed to determine the clinical importance of this interaction.

[1] Miceli JJ, et al. *Br J Clin Pharmacol.* 2000;49(suppl 1):65S.

* Asterisk indicates drugs cited in interaction reports.

Ziprasidone — *Cisapride*

Ziprasidone* (*Geodon*)	Cisapride*† (eg, *Propulsid*)

Significance	Onset	Severity	Documentation
1	□ Rapid ■ **Delayed**	■ **Major** □ Moderate □ Minor	□ Established □ Probable ■ **Suspected** □ Possible □ Unlikely

Effects The risk of life-threatening cardiac arrhythmias, including torsade de pointes, may be increased.

Mechanism Possibly synergistic or additive prolongation of the QTc interval.

Management ZIPRASIDONE is contraindicated in patients receiving CISAPRIDE.[1]

Discussion

Do not use ziprasidone with other drugs that prolong the QT interval. Ziprasidone causes dose-related prolongation of the QT interval and other drugs that prolong the QT interval (eg, cisapride)[2] have been associated with fatal arrhythmias.[1] Neither pharmacokinetic nor pharmacodynamic studies between ziprasidone and other drugs that prolong the QT interval have been conducted. However, an additive effect of ziprasidone with coadministration of other drugs that prolong the QT interval (eg, cisapride) cannot be excluded. Therefore, do not administer ziprasidone with other drugs that prolong the QT interval.[2] Sudden unexplained deaths have been reported in patients receiving ziprasidone at recommended doses. In addition to other agents that prolong the QT interval, certain factors may increase the risk of occurrence of torsade de pointes and sudden death in association with ziprasidone, including bradycardia, hypokalemia, hypomagnesemia, and congenital prolongation of the QT interval.

The basis for this monograph is information on file with the manufacturer. Because of the seriousness of the cardiac problems, clinical evaluation of this interaction in humans is not likely to be forthcoming.

[1] *Geodon* [package insert]. New York, NY: Pfizer Labs; August 2004.

[2] Thomas M, et al. *Br J Clin Pharmacol.* 1996;41:77.

* Asterisk indicates drugs cited in interaction reports.
† Available from the manufacturer on a limited-access protocol.

Ziprasidone — *Dofetilide*

Ziprasidone*
(*Geodon*)

Dofetilide*
(*Tikosyn*)

Significance	Onset	Severity	Documentation
1	☐ Rapid ■ **Delayed**	■ **Major** ☐ Moderate ☐ Minor	☐ Established ☐ Probable ■ **Suspected** ☐ Possible ☐ Unlikely

Effects The risk of life-threatening cardiac arrhythmias, including torsades de pointes, may be increased.

Mechanism Possibly synergistic or additive prolongation of the QTc interval.

Management ZIPRASIDONE is contraindicated in patients receiving DOFETILIDE.[1]

Discussion

Do not use ziprasidone with other drugs that prolong the QT interval. Ziprasidone causes dose-related prolongation of the QT interval, and other drugs that prolong the QT interval (eg, dofetilide)[2] have been associated with fatal arrhythmias.[1] Sudden, unexplained deaths have been reported in patients receiving ziprasidone at recommended doses. In addition to other agents that prolong the QT interval, certain factors may increase the risk of occurrence of torsades de pointes and sudden death in association with ziprasidone, including bradycardia, hypokalemia, hypomagnesemia, and congenital prolongation of the QT interval.

The basis for this monograph is information on file with the manufacturers. Because of the seriousness of the cardiac problems, clinical evaluation of this interaction in humans is not likely to be forthcoming.

[1] *Geodon* [package insert]. New York, NY: Pfizer Labs; 2001.

[2] *Tikosyn* [package insert]. New York, NY: Pfizer Labs; December 1999.

* Asterisk indicates drugs cited in interaction reports.

Ziprasidone — *Dolasetron*

Ziprasidone*
(*Geodon*)

Dolasetron*
(*Anzemet*)

Significance	Onset	Severity	Documentation
1	☐ Rapid	■ **Major**	☐ Established
	■ **Delayed**	☐ Moderate	☐ Probable
		☐ Minor	■ **Suspected**
			☐ Possible
			☐ Unlikely

Effects The risk of life-threatening cardiac arrhythmias, including torsades de pointes, may be increased.

Mechanism Possibly synergistic or additive prolongation of the QT interval.

Management ZIPRASIDONE is contraindicated in patients receiving DOLASETRON.[1]

Discussion

Do not use ziprasidone with other drugs that prolong the QT interval. Neither pharmacokinetic nor pharmacodynamic studies between ziprasidone and other drugs that prolong the QT interval have been conducted. However, an additive effect of ziprasidone with coadministration of other drugs that prolong the QT interval (eg, dolasetron) cannot be excluded. Therefore, ziprasidone should not be administered with other drugs that prolong the QT interval.[1] Sudden, unexplained deaths have been reported in patients receiving ziprasidone at recommended doses. In addition to other agents that prolong the QT interval, certain factors may increase the risk of occurrence of torsades de pointes and sudden death in association with ziprasidone, including bradycardia, hypokalemia, hypomagnesemia, and congenital prolongation of the QT interval.

The basis for this monograph is information on file with the manufacturer. Because of the seriousness of the cardiac problems, clinical evaluation of this interaction in humans is not likely to be forthcoming.

[1] *Geodon* [package insert]. New York, NY: Pfizer Labs; June 2002.

* Asterisk indicates drugs cited in interaction reports.

Ziprasidone — *Droperidol*

Ziprasidone* (*Geodon*)	Droperidol* (eg, *Inapsine*)

Significance	Onset	Severity	Documentation
1	□ Rapid ■ **Delayed**	■ **Major** □ Moderate □ Minor	□ Established □ Probable ■ **Suspected** □ Possible □ Unlikely

Effects The risk of life-threatening cardiac arrhythmias, including torsades de pointes, may be increased.

Mechanism Possibly synergistic or additive prolongation of the QT interval.

Management ZIPRASIDONE is contraindicated in patients receiving DROPERIDOL.[1]

Discussion

Do not use ziprasidone with other drugs that prolong the QT interval. Neither pharmacokinetic nor pharmacodynamic studies between ziprasidone and other drugs that prolong the QT interval have been conducted. However, an additive effect of ziprasidone with coadministration of other drugs that prolong the QT interval (eg, droperidol) cannot be excluded. Therefore, ziprasidone should not be administered with other drugs that prolong the QT interval.[1] Sudden, unexplained deaths have been reported in patients receiving ziprasidone at recommended doses. In addition to other agents that prolong the QT interval, certain factors may increase the risk of occurrence of torsades de pointes and sudden death in association with ziprasidone, including bradycardia, hypokalemia, hypomagnesemia, and congenital prolongation of the QT interval.

The basis for this monograph is information on file with the manufacturer. Because of the seriousness of the cardiac problems, clinical evaluation of this interaction in humans is not likely to be forthcoming.

[1] *Geodon* [package insert]. New York: NY: Pfizer Labs; June 2002.

* Asterisk indicates drugs cited in interaction reports.

Ziprasidone — *Halofantrine*

Ziprasidone*
(*Geodon*)

Halofantrine*
(*Halfan*)

Significance	Onset	Severity	Documentation
1	☐ Rapid	■ **Major**	☐ Established
	■ **Delayed**	☐ Moderate	☐ Probable
		☐ Minor	■ **Suspected**
			☐ Possible
			☐ Unlikely

Effects The risk of life-threatening cardiac arrhythmias, including torsades de pointes, may be increased.

Mechanism Possibly synergistic or additive prolongation of the QT interval.

Management ZIPRASIDONE is contraindicated in patients receiving HALOFANTRINE.[1]

Discussion

Do not use ziprasidone with other drugs that prolong the QT interval. Neither pharmacokinetic nor pharmacodynamic studies between ziprasidone and other drugs that prolong the QT interval have been conducted. However, an additive effect of ziprasidone with coadministration of other drugs that prolong the QT interval (eg, halofantrine) cannot be excluded. Therefore, ziprasidone should not be administered with other drugs that prolong the QT interval.[1] Sudden, unexplained deaths have been reported in patients receiving ziprasidone at recommended doses. In addition to other agents that prolong the QT interval, certain factors may increase the risk of occurrence of torsades de pointes and sudden death in association with ziprasidone, including bradycardia, hypokalemia, hypomagnesemia, and congenital prolongation of the QT interval.

The basis for this monograph is information on file with the manufacturer. Because of the seriousness of the cardiac problems, clinical evaluation of this interaction in humans is not likely to be forthcoming.

[1] *Geodon* [package insert]. New York: NY: Pfizer Labs; June 2002.

* Asterisk indicates drugs cited in interaction reports.

Ziprasidone — *Levomethadyl*

Ziprasidone*
(*Geodon*)

Levomethadyl*†

Significance	Onset	Severity	Documentation
1	☐ Rapid ■ **Delayed**	■ **Major** ☐ Moderate ☐ Minor	☐ Established ☐ Probable ■ **Suspected** ☐ Possible ☐ Unlikely

Effects The risk of life-threatening cardiac arrhythmias, including torsades de pointes, may be increased.

Mechanism Possibly synergistic or additive prolongation of the QT interval.

Management ZIPRASIDONE is contraindicated in patients receiving LEVOMETHADYL.[1]

Discussion

Do not use ziprasidone with other drugs that prolong the QT interval. Neither pharmacokinetic nor pharmacodynamic studies between ziprasidone and other drugs that prolong the QT interval have been conducted. However, an additive effect of ziprasidone with coadministration of other drugs that prolong the QT interval (eg, levomethadyl) cannot be excluded. Therefore, ziprasidone should not be administered with other drugs that prolong the QT interval.[1] Sudden, unexplained deaths have been reported in patients receiving ziprasidone at recommended doses. In addition to other agents that prolong the QT interval, certain factors may increase the risk of occurrence of torsades de pointes and sudden death in association with ziprasidone, including bradycardia, hypokalemia, hypomagnesemia, and congenital prolongation of the QT interval.

The basis for this monograph is information on file with the manufacturer. Because of the seriousness of the cardiac problems, clinical evaluation of this interaction in humans is not likely to be forthcoming.

[1] *Geodon* [package insert]. New York, NY: Pfizer Labs; June 2002.

* Asterisk indicates drugs cited in interaction reports.
† Not available in the United States.

Ziprasidone — *Mefloquine*

Ziprasidone* (*Geodon*)	Mefloquine* (eg, *Lariam*)

Significance	Onset	Severity	Documentation
1	☐ Rapid ■ **Delayed**	■ **Major** ☐ Moderate ☐ Minor	☐ Established ☐ Probable ■ **Suspected** ☐ Possible ☐ Unlikely

Effects The risk of life-threatening cardiac arrhythmias, including torsades de pointes, may be increased.

Mechanism Possibly synergistic or additive prolongation of the QT interval.

Management ZIPRASIDONE is contraindicated in patients receiving MEFLOQUINE.[1]

Discussion

Do not use ziprasidone with other drugs that prolong the QT interval. Neither pharmacokinetic nor pharmacodynamic studies between ziprasidone and other drugs that prolong the QT interval have been conducted. However, an additive effect of ziprasidone with coadministration of other drugs that prolong the QT interval (eg, mefloquine) cannot be excluded. Therefore, ziprasidone should not be administered with other drugs that prolong the QT interval.[1] Sudden, unexplained deaths have been reported in patients receiving ziprasidone at recommended doses. In addition to other agents that prolong the QT interval, certain factors may increase the risk of occurrence of torsades de pointes and sudden death in association with ziprasidone, including bradycardia, hypokalemia, hypomagnesemia, and congenital prolongation of the QT interval.

The basis for this monograph is information on file with the manufacturer. Because of the seriousness of the cardiac problems, clinical evaluation of this interaction in humans is not likely to be forthcoming.

[1] *Geodon* [package insert]. New York, NY: Pfizer Labs; June 2002.

* Asterisk indicates drugs cited in interaction reports.

Ziprasidone — *Pentamidine*

Ziprasidone*	Pentamidine*
(*Geodon*)	(eg, *Pentam*)

Significance	Onset	Severity	Documentation
1	☐ Rapid ■ **Delayed**	■ **Major** ☐ Moderate ☐ Minor	☐ Established ☐ Probable ■ **Suspected** ☐ Possible ☐ Unlikely

Effects The risk of life-threatening cardiac arrhythmias, including torsades de pointes, may be increased.

Mechanism Possibly synergistic or additive prolongation of the QT interval.

Management ZIPRASIDONE is contraindicated in patients receiving PENTAMIDINE.[1]

Discussion

Do not use ziprasidone with other drugs that prolong the QT interval. Neither pharmacokinetic nor pharmacodynamic studies between ziprasidone and other drugs that prolong the QT interval have been conducted. However, an additive effect of ziprasidone with coadministration of other drugs that prolong the QT interval (eg, pentamidine) cannot be excluded. Therefore, ziprasidone should not be administered with other drugs that prolong the QT interval.[1] Sudden, unexplained deaths have been reported in patients receiving ziprasidone at recommended doses. In addition to other agents that prolong the QT interval, certain factors may increase the risk of occurrence of torsades de pointes and sudden death in association with ziprasidone, including bradycardia, hypokalemia, hypomagnesemia, and congenital prolongation of the QT interval.

The basis for this monograph is information on file with the manufacturer. Because of the seriousness of the cardiac problems, clinical evaluation of this interaction in humans is not likely to be forthcoming.

[1] *Geodon* [package insert]. New York, NY: Pfizer Labs; June 2002.

* Asterisk indicates drugs cited in interaction reports.

Ziprasidone | *Phenothiazines*

Ziprasidone* (*Geodon*)	Chlorpromazine* (eg, *Thorazine*)	Thioridazine*

Significance	Onset	Severity	Documentation
1	☐ Rapid ■ **Delayed**	■ **Major** ☐ Moderate ☐ Minor	☐ Established ☐ Probable ■ **Suspected** ☐ Possible ☐ Unlikely

Effects The risk of life-threatening cardiac arrhythmias, including torsades de pointes, may be increased.

Mechanism Possibly synergistic or additive prolongation of the QT interval.

Management ZIPRASIDONE is contraindicated in patients receiving CHLORPROMAZINE, MESORIDAZINE, or THIORIDAZINE.[1]

Discussion

Do not use ziprasidone with other drugs that prolong the QT interval. Ziprasidone causes dose-related prolongation of the QT interval, and other drugs that prolong the QT interval (eg, phenothiazines)[2] have been associated with fatal arrhythmias.[1] Neither pharmacokinetic nor pharmacodynamic studies between ziprasidone and other drugs that prolong the QT interval have been conducted. However, an additive effect of ziprasidone with coadministration of other drugs that prolong the QT interval (eg, phenothiazines) cannot be excluded. Therefore, ziprasidone should not be administered with other drugs that prolong the QT interval.[2] Sudden, unexplained deaths have been reported in patients receiving ziprasidone at recommended doses. In addition to other agents that prolong the QT interval, certain factors may increase the risk of occurrence of torsades de pointes and sudden death in association with ziprasidone, including bradycardia, hypokalemia, hypomagnesemia, and congenital prolongation of the QT interval.

The basis for this monograph is information on file with the manufacturer. Because of the seriousness of the cardiac problems, clinical evaluation of this interaction in humans is not likely to be forthcoming.

[1] *Geodon* [package insert]. New York, NY: Pfizer Labs; June 2002.

[2] Thomas M, et al. *Br J Clin Pharmacol.* 1996;41:77.

* Asterisk indicates drugs cited in interaction reports.

Ziprasidone — *Pimozide*

Ziprasidone* (*Geodon*)	Pimozide* (*Orap*)

Significance	Onset	Severity	Documentation
1	☐ Rapid ■ **Delayed**	■ **Major** ☐ Moderate ☐ Minor	☐ Established ☐ Probable ■ **Suspected** ☐ Possible ☐ Unlikely

Effects The risk of life-threatening cardiac arrhythmias, including torsades de pointes, may be increased.

Mechanism Possibly synergistic or additive prolongation of the QTc interval.

Management ZIPRASIDONE is contraindicated in patients receiving PIMOZIDE.[1]

Discussion

Do not use ziprasidone with other drugs that prolong the QT interval. Ziprasidone causes dose-related prolongation of the QT interval, and other drugs that prolong the QT interval (eg, pimozide)[2] have been associated with fatal arrhythmias.[1] Neither pharmacokinetic nor pharmacodynamic studies between ziprasidone and other drugs that prolong the QT interval have been conducted. However, an additive effect of ziprasidone with coadministration of other drugs that prolong the QT interval (eg, pimozide) cannot be excluded. Therefore, ziprasidone should not be administered with other drugs that prolong the QT interval.[2] Sudden, unexplained deaths have been reported in patients receiving ziprasidone at recommended doses. In addition to other agents that prolong the QT interval, certain factors may increase the risk of occurrence of torsades de pointes and sudden death in association with ziprasidone, including bradycardia, hypokalemia, hypomagnesemia, and congenital prolongation of the QT interval.

The basis for this monograph is information on file with the manufacturer. Because of the seriousness of the cardiac problems, clinical evaluation of this interaction in humans is not likely to be forthcoming.

[1] *Geodon* [package insert]. New York, NY: Pfizer Labs; June 2002.

[2] Thomas M, et al. *Br J Clin Pharmacol.* 1996;41:77.

* Asterisk indicates drugs cited in interaction reports.

Ziprasidone — *Quinolones*

Ziprasidone	Quinolones	
Ziprasidone* (*Geodon*)	Gatifloxacin* (*Tequin*)	Moxifloxacin* (*Avelox*)
	Levofloxacin* (*Levaquin*)	Sparfloxacin* (*Zagam*)

Significance	Onset	Severity	Documentation
1	□ Rapid ■ **Delayed**	■ **Major** □ Moderate □ Minor	□ Established □ Probable ■ **Suspected** □ Possible □ Unlikely

Effects The risk of life-threatening cardiac arrhythmias, including torsades de pointes, may be increased.

Mechanism Possibly synergistic or additive prolongation of the QT interval.

Management ZIPRASIDONE is contraindicated in patients receiving GATIFLOXACIN, MOXIFLOXACIN, or SPARFLOXACIN and in patients receiving drugs that have demonstrated QT prolongation[1] (eg, LEVOFLOXACIN[2]).

Discussion

Neither pharmacokinetic nor pharmacodynamic studies between ziprasidone and other drugs that prolong the QT interval have been conducted. However, an additive effect of ziprasidone with coadministration of other drugs that prolong the QT interval (eg, sparfloxacin) cannot be excluded. Therefore, do not administer ziprasidone with other drugs that prolong the QT interval.[1] Levofloxacin administration has been associated with prolongation of the QT interval and infrequent cases of cardiac arrhythmias.[2] Sudden, unexplained deaths have been reported in patients receiving ziprasidone at recommended doses. In addition to other agents that prolong the QT interval, certain factors may increase the risk of torsades de pointes and sudden death in association with ziprasidone, including bradycardia, hypokalemia, hypomagnesemia, and congenital prolongation of the QT interval.

The effect of other quinolone antibiotics on QT prolongation needs to be assessed. The basis for this monograph is information on file with the manufacturer. Because of the seriousness of the cardiac problems, clinical evaluation of this interaction in humans is not likely to be forthcoming.

[1] *Geodon* [package insert]. New York, NY: Pfizer; June 2002.

[2] *Levaquin* [package insert]. Raritan, NJ: Ortho-McNeil Pharmaceuticals, Inc; February 2004.

* Asterisk indicates drugs cited in interaction reports.

Ziprasidone — *Tacrolimus*

Ziprasidone* (*Geodon*)

Tacrolimus* (*Prograf*)

Significance	Onset	Severity	Documentation
1	☐ Rapid ■ **Delayed**	■ **Major** ☐ Moderate ☐ Minor	☐ Established ☐ Probable ■ **Suspected** ☐ Possible ☐ Unlikely

Effects The risk of life-threatening cardiac arrhythmias, including torsades de pointes, may be increased.

Mechanism Possibly synergistic or additive prolongation of the QT interval.

Management ZIPRASIDONE is contraindicated in patients receiving TACROLIMUS.[1]

Discussion

Do not use ziprasidone with other drugs that prolong the QT interval. Neither pharmacokinetic nor pharmacodynamic studies between ziprasidone and other drugs that prolong the QT interval have been conducted. However, an additive effect of ziprasidone with coadministration of other drugs that prolong the QT interval (eg, tacrolimus) cannot be excluded. Therefore, ziprasidone should not be administered with other drugs that prolong the QT interval.[1] Sudden, unexplained deaths have been reported in patients receiving ziprasidone at recommended doses. In addition to other agents that prolong the QT interval, certain factors may increase the risk of occurrence of torsades de pointes and sudden death in association with ziprasidone, including bradycardia, hypokalemia, hypomagnesemia, and congenital prolongation of the QT interval.

The basis for this monograph is information on file with the manufacturer. Because of the seriousness of the cardiac problems, clinical evaluation of this interaction in humans is not likely to be forthcoming.

[1] *Geodon* [package insert]. New York, NY: Pfizer Labs; June 2002.

* Asterisk indicates drugs cited in interaction reports.

Zolmitriptan — *Beta-Blockers*

Zolmitriptan* (*Zomig*)	Propranolol* (eg, *Inderal*)

Significance	Onset	Severity	Documentation
5	☐ Rapid	☐ Major	☐ Established
	■ **Delayed**	☐ Moderate	☐ Probable
		■ **Minor**	☐ Suspected
			☐ Possible
			■ **Unlikely**

Effects Plasma concentrations of ZOLMITRIPTAN may be elevated, increasing the pharmacologic and adverse effects.

Mechanism Possibly caused by inhibition of ZOLMITRIPTAN metabolism.

Management Based on available data, the changes in ZOLMITRIPTAN single-dose pharmacokinetics would not be expected to be clinically important.

Discussion

In a double-blind, randomized, crossover study, the effects of propranolol on the pharmacokinetics and cardiovascular response to zolmitriptan were investigated in 14 healthy volunteers.[1] Subjects were given propranolol 160 mg or placebo daily for 7 days. Zolmitriptan 10 mg was administered with the last dose of propranolol. Concurrent propranolol administration increased the mean peak plasma concentration of zolmitriptan 38%, the AUC 56%, and the mean $t_{1/2}$ 29% (from 3.1 to 4 hr). The mean peak concentration and AUC of the active N-desmethyl metabolite were decreased 24% and 11%, respectively. The peak concentration and AUC of the inactive indole acetic acid metabolite were decreased 13%. There was a mean peak increase of 13 mm Hg in systolic pressure and an 11 mm Hg rise in diastolic pressure following zolmitriptan administration with or without propranolol. Adverse effects were mild-to-moderate in intensity, and none were serious.

Evaluation of this interaction with multiple-dose administration of zolmitriptan is warranted.

[1] Peck RW, et al. *Br J Clin Pharmacol.* 1997;44:595.

* Asterisk indicates drugs cited in interaction reports.

Zolpidem — *Azole Antifungal Agents*

Zolpidem	Azole Antifungal Agents	
Zolpidem* (eg, *Ambien*)	Fluconazole* (eg, *Diflucan*)	Posaconazole (*Noxafil*)
	Itraconazole* (eg, *Sporanox*)	Voriconazole* (*Vfend*)
	Ketoconazole* (eg, *Nizoral*)	

Significance	Onset	Severity	Documentation
2	☐ Rapid	☐ Major	☐ Established
	■ **Delayed**	■ **Moderate**	☐ Probable
		☐ Minor	■ **Suspected**
			☐ Possible
			☐ Unlikely

Effects Plasma concentrations and therapeutic effects of ZOLPIDEM may be increased. The effects on ZOLPIDEM appear to be greatest with KETOCONAZOLE.

Mechanism AZOLE ANTIFUNGAL AGENTS may interfere with the major route of ZOLPIDEM metabolism (ie, CYP3A4).

Management Monitor the patient's clinical response. The ZOLPIDEM dose may need to be decreased during coadministration of AZOLE ANTIFUNGAL AGENTS.

Discussion

The effects of the azole antifungal agents fluconazole, itraconazole, and ketoconazole on the pharmacokinetics and pharmacodynamics of zolpidem were studied in a randomized, double-blind, 5-way, crossover investigation.[1] Twelve healthy volunteers received an oral azole antifungal agent or placebo twice daily for 2 days (4 doses). Zolpidem 5 mg or placebo was administered with the third dose of the azole antifungal agent. Administration of zolpidem with ketoconazole resulted in a 41% decrease in the oral clearance of zolpidem and a prolongation in the elimination $t_{½}$ (from 1.9 to 2.4 hours), compared with placebo. Administration of zolpidem with fluconazole or itraconazole decreased the oral clearance of zolpidem 20% and 24%, respectively, but the differences were not statistically significant. Ketoconazole administration increased the electroencephalogram (EEG) and digit symbol substitution test (DSST) effects of zolpidem. However, administration of either fluconazole or itraconazole did not enhance the EEG or DSST effects of zolpidem. In a randomized, crossover study involving 10 healthy volunteers, administration of itraconazole 200 mg/day for 4 days and zolpidem 10 mg on day 4 increased the AUC of zolpidem 34%.[2] In 5 of 6 psychomotor tests assessed, itraconazole did not increase the pharmacodynamic effects of zolpidem. In healthy men, voriconazole increased the C_{max} and AUC of zolpidem 1.23- and 1.48-fold, respectively, and prolonged the $t_{½}$ from 3.2 to 4.1 hours.[3]

[1] Greenblatt DJ, et al. *Clin Pharmacol Ther.* 1998;64(6):661.
[2] Luurila H, et al. *Eur J Clin Pharmacol.* 1998;54(2):163.
[3] Saari TI, et al. *Br J Clin Pharmacol.* 2007;63(1):116.

* Asterisk indicates drugs cited in interaction reports. Based on pharmacologic and pharmacokinetic considerations, similar interactions may occur with other drugs that are listed.

Zolpidem — Caffeine

Zolpidem* (eg, *Ambien*)	Caffeine*

Significance	Onset	Severity	Documentation
4	■ **Rapid**	□ Major	□ Established
	□ Delayed	■ **Moderate**	□ Probable
		□ Minor	□ Suspected
			■ **Possible**
			□ Unlikely

Effects The pharmacodynamic effects of ZOLPIDEM (eg, sedation, performance impairment) may be partially reversed.

Mechanism Unknown.

Management Advise patients taking ZOLPIDEM that CAFFEINE ingestion may partially reverse the effects of ZOLPIDEM.

Discussion

The effects of the caffeine and zolpidem interaction were evaluated in 20 healthy volunteers.[1] Using a double-blind, single-dose, crossover design, each subject received zolpidem 7.5 mg or placebo combined with low-dose caffeine (250 mg), high-dose caffeine (500 mg), or placebo. Compared with placebo, caffeine increased the zolpidem C_{max} and AUC 30% to 40%, and decreased oral clearance 29%. In addition, caffeine partially reversed most of the pharmacodynamic effects of zolpidem (eg, sedation, performance impairment). Zolpidem did not affect the pharmacokinetics of caffeine. On average, 240 mL of brewed coffee contains 120 mg of caffeine.[2]

[1] Cysneiros RM, et al. *Clin Pharmacol Ther.* 2007;82(1):54.

[2] Wickersham RM, Novak KK, managing eds. *Drug Facts and Comparisons.* 60th ed. St. Louis, MO: Wolters Kluwer Health, Inc; 2006: 942.

* Asterisk indicates drugs cited in interaction reports.

Zolpidem | *Rifamycins*

Zolpidem* (eg, *Ambien*)	Rifabutin (*Mycobutin*)	Rifampin* (eg, *Rifadin*)

Significance	Onset	Severity	Documentation
3	☐ Rapid ■ **Delayed**	☐ Major ☐ Moderate ■ **Minor**	☐ Established ☐ Probable ■ **Suspected** ☐ Possible ☐ Unlikely

Effects Plasma concentrations and therapeutic effects of ZOLPIDEM may be reduced.

Mechanism RIFAMYCINS may increase the metabolism (CYP3A4) of ZOLPIDEM.

Management Monitor the clinical response of the patient. The dose of ZOLPIDEM may need to be increased during coadministration of RIFAMYCINS.

Discussion

The effects of rifampin on the pharmacokinetics and pharmacodynamics of zolpidem were studied in 8 healthy women.[1] Using a 2, randomized, crossover design, each subject received oral rifampin 600 mg/day or placebo for 5 days. On day 6, oral zolpidem 20 mg was given. Compared with placebo, rifampin administration decreased the AUC of zolpidem by 72%, the C_{max} by 60% (from 293 to 117 ng/mL), and the elimination $t_{1/2}$ by 36% (from 2.5 to 1.6 hours). Following rifampin administration, there was a reduction in the effects of zolpidem in all 6 pharmacodynamic tests, including the digit symbol substitution test, visual analog scale for subjective drowsiness and drug effect, critical flicker fusion test, Maddox wing test, and saccadic eye movement.

[1] Villikka K, et al. *Clin Pharmacol Ther.* 1997;62(6):629.

* Asterisk indicates drugs cited in interaction reports. Based on pharmacologic and pharmacokinetic considerations, similar interactions may occur with other drugs that are listed.

Zolpidem — *Ritonavir*

Zolpidem* (eg, *Ambien*)	Ritonavir* (*Norvir*)

Significance	Onset	Severity	Documentation
2	☐ Rapid	☐ Major	☐ Established
	■ **Delayed**	■ **Moderate**	☐ Probable
		☐ Minor	■ **Suspected**
			☐ Possible
			☐ Unlikely

Effects ZOLPIDEM plasma concentrations may be elevated, increasing the pharmacologic effects and risk of adverse reactions (eg, severe sedation, respiratory depression).

Mechanism Inhibition of the hepatic metabolism of ZOLPIDEM.

Management A dosage decrease may be needed for ZOLPIDEM when coadministered with RITONAVIR. Monitor the clinical response and adjust the ZOLPIDEM dose as needed.

Discussion

Ritonavir is expected to produce large increases in zolpidem plasma concentrations, which may lead to severe sedation and respiratory depression.[1] Because of the potential for extreme sedation and respiratory depression, the manufacturer of ritonavir warns that zolpidem should not be administered concomitantly with ritonavir.[1]

The basis for this monograph is information on file with the manufacturer. Published clinical data are needed to further assess this interaction.

[1] *Norvir* [package insert]. Abbott Park, IL: Abbott Laboratories; April 2010.

* Asterisk indicates drugs cited in interaction reports.

Zolpidem — *Serotonin Reuptake Inhibitors*

Zolpidem	Serotonin Reuptake Inhibitors	
Zolpidem* (*Ambien*)	Fluoxetine (*Prozac*)	Paroxetine (*Paxil*)
	Fluvoxamine (*Luvox*)	Sertraline* (*Zoloft*)

Significance	Onset	Severity	Documentation
3	☐ Rapid	☐ Major	☐ Established
	■ **Delayed**	☐ Moderate	☐ Probable
		■ **Minor**	■ **Suspected**
			☐ Possible
			☐ Unlikely

Effects The onset of action of ZOLPIDEM may be shortened and the effect increased.

Mechanism SERTRALINE may inhibit the metabolism of ZOLPIDEM.

Management Observe the patient for an increase in the effects of ZOLPIDEM.

Discussion

A study was conducted in 28 healthy female volunteers to determine whether there is a pharmacokinetic or pharmacodynamic interaction between zolpidem and sertraline.[1] In an open-label, randomized, fixed treatment sequence study, subjects received a single evening dose of zolpidem 10 mg alone or with chronic sertraline 50 mg/day in the morning. In addition, subjects received 5 consecutive evening doses of zolpidem with chronic sertraline. Compared with administration of zolpidem alone, administration of a single dose of zolpidem with chronic sertraline decreased the half-life of zolpidem approximately 20 minutes. After the fifth dose of zolpidem with chronic sertraline administration, peak plasma concentrations of zolpidem increased approximately 43%, and the time to reach the peak concentration was reduced approximately 53%. Following 5 doses of zolpidem with sertraline, the area under the plasma concentration-time curve of sertraline decreased 6%, and the peak concentration of the N-desmethyl metabolite of sertraline increased 13%. There was no effect on the next morning pharmacodynamics of zolpidem (ie, 9 hours after the administration of zolpidem), indicating no residual drug effects.

Additional studies are needed to determine the effects with longer term use of zolpidem.

[1] Allard S, et al. *J Clin Pharmacol.* 1999;39:184.

* Asterisk indicates drugs cited in interaction reports. Based on pharmacologic and pharmacokinetic considerations, similar interactions may occur with other drugs that are listed.

INDEX

The interactions in this text are assigned numbers according to the type and magnitude of their effect and the necessity of monitoring the patient or altering therapy to avoid potentially adverse consequences. This rating is determined by the ONSET of the effects of the interaction, the potential SEVERITY of the reaction, and the clinical DOCUMENTATION of the occurrence of the interaction. Entries appearing without a significance number are mentioned in the discussion section for the particular interaction. For further information on significance numbers, refer to pages xi and xiv-xvi.

[1] The interaction is potentially severe or life-threatening, and its occurrence has been suspected, established, or probable in well-controlled studies. Contraindicated drug combinations may also have this number.

[2] The interaction may cause deterioration in a patient's clinical status, and its occurrence has been suspected, established, or probable in well-controlled studies.

[3] The interaction causes minor effects, and its occurrence has been suspected, established, or probable in well-controlled studies.

[4] The interaction may cause moderate-to-major effects, but data are very limited.

[5] The interaction may cause minor-to-major effects, but the occurrence of an interaction is unlikely or there is no good evidence of an altered clinical effect.